P9-CQP-683

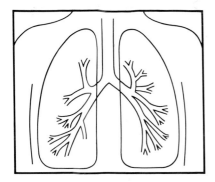

KENDIG'S

DISORDERS OF THE RESPIRATORY TRACT IN CHILDREN

FIFTH EDITION

Editor

VICTOR CHERNICK, M.D., F.R.C.P.(C)

Professor of Pediatrics, University of Manitoba;
Section Head of Respirology, Department of Pediatrics,
and Director, Cystic Fibrosis Clinic,
Children's Hospital of Winnipeg,
Winnipeg, Manitoba, Canada

Consulting Editor

EDWIN L. KENDIG, Jr., M.D., Sc.D.(Hon.)

Professor of Pediatrics, Medical College of Virginia
Health Sciences Division, Virginia Commonwealth University,
Richmond, Virginia;
Director, Child Chest Clinic,
Medical College of Virginia Hospitals;
Director Emeritus, Department of Pediatrics,
St. Mary's Hospital, Richmond, Virginia

1990

W.B. SAUNDERS COMPANY
Harcourt Brace Jovanovich, Inc.

Philadelphia   London   Toronto   Montreal   Sydney   Tokyo

W. B. SAUNDERS COMPANY
Harcourt Brace Jovanovich, Inc.

The Curtis Center
Independence Square West
Philadelphia, PA 19106

Library of Congress Cataloging-in-Publication Data

Kendig's disorders of the respiratory tract in children / editor,
Victor Chernick; consulting editor, Edwin L. Kendig, Jr.—5th
ed.   p.   cm.

Rev. ed. of: Disorders of the respiratory tract in children. 4th
ed. 1983.

Includes bibliographical references.

Includes index.

1. Pediatric respiratory diseases.   I. Chernick, Victor.
II. Kendig, Edwin L., 1911–   .   III. Title: Disorders
of the respiratory tract in children.
[DNLM: 1. Respiratory Tract Diseases—in infancy &
childhood.   WS 280 K331]

RJ431.K42 1990   618.92′2–dc20   90–8515

ISBN 0–7216–2214–3

Listed here is the latest translated edition of this book together with the language of the translation and
the publisher.

Spanish (4th edition)—Editorial Medica Panamericana, Rua Santa Izabel 267, CEP 01221 Vila Buarque,
Sao Paulo, Brazil

Editor: W. B. Saunders Staff
Developmental Editor: Hazel Hacker
Designer: Maureen Sweeney
Production Manager: Bill Preston
Manuscript Editor: Lee Ann Draud
Illustration Coordinator: Cecilia Kunkle
Indexer: Linda Van Pelt

Kendig's Disorders of the Respiratory Tract in Children, 5th ed.   ISBN   0–7216–2214–3

Copyright © 1990, 1983, 1977, 1972, 1967 by W. B. Saunders Company

All rights reserved. No part of this publication may be reproduced or transmitted in any form or by
any means, electronic or mechanical, including photocopy, recording, or any information storage and
retrieval system, without permission in writing from the publisher.

Printed in the United States of America

Last digit is the print number: 9   8   7   6   5   4   3   2   1

WS
280
K 331
1990

For Jasmine, Mandy, Eli, Zachary, and Erica—
those special little people

3 0001 00206 0046

21413 772

CONTRIBUTORS

Adekunle D. Adekile, M.B., B.S.
Associate Dean, Faculty of Health Sciences, Obafemi Awolowo University, Ile-Ife; Consultant Pediatrician, Department of Pediatrics, University Teaching Hospital, Ile-Ife, Nigeria.
The Lungs in Sickle Cell Disease

Stuart P. Adler, M.D.
Professor of Pediatrics, Medicine, and Microbiology, Medical College of Virginia, Health Sciences Division, Virginia Commonwealth University; Medical College of Virginia Hospitals, Richmond, Virginia.
Salmonella Pneumonia

William L. Albritton, M.D., Ph.D.
Professor and Head, Department of Microbiology, University of Saskatchewan College of Medicine; Active Staff, University Hospital, Saskatoon, Saskatchewan, Canada.
Q Fever; Varicella Pneumonia

Carl Alexander-Reindorf, M.D.
Clinical Associate Professor of Pediatrics, Georgetown University School of Medicine; Courtesy Attending Pediatrician, Georgetown University Hospital, Children's Hospital, and Howard University Hospital; Consultant Pediatrician, Child and Adolescent Program, St. Elizabeths Hospital, Washington, D.C.
The Lungs in Sickle Cell Disease

Adriano G. Arguedas, M.D.
Clinical Associate Instructor, University of California, Irvine, California College of Medicine, Irvine, California; Research Fellow, Pediatric Infectious Diseases, Miller Children's Hospital, Memorial Medical Center, and University of California, Irvine, Long Beach, California.
Bacterial Pneumonias

M. Innes Asher, M.B., Ch.B.
Senior Lecturer, School of Medicine, University of Auckland; Paediatrician, Auckland Hospital, Auckland Area Health Board, Auckland, New Zealand.
Lung Abscess

A. Avital, M.D.
Lecturer, Hadassah University Hospital, Mt. Scopus, Jerusalem, Israel; Fellow in Pediatric Respirology, University of Manitoba, Winnipeg, Manitoba, Canada.
Emphysema and Alpha₁-Antitrypsin Deficiency; Psittacosis

Felicia B. Axelrod, M.D.
Professor, Department of Pediatrics, New York University School of Medicine; Attending in Pediatrics, New York University Medical Center, New York, New York.
Familial Dysautonomia

Pierre H. Beaudry, M.D.
Professor and Chairman, Department of Paediatrics, University of Ottawa School of Medicine; Chief, Department of Paediatrics, Children's Hospital of Eastern Ontario, Ottawa, Ontario, Canada.
Lung Abscess

Marc O. Beem, M.D.
Professor Emeritus of Pediatrics, University of Chicago Pritzker School of Medicine, Chicago, Illinois.
Chlamydial Infections of Infants

Joseph A. Bellanti, M.D.
Professor of Pediatrics and Microbiology, and Director, International Center for Interdisciplinary Studies of Immunology, Georgetown University School of Medicine, Washington, D.C.
Host Defense Mechanisms

C. Warren Bierman, M.D.
Clinical Professor of Pediatrics, University of Washington School of Medicine; Chief, Division of Allergy, Children's Orthopedic Hospital and Medical Center, Seattle, Washington.
Asthma; Nonasthmatic Allergic Pulmonary Disease

Thomas F. Boat, M.D.
Professor and Chairman, Department of Pediatrics, University of North Carolina at Chapel Hill School of Medicine; Director of Pediatric Service, University of North Carolina Hospitals, Chapel Hill, North Carolina.
Lung Injury Caused by Pharmacologic Agents

Robert W. Bradsher, M.D.
Chief, Infectious Diseases, and Associate Professor of Medicine, University of Arkansas College of Medicine, Little Rock, Arkansas.
The Mycoses Other Than Histoplasmosis

James W. Brooks, M.D.
Professor of Surgery, Medical College of Virginia, Health Sciences Division, Virginia Commonwealth University; Attending General Thoracic Surgery, Medical College of Virginia, Richmond, Virginia.
Disorders of the Respiratory Tract Due to Trauma; Foreign Bodies in the Air Passages; Tumors of the Chest

Robert T. Brouillette, M.D.
Professor of Pediatrics, McGill University Faculty of Medicine; Division Head, Newborn Medicine, Montreal Children's Hospital, Montreal, Québec, Canada.
Disorders of Breathing During Sleep

Mark A. Brown, M.D.
Pediatric Pulmonary Fellow, University of Arizona College of Medicine; Staff Physician, University Medical Center, Tucson, Arizona.
Bronchiectasis

Michel A. Bureau, M.D., F.R.C.P.(C), F.C.C.P.
Dean and Professor of Pediatrics and Pneumology, Université de Sherbrooke Faculty of Medicine, Sherbrooke, Québec, Canada.
Chest Wall Diseases and Dysfunction in Children

Emmanuel Canet, M.D.
Assistant Professor of Pediatrics, Université de Sherbrooke Faculty of Medicine; Department of Pediat-

rics, Centre hospitalier universitaire de Sherbrooke, Sherbrooke, Québec, Canada.
Chest Wall Diseases and Dysfunction in Children

Victor Chernick, M.D., F.R.C.P.(C)
Professor of Pediatrics, University of Manitoba Faculty of Medicine; Section Head of Respirology, Department of Pediatrics, and Director, Cystic Fibrosis Clinic, Children's Hospital of Winnipeg, Winnipeg, Manitoba, Canada.
Emphysema and Alpha₁-Antitrypsin Deficiency; Liquid and Air in the Pleural Space; Measles and Giant Cell Pneumonia; Psittacosis

Wallace A. Clyde, Jr., M.D.
Professor of Pediatrics and Microbiology, University of North Carolina at Chapel Hill School of Medicine; Staff, University of North Carolina Children's Hospital, Chapel Hill, North Carolina.
Infections of the Respiratory Tract Due to Mycoplasma Pneumoniae

Dan Michael Cooper, M.D.
Associate Professor of Pediatrics, Department of Pediatrics, University of California, Los Angeles, UCLA School of Medicine, Los Angeles, California; Chief, Division of Respiratory and Critical Care, Department of Pediatrics, Harbor-UCLA Medical Center, Torrance, California.
Pulmonary Function Assessment in the Laboratory During Exercise

Anthony Corbet, M.D.
Associate Professor, Department of Pediatrics, Baylor College of Medicine; Staff Neonatologist, Texas Children's Hospital, St. Luke's Episcopal Hospital, Woman's Hospital of Texas, The Methodist Hospital, Ben Taub General Hospital; Houston, Texas.
Respiratory Disorders in the Newborn

Joanna R. Firth, M.D.
Clinical Instructor in Pediatrics, Jefferson Medical College of Thomas Jefferson University; Director, Pediatric Allergy Clinic, Albert Einstein Medical Center, Northern Division, Philadelphia, Pennsylvania.
Pulmonary Hemorrhage and Massive Hemoptysis

John A. Fleetham, M.B., B.S., F.R.C.P.(C)
Associate Professor of Medicine, University of British Columbia Faculty of Medicine; Head of Respiratory

Division, University Hospital, Vancouver, British Columbia, Canada.
Desquamative Interstitial Pneumonia and Other Variants of Interstitial Pneumonia; Usual Interstitial Pneumonia

Barry D. Fletcher, M.D.
Professor of Radiology and Pediatrics, University of Tennessee, Memphis, College of Medicine; Chairman, Diagnostic Imaging, St. Jude Children's Research Hospital, Memphis, Tennessee.
Diagnostic Imaging of the Respiratory Tract

W. Paul Glezen, M.D.
Professor of Microbiology and Pediatrics, Baylor College of Medicine; Adjunct Professor of Epidemiology, University of Texas Health Science Center at Houston; Attending Pediatrician, Harris County Hospital District; Courtesy Staff, Infectious Diseases, Texas Children's Hospital, Houston, Texas.
Diagnosis of Viral Respiratory Illness; Viral Pneumonia

Roni Grad, M.D.
Research Instructor, Department of Pediatrics, University of Arizona College of Medicine; Attending Physician, University Medical Center and Tucson Medical Center, Tucson, Arizona.
Acute Infections Producing Upper Airway Obstruction

Hilda L. Gritter, M.D., F.R.C.P.(C)
Assistant Professor, Department of Pathology, University of Manitoba Faculty of Medicine; Staff Pathologist, St. Boniface General Hospital, Winnipeg, Manitoba, Canada.
Langerhans Cell Histiocytosis

Michael M. Grunstein, M.D., Ph.D.
Professor of Pediatrics, University of Pennsylvania School of Medicine; Chief, Division of Pulmonary Medicine, Children's Hospital of Philadelphia, Philadelphia, Pennsylvania.
Pulmonary Function Tests in Infants

Gabriel G. Haddad, M.D.
Associate Professor, Yale University School of Medicine; Director, Section of Respiratory Medicine, Yale-New Haven Hospital, New Haven, Connecticut.
The Functional Basis of Respiratory Pathology

Thomas A. Hazinski, M.D.
Associate Professor of Pediatrics, Vanderbilt University School of Medicine; Director, Division of Pedi-

atric Pulmonary Medicine, and Co-Director, Cystic Fibrosis Center, Vanderbilt University Medical Center, Nashville, Tennessee.
Atelectasis; Bronchopulmonary Dysplasia

Douglas C. Heiner, M.D.
Professor of Pediatrics, University of California, Los Angeles, UCLA School of Medicine; Chief, Division of Immunology/Allergy, Harbor-UCLA Medical Center, Torrance, California.
Pulmonary Hemosiderosis

Marianna M. Henry, M.D.
Assistant Professor of Pediatrics, Department of Pediatrics, University of North Carolina at Chapel Hill School of Medicine; Attending Physician, University of North Carolina Hospitals, Chapel Hill, North Carolina.
Lung Injury Caused by Pharmacologic Agents

William A. Howard, M.D.
Clinical Professor Emeritus of Child Health and Development, George Washington University School of Medicine and Health Sciences; Chairman Emeritus, Division of Allergy and Immunology; Children's Hospital, National Medical Center, Washington, D.C.
Pulmonary Infiltrates with Eosinophilia; Tularemia; Visceral Larva Migrans

Walter T. Hughes, M.D.
Professor of Pediatrics, University of Tennessee Center for Health Sciences; Chairman, Department of Infectious Diseases, St. Jude Children's Research Hospital, Memphis, Tennessee.
Histoplasmosis; Pneumocystis Carinii *Pneumonitis*

Carl E. Hunt, M.D.
Professor and Chairman, Department of Pediatrics, Medical College of Ohio; Medical College Hospitals and Toledo Hospital, Toledo, Ohio.
Disorders of Breathing During Sleep

Laura S. Inselman, M.D.
Assistant Professor of Pediatrics, University of Connecticut Health Center, Farmington, Connecticut; Assistant Clinical Professor of Pediatrics, Yale University School of Medicine, New Haven, Connecticut; Clinical Director, Pediatric Pulmonology, Newington Children's Hospital, Newington, Connecticut.
Pulmonary Disorders in Pediatric Acquired Immune Deficiency Syndrome; Tuberculosis

Richard F. Jacobs, M.D.
Associate Professor of Pediatrics, University of Arkansas College of Medicine; Chief, Pediatric Infectious Diseases, Arkansas Children's Hospital, Little Rock, Arkansas.
The Mycoses Other Than Histoplasmosis

Melvin E. Jenkins, M.D.
Professor Emeritus, Howard University College of Medicine; Pediatrician, Howard University Hospital, Washington, D.C.
The Lungs in Sickle Cell Disease

Josef V. Kadlec, M.D., Ph.D.
Associate Professor of Pediatrics and Microbiology, Georgetown University School of Medicine; Member, International Center for Interdisciplinary Studies of Immunology, Georgetown University Medical Center, Washington, D.C.
Host Defense Mechanisms

Dorothy H. Kelly, M.D.
Associate Professor of Pediatrics, Harvard Medical School, Cambridge, Massachusetts; Associate Pediatrician and Associate Director of the Pediatric Pulmonary Unit, Massachusetts General Hospital, Boston, Massachusetts.
SIDS and Apnea of Infancy

Edwin L. Kendig, Jr., M.D., Sc.D.(Hon.)
Professor of Pediatrics, Medical College of Virginia, Health Sciences Division, Virginia Commonwealth University; Director, Child Chest Clinic, Medical College of Virginia Hospitals; Director Emeritus, Department of Pediatrics, St. Mary's Hospital, Richmond, Virginia.
Idiopathic Pulmonary Alveolar Microlithiasis; Sarcoidosis; Tuberculosis

Jerome O. Klein, M.D.
Professor of Pediatrics, Boston University School of Medicine; Director, Division of Pediatric Infectious Diseases, Boston City Hospital, Boston, Massachusetts.
Antimicrobial Therapy

Nathan L. Kobrinsky, M.D., BSc.(Med)
Clinical Professor of Oncology and Pediatrics, Department of Pediatrics, University of Saskatchewan College of Medicine; Head of Pediatric Hematology/ Oncology Programme, Saskatoon Cancer Centre and the Department of Pediatrics, University Hospital, Saskatoon, Saskatchewan, Canada.
Langerhans Cell Histiocytosis

Thomas M. Krummel, M.D.
Associate Professor of Surgery and Pediatrics, Chairman, Division of Pediatric Surgery, Department of Surgery, Medical College of Virginia, Health Sciences Division, Virginia Commonwealth University, Richmond, Virginia.
Congenital Malformations of the Lower Respiratory Tract; Disorders of the Respiratory Tract Due to Trauma; Foreign Bodies in the Air Passages

Barbara J. Law, M.D.
Section Head, Pediatric Infectious Diseases, and Associate Professor, Department of Pediatrics and Child Health, University of Manitoba Faculty of Medicine; Full-time Admitting Staff, Health Sciences Centre; Consultant, St. Boniface Hospital and St. Amant Centre, Winnipeg, Manitoba, Canada.
Pertussis

Richard J. Lemen, M.D.
Professor of Pediatrics, University of Arizona College of Medicine; Staff Physician, University Medical Center, Tucson, Arizona.
Bronchiectasis; Pulmonary Function Testing in the Office, Clinic, and Home

Henry Levison, M.D.
Professor of Pediatrics, University of Toronto Faculty of Medicine; Chief, Division of Respiratory Medicine, Hospital for Sick Children, Toronto, Ontario, Canada.
Cystic Fibrosis

Gerald M. Loughlin, M.D.
Associate Professor of Pediatrics, Johns Hopkins University School of Medicine; Chief, Eudowood Division of Pediatric Respiratory Sciences, Johns Hopkins Children's Center, Baltimore, Maryland.
Bronchitis

Stephen J. McGeady, M.D.
Director of Allergy and Clinical Immunology, Jefferson Medical College of Thomas Jefferson University; Medical Director, Jefferson Park Hospital, Philadelphia, Pennsylvania.
Pulmonary Hemorrhage and Massive Hemoptysis

Ian MacLusky, M.D.
Assistant Professor of Pediatrics, University of Toronto Faculty of Medicine; Director, Pulmonary Function and Sleep Laboratories, Hospital for Sick Children, Toronto, Ontario, Canada.
Cystic Fibrosis

Melvin I. Marks, M.D.
Professor and Vice Chair of Pediatrics, University of California, Irvine, California College of Medicine, Irvine, California; Medical Director, Miller Children's Hospital, Memorial Medical Center, Long Beach, California.
Bacterial Pneumonias

F. Stanford Massie, M.D.
Clinical Professor of Pediatrics, Medical College of Virginia, Health Sciences Division, Virginia Commonwealth University; Attending Staff, Medical College of Virginia, Virginia Commonwealth University, St. Mary's Hospital, Richmond, Virginia.
Nonasthmatic Allergic Pulmonary Disease

Jere Mead, M.D.
Cecil K. and Philip Drinker Professor of Environmental Physiology (Emeritus), Harvard School of Public Health, Cambridge, Massachusetts.
Age as a Factor in Respiratory Disease

Robert B. Mellins, M.D.
Professor of Pediatrics, and Director, Pediatric Pulmonary Division, Columbia University College of Physicians and Surgeons; Attending Physician, Babies Hospital, Columbia-Presbyterian Medical Center, New York, New York.
Lung Injury from Hydrocarbon Aspiration and Smoke Inhalation; Pulmonary Edema

Jerome H. Modell, M.D.
Professor and Chairperson, Department of Anesthesiology, University of Florida College of Medicine, Gainesville, Florida.
Drowning and Near-Drowning

Mark D. Montgomery, M.D.
Assistant Professor of Pediatrics, University of Calgary Faculty of Medicine; Staff Physician (Pediatric Pulmonologist), Children's Hospital of Calgary, Calgary, Alberta, Canada.
Pleurisy and Empyema

Rosa Lee Nemir, M.D.
Professor of Pediatrics, New York University School of Medicine; Director, Children's Chest Clinic, Bellevue Hospital, New York, New York.
Measles and Giant Cell Pneumonia

Jacqueline A. Noonan, M.D.
Professor and Chairman, Department of Pediatrics, University of Kentucky College of Medicine; Chief of Pediatrics, University of Kentucky Medical Center, Lexington, Kentucky.
Cor Pulmonale

Hugh M. O'Brodovich, M.D.
Associate Professor of Pediatrics, University of Toronto Faculty of Medicine, Research Institute, Hospital for Sick Children, Toronto; Staff Physician, Chest Division, Hospital for Sick Children, Toronto, Ontario, Canada.
The Functional Basis of Respiratory Pathology

Reynaldo D. Pagtakhan, M.D.
Professor of Pediatrics, University of Manitoba Faculty of Medicine; Associate Director, Pediatric Respirology, Children's Hospital, Winnipeg, Manitoba, Canada.
Intensive Care for Respiratory Disorders; Liquid and Air in the Pleural Space; Pleurisy and Empyema

Byung Hak Park, M.D.
Professor Emeritus, State University of New York at Buffalo, Buffalo, New York.
Chronic Granulomatous Disease of Childhood

Robert H. Parrott, M.D.
Professor of Pediatrics, George Washington University School of Medicine and Health Sciences; Director Emeritus, Children's National Medical Center, Washington, D.C.
Influenza

Robert F. Pass, M.D.
Professor of Pediatrics and Microbiology, University of Alabama School of Medicine; Staff, University Hospital and The Children's Hospital of Alabama, Birmingham, Alabama.
Cytomegalovirus

Hans Pasterkamp, M.D., F.R.C.P.(C)
Assistant Professor, Department of Pediatrics, University of Manitoba Faculty of Medicine; Section of Respirology, Children's Hospital of Winnipeg, Winnipeg, Manitoba, Canada.
The History and Physical Examination; Hydatid Disease of the Lung; Intensive Care for Respiratory Disorders

Mark S. Pasternack, M.D.
Assistant Professor of Pediatrics, Harvard Medical School, Cambridge, Massachusetts; Head, Pediatric Infectious Disease Unit, Massachusetts General Hospital, Boston, Massachusetts.
Legionnaires' Disease and Other Related Pneumonias

Edward N. Pattishall, M.D.
Research Assistant Professor of Pediatrics, University of North Carolina at Chapel Hill Medical School; North Carolina Memorial Hospital, Chapel Hill, North Carolina.
Sarcoidosis

David S. Pearlman, M.D.
Clinical Professor of Pediatrics, University of Colorado Medical School; Senior Clinical Staff, National Jewish Center for Immunology and Respiratory Medicine, Denver, Colorado.
Asthma

William E. Pierson, M.D.
Clinical Professor of Pediatrics and Environmental Health, University of Washington School of Medicine; Co-Director, Division of Allergy, Children's Hospital and Medical Center, Seattle, Washington.
Nonasthmatic Allergic Pulmonary Disease

Arnold C. G. Platzker, M.D.
Professor, Department of Pediatrics, University of Southern California School of Medicine; Head, Division of Neonatology and Pediatric Pulmonology, Children's Hospital of Los Angeles, Los Angeles, California.
Gastroesophageal Reflux and Respiratory Illness; Pulmonary Involvement in the Rheumatic Disorders of Childhood

Harris D. Riley, Jr., M.D.
Distinguished Professor of Pediatrics, University of Oklahoma College of Medicine; Attending Physician, Children's Hospital of Oklahoma, University of Oklahoma Health Sciences Center, Oklahoma City, Oklahoma.
Pulmonary Alveolar Proteinosis

Gilberto E. Rodriguez, M.D.
Associate Professor of Pediatrics, Medical College of Virginia, Health Sciences Division, Virginia Commonwealth University; Medical College of Virginia Hospitals, Richmond, Virginia.
Salmonella Pneumonia

Sami I. Said, M.D.
Professor of Medicine and Associate Head for Research, University of Illinois College of Medicine, Chicago, Illinois.
Metabolic and Endocrine Functions of the Lung

Arnold M. Salzberg, M.D.
Professor of Surgery and Pediatrics, Department of Surgery, Medical College of Virginia, Health Sciences Division, Virginia Commonwealth University, Richmond, Virginia.
Congenital Malformations of the Lower Respiratory Tract; Disorders of the Respiratory Tract Due to Trauma; Foreign Bodies in the Air Passages

Evelyn M. Saxon, B.S.
Senior Technologist and Supervisor at Virus Laboratory, Wyler Children's Hospital, Chicago, Illinois.
Chlamydial Infections of Infants

Craig M. Schramm, M.D.
Assistant Professor of Pediatrics, University of Pennsylvania School of Medicine; Division of Pulmonary Medicine, Children's Hospital of Philadelphia, Philadelphia, Pennsylvania.
Pulmonary Function Tests in Infants

Daniel C. Shannon, M.D.
Associate Professor of Pediatrics, Harvard-Massachusetts Institute of Technology Division of Health Sciences and Technology, Cambridge, Massachusetts; Director, Pediatric Pulmonary Unit, Massachusetts General Hospital, Boston, Massachusetts.
SIDS and Apnea of Infancy

Bruce Shuckett, M.D., F.R.C.P.(C)
Assistant Professor, Department of Radiology, University of Toronto Faculty of Medicine, Staff Radiologist, Hospital for Sick Children, Toronto, Ontario, Canada.
Langerhans Cell Histiocytosis

Bernhard H. Singsen, M.D.
Professor of Pediatrics, Jefferson Medical College of Thomas Jefferson University, Philadelphia, Pennsylvania; Attending Physician, Alfred I. DuPont Institute, Wilmington, Delaware.
Pulmonary Involvement in the Rheumatic Disorders of Childhood

David S. Smith, M.D.
Professor and Deputy Chairman, Department of Pediatrics, Temple University School of Medicine; Deputy Chairman, St. Christopher's Hospital for Children; Associate Staff, Nazareth Hospital, Philadelphia, Pennsylvania.
Pulmonary Hemorrhage and Massive Hemoptysis

Jennifer M. Sturgess, Ph.D.
Associate Professor, University of Toronto Faculty of Medicine; Consultant Scientist, Hospital for Sick Children, Toronto, Ontario, Canada.
The Immotile Cilia Syndrome

Harris R. Stutman, M.D.
Assistant Professor of Pediatrics, University of California, Irvine, California College of Medicine, Irvine, California; Director, Pediatric Infectious Disease Service, and Associate Director, Cystic Fibrosis Center, Miller Children's Hospital, Memorial Medical Center, Long Beach, California.
Bacterial Pneumonias

Morton N. Swartz, M.D.
Professor of Medicine, Harvard Medical School, Cambridge, Massachusetts; Chief, Infectious Disease Unit, Massachusetts General Hospital, Boston, Massachusetts.
Legionnaires' Disease and Other Related Pneumonias

Lynn M. Taussig, M.D.
Professor and Chairman, Department of Pediatrics, University of Arizona College of Medicine; Attending Physician and Chairman, Department of Pediatrics, University Medical Center; Attending Physician, Tucson Medical Center, Tucson, Arizona.
Acute Infections Producing Upper Airway Obstruction

William M. Thurlbeck, M.B., F.R.C.P.(C)
Professor of Pathology, University of British Columbia Faculty of Medicine; Pathologist, Children's Hospital; Consultant Pathologist, University Hospital, Vancouver, British Columbia, Canada.
Desquamative Interstitial Pneumonia and Other Variants of Interstitial Pneumonia; Usual Interstitial Pneumonia

Margaret A. Tipple, M.D.
Division of Viral and Rickettsial Diseases, Centers for Disease Control, Atlanta, Georgia.
Chlamydial Infections of Infants

Alexander O. Tuazon, M.D.
Assistant Professor, College of Medicine, University of the Philippines, Manila; Attending Pediatrician, Pediatric Pulmonology and Intensive Care, Philippine General Hospital, University of the Philippines, Manila, Manila, the Philippines.
Hydatid Disease of the Lung

J. A. Peter Turner, M.D., F.R.C.P.(C)
Professor Emeritus, Department of Pediatrics, University of Toronto Faculty of Medicine; Co-ordinator, Continuing Medical Education, Department of Pediatrics, Hospital for Sick Children, Toronto, Ontario, Canada.
The Immotile Cilia Syndrome

William W. Waring, M.D.
Professor of Pediatrics, and Chief, Section of Pulmonary Diseases, Department of Pediatrics, Tulane University School of Medicine; Senior Visiting Physician, Charity Hospital of Louisiana; Active Pediatric Staff, Tulane Medical Center Hospital, New Orleans, Louisiana.
Diagnostic and Therapeutic Procedures

Mary Ellen B. Wohl, M.D.
Associate Professor of Pediatrics, Harvard Medical School, Cambridge, Massachusetts; Chief, Division of Respiratory Diseases, and Senior Associate in Medicine, Children's Hospital, Boston, Massachusetts.
Age as a Factor in Respiratory Disease; Bronchiolitis

PREFACE

This new edition of *Kendig's Disorders of the Respiratory Tract in Children* continues the vision and philosophy established by Dr. Edwin L. Kendig, Jr., in the first edition published in 1967. The book is meant to provide information on almost any aspect of pediatric respiratory disease for the practitioner, resident, and intern in pediatrics; the chest physician; the roentgenologist; and the medical student. Since the last edition in 1983, subspecialty examinations in pediatric pulmonology have been established in both the American and Canadian medical systems, and the book should be a valuable text for trainees in the subspecialty.

Only 7 years have passed between the fourth and fifth editions. The explosion of medical information has required that all chapters be rewritten or carefully revised and updated. There are 28 new contributors who are leaders in their fields. In addition, seven chapters have been added that provide the most recent information on pulmonary function testing in infants, exercise testing in children, host defense mechanisms and their relevance to pediatric lung disease, psittacosis, hydatid cyst, pulmonary disorders in pediatric AIDS, and disorders of breathing during sleep.

With this edition there has been another major change as I assumed the position of editor. Fortunately, Ed Kendig has remained as consulting editor, and I am very grateful for his wise counsel, encouragement, and friendship, which were invaluable. One has to take on this arduous (and sometimes aggravating!) task to appreciate fully what he has accomplished in the past.

I am also grateful to Mr. Albert E. Meier, formerly of the W.B. Saunders Company, and Mrs. Hazel Hacker and Ms. Lee Ann Draud of the W.B. Saunders Company for their advice and help.

VICTOR CHERNICK, M.D.

CONTENTS

GENERAL CONSIDERATIONS

HUGH M. O'BRODOVICH, M.D., and
GABRIEL G. HADDAD, M.D.

1

THE FUNCTIONAL BASIS OF RESPIRATORY PATHOLOGY

A knowledge of the normal development and physiologic function of the lungs is required to understand the pathophysiology that is seen in disease. Historically our understanding of lung function was derived solely from clinical observation and postmortem histologic examination. The development of invasive and noninvasive techniques that were capable of assessing lung function in living subjects greatly improved our understanding of lung physiology on an "organ basis." There has been an explosion of knowledge in cellular and molecular biology. Clearly it is beyond the scope of a single chapter to discuss in detail these various levels of lung physiology. We shall indicate, however, some of the areas in which this relatively new knowledge has increased our understanding of how the lung develops and functions.

NORMAL LUNG ANATOMY AND CELL FUNCTION

A knowledge of normal lung anatomy is one of the basic requirements for understanding lung function in health and disease. Because detailed descriptions of lung anatomy are available elsewhere, this section will focus on selected aspects of gross and microscopic anatomy to enable the reader to understand the physiologic changes that occur in congenital and acquired lung disease.

AIRWAYS

The basic structure of the airways is already present at birth, and thus neonates and adults share a common bronchopulmonary anatomy (Fig. 1–1). Airways within the lung, however, are quite asymmetric at all ages. When airways divide, there is a variation in the size and number of branches (irregular dichotomous branching), and depending on the location there may be anywhere from 10 (hilar region) to 25 (basal region) airway divisions before the gas-exchanging units are reached. This airway variability has physiologic implications; for example, different pathways will have different resistances to airflow,

and a heterogeneous distribution of gases or inhaled particles may occur. As the bronchi branch and decrease in size, they lose their cartilage and become bronchioles. Ultimately, a terminal bronchiole opens up into the gas-exchanging area of the lung (Fig. 1–2).

The airways are lined with an epithelial membrane that gradually changes from ciliated pseudostratified columnar epithelium in the bronchi to a ciliated cuboidal epithelium near the gas-exchanging units. Ciliated cells predominate throughout this epithelium and are responsible for propelling mucus from the peripheral airways to the pharynx. This mucociliary transport system is an important defense mechanism of the lungs (see also "Nonrespiratory Aspects of the Lung"). The cilia form a dense, long carpet on top of the epithelial cells, and their coordinated to-and-fro action propels the mucous layer toward the oropharynx. Cilia are a derivative of the centrioles, and there are approximately 200 of them on the apex of each ciliated cell. The cilia are anchored within the cell with a basal body that is oriented in the direction of mucous movement. The shaft of the cilium has a central pair of single tubules that are connected via radial spokes to nine peripheral pairs of tubules. The tip of the cilium has tiny hooklets that probably help grab the gel component of the mucous layer and propel it forward. The cilium has a beat frequency of 12 ± 1 SD hertz and is coordinated both with other cilium on that cell and concurrently with the cilium on adjacent cells to yield a synchronized wave flowing up the airway. Primary ciliary dyskinesia (PCD) is a group of disorders that includes Kartagener syndrome and the erroneously named immotile cilia syndrome. In PCD there are defects within the tubules, in their inner or outer dynein arms, or in the radial arms that result in a disorganized movement of the cilia that precludes normal mucociliary transport and results in chronic bronchitis and repeated pneumonias (see Chapter 45).

Goblet cells are seen in the trachea and bronchi. They produce mucin within their rough endoplasmic reticulum and Golgi apparatus. Mucin is a viscous mixture of acid glycoproteins that contributes to the mucous layer. Goblet cells can increase in number in

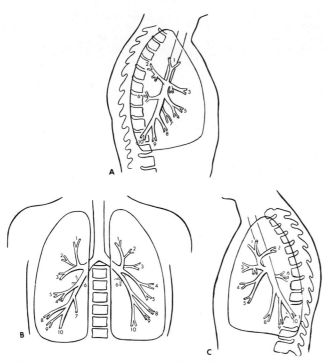

Figure 1–1. The nomenclature of bronchopulmonary anatomy, from a report by the Thoracic Society in 1950. (Adapted from Negus V: The Biology of Respiration. Baltimore, Williams & Wilkins Co, 1965.) A, right lateral view; B, anterior view; C, left lateral view.

Right lung
Upper lobe
1. Apical
2. Posterior
3. Anterior
Middle lobe
4. Lateral
5. Medial
Lower lobe
6. Apical
7. Cardiac (medial basal)
8. Anterior ⎫
9. Lateral ⎬ basal
10. Posterior ⎭

Left lung
Upper lobe
1. ⎫
2. ⎬ Apicoposterior
3. Anterior
4. ⎫
5. ⎬ Lingula
Lower lobe
6. Apical
7. ——absent
8. Anterior ⎫
9. Lateral ⎬ basal
10. Posterior ⎭

disorders such as chronic bronchitis, the result being mucous hypersecretion and increased sputum production. There are several other cell types found within the airways; however, their functional significance is less well understood. The basal cell, commonly seen within the pseudostratified columnar epithelium, is undifferentiated and may be a precursor of ciliated or secretory cells. The brush cell has a dense tuft of broad, short microvilli and is only very rarely seen within the conducting airways and alveolar space. Clara cells are seen exclusively within the bronchiolar region of the lung. Their physiologic role has been uncertain, but data suggest that they may play two important roles. First, because they contain but do not synthesize surfactant apoproteins, they may recycle surfactant within the distal lung unit. Second, they are capable of actively transporting sodium from their apical to their basal side and thus

may be involved in the reabsorption of fluid from the distal lung unit.

There are curious cells found within the airways that are believed to possess neuroendocrine properties. They are known under a variety of names, including Feyrter or Kulchitsky cells. Histochemical staining indicates that they contain a variety of vasoactive peptides, including serotonin and kinins, so these cells may belong to the class of amine precursor uptake and decarboxylation (APUD) cells. These neuroendocrine cells are innervated and are found more frequently, and in groups (neuroepithelial bodies), within the fetal airways or in pediatric disorders characterized by chronic hypoxemia (e.g., bronchopulmonary dysplasia).

Histologically the remainder of the airway consists of the lamina propria, with its network of blood vessels and nerves, and a variable amount of smooth muscle and cartilage. Within the lamina propria are found mast cells containing vasoactive peptides and amines, cells of the immune system (plasma cells, lymphocytes, and phagocytes), and mucous glands. These mucous glands are present in large and small bronchi and are the chief source of airway secretions. In the main stem bronchi, cartilage is present in C-shaped rings. However, as further branching occurs, progressively less cartilage is present, so that bronchi 2 mm in diameter have cartilage only at the origins of the bronchioles. Cartilage adds structural rigidity to the airway and thus plays an important role in maintaining airway patency, especially during expiration. Congenital deficiency of airway cartilage and hence airway instability has been associated with bronchiectasis (Williams-Campbell syndrome) and congenital lobar emphysema.

The smooth muscle content of the airway also varies with its anatomic location. In the largest airways a muscle bundle connects the two ends of the C-shaped cartilage. As the amount of cartilage decreases, the smooth muscle assumes a helical orientation and gradually becomes thinner, ultimately reaching the alveolar ducts. Muscle contraction increases airway rigidity in all airways and terminal respiratory units.

Although it has been widely assumed that the airway muscles of newborn infants are inadequate for bronchoconstriction, the data do not support this belief. Even premature infants have smooth muscle, and although the amount may be statistically less than that seen in adults, it is likely enough to constrict the infant's much more compliant airways. Indeed, pulmonary function test results have demonstrated that airway resistance can be altered with bronchodilating drugs. The belief that infants have little or no smooth muscle in their airways is even less tenable in such disorders as bronchopulmonary dysplasia and left-to-right congenital heart disease, in which hypertrophy of the airway smooth muscle has been demonstrated by morphometric measurement. Congenital deficiency of large-airway smooth muscle and elastic fibers is associated with marked dilation of the

Figure 1–2. The architecture of the lung. *A*, Fresh frozen cat lung. Segmental cartilaginous bronchus and branches. The pulmonary artery is close to the airway; the pulmonary vein is in a more peripheral location (×4). *B*, Fresh frozen cat lung (×4). Terminal bronchiole with many alveolar ducts arising from it. *C*, Thick section of cat lung. A single alveolar wall is in the plane of focus. Individual red blood cells in alveolar capillaries are clearly seen (×100). *D*, Guinea pig, fixed thin section. The terminal respiratory unit, with alveoli shown as outpouchings of the alveolar duct, arises from the terminal bronchiole at the top of the picture. Note that three vessels, probably pulmonary veins, mark the distal boundaries of the unit (×15). (Reproduced with permission from Dr. Norman Staub. All but *A* appeared in color in Anesthesiology *24*:831, 1963.)

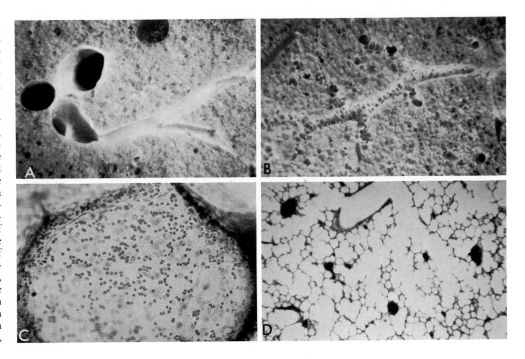

trachea and bronchi, which promotes retention of airway secretions and ultimately leads to recurrent pulmonary sepsis (Mounier-Kuhn syndrome).

TERMINAL RESPIRATORY UNIT

The terminal respiratory (gas-exchanging) unit consists of the structures distal to the terminal bronchiole: the respiratory bronchiole (bronchiole with alveoli budding from its wall), alveolar ducts, and alveoli. This unit is also known as an acinus and may be considered the basic functional unit of the lung. Terminal respiratory units are well suited for gas exchange. In the adult lung these units have a total gas volume of 2500 ml and a surface area of 80 sq m, yet all alveoli are within 5 mm of the closest terminal bronchiole. True alveoli are not spherical but more closely resemble hexagons with flat, sheet-like surfaces. Their average total depth ranges from 250 to 300 μ. Within the terminal respiratory units, two types of intercommunicating channels provide collateral ventilation for the gas-exchanging units. The alveolar pores of Kohn are holes in the alveolar wall of 3 to 13 μ in diameter that provide channels for gas movement between contiguous alveoli. These pores are not present in newborn lungs. The canals of Lambert are accessory channels that connect a small airway to an air space normally supplied by a different airway.

The alveoli are lined by two types of epithelial cells (Fig. 1–3). The type I epithelial cell is an extremely broad, thin (0.1 to 0.5 μ) cell that covers 95 per cent of the alveolar surface. It is a markedly differentiated cell possessing few organelles. The type II epithelial cells are more numerous than type I cells, but owing to their cuboidal shape, type II cells occupy only 5 per cent of the alveolar surface area (Table 1–1). They are characterized histologically by microvilli and osmophilic inclusion bodies.

The type II epithelial cell maintains homeostasis within the alveolar space in several ways. First, it is the source of pulmonary surfactant and as such indicates maturity of the lung; it decreases the surface tension at the alveolar air liquid interface. Second, this cell is likely the precursor of the alveolar type I cell and thus plays a key role in the repair process following lung injury. Third, it is capable of actively transporting ions against an electrochemical gradient and likely is involved in both fetal lung liquid secretion and, postnatally, the reabsorption of fluid from the air space following the development of alveolar pulmonary edema (see also "Fetal Lung Liquid Secretion"). Two pediatric disorders associated with the type II epithelial cell are (1) its lack of maturity and surfactant secretion in *hyaline membrane disease* and (2) its excessive and disordered secretion of surfactant in *alveolar proteinosis*.

The cell junctions (zonulae occludentes) between alveolar type I and II cells are very tight and restrict the movement of both macromolecules and small

Table 1–1. CELLULAR CHARACTERISTICS OF THE HUMAN LUNG

Cell Type	Total Cells (%)	Apical Surface Area (μm²)
Epithelium		
Alveolar type I	8.3	5098
Alveolar type II	15.9	183
Endothelium	30.2	1353
Interstitial	36.1	
Alveolar macrophages	9.4	

Data from Crapo JD, Barry BE, Gehr P et al: Am Rev Respir Dis 125:740–745, 1982.

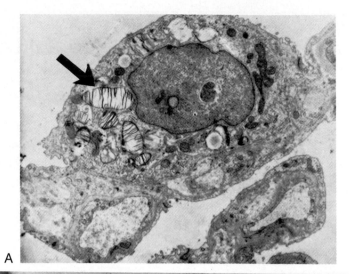

A

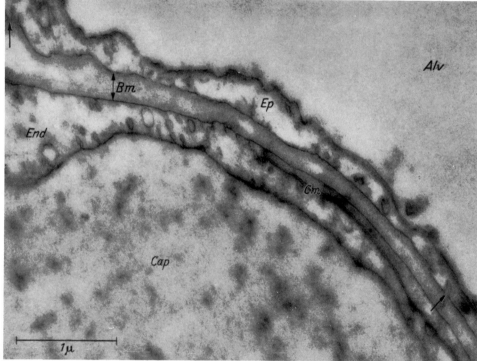

B

Figure 1–3. *A,* Electron micrograph of a type II epithelial cell. This particular cell is from a dog's lung but is similar to those found in all mammalian lungs. The air space is in the upper portion of the figure. The *arrow* points to the osmophilic inclusions that are thought to be associated with the alveolar lining substance. The cell rests on a basement membrane that separates it from the capillary endothelium in the lower part of the picture. (Courtesy of ES Boatman and HB Martin.) *B,* Normal human lung showing the attenuated alveolar cytoplasm of a type I epithelial cell. *Alv,* alveolus; *Ep,* cytoplasmic layer of an epithelial cell; *Bm* basement membrane; *End,* capillary endothelium; *Cm,* erythrocyte cell membrane; *Cap,* capillary. (Reproduced with permission from Schultz H: The Submicroscopic Anatomy and Pathology of the Lung. Berlin, Springer-Verlag, 1959.)

ions such as sodium and chloride. This tightness is an essential characteristic of the cells lining the alveolar space; it enables the active transport of ions. Also these tight junctions provide a margin of safety for patients susceptible to pulmonary edema: significant interstitial pulmonary edema can be present without alveolar flooding occurring, thus preserving gas exchange.

There is a thick side and a thin side to the alveolar capillary membrane. Gas exchange is thought to occur predominantly on the thin side, where there are only the alveolar epithelial cell, fused basement membranes, and endothelial cell (Fig. 1–3). The thick side consists of connective tissue, amorphous ground substance, and scattered fibroblasts. The thick side,

in addition to providing structural support, acts as a site of fluid and solute exchange.

PULMONARY VASCULAR SYSTEM

The lung receives blood from both ventricles. The entire right ventricular output enters the lung via the pulmonary arteries, and blood ultimately reaches the gas-exchanging units by one of the pulmonary arterial branching systems. Conventional arteries accompany the bronchial tree and divide with it, each branch accompanying the appropriate bronchial division. Supernumerary arteries do not travel with the airways but directly supply the gas-exchanging units.

These extra arteries actually outnumber the conventional ones and supply approximately one third of the pulmonary capillary bed. Their likely physiologic role is to act as a collateral circulation so that the lung can filter out blood-borne particles while maintaining an adequate blood supply. The pulmonary capillary bed is the largest vascular bed in the body and covers a surface area of 70 to 80 sq m. The network of capillaries is so dense that it is best thought of as a sheet of blood interrupted by small vertical supporting posts. The pulmonary veins return blood to the left atrium via conventional and supernumerary branches. By virtue of their larger numbers and thinner walls, the pulmonary veins provide a large reservoir for blood and help maintain a constant left ventricular output in the face of a variable pulmonary arterial flow.

The bronchial arteries, usually three in number, provide a source of well-oxygenated systemic blood to the lungs. This blood supply nourishes the walls of the bronchi, bronchioles, blood vessels, and nerves in addition to perfusing the lymph nodes and most of the visceral pleura. There are numerous communications between the bronchial arterial system and the remainder of the pulmonary vascular bed: approximately one third of the blood returns to the right atrium via bronchial veins, and the remainder drains into the left atrium via pulmonary veins. Although normally the bronchial arteries receive only 1 to 2 per cent of the cardiac output, they hypertrophy in chronically infected lungs, and blood flow may easily increase by more than tenfold. This is clinically important because virtually all hemoptysis originates from the bronchial vessels in such disorders as cystic fibrosis.

Histologically, the pulmonary arteries can be classified as elastic, muscular, partially muscular, or nonmuscular. The elastic pulmonary arteries are characterized by elastic fibers embedded in their muscular coat, whereas the smaller muscular arteries have a circular layer of smooth muscle bounded by internal and external elastic laminae. As arteries decrease further in size, only a spiral of muscle remains (partially muscular arteries), which ultimately disappears so that vessels still larger than capillaries have no muscle in their walls (nonmuscular arteries). In the adult lung, elastic arteries are greater than 1000 μ in diameter, and muscular arteries range from 150 to 100 μ. In the pediatric age group, histologic structure is not as easily determined from vessel size. Reid and co-workers have demonstrated that during growth of the lung a remodeling of the pulmonary vasculature occurs. Muscularization of the arteries lags behind multiplication of alveoli and appearance of new arteries. Therefore the patient's age must be considered before histologic structure can be assumed from vessel size within the pulmonary acinus (Fig. 1–4).

The endothelium of the pulmonary vascular system is continuous and nonfenestrated. As previously mentioned for the type II epithelium lining the air

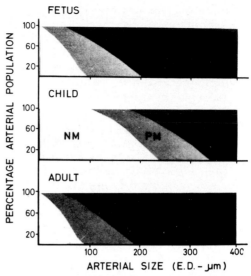

Figure 1–4. The populations of the three arterial types: muscular (*M*), partially muscular (*PM*), and nonmuscular (*NM*), in fetus, child, and adult. The distribution of structure in size is similar in fetus and adult, whereas during childhood NM and PM structures are found in much larger arteries. *E.D.*, external diameter. (Reproduced with permission from Reid LM: The pulmonary circulation: remodelling in growth and disease. Am Rev Respir Dis 119:531, 1979.)

space, it is now known that the endothelium is an intensely active cell layer and is not just serving a passive barrier function. The endothelial cell produces a glycocalyx that interacts with blood-borne substances and blood cellular elements, thereby influencing such homeostatic functions as hemostasis. The endothelium produces von Willebrand factor, which is part of the factor VIII complex and is necessary for normal platelet function. Similarly, there are enzymes located on the surface and within the cell itself that are capable of synthesizing, altering, or degrading blood-borne vasoactive products (see also "Nonrespiratory Aspects of the Lung"). The individual cells are separated by gaps of approximately 35 Å in radius, which allow the free movement of water and small ions but restrict the movement of proteins. The cells and the basement membrane on which they sit carry different net surface charges, which affect the movement of anionic macromolecules such as proteins and thus affect lung water and solute exchange (see Chapter 38). The capacity of the pulmonary endothelium and its basement membrane to restrict fluid and protein movement is impressive. It has been estimated that the amount of lung lymph flow is only 10 to 20 ml/hr despite a total blood flow of 300,000 ml/hr.

LYMPHATIC SYSTEM

There is an extensive interconnecting network of lymphatic vessels throughout the lung. The major function of this network is to collect the protein and water that has moved out of the pulmonary vascular space and to return it to the circulation, thus maintaining the lung at an appropriate degree of hydration. The lymphatic vessels travel alongside the blood vessels in the loose connective tissue of the pleura and bronchovascular spaces. It is likely—although controversy still exists regarding the issue—that there are no lymphatics within the alveolar wall itself and that juxta-alveolar lymphatics represent the beginning of the pulmonary lymphatic system. Histologically, the lymphatic capillaries consist of thin, irregular endothelial cells lacking a basement membrane. Occasionally, there are large gaps between endothelial cells that allow direct communication with the interstitial space. Larger lymphatic vessels contain smooth muscle in their walls that undergoes rhythmic contraction. This muscular contraction plus the presence of funnel-shaped, monocuspid valves ensures an efficient unidirectional flow of lymph. In addition to helping maintain lung water balance, the lymphatic system is one of the pulmonary defense mechanisms. It aids in removal of particulate matter from the lung, and aggregates of lymph tissue near major airways contribute to the host's immune response.

INNERVATION OF THE LUNG

The lung is innervated by both components of the autonomic nervous system. Parasympathetic nerves arise from the vagus nerve, and sympathetic nerves are derived from the upper thoracic sympathetic ganglia. These branches congregate around the hila of the lung to form the pulmonary plexus. Myelinated and nonmyelinated fibers then enter the lung tissues and travel along with and innervate the airways and blood vessels. Although the anatomic location of pulmonary nerves has been elucidated, their physiologic role in health and disease is incompletely understood. In general, the airways constrict in response to vagal stimulation and dilate in response to adrenergic stimulation. The pulmonary vasculature appears to be maximally dilated under normal conditions, and it is difficult to demonstrate any significant physiologic effect of either parasympathetic or sympathetic stimulation. The vascular response, however, is influenced by age and initial vascular tone: for example, in fetal lungs vagal stimulation results in significant vasodilation, but sympathetic stimulation results in marked vasoconstriction.

Sensory nerves from the lungs are vagal in origin and arise from slowly and rapidly adapting receptors and from C-fiber receptors. The slowly adapting (stretch) receptors, located in the smooth muscle of the airway, are stimulated by an increase in lung volume or transpulmonary pressure. They induce several physiologic responses including inhibition of inspiration (Hering-Breuer reflex), bronchodilation, increased heart rate, and decreased systemic vascular resistance. The rapidly adapting vagal (irritant) receptors are activated by a wide variety of noxious stimuli, ranging from mechanical stimulation of the airways to anaphylactic reactions within the lung

parenchyma. The rapidly adapting receptors induce hyperpnea, cough, and constriction of the airways and larynx. C-fiber receptors are the terminus of nonmyelinated vagal afferents. They include the J receptors that are located near the pulmonary capillaries and are stimulated by pulmonary congestion and edema; they evoke a sensation of dyspnea and induce rapid shallow breathing along with laryngeal constriction during expiration.

Humans and several other species have, in addition to the sympathetic and parasympathetic nervous system, a third nervous system within their lungs. The noncommittal name *nonadrenergic noncholinergic nervous system* has been chosen because its function and properties are not understood. Purines, substance P, and vasoactive intestinal polypeptide (VIP) have been suggested as possible neurotransmitters for this system.

INTERSTITIUM

The interstitium plays several roles in lung function in addition to providing a structural framework that consists of insoluble proteins. The ground substance influences cell growth and differentiation and lung water and solute movement. The cells contained within this region of the lung not only play their own individual roles that result from their contractile or synthetic properties but also can interact with other cells, such as the endothelium and epithelium, to alter the basic structure and function of the lung.

Most of the interstitial matrix of the lung is composed of type I collagen. Type I, along with the less common types II, III, IV, and V collagen, forms a structural, fibrous framework within the lung. The three principal components of this framework, which include the axial, peripheral, and septal fiber systems, are illustrated in Figure 1–5. Elastin, a contractile insoluble protein, provides elasticity and support to

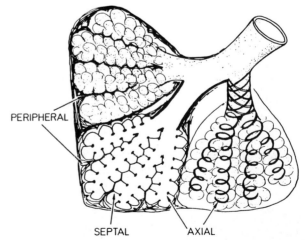

Figure 1–5. Schematic diagram of the fibrous support of the lung. See text for detail. (Reproduced with permission from Weibel ER and Bachofen H: News in Physiological Sciences 2:72–75, 1987.)

the structures. Both elastin and collagen are long-lived proteins within the interstitium that turn over very slowly. In diseases such as alpha$_1$-antitrypsin deficiency (in elastin) and pulmonary fibrosis (in collagen), there are marked qualitative and quantitative changes in these proteins. The remainder of the matrix is made up of proteoglycans and glycosaminoglycans. These carbohydrate-protein complexes can affect cell proliferation and differentiation in addition to their known effect on cell adhesion and attachment (e.g., laminin) and ability to diminish fluid movement (glycosaminoglycans).

Fibroblasts are capable of synthesizing collagen, elastin, and glycosaminoglycans and hence contribute significantly to the composition of the lung's interstitial space. They can be found within all of the interstitial regions of the lung, although their apparent structure may change. For example, because "myofibroblasts" contain obvious contractile elements, they may represent fibroblasts that are capable of contraction, or they may be cells that are intermediate between fibroblasts and smooth muscle cells. Similarly, it is likely that morphologically similar fibroblasts are not similar in terms of proliferative capacity and ability to synthesize various types of collagen. Data suggest that fibrotic lung diseases are characterized by the loss of the normal heterogenous fibroblast population and that there may be a selection for certain clones that promote inappropriate collagen deposition within the lung parenchyma.

Smooth muscle cells are contractile interstitial cells that influence the bronchomotor and vasomotor tone within the conducting airways and blood vessels. They are also seen within the free edge of the alveolar septa, and they form an alveolar entrance ring that is capable of constricting or dilating. The smooth muscle cells form bundles connected by nexus or gap junctions that enable electrical coupling and synchronous contraction. The pericyte is another interstitial cell that is found between the basement membrane and the endothelium. It is believed to be a precursor cell that can differentiate into a mature vascular smooth muscle cell.

There are a variety of interstitial cells that are concerned with immune and nonimmune defense of the lung. The interstitial macrophage and the alveolar macrophage are predominantly responsible for nonimmune defense, which they manage by ingesting particulate matter and removing it from the lung. These macrophages along with their alveolar counterparts are capable of secreting many compounds, including proteases and cytokines (substances capable of modulating the growth and function of other cells). B and T lymphocytes are present in the lung and especially within the bronchus-associated lymphoid tissue (BALT), where they contribute to the cellular and humorally mediated immune response.

Although not within the interstitium per se, there are large numbers of intravascular granulocytes that adhere to the pulmonary endothelium. Indeed, next to the bone marrow and spleen, there are more granulocytes within the lung than in any other organ. These granulocytes can be released into the systemic circulation during such stimuli as exercise or the infusion of adrenalin, and this demargination is responsible for the concomitant blood leukocytosis. These leukocytes are also in a prime location for movement into the lung should an infection or inflammatory stimulus occur. There is much evidence to suggest that the pulmonary granulocyte contributes to the pulmonary dysfunction seen in acute lung injury or adult respiratory distress syndrome.

GROWTH AND DEVELOPMENT OF THE LUNG

PRENATAL LUNG GROWTH

Intrauterine growth and development of the lung have been divided into various stages with names that reflect the respective histologic appearance of the lung, the region of the lung that is most obviously developing, or both. Obviously, all the regions of the lung are developing during the various stages; in addition, there are variations in growth rates among individual fetuses. Thus there is no exact differentiation between the various stages. Various investigators have described slightly different periods. However, the major reason for identifying these stages of development is to improve our understanding of how and why specific congenital lesions occur. Obviously, the child with unilateral lung agenesis must have had defective lung development much earlier than another child with a peripheral congenital lung cyst.

The five stages of lung development are (1) embryonic (day 26 to day 52), (2) pseudoglandular (day 52 to week 16), (3) canalicular (week 16 to 28), (4) saccular (week 28 to 36), and (5) alveolar (week 36 to term). This slight change in classification largely results from the observation that there are true alveoli present in the human lung before birth, with the first being seen at 29 to 32 weeks of gestation. This example illustrates the inexact nature of staging lung development, since the alveolar period does not "begin" until 36 weeks (Fig. 1–6).

The lung first appears in the embryonic period as a ventral outpouching of the primitive gut. The primary bronchi elongate into the mesenchyme and divide into the two main bronchi. In the pseudoglandular period the branching continues by means of a higher mitotic rate in the epithelium relative to the mesenchyme. The mesenchyme differentiates into cartilage, smooth muscle, and connective tissue around the epithelial tubes. By the end of the pseudoglandular period (16 weeks) all the major conducting airways including the terminal bronchioles have formed. The canalicular period is characterized by the development of respiratory bronchioles, each of which ends in two or three thin-walled dilations called terminal sacs or primitive alveoli. Vasculariza-

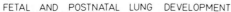

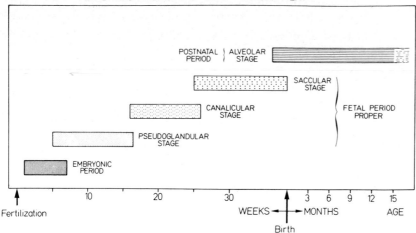

Figure 1–6. Various stages of lung development. The actual separation of individual stages is not discrete, and it overlaps. Note that the alveolar stage commences before birth. (Reproduced with permission from Burri PH: Annu Rev Physiol 46:617–628, 1984. © 1984 by Annual Reviews, Inc.)

tion of the lung interstitium intensifies, and the glandular appearance is lost as there is a decrease in the relative amount of connective tissue. Further differentiation of the respiratory portion of the lung takes place during the saccular period. During this period, there is for the first time close contact between the air space and the blood stream, as the pulmonary capillaries rapidly proliferate and the epithelium thins. Gas exchange is now possible although obviously not optimal. Elastic fibers, which will be important in subsequent true alveolar development, are beginning to be laid down. At this time cuboidal (type II) and thin (type I) epithelial cells line the air space. During the alveolar period further refinement takes place as tiny secondary septa form on the walls of the larger saccules. These outpouchings grow into the lumen and form the walls of true alveoli, thus further increasing the surface area available for gas exchange.

The development of the pulmonary vasculature coincides with the development of the airways. During the embryonic period the main pulmonary artery arises from the sixth branchial arch and nourishes the developing lung bud. Throughout the pseudo-glandular period, arteries are evident alongside the conducting airways. In addition to the conventional arteries that branch and travel with the airways, supernumerary arteries are evident by 12 weeks of gestation. By 16 weeks of gestation all preacinar arterial branches have formed; although these will increase in size and length, no new preacinar branches will appear. During the canalicular period the lung develops a rich vascular supply that is closely associated with the respiratory bronchioles. As saccules begin to develop during the saccular period, capillaries can be found within the walls of the air spaces in close contact with the epithelium. Gas exchange can now occur.

The maturation of surfactant production has been studied intensively since Avery and Mead's discovery that prematurely born infants with hyaline membrane disease had abnormal surface tension at the air-liquid interface. It is now known that the source

of pulmonary surfactant is the mature type II epithelial cell. When the type II epithelial cell first appears within the lung during the saccular stage, however, it is immature and contains much intracellular glycogen. Many drugs and hormones, including steroids, thyroid and peptide hormones, can influence surfactant biosynthesis and accelerate lung maturation. One intriguing observation is the interaction of the pulmonary fibroblast with the type II epithelial cell. The fibroblast can secrete a factor that induces the type II cell to rapidly synthesize and secrete surfactant (see subsequent discussion). Surfactant itself is a mixture of phospholipids (predominantly dipalmityl phosphatidylcholine but also contains lesser amounts of other phospholipids, such as phosphatidylinositol and phosphatidylglycerol) and lipophilic proteins. These surfactant-associated proteins (SPs) are important for normal surfactant function, because their exclusion from surfactant preparations prevents normal in vivo performance. There are at least three families of SP: SP-A has a molecular weight of approximately 35,000 daltons; this family, along with SP-B, with molecular weight of approximately 15,000 daltons, does not appear to be necessary for in vivo surfactant performance. Instead SP-A and SP-B may play a role in the recycling of surfactant within the distal lung unit. In contrast, SP-C, which has a molecular weight of approximately 3500 daltons, is essential for in vivo performance of surfactant. Identification of the genes responsible for the synthesis of these SPs will shortly enable their large-scale production, which, when combined with synthetic phospholipids, can be used in the treatment of respiratory distress syndromes.

The control of lung development is complex and is now known to be strongly influenced by interactions between the pulmonary epithelium and mesenchyme. Epithelium isolated in vitro does not undergo morphogenesis; when it is recombined with pulmonary mesenchyme, development resumes. In a similar manner, it has been demonstrated that the mesenchymal signals can be organ specific. For example, submandibular mesenchyme can induce

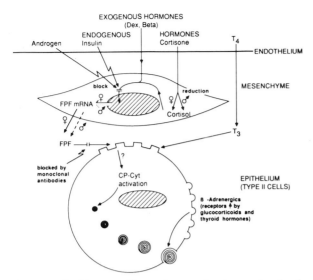

Figure 1–7. Diagram illustrating mechanisms whereby hormones regulate the development of pulmonary surfactant during fetal life. *FPF*, fibroblast pneumonocyte factor; *Dex*, dexamethasone; *Beta*, betamethasone; T_3, triiodothyronine; T_4, thyroxine; *CP-Cyt*, cholinephosphate cytidyltransferase. (Reproduced with permission from Post M and van Golde LMG: Biochim Biophys Acta 947:249–286, 1988.)

mammary gland epithelium to express submandibular epithelium gene products. Thus defects in lung epithelial development could conceivably result from abnormalities within the mesenchymal rather than the epithelial structures.

The mesenchyme's influence on lung development can be classified as instructive (directive) or permissive. The former influence instructs the epithelium to take a specific developmental pathway (e.g., to differentiate into a type II versus a ciliated epithelial cell). In contrast, permissive inductions allow an already committed cell to express its capabilities (e.g., a type II cell to start secreting surfactant).

Mesenchymal and epithelial interactions may, in some circumstances, depend on direct cell-to-cell communication. Morphologic studies have demonstrated that during the later stages of lung development the epithelial cells extend foot processes through the basement membrane and contact interstitial cells. In other circumstances, secreted factors might influence cellular differentiation. One example of this last process is fibroblast pneumonocyte factor (FPF). If type II cells are exposed in vitro to corticosteroids there is no induction of surfactant synthesis. In contrast, if fibroblasts are exposed to steroids, they release FPF, which in turn causes type II cell maturation and surfactant release (Fig. 1–7).

FETAL LUNG LIQUID SECRETION

Fetal lung liquid secretion is essential for normal lung development. Exactly when the lung begins to secrete fluid is unknown, but the secretion is well established by the second half of gestation and is produced at a rate of 4 to 5 ml/kg/hr. Analysis of fetal lung liquid has demonstrated that it is neither a mere ultrafiltrate of plasma nor aspirated amniotic fluid. The lung fluid relative to plasma has higher concentrations of chloride ($\sim$155 mM) and potassium ($\sim$6 mM), similar sodium concentration, and markedly lower bicarbonate ($\sim$3 mM) concentration. The lung liquid protein concentration is so low that it is comparable to cerebrospinal fluid ($\sim$0.03 g/dL). Olver and others have demonstrated that this fetal lung liquid secretion is dependent on the active transport of electrolytes into the air space (Olver, Ramsden, Strang, and Walters, 1986).

There are two requirements for the active secretion of fluid into the developing air spaces (Fig. 1–8). First, there must be an electrochemical gradient for ion movement that will carry water with it. The source of energy for the active transport is the sodium-potassium ATPase located on the basolateral epithelial cell membrane. As the pump extrudes sodium out of the cell, there is a linked re-entry of this sodium along with chloride (and perhaps potassium) back into the cell down sodium's electrochemical gradient. The intracellular chloride concentration rises, and it exits out into the air space through chloride channels in the apical membrane, driven out by the electrical gradient (the inside of the cell membrane is negative relative to the lumen). The second requirement for ion transport is a very tight epithelial membrane, which is necessary to establish these gradients and to prevent rapid backward flow of ions and water between the cells. This requirement is met by the extremely tight interepithelial junctions that restrict the movement of these small ions. Data from fetal sheep suggest that the air space's epithelium is tight and remarkably constant between 50 per cent of gestation and term.

THE LUNG AT BIRTH

Many dramatic changes must occur in the lungs during the transition from intrauterine to extrauter-

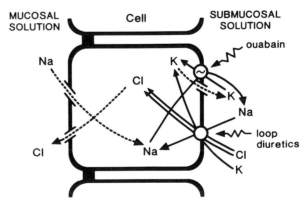

Figure 1–8. A model of pathways for active transport of electrolytes by a pulmonary epithelial cell. In fetal life, chloride (*Cl*) secretion predominates and presumably occurs via the apical Cl channel. After birth sodium (*Na*) absorption is dominant. Ouabain inhibits the Na-K ATPase pump, whereas loop diuretics can inhibit the Na:K:2Cl cotransporter, thus impeding Cl secretion. See text for details. (Reproduced with permission from Welsh M: Physiol Rev 67:1143–1184, 1987.)

ine life. The lung's epithelium must change from fluid secretion to fluid absorption, the distal lung units must fill with and retain the inhaled air, and blood flow must increase approximately twentyfold.

Just before birth the lungs contain approximately 30 ml/kg of fetal lung liquid. At the time of birth it is essential that fetal lung liquid secretion decrease so that the lung liquid can be cleared to allow for normal gas exchange. The control mechanisms for this decrease in secretion are incompletely understood, but evidence suggests that catecholamines released before or during the birth process will decrease secretion, possibly by inhibiting chloride ion transport, opening sodium channels in the apex of the epithelial cell, thereby converting it into a sodium reabsorbing membrane, or both. It has also been demonstrated that this effect of catecholamines is dependent on gestational age. In the more immature fetus, beta agonists have little effect on lung liquid secretion, and thus the immature fetus may have greater difficulty clearing the air space fluid when making the transition to breathing air. The process of labor itself will increase the amount of sodium-potassium ATPase activity in the type II epithelial cells; which aspect of labor is important is unknown. Fetal lung liquid is cleared at birth by several mechanisms; approximately one third is squeezed out during the birth process, and the remainder is absorbed by the epithelium; the fluid is then taken up by pulmonary vessels or cleared by the lymphatics. Failure of normal lung water clearance at birth is simply one type of pulmonary edema, and it results in respiratory distress (wet lung syndrome or transient tachypnea of the newborn).

The assessment of lung function in early stages of development is based chiefly on measurement in lambs, which provides insight into the direction of changes that occur with time, although exact analogies to the human subject are speculative. The distensibility of the lung early in gestation is much less than at term. When peak volumes are expressed as milliliters per gram of lung tissue, it is evident that the potential air space is small with respect to lung mass. The ability to retain air at end-expiration, which depends on the presence of the pulmonary surfactant, does not appear until later in the canalicular stage of development. In the lamb it appears between days 120 and 130 of a 147-day gestation. In the human it appears probably between the twentieth and the twenty-fourth week of gestation, with a wide distribution over this period.

In utero, little blood flows through the lung despite a relatively high perfusion pressure. Although during the last trimester, concomitant with surfactant production, blood flow increases to 7 per cent of the cardiac output, it is only at birth that marked increases in the capacity and distensibility of the pulmonary vasculature occur. Several mechanisms are responsible for the changes in circulation. Inflation of the lung with air results in mechanical distention of the vessels, and improvement in oxygenation re-

moves hypoxic vasoconstriction. In addition, the rise in PaO_2 induces granulocytes in the lung to release massive quantities of kinin. This kinin alters the tissue concentrations of prostaglandins and helps to mediate the vasoconstriction of the ductus arteriosus and umbilical vessels and to dilate the pulmonary vascular bed. With increasing postnatal age, vascular muscle regresses so that the wall-lumen ratio decreases. After about 10 days of extrauterine life the lumens are wider, regardless of the gestational age of the baby. The events of birth have little effect on other aspects of lung development, including histochemical maturation.

POSTNATAL LUNG GROWTH

The postnatal growth of the lung continues into the adolescent years and perhaps beyond. It is important to remember that the lung of the newborn is not a miniature of the lung of the adult; during growth tracheal diameter approximately triples, alveolar dimensions increase about fourfold, and alveolar numbers increase about tenfold while body mass increases about twentyfold. Other anatomic relationships of the infant's and child's lungs are similar to those in the adult's lung (see Figs. 1–1 and 1–2). The internal surface area of the lung maintains a close relationship to body mass (approximately 1 sq m per kg of body weight), and the proportion of total lung weight represented by each lobe is remarkably constant from infancy to adulthood. Average values of lung lobe weight expressed as a percentage of total lung weight are as follows: right upper lobe 19.5 per cent, right middle lobe 8.3 per cent, right lower lobe 25.3 per cent, left upper lobe 22.5 per cent, and left lower lobe 24.6 per cent.

The preacinar blood vessels and airways have developed by 16 weeks of gestation, and although they do increase in size after birth, the majority of postnatal lung growth involves the terminal respiratory unit.

New secondary septa continue to appear on the walls of the saccules and grow into the air space, thus creating more true alveoli. Alveoli continue to increase in number through segmentation of these primitive alveoli and through transformation of terminal bronchioles into respiratory bronchioles, a process known as alveolarization. The number of alveoli rapidly increases from 20 million to 200 million by the third year of life, but then alveolar multiplication slows.

There is not agreement about when alveolar multiplication ceases (2 versus 8 years), but few if any new alveoli develop after 8 years of age. Further growth of the air space then occurs through increases in alveolar dimensions. In the mature adult lung the number of alveoli varies from 200 million to 600 million, and an individual alveolus is 250 to 350 μ deep. The reason for the variable number of alveoli in the adult lung is unknown; the number may be genetically determined or may depend on the subject's height or the age at which alveolar multiplication ceased.

As alveolar multiplication occurs new blood vessels appear within the acinus, so the ratio between the numbers of alveoli and arteries remains relatively constant throughout childhood. Branching of conventional arteries continues until 18 months of age, whereas supernumerary arteries continue to appear until 8 years of age.

Throughout childhood there is an increase in the concentration of arteries to alveoli. The alveolar to arterial ratio is 20:1 in the newborn, 12:1 in a 2-year-old child, and 8-10:1 in the older child. The muscularization of the arteries lags behind during childhood, with a return to muscularization of more peripheral arteries by adult life (see Fig. 1–8).

VENTILATION

The principal function of the lung is to perform gas exchange, that is, to enrich the blood with oxygen and cleanse it of carbon dioxide. An essential feature of normal gas exchange is that the volume and distribution of ventilation are appropriate. Ventilation of the lung depends on the adequacy of the respiratory pump (muscles and chest wall) and the mechanical properties of the airways and gas-exchanging units.

It is traditional and useful to consider mechanical events as belonging to two main categories: the static-elastic properties of the lungs and chest wall and the flow-resistive or dynamic aspects of moving air. Changes in one category may be associated with compensatory changes in the other. Thus many diseases affect both static and dynamic behavior of the lungs. Often the principal derangement is in the elastic properties of the tissues or in the dimensions of the airways, and the treatment or alleviation of symptoms depends on distinguishing between them.

Before we discuss the mechanical aspects of lung function and gas exchange it is important to review several basic physical laws concerning the behavior of gases and also the related abbreviations and symbols that will be used.

DEFINITIONS AND SYMBOLS

The principal variables for gases are as follows:

V = gas volume
$\dot{V}$ = volume of gas per unit time
P = pressure
F = fractional concentration in dry gas
R = respiratory exchange ratio, $\dot{V}$ carbon dioxide/$\dot{V}$ oxygen
f = frequency
D_L = diffusing capacity of lung

The designation of which volume or pressure is cited requires a small capital letter after the principal variable. Thus V_{O_2} = volume of oxygen; P_B = barometric pressure.

I = inspired gas
E = expired gas
A = alveolar gas
T = tidal gas
D = dead space gas
B = barometric pressure

When both location of the gas and its species are to be indicated, the order is $V_{I_{O_2}}$, which means the volume of inspired oxygen.

STPD = standard temperature, pressure, dry (0°C, 760 mm Hg)
BTPS = body temperature, pressure, saturated with water vapor
ATPS = ambient temperature, pressure, saturated with water vapor

The principal designations for blood are as follows:

S = percentage saturation of gas in blood
C = content of gas per 100 ml of blood
Q = volume of blood
$\dot{Q}$ = blood flow per minute
a = arterial
$\bar{v}$ = mixed venous
c = capillary

All sites of blood determinations are indicated by lower-case initials. Thus Pa_{CO_2} = partial pressure of carbon dioxide in arterial blood. $P\bar{v}_{O_2}$ = partial pressure of oxygen in mixed venous blood. Pc_{O_2} = partial pressure of oxygen in a capillary.

Properties of Gases. Gases behave as an enormous number of tiny particles in constant motion. Their behavior is governed by the gas laws, which are essential to the understanding of pulmonary physiology.

Dalton's law states that the total pressure exerted by a gas mixture is equal to the sum of the pressures of the individual gases. The pressure exerted by each component is independent of the other gases in the mixture. For instance, at sea level, air saturated with water vapor at a temperature of 37°C has a total pressure equal to the atmospheric pressure (P_B = 101.3 kilopascals or 30 in of mercury or 760 mm Hg), with the partial pressures of the components as shown in Equation 1, below.

The gas in alveoli contains 5.6 per cent carbon dioxide, BTPS. If P_B = 760 mm Hg, then:

$$PA_{CO_2} = 0.056 (760 - 47) = 40 \text{ mm Hg}$$

The terms *partial pressure* and *tension* are interchangeable for gases.

Boyle's law states that at a constant temperature the volume of any gas varies inversely as the pressure to which the gas is subjected: $PV = k$. Because respiratory volume measurements may be made at different barometric pressures, it is important to know the

Equation 1:

$$P_B = 760 \text{ mm Hg} = P_{H_2O} (47 \text{ mm Hg}) + P_{O_2} (149.2 \text{ mm Hg}) + P_{N_2} (563.5 \text{ mm Hg}) + P_{CO_2} (0.3 \text{ mm Hg})$$

barometric pressure and to convert to standard pressure, which is considered to be 760 mm Hg.

Charles's law states that if the pressure is constant, the volume of a gas increases in direct proportion to the absolute temperature. At absolute zero ($-273°C$), molecular motion ceases. With increasing temperature, molecular collisions increase, so that at constant pressure, volume must increase.

In all respiratory calculations, water vapor pressure must be taken into account. The partial pressure of water vapor increases with temperature but is independent of atmospheric pressure. At body temperature ($37°C$), fully saturated gas has a P_{H_2O} of 47 mm Hg.

Gases may exist in physical solution in a liquid, escape from the liquid, or return to it. At equilibrium, the partial pressure of a gas in a liquid medium exposed to a gas phase is equal in the two phases *(Henry's law)*. Note that in blood the sum of the partial pressures of all the gases does not necessarily equal atmospheric pressure. For example, in venous blood P_{O_2} has fallen from the 100 mm Hg of the arterial blood to 40 mm Hg—, while P_{CO_2} has changed from 40 to 46 mm Hg. Thus the sum of the partial pressures of O_2, CO_2, and N_2 in venous blood equals 655 mm Hg.

According to *Henry's law of diffusion*, the diffusion rate for gases in a liquid phase is directly proportional to their solubility coefficients. For example, in water:

$$\frac{\text{Solubility of } CO_2}{\text{Solubility of } O_2} = \frac{0.592}{0.0244} = \frac{24.3}{1}$$

Therefore, carbon dioxide diffuses more than 24 times as fast as oxygen.

The diffusion rate of a gas in the gas phase is inversely proportional to $\sqrt{\text{molecular weight}}$ *(Graham's law)*. Therefore, in the gas phase:

$$\frac{\text{rate for } CO_2}{\text{rate for } O_2} = 0.85$$

That is, carbon dioxide diffuses slower in the gas phase than oxygen.

Combining Henry's and Graham's laws for a system with both a gas phase and a liquid phase, e.g., alveolus and blood: carbon dioxide diffuses $24.3 \times 0.85 = 20.7$ times as fast as oxygen.

ELASTIC RECOIL OF THE LUNG AND CHEST WALL

The lung is an elastic structure that tends to decrease its size at all volumes. The chest wall is also an elastic structure, but in contrast to the lung, it tends to push outward at low volumes and inward at high volumes. These phenomena are illustrated when air is introduced into the pleural space: the lung collapses and the chest wall springs outward.

The elasticity of the lung depends on the structural components (although elastic fibers are not essential for normal performance), the geometry of the terminal air spaces, and the presence of an air-liquid interface. When a lung is made airless and is then inflated with liquid, the elastic recoil at large volumes is less than half that of a lung inflated to the same volume with air. Thus, the most significant determinant of the elastic properties of the lung is the presence of an air-liquid interface.

The increase of elastic recoil in the presence of an air-liquid interface results from the forces of surface tension. What is surface tension? When molecules are aligned at an air-liquid interface, they lack opposing molecules on one side. The intermolecular attractive forces are then unbalanced, and the resultant force tends to move molecules away from the interface. The effect is to reduce the area of the surface to a minimum. In the lungs the forces at the air-liquid interface operate to reduce the internal surface area of the lung, and thus they augment elastic recoil. A remarkable property of the material at the alveolar interface, the alveolar lining layer or pulmonary surfactant, is its ability to achieve a high surface tension at large lung volumes and a low surface tension at low volumes. Surfactant is a phospholipid-protein complex that when compressed forms insoluble, folded-surface films of low surface tension. The ability to achieve a low surface tension at low lung volumes tends to stabilize the air spaces and prevent their closure.

The exact method of lung stabilization and the concomitant role of surfactant in this stabilization

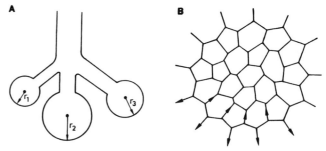

Figure 1–9. *A,* Classic model of the distal lung unit, in which individual alveoli would be controlled by Laplace's law: $P = 2\gamma/r$. Small alveoli would empty into large alveoli. *B,* Interdependence model of the lung, in which alveoli share common planar and not spherical walls. Any decrease in the size of one alveolus would be stabilized by the adjacent alveoli. (Reproduced with permission from Weibel ER and Bachofen H: News in Physiological Sciences 2:72–75, 1987.)

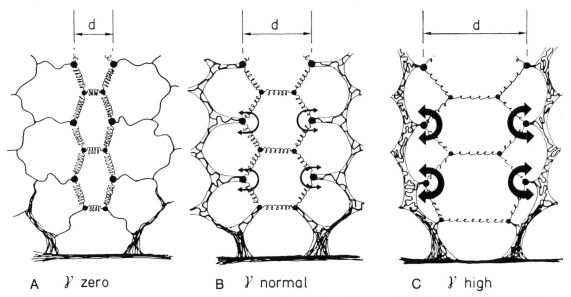

A γ zero   B γ normal   C γ high

Figure 1–10. Geometry of the alveolar duct with changes in surface tension. *A* is comparable to a fluid-filled lung in which surface tension (γ) is zero and diameter of the alveolar duct (*d*) is small relative to the size when filled with air (*B*). When surface tension is increased (*C*), the alveolar septa diminish in length in response to the increased force (*heavy arrows*) and the alveolar duct distends markedly. (Reproduced from Weibel ER and Bachofen H: News in Physiological Sciences 2:72–75, 1987.)

can be debated. The classic interpretation is that without surfactant the smaller alveoli would tend to empty into the larger alveoli in accordance with the Laplace relationship, which relates the pressure across a surface (P) to surface tension (T) and radius (r) of curvature. For a spherical surface, $P = 2T/r$. The smaller the radius, the greater is the tendency to collapse.

The difficulty with this hypothesis is that the individual lung units are drawn as independent but communicating bubbles or spheres (Fig. 1–9). This is not the structure of the lung! First, the alveolar walls are planar, not spherical. More important, the inside wall of one alveolus is the outside wall of the adjacent alveolus. This last explanation has been utilized to develop the interdependence model of lung stability (see Fig. 1–9), but it too has certain limitations. Weibel and Bachofen (1987) have proposed that the surface and tissue forces interact to

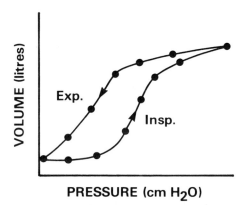

Figure 1–11. Pressure-volume curve of a normal lung. Pleural pressure and lung volume are simultaneously determined during brief breath-holds. Lung compliance is calculated from data obtained on the expiratory portion of the pressure-volume curve.

maintain the lungs' inherent structure, with the fibrous components playing an important role (Fig. 1–10).

The elastic recoil of the lung is responsible for the lung's tendency to pull away from the chest wall with the resultant subatmospheric pressure in the pleural space. Lung recoil can therefore be derived from measurement of the pleural pressure when no airflow is occurring and alveolar pressure is zero. (The pressure measurement is taken with the patient holding his breath for a brief period with the glottis open.) Measurement of pleural pressure can be done in vivo with great difficulty; alternatively, and more safely, the pressure within the esophagus can be used as an index for mean pleural pressure. This is a reasonable assumption as long as there is no paradoxical rib cage movement. However, it is not a reasonable assumption for premature infants, term infants in rapid eye movement (REM) sleep, and older infants with severe lung disease. For these infants no average pleural pressure exists, and calculations of resistance and compliance will not be accurate using this method. When pleural pressure is estimated with an esophageal balloon, one must be careful to avoid artifacts resulting from the gravitational pressure of the mediastinum. For this reason these measurements are best performed with the patient in the upright or lateral rather than the supine position. Once a series of pressure measurements has been made during brief breath-holds at different lung volumes, a pressure-volume curve of the lung can be constructed (Fig. 1–11).

COMPLIANCE OF THE LUNG AND CHEST WALL

The pressure-volume curve of the lung describes the two elastic properties of the lung, elastic recoil and lung compliance. *Elastic recoil* is the pressure generated at a given lung volume, whereas *compliance* is the slope of the pressure-volume curve, or the volume change per unit of pressure:

$$\text{Compliance} = \frac{\Delta\text{volume}}{\Delta\text{pressure}} = \frac{\text{liters}}{\text{cm } H_2O}$$

Compliance depends on the initial lung volume from which the change in volume is measured and the ventilatory events immediately preceding the measurement as well as the properties of the lung itself. At large lung volumes compliance is lower, because the lung is nearer its elastic limit. If the subject has breathed with a fixed tidal volume for some minutes, portions of the lung are not participating in ventilation, and compliance may be reduced. A few deep breaths, with return to the initial volume, will increase compliance. Thus a careful description of associated events is required for correct interpretation of the measurement.

Changes in lung compliance occur with age (Table 1–2). Of course, the smaller the subject, the smaller is the change in volume, so that $\Delta V/\Delta P$ is close to 6 ml/cm H_2O in infants, and is 125 to 190 ml/cm H_2O in adults. It is more relevant to a description of the elastic properties of the lung to express the compliance in relation to a unit of lung volume such as the functional residual capacity (FRC). Note that with age, as shown in Table 1–2, the compliance of the lung/FRC, or the specific compliance, changes much less.

It is worth re-emphasizing that total lung compliance is a function not only of the lung's tissue and surface tension characteristics but also of its volume. This is especially important to remember when compliance has been measured in newborn infants with respiratory distress syndromes (RDSs). The total compliance is a composite of the lung's elastic properties and the number of open lung units. In RDS sudden changes in total measured compliance (if uncorrected for simultaneously measured lung gas volume) will predominately, if not exclusively, reflect the opening and closing of individual lung units.

Lung compliance may also be measured during quiet breathing with pressure and volume being recorded at end-inspiration and end-expiration. The resultant value is the *dynamic lung compliance*. Al-

though dynamic lung compliance does reflect the elastic properties of the normal lung, it is also influenced by the pressure required to move air within the airways. Therefore, dynamic lung compliance increases with increased respiratory rate and with increased airway resistance. Airflow is still occurring within the lung after it has ceased at the mouth, and pleural pressure reflects both the elastic recoil of the lung and the pressure required to overcome the increased airway resistance. Indeed, dynamic lung compliance can be used as a sensitive test of obstructive airway disease.

Compliance of the chest wall can be measured by considering the pressure difference between the pleural space or esophagus and the atmosphere, per change in volume. Significant changes in thoracic compliance occur with age (Fig. 1–12). In the range of normal breathing, the thorax of the infant is nearly infinitely compliant. The pressures measured at different lung volumes are about the same across the lung as those measured across lung and thorax together. The functional significance of the neonatal thorax's high compliance is observed when there is lung disease. The necessarily greater inspiratory effort and more negative pleural pressure can "suck" in the chest wall, resulting in less effective gas exchange and a higher work of breathing.

With advancing age the thorax becomes relatively stiffer. Changes in volume-pressure relations are profitably considered only if referred to a reliable unit, such as a unit of lung volume or a percentage of total lung capacity. Considered on a percentage basis, compliance of the thorax decreases with age. How much of this change is contributed by changes in tissue properties, such as increasing calcification of ribs and connective tissue changes, and how much is a disproportionate growth of the chest wall relative to the lung remains unclear (see Fig. 1–12).

LUNG VOLUMES

Definition. The concept of lung volumes and capacities, rather than a single volume, derives from the fact that sometimes more or less air is moved, that some air is always present in normal lungs, and that it is useful to apply labels to the portions of the total gas volume under discussion. The partition of commonly used lung volumes can be understood by studying Figure 1–13. The spirogram on the left represents the volume of air breathed in and out by a normal subject. The first portion of the tracing illustrates normal breathing and is called the tidal volume (V_t). The subject then makes a maximal inspiration followed by a maximum expiration: the volume of expired air is the vital capacity (VC). The volume of air that still remains in the lung after a maximal expiration is the residual volume (RV), whereas the volume of air remaining in the lung after a normal passive expiration is the functional residual capacity (FRC). The maximum amount of

Table 1–2. LUNG COMPLIANCE (C_L) WITH AGE

	ml/cm H_2O	C_L/FRC
Newborns		
3 hours	4.75 ± 1.67	0.041 ± 0.01
24 hours	6.24 ± 1.45	0.055 ± 0.01
Infants		
1 month–2 years	7.9	0.038
Children		
Average age 9 years	77	0.063
Young adult males	184	0.050
Young adult females	125	0.053
Adults over 60 years	191	0.041

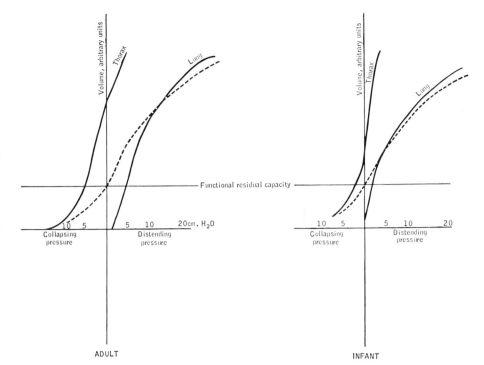

Figure 1–12. Pressure-volume relations of lungs and thorax in an adult and an infant. The *dashed line* represents the characteristic of lungs and thorax together. Transpulmonary pressure at the resting portion (functional residual capacity) is less in the infant, and thoracic compliance is greater in the infant.

air that a subject can have in the lungs is called the total lung capacity (TLC). In healthy young subjects TLC correlates best with subject height.

The volumes and capacities of the lungs are determined by many factors including muscle strength, static-elastic characteristics of the chest wall and lungs, airway status, and patient age and cooperation. Total lung capacity is reached when the force generated by maximal voluntary contraction of the inspiratory muscles equals the inward recoil of the lung and chest wall. Functional residual capacity occurs when the respiratory muscles are relaxed and no external forces are applied; it is therefore the volume at which the inward recoil of the lung is exactly balanced by the outward recoil of the chest wall (see Fig. 1–12).

In healthy children and young adults, end-expiratory lung volume is equivalent to FRC. This is not the case in infants, who breathe at a lung volume higher than FRC. This higher volume seems to be a sensible solution to the infants' problem of having a closing volume that exceeds FRC. An infant maintains the expiratory lung volume higher than FRC by a combination of postinspiratory diaphragmatic activity and laryngeal adduction.

The factors determining RV vary with age: in adolescents and young adults RV occurs when the expiratory muscles cannot compress the chest wall further. In young children and older adults RV is a function of the patency of small airways and the duration of expiratory effort.

Measurement. Tidal volume and vital capacity can be determined by measuring the expired volume. The measurement of functional residual capacity and residual volume requires another approach. Because both volumes include the air in the lungs that the patient does not normally exhale, they must be measured indirectly. One method uses the principle of dilution of the unknown volume with a known concentration of a gas that is foreign to the lung and only sparingly absorbed, such as helium. The patient breathes from a container with a known volume and concentration of helium in oxygen-enriched air. After sufficient time has elasped for the gas in the lung to mix and equilibrate with the gas in the container, the concentration of helium in the container is remeasured. Because initial volume × initial concentration of helium = final volume × final concentration of helium, the final volume, which includes gas in the lungs, can be calculated.

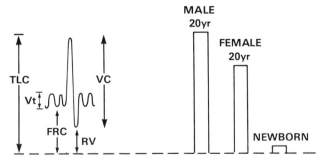

Figure 1–13. The lung volumes. The spirogram (*left*) demonstrates normal breathing followed by a maximal inspiratory effort and a maximal expiratory effort. *TLC*, total lung capacity (6.0 liters in an average male, 4.2 liters in an average female, and 160 ml in an average 3-kg infant: see histograms on right); *FRC*, functional residual capacity; *VC*, vital capacity; *RV*, residual volume; *Vt*, tidal volume.

If some of the gas is "trapped" within the lungs, its volume will not be reflected in the helium dilution measurement. There is, however, a method of measuring total gas volume within the thorax that depends on the change in volume that occurs with compression of the gas when breathing against an obstruction. Practically, this measurement requires the patient to be in a body plethysmograph and to pant against a closed shutter. The change in pressure can be measured in the mouthpiece; the change in volume can be recorded with a spirometer attached to the body plethysmograph: $V = P\Delta V/\Delta P$. This method has the advantage of being able to be repeated several times a minute. It has the disadvantage of including some abdominal gas in the measurement.

There have also been concerns about the validity of the plethysmographic technique in patients with obstructive lung disease. This issue has not yet been resolved, because the technique has been reported to overestimate the lung volume in adults but underestimate the lung volume in infants with obstructive lung disease.

Interpretation. The measurement of lung volumes and capacities provides an objective assessment of the patient with respiratory symptoms. This objectivity, however, must be tempered with a dose of realism when results are being interpreted. Although patient cooperation and technical problems can always be sources of error, the major difficulty in detecting abnormalities in lung volumes is that the range of normal values is so large. For example, the mean TLC for a child 140 cm tall is 3.2 L; however, the statistical range of normal (mean ± 2 SD) is from 1.9 to 4.3 L. This range of normal values, when expressed as per cent predicted, is even greater for younger children or smaller lung volumes (such as RV). Owing to this wide range of normality, care must be exercised in the interpretation of lung volumes. Measurement of lung volumes is of greatest benefit when repeated over several months to assess the progress of a chronic respiratory illness and the efficacy of treatment.

The vital capacity (VC) is one of the most valuable measurements that can be made in a functional assessment, because it is highly reproducible and has a relatively narrow range of normal values. It can be decreased by a wide variety of disease processes, including muscle weakness, loss of lung tissue, obstruction of the airway, and decreased compliance of the chest wall. Vital capacity is therefore not a useful tool to discriminate between types of lesions. Its chief role is to assign a value to the degree of impairment and to document changes that occur with therapy or time. In order to decide whether obstructive or restrictive lung disease is present, it is useful to measure expiratory flow rates (see Chapters 7 and 8) and to observe the pattern of abnormalities in the other lung volumes. In obstructive lung disease, e.g., asthma, the smallest lung volumes are affected first: RV increases owing to abnormally high airway resistance at low lung volumes, and as the disease progresses the FRC increases. Although the increase in FRC (hyperinflation) may rarely be due to loss of lung recoil, the overdistention is usually compensating for partial lower airway obstruction. When the lung volume is increased, intrathoracic airways enlarge, and widespread partial obstruction may be partially relieved by the assumption of a larger resting lung volume. Whereas the total lung capacity is only rarely affected in obstructive disease, TLC and VC are the first lung volumes to be affected in restrictive diseases of the chest wall (e.g., kyphoscoliosis) or lung (e.g., fibrosing alveolitis). Airway disease is not usually a significant feature of restrictive disease, so RV and FRC tend to be normal.

REGIONAL LUNG VOLUMES

During normal breathing, different areas of the lung have different regional lung volumes; the upper air spaces are inflated more than the lower air spaces. Because static-elastic properties are fairly constant throughout the lung, these different regional lung volumes result from the gradient of pleural pressure that exists from the top to the bottom of the lung. Although gravitational forces are thought to be largely responsible, the mechanisms responsible for this pleural pressure gradient are incompletely understood. In the erect adult lung the pleural pressure is -8 cm H_2O at the apex and only -2 cm H_2O at the base. The significance of this phenomenon is that when a subject breathes in, the lowermost lung units will receive the majority of the inspired air (Fig. 1–14). This is advantageous because the majority of pulmonary blood flow also goes to the base of the lung, and thus blood flow and ventilation patterns are matched.

DYNAMIC (FLOW-RESISTIVE) PROPERTIES OF THE LUNG

Gas Flow Within Airways

The respiratory system must perform work to move gas into and out of the lungs. Because air moves into the lungs during inspiration and out of the lungs during expiration, and because the velocity of airflow increases from small airways to large airways, energy must be expended to accelerate the gas molecules. The respiratory system's resistance to acceleration (inertance) is minimal during quiet breathing and will not be considered further. In contrast, however, frictional resistance to airflow accounts for one third of the work performed during quiet breathing. The magnitude of pressure loss due to friction is determined by the pattern of flow. Flow may be laminar (streamlined) or turbulent, and which pattern exists depends on the properties of the gas (viscosity, density), the velocity of airflow, and the radius of the airway. In general, there is laminar flow in the small peripheral airways and turbulent flow in the large central airways.

The laws governing the frictional resistance to flow of gases in tubes apply to pulmonary resistance. The equation for calculating the pressure gradient required to maintain a laminar flow of air through a tube is given by Poiseuille's law:

$$P = \dot{V}\left(\frac{8l\eta}{\pi r^4}\right)$$

where P is pressure, $\dot{V}$ is flow, l is length, r is radius of the tube, and η is the viscosity of the gas. The viscosity of air is 0.000181 poise at 20°C, or only 1 per cent that of water. Because resistance = pressure/flow, it is clear that the most important determinant of resistance in small airways will be the radius of the tube, which is raised to the fourth power in the denominator of the equation.

The pressure required to maintain turbulent flow is influenced by airway diameter and gas density and is proportional to the square of the gas velocity. The effect of gas density on turbulent flow has both diagnostic and therapeutic implications. In patients with obstructive airway disease, for instance, the major site of obstruction (large vs. small airways) can be determined by measuring expiratory flow rates when helium (a low-density gas) has been substituted for nitrogen. Children with viral laryngotracheobronchitis have marked narrowing of the subglottic area, which greatly increases the resistance to airflow. The pressure required to overcome this increased resistance in the large airways, and hence the work of breathing, can be decreased by administering a low-density gas mixture (70 per cent helium, 30 per cent oxygen).

Measurement of Resistance

Resistance (R) is calculated from the equation

$$R = \frac{\text{driving pressure}}{\text{airflow}}$$

The pressure is measured at the two ends of the system—in the case of the lung, at the mouth and at the alveoli—and the corresponding flow is recorded. Alveolar pressure presents the greatest problem. If pleural pressure is substituted, the result is a measure of both airway and lung tissue viscous resistance (total nonelastic resistance). In health, tissue viscous resistance is about 20 per cent of the total.

Several methods have been used to measure alveolar pressure. The most common method employs a body plethysmograph. The subject sits in the airtight box and breathes through a tube connected to a pneumotachometer, an apparatus that measures airflow. When a shutter occludes the tube and airflow ceases, the mouth pressure is assumed to be equal to the alveolar pressure. Airway resistance can then be calculated because airflow, alveolar pressure, and ambient pressure are known.

Total pulmonary resistance can be measured in infants and children by the forced oscillation technique. This measurement includes airway resistance plus the tissue viscous resistance of the lung and chest wall. Nasal resistance is also included in the measurement if the infant is breathing through the nose. Although there are theoretical objections to this technique, it has several advantages. It does not require a body plethysmograph, estimates of pleural pressure, or patient cooperation, and it can be done quickly enough to be used on ill patients. A sinusoidal pressure applied at the upper airway changes the airflow, and the ratio of pressure change to flow change is used to calculate resistance. When the forced oscillations are applied at the so-called resonant frequency of the lung (believed to be 3 to 5 cycles/sec), it is assumed that the force required to overcome elastic resistance of the lung and the force required to overcome inertance are equal and opposite, so that all of the force is dissipated in overcoming flow resistance. This technique has demonstrated that infants with bronchiolitis have about a twofold increase in inspiratory pulmonary resistance and a threefold increase in expiratory resistance.

Several new techniques have been developed that are capable of measuring lung function in infants and young children. Each has its advantages, underlying assumptions, and limitations, and these techniques are discussed in detail in Chapter 6. (See also England, 1988).

Sites of Airway Resistance

The contribution of the upper airway to total airway resistance is substantial. The average nasal resistance of infants by indirect measurement is 13 cm H_2O/L/sec, or nearly half of the total respiratory resistance, as is the case in adults. It is hardly surprising that any compromise of the dimensions of the nasal airways in an infant who is a preferential nose breather will result in retractions and labored breathing. Likewise, even mild edema of the trachea or larynx will impose a significant increase in airway resistance.

In the adult lung, about 80 per cent of the resistance to airflow resides in airways greater than 2 mm in diameter. The vast number of small peripheral airways provides a large cross-sectional area for flow and therefore contributes less than 20 per cent to the airway resistance. Thus these airways may be the sites of disease that may severely impair ventilation of distal air spaces without appreciably altering the total airway resistance. In the infant lung, however, small peripheral airways may contribute as much as 50 per cent of the total airway resistance, and this proportion does not decrease until about 5 years of age. Thus the infant and young child are particularly severely affected by diseases that affect the small airways, e.g., bronchiolitis (see Chapter 9).

Factors Affecting Airway Resistance

Airway resistance is determined by the diameter of the airways, the velocity of airflow, and the physical properties of the gas breathed. The diameter is determined by the balance between the forces tending to narrow the airways and the forces tending to widen them. One of the forces tending to narrow the airways is exerted by the contraction of bronchial smooth muscle. The neural regulation of bronchial smooth muscle tone is mediated by efferent impulses through autonomic nerves. Sympathetic impulses relax the airways, and the parasympathetic impulses constrict them. Bronchi constrict reflexly from irritating inhalants such as sulfur dioxide and some dusts; by arterial hypoxemia and hypercapnia; by embolization of the vessels; by cold; and by some vasoactive mediators, such as acetylcholine, histamine, and bradykinin. They dilate in response to an increase in systemic blood pressure through baroreceptors in the carotid sinus and to sympathomimetic agents such as isoproterenol and epinephrine. The large airways are probably in tonic contraction in health, because in unanesthetized adults, atropine or isoproterenol will decrease airway resistance by nearly 50 per cent.

Airway resistance changes with lung volume, but not in a linear manner. Increasing the lung volume to above FRC only minimally decreases airway resistance. In contrast, as lung volume decreases from FRC, resistance rises dramatically and approaches infinity at RV. Although alterations in bronchomotor tone play a role, it is the decrease in lung elastic recoil as lung volume declines that is the predominant mechanism for the change in airway resistance. The

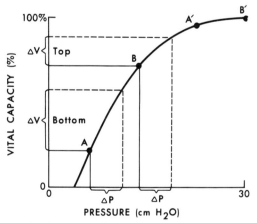

Figure 1–14. Pressure-volume curve of a normal lung (*heavy solid line*). At functional residual capacity, distending pressure is less at the bottom than at the top; accordingly, alveoli at the bottom (*A*) are smaller (i.e., lower per cent regional vital capacity) than those at the top (*B*). When a given amount of distending pressure (ΔP) is applied to the lung, alveoli at the bottom increase their volume (ΔV) more than alveoli at the top, owing to the varying steepness of the pressure-volume curve. When fully expanded to total lung capacity (100 per cent VC), alveoli at the bottom (*A′*) are nearly the same size as alveoli at the top (*B′*), because both points lie on the flat portion of the curve. (Reproduced with permission from Murray JF: The Normal Lung. Philadelphia, WB Saunders Co, 1976.)

recoil of the lung provides a tethering or "guy wire" effect on the airways that tends to increase their diameter. Children of different ages will have different airway resistances owing to the different sizes of their lungs. Therefore, the measurement of airway resistance or its reciprocal, airway conductance, is usually corrected by dividing the airway conductance by the simultaneously measured lung volume. The resultant *specific airway conductance* is remarkably constant regardless of the subject's age or height.

Dynamic Airway Compression

During a forced expiration both the pleural and the peribronchial pressures become positive and tend to narrow the airways; forces tending to keep airways open are the intraluminal pressure and the tethering action of the surrounding lung. During active expiration, however, the intraluminal pressure must decrease along the pathway of airflow from the alveoli to the mouth, where it becomes equal to atmospheric pressure. Therefore, at some point in the airway, intraluminal pressure must equal pleural pressure—the equal pressure point (EPP). Downstream from the EPP, pleural pressure exceeds intraluminal pressure and thus is a force that tends to narrow the airways. Indeed, during periods of maximum expiratory flow, pleural pressure exceeds the critical closing pressure of the airways, which become narrowed to slits. Despite the cartilaginous support of the larger airways, the membranous portion of the wall of the trachea and large bronchi invaginates under pressure to occlude the airways. Maximum flow under this circumstance is therefore determined by the resistance of the airways located upstream from the EPP, and the driving pressure is the difference between the alveolar pressure and the pressure at the EPP. In disease states in which there is an increased airway resistance, the EPP moves toward the alveoli because of the greater intraluminal pressure drop. Thus small airways are now compressed during forced expiration with severe flow limitation. With the measurement of pressure-flow and flow-volume curves during forced expiration, it is possible to calculate resistance upstream and downstream from the point of critical closure, or EPP. Increasing the lung volume increases the tethering action of the surrounding lung on the airways, and therefore close attention must be paid to the lung volume at which resistance measurements are made during these studies.

DISTRIBUTION OF VENTILATION

The distribution of ventilation will be influenced by several factors of normal lungs. The pleural pressure gradient results in a greater amount of the tidal volume going to the dependent areas of the lung (see Fig. 1–14). In addition, the rate at which an area of the lung fills and empties is related to both airway resistance and compliance. A decrease in airway dimension increases the time required for air to reach the alveoli; a region of low compliance receives less ventilation per unit of time than an area with high compliance. The product of resistance × compliance (time constant) is approximately the same in health for all ventilatory pathways. The unit of this product is time. Note:

$$\text{Resistance} = \frac{\text{pressure}}{\text{flow}} = \frac{\text{cm } H_2O}{L/\text{sec}}$$

and

$$\text{Compliance} = \frac{\Delta \text{volume (L)}}{\Delta \text{pressure (cm } H_2O)}$$

The product, then, is a unit of time, analogous to the time constant in an electrical system, that represents the time taken to accomplish 63 per cent of the volume change.

As mentioned previously, peripheral airways contribute little to overall airway resistance after the age of 5 years. However, in the presence of small-airway disease, some areas of the lung have long time constants but those of others are normal. This is particularly evident as the frequency of respiration increases. With increasing frequency, air goes to those areas of the lung with short time constants. These areas then become relatively overdistended, and a greater transpulmonary pressure is required to inspire the same volume of air because alveoli in these relatively normal areas are reaching their elastic limit. Thus a decreased dynamic compliance with increasing frequency of respiration has been used as a test of small-airway disease and indeed may be the only mechanical abnormality detectable in the early stages of diseases such as emphysema and cystic fibrosis.

Airway closure occurs in dependent areas of the lung at low lung volumes. The lung volume above RV at which closure occurs is called the closing volume. In infants, very young children, and older adults, airway closure occurs at FRC and therefore is present during normal tidal breathing. This results in intermittent inadequate ventilation of the respective terminal lung units and leads to abnormal gas exchange, notably to the lower Pa_{O_2} seen in these age groups. It also explains why oxygenation usually can be improved by placing the patient so that the good lung is uppermost in the infant with unilateral lung disease (in young healthy adults the opposite is true).

PULMONARY CIRCULATION

PHYSIOLOGIC CLASSIFICATION OF PULMONARY VESSELS

The pulmonary circulation is the only vascular bed to receive the entire cardiac output. This unique characteristic enables the pulmonary vascular bed to perform a wide variety of homeostatic physiologic functions. It provides an enormously large (80 sq m) yet extremely thin film of blood for gas exchange, filters the circulating blood, controls the circulating concentrations of many vasoactive substances, and provides a large surface area for the absorption of lung liquid at birth. The nomenclature of the pulmonary vessels is at times confusing because the anatomic classification of the vessels often does not correspond to their physiologic role.

Pulmonary vessels have been classified physiologically as extra-alveolar and alveolar vessels, fluid-exchanging vessels, and gas-exchanging vessels. When the outside of a vessel is exposed to alveolar pressure it is classified as an alveolar vessel (capillaries within the middle of the alveolar septum), whereas extra-alveolar vessels (arteries, veins, and capillaries at the corner of alveolar septa) are intrapulmonary vessels that are subjected to a more negative pressure resulting from and approximating pleural pressure. The diameter of the extra-alveolar vessels is therefore greatly affected by lung volume, expanding as inspiration occurs. Although extra-alveolar vessels and alveolar vessels are subjected to different mechanical pressures, they are both classified as fluid-exchanging vessels because both leak water and protein and both can contribute to the production of pulmonary edema. The anatomic location of gas-exchanging vessels is unclear but is likely limited to the capillaries and smallest arterioles and venules.

PULMONARY VASCULAR PRESSURES

The pressure within the pulmonary circulation is remarkably low, considering that it receives the entire cardiac output (5 L/min in the adult human). Beginning a few months after birth, pulmonary arterial pressures are constant throughout life, with the average mean pulmonary arterial pressure being 15 mm Hg and the systolic and diastolic pressures being 22 and 8 torr, respectively. The pulmonary venous pressure is minimally higher than the left atrial pressure, which averages 5 mm Hg. The pressure within human lung capillaries is unknown, but work in isolated dog lungs suggests it is 8 to 10 mm Hg, approximately halfway between the mean arterial and venous pressures. These values refer to pressures at the level of the heart in the supine position; because of gravity, pulmonary arterial pressures will be near zero at the apex of the upright adult lung and close to 25 mm Hg at the base. This fact helps to explain the well-known observation that the majority of pulmonary blood flow goes to the lung bases. Depending on their location, vessels have different pressures on their outside walls. As defined previously, the alveolar vessels are exposed to alveolar pressure, which fluctuates during the respiratory cycle but will average out close to zero. In contrast, the extra-alveolar vessels are exposed to a negative fluid pressure on their outer walls, estimated to be between -6 and -9 cm H_2O. The pressure on the outside of the pulmonary vessel is not a trivial matter, because the transmural pressure (inside pressure–outside pressure), rather than the intravascular pressure, is the pertinent hydrostatic pressure influencing vascular distention and the transvascular movement of water and protein.

PULMONARY VASCULAR RESISTANCE

The resistance to blood flow through the lungs can be calculated by dividing the pressure across the lungs by the pulmonary blood flow.

$$R = \frac{\text{mean PA pressure} - \text{mean LA pressure}}{\text{pulmonary blood flow}}$$

A decrease in resistance to blood flow can occur only through (1) an increase in the blood vessels' diameters or (2) an increase in the number of perfused vessels, that is, an increase in the cross-sectional diameter of the pulmonary vascular bed. The diameter of an already open pulmonary vessel can be increased by decreasing the muscular tone of the vessel wall (e.g., with a vasodilating agent) or by increasing the transmural pressure (e.g., through increased pulmonary arterial (PA) or left atrial (LA) pressure). Previously unperfused pulmonary vessels may be opened up ("recruited") when their transmural pressure exceeds their critical opening pressure. This occurs when intravascular pressures are raised or when a vasodilator has decreased the vessels' critical opening pressure. An increase in cardiac output decreases the calculated pulmonary vascular resistance (PVR). This is important to remember when discussing vasodilating drugs; studies have been performed in which drugs were found to increase cardiac output substantially and to increase pulmonary arterial pressures minimally so that the calculated PVR falls. This permissive fall in resistance does not ensure that a particular drug has any direct vasodilating action at all, because the entire fall in PVR may have resulted from the drug's cardiac effects.

The interrelationship between lung volume and PVR is complex and is influenced by pulmonary blood volume, cardiac output, and initial lung volume. The principal reason for this complex relationship is that a change in lung volume has opposite effects on the resistances of the extra-alveolar and alveolar vessels. As the lung is inflated, the radial traction on the extra-alveolar vessels increases their diameter, whereas the same rise in lung volume increases the resistance to flow through the alveolar vessels (which constitutes 35 to 50 per cent of the total PVR). It is reasonable to say, however, that PVR is at its minimum at FRC, and any change in lung volume (increase or decrease) will increase the PVR (Fig. 1–15).

Active changes in the PVR can be mediated by neurogenic stimuli, vasoactive compounds, or chem-

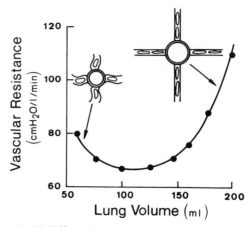

Figure 1–15. Effect of lung volume on pulmonary vascular resistance when the transmural pressure of the capillaries is held constant. At low lung volumes, resistance is high because the extra-alveolar vessels become narrow. At high volumes, the capillaries are stretched, and their caliber is reduced. (Reproduced with permission from West JB: Respiratory Physiology—the Essentials. © 1974, Williams & Wilkins Co, Baltimore.)

ical mediators. The normal adult pulmonary circulation appears to be maximally dilated, since no stimulus has been found that can further dilate the pulmonary vessels. In contrast, the neonatal lung or the vasoconstricted adult lung vasodilates in response to a variety of agents, including acetylcholine, beta-agonist drugs, bradykinin, prostaglandin E, and prostacyclin.

The pulmonary circulation can undergo significant vasoconstriction, which is surprising in view of the paucity of muscle in the postnatal lung vessels. Hypoxia is the most common potent pulmonary vasoconstricting agent. Hypoxic vasoconstriction, which occurs when the alveolar P_{O_2} falls below 50 to 60 mm Hg, is a local response independent of neurohumoral stimuli. Although many suggestions have been made, the exact mechanism of hypoxia-induced vasoconstriction is unknown. Acidosis acts synergistically with hypoxia to constrict the pulmonary vessels; however, it is unlikely that CO_2 alone has any direct effect on the pulmonary circulation in humans. Stimulation of the pulmonary sympathetic nerves results in a weak vasoconstrictive response in the dog lung but little or no response in the normal human adult pulmonary circulation. Vasoactive substances such as histamine, fibrinopeptides, prostaglandins of the F series, and leukotrienes are capable of constricting the pulmonary vascular bed. It had been believed that vasoconstriction in the pulmonary circulation took place predominantly, if not exclusively, within the arterial section of the vascular bed. It has been demonstrated that other regions of the bed may narrow in response to stimuli. For example, hypoxia can constrict the pulmonary venules of newborn animals and might increase resistance within the capillary bed by inducing constriction of Kapanci cells that are located within the interstitium of the alveolar-capillary membrane.

DISTRIBUTION OF BLOOD FLOW

Blood flow is uneven within the normal lung and decreases from the basal to apical regions. Gravitational forces are likely responsible for this phenomenon, because the intravascular pressure of a given blood vessel is determined by the pulmonary arterial pressure immediately above the pulmonary valve and the blood vessel's vertical distance from the pulmonary valve. Thus with increasing height above the heart, the pulmonary arterial pressure decreases and less perfusion occurs. The opposite occurs for vessels located in the lung bases, and together these gravitational effects are responsible for a pressure difference of 23 mm Hg between apical and basal pulmonary arteries.

These regional differences in lung perfusion are best understood in terms of West's zones of perfusion (Fig. 1–16). West's *Zone I* occurs when mean pulmonary arterial pressure is less than or equal to alveolar pressure, and as a result no blood flow occurs (except perhaps during systole). Zone I conditions are present in the apices of some upright adults and result in unperfused yet ventilated lung units (alveolar dead space). Moving down from the lung apices, pulmonary arterial pressure becomes greater than alveolar pressure, with the latter being greater than venous pressure. These are *Zone II* conditions, and blood flow is determined by the difference between arterial and alveolar pressures and is not influenced by venous pressure; an appropriate analogy would be that of a vascular "waterfall" in which the flow rate is independent of the height of the falls. In *Zone III*, left atrial pressure exceeds alveolar pressure and flow is determined in the usual manner, i.e., by the arterial-venous pressure gradient.

METHODS OF EVALUATING THE PULMONARY CIRCULATION

The chest radiograph remains the most widely used tool for determining the possible presence of

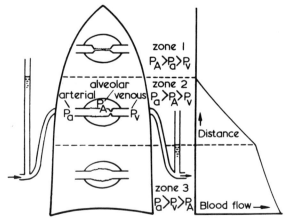

Figure 1–16. Model to explain the uneven distribution of blood flow in the lung based on the pressures affecting the capillaries. (Reproduced with permission from West JB, Dollery CT, and Naimark A: Distribution of blood flow in isolated lung: relation to vascular and alveolar pressures. J Appl Physiol 19:713, 1964.)

pulmonary vascular disease. Prominence of the pulmonary outflow tract and increased or decreased vascular markings may be noted radiographically. Regional pulmonary angiography further delineates localized disturbance in blood flow, although the procedure requires cardiac catheterization. Direct measurements of pulmonary artery and "wedge" pressures add further information. Occasionally, drugs can be infused into the pulmonary artery to evaluate the potential reversibility of pulmonary hypertension.

Noninvasive quantitative assessments of the pulmonary circulation are now available. Echocardiography is able not only to assess the structure and function of the right ventricle but also to provide a reasonable estimate of right ventricular pressure by assessing the small retrograde flow through the tricuspid valve that frequently occurs in significant pulmonary hypertension. Quantitative assessment of regional pulmonary blood flow can be made with intravenous injections of macroaggregates of albumin labeled with [99m]technetium. The macroaggregates occlude a very small portion of the pulmonary vascular bed. The amount of regional blood flow can be determined by imaging the lungs with a large field of view gamma camera and determining the count rate with a computer. The perfusion lung scintigram can be combined with a ventilation scintigram performed with either a radioactive gas (e.g., ^{133}Xe or [81m]Kr) or a radiolabeled (^{99m}Tc-DTPA) submicronic aerosol that is distributed like a gas.

MUSCLES OF RESPIRATION

The importance of the muscles of respiration derives from the fact that these muscles, like the myocardium, can fail under abnormal circumstances and can induce or contribute to an impending or existing ventilatory failure. Although respiratory muscle fatigue has been suspected by clinicians at the bedside for a long time, it was only later demonstrated in human adults and newborn infants.

The principal muscle of respiration is the diaphragm, a thin musculotendinous sheet that separates the thoracic from the abdominal cavity. In adults its contraction causes descent of its dome and aids in elevation of the lower ribs. If the airway is occluded during normal breathing, the adult diaphragm is capable of generating airway pressures up to 150–200 cm H_2O during a maximal inspiratory effort. Some work indicates that the diaphragm has two separate but related functions. The costal part of the diaphragm (largely innervated by C_5) acts to stabilize and elevate the lower rib cage during contraction. The vertebral (crural) portion (largely innervated by C_3), a much thicker muscle, descends with contraction and is largely responsible for the volume change that occurs.

Other skeletal muscles located in the chest or abdominal wall, such as the intercostals, the scalenes, and the abdominal muscles, can play an important role in ventilation. During normal breathing, most of the accessory muscles are silent. However, during abnormal conditions or disease states, these muscles are recruited to stabilize the chest or abdominal wall so that the diaphragm may be more efficient. In addition, it has been demonstrated that the external intercostal muscles contract in acute asthmatic attacks not only during inspiration but also during expiration; this contraction maintains a higher lung volume and hence increases airway diameter. When airways are occluded during inspiration, abdominal muscles contract powerfully during expiration, pushing the abdominal contents and diaphragm toward the thoracic cavity. This action lengthens diaphragmatic fibers and enhances the capability of the diaphragm to generate force during the subsequent inspiration (length-tension curve).

The upper airways must be kept patent during inspiration, and therefore the pharyngeal wall muscles, genioglossus, and arytenoid muscles are properly considered muscles of respiration. There is an increase in neural output to these muscles immediately before diaphragmatic contraction during inspiration. The newborn also contracts these muscles during expiration to provide an expiratory outflow resistance and thus keeps end-expiratory volume greater than the FRC.

Respiratory muscles, whether the diaphragm, upper airway, intercostal, or abdominal muscles, are not homogeneous muscles in terms of their cellular structure, blood supply, metabolism, and recruitment patterns. Adult mature skeletal muscles have a mixture of fibers, and respiratory muscles are no different. The adult diaphragm, for instance, is made of fast- and slow-twitch fibers. Slow-twitch fibers are oxidative, and fast-twitch fibers are either glycolytic or moderately oxidative. Slow-twitch fibers are fatigue resistant; they are recruited first during a motor act; they generate low tensions; and they usually have a higher capillary to fiber ratio than fast fibers. Fast-twitch fibers can be either fatigue resistant (fast, moderately oxidative) or fast fatiguing (fast glycolytic); they are recruited during motor acts that require large force output. Thus during normal quiet breathing, it is presumed that only the slow-twitch fibers in the diaphragm are active. In contrast, at the height of an acute attack of croup, asthma, or bronchiolitis during which muscle contractions are strong, both fiber types can be active, with the fast fibers generating the bulk of the force.

Muscle fiber composition, innervation, and metabolism are different in early life. The process of muscle fiber differentiation and interaction with the central nervous system is a continuous process, starting in utero and continuing postnatally. For example, slow oxidative fibers increase in utero and postnatally, whereas fast glycolytic fibers decrease postnatally. Polyneuronal innervation transforms into one motoneuron = one muscle fiber—the adult type of innervation—postnatally. Whether the young infant's

ability to resist muscle fatigue is jeopardized by premature muscle fiber composition, innervation, and metabolism is not known and deserves further investigation.

Many factors predispose respiratory muscles to fatigue. Factors that increase fuel consumption (e.g., increased loads with disease); limit fuel reserves (e.g., malnutrition); alter acid-base homeostasis (e.g., acidosis); modify the oxidative capacity, glycolytic capacity, or both of the muscle (e.g., decreased activity of the muscle and possible atrophy after prolonged artificial ventilation); and decrease the oxygen availability to the muscle (e.g., anemia, low cardiac output states, hypoxemia) all predispose the diaphragm to failure. In addition, changes in the external milieu of the muscle cell such as low phosphate levels or the presence of certain drugs (e.g., anesthetics) can limit the contractile ability and lead to premature muscle fatigue.

Diaphragmatic muscle function can be assessed clinically by observing the movements of the abdominal wall. During normal inspiration and with the contraction of the diaphragm, the abdominal contents are pushed away from the thorax. Because the abdominal wall is normally compliant during inspiration, the abdominal wall moves out to accommodate the increased pressure from the contracting diaphragm. With diaphragmatic fatigue, weakness, or paralysis, it is possible to observe an inward motion of the abdominal wall. Through the action of other respiratory muscles (intercostals), a drop in pressure occurs in the thorax during inspiration. Because of the "passive" behavior of the fatigued diaphragm, this pressure drop is transmitted to the abdomen; hence the movement of the abdominal contents toward the thoracic cavity.

In the laboratory, respiratory muscle function can be assessed using a number of techniques and tests, some more direct than others. Maximum airway pressure and fluoroscopic evaluation of the diaphragm are less invasive but may have less resolution than transdiaphragmatic pressure (P_{di}, measured using balloon catheters across the diaphragm). Both the P_{di} and electromyographic measurements can be useful in assessing change of muscle function over time, for example, when fatigue is suspected or after extubation and assisted ventilation.

To consider the main respiratory muscles—the diaphragm and the intercostal muscles—as the only respiratory muscles for breathing is insufficient, especially during stressful conditions or disease states. A number of muscles such as the alae nasi, the pharyngeal wall muscles, the genioglossus, the posterior cricoarytenoid, and the thyro-arytenoid can play major roles in airway patency and hence in ventilatory output. Data indicate that upper airway muscles are strongly recruited during obstructive disease or during inspiratory occlusion, and that blood flow increases considerably to some of them (e.g., genioglossus). How prone these muscles are to fatigue under increased loads is unknown. How different these muscles are in terms of their structure, metabolism, and function in the neonate versus the adult is unclear and needs further research.

Because of the number of muscles involved, their location, and their function, the coordination of respiratory muscles becomes increasingly complex. The motor act of respiration should no longer be viewed as the result of one or two muscles contracting during inspiration and relaxing during expiration. At rest and even more so during disease states, the active coordination of various muscles becomes functionally very important. Defecation, sucking, and talking all involve the activation of several muscles that are shared by the respiratory apparatus for generating adequate ventilation. In some cases, obstructive apneas can actually be the result of muscle incoordination, with the diaphragm contracting when upper airway muscles that normally hold the airway open are relaxed.

GAS EXCHANGE

The vital process of gas exchange occurs in the terminal respiratory unit. The previous sections of this chapter deal with the problems of moving air and blood to and from these gas-exchanging units. This section focuses on the fate of gas once it is introduced into the lungs, how it is transferred from the alveolar space to the blood stream, and how ventilation and perfusion are matched.

In Figure 1–17 the partial pressures of oxygen and carbon dioxide are depicted at various stages of the pathway from ambient air to the tissues. Because nitrogen is inert, changes in its partial pressure in the gas phase depend on changes in the partial pressures of oxygen and carbon dioxide, gases that are utilized and excreted, respectively. In contrast, P_{N_2} in blood and tissue is identical because nitrogen is inert. The rather complex influences of dead space, alveolar ventilation, ventilation-perfusion relationships, and tissue metabolism on the partial pressures of oxygen and carbon dioxide are discussed in some detail, and frequent reference to Figure 1–17 is useful in clarifying some of the concepts.

ALVEOLAR VENTILATION

Dead Space

A portion of each inspired breath remains in the conducting airways (consisting of the nose, mouth, pharynx, larynx, trachea, bronchi, and bronchioles), where no significant exchange of oxygen and carbon dioxide with blood takes place. The volume of the conducting airways is called the anatomic dead space ($V_{D_{anat}}$) and is filled by about 25 per cent of each tidal volume (V_T). The remainder of each V_T goes to the alveoli, where rapid exchange of oxygen and carbon dioxide occurs, and the proportion of ventilation that

undergoes gas exchange is known as the alveolar ventilation (V_A). When some alveoli are relatively underperfused with blood, as in some disease states, a proportion of alveolar air does not undergo gas exchange but acts as if it were in a dead space. It is called the alveolar dead space ($V_{D_{alv}}$). Thus:

$$V_T = V_{D_{anat}} + V_{D_{alv}} + V_A$$

$V_{D_{anat}} + V_{D_{alv}}$ is called the physiologic dead space ($V_{D_{phys}}$).

In health, anatomic dead space and physiologic dead space are nearly identical, since the distribution of air and blood in alveoli is nearly uniform. Anatomic dead space in milliliters is roughly equal to the weight of the subject in pounds (for a 7-lb baby, 7 or 8 ml; for an adult, 150 ml) and is normally less than 30 per cent of V_T. In the normal premature infant, anatomic dead space is slightly higher than 30 per cent and physiologic dead space may be higher than 40 per cent. In the infant with respiratory distress, physiologic dead space may be more than 70 per cent of the tidal volume.

Anatomic dead space may be measured by making use of the argument originally developed by Bohr, which is expressed in Equation 2:

Equation 2:

$$V_{CO_2} \text{ per breath} = V_{CO_2} \text{ dead space} + V_{CO_2} \text{ alveoli}$$

The volume of carbon dioxide is equal to the volume of a compartment × the fractional concentration of carbon dioxide. Thus:

$$F_{E_{CO_2}} V_E = F_{D_{CO_2}} V_D + F_{A_{CO_2}} V_A$$

Because the dead space at end-inspiration is filled with air containing no significant amount of carbon dioxide,

$$F_{D_{CO_2}} V_D = 0;$$

and because $V_A = V_E - V_D$,

$$F_{E_{CO_2}} V_E = F_{A_{CO_2}} (V_E - V_D),$$

$$F_{A_{CO_2}} V_D = (F_{A_{CO_2}} - F_{E_{CO_2}}) V_E,$$

and

$$V_{D_{anat}} = \frac{(F_{A_{CO_2}} - F_{E_{CO_2}}) V_E}{F_{A_{CO_2}}}.$$

Because

$$P_{A_{CO_2}} = F_{A_{CO_2}} \times (P_b - 47)$$

and

$$P_{A_{CO_2}} = P_{a_{CO_2}},$$

$$V_{D_{phys}} = \left(\frac{P_{a_{CO_2}} - P_{E_{CO_2}}}{P_{a_{CO_2}}} \right) V_E$$

The concentration of carbon dioxide in the alveolus ($F_{A_{CO_2}}$) can be measured from an end-tidal sample, which represents the average alveolar carbon dioxide concentration. V_E is measured by collecting expired gases, and $F_{E_{CO_2}}$ can be measured using an aliquot of mixed expired air. The amount of dilution

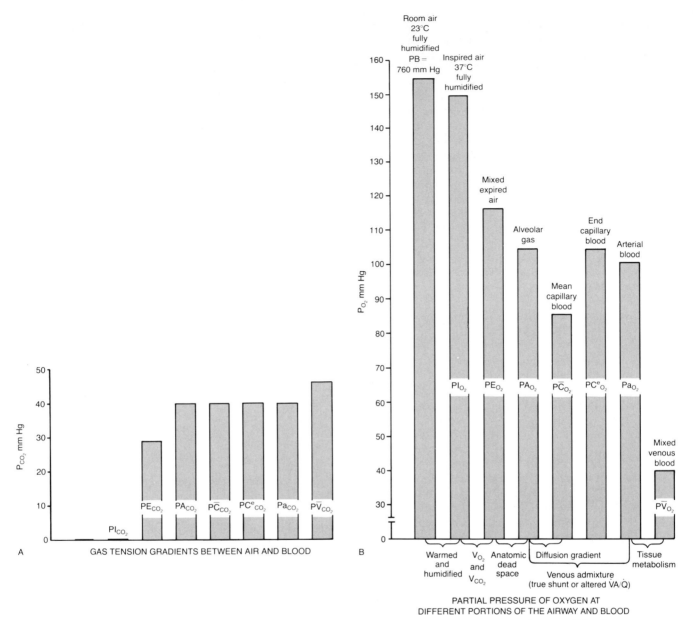

Figure 1–17. Partial pressures of oxygen and carbon dioxide in different portions of the airway and blood.

of FA_{CO_2} is proportional to the size of the dead space; the larger it is, the lower is FE_{CO_2}. For physiologic dead space, the partial pressure of carbon dioxide in arterial blood is used instead of the end-expired sample. A discrepancy in the two determinations, using end-tidal versus arterial blood, implies that portions of the lung are being ventilated and not perfused. That is, PA_{CO_2} is diluted by alveolar dead space and is therefore lower than Pa_{CO_2}.

Another method of measuring the anatomic dead space, Fowler's method, requires that a single breath of oxygen be inspired. On expiration both the volume of expired gas and the percentage of nitrogen are measured. The first portion of the expired gas comes from the dead space and contains little or no nitrogen. As the breath is expired, the percentage of nitrogen increases until it "plateaus" at the alveolar concentration. By assuming that all the initial part of the breath comes from the anatomic dead space and all the latter portion from the alveoli, the anatomic dead space can be calculated. The same measurements can be made by monitoring the expired carbon dioxide concentration.

In practice, anatomic dead space is difficult to define accurately, because it depends on lung volume (greater at large lung volumes when the airways are more distended) and on body position (smaller in supine position). It is now quite clear that V_{Dphys} must be defined according to the gas being measured. Because oxygen is more diffusible in the gas phase than is carbon dioxide, physiologic dead space using oxygen or various inert gases is different from the CO_2 dead space. However, V_{Dphys} measurements using CO_2 are helpful in assessing patients because they do reflect the portion of each breath that participates in gas exchange, particularly with respect to CO_2.

From the foregoing discussion, it is apparent that a tidal volume must be chosen that will allow adequate alveolar ventilation. For example, an adult might breathe 60 times a minute with a tidal volume of 100 ml for a minute ventilation of 6L. Nevertheless, alveolar ventilation under these circumstances is zero, because the dead space is ventilated. In selecting suitable volumes and rates for patients on respirators, it is useful to approximate normal values and to consider adequate alveolar ventilation rather than total ventilation.

Alveolar Gases

The amount of alveolar ventilation per minute must be adequate to keep the alveolar P_{O_2} and P_{CO_2} at values that will promote the escape of carbon dioxide from venous blood and the uptake of oxygen by pulmonary capillary blood. In health this means that PA_{O_2} is approximately 105 to 110 mm Hg and PA_{CO_2} is 40 mm Hg (Fig. 1–18).

Inspired air has an FI_{O_2} of 0.2093, and it is "diluted" in the alveoli by the FRC of air containing carbon dioxide and water vapor, so the partial pressure of oxygen in alveolar gas must be less than that of the inspired air (see Dalton's law, p. 13). PA_{O_2} must be calculated from the alveolar air equation, which is given later. When oxygen consumption equals carbon dioxide production, then:

$$PA_{O_2} = PI_{O_2} - PA_{CO_2}$$

$$PI_{O_2} = 0.2093 \times (P_b - 47 \text{ mm Hg}) = 150 \text{ mm Hg}.$$

If PA_{CO_2} is 40 mm Hg, then PA_{O_2} is 110 mm Hg. Usually the respiratory exchange ratio (R) is 0.8, or more oxygen is consumed than carbon dioxide eliminated, thereby decreasing PA_{O_2} slightly more than would be expected from the dilution of PA_{CO_2}. To account for changes in R, a useful form of the alveolar air equation for clinical purposes is

$$PA_{O_2} = PI_{O_2} - \frac{PA_{CO_2}}{R}$$

When PA_{CO_2} is 40 and R is 0.8, PA_{O_2} is 99 mm Hg. Note that 40 per cent oxygen raises PA_{O_2} to 235 mm Hg because FI_{O_2} is now 0.40 instead of 0.2093, as is the case when inhaling room air.

Because the partial pressures of alveolar gases must always equal the same total pressure, any increase in one must be associated with a decrease in the other. For example, If Pa_{CO_2} is 80 mm Hg and the patient is breathing room air, assuming an R of 0.8, the highest that PA_{O_2} can be is 50 mm Hg.

Arterial P_{O_2} is markedly affected by the presence of right-to-left shunts, and therefore it is not a good measurement of the adequacy of pulmonary ventilation. Pa_{CO_2} is minimally affected in the presence of shunts because $P\bar{v}_{CO_2}$ is 46 mm Hg and Pa_{CO_2} is 40 mm Hg. If one third of the cardiac output is shunted, this raises Pa_{CO_2} to only 42 mm Hg. Thus the arterial P_{CO_2} is the optimum measurement of the adequacy of alveolar ventilation. When alveolar ventilation halves, Pa_{CO_2} doubles; when alveolar ventilation doubles, Pa_{CO_2} halves. Hyperventilation is defined as a Pa_{CO_2} less than 35 mm Hg, and hypoventilation as a Pa_{CO_2} greater than 45 mm Hg. Some of the causes of hypoventilation are listed in Table 1–3.

DIFFUSION

Principles. The barriers through which a gas must travel when diffusing from an alveolus to the blood include the alveolar epithelial lining, basement membrane, capillary endothelial lining, plasma, and red blood cell. As observed on electron micrographs of lung tissue, the thinnest part of the barrier is 0.2 μ but may be as much as three times this thickness.

Fick's law of diffusion, modified for gases, states:

$$Q/\text{min} = \frac{K\ S\ (P_1 - P_2)}{d}$$

The amount of gas (Q) diffusing through a membrane is directly proportional to the surface area available for diffusion (S), the pressure difference of the two gases on either side of the membrane, and a constant (K) that depends on the solubility coefficient of the gas and the characteristics of the particular membrane and liquid used, and is inversely proportional to the distance (d) through which the gas has to diffuse. In the lung of a given subject, exact values for K, S, and d are unknown. Therefore, for the lung, Bohr and Krogh suggested "diffusion capacity" (DL). DL is simply the inverse of the total resistance to diffusion and can be expressed as the sum of the individual component resistances:

$$\frac{1}{DL} = \frac{1}{DM} + \frac{1}{\theta V_c}$$

where 1/DM is the resistance to diffusion of the gas across the alveolar-capillary membrane, plasma, and red blood cell membrane, θ is the reaction rate of

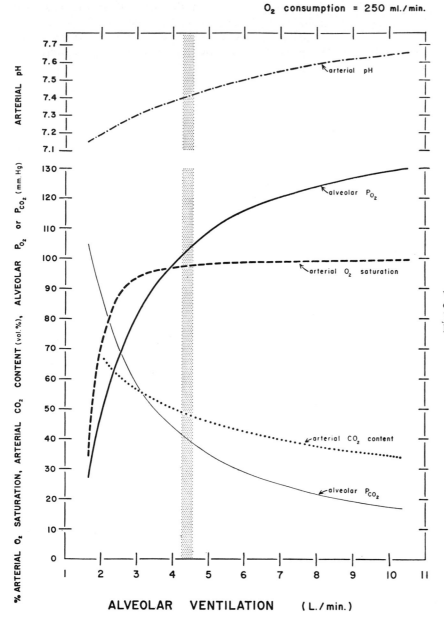

O₂ consumption = 250 ml./min.

Figure 1–18. The effect of changing alveolar ventilation on alveolar gas and arterial blood oxygen, carbon dioxide, and pH. (From Comroe JH Jr et al: The Lung. 2nd ed. Chicago, Year Book Medical Publishers, Inc, 1963.)

the gas with hemoglobin, and V_c is the pulmonary capillary blood volume.

Measurement. Carbon dioxide and oxygen have been used to measure the D_L. Although the diffusing capacity of the lung for oxygen ($D_{L_{O_2}}$) has been measured, the process is both complicated and fraught with technical problems because the average capillary oxygen tension must be determined. For this reason, and because a defect in $D_{L_{O_2}}$ is rarely the cause of hypoxemia, it is not used in the clinical setting. Carbon monoxide (CO), however, has been used extensively in children to test diffusing capacity. The advantage of using carbon monoxide is its remarkable affinity for hemoglobin, some 210 times that of oxygen, and therefore the capillary P_{CO} is negligible and offers no back pressure for diffusion. To calculate the $D_{L_{CO}}$, one need know only the amount of CO taken up per unit time and the $P_{A_{CO}}$.

Many techniques have been developed to measure the $D_{L_{CO}}$, but only two are discussed. The measurement of steady-state $D_{L_{CO}}$ is performed by having the patient breathe a gas mixture containing 0.1 per cent CO for several minutes. Although this measurement requires only a little patient cooperation, its disadvantage is that the value obtained is strongly influenced by maldistribution of the inspired air; if the inhaled gas mixture is not distributed properly to all parts of the lung, the measured $D_{L_{CO}}$ will be decreased but not because of changes in D_M, θ, or V_c.

The second technique, the measurement of single-breath $D_{L_{CO}}$, is virtually unaffected by airway disease. In this test the subject takes a single large breath (from RV to TLC) of a CO-containing gas mixture. Following a 10-second breath-hold, the expired gases are collected so that $P_{A_{CO}}$ can be determined.

Table 1–3. ILLUSTRATIVE CAUSES OF HYPOVENTILATION

Respiratory Center Depression
General anesthesia; excessive doses of drugs such as morphine, barbiturates, or codeine; severe or prolonged hypoxia, cerebral ischemia, high concentrations of CO_2; electrocution; cerebral trauma; increased intracranial pressure

Conditions Affecting the Airways and Lung

UPPER OR LOWER AIRWAY OBSTRUCTION
Foreign body, large tonsils and adenoids, vocal cord paralysis, croup, endobronchial tuberculosis, chronic bronchitis, emphysema, asthma, bronchiectasis, cystic fibrosis, bronchiolitis

DECREASED LUNG COMPLIANCE
Vascular diseases such as emboli, polyarteritis, mitral stenosis; parasitic infiltrations; interstitial disease such as sarcoid, Hamman-Rich syndrome, pneumoconioses, lupus, rheumatoid arthritis, berylliosis, histiocytosis X, radiation fibrosis, idiopathic pulmonary hemosiderosis

EXTENSIVE LOSS OF FUNCTIONING LUNG TISSUE
Atelectasis, tumor, pneumonia, cystic fibrosis, surgical resection

LIMITATION OF MOVEMENT OF LUNGS
Pleural effusion, pneumothorax, fibrothorax

Conditions Affecting the Thorax

DECREASED CHEST WALL COMPLIANCE
Arthritis, scleroderma, kyphoscoliosis, fractured ribs, thoracoplasty, thoracotomy, pickwickian syndrome, phrenic nerve paralysis

DISEASES OF RESPIRATORY MUSCLES
E.g., muscular dystrophy

PARALYSIS OF RESPIRATORY MUSCLES
Poliomyelitis, peripheral neuritis, spinal cord injury, myasthenia gravis; curare, succinylcholine botulinus, and nicotine poisonings

The difference between these two techniques is exemplified by the patient with acute asthma, in whom the steady-state DL_{CO} value will be decreased, whereas the single-breath DL_{CO} value will be normal or increased. Another advantage of the single-breath DL_{CO} method results from the inclusion of helium in the inspired gas. This inert gas allows the DL_{CO} to be corrected for the alveolar volume in which it was distributed, a measurement known as K_{CO}.

$$K_{CO} = \frac{DL_{CO} \text{ single-breath}}{\text{alveolar volume}}$$

The K_{CO} is the most useful parameter for comparing the DL of children of different ages and hence different lung volumes (Fig. 1–19). In addition, the K_{CO} helps differentiate among simple loss of lung units (atelectasis), a decrease in pulmonary blood volume (emphysema), and the (albeit rarely seen) true diffusion defect.

The DL_{CO} increases throughout childhood, is related to lung growth, and correlates best with subject height or body surface area. Clinically, a reduction in DL_{CO} may occur for many reasons, including surgical lung resection, diffuse lung disease (pulmonary fibrosis, cystic fibrosis), and emphysematous destruction of the alveolar-capillary membrane. In addition, anemia by itself decreases the DL_{CO} (equations to correct the DL_{CO} for anemia are available)

(Single-breath carbon monoxide, 1987). Increases in DL_{CO} rarely occur and usually result from pulmonary vascular engorgement (increased V_c) or pulmonary hemorrhage (e.g., Goodpasture syndrome and idiopathic pulmonary hemosiderosis).

It is important to reinforce the point that impaired diffusion of oxygen from the alveolar air to the pulmonary capillary is rarely, if ever, the cause of a low Pa_{O_2}. Hypoxemia in pulmonary diseases usually results from alveolar hypoventilation or an imbalance between ventilation and perfusion of lung units. Thus low DL_{CO} values almost always reflect abnormalities in gas exchange rather than true diffusion defects.

SHUNT AND VENTILATION-PERFUSION RELATIONSHIPS

There are four pulmonary causes of arterial hypoxemia. Two of these, alveolar hypoventilation and diffusion defects, have already been discussed in this section. The remaining two, intrapulmonary shunt and ventilation-perfusion defects, result from abnormalities in the distribution of the ventilation and perfusion of the gas-exchanging units.

Shunt refers to blood that reaches the systemic circulation without coming in direct contact with a ventilated area of the lung. Because this blood is deoxygenated it depresses the Pa_{O_2}. There are several causes of shunt. In normal lungs a small amount of shunt is present, because the thebesian veins and a portion of the bronchial vascular flow drain into the left side of the heart. Pathologic shunts result when abnormal vascular channels exist, as in cyanotic congenital heart disease or pulmonary arteriovenous fistula. Shunt, however, most commonly occurs in diseased lungs in which alveoli are not ventilated but

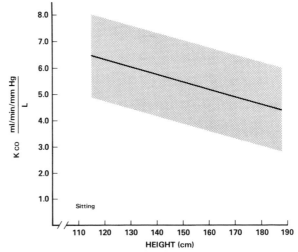

Figure 1–19. Diffusion constant for the transfer of carbon monoxide (K_{CO}) as a function of height in subjects 6 to 30 years of age. Stippled areas indicate 95 per cent confidence limits. (Adapted from O'Brodovich HM et al: Am Rev Respir Dis 125:670, 1982.)

are still being perfused. This condition, known as intrapulmonary shunting, occurs in a variety of lung diseases including pulmonary edema, atelectasis, and pneumonia.

A characteristic feature of shunt is that the resultant hypoxemia cannot be corrected by breathing pure oxygen, a reasonable consequence because, by definition, shunted blood does not pass ventilated lung units. This characteristic can be a useful clinical tool; if the Pa_{O_2} is less than 500 mm Hg while the subject is breathing 100 per cent oxygen, a significant shunt is present. If mixed venous (pulmonary arterial) blood is available for measurement, the amount of shunt can be calculated at any inspired oxygen concentration using the shunt equation: the amount of oxygen in arterial blood = the amount of oxygen in blood that has passed through pulmonary capillaries ($\dot{Q}_c$) + the amount of oxygen in shunted blood ($\dot{Q}_s$), and the amount of oxygen = the content of oxygen per liter (C_{O_2}) × the blood flow ($\dot{Q}$). Therefore,

$$Ca_{O_2} \cdot \dot{Q}_t = Cc_{O_2} \, \dot{Q}_c + C\bar{v}_{O_2}\dot{Q}_s$$

(where $\dot{Q}_t$ is total blood flow).

Since $\dot{Q}_c = \dot{Q}_t - \dot{Q}_s$,

$$Ca_{O_2}\dot{Q}_t = Cc_{O_2}\dot{Q}_t - Cc_{O_2}\dot{Q}_s + C\bar{v}_{O_2}\dot{Q}_s$$

and

$$\frac{\dot{Q}_s}{\dot{Q}_t} = \frac{Cc_{O_2} - Ca_{O_2}}{Cc_{O_2} - C\bar{v}_{O_2}}$$

where $\dot{Q}_s/\dot{Q}_t$ is the fraction of the total cardiac output that is shunted.

Arterial hypoxemia most commonly results from a mismatch of ventilation and perfusion within the lung. When a lung unit receives inadequate ventilation relative to its blood flow, insufficient oxygen is delivered to the alveolus. The alveolar P_{O_2} then decreases and the oxygen content of the end capillary blood falls. In contrast to what occurs in shunt, administration of an enriched oxygen mixture will correct the hypoxemia due to ventilation perfusion mismatches, because oxygen delivery is increased to the alveolus and hence to the pulmonary capillary blood.

Whatever the absolute amount of regional ventilation and perfusion, the lung has intrinsic regularity mechanisms that are directed toward the preservation of normal $\dot{V}_A/\dot{Q}$ ratios. When $\dot{V}_A/\dot{Q}$ is high, the low carbon dioxide concentration results in local constriction of airways and tends to reduce the amount of ventilation to the area. When $\dot{V}_A/\dot{Q}$ is low, the high alveolar carbon dioxide concentration results in low airway dilation and tends to increase ventilation to the area. Furthermore, a low $\dot{V}_A/\dot{Q}$ with an associated low alveolar oxygen concentration causes regional pulmonary vasoconstriction and produces a redistribution of blood flow to healthier lung units. These effects on airways and vessels from changing gas tensions tend to preserve a normal $\dot{V}_A/$ $\dot{Q}$, but they are limited mechanisms, and derangements are not uncommon.

GAS TRANSPORT TO THE SYSTEMIC VASCULATURE

OXYGEN TRANSPORT

Once oxygen molecules have passed from the alveolus into the pulmonary capillary, they are transported in the blood in two ways. A small proportion of the oxygen exists as dissolved oxygen in the plasma and water of the red blood cell. For 100 ml of whole blood equilibrated with a P_{O_2} of 100 mm Hg, 0.3 ml of oxygen is present as dissolved oxygen. If this represented the total oxygen-carrying capacity of blood, cardiac output would have to be greater than 80 L/min to allow 250 ml of oxygen to be consumed per minute. During 100 per cent oxygen breathing, Pa_{O_2} is approximately 650 mm Hg, and 100 ml of blood contains 2.0 ml of dissolved oxygen; a cardiac output of about 12 L/min would be required if no hemoglobin were present and if the tissues could extract all of the oxygen.

Because 1 g of hemoglobin can combine with 1.34 ml of oxygen, between 40 and 70 times more oxygen is carried by hemoglobin than by the plasma, enabling the body to achieve a cardiac output at rest of 5.5 L/min with an oxygen uptake of 250 ml/min.

The potential usefulness of hyperbaric oxygen (i.e., oxygen under very high pressures) for a variety of clinical conditions is due to the fact that at a pressure of 3 atmospheres (absolute) (PA_{O_2} about 1950 mm Hg) approximately 6.0 ml of oxygen is dissolved in 100 ml of whole blood, and this amount can meet the metabolic demands of the tissues under resting conditions even when no hemoglobin is present.

The remarkable oxygen-carrying properties of blood depend not on the solubility of oxygen in plasma but on the unusual properties of hemoglobin. Figure 1–20 illustrates the oxyhemoglobin dissociation curve, showing that hemoglobin is nearly 95 per cent saturated at a P_{O_2} of 80 mm Hg. The steep portion of the curve, up to about 50 mm Hg, permits large amounts of oxygen to be released from hemoglobin with small changes in P_{O_2}. Under normal circumstances, 100 per cent oxygen breathing will raise the amount of oxygen carried by the blood by only a small amount, because at a P_{O_2} of 100 mm Hg, hemoglobin is already 97.5 per cent saturated. Even with air breathing one is on the flat portion of the curve. The presence of a right-to-left shunt markedly affects P_{O_2} but may reduce the percentage saturation only minimally. For example, a 50 per cent shunt with venous blood containing 15 ml of oxygen/100 ml will reduce the oxygen content of 100 ml of blood only from 20 ml to 17.5 ml. The blood is still 88 per cent saturated, but Pa_{O_2} is now 60 mm Hg instead of 100 mm Hg. Thus the change in oxygen content is linearly related to the amount of

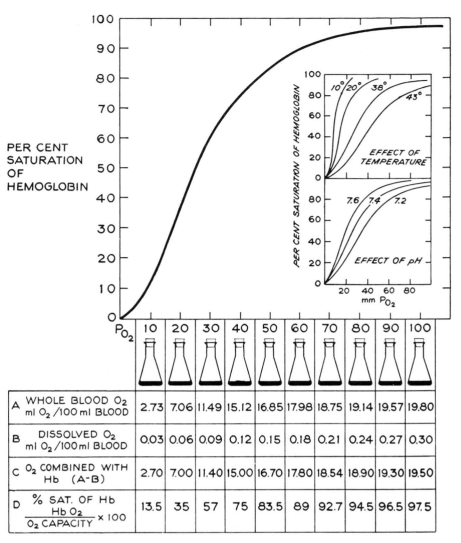

Figure 1–20. Oxyhemoglobin dissociation curves. The large graph shows a single dissociation curve, applicable when the pH of the blood is 7.40 and temperature is 38°C. The blood oxygen tension and saturation of patients with carbon dioxide retention, acidosis, alkalosis, fever, or hypothermia will not fit this curve because it shifts to the right or left when temperature, pH, or P_{CO_2} is changed. Effects on the oxyhemoglobin dissociation curve of change in temperature (*upper right*) and in pH (*lower right*) are shown in the smaller graphs. A small change in blood pH occurs regularly in the body; i.e., when mixed venous blood passes through the pulmonary capillaries, P_{CO_2} decreases from 46 to 40 mm Hg, and pH rises from 7.37 to 7.40. During this time, blood changes from a pH of 7.37 dissociation curve to a pH of 7.40 dissociation curve. (From Comroe JH: Physiology of Respiration. Chicago, Year Book Medical Publishers, Inc, 1965.)

P_{O_2}	10	20	30	40	50	60	70	80	90	100
A WHOLE BLOOD O_2 ml O_2/100 ml BLOOD	2.73	7.06	11.49	15.12	16.85	17.98	18.75	19.14	19.57	19.80
B DISSOLVED O_2 ml O_2/100 ml BLOOD	0.03	0.06	0.09	0.12	0.15	0.18	0.21	0.24	0.27	0.30
C O_2 COMBINED WITH Hb (A-B)	2.70	7.00	11.40	15.00	16.70	17.80	18.54	18.90	19.30	19.50
D % SAT. OF Hb $\frac{Hb\,O_2}{O_2\,CAPACITY} \times 100$	13.5	35	57	75	83.5	89	92.7	94.5	96.5	97.5

right-to-left shunt, but the change in P_{O_2} is not, because the oxyhemoglobin dissociation curve is S-shaped. It is also apparent that at levels greater than 60 mm Hg, Pa_{O_2} is a more sensitive measure of blood oxygenation because neither percentage saturation nor oxygen content changes as much as P_{O_2} in this range. However, at P_{O_2} below about 60 mm Hg, relatively small changes of P_{O_2} produce large changes in saturation and content, and in this range the measurement of content may be more reliable than the measurement of P_{O_2}.

The oxyhemoglobin dissociation curve is affected by changes in pH, P_{CO_2}, and temperature. A decrease in pH, an increase in P_{CO_2} (Bohr effect), or an increase in temperature shifts the curve to the right, particularly in the 20 to 50 mm Hg range. Thus for a given P_{O_2} the saturation percentage is less under acidotic or hyperpyrexic conditions. In the tissues, carbon dioxide is added to the blood, and this facilitates the removal of oxygen from the red blood cells. In the pulmonary capillaries, carbon dioxide diffuses out of the blood, facilitating oxygen uptake by hemoglobin. An increase in temperature has an effect similar to that of an increase in P_{CO_2} and thus facili-

tates oxygen removal from the blood by the tissues. Note that a patient who is pyrexic with carbon dioxide retention could not have a normal oxygen saturation during air breathing because of the Bohr and temperature effects on the oxyhemoglobin dissociation curve.

The erythrocyte concentration of D-2,3-diphosphoglycerate (DPG) plays a major role in shifting oxyhemoglobin dissociation curves. DPG and hemoglobin are present in about equimolar concentrations in adult human red blood cells. There is strong binding between DPG and the β chain of hemoglobin, and this complex is highly resistant to oxygenation. Shifts of the dissociation curve to the right associated with an increased DPG concentration—for example, in anemia—facilitate the release of oxygen to the tissues. Because erythrocyte DPG concentration can change within a matter of hours, a regulatory role for DPG in maintaining optimal tissue oxygenation has been suggested.

The fetal oxyhemoglobin dissociation curve is to the left of the adult curve at a similar pH. Thus at a given P_{O_2}, fetal hemoglobin contains more oxygen than adult hemoglobin. This property ensures that

Table 1–4. EFFECT OF TEMPERATURE AND ACUTE RESPIRATORY ACIDOSIS AND ALKALOSIS ON HEMOGLOBIN OXYGEN AFFINITY

Temperature*	P_{50}	P_{90}
28° C	16.5	35
32° C	20.5	44
40° C	32.0	68

Respiratory Acidosis and Alkalosis† pH	P_{CO_2}	P_{50}	P_{90}
7.56	20	22	48
7.48	30	24.5	52.5
7.40	40	27	58
7.32	50	29.5	63
7.26	60	31	67

P_{50} and P_{90}: P_{O_2} at which 50 per cent or 90 per cent of the hemoglobin is saturated.
*P_{CO_2} = 40 mm Hg, pH = 7.40.
†Temperature = 37° C.
(Data from Rebuck AS and Chapman KR: Am Rev Respir Dis 137:962–963, 1988.)

an adequate amount of oxygen will reach fetal tissues, since the fetus in utero has a Pa_{O_2} of about 30 mm Hg. The different affinity of fetal hemoglobin for oxygen results from its interaction with DPG. Both fetal and adult red blood cells have similar intracellular concentrations of DPG, but fetal hemoglobin, which has a γ chain instead of a β chain, interacts less strongly with this molecule; therefore the fetal oxyhemoglobin curve is to the left of the adult curve. Fetal hemoglobin disappears from the circulation shortly after birth, and by a few months of age less than 2 per cent is present. Normal fetal development is not dependent on differences in maternal and fetal hemoglobins, because in some species they are identical.

Abnormal hemoglobins differ in their oxygen-carrying capacity. For example, hemoglobin M is oxidized by oxygen to methemoglobin, which does not release oxygen to the tissues; a large amount is incompatible with life. The formation of methemoglobin by agents such as nitrates, aniline, sulfon-

Table 1–5. FOUR TYPES OF HYPOXIA AND SOME CAUSES

Hypoxemia (low P_{O_2} and low oxygen content)
Deficiency of oxygen in the atmosphere
Hypoventilation (see Table 1–3)
Uneven distribution of alveolar gas and/or pulmonary blood flow
Diffusion impairment
Venous to arterial shunt

Deficient Hemoglobin (normal P_{O_2} and low oxygen content)
Anemia
Carbon monoxide poisoning

Ischemic Hypoxia (normal P_{O_2} and oxygen content)
General or localized circulatory insufficiency
Tissue edema
Abnormal tissue demands

Histotoxic Anoxia (normal P_{O_2} and oxygen content)
Poisoning of cellular enzymes so that they cannot use the available oxygen (e.g., cyanide poisoning)

amides, acetanilid, phenylhydrazine, and primaquine may also be life threatening. Congenital deficiency of the enzyme hemoglobin reductase is also associated with large amounts of methemoglobin, and affected patients are cyanotic in room air. Sulfhemoglobin is, likewise, unable to transport oxygen. Carbon monoxide has 210 times more affinity for hemoglobin than oxygen, so it is important to note that P_{O_2} may be normal in carbon monoxide poisoning but oxygen content will be reduced markedly.

Thus a variety of factors may affect the position of the oxyhemoglobin dissociation curve. The position of the curve may be described by measuring the P_{O_2} at which there is 50 per cent saturation, the so-called P_{50}. When the curve is shifted to the left, the P_{50} is low; when the curve is shifted to the right, P_{50} is elevated. Although the P_{50} is the traditional method of describing the affinity of hemoglobin for oxygen (see Fig. 1–20) a more appropriate clinical measurement is the P_{90}. This is the Pa_{O_2} at which the hemoglobin is 90 per cent saturated and, as outlined below, corresponds to the goal of oxygen therapy (Table 1–4).

Oxygen Delivery to Tissues

The cardiopulmonary unit not only must oxygenate the blood but also must transport oxygen to the systemic tissues in adequate amounts. The total oxygen delivery to the systemic tissues is determined by the Pa_{O_2}, the amount of saturated hemoglobin, and the left ventricular output, as expressed in Equation 3. For an average adult with a Pa_{O_2} of 100 mm Hg, a hemoglobin (Hb) concentration of 15 g/100 ml (97.5 per cent saturation), and a cardiac output (C.O.) of 5 L/min, approximately 1000 ml of oxygen are delivered to systemic tissues each minute! This large delivery of oxygen provides a significant margin of safety, because under normal circumstances the systemic tissues use only one fourth of the available oxygen; mixed venous Pa_{O_2} is 40 mm Hg and hemoglobin is 73 per cent saturated. The systemic oxygen transport equation is useful to emphasize a therapeutic principle: the three practical ways to improve oxygenation of peripheral tissues are to increase hemoglobin saturation, to increase hemoglobin concentration, and to augment cardiac output.

Cyanosis is one clinical sign of inadequate oxygenation of systemic tissues. The degree of visible cyanosis depends on the amount of unsaturated hemoglobin present in the blood perfusing the superficial vessels. In polycythemia adequate amounts of oxygen may be present, but the patient appears cyanotic because not all the hemoglobin is saturated. Conversely, in anemia, the patient may be inadequately oxygenated without appearing cyanotic. The clinical assessment of oxygenation is hazardous in part because poor peripheral circulation may result in peripheral cyanosis when the arterial blood is well oxygenated. Thus the most reliable estimate of the oxygen content of arterial blood requires direct meas-

Equation 3:

oxygen delivery = [blood oxygen content] [cardiac output]*

$$= 10 \cdot \left[\left(\frac{0.003 \text{ ml}}{\text{mm Hg}/100 \text{ ml}} \right) (\text{Pa}_{O_2}) + \left(\frac{1.34 \text{ ml O}_2}{\text{g Hb}} \right) \left(\text{Hb} \frac{\text{g}}{100 \text{ ml}} \right) (\% \text{ saturation}) \right] [\text{C.O.}]$$

---

*Note: To maintain consistency of units, blood oxygen content (expressed per 100 ml blood) must be multiplied by 10, because cardiac output is expressed in L/min.

urement, because neither hypoxemia nor hyperoxemia can be assessed reliably by clinical observation.

OXYGEN THERAPY

Increased Inspired Mixtures

Increased inspired mixtures of oxygen are required when tissue oxygenation is inadequate. The response to increased inspired oxygen depends on which cause of hypoxia is present (Table 1–5). Most of the conditions characterized by hypoxemia respond well to added oxygen. Patients with venoatrial shunts will respond less well, because the shunted blood does not perfuse alveoli. Even so, tissue oxygenation may be improved slightly by the addition of oxygen to the blood, which does undergo gas exchange in the lung. A direct attack on the underlying disorder in anemia, ischemia, and poisonings is clearly indicated; oxygen therapy may be a life-saving measure during the time required to treat the disease.

Oxygen therapy can be utilized to facilitate the removal of other gases loculated in body spaces, such as air in pneumothorax, pneumomediastinum, and ileus. High inspired oxygen mixtures effectively wash out body stores of nitrogen. With air breathing, the blood that perfuses the tissue spaces has an arterial oxygen tension of 100 mm Hg and a venous tension of 40 mm Hg. With oxygen breathing, although arterial tensions rise to 600 mm Hg, venous oxygen tensions do not rise above 50 to 60 mm Hg because of oxygen consumption and the shape of the dissociation curve. With air breathing, arterial and venous

nitrogen tensions are the same, about 570 mm Hg. If the loculated gas were air at atmospheric pressure, the gradient for the movement of nitrogen to the blood would be very small. After nitrogen washout, with oxygen breathing, the lack of high elevation in venous oxygen tension permits movement of both nitrogen and oxygen into the blood. The increased pressure differences increase the rate of absorption of loculated air some fivefold to tenfold.

Administration of Oxygen

There are several methods of delivering enriched oxygen gas mixtures to nonintubated patients. Known concentrations of oxygen can be piped into chambers that surround the infant's head, such as an oxygen tent or a head box. Usually these chambers allow significant leakage of gases, so it is imperative that the O_2 concentration be measured inside the chamber near the patient's face. Another method is to run pure oxygen through nasal prongs or cannulae at specified flow rates. Although this method can be efficacious in improving the Pa_{O_2}, it must be remembered that it does not provide a constant FI_{O_2} during the breath, nor can the FI_{O_2} be accurately calculated or measured. The reason is that patients will "beat the system," because their inspiratory flow rates exceed the rate at which the pure oxygen is being piped toward their faces. A simple calculation illustrates the point. If a 70-kg man breathes at 30 breaths per minute with an inspiratory to expiratory time ratio of 1:1, his duration of inspiration will be 1 sec. Given a tidal volume of 0.5 L, his average inspiratory flow rate will be 0.5 L/sec or 30 L/min. Given that nasal

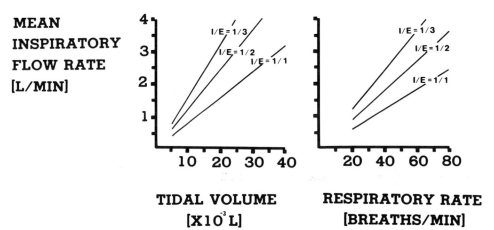

Figure 1–21. Mean inspiratory flow rate in infants with respiratory rates of 40/min (*left*) or with tidal volume of 15 ml (*right*). I/E is the ratio of the duration of inspiration to the duration of expiration. Peak flow rates during tidal volume breathing will be greater.

CALCULATED TOTAL GAS FLOW

WITH VENTURI MASKS

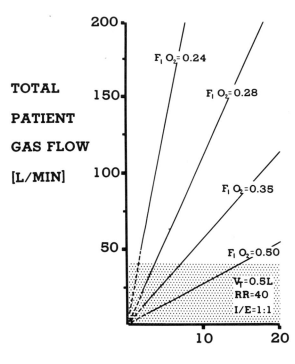

Figure 1–22. Calculated total gas flow that is delivered to the patient using various Venturi valves designed to deliver specified oxygen concentrations. Note that $F_{I_{O_2}}$ is constant regardless of the flow rate of pure oxygen (x axis) that is delivered to the valve.

prongs are usually set at 2–6 L/min for the average 70-kg man, it is immediately obvious that his initial portion of inspiration will be 100 per cent oxygen but that the percentage will fall quickly toward that of room air by the end of inspiration. This pattern is not only applicable to adults but is equally applicable to infants (Fig. 1–21).

Thus although one can "guestimate" what flow rate of oxygen the patient will require to normalize the blood oxygen tension, the actual $F_{I_{O_2}}$ will vary within and between breaths, especially if the patient changes the depth or pattern of breathing (see Fig. 1–21). Recognizing these difficulties, Campbell in 1960 developed the concept of controlled oxygen therapy, using high flow rates of enriched oxygen gas mixtures. This therapy utilizes the Venturi principle by flowing pure oxygen through a Venturi valve that permits entrainment of room air. The amount of room air that is entrained is dependent on the size of the opening in the valve and thus determines the oxygen concentration of the final gas mixture that goes to the patient. Figure 1–22 demonstrates the very high flow rates that are achievable with such

systems. The advantages are clear: the patient has difficulty beating the system; changes in the gas-exchanging characteristics of the lungs can be followed because the $F_{I_{O_2}}$ is accurately known; and the high flow rates allow the mask to be placed *loosely* on the face, thereby increasing patient comfort.

It must also be emphasized that oxygen requirements can be influenced by the state of wakefulness. This is especially important in severe chronic lung disease (Fig. 1–23).

Hazards of High Oxygen Mixtures

Hypoxemia in conditions associated with alveolar hypoventilation, such as chronic pulmonary disease and status asthmaticus, may be overcome by enriched oxygen mixtures without concomitant lessening of the hypercapnia. The patient may appear pink but become narcotized under the influence of carbon dioxide retention. In chronic respiratory acidosis, respiration may be maintained chiefly by the hypoxic drive.

With the institution of oxygen therapy, there is usually a small drop in minute ventilation as the hypoxic stress is relieved with a concomitant small increase in the Pa_{O_2}. Rarely, a patient with chronic respiratory failure may cease breathing if excessive oxygen is given. It is therefore essential to measure the pH and Pa_{CO_2} in addition to the Pa_{O_2} or saturation in these groups of patients. The goal of oxygen therapy is to give just enough oxygen to return the arterial oxygen saturation to 90 per cent.

Excessive oxygenation of the blood can be dangerous. Human volunteers in pure oxygen at one atmosphere experience symptoms in about 24 hours, chiefly substernal pain and paresthesias. Laboratory animals exposed for longer periods die of pulmonary congestion and edema in 4 to 7 days. The toxicity of oxygen is directly proportional to its partial pressure. Symptoms occur within minutes under hyperbaric conditions and yet are not present after 1 month in pure oxygen at one-third atmosphere. Some of the acute effects of oxygen are a slight decrease of minute ventilation and cardiac output and constriction of retinal and cerebral vessels and the ductus arteriosus. Retinal vasoconstriction does not seem to be a significant problem in mature retinas that are fully vascularized. In premature infants, however, the vasoconstriction may lead to ischemia. After the cessation of oxygen therapy, or with maturation of the infant, neovascularization of the retina occurs. The disorderly growth and scarring may cause retinal detachments and fibroplasia, which appears behind the lens; hence, the name *retrolental fibroplasia* or *retinopathy of prematurity* as it is now known. Experimental data have shown that the retinal disease is worse in newborn kittens that are made mildly hypoxemic or normoxemic after exposure to high oxygen, relative to kittens that have been kept in slightly enriched oxygen environment following hyperoxic exposure. This suggests that an overaggressive approach to

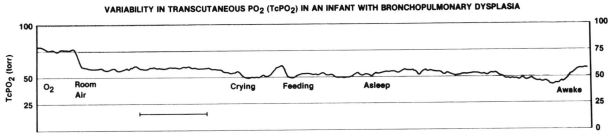

Figure 1–23. This infant with bronchopulmonary dysplasia had adequate oxygenation on room air while awake but desaturated to unacceptable levels after falling asleep. Bar indicates 5 minutes.

decreasing the level of oxygen therapy in premature infants may actually enhance rather than decrease the risk of severe retinal disease.

As the care of premature infants with acute lung disease has improved, the survival rate has increased impressively. Regrettably, chronic lung disease of prematurity or bronchopulmonary dysplasia has emerged (Chapter 14). At the present time it is difficult, if not impossible, to determine the relative contributions of prematurity, ventilator-induced barotrauma, oxygen toxicity, and the preceding acute lung injury in the evolution of this serious disorder. It does seem prudent, however, to minimize the $F_{I_{O_2}}$ in these patients, given the damage that occurs in totally normal lungs exposed to very high concentrations of oxygen.

CARBON DIOXIDE TRANSPORT AND ACID-BASE BALANCE

Buffering and Transport

Acids are normally produced in the body at the rates of 15 to 20 moles (mol) of carbonic acid and 80 mmol of fixed acids per day. For the cells to maintain their normal metabolic activity, the pH of the environment of the cells must be close to 7.40. The understanding of the regulation of hydrogen ion concentration requires knowledge of the buffering action of the chemical constituents of the blood and of the role of the lungs and kidneys in the excretion of acids from the body.

The most important constituents for acid-base regulation are the sodium bicarbonate and carbonic acid of the plasma, the potassium bicarbonate and carbonic acid of the cells, and hemoglobin.

The concentration of carbonic acid is determined by the partial pressure of carbon dioxide and the solubility coefficients of carbon dioxide in plasma and in red blood cell water. Carbonic acid in aqueous solution dissociates as follows:

$$CO_2 + H_2O \rightleftarrows H_2CO_3$$
$$H_2CO_3 \rightleftarrows H^+ + HCO_3^-$$

The law of mass action describes this reaction:

$$\frac{[H^+][HCO_3^-]}{[H_2CO_3]} = K$$

In plasma, K has the value of $10^{-6.1}$. An equivalent form of this equation is

$$pH = pK + \log\frac{[HCO_3^-]}{H_2CO_3}$$

By definition, $pH = -\log[H^+]$; $pK = -\log K = 6.1$ for plasma. Applied to plasma, in which dissolved carbon dioxide exists at a concentration 1000 times that of carbonic acid, the equation becomes

$$pH = 6.1 + \log\frac{[HCO_3^-]}{0.03P_{CO_2}}$$

This form of the equation is known as the Henderson-Hasselbalch equation. A clinically useful form of this equation is

$$\frac{H^+}{(nmol/L)} = 24 \times \frac{P_{CO_2}}{HCO_3^-}$$

Thus at a normal bicarbonate concentration of 24 mEq/L, when Pa_{O_2} is 40 mm Hg, hydrogen ion concentration is 40 nmol/L.

Just as oxygen has a highly specialized transport mechanism in the blood to ensure an adequate delivery to tissues under physiologic conditions, carbon dioxide produced by the tissues has a special transport system to carry it in the blood to the lung, where it is expired. The amount of carbon dioxide in blood is related to the P_{CO_2} in a manner shown in Figure 1–24. Unlike the relation of oxygen content to P_{O_2}, the relation of carbon dioxide content to P_{CO_2} is nearly linear; therefore, doubling alveolar ventilation halves Pa_{CO_2}, and halving alveolar ventilation doubles Pa_{CO_2}. Oxygenated hemoglobin shifts the carbon dioxide dissociation curve to the right (Haldane effect), so that at a given P_{CO_2} there is a lower carbon dioxide content. This effect aids in the removal of carbon dioxide from the blood in the lung when venous blood becomes oxygenated. The average arterial carbon dioxide tension (Pa_{CO_2}) is adults is 40 mm Hg and in infants is closer to 35 mm Hg; venous levels in both are normally 6 mm Hg higher. The small difference between arterial and venous P_{CO_2} is why the effect of venous admixture on arterial P_{CO_2} is very small.

The processes involved in the uptake of carbon dioxide in the blood and tissues are as follows:

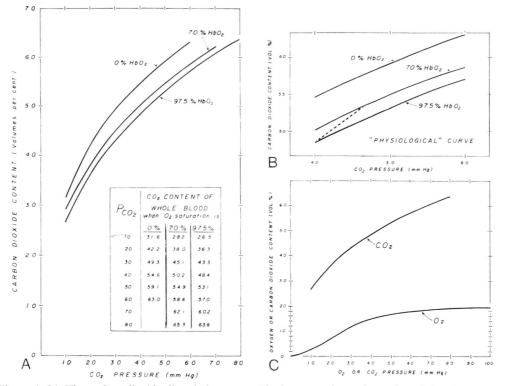

Figure 1–24. The carbon dioxide dissociation curve. The large graph (*A*) shows the relation between P_{CO_2} and carbon dioxide content of whole blood; this relation varies with changes in saturation of hemoglobin with oxygen. Thus, P_{CO_2} of the blood influences oxygen saturation (Bohr effect), and oxygen saturation of the blood influences carbon dioxide content (Haldane effect). The oxygen-carbon dioxide diagram gives the correct figure for both carbon dioxide and oxygen at every P_{O_2} and P_{CO_2}. *B,* Greatly magnified portion of the large graph to show the change that occurs as mixed venous blood (70 per cent oxyhemoglobin, P_{CO_2} 46 mm Hg) passes through the pulmonary capillaries and becomes arterial blood (97.5 per cent oxyhemoglobin, P_{CO_2} 40 mm Hg). Dashed line is a hypothetical transition between the two curves. *C,* Oxygen and carbon dioxide dissociation curves plotted on same scale to show the important point that the oxygen curve has a steep and a flat portion and that the carbon dioxide curve does not. (From Comroe JH Jr et al: The Lung. 2nd ed. Chicago, Year Book Medical Publishers, Inc, 1963.)

1. Carbon dioxide diffuses into the blood from the tissue. Some carbon dioxide is dissolved in the plasma water in physical solution.

2. Carbon dioxide hydrates slowly in the plasma to form a small amount of carbonic acid.

3. Most of the carbon dioxide enters the red blood cells. A small amount is dissolved in the water of each red cell. A fraction combines with hemoglobin to form a carbamino compound.

4. A larger fraction in the red blood cell hydrates rapidly, because of the presence of carbonic anhydrase, to form carbonic acid, which dissociates into H^+ plus HCO_3^-.

5. Bicarbonate diffuses into plasma because of the concentration gradient, and Cl^- ions enter the cell to restore electrical neutrality.

Hemoglobin is important in the transport of carbon dioxide because of two properties of the molecule. First, it is a good buffer, permitting blood to take up carbon dioxide with only a small change in pH. Second, hemoglobin is a stronger acid when oxygenated than when reduced; thus when oxyhemoglobin is reduced, more cations are available to

neutralize HCO_3^-. Carbon dioxide exists in two forms in the red blood cell because of this property of hemoglobin, as bicarbonate ion and as hemoglobin carbamate ($HbNHCOO^-$).

$$KHbO_2 + H_2CO_3 \rightleftarrows HHb + O_2 \uparrow + KHCO_3$$

$$KHbO_2NH_2 + CO_2 \rightleftarrows HHb \cdot NHCOOK + O_2 \uparrow$$

An enzyme in the red cell, carbonic anhydrase, accelerates the reaction

$$CO_2 + H_2O \rightleftarrows H^+ + HCO_3^-$$

some 13,000 times. A concentration gradient between red cell and plasma causes the bicarbonate ion to leave the red cell. Because the red blood cell membrane is relatively impermeable to Na^+ and K^+, the chloride ion and water move into the red cell to restore electrical neutrality (chloride shift or Hamburger shift). Thus although the larger portion of the buffering occurs within the red cell, the largest amount of carbon dioxide is in the plasma as HCO_3^-

(Table 1–6). The shift of chloride and HCO_3^- was previously thought to be passive, that is, to occur by diffusion due to a concentration gradient. It is now known to be an active process dependent on a specific transport protein within the red blood cell membrane. This anion transport occurs rapidly with a half-time of 50 ms.

In the lung a process the reverse of that just described takes place, because carbon dioxide diffuses out of the blood and into the alveoli. Diffusion of CO_2 is rapid, so the equilibrium between the P_{CO_2} of the pulmonary capillary and that of alveolar air is promptly achieved. About 30 per cent of the CO_2 that is exchanged is given up from hemoglobin carbamate. When hemoglobin is oxygenated in the pulmonary capillary, chloride and water shift out of the red cell, and bicarbonate diffuses in to combine with hydrogen ion to form H_2CO_3, which is in turn dehydrated to form carbon dioxide. Carbon dioxide then diffuses out of the cell into the plasma and alveolar gas.

Although red blood cells from newborn infants have less carbonic anhydrase activity than adult cells, no defect in carbon dioxide transport is apparent. However, when breathing 100 per cent oxygen, there is less reduced hemoglobin present in venous blood, and therefore less buffering capacity for H^+ is present, leading to an increased P_{CO_2}. This is an important consideration during hyperbaric oxygenation, when the venous blood may remain almost completely saturated with oxygen, H^+ is less well buffered, and tissue P_{CO_2} rises.

Acid-Base Balance

To understand acid-base balance within the body it is important to differentiate between the processes that promote a change in acid-base state and the end result of all these primary and secondary processes. *Acidemia* and *alkalemia* refer to the final acid-base status within the blood (hence the suffix -*emia*). Two processes can promote the development of acidemia: metabolic acidosis (loss of HCO_3^- or gain of H^+) and respiratory acidosis (increase in P_{CO_2}, which increases

H^+ via carbonic acid). Two processes can promote the development of alkalemia: metabolic alkalosis (gain of HCO_3^- or loss of H^+) and respiratory alkalosis (decrease in P_{CO_2}). Obviously, if there is a primary acidotic process, the body will try to maintain homeostasis by promoting a secondary alkalotic process and vice versa. Therefore, to understand the patient's acid-base balance, one must first measure the pH of the blood, and if it is abnormal, determine what primary and secondary (or compensatory) processes are involved. This is illustrated in Table 1–7; note, however, that the HCO_3^- shown in Table 1–7 is the *standard* HCO_3^- (see "Differences Between Additions of CO_2 to Blood in Vitro and in Vivo").

Metabolic acidosis occurs in such conditions as diabetes (in which there is an accumulation of keto acids); renal failure, when the kidney is unable to excrete hydrogen ion; diarrhea from loss of base; and tissue hypoxia associated with lactic acid accumulation. When pH falls, respiration is stimulated so that P_{CO_2} will fall and tend to compensate for the reduction in pH. This compensation is usually incomplete, and pH remains below 7.35. The pH, carbon dioxide content ($HCO_3^- + P_{CO_2}$), HCO_3^-, and P_{CO_2} are all reduced.

Metabolic alkalosis occurs most commonly after excessive loss of HCl due to vomiting (as in pyloric stenosis) or after an excessive citrate or bicarbonate load. The carbon dioxide content is elevated, and the P_{CO_2} will be normal or elevated, depending on the chronicity of the alkalosis.

Acute respiratory acidosis is secondary to respiratory insufficiency and accumulation of carbon dioxide within the body. The associated acidosis may be compensated for by renal adjustments that promote retention of HCO_3^-. Compensation may require several days. Patients with chronic respiratory acidosis, in whom therapy may improve alveolar ventilation, often have a rapid fall of Pa_{CO_2}. The adjustment in bicarbonate may be much slower, with a resultant metabolic alkalosis of several days' duration. Such a sequence of events has been noted in emphysema and cystic fibrosis.

Similarly, acute respiratory alkalosis, for example, secondary to fever, psychogenic hyperventilation, or a pontine lesion with meningoencephalitis, is associated with high pH, low P_{CO_2}, and normal bicarbonate level. Renal compensation in time leads to excretion of bicarbonate and return of pH toward normal.

It is important to point out that the lung excretes some 300 mEq/kg of acid per day in the form of carbon dioxide, and the kidney excretes 1 to 2 mEq/kg per day. Thus the lung plays a large role in the acid-base balance of the body, in fact providing rapid adjustment when necessary. The Henderson-Hasselbalch equation may be thought of as

$$pH \alpha \frac{kidney}{lung}$$

Table 1–6. CARBON DIOXIDE IN THE BLOOD

	Arterial Blood		Venous Blood	
	MM/L BL	%	MM/L BL	%
Total	21.9		24.1	
Plasma				
Dissolved CO_2	0.66	3	0.76	3
HCO_3^-	14.00	64	15.00	63
Cells				
Dissolved CO_2	0.44	2	0.54	2
HCO_3^-	5.7	26	6.1	25
$HbNHCOO^-$	1.2	5	1.8	7

The table gives normal values of the various chemical forms of CO_2 in blood with an assumed hematocrit level of 46. Approximately twice as much CO_2 exists in the plasma as in the red blood cells, chiefly as HCO_3^-.

Table 1–7. BLOOD MEASUREMENTS IN VARIOUS ACID-BASE DISTURBANCES

	pH	Pa_{CO_2} (mm Hg)	Standard HCO_3^- (mEq/L)	CO_2 Content (mEq/L)
Metabolic acidosis	↓	↓	↓	↓
Acute respiratory acidosis	↓	↑	↔	Slight ↑
Compensated respiratory acidosis	(↔ or slight ↓)	↑	↑	↑
Metabolic alkalosis	↑	Slight ↑	↑	↑
Acute respiratory alkalosis	↑	↓	↔	Slight ↓
Compensated respiratory alkalosis	(↔ or slight ↑)	↓	↓	↓
Normal values	7.35–7.45	35–45	24–26	25–28

Difference Between Additions of CO_2 to Blood in Vitro and in Vivo

An appreciation of the difference between the so-called in vitro and in vivo CO_2 dissociation curves is necessary to clarify the confusion that has arisen regarding the interpretation of measurements of acid-base balance, particularly during acute respiratory acidosis (acute hypoventilation). When blood in vitro is equilibrated with increasing concentrations of CO_2, bicarbonate concentration also increases because of the hydration of carbon dioxide. If, for example, blood with a P_{CO_2} of 40 mm Hg and a bicarbonate concentration of 24 mEq/L were equilibrated with a P_{CO_2} of 100 mm Hg, the actual bicarbonate concentration would be measured as 34 mEq/L. In the commonly used Astrup nomogram, a correction for this increased bicarbonate due to CO_2 alone is made, and the standard bicarbonate (bicarbonate concentration at P_{CO_2} of 40 mm Hg) is considered to be 24 mEq/L, or a base excess of zero. With this correction, one can readily see that the metabolic (renal) component of acid-base balance is normal. However, confusion has arisen because the in vitro correction figures have been incorrectly applied to the situation in vivo. Unlike equilibration in the test tube, the additional bicarbonate generated during in vivo acute hypercapnia not only is distributed to water in red cells and plasma but also equilibrates with the interstitial fluid space; that is, bicarbonate ion equilibrates with extracellular water. If the interstitial fluid represents 70 per cent of extracellular water, then 70 per cent of the additional bicarbonate generated will be distributed to the interstitial fluid. Thus an arterial sample taken from a patient with an acute elevation of P_{CO_2} to 100 mm Hg would have an actual bicarbonate concentration of 27 mEq/L. If 10 mEq/L were subtracted according to the in vitro correction, the standard bicarbonate would be reported as 17 mEq/L, or a base excess of −7, indicating the presence of metabolic as well as respiratory acidosis. This conclusion would be incorrect, however; the bicarbonate concentration in vivo is appropriate for the P_{CO_2}. The situation is worse in the newborn infant because of the high hematocrit and large interstitial fluid space. Base excess values of as much as −10 mEq/L (standard bicarbonate 14 mEq/L) may be calculated despite the fact that the in vivo bicarbonate concentration is appropriate for the particular P_{CO_2} and there is no metabolic component to the acidosis. Thus the appropriate therapy is to increase alveolar ventilation and not to administer bicarbonate.

TISSUE RESPIRATION

Aerobic Metabolism

The ultimate function of the lung is to provide oxygen to meet the demands of the tissues and to excrete carbon dioxide, a by-product of metabolic activity. Thus respiratory physiologists have been concerned with the assessment of respiration at the tissue level and the ability of the cardiopulmonary system to meet the metabolic demands of the body.

One method is to measure the amount of oxygen consumed by the body per minute ($\dot{V}_{O_2}$). This is equal to the amount necessary to maintain the life of the cells at rest, plus the amount necessary for oxidative combustion required to maintain a normal body temperature, as well as the amount used for the metabolic demands of work above the resting level. The basal metabolic rate is a summation of many component energy rates of individual organs and tissues and is defined as the amount of energy necessary to maintain the life of the cells at rest, under conditions in which there is no additional energy expenditure for temperature regulation or additional work.

In practice, $\dot{V}_{O_2}$ is measured after an overnight fast, the subject lying supine in a room at a comfortable temperature. This "basal" metabolic rate has a wide variability (± 15 per cent of predicted $\dot{V}_{O_2}$). Since absolutely basal conditions are difficult to ensure, the measurement of basal metabolic rate is not widely used at present.

The performance of the cardiopulmonary system can be more adequately assessed and compared with normal measurements under conditions of added work, such as exercise. During exercise, healthy subjects demonstrate an improvement in pulmonary gas exchange, cardiac output, and tissue oxygen extraction. Performance can be increased by physical fitness, and athletes are able to increase their cardiac output by sixfold or sevenfold. Athletic conditioning also increases the diffusing capacity of the lung and, in some manner not understood, increases the efficiency of oxygen extraction from the blood in the tissues at a given cardiac output. Fewer studies have been done in children, but in general the relation among work capacity, ventilation, and oxygen consumption is the same as that in the adult. The maximal $\dot{V}_{O_2}$ that can be achieved increases throughout childhood, reaches its peak of 50 to 60 ml per minute per kilogram between 10 and 15 years of age, and thereafter declines slowly with age.

At the tissue level, the ability of a given cell to receive an adequate oxygen supply depends on the amount of local blood flow, the distance of the cell from the perfusing capillary, and the difference between the partial pressures of oxygen in the capillary and in the cell. The critical mean capillary P_{O_2} appears to be in the region of 30 mm Hg for children and adults. Exercising muscle has 10 to 20 times the number of open capillaries as resting muscle does.

The body's response to exercise therefore is complex and depends on the amount of work, the rate at which the workload is increased, and the subject's state of health and degree of physical fitness. A detailed description of the physiologic response to exercise and its use in diagnosing cardiorespiratory disease is beyond the scope of this chapter, but exercise testing is now an essential tool in clinical medicine.

Anaerobic Metabolism

The adequacy of oxygen supply to the tissues has been assessed by measuring blood lactate, a product of anaerobic metabolism (Embden-Meyerhof pathway). When there is an insufficient oxygen supply to the tissues due to either insufficient blood flow or a decrease in blood oxygen content, lactic acid concentration within the tissues and blood rises. In the blood this accumulation leads to a metabolic acidosis.

During moderate to heavy muscular exercise, cardic output cannot meet the demands of the muscles, and an oxygen debt is incurred, which is repaid on cessation of exercise. During this period lactic acid accumulates, and therefore rigorous exercise is often associated with metabolic acidosis. There is an excellent correlation between the serum lactate level and the oxygen debt. Oxygen debt is not measurable at rest and is difficult to measure during exercise, but the adequacy of tissue oxygenation appears to be accurately reflected in the serum lactate level. In adult humans, blood lactate is less than 1 mEq/L but may rise to 10 to 12 mEq/L during very heavy exercise.

Relation Between $\dot{V}_{O_2}$ and $\dot{V}_{CO_2}$

In the normal subject in a steady state, the amount of carbon dioxide excreted by the lung per minute depends on the basal metabolic activity of the cells and the type of substrate being oxidized. The volume of carbon dioxide exhaled divided by the amount of oxygen consumed is known as the ventilatory respiratory quotient (R). For the body as a whole the ratio is 1 if primarily carbohydrate is being metabolized, 0.7 if fat, and 0.8 if protein. Normally the ratio is 0.8 at rest, approximately 1.0 during exercise, and greater than 1 at exhaustion. The ventilatory respiratory quotient may vary considerably with changes in alveolar ventilation and metabolism and therefore must be measured in the steady state, i.e., with a steady alveolar ventilation and a steady metabolic rate. For an individual organ, the metabolic respiratory quotient (R.Q.) is nearly constant but may vary from 0.4 to 1.5, depending on the balance of anabolism and catabolism in that organ. Thus the measurement of R represents the result of many component metabolizing organs and tissues. In the first few days after birth, R falls from nearly 1 to 0.7, indicating a loss of carbohydrate stores; when feeding has started, R approaches 0.8.

With breath-by-breath CO_2 and O_2 concentrations, R can now be calculated on a breath-by-breath basis. Using this technique it is possible to define more precisely the workload at which anaerobic metabolism begins (threshold for anaerobic metabolism). As lactic acid begins to accumulate in the blood, the carbon dioxide dissociation curve shifts to the right, and there is a sudden increase in expired CO_2. R therefore suddenly increases from about 1.0 to above 1.0. It has been shown that the threshold for anaerobic metabolism in both adults and children can be increased by training. This technique is particularly useful in children, because it does not require blood sampling and can be readily applied to cooperative subjects with a variety of pulmonary and cardiac problems.

REGULATION OF RESPIRATION

Over the past 20 years, the classic concepts regarding the respiratory control system have been challenged and broadened in many areas. It is appropriate for pediatricians to have an understanding of the normal respiratory control mechanisms, because alterations in respiratory frequency or alveolar ventilation are common to many diseases in infancy and childhood.

The study of the regulation of respiration centers around three main ideas: (1) the generation and maintenance of a respiratory rhythm, (2) the modulation of this rhythm by a number of sensory feedback loops and reflexes, and (3) the recruitment of respiratory muscles that can contract appropriately for gas exchange. The central controller requires reflexes to make "on-line" adjustments of the pattern of breathing not only to minimize energy costs but also to adapt to a variety of conditions and situations. These conditions may be behavioral, nonhomeostatic (e.g., sucking, speech production), and homeostatic (metabolic rate, oxygenation).

CENTRAL PATTERN GENERATION

It is clear now that the central nervous system, and in particular the brainstem, has the inherent ability to function as the respiratory "sinus node," or the central pattern generator (CPG). Although not well defined, the CPG for breathing is most likely composed of several groups of cells in the brainstem that have the property of a pacemaker. By analogy with rhythmic oscillatory systems, such as locomotion in vertebrates or other rhythmic behavior in invertebrates, this property of pacemaking is thought to be brought about in one of two ways: (1) Endogenous burster cells in the brainstem may have an inherent pacemaker property. These cells fire rhythmically in the absence of input or drive by virtue of their membrane properties and ion currents. (2) Alternatively, none of the respiratory-related cells may have the capability of bursting without synaptic input, but it is by virtue of their interconnections and their network properties that the output of the respiratory system oscillates rhythmically.

Whether respiratory pacemaking is the result of endogenous burster neurons or of synaptically driven neurons, two other properties have to be added to the respiratory CPG to explain its function. First, because both peripheral input (e.g., stretch receptors from the lungs and oxygen receptors from the carotid bodies) and central input (e.g., hypothalamus, amygdala) converge on the brainstem and make synapses with respiratory neurons, the CPG has to be able to integrate input from phasic or tonic excitatory or inhibitory influences. Moreover, because phrenic output is absent between inspiratory efforts, an inspiratory off-switch mechanism must be incorporated in the system. This off-switch mechanism is excited by the generator and in turn inhibits the CPG for the duration of expiration.

Little is known about the interconnections of the various respiratory groups of cells or nuclei or about the respiratory CPG. We know, however, that the medullary respiratory-related neurons are concentrated in two columns of cells that are not totally separate, one dorsally and the other ventrally located. Most cells in these two columns are located rostral to the obex, the dorsal column being just lateral to the central canal or the floor of the fourth ventricle and the ventral being lateral and ventral to the dorsal column.

Pontine neurons located in the rostral pons (pneumotaxic nucleus) also play an important role in shaping respiratory output. Sectioning the pons below this group of neurons induces a slower and deeper respiration. Although inherent rhythmicity cannot be ruled out totally for other pontine cell groups, the pneumotaxis (rostral) pontine cells cannot spontaneously generate respiratory rhythmicity.

The respiratory control areas are also influenced by higher centers. Tachypnea, associated with fever or changes in behavioral states or emotion, is presumably mediated by the influence of the hypothalamus, cortex, or the limbic system on the brainstem centers. Furthermore, voluntary control of ventilation has been demonstrated in adult humans and is based on the influence of forebrain structures on brainstem or spinal cord nuclei.

The main investigative problem in this area, which is precisely how the respiratory CPG works, still remains unsolved. The following sets of questions must be addressed: (1) Which groups of neurons are involved in the genesis of the respiratory act? What is their precise function in periodic oscillating motor behavior? (2) What are their network properties? How are these groups of cells physiologically and anatomically connected? For example, are they reciprocally inhibited or reciprocally excited? (3) What are the synaptic properties of the various cells, that is, the sign, nature, and strength of their synapses? (4) What are the membrane and subcellular properties of these cells? The last question is important because membrane currents determine the repetitive firing properties of neurons, and these in turn can determine the overall output of the network.

SENSORY FEEDBACK SYSTEM

The respiratory system is endowed with a wealth of afferent pathways to maintain control over several functional variables and adjust them at appropriate times. These pathways inform the central pattern generator about instantaneous changes that take place in, for example, the lungs, the respiratory musculature, the blood (acid-base), and the environment. The terms *sensory* and *afferent* refer not only to peripheral but also to central systems converging on the brainstem respiratory neurons.

Studies performed on adult animals have strongly suggested that the afferent receptor system is important not only to signal changes but also to provide an excitatory driving influence on the CPG. This sensory system might be even more significant in early life than in more mature subjects. The best illustration is in the newborn infant, who begins to breathe spontaneously in association with various sensory stimuli of the birth process.

Upper Airways and Lung Receptors

Cutaneous or mucocutaneous stimulation of the area innervated by the trigeminal nerve (e.g., face, nasal mucosa) decreases respiratory frequency and may lead to generation of respiratory pauses. These respiratory effects become less important with age, their strengths are species specific, and they depend on the state of consciousness. Because cortical inhibition of the trigeminal afferent impulses is more pronounced during REM sleep, trigeminal stimulation has a greater effect on respiration during quiet (non-REM) sleep.

The laryngeal receptor reflex is probably the most inhibitory reflex on respiration known. Sensory receptors are present in the epithelium of the epiglottis and upper larynx. Introduction into the larynx of small amounts of water or solutions with low concentrations of chloride results in apnea. The duration and severity of the respiratory changes depend on the behavioral state and are exacerbated by the presence of anesthesia. They are also worse if the subject is anemic, hypoglycemic, or a premature infant. In the unanesthetized subject, the reflex effects are almost purely respiratory and are mediated by the superior laryngeal nerve, which joins the vagal trunk after the nodose ganglion.

Stretch, irritant, and J receptors (vagal) are present in the tracheobronchial tree and lung interstitial space and were described previously in this chapter. These play an important role in informing the central nervous system about the status of lung volume, tension across airways, and lung interstitial pressure. The secondary neurons (where vagal afferents first synapse) are located in the nucleus tractus solitarius in the medulla. Stretch receptors, when stimulated by inflation of the lungs, prolong expiratory duration and delay the start of the next inspiration. However, the effect of lung inflation on the activity of inspiratory neurons in the medulla is not uniform. Some of the neurons are inhibited but others are excited, and it is on the basis of lung inflation that some have categorized brainstem neurons. Stimulation of vagal afferents at low current intensities (i.e., stretch receptor afferents) inhibits inspiration, hence the term inspiration-inhibiting reflex. Cooling the whole vagus nerve, thus eliminating stretch, irritant, and J receptors, induces an increase in the duration of both inspiration and expiration and in tidal volume. J receptors appear to be stimulated by lung edema. They produce tachypnea with interspersed short periods of respiratory pauses.

Vagal afferents carrying impulses from the lungs and airways have to be differentiated from vagal axons of vagal motoneurons, also located in the dorsal medulla (dorsomedial nucleus of the vagus, DMNX) or in the ventral medulla (part of the nucleus ambiguus). Vagal motoneurons, which innervate upper airway musculature, are important in determining the tone of these muscles and thus the patency of the upper airways. The interconnections between these neurons and others in the medulla are not well defined, but later studies have indicated that vagal motoneurons are relatively small, have high input resistance, and are probably recruited with relatively small synaptic currents.

O_2 and CO_2

The respiratory control system also receives information about O_2 and CO_2 tensions from sensory receptors located in specialized neural structures in blood vessels, airways, and the central nervous system. These tensions seem to be sensed, compared with "programmed" values, and acted on by the controller to increase or decrease ventilation accordingly. Although these structures help maintain acid-base homeostasis in the blood and the cerebrospinal fluid (CSF), one could view the brainstem ventilatory control apparatus as a way the brain adjusts its own

CSF acid-base medium for neuronal function at large.

The exact location of the central chemoreceptors is uncertain. Evidence suggests that chemoreceptive tissue is located superficially along the ventral lateral medulla. Direct stimulation of this area by an increase in P_{CO_2} or H^+ concentration produces an increase in ventilation, and conversely, a decrease in P_{CO_2} or H^+ concentration causes a depression of ventilation. It has been suggested that this area is influenced primarily by the acid-base composition of CSF and that the delay in ventilatory response to changes in arterial P_{CO_2} and bicarbonate is due to the time required to change the CSF H^+ concentration. Carbon dioxide, which diffuses into the CSF in a few minutes, has a rapid effect on the central chemoreceptors. Changes in blood bicarbonate are much less rapidly reflected in the CSF (24 to 48 hours). Thus with acute metabolic acidosis, arterial P_{CO_2} falls along with CSF P_{CO_2}. Hyperventilation is produced by the H^+ stimulation of peripheral chemoreceptors, but this stimulus is inadequate to compensate fully for the metabolic acidosis because of inhibition from the decreased H^+ concentration in the CSF. After 24 hours, CSF bicarbonate falls and restores CSF pH to normal. There is a further fall in arterial P_{CO_2}, and arterial pH returns toward normal. From these observations it has been suggested that the control of alveolar ventilation is a function of the central chemoreceptors, which are under the influence of CSF or brain interstitial fluid H^+, acting in association with the peripheral chemoreceptors, which are directly under the influence of the arterial blood.

The peripheral chemoreceptors are found in the human along the structures associated with the branchial arches. Two sets of chemoreceptors appear to be of greatest physiologic importance: (1) the carotid bodies, located at the division of the common carotid artery into its internal and external branches, and (2) the aortic bodies, which lie between the ascending aorta and the pulmonary artery. Afferent nerves from the carotid body join the glossopharyngeal (IX) nerve; those from the aortic bodies join the vagosympathetic trunk along with the recurrent laryngeal nerves.

The carotid and aortic bodies are responsive primarily to changes in oxygen tension. At rest they are tonically active, signifying that some ventilatory drive exists even at a Pa_{O_2} of 100 mm Hg. Inhalation of 33 per cent oxygen reduces ventilation; inhalation of low oxygen mixtures is associated with a significant increase in ventilation when the Pa_{O_2} is less than 60 mm Hg. Potentiation of the hypoxic stimulus is achieved by an increase in Pa_{CO_2}. For example, at a Pa_{CO_2} of 50 mm Hg, ventilation is significantly increased when Pa_{O_2} is lowered to 80 mm Hg. Hypoxia and hypotension presumably act together to decrease the oxygen supply of the chemoreceptor tissue, resulting in a greater ventilatory response to hypoxia.

The response of the peripheral chemoreceptors to P_{CO_2} is rapid (within seconds), and ventilation increases monotonically with Pa_{CO_2}. This increase in ventilation can be substantial (twofold to threefold), with a 5 to 10 mm Hg increase in Pa_{CO_2}. More important than the amplitude may be the rate of the change in Pa_{CO_2}. Further evidence supports the hypothesis that the carotid bodies respond more to an oscillating Pa_{CO_2} than to a steady Pa_{CO_2} at the same mean level, because these chemoreceptors adapt to a constant stimulus in the same manner as to thermal or touch sensory receptors of the skin. Part of the hyperventilation of exercise may be accounted for on this basis, because oscillations of arterial P_{CO_2} of about 7 mm Hg accompany moderate exercise. Another important concept related to carotid body function is the "gated" nature of its responsiveness. Stimulation of the carotid sinus nerve has no effect during expiration, only during inspiration. The peripheral chemoreceptors play a minor role in the stimulation of respiration when there is central depression, and respiration is maintained for the most part by the hypoxic drive alone.

The peripheral chemoreceptors, also responsive to changes in arterial pH, increase ventilation in association with a fall of 0.1 pH unit and produce a twofold to threefold increase with a fall of 0.4 pH unit. Some investigators believe that the peripheral chemoreceptor response is mediated through changes in intracellular hydrogen ion concentration.

Other Reflexes

A variety of peripheral reflexes are known to influence respiration. Hyperpnea may be produced by stimulation of pain and temperature receptors or mechanoreceptors in limbs. Visceral reflexes, such as those resulting from distention of gallbladder or traction on the gut, are usually associated with apnea. Afferent impulses from respiratory muscles (e.g., intercostals) may play a role in determining the optimum response of the muscles of ventilation to various respiratory stimuli. In newborn infants an inspiratory gasp may be elicited by distention of the upper airways. This reflex is mediated by the vagus nerve and is known as the Head reflex. It has been suggested that this inspiratory gasp reflex is important in the initial inflation of the lungs at birth.

The Newborn Infant

There is special interest in the control of breathing in the newborn period because it is the period of transition from the intrauterine state, when the lungs are not required for gas exchange, to extrauterine existence, which depends on the lung as the organ of gas exchange.

A number of studies have demonstrated that the responsiveness to stimuli in newborn infants is different from that of older or mature adult subjects. Although the exact mechanisms for these differences have generally been elusive, the rapid maturational changes that occur in key control systems could serve as the bases for the different responses seen in early life.

Infants, like adults, increase ventilation in response to inspired carbon dioxide. However, a comparison of ventilation per kg in infants (premature and full-term) and adults shows that all infants breathe more at a given P_{CO_2} than adults do. Presumably this is because infants have a higher CO_2 production per kg and a lower buffering capacity of the blood. Yet the change in ventilation per mm Hg change in P_{CO_2} is the same in full-term infants and adults, suggesting that their neurochemical apparatus have the same sensitivity but that the ventilatory response is a function of body mass. This concept has been challenged; it has been pointed out that the ventilatory response to CO_2 may be impaired because of mechanical factors, such as stiffness of a lung, or because of a very compliant chest wall. However, measurements of respiratory center output by mouth pressure during brief airway occlusion (presumably eliminating mechanical factors) indicate that premature infants may not respond as well as the full-term infant or adult to inspired CO_2. Maturation of this response is a function of gestational as well as postnatal age.

Peripheral chemoreceptors are functional in newborn infants, as demonstrated by a slight decrease in $\dot{V}E$ with 100 per cent oxygen breathing. The effect of hypoxia as a stimulant may differ in the first 12 hours of life; 12 per cent oxygen in the first 12 hours of life fails to stimulate ventilation. Presumably, the atypical response reflects the persistence of fetal shunts that affect the oxygen tensions of blood perfusing that carotid body. In addition, the newborn infant has been found to increase ventilation only transiently in response to a hypoxic stimulus, whereas the adult will have a sustained increase in ventilation.

The mechanisms responsible for this different response to hypoxia in the newborn are not well understood. It has been suggested that the biphasic hypoxic response is multifactorial. Several groups of investigators have examined this question, and it is clear now that the drop in ventilation in phase 2 of the biphasic response may be due to one or more of the following: (1) reduction in dynamic lung compliance, (2) reduction in chemoreceptor activity during sustained (more than 1–2 min) hypoxia, (3) central neuronal depression due to either an actual drop in excitatory synaptic drive other than carotid input or changes in neuronal membrane properties reducing excitability, and (4) decrease in metabolic rate. These studies are not conclusive with respect to the relationship between the drop in ventilation and respiratory failure. Animal studies have failed so far to show that hypercapnia results from the decrease in ventilation.

Whether this decrease in respiration during phase 2 is mediated by certain neurotransmitters is not clear. Adenosine, prostaglandins, and endorphins have been tested as potential mediators, but results have not been conclusive. It is known, however, that endorphins may play an important modulator role during severe hypoxia in animals or humans, in newborns or adults. Primary apnea, for example, is markedly shortened with naloxone in asphyxiated newborn animals.

Of exquisite importance is the fact that newborn animals rely on carotid body function for O_2 responsiveness and survival more than adults do. This may seem paradoxical to conventional teaching. However, a number of newborn animal species (lambs, rats, piglets) have died within days to weeks of carotid body denervation when performed during a certain time window in early life. This does not happen in the more mature animal.

Other key systems are also maturing in the newborn and may be important to the overall output of the respiratory system. For example, it is well known that the chest wall in the newborn infant is very compliant. During REM sleep, when intercostal muscles are inhibited and chest wall stability is jeopardized, a load is added on the respiratory muscles. Whether this leads to respiratory muscle fatigue or predisposes the infant to it depends on a number of variables including oxygenation, cellular composition of the respiratory muscles, general nutritional status, hemoglobin content, cardiovascular function, electrolyte concentrations, phosphate and acid-base status, and the presence or absence of anesthetics or depressant drugs.

Although the maturation of the central nervous system and its activities have been thought to be at the basis of some responses observed in early life, very few studies have been done to test this hypothesis. Studies have demonstrated that neurons in the medulla oblongata of newborn animals have different electrophysiologic properties than the neurons of adult animals. This finding may have profound implications on the capabilities of neurons for synaptic integration and repetitive firing in early life.

DERANGEMENTS OF RESPIRATORY REGULATION

Periodic Breathing. Periodic breathing is commonly seen in otherwise normal premature infants and rarely seen in full-term infants. It is characterized by a period of apnea lasting from 3 to 10 sec followed by a period of ventilation for 10 to 15 sec. The average respiratory rate is 30 to 40 per min; the rate during the ventilatory interval is 50 to 60 per min. It is rarely seen during the first 24 hours of life and disappears by 38 to 40 weeks postconceptual age. Periodic breathing may appear intermittently, interspersed with long periods of regular breathing. During periodic breathing infants appear more wakeful, with tremors of the tongue and extremities and movements of the eyes. This resembles the REM stage of sleep in the adult, which can also be associated with periodic or Cheyne-Stokes respiration. Also, as in the adult with Cheyne-Stokes respiration, periodic breathing is associated with mild hyperven-

tilation, resulting in slightly alkalotic arterial blood (mean pH 7.44) compared with regular breathing (mean pH 7.39). Average arterial P_{CO_2} is approximately 3 to 4 mm Hg lower during periodic breathing. During the apneic period P_{CO_2} increases by 6 to 7 mm Hg, and the increased cyclic change in Pa_{CO_2} may be responsible for the slight hyperventilation.

The cause of periodic breathing is unknown. Some believe that it is the result of an immature brainstem. It is interesting to note that Cheyne-Stokes breathing, which is a form of periodic breathing, is prevalent in the elderly, who are at the other end of the age spectrum.

Respiratory Pauses and Apneas

The term *apnea* has been variously defined by different investigators and clinicians. Pauses of more than 2 to 3 sec, 6 sec, 10 sec, 15 sec, or 20 sec have all been considered apneas. Because long respiratory pauses are more likely to be associated with life-threatening alterations in cardiovascular, metabolic, and neurologic functions, it may be more appropriate to categorize or define respiratory pauses by the presence or absence of associated changes. In addition, because infants have higher O_2 consumption per unit of body weight and a relatively smaller lung volume and O_2 stores than adults, it is possible that relatively short pauses (up to several sec) that are not clinically important in the adult can induce consequential clinical effects in the newborn infant. Evidence in young animals has shown that hemoglobin saturation starts to decrease within 5 to 10 sec of a pause. By 20 to 30 sec, electroencephalographic changes have started to occur, and by 60 sec after the start of the pause, the electroencephalogram is almost isoelectric. Although the study of the sequence of events during prolonged apneas may not be feasible in infants for ethical reasons, it is important at this stage to investigate the pauses that are considered clinically "safe" and possibly redefine what constitutes a prolonged apnea that needs attention.

Although the pathogenesis of respiratory pauses is controversial, there is a consensus about some observations. For example, normal infants, children, and adult humans exhibit respiratory pauses and apneas, mostly during sleep. Pauses are more frequent during REM sleep, and the average pause is longer in quiet sleep. Paradoxical as it may seem, the presence of respiratory pauses and breathing irregularities is a healthy sign; the complete absence of such pauses may be indicative of respiratory control abnormalities.

Prolonged apneas, in comparison, can be life threatening. Some of these apneas, called apneic spells, are associated with overt clinical symptoms of distress, including cyanosis and marked bradycardia. These spells occur generally in premature infants, suggesting serious underlying disease and requiring treatment. The lack of air movement in the chest and apnea can be related to either an obstructive condition or a failure to generate breathing. Obstruction has been described in infants, and it occurs mostly during sleep. The site of obstruction can vary; most often it is at the level of the posterior pharyngeal wall. In infants and children this obstruction can be due to enlarged tonsils and adenoids, excess fat in the pharyngeal wall, reduced tone in a large genioglossus muscle, or short retracted jaws. Obstruction can also occur in the nose or in the larynx.

Failure to generate breathing, called *central apnea*, is probably due to either failure of the excitatory mechanisms or the drive to terminate a normally occurring respiratory pause, or active inhibition or obstruction of central mechanisms that initiate breathing. Examples of conditions that are associated with central apnea include activation of laryngeal receptors (e.g., during aspiration); hypoventilation syndromes; carotid body immaturity or degeneration (loss of excitatory input); presence of anesthetics or depressant drugs; and, in certain instances, seizures.

Upper Airway Obstruction (UAO). This condition occurs mostly in sleep and is being recognized with increased frequency in children, from infancy to adolescence. In contrast to the pathophysiology of UAO in adults, anatomic abnormalities often prove to be the cause of UAO in children. Such abnormalities include malformations (Crouzon disease), micrognathia (Pierre Robin syndrome), and muscular hypotonia. The usual site of obstruction is the oropharynx, between the pharyngeal wall, the soft palate, and the tongue. In some UAO episodes it is possible, as has been shown in studies of animals, that the basis for obstruction is the difference in Pa_{CO_2} or Pa_{O_2} sensitivity between the diaphragm and upper airway muscles.

Snoring is commonly present with UAO in children. Pauses are usually terminated by a loud snore and arousal. In older children, disturbed sleep habits include restlessness and arousals during the night, enuresis, failure to thrive, developmental delays, and poor school performance. Long-standing UAO can first become evident with right ventricular failure and cor pulmonale. Treatment varies, depending on the underlying cause of obstruction.

Sudden Infant Death Syndrome (SIDS). This syndrome is not uncommon, occurring between the ages of 1 month and 1 year, with a peak incidence at about 3 months of age. The terminal episode is presumed to occur during sleep. Thus investigators have been led to suspect that SIDS results from a conglomeration of events, some related to abnormal or immature control systems and others to environmental factors. The pathophysiology of SIDS seems to involve the cardiorespiratory control system, and abnormalities in the autonomic nervous system and in arousal from sleep have been proposed (see Chapter 70).

Dysautonomia (Riley-Day Syndrome). This rare disease, first recognized in 1949, is characterized by some degree of mental and physical retardation, deficient lacrimation, excessive sweating, transient hypertension, postural hypotension, attacks of cyclic vomiting, absence of the knee jerk reflex and of tongue papillae, and blotchy skin. It occurs predominantly in Jewish children and may or may not be associated with mental deficiency. Recurrent pulmonary infiltrations are thought to be the result of a defective swallowing mechanism with associated aspiration. Studies of the control of breathing in these patients show that they are less responsive than normal subjects to changes in Pa_{CO_2} and oxygen tensions, perhaps because of peripheral chemoreceptor dysfunction. Since they do not have a normal ventilatory drive prompted by changes in arterial P_{CO_2} and P_{O_2}, protection from high altitude and a warning against breath-holding during swimming may be important considerations.

NONRESPIRATORY ASPECTS OF THE LUNG

LUNG WATER AND SOLUTE MOVEMENT

There is a continuous movement of water and solutes (salts, proteins) out of the vascular spaces and into the interstitium of the lung. Under normal conditions the amount of fluid moved is minimal, and it is promptly returned to the vascular space via the pulmonary lymphatics or reabsorbed in downstream venules or within the bronchovascular sheath.

The factors influencing the movement of water across vessel walls were first clearly stated by Starling, and later investigators developed the equation that bears his name. In simple terms, this equation states that water moves in response to the net pressure gradient across the vessel wall, which is determined by the sum of the transvascular hydrostatic pressure and the effective transvascular oncotic pressure gradient.

Although it is generally agreed that water moves across the capillary endothelium both through and between cells, the pathways for solute movement are currently in dispute. The smallest solutes and proteins (albumin) are able to pass through the interendothelial junctions, but the pathway for larger proteins is unknown. The large proteins may pass through large pores (which no one has ever seen) or may be transported passively in endothelial vesicles that move in a diffusive fashion. Despite the lack of knowledge regarding anatomic pathways, physiologic data suggest that protein movement in the lung involves both diffusion and convective flow; *diffusion* is the passive movement of a molecular species down its own concentration gradient, whereas *convective* or *bulk flow* refers to the dragging of molecules along with water flow, much like logs in a river.

When water and protein movement within the lung is increased so that clearance mechanisms are overwhelmed, fluid accumulates within the lung (edema). Several hundred clinical conditions or diseases have been associated with pulmonary edema, but there are really only two mechanisms involved. Edema can occur from an increase in the transvascular pressure gradient, from an increase in vascular permeability (the ease with which water and protein cross the endothelial membrane), or, as commonly happens, from a combination of both. The pathogenic mechanisms, physiologic consequences, and therapy of pulmonary edema are discussed in detail in Chapter 38.

DEFENSE MECHANISMS OF THE LUNG

Each day the average adult inhales more than 9000 L of air. The respiratory tract therefore provides a major source of contact between humans and their environment and must contain an elaborate defense mechanism to protect itself against such damaging agents as bacteria and other particles or noxious gases that may pollute the atmosphere.

The lung defenses against noxious gases are poor and include reflex apnea on exposure to an irritant gas, absorption of a gas such as sulfur dioxide on the moist epithelial surface of the nasal cavity or tracheobronchial tree, and local detoxification.

The respiratory tract is better equipped to deal with inhaled particles. Because of turbulence and inertial impaction, particles larger than 10 μ in diameter are largely filtered out in the nose; those between 2 and 10 μ settle out onto the mucous blanket of the tracheobronchial epithelium. Ninety per cent of the particles larger than 2 to 3 μ settle out on the mucociliary blanket. Smaller particles in the range of 0.5 to 3 μ penetrate to the alveolar ducts and alveoli. Smaller particles show no appreciable deposition and are exhaled. Humidification of incoming air causes hygroscopic particles to increase in size and thus to land at a higher point in the tracheobronchial tree.

Once deposited, particles are subject to several excretory transport mechanisms. The mucous lining layer is propelled by ciliary activity at the rate of 10 to 20 mm/min, so 90 per cent of the material deposited on the tracheal mucosa is physically cleared within an hour. Particles deposited distal to the ciliated columnar epithelium are cleared much more slowly and depend on the rate of phagocytosis by alveolar or interstitial macrophages and the rate of fluid transport from alveoli to the mucociliary blanket. Fluid transport is probably the mechanism for the clearance of about 50 per cent of the deposited material in 24 hours. The second phase of alveolar clearance has a half-life of 100 hours and may reflect interstitial fluid flow mechanisms. The third phase has a half-life of 60 to 100 days and is likely due to movement of particles to perivascular channels where removal is very slow.

Ciliary activity carries particles and macrophages on the mucous lining layer of the respiratory epithelium to larger bronchi, where the cough reflex is important in clearance. Ciliary activity is influenced by numerous agents. Ciliary motion is stimulated by acetylcholine, β agonists, inorganic ions, weak acids, and low concentrations of local anesthetics. It is inhibited by low humidity, alcohol, cigarette smoke, oxygen, and other noxious gases.

In addition to these transport mechanisms, the lung is capable of detoxifying potentially injurious particles such as bacteria. Phagocytosis by alveolar macrophages and tissue histiocytes is the major defensive response to particles smaller than 3 μ and has been shown to be impaired by smoking, air pollutants such as ozone, and high concentrations of oxygen. Immunoglobulins, such as IgA in normal lung and IgM and IgG in inflamed lung, appear to have opsonic activity and thus to enhance phagocytosis. In addition, studies have indicated that IgA on epithelial surfaces, e.g., the respiratory tract, contains specific neutralizing antibodies and is the major determinant of immunity against viral infection. IgA is actively secreted onto respiratory epithelium and requires the addition of a secretory "piece" (S) to two molecules of circulating IgA. Deficient secretory IgA has been described in normal newborn infants and in patients with recurrent sinopulmonary infection or ataxia telangiectasia.

METABOLIC FUNCTIONS OF THE LUNG

The lungs have important nonrespiratory functions, including phagocytosis by alveolar macrophages, filtering of microemboli from blood, biosynthesis of surfactant phospholipids, and excretion of volatile substances. An equally important nonrespiratory function is the pharmacokinetic function of the pulmonary vascular bed: the release, degradation, and activation of vasoactive substances. The lung is ideally situated for regulating the circulating concentrations of vasoactive substances, as it receives the entire cardiac output and possesses an enormous vascular surface area. As Table 1–8 illustrates, the pulmonary vascular bed not only handles a wide variety of compounds (amines, peptides, lipids) but in addition is highly selective in its metabolic activity. For example, norepinephrine is metabolized by the lung, whereas epinephrine, which differs from it only by a methyl group, is unaffected by passage through the pulmonary circulation.

The physiologic consequences of the metabolic functions of the lung can be illustrated by angiotensin-converting enzyme (ACE). A peptidase located on the surface of the endothelial cell, ACE is responsible for the degradation of bradykinin, a potent vasodilator and edematogenic peptide, and for the conversion of angiotensin I to angiotensin II, a potent vasoconstrictor. Angiotensin II production influences

Table 1–8. HANDLING OF BIOLOGICALLY ACTIVE COMPOUNDS BY THE LUNG

Metabolized at the endothelial surface without uptake	Bradykinin Angiotensin I Adenine nucleotides
Metabolized after uptake by the endothelial cell	Serotonin Norepinephrine Prostaglandins E and F
Unaffected by passage through the lung	Epinephrine Dopamine Angiotensin II Vasopressin PGA
Released by the lung	Prostaglandins (e.g., prostacyclin) Histamine SRS-A ECF-A Kallikrein

systemic blood pressure at all ages but is especially important during the neonatal period, because sympathetic innervation is incompletely developed.

Consideration of these and other metabolic functions of the lung have only lately been actively investigated. They are of obvious importance not only in understanding the mechanisms of pulmonary disease but also in the development of specific therapeutic measures. The metabolic and endocrine functions of the lung are dealt with in greater detail in Chapter 2.

REFERENCES

Normal Lung Anatomy and Cell Function

Barnes PF: Neural control of airways in health and diseases. Am Rev Respir Dis 134:1289, 1986.

Derenne JP, Macklem PT, and Roussos C: The respiratory muscles: mechanics, control and pathophysiology. Am Rev Respir Dis 118:(Part I), 119, (Part II), 373, 1978.

Van Hayek H: The Human Lung. Krahl VE (trans). New York, Hafner Publishing Co, 1960.

Weibel ER: Morphometry of the Human Lung. New York, Academic Press, 1963.

Weibel ER: Lung cell biology. In Fishman AP (ed): The Respiratory System: Handbook of Physiology. Sec 3, vol 1. (American Physiologic Society.) Baltimore, Williams & Wilkins Co, 1985.

Growth and Development of the Lung

Burri PH: Development and growth of the human lung. In Fishman AP (ed): The Respiratory System: Handbook of Physiology. Sec 3, vol 1. (American Physiologic Society.) Baltimore, Williams & Wilkins Co, 1985.

Olver RE, Ramsden CA, Strang LB, and Walters DV: The role of amiloride blockable sodium transport in adrenaline induced lung liquid reabsorption in the fetal lamb. J Physiol 376:321, 1986.

Polger G and Weng TR: The functional development of the respiratory system. Am Rev Respir Dis 120:625, 1979.

Post M, O'Brodovich H, Rabinovitch M, et al: Strategies for regulation of growth and development: lessons from the pulmonary alveolar region. Physiol Rev (in press).

Reid LM: The pulmonary circulation: remodelling in growth and disease. Am Rev Respir Dis 119:531, 1979.

Van Golde L, Batenburg JJ, and Robertson P: The pulmonary surfactant system: biochemical aspects and functional significance. Physiol Rev 68:374, 1988.

Ventilation

Bates DV: Respiratory Function in Disease. 3rd ed. Philadelphia, WB Saunders Co, 1989.

Bryan AC and Wohl MD: Respiratory mechanics in children. In Fishman AP (ed): The Respiratory System: Handbook of Physiology. Sec 3, vol 3. (American Physiologic Society.) Baltimore, Williams & Wilkins Co, 1986.

England S: Current techniques for assessing pulmonary function in the newborn and infant: advantages and limitations. Pediatr Pulmonol 4:48, 1988.

Murray JF: The Normal Lung. 2nd ed. Philadelphia, WB Saunders Co, 1986.

Nunn VF: Applied Respiratory Physiology. London, Butterworths, 1977.

Pulmonary terminology and symbols—report of the ACCPATS joint committee on pulmonary nomenclature. Chest 67:5, 1975.

Weibel ER and Bachofen H: How to stabilize the alveoli: surfactant or fibers. News in Physiological Sciences 2:72, 1987.

West JB: Ventilation/Bloodflow and Gas Exchange. Oxford, Blackwell Scientific Publications, 1970.

Pulmonary Circulation

Barer GR: The physiology of the pulmonary circulation and methods of study. Pharmacol Ther 2:247, 1976.

Culver BH and Butler J: Mechanical influences on the pulmonary circulation. Ann Rev Physiol 42:187, 1980.

Hughes JMB: Pulmonary circulation and fluid balance. In Widdicombe JG (ed): Respiratory Physiology. Vol II. (International Review of Physiology Ser, vol 14.) Baltimore, University Park Press, 1977.

Moser KM: Pulmonary Vascular Diseases. (Lung Biology in Health and Disease Ser, vol 14.) New York, Marcel Dekker, Inc, 1979.

Permutt S: Mechanical influences on water accumulation in the lung. In Fishman AP and Renkin E (eds): Pulmonary Edema. (American Physiologic Society.) Baltimore, Williams & Wilkins Co, 1979.

Muscles of Respiration

Grassino A and Macklem PT: Respiratory muscle fatigue and ventilatory failure. Ann Rev Med 35:625, 1984.

Haddad GG and Akabas SR: Adaptation of respiratory muscles to acute and chronic stress: considerations on energy and fuels. Clinics in Chest Medicine 7:70, 1986.

Gas Exchange

Single-breath carbon monoxide diffusing capacity (transfer factor). Recommendations for a standard technique. Am Rev Respir Dis 136:1299, 1987.

Gas Transport to the Systemic Vasculature

Astrup P et al: The acid-base metabolism. A new approach. Lancet 1:1035, 1960.

Davenport H: The ABC of Acid Base Chemistry. 4th ed. Chicago, University of Chicago Press, 1958.

Jones NL: Blood gases and acid-base physiology. New York, Thieme-Stratton, 1980.

Winters RW: Terminology of acid-base disorders. Ann Intern Med 63:873, 1965.

Regulation of Respiration

Berger AJ et al: Regulation of respiration. N Engl J Med 297:92, 1977.

Haddad GG and Mellins RB: The role of airway receptors in the control of respiration in infants: a review. J Pediatr 91:281, 1977.

Phillipson EA: Control of breathing during sleep. Am Rev Respir Dis 118:909, 1978.

Nonrespiratory Aspects of the Lung
Bakhle YS and Vane JR (eds): Metabolic Functions of the Lung. New York, Marcel Dekker, Inc, 1977.
Brain JD, Proctor DV, and Reid LM (eds): Respiratory Defense Mechanisms. New York, Marcel Dekker, Inc, 1978.
Parker JC, Guyton AC, and Taylor AC: Pulmonary transcapillary exchange and pulmonary edema. In Guyton AC and Young DB (eds): Cardiovascular Physiology. Vol III. (International Review of Physiology Ser, vol 18.) Baltimore, University Park Press, 1979.
Staub NC (ed): Lung Water and Solute Exchange. New York, Marcel Dekker, Inc, 1978.

2

SAMI I. SAID, M.D.

METABOLIC AND ENDOCRINE FUNCTIONS OF THE LUNG

In examining the mechanisms and effects of pulmonary diseases (in children or in adults), it is helpful to view the lung not merely as an organ that performs the vital functions of ventilation and gas exchange but also as an organ with multiple metabolic and endocrine activities. These activities play an important role in the maintenance of the normal structure and function of the lung and in the pathogenesis or mediation of many pulmonary disorders.

SOME PULMONARY CELLS IMPORTANT IN METABOLIC FUNCTION AND DYSFUNCTION

The lung is made up of numerous cell types. Some of these are listed here, along with an outline of their metabolic activities and comments on their probable function or role in disease.

Large Alveolar Cell (great alveolar cell, type II alveolar cell, granular pneumonocyte). Having an abundant cytoplasm that is rich in mitochondria, endoplasmic reticulum, and lamellated, electron-dense inclusion bodies (Fig. 2–1), this cell is credited with the biosynthesis and secretion of alveolar surfactant. Immaturity of or massive injury to this cell is associated with large-scale atelectasis, as in the respiratory distress syndrome (hyaline membrane disease). This is also the one alveolar epithelial cell that can proliferate in response to alveolar injury.

Flat Alveolar Cell (small, type I pneumonocyte). By contrast, this cell has a thin shell of cytoplasm with few cytoplasmic organelles (see Fig. 2–1) and no known specific metabolic activity. Flat epithelial cells constitute the major portion of the alveolar surface area and are vulnerable to the toxic effects of high PO_2 and inhaled chemical irritants but are incapable of mitotic division. Regeneration of type I cells takes place by means of division and subsequent transformation of type II cells.

Alveolar Macrophage. The lung's chief defense against invading bacteria and other foreign particles, this cell functions like other phagocytic cells (e.g., the monocyte) but has distinguishing morphologic and metabolic features (Fig. 2–2). The proteolytic and other hydrolytic enzymes normally contained within the lysosomal granules of these cells may, if released, cause profound lung damage and destruction.

Endothelial Cell. Although unimpressive in appearance, this cell (Fig. 2–3) is strategically positioned and functionally equipped to play a key role in the pulmonary metabolism of vasoactive hormones, e.g., the activation of angiotensin I to angiotensin II, the inactivation of bradykinin, and the production of prostacyclin. Injury to the endothelium is the primary lesion in high-permeability pulmonary edema.

Mast Cell. Located in the bronchial mucosa (Fig. 2–4) and the alveolar wall, around small blood vessels, and in the pleura, the mast cell is packed with metachromatic, electron-dense granules that contain biogenic amines, heparin, and various other biologically active substances, including lipids, peptides, and enzymes. The mast cell is the chief target cell for immediate hypersensitivity reactions typical of hay fever and extrinsic asthma.

Smooth Muscle and Other Contractile Elements. The tracheobronchial tree is supplied by smooth muscle fibers, arranged in longitudinal and helical patterns. Spirals of smooth muscle extend to the respiratory bronchioles and to the openings of alveolar ducts. Although there is no smooth muscle in alveoli, alveolar walls contain special "contractile interstitial cells." The smooth muscle fibers contract or relax in response to neurohumoral influences. Their contraction results in the constriction of larger airways and the constriction and shortening of smaller airways. Contraction of alveolar ducts causes expul-

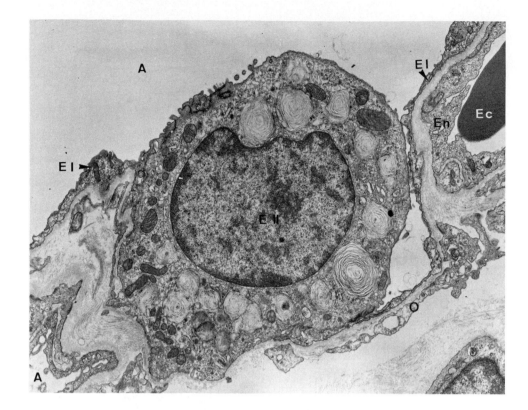

Figure 2–1. Alveolar epithelial type II cell *(E II)* showing numerous lamellar bodies. Shown also are epithelial type I cells *(E I)* and a capillary. *A*, Alveolar space; *Ec*, erythrocyte in capillary; *En*, endothelium. (Human lung, × 13,340.) (Courtesy of Drs. ER Weibel, M Bachofen, and Joan Gil.)

sion of alveolar air and reduction of pulmonary compliance. Airway smooth muscle is innervated by adrenergic and cholinergic fibers, as well as by other nerves that are neither adrenergic nor cholinergic; they are probably peptidergic, i.e., they contain neuropeptides. "Irritability" and hypertrophy of bronchial smooth muscle are characteristic changes that occur in bronchial asthma.

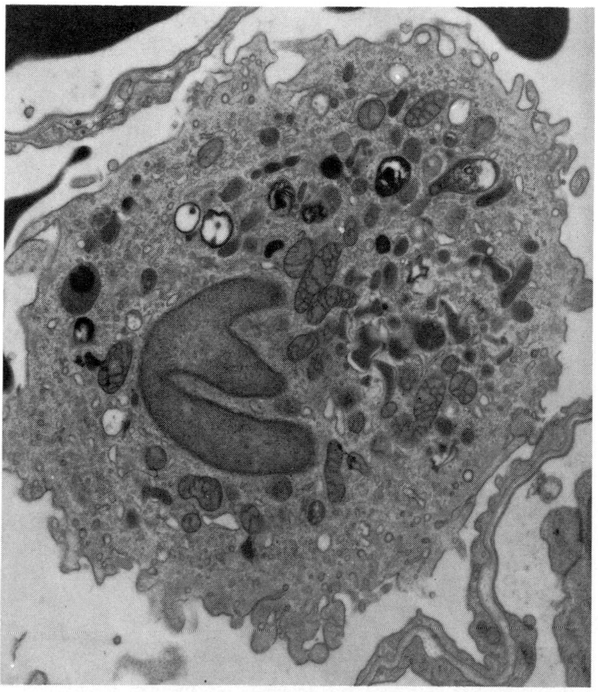

Mucus-Secreting and Other Glandular Cells. Normal bronchial secretion results from contributions from cells secreting mucus and others secreting serous fluid. Abnormalities in bronchial secretion could result from alterations in the proportions or properties of these two constituents. Examples are increased mucus production, as in chronic bronchitis (in which goblet cells are increased in number and size and may extend to terminal bronchioles); decreased water content, as from excessive evaporation through a tracheostomy; and qualitative changes, as in cystic fibrosis.

Ciliary Epithelium. Ciliated epithelial cells (Fig. 2–5), extending distally just short of the alveolar ducts, provide the coordinated, rhythmic force that propels the overlying "mucus blanket" toward the upper respiratory passages and the oropharynx.

Connective Tissue. Comprising ground substance (proteoglycans), elastin, elastic fibers, collagen, and reticulin, connective tissue is present in the airways, lung parenchyma, and blood vessels (see Fig. 2–3). Normal connective tissue provides structural support for the lung and airways. Abnormalities of connective tissue are of central importance in certain lung diseases, especially emphysema and interstitial fibrosis (fibrosing alveolitis).

Neuroendocrine Cells. In addition to the mast cells, which have neuroendocrine properties and characteristics, the lung contains cellular elements that synthesize, store, or secrete neurohumoral products. Among these cells is the *Kulchitsky cell.* Morpho-

Figure 2–2. Alveolar macrophage. (Rat lung, × 3400.) (Courtesy of Dr. Rolland C Reynolds.)

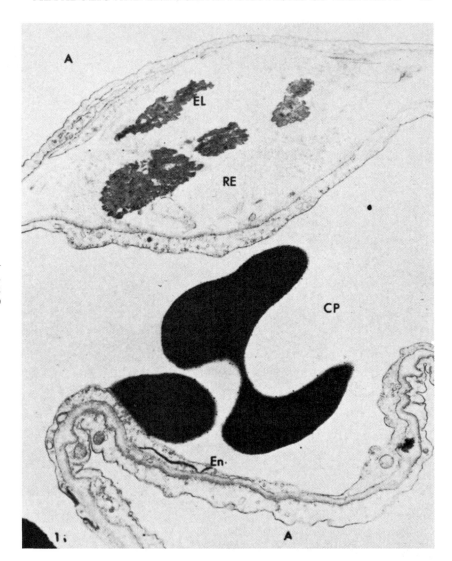

Figure 2–3. Portion of alveolar-capillary septum, showing capillary *(CP)*, endothelium *(En)*, and connective tissue. *EL*, Elastin; *RE*, reticulin; *A*, alveolar space. (Human lung, × 8400.) (Courtesy of Dr. Rolland C Reynolds.)

logically similar to the cell of the same name in the gastrointestinal tract, the pulmonary Kulchitsky cell is believed to give rise to bronchial carcinoid tumors as well as to oat cell carcinoma.

Other neuroendocrine cells have been referred to as *APUD cells*, an acronym derived from certain cytochemical features they have in common: *a*mine content, amine-*p*recursor *u*ptake, and *d*ecarboxylation (Fig. 2–6). The APUD cells occur in many organs that are apparently unrelated, e.g., pituitary, thyroid (C cells), pancreatic islets, adrenal medulla, stomach, and small intestine. In addition to the histochemical features that earned them their name, these cells in all organs contain characteristic electron-dense granules, are able to secrete polypeptide hormones, and probably arise from the neural ectoderm. The APUD cells are demonstrable in fetal, newborn, and mature lungs.

Clusters of cells with a probable neuroendocrine function have been described in bronchial and bronchiolar epithelium. These groups of cells, called *neuroepithelial bodies*, are ultrastructurally similar to the APUD cells and contain argyrophilic, serotonin-rich granules that are depleted in response to hypoxia.

The likely neuroendocrine role of neuroepithelial bodies is further suggested by their rich afferent and efferent innervation.

SOME METABOLIC AND ENDOCRINE FUNCTIONS OF THE LUNG

Biosynthesis and Secretion of Alveolar Surfactant

The alveoli of human and other mammalian lungs are lined with a thin layer of surface-active material that regulates surface tension of the air-liquid interface. Investigation into the composition, biosynthesis, cellular origin, secretion, and metabolism of surfactant was a major stimulus to the study of other aspects of pulmonary metabolism.

The main component of alveolar surfactant is a saturated phospholipid—dipalmitoyl lecithin or dipalmitoylphosphatidylcholine—which is present together with other phospholipids, neutral lipids, and a specific protein. The main mechanism for de novo

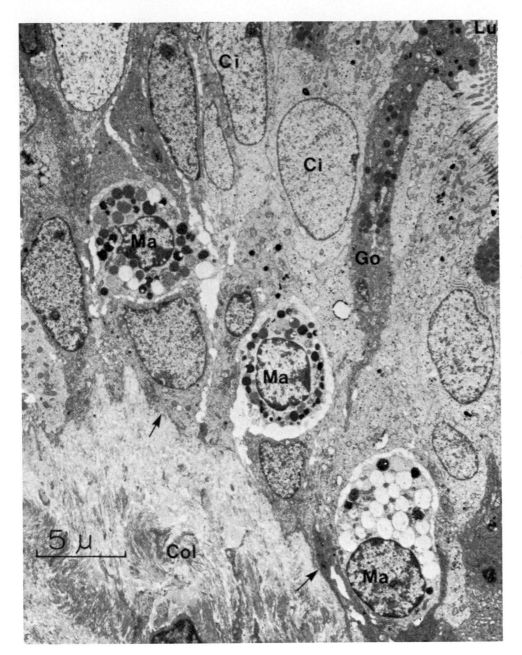

Figure 2–4. Section of lung biopsy specimen from an asthmatic patient showing mast cells *(Ma)* within the bronchial mucosa. The mast cells are wedged between ciliated *(Ci)* and goblet *(Go)* cells and are distributed along the basement membrane *(arrows)*. *Col*, Collagen deposit beneath the basement membrane; *Lu*, lumen (× 6000). (Courtesy of Dr. Ernest Cutz. Reproduced with permission from Lichtenstein LM and Austen KF (eds): Asthma: Physiology, Immunopharmacology and Treatment. Vol 2. New York, Academic Press, 1977.)

synthesis of this phospholipid is the phosphorylation of choline followed by its conversion to cytidine diphosphate choline and the incorporation of the latter compound with a diglyceride molecule to form phosphatidylcholine (lecithin). Another biosynthetic pathway, the formation and subsequent methylation of phosphatidylethanolamine, appears to be of minor importance in the human lung.

Surfactant is synthesized and secreted by the large alveolar cell. The primary function of surfactant is to stabilize the alveoli by preventing excessive increases or unevenness in alveolar surface forces. Reduction of surface tension by surfactant decreases the pressure required to fill the alveoli during inspiration and helps to maintain alveolar patency at a given pressure during expiration. Surfactant is also a factor in guarding against transudation of fluid

into the alveoli. Thus its absence or deficiency predictably leads to large-scale atelectasis and pulmonary edema.

The formation and maintenance of normal surfactant depends on several factors, including the maturity of the great alveolar cells and their biosynthetic enzyme systems, the adequacy of blood flow to the alveolar walls (normally from the pulmonary arterial circulation), a normal rate of turnover, and the absence of inhibitors. Surfactant synthesis is influenced by certain hormones: glucocorticoids and thyroid hormone (or thyrotropin-releasing hormone) in pharmacologic doses can accelerate the maturation of the large alveolar cells and the secretion of surfactant in fetal lungs (see "Metabolic Basis of Pulmonary Disease"). The possible effect of innervation on the functioning of alveolar cells is unknown.

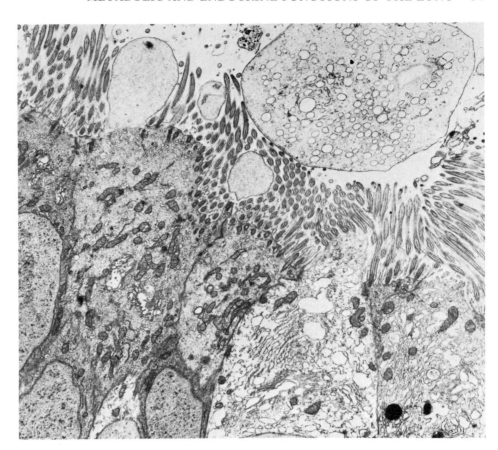

Figure 2–5. Ciliated bronchial epithelium. A goblet cell is seen in section. (Human lung, × 8000.) (Courtesy of Dr. Rolland C Reynolds.)

Numerous clinical and experimental situations are associated with the inadequacy of surfactant. This inadequacy could be due mainly to insufficient formation, e.g., in prematurity; to inactivation, as by certain constituents of serum, e.g., in pulmonary edema; or to both factors, e.g., after pulmonary arterial occlusion or in the respiratory distress syndrome (RDS) of infants or adults. Excessively rapid depletion and incomplete regeneration of surfactant may complicate breathing at the extremes of lung volumes. Surfactant deficiency is the primary and principal defect in neonatal RDS, but its relative importance in the other conditions is difficult to ascertain. Even if it is not the predominant lesion, however, surfactant deficiency, whenever present, is certain to contribute to compromised lung function.

Defense Against Infectious Agents and Other Foreign Particles

This important function depends on the combined effects of the following mechanisms.

Phagocytosis. The ability of alveolar macrophages to defend the lung effectively against infectious agents depends on a complex interaction of biochemical pathways. These pathways provide the energy for oxidative metabolism and "trigger" the macrophages to synthesize and release a host of chemicals, including arachidonate metabolites; reactive oxygen radicals; and proteolytic enzymes, especially elastase and collagenase.

Mucociliary Transport. The mucociliary transport system is designed to remove both healthy and pathologic secretions from the airways, thus facilitating effective gas transport to and from the alveoli. Mucus transport is also responsible for the removal of inhaled particles. The effective transport of secretions depends on the coordination of the beating cilia and their interaction with the overlying viscoelastic layer of mucus. The usual response of this system to low levels of irritants is the stimulation of both ciliary beating and mucus production. When the level of irritants is high, inhaled substances can inhibit the proper functioning of the mucociliary transport system, leading to the retention of secretions. Persistent exposure to irritants such as cigarette smoke or the oxides of sulfur can cause the clearance of secretions to become erratic, which may mark the genesis of acute bronchitis. Exposure of sensitive individuals to specific antigens can cause not only bronchoconstriction but also a prolonged inhibition of mucociliary transport. Infectious organisms, such as *Mycoplasma pneumoniae* and influenza A virus, can damage the mucociliary transport system. When this happens, mucus is cleared from the airways by coughing. Despite the apparent importance of ciliary functioning, its absence, as in patients with Kartagener syndrome, is not incompatible with life.

Immune Mechanisms. Among these are blood-borne immunoglobulins; local (secretory) immunoglobulins, principally IgA; and inflammatory cell secretions that promote or modulate inflammation. Known as cytokines, these secretions include tumor necrosis factor (also known as cachectin), now be-

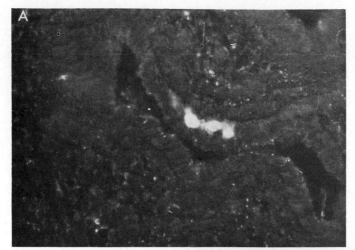

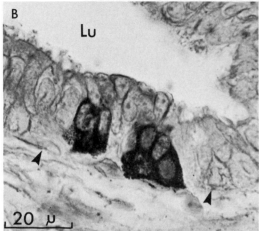

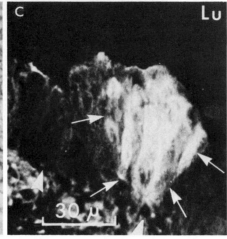

Figure 2–6. *A,* Amine precursor uptake decarboxylation (APUD) cell in lung of human fetus, crown-rump length of 95 mm. Cell was demonstrated by formaldehyde-induced fluorescence, which depends on the presence of catecholamines (× 40). (Courtesy of Dr. Esther Hage.) *B,* Group of argyrophilic cells forming a "neuroepithelial body" within the bronchial mucosa of a human lung. The cells are resting on the basement membrane *(arrows)* and do not extend to the lumen *(Lu).* (Grimelius' silver nitrate stain, × 1000.) *C,* Intensely fluorescent, amine-containing cells *(arrows)* within the bronchial mucosa of a rabbit lung. The apical surfaces of these cells are in contact with the lumen *(Lu).* (L-DOPA incubation, formaldehyde-induced fluorescence, × 640.) (*B* and *C* courtesy of Dr. Ernest Cutz. Reproduced with permission from Lichtenstein LM and Austen KF (eds.): Asthma: Physiology, Immunopharmacology and Treatment. Vol. 2. New York, Academic Press, 1977.)

lieved to be the most important mediator of septic shock, and several other polypeptides called interleukins.

Metabolism, Synthesis, and Release of Vasoactive Hormones

The lung has the only capillary bed through which the entire blood flow passes, making the pulmonary microcirculation uniquely suited to exercise a controlling influence on blood-borne biologically active substances. These compounds have many and diverse actions on all smooth muscle organs, such as the pulmonary and systemic blood vessels, the bronchi and alveolar ducts, the gastrointestinal system, and the uterus. In addition to affecting vascular and nonvascular smooth muscle, biologically active compounds usually also affect other functions throughout the body, including exocrine and endocrine secretion, lipid and carbohydrate metabolism, and tissue cyclic nucleotide levels.

The pulmonary handling of a given active agent can modulate its physiologic or pharmacologic effects. A summary of the metabolic alterations of some vasoactive agents by the lung is given in Table 2–1. The conversion of angiotensin I to angiotensin II (up to 50 times more active than its precursor) is an

example of biologic activation by passage through the pulmonary circulation. The angiotensin-converting activity of the lung is many times greater than that of plasma. Many vasoactive materials are partially or completely inactivated by the lung. Among those that are almost completely removed or inactivated are serotonin (5-hydroxytryptamine); bradykinin; adenosine 5'-triphosphate (ATP); and prostaglandins E_1, E_2, and $F_2\alpha$. Norepinephrine and histamine are taken up to lesser degrees. Vasoactive hormones that pass through the lung without significant loss or gain in activity include epinephrine, prostaglandins A_1 and A_2, prostacyclin (PGI_2), angiotensin II, vasopressin (ADH), and vasoactive intestinal peptide (VIP).

Table 2–1. PULMONARY METABOLISM OF VASOACTIVE HORMONES

Activation
  Angiotensin I to angiotensin II
Inactivation
  Highly effective: Bradykinin, serotonin (5-hydroxytryptamine),
    PGE and $PGF_{2\alpha}$
  Partial: Norepinephrine, (?)histamine
Little or No Change
  Epinephrine, angiotensin II, vasopressin (ADH), PGA, PGI_2, VIP

PGE, prostaglandin E; $PGF_{2\alpha}$, prostaglandin $F_{2\alpha}$; PGA, prostaglandin A; PGI_2, prostacyclin; VIP, vasoactive intestinal peptide.

Pulmonary metabolism of vasoactive hormones is highly selective. One member of a given group of substances—e.g., catecholamines, prostaglandins, or kinins—may be removed during passage, whereas another member of the same group is permitted to go through without change. In the case of compounds such as serotonin, norepinephrine, and PGE_2, loss of activity in passage across the lung is mainly due to uptake and transport, followed by enzymatic inactivation. With other compounds, such as bradykinin, the inactivation is by enzymatic action at the endothelial surface. Economy is another feature of the metabolism of vasoactive substances by the lung. For example, the same enzyme that inactivates the vasodepressor bradykinin can also activate angiotensin I.

The pulmonary endothelial cell, in intimate contact with blood, is the principal site of these metabolic alterations. The pinocytotic vesicles of this cell, many of which communicate directly with the capillary lumen, take up ATP and other adenine nucleotides, bradykinin, and angiotensin I. Endothelial cells also produce one or more substances (endothelium-derived relaxant factors) that mediate the relaxant effect of several vasodilators, including acetylcholine, ATP and bradykinin, and a very potent vasoconstrictor peptide known as endothelin.

Under certain pathologic influences, the lung may discharge into the circulation in large quantities substances it is capable of synthesizing. In anaphylaxis, for example, the lung releases histamine, prostaglandins, thromboxane A_2, leukotrienes, bradykinin, and other pharmacologically active compounds. In other conditions, including pulmonary embolism, mechanical hyperventilation, respiratory alkalosis, alveolar hypoxia, and pulmonary edema, the pulmonary synthesis and release of potent chemicals is stimulated (Table 2–2). These chemicals may contribute to such complications as systemic hypotension, pulmonary hypertension, pulmonary edema, and bronchial and alveolar duct constriction (see "Metabolic Basis of Pulmonary Disease").

METABOLIC BASIS OF PULMONARY DISEASE

Knowledge of altered metabolic function has improved our understanding of the pathogenesis and the pathophysiology of certain pulmonary disorders. In some instances, it has also led to new methods of treatment. A few illustrations follow.

Hyaline Membrane Disease

Hyaline membrane disease (HMD) is currently estimated to affect approximately 1 per cent of newborn babies in the world annually. The incidence is directly related to the degree of prematurity, judged by gestational age or by birth weights below 2500 g,

Table 2–2. NATURE AND ACTIONS OF VASOACTIVE AGENTS

Agent	Action
BIOGENIC AMINES	
Histamine	Bronchoconstriction, alveolar duct constriction, increased permeability
Serotonin (5-HT)	
POLYPEPTIDES	
Bradykinin	Vasodilation, increased permeability
Angiotensin	Vasoconstriction, raised blood pressure, aldosterone release
VIP	Vasodilation, bronchodilation
ANP	Vasodilation
Neurokinins	Bronchoconstriction
PROTEINS (ENZYMES)	
Elastase and Collagenase	Destruction of lung tissue
LIPIDS	
PGD_2, $PGF_{2\alpha}$	Bronchoconstriction
PGE_2	Bronchial relaxation
Thromboxanes	Bronchoconstriction, platelet aggregation
Prostacyclin (PGI_2)	Inhibition of platelet aggregation, vasodilation
Leukotrienes	Bronchoconstriction, pulmonary vasoconstriction, pulmonary edema
PAF	

ANP, atrial natriuretic peptide; VIP, vasoactive intestinal peptide; PAF, platelet-activating factor.

and may reach as high as 80 per cent at the lowest birth weights.

Dramatic advances have been made in the prenatal diagnosis, prevention, and treatment of HMD. Not only the incidence of HMD has decreased, but its mortality has been reduced even more strikingly. Today most infants with a birth weight greater than 1000 g are expected to survive if they are given appropriate care. These advances have resulted directly from (1) the discovery of the association and causal relationship between HMD and a deficiency of pulmonary surfactant; (2) the identification of the main surface-active components; (3) the elucidation of the biosynthetic pathways of surfactant by the mature and developing lung; (4) the demonstration that amniotic fluid lipids can reveal evidence of pulmonary prematurity and thus of increased risk of RDS; (5) the availability of measures to prolong preterm gestation; (6) the ability to accelerate lung maturation by pharmacologic agents; (7) the use of fetal monitoring to recognize and treat fetal distress; (8) the introduction of more effective methods of intensive care and positive-pressure ventilation of preterm babies; and (9) the observation that supplemental therapy with surfactant can restore normal gas exchange and lung mechanics in HMD.

Fetal lung maturity can be predicted from the ratio of lecithin to sphingomyelin (L/S) in amniotic fluid. At a ratio of 2 or higher, HMD is extremely unlikely (less than 1 per cent), whereas a ratio of less than 2 implies an increased risk of HMD. The appropriate therapeutic response to a diagnosis of fetal lung immaturity is to delay delivery, if possible, or to use pharmacologic agents to enhance lung maturation. The approach using pharmacologic agents is based

Table 2–3. SOME POSSIBLE EFFECTS OF ALTERED
PULMONARY METABOLISM OF
VASOACTIVE HORMONES

Pulmonary
Bronchoconstriction, alveolar duct constriction; pulmonary
vasoconstriction; inflammation; increased capillary
permeability; platelet aggregation.
Systemic
Peripheral vasodilation, hypotension and shock; (?)hypertension;
(?)other.

on observations that cortisol receptors are present in fetal lung cells and that glucocorticoids can induce key enzymes of lecithin biosynthesis. Experimental and clinical trials show that intramuscular administration of the glucocorticoid betamethasone more than 24 hours before delivery to expectant mothers with less than 32 completed weeks of gestation reduces the incidence and severity of HMD.

The most important therapeutic advance has been the successful treatment of HMD by intratracheal instillation of natural or synthetic surfactant. Earlier attempts to treat HMD by aerosols of dipalmitoyl-phosphatidylcholine were unsuccessful, but renewed efforts at replacement therapy by intratracheal instillation of liquid suspensions of natural surfactant improved gas exchange, lung stability, and survival of immature animals. The same approach was later tried with favorable results in infants. Synthetic surfactant, which does not contain proteins, appears to be as effective as natural surfactant.

Bronchial Asthma

In bronchial asthma, the basic disease process is an interaction of inhaled, extrinsic antigens with tissue mast cells and basophil leukocytes in the presence of specific antibodies of the IgE class. This union sets off a cascade of metabolic reactions inside the mast cells, culminating in the release of biologically active mediators that bring about episodic bronchoconstriction, increased mucus secretion, and inflammatory cell infiltration.

The identities of these mediators, their interactions, and the factors governing their formation, release, and degradation are major topics of investigation. Much has been learned, some of it directly applicable to the treatment and prevention of this disease, but our knowledge remains incomplete. The best known of these mediators is histamine. It is concentrated within the granules of the mast cells and basophils, may be released from these cells or from lung tissue with appropriate immunologic challenge, and can induce some of the changes characteristic of an asthmatic attack—bronchoconstriction and increased systemic microvascular permeability. But histamine is not the most important mediator, for it is well known that antihistaminics (antagonists of H_1 receptors) are practically useless in the treatment of asthma.

A variety of other chemical mediators are now known to be released in the immediate hypersensitivity state (and other inflammatory states), only some of which have been fully characterized. These mediators include (1) the arachidonic acid metabolites prostaglandins D_2, E_2, and $F_2\alpha$; thromboxane A_2; and leukotrienes B_4, D_4, and E_4, formerly known as the "slow-reacting substance of anaphylaxis"; (2) the potent phospholipid platelet-activating factor; (3) a variety of biologically active peptides, especially neurokinins; and (4) proteolytic enzymes. These and other products contribute to the production of the cardinal features of asthma: airway constriction, airway hyperreactivity, and bronchial inflammation.

The importance of bronchial epithelium in airway hyperreactivity has been recognized. The presence of intact epithelium is required for full bronchial relaxation by many agonists, and bronchial epithelial injury is a common feature in asthma.

Emphysema

Evidence from studies of animals and humans has now validated what was labeled a hypothesis in earlier editions of this book: that an underlying mechanism

Table 2–4. HORMONAL SECRETION BY PULMONARY TUMORS: PARANEOPLASTIC SYNDROMES

Hormone	Syndrome	Lesion
ACTH	Hypokalemic alkalosis, edema, Cushing syndrome	Oat cell carcinoma, adenoma
ADH (arginine vasopressin)	Hyponatremia (SIADH)	Oat cell carcinoma, adenoma; also, tuberculosis, pneumonia, aspergillosis
PTH or related peptide	Hypercalcemia	Squamous cell carcinoma, adenocarcinoma, and large-cell undifferentiated carcinoma
Gonadotropins	Gynecomastia (adults), precocious puberty (children)	Large-cell anaplastic carcinoma
Calcitonin	No clinical findings	Adenocarcinoma, squamous cell and oat cell carcinoma
VIP or related peptide	Watery diarrhea or no symptoms	Squamous cell, oat cell, or large-cell carcinoma
Growth hormone(?)	Hypertrophic osteoarthropathy	Squamous cell carcinoma
Serotonin, kinins (and PGs)	"Carcinoid"	Bronchial adenoma, oat cell carcinoma
Insulin-like peptide	Hypoglycemia	Mesenchymal cell tumors
Glucagon or related peptide	Diabetes	Fibrosarcoma
Prolactin	Galactorrhea (or no symptoms)	Anaplastic cell carcinoma
Combination of above	Multiple syndromes	Anaplastic cell carcinoma

ACTH, adrenocorticotropic hormone; SIADH, syndrome of inappropriate secretion of antidiuretic hormone; PTH, parathyroid hormone; PGs, prostaglandins; VIP, vasoactive intestinal polypeptide.

of emphysema is an excess of proteolytic enzymes with a potential for attacking lung connective tissue relative to protease inhibitors available for counteracting these enzymes. This concept has greatly aided our understanding of this disease and has provided promise for effective therapy.

Severe alpha$_1$-antitrypsin deficiency, an autosomal recessive disorder in which serum alpha$_1$-antitrypsin levels are less than 35 per cent of normal, is associated with panacinar emphysema. This type of emphysema, accounting for 2 per cent of all cases of emphysema in the United States, results from a lack of antineutrophil elastase protection in the lower respiratory tract. The disease is slowly progressive but can be accelerated by cigarette smoking.

Alpha$_1$-antitrypsin, a glycoprotein produced by hepatocytes and mononuclear phagocytes, is the dominant human inhibitor of neutrophil elastase, the most powerful protease in the lower respiratory tract. In alpha$_1$-antitrypsin deficiency, the lack of protection of alveolar walls against the elastase produced by neutrophils in the pulmonary microcirculation results in the continuing destruction of lung parenchyma.

It has now been demonstrated that infusions of human alpha$_1$-antitrypsin over a period of months can replenish the missing protease inhibitor and thus restore the anti-elastase protective shield of the lung. This therapy, together with abstention from cigarette smoking, provides an effective and a rational approach to the management of alpha$_1$-antitrypsin deficiency.

Vascular Disorders

In a number of disorders of the pulmonary circulation, various vasoactive (and otherwise biologically active) substances may be released from the lung. This release, along with possible impairment of normal pulmonary inactivation of these substances, could have important effects on the lung and on the systemic circulation (Table 2–3) and thus could play an important contributory role in the pathogenesis of such vascular disorders as pulmonary thromboembolism, pulmonary microembolism (intravascular platelet aggregation), pulmonary edema, and RDS.

Paraneoplastic Syndromes

Hypersecretion of hormones by tumors may result in a variety of endocrine syndromes. These hormones are usually polypeptides, and the tumors are most often bronchogenic in adults or neurogenic in children. Table 2–4 gives a listing of the more common endocrine syndromes, together with the associated hormonal secretions and anatomic lesions.

Cystic Fibrosis

One of the more common fatal diseases of children, this is an inherited disorder of all exocrine glands. Death usually results from respiratory insufficiency. The basic underlying defect remains unknown, but significant advances have been made on two fronts. First, a metabolic defect has been identified in chloride movement across epithelial surfaces, such as nasal and bronchial mucosae and sweat glands. This chloride block explains the characteristically high chloride levels in the sweat of cystic fibrosis patients and other electrolyte abnormalities. Second, much progress has been made toward localizing the cystic fibrosis gene. Complete delineation of the genetic defect in this disease may clear the way for definitive corrective treatment.

REFERENCES

Avery ME: Pharmacological approaches to acceleration of fetal lung maturation. Br Med Bull 31:13, 1975.
Farrell PM (ed): Lung Development: Biological and Clinical Perspectives, Vol 1 Biochemistry and Physiology; Vol 2 Neonatal Respiratory Distress, New York, Academic Press, 1982.
Hitchcock KR: Lung development and the pulmonary surfactant system: hormonal influences. Anat Rec 98:13, 1980.
Jobe A and Ikegami M: Surfactant for the treatment of respiratory distress syndrome. Am Rev Respir Dis 136:1256, 1987.
Odell WD and Wolfsen AR: Paraendocrine syndromes of cancer. Ann Intern Med 34:325, 1989.
Ryan US (ed): Pulmonary Endothelium in Health and Disease. Monographs on Lung Biology in Health and Disease, Vol 32. New York, Marcel Dekker, Inc, 1987.
Said SI: Metabolic functions of the pulmonary circulation. Circ Res 50:325, 1982.
Said SI: Influence of neuropeptides on airway smooth muscle. Am Rev Respir Dis 136:S5258, 1987.
Watkins WD (ed): Prostaglandins, thromboxane and leukotrienes in pulmonary disease. In Prostaglandins in Clinical Practice, New York, Raven Press, 1989.
Welsh MJ and Fick RB: Cystic fibrosis. J Clin Invest 80:1523, 1987.
Wewers MD, Casolaro MA, Sellers SE et al: Replacement therapy for alpha$_1$-antitrypsin deficiency associated with emphysema. N Engl J Med 316:1055, 1987.

3

HANS PASTERKAMP, M.D., F.R.C.P.(C)

THE HISTORY AND PHYSICAL EXAMINATION

At the end of the twentieth century, the diagnosis of disease is still made after a detailed medical history has been taken and a thorough physical examination has been made. For the majority of patients in many areas of the world, additional information from laboratory tests and other data are of rather limited availability. Modern science and technology have changed the situation considerably in the industrialized nations of the world, but we are paying a high price. Cost containment in health care has become essential, and physicians have to be skillful in their history taking and physical examination techniques to collect a maximum of information before ordering expensive medical-technical investigations.

The diagnosis of disease in children even more than in older patients has to rely on the patient's history and on observations gathered during the physical examination. Young children cannot follow instructions and participate in formal physiologic testing, and physicians hesitate before subjecting their pediatric patients to invasive diagnostic procedures. Diseases of the respiratory tract are among the most common in children, and in the majority of cases they can be correctly identified from medical history data and physical findings alone. The following review of the medical history and physical examination in children with respiratory disease includes some observations that were made with the help of modern technology. These technologic aids do not lessen the value of subjective perceptions but rather emphasize how new methods may further our understanding, sharpen our senses, and thereby advance the art of medical diagnosis.

THE HISTORY

General Principles

The medical history should be taken in an environment with comfortable seating for all, a place for clothing and belongings, and some toys for younger children. Formula should be on hand to help quiet infants and toddlers. Privacy has to be assured, without the usual interruptions by phone calls and other distractions. The physician should see one child at a time because the presence of young siblings or other children in the room tends to be distracting. Most physicians will find it necessary to make some notes while taking the history, but this writing should not interrupt the flow of the interview. Data that should be recorded at the beginning include the patient's name and address, the parents' or guardians' home and work phone numbers, the name of the referring physician, and information on the kindergarten or school if this is relevant. In many cases the history will be given by someone other than the patient, but the physician should still ask even young children directly about their complaints. The patient's own descriptions and those of the parents should be quoted. When asking about the history of the present illness, the physician should encourage a clear and chronologic narrative account. Questions should be open ended, and at intervals the physician should give a verbal summary to confirm and clarify the information. Past medical data and system review are usually obtained by answers to direct questions.

Structure of the Pediatric History

The source of and the reason for referral should be noted. On occasion, the referral may have been made by someone other than the patient or the parents, such as a school teacher, a relative, or a friend. The *chief complaint* and the person most concerned about it should be identified. The *illness at presentation* should be documented in detail regarding its onset and duration, the environment and circumstances under which it developed, its manifestations and their treatments, and its impact on the patient and the family. Symptoms should be defined by their qualitative and quantitative characteristics as well as by their timing, location, aggravating or alleviating factors, and associated manifestations. Relevant past medical and laboratory data should be included in the documentation of the present illness.

This general approach is also applicable when the emphasis is on a single organ system, such as the respiratory tract. The onset of disease may have been gradual, e.g., with some interstitial lung diseases, or sudden, e.g., with foreign body aspiration. The phy-

56

sician should ask about initial manifestations and who noticed them first. The age at first presentation is important because respiratory diseases that manifest soon after birth are more likely to have been inherited or to be related to congenital malformations. Depending on the duration of symptoms, the illness will be classified as acute, subacute, chronic, or recurrent. These definitions are arbitrary, but a disease of less than 3 weeks duration is generally called *acute,* between 3 weeks and 3 months *subacute,* and longer than 3 months *chronic.* If symptoms are clearly discontinuous, with documented intervals of well-being, the disease is *recurrent.* This distinction is important because many parents may perceive their child as being chronically ill, not realizing that young normal children may have six to eight infections of the upper respiratory tract per year.

Respiratory diseases are often affected by *environmental factors.* There should be a careful search for seasonal changes in symptoms to uncover possible allergic causes. Exposure to noxious inhalative agents, for example, from industrial pollution or more commonly from indoor pollution by cigarette smoke, can sustain or aggravate a patient's coughing and wheezing. Similarly, a wood-burning stove used for indoor heating may be a contributing factor. The physician should therefore obtain a detailed description of the patient's home environment. Are there household pets, such as dogs, cats, and hamsters, or birds, such as budgies, pigeons, or parrots? What are the plants in and around the house? Are there animal or vegetable fibers in the bedclothes or in the floor and window coverings (wool, feathers, or eiderdowns)? Are there systems in use for air conditioning and humidification?

There may be a relation between respiratory symptoms and daily activities. Bodily exercise is a common *trigger factor* for cough and wheezing in many patients with hyperreactive airways. A walk outside in cold air may have similar effects. Diurnal variation of symptoms may be apparent, and attention should be paid to changes that occur at night. These changes may also be related to airway cooling, or they may reflect conditions that are worse in the recumbent position, such as postnasal drip or gastroesophageal reflux. Food intake may bring on symptoms of respiratory distress when food is aspirated or when food allergies are present.

A large proportion of children presenting with respiratory symptoms will be suffering from infection, most often viral. It is important to know whether other family members or persons in regular contact with the patient are also affected. When unusual infections are suspected, questions should be asked about recent travel to areas where exotic infective organisms may have been acquired. Drug abuse by parents or by older patients and others with high-risk life styles may lead the physician to consider the possibility of the acquired immune deficiency syndrome (AIDS).

Parents and older children should give their own descriptions of respiratory disease manifestations. Common signs and symptoms are fever, cough and sputum production, wheezing or noisy breathing, dyspnea, cyanosis, finger clubbing, and chest pain. Most of these are discussed in more detail at the end of this chapter.

The *previous medical history* will provide an impression of the general health status of the child. First, the *birth history* should be reviewed, including prenatal, natal, and neonatal events. The physician should inquire about the course of pregnancy, in particular whether the mother and fetus suffered from infections; metabolic disorders; or exposure to noxious agents, such as nicotine. The duration of pregnancy, possible multiple births, and circumstances leading to the onset of labor should be noted. Difficult labor and delivery may cause respiratory problems at birth (e.g., asphyxia and meconium aspiration), and the physician should ask about birth weight and Apgar scores. The neonatal course has to be reviewed carefully because many events during this period may have an impact on the patient's respiratory status in later years. Were there any signs of neonatal respiratory distress, such as tachypnea, retractions, and cyanosis? Treatment with oxygen or endotracheal intubation should be recorded. Some extrathoracic symptoms provide valuable clues for diagnosis, such as the presence of eczema in atopic infants or neonatal conjunctivitis in a young patient with chlamydia pneumonia, particularly if there was a documented infection of the mother.

Much is learned from a detailed *feeding history,* which should include the amount, type, and schedule of food intake. The physician should ask whether the child was fed by breast or bottle. For the newborn and young infant, feeding is a substantial physical exercise and may, in the presence of respiratory disease, lead to distress, much as climbing stairs does in the older patient. The question of exercise tolerance in an infant is therefore asked by inquiring how long it takes the patient to finish a meal. The caloric intake of infants with respiratory disease is often reduced despite an increased caloric consumption, which is necessary to support the work of breathing. This reduced caloric intake commonly results in a failure to thrive. Older patients with chronic respiratory disease and productive cough may suffer from a continuous exposure of their taste buds to mucopurulent secretions and may quite understandably lose their appetites, but medical treatment, e.g., with certain antibiotics, may have similar effects. Patients with food hypersensitivity may react with bronchospasm or even with interstitial lung disease on exposure to the allergen (e.g., to milk). Physical irritation and inflammation occur if food is aspirated into the respiratory tract. This happens frequently in patients with debilitating neurologic diseases and deficient protective reflexes of the upper airways.

The *physical development* of children with chronic respiratory diseases may be retarded. Malnutrition in the presence of increased caloric requirements is common, but the effects of some long-term medical treatments (e.g., with steroids) should also be considered. Previous measurements of body growth should be obtained and plotted on standard nomograms. *Psychosocial development* may be affected if chronic lung diseases, such as asthma or cystic fibrosis, limit attendance and performance at school or if behavioral problems arise in children and adolescents subjected to chronic therapy. More severely affected patients may also be delayed in their sexual development.

Many diseases of the respiratory tract in children have a *genetic component*, either with a clear mendelian mode of inheritance (e.g., autosomal recessive in cystic fibrosis, homozygous deficiency of alpha$_1$-antitrypsin, sex-linked recessive in chronic granulomatous disease, and autosomal dominant in familial interstitial fibrosis) or with a genetic contribution to the cause. Examples of familial aggregation of respiratory disease are chronic bronchitis and bronchiectasis or familial emphysema in patients with heterozygous alpha$_1$-antitrypsin deficiency, in which the susceptibility of the lung to the action of irritants (e.g., cigarette smoke) is increased. A mixed influence of genetic and environmental factors exists in polygenic diseases, such as asthma or allergic rhinitis.

When inquiring about the *family history*, the physician should review at least two generations on either side. The parents should be asked whether they are related by blood, and information should be obtained about any childhood deaths in the family. The health of the patient's siblings and also of brothers and sisters of both parents should be documented. Particular attention should be paid to histories of asthma, allergies and hay fever, chronic bronchitis, emphysema, tuberculosis, cystic fibrosis, and sudden unexpected infant death.

A detailed report of *prior tests and immunizations* should be obtained. Quite often this requires communication with other health care providers. Results of screening examinations (e.g., tuberculin and other skin tests, chest radiographs, and sweat chloride measurements) should be noted. Similarly, childhood illnesses, immunizations, and possible adverse immunization reactions should be documented. If the history is positive for *allergic reactions*, these have to be confirmed and defined. Previous hospital admissions and their indications should be listed, and the physician should document the patient's *current medications* and their efficacy. Many patients and parents have a surprisingly incomplete recollection of the names and nature of prescribed medications. If possible, the drug containers and prescriptions should be reviewed. The physician may use the opportunity to discuss the pharmacologic information and the technique of drug administration, particularly with inhaled bronchodilator medications.

One of the most important goals in taking a history is to become more aware of the particular *psychological and social situation* of the patient. It is impossible to judge current complaints or responses to medical interventions without an individual point of reference for each patient. The physician should encourage the child and the parents to describe a typical day at home, day care, kindergarten, or school. This will provide valuable information about the impact of the illness on daily routines, the financial implications, the existing or absent social support structures, and the coping strategies of the family. Compliance with medical treatment is rarely better than 50 per cent, and physicians are generally unable to predict how well their patients follow and adhere to therapeutic regimens. Compliance can improve if the patient and the parents gain a better understanding of the disease and its treatment. It is important to recognize prior experiences that the family may have had with the health care system and to understand individual religious and health beliefs. Particularly in children with chronic respiratory ailments whose symptoms are not being controlled or prevented, the effort and unpleasantness, e.g., of chest physiotherapy, may limit the use of such interventions. The physician should also consider the social stigma associated with visible therapy, especially among peers of the adolescent patient.

A *review of organ systems* is usually the last part of the history and may actually be completed during the physical examination. Although the emphasis is on the respiratory system, questions about the general status of the child will be about appetite, sleep, level of activity, and prevailing mood. Important findings in the region of head and neck are nasal obstruction and discharge, ear or sinus infection, conjunctival irritation, sore throat, and swallowing difficulty. The respiratory manifestations of coughing, noisy breathing, wheezing, and cyanosis are discussed in detail the end of this chapter. Cardiovascular findings may include palpitations and dysrhythmia in hypoxic patients; there may be edema formation and peripheral swelling with cor pulmonale. Effects of respiratory disease on the gastrointestinal tract may appear with cough-induced vomiting and abdominal pain. There may be a direct involvement with diarrhea, cramps, and fatty stools in patients with cystic fibrosis. The physician should ask about hematuria and about skin manifestations, such as eczema or rashes, and about swellings and pain of lymph nodes or joints. Finally, neurologic symptoms, such as headache, lightheadedness, or paraesthesia may be related to respiratory disease and cough paroxysms or hyperventilation.

THE PHYSICAL EXAMINATION

Traditionally, the physical examination is divided into inspection, palpation, auscultation, and percussion. The sequence of these steps may be varied depending on the circumstances, particularly in the assessment of the respiratory tract in children. The classic components of the physical examination and some modern aids and additions are discussed in the following sections.

INSPECTION

Much can be learned from simple observation, particularly during those precious moments of sleep in the young infant or toddler, who when awake can be a challenge even for the skilled examiner. First, the *pattern of breathing* should be observed. This includes the respiratory rate, rhythm, and effort. The *respiratory rate* decreases with age and shows its greatest variability in newborns and young infants (Fig. 3–1). The rate should be counted over at least 1 min, ideally several times for the calculation of average values. Because respiratory rates differ among sleep states and become even more variable during wakefulness, a note should be made describing the behavioral state of the patient. Observing abdominal movements or listening to breath sounds with the stethoscope placed before the mouth and nose may help in counting respirations in patients with very shallow thoracic excursions.

Longitudinal documentation of the respiratory rate during rest or sleep is important for the follow-up of patients with chronic lung diseases, even more so for those too young for standard pulmonary function tests. Abnormally high breathing frequencies or *tachypnea* can be seen in patients with decreased compliance of the respiratory apparatus and in those with metabolic acidosis. Other causes of tachypnea are fever, anemia, exertion, intoxication (salicylates), and anxiety and psychogenic hyperventilation. The opposite, an abnormally slow respiratory rate or *bradypnea*, can occur in patients with metabolic alkalosis or central nervous system depression. The terms *hyperpnea* and *hypopnea* refer to abnormally deep or shallow respirations. At given respiratory rates, this determination is a subjective clinical judgment and is

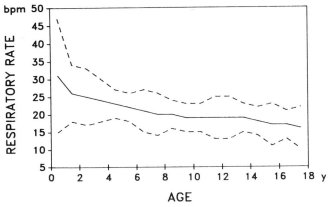

Figure 3–1. Mean values *(solid line)* ± 2 SD *(dashed lines)* of the normal respiratory rate at rest. There is no significant difference between the sexes, and the regression line represents data from both boys and girls. The respiratory rate decreases with age and shows the greatest normal variation during the first 2 years of life. (Data from Iliff A and Lee VA: Child Devel 23:237, 1952.)

not easily quantified unless the pattern is obvious, such as the Kussmaul type of breathing in patients with diabetic ketoacidosis.

Significant changes in the *rhythm* of breathing occur during the first months of life. Respiratory pauses of less than 10 sec are common in infants under 3 months of age. If these pauses occur in groups of three or more that are separated by less than 20 sec of respiration, the pattern is referred to as *periodic breathing.* This pattern is very common in premature infants after the first days of life. In full-term infants, periodic breathing is usually observed between 1 week and 2 months of age and is normally absent by 6 months. Apnea with cessation of air flow lasting more than 15 sec is abnormal at all times and may be accompanied by bradycardia and cyanosis. Other abnormal patterns include Cheyne-Stokes breathing, which occurs as cycles of increasing and decreasing tidal volumes separated by apnea, e.g., in children with congestive heart failure and increased intracranial pressure. Biot breathing consists of irregular cycles of respiration at variable tidal volumes interrupted by apnea and is an ominous finding in patients with severe brain damage.

After noting the rate and rhythm of breathing, the physician should look for signs of increased *respiratory effort.* The older child will be able to communicate the subjective experience of difficult breathing, or *dyspnea.* Objective signs that reflect distressed breathing are chest wall retractions; visible use of accessory muscles and the alae nasi; orthopnea; and paradoxical respiratory movements. The more negative intrapleural pressure during inspiration against a high airway resistance leads to retraction of the pliable portions of the chest wall, including the inter- and subcostal tissues and the supraclavicular and suprasternal fossae. Conversely, bulging of intercostal spaces may be seen when pleural pressure becomes greatly positive during a maximally forced expiration. Retractions are more easily visible in the newborn infant, in whom intercostal tissues are thinner and more compliant than in the older child.

Visible contraction of the sternocleidomastoid muscles and indrawing of supraclavicular fossae during inspiration are among the most reliable clinical signs of airway obstruction. In young infants, these muscular contractions may lead to head bobbing, which is best observed when the child rests with the head supported slightly at the suboccipital area. If no other signs of respiratory distress are present in an infant with head bobbing, however, central nervous system disorders, such as third ventricular cysts, should be considered. Older patients with chronic airway obstruction and extensive use of accessory muscles may appear to have a short neck because of hunched shoulders. Orthopnea exists when the patient is unable to tolerate a recumbent position.

Flaring of the alae nasi is a sensitive sign of respiratory distress and may be present when inspiration is abnormally short, e.g., under conditions of chest pain. Nasal flaring enlarges the anterior nasal passages and reduces upper and total airway resistance. It may also help to stabilize the upper airways by preventing large negative pharyngeal pressures during inspiration.

The normal movement of chest and abdominal walls is directed outward during inspiration. Inward motion of the chest wall during inspiration is called *paradoxical breathing*. This is seen when the thoracic cage loses its stability and becomes distorted by the action of the diaphragm. Classically, paradoxical breathing with a seesaw type of thoracoabdominal motion is seen in patients with paralysis of the intercostal muscles, but it is also commonly seen in premature and newborn infants who have a very compliant rib cage. Inspiratory indrawing of the lateral chest is known as Hoover's sign and can be observed in patients with obstructive airway disease. Paradoxical breathing also occurs during sleep in patients with upper airway obstruction. The development of paradoxical breathing in an awake, nonparalyzed patient beyond the newborn period usually indicates respiratory muscle fatigue and impending respiratory failure.

Following inspection of the breathing pattern, the examiner should pay attention to the *symmetry* of respiratory chest excursions. Unilateral diseases affecting lungs, pleura, chest wall, or diaphragm may all result in asymmetric breathing movements. Trauma to the rib cage may cause fractures and a "flail chest" that shows local paradoxical movement. Pain during respiration usually leads to "splinting" with flexion of the trunk toward and decreased respiratory movements of the affected side. The signs of hemidiaphragmatic paralysis may be subtle and are usually more noticeable in the lateral decubitus position with the paralyzed diaphragm placed up. This position tends to accentuate the paradoxical inward epigastric motion on the affected side.

Other methods to augment inspection of chest wall motion use optical markers. In practice, this technique is done by placing both hands on either side of the patient's lateral rib cage with the thumbs along the costal margins. Divergence of the thumbs during expansion of the thorax aids in the visual perception of the range and symmetry of respiratory movements. A more accurate method of documenting the vectors of movement at different sites (but one that is not yet practical for bedside evaluation) is to place a grid of optical markers on the chest surface and film their positional changes during respiration relative to a steady reference frame. A similar concept is used in optical studies of chest deformities. Projection of raster lines onto the anterior chest surface allows stereographic measurement of deformities, such as pectus excavatum, and augments the visual image of the surface shape (Fig. 3–2). In practice and without such tools, however, the physician should inspect the chest at different angles of illumination to enhance the visual perception of chest wall deformities. Their location, size, symmetry, and change with respiratory or cardiac movements should be noted.

The *dimensions of the chest* should be measured. Chest size and shape are influenced by ethnic and geographic factors that should be taken into account when measurements are compared to normative data. Andean children who live at high altitudes, for example, have larger chest dimensions relative to stature than children in the United States. The chest circumference is usually taken at the mamillary level during midinspiration. In practice, mean readings during inspiration and expiration should be noted (Fig. 3–3). At birth and until 6 months of age, head circumference is larger than chest circumference. Malnutrition can delay the time at which chest circumference begins to exceed head circumference.

To document chest shape, the lateral or transverse diameter and the anteroposterior (A-P) diameter should be measured (Fig. 3–4A–D). The lateral diameter is taken with a caliper at the nipple level during the middle phase of quiet respiration. The A-P diameter is similarly measured at the junction of the fourth rib with the sternum (this is the nipple level except in girls after complete development of the breasts). Patients should be standing during the measurement, and the caliper instrument has to be held parallel to the floor. The ratio of the A-P and lateral chest diameters is the thoracic index. This index shows a wide range of normal (Table 3–1) but can be a useful parameter for serial measurements in children with chronic obstructive lung disease. In these patients, a barrel-shaped chest with increased A-P diameter and a thoracic index close to or even greater than 1.0 can develop as a result of chronic hyperinflation.

Inspection of the patient should then focus on the extrathoracic regions. Many observations on the examination of the head and neck provide valuable clues to the physical diagnosis. Bluish coloration of the lower eyelid ("allergic shiners"); a bilateral fold of skin just below the lower eyelid ("Dennie line"); and a transverse crease from "allergic salutes," running at the junction of the cartilaginous and bony portion of the nose, may all be found in atopic individuals. The nose should always be examined, and bilateral patency should be documented by occluding each side while feeling and listening for airflow through the other nostril. Even without a speculum one can assess the anterior half by raising the nose tip with one thumb and shining a light into the nasal passageways. Color and size of the mucosa should be noted. Nasal polyps are not uncommon in patients with cystic fibrosis. These polyps may also be familial or associated with aspirin intolerance.

The oropharynx should be inspected for its size and signs of malformation, such as cleft palate, and for signs of obstruction by enlarged tonsils. Evidence of chronic ear infections should be documented, and the areas over frontal and maxillary paranasal sinuses should be tested for tenderness. Inspection of the skin is important and may reveal the eczema of atopy. The finding of a scar that typically develops at the site of a successful bacillus Calmette-Guérin (BCG)

Figure 3–2. Optical markers augment the visual perception of chest wall deformities. In this example of rasterstereography, lines are projected onto the anterior thorax, and the surface image is computed as a regular network. The change of the funnel chest deformity before *(A)* and after surgery *(B)* is easily appreciated. In practice and at the bedside, the physician should inspect at different angles of illumination to enhance the visual perception of chest wall deformities. (Reproduced with permission from Hierholzer E and Schier F: Z Kinderchir 41:267–271, 1986.)

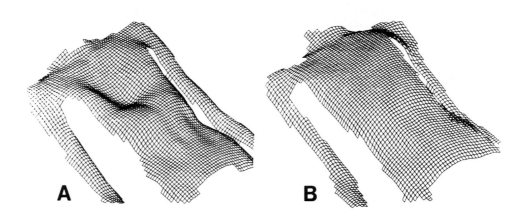

vaccination may be relevant. Common physical findings such as cyanosis, clubbing, and the cardiovascular signs of pulmonary disease are discussed in more detail at the end of this chapter.

PALPATION

Palpation follows chest inspection to confirm observed abnormalities, such as swellings and deformations; to identify areas of tenderness or lymph nodal enlargement; to document the position of the trachea; to assess respiratory excursions; and to detect changes in the transmission of voice sounds through the chest. Chest palpation may offer the first physical contact with the patient, and it is very important for the physician to perform this procedure with warm hands.

Palpation should be done in an orderly sequence. Commonly one begins with an examination of the head and neck. Cervical lymphadenopathy and ten-

derness over paranasal sinuses should be noted. Palpation of the oropharynx may be indicated to find malformations such as submucosal clefts or to identify causes of upper airway obstruction. The position of the trachea must be documented in every patient. This is a very important part of the physical chest examination because tracheal deviation most often indicates significant intra- or extrathoracic abnormalities.

In the older child, the tracheal position is assessed by placing the index and the ring fingers on both sternal attachments of the sternocleidomastoid muscles. The trachea is then felt between these landmarks with the middle finger on the suprasternal notch. In small children, palpation is done with one index finger sliding gently inward over the suprasternal notch. Looking for asymmetry, the physician should always make sure that the patient is in a straight position, and deformities, such as scoliosis, should be taken into account.

A very slight deviation of the trachea toward the

Figure 3–3. Normal distribution of chest circumference from birth to 14 years. Tape measurements are made at the mamillary level during midinspiration. Before plotting the values on the graph, one should add 1 cm for males and subtract 1 cm for females between 2 and 12 years of age. (Reproduced with permission from Feingold M and Bossert WH: Birth Defects 10(13): 14, 1974.)

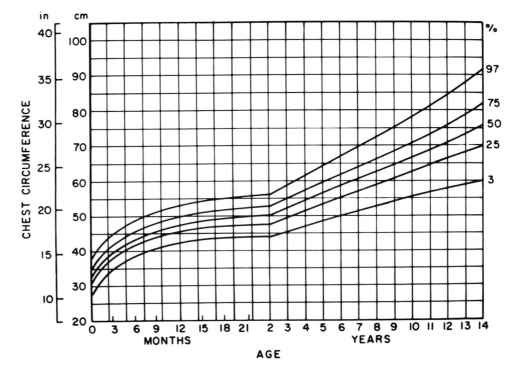

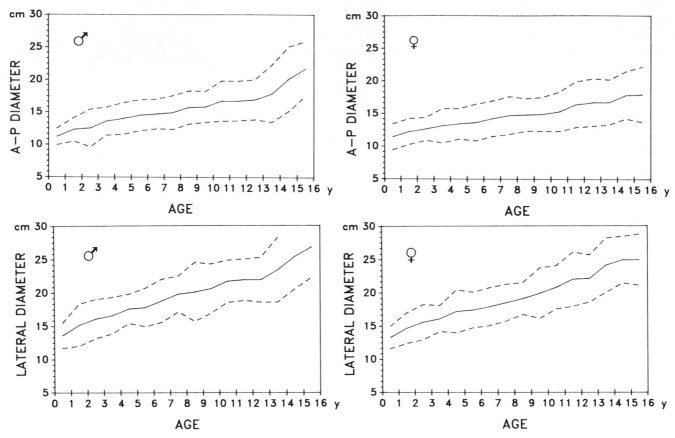

Figure 3–4. Mean values *(solid line)* ± 2 SD *(dashed lines)* of the normal distribution of anteroposterior *(A-P)* and lateral chest diameters in boys and girls. Caliper measurements are made at the mamillary level during midinspiration. (Data from Lucas WP and Pryor HB: J Pediatr 6:533–545, 1935.)

right is normal. Marked deviations may indicate a pulling force toward the side of displacement (e.g., atelectasis) or a pushing force on the contralateral side (e.g., pneumothorax). The physician should note whether the displacement is fixed or whether there is a pendular movement of the trachea during inspi-

ration and expiration that may suggest obstruction of a large bronchus. Posterior displacement of the trachea may occur with anterior mediastinal tumors or barrel chest deformities, whereas an easily palpable anteriorly displaced trachea is sometimes seen with mediastinitis. In patients with airway obstruction

Table 3–1. THORACIC INDEX (TI) (RATIO OF A-P AND LATERAL CHEST WALL DIAMETERS) FOR GIRLS AND BOYS

	Girls				Boys			
	Number of		Range			Number of		Range	
Age (yr)	Subjects	TI	Min	Max	Age (yr)	Subjects	TI	Min	Max
<1	106	0.841	0.637	1.040	<1	109	0.805	0.632	0.936
1	163	0.831	0.688	0.929	1	170	0.814	0.639	0.933
2	150	0.812	0.735	1.000	2	154	0.804	0.700	0.900
3	148	0.812	0.765	0.914	3	162	0.807	0.609	0.906
4	163	0.781	0.684	0.900	4	153	0.796	0.666	0.882
5	164	0.783	0.686	0.880	5	161	0.800	0.633	0.933
6	170	0.783	0.664	0.909	6	175	0.786	0.695	0.895
7	162	0.765	0.675	0.914	7	163	0.785	0.684	0.882
8	173	0.776	0.650	0.944	8	166	0.781	0.700	0.895
9	158	0.754	0.650	0.900	9	157	0.756	0.650	0.944
10	232	0.748	0.619	0.842	10	218	0.775	0.640	0.857
11	194	0.738	0.537	0.738	11	193	0.784	0.660	0.944
12	258	0.743	0.604	0.950	12	260	0.753	0.652	0.905
13	265	0.694	0.638	0.773	13	264	0.766	0.500	0.909
14	183	0.794	0.771	0.861	14	106	0.793	0.714	0.845
15	151	0.730	0.600	0.863	15	119	0.732	0.600	0.808

Data from Lucas WP and Pryor HB: J Pediatr 6:533, 1935.

and respiratory distress, retractions of the suprasternal fossa may be seen, and a "tracheal tug" may be felt by the examiner.

Placing the hands on both sides of the lateral rib cage, the physician should feel for symmetry of chest expansion during regular and deep breathing maneuvers. Slight compression of the chest in the transverse and anteroposterior directions may help to localize pain from lesions of the bony structures. Voice-generated vibrations are best felt with the palms of both hands just below the base of the fingers placed over corresponding sites on the right and left hemithorax. Asymmetric transmission usually indicates unilateral intrathoracic abnormalities. The patient is asked to produce low-frequency vibrations of sufficient amplitude by saying "ninety-nine" in a loud voice. In young infants, crying may produce the vibrations that are felt as tactile fremitus over the chest wall. This fremitus is decreased if an accumulation of air or fluid in the pleural space reduces transmission. Small consolidations of the underlying lung will not diminish the tactile fremitus as long as the airways remain open, whereas collapse of the airways and atelectasis will reduce the transmission of vibratory energy if larger portions of the lung are affected.

AUSCULTATION

Auscultation is arguably the most important part of the physical chest examination. The subjective perception of respiratory acoustic signs is influenced by the site and mode of sound production; by the modification of sound on its passage through lung, chest wall, and stethoscope; and finally by the auditory system of the examiner. Knowledge about these factors is necessary to appreciate fully the wealth of information that is contained in the acoustic signs of the thorax.

Thoracic Acoustics

Observations on sound generation in airway models and electronic analyses of respiratory sounds suggest a predominant origin from complex turbulences within the central airways. During inspiration, a jet mechanism of sound production just below the larynx appears to contribute a large component of clinically observed breath sounds. During expiration, a smaller component of sound may originate from the convergence of airstreams at airway bifurcations. It is possible that there are nonturbulent mechanisms of sound generation within small bronchi, but their contribution to the sounds heard over the chest remains to be defined. Whether flow becomes turbulent depends on the airway diameter and on the linear velocity, density, and viscosity of the gas. Therefore, breathing air at different flows through central airways of unchanged dimensions will produce sounds that are a function of airflow. When gas density is reduced to 35 per cent of that of air by breathing a mixture of 80 per cent helium and 20 per cent oxygen, tracheal sound intensity is reduced significantly, but lung sounds at the same time remain relatively unchanged. This supports the concept that inspiratory lung sounds are not simply a consequence of the turbulence in central airways. The propagation of sound depends on the tissue density, which in turn depends on lung volume. At total lung capacity, sound travels through the lung with a speed of 60 m/sec, whereas sound propagation slows to one tenth of that in air, or 25 m/sec, through atelectatic areas.

Adventitious respiratory sounds usually indicate respiratory disease. *Wheezes* are musical, continuous (more than 200 msec duration) sounds that originate from oscillations in narrowed airways. The frequency of the oscillation depends on the mass and elasticity of the airway wall as well as on local airflow. Widespread narrowing of airways in asthma leads to various pitches or "polyphonic" wheezing, whereas a fixed obstruction in a larger airway produces a single wheeze or "monophonic" wheezing. Expiratory wheezing is directly related to flow limitation and can be produced by normal subjects during forced expiratory maneuvers. The situation is less clear for wheezing during inspiration, which is common in asthma but cannot be produced by healthy subjects unless it originates from the larynx.

Crackles are nonmusical, discontinuous (less than 20 msec duration) lung sounds. Crackle production requires the presence of air-fluid interfaces and occurs either by air movement through secretions or by sudden equalization of gas pressure. Another mechanism may be the release of tissue tension during sudden opening or closing of airways. Crackles are perceived as fine or coarse, depending on the duration and frequency of the brief and dampened vibrations created by these mechanisms. There may be a musical quality to the sound if a short oscillation occurs at the generation site. This has been called *tinkling crackle* or *squawk* and is sometimes heard during late inspiration in patients with interstitial lung diseases. Fine crackles during late inspiration are common in restrictive lung diseases and in the early stages of congestive heart failure, whereas coarse crackles during early inspiration and during expiration are frequently heard in chronic obstructive lung disease. Fine crackles are usually inaudible at the mouth, whereas the coarse crackles of widespread airway obstruction can be transmitted through the large airways and may be heard as clicks through the stethoscope. Some crackles over the anterior chest may occur in normal subjects who were breathing at low lung volumes, but they will disappear after a few deep breaths.

Several other abnormal respiratory sounds are not generated in intrathoracic airways. *Pleural rubs* originate from mechanical stretching of the pleura, which causes vibration of the chest wall and local pulmonary parenchyma. These sounds can occur during both inspiration and expiration. Their character is like that of creaking leather and is similar in some ways to pulmonary crackles. *Stridor* refers to a musical sound of single pitch that is produced by oscillations of critically narrowed extrathoracic airways. It is therefore most commonly heard during inspiration. *Grunting* is an expiratory sound, usually low pitched and with musical qualities. It is produced in the larynx when vocal cord adduction is used to generate positive end-expiratory pressures, such as in premature infants with immature lungs and surfactant deficiency. *Snoring* originates from the flutter of tissues in the oropharynx and has less musical qualities. It may be present during both inspiration and expiration.

There may also be *cardiorespiratory sounds.* These are believed to occur when cardiac movements cause regional flows of air in the surrounding lung. Because of its synchronicity with the heart beat, this sound may be mistaken for a cardiac murmur. It can be identified by its vesicular sound quality and its exaggeration during inspiration and in different body positions.

Sounds recorded from the inside of airways are quite different from those heard over the chest. The loss of sound energy on its passage through the lung tissue and chest wall depends on the path length and the characteristics of the tissues. In particular, if sound absorption in the tissue is frequency dependent, the transmission path will color the sound. During sound passage through the lung, for example, higher frequencies are absorbed, whereas sounds transmitted from the trachea to the neck do not exhibit such low-pass filtering. Respirosonography demonstrates that tracheal sounds recorded over the neck have higher frequency components and a louder expiration than vesicular lung sounds recorded over the posterior chest (Figs. 3–5 and 3–6). Lung sounds in newborn infants travel a shorter distance and may meet less attenuation at the chest wall. They contain higher frequencies and have a more noticeable expiration (Fig. 3–7). These respiratory sounds share characteristics of tracheal/bronchial and vesicular lung sounds and are therefore called *bronchovesicular.*

At the boundary between different tissues, *reflection* of sound may occur and sound transmission may decrease, depending on the matching or mismatching of the tissue impedances. Many of the acoustic signs of the chest are explained on the basis of impedance matching alone. The stethoscope is basically an impedance transformer that reduces sound reflection at a mismatched interface, namely, body surface to air. Because it is the only part of the sound transmission pathway that can be kept constant, the physician should always use the same stethoscope. The choice of a bell- or a diaphragm-type stethoscope depends on individual preference. Diaphragm chest pieces can be placed more easily and with less pressure on small chests with narrow intercostal spaces. Compared with bell-type stethoscopes, however, they tend to emphasize higher frequencies and may not

as easily transmit the components below 100 Hz. Such low frequencies are quite prominent in normal respiratory sounds but may not be appreciated by the listener because the human auditory threshold increases steeply at low frequencies.

Technique of Auscultation

Ideally, auscultation of the chest should be performed in a quiet room; however, with pediatric patients the usual setting may be anything but quiet. Fortunately, the human auditory system allows selective evaluation of acoustic signals even when they are masked by much louder surrounding noises. This psychoacoustic phenomenon, known as the "cocktail party effect," at present cannot be reproduced by modern electronic techniques, which is but one of the reasons for the lasting popularity of the stethoscope.

This instrument, the most widely used in clinical medicine since its introduction 170 years ago, carries symbolic value for the health care profession, much like a modern staff of Aesculapius. Every child knows that doctors have stethoscopes. The physician should use this to advantage when assessing pediatric patients by encouraging children to listen themselves to their heartbeats and breathing sounds. Even infants may be fascinated as long as the stethoscope is shiny. Ice cold chest pieces, however, scare off most patients. Therefore, before placing it on the chest, the physician should check with the child as to whether the chest piece is "too cold" by putting it on the patient's hand or arm and, if necessary, "rub it warm" before proceeding with the chest examination.

The patient should be in a straight position during auscultation because incurvature of the trunk may lead to artificial side differences of sound production and transmission. In newborns and young infants, a straight position may be best achieved when they are supine. Infants and toddlers will often be assessed while their parents hold them on their laps. Beginning auscultation on the back of these young patients will provoke less anxiety than a frontal approach. Older children can be examined in the sitting or standing position. The number of sites over the chest that are assessed during auscultation will be determined by the clinical situation. Ideally, all segments of the lung should be listened to, but this may not be possible, particularly in very young children. Because the intensity of respiratory sounds is related to airflow, sufficiently deep respirations (with flow > 0.5 L/sec) are needed for a good sound signal. An older patient will cooperate and breathe deeply through an open mouth. Younger children may be motivated if one asks them to "pant like a puppy dog." With infants, however, one may have to rely on sounds made during sighs or deep inspirations in between crying.

The physician should make note of the lung sound intensity over different areas of the chest in a qualitative way, keeping in mind that this intensity reflects

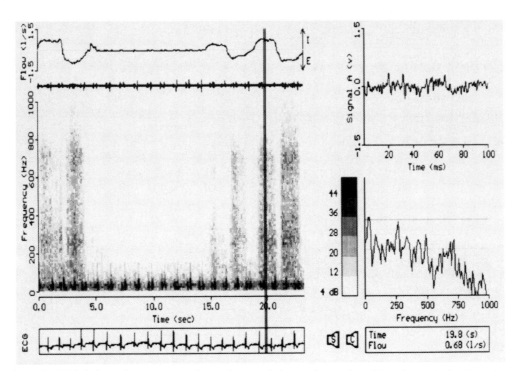

Figure 3–5. Digital respirosonogram of sounds recorded over the trachea. Time is on the horizontal axis, frequency is on the vertical axis, and sound intensity is shown on a scale from black (loud) to white (low). Airflow is plotted at the top. The sonogram illustrates the normal range of tracheal sounds, from less than 100 Hz to approximately 1000 Hz during both inspiration and expiration. There is a distinct pause between the respiratory phases. In this example, the subject was holding his breath for several seconds. During this respiratory pause, heart sounds below 200 Hz are easily identified by their temporal relation to the simultaneously recorded electrocardiogram (ECG). Inspiratory sounds during a 100 ms interval (enclosed by the vertical double bar at 19.8 sec) are shown in detail at the top right (expanded time-amplitude plot) and at the bottom right (power spectrum, calculated by fast Fourier transformation).

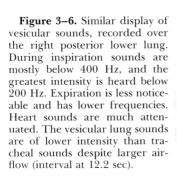

Figure 3–6. Similar display of vesicular sounds, recorded over the right posterior lower lung. During inspiration sounds are mostly below 400 Hz, and the greatest intensity is heard below 200 Hz. Expiration is less noticeable and has lower frequencies. Heart sounds are much attenuated. The vesicular lung sounds are of lower intensity than tracheal sounds despite larger airflow (interval at 12.2 sec).

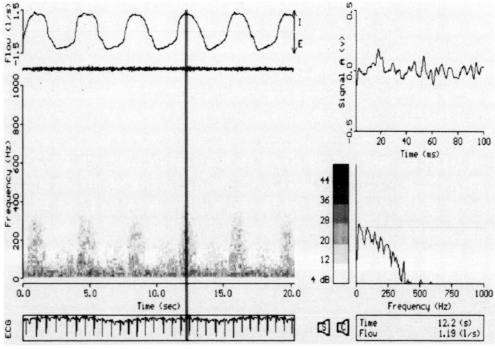

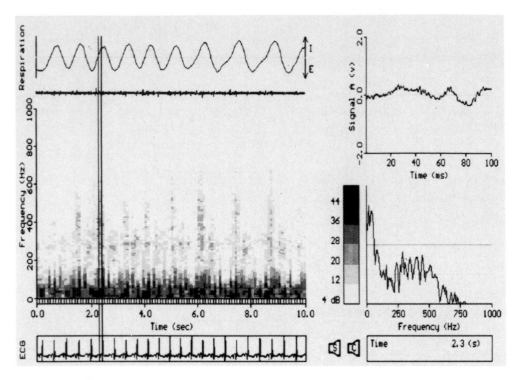

Figure 3–7. Bronchovesicular lung sounds over the right anterior upper lobe in a healthy preterm infant. Respiration was sensed by nasal thermistor and is shown at the top with an upward slope during inspiration. Inspiratory sounds have a frequency range somewhere between vesicular and bronchial/tracheal sounds, and expiration is more noticeable than that in vesicular sounds. Most of the sound intensity is heard below 500 Hz (interval at 2.3 sec).

both local sound generation and sound transmission characteristics of the thorax. It is therefore not correct to speak of local "air entry" when one actually refers to local breath sound intensity. Obviously, a qualitative distinction between absence or presence of local breath sounds will be easier than attempts at quantification. Also, when the stethoscope is placed over any given location, it is not known how large an area of the underlying lung is actually being assessed. In adult subjects, moving the chest piece of the stethoscope by 10 cm will position it to receive sound from entirely different lung units, but similar data for children are not available.

Assessment of regional ventilation by thoracic acoustic signs becomes more meaningful when two sites are compared simultaneously. This can be done by differential auscultation, using a stethoscope modification that can be easily produced (Fig. 3–8). A variant of this setup, using two chest pieces that are taped on either side of the chest and connected by flexible tubing to a three-way stopcock, has been described for auscultation in the neonatal nursery. Comparative auscultation is absolutely essential for airway management in the emergency room and intensive care unit for assessment of endotracheal tube position or for identification of the side of a pneumothorax. Listening simultaneously to two homologous sites over both lungs may also help to detect local abnormalities. Atelectatic areas will transmit sound more slowly than inflated lung tissue, but the resulting phase shift is too small to be detectable on subjective auscultation. With local airway narrowing, however, the maximum sound intensity over the affected side may become sufficiently delayed to be perceived as "phase heterophony." In some cases,

breath sounds may still be audible over the affected side after inspiratory efforts have ceased. This "posteffort" breath sound is a sign of incomplete airway obstruction.

There are special circumstances in which only the presence or absence of breath sounds is of interest, e.g., during transportation of critically ill patients in noisy vehicles and during resuscitation in the emergency department. Under these conditions, and when a firm attachment of the chest piece is important, a

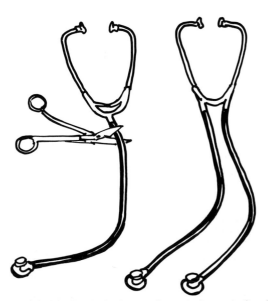

Figure 3–8. Simple method to make a stethoscope for differential auscultation. Care should be taken to use two identical stethoscopes and to cut the tubing for both sides at equal lengths. (See Ackerman NB, Bell RE, and deLemos RA: Clin Pediatr 21:566–567, 1982.)

self-adhering stethoscope, based on negative suction pressure within the bell of the chest piece, may be applied. Because of the resulting changes to tissue impedance and chest wall coupling, however, such stethoscopes will influence in an unpredictable way the frequency characteristics of transmitted lung sounds.

Respiratory sounds should be documented according to their location and character. Normal projections of lobar borders to the surface of the chest are shown in Figure 3–9. These may be distorted by local pulmonary disease, and mapping of respiratory sounds should therefore be done with reference to external anatomic landmarks (Fig. 3–10). The examiner should be familiar with the segmental structure of the underlying lung.

Respiratory sound characteristics include the intensity (amplitude), pitch (predominant frequency), and timing during the respiratory cycle. Also, sounds will have a particular timbre caused by the presence of resonances and overtones. Unfortunately, the terminology in use for the description of respiratory sounds is still confusing and imprecise. During a symposium on lung sounds in Tokyo in 1985, an attempt was made to achieve a global and uniform nomenclature for breath sounds. The resulting recommendations for classification of adventitious lung sounds are summarized in Figure 3–11.

A basic grouping into musical, continuous sounds of long duration and nonmusical, discontinuous sounds of short duration is made, with the former being referred to as *wheezes* and the latter as *crackles*.

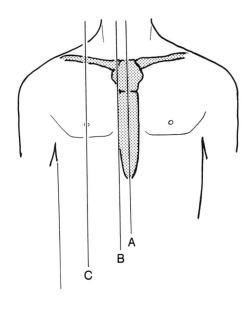

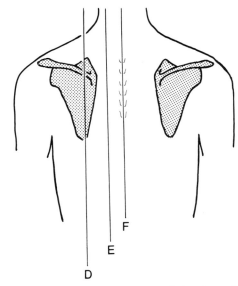

Figure 3–10. Vertical reference lines of the chest. The center line is indicated anteriorly by the suprasternal notch *(A)* and posteriorly by the spinous processes *(F)*. The sternal *(B)* and midclavicular *(C)* lines over the front and the scapular *(D)* and paravertebral *(E)* lines over the back provide longitudinal landmarks of the thorax. From a lateral view, the midaxillary line is used for orientation. Horizontal reference points are the supra- and infraclavicular fossae, Ludwig's angle (junction of the second rib at the sternum), the mammillae (normally at the fourth rib), and the epigastric angle. Posteriorly, the prominent spinous process of the seventh cervical vertebra and the supra- and infraspinous fossae of the scapulae provide markers for orientation.

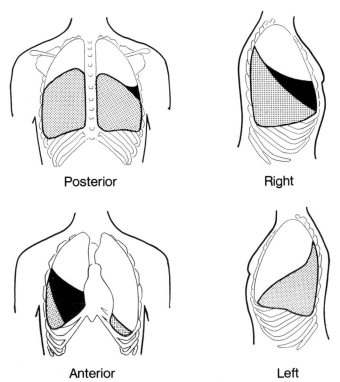

Figure 3–9. Projections of the pulmonary lobes on the chest surface. The upper lobes are white, the right-middle lobe is black, and the lower lobes are dotted.

Furthermore, musical adventitious sounds or wheezes may be classified as high or low pitched. Some use the term *rhonchus* for low-pitched wheezes (<200 Hz), whereas others describe the poorly characterized "secretion sounds," which share musical and nonmusical qualities, as rhonchi. Crackles are subclassified as fine or coarse. Regular breath sounds include tracheal/bronchial, bronchovesicular, and vesicular/normal sounds. Finally, other respiratory sounds should be specified, e.g., pleural rubs, expi-

LUNG SOUND NOMENCLATURE

	English	French	German	Japanese	Portuguese	Spanish
Discontinuous						
Fine (high pitched, low amplitude, short duration)	Fine crackles	Râles crepitants	Feines Rasseln	捻髪音	Estertores finos	Estertores finos
Coarse (low pitched, high amplitude, long duration	Coarse crackles	Râles bulleux ou Sous-crepitants	Grobes Rasseln	水泡音	Estertores grossos	Estertores gruesos
Continuous						
High pitched	Wheezes	Râles sibilants	Pfeifen	ふえ(捩)音	Sibilos	Sibilancias
Low pitched	Rhonchus	Râles ronflants	Brummen	いびき(捩)音	Roncos	Roncus

Figure 3–11. Recommendation from the 1985 International Symposium on Lung Sounds in Tokyo for a unified nomenclature of adventitious sounds. (Reproduced with permission from Cugell DW: Lung sound nomenclature. Am Rev Respir Dis 136:1016, 1987.)

ratory grunting, and inspiratory stridor. Historical terms such as *rales* and *crepitations* should be abandoned, and flowery descriptions such as "raspy" or "blowing" breath sounds should not be used because these adjectives are even less well defined than the suggested terms.

Several auscultatory signs are based on the transmission of voice sounds. Speech sounds have a fundamental note of about 130 Hz in men and 230 Hz in women, with overtones from 400 to 3500 Hz. Vowels are produced when particular pairs of overtones or formants are generated. On passage through the lung, the higher frequency formants are filtered, and speech heard over the chest becomes a meaningless mumble. With consolidation and transmission of higher frequency components, however, speech may become intelligible. This occurs with normal speech (*bronchophony*) and with whispered voice (*pectoriloquy*). There may be a change in vowels from *e* to *a* over areas of lung consolidation. The acoustic basis for these phenomena is the same as for bronchial breath sounds. The American Thoracic Society and the American College of Chest Physicians recommend the term *egophony* for all of these findings.

PERCUSSION

Percussion is used to set tissues into vibration with an impulsive force so that their mechanical and acoustic response can be studied. If the vibrations are undamped and continue for a significant amount of time, the perceived sound will be resonant or "tympanic," whereas rapid attenuation of the vibrations will lead to a flat or "dull" percussion note. The former occurs when there is a large acoustic mismatch, e.g., tissue overlying an air-filled cavity, whereas the latter occurs when the underlying tissue is similar to the surface tissue and vibratory energy propagates away quickly. Structures that absorb energy when struck by a sound at their natural frequency continue vibrating after the initial sound is gone and are called resonant. The fundamental resonance of the thorax depends on body size and is about 125 Hz for adult males, between 150 and 175 Hz for adult females, and between 300 and 400 Hz for small children.

Chest percussion in children is performed by light tapping with the index or middle finger (the plexor) on the terminal phalanx of the other hand's middle finger (the pleximeter). The pleximeter should be placed firmly but not hard, and care should be taken that other fingers do not touch the chest wall, which may cause artificial damping of the percussion note. Percussion should be gentle, with quick perpendicular movements of the plexor originating from the wrist (Fig. 3–12). The physician should explain the procedure, particularly to the younger patient who otherwise might feel threatened. The patient should be relaxed during the examination because tension of the chest wall muscles may alter the percussion note. More important, chest deformities and scoliosis in particular will have a significant effect on percussory findings.

Symmetric sites over the anterior, lateral, and posterior surface of the chest should be compared in an orderly fashion. As with chest auscultation, findings should be reported with reference to standard external landmarks (see Fig. 3–10). The ribs and vertebral spinous processes are used for horizontal mapping. The level at which the tympanic lung resonance changes to a dull percussion note should be defined

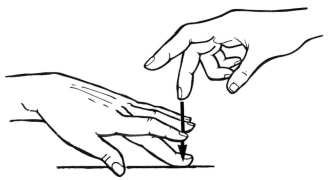

Figure 3–12. Percussion in children should be done with gentle perpendicular movements from the wrist and tapping of the plexor finger *(right)* on the terminal phalanx of the pleximeter finger *(left)*. The contact area of the pleximeter on the chest should be small, and other fingers should not touch the surface to avoid damping of the percussory vibrations.

over the posterior chest during maximal inspiration and expiration to delineate the lung borders and their respiratory excursions.

Subjective assessment of percussion note differences includes both acoustic and tactile perception. Tympanic, lower-pitched percussion notes mean less-damped vibrations of longer duration, which are felt by the pleximeter finger. Dull sounds with higher frequencies correspond to vibrations that die away quickly. Dullness replaces the normal chest percussion note when fluid accumulates in the pleural space or when consolidation close to the chest wall occurs in the underlying pulmonary parenchyma. Similar to the vibrations generated by percussion, the vibrations from the patient's voice ("say 'ninety-nine' ") will also not be felt under these circumstances. However, the tactile fremitus is equally absent over areas of pneumothorax, whereas the percussion note may have a hyperresonant quality.

Conventional percussion cannot detect small pulmonary lesions located deeply within the thorax. Auscultatory percussion has been proposed to overcome this limitation. This technique combines light percussion of the sternum with simultaneous auscultation over the posterior chest. A decrease in sound intensity is believed to indicate lung disease. The method is of little value, however, because it has been shown convincingly that even large intrathoracic lesions can remain undetected. This problem is understandable, considering that percussion sounds either may be totally absorbed within the lung or may travel as transverse waves along the thoracic bones. Propagation along the thoracic bones is believed to explain the "coin sound," a sign that is used to detect a pneumothorax. It is elicited by creating a high-pitched sound impulse that propagates into the body, using a coin placed flat on the chest, which is then struck with another coin edge on. On auscultation of the opposite side of the thorax, a distinct click is heard if air separates the ribs from the lung and sound travels along these bones. Under normal circumstances with ribs and parenchyma in contact, however, the sound will be absorbed strongly and no click will be heard.

TASTE AND SMELL

A complete physical examination extends beyond the perception of vision, hearing, and touch. Olfactory impressions should also be documented, even if they are subtle. Malodorous breath is easily noticed and may, particularly if chronic, indicate infections within the nasal or oral cavity, e.g., paranasal sinusitis, nasal foreign body, and dental abscess. Bad breath may also originate from intrathoracic infections, such as lung abscess or bronchiectasis. Nowadays physicians rarely use their tastebuds to make a medical diagnosis. One particular disease of the respiratory tract in children, however, lends itself to gustatory diagnosis. Most often the discovery is made by the mother of a patient with cystic fibrosis who notices that the skin of her child tastes abnormally salty.

COMMON SIGNS AND SYMPTOMS OF CHEST DISEASE IN CHILDREN

There are several common complaints and presentations of children with chest diseases that deserve a more detailed description. In particular, cough and sputum production, noisy breathing, wheezing, cyanosis, digital clubbing, cardiovascular signs, and chest pain should be discussed.

COUGH AND SPUTUM PRODUCTION

Cough is not an illness by itself, but it is a cardinal manifestation in many chest diseases. Cough is probably the single most common complaint in children presenting to the physician. The act of coughing is a reflex aimed at removal of mucus and other material from the airways that follows the stimulation of cough or irritant receptors. These receptors are located anywhere between the pharynx and the terminal bronchioles. They send their afferent impulses via branches of the glossopharyngeal and vagus nerves to the cough center in the upper brainstem and pons. The efferent signals travel from the cough center via vagus, phrenic, and spinal motor nerves to the larynx and diaphragm as well as to the muscles of chest wall, abdomen, and pelvic floor. Cortical influences allow the voluntary initiation or suppression of cough.

There are three phases of coughing: (1) deep inspiration; (2) closure of the glottis, relaxation of the diaphragm, and contraction of expiratory muscles; and (3) sudden opening of the glottis. During the second phase, intrathoracic pressures up to 300 mm Hg can be generated and may be transmitted to the vascular and cerebrospinal spaces. Airflow velocity during the third phase is highest in the central airways and may reach three fourths the speed of sound. This speed depends on the sudden opening of the glottis and influences the success of expectoration. Patients with glottic dysfunction and those with tracheostomies may therefore have a less effective cough.

Stimuli that cause coughing may originate centrally, such as in psychogenic cough, or they may be pulmonary, located either in the major airways or in the pulmonary parenchyma. Also, cough can be provoked by nonpulmonary causes, such as irritation of pleura, diaphragm, or pericardium and even through stimulation of Arnold's nerve (a branch of the vagus) by wax or foreign bodies in the external ear.

A detailed history should define the nature of the cough, whether it is dry, hacking, or brassy, and whether it is productive by sound and appearance. In young children, expectoration is unusual, but if observed, the quantity and quality of sputum should be noted. In particular, the physician should inquire about the color and odor of the expectorate and about the presence of blood in the sputum. The yellow-green color of purulent sputum results from the cellular breakdown of leukocytes and the liberation of myeloperoxidase from these cells. This finding indicates a retention of secretions and does not necessarily reflect an acute infection.

The timing of coughing is important, and its relationship to daily routines should be sought. Cough during or after feeding occurs with aspiration. Nighttime cough may be related to asthma or to postnasal drip, whereas productive cough early in the morning is typical for bronchiectasis. Cough following exercise or exposure to cold air points toward airway hyperreactivity. Seasonal worsening or coughing on exposure to potential allergens should be documented, as well as the association of coughing and wheezing. The physician should ask about active and passive smoking, keeping in mind that, regrettably, there are quite a few children between 8 and 15 years who smoke regularly.

A detailed diary kept by the parents or the patient to note the frequency and timing of cough may prove invaluable. Tape recording and analysis of cough sounds, a so-called tussigraphy, may prove to be useful for objective quantification. Some acoustic characteristics of cough are quite specific for certain diseases, such as the sound of a barking seal in viral croup or the whooping noise in pertussis. In patients with chronic cough, the physician should weigh the possible causes in view of their prevalence at different ages (Table 3–2). Also, complications of severe coughing paroxysms, such as pneumothorax, cough syncope, or nonsyncopal neurologic manifestations, should be considered. Regarding the last, the physician should inquire about lightheadedness, headache, visual disturbance, paresthesia, and tremor.

NOISY BREATHING

Quite frequently a child is brought to the physician's attention because of abnormal breathing noises. This noise may be a nonmusical hiss, much like the one produced in normal subjects at increased rates of ventilation, or it may have the musical qualities of stridor and snoring. Also, bubbling and crackling noises may be heard, and the tactile perception may contribute to the impression of a "rattly" chest in these patients.

Attention should be focused on the noise-generating structures of the extrathoracic airways that are located at points of anatomic narrowing, e.g., the nasal vestibule, the posterior nasal orifices, and the glottis. The most common cause of noisy breathing in toddlers and young children is nasopharyngeal obstruction; in young infants, laryngomalacia is a leading cause. It is uncertain to what degree sounds from large intrathoracic airways contribute to the noise of breathing. Placing the stethoscope within the airstream, one hears predominantly those sounds that are produced locally in the mouth and larynx. Noisy breathing is a common finding in patients with asthma and bronchitis and does not necessarily reflect intrathoracic airway pathology because the upper airways are also frequently affected in these patients.

To clarify the causes of noisy breathing, the parents or patient should describe their own perceptions of the noise: does it occur during inspiration, expiration, or both? Is it just an exaggeration of the normal breath sound noise, or does it have musical qualities? Did an episode of choking precede the onset of noisy breathing? Is the abnormal sound more prominent during certain activities, such as exercise? At what times of day or night and in which body positions is it most noticeable? The physician should also inquire about associated respiratory distress, cough, sputum production, and dyspnea.

Children may suffer from partial obstruction of the upper airways during sleep; complete obstruction, which is found in adult patients with sleep apnea, is less common. Invariably, these children are heavy snorers at night, whereas normal children's snoring is largely confined to times of upper respiratory tract infection. Usually enlarged adenoids and tonsils cause the breathing disturbance. The physician should inquire about the typical signs and symptoms found in patients with increased work of breathing and abnormal sleep patterns at night (Table 3–3).

In the older child and adolescent, the physician should first inspect the nasal passageways and proceed to an examination of the oropharynx before auscultation of the neck and thorax. The acoustic signs should be checked while the patient breathes first with the mouth open, then with it closed. In younger children, examination of the nose and mouth is widely unpopular and often results in agitation and crying. It is better to start with auscultation before inspection in these children. Noisy breathers should be examined when they are sitting or standing upright and when they are lying down because upper airway geometry is position dependent and may influence the respiratory sounds. The examiner should also note abnormal crying or speech in the patient, as this may point to laryngeal disease.

Table 3–2. CAUSES OF CHRONIC COUGH

Infant	Preschool	School Age/Adolescence
CONGENITAL ANOMALIES	FOREIGN BODY	REACTIVE
Tracheoesophageal fistula	INFECTIONS	Asthma
Neurologic impairment	Viral	Postnasal drip
INFECTIONS	Mycoplasma	INFECTIONS
Viral (RSV, CMV)	Bacterial	Mycoplasma
Chlamydia	REACTIVE	IRRITATIVE
Bacterial (pertussis)	Asthma	Smoking
CYSTIC FIBROSIS	CYSTIC FIBROSIS	Air pollution
	IRRITATIVE	PSYCHOGENIC
	Passive	
	smoking	

Data modified from Eigen H: Pediatr Clin North Am 29:67, 1982.

WHEEZING

Wheezing is a common respiratory symptom and refers to musical, adventitious lung sounds that are often heard by the patient as well as the physician. Stridor is even more noticeable. Essentially, it is a very loud inspiratory wheeze originating from extrathoracic airways. When asking the patient or the parents about wheezing and stridor, one should keep in mind that the use of lung sound terminology among nonprofessionals is no better standardized than it is among health care providers. Therefore, the physician should inquire about musical, whistling noises during respiration, and if necessary, demonstrate stridor or the forced expiratory wheeze that can be produced even by healthy individuals.

Most typically, wheezing is associated with hyperreactive airway disease, but any critical narrowing of the airways can produce wheezing. Table 3–4 lists conditions other than asthma that may be associated with wheezing and stridor. The wheezing typical in asthma originates from oscillations of airways at many sites. On auscultation, one hears many different tones simultaneously, which is called *polyphonic wheezing.* Obstruction of a single airway can produce a single *monophonic wheeze* or, in the obstruction of extrathoracic airways, *stridor.* Both inspiratory and expiratory wheezes are present in the majority of asthmatic patients. Expiration may be prolonged in very severe airway obstruction. This prolongation may be so extreme that airflow is minimal, and thus wheezing is absent. Respiration under these circumstances is ominously silent, and the patient may have carbon dioxide retention and cyanosis. In less severe cases, however, the proportion of inspiration and expiration occupied by wheezing correlates with the degree of airflow obstruction. Objective and reproducible wheeze quantification can be achieved by computer-assisted techniques, but in practice the quantification of wheezing severity is made by subjective assessment at the bedside.

Wheezes are often high pitched and will therefore attenuate during their passage through lung tissue, particularly if the lungs are hyperinflated. Auscultation over the neck may give a better impression of respiratory sounds and should be included as a part

Table 3–3. CLINICAL SYMPTOMS IN CHILDREN WITH HEAVY NOCTURNAL SNORING

Nighttime Manifestations
Profuse nocturnal sweating
Restless sleep
Abnormal movements during sleep
Special sleeping position
Enuresis

Problems with Growth and Nutrition
Anorexia
Weight < 3rd percentile
Nausea with or without vomiting

Behavioral and Learning Problems
Hyperactivity
Aggression
Social withdrawal

Minor Motor Problems
Lack of coordination
Clumsiness

Other Manifestations
Frequent upper airway infections
Frequent morning headaches
Excessive daytime somnolence

Data modified from Guilleminault C, Winkle R, Korobkin R, and Simmons B: Eur J Pediatr 139:165, 1982.

Table 3–4. CAUSES OF WHEEZING AND STRIDOR OTHER THAN ASTHMA

Malformation
Cardiovascular anomalies (e.g., vascular ring)
Airway anomalies (e.g., web, cyst, hemangioma, malacia, stenosis)
Esophageal anomalies (e.g., enteric cyst)
Inflammation
Tracheitis
Bronchitis
Bronchiolitis
Bronchiectasis
Cystic fibrosis
Compression
EXTRINSIC
Esophageal foreign body
Lymphadenopathy
Malignancy
INTRINSIC
Endobronchial foreign body
Tumor (rare)

Extrathoracic Disease
Laryngitis
Epiglottitis
Vocal cord paralysis
Retropharyngeal abscess
Peritonsillar abscess
Laryngomalacia
Polyps, adenoids
Other
Metabolic disturbances (e.g., hypocalcemia, hypokalemia)
Psychosomatic illness (e.g., emotional laryngeal wheezing, factitious asthma)

of the routine physical examination (Fig. 3–13). Tracheal auscultation to determine if and when there is wheezing after methacholine inhalation challenge can be used instead of spirometry in young children who are thought to have bronchial hyperreactivity. Listening to respiratory sounds over the neck may also help to identify patients who are thought to be asthmatic but who generate the wheezing noises solely in the larynx. These are usually older children and adolescents who may have severe emotional problems or who suffer from vocal cord dysfunction.

CYANOSIS

Cyanosis refers to a blue color of the skin and mucous membranes due to excessive concentrations of reduced hemoglobin in capillary blood. The oxygen content of capillary blood is assumed to be midway between that of arterial and that of venous blood. Areas with a high blood flow and a small arteriovenous oxygen difference, e.g., the tongue and mucous membranes, will not become cyanotic as readily as those with a low blood flow and a large arteriovenous oxygen difference, e.g., the skin of cold hands and feet. A distinction is therefore made between *peripheral cyanosis,* which is confined to the skin of the extremities, and *central cyanosis,* which includes the tongue and mucous membranes. The absolute concentration of reduced hemoglobin in the capillaries necessary to produce cyanosis is between 4 and 6 g/100 ml of blood. This level is usually present when the concentration of reduced hemoglobin in arterial blood exceeds 3 g/100 ml. Clinical cyanosis will occur at different levels of arterial oxygen saturation, depending on the amount of total hemoglobin (Fig. 3–14).

Physiologically, there are five mechanisms that can cause arterial hemoglobin desaturation in the patient who breathes room air at normal altitude: (1) alveolar hypoventilation, (2) diffusion impairment, (3) right-to-left shunting, (4) mismatch of ventilation and perfusion, and (5) inadequate oxygen transport by hemoglobin. Clinically, diffusion impairment is of little importance as a single cause. Imbalance of ventilation and perfusion is by far the most common mechanism and is correctable by administration of 100 per cent oxygen. The physician should therefore look for a change in cyanosis while the patient breathes oxygen.

Cyanosis is best observed under daylight and with the patient resting in a comfortably warm room. The distribution of cyanosis and the state of peripheral perfusion should be noted. Patients with decreased cardiac output and poor peripheral perfusion can be cyanotic despite a normal arterial hemoglobin saturation. Some patients may become cyanotic only during exercise, a not uncommon response when restrictive lung disease reduces the pulmonary capillary bed and the transit time of erythrocytes becomes too short for full saturation during episodes of increased cardiac output. Congenital heart disease in infants may lead to *differential cyanosis,* which affects only the lower part of the body, e.g., in patients with preductal coarctation of the aorta. Less commonly, only the upper part of the body is cyanotic, e.g., in patients with transposition of the great arteries, patent ductus arteriosus, or pulmonary hypertension.

The clinical impression of cyanosis is usually confirmed by an analysis of blood gases or pulse oximetry. Pulse oximetry, however, will not take into account the presence of abnormal hemoglobin. For example, in methemoglobinemia the oxygen carrying capacity of blood is reduced and patients may appear lavender blue, but pulse oximetry may overestimate Sa_{O_2}. The blood of newborn infants, conversely, can be well saturated and not cyanotic at lower arterial

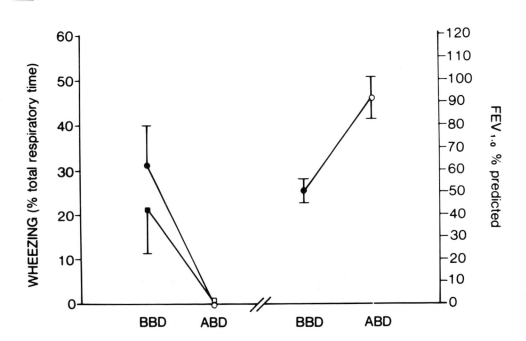

Figure 3–13. Example of the relation between wheezing *(left side)* and flow limitation *(right side)*. Computer analysis of lung sounds *(squares)* and tracheal sounds *(circles)* before *(BBD)* and after *(ABD)* bronchodilator treatment is shown for six children with acute asthma (bars indicate SD). Severity is measured as the proportion of the respiratory cycle occupied by wheezing. Before bronchodilation the average forced expiratory volume in 1 second ($FEV_{1.0}$) is 53 per cent of predicted values, and there is wheezing, more over the trachea than over the lung. After bronchodilation $FEV_{1.0}$ becomes normal and wheezing disappears (Pasterkamp H: Unpublished data).

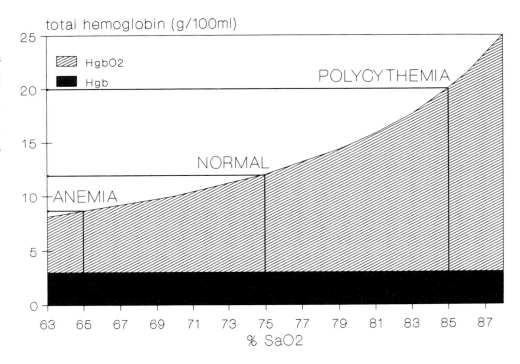

Figure 3–14. Cyanosis requires at least 3 g/100 ml of reduced hemoglobin *(Hgb)* in arterial blood or 4 to 6 g/100 ml in capillary blood. The arterial oxygen saturation (Sa_{O_2}) at which cyanosis occurs is dependent on the amount of total Hgb. As illustrated, a child with 3 g/100 ml of Hgb *(solid area)* plus 9 g/100 ml of oxyhemoglobin $(HgbO_2)$ *(shaded area)* has an Sa_{O_2} of 75 per cent. In the anemic patient (i.e., total Hgb of 8 g/100 ml) with Hgb of 3 g/100 ml, Sa_{O_2} will drop much lower (to 65 per cent in this example) before cyanosis occurs, whereas in the patient with polycythemia (i.e., total Hgb of 20 g/100 ml), cyanosis appears at a higher Sa_{O_2} (85 per cent).

oxygen tensions because of the different oxygen-binding curve of fetal hemoglobin. In the patient with hypoxemia who does not present with cyanosis, the physician has to pay particular attention to other *clinical signs and symptoms of hypoxia.* These include tachypnea and tachycardia, exertional dyspnea, hypertension, headache, and behavioral changes. With more severe hypoxia there may be visual disturbance, somnolence, hypotension, and ultimately coma. In addition, the patient may have an elevated level of carbon dioxide. Depending on how rapidly and to what extent the level of carbon dioxide has risen, the *clinical signs of hypercarbia* will largely reflect vascular dilation. These signs include flushed, hot hands and feet; bounding pulses; confusion or drowsiness; muscular twitching; engorged retinal veins; and, in the most severe cases, papilledema and coma.

DIGITAL CLUBBING

Digital clubbing refers to a focal enlargement of the connective tissue in the terminal phalanges of fingers and toes, most noticeably on their dorsal surfaces. This sign was first described by Hippocrates, and the term *Hippocratic fingers* is used by some to denote simple digital clubbing. The pathogenesis of clubbing is still unclear. In view of the great variety of acute and chronic diseases associated with digital clubbing, two main theories are proposed. The first suggests a neurogenic mechanism in which impulses from the diseased organ travel via the vagus nerve and induce clubbing through an undetermined reflex that includes vasodilation. The second assumes the appearance of a humoral substance that is normally present in the venous circulation. In this model, failure to remove or inactivate this substance on its passage through the lung or overproduction of the

substance in chronic inflammatory gastrointestinal diseases would be causative factors for clubbing. Prostaglandins $F_{2\alpha}$ and E have been suggested as vasodilator substances in patients with cystic fibrosis.

Clubbing of the digits may be idiopathic, acquired, or hereditary. Cystic fibrosis, bronchiectasis, and empyema are the most common pulmonary causes of acquired digital clubbing in children. Clubbing is also seen infrequently in extrinsic allergic vasculitis, pulmonary arteriovenous malformations, bronchiolitis obliterans, sarcoidosis, and chronic asthma. Table 3–5 shows a list of nonpulmonary diseases associated with clubbing. A systemic disorder of bones, joints, and soft tissues known as *hypertrophic osteoarthropathy (HOA)* includes digital clubbing. In the majority of cases, HOA is associated with bronchogenic carcinoma and other intrathoracic neoplasms, but the pediatrician may see HOA in patients with severe cystic fibrosis or chronic empyema and lung abscess. In addition to clubbing, these patients may have periosteal thickening; symmetric arthritis of ankles, knees, wrists, and elbows; neurovascular changes of hands and feet; and increased thickness of subcutaneous soft tissues in the distal portions of arms and legs. The primary idiopathic or hereditary form of HOA—pachydermoperiostosis—appears with prominent furrowing of the forehead and scalp. Approximately half of the reported cases have a positive family history. Genetic studies suggest an autosomal dominant inheritance with variable expression and a predilection for males.

Digital clubbing not only is an important indicator of pulmonary disease but also may reflect the progression or resolution of the causative process. Pulmonary abscess and empyema may lead to digital clubbing over the course of only a few weeks. In this case, clubbing will resolve if effective treatment is instituted before connective tissue changes become fixed. Interestingly, even long-standing finger club-bing seems to resolve in patients after successful heart and lung transplantation. In patients with cystic fi-brosis, progression of finger clubbing suggests a suboptimal control of chest infections. It is therefore useful to quantify the degree of digital clubbing. Measurements have focused on the hyponychial (Lovibond) angle and on the phalangeal depth ratio (Fig. 3–15). Changes of the hyponychial angle are quantified on "shadowgrams"—projections of the fin-ger's lateral profile onto a magnifying screen—whereas the phalangeal depth ratio is measured from plaster casts. In addition, capillaroscopy may be used to study under magnification the abnormal plexus formed in the capillary bed in patients with finger clubbing (Baughman RP et al, unpublished observa-tions).

For routine clinical practice, the sign described by Schamroth, a cardiologist who himself developed finger clubbing during several attacks of infective endocarditis, is a most useful method of measuring finger clubbing (see Fig. 3–15). Another way is to place a plastic caliper with minimal pressure over the interphalangeal joint. If it is easy to slide the caliper from this joint across the nail fold, the distal phalan-geal diameter (DPD) to interphalangeal diameter (IPD) ratio must be less than 1, and the patient has no clubbing.

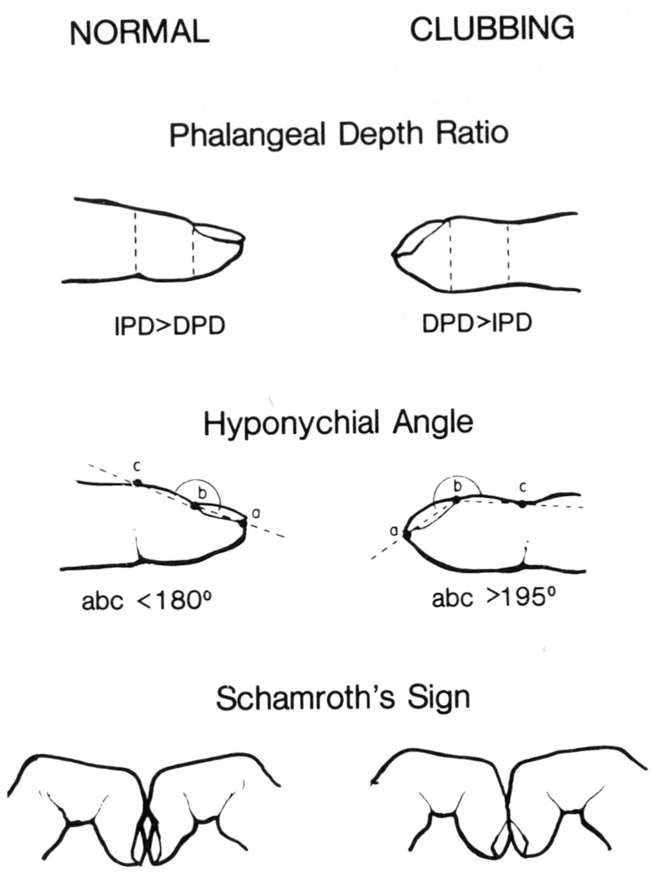

CARDIOVASCULAR SIGNS

Pulmonary heart disease, or *cor pulmonale*, is a consequence of acute or chronic pulmonary hyper-

Table 3–5. NONPULMONARY DISEASES ASSOCIATED WITH CLUBBING

Cardiac
  Cyanotic congenital heart disease
  Subacute bacterial endocarditis
  Chronic congestive heart failure
Hematologic
  Thalassemia
  Congenital methemoglobinemia (rare)
Gastrointestinal
  Crohn disease
  Ulcerative colitis
  Chronic dysentery, sprue
  Polyposis coli
  Severe GI hemorrhage
  Small bowel lymphoma
  Liver cirrhosis (including α_1-antitrypsin deficiency)
Other
  Thyroid deficiency (thyroid acropathy)
  Chronic pyelonephritis (rare)
  Toxic (e.g., arsenic, mercury, beryllium)
  Lymphomatoid granulomatosis
  Fabry disease
  Raynaud disease, scleroderma
Unilateral Clubbing
  Vascular disorders (e.g., subclavian arterial aneurysm, brachial arteriovenous fistula)
  Subluxation of shoulder
  Median nerve injury
  Local trauma

Figure 3–15. Finger clubbing can be measured in different ways. The ratio of the distal phalangeal diameter (*DPD*) over the interphalangeal diameter (*IPD*), or the phalangeal depth ratio, is less than 1 in normal subjects but increases to greater than 1 with finger clubbing. The DPD/IPD can be measured with calipers or more accurately with finger casts. The hyponychial angle can be measured from lateral projections of the finger contour on a magnifying screen and is usually less than 180 degrees in normal subjects but greater than 195 degrees in patients with finger clubbing. For bedside clinical assessment, Schamroth's sign is useful. The dorsal surfaces of the terminal phalanges of similar fingers are placed together. With clubbing, the normal diamond-shaped aperture or "window" at the bases of the nail beds disap-pears, and a prominent distal angle forms between the end of the nails. In normal subjects this angle is minimal or nonexistent.

tension and appears as right ventricular enlargement. The progression of chronic cor pulmonale to ultimate right ventricular failure is accompanied by certain physical signs. Initially, the right ventricular systolic pressure and muscle mass increase as pulmonary artery pressure rises. During this stage, cardiac aus-cultation may be normal or may reveal an increased pulmonary component of the second heart sound, caused by an increase in diastolic pulmonary arterial pressure. The physician should look for a parasternal right ventricular heave. As pulmonary hypertension progresses, there is an increase in right ventricular end-diastolic volume. Dilation of the main pulmonary artery and right ventricular outflow tract lead to systolic pulmonary ejection clicks and murmurs. Di-astolic murmurs appear when pulmonary or tricuspid valves or both become insufficient. Third and fourth heart sounds at the left lower sternal border are signs of decreased right ventricular compliance. Most of these right-sided cardiovascular findings are accentuated during inspiration, which augments venous return. Finally, cardiac output falls while end-diastolic pressure and volume increase further in the failing right ventricle.

Clinical findings at this stage include hepatic engorgement, jugular venous distention, and peripheral edema. Occasionally, there may be cyanosis and intracardiac right-to-left shunting through a patent foramen ovale. The physician should exclude the possibility of congenital cardiac defects or acquired left-sided heart disease before making the diagnosis of cor pulmonale. Hyperinflation of the lungs should be taken into account as a cause of the attenuation of cardiovascular sounds and the lowering of the subcostal liver margin, which may be misinterpreted as hepatic enlargement.

Complete assessment of the cardiovascular system includes a careful auscultation and palpation of the pulse to detect *cardiac arrhythmia*. This problem is not uncommon in patients with chronic lung disease and may appear as sinus or paroxysmal supraventricular tachycardia, atrial premature contractions, or ventricular ectopic beats. Causes include hypoxemia, acid-base imbalance, and enlargement of the right heart, but effects of common drugs such as aminophylline, beta sympathomimetics, or diuretics should not be overlooked.

During quiet spontaneous respiration there is a phasic variation of arterial blood pressure. The widening of this normal respiratory variation is known as *pulsus paradoxus*. Increased respiratory resistance may exaggerate the normal inspiratory-expiratory difference in left ventricular stroke volume. This is mediated by effects of intrathoracic pressures on ventricular preload. Clinically, pulsus paradoxus is first assessed by palpation of the radial pulse and then is measured at the brachial artery with a sphygmomanometer as the difference in systolic pressure between inspiration and expiration. The pressure cuff is deflated from above systolic level, and the highest pressure during expiration at which systolic pulse sounds are heard is recorded. Similarly, the highest pressure at which every pulse is just audible throughout inspiration is also noted. In general, a drop of greater than 10 mm Hg during inspiration is taken as clinically significant. This finding is used in the assessment of patients with asthma, but systolic blood pressure fluctuations are influenced by breathing pattern, and the correlation of pulsus paradoxus with objective measurements of airway obstruction is poor.

CHEST PAIN

Chest pain is relatively common in older children and adolescents but may also present in younger children. The occurrence rate in an emergency department approaches 2.5 per 1000 patient visits, and chest pain accounts for an estimated 650,000 physician visits of patients between the ages of 10 and 21 years in the United States. Chest pain in children is most often benign and self-limited. Typical origins are musculoskeletal problems and idiopathic, dysfunctional, and psychogenic causes (Table 3–6). Younger children more frequently have underlying cardiorespiratory problems, whereas children over the age of 12 years are more likely to have psychogenic pain.

The history is most important in the assessment of these patients, who usually have few physical findings and rarely any laboratory data of diagnostic value. The physician should recognize a clinical profile suggestive of psychogenic pain but should also keep

Table 3–6. CAUSES OF CHEST PAIN IN CHILDREN

Thorax	**Cardiovascular System**
Costochondritis	Structural lesions (e.g., mitral valve prolapse,
Tietze syndrome	idiopathic hypertrophic subaortic stenosis
Muscular disease	[IHSS], coronary disease)
Precordial catch	Acquired cardiac disease (e.g., carditis,
Trauma	arteritis, tumor involvement)
Connective tissue disorders	Arrhythmia
Xiphoid-cartilage syndrome	**Esophagus**
Rib tip syndrome	Gastroesphageal reflux
Leukemia	Foreign body
Herpes zoster	Achalasia
Breast development or disease (e.g., gynecomastia, mastitis)	**Vertebral Column**
Lungs, Pleura, and Diaphragm	Deformities (e.g., scoliosis)
Asthma	Vertebral collapse
Cystic fibrosis	**Psychogenic Causes**
Infection (e.g., bronchitis, pneumonia, epidemic pleurodynia)	Anxiety
Inhalation of irritants (e.g., chemical pneumonitis, smoking)	Hyperventilation
Stitch (associated with exercise)	Unresolved grief
Foreign body	Identification with another person suffering
Pneumothorax	chest pain
Pleural disease (e.g., pleurisy, effusion)	
Diaphragmatic irritation (e.g., subphrenic abscess, gastric distention)	
Sickle cell anemia	

in mind that psychogenic and organic causes are not mutually exclusive. A substantial number of patients have a family history of chest pain. Parents of younger children should explain how they know that their child is in pain. It is important to determine whether sleep is affected, because organic pain is more likely than psychogenic pain to awaken the patient or to prevent the child from falling asleep. The duration of symptoms may be an indicator; acute, short-lasting pain is more likely to be organic than pain of many months duration. Localized, sharp, and superficial pains suggest an origin in the chest wall, whereas diffuse, deep, substernal, and epigastric pains are likely to be visceral, originating in the thorax if the pain affects dermatomes T1 to T4 and in the diaphragm or abdomen if it affects dermatomes T5 to T8. The physician should inquire about cough or asthma, recent exercise or trauma, heart disease in the patient and the family, cigarette smoking, and emotional problems.

A close inspection and careful palpation of the chest and abdomen are essential. Common abnormal findings include chest wall tenderness, fever, or both. The physician should use pressure on the stethoscope to elicit local tenderness while the patient is distracted by the auscultation. Cardiac murmurs and clicks may be found in patients with mitral valve prolapse. The presence of systemic signs such as weight loss, anorexia, or syncopal attacks will direct the attention to organic causes.

REFERENCES

General Reading

Athreya BH, Silverman BK (eds): Pediatric Physical Diagnosis. East Norwalk, Conn, Appleton-Century-Crofts, 1985.

Bates B (ed): A Guide to Physical Examination. Philadelphia, JB Lippincott Co, 1983.

Boyle WE and Hoekelman RA: The pediatric history. In Hoekelman RA (ed): Primary Pediatric Care. St. Louis, CV Mosby Co, 1987.

Glauser FL (ed): Signs and Symptoms in Pulmonary Medicine. Philadelphia, JB Lippincott Co, 1983.

Inspection of the Respiratory System

Carlo WA, Martin RJ, Bruce EN et al: Alae nasi activation (nasal flaring) decreases nasal resistance in preterm infants. Pediatrics 72:338, 1983.

Carse EA, Wilkinson AR, Whyte PL et al: Oxygen and carbon dioxide tensions, breathing and heart rate in normal infants during the first six months of life. J Dev Physiol 3:85, 1981.

Commey JO and Levison H: Physical signs in childhood asthma. Pediatrics 58:537, 1976.

Feingold M and Bossert WH: Normal values for selected physical parameters. Birth Defects 10:14, 1974.

Gilmartin JJ and Gibson GJ: Mechanisms of paradoxical rib cage motion in patients with chronic obstructive pulmonary disease. Am Rev Respir Dis 134:683, 1986.

Hierholzer E and Schier F: Rasterstereography in the measurement and postoperative follow-up of anterior chest wall deformities. Z Kinderchir 41:267, 1986.

Iliff A and Lee VA: Pulse rate, respiratory rate and body temperature in children between two months and eighteen years of age. Child Dev 23:237, 1952.

Lees MH: Cyanosis of the newborn infant. J Pediatr 77:484, 1970.

Lucas WP and Pryor HB: Range and standard deviations of certain physical measurements in healthy children. J Pediatr 6:533, 1935.

Robotham JL: A physiological approach to hemidiaphragm paralysis. Crit Care Med 7:563, 1979.

Staats BA, Bonekat HW, Harris CD, and Offord KP: Chest wall motion in sleep apnoea. Am Rev Respir Dis 130:59, 1984.

Stinson S: The physical growth of high altitude bolivian Aymara children. Am J Phys Anthropol 52:377, 1980.

Respiratory Sounds

Ackerman NB, Bell RE, and deLemos RA: Differential pulmonary auscultation in neonates. Clin Pediatr 21:566, 1982.

Austrheim O and Kraman SS: The effect of low density gas breathing on vesicular lung sounds. Respir Physiol 60:145, 1985.

Baughman RP and Loudon RG: Quantitation of wheezing in acute asthma. Chest 86:718, 1984.

Baughman RP and Loudon RG: Sound spectral analysis of voice transmitted sound. Am Rev Respir Dis 134:167, 1986.

Bohadana AB, Coimbra FTV, and Santiago JRF: Detection of lung abnormalities by auscultatory percussion: a comparative study with conventional percussion. Respiration 50:218, 1986.

Cole WHJ: Description of a self-adherent stethoscope. Med J Aust 2:252, 1969.

Cugell DW: Lung sound nomenclature. Am Rev Respir Dis 136:1016, 1987.

Efron R: Central auditory processing. III. The "cocktail party effect" and anterior temporal lobectomy. Brain Lang 19:254, 1983.

Forgacs P: Lung Sounds. London, Baillière Tindall, 1978.

Gavriely N, Palti Y, and Alroy G: Spectral characteristics of normal breath sounds. J Appl Physiol 50:307, 1981.

Gavriely N, Palti Y, Alroy G, and Grotberg JB: Measurement and theory of wheezing breath sounds. J Appl Physiol 57:481, 1984.

Ginott N, Barnea E, Monosevitch M, and Buncher R: New vacuum stethoscope for immediate monitoring and recording of resuscitation in newborns. Isr J Med Sci 16:447, 1980.

Guilleminault C, Winkle R, Korobkin R, and Simmons B: Children and nocturnal snoring: evaluation of the effects of sleep related respiratory resistive load and daytime functioning. Eur J Pediatr 139:165, 1982.

Hopkins RL: Differential auscultation of the acutely ill patient. Ann Emerg Med 14:589, 1985.

Kanga JF and Kraman SS: Comparison of the lung sound frequency spectra of infants and adults. Pediatr Pulmonol 2:292, 1986.

Kraman SS (ed): Lung sounds. Semin Respir Med 6:157, 1985.

Morrison RB: Post-effort breath sound. Tex Med 67:72, 1971.

Murphy RLH: Auscultation of the lung: past lessons, future possibilities. Thorax 36:99, 1981.

Pasterkamp H, Carson C, Daien D, and Oh Y: Digital respirosonography—new images of lung sounds. Chest 96:1405, 1989.

Pasterkamp H, Montgomery M, and Wiebicke W: Nomenclature used by health care professionals to describe breath sounds in asthma. Chest 92:346, 1987.

Schwartz N and Eisenkraft JB: Continuous auscultation of heart and bilateral breath sounds. Pediatrics 81:745, 1988.

Waring WW: Physical examination of children. Quantitative extensions. In Sackner MA (ed): Diagnostic Techniques in Pulmonary Disease. New York, Marcel Dekker, Inc, 1980.

Pulsus Paradoxus

Blaustein AS, Risser TA, Weiss JW et al: Mechanisms of pulsus paradoxus during resistive respiratory loading and asthma. J Am Coll Cardiol 8:529, 1986.

Carden DL, Nowak RM, Sarkar D, and Tomlanovich MC: Vital signs including pulsus paradoxus in the assessment of acute bronchial asthma. Ann Emerg Med 12:80, 1983.

Martin J, Jardim J, Sampson M, and Engel LE: Factors influencing pulsus paradoxus in asthma. Chest 80:543, 1981.

Digital Clubbing

Bentley D, Moore A, and Schwachman H: Finger clubbing: a quantitative survey by analysis of the shadowgraph. Lancet 2:164, 1976.

Hansen-Flaschen J and Nordberg J: Clubbing and hypertrophic osteoarthropathy. Clin Chest Med 8:287, 1987.

Lemen RJ, Gates AJ, Mathe AA et al: Relationships among digital clubbing, disease severity, and serum prostaglandins F_{2alpha} and E concentrations in cystic fibrosis patients. Am Rev Respir Dis 117:639, 1978.

Pitts-Tucker TJ, Miller MG, and Littlewood JM: Finger clubbing in cystic fibrosis. Arch Dis Child 61:576, 1986.

Schamroth L: Personal experience. S Afr Med J 50:297, 1976.

Waring WW, Wilkinson RW, Wiebe RA et al: Quantitation of digital clubbing children. Measurements of casts of the index finger. Am Rev Respir Dis 104:166, 1971.

Cough and Wheezing

Avital A, Bar-Yishay E, Springer C, and Godfrey S: Bronchial provocation tests in young children using tracheal auscultation. J Pediatr 112:591, 1988.

Eigen H: The clinical evaluation of chronic cough. Pediatr Clin North Am 29:67, 1982.

Mountain RD and Sahn SA: Clinical features and outcome in patients with acute asthma presenting with hypercapnia. Am Rev Respir Dis 138:535, 1988.

Pasterkamp H, Wiebicke W, and Fenton R: Subjective assessment vs computer analysis of wheezing in asthma. Chest 91:376, 1987.

Shim CS and Williams MH: Relationship of wheezing to the severity of asthma. Arch Intern Med 143:890, 1983.

Stanwick RS, Fish DG, Manfreda J et al: Where Manitoba children obtain their cigarettes. Can Med Assoc J 137:405, 1987.

Stern RC, Horwitz SJ, and Doershuk CF: Neurologic symptoms during coughing paroxysms in cystic fibrosis. J Pediatr 112:909, 1988.

Chest Pain

Coleman WL: Recurrent chest pain in childhood. Pediatr Clin North Am 31:1007, 1984.

Selbst SM: Chest pain in children. Pediatrics 75:1068, 1985.

Selbst SM, Ruddy RM, Clark BJ et al: Pediatric chest pain: a prospective study. Pediatrics 82:319, 1988.

Cyanosis

Watcha MF, Connor MT, and Hing AV: Pulse oximetry in methemoglobinemia. Am J Dis Child 143:845, 1989.

4

WILLIAM W. WARING, M.D.

DIAGNOSTIC AND THERAPEUTIC PROCEDURES

It is possible to divide all procedures pertaining to respiratory disease into the categories of prophylaxis, diagnosis, and therapy. Only those that are believed to deserve special comment are discussed in this chapter. (Radiologic procedures are discussed in Chapter 5, and pulmonary function testing is covered in Chapters 6, 7, and 8.) Some procedures can be performed without assistance by any physician, and other procedures require specialized skills or other physicians or laboratory workers.

DIAGNOSTIC PROCEDURES

BRONCHOSCOPY

Bronchoscopy is a procedure performed to visualize and manipulate the larger branches of the tracheobronchial tree. The trachea and main bronchi can thus be directly approached in a child of any age. With a conventional rigid bronchoscope, the lower lobe bronchi, the orifices of the upper and middle lobe bronchi, and those of the lower lobe segmental bronchi are accessible in most instances, depending on the size of the patient and the type and size of the instrument.

The availability within the past 15 years of the flexible fiberoptic bronchoscope has revolutionized adult pulmonology, in which its chief application is the detection of carcinoma of the lung. However, the use of this instrument with pediatric patients has been delayed because of the need for scope miniaturization, which at last has been effected. The new pediatric fiberoptic bronchoscope is now a well-established instrument for the detection of a variety of upper and lower airway problems in infants and children of all sizes.

The technologic achievement common to all flexible fiberoptic bronchoscopes is their ability to transmit light and images around corners. An excellent review has been written by Wood and Postma (1988) on the relative merits of and indications for the use of rigid and flexible bronchoscopy in children. The flexible bronchoscope used to be relatively large in diameter because it contained a channel for suction, instillation of therapeutic solutions, and passage of brushes or biopsy forceps. However, the standard pediatric fiberoptic bronchoscope has a 1.2-mm suction channel and an external diameter of only 3.6 mm. Indeed, there is now available a directable ultrathin fiber bronchoscope with an external diameter of only 2.7 mm.

Advances have also been made in rigid bronchoscopic systems, including the Storz scopes with fiberoptic light sources, glass-rod telescopes, and *internal* lumens as small as 2.5 mm. Both rigid and flexible bronchoscopes can be adapted for video monitoring and taping with subsequent slow-motion and "freeze"-mode playback. It is now apparent that the two types of instrument complement each other, and although there are situations in which either may be used, there are clear-cut instances in which one is the instrument of choice. Table 4–1 lists important differences between the rigid and flexible bronchoscopes and their applications.

Rigid bronchoscopy is a more formidable procedure, usually requiring general anesthesia in an operating room. In the United States it has traditionally been the tool of pediatric surgeons and otolaryngologists. Flexible bronchoscopy can usually be performed under heavy sedation and with local anesthesia. Not ideally, it can be performed in a patient's bed when it is impossible or inadvisable to move the child.

Because of its wide application to diagnosis of airway problems in infants and children and its relative simplicity, increasing numbers of pediatric pulmonologists have begun to use the new instrument. Most pediatric pulmonary fellowship training programs now include a requirement for experience with, if not mastery of, fiberoptic bronchoscopy in their curricula. Nevertheless, considerable skill and experience are required to obtain the maximum benefit from this instrument, because the anatomy of the upper airways and tracheobronchial tree can be confusing. Established landmarks can be altered by volume shifts within the thorax. Prolonged or clumsy bronchoscopy may traumatize the larynx and may be followed by dangerous edema and upper airway obstruction. During bronchoscopy, the patient's color, pulse, and respirations should be carefully monitored, because dangerous hypoxemia may occur in children with severe unilateral or bilateral pulmonary disease. The solid construction of the fiberoptic bronchoscope may not permit adequate ventilation, and in infants and small children it is important to hold subglottic inspection to a minimum. The use of a pulse oximeter can be particularly helpful during bronchoscopy.

Bronchoscopy is performed when disease is known or presumed to involve the bronchi observable thereby and when less invasive diagnostic and therapeutic procedures have failed. Because the flexible scope is usually passed through the nose, bronchoscopy by this method includes nasopharyngoscopy and laryngoscopy. Indeed, several of the indications for use of the flexible scope involve the upper airway (evaluation of snoring, stridor, or other evidence of obstruction). Both instruments permit identification and localization of foreign bodies and of the origin of bleeding or purulent secretions and the removal of fluid for culture or other analysis. (See also "Diagnostic Bronchoalveolar Lavage.") Transbronchial biopsy requires the rigid scope or adult flexible scope and for that reason is not frequently performed on children by pediatric pulmonologists. Anomalies and sites of compression or stenosis can be identified definitively.

Rigid bronchoscopy is the established instrument for removing aspirated foreign bodies from the major airways, although the locations and numbers of such objects can be defined by the flexible scope. Foreign body removal is facilitated by a preoperative assessment of the nature, number, and locations of foreign objects. This type of information is generated by a probing history, a careful physical examination, inspiration and expiration chest roentgenograms, and, frequently, fluoroscopy. A skilled team composed of a pediatric pulmonologist and an endoscopist, working together before, during, and after bronchoscopic removal of a foreign body, can make the difference between a smooth, complete recovery and a traumatic experience.

Tenacious or mucopurulent secretions may be directly aspirated through a bronchoscope with relief of atelectasis or obstructive overinflation. Simultaneous atelectasis of the right middle and right lower lobes almost always indicates obstruction of the bronchus intermedius, a particularly common site for the lodging of foreign bodies. Disease of the upper lobes or right middle lobe is generally less susceptible to rigid bronchoscopic attack because of the awkward locations and orientations of these lobar bronchi, although they can be easily approached with the flexible scope.

Localized lobar or segmental lavage may assist in removing mucoid bronchial plugs, which may lie beyond the sight of the rigid bronchoscopist. Multiple bronchial lavage has been employed, especially in patients with cystic fibrosis, with both rigid and flexible bronchoscopes, although there is still disagreement over its indication and efficacy.

Table 4–1. BRONCHOSCOPY: RIGID VERSUS FLEXIBLE

	Rigid	Flexible
Applicable ages	Almost all	All
Instrument size	2.5–10 mm *internal* lumen	*External* diameter (mm): 2.7 ultrathin 3.5 pediatric 4.7–6.3 adult
Optics	Poor without tele Excellent with tele	Good
Approach	Through mouth or tracheostomy stoma	Through nose, mouth, stoma, or tube
Penetration	Less peripheral	More peripheral
Lavage, aspiration	Easy	Not possible with smallest scope
Diagnosis	Less broad	Broader, easier
Therapy (tissue or FB removal)	Yes	Very limited

FB, foreign body; tele, telescope.

Judgment about timing may have to be made for both diagnostic and therapeutic bronchoscopy. For example, in known foreign body aspirations of longer than acute duration, a judicious delay of 2 or 3 days for good medical preparation (antibiotics, expectorants, aerosols) may make a subsequent bronchoscopy both safer and more likely to retrieve the offending foreign body than would have been the case with immediate intervention.

In acute atelectasis of either lower lobe, as in infants with otherwise uncomplicated pneumonia, it is safe to try vigorous medical therapy for 1 week before resorting to bronchoscopy. A shorter delay seems reasonable when both the middle and lower lobes on the right collapse; collapse of an entire lung usually calls for prompt intervention. Regardless of the duration of the collapse, one or more bronchoscopies should be performed before abandoning therapy or considering surgical intervention. Failure to recognize lobar collapse during pneumonia and to take the medical and bronchoscopic steps to rectify it is an established cause of preventable bronchiectasis in children.

In childhood, indications for bronchoscopy, either rigid or flexible, include stridor (e.g., laryngomalacia), atelectasis, pneumonia (especially in immunocompromised patients), persistent wheezing (in bronchodilator-unresponsive patients), hemoptysis (especially during active bleeding), foreign body aspiration, difficult intubations, tracheostomy evaluation, and others (e.g., suspected tracheoesophageal fistula, hoarseness, prolonged intubation).

The complications of bronchoscopy include subglottic edema (rare with flexible bronchoscopy), bronchial tears, pneumothorax, bleeding, hypoxia, cardiac arrhythmia, and anesthetic or drug complications. Higher risk patients are more likely to undergo rigid bronchoscopy. Procedures such as foreign body removal are inherently more risky. Flexible fiberoptic bronchoscopy, when carefully performed by skilled personnel with appropriate monitoring of the patient, has very low risks.

DIAGNOSTIC BRONCHOALVEOLAR LAVAGE

The role of diagnostic bronchoalveolar lavage (BAL) in children is still under investigation, although in adults it is used both in the investigation of noninfectious interstitial lung diseases and in the identification of infectious agents in immunocompromised patients. These important diagnostic functions have usually been thought to require open-lung biopsy in children. The advantages of diagnostic BAL compared with open-lung biopsy are its lesser degree of invasiveness and, as a result, its relatively simple repeatability.

The development of the pediatric fiberoptic bronchoscope has made possible the application of BAL to very small children. Children with tracheostomies or those on mechanical ventilators may be submitted to diagnostic BAL with special ease.

The technique, most frequently performed under local anesthesia, usually involves passage of the fiberoptic bronchoscope through the nose with its subsequent wedging in a lobar, segmental, or subsegmental bronchus. Aliquots of 5 to 30 ml of warmed normal saline solution are instilled and withdrawn repeatedly (5 to 7 times) over a period of 10 to 15 min. Examination of withdrawn fluid can include standard cultures for bacterial, viral, and mycobacterial pathogens; staining of centrifuged cells by Giemsa, silver methenamine, and Papanicolaou techniques; and evaluation for respiratory syncytial virus by the enzyme-linked immunosorbent assay (ELISA) technique.

The few reported studies of BAL in children have shown promising results. In patients with AIDS and other immunodeficiency diseases, BAL has been helpful in the diagnosis of infections with *Pneumocystis carinii,* cytomegalovirus, *Aspergillus fumigatus, Candida albicans, Legionella pneumophila,* and other pathogens. In one series (de Blic, 1987), BAL yielded a specific diagnosis in 60 per cent of 67 immunocompromised children. In another (Milburn, 1987), the procedure provided a positive diagnosis in 32 episodes of pneumonia in 24 child and adult recipients of bone marrow transplants—a diagnostic yield of 80 per cent.

Clinical investigators generally agree that diagnostic BAL with a fiberoptic bronchoscope is safe and well tolerated in children. It should be considered as a first-line investigation before open lung biopsy.

LUNG PUNCTURE

This rather old-fashioned diagnostic procedure probably deserves wider selective application, because it can yield information not otherwise easily obtained. Lung puncture has been used to obtain a lung aspirate for either histologic study or culture. The technique is simple. A short-bevel 20-gauge needle is attached to a 10-ml syringe containing 1 ml of sterile isotonic saline solution. *It is essential that the saline contain no bacteriostatic agent.* An intercostal space is locally anesthetized, and a quick stab is made through the space, across the pleurae, and into the lung to a depth of 3 to 4 cm. The saline is injected to assure patency of the needle, and negative pressure is produced in the syringe-needle system by withdrawing the plunger of the syringe. Simultaneously, the needle is withdrawn so that tissue fluid is drawn into the needle and syringe. The needle remains in the lung only a few seconds, preferably for less than one respiratory cycle. The contents of the needle and syringe may then be smeared on slides for special staining or may be transferred to a liquid culture medium by drawing up the medium into the syringe through the aspirating needle and then returning it to its original container. If the sample is sufficient, both may be accomplished. The method has been used successfully to isolate viruses, mycoplasma, and tubercle bacilli in addition to conventional bacterial pathogens. In the absence of the means to perform a diagnostic BAL, lung puncture can play a most useful role.

The procedure has theoretical dangers: pulmonary hemorrhage, empyema, and pneumothorax. In practice, the only complications have been transient, slight pneumothorax when the tap has been made into air-containing lung and rare minimal hemoptysis. One death related to the procedure has been reported by Sapington and Favorite (1936) in a series of 2000 lung taps. Pneumothorax can usually be avoided by choosing a densely consolidated segment for puncture.

LUNG BIOPSY

Biopsy of the lung is occasionally necessary when protracted pulmonary disease cannot be explained by other means, although careful and intelligent use of less extreme diagnostic procedures, especially diagnostic BAL (see above) makes it commonly unnecessary. Transbronchial biopsy through the fiberoptic bronchoscope has not been utilized extensively in the pediatric age range. When indicated, lung biopsy is usually performed under general anesthesia with an endotracheal airway, by which normal pulmonary ventilation is maintained and collapse of the lung is prevented. Open thoracotomy is performed at a site of known involvement, and sufficient pulmonary tissue is removed for all required studies. The site of biopsy should be agreed on by the pulmonologist and the surgeon. The inferior lingula is easy to biopsy, but the histology of this segment is often atypical. Therefore, it is preferably avoided. Often biopsy of more than one site is a good idea because tissue at different stages of disease involvement can then be studied. Even critically ill (hypoxic, anemic, thrombocytopenic, leukopenic) patients have successfully withstood open lung biopsy. Percutaneous lung biopsy with a Vim-Silverman or Franklin-Silverman needle and by trephine has been reported in adults but is not at present recommended for infants and children.

PNEUMOPERITONEUM

The injection of 200 to 300 cc of air into the peritoneal cavity sharply demarcates the position of the diaphragm on subsequent chest roentgenography of the erect patient. It is occasionally useful in differentiating eventration of the diaphragm from supradiaphragmatic lesions, such as extralobar sequestration. In cases of this type, confirmation of an asymptomatic localized eventration might obviate a formal surgical exploration.

ARTERIAL PUNCTURE

The quantitation of hypoxemia and hypercapnia requires precise analyses of the partial pressures of oxygen (P_{O_2}) and carbon dioxide (P_{CO_2}) in arterial blood—that is, blood that has been acted on by the lungs but in which the gaseous composition has not yet been altered by passage through the tissues. "Arterialized" capillary or venous blood has been used, but significant underestimates of P_{O_2} may result, especially in critically ill patients with poor peripheral perfusion. Blood gas analyzers are universally available in hospitals; therefore, pediatricians should be able both to obtain an anaerobic sample of arterial blood and to interpret blood gas data from the laboratory.

Vessels that can be sampled include the temporal (in neonates), brachial, radial, and femoral arteries. The brachial and radial vessels are to be preferred in older infants and children, and use of the femoral artery should be avoided because of post-tap arterial spasm.

Radial arteriopuncture is a relatively simple and safe procedure at all ages, although it is wise to test the efficacy of the ulnar collateral arterial supply by compressing the radial artery and noting that the palm does not blanch. A 2-ml glass syringe (with a plunger that slides easily in the barrel) and an attached small-gauge needle (23 to 24 gauge) are rinsed with a solution of the sodium heparin (1000 units/ml), leaving only the dead space of the syringe and needle filled. Alternately, one may use 23-gauge needle with an attached catheter ("butterfly"), the dead space of which has been filled with heparinized saline. A heparinized syringe is attached later when blood flow has been established.

I prefer to use local anesthesia (2 per cent lidocaine *without* epinephrine) in small volume so as not to disturb the vessel position or size. The puncture is made at an angle of about 45 degrees between the tips of the operator's index and middle fingers. Occlusion of the vessel with the downstream finger helps to dilate the artery (Fig. 4–1). The needle is pointed upstream with the bevel pointed down. As the artery is entered, blood will appear in the syringe

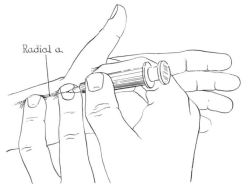

Figure 4–1. Radial arteripuncture. See text for details. (From Waring WW and Jeansonne LO III: Practical Manual of Pediatrics. 2nd ed. St. Louis, CV Mosby Co, 1982.)

(or catheter), which will fill slowly and spontaneously if the plunger is properly fitted and moistened with heparin. One should attempt to collect a full 2 ml of blood, since significant errors in P_{CO_2} occur with small samples that are diluted by dead-space heparin. The needle is removed as soon as the sample is collected, and any small air bubbles are immediately expelled. The system is then sealed by embedding the needle tip in a rubber stopper. Heparin and blood sample are mixed by vigorous rotary movement of the syringe between the palms, and the syringe is dropped into a small pan containing ice and water. Analyses should be made within minutes after collection for greatest accuracy. Firm pressure is maintained at the puncture site for 3 to 4 minutes to ensure sealing of the vessel wall.

The laboratory is usually prepared to report P_{O_2}, P_{CO_2}, and pH as well as to calculate certain secondary parameters, such as standard bicarbonate, base excess, and arterial oxygen saturation.

For patients past the neonatal period, I have found Table 4–2 of value in interpreting blood gas results. The monograph of Shapiro (1977) should be con-

sulted for further details on blood gas analysis and interpretation.

The continuing development of medical instrumentation may under certain circumstances obviate the need for arterial puncture. Such instruments include rapidly responding CO_2 analyzers for end-tidal P_{CO_2} measurement, oximeters (ear and especially pulse) for estimates of arterial oxygen saturation, and transcutaneous P_{O_2} and P_{CO_2} electrodes. Depending on age and clinical circumstances, the choice of one or more of these noninvasive instruments may be preferred to arterial blood sampling.

THERAPEUTIC PROCEDURES

BRONCHIAL (POSTURAL) DRAINAGE AND PHYSICAL THERAPY

These methods of treating bronchial disease receive considerable emphasis here because they are neither practiced as effectively nor used as frequently as they should be. Bronchial drainage is indicated in any clinical situation in which excessive fluid in the bronchi is not being removed by normal ciliary activity and cough. Determination of the presence of excessive bronchial fluid and its localization are most easily accomplished by segmental auscultation of the lungs. Persistent crackles in a given segment or lobe constitute a sufficient indication in themselves of the need for drainage of the involved bronchi.

Examination of the anatomy of the tracheobronchial tree (Fig. 4–2) indicates that in the erect position the segments of the middle lobe, of the lingular division of the left upper lobe, and of both lower lobes normally must drain against gravity. Only the segments of the right upper lobe and the nonlingular portions of the left upper lobe receive gravitational assistance in the erect human. Normally, such a situation does not interfere with the body's ability to maintain patency of the tracheobronchial tree. Special loads, however, may be placed on the clearing mechanisms of the relatively small bronchi of children by viscous or excessive mucus and pus. It is axiomatic that infection is ultimately superimposed on bronchial obstruction due to any cause and that infection increases obstruction. Although bronchial drainage may not be the principal or sole therapy, it can be of invaluable assistance. After bronchoscopic removal of a foreign body, after administration of a bronchodilator to an asthmatic child, or during the resolution of a pneumonia, excessive fluid may remain in one or more lobar or segmental bronchi. The affected bronchi can be identified by the topographic distribution of crackles as well as by roentgenograms. The physician then can determine the position in which to place the patient that best promotes drainage of the involved bronchi (Figs. 4–3 and 4–4).

Bronchial drainage is carried out three or four times daily, usually before meals and at bedtime, for

Table 4–2. BLOOD GAS AND ACID-BASE INTERPRETATION

pH
(Normal = 7.350–7.450)

ACIDOSIS		ALKALOSIS	
Mild:	7.300–7.350	Mild:	7.450–7.500
Mod.:	7.250–7.300	Mod.:	7.500–7.550
Severe:	<7.250	Severe:	>7.550

P_{CO_2}
(Normal = 35–45 mm Hg)

HYPERCAPNIA		HYPOCAPNIA	
Mild:	45–50	Mild:	30–45
Mod.:	50–60	Mod.:	25–30
Severe:	>60	Severe:	<25

P_{O_2}
(Sea level, room air, normal = >85 mm Hg)

HYPOXEMIA	
Mild:	55–85
Mod.:	40–55
Severe:	<40

Standard Bicarbonate
(Normal = 22–28 mEq/L)

DEPRESSION		ELEVATION	
Mild:	19–22	Mild:	28–31
Mod.:	17–19	Mod.:	31–35
Severe:	< 17	Severe:	>35

Base Excess
(Normal = −3 to +4)

Depression		Elevation	
Mild:	−3 to −7	Mild:	+4 to +8
Mod.:	−7 to −10	Mod.:	+8 to +12
Severe:	< −10	Severe:	> +12

Text continued on page 87

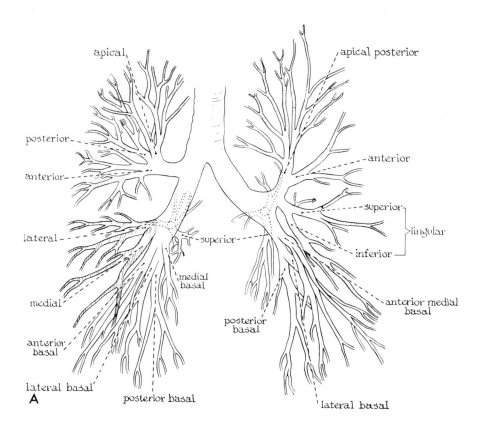

apical

apical posterior

posterior

anterior

anterior

superior

lingular

lateral

inferior

superior

medial basal

medial

anterior medial basal

anterior basal

posterior basal

lateral basal

A

posterior basal

lateral basal

Figure 4–2. Distribution of lobar and segmental bronchi. Upper lobe bronchi are stippled, middle lobe bronchi are diagonally lined, and lower lobe bronchi are outlined only. Segmental bronchi are labeled. *A,* Anteroposterior projection. *B,* Lateral projection of right bronchi, as viewed from the mediastinum.

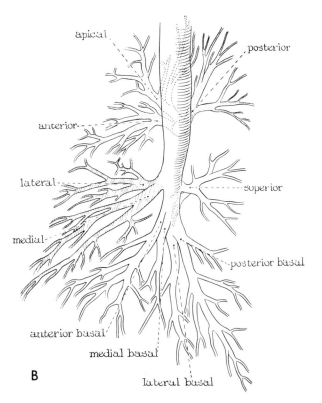

apical

posterior

anterior

lateral

superior

medial

posterior basal

anterior basal

medial basal

lateral basal

B

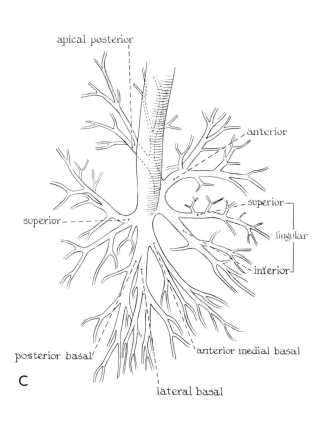

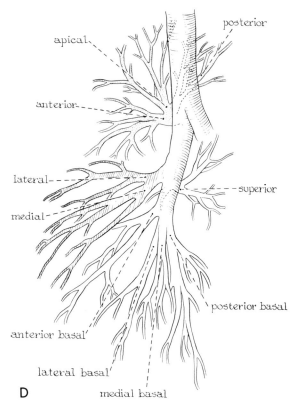

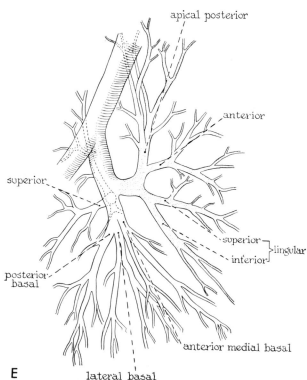

Figure 4–2 *Continued C,* Lateral projection of left bronchi, as viewed from the mediastinum. *D,* Right posterior oblique projection of right bronchi. *E,* Left posterior oblique projection of left bronchi.

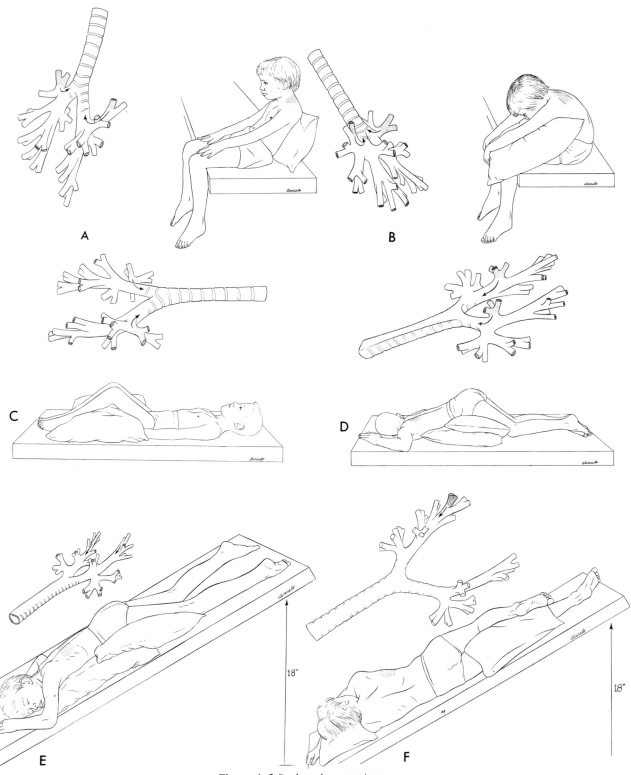

Figure 4–3 *See legend on opposite page*

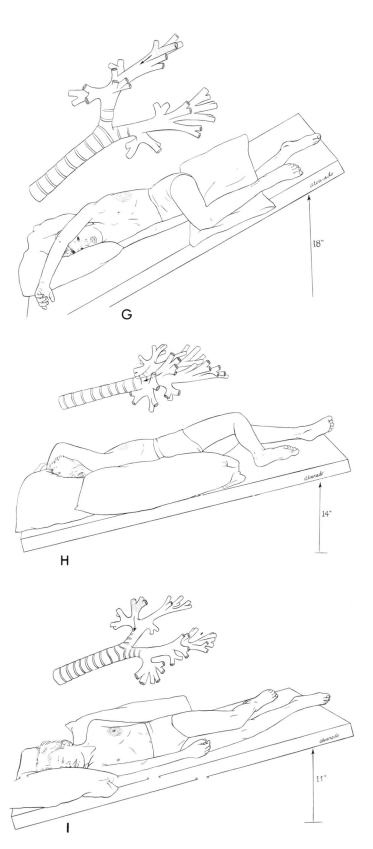

Figure 4–3. Bronchial drainage positions for the major segments of all lobes in a child. In each position, a model of the tracheobronchial tree is projected beside the picture of child to show the segmental bronchus being drained (*stippled area*) and the flow of secretions out of the segmental bronchus (*arrow*). The drainage platform is padded but firm, and pillows are liberally used to maintain each position with comfort. The platform is horizontal unless otherwise noted. A stippled area on the child's chest indicates the area to be "cupped" or vibrated by the therapist (see text). *A,* Apical segment of right upper lobe and apical subsegment of apical-posterior segment of left upper lobe. Drainage moves secretions into main bronchi (*curved arrows*), from which they can be more easily expelled. *B,* Posterior segment of right upper lobe and posterior subsegment of apical-posterior segment of left upper lobe. Drainage moves secretions into main bronchi (*curved arrows*), from which they can be more easily expelled. *C,* Anterior segments of both upper lobes. The child should be rotated slightly away from the side being drained. *D,* Superior segments of both lower lobes. Although the platform is flat, pillows are used to raise the buttocks moderately. *E,* Posterior basal segments of both lower lobes. The platform is tilted as shown. *F,* Lateral basal segment of the right lower lobe. The platform is tilted as shown. Drainage of the lateral basal segment of the left lower lobe would be accomplished by a mirror image of this position (right side down). *G,* Anterior basal segment of the left lower lobe. The platform is tilted as shown. *H,* Right middle lobe. The platform is tilted as shown. *I,* Lingular segments of the left upper lobe (homologue of the right middle lobe). The platform is tilted as shown.

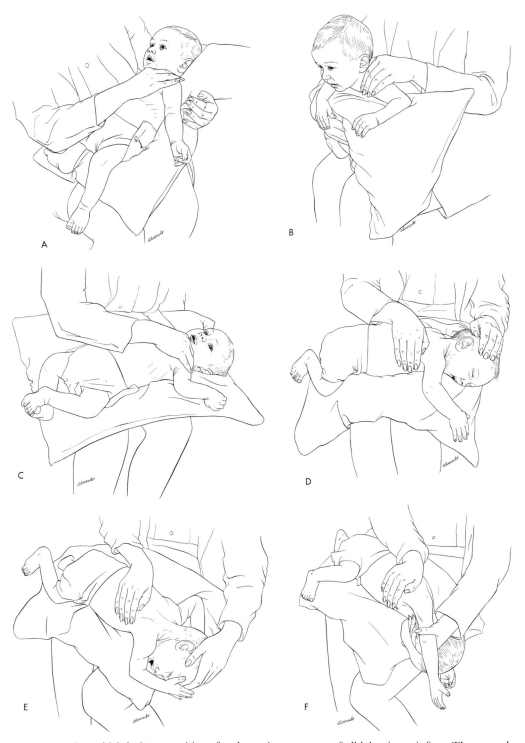

Figure 4–4. Bronchial drainage positions for the major segments of all lobes in an infant. The procedure is most easily carried out in the therapist's lap. The therapist's hand on the chest indicates the area to be "cupped" or vibrated (see text). *A,* Apical segment of the left upper lobe. *B,* Posterior segment of the left upper lobe. *C,* Anterior segment of the left upper lobe. *D,* Superior segment of the right lower lobe. *E,* Posterior segment of the right lower lobe. *F,* Lateral segment of the right lower lobe.

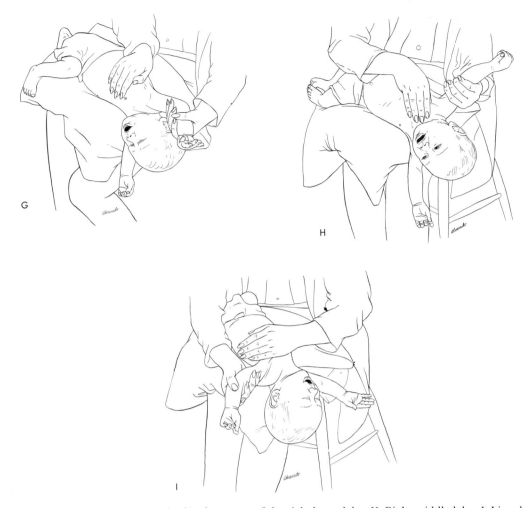

Figure 4–4 *Continued G,* Anterior basal segment of the right lower lobe. *H,* Right middle lobe. *I,* Lingular segments of the left upper lobe.

periods not exceeding 30 min. Up to four positions may be used, because more than this number tends to exceed reasonable limits of cooperation. The exact arrangements for drainage vary with the situation: the physical therapy department, bed, or treatment room if the child is hospitalized; the bedroom if the child is at home. Infants may be positioned on the lap and legs of a parent, and small children may be effectively drained while lying on a padded ironing board.

Children with chronic bronchial disease, such as cystic fibrosis or bronchiectasis, may require daily periods of drainage over many months. They will profit from specially constructed tables or platforms, the surfaces of which can be padded for comfort and adjusted to the different angles required to drain all involved segments (Fig. 4–5). Comfort is important because adequate drainage depends on relaxation and cooperation in each position for 5 to 15 min. Utilization of chest physical therapy in a specific patient may be discontinued when auscultation reveals that no excessive bronchial fluid remains and when the chest roentgenogram indicates clearing of the disease.

In all cases, the exact positions, as well as their order, duration, and frequency, should be explained to the person (parent, nurse, or therapist) who will be working with the child. At least one treatment should be demonstrated on the patient to parents or others who are unfamiliar with the techniques. Positions for drainage are varied subsequently by the physician in accordance with shifting patterns of bronchial disease. The family should have diagrams

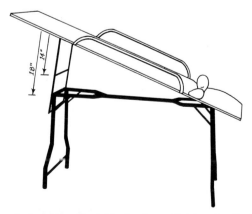

Figure 4–5. Adjustable table for bronchial (postural) drainage (Greater Cleveland Cystic Fibrosis Chapter, 2490 Lee Boulevard, Suite 301, Cleveland Heights, Ohio 44118). The surface measures 15½″ × 71″ and is padded but firm. The top adjusts from horizontal to two inclinations, a shallow one for the lingula and the right middle lobe and a deep one for the basal segments of the lower lobes.

to which reference may be made until they are thoroughly familiar with the prescribed positions.

If bronchorrhea is diffuse without any specific localization, it is reasonable to emphasize positions that will drain major dependent bronchi when the child is in the erect position; the posterior basal segments, the middle lobe, and the lingula, in that order. Drainage positions for the upper lobes may also be of importance for predominantly recumbent infants.

Certain physical therapeutic maneuvers are of great help when combined with bronchial drainage. Indeed, the modern concept of bronchial drainage implies the use of such maneuvers in addition to simple positioning of the patient. Viscid secretions may not drain from bronchi by gravity alone. The analogy of a freshly opened bottle of catsup is often used to explain this concept: although the bottle is inverted, i.e., properly positioned for drainage, no catsup may flow until it is ejected by repeated blows on the bottom of the bottle; once started, however, flow may continue with little further agitation.

The maneuvers that may assist the removal of fluid by gravity include deep breathing, reinforced cough, thoracic "squeezing," "cupping," and vibration. Each is briefly described.

After being placed in position for drainage and being encouraged to relax, the child is asked to take several deep breaths. Because deep inspiration enlarges the tracheobronchial tree, air may penetrate around and through secretions that would not be affected by usual tidal volumes. Expiration following such a deep breath may carry secretions in the desired direction and may even initiate a productive cough.

The child should be taught not to suppress a cough and not to waste energy with repeated feeble, and therefore ineffective, coughs. Instead, the child should take a deep breath and cough once or twice forcefully. Such anticipated coughs can be reinforced by the hands of the operator encircling and synchronously compressing the sides of the lower half of the chest. The cough may thus be less fatiguing and more effective. Many children are not able to cough well in a dependent position. These children should be allowed to sit up after several minutes of drainage for a further trial of repeated, reinforced coughs. Sputum produced should be spit out into a container so that the productivity of the treatment can be demonstrated to both the child and the physician.

With the child in a bronchial drainage position, another maneuver, the "squeeze," may be tried. The child is asked to take a deep breath and then to exhale through the mouth as completely and rapidly as possible, as would be done for a forced expiratory volume determination. The depth of expiration is increased by brief, firm pressure from the operator's hands compressing the sides of the thorax. The goal is to decrease maximally the volume of the tracheobronchial tree. Secretions may thus be expressed from the "open ends" of the bronchi, similar to the squeezing of toothpaste from a tube. The subsequent inspiration may be followed by a most productive cough, which should again be "reinforced" by the operator.

The maneuver known as "cupping" or "clapping" is performed intermittently several times in each drainage position. One or both of the cupped hands of the operator vigorously and repeatedly strike *that part of the chest under which the segments being drained are located.* Although "cupping" should be vigorous, it is painless if performed properly. The patient should wear a light cotton undershirt to avoid irritation of the skin of the chest. Care should be taken not to slap the chest with the fingers or palm but to make the cupped hand conform exactly to the contour of the chest wall. No jewelry should be worn on the hands of the therapist. The entire circumference of the hand should touch the chest at the same instant. A proper "cupping" emits a definitely hollow sound. The effect of "cupping" is related partly to the compression of air between the operator's hand and the patient's chest wall. This compression wave is presumably transmitted to the underlying bronchi and aids the gravitational flow of secretions from them.

Vibration is a more difficult procedure and, therefore, is usually effectively executed only by a therapist. A rapid vibratory impulse is transmitted through the chest wall from the flattened hands of the operator by an almost isometric contraction of forearm flexor and extensor muscles. Vibration may be used directly over the involved area, or it may be applied to the sides of the chest in performing the chest "squeeze" maneuver.

If the operator is a parent, he or she can easily be taught the maneuvers of deep breathing, reinforced coughing, and "cupping." More advanced techniques should be reserved for the trained therapist or for the intelligent parent with a child who will require bronchial drainage over months or years.

Danish clinicians have recommended positive expiratory pressure as an aid to chest physical therapy in cystic fibrosis. Resistance to expiration is provided by a face mask and a one-way valve with attachable connections to provide variable resistances.

Because bronchial drainage is both fatiguing and time consuming, efforts have been made to introduce mechanical vibration of various types as a substitute for cupping and vibrating. These have ranged from simple "barber shop" massage-vibrators, through modified saber-saws with a piston and padded cushion replacing the blade, to larger percussion devices designed for hospital use. The evaluation of such equipment is extremely difficult. It probably ranges from ineffective to less effective than a trained therapist. Nevertheless, the more rugged of these devices are probably of value and can be employed by adolescents away from home or by children whose parents are unable to carry out the procedure at home because of conflicting work hours, arthritis, or other reasons.

Bronchial drainage has also been advocated as a means of removing aspirated foreign bodies from the tracheobronchial tree. The method is hazardous, however, and is not recommended except for removal of very small fragments. It should never be employed outside a hospital intensive care setting, in which emergency endoscopy is immediately available.

The efficacy of conventional physical therapy in delaying the decline in pulmonary function of patients with cystic fibrosis has been reported in a 3-year prospective study from Toronto by Reisman and associates (1988). Although many investigators believe that drainage procedures of the types described previously are effective in clinical situations associated with bronchorrhea, there is a division of opinion as to their prophylactic value in patients who are expected, because of their disease (cystic fibrosis), to develop chronic bronchitis and bronchiectasis. Nevertheless, some physicians routinely prescribe prophylactic bronchial drainage as soon as a diagnosis of cystic fibrosis is made, even in the absence of any evidence of pulmonary disease.

BREATHING EXERCISES

Breathing exercises have not been widely applied in children but may be of value in certain patients, including those with kyphoscoliosis, cystic fibrosis, asthma, and bronchiectasis, as well as those who have had extensive resections of diseased lung. There are few data available with which to argue the efficacy of the various breathing exercise programs. If applied, however, exercises should be a part of a total therapeutic program that frequently also includes correction of posture, bronchial drainage, and various types of inhalation therapy.

Goals of the exercises include (1) development of more effective diaphragmatic and lower costal breathing; (2) relaxation of all muscles, but especially those of the upper part of the chest, shoulder girdle, and neck; and (3) attainment of a good, easy posture.

AEROBIC EXERCISE AND FITNESS

There has been considerable interest in and research on aerobic exercise and conditioning in children with chronic or recurrent lung disease. There are obvious psychologic benefits for such children if their physical limitations can be partially circumvented to make them more like their healthy peers. The data on the effects and role of aerobic fitness in both cystic fibrosis and asthma have been reviewed by Orenstein (1988). It is not known whether exercise can replace chest physical therapy and postural drainage treatments in patients with cystic fibrosis. However, such programs can increase the physical working capacity of such patients, which will have obvious ramifications for the quality of their lives. Like children with cystic fibrosis, asthmatics can in-

crease their working capacity, and, if treated before each exercise session with a bronchodilator, they can also improve their aerobic fitness. There is no evidence that exercise has any appreciable effect on exercise-induced bronchospasm.

RESPIRATORY THERAPY

The term *respiratory therapy* is an ever-enlarging one that covers the theory and practice of treating a patient by making certain changes in the composition, volume, or pressure of inspired gases; by adapting to his needs all types of equipment, including respirators; and by judiciously combining ventilatory and respiratory physical therapy support. A full discussion of respiratory therapy and its application to children would require a text in itself. Only certain aspects of this field can be alluded to here, but the physician caring for children with respiratory disease is urged to become familiar with the goals and methods of respiratory therapy and with a few specific items of equipment.

Oxygen Therapy

Although extensively used in hospitals for many years in the treatment of children with pulmonary disease, oxygen therapy is moving increasingly from the hospital to the home for infants with bronchopulmonary dysplasia or for older children and adolescents with severe chronic pulmonary disease, especially cystic fibrosis. In one series of 137 patients, Givan and Wylie (1986) noted that about one third required oxygen at home for bronchopulmonary dysplasia, another one third for cystic fibrosis and heart disease, and the remaining one third for mixed causes, including interstitial lung disease, aspiration syndromes, sleep hypoventilation, neuromuscular disease, upper airway obstruction, and hypoplastic lung disease.

Oxygen should be given when significant reductions in its partial pressure in arterial blood are present and when such reductions can be significantly elevated by increasing alveolar oxygen concentrations. Children with anatomic right-to-left shunts, such as those with tetralogy of Fallot, may neither require nor benefit from oxygen. The presence of cyanosis remains the best single clinical criterion for supplemental oxygen. It is a late sign, however, because a considerable drop in the partial pressure of oxygen in arterial blood must occur before cyanosis is detectable. Oxygen alone will not relieve dyspnea, and, depending on the cause of dyspnea, a more rational therapy might be a bronchodilator administered by metered dose inhaler or nebulizer.

When oxygen is indicated, it may be given by mask, face tent, nasal catheter or cannula, head hood, intermittent positive pressure breathing apparatus, or conventional oxygen tent. The method of choice depends on the ventilatory status of the child, the percentage of oxygen desired in the inspired air, and the anticipated duration of need. For most clinical circumstances, an inspired oxygen concentration of 30 to 50 per cent (FIO_2 of 0.3 to 0.5) is satisfactory. There has been a steadily increasing use of nasal or nasopharyngeal delivery systems (cannula or catheter), which separate the child from the environment less than other methods, require the least possible oxygen usage, and, of the various delivery systems, seem to be best tolerated. Attempts have been made to estimate FIO_2 in the use of both a nasal cannula and a nasopharyngeal catheter in infants.

The use of oxygen at home has been facilitated by the variety of ways (and concentrations) in which it can be supplied there, including compressed gas in various sized cylinders (100 per cent), liquid oxygen (100 per cent), oxygen concentrators (about 90 per cent), and oxygen enrichers (30 to 40 per cent). A combination of systems may be required both for continuous nocturnal use and for essentially unimpeded mobility during the day. With the exception of the oxygen enricher, the systems mentioned provide dry oxygen, which should be humidified before delivery to the patient. In the hospital, it is possible both to warm and to saturate inspired gas with water. This is seldom practical at home, however, where a simple bubble aerator is usually used to provide about 40 per cent humidification.

In bronchopulmonary dysplasia optimal cardiopulmonary support of the older infant requires maintenance of arterial oxygen saturations (SaO_2) of 90 to 95 per cent, and nasal cannula flow rates are set at the lowest flow that will achieve such saturations. Oxygen requirements are greater during sleeping and eating than during the awake and quiet state. Accordingly, oxygen flows may require adjustment for these changes in activity. Oxygen needs can be assessed during periodic brief hospitalizations or in the clinic by means of pulse oximetry. In older children with stable pulmonary disease due to cystic fibrosis it has been shown that nocturnal low-flow oxygen is effective in alleviating nocturnal hypoxemia.

Oxygen concentrations of inspired gas can be determined by devices that employ principles of thermal conductivity, paramagnetic susceptibility, and membrane diffusion in an electrode. It is also possible to monitor arterial oxygen saturation by ear or pulse oximetry or by partial pressure within the patient himself by a transcutaneous PO_2 probe or by conventional blood gas analysis.

The administration of oxygen, either at home or in the hospital, should not be continued after indications for its use no longer exist. This seldom occurs in the older patient with cystic fibrosis and diffuse interstitial fibrosis. However, in infants with bronchopulmonary dysplasia, oxygen may be tapered off and finally discontinued when the infant has shown an ability to maintain arterial oxygen saturations above 95 per cent. Even so, it is a cautious practice to maintain minimal oxygen flows during the night for 1 or 2 months longer than saturations would dictate in such patients.

To the extent that oxygen reduces the partial pressure of nitrogen in alveoli, it increases the rate of lung collapse in the event of airway obstruction. Excessive and prolonged concentrations are related to the production of retrolental fibroplasia and play a significant role in bronchopulmonary dysplasia in newborn infants. Moreover, the lung can be injured at *any* age by excessive and prolonged inspired oxygen concentrations.

Aerosol Therapy

Aerosol therapy is designed to prevent or treat respiratory disease by the inhalation and subsequent deposition of air-borne water particles. In addition, these particles may contain specific bronchodilating, decongestant, mucolytic, antimicrobial, or other agents. Particle sizes range from a fraction of a micron in diameter to droplets larger even than 50 microns. Aerosol therapy may be either intermittent and brief (a single inhalation) or continuous and prolonged (hours at a time). The former technique is usually employed for the purpose of delivering a specific pharmacologic agent to the respiratory tract. The latter is always used to deliver water to the airways, usually with the goal of thinning secretions. The kind of equipment chosen for aerosol therapy largely depends on whether the physician wants to treat the patient continuously (hours at a time) or intermittently (for 20 or 30 min).

It is implicit in all forms of aerosol therapy that the nebulized material is distributed in accordance with gas flow patterns within the lung. Unventilated areas of the lung thus receive none of the aerosol; this is important in obstructive lung disease, especially if atelectasis is present.

Aerosols for clinical use are produced by nebulizers, which act as repositories for the solution to be nebulized and generate visible aerosol mists when connected to a source of gas under pressure (oxygen cylinder, hand bulb, or powered oil-free air compressor). By suitable internal construction, a nebulizer can be made to baffle out large particles and deliver a spectrum of particles over the desired range of diameters.

Water may exist in inspired air either in the form of vapor or in the form of droplets. Regardless of its initial water content or initial temperature, inspired air is warmed to body temperature and essentially is fully saturated with water in the upper respiratory tract. The alveoli thus receive air containing about 44 mg of water in invisible vapor form per liter of gas. Air holds more water when fully saturated at 37°C than at room temperature, so full saturation of inspired air under ordinary conditions can occur only by an obligatory transfer of water from the mucosa of the respiratory tract. Only about 20 to 25 per cent of the heat and water transferred to inspired air is normally recovered during expiration. This obligatory transfer can be diminished, however, by warming and fully saturating inspired air. Additionally, if water is added to inspired gas in the form of particles, it is possible to achieve a positive net delivery of water to the respiratory tract.

Aside from the total water output of the nebulizers, the distribution of the aerosol mass into various sizes of particles is certainly a critical factor in considering levels of deposition. Particles larger than 10 μ probably do not penetrate beyond the upper airway, whereas intermediate particles (measuring 1 to 10 μ) achieve deeper penetration, and submicronic (smaller than 1 μ) particles in theory reach the alveolar level. The largest particles are deposited by inertial impaction, the intermediate are deposited by sedimentation, and the smallest are subject to diffusion forces.

In asthma, continuous water mist tent therapy seems to have a variable effect and is not recommended. Intermittent aerosol therapy for the purpose of delivering a specific bronchodilating agent, such as isoproterenol or albuterol, has a definite beneficial effect, promptly improving airway mechanics but paradoxically, in some patients, causing increased unevenness in ventilation-perfusion relationships. Aerosolized racemic epinephrine, delivered either by intermittent positive pressure apparatus or by nonpressure nebulizer, has been advocated for the treatment of infectious croup and postintubation laryngeal edema and tracheitis.

Aerosol therapy also appears to have an important role in maintaining normal airway patency in patients with tracheostomies and in patients with other types of artificial airways, such as orotracheal or nasotracheal tubes, especially if they are also being mechanically ventilated. However, in most cases, aerosols are not required if inspired gas can be delivered fully saturated with water at body temperature.

Intermittent inhalation of aerosols of 20 per cent or less N-acetylcysteine has been advocated and widely used for a mucolytic action. Although testimonial evidence supports its beneficial action, studies have failed to show improvement in pulmonary function after its aerosolization.

Aerosol therapy does not appear to have a beneficial role in the treatment of respiratory distress syndrome or bronchiolitis of viral cause in infancy.

With regard to the harmful effects of aerosol therapy, there has been strong circumstantial evidence relating excessive use of concentrated isoproterenol aerosols and asthma deaths. In addition, failure to control bacterial growth in aerosol equipment or in nebulized solutions has led to serious and even fatal gram-negative bacterial infections in immunocompromised patients. Parents should be given detailed instructions on how to clean respiratory therapy equipment at home. The availability of disposable equipment has undoubtedly been valuable in reducing nosocomial infections.

There is general agreement that the coupling of aerosol therapy and chest physical therapy is probably beneficial.

Air compressor–driven nebulizers have been commonly used to administer bronchodilating agents to children with asthma or cystic fibrosis (with reactive airways). The chief advantage of such a delivery system is the lack of need for cooperation. As a result, aerosols can be administered to crying, dyspneic infants with relative ease. Effective delivery depends on (1) a compressor that will provide a gas flow of approximately 6 L/min and (2) a dilution of the agent in the nebulizer to a volume of 3 to 4 ml. In many emergency rooms, the oxygen-driven nebulizer with a beta₂ agent has replaced subcutaneous epinephrine as the initial treatment of status asthmaticus.

The safety and efficacy of nebulized beta₂ agonists (metaproterenol, terbutaline) have been evaluated retrospectively in a group of 22 inner-city children with severe, perennial, reversible asthma. There were significant reductions in the number of emergency room visits, hospital admissions, and required courses of oral prednisone after initiation of such home nebulizer therapy.

The development of new, selective beta₂ agonists (terbutaline, albuterol), the anticholinergic ipratropium bromide, cromolyn sodium, and topical corticosteroids (beclomethasone dipropionate, triamcinolone) to control reactive airways disease has led to studies on how best to administer them. These studies, done first on adults and later on older children, have shown that the metered dose inhaler (MDI), especially with a spacer, has begun to supplant the traditional compressor and nebulizer.

The MDI has the great advantages of being compact, portable, and inconspicuous. Because it is self-powered and drug dosage is automatic, no bulky compressor or medication measuring is required. It is the device of choice for children over 6 to 7 years of age. Although differences of opinion exist on the best way to use the MDI, the usual technique involves (1) shaking the inhaler and then removing its cap, (2) holding the inhaler upright and exhaling fully, (3) closing the lips around the mouthpiece, (4) activating (by pressing) the inhaler while inspiring deeply and slowly, and (5) holding one's breath at full inspiration for at least 10 sec. If the dose is to be repeated, the patient waits for about 1 min and then repeats the above steps. Some recommend, in place of step 3, activating the inhaler a few centimeters in front of the open mouth after inspiration has begun. Whichever method is chosen, the technique calls for what has been called "hand-lung coordination," which is frequently lacking in small children and even in some adults.

In part to circumvent hand-lung uncoordination, spacers have been developed that can be inserted between the MDI and the mouth of the patient. The inhaler is activated, delivering the dose into the spacer, from which the patient slowly inhales. Because large particles of medication are retained in the spacer (rather than being ineffectively deposited in the oropharynx), many recommend that all patients use spacers when inhaling corticosteroids. This tends to reduce the incidence of both oropharyngeal candidiasis and hoarseness that have been associated with long-term use of these agents.

An additional application of spacers has been in younger children in whom the compressor-nebulizer technique for aerosol therapy has been thought to be necessary. Sly and associates (1988) have shown that the MDI and spacer (Aerochamber) can be effective in asthmatic children as young as 3 years of age.

THERAPEUTIC BRONCHOALVEOLAR LAVAGE

The instillation of varying quantities of liquids into the tracheobronchial tree has been advocated in adults for the treatment of pulmonary alveolar proteinosis and obstructive pulmonary diseases (chronic bronchitis and status asthmaticus). In children, the technique was first advocated for cystic fibrosis more than 20 years ago. The techniques have varied widely and have ranged from limited lobar lavage through multifocal bilateral lavages to total unilateral bronchoalveolar lavage (with a Carlens catheter to ventilate the contralateral lung).

The purpose of lavage in cystic fibrosis is to wash out trapped accumulations of mucopus from extensively bronchiectatic airways. Patients have been selected in various ways. Usually patients include children with (1) failure of response to conventional but vigorous medical therapy; (2) diffuse pulmonary disease, presumably bronchiectasis; and (3) decreased pulmonary function without respiratory failure.

Both transient decreases in pulmonary function and postlavage pneumonias are commonly observed. Therapeutic BAL should not be attempted in critically or terminally ill patients or in the absence of expert pediatric anesthetic assistance and intensive care facilities.

Although it is quite possible that selective lavage is an effective form of therapy in cystic fibrosis, the controlled prospective studies to establish its efficacy in cystic fibrosis have not been performed. After reviewing all available data, Sherman (1986) concluded that evidence at that time did not support the use of therapeutic BAL in cystic fibrosis unless that use would be in a manner to obtain objective, controlled data.

PLEURAL SPACE DRAINAGE AND DECOMPRESSION

The insertion of a soft catheter between the ribs for draining or decompressing the pleural space is commonly employed, especially in neonates with pneumothorax resulting from pulmonary interstitial emphysema and mechanical ventilation. In older infants empyema or pyopneumothorax, complica-

tions of bacterial pneumonia, may require such therapy. In children and young adults with cystic fibrosis, the rupture of pulmonary apical bullae may produce life-threatening pneumothorax. Depending on the circumstances, tube placement may be effected without moving the patient or may be semielectively carried out in a treatment room or an operating room. Such drainage serves to remove fluid or gas that may restrict pulmonary function, unduly prolong a septic process, or cause fibrotic imprisonment of the lung in a partially collapsed state.

Soft rubber catheters are generally used, because they are available in a variety of sizes and have the desirable combination of flexibility and relative incompressibility. Several additional holes are cut near the tip so that drainage will not be stopped by occlusion of a single orifice. The catheter is secured to the chest wall and is usually connected to a drainage-suction system that is simultaneously capable of removing large volumes of gas, collecting effluvia, and applying a negative pressure of 15 to 18 cm H_2O at the catheter holes.

The insertion of such tubes is always indicated in pyopneumothorax and tension pneumothorax. Their application to empyema without pneumothorax is less absolute, because some prefer to use intermittent thoracentesis to drain empyemas in children. It is true that almost all pleural effusions in the course of acute pneumonias in childhood can be easily drained by one or two needle aspirations, since they are thin and usually sterile. But if the fluid is frankly purulent and is present in more than trace quantities, needle drainage is usually inadequate, and the more effective tube should be inserted. Tube placement is dependent on the type and site of pathology in each case. Pneumothorax decompression usually requires an anterior upper thoracic insertion site, whereas drainage of fluid usually requires a posterolateral insertion.

In empyema without bronchopleural fistula, the tube should remain until drainage has ceased and the patient's temperature is essentially normal. In late empyema, the tendency of the pus to loculate in various parts of the pleural space may require repositioning of the catheter or insertion of another catheter. In most patients it is possible to discontinue pleural drainage after 1 week. In pyopneumothorax, the tube must remain until the bronchopleural fistula has closed; in some cases this may require 3 weeks or more of suction. Depending on the adequacy of antibiotic therapy, it is usually possible to remove the tube in less than 10 days when closure of the fistula is indicated by cessation of bubbling of the underwater portion of the system. Before removing the tube in pyopneumothorax, it is wise to clamp it for 24 hours, at the end of which time a chest roentgenogram should be taken to ascertain whether the fistula is truly closed.

In patients with cystic fibrosis and pneumothorax, some decision is generally required regarding what means, if any, will be employed to prevent a recurrence of lung rupture. These include instillation of pleurodesing agents through the tube before it is removed.

BRONCHOTOMY

Occasionally a lobar or segmental bronchus may harbor obstructing material that can be removed only by a direct surgical attack on the involved bronchus at the point of obstruction. Successful bronchotomy demands exact anatomic localization of the pathologic process before operating. It is usually possible to achieve such precision by combining information from physical examination, chest roentgenography, bronchoscopy, and bronchography. It is presumed that the lung distal to the point of obstruction is not permanently damaged, because if it were, the treatment of choice would be segmental or lobar resection.

TRACHEOSTOMY

Tracheostomy may be a life-saving procedure, the indications for which have been divided into six categories: (1) mechanical obstruction of the upper airway (croup, epiglottitis, foreign body, laryngeal paralysis); (2) disease of the central nervous system (head injury, craniotomy, drug depression); (3) neuromuscular disease (poliomyelitis, tetanus, myasthenia gravis, amyotonia congenita); (4) secretional obstruction (debility with weak cough, painful thoracic or abdominal incision); (5) intrinsic acute or chronic disease with disturbances of gas diffusion or distribution (blunt chest injuries, smoke inhalation, widespread pneumonia); and (6) prophylaxis (radical head and neck surgery). The availability of endotracheal tubes that are well tolerated for prolonged periods, the ever-increasing expertise of pediatricians and anesthesiologists in intubation techniques, and the development of pediatric intensive care units have challenged the use of tracheostomy for several of its previously well-established indications. It is safe to say that tracheostomy currently is performed rarely for acute airway obstruction in which the need for an artificial airway is anticipated not to exceed a few days or weeks. Nevertheless, it remains the airway of choice for most congenital upper airway anomalies, neoplasms, airway burns, and instances of severe trauma to the larynx or upper trachea.

The procedure is almost always done on an elective basis, and even in an emergency, an endotracheal airway (bronchoscope or endotracheal tube) can almost always be inserted before the operation. Although opinions differ on the best surgical techniques, many surgeons prefer a horizontal skin incision with a vertical tracheal incision in the third to fifth tracheal rings without resection of cartilage. The addition of traction sutures facilitates the prompt reinsertion of a tracheostomy tube in the event of accidental decannulation during the first week or two after surgery.

Aberdeen's development, more than 20 years ago, of tracheostomy tubes anatomically designed to fit the necks and tracheas of infants and children was a milestone in the history of pediatric tracheostomy. His use of polyvinylchloride (PVC) permitted a degree of flexibility that enhanced the conforming design of these tubes, increased their comfort, and reduced some of the most serious complications of tracheostomy. Although still available, the silver Hollinger and metal Jackson tracheostomy tubes are being used less often as the Aberdeen-type tubes of PVC (Shiley, Franklin/Searle, Portex) or silicone (Dow Corning) have become available.

Cuffed tubes of all types are generally considered more hazardous because of the greater chance of tracheal damage that can result in scarring with stenosis. Conventional flexible endotracheal tubes of the anesthesia type, either cuffed or uncuffed, are not recommended for tracheostomy because of possible plugging at the tip and difficulties in maintaining proper positioning.

The size of the tube can be preselected, but for all patients the tube must be large enough for effortless gas exchange without excessive pressure inside the trachea. The operator should have tubes both larger and smaller than the size anticipated. The smaller sizes are available in various lengths and bevel angles. Prompt postoperative anteroposterior and lateral roentgenograms are essential; they allow the physician to determine the exact position of the tube (if radiopaque) with respect to the trachea and carina and then to make any necessary adjustments or revisions. They also reveal the presence and extent of pneumothorax and pneumomediastinum.

Accidental decannulation is probably the most common serious complication of tracheostomy, the prevention of which depends on proper securing of the tube itself and selection of appropriate hardware with which to connect the tube to a source of inspired and humidified gas. Downes and Schreiner (1985) have termed this combination of tracheostomy tube and connecting tubing the *tracheostomy system* and have listed the attributes of an ideal tracheostomy system: (1) the tube itself must conform to the trachea and soft tissues, must not collapse or kink, must be composed of material with minimal tissue toxicity, and must be wholly or partly (its tip) radiopaque; (2) its neckplate must conform to the infant's or child's neck and have reinforced eyelets to prevent tearing from the various ties that secure its tracheal placement; (3) its connection to the gas source must be by a swivel attachment that is low profile and double in its action, with a flexible, short, nonkinkable extension tube; and (4) the system must have a suction port (with cap) in line with the lumen of the tube. Optional tube features for this "ideal" system include a beveled tube tip (30 degrees or less), removable inner cannula, and stylet.

The postoperative care of a child with a tracheostomy is crucial. He requires psychologic and physical support, which is best supplied by the constant attendance of a nurse experienced in tracheostomy care in a pediatric intensive care unit. Vital signs must be regularly monitored, but continuous monitoring of arterial oxygen saturation by a pulse oximeter with a "low" saturation alarm is recommended. The trachea should be suctioned gently by special sterile catheters. The attendant must be aware of the need to suction the oropharynx occasionally, because vomitus and secretions accumulating there may be aspirated into the lungs between a loose-fitting cannula and the inner wall of the trachea.

A spare tube and stylet of the proper size should be kept at the bedside in the event that the tube becomes dislodged and requires replacement. A cannula dislodged during the first 2 days may be extremely difficult to replace. A good light, soft-tissue "spreaders," and skill are required immediately in such a circumstance. After a few days, a tract is usually sufficiently established to allow easy reinsertion.

Provision should be made for humidifying inspired gas, because the wetting, warming, and filtering functions of the upper airway are now inoperative. Although plastic "collars" that allow aerosols to be delivered directly to a tracheostomy are available, they may not work for infants or young children; hence the need of a customized tracheostomy "system," as outlined above.

The tracheostomy tube should be removed as soon as it is no longer needed. In general, the longer a tube remains in the trachea, the more difficult will be the process of decannulation. Disease processes of short duration (foreign body) usually permit prompt removal of the tube, whereas others of a chronic nature (anomalies) may take much longer.

Although opinions differ on the best way to remove a tube, the more common practice is to reduce the size of the cannula daily. When a small tube (perhaps two or more sizes smaller than the original) has been used without difficulty, it is then plugged. If the child has no difficulty after 24 hours, the plugged tube may be removed. Subsequent air leaks through the wound nearly always cease within 72 hours. In small infants, the parent may partially occlude the tracheostomy tube with a finger while rocking and cuddling the baby. The infant may thus be slowly adapted to decannulation.

The complications of tracheostomy can be divided into immediate (operative) and late (postoperative) categories. Operative complications, usually in children less than 5 years old, include wound bleeding, pneumothorax, pneumomediastinum, tracheoesophageal fistula, subcutaneous emphysema, cardiac or respiratory arrest, and apnea immediately after provision of a good airway. Late complications include infection, atelectasis, cannula occlusion, tracheal bleeding, expulsion of the cannula, tracheal ulceration and granulation, tracheal stenosis, aerophagia, and delayed healing of the stoma.

DIAPHRAGMATIC PACING

Stimulation of the phrenic nerve to produce regular contractions of the diaphragm (pacing) has been used in infants with central hypoventilation and in children with spinal cord injuries. Successful pacing of the diaphragm means that a child may not require mechanical ventilation to breathe or may require it much less than without pacing. Pacing can thus contribute to effective ambulation and rehabilitation. Many aspects of its use and application remain controversial, although there appears to be less concern now than in the past over ill effects—either to the muscle of the diaphragm or to the phrenic nerve itself. Careful selection of candidates is essential for good long-term results.

RESECTION OF LUNG TISSUE

Advances in diagnostic and surgical methods have made it possible to remove diseased segments or lobes, as well as an entire lung. Such operations are indicated when it has been established (1) that the disease is creating significant present or potential morbidity; (2) that the disease is not treatable by other means; (3) that the disease is sufficiently localized that lung resection will leave adequate pulmonary reserve; and (4) that the resection is technically feasible and does not constitute a risk out of proportion to that of the disease itself.

Surgery should be preceded by appropriate diagnostic studies to define the anatomic and physiologic extent of the disease, as well as the state of the lung to be left after resection. Most helpful are computed tomography, ventilation and perfusion scans, and pulmonary function tests. Bronchograms have been traditionally employed, but the aforementioned scanning techniques have largely supplanted their use.

The most common indication for resection is bronchiectasis, with or without atelectasis, although asymptomatic bronchiectasis, especially of an upper lobe, and so-called cylindrical bronchiectasis almost never require resection. Other indications include anomalies, tuberculosis, and neoplasms.

Postoperative complications are common in small children, especially atelectasis and pneumonia. Unless these complications can be avoided or promptly handled by enlightened management, the procedure may be responsible for more harm than good. Scrupulous attention should be given to maintaining good tracheobronchial toilet. This usually requires continuous or intermittent aerosol therapy and physical therapy (e.g., bronchial drainage, breathing exercises, controlled cough, thoracic "cupping") and may necessitate bronchoscopy, tracheostomy, and mechanical ventilation.

LUNG TRANSPLANTATION

Perhaps the definitive pulmonary therapeutic procedure is to remove a lung that is hopelessly diseased and replace it with a normal lung. Candidates for transplants include patients with end-stage lung disease, such as cystic fibrosis, sarcoidosis, emphysema, histiocytosis X, bronchiectasis, and interstitial fibrosis of various causes. Since 1981 there have been more than 250 heart-lung transplants, the majority of which have been done in adults with pulmonary vascular or coronary heart disease. Results generally suggest that the bronchial epithelium can continue its secretory functions after transplantation. Survival at 1 year has been approximately 60 per cent and at 5 years 20 per cent. Triple immunosuppressive therapy is thought to be important (cyclosporine, prednisone, azathioprine) after the transplant; graft rejection is usually manifested by bronchiolitis obliterans.

Especially in England, heart-lung transplants have been done to combat end-stage lung disease in patients with cystic fibrosis. Scott (1988) and his team performed transplants in six such patients with severe pulmonary disease and cor pulmonale. Five at the time of his report in July 1988 had normal lung function 3 to 29 months after surgery. Interestingly, these investigators assert that the costs of assessment, surgery, and 1 year's treatment and follow-up after heart-lung transplantation are similar to those of medical treatment for such patients. Regardless, the chief limiting factor for heroic surgery of this type will continue to be the scarcity of suitable donor organs.

REFERENCES

Bronchoscopy

Fan LL, Sparks LM, and Dulinski JP: Applications of an ultrathin flexible bronchoscope for neonatal and pediatric airway problems. Chest 89:673, 1986.

Godfrey S, Springer C, Maayan C et al: Is there a place for rigid bronchoscopy in the management of pediatric lung disease? Pediatr Pulmonol 3:179, 1987.

Godfrey S: Bronchoscopy in childhood. Br J Dis Chest 81:225, 1987.

Sherman JM: Rigid or flexible bronchoscopy in children (guest editorial). Pediatr Pulmonol 3:141, 1987.

Wood RE and Postma D: Endoscopy of the airway in infants and children. J Pediatr 112:1, 1988.

Diagnostic Bronchoalveolar Lavage

Bye MR, Bernstein L, Shah K et al: Diagnostic bronchoalveolar lavage in children with AIDS. Pediatr Pulmonol 3:425, 1987.

de Blic J, McKelvie P, Le Bourgeois M et al: Value of bronchoalveolar lavage in the management of severe acute pneumonia and interstitial pneumonitis in the immunocompromised child. Thorax 42:759, 1987.

Frankel LR, Smith DW, and Lewiston NJ: Bronchoalveolar lavage for diagnosis of pneumonia in the immunocompromised child. Pediatrics 81:785, 1988.

Milburn HJ, Prentice HG, and du Bois RM: Role of bronchoalveolar lavage in the evaluation of interstitial pneumonitis in recipients of bone marrow transplants. Thorax 42:766, 1987.

Lung Puncture

Finland M: Diagnostic lung puncture. Pediatrics 44:471, 1969.

Gellis, SS, Reinhold JLD, and Green S: Use of aspiration lung puncture in diagnosis of idiopathic pulmonary hemosiderosis. Am J Dis Child 85:303, 1953.

Hughes JR, Sinha DP, Cooper MR et al: Lung tap in childhood. Bacteria, viruses, and mycoplasmas in acute lower respiratory tract infections. Pediatrics 44:477, 1969.

Klein JO: Diagnostic lung puncture in the pneumonias of infants and children. Pediatrics 44:486, 1969.

Sapington SW, and Favorite GO: Lung puncture in lobar pneumonia. Am J Med Sci 191:225, 1936.

Lung Biopsy

Roback SA, Weintraub WH, Nesbit M et al: Diagnostic open lung biopsy in the critically ill child. Pediatrics 52:605, 1973.

Weng TR, Levison H, Wentworth P et al: Open lung biopsy in children. Am Rev Resp Dis 97:673, 1968.

Arterial Puncture

Olszowka AJ, Rahn H, and Farhi LE: Blood Gases: Hemoglobin, Base Excess and Maldistribution. Philadelphia, Lea & Febiger, 1973.

Shapiro BA: Clinical Application of Blood Gases. 2nd ed. Chicago, Year Book Medical Publishers, 1977.

Bronchial Drainage and Physical Therapy

Cotton EK, Abrams G, Vanhoutte J, and Burrington J: Removal of aspirated foreign bodies by inhalation and postural drainage. Clin Pediatr 12:270, 1973.

Falk M, Kelstrup M, Andersen JB et al: Improving the ketchup bottle method with positive expiratory pressure, PEP, in cystic fibrosis. Eur J Respir Dis 65:423, 1984.

Gaskell DV, and Webber BA: The Brompton Hospital Guide to Chest Physiotherapy. 2nd ed. London, Blackwell Scientific Publications, 1973.

Mellins RB: Pulmonary physiotherapy in the pediatric age group. Am Rev Resp Dis 110 (Suppl):137, 1974.

Reisman JJ, Rivington-Law B, Corey M et al: Role of conventional physiotherapy in cystic fibrosis. J Pediatr 113:632, 1988.

Tecklin JS and Holsclaw DS: Evaluation of bronchial drainage in patients with cystic fibrosis. Phys Ther 55:1081, 1975.

Thacker EW: Postural Drainage and Respiratory Control. London, Lloyd-Luke (Medical Books), Ltd, 1959.

Aerobic Exercise and Fitness

Fitch KD, Blitvich JD, and Morton AR: The effect of running training on exercise-induced asthma. Ann Allergy 57:90, 1986.

Orenstein DM: Exercise tolerance and exercise conditioning in children with chronic lung disease. J Pediatr 112:1043, 1988.

Szentagothai K, Gyene I, Szocska M, and Osvath P: Physical exercise program for children with bronchial asthma. Pediatr Pulmonol 3:166, 1987.

Oxygen Therapy

Campbell AN, Zarfin Y, Groenveld M, and Bryan MH: Low flow oxygen therapy in infants. Arch Dis Child 58:795, 1983.

Fan LL and Voyles JB: Determination of inspired oxygen delivered by nasal cannula in infants with chronic lung disease. J Pediatr 103:923, 1983.

Givan DC and Wylie P: Home oxygen therapy for infants and children. Indiana Med 79:849, 1986.

Hudak BB, Allen MC, Hudak ML, and Loughlin GM: Home oxygen therapy for chronic lung disease in extremely low-birth-weight infants. Am J Dis Child 143:357, 1989.

Shann F, Gatchalian S, and Hutchinson R: Nasopharyngeal oxygen in children. Lancet 2:1238, 1988.

Spier S, Rivlin J, Hughes D, and Levison H: The effect of oxygen on sleep, blood gases, and ventilation in cystic fibrosis. Am Rev Respir Dis 129:712, 1984.

Aerosol Therapy

Canny GJ and Levison H: Aerosols—therapeutic use and delivery in childhood asthma. Ann Allergy 60:11, 1988.

Sly RM, Barbera JM, Middleton HB, and Eby DM: Delivery of albuterol by aerochamber to young children. Ann Allergy 60:403, 1988.

Summer W, Elston R, Tharpe L et al: Aerosol bronchodilator delivery methods. Relative impact on pulmonary function and cost of respiratory care. Arch Intern Med 149:618, 1989.

Zimo DA, Gaspar M, and Akhter J: The efficacy and safety of home nebulizer therapy for children with asthma. Am J Dis Child 143:208, 1989.

Therapeutic Bronchoalveolar Lavage

Hacket PR and Reas HW: A radical approach to therapy for the pulmonary complications of cystic fibrosis. Anesthesiology 26:248, 1965.

Kylstra JA, Rausch DC, Hall KD, and Spock A: Volume-controlled lung lavage in the treatment of asthma, bronchiectasis, and mucoviscidosis. Am Rev Resp Dis 103:651, 1971.

Ramirez-R J, Kieffer RF, and Ball WC: Bronchopulmonary lavage in man. Ann Intern Med 63:819, 1965.

Sherman JM: Bronchial lavage in patients with cystic fibrosis. A critical review of current knowledge. Pediatr Pulmonol 2:244, 1986.

Tracheostomy

Aberdeen E: Mechanical pulmonary ventilation in infants: trache-ostomy and tracheostomy care in infants. Proc R Soc Med 58:900, 1965.

Downes JJ and Schreiner MS: Tracheostomy tubes and attachments in infants and children. Int Anesthesiol Clin 23:37, 1985.

Diaphragmatic Pacing

Glenn WWL: Pacing the diaphragm in infants. Ann Thoracic Surg 40:319, 1985.

Transplantation

Reitz BA: Heart-lung transplantation (editorial). Chest 93:450, 1988.

Scott J, Higenbottam T, Hutter J et al: Heart-lung transplantation for cystic fibrosis. Lancet 2:192, 1988.

Veith FJ: Lung transplantation in perspective (editorial). New Engl J Med 314:1186, 1986.

5

BARRY D. FLETCHER, M.D.

DIAGNOSTIC IMAGING OF THE RESPIRATORY TRACT

The purpose of this chapter is to explain some of the basic concepts used in the interpretation of chest radiographs as well as to discuss the use of more sophisticated imaging modalities, including computed tomography (CT) and magnetic resonance imaging (MRI) in the diagnosis of pediatric respiratory disorders. Minor modifications of the principles of radiologic interpretation found in standard textbooks directed toward diagnosis of disease in the adult are necessary. Obviously, a complete course in pulmonary radiology cannot be offered here. I have, therefore, based my choice of the subjects to follow on their importance in the day-to-day practice of radiology as well as on the frequency with which the meaning and importance of certain radiologic findings are queried by clinical colleagues. Specific disease entities will be discussed when they illustrate the more important anatomic or pathophysiologic principles necessary for successful radiologic diagnosis, but detailed accounts of these disorders that are found in other sections of this book will not be duplicated here.

Chest radiographs remain the predominant method of diagnosing respiratory tract disease, particularly when the lung parenchyma or pleura is involved. Other methods, notably CT and MRI, are becoming more important in imaging the chest. Indeed, fluoroscopy, esophagography, bronchography, and conventional tomography are now less commonly employed, although they are still valuable in selected cases. Radionuclide scintigrams are not commonly employed in children. This chapter will focus, therefore, on the most frequently used modalities: chest radiography, CT, and MRI.

RADIATION HAZARDS

Protection of the immature gonads of the infant and child is essential. The thyroid gland, ocular lens, and bone marrow are also relatively radiosensitive structures and therefore deserve protection as well. Unnecessary exposure of both patients and health care personnel to diagnostic radiation occurs frequently and is related to overexposure of radiographs, overutilization of radiologic services, improper collimation of the x-ray beam, and absence of appropriate lead shielding. The overall x-ray dose during childhood can be further reduced by eliminating the practice of routine chest screening and hospital admission radiographs and by curtailing the custom of routine preoperative chest radiographs (Brill et al, 1973).

IMAGING METHODS

FLUOROSCOPY

Fluoroscopy is performed by employing an image intensifier, which electronically increases the brightness level so that the image can be displayed on a television monitor. *Spot films* are radiographs made at desired times during fluoroscopy. Cinefluoroscopy can also be carried out, but it requires an increased radiation dosage, particularly when high frame speeds are employed. A decline in the use of cinefluoroscopy has coincided with the increased resolution now attainable with modern image tubes, television systems, and video tapes. Photofluorography, with 70- to 105-mm film exposed directly from the output phosphor of the image intensifier, produces high-quality films with considerably lower radiation exposure than spot films. The entire examination can be recorded on video tape for later review. Fluoroscopy is principally used to study diaphragmatic excursion and to examine the barium-filled esophagus. It is a useful method of assessing regional ventilation, particularly in patients with emphysema due to airway obstruction associated with such conditions as endobronchial foreign bodies and hyperlucent lung syndrome. Fluoroscopy may be performed to evaluate swallowing in patients with suspected aspiration pneumonia (see also pages 98 and 100).

RADIOGRAPHY

The methods of obtaining chest films vary for infants and children. Except for a routine follow-up of chronic disease, when a frontal projection may be sufficient, lateral views should be obtained. In x-ray departments, generators that provide high milliamperage and, conversely, very short exposure times are now commonly available. "Rare earth" intensifying screens have come into wide use in radiology departments. They permit even more rapid exposures, in the range of a few milliseconds, with a consequent reduction in radiation dose, although there is a slight decrease in image quality (Brodeur et al, 1981).

In the newborn nursery, radiographs are usually exposed with the baby in the incubator, using portable x-ray equipment. We have found that a vertical beam anteroposterior (AP) view taken through the Plexiglas cover and a lateral view made with a horizontally directed beam require the least handling of fragile newborn infants. Metallic devices such as electrocardiogram electrodes, which may obscure significant portions of the chest, should be removed.

In the older infant, AP supine and vertical beam lateral views can be obtained in the x-ray department. Because the patient is radiographed on the x-ray table, the tube to film distance is considerably decreased from the usual 6 ft used for older children. The distorting effect of magnification at the shorter distance is not significant in these patients, and shorter exposure times can be achieved. Upright views of the chest can be obtained in cooperative young children with the use of various supporting devices that usually fix the child in a sitting position.

These, however, will not completely eliminate slumping of the body in the younger child, so the recumbent position described previously is preferable in those up to 2 to 3 years of age. After the patient is able to sit or stand unsupported, conventional posteroanterior (PA) and lateral radiographs can be made at a distance of 72 in (Fig. 5–1).

Special Views

Oblique views aid in the spatial perception of thoracic lesions and are frequently used in assessing cardiac chambers. These projections are also sometimes helpful in evaluating the lungs of patients with severe chest wall deformities or scoliosis. Evaluation of pneumothorax and pleural effusion is facilitated by lateral decubitus views, which are made with a horizontal x-ray beam and the patient lying on one side (see also page 109). A frontal projection of the chest made at the end of expiration is used chiefly to demonstrate air trapping in patients with suspected foreign body aspiration. Because exact timing of the exposure may be difficult in these patients, fluoroscopic evaluation is more precise. Apical-lordotic views are made in the AP position with an exaggerated extension of the spine. These are helpful for the visualization of upper lobe lesions and the demonstration of middle lobe disease (see Fig. 5–39B).

High kilovoltage (KV) films refers to radiographs on which increased penetration of the x-rays results in a relative decrease in radiographic density of the bones, thus accentuating the air-containing structures such as the trachea and major bronchi (see Fig. 5–10). The assessment of airway narrowing, bronchial anomalies, and mediastinal masses is, therefore, facilitated.

Digital Radiography

Digital images, which are common to CT and MRI, are now being applied to chest radiography (Kundel, 1986). The digital images may be derived directly or from a conventional (analog) radiograph. Although the resolution of digital radiographs may not be as great as that of conventional chest films, digital images can be enhanced by altering contrast and other image parameters. The ability to manipulate the images is an important advantage of digital radiography in pediatrics because it means that examinations will not have to be repeated because of faulty radiographic technique.

TOMOGRAPHY

Tomograms or laminograms are produced by simultaneous motion of the tube and film at varying levels so that all structures not included in a predetermined plane are blurred. The structures that remain stationary are, therefore, viewed independently of superimposed tissues. For studies of the

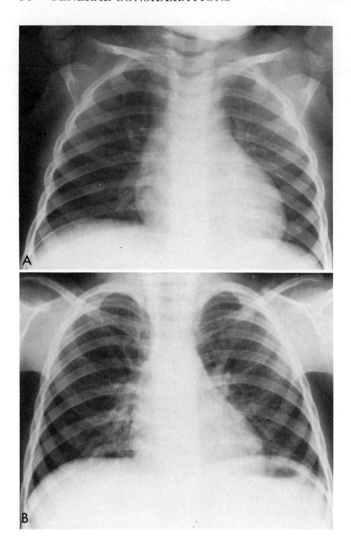

Figure 5–1. Normal chest radiographs of the same patient. Note the differences in heart size in *A*, anteroposterior supine position, and *B*, posteroanterior erect position made with a longer focal-film distance.

lungs, thick sections approximating 1 cm are commonly used. Computed tomography has largely supplanted conventional tomography, especially for the evaluation of mediastinal lesions and lung metastases (see page 100).

ESOPHAGOGRAPHY

This is a valuable adjunct to diagnosis of chest diseases and is used principally to define mediastinal masses that may cause esophageal displacement, as well as swallowing disorders and malformations such as tracheoesophageal fistula. Colloidal barium is preferred over water-soluble contrast media, because it is more palatable and less irritating if it enters the tracheobronchial tree. The barium esophagram is usually performed under fluoroscopic control.

The esophagram is also widely utilized in the patient with "near-miss" sudden infant death syndrome (near-SIDS) and the patient in whom aspiration is suspected as a cause of recurrent or chronic pneumonia. The patient is fed a volume of barium similar to that of a usual feeding. The swallowing

mechanism and esophageal peristaltic activity are observed carefully. Gastroesophageal reflux may occur spontaneously or may be elicited by swallowing while sucking. Reflux is graded according to its severity and whether aspiration has occurred into the tracheobronchial tree (McCauley et al, 1978).

Radioisotope methods are also used to evaluate gastroesophageal reflux and aspiration into the lungs (see page 100).

BRONCHOGRAPHY

Bronchography is used less frequently than previously, and its value has been seriously questioned (Avery, 1970). In the past, bronchography was commonly employed in the evaluation of chronic lung disease, and its decline has coincided with the diminishing need for surgical therapy and the availability of greater information from other methods, especially computed tomography (Fig. 5–2). Bronchography can be safely carried out using small amounts of propyliodone (Dionosil). An opaque catheter is inserted via an orotracheal tube and is positioned

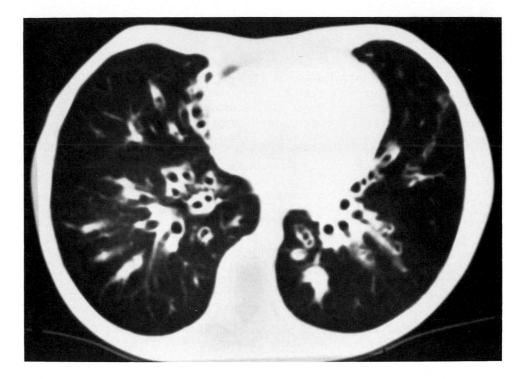

Figure 5–2. Computed tomographic section of the chest, showing severe central bronchiectasis in a child with chronic pulmonary disease of unknown origin. (Courtesy of Dr. Jerald P Kuhn.)

under fluoroscopic control. A small amount of contrast medium is then injected. Separate examination of each lung is recommended, particularly if pulmonary function is abnormal. Selective opacification of lobar and segmental bronchi is a useful adjunct to bronchoscopy for assessment of bronchi distal to the visual limits of the bronchoscope.

ANGIOGRAPHY

Aside from the investigation of various anomalies of the pulmonary vasculature (Gooding, 1974), pulmonary angiography has not found many applications in children. Fellows and colleagues (1975) have used bronchial arteriography to localize sites of hemoptysis in patients with cystic fibrosis in whom bronchoscopy could not be done. Franken and co-workers (1973) have pointed out the advantages of pulmonary angiography over bronchography in the investigation of causes of unequal aeration of the lungs. A newer technique called *digital subtraction angiography* makes use of an intravenous rather than intra-arterial injection of contrast medium (Fletcher, 1982, 1984). Systemic or pulmonary arteries can be visualized by "subtracting" an image made before arrival of the contrast material (Fig. 5–3).

Dynamic CT techniques, which provide serial scans during rapid intravenous administration of contrast material, are capable of providing similar information.

RADIOISOTOPE SCANNING

Lung scans are useful in the detection of abnormalities of perfusion or ventilation that may not be recognizable on radiographs. Modern perfusion scans are made using intravenous injections of human serum albumin microspheres or macroaggregated albumin (MAA) labeled with technetium 99m. The particles are nearly all extracted during their first pass through the pulmonary circulation. The most commonly used radiopharmaceutical for ventilation scans is ^{133}Xe gas. ^{81m}Kr, which has an extremely short half-life, has come into use for assessment of ventilation (Li et al, 1979). Airway obstruction may be demonstrated by inhalation of technetium-labeled aerosols produced by ultrasonic nebulization (Gates et al, 1976). Gallium-67 scintigrams may be positive in acquired immune deficiency syn-

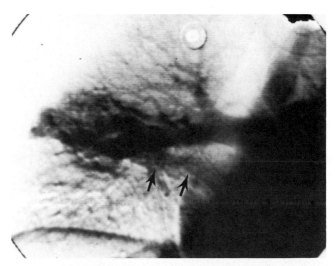

Figure 5–3. Digital subtraction angiography employing intravenous injection of contrast material shows a pulmonary arteriovenous malformation. Pulmonary venous return *(arrows)* is to the left atrium.

drome (AIDS) patients with *Pneumocystis carinii* infection, even when radiographs appear normal (Barron, 1985).

There are numerous pediatric applications of radionuclide lung scans. Advances in this field have been reviewed by Papanicolaou and Treves (1980). Perfusion scans demonstrate defects in pulmonary arterial distribution that may occur with congenital malformations of the pulmonary arteries (Pendarvis and Swischuk, 1969) or pulmonary emboli. Sequestered lung tissue perfuses during the systemic rather than the pulmonary arterial phase because of its anomalous arterial supply (Gooneratne and Conway, 1976). Abnormalities of regional ventilation also produce defects in the distribution of pulmonary blood flow. These defects have been shown in such disorders as asthma (Fig. 5–4), lobar interstitial emphysema (Leonidas et al, 1978), and endobronchial foreign body. The perfusion defect due to a foreign body may not be apparent within the first 24 hours after aspiration (Rudavsky et al, 1973).

Ventilation scanning is often combined with a perfusion study and is useful in assessing lung function in such disorders as cystic fibrosis, congenital lobar emphysema, hyperlucent lung syndrome, and postoperative diaphragmatic hernia.

Radionuclide methods of studying gastroesophageal reflux and tracheobronchial aspiration make use of a technetium 99m–labeled milk or juice feeding and sequential imaging. Heyman and associates (1979) found this test to be more sensitive than barium studies (see page 98). It duplicates physiologic conditions with a relatively small absorbed radiation dose.

COMPUTED TOMOGRAPHY

In the few years since the introduction of body CT as a clinical tool, remarkable progress has been made in image quality and scanning speed. Excellent scans can now be obtained, even in newborn infants with rapid respiratory rates.

Newer CT scanners have acquisition times of 2 to 5 seconds. For the chest, contagious axial scans approximately 5 to 10 mm thick are made from just below the level of the diaphragm to the clavicles. Sedation or immobilization is usually necessary for younger children. General anesthesia is not required or recommended. Feedings should be withheld for 3 to 4 hours before the examination, because intravenous contrast medium is often administered to opacify the cardiac chambers and great vessels.

Kirks and Korobkin (1980) found that the most common indications for chest CT were to evaluate suspected metastases and to define the location and extent of a known lesion. Computed tomography is also very helpful in assessing the response of primary or secondary malignant lesions to therapy. It is possible to define lesions located anywhere within the chest wall, pleural space, mediastinum, or lung parenchyma.

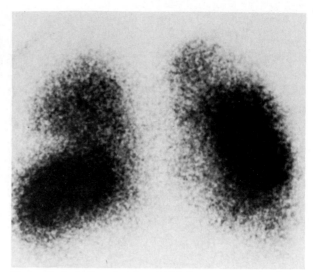

Figure 5–4. A [99m]technetium-MAA isotope scan showing perfusion defects in the lungs of an asthmatic patient.

The increased contrast enhancement inherent in CT allows discrimination between changes in tissue density in the range of 0.5 to 1 per cent. This ability to discriminate allows one to predict the type of tissue—blood, fat, or necrotic material—within a lesion. It is also helpful in differentiating inflammatory parenchymal masses from tumors by demonstrating small air-containing cavities not visible radiographically and by showing normal pulmonary vascular perfusion of the mass after a rapid intravenous injection of contrast medium (Shurin et al, 1981) (Fig. 5–5).

Other potentially important applications of CT in the pediatric age group include the localization of aspirated foreign bodies in the tracheobronchial tree (Berger et al, 1980) and definition of the anatomy of aortic arch malformations and resultant tracheal compression (McLoughlin et al, 1981).

High-resolution CT is employed to evaluate interstitial lung disease (Zerhouni et al, 1985). At least in adults, it is possible to demonstrate structures as small as the secondary pulmonary lobule (Bergin et al, 1988). This type of CT imaging is performed by obtaining thin (1.0 to 2.0 mm) sections using a high-spatial-frequency reconstruction algorithm, normally reserved for bone imaging (Mayo et al, 1987) (Fig. 5–6).

Radiation doses for complete CT scans of the chest vary somewhat according to the type of equipment (Brasch et al, 1978). In general, the dose is comparable to that for conventional whole lung tomography and is significantly less than that received during pulmonary angiography.

MAGNETIC RESONANCE IMAGING

Magnetic resonance imaging is the newest technique for the evaluation of pediatric chest disorders. This imaging modality makes use of the ability of

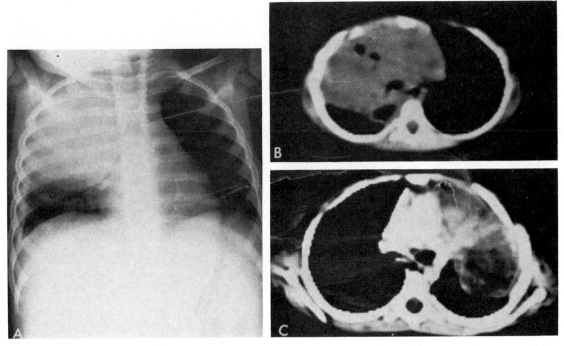

Figure 5–5. *A,* A posteroanterior chest radiograph demonstrates a large right upper chest mass with deviation of the trachea to the left and a right pleural effusion. *B,* The computed tomogram done on the same day shows numerous air-filled cavities not visible on the plain films. This evidence of communication with the tracheobronchial tree suggests inflammatory consolidation of the lung rather than a tumor. *C,* A computed tomogram of another patient with a large left inflammatory chest mass demonstrates pulmonary vessels traversing the lesion after intravenous injection of a bolus of contrast medium. The area of decreased attenuation seen posteriorly suggests an abscess. A neoplasm would be expected to displace or destroy pulmonary vessels. (Reproduced with permission from Shurin SB, Haaga JR, Wood RE et al: Computed tomography for the evaluation of thoracic masses in children. JAMA 246:65, 1981. Copyright 1981. American Medical Association.)

hydrogen atoms (protons) to resonate at a specific frequency when subjected to an electromagnetic field. The protons act as tiny magnets that align in the direction of a strong magnetic field. Application of weaker, rotating fields and radio frequency pulses causes the protons to spin or precess at specific frequencies. The resonance radio frequency signals or "echoes" can then be detected, and images are formed by computerized encoding of phase and spatial information.

Signal strength and consequent image brightness of a given tissue depend on its abundance of protons and their relaxation times, T1 and T2. T1 relaxation depends on the interactions of the spinning protons within their molecular environment, whereas T2 is the time required for the spinning nuclei to dephase relative to each other. Either of these tissue parameters, which exhibit some specificity in anatomic structures and disease processes, can be emphasized by altering the radio frequency pulses. Thus MRI is able to provide certain biologic information unavailable with previous imaging methods. In addition, MR images can be made in longitudinal (sagittal and coronal) as well as axial (transverse) planes. Magnetic resonance imaging is also valuable for imaging the mediastinum because flowing blood within a vessel or cardiac chamber appears dark in contrast to the brighter surrounding tissues (Brasch et al, 1984).

We have used MRI extensively for evaluating congenital cardiovascular malformations, such as vascular rings, pulmonary artery abnormalities, tracheobronchial airway obstruction, and mediastinal masses (Fletcher, Dearborn, and Mulopulos, 1986; Fletcher and Jacobstein, 1986). Some degree of tissue char-

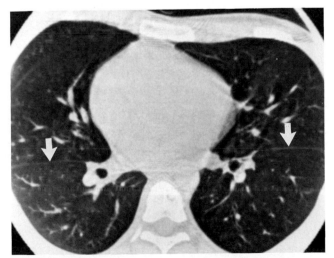

Figure 5–6. High-resolution computed tomography of a normal chest. Note the distinct branching pattern of the small peripheral pulmonary arteries and the clearly defined major fissures (*arrows*).

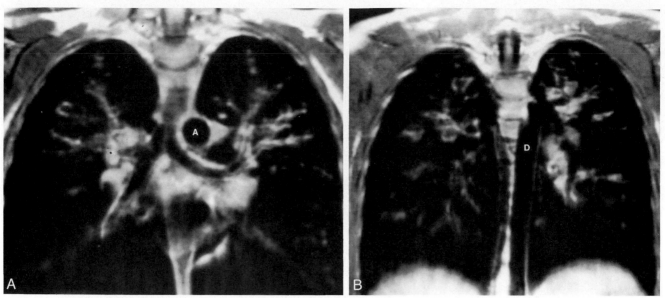

Figure 5–7. *A,* A T1-weighted coronal magnetic resonance image through the middle mediastinum of a patient with cystic fibrosis shows bright, enlarged hilar and subcarinal lymph nodes. The major bronchi are well shown. (A, Aortic arch.) *B,* Bright mucus plugs are demonstrated in the dilated upper lobe bronchi on a more posterior magnetic resonance imaging section. (D, descending aorta.)

acterization is also possible, allowing one to diagnose hemorrhagic lesions, cysts, and fatty tumors, such as lipomas and teratomas. Others have utilized MRI to distinguish between inflammatory lesions and fibrosis on the bases of T2 characteristics (Cohen et al, 1986) and to differentiate mucus plugs from fibrosis and atelectasis in patients with cystic fibrosis (Gooding et al, 1984) (Fig. 5–7).

A particular advantage of using MRI in children is that it does not require a dose of ionizing radiation; its disadvantages, however, are that it has a relatively long imaging time and is extremely sensitive to motion. In addition, the spatial resolution of MRI is not as great as with CT, and therefore it is less capable of disclosing pulmonary parenchymal abnormalities, such as interstitial disease and metastases.

INTERVENTION

Wesenberg and Struble (1972) have recommended selective bronchial catheterization and lavage under fluoroscopic control for newborn infants with lobar atelectasis. Fluoroscopic visualization may also be helpful in locating sites for needle aspiration and biopsy. The needle may also be guided by means of CT.

ULTRASONOGRAPHY

Because transmission of sound waves is poor in air and the rib cage produces reverberation artifacts, this imaging technique is of limited usefulness in the diagnosis of respiratory disorders. However, in patients with complete opacification of a hemithorax

the nature of the pathologic process may be demonstrated, and ultrasonography is a simple method of differentiating pleural effusion from pulmonary consolidation as well as of assessing diaphragmatic position and excursion. The cystic or solid nature of some intrathoracic masses can also be determined by ultrasound (Haller et al, 1980).

TECHNICAL FACTORS AFFECTING INTERPRETATION OF CHEST RADIOGRAPHS

EXPOSURE

The quantity and quality of the x-ray exposure are determined by two factors: kilovoltage (KV), which controls the penetration of the beam, and milliamperage (MA), on which contrast depends. On a well-exposed frontal view of the chest, the vertebrae should be seen fairly clearly; at the same time, water-density structures, such as the pulmonary vascular markings, should be visible easily. Excess contrast results in a radiograph in which the bones and soft tissue structures appear chalk-like with considerable loss of detail.

MOTION

The most common cause of loss of image sharpness is respiratory motion due to ineffective immobilization of the child and lengthy exposure times. This technical fault is indicated by blurring of the diaphragmatic domes and intrapulmonary structures. With contemporary equipment, motion artifacts are now uncommon in pediatric radiography.

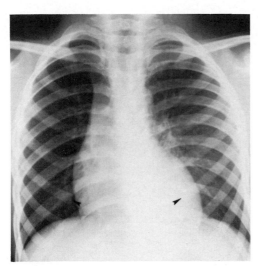

Figure 5–8. The thorax is mildly rotated toward the right posterior oblique position. The anterior ends of the fifth ribs are marked. Note the relative lucency of the right lung.

ROTATION

Because the spinous processes of children have varying degrees of ossification, and because some twisting of the upper thorax frequently occurs during radiography, it is not practical to compare the distance between the proximal ends of the clavicles and the spinous processes as is done in adults. Rotation can be judged more effectively by comparing the position of the anterior ends of the lower ribs (Fig. 5–8). Rotation produces considerable diagnostic confusion. For example, on AP radiographs, rotation of the thorax toward the right causes the mediastinum to be projected in the right hemithorax; the right lung appears more lucent, and the left hila, pulmonary vessels, and anterior rib ends are magnified. On lateral views, variable lengths of the posterior rib ends can be seen if the patient is rotated.

RESPIRATORY CYCLE

The level to which the diaphragmatic domes descend on full inspiration depends to some extent on the age of the child. The degree of inspiratory effort is usually judged according to the position of the top of the right diaphragmatic dome with respect to the adjacent rib. In general, if the right diaphragmatic dome is projected at the level of the sixth rib anteriorly and the ninth to tenth ribs posteriorly, a satisfactory inspiratory film has been made. In normal newborn infants the right hemidiaphragm usually descends to the level of the eighth posterior rib (Edwards et al, 1981). Expiration films result in crowding of the bronchovascular markings and are a common cause of "false-positive" diagnosis of pulmonary abnormalities.

MAGNIFICATION

A certain amount of magnification occurs when the focus to object distance is short, as it is in portable and AP recumbent chest films. In small children, the amount of magnification is not detrimental (see Fig. 5–1A), but in the larger patient considerable distortion occurs owing to artifactual enlargement of intrathoracic structures, especially those closest to the x-ray tube.

Sharpness of a magnified image can be maintained by reducing the diameter of the x-ray beam. X-ray tubes with focal spots of 0.2 to 0.3 mm in diameter are available that allow more information to be obtained by magnifying the image while preserving its clarity. This technique is sometimes used for neonatal chest radiography.

The experienced observer develops a systematic approach to the interpretation of chest radiographs, which is designed to ensure that assessment is complete in the face of an apparently normal appearance and that additional information is not overlooked when there is an obvious lesion. Individual systems of examination may differ considerably, but all are designed to promote accurate observation of all structures displayed on the films. One such personal approach is offered in Table 5–1 for use and modification by the reader.

Table 5–1. BASIC APPROACH TO ASSESSMENT OF CHEST RADIOGRAPHS

Technique
Are the views appropriate for the information sought?
Are there technical variations or faults that might influence your interpretation?

Chest Wall
Does the appearance of the soft tissues suggest any disturbance of growth or nutrition?
Are there congenital or acquired defects of the ribs or spine?
Are the spine and sternum intact on lateral view?

Diaphragm
Are the diaphragmatic outlines intact, or is there a positive silhouette sign?
Are the diaphragmatic domes in normal position?

Pleura
Are the costophrenic angles sharply outlined?
Is there a pneumothorax?
Are the fissures in normal position?

Mediastinum
Is the mediastinum in normal position?
Is the heart large? If so, is the enlargement real (cardiomegaly) or only apparent (thymus shadow or expiration film)?
Is the aortic arch on the left?
Are the heart borders clearly visible?
Are the major airways normal?

Hila and Pulmonary Vessels
Are the hila normal in size and position?
Are the pulmonary vessels normal in caliber and sharply defined?

Lungs
Are there any abnormal densities?
Is there an air bronchogram?
Is there a positive silhouette sign?
Is the area behind the heart normal?
Are there Kerley lines?
Is there a "spine sign"?
Are there any areas of hyperaeration or atelectasis?

RADIOLOGY OF THE NECK AND THORACIC INLET

Technique

Frequently, the lower neck is exposed on routine AP and lateral radiographs. Whereas excessive exposure of radiosensitive organs, such as the thyroid, should be avoided on a routine basis, a glimpse of the cervical airway can be very helpful in determining a cause of respiratory distress. When an obstructive airway lesion is suspected clinically, high KV radiographs provide excellent visualization. Dunbar (1970) utilizes AP and lateral views taken during inspiration and expiration. Joseph and co-workers (1976) have worked out a method for high KV magnification radiography of the neck.

For specific purposes, a barium esophagram may be a useful additional examination (see page 98).

Normal Appearance

The amount of air contained in the pharynx varies with the respiratory cycle and is expelled with swallowing. When the vallecula is filled with air and the pyriform sinuses are distended, the epiglottis is distinctly outlined. Enlarged palatine tonsils can be seen, superimposed on the pyriform sinuses in lateral projection (Fig. 5–9).

When the laryngeal ventricle is filled with air, it is recognizable on AP or lateral projections as a lucent elliptic shadow situated at approximately the same level as the inferior angle of the pyriform sinuses. The subglottic portion of the trachea is seen on AP views as an arch-like structure. Below this, the trachea should be of uniform caliber to the level of the thoracic inlet, where its AP diameter may normally decrease by up to 50 per cent in a struggling or crying infant. There is little change in caliber with quiet breathing.

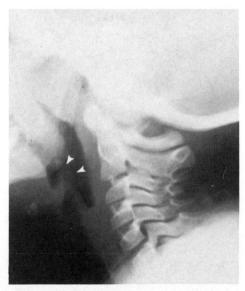

Figure 5–9. A lateral view of the neck, showing prominent adenoid tissue and palatine tonsils. The epiglottis (*arrows*) is normal in size (compare with Fig. 5–13).

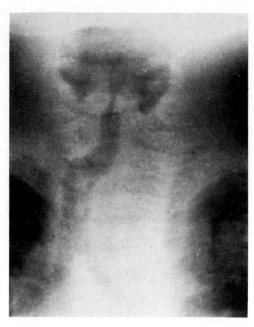

Figure 5–10. A high KV film of a normal infant's neck, showing deviation of the trachea to the right. Note the arch-like appearance of the normal subglottic portion of the trachea.

In babies and young children, the cervical trachea is redundant and, therefore, may buckle anteriorly and to the right, particularly if the neck is flexed (Fig. 5–10). Occasionally, this normal finding may lead to the erroneous diagnosis of a cervical mass. The normal trachea will, however, straighten when the neck is extended.

Immediately below the thoracic inlet, the trachea deviates to the right owing to the normal left-sided aortic arch. Because the infant is held in a somewhat exaggerated lordotic position, the carina is projected high in the thorax, immediately below the aortic "knob."

Signs of Respiratory Distress

Besides direct visualization of the obstructed airway, a number of other findings are helpful in deciding whether respiratory distress is due to airway obstruction or pulmonary disease. Upper airway obstruction should be suspected when (1) tracheal collapse occurs with quiet breathing, (2) the pharynx is distended (Meine et al, 1974), (3) a paradoxical change in heart size occurs during respiration (i.e., the transverse cardiac diameter is smaller on expiration than on inspiration) (Capitanio and Kirkpatrick, 1973), (4) the lung volume is decreased, (5) a large amount of swallowed air is present in the esophagus (Fig. 5–11), or (6) indrawing of the anterior chest wall occurs.

It is worthwhile to note that the last two findings also occur in neonates with respiratory distress syndrome because they tend to swallow air (Keats and Smith, 1974).

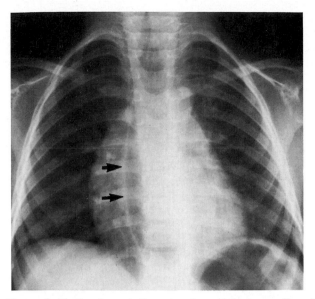

Figure 5–11. Esophageal distention *(arrows)* due to swallowed air and decreased lung volume in acute epiglottitis.

CROUP

On occasions when the clinical diagnosis is in doubt, the diagnosis of laryngotracheobronchitis can be made because of its distinctive radiologic appearance. The normal subglottic arch becomes obliterated because of submucosal edema, so that a diffuse narrowing, in the shape of an inverted "V," is seen on AP projections (Fig. 5–12). Distention of the supraglottic airway and secondary tracheal collapse may be visible on lateral views. However, there is no direct correlation of severity between the radiologic and the clinical findings (DeLevie et al, 1972). Edema due to tracheal intubation produces a similar appearance, as does congenital subglottic stenosis (Grünebaum, 1975). Subglottic hemangiomas are usually asymmetric and cause a more discrete indentation of the trachea.

EPIGLOTTITIS

Lateral radiographs of the neck are extremely helpful in confirming this diagnosis. Although radiography is less traumatic than direct visualization, attempts to put the child in a recumbent position may trigger further airway obstruction. For this reason, a lateral radiograph is made, with the patient sitting. In epiglottitis, marked swelling of the epiglottis and aryepiglottic folds is evident (Fig. 5–13).

MASSES

Tumors arising from the retropharyngeal and retrotracheal soft tissues compress the trachea, as do large foreign bodies that have become lodged in the cervical esophagus (Smith et al, 1974) (Fig. 5–14). The latter diagnosis can be established by means of a barium swallow.

Retropharyngeal cellulitis causes posterior compression of the pyriform sinuses and anterior deviation of the trachea. Except in the case of traumatic perforation, an air-containing retropharyngeal abscess is rarely encountered.

Cross-sectional imaging using CT or MRI often allows a more definitive evaluation of mass lesions involving the cervical airway. A more precise estimate of the degree to which the airways have been compromised can also be gained. Ultrafast or "cine CT," which is available in only a few centers, is capable of

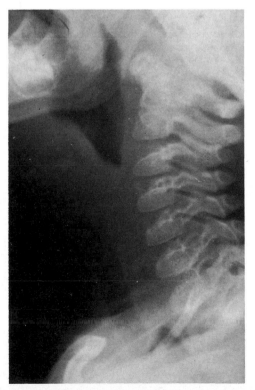

Figure 5–13. Marked swelling of the epiglottis and aryepiglottic folds in a patient with acute epiglottitis. The supraglottic portion of the trachea is obliterated (compare with Fig. 5–9).

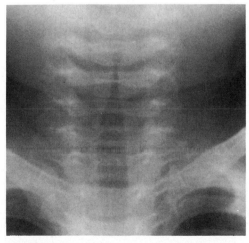

Figure 5–12. Subglottic narrowing due to croup.

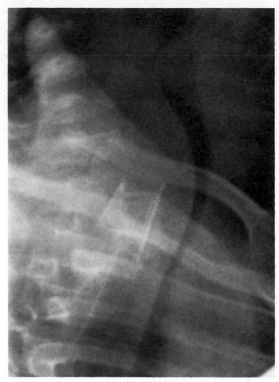

Figure 5–14. A slightly opaque retrotracheal foreign body is demonstrated on a 105-mm lateral "spot" film of the neck of an infant. The trachea is narrowed and displaced anteriorly. The foreign body, the removable top of a soft drink can lodged within the esophagus, resulted in respiratory distress as well as feeding problems.

recording dynamic changes of the larynx (Brasch et al, 1987). Mediastinal lesions affecting the airway will be considered in more detail on page 113.

CONGENITAL LARYNGEAL STRIDOR

Anteroinferior displacement and buckling of the aryepiglottic folds and posterior deflection of the epiglottis have been convincingly demonstrated in congenital laryngeal stridor by Dunbar (1970). These changes occur on inspiration simultaneously with inspiratory stridor. In the absence of stridor at the time of fluoroscopy, however, no abnormalities will be seen.

THE CHEST WALL AND DIAPHRAGM

Chest Wall

The changes in configuration of the chest wall that occur with growth are reflected on both AP and lateral chest radiographs. During infancy, the thorax is circular, and its AP diameter is greater than its transverse diameter. The latter becomes relatively larger as the child grows. The ribs of the infant are

aligned horizontally. On the supine radiograph, which is often obtained with the patient in an exaggerated lordotic position, the anterior rib ends may be projected over or even slightly above the posterior aspects of the ribs. In this position, the clavicles are projected well above the first ribs.

The shape of the chest wall may also reflect the volume of the lungs. Hyperaeration produces anterior bowing of the sternum and an increase in the AP diameter of the chest as well as flattening of the diaphragmatic domes. A decrease in lung volume is accompanied by a reduction in width of the intercostal spaces. A "bell-shaped" thorax may be the result of pulmonary hypoplasia or muscular weakness (Fig. 5–15).

Several misleading images can be produced by structures of the chest wall. In babies, skin folds on the back produce slightly curved lines that may simulate pneumothorax. Recognition of pulmonary vessels peripheral to these lines and careful examination of their course will usually clarify this artifact. On lateral radiographs made with the patient's arms extended over the head, the axillary folds are prominent and produce a homogeneous density overlying the posterior aspect of the chest that may be mistaken for an intrathoracic abnormality. Also on lateral projection, the density cast by the scapulas may simulate a posterior mediastinal mass (Alazraki and Friedman, 1972). The scapulae also overlie the upper lung fields on AP projections, and their shadows may be mistaken for pneumonia or pleural effusion.

The Spine on Chest X-Rays

The thoracic and upper lumbar spine is well visualized on adequately exposed chest radiographs, and examination of these vertebrae is one of the most important aspects of chest radiology. The vertebral bodies are particularly well demonstrated on lateral

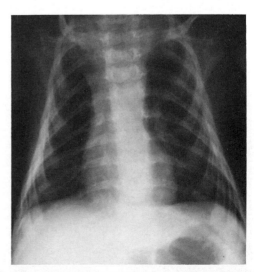

Figure 5–15. The thorax is bell shaped due to Werdnig-Hoffmann disease.

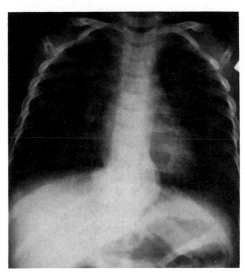

Figure 5–16. A lower thoracic paraspinal mass due to tuberculosis.

views, enabling assessment of congenital and acquired disorders, such as fusion and compression. On frontal projection, recognition of a significant scoliosis may be as important as the observation of intrathoracic disease. Significant disturbance of segmentation of the vertebrae and defects in their bodies or neural elements occur with such anomalies as enteric duplications, intraspinal lesions, and meningomyelocele. Inflammatory processes, such as tuberculosis (Fig. 5–16), and neoplasms, such as neuroblastoma, may produce paraspinal masses.

Diaphragm

The diaphragm descends on full inspiration, so the higher right diaphragmatic dome is projected at the level of the ninth to tenth ribs posteriorly. Consistent elevation of both diaphragmatic domes occurs when there is abdominal distention or a large intra-abdominal mass. A large amount of gas in the stomach elevates the left hemidiaphragm. The colon is sometimes interposed between the liver and right diaphragmatic dome (Fig. 5–17). Elevation of a hemidiaphragm is seen in phrenic nerve paralysis and eventration. Paradoxical movement occurs in either condition, whereas a subphrenic abscess usually causes a decrease or absence of excursion of the adjacent hemidiaphragm.

It is very helpful to be able to differentiate between the right and left hemidiaphragms on lateral views of the chest. Their relative height may be misleading owing to variations in position of the central x-ray beam. Identification of the gastric air bubble is helpful, because it cannot be projected above the left hemidiaphragm. Also, because of the levoposition of the heart, the superior surface of the left hemidiaphragm is obscured anteriorly (see "Silhouette Sign," page 119), whereas the outline of the right hemidiaphragm can be traced to the anterior chest wall.

THE PLEURA AND FISSURES

The lungs are surrounded by two layers of pleura—the visceral and parietal—between which there is a potential space. The fissures are formed by two apposed layers of visceral pleura that separate the lobes. When the x-ray beam is directed tangentially to them, the fissures can be visualized as thin curvilinear densities.

The oblique or major fissures run from the posterior surface of the lungs, at about the level of the fourth thoracic vertebra, downward and anteriorly,

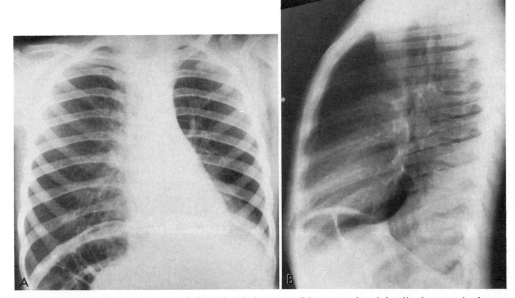

Figure 5–17. The hepatic flexure of the colon is interposed between the right diaphragmatic dome and the liver. The haustral markings serve to distinguish the colon from free intraperitoneal air. Left lower lobe atelectasis has caused a leftward shift of the heart, loss of the left diaphragmatic outline, and posterior displacement of the major fissure.

where their pleural surfaces become continuous with the visceral pleura of the diaphragmatic surfaces of the lungs. For purposes of anatomic localization, the right major fissure usually extends more anteriorly at its inferior end than does the left.

On occasion, the inferior portion of the major fissure may have a more vertical course than normal, allowing it to be visualized on frontal projections. This finding occurs particularly in association with cardiomegaly.

The minor or horizontal fissure extends from the right major fissure at approximately its midpoint to the anterior surface of the lung, thus dividing the upper and middle lobes. The juncture of the two fissures is an important landmark on lateral chest radiographs, because it serves to identify the right lung. The minor fissure may be absent, bilateral, or left-sided, particularly with congenital heart disease and abnormal situs (Landing et al, 1971).

The azygos fissure (Fig. 5–18) is the most frequently visualized accessory fissure. It is seen as a curvilinear density coursing downward and medially from the apex of the lung, blending inferiorly with the teardrop-shaped density that is formed by the azygos vein. The vein is surrounded by both visceral and parietal pleura. The azygos "lobe," which is the portion of the lung medial to the fissure, may occasionally appear to be opaque. This opacity is more likely caused by the pleural layers than by disease within the accessory "lobe."

Occasionally, two other accessory fissures are visible radiographically (Godwin and Tarver, 1985). The superior accessory fissure is seen on the lateral view as a horizontal line extending posteriorly from the

major fissure to the posterior pleural surface of the lung. It separates the superior segment of the lower lobe from the basilar segments. The inferior accessory fissure is an oblique line lateral to the medial basilar segment and is seen near the cardiophrenic angle on frontal projections. Both of these fissures are more commonly seen in the right lung.

A left minor fissure that separates the lingula from the remainder of the left upper lobe is occasionally seen. Normal segmental anatomy is usually preserved.

PLEURAL EFFUSION

Intrapleural fluid accumulates primarily below the diaphragmatic surface of the lung and then extends posteriorly, causing the posterior costophrenic angle to be blunted on lateral views. Small amounts of pleural fluid can also be detected between the convex surface of the lung and the chest wall on lateral decubitus views. Larger accumulations are readily visible on frontal projections because of blunting of the lateral costophrenic angles. Fluid also may be seen in the mediastinal pleural space as a triangular density to the left of the lower thoracic spine and may accumulate between the visceral pleural layers of the fissures. A variable proportion of the superior surface of the hemidiaphragm becomes obliterated, depending on the size of the effusion. Superiorly, the intrapleural fluid seems to terminate as a concave meniscus.

Because many small children are radiographed in the supine position, pleural fluid tends to collect posteriorly. If the amount of fluid is large enough, it causes an increase in the density of the hemithorax (Fig. 5–19B). The fluid may also cap the lung apex because of the lordotic position of the supine patient.

Any type of pleural fluid, i.e., exudate, transudate, blood, or even chyle, produces similar radiographic densities. However, empyema due to staphylococcus should be suspected in an infant with a large unilateral effusion. A lack of change in the configuration of pleural effusion with alteration of the position of the patient suggests loculation or organization. The presence of a horizontal air-fluid level rather than a meniscus superiorly indicates a hydropneumothorax.

Because the distribution of pleural effusion is also related to lung elasticity, atypical configurations occur when there is underlying pulmonary disease. A large volume of intrapleural fluid obscures the ipsilateral lung and causes the mediastinum to shift to the opposite side. Absence of shift, then, indicates the presence of atelectasis of the underlying lung.

SUBPULMONIC EFFUSION

With the patient erect, fluid accumulates below the visceral pleura of the diaphragmatic surface of the lung. When it reaches a large enough proportion,

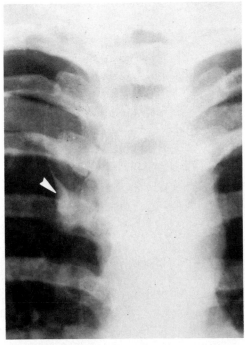

Figure 5–18. The azygos fissure extends inferiorly to envelop the aberrantly positioned azygos vein (*arrow*).

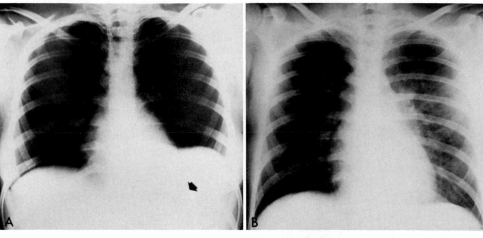

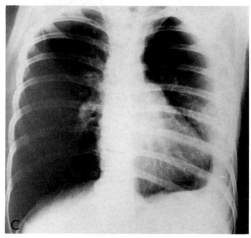

Figure 5–19. *A,* The anteroposterior view of the chest shows an apparently elevated left diaphragmatic dome, which is separated from the stomach bubble *(arrow). B,* In the supine position, the left pleural effusion has caused a diffuse increase in density of the hemithorax. *C,* The left lateral decubitus view demonstrates the extent of the subpulmonic effusion.

the fluid on which the lung is floating will visibly widen the space between the visceral and diaphragmatic pleura. The superior aspect of the fluid then resembles a hemidiaphragm, but its "dome" tends to be more lateral in position than the normal diaphragmatic dome. Moreover, there is a wider than normal distance between the inferior surface of the lung and the gastric air bubble on the left side. The presence of an infrapulmonary collection of fluid can be confirmed readily by lateral decubitus views (Fig. 5–19).

PNEUMOTHORAX

The presence of air outside the visceral pleura on the convex aspect of the lung indicates a pneumothorax (Fig. 5–20). In older children, this pleural surface is usually readily visible.

Visualization of the visceral pleural line, which is necessary to establish the diagnosis of pneumothorax, can be improved on an expiratory film, because the amount of intrapleural air is *relatively* increased on expiration. Loss of volume of the ipsilateral lung also occurs with pneumothorax, but until atelectasis becomes severe, the density of the lung does not increase markedly. This lack of change is due to diminished perfusion and thus a diminution in the

radiographic density produced by the vascular structures within the poorly ventilated lung (Fig. 5–21).

Intrapleural air is often less obvious on radiographs of supine infants, because the air tends to rise

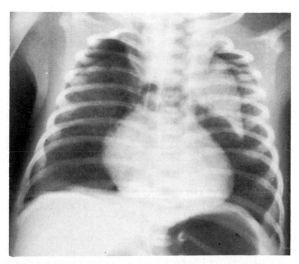

Figure 5–20. Bilateral pneumothoraces are indicated by air outlining the visceral pleura of the lung apices. A pneumomediastinum is also present, separating the inferior surfaces of the thymic lobes from the pericardium.

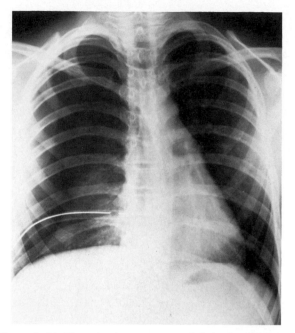

Figure 5–21. There is a large amount of air in the right pleural space in spite of thoracostomy drainage. The lung remains lucent although decreased in volume. There is a slight mediastinal shift to the left.

over the anterior surface of the lung. In these patients, lateral decubitus views may be necessary to demonstrate the presence and extent of a pneumothorax (MacEwan et al, 1971). This method is helpful even in the presence of bilateral pneumothoraces. Also, a collection of intrapleural air medial to the lung may simulate a pneumomediastinum (Moskowitz and Griscom, 1976) and may stretch the pleura so that it herniates across the midline (Fletcher, 1978) (Fig. 5–22). In medial pneumothorax, however, air does not collect between the thymus and the pericardium as it does in pneumomediastinum.

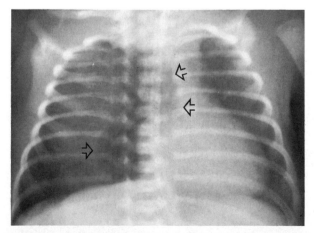

Figure 5–22. Intrapleural air *(arrows)* is outlined medial to the right lung on an anteroposterior portable film taken with the patient recumbent. (Reproduced with permission from Fletcher BD: Medial herniation of the parietal pleura: a useful sign of pneumothorax in neonates. AJR 130:469, 1978. © 1978, American Roentgen Ray Society.)

THE MEDIASTINUM

The mediastinum includes those structures that are encased in the parietal pleura between the two lungs. The pleural reflections of a number of mediastinal structures can be visualized on plain chest radiographs. It is beyond the scope of this chapter to discuss mediastinal anatomy in detail. The heart and thymus, however, are frequently sources of confusion in the interpretation of chest radiographs, and some of their features are described subsequently. Other anatomic details are shown in Figure 5–23.

The mediastinum is arbitrarily divided, for descriptive purposes, into three compartments: the anterior, which contains lymph nodes and the thymus gland; the middle, which contains the heart and great vessels, esophagus, trachea, and major bronchi; and the posterior, which contains the descending aorta, azygos venous system, and sympathetic chain.

Anterior Mediastinum

The major structure of the anterior mediastinal compartment, the thymus, is a source of endless confusion because of its protean configuration. Although the thymus gland continues to grow throughout childhood until prepubescence, it is relatively most prominent in the infant and small child, in whom it can simulate a mediastinal tumor or cardiomegaly. Unfortunately, no modality exists that is capable of distinguishing a large, but otherwise normal, thymus from a lymphomatous anterior mediastinal mass (Fig. 5–24) with absolute certainty. A lobular contour, anterior mediastinal lymphadenopathy, and extension of the mass posterior to the superior vena cava suggests the presence of neoplastic tissue. A number of radiologic characteristics, however, help to elucidate this polymorphous structure:

SAIL SIGN. The thymus projects laterally to (usually to the right of) the upper mediastinum, and its shape is reminiscent of a triangular sail. Its sharply defined lateral and lower borders as well as the absence of an air bronchogram help to distinguish it from upper lobe consolidation (Fig. 5–25).

WAVE SIGN. Because the edge of the thymus is indented by the costal cartilages, its lateral border sometimes has a wave-like contour.

RETRACTION. Under fluoroscopy, the edge of the thymus can be seen to retract momentarily during a deep inspiration. At this time, the wave-like configuration of its lateral border becomes apparent.

ABSENCE OF MEDIASTINAL DISPLACEMENT. The thymus is a compliant structure and, with rare exceptions, such as severe hyperplasia or posterior ectopy, should not compress or displace adjacent structures.

ANTERIOR POSITION. On lateral projections, the gland tends to obliterate the space between the posterior border of the sternum and the anterior surface of the right ventricle. The lateral view is, therefore, very helpful in making the correct diagnosis (Fig. 5–26).

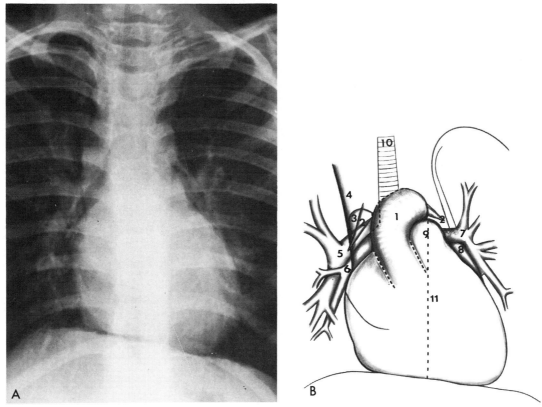

Figure 5–23. *A* and *B*, Normal mediastinal structures outlined by a small pneumomediastinum. *1*, Aorta; *2*, thymus; *3*, azygos vein; *4*, superior vena cava; *5*, right pulmonary artery; *6*, right bronchi; *7*, left pulmonary artery; *8*, left bronchus; *9*, main pulmonary artery; *10*, trachea; *11*, descending aorta.

Figure 5–24. A sagittal magnetic resonance image demonstrates a bright anterior mediastinal mass in a teen-ager with lymphoma. The appearance of the mass is indistinguishable from that of the thymus in a younger child. Note the relationship of the ascending aorta *(A)*, the innominate artery *(a)*, and left innominate vein *(V)* to the trachea *(t)*. *LA*, Left atrium; *P*, right pulmonary artery.

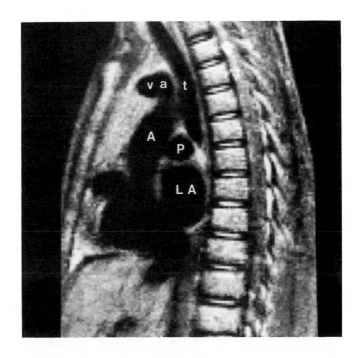

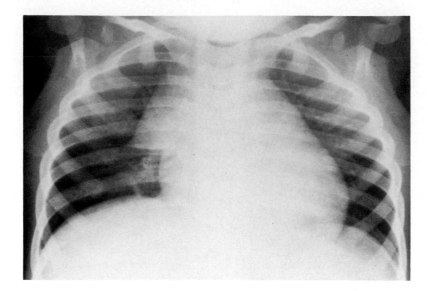

Figure 5–25. Thymic "sail sign."

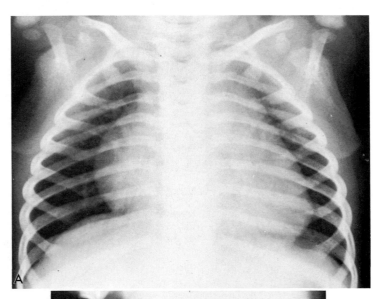

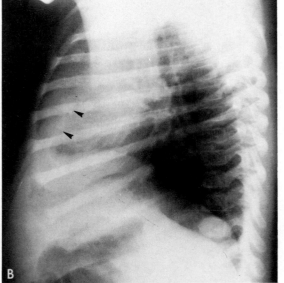

Figure 5–26. *A,* Apparent cardiomegaly due to a large thymus on the anteroposterior projection. *B,* The lateral view shows a normal retrocardiac space. The anterior density is caused by the thymus *(arrows).*

EFFECT OF STEROIDS. Exogenous steroids were sometimes used diagnostically to promote involution of the gland and thus to exclude a mediastinal mass. Such testing is now rarely used.

Absence of the Thymus. Along with anomalies of the aortic arch and absence of the parathyroids, the thymus may also be missing, as in the DiGeorge syndrome. The thymus is also dysplastic in a number of immunodeficiency diseases. Thymic involution occurs with stress, so absence of the gland cannot usually be diagnosed with certainty on chest radiographs. Conversely, definite identification of thymic tissue may be helpful in assessment of immune disorders.

Later CT studies have shown that the thymus persists well into adult life as a thin, anterior mediastinal structure, the shape of which resembles an arrowhead. It also becomes more lucent with age because of the infiltration of fat (Moore et al, 1983).

Middle Mediastinum

The heart and pericardium are the major components of the middle mediastinum. In infants, cardiac morphologic features are difficult to assess because of the thymus, which drapes over the anterior aspect of the pericardium. In addition, the heart is more transverse in position, and the right cardiac border, which is formed by the right atrium, is relatively prominent. The ratio of the transverse diameter of the heart to that of the thorax is usually given as 0.5 or less for the child. A ratio of 0.6 or more almost always indicates a cardiac abnormality in an infant. Considerable variation in these measurements occurs in normal infants and children. These variations are related to the phase of the respiratory and cardiac cycles during which the radiographic exposure is made as well as to the variable size of the thymus. Edwards and colleagues (1981) have made detailed measurements of cardiothoracic ratios in infants during the first week after birth. They found that the least variability occurred when they compared the maximum width of the cardiac silhouette with the transverse diameter of the bony thorax measured either at the inner aspects of the eighth ribs or at the widest internal width of the bony thorax. The ratios obtained were less than 0.57 in infants with normal lungs and less than 0.60 in those with abnormal lungs.

Cardiomegaly is frequently simulated by a large thymus or on AP radiographs taken during expiration. Because the heart must enlarge multidirectionally, a lateral view of the chest allows a correct interpretation (see Fig. 5–26).

The arch of the azygos vein casts an oval shadow on a frontal projection at the right tracheobronchial junction. It varies in size with posture, respiration, and disease states involving right-sided heart function. It is, however, not consistently visible in infants and younger children, and according to Wishart (1972), the arch can be so variable that correlation of its width with pathologic states is uncertain.

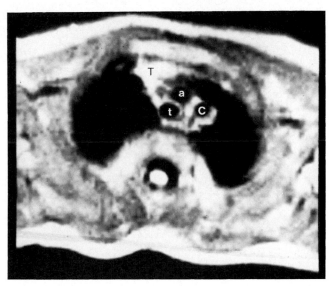

Figure 5–27. An axial magnetic resonance image of the chest of an infant shows the normal rounded appearance of the trachea *(t)* in the superior mediastinum. The innominate artery *(a)*, left carotid artery *(C)*, and thymus *(T)* are also visible. (Reproduced with permission from Fletcher BD, Dearborn DG, and Mulopulos GP: MR imaging in infants with airway obstruction: preliminary observations. Radiology 160:245–249, 1986.)

Trachea and Major Bronchi

The ability of CT to image in transverse section has resulted in improved appreciation of the dimensions and shape of the trachea in the infant and child (Griscom, 1982; Effman et al, 1983). At most levels, the intrathoracic trachea appears nearly circular in cross section, with some loss of roundness near the larynx and carina. Some tracheas are also indented by the aortic arch and flattened posteriorly. The normal infant trachea tends to be less round than that of the older child (Griscom, 1983). Computed tomography permits precise estimation of cross-sectional tracheal area in patients with mediastinal masses, such as lymphoma (Kirks et al, 1983), and tracheal stenosis due to complete tracheal rings (Berdon et al, 1984). Magnetic resonance imaging is capable of displaying the trachea and mediastinal vessels without the use of exogenous contrast materials (Fletcher, Dearborn, and Mulopulos, 1986) (Fig. 5–27).

Because of their oblique anatomic course, the major bronchi are less satisfactorily visualized by cross-sectional imaging methods than the trachea. In many children with suspected tracheobronchial compression due to mediastinal masses, high KV radiography, fluoroscopy, and conventional tomography continue to be useful methods of estimating major airway obstruction (Mandell et al, 1982).

Vascular Rings

Vascular rings encircling the trachea may be responsible for symptoms of airway obstruction. Two common types of vascular rings are double aortic arch and right aortic arch with an aberrant left

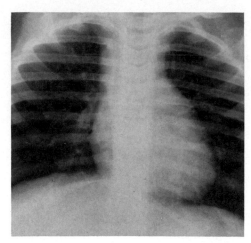

Figure 5–28. The "mass" to the right of the trachea is produced by a right aortic arch. The pleural reflection of the descending thoracic aorta is also clearly visible adjacent to the right lateral vertebral border.

subclavian artery. In the latter disorder, traction by the ligamentum arteriosum contributes to tracheal compression. In either of these types of vascular rings, radiographs demonstrate deviation of the trachea to the left by the right-sided aortic arch component. Unlike mirror-image aortic arches, which are frequently associated with congenital heart disease, such as tetralogy of Fallot, vascular rings are frequently a cause of tracheal compression and are found in otherwise normal children. Abnormal tracheal deviation should therefore be sought on chest radiographs of a child with signs and symptoms of upper airway obstruction (Fig. 5–28). The diagnosis of the vascular ring can be confirmed by means of a barium esophagogram, and the exact type of anomaly may be demonstrated by angiography (Tonkin et al,

1980) or CT (Frye et al, 1987). There is currently considerable interest in noninvasive diagnosis of these anomalies using MRI (Fletcher, Dearborn, and Mulopulos, 1986; Bisset et al, 1987) (Fig. 5–29).

Posterior Mediastinum

The posterior mediastinum should be assessed to detect neurogenic tumors, which displace the paravertebral pleural reflections. These lesions are best evaluated by means of CT or MRI (Siegel et al, 1986) (Fig. 5–30).

The left lateral border of the descending aorta may be clearly visible during childhood but usually cannot be seen in the infant. Chest radiographs taken in the immediate newborn period often show a small mass to the left of the upper mediastinum. This shadow, which is due to the closing ductus arteriosus, has been termed the *ductus bump.*

PNEUMOMEDIASTINUM

When an alveolar rupture occurs, the extravasated gas traverses the pulmonary interstitium to enter the mediastinum. On frontal projections, the air may be visible as an increased lucency adjacent to the heart borders. More often, however, the only direct evidence of pneumomediastinum is elevation of the thymic lobes away from the pericardium. This has been termed the *spinnaker-sail sign* (see Fig. 5–20). Extension of air into the neck occurs less frequently in infants than in older children. Occasionally, other mediastinal structures, such as the aortic arch, azygos vein, main pulmonary artery, and superior vena cava, may also be outlined by mediastinal air (see Fig. 5–23).

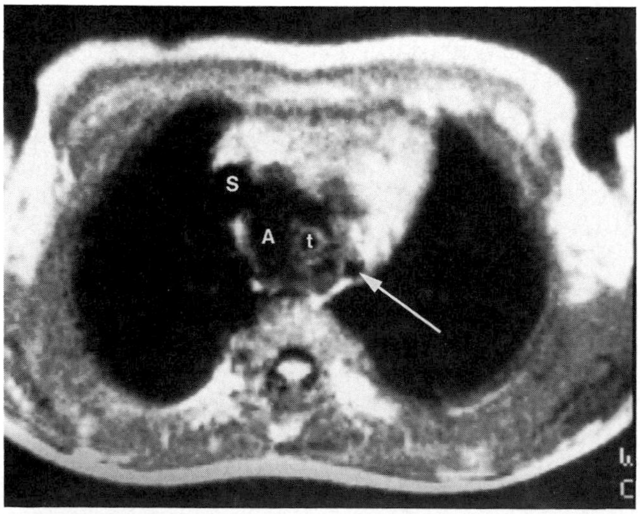

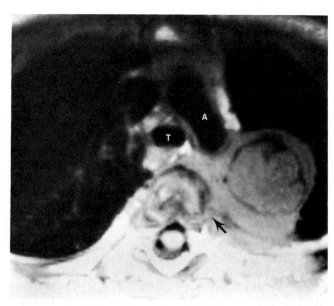

Figure 5–29. An axial magnetic resonance image of an infant with a vascular ring shows a right aortic arch (A) displacing the narrowed trachea (t) to the left. The ring encircles the trachea and gives rise to the left subclavian artery (arrow). S, Superior vena cava. (Reproduced with permission from Fletcher BD, Dearborn DG, and Mulopulos GP: MR imaging in infants with airway obstruction: preliminary observations. Radiology 160:245–249, 1986.)

Figure 5–30. An axial magnetic resonance image shows a large left paraspinal neuroblastoma extending into the intervertebral foramen (arrow) and spinal canal. The dark rings represent calcification within the tumor mass. A, Aortic arch; T, trachea.

In the much less common *pneumopericardium,* gas completely surrounds the epicardium and is thus visible in the pericardial sac between the central tendon of the diaphragm and inferior heart border as well as within the pericardial reflections over the great vessels. In contrast to the thymus's position in mediastinal emphysema, the gland remains approximated to the pericardium.

MEDIASTINAL MASSES

Because of the extrapleural position of a mediastinal mass, its surface adjacent to the lung is sharply defined. Its superior and inferior extremities tend to taper. Mediastinal masses can also be differentiated from lesions arising in the pulmonary parenchyma by the lack of an air bronchogram. A mass may displace mediastinal structures, such as the trachea (Fig. 5–31).

THE BRONCHI

Air Bronchogram

Air bronchogram refers to the air-containing bronchi that become visible when the surrounding lung parenchyma is opacified because of alveolar consolidation or atelectasis (Fig. 5–32). It is perhaps the most revealing sign of pulmonary parenchymal disease. An air bronchogram is not seen in abnormalities of the pleura or in lesions arising in the mediastinum. For obvious reasons, an air bronchogram is not visible within solid parenchymal tumors or fluid-containing pulmonary cysts. However, the main stem and segmental bronchi can produce an "air bronchogram" in the absence of parenchymal disease, because of their contiguity with other water-density hilar structures and the normal thickness of their walls.

In the absence of major pulmonary disease, the bronchial lumens are sometimes outlined along a portion of their length or on cross section. These

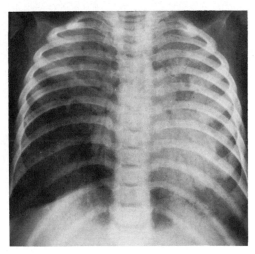

Figure 5–32. Bilateral, diffuse air bronchograms caused by *Pneumocystis carinii* pneumonia.

findings, which are most prominent in the lung bases, are thought to be due to bronchial wall thickening or "peribronchial infiltration" and are usually diagnosed as bronchitis or mild bronchopneumonia. However, the exact implications of these roentgen findings remain unclear.

BRONCHIECTASIS

Bronchiectasis is associated with chronic pulmonary infection and is particularly severe in the lungs of patients with cystic fibrosis of the pancreas. Foreign body aspiration, aspergillosis, ciliary dysmotility, and immunodeficiency disorders should also be considered as possible causative agents in localized chronic pulmonary disease with bronchiectasis.

In chronic pneumonia, loss of lung volume may lead to secondary bronchial dilation. A central bronchial obstruction need not be present. Bronchograms may demonstrate a lack of normal tapering of the bronchi and incomplete peripheral filling, but irreversible saccular bronchiectasis is rarely present.

In cystic fibrosis, bronchiectasis is eventually recognizable on plain films because of either mucus filling of the dilated bronchi or peribronchial disease. On bronchography, the extent of bronchiectasis in affected patients is often found to be much greater than was suspected from the evidence on the plain films (Fig. 5–33). In severe bronchiectasis from any cause, large mucus plugs may form and simulate mass lesions (Fig. 5–34).

Further abnormalities of the bronchial tree are discussed in the sections on decreased lung volume.

THE HILA AND PULMONARY VESSELS

The right and left pulmonary arteries and the upper lobe veins are mainly responsible for the

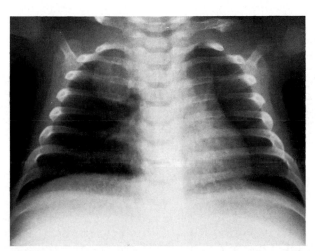

Figure 5–31. A neuroblastoma arising from the right posterior mediastinum has produced a tracheal shift to the left. Calcification is faintly visible at the lower margin of the tumor.

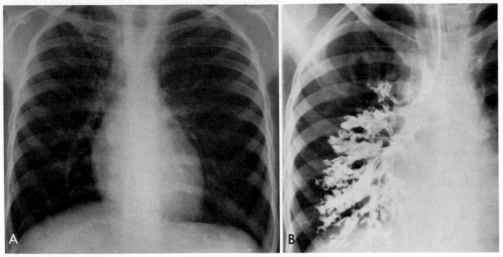

Figure 5–33. *A,* Bronchiectasis seems to be most marked in the right upper lobe of this patient with cystic fibrosis. *B,* On bronchography, extensive middle and lower lobe bronchiectasis becomes obvious. The upper lobe bronchi are incompletely filled.

radiographic density of the hila. The major bronchi are projected as tubular lucencies. The lower lobe veins return to the left atrium below the hila. The bronchopulmonary lymph nodes are recognizable only if they enlarge. The right hilum, because of the configuration of the heart, may appear slightly more prominent than the left. Spurious differences in size of the hila can occur because of magnification when

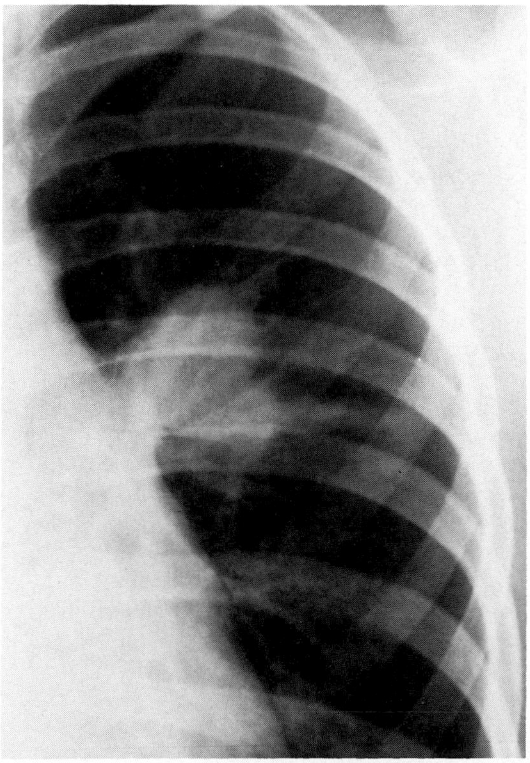

Figure 5–34. Bronchial mucus plugs due to aspergillosis appear as well-defined nodular densities involving the proximal bronchi. Note the finger-like projections of mucus extending into the more distal bronchi.

the chest is rotated. The left hilum is normally slightly higher than the right.

ASSESSMENT OF HILAR SIZE

This is a largely subjective step in the evaluation of chest radiographs. The hila are decreased in size in cyanotic congenital heart disease, such as tetralogy of Fallot, and in hypoplasia or absence of a pulmonary artery. Enlargement of the pulmonary arteries is most commonly associated with left-to-right shunt. Coussement and Gooding (1973) found that, in the presence of a left-to-right shunt, the diameter of the right descending pulmonary artery, as measured on frontal projections, was never less than that of the trachea.

Enlargement of the bronchopulmonary nodes imparts a lobular appearance to the border of the hilum that faces the lung. This appearance is in contrast to the linear or slightly concave aspect presented by the pulmonary arteries. A well-exposed, nonrotated lateral view is very helpful in the assessment of changes in the size of the hila (Fig. 5–35).

Computed tomography and MRI are also sensitive methods of detecting enlarged hilar lymph nodes (Heelan et al, 1985) (Fig. 5–36). Magnetic resonance imaging is capable of distinguishing hilar masses from enlarged vessels without the use of intravenous contrast enhancement.

THE PULMONARY VASCULATURE

The pulmonary arteries and veins are responsible for the majority of the linear densities seen in the lungs. On plain chest radiographs and on tomograms, the arteries and veins can be distinguished, because the arteries branch from the hilus segmen-

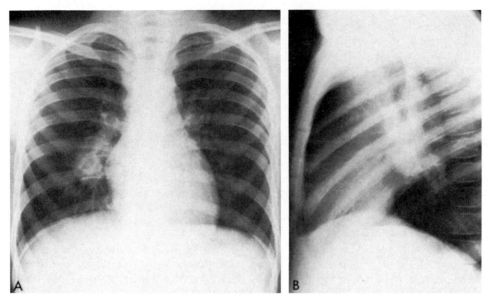

Figure 5–35. The enlargement of bronchopulmonary nodes in the right hilum *(A)* is well visualized on the lateral projection *(B)*.

tally with the bronchi and arch laterally and downward in a "weeping willow" pattern. The upper lobe veins course toward the heart in a position lateral to the arteries, and the lower lobe veins are nearly horizontal in their course to the left atrium.

Pulmonary Arteries

The size of the pulmonary arteries roughly correlates with the amount of flow. In a study by Schwarz and co-workers (1970), the presence of a left-to-right shunt was diagnosed with 100 per cent accuracy only when the pulmonary–systemic shunt ratio was greater than 2.2:1. Small shunts (Qp-Qs less than 1.4:1) were not appreciated in 45 to 58 per cent of the cases. In assessing increased flow to the lungs, it

is helpful to concentrate on the size of the arteries in the middle third of each lung. In the lung periphery, a fine reticular pattern may be seen as the smaller arterial branches become visible owing to engorgement.

Pulmonary arterial hypertension is recognizable when there is an exaggerated discrepancy between the calibers of the central and peripheral pulmonary arteries.

Decreased arterial flow associated with cyanotic congenital heart disease results in hyperlucent lungs with decreased vascular markings.

The main pulmonary artery and its main branches can also be studied by means of dynamic, contrast-enhanced CT and by MRI (Fig. 5–37). In patients with pulmonary hypertension, MRI may show en-

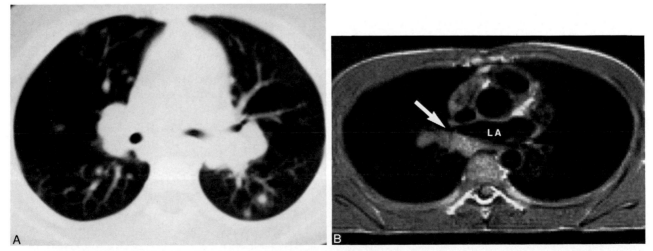

Figure 5–36. *A,* A computed tomogram scan demonstrates bilateral hilar node enlargement. *B,* An axial magnetic resonance image of another patient shows a tumor extending into the right hilum, compressing the posterior wall of the left atrium *(LA)* and the right pulmonary vein *(arrow).*

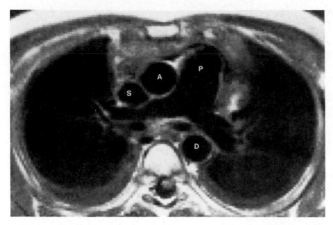

Figure 5–37. An axial magnetic resonance image demonstrates a normal main pulmonary artery (*P*) and its right and left branches. The ascending aorta (*A*), descending aorta (*D*), and superior vena cava (*S*) are also shown.

hancement of the pulmonary arterial blood because of slow flow.

Bronchial Arteries

On plain films, the bronchial arteries are not visible at their point of origin from the descending aorta. Their intrapulmonary branches, however, may be recognized as fine, reticular densities in the central and basilar portions of the lungs of patients whose pulmonary arterial flow is reduced owing to cyanotic congenital heart disease.

Pulmonary Veins

The caliber of the pulmonary veins increases as they become engorged. They can be distinguished from pulmonary arteries by their somewhat tortuous course, which can be traced to the periphery of the lungs. Pulmonary veins can also be recognized as such by their lack of peripheral tapering and absence of artery-like branching as well as by the more horizontal path of those in the lower lobe. An increase in pulmonary venous pressure is reflected by distention of the veins in the upper lung zones due to spasm of the veins in the lung bases.

THE LUNG PARENCHYMA

PULMONARY EDEMA

Leakage of fluid from the pulmonary microvascular bed results in interstitial pulmonary edema. An early sign of fluid in the perivascular interstitial space is a loss of definition of the pulmonary veins. This sign is best appreciated in the middle third of the lungs and is probably more reliable than loss of definition of hila, or "hilar haze."

Interstitial edema is also manifested radiologically by Kerley A and B lines, which are caused by fluid

in the interlobular septa (Heitzman and Ziter, 1966) (Fig. 5–38A). The A lines are thin linear densities that tend to radiate upward from the hila. The B lines are short horizontal linear densities that extend for a short distance into the lung from the pleural surface. They may be difficult to identify on the AP view of the lungs of a small infant and occasionally are better seen in the retrosternal area on a lateral view. In pulmonary edema, the fissures of the lungs also may appear thickened because of subpleural edema or fluid within the fissure.

Alveolar edema, which may be preceded by interstitial edema, fills the air spaces and produces ill-defined homogeneous shadows of water density through which an air bronchogram may be visible (Fig. 5–38B). The typical picture of alveolar edema is one in which the medial aspects of both lungs are homogeneously opacified and the lung periphery is spared. However, variations are numerous; a common example is pulmonary edema that is predominantly right-sided, which may be related to differences in respiratory motion of the two lungs because of the patient's position or because of differences in pulmonary lymphatic drainage. When there is underlying chronic lung disease, the patterns of pulmonary edema may be very atypical. Pulmonary edema serves as a model for the study of other types of air space and interstitial disease to be discussed later.

PATTERNS OF PULMONARY DISEASE

Alveolar (air space) disease refers to any disorder in which the air spaces of the lung become filled with a substance of water density. Thus, although pneumonia is often used as the prototype, other materials, such as edema fluid, pus, and blood, can produce identical radiographic appearances. When the process involves both the air spaces and the interstitium, the shadows cast by the air space or alveolar consolidation usually predominate.

Alveolar lesions are recognized by their ill-defined, fluffy margins; a tendency to coalesce; large areas of involvement; and, if the airways are clear of fluid, an air bronchogram (Felson, 1967) (see Fig. 5–32). The "air alveologram" is another feature of pneumonia that imparts a mottled appearance because of numerous small lucencies cast by uninvolved groups of alveoli.

Pneumonia may be lobar or segmental in distribution, although many (probably most) pneumonias of childhood are nonsegmental. This finding can be explained by a tendency for the disease to spread circumferentially from lobule to lobule via the intra-alveolar pores of Kohn (Fraser and Wortzman, 1959).

Localization of Disease

For purposes of physiotherapy, bronchoscopy, and surgery, the exact localization of pulmonary densities

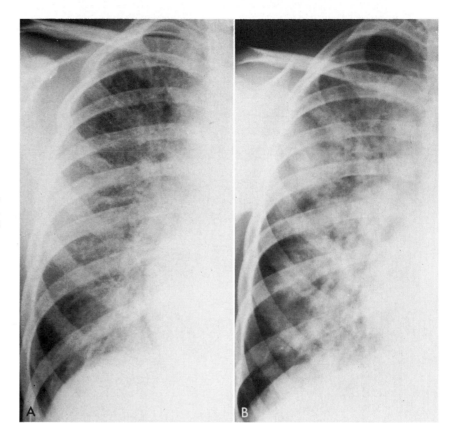

Figure 5–38. *A,* Reticular pattern with Kerley "A" and "B" lines in interstitial edema. *B,* At a later date, the same patient developed a "fluffy" coalescent pattern of alveolar edema.

becomes necessary. Although, as noted previously, disease may not be confined to a segment or even a lobe, when it does correspond to the anatomy of the bronchial tree, its distribution can be determined. It is helpful to localize pulmonary consolidation by contiguity with a fissure; for example, consolidation limited on its inferior aspect by the minor fissure must involve the contiguous (anterior) segment of the upper lobe.

Silhouette Sign

Silhouette sign refers to the finding that the borders of contiguous structures of similar radiodensity are obscured by one another. The concept can then be applied to a disease process that produces a water density when it is in contact with structures of similar density, such as the heart, aortic arch, and superior surface of the diaphragm. A silhouette sign is present when the contiguous borders of these structures are lost. This sign is used most frequently for localization of disease to the right middle lobe and lingula, in which the right and left heart borders, respectively, are obscured (Fig. 5–39). If disease is localized in the basilar segments of the lower lobes, the adjacent diaphragmatic surfaces are usually obliterated. The right upper mediastinal border may be lost owing to disease in the anterior segment of the right upper lobe, and a density in the apicoposterior segment of the left upper lobe may mask the aortic knob.

Absence of a silhouette sign can also be helpful. For example, a lesion in the superior segment of a lower lobe is projected through the hilum and may be mistaken for perihilar pneumonia or hilar enlargement. Careful observation will reveal the borders of the hilum distinctly visible through the density, because this segment is separated from the more anterior hilum by normally aerated lung (Fig. 5–40).

The silhouette sign is occasionally erroneously identified when the right heart border is obscured by a normal pulmonary artery or by the parasternal soft tissues of the anterior chest wall in patients with pectus excavatum.

Errors of Interpretation

Poor definition of the right heart border is particularly prevalent in infants and is often explained by overlying thymic tissue or poor resolution of the numerous pulmonary vessels in the area. Overdiagnosis of abnormalities based on such a finding is probably fairly common, although Culham (1981) investigated this "no man's land" of pediatric pulmonary diagnosis by CT and found that pleural or pulmonary abnormalities explained the lack of definition of the right heart border in seven of eight cases. Computed tomography, however, is not routinely recommended for this purpose. A well-exposed AP film of a recumbent patient taken during maximum inspiration will often rule out or confirm the presence of disease in this area.

Consolidations in the left lung behind the heart are often overlooked because of the large similar density produced by the ventricles. This fault in

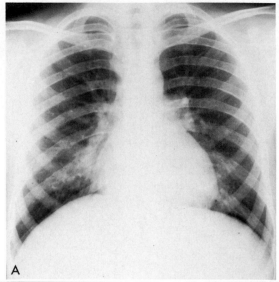

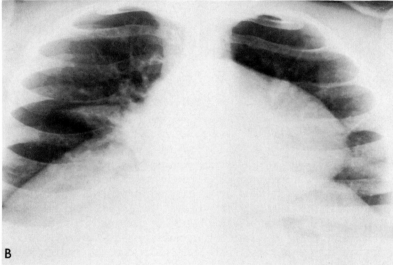

Figure 5–39. *A,* Obliteration of the right heart border indicates middle lobe disease. *B,* The anteroposterior lordotic view of the same patient shows a wedge-shaped atelectatic middle lobe.

Figure 5–40. A round mass due to pneumonia is superimposed over the right hilum. The disease, which is in the superior segment of the right lower lobe, does not create a positive silhouette with the hilum or heart border because of its posterior location (compare with Fig. 5–39).

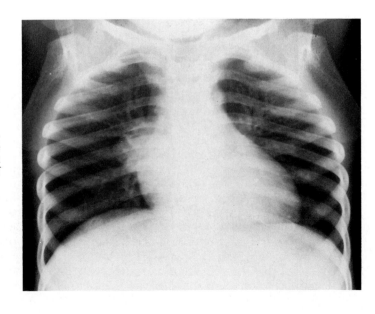

diagnosis is usually the combined product of under-exposure of the chest film and lack of observer perception. Because these pneumonias involve the posterior aspects of the lung bases, they are revealed on a well-positioned lateral view, which shows an apparent increase in density of the lower thoracic vertebrae just above the posterior cardiophrenic angle. The lower thoracic vertebrae normally appear more lucent than the upper because of the large volume of superimposed lung and the absence of overlying axillary and scapular shadows. Therefore, an interruption of this sequence of densities, which might be termed a *spine sign,* indicates the presence of pulmonary disease (Fig. 5–41).

Opaque structures, such as the liver, immediately inferior to the diaphragm, may also mask pulmonary lesions in the posterior sulcus of the lung base. For this reason, we add a coned-down, overpenetrated

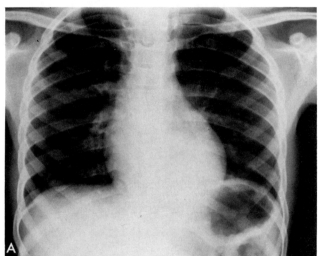
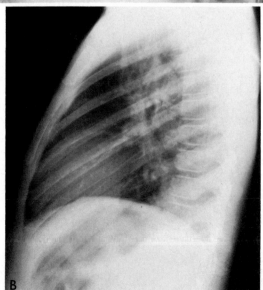

Figure 5–41. *A,* The left basilar pneumonia has created an increase in density behind the heart on the left. *B,* On the lateral projection, the pneumonia is superimposed over the lower thoracic vertebrae.

AP view of the lower thorax and upper abdomen (Bein, 1979) to our routine chest radiographs when searching for pulmonary metastases. Alternatively, right and left anterior oblique views may be added.

Interstitial Patterns

Felson (1979) recognizes eight distinctive lung patterns that, to the experienced radiologist, can be very helpful in narrowing the differential diagnosis. It is especially practical to distinguish between an alveolar pattern of disease (previously discussed) and an interstitial pattern, but pulmonary disease is rarely confined to either the interstitial or alveolar spaces. This statement is particularly important to remember when examining patients with pneumonia. The commonly held belief that viral pneumonias are predominately interstitial is quite inaccurate and can lead one to an entirely erroneous diagnosis.

Interstitial pulmonary edema is a prime example of an interstitial pulmonary pattern (see Fig. 5–38A). Normal pulmonary vascular markings are obliterated by perivascular edema. Kerley lines, due to edema of the interlobular septa, account for the diffuse linear markings. In spite of the increase in lung density caused by the interstitial fluid, no air bronchogram is visible.

When the parenchymal or interalveolar interstitium is involved, a reticulonodular pattern is produced. A diffuse cloudy or "ground-glass" appearance of the lungs has also been attributed to involvement of the parenchymal interstitium. *Honeycomb lung,* which is often associated with histiocytosis, implies a reticular pattern in which small cysts are visible. Interstitial patterns in infants and children may be produced by such diseases as pulmonary hemosiderosis, histiocytosis, collagen-vascular diseases, tuberculosis, sarcoid, lymphangiectasia, and hypersensitivity pneumonitis. Examples of interstitial patterns are shown in Figures 5–42 through 5–44.

On high-resolution CT, a variety of findings are characteristic of interstitial disease. These include thickened, irregular pleural and fissural surfaces, ground-glass pulmonary densities, emphysematous areas, nodules of various sizes, and reticular densities (Naidich et al, 1985; Zerhouni et al, 1985).

Pneumonia

The usefulness of the chest radiograph overshadows even that of the stethoscope in the diagnosis of pneumonia. Indeed, the need to evaluate pulmonary infections is the major indication for chest radiography during childhood. Radiologists have long sought to specify infectious causative agents on the basis of radiographic patterns, and particular emphasis has been placed on differentiating bacterial and viral pneumonias by equating viral disease with interstitial patterns and bacterial infection with air space involvement. Although infections usually produce a combination of air space and interstitial abnormali-

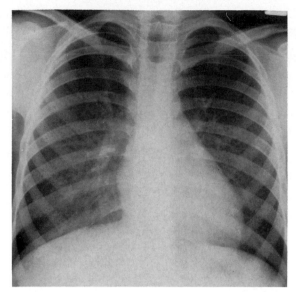

Figure 5–42. The bilateral "ground-glass" appearance of the lungs is due to interstitial disease associated with hypersensitivity reaction. There is no air bronchogram.

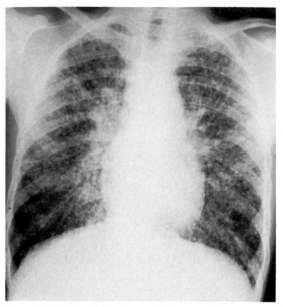

Figure 5–44. A nodular interstitial pattern due to sarcoid.

ties, certain generalizations can be helpful in distinguishing bacterial and viral disease (Griscom, 1988).

Bacterial pneumonias usually produce air space disease with lobar or segmental lung opacities. Pleural effusions may occur, including empyema, which is prevalent in staphylococcal and other purulent infections. Plugging of the small airways may lead to the formation of pneumatoceles.

An unnerving appearance of bacterial pneumonias is their occasional presentation as a spherical density.

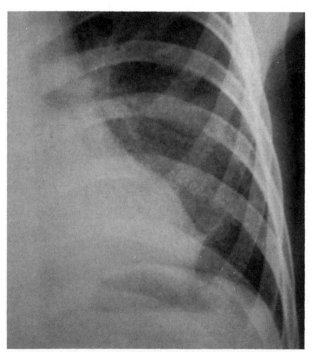

Figure 5–43. Fine reticular pattern, best seen in the left lower lobe, in a patient with desquamative interstitial pneumonitis.

If an air bronchogram is not present, the specter of tumor arises. The edges of these "round pneumonias" are usually not as well defined as those of a neoplasm, however, and the pneumonia usually does not appear as a circular shadow on both AP and lateral radiographs. Follow-up radiography a few days later will usually reveal the true nature of the lesion (Fig. 5–45).

Viral pneumonias, in comparison, usually produce more generalized interstitial patterns with less marked opacification. They frequently occur with bronchial wall thickening, peribronchial "cuffing," and nonconfluent patchy opacifications. When small airways are involved, as with respiratory syncytial viral infection, there is often pulmonary hyperinflation with anterior bowing of the sternum and flattening of the diaphragm (Osborne, 1978).

Other organisms may be suspected when they produce characteristic patterns. For example, hilar and paratracheal adenopathy is frequently associated with primary tuberculosis; mycoplasma pneumonia often produces lobar or segmental opacities in children with minor symptomatology, and group B streptococcal pneumonia in the newborn may be indistinguishable from the reticulogranular pattern of hyaline membrane disease.

DECREASED LUNG VOLUME

Atelectasis

Basically, collapse of lung parenchyma occurs from one of two causes: (1) obstruction of an airway and resorption of gas from the alveolus, or (2) compression by fluids or gas in the pleural space or by an intrathoracic mass. Atelectasis may involve varying amounts of lung parenchyma, depending on the size

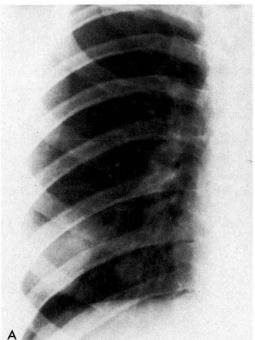

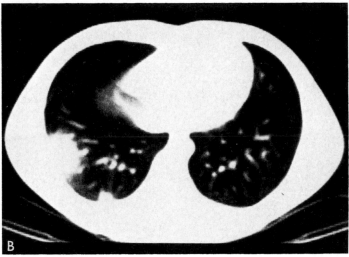

Figure 5–45. Two round pulmonary nodules are seen on a plain chest radiograph *(A)* and computed tomogram *(B)*. The slight pleural reaction adjacent to the large mass suggested the inflammatory nature of the process. A biopsy was performed on the lesions, which resolved with antibiotic therapy.

and numbers of airways that are occluded. Thus atelectasis may involve an entire lung or one or more lobes, segments, or subsegments. Small linear areas of increased density due to hypoventilation and atelectasis are frequently seen in the posterior lung bases on CT images.

Lobar collapse is identified by an increase in density of the involved lung and rearrangement of the position of the interlobar fissures. For example, the major fissures shift posteriorly when the lower lobes collapse (see Fig. 5–17*B*). Right upper lobe atelectasis causes the minor fissure to rotate upward and medially. The major fissure is retracted upward and anteriorly when the left upper lobe becomes atelectatic. Loss of volume of the middle lobe results in a laterally tapering, wedge-shaped density bounded by the major and minor fissures, which can be elegantly demonstrated by means of an AP lordotic view (see Fig. 5–39*B*).

Lobar collapse may be incomplete. The degree of atelectasis is modified by the rate of resorption of gas from the alveolus, the chronicity of obstruction, and the presence of pre-existing parenchymal disease. An air bronchogram will be seen as the alveoli collapse. Just as in pulmonary consolidation, a silhouette sign develops as the dense atelectatic lung parenchyma obliterates the margins of the adjacent mediastinal and diaphragmatic structures.

Lobar atelectasis also results in a number of recognizable secondary signs, which vary to some degree according to the site of involvement: (1) narrowing of the intercostal spaces on the ipsilateral side, (2) elevation of the hemidiaphragm adjacent to a lower lobe collapse, (3) upward displacement of the hilum in upper lobe atelectasis and downward displacement in lower lobe collapse, (4) shift of the cardiac silhou-

ette or trachea toward the atelectatic lobe, and (5) compensatory hyperinflation of uninvolved portions of lung or of the opposite lung. The last two indirect effects of lobar collapse require further comment. Tracheal shift may be detected clinically and radiologically when upper lobe atelectasis occurs in older children and adults. However, shift of the trachea alone is a less valuable sign in infants because of the natural redundancy of the trachea and its tendency to buckle to the right. Instead, when an upper lobe is atelectatic, the entire mediastinum appears to tilt toward the collapsed lobe. Furthermore, when there is reduction in volume of a lower lobe, shift of the heart toward the side of collapse occurs especially readily in infants because of the marked elasticity of their mediastinal structures.

Compensatory hyperinflation of uninvolved lobes of the same lung or of the other lung is recognized by hyperlucency and splaying of the affected pulmonary vessels. Actual herniation of lung across the upper mediastinum toward the affected hemithorax is common. Occasionally, confusion may arise between primary and compensatory emphysema. This is discussed in the section on increased lung volume.

In terms of displacement of intrathoracic structures, atelectasis at the segmental or subsegmental level does not cause a significant change. Both are recognized by an increase in density of the involved lung parenchyma. Segmental collapse produces a wedge-shaped density, the apex of which is directed toward the hilum. Plate-like areas of subsegmental atelectasis appear as short horizontal linear streaks above the diaphragmatic domes. These tend to occur in disorders in which there is diminished diaphragmatic motion and are not frequently seen in children.

Acute asthma is one example of disease in which

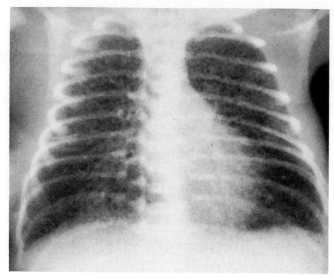

Figure 5–46. The reticulogranular pattern of hyaline membrane disease. In this patient, the lungs are unusually voluminous.

multiple areas of segmental and subsegmental atelectasis occur. The diffuse streaky densities that result may be incorrectly diagnosed as pneumonia. The proper diagnosis is usually clarified by follow-up films made a day or two after the acute attack. Two other situations in which diffuse atelectasis of both lungs occurs also deserve special mention.

The first is hyaline membrane disease, in which there is a deficiency of surfactant and, therefore, an increase in surface tension, leading to alveolar collapse. The classic reticulogranular pattern seen radiologically is produced by overdistention of small airways and some of the air spaces, in contrast to the densities produced by other areas of parenchymal collapse (Recavarren et al, 1967) (Fig. 5–46). This pattern bears some resemblance to the "air alveologram" discussed on page 118. Homogeneous opacification of the lungs in hyaline membrane disease signifies even more extensive parenchymal atelectasis.

A second situation in which massive and rapid collapse of both lungs can occur is when the alveoli contain high concentrations of inspired oxygen. Occlusion of the endotracheal tube in a newborn infant or a period of apnea in a child of any age results in rapid resorption of oxygen at the alveolar-capillary level and consequent atelectasis of both lungs within minutes (Fletcher and Avery, 1973).

Atelectasis versus Dysgenesis

Congenital absence of a lung or lobe simulates atelectasis, and bronchography or angiography may be necessary for a correct diagnosis. When the entire lung is absent, the hemithorax is completely opaque and is occupied by the mediastinum. The decrease in hemithorax size, however, may not be as marked as when massive atelectasis occurs. Hypoplasia may also be accompanied by an increase in extrapleural alveolar tissue, which on lateral radiographs creates

a substernal opacity extending from the thoracic inlet to the diaphragm (Felson, 1972). This opaque stripe is somewhat similar to that produced by collapse of the left upper lobe.

Pneumothorax and pneumomediastinum, indirect signs of pulmonary hypoplasia in newborns, are prevalent in infants born with renal malformations and Potter syndrome (Stern et al, 1972).

INCREASED LUNG VOLUME

An increase in volume of a lobe or lung is usually due to an increase in the amount of gas contained within the alveoli. Only occasionally is the lung increased in density as well as volume, as in the case of *Klebsiella* pneumonia, bronchial obstruction in the fetal lung, and rare malformations and cysts.

Hyperaeration may be unrelated to primary pulmonary disease when it results from acidosis or is associated with cyanotic congenital heart disease. However, obstruction or spasm of small airways, as in emphysema or bronchiolitis, will cause diffuse bilateral pulmonary hyperaeration. Consideration of several disorders that cause a localized increase in lung volume is in order here.

Bronchial Foreign Body

Obstructive emphysema due to an inhaled foreign body results from a ball-valve mechanism by which the foreign body allows the passage of air distal to it but impedes its egress. The resultant voluminous lung or lobe produces a shift of the mediastinum to the opposite side. When these findings are present on routine chest radiographs, they do not constitute a diagnostic problem. However, when a patient presents with clinical features of airway obstruction and abnormal findings are minimal or absent on routine radiographs, expiration films and fluoroscopy are required. The important feature of this type of bronchial occlusion is the inability of the abnormal lung to deflate, which causes the mediastinum to shift away from the obstructed side on expiration.

Congenital Lobar Emphysema

This disorder, which causes an increase in volume of a lobe, also shifts the mediastinum toward the unaffected side. This change, plus partial compression atelectasis of the adjacent portions of the ipsilateral lung (Fig. 5–47), accounts for varying degrees of respiratory distress. The size of the emphysematous lobe is unchanged throughout the respiratory cycle.

Idiopathic Hyperlucent Lung (Swyer-James-MacLeod Syndrome)

It seems appropriate to include this entity here, for although the involved lung is slightly smaller than

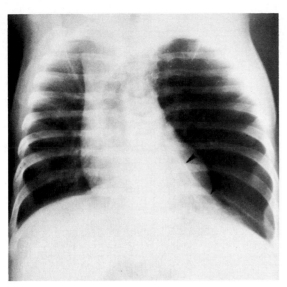

Figure 5–47. Lobar emphysema involving the left upper lobe caused compression atelectasis of the left lower lobe *(arrows)* and produced a marked shift of the mediastinum to the right.

normal, air is trapped within it. No central bronchial obstruction is present, but the peripheral bronchi are "pruned" because of pre-existing obliterative bronchiolitis. The hyperlucency is caused by overdistended alveoli and diminished pulmonary arterial flow (Cumming et al, 1971). Despite the slight hypoplasia of the involved lung, the associated air trapping causes a shift of the mediastinum toward the contralateral side on expiration.

Compensatory Emphysema

On routine chest radiography, it may be difficult to differentiate between hyperaeration of a lobe or lung due to obstructive emphysema and overinflation due to compensatory emphysema associated with atelectasis elsewhere. This can be resolved by fluoroscopy. Because air is not trapped on expiration in an otherwise normal lung that is voluminous owing to compensatory emphysema, it therefore will increase in density and decrease in volume on expiration.

REFERENCES

Alazraki NP, and Friedman PJ: Posterior mediastinal "pseudomass" of the newborn. Am J Roentgenol 116:571, 1972.

Avery ME: Bronchography: outmoded procedure? Pediatrics 46:333, 1970.

Barron TF, Birnbaum NS, Shane LB et al: Pneumocystis carinii pneumonia studied by gallium-67 scanning. Radiology 154:791, 1985.

Bein ME: Plain film diaphragm view as adjunct to full lung tomography. AJR 133:217, 1979.

Berdon WE, Baker DH, Wung J-T et al: Complete cartilage-ring tracheal stenosis associated with anomalous left pulmonary artery: the ring-sling complex. Radiology 152:57, 1984.

Berger PE, Kuhn JP, and Kuhns LR: Computed tomography and the occult tracheobronchial foreign body. Radiology 134:133, 1980.

Bergin C, Roggli V, Coblentz C et al: The secondary pulmonary lobule: normal and abnormal CT appearances. AJR 151:21, 1988.

Bissett GS, Strife JL, Kirks DR et al: Vascular rings: MR imaging. AJR 149:251, 1987.

Brasch RC, Boyd DP, and Gooding CA: Computed tomographic scanning in children: comparison of radiation dose and resolving power of commercial CT scanners. AJR 131:95, 1978.

Brasch RC, Gooding CA, Lallemand DP et al: Magnetic resonance imaging of the thorax in childhood. Radiology 150:463, 1984.

Brasch RC, Gould RG, Gooding CA et al: Upper airway obstruction in infants and children: evaluation with ultrafast CT. Radiology 165:459, 1987.

Brill PW, Ewing ML, and Dunn AA: The value (?) of routine chest radiography in children and adolescents. Pediatrics 52:125, 1973.

Brodeur AE, Silberstein MJ, Graviss ER et al: Three-tier rare-earth imaging system. AJR 136:755, 1981.

Capitanio MA and Kirkpatrick JA: Obstructions of the upper airway in children as reflected on the chest radiograph. Radiology 107:159, 1973.

Cohen MD, Siddiqui A, Weetman R et al: Hodgkin disease and non-Hodgkin lymphomas in children: utilization of radiological modalities. Radiology 158:499, 1986.

Coussement AM, and Gooding CA: Objective radiographic assessment of pulmonary vascularity in children. Radiology 109:649, 1973.

Culham JAG: The right heart border in infancy. Radiology 139:381, 1981.

Cumming GR, MacPherson RI, and Chernick V: Unilateral hyperlucent lung syndrome in children. J Pediatr 78:250, 1971.

DeLevie M, Nogrady MB, and Spence L: Acute laryngotracheobronchitis (croup): correlation of clinical severity with radiologic and virologic findings. Ann Radiol 15:193, 1972.

Dunbar JS: Upper respiratory tract obstruction in infants and children. Am J Roentgenol 109:227, 1970.

Edwards DK, Higgins CB, and Gilpin EA: The cardiothoracic ratio in newborn infants. AJR 136:907, 1981.

Effmann EL, Fram EK, Vock P et al: Tracheal cross-sectional area in children: CT determination. Radiology 149:137, 1983.

Fellows KE, Stigol L, Shuster S et al: Selective bronchial arteriography in patients with cystic fibrosis and massive hemoptysis. Radiology 114:551, 1975.

Felson B: The roentgen diagnosis of disseminated pulmonary alveolar diseases. Semin Roentgenol 2:3, 1967.

Felson B: Pulmonary agenesis and related anomalies. Semin Roentgenol 7:17, 1972.

Felson B: A new look at pattern recognition of diffuse pulmonary disease. AJR 133:183, 1979.

Fletcher BD: Medial herniation of the parietal pleura: a useful sign of pneumothorax in supine neonates. AJR 130:469, 1978.

Fletcher BD: Digital x-ray-imaging techniques in pediatric diagnosis. Am J Dis Child 136:771, 1982.

Fletcher BD and Avery ME: The effects of airway occlusion after oxygen breathing on the lungs of newborn infants: radiologic demonstration in the experimental animal. Radiology 109:655, 1973.

Fletcher BD, Dearborn DG, and Mulopulos GP: MR imaging in infants with airway obstruction: preliminary observations. Radiology 160:245, 1986.

Fletcher BD and Jacobstein MD: MRI of congenital abnormalities of the great arteries. AJR 146:941, 1986.

Fletcher BD, Jacobstein MD, and Morrison SC: Intravenous digital subtraction angiography (IVDSA) in children. Pediatr Radiol 14:423, 1984.

Franken EA Jr, Hurwitz RA, and Battersby JS: Unequal aeration of the lungs in children: the use of pulmonary angiography. Radiology 109:401, 1973.

Fraser RG and Wortzman G: Acute pneumococcal lobar pneumonia: the significance of nonsegmental distribution. J Can Assoc Radiol 10:37, 1959.

Frey EE, Sato Y, Smith WL et al: Cine CT of the mediastinum in pediatric patients. Radiology 165:19, 1987.

Gates GF, Dore EK, Markarian M, and Takanaka J: Radionuclide imaging of airway obstruction following assisted ventilation. Am J Dis Child 130:1222, 1976.

Godwin JD and Tarver RD: Accessory fissures of the lung. AJR 144:39, 1985.

Gooding CA: Pulmonary angiography. In Gyepes MT (ed): Angiography in Infants and Children. New York, Grune & Stratton, 1974.

Gooding CA, Lallemand DP, Brasch RC et al: Magnetic resonance imaging in cystic fibrosis. J Pediatr 105:384, 1984.

Goodman LR, Foley WD, Wilson CR et al: Digital and conventional chest images: observer performance with film digital radiography system. Radiology 158:27, 1986.

Gooneratne N and Conway JJ: Radionuclide angiographic diagnosis of bronchopulmonary sequestration. J Nucl Med 17:1035, 1976.

Griscom NT: Computed tomographic determination of tracheal dimensions in children and adolescents. Radiology 145:361, 1982.

Griscom NT: Cross-sectional shape of the child's trachea by computed tomography. AJR 140:1103, 1983.

Griscom NT: Pneumonia in children and some of its variants. Radiology 167:297, 1988.

Grünebaum M: The roentgenologic investigation of congenital subglottic stenosis. Am J Roentgenol 125:877, 1975.

Haller JO, Schneider M, Kassner EG et al: Sonographic evaluation of the chest in infants and children. AJR 134:1019, 1980.

Heelan RT, Martini N, Westcott JW et al: Carcinomatous involvement of the hilum and mediastinum: computed tomographic and magnetic resonance evaluation. Radiology 156:111, 1985.

Heitzman ER and Ziter FM Jr: Acute interstitial pulmonary edema. Am J Roentgenol 98:291, 1966.

Heyman S, Kirkpatrick JA, Winter HS et al: An improved radionuclide method for the diagnosis of gastroesophageal reflux and aspiration in children (milk scan). Radiology 131:479, 1979.

Joseph PM, Berdon WE, Baker DH et al: Upper airway obstruction in infants and small children: improved radiographic diagnosis by combining filtration, high kilovoltage and magnification. Radiology 121:143, 1976.

Keats TE and Smith TH: Air esophagogram: a sign of poor respiratory excursion in the neonate. Am J Roentgenol 120:300, 1974.

Kirks DR: Practical techniques for pediatric computed tomography. Pediatr Radiol 13:148, 1983.

Kirks DR, Fram EK, Vock P et al: Tracheal compression by mediastinal masses in children: CT evaluation. AJR 141:647, 1983.

Kirks DR and Korobkin M: Chest computed tomography in infants and children. Pediatr Radiol 10:75, 1980.

Kundel HL: Digital projection radiography of the chest. Radiology 158:274, 1986.

Landing BH, Lawrence T-YK, Payne VC Jr, and Wells TR: Bronchial anatomy in syndromes with abnormal visceral situs, abnormal spleen and congenital heart disease. Am J Cardiol 28:456, 1971.

Leonidas JC, Moylan FMB, Kahn PC et al: Ventilation-perfusion scans in neonatal regional pulmonary emphysema complicating ventilatory assistance. AJR 131:243, 1978.

Li DK, Treves S, Heyman S et al: Krypton-81m: a better radiopharmaceutical for assessment of regional lung function in children. Radiology 130:741, 1979.

McCauley RGK, Darling DB, Leonidas JC, and Schwartz AS: Gastroesophageal reflux in infants and children: a useful classification and reliable physiologic technique for its demonstration. AJR 130:47, 1978.

MacEwan DW, Dunbar JS, Smith RD, and Brown BStJ: Pneumothorax in young infants—recognition and evaluation. J Can Assoc Radiol 22:264, 1971.

McLoughlin MJ, Weisbrod G, Wise DJ et al: Computed tomography in congenital anomalies of the aortic arch and great vessels. Radiology 138:399, 1981.

Mandell GA, Lantieri R, and Goodman LR: Tracheobronchial compression in Hodgkin lymphoma in children. AJR 139:1167, 1982.

Margulis AR: The lesions of radiobiology for diagnostic radiology. Am J Roentgenol 117:741, 1973.

Mayo JR, Webb WR, Gould R et al: High-resolution CT of the lungs: an optimal approach. Radiology 163:507, 1987.

Meine FJ, Lorenzo RL, Lynch PF et al: Pharyngeal distention associated with upper airway obstruction. Radiology 3:395, 1974.

Milne ENC and Gillan GG: Technique for improving neonatal chest roentgenograms. Appl Radiol 10:45, 1981.

Moore AV, Korobkin M, Olanow W et al: Age-related changes in the thymus gland: CT-pathologic correlation. AJR 141:241, 1983.

Moskowitz PS and Griscom NT: The medial pneumothorax. Radiology 120:143, 1976.

Naidich DP, Zerhouni EA, Hutchins GM et al: Computed tomography of the pulmonary parenchyma. Part 1: distal air-space disease. J Thorac Imaging 1:39, 1985.

Neches WH, Williams RL, and McNamara DG: Pulmonary angiographic findings in infantile lobar emphysema. Am J Dis Child 123:171, 1972.

Osborne D: Radiologic appearance of viral disease of the lower respiratory tract in infants and children. AJR 130:29, 1978.

Papanicolaou N and Treves S: Pulmonary scintigraphy in pediatrics. Semin Nucl Med 10:259, 1980.

Pendarvis BC and Swischuk LE: Lung scanning in the assessment of respiratory disease in children. Am J Roentgenol 107:313, 1969.

Recavarren S, Benton C, and Gall EA: The pathology of acute alveolar disease of the lung. Semin Roentgenol 2:22, 1967.

Rees AM, Roberts CJ, Bligh AS et al: Routine preoperative chest radiography in non-cardiopulmonary surgery. Br Med J 1:1333, 1976.

Rose RW and Ward BH: Spherical pneumonias in children simulating pulmonary and mediastinal masses. Radiology 106:179, 1973.

Rudavsky AZ, Leonidas JC, and Abramson AL: Lung scanning for the detection of endobronchial foreign bodies in infants and children. Radiology 108:629, 1973.

Schaner EG, Chang AE, Doppman JL et al: Comparison of computed and conventional whole lung tomography in detecting pulmonary nodules: a prospective radiologic pathologic study. AJR 131:51, 1978.

Schwarz ED, Dorst JP, Kuhn JP et al: Reliability of roentgenographic evaluation of ventricular septal defects in children. Johns Hopkins Med J 127:164, 1970.

Shurin SB, Haaga JR, Wood RE et al: Computed tomography for the evaluation of thoracic masses in children. JAMA 246:65, 1981.

Siegel MJ, Nadel SN, Glazer HS et al: Mediastinal lesions in children: comparison of CT and MR. Radiology 160:241, 1986.

Smith PC, Swischuk LE, and Fagan CJ: An elusive and often unsuspected cause of stridor or pneumonia (the esophageal foreign body). Am J Roentgenol 122:80, 1974.

Stern L, Fletcher BD, Dunbar JS et al: Pneumothorax and pneumomediastinum associated with renal malformations in newborn infants. Am J Roentgenol 116:785, 1972.

Tonkin IL, Elliott LP, Bargeron LM Jr: Concomitant axial cineangiography and barium esophagography in the evaluation of vascular rings. Radiology 135:69, 1980.

Wesenberg RL and Struble RA: Selective bronchial catheterization and lavage in the newborn. Radiology 105:397, 1972.

Wishart DL: Normal azygos vein width in children. Radiology 104:115, 1972.

Wittenborg MH, Gyepes MT, and Crocker D: Tracheal dynamics in infants with respiratory distress, stridor and collapsing trachea. Radiology 88:653, 1967.

Zerhouni EA, Naidich DP, Stitik FP et al: Computed tomography of the pulmonary parenchyma. Part 2: interstitial disease. J Thorac Imaging 1:54, 1985.

CRAIG M. SCHRAMM, M.D., and
MICHAEL M. GRUNSTEIN, M.D., Ph.D.

6

PULMONARY FUNCTION TESTS IN INFANTS

The morphologic sequences of postnatal airway and lung parenchymal growth and development (see Chapter 1), together with maturational changes in the mechanical properties of the chest wall (Agostoni, 1959), result in significant ontogenetic alterations in the mechanical properties of the respiratory system during infancy and early childhood. Because of the lack of subject cooperation with the voluntary maneuvers required to perform standard techniques of lung function assessment, studies of pulmonary function in infants and children up to the age of 7 years have been relatively few in number, generally difficult to conduct, and often not suitable for use in ill patients. However, considerable progress has been made with the recent development of innovative approaches to measure lung function in infants and young children. This chapter focuses on various current methods of pulmonary function testing in infants and discusses the physiologic bases of the techniques and the measurements reported in relation to information known about the mechanical properties of the lung and respiratory system in infancy and early childhood.

LUNG VOLUMES

A principal maturational process that influences measurement of the static mechanical properties of the respiratory system is the progressive increase in the elastic recoil of the chest wall. As shown in Figure 6–1, the newborn's chest wall, relative to the lung, is almost infinitely compliant above the resting lung volume, and accordingly its elastic recoil is minimal (Agostini, 1959). During childhood maturation a progressive increase occurs in the elastic recoil of both the lung and the chest wall, although it is the decrease in chest wall compliance that contributes proportionately more to the net reduction in the compliance of the total respiratory system. In part, the increase in the elastic recoil of the chest wall is attributed to ossification of various cartilaginous structures of the rib cage, a process that continues from birth until completion of the adolescent growth spurt (Sharp et al, 1970). In addition, assumption of the upright posture in early childhood and the subsequent axial growth of the abdomen impart increasingly negative pressure on the abdominal surface of the diaphragm (Bryan et al, 1977), thereby further contributing to chest wall recoil.

FUNCTIONAL RESIDUAL CAPACITY

The passive balance of the oppositional forces resulting from the outward elastic recoil of the chest wall and the inward elastic recoil of the lung determines the static resting volume of the lung, defined as the functional residual capacity (FRC). In the adult, FRC amounts to approximately 50 per cent of the total lung capacity (TLC) in the upright position and 30 to 40 per cent of TLC in the supine position (see Fig. 6–1). In contrast, the balance of the elastic recoil forces of the lung and chest wall in the infant predicts a supine FRC of only approximately 10 per cent of TLC, a level that is incompatible with appropriate stability and patency of the peripheral airways and air spaces and, hence, with even gas exchange. To promote more even gas exchange, infants have been shown to maintain their dynamic FRC above the passively determined level by incorporating breathing strategies that limit the expiratory flow rate (i.e., expiratory braking) or the duration of expiration relative to the passive expiratory time constant of the respiratory system (i.e., the product of compliance and resistance) or both. Figure 6–2 demonstrates that the typically abrupt termination of expiratory flow that occurs with the initiation of inspiration during spontaneous breathing can result in a substantial increase in the dynamic and expiratory lung volume (i.e., dynamic FRC) above the passive level. Similarly, expiratory braking secondary to persistence of tonic inspiratory activity in the diaphragm and intercostal muscles during the expiratory phase (Muller et al, 1979) or glottic narrowing associated with enhanced expiratory laryngeal adductor activity (Fisher et al, 1982; Kosch and Stark, 1984) both serve to establish a higher dynamic FRC. The net result of these breathing strategies is that measured values of dynamic FRC in infants (see

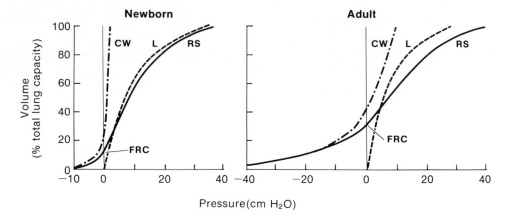

Figure 6–1. A comparison of static pressure-volume curves of the lung (L), chest wall (CW), and total respiratory system (RS) in newborns and adults. In contrast to the adult, the neonate has a highly compliant chest wall relative to the lung, in association with a relatively reduced functional residual capacity (FRC) (From Agostoni E: J Appl Physiol 14:909, 1959.)

subsequent discussion) remain approximately 40 per cent of anatomic estimates of their TLC (Fagan, 1976). It is not known at what age the FRC is no longer determined dynamically and depends solely on the balance of the passive recoil forces of the lung and chest wall. Nevertheless, given its relative consistency in proportion to TLC, the dynamic FRC appears to be a representative measure of lung volume throughout childhood.

The determination of lung volume is important for assessing lung growth and for standardizing measurements of pulmonary mechanics. Indeed, because the measurements of compliance and resistance are both volume dependent, relating compliance and resistance (or its reciprocal, conductance) to FRC permits valid comparisons between infants and children of different sizes and ages or between different

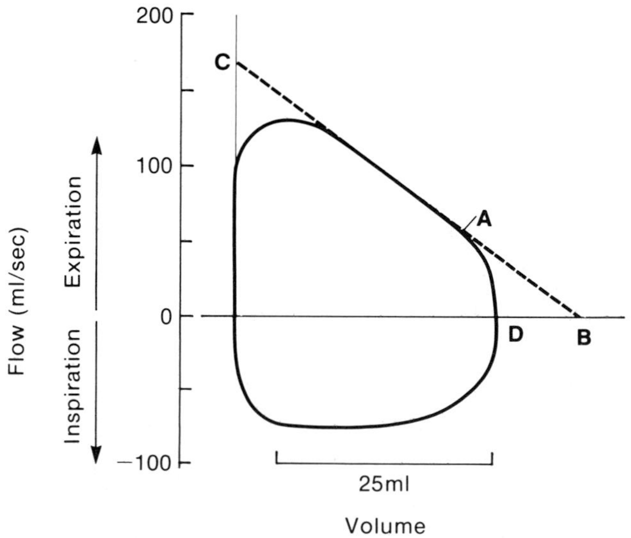

states or conditions in the same child. Two distinct approaches adapted for measurement of FRC in infants are the gas dilution methods and body plethysmography. A calculation of FRC by gas dilution may differ from one that has been determined by plethysmography because of the presence of trapped or poorly accessible gas within the lungs, which is measured by body plethysmography but not by gas dilution. Accordingly, to the extent that the quantity of such poorly accessible gas may be appreciable in infancy (Nelson et al, 1963; Ronchetti et al, 1975; Sjoqvist et al, 1984), the measurement of FRC by gas dilution will be less than the volume determined by body plethysomography, which is customarily designated the thoracic gas volume (TGV).

Gas Dilution Methods

Functional residual capacity has been measured in infants and young children by both closed-circuit and open-circuit gas dilution techniques. In the closed-circuit method, the sleeping infant, starting from FRC, rebreathes via a face mask from a bag or reservoir containing a known volume and concentration of an inert gas (usually helium, He) until the administered gas is completely mixed between the bag and the subject's lungs. The bag volume is kept constant by adding O_2 to account for the O_2 lost because of oxygen consumption (e.g., between 8 and 11 ml/kg/min in the newborn) (Sjoqvist et al, 1984; Cook et al, 1955) and by absorbing CO_2. Removal of CO_2 is also necessary to avoid retention of the gas in the closed circuit and, hence, to prevent any hyperventilation that can potentially alter the FRC level. By measuring the initial (He_i) and final equilibrium (He_f) helium concentrations, knowing the reservoir volume (V_r), and subtracting the dead space of the system (V_D), the lung volume at FRC is determined from the following equation:

Equation 1

$$\text{FRC} = V_r \times \frac{He_i - He_f}{He_f} - V_D$$

An alternate method for measuring FRC is the

Figure 6–2. A representative flow-volume curve obtained during quiet breathing in a supine infant. The loop runs clockwise. The dashed line *CB* is the linear portion of the curve, and the reciprocal of its slope represents the passive time constant (τ_{rs}) of the respiratory system. *A*, point at which expiratory flow is abruptly reduced because of the initiation of an active inspiration; *B*, the relaxation volume (i.e., passive functional residual capacity [FRC] level); *C*, extrapolated maximal expiratory flow rate; *D*, dynamic FRC level.

open-circuit washout technique in which the N_2 in an infant's lungs is flushed out with 100-per cent O_2 (or a He:O_2 mixture) and collected in a reservoir previously flushed with O_2 so that it is N_2-free. The gas collection is performed over several minutes, until the final alveolar N_2 concentration ($F_{Af}N_2$) is 0.01 to 0.02. By then measuring the N_2 concentration in the reservoir at equilibrium (F_rN_2), FRC can be determined from the following equation:

Equation 2

$$FRC = (V_r + V_D) \times \frac{F_rN_2}{F_{Ai}N_2 - F_{Af}N_2}$$

where $F_{Ai}N_2$ is the initial alveolar N_2 concentration (0.796 if the subject is initially breathing room air). Corrections can be made for the small amount of N_2 in "pure" O_2 and for the estimated amount of N_2 diffusing from blood and tissues because of the low alveolar N_2 concentration. The latter represents a small volume over a 2- to 3-min collection period in infants, usually causing FRC to be overestimated by no more than 5 per cent (Sjoqvist et al, 1984; Gerhardt et al, 1986).

The time required to achieve complete gas mixing or washout depends on the relationships among tidal volume, respiratory rate, system dead space, initial bag volume in the rebreathing system, and any slowly ventilated areas of the lung. Although 1 to 2 min may be adequate for achieving gas equilibration in well infants, gas mixing can remain incomplete in infants who have lung units that are poorly ventilated even after 5 min of rebreathing (Ronchetti et al, 1975). With prolonged collection times, a bulky reservoir is needed to collect the expired gas for the aforementioned calculations. Moreover, several measurements of bag gas concentration are needed to assess accurately when true equilibrium occurs. The development of rapid-response N_2 analyzers and on-line computer determination of instantaneous expiratory volumes and fractional N_2 concentrations have enabled the measurement of FRC without the need for voluminous gas collection. Moreover, by continuously monitoring the instantaneous expiratory N_2 concentration (F_EN_2), the time to complete the washout is readily apparent.

With the previously mentioned open-circuit integration techniques, FRC is related to the cumulative volume of expired N_2 (V_EN_2) by the following equation:

Equation 3

$$FRC = \frac{V_EN_2}{F_{Ai}N_2 - F_{Af}N_2}$$

Additional information on the uniformity of ventilation may be obtained by plotting instantaneous F_EN_2 against the cumulative alveolar ventilation to that time. As with any of the previous calculations, the values for FRC are obtained at ambient temper-

ature, pressure, and saturation (ATPS), and the measurements are corrected to body temperature and ambient pressure, saturated (BTPS) conditions to more accurately represent the volume as it exists within the lungs. This adjustment to BTPS is given by

Equation 4

$$V_{BTPS} = V_{ATPS} \times \frac{310}{T} \times \frac{P_B - P_{H2O}}{P_B - 47}$$

where V_{ATPS} is the measured volume (here, FRC), T is the ambient temperature in degrees Kelvin (273 + T, °C), P_B is the barometric temperature, and P_{H2O} is water vapor pressure at ambient temperature (i.e., 47 mm Hg at 37°C).

As compiled in Table 6–1, the data from several studies employing gas dilution methods in infants yield FRC measurements of 20 to 25 ml/kg of body weight or 1.3 to 1.4 ml/cm of body length. In the first maturational study to investigate the effects of growth and aging on lung volume, Cook and co-workers (1958) measured FRC by the He-dilution closed-circuit technique in 23 normal newborn infants and 85 children between the ages of 5 and 17 years. When comparing their values to the FRC determinations by He-dilution made in young adults by Blair and Hickam (1955), Cook and colleagues found that FRC (in ml) was approximately proportional to the third power of body length (in cm) at all ages, with the regression line given by

$$FRC = 0.00114 \times (length)^{2.86}$$

Gerhardt and colleagues (1986) studied 50 healthy children from age 1 week to 5 years with a modified integrated N_2 washout technique employing a continuous background flow of He:O_2 and found a similar relationship, given by

$$FRC = 0.000937 \times (length)^{2.78}$$

These investigators also found that FRC was linearly related to body weight (in kg) over this age range, whereby

$$FRC = 20.4 \times (weight) - 14.8.$$

Body Plethysmography

Body plethysmography, as originally described by DuBois and co-workers (1956), has been employed for more than 30 years to measure TGV. The technique is based on Boyle's law, which states that the volume of a gas varies inversely to the pressure applied to it. Thus, as shown in Figure 6–3, when the breathing of an infant placed in an air-tight chamber is occluded at end-expiration, continued respiratory efforts against the occlusion cause the intrathoracic gas to be alternately compressed and

Table 6–1. FUNCTIONAL RESIDUAL CAPACITY (FRC) VALUES IN NEWBORNS AND OLDER INFANTS

Study	Methods	Subjects*	FRC (ml/kg)	FRC (ml/cm)	TGV (ml/kg)
NEWBORNS					
Cook, Helliesen, and Agathon	C C He	Term (33)		1.55 ml/cm	
Nelson et al	O C N Plethys	Preterm–71 days (23)	31.3 ± 11.3 (all) 25.7 ± 8.8 (>2.5 kg)		40.6 ± 13.1 (all) 30.2 ± 6.7 (> 2.5 kg)
Berglund and Karlberg	C C He	Term (12)	24.8 ± 3.9		
Krauss & Auld	C C He	Healthy preterm (23) RDS preterm (22)		1.3 ± 0.4 0.9 ± 0.3	
Ronchetti et al	C C N Plethys	Healthy preterm (8) RDS preterm (4)	29.4 ± 4.6 29.3 ± 7.5	1.41 ± 0.25 1.43 ± 0.46	37.5 ± 3.6 ml/kg 44.4 ± 10.2 cc/kg
Hanson and Shinozaki	Int N	Term ≤24 hrs (18)	18.6 ± 1.5		
INFANTS					
Gerhardt et al	Int N	1–60 mo (25)	18.5 ± 2.7		

*Number of study subjects given in parentheses.
C C, closed circuit; O C, open circuit; Int, integrated; Plethys, plethysmography; N, nitrogen; He, helium; TGV, thoracic gas volume.

decompressed, with resulting changes in volume. The TGV in BTPS units is determined by relating these changes in volume (reflected as changes in plethysmographic pressure, ΔP_{box}) to the corresponding changes in alveolar pressure, which is assumed to be equal to mouth pressure (ΔP_m) during the occlusion, according to the expression

Equation 5

$$TGV = (P_B - P_{H_2O} \times \frac{\Delta P_{box}}{\Delta P_M} \times \frac{B_f}{M_f}$$

where P_B and P_{H_2O} are the barometric and water vapor pressures in cm H_2O, respectively, and B_f and M_f are calibration factors for the box volume and mouth pressure, respectively. Older children are re-

quested to pant against the closed shutter in order to minimize temperature, saturation, and respiratory coefficient variation, as well as to improve the signal-to-drift ratio (DuBois et al, 1956). Obviously such cooperation cannot be obtained from infants, and this problem has prompted investigators to incorporate rebreathing reservoirs of heated and humidified air within the infant plethysmograph to minimize these errors (Radford, 1974; Stocks et al, 1977).

As listed in Table 6–2, values for TGV in healthy term newborns have averaged 30 to 35 ml/kg. Extending these determinations in 52 infants and children through the first 5 years of life, Doershuk and colleagues (1970) reported a mean (± SD) TGV value of 32.4 ± 5 ml/kg. As noted in Figure 6–4, the TGV (in ml) was also related as a power function of body length (in cm), according to the equation

$$TGV = 0.0157 \times (length)^{2.238}$$

The regression function was largely similar to that also obtained by Doershuk and colleagues (1970) in a study of 88 subjects ranging in age from 6 to 18 years (where $TGV = 0.01292 \times [length]^{2.352}$). In part, the small difference in these two regression functions may be explained by the body position of the subjects studied: FRC is 20 to 30 per cent less in the supine position (as measured in infants) than in the sitting position (as measured in older children).

GAS TRAPPING AND HOMOGENEITY OF VENTILATION

By either method of measurement, the end-expiratory lung volume determined during spontaneous breathing appears to remain roughly proportionate to body size from the newborn period to early adulthood. Of interest, whereas the values of TGV and FRC are nearly equal in healthy adults, FRC measurements are generally significantly less than TGV values in healthy newborn infants. In studies on paired gas-dilution and plethysmographic determinations, TGV has uniformly been found to be greater

$$TGV = (P_B - P_{H_2O}) \times \frac{\Delta P_{box}}{\Delta P_M} \times \frac{B_f}{M_f}$$

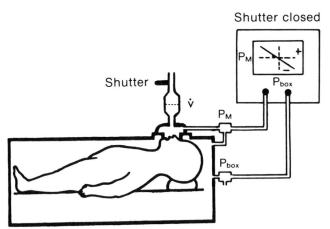

Figure 6–3. The body plethysmographic technique for the determination of thoracic gas volume (TGV). Following an initial determination of the calibration factors for box volume (B_f) and mouth pressure (M_f), the relationship between box pressure (P_{box}) and mouth pressure (P_M) is displayed, and the inverse slope of this relationship during shutter closure (i.e., $\Delta P_{box}/\Delta P_M$) is measured. The TGV is then calculated according to the above equation.

Table 6–2. THORACIC GAS VOLUME (TGV) VALUES IN NEWBORNS AND OLDER INFANTS

Study	Methods	Subjects*	TGV (ml/kg)	FRC (ml/kg)
NEWBORNS				
Nelson et al	O C N	Preterm–71 days (23)	40.6 ± 13.1 (all)	31.3 ± 11.3 (all)
	Plethys		30.2 ± 6.7 (>2.5 kg)	25.7 ± 8.8 (>2.5 kg)
Ronchetti et al	C C N	Healthy preterm (8)	37.5 ± 3.6	29.4 ± 4.6
	Plethys	RDS preterm (4)	44.4 ± 10.2	29.3 ± 7.5
Auld et al	Plethys	Term (10)	33.8 ± 7.3	
Chu et al	Plethys	Term (31)	38.0 ± 5.2	
		Preterm (29)	47.8 ± 10.3	
Doershuk and Matthews	Plethys	Term (51)	29.0 ± 6.0	
Howlett	Plethys	1–8 wks (24)	35.5 ± 1.8	
Stocks, Levy, and Godfrey	Plethys	Preterm–10 mo (55)	35.1 ± 3.0	
INFANTS				
Radford	Plethys	1–10 mo (10)	34.9 ± 5.8	
Krieger	Plethys	1–24 mo (24)	27.4 ± 4.3	
Phelan and Williams	Plethys	4–46 wks (24)	30.2 ± 3.3	
Doershuk et al	Plethys	1–60 mo (52)	32.4 ± 5.0	

*Numbers of study subjects given in parentheses.
C C, closed circuit; O C, open circuit; Plethys, plethysmography; N, nitrogen; FRC, functional residual capacity.

than FRC by about 8 to 9 ml/kg in healthy premature infants (Nelson et al, 1963; Ronchetti et al, 1975), compared with a difference of about 15 ml/kg in premature infants with respiratory distress syndrome (Ronchetti et al, 1975). Although analogous studies have not been conducted in older children, the mean weight-specific FRC reported in 24 term infants varying in age from 1 to 60 months was 18.6 ± 2.8 ml/kg (Gerhardt et al, 1987). Compared with the average TGV value of 32.4 ± 5 ml/kg found by Doershuk and co-workers (1970) in children of similar ages, gas-dilutional FRC measurements appear to average

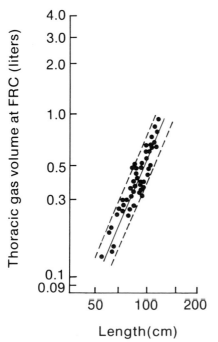

Figure 6–4. A log-log plot of thoracic gas volume versus body length for 52 children aged 1 week to 5 years. *Dashed lines* represent 2 SD from the mean regression fit *(solid line)*. (From Doershuk CF, Downs TD, Matthew LW, and Lough MD: Pediatr Res 4:165, 1970.)

10 to 15 ml/kg less than plethysmographic TGV values from birth through 5 years of age. As noted previously, the difference between TGV and FRC generally has been interpreted as indicating the presence of trapped or very slowly equilibrating gas secondary to airway closure at low lung volumes.

Such ventilatory inhomogeneity is evident by analysis of integrated, multibreath N_2 washout curves, which demonstrate in all "healthy" newborns a biphasic distribution. This biphasic distribution typically consists of an initial large, fast space and a later slow space that appears in the 4 to 7 per cent N_2 range and usually accounts for 10 to 20 per cent of the infant's total alveolar ventilation (Hanson and Shinozaki, 1970). The distribution of ventilation appears to remain inhomogeneous through the ages of 3 to 6 years (Wall et al, 1988). To the extent that sedation, usually necessary to obtain pulmonary function measurements beyond the immediate newborn period, may depress the mechanisms maintaining an elevated dynamic FRC in infants, airway closure in the supine infant at lower lung volumes may be potentiated during the testing procedure. Ontogenetic studies comparing dynamic TGV and FRC measurements to the passive FRC values are lacking.

The TGV measurements can be obtained within seconds and may be repeated frequently within a short period of time. The need, however, for intricate and somewhat cumbersome equipment, as well as the complicated subject preparation required to properly conduct body plethysmographic measurements, have largely confined these determinations to relatively few research institutions. In contrast, although the procedures for obtaining gas-dilution FRC measurements are considerably slower, the open-circuit integrator techniques are relatively simple and portable and, hence, more readily applied at the bedside and on distressed infants. As the latter techniques become more routinely employed in the assessment of pulmonary function in infants, the information obtained will provide us with a sounder understanding of the interaction of lung growth with lung mechanics in health and disease.

TOTAL LUNG CAPACITY

Total lung capacity (TLC) is an effort-dependent measurement and, therefore, cannot be obtained readily in infants. Post-mortem studies have demonstrated that lung volume is linearly related to body length during childhood and that the length-specific lung volume (i.e., V_L/CHL, where CHL is the crown-heel length) increases with age (Thurlbeck, 1982). As illustrated in Figure 6–5, throughout most of childhood, for any given age and stature, boys have larger lung volumes than girls, the result of an increased number of alveoli and respiratory bronchioles. These sex-dependent differences are apparently absent below 2 years of age.

Because, apart from effort per se, the in vivo determination of TLC is also dependent on the strength of the respiratory muscles, the maturational increase in the force of contraction of the inspiratory muscles contributes to the overall increase in the functional measurement of TLC. Thus the enhancement of TLC with age is attributed to an increase in the inspiratory muscle strength of the growing child, as well as to the maturational increase in anatomic lung volume.

LUNG COMPLIANCE

STATIC MEASUREMENTS

Static lung compliance is defined as the change in lung volume associated with a given change in trans-

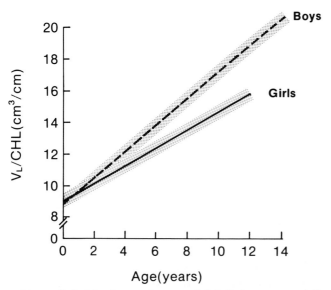

Figure 6–5. The lung volume at full inflation corrected for crown-heel length (V_L/CHL) is greater in males than in females. This sex difference becomes significant at 2 to 3 years of age. The stippled areas represent mean ±2 SD. V_L, lung volume at full inflation; *CHL*, crown-heel length. (From Thurlbeck WM: Thorax 37:564, 1982.)

pulmonary pressure (i.e., $\Delta V/\Delta P$). Because of the curvilinearity of the static pressure-volume (P-V) relationship of the lung, the measurement of lung compliance clearly depends on the lung volume at which the measurement is made. For this reason, measurements of static lung compliance are rarely obtained; rather, static lung recoil is often determined by assessing the entire P-V characteristics of the lung. Deflation P-V curves are typically measured during stepwise, quasi-static decreases in lung volume from TLC. The placement of an intraesophageal balloon is used to estimate transpulmonary pressure (i.e., the difference between airway and intraesophageal pressure), and volume is measured concomitantly in a body plethysmograph, at the mouth with a spirometer, or by integration of the flow signal from a pneumotachograph. Following inhalation to TLC, the airway is intermittently occluded by closure of a shutter on five to seven occasions during the subsequent course of a very slow deflation of the lungs to FRC. Based on a series of measurements of volume and transpulmonary pressure, the quasi-static lung P-V curve is graphically constructed, with lung volume typically expressed as a percentage of the subject's TLC or, for purposes of cross-sectional studies of age or disease, as a percentage of the predicted normal TLC. Apart from graphic representation, the approaches used to quantify the elastic recoil of the lung include determinations of the transpulmonary pressures at a given absolute, relative, or predicted lung volume; several studies have also utilized different mathematic expressions to characterize the entire P-V curve.

Although quasi-static lung P-V relationships have been measured in older children and adults as previously described, in vivo studies of the static P-V curves in children under 6 years of age are lacking because their cooperation cannot be guaranteed. Ontogenetic information has been extrapolated from investigations performed by Fagan (1976, 1977) on excised lungs from infants varying in age from 33-week gestation newborns to 2 year olds. Over this age range, there occurs a marked change in the overall shape of the P-V curve when lung volume is expressed as a fraction of maximal volume (V_{max}) obtained at 30 cm H_2O distending pressure. As demonstrated in Figure 6–6A, lungs from older infants are less compliant and thus depict a greater elastic recoil (i.e., shifted to the right) relative to lungs from premature infants. This maturational trend appears to continue throughout childhood, with a further decrease in compliance and increase in elastic recoil pressure at TLC determined in children from 6 to 18 years of age (Fig. 6–6B) (Zapletal et al, 1976). This progressive decrease in lung compliance is presumably due to age-dependent alterations in the total number and size of the alveoli, as well as the amount, distribution, and structure of elastin, collagen, and smooth muscle in the developing lung.

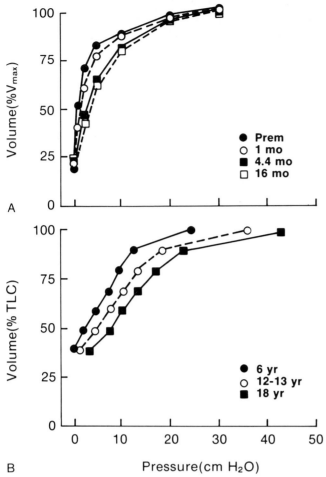

A

B

Figure 6–6. *A,* Pressure-volume curves obtained in excised lungs from premature (33-weeks' gestation), 1-, 4.4-, and 16-month-old infants. (From Fagan DG: Thorax 31:534, 1976; Fagan DG: Thorax 32:198, 1977.) *B,* Pressure-volume curves obtained in children averaging 6, 12 to 13, and 18 years of age. V_{max}, maximum volume; *TLC,* total lung capacity. (From Zapletal A, Paul T, and Samanek M: J Appl Physiol 40:953, 1976.)

DYNAMIC MEASUREMENTS

Although static lung compliance (C_L) is not readily measured in infants and young children, it may be approximated by the determination of dynamic lung compliance (C_{dyn}) during quiet breathing. To obtain the measurement of C_{dyn}, the infant is typically studied in the supine position while sedated. Mean pleural pressure is estimated by intraesophageal pressure, which is recorded using either a water-filled catheter or an air-filled balloon appropriately positioned in the lower third of the esophagus such that the ratio of instantaneous change in intra-esophageal-to-mouth pressure ($\Delta P_{es}/\Delta P_{m}$) generated during an airway occlusion is close to unity (Beardsmore, 1980). Tidal volume breathing is occasionally monitored in a plethysmograph but is more often determined by integration of the flow signal from a pneumotachograph attached to the subject via a face mask. The C_{dyn} is then represented by the ratio of tidal volume to the absolute change in transpulmonary pressure

($P_{tp} = P_{es} - P_{m}$) obtained between the points of zero flow occurring at the termination and onset of a tidal inspiration (Fig. 6–7). The measurement of C_{dyn} may then be expressed as a function of body weight or length or of lung volume. The latter normalization to lung volume (e.g., C_{dyn}/FRC) is termed the specific dynamic compliance (SC_{dyn}).

Several investigators have applied the aforementioned technique to neonates and young children and have reported average values for C_{dyn} ranging from 1.1 to 2.0 cc/kg/cm H_2O, and for SC_{dyn} ranging from 0.038 to 0.062 ml/cm H_2O/ml FRC, as listed in Table 6–3. Krieger (1963) found SC_{dyn} to remain constant throughout the first 2 years of life, averaging 0.038 ml/cm H_2O/ml FRC (Fig. 6–8). In contrast, Cook and co-workers (1958) found an identical SC_{dyn} of 0.057 ml/cm H_2O/ml FRC in 33 healthy newborns and in 85 children from 5 to 17 years of age. The discrepancy in the measurements of SC_{dyn} between these studies may be the result of methodologic differences, as the former study employed air-filled esophageal balloons and predicted values for FRC, whereas the latter employed water-filled esophageal catheters and actual FRC measurements.

Insofar as the previously mentioned approach used to measure C_{dyn} (also pulmonary resistance; see the subsequent discussion) relies on accurate estimation of the mean pleural pressure, several investigators have called attention to the difficulties inherent in utilizing esophageal pressure measurements in newborn infants (Beardsmore et al, 1980; Asher et al, 1982; LeSouef et al, 1983; Thomson et al, 1983; Heaf et al, 1986). Balloons have been reported to be superior to catheters, and the characteristics of the ideal balloon for use in infants are described as being thin-walled (0.045 to 0.075 mm), long (35 to 50 mm), wide (7.6 mm diameter), and filled with 0.5 to 0.8 ml

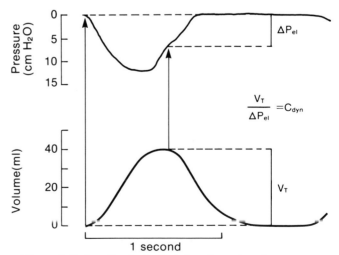

Figure 6–7. A method of calculating dynamic pulmonary compliance (C_{dyn}). As demonstrated in this schematic representation of simultaneous esophageal pressure (P_{el}) and volume recordings, C_{dyn} is determined by the ratio of tidal volume (V_T) to the change in P_{el} measured between points of no flow at end-inspiration and end-expiration.

Table 6–3. COMPLIANCE VALUES IN NEWBORNS AND OLDER INFANTS

Study	Methods*	Subjects†	C_{dyn}	SC_{dyn}	C_{rs}	SC_{rs}
NEWBORNS						
Cook et al	Es Cath	Term (13)	1.73 ± 0.70			
Cook et al	Es Cath	Term (33)		0.057		
Swyer et al	ES Cath	Term (15)	1.69 ± 0.62			
Chu et al	Es Ball	Term (31)	2.0 ± 0.4	0.053 ± 0.009		
		Preterm (29)	1.9 ± 0.6	0.040 ± 0.013		
Olinsky et al	Es Ball	Healthy preterm (12)	1.11 ± 0.26	0.047 ± 0.013		
	Insp Occl				1.53 ± 0.32	0.064 ± 0.010
Davis et al	Es Ball	Healthy preterm (8)	1.35 ± 0.31			
	Exp Occl				1.19 ± 0.25	
Howeltt	Es Ball	1–8 wks (24)		0.062 ± 0.004		
Mortola et al	Exp Occl	Term (10)			$1.1 \pm 0.4\ddagger$	
LeSouef et al	Exp Occl	Term (8)			$1.2 \pm 0.5\ddagger$	
Thomson et al	Exp Occl	Healthy newborns (20) + post RDS (14)			1.14 ± 0.26	
Tepper et al	Wght Spir	Term (7)			1.11 ± 0.16	
INFANTS						
Phelan & Williams	Es Ball	4–46 wks (24)	1.66 ± 0.26	0.056 ± 0.010		
Grustein et al	EVC Occl	6–18 mos (8)			1.61 ± 0.48	
Krieger	Es Ball	1–24 mos (24)		0.038 ± 0.010		

*Methods abbreviations: Es, esophageal; Cath, catheter; Ball, balloon; Insp, inspiratory; Exp, expiratory; Occl, occlusion; Wght Spir, weighted spirometer; EVC, expiratory volume clamp
†Number of study subjects given in parentheses
Compliance values in ml/kg/cm H_2O; specific compliance values in ml/cm H_2O/ml FRC
‡Average values calculated from mean $\pm$ SD Crs (ml/cm H_2O) divided by average weight

of air (Beardsmore et al, 1980). Even with the best technique of balloon placement, however, it appears to be impossible to estimate reliably the mean pleural pressure in certain infants. When a compliant rib cage is distorted during inspiration, as is often the case in premature infants (Fig. 6–9) (LeSouef et al, 1983), intubated infants (Thomson et al, 1983; Heaf et al, 1986), term infants in rapid eye movement (REM) sleep (see Fig. 6–9) (LeSouef et al, 1983), and older infants with respiratory neuromuscular (Beardsmore et al, 1980) or obstructive lung disease

(Heaf et al, 1986), pleural pressure swings may be heterogeneously distributed within the thorax. Under these conditions, the esophageal pressure measured in a given site in the thorax may not reliably reflect the average pleural pressure, thereby potentially leading to an erroneous interpretation of the measurements made.

An additional consideration in the interpretation of C_{dyn} is that it is, by definition, measured during active breathing and thus includes a small resistive component. Moreover, infants appear to exhibit frequency dependence of compliance (Fig. 6–10) such that, at greater respiratory frequencies, C_{dyn} becomes progressively less than static lung compliance (C_{stat}). This finding occurs because of the presence of heterogeneous time constants within the lung, a phenomenon that is attributed to chest wall distortion resulting in uneven distribution of pleural pressure, peripheral airway closure at low lung volumes, or poor collateral ventilation in infancy. Consequently, lung regions having relatively higher resistances or greater compliances fill more slowly, and, during rapid breathing, the regions that are slower to expand may be incompletely filled at the moment the infant starts to exhale. Under these circumstances, the total volume of air dynamically entering the lung in response to a given change in transpulmonary pressure becomes less than that predicted on the basis of the measurement of static lung compliance.

RESPIRATORY SYSTEM COMPLIANCE

STATIC MEASUREMENTS

The individual elastances of the lung (E_L) and chest wall (E_{cw}) are added in series to determine the net

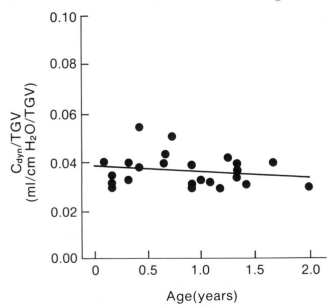

Figure 6–8. Changes in specific dynamic compliance (SC_{dyn} = C_{dyn}/TGV) as a function of age. Note that SC_{dyn} remains relatively constant throughout the first 2 years of life. SC_{dyn}, specific dynamic compliance; C_{dyn}, dynamic lung compliance; TGV, thoracic gas volume. (Data from Krieger I: Am J Dis Child 105:439, 1963.)

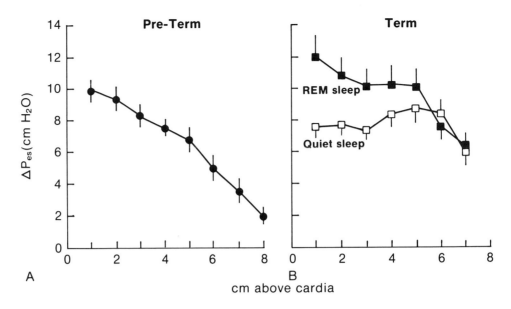

Figure 6–9. *A*, Caudocephalad profile of esophageal pressure changes (P_{es}) for breaths of equal magnitude in ten preterm infants. Note the fivefold variation in P_{es} with changes in the esophageal balloon position. *B*, Caudocephalad profile of P_{es} in four full-term infants during quiet sleep *(open squares)* and during rapid eye movement (REM) sleep *(closed squares)*. Because of the loss of chest wall tone in REM sleep, there occurs greater variation in P_{es} with changes in balloon position when compared to quiet sleep. Values are ± the standard error of the mean. (From Le-Souef PN, Lopes JM, England SJ et al: J Appl Physiol 55:353, 1983.)

elastance of the respiratory system ($E_{rs} = E_L + E_{cw}$). Because compliance is the reciprocal of elastance, the relationship is also given by the expression

Equation 6

$$1/C_{rs} = 1/C_L + 1/C_{cw}$$

where C_L is the static compliance of the lung, C_{cw} is the compliance of the chest wall, and C_{rs} is the static compliance of the respiratory system. Whereas in children aged 5 to 16 years E_L represents approximately 60 per cent of the total E_{rs} (Fisher et al, 1982), E_L accounts for about 85 per cent of the total elastic recoil in newborns (Reynolds and Etsten, 1966; Davis et al, 1988). Thus C_{rs} more closely approximates C_L

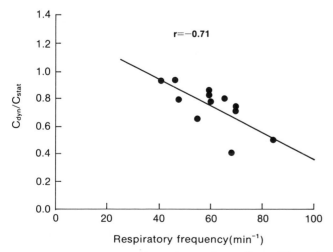

Figure 6–10. Frequency dependence of compliance. The ratio of dynamic compliance (C_{dyn}) to static compliance (C_{stat}) decreases with increasing respiratory frequency in 12 healthy premature infants. (From Olinsky A, Bryan AC, and Bryan MH: S Afr Med J 50:128, 1976.)

in newborns and young children. To obtain truly passive measurements of C_{rs}, earlier investigations studied children undergoing general anesthesia and neuromuscular blockade. Based on passive inflations of the lungs with a syringe, absolute values for C_{rs} were found to increase with age and to be related closely to the cube of height from the newborn period to adulthood. However, when adjusted for lung size (i.e., TLC or FRC), the volume-specific C_{rs} values were found to decrease from 0.043 to 0.037 ml/cm H_2O/ml FRC between 5 and 15 years of age (Figs. 6–11 and 6–12), paralleling ontogenetic changes in C_L (see Fig. 6–6).

In light of the complexities inherent in measuring static C_L in spontaneously breathing infants, several investigators have turned to the measurement of C_{rs}. Two noninvasive approaches that have been developed to circumvent the need for neuromuscular blockade in the determination of static C_{rs} are discussed later.

Weighted-Spirometer Method

The weighted-spirometer method (Cherniack and Brown, 1965) has been adapted by Tepper and co-workers (1984) for the measurement of C_{rs} in sedated infants. While lying in the supine position, the infant breathes via a face mask into a modified water-sealed spirometer connected to a CO_2 absorber and a variable O_2 supply. After a constant end-expiratory level is established by adjusting the O_2 flow, a weight is placed on the spirometer bell to produce a continuous positive pressure within the respiratory-spirometer circuit, thereby increasing the infant's end-expiratory volume (schematically illustrated in Fig. 6–13). The ratio of the increase in end-expiratory volume (ΔV) to the increase in end-expiratory pres-

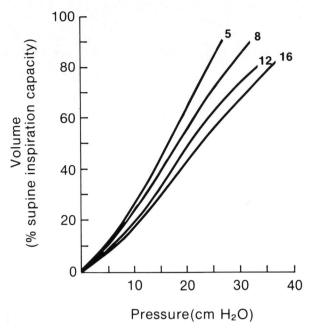

Figure 6–11. Shifts in the deflation volume-pressure relationship of respiratory system compliance with age. Volume is expressed as a function of supine inspiration capacity. Mean ages in years are noted above the curves. (From Sharp M, Druz W, and Balgot R: J Appl Physiol 29:775, 1970.)

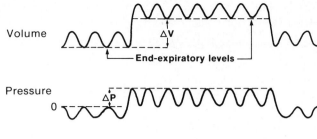

Calculations:
Total respiratory system compliance (C_{rs}) $= \dfrac{\Delta V}{\Delta P} - C_{circuit}$

Figure 6–13. A schematic diagram demonstrating the calculation of total respiratory system compliance by the weighted-spirometer method. A weight is applied to the spirometer bell after the third breath, generating a positive airway pressure (ΔP) and a corresponding increase in end-expiratory volume (ΔV). (From Tepper RS, Pagtakhan, and Taussig LM: Am Rev Respir Dis 130:461, 1984.)

sure (ΔP) determines the quasi-static compliance of the total system. Subtraction of circuit compliance yields C_{rs}, which averaged (mean ± SD) 1.11 ± 0.16 ml/kg/cm H_2O in seven term newborns compared with 0.60 ± 0.08 in five infants with bronchopulmonary dysplasia (Tepper et al, 1984). When comparing the values reported for C_{rs} by the weighted-spirometer method (Greenough et al, 1986) with those obtained in intubated, paralyzed children (Sharp et al, 1970), it can be seen in Figure 6–14 that the two methods yield similar results throughout

the first 2 years of life but that discrepancies exist in older children. These discrepancies may be attributed to the effect of anesthesia and respiratory muscle paralysis on lung compliance (Rich et al, 1979; Westbrook et al, 1973) and possibly to certain assumptions underlying the weighted-spirometer technique. These assumptions include that the pattern of airway-alveolar distention produced by the application of positive pressure to the upper airway is identical to that occurring during normal breathing and that the chest wall muscles are completely relaxed at end-expiration during steady-state positive-pressure breathing (Tepper et al, 1984). The observation noted previously that infants maintain their dynamic FRC above the passively determined level suggests that their respiratory muscles may not be fully re-

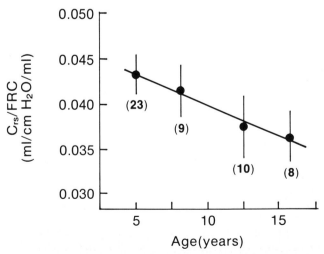

Figure 6–12. Specific respiratory system compliance (C_{rs}/FRC) versus age. Data expressed as means ± the standard error of the mean. Equation of regression line: C_{rs}/FRC = 0.047 − 0.0068 (age). (Data from Sharp M, Druz W, and Balgot R: J Appl Physiol 29:775, 1970, with C_{rs} values measured by the authors and FRC values calculated by the authors as predicted for heights.)

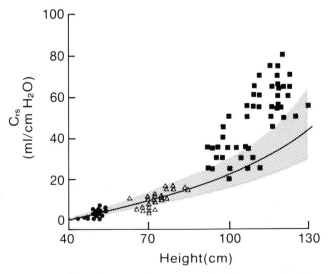

Figure 6–14. Changes in total respiratory system compliance (C_{rs}) as a function of height during the first 8 years of life. Individual data denote newborns *(filled circles)*, infants *(open triangles)*, and older children *(filled squares)* (From Greenough A, Stocks J, Nothen U, and Helms P: Pediatr Pulmonol 2:321, 1986.) The solid curve and shaded region represent mean values (±2 SD) of C_{rs} obtained from the regression function reported by Sharp and associates (1970) in intubated, anesthetized/paralyzed children.

laxed at end-expiration, with or without added airway pressure. Accordingly, this method may underestimate true C_{rs} in such infants. The weighted-spirometer method, however, appears particularly useful in older children who do not demonstrate dynamic FRC augmentation and who lack an active Hering-Breuer reflex, because integrity of the latter reflex is necessary for the determination of C_{rs} using the "occlusion" techniques discussed later.

Airway Occlusion Methods

Considerable training is needed for older children to relax their respiratory muscles against an airway occlusion in order to obtain quasi-static P-V curves. In contrast, infants, relative to adults, have a potent Hering-Breuer reflex that produces apnea (i.e., respiratory muscle relaxation) when the airway is occluded at lung volumes above FRC. In light of this reflex response, it is assumed that the elevated brief plateaus in airway pressure accompanying airway occlusion represent the static elastic recoil pressures of the respiratory system. Olinsky and colleagues (1976) were the first to employ multiple inspiratory occlusions in infants to generate P-V relationships within the tidal breathing range. Subsequently, Mortola and co-workers (1982) modified the technique by producing expiratory occlusions over the tidal range, recognizing that the inspiratory muscles are naturally inhibited during expiration and that expiratory muscles are usually inactive during normal tidal breathing. Thus expiratory occlusions were believed more likely to generate truly passive pressure plateaus.

In applying the airway occlusion technique, the sedated infant breathes quietly through a face mask attached to a pneumotachograph. The airway is occluded for a single breath at end-inspiration and, on different occasions, at various lung volumes during tidal expiration. As shown in Figure 6–15, during each occlusion, mouth pressure (P_m) rises until it reaches a stable plateau, at which point P_m represents the passive elastic recoil pressure of the respiratory system corresponding to the fixed occluded volume. The presence of any significant activity in either the inspiratory or the expiratory muscles can be readily seen as negative or positive deflections in P_m, respectively, from the plateau pressure. By relating the brief occlusion plateaus to the corresponding changes in lung volume within the tidal volume range, the resultant P-V relationship is closely approximated by a straight line, wherein the slope (i.e., $\Delta V/\Delta P_m$) denotes the C_{rs}. As further shown in Figure 6–15, the volume-intercept obtained at $P_m = 0$ is typically less than the zero-volume point, which denotes the dynamic end-expiratory lung volume. The volume difference represents the magnitude of increase in the end-expiratory volume above the passive FRC, a phenomenon attributed to the abrupt termination of expiratory flow by the initiation of an active inspiration during spontaneous breathing (see Fig. 6–2).

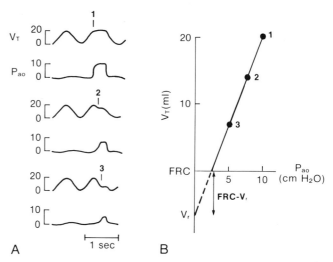

Figure 6–15. A determination of total respiratory system compliance (C_{rs}) by the airway occlusion method. *A,* Recorded changes in lung volume (V_T; in ml) and airway pressure (P_{ao}; in cm H_2O) during one spontaneous breath and occlusion during the expiratory phase of the next breath. In the three examples shown, occlusions are performed at end-inspiration *(1),* in the first third of expiration *(2),* and in the last third of expiration *(3).* With each occlusion, P_{ao} rises to a plateau, corresponding to the recoil pressure of the respiratory system at that volume. *B,* A plot of the changes in lung volume above the functional residual capacity (FRC) against the corresponding changes in P_{ao}, as obtained in *A.* The slope represents C_{rs}, and the volume intercept represents the resting static volume (V_r) below the dynamic FRC. (From Mortola JP and Saetta M: Pediatr Pulmonol 3:123, 1987.)

LeSouef and co-workers (1984) further modified the occlusion technique by determining the airway pressure generated during single-breath occlusions performed at end-inspiration and relating the measured pressure to the corresponding volume derived by extrapolation of the subsequent passive expiratory flow-volume relationship to zero flow (i.e., as per Fig. 6–2). When applied to intubated newborns, it was demonstrated that premature neonates with respiratory disease had a lower mean ($\pm SD$) C_{rs} value of 0.76 (± 0.34) ml/cm H_2O than did neonates of comparable age and weight but without respiratory distress, in whom C_{rs} averaged 1.31 (± 0.28) ml/cm H_2O (LeSouef, 1984). The average weight-specific measurement of C_{rs} in the latter group of premature infants (i.e., mean C_{rs}/mean body weight = 1.16 ml/kg/cm H_2O, at an average gestational age of 28 weeks) was similar to the mean ($\pm SD$) C_{rs} value of 1.19 (± 0.27) ml/kg/cm H_2O reported in a study of 34 healthy infants throughout the first year of life (Thomson et al, 1985).

Because of attenuation of the Hering-Breuer reflex during maturation, the occlusion method described earlier has generally been used only on newborns, sedated infants, or anesthetized patients in whom the reflex response may be potentiated. Reports of the weight-specific values for C_{rs} have averaged 1.0 to 1.5 ml/kg/cm H_2O, as shown in Table 6–3. In older children, the mean ($\pm SD$) specific respiratory compliance (i.e., C_{rs}/FRC) determined by passive lung

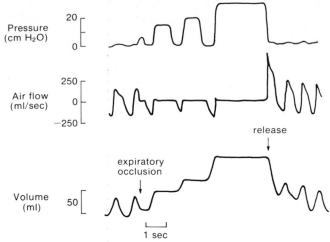

Figure 6–16. A schematic record demonstrating the application of the expiratory volume-clamp technique on tracings of volume, airflow, and airway pressure. Occlusion of the expiratory valve was initiated during a spontaneous midexpiration and was sustained for three subsequent expirations, resulting in a cumulative increase in lung volume and increasing plateaus in airway pressure. Expiratory occlusion was released during the fourth expiratory phase.

inflation during anesthesia and paralysis appears to decrease slightly from 0.043 ± 0.002 ml/cm H_2O/ml FRC in 5 year olds to 0.037 ± 0.003 ml/cm H_2O/ml FRC in 15 year olds (Sharp et al, 1970).

Expiratory Volume-Clamp Method

Because of intersubject variability in the strength of the Hering-Breuer reflex, the respiratory pauses elicited with airway occlusions in the tidal volume range may be too short to allow for complete respiratory muscle relaxation and, hence, accurate estimation of the static recoil pressures of the respiratory system (Thomson et al, 1985; Stocks et al, 1987). Moreover, the values of C_{rs} obtained with tidal volume occlusions are based on measurements confined to a relatively low lung volume range. In addressing these issues, the airway occlusion technique was modified by Grunstein and colleagues (1987) to extend the measurements of the passive inflation P-V relationship of the respiratory system to encompass a wider lung volume range by progressive recruitment of the Hering-Breuer reflex. This method (i.e., expiratory volume-clamp technique) is based on having the sedated infant breathe through a two-way valve system partitioned into separate inspiratory and expiratory ports. During spontaneous respiration, the expiratory valve is intermittently occluded for three to five breaths, and each successive unobstructed inspiration results in a sequential cumulative increase in lung volume, which ultimately approaches 60 to 80 per cent of TLC. As depicted in Figure 6–16, the cumulative increase in lung volume is associated with progressive recruitment of the Hering-Breuer reflex, a phenomenon that results in lengthening of the duration of the apneic pauses and facilitation of

complete relaxation of the respiratory muscles. Over the extended volume range, the passive inflation P-V relationship of the respiratory system was found to be most closely approximated by the binomial expression

Equation 7

$$V = aP^2 + bP + c$$

wherein c denotes the volume difference between the dynamic and passive FRC, and the constants a and b are indices that describe the curvilinearity and steepness of the P-V relationship, respectively (Fig. 6–17A). Rearranging the previous expression into its linear transform, the cord compliance (i.e., [V − c]/P) obtained at any given pressure (P) is given by

Equation 8

$$C_{\overline{rs}} = aP + b$$

Equation 8 indicates that the inflation cord compliance varies linearly as a function of the inflation pressure (Fig. 6–17B). The mean (±SD) weight-

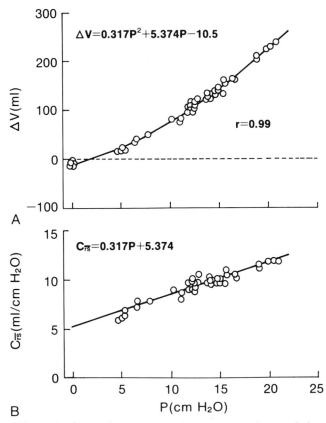

Figure 6–17. *A*, The representative pressure-volume relationship obtained in a normal 1-year-old infant using the expiratory volume-clamp technique. The relationship is fit by the polynomial function V = aP² + bP + c, where *c* represents the difference between the passive and dynamic functional residual capacity (FRC) levels (i.e., the "zero" volume point). Points at 0 pressure were determined by extrapolation of tidal flow-volume curves to zero flow, as in Figure 6–2. *B*, The chord compliance determined for each data point varies linearly with P. (From Grunstein MM, Springer C, Godfrey S et al: J Appl Physiol 62:2107, 1987.)

specific value of the cord compliance obtained at a pressure of 20 cm H_2O (i.e., $C_{\overline{rs}20}$) using this method in normal infants amounted to 1.61 ± 0.48 cc/kg/cm H_2O (Grunstein et al, 1987), a value similar to the average passive $C_{\overline{rs}}$ of 1.45 ± 0.27 ml/kg/cm H_2O measured at P = 20 cm H_2O in paralyzed infants (Nightingale and Richards, 1965). Because of augmentation of the Hering-Breuer reflex at higher lung volumes, the technique was found applicable in children up to 4 years of age, with values of $C_{\overline{rs}20}$ remaining a constant function of body weight throughout that age range (Fig. 6–18).

ACTIVE MEASUREMENTS

To achieve and maintain a given tidal volume during active breathing, the force generated by the contracting inspiratory muscles must overcome various dynamic impedances in addition to those attributed to the passive mechanical properties of the respiratory system (elastic and flow resistive). These additional impedances to lung expansion include chest wall distortion and the mechanical properties of the contracting respiratory muscles, which are reflected in their force-length and force-velocity

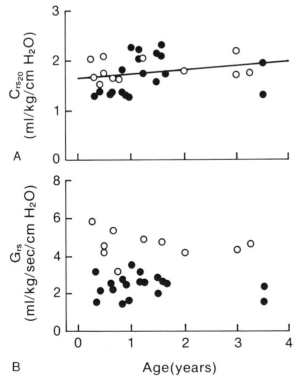

Figure 6–18. A, Weight-specific values of $C_{\overline{rs}20}$ as a function of age. Note: $C_{\overline{rs}20}$/kg does not change with age over the first 4 years of life and is similar in children with reactive airway disease *(closed figures)* and normal children *(open figures)*. The regression line for all the infants is given by $C_{\overline{rs}20}$/kg = 1.65 + 0.08 (years). B, Corresponding weight-specific values for respiratory system conductance (Grs) as a function of age. Note that Grs/kg does not substantially change over the first 4 years of life in normal children but is significantly lower at any age in children with reactive airway disease.

characteristics. As noted earlier, infants have a high chest wall compliance relative to that of the lung. This situation results in a lowered passive FRC and predisposes the respiratory system to undergo chest wall distortion during active inspiration, because the generation of a negative intrapleural pressure by the contracting inspiratory muscles tends to draw the highly compliant chest wall in an inward (i.e., paradoxical) direction. The consequence of such inward chest wall movement is that a fraction of the inspiratory muscle activity is uncoupled from lung expansion, resulting in a decrease in the magnitude of the tidal volume. Accordingly, for a given volume, the inspiratory muscles must generate pressures greater than those predicted purely on the basis of the passive P-V characteristics of the lungs and chest wall. Thus it is expected that the active compliance of the respiratory system should be less than the static compliance.

A noninvasive approach has been developed to estimate the active or "effective" compliance of the respiratory system (C'_{rs}) during dynamic breathing (Zin et al, 1982). When the airway is occluded at end-expiration, the airway opening pressure (P_{ao}) generated during the following obstructed inspiratory effort represents the mechanical transformation of the central inspiratory output to the respiratory muscles. Moreover, based on the consideration that the neural output of the first occluded inspiration is similar to that of the preceding unoccluded breaths (Whitelaw et al, 1975), a finding supported by studies on sleeping infants (Carlo et al, 1985), the measurements of P_{ao} at given time intervals from the onset of the inspiratory effort may be used to estimate the total instantaneous pressure required to inflate the respiratory system during an active inspiration. By relating the values of P_{ao} to the corresponding measurements of instantaneous flow ($\dot{V}$) and volume (V) obtained during the course of the preceding unobstructed inspiration, the active compliance (C'_{rs}) and resistance (R'_{rs}) may be determined according to the following equation of motion of the respiratory system (Zin et al, 1982):

Equation 9
$$P_{ao} = (1/C'_{rs}) \cdot V + R'_{rs} \cdot \dot{V}$$

Dividing the components of the above expression by $\dot{V}$ yields

Equation 10
$$P_{ao}/\dot{V} = (1/C'_{rs}) \cdot V/\dot{V} + R'_{rs}$$

According to equation 10, graphic representation of the relationship between $P_{ao}/\dot{V}$ (y axis) and $V/\dot{V}$ (x axis) depicts a straight line, wherein the slope represents the active elastance (i.e., $1/C'_{rs}$) and the y intercept represents the active resistance of the respiratory system (Fig. 6–19). The C'_{rs} was found to increase significantly in ten healthy term newborns from a mean ($\pm$SD) value of 1.87 ± 0.54 ml/cm H_2O

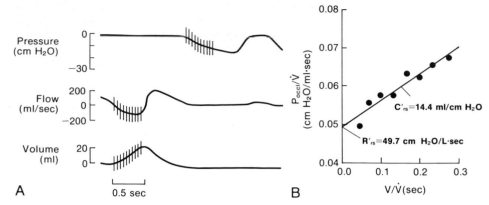

Figure 6–19. Measurement of active compliance (C'_{rs}) and resistance (R'_{rs}) of the respiratory system. *A*, the schematic record of airway pressure (P_{occl}), air flow ($\dot{V}$), and volume (V) in a sleeping infant. After one control breath, the airway is occluded at end-expiration. During the ensuing occluded inspiratory effort, P_{occl} is measured every 0.05 sec, along with the corresponding values of $\dot{V}$ and V of the preceding breath. *B*, $P_{occl}/\dot{V}$ versus $V/\dot{V}$ plot constructed on the basis of the values obtained in *A*. The slope of the relationship represents E'_{rs} (i.e., $1/C'_{rs}$), and the y-intercept represents R'_{rs} according to equation 10 in the text.

at 10 to 90 min of life to a value of 2.51 ± 1.15 ml/cm H_2O at 1 to 5 days of life (Mortola et al, 1982). Moreover, the measurement of C'_{rs} at the age of 1 to 5 days was found to be approximately 65 per cent of the passive C_{rs}, a value somewhat lower than the average C'_{rs}/C_{rs} ratio of 74 per cent reported in adults (Behrakis et al, 1983). The corresponding values of R'_{rs} and R_{rs} were found to be similar in infants (Mortola et al, 1982) as well as in adults (Behrakis et al, 1983).

The accuracy of the previously discussed method to measure C'_{rs} in infants may be limited in light of two primary considerations. First, infants characteristically maintain a dynamically elevated FRC, and hence during active inspiration an initial component of the inspiratory output is lost to offset the intrinsic passive recoil of the respiratory system. Second, in the presence of chest wall distortion during airway occlusion, contraction of the inspiratory muscles is nonisometric, resulting in an underestimate of the measurement of $1/C'_{rs}$. Notwithstanding these limitations, the aforementioned approach appears useful in that it is noninvasive and provides some reasonable estimates of the active mechanical properties of the respiratory system.

RESISTANCE

In addition to overcoming the elastic impedance of the respiratory system, the force generated by the contracting inspiratory muscles must also overcome the impedance attributed to the resistance to gas flow through the airways (R_{aw}), as well as to the frictional or viscous resistances of the lung (R_L) and chest wall (R_{cw}). The measurement of R_{aw} is dependent on the caliber of the airways in addition to the viscosity of the respired gas and its degree of flow turbulence. Moreover, to the extent that airway diameter varies in proportion to the degree of lung expansion, R_{aw}

is also dependent on lung volume, and it falls significantly as lung volume is increased. In contrast, it has been demonstrated that airway conductance (G_{aw}; i.e., $1/R_{aw}$) varies linearly with lung volume. Accordingly, the measurement of specific airway conductance (SG_{aw}; i.e., G_{aw}/FRC) provides a useful estimate of the volume-dependence of resistance and is routinely determined in studies of pulmonary function in older children and adults.

Whereas R_{aw} and SG_{aw} are typically assessed in older children applying the body plethysmographic approach (see later discussion), the technical demands inherent in adapting the latter technique for use in young children have fostered the development of alternative approaches to measure resistance in infants. Depending on the methods used, measurements of resistance have included determination of the R_{aw}, the total pulmonary resistance (R_{tp}; i.e., $R_{aw} + R_L$), and the active or passive respiratory system resistance (R'_{rs} or R_{rs}), where $R_{rs} = R_{aw} + R_L + R_{cw}$. In adults, the tissue frictional resistances are relatively minor, with R_L and R_{cw} constituting less than 10 and 20 per cent, respectively, of the total respiratory resistance during nasal breathing (Murray, 1986). Although Polgar and String (1966) reported that R_L averaged 24 per cent of R_{tp} in ten term newborns, a value amounting to twice that obtained in normal adults, subsequent investigators have found that simultaneous measurements of R_{aw} and R_{tp} are nearly identical and have suggested that R_L is minimal in neonates as well (Helms, 1982; Stocks et al, 1985).

Largely because of the use of different techniques of measurement, absolute values for resistance in infants and young children remain unsettled. Furthermore, difficulties in comparing the resistance values in older children and adults with those of infants arise because older children and adults are typically studied in the upright position, fully conscious, and breathing through a mouthpiece, whereas infants are generally studied supine, sedated, and breathing nasally. As in adults, nasal resistance in infants is substantial, constituting anywhere between 20 and 70 per cent of the total airway resistance in healthy newborns (Polgar and Kong, 1965). The different parameters of resistance and the methods currently employed in their measurement are discussed later.

RESPIRATORY SYSTEM RESISTANCE

ACTIVE MEASUREMENTS

As per Figure 6–19, measurement of the active inspiratory resistance (R'_{rs}) is represented by the y intercept in the plot of the $P_{ao}/\dot{V}$ versus $\dot{V}/\dot{V}$ relationship. To date, use of this approach to determine R'_{rs} has not been applied to older infants; however, the value of R'_{rs} reported in a group of healthy newborn infants averaged (mean ± SD) 45.0 ± 21.6 cm H_2O/L • sec, a value similar to the estimated passive inspiratory R_{rs} in the same infants (Mortola et al, 1982). The latter parameter was derived from analysis of the passive expiratory flow-volume loop (see later discussion) and included the assumption that inspiratory resistance represents approximately 70 per cent of expiratory resistance during infancy (Cook et al, 1957). This similarity between the active and passive measurements of R_{rs} persists into adulthood (Behrakis et al, 1983) and suggests that the force-velocity relationship of the contracting inspiratory muscles does not significantly contribute to the net active flow impedance of the respiratory system.

PASSIVE MEASUREMENTS

Airway Occlusion Methods

The passive respiratory system resistance (R_{rs}) can be determined by analysis of the expiratory flow-volume relationship obtained following the release of an airway occlusion at end-inspiration (i.e., when the respiratory muscles are presumably inactivated by stimulation of the Hering-Breuer reflex) (Siafakas, 1981). As illustrated in Figure 6–2, the passive expiratory flow-volume curve may often be closely approximated by a linear relationship, wherein the slope defines the passive time constant of the respiratory system (τ_{rs}). Indeed, the determination of τ_{rs} is based on the time (t) − related decreases in volume (V) and flow ($\dot{V}$), which are represented by the following exponential functions, respectively:

Equation 11

$$V = V_o \cdot e^{-t/\tau_{rs}}$$

and

Equation 12

$$\dot{V} = - (V_o/\tau_{rs}) \cdot e^{-t/\tau_{rs}}$$

where V_o is the total expired volume. The quotient $-V/\dot{V}$, obtained by dividing equation 11 by equation 12, defines τ_{rs}.

Because τ_{rs} represents the product of respiratory system resistance and compliance, knowledge of C_{rs} (obtained as per Fig. 6–15 or 6–17) and τ_{rs} allows for calculation of the passive resistance of the respiratory system (i.e., $R_{rs} = \tau_{rs}/C_{rs}$) or its reciprocal, respiratory system conductance ($G_{rs} = C_{rs}/\tau_{rs}$). The mean (±SD) values of R_{rs} reported in a group of term newborns amounted to 58.7 (±27.0) cm H_2O/L • sec, which corresponds to an average G_{rs}/mean body weight value of 5.0 ml/kg/sec/cm H_2O (Mortola et al, 1982). A modification of the previously mentioned approaches for determining R_{rs} was applied in intubated newborns using a single breath method (Le-Souef et al, 1984). The latter determination of R_{rs} is based on relating the peak pressure obtained during an airway occlusion at end-inspiration to the corresponding peak flow extrapolated from the slope of the subsequent released, passive expiratory flow-volume relationship (see Fig. 6–2). The extended passive flow-volume curves obtained following release of a volume-clamp maneuver were also approximated by a linear function (Fig. 6–20), with an extended slope generally similar to that obtained in the tidal volume range. Indeed, a similar mean (±SD) G_{rs}/body weight value of 5.5 (±2.3) ml/kg/sec/cm H_2O was reported using the volume-clamp technique in healthy 1- to 18-month-old infants (Grunstein et al, 1987). The last measurement appears to remain fairly constant throughout the first 4 years of life (see Fig. 6–18B).

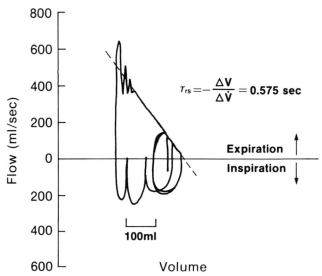

Figure 6–20. Flow-volume relationships obtained during both tidal breathing and application of the expiratory volume-clamp (EVC) test. Two smaller and complete (i.e., inspiration and expiration) flow-volume loops represent unobstructed tidal breaths, whereas three successive inspiratory loops obtained during the EVC maneuver are associated with cumulative increases in volume. The larger expiratory flow-volume relationship depicts that obtained during subsequent release of expiratory obstruction. (From Grunstein MM, Springer C, Godfrey S et al: J Appl Physiol 62:2107, 1987.)

The aforementioned approaches for determining R_{rs} are dependent on obtaining a linear expiratory flow-volume relationship, which implies a uniform time constant of the respiratory system (single resistance and compliance). Infants with inhomogeneous pulmonary disease, however, may demonstrate significant concavity of their tidal flow-volume curves, implying the presence of heterogeneity in the distribution of time constants within the lungs.

Forced Oscillatory Technique

The R_{rs} may also be derived from measurement of the mechanical impedance of the respiratory system (Z_{rs}) using the forced oscillatory technique (DuBois et al, 1955; Fisher et al, 1968), whereby air pressure and flow are simultaneously recorded at the mouth during the administration of rapid, sinusoidal airflow cycles (above 3 cycles/sec) generated by a piston or loud-speaker positioned at the mouth or across the chest wall. The Z_{rs} (in cm H_2O/L • sec can be defined by the equation

Equation 13

$$Z_{rs} = \sqrt{R_{rs}^2 + (2\pi fL - \frac{1}{2\pi fC})^2}$$

where L is inertance in cm H_2O/L • sec^2, C is respiratory system compliance in L/cm H_2O, and f is the oscillatory frequency in cycles/sec. The inertial forces or reactance of the lungs, thorax, and airway gas (given by the $2\pi fL$ term) increase as the oscillatory frequency increases. In contrast, the elastic forces or reactance opposing volume change in the lungs and thorax (given by the $1/[2\pi fC]$ term) decreases as the oscillatory frequency is enhanced. In practice, mouth pressure is displayed against airflow on an oscilloscope, and the oscillatory frequency is varied until the P-V loop closes, at what is termed the resonant frequency (usually 5 to 7 cycles/sec in adults [Fisher et al, 1968] and children [Cogswell, 1973]). The inertial and elastic reactances are nearly equal at the resonant frequency and, according to equation 13, Z_{rs} (i.e., the slope of the P-V relationship) approximates R_{rs}. In adapting this technique for use in infants, Wohl and associates (1969) found that the inspiratory and expiratory oscillatory R_{rs} values were equal and averaged (mean ± SD) 46 (±17) cm H_2O/L • sec during the first 15 months of life. The last value corresponds to a weight-specific G_{rs} of 3.7 (±1.7) ml/kg/sec/cm H_2O. As anticipated from the increase in airway caliber with age, the forced oscillatory R_{rs} progressively decreases during growth (Hantos et al, 1985). Moreover, the oscillatory values of G_{rs} were found to be significantly lower in infants with bronchiolitis (inspiratory $G_{rs}BW$ 2.4 ± 1.3 and expiratory G_{rs}/BW 1.2 ± 0.8 ml/kg/sec/cm H_2O) (Wohl et al, 1969); however, the reactance terms may

contribute to the oscillatory impedance measurements in nonuniformly diseased lungs, thereby causing Z_{rs} to overestimate R_{rs}.

TOTAL PULMONARY RESISTANCE

As noted previously, the total pulmonary resistance (R_{tp}) represents the sum of R_{aw} and R_L, and R_{tp} may be determined in infants by placement of an intraesophageal balloon or catheter, as described for the measurement of dynamic lung compliance. From continuous recordings of esophageal pressure (P_{es}), airflow ($\dot{V}$), and volume (V), the last derived by integration of the flow signal from a pneumotachograph, R_{tp} is conventionally calculated at the midtidal volume points of inspiration and expiration by dividing the ΔP_{es} at those points by the corresponding absolute difference between the inspiratory and expiratory flows (i.e., $\Delta \dot{V}$), as depicted in Figure 6–21. Using this approach, R_{tp} was found to average (mean ± SD) 21 (±4) to 29 (±13) cm H_2O/L • sec in healthy term newborns (Howlett, 1972; Krieger, 1963; Cook et al, 1957; Swyer et al, 1960) and to remain constant at 22 (±5) to 29 (±20) cm H_2O/L • sec over the first 1 to 2 years of life (Phelan and Williams, 1969; Krieger, 1963). Moreover, when corrected for lung size, the specific expiratory pulmonary conductance (i.e., $SG_{ep} = [R_{ep}]$/FRC) was reported to be relatively high in newborn infants (0.44 ± 0.11 ml/sec/cm H_2O/ml FRC) as compared with the mean value of 0.17 (±0.08) ml/sec/cm H_2O/ml FRC obtained in children 1 to 60 months of age (Gerhardt et al, 1987).

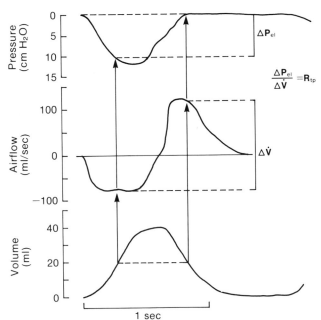

Figure 6–21. A method for calculating dynamic total pulmonary resistance (R_{tp}). As demonstrated in this schematic representation of simultaneous esophageal pressure (P_{el}), airflow ($\dot{V}$), and volume (V) recordings, R_{tp} is determined by P_{el} divided by $\dot{V}$ obtained between points of isovolume during inspiration and expiration.

AIRWAY RESISTANCE

The measurement of airway resistance (R_{aw}) is based on determination of the difference between alveolar pressure (P_{alv}) and airway opening pressure (P_{ao}) divided by the airflow ($\dot{V}$) (i.e., $[P_{alv} - P_{ao}]/\dot{V}$). With the subject spontaneously breathing in a body plethysmograph, simultaneous changes in $\dot{V}$ and plethysmographic pressure (P_{box}) are recorded on an x-y oscilloscope, and the slope of this relationship is recorded. The airway is then occluded, and simultaneous changes in volume (reflected as changes in P_{box}) and mouth pressure (P_m, which is assumed to equal P_{alv}) are monitored, as for the determination of TGV (DuBois et al, 1956). Provided that the ratio of lung to plethysmographic gas volume remains constant, the P_{alv} corresponding to a given P_{box} remains constant, whether or not flow is interrupted (Fig. 6–22). Accordingly, derivation of R_{aw} is obtained by dividing the slope of P_m/P_{box} by the slope of $\dot{V}/P_{box}$:

Equation 14

$$R_{rs} = \frac{\Delta P_{alv}}{\dot{V}} = \frac{\Delta P_m}{\dot{V}} = \frac{\Delta P_m/\Delta P_{box}}{\dot{V}/\Delta P_{box}} - R_{equipment}$$

In older children and adults, the measurements of R_{aw} are standardized to a given flow rate, traditionally 0.5 L/sec. Because the flow rates in infants vary considerably, measurements of R_{aw} in young children have been obtained at a similar phase of respiration, arbitrarily chosen as two thirds of maximum inspiratory flow (Radford, 1974; Stocks et al, 1977). Using body plethysmography, Doershuk and colleagues (1970) determined that the mean ($\pm$SD) R_{aw} diminished from 20.3 ($\pm$6.9) cm $H_2O/L \cdot$ sec in infants during the first year of life to 11.2 ($\pm$3.0) cm $H_2O/L \cdot$ sec over the next 4 years of age.

Direct comparison of R_{aw} at different ages is limited, however, because R_{aw} is nonlinearly related to lung volume. G_{aw} does vary directly with lung volume, however, so SG_{aw} (i.e., G_{aw}/FRC) has been used as a

volume-corrected measurement to assess the changes in airway caliber during lung growth and development. In accord with the concept of dysanaptic lung development, as described by Stocks and Godfrey (1977), SG_{aw} decreases from a range of 0.28 to 0.59 ml/sec/cm H_2O/ml FRC in premature infants to mean ($\pm$SD) levels of 0.31 ($\pm$0.04) and 0.27 ($\pm$0.04) ml/sec/cm H_2O/ml FRC in term and 1- to 11-month-old infants, respectively. Moreover, the changing relationship between G_{aw} and lung volume continues during early childhood, such that airway caliber is relatively larger in relation to lung volume in the newborn infant. During the course of subsequent childhood development, however, airway size grows more slowly in proportion to the increase in lung alveolar volume. Further enhanced airway growth continues during adolescence, resulting in stable adult values for SG_{aw}.

MAXIMAL FORCED EXPIRATORY FLOW

Because of the presence of dynamic compression of the intrathoracic airways during forced exhalation, the maximum expiratory flow rates achieved at lung volumes below 70 per cent of TLC are largely independent of effort and are determined by the elastic recoil pressure of the lung and the airway resistance upstream to the site of airway compression (Mead et al, 1967). Although maximal (i.e., from TLC to residual volume) or partial (i.e., not encompassing the entire vital capacity) expiratory flow-volume curves are easily elicited and routinely measured in adults and older children, forced expiratory flow rates could not be determined in uncooperative infants until recently. Two innovative techniques have been developed, however, to elicit forced expirations in infants, which consist of applying either a positive pressure to the thorax and abdomen or a negative pressure to the airway opening.

NEGATIVE PRESSURE-INDUCED DEFLATION TECHNIQUE

Motoyama and co-workers introduced a method whereby maximum expiratory flow-volume curves are generated by means of the sudden application of a negative pressure to rapidly deflate the lungs of infants and older children ventilated through an endotracheal tube (1977, 1987). In applying this technique, a constant volume history is initially set by three standard inflations to TLC with a static pressure of +40 cm H_2O. After a fourth such inflation, the subject's airway opening is quickly switched to a 40-L negative-pressure reservoir set at −40 cm H_2O and, thereby, the lungs are rapidly deflated until expiratory flow ceases (i.e., to residual volume) or for up to 3 sec. From the resultant maximum expiratory flow-volume relationship (MEFV), the forced vital

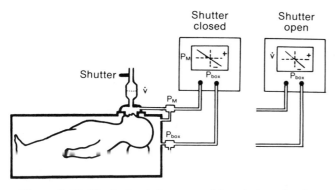

Figure 6–22. The body plethysmographic technique for determination of airway resistance (R_{aw}). The relationship between mouth pressure (P_M) − box pressure (P_{box}) and airflow ($\dot{V}$) − P_{box} are separately obtained with the shutter closed and open, respectively. The R_{aw} is then calculated by the ratio of the two slopes, according to equation 14 in the text.

capacity (FVC) and the maximal flow at 25 per cent of FVC from RV (i.e., $\dot{V}max_{25}$) are determined. Using this approach, premature infants without lung disease were found to have a mean ($\pm SD$) FVC of 58.3 (± 13.6) ml/kg and $\dot{V}max_{25}$ of 95.0 (± 26.8) ml/kg/sec. Both the measurements were significantly greater than those obtained in 32 premature infants with lung disease, in whom the FVC and $\dot{V}max_{25}$ values averaged 30.9 (± 13.6) ml/kg and 17.2 (± 14.4) ml/kg/sec, respectively (Motoyama et al, 1987). When corrected for lung volume, the range of $\dot{V}max_{25}$/FRC was significantly higher in infants (0.97 to 1.11 FRC/sec) than in older children (0.50 to 0.85 FRC/sec) up to 17 years of age (Motoyama, 1977), suggesting the presence of larger airways relative to lung volume in the younger children.

CHEST COMPRESSION TECHNIQUE

In contrast to the above deflation technique applied to intubated patients, an effective approach to generate partial expiratory flow-volume (PEFV) curves in spontaneously breathing infants and young children was developed by Adler and Wohl (1978) and refined by Taussig and co-workers (1982; Godfrey et al, 1983; Tepper et al, 1986; Morgan et al, 1988). In its current use, this method utilizes the sudden application of a positive pressure to the thorax and abdomen to establish a maximum forced exhalation. The exhalation is accomplished with the use of an inflatable plastic cuff or "jacket" wrapped around the trunk of a sedated, supine infant. The encircling jacket is attached to a reservoir of compressed air, with a volume of at least ten times that of the cuff to ensure a relatively constant applied pressure during the forced expiratory maneuver (Morgan et al, 1988). Spontaneous respiration is recorded with a pneumotachograph attached to the infant's nose and mouth via a face mask. When the subject's resting end-expiratory volume has remained constant for several breaths, a pressure-release valve connecting the jacket to the reservoir is opened at end-tidal inspiration. Within 70 to 100 ms, 95 per cent of the peak cuff inflation pressure is exerted around the subject's thorax and abdomen, and a PEFV curve is generated by maintenance of the pressure for 1 to 2 sec. The pressure-release valve is then closed and a relief valve is opened to decompress the surrounding cuff pressure. Although vital capacity is unknown in these infants, the fact that the forced expiratory volume normally proceeds below the spontaneous end-expiratory level allows the PEFV curve to be quantified by measuring the flow at FRC. Because the fraction of the pressure that is delivered to the infant's pleural space is unpredictable and because pressures that are either too high or too low may generate suboptimal flows (LeSouef et al, 1986), the forced expiratory maneuver is repeated at increasing pressures until a maximal flow (i.e., $\dot{V}_{max}$FRC) is obtained. If FRC or TGV is measured concomitantly,

values for $\dot{V}_{max}$FRC may then be standardized in terms of volume units (e.g., FRC/sec). Such volume correction is essential when interpreting changes in $\dot{V}_{max}$FRC that occur with maturation, disease states, or following therapeutic interventions, because any observed variations in $\dot{V}_{max}$FRC may be related to changes in lung volume apart from any direct alterations in airway caliber per se.

Flow limitation typically occurs in neonates subjected to 30 to 44 cm H_2O of externally applied pressure, levels that are estimated to generate pleural pressures of approximately 8 to 10 cm H_2O (Taussig et al, 1982). Of interest, flow limitation is also reached in adults at similar pleural pressures (approximately 10 cm H_2O) (Mead, 1980). At such pressures, mean ($\pm SD$) $\dot{V}_{max}$FRC values of 185 (± 18) and 186 (± 55) ml/sec have been measured in healthy term neonates (Adler and Wohl, 1978; Taussig et al, 1982), the latter amounting to 1.90 (± 0.58) TGV/sec. Volume-specific airflow at FRC appears to be maximal in the neonatal period and decreases by 1 month of age to a range of 1.1 to 1.6 FRC/sec that is maintained throughout subsequent childhood (Tepper et al, 1986; Silverman et al, 1986; Masters et al, 1987; Buist et al, 1980). Substantially lower $\dot{V}_{max}$/FRC values of 0.3 to 0.7 FRC/sec have been reported in infants with bronchiolitis, cystic fibrosis, and bronchopulmonary dysplasia (Godfrey et al, 1983; Hoskyns et al, 1987). Between 1 and 13 months of age, $\dot{V}_{max}$FRC (in FRC/sec) has been shown to be significantly correlated with SG_{rs} (in ml/sec/cm H_2O/ml FRC), both in healthy infants as well as in those with respiratory disease (Hoskyns et al, 1987), according to the overall expression

$$\dot{V}_{max}FRC = 6.37 \, (SG_{rs}) - 0.15$$

LeSouef and associates have suggested that additional information may be obtained from the shape of the PEFV curves produced by chest compression in infants (1988). The investigators noted that convex curves (e.g., curve A, Fig. 6–23) tended to denote better respiratory function and were found more commonly in healthy infants. In contrast, significantly concave curves (e.g., curve B, Fig. 6–23) were associated with flow limitation during normal tidal expiration, perhaps reflecting the consequence of hyperinflation or exaggerated dynamic compression of airways in infants with impaired respiratory function. In support of the concept of airway compression, LeSouef and associates have previously demonstrated that PEFV curves in normal infants can change from convex to straight to concave as the applied compression pressure is increased (1986).

Additional research is needed in applying the aforementioned methodology to address such issues as varying passive and dynamic FRC levels; standardization of applied pressures and lung volume histories; flow limitation by isovolume pressure-flow curve analysis; and reflex responses elicited by sudden chest compression, including glottic closure (Silverman et

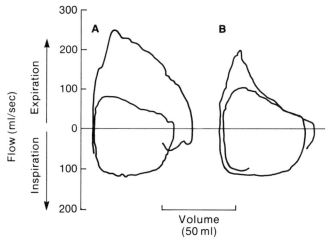

Figure 6–23. A comparison of representative partial forced-expiratory flow-volume curves obtained during chest compression in infants with differing respiratory function. The shape of the forced expiratory flow-volume curve is concave in the infant with impaired airway function *(curve B)* but convex in the infant with better respiratory function *(curve A)*. Note that in both examples a smaller tidal loop and a larger forced expiratory flow-volume curve are depicted. (From LeSouef PN, Hughes DM, and Landaw LI: Am Rev Respir Dis 138:590, 1988.)

al, 1986; Hoskyns et al, 1987) and stimulation of inspiratory activity (Hoskyns et al, 1987). Notwithstanding the last mentioned issues, the partial forced expiratory maneuvers applied to infants have the potential to provide valuable clinical information about the developing lungs in health and disease.

CONCLUSION

There has been a resurgence in the development of new and innovative approaches to measure pulmonary function in infants and young children. Although it is apparent that further important research into the standardization and automation of the current procedures must precede any substantial progress in their use on a routine basis, a number of the techniques developed to date hold great promise for physicians seeking to diagnose and intervene earlier in the course of an infant's lung disease. Clearly, further experience with the various techniques and measurements of respiratory mechanics will better define normal values and will determine which methods are best suited for following infants with pulmonary disease. Ultimately, it will be important to discern how the approaches used to assess infant pulmonary function compare with the more conventional parameters of lung function obtained in the older child and adult.

REFERENCES

Adler S and Wohl ME: Flow-volume relationship at low lung volumes in healthy term newborn infants. Pediatrics 61:636, 1978.

Agostoni E: Volume-pressure relationships of the thorax and lung in the newborn. J Appl Physiol 14:909, 1959.

Asher MI, Coates AL, Collinge JM, and Milic-Emili J: Measurement of esophageal pressure in neonates. J Appl Physiol 52:491, 1982.

Auld PAM, Nelson NM, Cherry RB et al: Measurement of thoracic gas volume in the newborn infant. J Clin Invest 42:476, 1963.

Beardsmore CS, Helms P, Stocks J et al: Improved esophageal balloon technique for use in infants. J Appl Physiol 49:735, 1980.

Behrakis PK, Higgs BD, Baydur A et al: Active inspiratory impedance in halothane-anesthetized humans. J Appl Physiol 54:1477, 1983.

Berglund G and Karlberg P: Determination of the functional residual capacity in newborn infants. Acta Pediatr 45:541, 1956.

Blair E and Hickam JB: Effect of change in body position on lung volume and intrapulmonary gas mixing in normal subjects. J Clin Invest 34:383, 1955.

Bryan AC, Mansell AL, and Levison H: Development of the mechanical properties of the respiratory system. In: Hodson WA (ed): Development of the Lung. Lung Biology in Health and Disease. Vol 6. New York, Marcel Dekker, Inc, 1977.

Buist AS, Adams BE, Sexton GJ, and Aczam AH: Reference values for functional residual capacity and maximal expiratory flow in young children. Am Rev Respir Dis 122:983, 1980.

Carlo WA, Miller MJ, and Martin RJ: Differential response of respiratory muscles to airway occlusion in infants. J Appl Physiol 59:847, 1985.

Cherniack RM and Brown E: A simple method for measuring total respiratory compliance: normal values for males. J Appl Physiol 20:87, 1965.

Chu JS, Dawson P, Klaus M, and Sweet AY: Lung compliance and lung volume measured concurrently in normal full-term and premature infants. Pediatrics 34:525, 1964.

Cogswell JJ: Forced oscillation technique for determination of resistance to breathing in children. Arch Dis Child 48:259, 1973.

Cook CD, Cherry RB, O'Brien D et al: Studies of respiratory physiology in the newborn infant. I. Observations on normal premature and full-term infants. J Clin Invest 34:975, 1955.

Cook CD, Helliesen PJ, and Agathon S: Relation between mechanics of respiration, lung size and body size from birth to young adulthood. J Appl Physiol 13:349, 1958.

Cook CD, Sutherland JM, Segal S et al: Studies of respiratory physiology in the newborn infant. III. Measurements of mechanics of respiration. J Clin Invest 36:440, 1957.

Davis GM, Coates AL, Papageorgiou A, and Bureau MA: Direct measurement of static chest wall compliance in animal and human neonates. J Appl Physiol 65:1093, 1988.

Doershuk CF, Downs TD, Matthews LW, and Lough MD: A method for ventilatory measurements in subjects 1 month–5 years of age: normal results and observations in disease. Pediatr Res 4:165, 1970.

Doershuk CF and Matthews LW: Airway resistance and lung volume in the newborn infant. Pediatr Res 3:128, 1969.

DuBois AB, Botelho SY, Bedell GN et al: A rapid plethysmographic method for measuring thoracic gas volume: a comparison with a nitrogen washout method for measuring functional residual capacity in normal subjects. J Clin Invest 35:322, 1956.

DuBois AB, Botelho SY, and Comroe JH Jr: A new method for measuring airway resistance in man using a body plethysmograph: values in normal subjects and in patients with respiratory disease. J Clin Invest 35:327, 1956.

DuBois AB, Brody AW, Lewis DH, and Burgess BF Jr: Oscillation mechanics of lungs and chest in man. J Appl Physiol 8:587, 1955.

Fagan DG: Post-mortem studies of the semistatic volume-pressure characteristics of infants' lungs. Thorax 31:534, 1976.

Fagan DG: Shape changes in static V-P loops for children's lungs related to growth. Thorax 32:198, 1977.

Fisher AB, DuBois AB, and Hyde RW: Evaluation of the forced oscillation technique for the determination of resistance to breathing. J Clin Invest 47:2045, 1968.

Fisher JT, Mortola JP, Smith JB et al: Respiration in newborns: development of the control of breathing. Am Rev Respir Dis 125:650, 1982.

Gerhardt T, Hehre D, Feller R et al: Pulmonary mechanics in normal infants and young children during first 5 years of life. Pediatr Pulmonol 3:309, 1987.

Gerhardt T, Reifenberg L, Hehre D et al: Functional residual capacity in normal neonates and children up to 5 years of age determined by a N_2 washout method. Pediatr Res 20:668, 1986.

Godfrey S, Bar-Yishay E, Arad I et al: Flow-volume curves in infants with lung disease. Pediatrics 72:517, 1983.

Greenough A, Stocks J, Nothen U, and Helms P: Total respiratory compliance and functional residual capacity in young children. Pediatr Pulmonol 2:321, 1986.

Grunstein MM, Springer C, Godfrey S et al: Expiratory volume clamping: a new method to assess respiratory mechanics in sedated infants. J Appl Physiol 62:2107, 1987.

Hanson JS and Shinozaki T: Hybrid computer studies of ventilatory distribution and lung volume. I. Normal newborn infants. Pediatrics 46:900, 1970.

Hantos Z, Daroczy B, and Gyurkovits K: Total respiratory impedance in healthy children. Pediatr Pulmonol 1:91, 1985.

Heaf DP, Turner H, Stocks J, and Helms P: The accuracy of esophageal pressure measurements in convalescent and sick intubated infants. Pediatr Pulmonol 2:5, 1986.

Helms P: Problems with plethysmographic estimation of lung volume in infants and young children. J Appl Physiol 53:698, 1982.

Hoskyns EW, Milner AD, and Hopkin IE: Validity of forced expiratory flow volume loops in neonates. Arch Dis Child 62:895, 1987.

Howlett G: Lung mechanics in normal infants with congenital heart disease. Arch Dis Child 47:707, 1972.

Kosch PC and Stark AR: Dynamic maintenance of end-expiratory lung volume in full-term infants. J Appl Physiol 57:1126, 1984.

Krauss AN and Auld PAM: Measurement of functional residual capacity in distressed neonates by helium rebreathing. J Pediatr 77:228, 1970.

Krieger I: Studies on mechanics of respiration in infancy. Am J Dis Child 105:439, 1963.

LeSouef PN, England SJ, and Bryan AC: Passive respiratory mechanics in newborns and children. Am Rev Respir Dis 129:552, 1984.

LeSouef PN, Hughes DM, and Landau LI: Effect of compression pressure on forced expiratory flow in infants. J Appl Physiol 61:1639, 1986.

LeSouef PN, Hughes DM, and Landau LI: Shape of forced expiratory flow-volume curves in infants. Am Rev Respir Dis 138:590, 1988.

LeSouef PN, Lopes JM, England SJ et al: Influence of chest wall distortion on esophageal pressure. J Appl Physiol 55:353, 1983.

Masters IB, Seidenberg J, Hudson I et al: Longitudinal study of lung mechanics in normal infants. Pediatr Pulmonol 3:3, 1987.

Mead J: Dysanapsis in normal lungs assessed by the relationship between maximal flow, static recoil, and vital capacity. Am Rev Respir Dis 121:339, 1980.

Mead J, Turner JM, Macklem PT, and Little JB: Significance of the relationship between lung recoil and maximum expiratory flow. J Appl Physiol 22:95, 1967.

Morgan WJ, Geller DE, Tepper RS, and Taussig LM: Partial expiratory flow-volume curves in infants and young children. Pediatr Pulmonol 5:232, 1988.

Mortola JP and Saetta M: Measurements of respiratory mechanics in the newborn: a simple approach. Pediatr Pulmonol 3:123, 1987.

Mortola JP, Fisher JT, Smith B et al: Dynamics of breathing in infants. J Appl Physiol 52:1209, 1982.

Motoyama EK: Pulmonary mechanics during early postnatal years. Pediat Res 11:220, 1977.

Motoyama EK, Fort MD, Klesh KW et al: Early onset of airway reactivity in premature infants with bronchopulmonary dysplasia. Am Rev Respir Dis 136:50, 1987.

Muller N, Volgyesi G, Becker L et al: Diaphragmatic muscle tone. J Appl Physiol: Respirat Environ Exercise Physiol 47:279, 1979.

Murray JF: The Normal Lung. Philadelphia, WB Saunders Co, 1986.

Nelson NM, Prod'hom LS, Cherry RB et al: Pulmonary function in the newborn infant. V. Trapped gas in the normal infant's lung. J Clin Invest 42:1850, 1963.

Nightingale DA and Richards CC: Volume-pressure relations of the respiratory system of curaraized infants. Anesthesiology 26:710, 1965.

Olinsky A, Bryan AC, and Bryan MH: A simple method for measuring total respiratory system compliance in newborn infants. S Afr Med J 50:128, 1976.

Phelan PD and Williams HE: Ventilatory studies in healthy infants. Pediatr Res 3:425, 1969.

Polgar G and Kong GP: The nasal resistance of newborn infants. J Pediatr 67:557, 1965.

Polgar G and String ST: The viscous resistance of the lung tissues in newborn infants. J Pediatr 69:787, 1966.

Radford M: Measurement of airway resistance and thoracic gas volume in infancy. Arch Dis Child 49:611, 1974.

Reynolds RM and Etsten BE: Mechanics of respiration in apneic anesthetized infants. Anesthesiology 27:13, 1966.

Rich CR, Rehder K, Knopp TJ, and Hyatt RE: Halothane and enflurane anesthesia and respiratory mechanics in prone dogs. J Appl Physiol 46:646, 1979.

Ronchetti R, Stocks J, Keith I, and Godfrey S: An analysis of a rebreathing method for measuring lung volume in the premature infant. Pediatr Res 9:797, 1975.

Sharp M, Druz W, Balgot R et al: Total respiratory compliance in infants and children. J Appl Physiol 29:775, 1970.

Siafakas NM, Peslin R, Bonora M et al: Phrenic activity, respiratory pressures, and volume changes in cats. J Appl Physiol 51:109, 1981.

Silverman M, Prendiville A, and Green S: Partial expiratory flow-volume curves in infancy: technical aspects. Bull Eur Physiopathol Respir 22:257, 1986.

Sjoqvist BA, Sandberg K, Hjalmarson O, and Olsson T: Calculation of lung volume in newborn infants by means of a computer-assisted nitrogen washout method. Pediatr Res 18:1160, 1984.

Stocks J and Godfrey S: Specific airway conductance in relation to postconceptional age during infancy. J Appl Physiol 43:144, 1977.

Stocks J, Levy NM, and Godfrey S: A new apparatus for the accurate measurement of airway resistance in infancy. J Appl Physiol 43:155, 1977.

Stocks J, Nothen U, Sutherland P et al: Improved accuracy of the occlusion technique for assessing total respiratory compliance in infants. Pediatr Pulmonol 3:71, 1987.

Stocks J, Thomson A, and Silverman M: The numerical analysis of pressure-flow curves in infancy. Pediatr Pulmonol 1:19, 1985.

Swyer PR, Reiman RC, and Wright JJ: Ventilation and ventilatory mechanics in the newborn. J Pediatr 56:612, 1960.

Taussig LM, Landau LI, Godfrey S, and Arad I: Determinants of forced expiratory flows in newborn infants. J Appl Physiol 53:1220, 1982.

Tepper RS, Morgan WJ, Cota K et al: Physiologic growth and development of the lung during the first year of life. Am Rev Respir Dis 134:513, 1986.

Tepper RS, Pagtakhan RD, and Taussig LM: Noninvasive determination of total respiratory system compliance in infants by the weighted-spirometer method. Am Rev Respir Dis 130:461, 1984.

Thomson A, Elliot J, Beardsmore CS, and Silverman M: The total compliance of the respiratory system during the first year of life. Bull Eur Physiopathol Respir 21:411, 1985.

Thomson A, Elliott J, and Silverman M: Pulmonary compliance in sick low birthweight infants. Arch Dis Child 58:891, 1983.

Thurlbeck WM: Postnatal lung growth. Thorax 37:564, 1982.

Wall MA, Misley MC, and Brown A: Changes in ventilation homogeneity from preschool through young adulthood as determined by moment analysis of nitrogen washout. Pediatr Res 23:68, 1988.

Westbrook PR, Stubbs SE, Sessler AD et al: Effects of anesthesia and muscle paralysis on respiratory mechanics in normal man. J Appl Physiol 34:81, 1973.

Whitelaw WA, Derenne JP, and Milic-Emili J: Occlusion pressure as a measure of respiratory center output in conscious man. Respir Physiol 23:181, 1975.

Wohl MEB, Stigol LC, and Mead J: Resistance of the total respiratory system in healthy infants and infants with bronchiolitis. Pediatrics 43:495, 1969.

Zapletal A, Paul T, and Samanek M: Pulmonary elasticity in children and adolescents. J Appl Physiol 40:953, 1976.

Zin WA, Pengelly LD, and Milic-Emili J: Single-breath method for measurement on respiratory mechanics in anesthetized animals. J Appl Physiol 52:1266, 1982.

7

RICHARD J. LEMEN, M.D.

PULMONARY FUNCTION TESTING IN THE OFFICE, CLINIC, AND HOME

The introduction of simple to operate pulmonary function equipment has expanded the usefulness of pulmonary function tests for the assessment of patients with pulmonary diseases. For the first time, accurate, reproducible pulmonary function studies can be obtained outside of sophisticated pulmonary function laboratories in tertiary care facilities. These simple tests rely on data generated from a forced expiratory vital capacity maneuver, which can be performed reliably by most children 5 years of age or older. The general uses of pulmonary function studies are summarized in Table 7–1. Methods of conducting these studies in the physician's office, clinic, and home, and methods of interpreting these data are the concern of this chapter.

SPECIAL CONSIDERATIONS WHEN TESTING CHILDREN

Children can be frustratingly uncooperative; they have a limited attention span, and, especially if ill at ease, they are easily distracted. A common mistake is to test children in a place where distractions may be frequent and where personnel are not accustomed to studying children. The results of testing under these conditions may vary greatly, and allowances must be made in interpreting such results. Special considerations that are most important for optimal pulmonary test function results in children are (1) a pleasant environment, (2) trained personnel, and (3) trained patients.

The tester must be patient, friendly, and able to relate well to children. The ideal tester is an office or a clinic nurse, parent, or physician, any or all of whom can be trained easily to conduct these tests. Patients must be trained as well. We use the following method: Before the study begins, the child practices a slow inspiration with a breath-hold of 1 to 2 sec at full inflation. This maneuver is demonstrated by the tester and practiced by the child; then, full deflation is demonstrated and practiced. Next, the maximal vital capacity maneuver is practiced, beginning with a slow full inflation, followed by a brief breath-hold, and then a sudden, sustained, maximal expiratory effort lasting at least 3 sec. Instructions to the child may take this form: "Let's make believe it's your birthday and you have to blow out all the candles with only one breath. Take a deep breath, more, more, more. Now *Blow!* More, more, more, squeeze, squeeze, squeeeeeze. . . . That's it! Good for you! Now let's see if you can do even better!"

Table 7–1. USES OF PULMONARY FUNCTION STUDIES IN CHILDREN

Clinical

PATIENT MANAGEMENT
    To follow the course of pulmonary disease
    To evaluate the response to therapy
    To regulate the duration and form of therapy

DIAGNOSIS
    To characterize pulmonary diseases physiologically
    To quantify disease severity
    To evaluate the risks of diagnostic or therapeutic procedures
    To suggest disease etiology
    To indicate specific therapy

Research
    To study changes in lung function with age
    To investigate acute and chronic factors on lung growth

Most children perform the maximal vital capacity maneuver reliably after 4 to 5 min of practice, but some, especially those less than 6 years old, require longer practice periods. Other good motivational techniques include computerized spirometers with graphics displays, such as inflating balloons or birthday candles; these provide incentive for the child to exhale fully. Stop the test if the child is sick or uncooperative and disregard all data. Cooperative children who still have not mastered the procedure benefit from the experience, but the data are not reported.

Criteria for determining that children have performed maximal expiratory vital capacity maneuvers with acceptable results are listed in Table 7–2. These criteria can be determined only from "hard copies" of the tracings at sufficient amplitude. Usually, children less than 10 years of age perform better if they are standing; it does not seem to matter if older children are standing or sitting during the procedure. The level of cooperation and difficulties such as fatigue and coughing should be included in the report. The environment must be pleasant and free of distractions. Most patients perform better if they are alone and at ease with the tester.

EQUIPMENT

Minimum specifications for spirometers for clinic and office use were proposed by the American Thoracic Society (ATS) (1979). These specifications were modified for children in 1980 (Table 7–3) (Taussig et al, 1980). A partial list of spirometers found to meet the ATS standards is shown in Table 7–3. Details of their operational characteristics can be found elsewhere (Enright and Hyatt, 1987).

Studies in our laboratory suggest that spirometers for children's studies should have flat dynamic response up to 12 Hz for flow and 6 Hz for volume if they are to record flows and volumes accurately during a maximum expiratory vital capacity maneuver (Lemen et al, 1982). Any spirometer must calculate or display the forced vital capacity (FVC), forced expiratory volume in 1 sec (FEV_1) and its ratio to FVC (FEV_1/FVC), and peak expiratory flow (PEF). These pulmonary function tests are the most reproducible of all spirometric measurements, useful for longitudinal studies and easiest to perform (Nickerson et al, 1980). As illustrated in Table 7–4, healthy children and adolescents (aged 7 to 16 years) perform

Table 7–3. COMPARISON OF OFFICE SPIROMETERS

Model, Manufacturer	Price ($)	Type	Auto	Graph
Vitalograph R, Vitalograph	1150	MV		§
VS 400, Puritan Bennett	1190	MV		§
Pulmonaire 10, Jones	1195	MV		
SM-1, Spirometrics	1295	MV		§
Survey I, Collins	1595	MV		
Model 822, SensorMedics	1900	MV		
SpiroComp, CDX Corporation	2900	AF	*	‡
3M/Mayo PF2001, CDX/Mayo	2940	AF	*	‡
SpiroScreen, SpectraMed, (Gould/SRL)	2950	AF	*	
Spiromate AS-500, Riko	2995	AF	*	
Jones Datamite III, Jones	3495	AV	*	
Spiro Analyzer ST-100, FIC	3500	AF	*	
SM-III, Spirometrics	3750	AV	*	§
Vitalograph-Compact, Vitalograph	3795	AF	*	
Eagle IIs, Collins	3950	AV	*	‡
UCI-500, Vacumetrics	3995	AV	†	§
SpiroScan 1000, Brentwood	4290	AF	*	‡
S400, Spirotech	4500	AV	*	§
PB 900, Puritan Bennett	4750	AF	*	‡
MultiSpiro-PC, MED	4990	AF	†	‡
Pulmo Screen II, S & M	4990	AV	†	§

*Automated by dedicated microcomputer.
†Personal computer (PC).
‡Meets the minimum recommended size of flow-volume (FV) or volume-time (VT) graph.
§Standard 8.5- × -11-in chart.
Price, 1986 retail price.
MV, manual volume; AF, automated flow; AV, automated volume.
(Modified from Enright P and Hyatt RE: Office Spirometry: A Practical Guide to the Selection and Use of Spirometers. Philadelphia, Lea & Febiger, 1987. Used with permission.)

pulmonary function studies as reproducibly as healthy adults (aged 16 to 35 years). The coefficients of variation were no different for FVC, FEV_1, PEF, or maximal expiratory flow at 50 per cent expired vital capacity ($\dot{V}max_{50\%}$). Thus reliable measurements of FVC, FEV_1, and the forced expiratory flow over the middle half of the vital capacity ($FEF_{25-75\%}$) may be made if these spirometers have reasonable frequency responses and linear flow and volume calibrations. Unfortunately, manufacturers' stated calibration specifications cannot always be relied on because equipment may have been damaged during transport or may malfunction for other reasons. Techniques of calibration should be explained in the equipment manual; if not, they are well described elsewhere (Enright and Hyatt, 1987).

Pulmonary function equipment for home use is limited to peak flow meters. Several new and inex-

Table 7–2. CRITERIA FOR ACCEPTABLE MAXIMAL EXPIRATORY VITAL CAPACITY MANEUVERS

Appropriate curve shape
Artifact-free results (no coughing, premature termination, or delayed onset)
Sustained expiration for at least 3 sec
At least three forced vital capacities within 10 per cent of the largest effort
Satisfactory performance as observed by the tester

Table 7–4. BETWEEN-SUBJECT COEFFICIENT OF VARIATION OF SIX TO EIGHT REPEATED TRIALS IN NORMAL SUBJECTS

Test	Coefficient of Variation (%)	
	≤16 Years of Age	>16 Years of Age
FVC	3.3	2.4
FEV_1	4.0	3.1
Peak flow	3.4	3.9
$\dot{V}max_{50\%}$	6.3	4.0

pensive peak flow meters (Table 7–5) have been introduced for home use in the last few years. These devices work for children and adults, and different-sized mouthpieces can be purchased.

TECHNIQUE

During a maximal vital capacity maneuver, expired volume-time (VT) curves are recorded as illustrated in Figure 7–1. A "good" expiratory curve starts with a steep slope that is nearly linear, then tails off markedly near end-expiration. A brief delay at the onset of full expiration is common. Time zero is determined by extrapolating the steep initial portion of the curve to the maximal inspiratory line (see Fig. 7–1). The FVC, the maximum volume of expired air, is read directly from the tracings at ambient temperature and pressure saturated with water vapor (ATPS). The volume of gas expired from the lungs at body temperature, saturated with water vapor (BTPS), may be 8 to 10 per cent greater than the volume measured in a spirometer at room temperature. To be correct, expired volume and airflow must be corrected to BTPS conditions; however, many physicians do not correct for BTPS conditions because their testing areas have controlled environments with little temperature variation.

Two measurements of average flow are easily obtained from the VT curve. First, the FEV_1 is the expired volume (BTPS) during the first second of a maximal expiratory effort (see Fig. 7–1). The FEV_1 is usually expressed as a percentage of FVC to correct for size differences between patients. Second, the forced expiratory flow over the middle half of the FVC should be determined, as illustrated in Figure 7–2, for a normal child (A) and for a patient with cystic fibrosis (B). A straight line, connecting points on the curve at 25 and 75 per cent of the FVC, is extended to intersect two vertical lines 1 sec apart. The $FEF_{25-75\%}$ is the expired volume (BTPS) determined from the slope of the line in liters (ATPS) per sec.

Flow-volume (FV) curves of instantaneous flow against lung volume are recorded also during a maximal vital capacity maneuver. The maximal expiratory vital capacity maneuver is followed by a maximal inspiratory maneuver to full inflation. Typical FV curves for a normal child and a patient with

mild obstructive airway disease are illustrated in Figure 7–3. Peak expiratory flow (PEF); maximal expiratory flow at 25, 50, and 75 per cent of expired vital capacity ($\dot{V}max_{25\%,\ 50\%,\ 75\%}$); and maximal inspiratory flow at 50 per cent vital capacity ($MIF_{50\%}$) are read directly from the recordings. An automatic timer with markers at 1 and 3 sec as indicated by the transient decreases in flow (Fig. 7–3A and B) permits calculations of the FEV_1/FVC ratio and the approximate duration of expiration.

Maximal expiratory flow is linearly related to expired volume in normal subjects (Fig. 7–3A) at all lung volumes more than 25 per cent below full inflation. Curvilinearity of this portion of the curve as illustrated in Figure 7–3B by the degree that expired flow deviates from a straight (dashed) line is associated with airway disease. The curvilinearity score—the ratio of the actual flow at 50 per cent expired vital capacity (VC) to the flow predicted from the straight line—is a measure of curvilinearity.

If patient effort and cooperation are maximal, the PEF and FVC of four to six FV curves should be reproducible within 5 per cent of their maximum. The PEF should be achieved rapidly with only 25 per cent or less of the VC expired from maximum inflation. Flow-volume curves obtained while the patient is coughing repeatedly during expiration should achieve the same flows (allowing for some flow transients) at lung volumes more than 25 per cent below the full inflation flows obtained during normal performance.

INTERPRETATION

The interpretation of the data is best if the patient's medical history, the degree of effort, and the lesion's anatomic location and severity are known. Some data require a maximal effort from the patient to produce; others do not. Figure 7–3A illustrates the parts of the maximal vital capacity maneuver that are dependent on or independent of effort. The effort-dependent tests, such as PEF or $\dot{V}max_{25\%}$, are expiratory tests that are measured at high lung volumes, the first 25 per cent of the expired vital capacity from full inflation, and inspiratory tests that are measured at all lung volumes. The effort-independent tests are those tests that are measured at low lung volumes, the lower 75 per cent of the expired vital capacity.

Table 7–5. COMPARISON OF PEAK FLOW METERS

	Mini-Wright(1)	Low Range Mini-Wright(2)	Assess(3)	Peak Flow Monitor
Age (years)	6+	4–8	7+	2½+
Reliability	excellent	excellent	excellent	excellent
Ease of reading	excellent	excellent	good	good
Ease of use	excellent	excellent	excellent	good
Approx. cost	$29.95	$35.95	$19.95	$12.95

(1) Clement Clarke, Inc., 3128 East 17 Avenue, Suites C and D, Columbus, Ohio 43219
(2) Healthscan Products, Inc., 908 Pompton Avenue, Cedar Grove, NJ 07009
(3) Biotrine Corporation, 52 Dragon Court, Woburn, MA 01801
(Modified from Plaut TF: Children with Asthma: A Manual for Parents. 2nd ed. Amherst, Mass, Pedipress, Inc, 1988. Used with permission.)

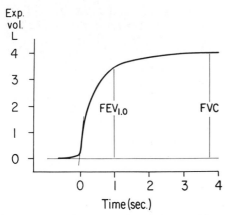

Figure 7–1. Volume-time curve for a 12-year-old normal boy. Zero time is determined by extrapolating the steepest part of the curve to the full inflation line. The forced expiratory volume in 1 sec ($FEV_{1.0}$) and the forced expiratory vital capacity (FVC) are read directly from the tracings at ambient temperature and pressure, saturated with water vapor (ATPS), and converted to body temperature and ambient pressure, saturated with water vapor (BTPS), conditions.

Effort-independent tests, such as the $\dot{V}max_{50\%}$, are not increased by more than moderate levels of effort; therefore, small differences in maximal effort among children have little influence on these results. Effort-independent tests are influenced more by the lung's static properties, dynamic compression of the airways, and resistance of the peripheral airways than by small differences in maximal effort.

Mild obstruction of the central airways (larynx, trachea, and main stem bronchi) reduces expiratory flows at high lung volumes and flows during inspiration. As the degree of obstruction increases, expiratory flow is reduced at progressively lower lung volumes. The relationship of reduced inspiratory flow to expiratory flow at midvital capacity ($\dot{V}max_{50\%}$/$MIF_{50\%}$) depends on the location of the lesion in the extrathoracic or intrathoracic central airways, as illustrated in Figure 7–4. Because these flows are at

least partly effort dependent, evidence that the patient performed with maximal effort is essential to the interpretation of these results. Increased resistance of peripheral airways is the most common cause of reduced expiratory flow at low lung volumes, as illustrated in Figure 7–3B.

There is still a difference of opinion concerning the report of results as the "best" or "average." The Snowbird report (American Thoracic Society, 1979) suggested that the "best" FVC and FEV_1 should be reported from any curve with the largest FVC or FEV_1. The single curve with the largest sum of the FVC and FEV_1 should be selected for measurement of $FEF_{25-75\%}$ and instantaneous flows (i.e., $\dot{V}max_{25\%}$, $_{50\%}$, and $_{75\%}$). The best seems valid for effort-dependent indices because it represents the patient's strongest effort. It can be argued, however, that the average is more typical of the patient's usual performance and may be more appropriate for indices that are effort independent. In addition, the interpretation of sequential studies in one individual requires an estimate of the within-individual variation of that index. In our laboratory, indices are reported from the best effort, and the average results are used to interpret sequential studies.

The discrimination of normal from abnormal pulmonary function results can be done in three ways: (1) by comparing a patient's results as percentage of (or standard deviation from) the mean predicted results for a normal population, (2) by considering the interrelationships of different pulmonary function indices, and (3) by considering their change with time.

The least discriminating method is to compare the results of each test with its predicted value for a normal population. The normal values used in our laboratory are summarized in Table 7–6. The large variability among individuals for each test is apparent from the large percentage of the mean predicted value that is equal to 1 standard deviation (SD). These

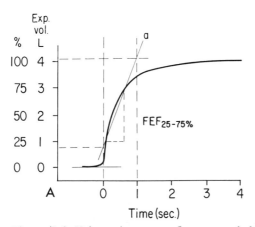

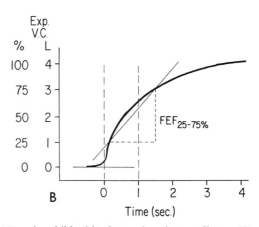

Figure 7–2. Volume-time curves for a normal child *(A)* and a child with obstructive airways disease *(B)*. The average slope is determined by connecting points on the curve at 25 and 50 per cent expired vital capacity *(line a)*. The forced expiratory flow over the middle half of the vital capacity ($FEF_{25-75\%}$) in liters per second (ATPS) is read directly from the tracing by extending line *a* to intercept two vertical lines *(dashed)* 1.0 sec apart.

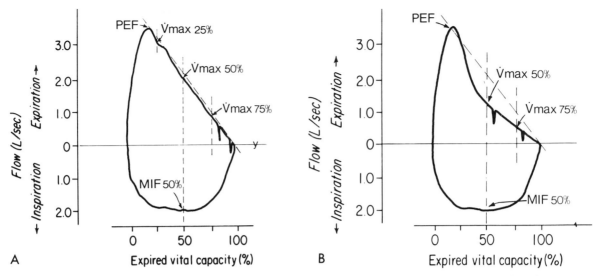

Figure 7–3. Flow-volume curves for a normal child *(A)* and a child with moderate obstructive airways disease *(B)*. See text for explanation.

differences can be eliminated by expressing the results as SD from the mean predicted values or as Z scores; however, discrimination between normal and abnormal results by this method is still limited because a patient's position in the normal population before the onset of illness is not known. For example, if a patient's normal FVC was +1.95 SD, the disease process would have to reduce the FVC by 42 per cent before it would be clearly below the normal limit of −1.95 SD for predicted values. However, if a child's normal FVC was −1.95 SD, a small decrease in FVC due to disease would result in clearly reduced values.

The FEV$_1$/FVC ratio may be reduced in obstructive disease but is usually normal or higher in restrictive disease. Reductions of PEF and $\dot{V}max_{25\%}$ are more sensitive indicators of obstruction of the central airways than is the FEV$_1$/FVC ratio because part of the FEV$_1$ occurs over low lung volumes, which reflect peripheral airway function. The PEF and $\dot{V}max_{25\%}$ usually are reduced in severe peripheral airway disease, but some patients may have normal values because of initially high-flow transients that occur before airway closure. In contrast, FEV$_1$ is influenced partially by severe central airway disease; therefore, the FEV$_1$/FVC may be normal early in the course of diseases that affect either the central or the peripheral airways. The FEF$_{25-75\%}$ measures the average flow over the middle half of the FVC and is less influenced by central airway disease than is the FEV$_1$/FVC ratio.

Following the changes in these indices that occur with time is more informative than single measurements because changes in pulmonary function (improved or worsening) are easier to detect than simply discriminating between normal and abnormal for the reasons indicated previously. The variation within individuals in these indices is considerably less than the variation among individuals, both in normal subjects and patients with stable pulmonary disease (Nickerson et al, 1980) (see Table 7–6). Children tend to "seek their own level" within the normal population, as illustrated in Figure 7–5 for one patient with mild but stable obstructive pulmonary disease. A significant change in pulmonary function has occurred when the subject's test results change (owing to the disease process or to therapy) more than the subject's normal variability. We calculate that required change (Δ) by using a modification of the equation to determine sample size, as shown in the following equation:

$$\Delta = \frac{(t_{0.05, n-1} + t_{0.10, n-1})\,S}{\sqrt{n}}\cdot\frac{S}{\bar{X}}\cdot 100$$

Figure 7–4. Maximal expiratory and inspiratory flow-volume curves *(A)* in fixed obstruction (e.g., postintubation tracheal stenosis) of the central airways (larynx, trachea, main stem bronchi). Variable obstruction of the extrathoracic *(B)* or intrathoracic *(C)* central airway produces flow patterns characteristic of dynamic changes in airway diameter during inspiration or expiration in these regions.

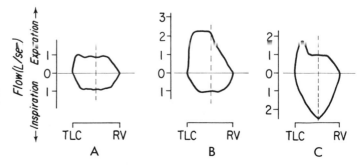

Table 7–6. SUMMARY OF NORMAL DATA FOR OUR LABORATORY

Index	Group	Predictive Equation	%X̄ for 1.0/SD
PEF* (L/min)	Female		
	MA	$9.28 \times 10^{-3} \times H^{2.12}$	15
	White	$1.63 \times 10^{-2} \times H^{2.00}$	14
	Black	$4.59 \times 10^{-3} \times H^{2.25}$	16
	Male		
	MA	$8.21 \times 10^{-3} \times H^{2.15}$	15
	White	$3.15 \times 10^{-3} \times H^{2.33}$	14
	Black	$2.26 \times 10^{-3} \times H^{2.39}$	19
FVC* (L)	Female		
	MA	$1.25 \times 10^{-3} \times H^{2.92}$	14
	White	$2.57 \times 10^{-3} \times H^{2.78}$	14
	Black	$8.34 \times 10^{-4} \times H^{2.98}$	15
	Male		
	MA	$1.06 \times 10^{-3} \times H^{2.97}$	13
	White	$3.58 \times 10^{-4} \times H^{3.18}$	13
	Black	$1.07 \times 10^{-3} \times H^{2.93}$	17
FEV* (L)	Female		
	MA	$1.61 \times 10^{-3} \times H^{2.85}$	14
	White	$3.79 \times 10^{-3} \times H^{2.68}$	14
	Black	$1.14 \times 10^{-3} \times H^{2.89}$	15
	Male		
	MA	$1.73 \times 10^{-3} \times H^{2.85}$	13
	White	$7.74 \times 10^{-4} \times H^{3.00}$	13
	Black	$1.03 \times 10^{-3} \times H^{2.92}$	17
FEF$_{25-75\%}$* (L/min)	Female		
	MA	$1.20 \times 10^{-3} \times H^{2.40}$	24
	White	$3.79 \times 10^{-3} \times H^{2.16}$	28
	Black	$1.45 \times 10^{-3} \times H^{2.34}$	30
	Male		
	MA	$9.13 \times 10^{-4} \times H^{2.45}$	25
	White	$7.98 \times 10^{-4} \times H^{2.46}$	26
	Black	$3.61 \times 10^{-4} \times H^{2.60}$	36
Flow-volume curve†			
V̇max$_{50\%}$ VC − (L/sec)	Male	$(0.113 \times in) - 3.653$	13
	Female	$(0.109 \times in) - 3.336$	15
V̇max$_{25\%}$ VC − (L/sec)	Male	$(0.040 \times in) - 1.167$	13
	Female	$(0.057 \times in) - 1.960$	16

*Normal data with height in cm from Hsu et al 1979.
†Normal data with height in in from Taussig (unpublished data).
MA, Mexican American.

where n is the number of trials per subject (usually three or four). The alpha and beta percentage points are 0.05 and 0.10, respectively, of the sample distribution (Z) and are replaced by the t value, with 3 to 4 degrees of freedom, because we estimate the population SD (S). The upper or lower limits for each test in each subject (significant improvement or worsening) are calculated as $\bar{x} \pm (\Delta/100)(\bar{x})$.

An example of calculations of required change for significance by our method follows: Subject A has 6 FVC measurements of 1.35, 1.55, 1.60, 1.40, 1.52, and 1.60 liters. The mean value is 1.50 liters, and the SD is 0.11. The t values with alpha 0.05 and beta 0.10 and 5 degrees of freedom are found in standard statistical tables to be 2.571 and 2.015, respectively. The calculated change is 14 per cent; thus, if the lower limit is less than 1.2881, or greater than 1.71 liters, you can be confident that a significant change has occurred, and you will be correct 95 per cent of

the time. If a new value is larger than 1.29 liters and less than 1.71 liters, you can be confident that no change has occurred, and you will be correct 90 per cent of the time.

We believe that this method is rapid, simple, and improves the accuracy of pulmonary function interpretations. It also normalizes differences among laboratories and subjects. These calculations can be done in less than 5 min using a "t" table and a pocket calculator with mean, SD, and square root functions. A summary of the per cent change required for significance in a group of normal subjects and a group of cystic fibrosis patients is shown in Table 7–7.

This method can also be used to determine positive responses to inhaled bronchodilators. Figure 7–6 illustrates the VT curves of a 7-year-old boy with asthma before and after inhalation of nebulized isoproterenol. His FVC and FEV₁ increased by 3 per cent and 43 per cent, respectively, to normal values

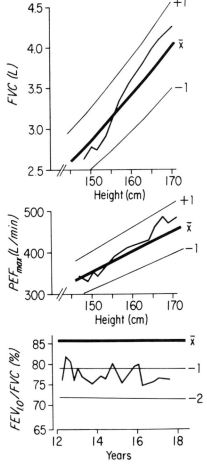

Figure 7–5. Sequential changes in forced vital capacity (FVC), peak expiratory flow (PEF), and the ratio of the forced expiratory volume in 1 sec to the forced vital capacity (FEV$_{1.0}$/FVC) in a boy with mild but stable obstructive airways disease associated with cystic fibrosis. The variability of repeated measurement was less than the variability among individuals for the normal population (mean ± 2 SD). Changes in these variables of more than 1.0 SD for the population suggest a significant change in pulmonary function.

Table 7–7. PER CENT CHANGE WITHIN SUBJECTS REQUIRED FOR SIGNIFICANCE

Test	Normal Subjects ($\Delta\%$)		Patients with Cystic Fibrosis ($\Delta\%$)	
	Mean	Max	Mean	Max
FVC	5	>8	15	>23
FEV_1	8	>15	13	>23
FEV_1/FVC	4	>10	9	>18
PEF	8	>15	15	>40
$FEF_{25-75\%}$	8	>13	16	>28
$\dot{V}max_{25\%}$	8	>14	15	>31
$\dot{V}max_{50\%}$	9	>19	16	>44
$\dot{V}max_{75\%}$	12	>20	26	>45

Mean, average per cent change for the group studied; *Max*, subject's results with the largest per cent change needed for significance for each test.

after isoproterenol inhalation. Both changes were larger than the per cent change for significance for that individual; however, compared with a normal group (see Table 7–7), the change in FVC was not different. This example demonstrates the power of estimates of each person's per cent change for significance instead of comparisons with group data. Because repeated testing in some patients yields "reproducible" results (almost no variation), a significant change in pulmonary function in such a patient is much smaller than in a patient in whom repeated testing yields highly variable normal results.

A different response to isoproterenol inhalation is illustrated by the FV curves in Figure 7–7. In this 9-year-old boy, isoproterenol inhalation increased FVC and PEF significantly by 3.8 and 4.4 SD, respectively. However, FEV_1 increased less than FVC did; thus the FEV_1/FVC ratio was reduced after bronchodilation. The FVC and PEF were within normal predicted values (± 2 SD) after bronchodilation, but flow at low lung volumes remained reduced, as indicated by its curvilinearity and a curvilinearity score of 0.34. These results suggest that smooth muscle constriction of the peripheral airways was only partially relieved or that some other factor (e.g., airway mucus and

edema) may have been responsible for the reduced flows. The use of home peak-flow meters to evaluate diurnal and day-to-day variations in lung function has greatly assisted asthma management. Most patients agree to record peak flow several times each day. Peak flow also is useful in determining responses to inhaled adrenergic agents or spontaneous worsening of the disease. The technique for home peak-flow meters is the same as that for the maximal expired vital capacity maneuver, except that it is less important to have a full deflation (which children younger than 6 years old infrequently master anyway).

Within a short time children will know their "personal best" peak flow. Comparisons with normal reference data (see Table 7–6) are useful; however, longitudinal peak-flow measurements, as illustrated in Figure 7–5, are more useful. As long as peak-flow values remain within 15 per cent of the personal best (see Table 7–7), the changes are within normal variation. If peak flow decreases more than 15 per cent, a significant change has occurred and therapeutic intervention or a visit to the physician or emergency room may be indicated.

In summary, pulmonary function testing in the office, clinic, and home is inexpensive, accurate, and easy to perform. These tests provide important objective data that can be valuable in evaluating patients with a variety of pulmonary diseases. Longitudinal pulmonary function tests are much better for detecting significant worsening or improvement of lung function than single studies that are compared with population reference standards. Pediatricians are accustomed to monitoring their patients' height, weight, blood pressure, and temperature with each visit. Longitudinal measurements for pulmonary function can be incorporated easily into the routine check-in procedures and provide valuable additional information about normal lung growth and the early detection of disease.

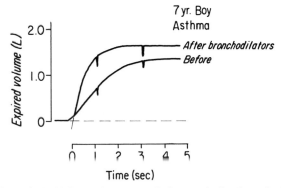

Figure 7–6. Volume-time curves before and after bronchodilator inhalation. The FVC and $FEV_{1.0}$/FVC are normal after use of the bronchodilator, suggesting that airway smooth muscle constriction was responsible for the reduced $FEV_{1.0}$ and FVC before bronchodilators.

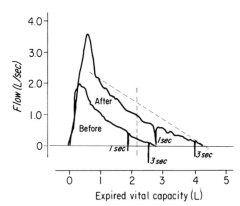

Figure 7–7. Flow-volume curves in an asthmatic 14-year-old boy. Inhalation of bronchodilators (*after*) resulted in an increase in PEF_{max} and flows at low volumes, as illustrated by $FEF_{50\%}$ (*vertical dashed line*). Reduced flows after inhalation of bronchodilators are indicated by the curvilinearity of flows at low lung volume compared with their predicted flows (*diagonal dashed line*).

REFERENCES

American Thoracic Society: ATS Statement—Snowbird workshop on standardization of spirometry. Am Rev Respir Dis 119:831, 1979.

Committee Recommendations: The assessment of ventilatory capacity. Statement of the Committees on Environmental Health and Respiratory Physiology. American College of Chest Physicians. Chest 67:95, 1975.

Cotes JE: Lung Function: Assessment and Application in Medicine. 3rd ed. Oxford, Blackwell Scientific Publications, 1975.

Drew CDM and Hughes DTD: Characteristics of the Vitalograph spirometer. Thorax 24:703, 1969.

Enright P and Hyatt RE: Office Spirometry: A Practical Guide to the Selection and Use of Spirometers. Philadelphia, Lea & Febiger, 1987.

Fitzgerald MX, Smith AA, and Gaensler EA: Evaluation of "electronic" spirometers. N Engl J Med 289:1283, 1973.

Hsu KHK, Jenkins DE, Hsi BP et al: Ventilatory functions of normal children and young adults—Mexican-American, white and black. I. Spirometry. J Pediatr 95:14, 1979; II. Wright peak flowmeter. J Pediatr 95:192, 1979.

Hyatt RE and Black LF: The flow-volume curve. A current perspective. Am Rev Respir Dis 107:191, 1973.

Kory RC and Hamilton LH: Evaluation of spirometers used in pulmonary function studies. Am Rev Respir Dis 87:228, 1963.

Kryger M, Bode F, Antic R, and Anthonisen N: Diagnosis of obstruction of the upper and central airways. Am J Med 61:85, 1976.

Landau LI, Taussig LM, Macklem PT, and Beaudry PH: Contribution of inhomogeneity of lung-units to the maximal expiratory flow-volume curve in children with asthma and cystic fibrosis. Am Rev Respir Dis 111:725, 1975.

Lemen R: Office pulmonary function testing in children. Audio-Digest, Vol 21, December 23, 1975.

Lemen R, Gerdes C, Wegmann M, and Perrin K: Frequency content of maximal expiratory vital capacity curves. J Appl Physiol 53(4):1005, 1982.

Levison H and Godfrey S: Cystic fibrosis. In Mangos J and Talamo R (eds): Projections into the Future. New York, Stratton Intercontinental Medical Book Corp, 1976.

Macklem PT: Airway obstruction and collateral ventilation. Physiol Rev 51:368, 1971.

Mead J: Mechanical properties of lungs. Physiol Rev 41:281, 1961.

Mead J, Turner JM, Macklem PT, and Little JB: Significance of the relationship between lung recoil and maximum expiratory flow. J Appl Physiol 22:95, 1967.

Miller RD and Hyatt RE: Evaluation of obstructing lesions of the trachea and larynx by flow-volume loops. Am Rev Respir Dis 108:475, 1973.

Nickerson B, Lemen R, Gerdes C et al: Within-subject variability and percent change for significance of spirometry in normal subjects and in patients with cystic fibrosis. Am Rev Respir Dis 122:859, 1980.

Polgar G and Promadhat V: Pulmonary Function Testing in Children: Techniques and Standards. Philadelphia, WB Saunders Co, 1971.

Taussig LM, Chernick V, Wood R et al: Standardization of lung function testing in children. J Pediatr 97:668, 1980.

Wang CS, Boyington DG, and Krumholz RA: Comparison of spirometry measurements using McKesson vitalor and Collins spirometer. Dis Chest 55:258, 1969.

Zapletal A, Motoyama EK, Van De Woestijne KP et al: Maximal expiratory flow volume curves and airway conductance in children and adolescents. J Appl Physiol 26:308, 1969.

8

DAN MICHAEL COOPER, M.D.

PULMONARY FUNCTION ASSESSMENT IN THE LABORATORY DURING EXERCISE

For both healthy children and those with chronic diseases, the ability to engage in play, exercise, and other physical activities is an essential component of daily life. For the pediatrician, precise assessment of the cardiorespiratory and metabolic responses to exercise is an invaluable tool in diagnosing disease, assessing its impact, and making recommendations of specific programs of physical activity (Table 8–1). As has been noted in previous chapters, analysis of static pulmonary function can yield important information about the capability of the respiratory system in children. But testing the mechanical properties of the lung at rest does not reveal the consequences of disease on metabolic function when the organism is stressed. To accomplish this, *respiration* in its fullest sense must be assessed. By measuring gas exchange at the mouth (oxygen uptake—$\dot{V}O_2$, carbon dioxide output—$\dot{V}CO_2$, and ventilation—$\dot{V}_E$) and heart rate responses to exercise-induced increases in metabolism, the relationship between respiration at the cells and respiration of the whole organism can be evaluated. This chapter reviews the cardiorespiratory response to exercise in healthy children and the ways in which specific diseases affect these responses. In addition, techniques for noninvasive measurements of gas exchange in children and promising methodologies that are still in the research and development stage are highlighted.

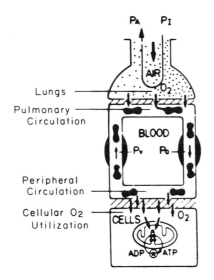

Figure 8–1. Model of the respiratory system indicating the pathway of O_2 flow from the environment to the mitochondria. Assessing respiration at the mouth during exercise is a means of measuring the integrated physiologic response to increases in metabolic rates occurring at the cells. (Reproduced with permission from Taylor CR and Weibel ER: Respir Physiol 44:1, 1981.)

* Pulmonary blood flow response

* Circulatory system parameters (resistance, heart muscle function)

* "Signal" response time (neural? humoral?)

* Inherent muscle cell response characteristics (O_2 stores, O_2 tension gradients)

THE CARDIORESPIRATORY RESPONSE TO EXERCISE

Consider the important acts of fleeing from a predator or, in more modern terms, running to avoid an oncoming car. When sudden and large increases in metabolic demand are imposed by physical activity, the whole organism can function successfully only by means of an *integrated* response among several organ systems. At the very onset of exercise, before there has been sufficient time for an increase in environmental oxygen uptake, the healthy human must have sufficient stores of oxygen and high-energy phosphates, nonaerobic metabolic capability, and supplies of substrate to perform significant amounts of physical activity. As exercise proceeds, cardiac output increases and blood flow is diverted to the working muscles without compromising the critical flow of oxygen and glucose to the brain. Ventilation and pulmonary blood flow must increase to match pre-

cisely the energy demand of the working muscles so that homeostasis for Pa_{CO_2} and pH are maintained. There must be a sufficient increase in substrate availability (glucose, fat, protein) without depleting the peripheral blood glucose stores. In addition, the heat produced during exercise must be dissipated so that homeostasis for body temperature is maintained. In summary, events at the cell are *closely linked* to events at the heart and lungs; Taylor and Weibel (1981) diagrammed this relationship schematically, as shown in Figure 8–1.

The current understanding of muscle energetics rests on the concept that the concentration of adenosine triphosphate (ATP) is held constant in the muscle cell (McMahon, 1984). Chemical bond energy is converted to mechanical energy through the reaction

$$ATP \rightarrow ADP + P_i + energy$$

where ADP is adenosine diphosphate and P_i is inorganic phosphate. Then ADP is rephosphorylated by the reaction

$$ADP + PCr \leftrightarrows ATP$$

where PCr is phosphocreatinine. Concentrations of ATP are constant throughout most of exercise except at the heaviest work rates, but the changes in PCr and P_i can now be examined in vivo and in vitro with the technique of magnetic resonance spectrometry. An example of the changes in the intracellular levels of PCr and P_i during exercise is shown in Figure 8–2 (Idstrom et al, 1985). Oxygen is linked to the rephosphorylation of ATP in the mitochondria. Electrons derived from catabolism of carbohydrates, fatty acids, or amino acids in the cytosol are shuttled to the mitochondria and provide the energy for the ultimate production of ATP. Following the Krebs cycle, molecular oxygen combines with electrons and protons in the cyto-

Table 8–1. EXAMPLES OF CURRENT CLINICAL USES OF EXERCISE IN CHILDREN

Diagnostic

Elucidation of bronchial reactivity (Godfrey et al, 1975).

Growth hormone deficiency (Shanis and Moshang, 1976).

Preparticipation sports physical in children (Driscoll, 1985).

Establishing reduced physical activity as an etiology for obesity (Reybrouck et al, 1987).

Evaluating fitness and the efficacy of therapy in patients with a variety of congenital heart diseases (Bar-Or, 1983, pp 126–167).

Determination of optimal hematocrit in patients with congenital anemia (Cooper, Hyman, Weiler-Ravell et al, 1985).

Quantifying the functional disability caused by chronic diseases of childhood and developing an "exercise prescription."

Therapeutic

Training respiratory muscles in patients with chronic lung disease (Orenstein, 1988).

Stabilization of glycemia in insulin-dependent diabetes (Stratton et al, 1987).

An adjunct to diet in the treatment of childhood obesity (Epstein et al, 1985).

Nonpharmacologic treatment of juvenile hypertension (Hagberg et al, 1983).

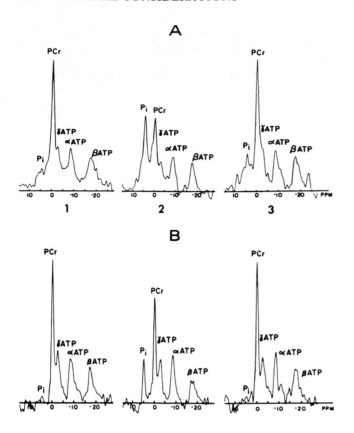

Figure 8–2. Nuclear magnetic resonance, phosphorus 31 spectra from a perfused *(A)* and an in vivo *(B)* rat hind limb obtained at rest *(1)*, during contractions *(2)*, and during recovery from contractions *(3)*; 60 scans accumulated in 1 min for each spectrum. Note that during contractions inorganic phosphate (P$_i$) increases and phosphocreatinine (PCr) decreases. (Reproduced with permission from Idstrom JP, Subramanian V, Chance B et al: Am J Physiol 248:H40, 1985.)

Figure 8–3. Cardiac output in relation to oxygen consumption in boys and girls estimated by the indirect (CO$_2$) Fick method. The equation for the line is $\dot{Q} = 6.3 \times \dot{V}O_2 + 3.3 \pm 0.9$ (SEY). $\dot{Q}$, cardiac output; $\dot{V}O_2$, oxygen uptake; *(SEY)*, standard error of estimate. (From Godfrey S: Exercise Testing in Children. Philadelphia, WB Saunders Co, 1974.)

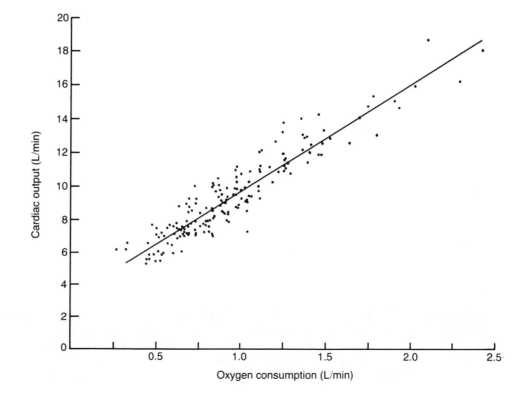

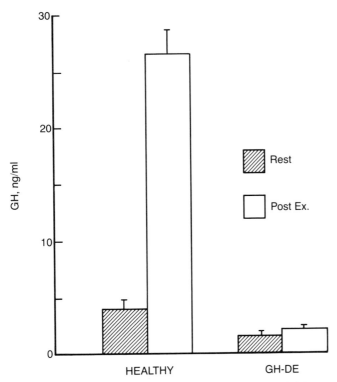

Figure 8–4. Exercise in diagnosis of growth hormone deficiency. Thirty-two healthy, short-statured 3- to 15-year-old children and five children with growth hormone deficiency (GH-DE) performed a 20-min exercise, 2 hr after receiving orally 24 to 40 mg of propanolol. Blood was sampled immediately after exercise. Vertical lines denote 1 standard error of the mean. (Data from Shanis BS and Moshang T: Pediatrics 57:712, 1976, as diagrammed by Bar-Or O: Pediatric Sports Medicine. New York, Springer Verlag, 1983.)

chrome chain, and water and CO_2 are released. The complete oxidation of one glucose molecule results in the production of 36 ATP molecules. When oxygen is not available to the mitochondrial cytochromes, sufficient ATP molecules can be regenerated to continue muscular activity, but this *anaerobic* process results in the production of lactic acid. For each molecule of glucose, only two ATP molecules are produced during anaerobic metabolism, an "expensive" way to produce new ATP. Aerobic processes are responsible for most of the ATP required during normal physical activity, but at the onset of exercise, or during high-intensity physical activity, the relative contribution of anaerobic metabolism increases.

Breathing increases during exercise. The stimulus for exercise hyperpnea is, to a large extent, the increased production of CO_2 at the cells (Phillipson et al, 1981; Whipp, 1983). Thus during progressive exercise, the relationship between $\dot{V}_E$ and $\dot{V}CO_2$ is significantly closer than is the relationship between $\dot{V}_E$ and $\dot{V}O_2$ (Wasserman et al, 1967). The concentration of CO_2 in the arterial blood (measured as the Pa_{CO_2}) is held constant throughout most of progressive exercise despite large increases in metabolically produced CO_2. The robust nature of Pa_{CO_2} homeostasis is reflected in healthy subjects at higher work intensities when additional CO_2 is liberated from the chemical combination of lactic acid (produced from

anaerobic metabolism) and the ubiquitous buffer bicarbonate. During this phase of isocapnic buffering (Wasserman et al, 1981), Pa_{CO_2} and pH remain constant as $\dot{V}_E$ increases in proportion to $\dot{V}CO_2$. Only at very high work intensities, when the pH begins to fall and the peripheral chemoreceptors are additionally stimulated, does hyperventilation occur and Pa_{CO_2} fall.

Increased alveolar ventilation alone can increase $\dot{V}CO_2$ but has little effect on $\dot{V}O_2$ in the healthy individual. Beyond a PO_2 of about 60 mm Hg, the "flat" portion of the oxyhemoglobin dissociation curve prevents significant amounts of molecular oxygen from being added to blood leaving the pulmonary vasculature even when the PO_2 increases. Thus the increase in $\dot{V}O_2$ known to occur with exercise is dependent on the increases in the pulmonary blood flow (cardiac output) and the return to the lungs of desaturated blood (i.e., a widening of the arteriovenous O_2 difference). During progressive exercise, cardiac output rises in a roughly linear manner with $\dot{V}O_2$ in both adults and children (Fig. 8–3). The increase in cardiac output is brought about both by changes in heart rate and stroke volume. It appears that stroke volume achieves its maximum early in progressive exercise, while heart rate continues to increase. At lower work intensities, the increase in heart rate results from an inhibition of parasympathetic tone (Ekblom et al, 1973), but at higher work rates, heart rate is probably stimulated by the increase in epinephrine.

The processes outlined summarize the general pattern of energy metabolism for virtually all mammalian species. For the pediatrician, the cardiorespiratory responses to exercise must be viewed within the context of growth and development. Thus in addition to determining the mechanisms responsible for a physiologic limitation caused by a particular disease, the child health care worker is concerned with the impact such a limitation may have on the process of growth in general. The biologic role of physical activity in the life of the child may actually differ from its role in the life of the adult. It is a generally held belief (with some corroboration in animal studies) that children are much more physically active than are adults. Exercise can stimulate or inhibit a number of growth-related mediators. Most intriguing to the pediatrician is the pronounced effect of exercise on human growth hormone release (Hunter et al, 1965), and exercise testing has been used in children to diagnose growth hormone deficiency (Shanis and Moshang, 1976) (Fig. 8–4). These observations suggest that physical activity may play a regulatory role in the actual process of normal growth, but the biologic role of physical activity in the life of children is, as yet, not known.

THE PHYSIOLOGIC RESPONSE TO EXERCISE IN CHILDREN

PROGRESSIVE EXERCISE TESTS

In Table 8–2 the gas exchange and heart rate variables of exercise testing in children are briefly

Table 8–2. CARDIORESPIRATORY AND METABOLIC INFORMATION AVAILABLE FROM EXERCISE TESTING

Term	Symbol	Definition
Maximal oxygen uptake	$\dot{V}O_{2max}$	A plateau or decrease in $\dot{V}O_2$ despite a continuing increase in work rate. Care must be taken to distinguish the peak $\dot{V}O_2$ (the largest $\dot{V}O_2$ achieved by the subject) from the true $\dot{V}O_{2max}$.
Anaerobic, lactate, or ventilatory threshold	AT, LT, VAT	The point during progressive exercise when lactate concentration begins to increase in the blood. The usual gas exchange manifestations of the AT are hyperventilation with respect to $\dot{V}O_2$ (increase in $\dot{V}_E/\dot{V}O_2$ and end-tidal PO_2), which occurs when $\dot{V}_E/\dot{V}CO_2$ and end-tidal PCO_2 are constant.
Work efficiency, O_2 cost of exercise	—	These variables are determined from the relationship of $\dot{V}O_2$ to the work rate.
Response time of gas exchange adaptations to exercise (mean response time, time constant)	RT, MRT, τ	The mathematically derived descriptor of the time required for $\dot{V}O_2$, $\dot{V}_E$, and $\dot{V}CO_2$ to achieve a steady state in response to a work rate input.
Ventilatory response to exercise	$\Delta\dot{V}_E/\Delta\dot{V}CO_2$	Slope of the linear portion of the relationship between $\dot{V}_E$ and $\dot{V}CO_2$ during progressive exercise. (n.b., the ventilatory equivalent of CO_2 is the ratio $\dot{V}_E/\dot{V}CO_2$ and is not the same as the slope.)
Respiratory compensation point	RCP	The point during AT exercise when hyperventilation for $\dot{V}CO_2$ occurs. Presumably, the RCP occurs when the bicarbonate is no longer able to adequately buffer the lactic acid produced during high-intensity exercise and pH changes. This stimulates the peripheral chemoreceptors.
Oxygen pulse	O_2-pulse	The ratio $\dot{V}O_2$/HR. This ratio represents the amount of oxygen extracted per heart beat, which is not the same as the slope of the $\dot{V}O_2$-heart rate relationship during progressive exercise.
$\dot{V}O_2$ to heart rate relationship	$\Delta\dot{V}O_2/\Delta HR$	This ratio represents the slope of the linear portion of the relationship between $\dot{V}O_2$ and HR during progressive exercise.
Exercise-induced bronchospasm	EIB	A fall of at least 15 per cent in the ratio FEV_1/FVC following a bout of exercise.

outlined. The gas exchange response to progressive, cycle ergometer exercise in a healthy 7-year-old boy tested in our laboratory is shown in Figure 8–5. Following a period of unloaded pedaling (0 watt), the work rate increases in a linear manner. This protocol is known as a *ramp* work rate input (Whipp et al, 1981) and is one of several types of progressive exercise tests that can be used in children (Bar-Or, 1983). Gas exchange is collected breath by breath and is displayed on-line. Note that the increase in $\dot{V}O_2$ does not immediately follow the onset of exercise. The response time of $\dot{V}O_2$ (RT) is determined by the cellular, circulatory, and respiratory adaptations to the increase in energy demand in the muscle tissue. Following this delay, $\dot{V}O_2$ typically rises in a linear manner with increasing work rate. However, the $\dot{V}O_2$ response may either "bend up" or "bend down" depending on the magnitude of change of the work rate input (Hansen et al, 1988). In the data shown in Figure 8–5, there was a plateau in $\dot{V}O_2$ at the end of exercise despite a continuing increase in the work rate. The appearance of a plateau classically defines the $\dot{V}O_{2max}$. It is important to distinguish the $\dot{V}O_{2max}$ (i.e., when a plateau or reduction in $\dot{V}O_2$ occurs despite an increasing work rate) from the peak $\dot{V}O_2$ (i.e., the highest $\dot{V}O_2$ achieved by a particular subject).

From cross-sectional population studies, the $\dot{V}O_{2max}$ changes in roughly direct proportion with body weight (Åstrand, 1952; Cooper et al, 1984a) (Figure 8–6, Table 8–3). This finding is at odds with the empirically observed "three-fourths power law"—demonstrated most commonly in Kleiber's "mouse-to-elephant" curve (Kleiber, 1975)—and with the so-called surface area law,* which states that in mammals metabolic rates (n.b., the $\dot{V}O_{2max}$ can be considered a metabolic rate) must scale to the two-thirds power of body mass (Gray, 1981). The finding of a *direct* relationship between $\dot{V}O_{2max}$ and body weight in children (i.e., a scaling factor of one) suggests that the mechanism that links structure and function during the growth process *within* a species is different from the processes that determine the relationship between metabolic rates and body size in mature animals of different species (Cooper, 1988).

The relationship between $\dot{V}O_2$ and work rate is known as the *oxygen cost* of performing a particular exercise. The *work efficiency* quantifies the proportion of the total energy turnover used specifically for mechanical work; it can also be calculated from the $\dot{V}O_2$ work rate relationship by converting the $\dot{V}O_2$ into units of energy (Whipp and Wasserman, 1969).

---

*The surface area law stemmed from the belief that for mammals, all metabolic rates were determined by the rate of heat loss and heat production. Because heat loss was determined largely by the ratio of surface area to body mass and because for spheres and cylinders (geometrically close to the shape of animals) the ratio of surface area to body mass scaled to the two-thirds power of body mass, it was concluded that metabolic rate must be proportional to body mass to the two-thirds power.

Table 8–3. PREDICTED MAXIMUM $\dot{V}O_2$ AND AT IN NORMAL CHILDREN FOR CYCLE ERGOMETRY

	Boys ≤ 13 (n = 37)	Boys > 13 (n = 21)	Girls ≤ 11 (n = 24)	Girls > 11 (n = 27)
$\dot{V}O_2$max, ml/min/kg (mean ± SD)	42 ± 6	50 ± 8*	38 ± 7	34 ± 4
AT, ml/min/kg (mean ± SD)	26 ± 5	27 ± 6	23 ± 4	19 ± 3†

*Higher than the other groups (p < .05).
†Lower than the other groups (p < .05).
(Data from Cooper DM, Weiler-Ravell D, Whipp BJ, and Wasserman K: J Appl Physiol 56:628, 1984a.)

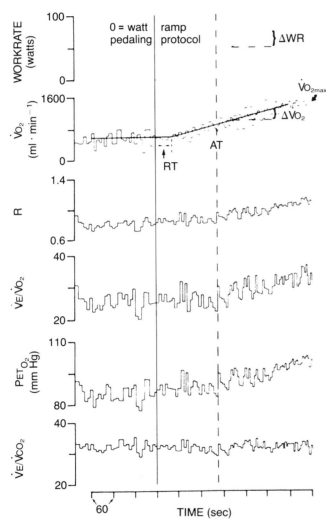

Figure 8–5. Breath-by-breath response of gas exchange to ramp exercise protocol in a 7-year-old boy. After a period of 0-watt pedaling, work rate increases *(ΔWR)* in a linear manner. Note the lag in the response time *(RT)* of O_2 uptake after WR has started (RT-$\dot{V}O_2$), the linear increase of $\dot{V}O_2$ as WR increases, and the plateau of $\dot{V}O_2$ during increasing WR ($\dot{V}O_{2max}$). Anaerobic threshold *(AT)* is determined by identifying $\dot{V}O_2$, where respiratory exchange ratio *(R)*, ventilatory equivalent for O_2 ($\dot{V}_E/\dot{V}O_2$), and end-tidal O_2 (PET_{O_2}) abruptly increase while ventilatory equivalent for CO_2 ($\dot{V}E/\dot{V}CO_2$) and end-tidal CO_2 (PET_{CO_2}) (not shown) remain unchanged or decrease. Work efficiency is determined from ratio of ΔWR to $\Delta\dot{V}O_2$. (From Cooper DM, Weiler-Ravell D, Whipp BJ, and Wasserman K: J Appl Physiol 56:628, 1984a.)

This conversion can be done by assuming a particular value for the metabolic respiratory exchange ratio (the ratio $\dot{V}CO_2/\dot{V}O_2$ resulting from the oxidation of a particular substrate) and by assuming that energy metabolism is fully aerobic. The work efficiency and the O_2 cost can be calculated by finding the slope of the $\dot{V}O_2$–work rate relationship ($\Delta\dot{V}O_2/\Delta WR$). In healthy children the oxygen cost for exercise below the anaerobic threshold is the same as that in adults, 10 ml/min/watt, corresponding to a work efficiency of 29 per cent (Cooper et al, 1984a). The remaining energy is largely dissipated as heat.

Respiratory Exchange Ratio and Anaerobic Threshold

Although $\dot{V}CO_2$ increases with progressive exercise, its pattern is not identical to that of $\dot{V}O_2$. Note in Figure 8–5 that the respiratory exchange ratio measured at the mouth (R, the ratio of $\dot{V}CO_2$ to $\dot{V}O_2$) is constant at the beginning of exercise but begins to increase well before maximal exercise, indicating that $\dot{V}CO_2$ is increasing at a faster rate than $\dot{V}O_2$. The mechanism for the rise in R is the increased production of lactic acid, most likely consequent to anaerobic metabolism occurring at the muscle cells (Wasserman et al, 1973). The buffering of the hydrogen ions releases additional CO_2. Because ventilation is stimulated by the flow of CO_2 to the respiratory centers, $\dot{V}_E$ increases as well. Thus, as shown in Figure 8–5, the ratio of $\dot{V}_E$ to $\dot{V}O_2$ rises. The hyperventilation for $\dot{V}O_2$ results in an increase in the end-tidal PO_2 (PET_{O_2}). But because $\dot{V}_E$ and $\dot{V}CO_2$ increase proportionally, the ratio of these two variables remains constant. This constellation of findings—an increase in R, $\dot{V}_E/\dot{V}O_2$, and PET_{O_2} while $\dot{V}_E/\dot{V}CO_2$ and PET_{CO_2} remain constant—constitutes the noninvasive measurement of the anaerobic or lactate threshold (AT). The AT in adults occurs at a metabolic rate (expressed as the $\dot{V}O_2$) equivalent to 40 to 60 per cent of the subject's maximal $\dot{V}O_2$, but this ratio is higher in children (Figs. 8–7 and 8–8) (Cooper et al, 1984a, Reybrouck et al, 1985). Because the ratio of the AT to the $\dot{V}O_{2max}$ can be increased as a consequence of training programs (Davis et al, 1979), one possible explanation is that children are generally "fitter" than adults. This explanation, however, has not yet been substantiated.

A number of theories have been proposed to explain the phenomenon of increasing blood lactate concentrations during progressive exercise (Katz and Sahlin, 1988; Walsh and Banister, 1988). The most

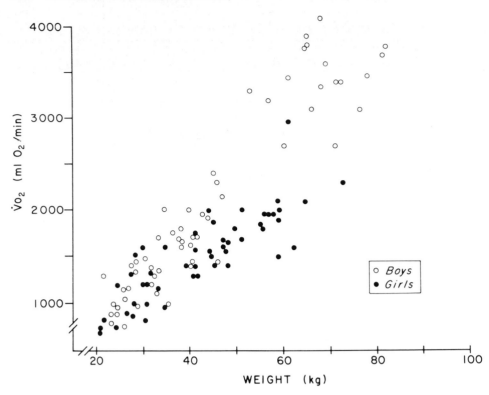

Figure 8–6. Maximum O_2 uptake ($\dot{V}O_{2max}$) as a function of weight in 109 normal children. $\dot{V}O_{2max}$ increases systematically with increasing body weight. Linear regression equations for $\dot{V}O_{2max}$ (ml/min) as a function of body weight (kg) were for boys, $Y = 52.8 \cdot X - 303.4$, $r = .94$; for girls, $Y = 28.5 \cdot X + 288.2$, $r = 0.84$; and for the group as a whole, $Y = 45.6 \cdot X - 197.9$, $r = 0.86$. The difference in the slope between boys and girls was significant. (From Cooper DM, Weiler-Ravell D, Whipp BJ, and Wasserman K: J Appl Physiol 56:628, 1984a.)

prominent theories are (1) an oxygen lack at the muscle tissue level that results in anaerobic metabolism and an increase in lactate production relative to uptake; (2) a reduction in lactate uptake *independent* of oxygen availability; and (3) an increase in lactate production due to a systematic switching of muscle fiber types to the predominately fast-twitch, glycolytic type.

Studies of the AT have been made in large numbers of children using both treadmill and cycle ergometer exercise (see Fig. 8–7) (Cooper et al, 1984a;

Reybrouck et al, 1985; Washington et al, 1988). As noted, the AT in children represents a larger proportion of the $\dot{V}O_{2max}$ than the AT in adults. There is evidence that the AT in both children and adults is related to oxygen availability. As shown in Figure 8–9, blood transfusions in children with β-thalassemia major resulted in increases of the AT. And both children and adults have reduced ATs under conditions of low FI_{O_2} breathing (Springer et al, 1989; Cooper et al, 1986).

The speed with which the work rate increases

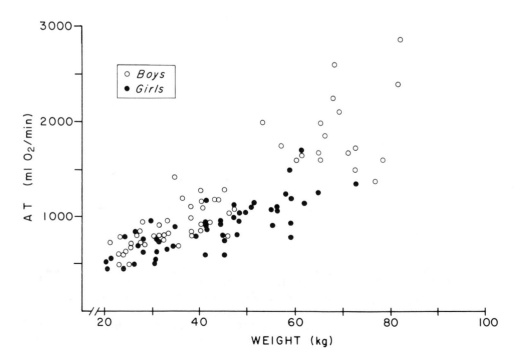

Figure 8–7. Anaerobic threshold *(AT)* as a function of weight in 109 normal children. Anaerobic threshold increased systematically with increasing weight. Linear regression equations for AT (ml/min) as a function of body weight (kg) were for boys, $Y = 27.3 \cdot X - 23.2$, $r = 0.78$; for girls, $Y = 16.1 \cdot X + 195$, $r = 0.82$; and for the group as a whole, $Y = 23.9 \cdot X - 4.3$, $r = 0.79$. The difference in the slope between boys and girls was significant. (From Cooper DM, Weiler-Ravell D, Whipp BJ, and Wasserman K: J Appl Physiol 56:628, 1984a.)

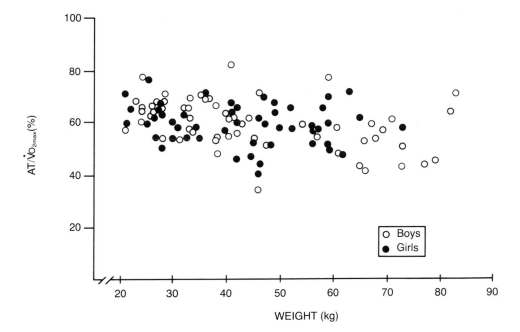

Figure 8–8. Ratio of anaerobic threshold to maximal O_2 uptake (AT/$\dot{V}O_{2max}$) (%) as a function of weight in 109 normal children. The ratio decreased slightly, but significantly, with increasing body size. Regression equation Y = −0.16 • X + 67. (From Cooper DM, Weiler-Ravell D, Whipp BJ, and Wasserman K: J Appl Physiol 56:628, 1984a.)

during progressive exercise testing can influence the gas exchange response. In choosing the appropriate increment time and magnitude (or slope in the case of a ramp-type input), several factors must be consid-

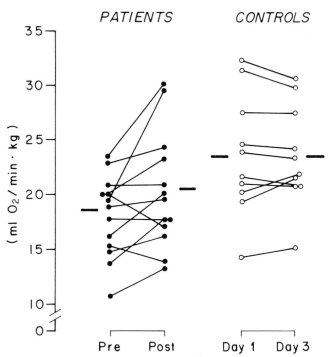

Figure 8–9. Anaerobic threshold in patients with anemia (thalassemia major or Blackfan-Diamond anemia) *(closed circles)* before and after transfusion, and in normal controls *(open circles)* on days 1 and 3. The results have been normalized to body weight. The horizontal bars represent the mean values. Anaerobic threshold increased in patients by a small but significant amount following transfusion. No difference was observed in the controls between days 1 and 3. In addition, AT in the patients was below normal in the majority of patients both before and after transfusion. (From Cooper DM, Hyman CB, Weiler-Ravell D et al: Pediatr Res 19:1215, 1985.)

ered, the first being the response time and delays that are known to occur in the gas exchange response. Because these times are different for $\dot{V}O_2$ and $\dot{V}CO_2$, care must be taken to ensure that the observed changes in variables, such as R (the ratio $\dot{V}CO_2/\dot{V}O_2$), do not result from these dynamic delays. If, for example, the slope is too steep for the capabilities of the subject being tested, then an increase in R may be observed that is not related to the production of lactic acid but that results from differences in the dynamics of the gas exchange responses. In general, a duration of about 10 to 15 min for a progressive exercise test in healthy children and adults is optimal. For children 6 to 8 years old, a ramp slope of 5 watts/min is used. For older children, 10 to 30 watt/min ramp slopes are used. The selection of the magnitude of the work rate input often involves an educated guess on the part of the investigator and requires some experience in assessing the capability of a particular child.

Coupling of Ventilation and CO_2 Production

Progressive exercise provides a relatively simple way to gauge the coupling of ventilation with $\dot{V}CO_2$ (Fig. 8–10). The alveolar gas equation suggests that the relationship is determined by the CO_2 set-point (i.e., the level at which Pa_{CO_2} is regulated) and the ratio of dead space to tidal volume (V_D/V_T):

$$\dot{V} = [863 \times Pa_{CO_2}^{-1} \times (1 - V_D/V_T)^{-1}] \times \dot{V}CO_2$$

As shown in Figure 8–10, there is a linear relationship between $\dot{V}_E$ and $\dot{V}CO_2$ for most of the progressive test (Cooper, Kaplan, Baumgarten et al, 1987). Factors such as elevated Pa_{CO2} will tend to lower the magnitude of the slope, whereas a high V_D/V_T will render the slope steeper. The rate of increase in $\dot{V}_E$

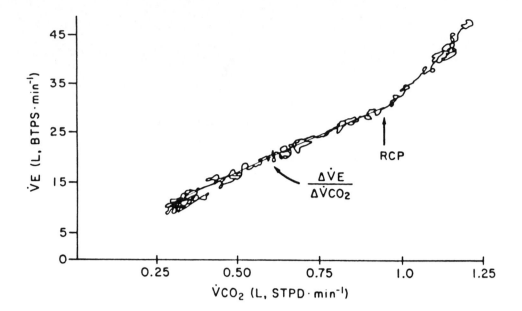

Figure 8–10. Breath-by-breath measurement of $\dot{V}_E$ as a function of $\dot{V}{CO_2}$ in an 8-year-old child during a progressive exercise protocol (ramp test). *Solid line* indicates the best-fit line from 1 min after the onset of the ramp to the respiratory compensation point *(RCP)* as indicated. The slope of the line is given as $\Delta\dot{V}_E/\Delta\dot{V}{CO_2}$. (From Cooper DM, Kaplan MR, Baumgarten L et al: Pediatr Res 21:568, 1987.)

may exceed that of $\dot{V}{CO_2}$ at very high work rates (true hyperventilation then ensues and Pa_{CO_2} falls) when buffering of lactic acid is no longer sufficient to prevent a rise in blood pH. The point at which ventilation increases out of proportion to $\dot{V}{CO_2}$ is known as the *respiratory compensation point*. We have found it helpful to quantify the relationship between $\dot{V}_E$ and $\dot{V}{CO_2}$ by calculating the slope of the best fit line through the linear portion of the relationship (see Fig. 8–10). Normal values have now been estab-

lished for this parameter and are shown in Figure 8–11. The slope of the relationship ($\Delta\dot{V}_E/\Delta\dot{V}{CO_2}$) decreases with increasing size among children and teen-agers. Younger children need to breathe more than adults for a given increase in metabolic rate (i.e., $\Delta\dot{V}{CO_2}$). Whether this difference results from lower CO_2 stores in children (associated with apparently lower Pa_{CO_2}) has not yet been determined.

In dealing with children, it is obviously advantageous to avoid invasive procedures, such as arterial

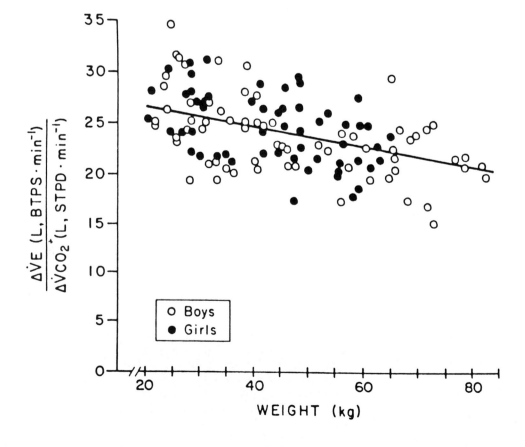

Figure 8–11. Slope of the $\dot{V}_E - \dot{V}{CO_2}$ relationship as a function of body weight in 128 normal boys *(open circles)* and girls *(closed circles)*, ranging in age from 6 to 18 years. There was a small but significant negative correlation between the slope and body weight. (From Cooper DM, Kaplan MR, Baumgarten L et al: Pediatr Res 21:568, 1987.)

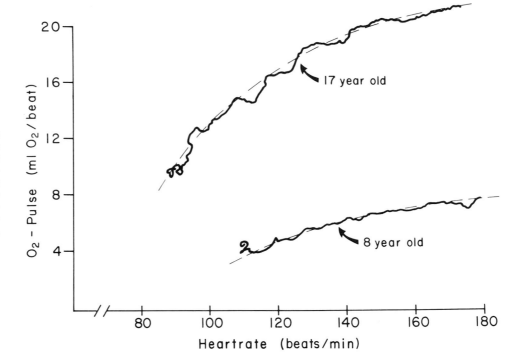

Figure 8–12. The O_2-pulse ($\dot{V}O_2$/HR) as a function of heart rate during progressive exercise in an 8-year-old and a 17-year-old subject. The O_2-pulse curve considered in this way is hyperbolic. (From Cooper DM, Weiler-Ravell D, Whipp BJ, and Wasserman K: Pediatr Res 18:845, 1984b.)

catheterization during exercise testing. But important indices of respiratory function, such as V_D/V_T (see the aforementioned alveolar gas equation), depend on measurement of arterial blood gases. Attempts have been made to estimate the arterial P_{CO_2} using the end-tidal CO_2 concentration. This approach has been taken with children most frequently by using the empirically derived equation of Jones and colleagues (1979). Cumming (1981) has proposed that the mean alveolar P_{CO_2} can be calculated from the relationship between the expired CO_2 volume and the total exhaled volume; Whipp and co-workers (in press) developed a computer-based methodology to estimate mean alveolar P_{CO_2} on a breath-by-breath basis during exercise. Preliminary studies suggest that this last method is the most accurate means of estimating the variations of Pa_{CO_2} in a given individual. The accuracy of the end-tidal estimations is known to be far worse in patients with lung disease, and validation of these techniques has not yet been done in children.

Relationship between Oxygen Consumption and Heart Rate

Much information can be gained from calculating the relationship between $\dot{V}O_2$ and heart rate (HR). The Fick equation holds that

$$\dot{V}O_2 = SV \cdot HR \cdot (a - \bar{v}) O_2$$

where SV is the stroke volume and $(a - \bar{v})O_2$ is the arteriovenous oxygen difference. The relationship between $\dot{V}O_2$ and HR can therefore yield indirect information on the changes occurring in stroke volume and the widening of the arteriovenous difference. During progressive exercise, the $\dot{V}O_2$ to HR relationship can be viewed in two ways. First, the O_2-pulse (Fig. 8–12) represents the instantaneous ratio $\dot{V}O_2$/HR and when plotted against time is typically hyperbolic in shape (Cooper et al, 1984b). But because of its curvilinear nature, the O_2-pulse response is difficult to quantify. Another approach is to consider the slope of the linear portion of the $\dot{V}O_2$-HR relationship (Cooper et al, 1984b) as shown in Figure 8–13. The slope of this response changes systematically with age, as demonstrated in Figure 8–13. In adult patients with congestive heart disease, a given increase in $\dot{V}O_2$ is accompanied by a more rapid heart rate response, most likely indicating a reduction in stroke volume (Wasserman et al, 1987).

CONSTANT WORK RATE TESTS

The vast majority of investigations focused on exercise in children utilize the *maximal oxygen uptake* as the primary parameter of the overall exercise response.* Although the notion of a true physiologic boundary is an attractive one, the clinical usefulness of the $\dot{V}O_{2max}$ is hampered by a number of factors.

---

*Another "maximal response" occasionally used in children is the maximal voluntary ventilation (MVV), which represents the most ventilation that a subject can perform while in the resting state. The maximal V_E during exercise is about 65 to 75 per cent of the MVV. Some investigators have suggested that this difference indicates a "ventilatory reserve." However, the lung during maximal exercise has an increased blood volume, and the mechanics of breathing during these rest and high-intensity exercise periods may not be completely comparable.

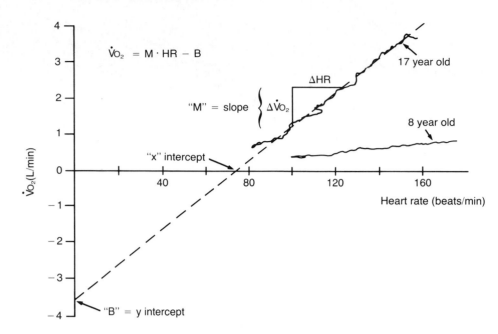

Figure 8–13. The relationship between $\dot{V}O_2$ and heart rate (HR) during progressive exercise in an 8-year-old and a 17-year-old subject. Linear regression techniques were used to evaluate the linear portion of the $\dot{V}O_2$-HR relationship. The subjects were compared by calculating (1) the slope of the line M ($\Delta\dot{V}O_2/\Delta HR$); (2) the y intercept $B;$ and (3) the x intercept, as illustrated. (From Cooper DM, Weiler-Ravell D, Whipp BJ, and Wasserman K: Pediatr Res 18:845, 1984b.)

First, the achievement of a plateau requires a great deal of effort on the part of the subject and vigorous verbal encouragement on the part of the investigator. Despite such efforts, only a minority of healthy, well-motivated children achieve true plateaus (28 per cent in studies done in my laboratory [Cooper et al, 1984a]). Second, the metabolic consequences of high-intensity exercise include increasing metabolic acidosis and elevated levels of catecholamines. Besides producing the sensation of discomfort and dyspnea, one must wonder whether the metabolic state of high-intensity exercise is truly advisable for children with abnormalities of the cardiac or respiratory systems.

In certain situations, constant work rate exercise tests can be at least as useful as progressive tests. In particular, when designing programs of exercise as a rehabilitative tool in children, the investigator needs to find those levels of exercise that can be sustained by the child for a reasonable period of time. From a protocol in which the child exercises at two different work rates for a period of 6 to 8 min each (e.g., 20 watts and 40 watts), the investigator can determine the oxygen cost, the $\Delta\dot{V}_E/\Delta\dot{V}CO_2$, and the $\Delta\dot{V}O_2/\Delta HR$. For example, to determine the $\Delta\dot{V}_E/\Delta\dot{V}CO_2$ from two 6-min constant work rate tests, one would use the *steady-state* values for each variable obtained over the last 3 min of sampling. The last 3 min are counted

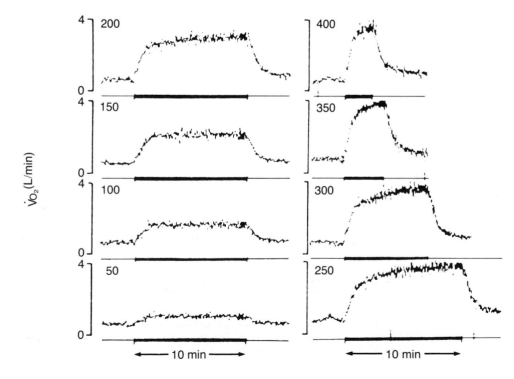

Figure 8–14. Oxygen uptake related to time for eight levels of constant work rate cycle ergometer exercise, starting from unloaded cycling. The work rate (watts) for each study is shown in the respective panel. The bar on the x-axis indicates the period of the imposed work rate. The $\dot{V}O_2$ asymptote (steady state) is significantly delayed for work above the anaerobic threshold. (From Whipp BJ and Mahler M: Pulmonary Gas Exchange. New York, Academic Press, 1980.)

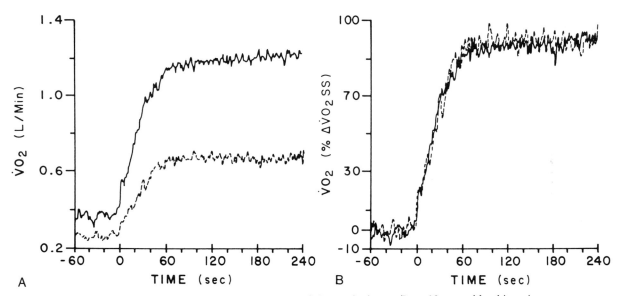

Figure 8–15. *Dashed lines,* group mean response of O_2 uptake in ten 7- to 10-year-old subjects in rest-to-exercise transitions; *solid lines,* ten 16- to 18-year-old subjects. Time is plotted on the *x*-axis; *time 0* indicates the onset of exercise. *A,* $\dot{V}O_2$ in L/min is plotted on the *y* axis; *B,* per cent change from rest to steady state ($\Delta \dot{V}O_{2ss}$) is plotted on the *y*-axis. Time constants did not differ between the two groups. (From Cooper DM, Berry C, Lamarra N, and Wasserman K: J Appl Physiol 59:211, 1985.)

because in the transition between rest and exercise (or between two different levels of exercise) it may take as long as 3 min to achieve a true steady-state value. The calculation would then be

$$\Delta \dot{V}_E / \Delta \dot{V}CO_2 =$$

$$\frac{\dot{V}_E(ss, \text{ higher work rate}) - \dot{V}_E(ss, \text{ lower work rate})}{\dot{V}CO_2(ss, \text{ higher work rate}) - \dot{V}CO_2(ss, \text{ lower work rate})}$$

where ss indicates the steady-state value for each variable.

When constant work rate exercise is performed below a subject's AT, $\dot{V}O_2$, $\dot{V}CO_2$, and $\dot{V}_E$ rapidly achieve a steady state. In contrast, when exercise is performed at work rates above the subject's *AT,* the achievement of steady-state exercise values takes longer; if the work rate is sufficiently high, a steady state may not be achieved at all (Fig. 8–14). Thus the constant work rate protocol can be used to determine whether a particular work rate is above or below the child's anaerobic threshold.

Additional information can be gained from constant work rate tests by focusing on the changes occurring at the onset of exercise. In the transition between rest and constant work rate exercise, the heart, lungs, and blood vessels must rapidly adapt to the large increases in metabolic rate that occur in the muscle cells. As noted, these adaptations of blood flow and ventilation must occur without compromising simultaneous oxygen delivery to the brain and other vital organs. For below-AT exercise, the time courses of $\dot{V}O_2$, $\dot{V}CO_2$, and $\dot{V}_E$ at the onset of exercise are described well by a single exponential equation and can be characterized by the time constant (τ), which indicates the time required to reach 62.5 per

cent of the rest-to-steady-state exercise value. Making these measurements in young children is not easy. Much patience is required on the part of the investigator because multiple transitions are required to reduce the noise-to-signal ratio, and these repetitions can quickly tax the attention span of younger children. Also, breath-by-breath systems are needed to achieve a sufficiently high density of data to allow for accurate curve fitting of the gas exchange data.

For exercise below the AT, the temporal response of O_2 at the onset of exercise is precisely the same in children and adults despite the large differences in body size and $\dot{V}O_{2max}$ (Cooper, Berry, Lamarra, and Wasserman, 1985) (Fig. 8–15). This finding suggests that there exist certain *homeostatic* properties of growth; changes in the relationships among the heart, lung, and blood systems must occur in such a way that the temporal coupling among them is preserved throughout childhood. It is noteworthy that when one component of this interrelated response is damaged, as can occur in congenital heart disease, then the ability to increase $\dot{V}O_2$ at the onset of exercise can become severely impaired, as shown in Figure 8–16.

In contrast to $\dot{V}O_2$, the time constants for $\dot{V}_E$ and $\dot{V}CO_2$ are 35 to 40 per cent faster in younger children than in adults (Cooper, Kaplan, Baumgarten et al, 1987). This disparity in temporal responses is surprising because the CO_2 produced is directly related to the O_2 consumed. The faster CO_2 response suggests relatively smaller capacitance (storage) of CO_2 in children than in adults. The relatively smaller CO_2 stores in children may, in turn, be related to lower tissue PCO_2 and hematocrit values. In addition, there is evidence that certain aspects of respiratory control, specifically, the peripheral chemoreceptor response

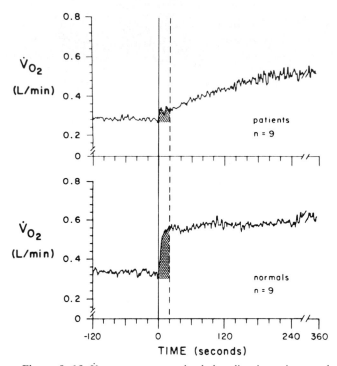

Figure 8–16. $\dot{V}_{O_2}$ response to unloaded cycling in patients and normal subjects. Data from six transitions from each of nine patients are averaged in the top panel and from nine normal subjects in the bottom panel. Exercise begins at time 0. The shaded area indicates the portion of the response occurring in the cardio-dynamic phase of the exercise response. (From Sietsema KE, Cooper DM, Perloff JK et al: Dynamics of oxygen uptake during exercise in adults with cyanotic congenital heart disease. Circulation 73:1137, 1986. Reproduced by permission of the American Heart Association, Inc.)

to hypoxia, is not the same in younger children as in adults (Springer et al, 1988; Springer et al, 1989). The ways in which CO_2 transport matures during growth or adapts to chronic diseases of children have yet to be fully elucidated.

HIGH- AND LOW-INTENSITY EXERCISE

The metabolic and gas exchange responses to exercise do not bear a simple, linear relationship to the work rate input. The $\dot{V}_{O_2}$ response during progressive exercise tests can vary according to the magnitude of the work rate input (Hansen et al, 1988). This variability appears to be dependent on a number of factors, one of the important ones being the rate of lactic acid accumulation. Investigations demonstrate the existence of at least two distinct domains of exercise intensity, and these may represent useful ways to categorize the metabolic consequences of exercise. With low-intensity exercise (i.e., below the subject's AT), lactic acid concentrations are constant, and there are no marked increases in catecholamines. In contrast, high-intensity exercise is accompanied by large increases in epinephrine and norepinephrine and by progressive lactic acidosis (Escourrou et al, 1984; Cooper, Barstow, Lee, and Bergner, 1987).

As a consequence, when *constant* work rate exercise is performed above a subject's AT, the $\dot{V}_{O_2}$ *will continue to increase* (see Fig. 8–14), but when constant work rate exercise is performed below a subject's AT, the $\dot{V}_{O_2}$, $\dot{V}_{CO_2}$, and $\dot{V}_E$ responses will achieve a steady state.

It appears, then, that performing exercise above the AT requires an additional amount of metabolic work that is not obligatory during low-intensity exercise. Programs of physical training can raise the work rate at which the AT occurs (Davis et al, 1979) and can result in increases of each of the following: muscle mass, mitochondrial density, levels of oxidative enzymes, and muscle capillarization (Åstrand and Rodahl, 1977). By reducing the metabolic acidosis accompanying a particular work rate, the perception of discomfort and dyspnea may be alleviated. In considering children with chronic lung disease, this effect on the *peripheral* muscles may be as important as any putative effect on the respiratory muscles, because reduction in the CO_2 load to a respiratory system with impaired capability of CO_2 excretion may allow the affected individual to sustain exercise and activity for longer periods of time (Casaburi and Wasserman, 1986).

THE PROBLEM OF SIZE

The evaluation and diagnosis of disease using exercise testing require knowledge of adaptive mechanisms at both the cellular and the organ-system level. In children, interpretation of these adaptations is confounded by the rapid change in body size and development that characterizes the growth process. For example, how can one appropriately compare the maximal oxygen uptake achieved by a 6-year-old child with that achieved by an 18 year old? Underlying the problem of *sizing* is the more fundamental question of how metabolic function relates to the changes in body size and development that occur during the growth process. As noted earlier, certain of the aerobic responses to exercise are independent of size or age in healthy subjects (e.g., work efficiency, time constant of the oxygen uptake response), but other responses are directly dependent on body size (e.g., $\dot{V}_{O_2max}$, anaerobic threshold). The interested reader may find a more basic discussion of these issues in the investigations of Cooper (1988), McMahon (1984), and Heusner (1982a, 1982b).

There is no perfect way to normalize the effects of body size on cardiorespiratory responses to exercise. The clinician will always be confronted with abnormalities in the growth process brought on by nutritional and hormonal factors or chronic disease that distort the normal relationship among age, height, and weight. Under these conditions, the appropriate cardiorespiratory response to exercise becomes difficult to define. Should an obese 6 year old who weighs as much as a normal 12 year old be expected to have the same $\dot{V}_{O_2max}$ as the older child? Some investigators have used body weight to compare lean and obese subjects and have found that obese children demonstrated low anaerobic thresholds per kg of body weight (Reybrouck et al, 1987). Based on this type of observation, it has been suggested that obese children are unfit and are less physically active than leaner children; however, if the exercise responses are normalized to body height (e.g., $\dot{V}O_{2max}$/cm) or lean body mass, then the degree of abnormality in the obese subject is significantly reduced. This determination is important. If the obese child is deemed "inactive," then the therapeutic approach ought to include programs of exercise. Such programs are expensive, and they require behavioral changes and extensive supervision. For the obese child who is as physically active as the leaner child, additional increases in physical activity may prove to be an impossible task.

In many areas of pediatrics, body surface area (BSA) has been used to calculate drug dosages, energy expenditure, and the like. The use of the BSA stems from the so-called surface area law, which, as noted, was a popular concept in comparative physiology in the nineteenth century (Gray, 1981). Much controversy surrounds the idea that metabolic rates in homeothermic animals are determined by the rate of heat loss, which in turn is dependent on the ratio of surface area to body mass. Moreover, the BSA is a derived value based on the actually measured height and weight and then calculated using a set of assumptions that have not been tested rigorously. Body weight and height are each simple and highly accurate assessments of body size. In children, the correlation between height and weight is much higher than in adults (Cooper et al, 1984a), probably because obesity in children is far less prevalent. Because the major metabolizing tissue during exercise is muscle, many investigators have attempted to measure lean body mass as an estimate of muscle mass. Several techniques have been developed to collect such data, ranging from cumbersome underwater weighing to the use of calipers to measure skinfold thickness (Lohman et al, 1984). Given the wide array of choices and the lack of a single "gold standard" for normalization, it behooves each investigator and clinician to define precisely how normalization was accomplished and how the rationale for using any particular approach evolved.

Another frequently used concept that lacks a universally accepted working definition is *fitness.* Fitness refers to a *task-specific* capability of the cardiorespiratory system but is often used as a global indicator of the exercise response. In adults and children, the ability to perform a particular muscular activity is, to some extent, dependent on the individual's history of participation in that activity. Sedentary individuals can improve their running distances or times in training programs. Thus the terms *fit* and *trained* are often interchanged. The lack of precision in terminology can be confusing. For example, are differences in the AT and $\dot{V}O_{2max}$ often observed between boys and girls indicative of differences in *fitness,* or do they represent gender-related biological differences in mechanisms of O_2 transport? Is the normally active 6-year-old boy less *fit* than another boy whose parents are grooming him to run a marathon? As with strategies for normalization, the investigator and clinician must attempt to be as specific as possible in applying the concept of fitness to a particular child.

METHODS OF ASSESSING EXERCISE RESPONSES IN CHILDREN

A variety of methodologies can be used successfully to measure cardiorespiratory or metabolic responses in children. The two most common testing devices are the cycle ergometer and the treadmill. In cycle ergometry, the work rate input is determined by the load on the cycle's flywheel, and the subject pedals at a constant rate. In treadmill exercise, external work rate is increased by various combinations of increasing treadmill speed and incline. Consequently, the fundamental difference between these two input devices is that with the cycle ergometer, the work rate (power) input is known precisely, but with treadmill exercise the external work rate can only be estimated. Hence, when one is attempting to relate gas exchange responses to specific work rates, the cycle ergometer is easier to use. Moreover, in studies of the transition between one level of exercise and another, changing the work rate on the cycle ergometer is effected simply by changing the load on the flywheel, whereas changing the work rate on the treadmill involves adjusting the incline or treadmill speed. These changes often evoke an anxiety response and may change the muscle groups involved in the exercise.

There are certain disadvantages to cycle ergometer exercise. The child is asked to maintain a constant pedaling rate, which is difficult for younger children unfamiliar with bicycles, particularly when they must maintain low work rates. Variability in pedaling rate with a constant external load will result in variability in work rate. This variability can be compensated for by specially designed ergometers in which the external load is adjusted to the pedaling rate to maintain a constant work rate. Another disadvantage is that not every child is adept at bicycle riding, and the investigator must always be aware that cardiorespiratory responses are task specific. In other words, a trained swimmer may be quite fit yet may perform poorly on a cycle ergometer.

Special skills are required of the clinician to achieve successful exercise testing in children. Younger subjects succumb easily to the barrage of sensory input in the laboratory and have difficulty focusing on the exercise task at hand. They will come off the mouthpiece, vary pedaling rates, or change running speeds on the treadmill. In addition, siblings often accompany the subject to be tested and provide additional distraction. In our laboratory, we have attempted to deal with these problems in a systematic manner.

There are always at least two trained individuals conducting the test; the role of one investigator is to stay with the subject at all times. Usually, gentle, continuous verbal encouragement will help the child focus on the task at hand. We have also found that the use of video cassettes and computer games is very helpful in occupying a sibling or the subject during breaks in the testing period.

Gas exchange analysis systems for measurement during exercise testing are of two general types: continuous measurement (breath-by-breath) and discrete measurement (requiring mixing chambers of the exhaled gas). Both systems can yield useful and accurate information on cardiorespiratory responses to exercise. For investigations of the dynamic or kinetic responses of gas exchange to various work rate inputs, breath-by-breath systems offer the advantage of providing a sufficiently high density of data to permit subsequent mathematic analysis (e.g., curve fitting) that would be unavailable otherwise. Some commercial systems can be adapted to the needs of children (by reducing system dead space, allowing a smaller crank radius for pedaling, providing adjustable seats). And although the mass spectrometer is still advantageous as a gas analyzer (rapid response, small sampling volume), advances in discrete gas analyzer technology have made these devices quite suitable for most systems designed for breath-by-breath analysis.

SAFETY OF EXERCISE TESTING IN CHILDREN

Several investigators have examined the safety of maximal exercise testing in children. Alpert and co-workers (1983) reviewed 1730 studies performed in their laboratory over a 9-year period in which children performed cycle ergometry testing to fatigue. Included in their sample was a large number of children with congenital heart disease. There were no deaths, and the total complication rate was 1.79 per cent. Complications included chest pain, dizziness or syncope, and decreased blood pressure. Hazardous arrhythmias occurred in only 0.46 per cent of the subjects. In my laboratory, more than 200 healthy children have undergone progressive exercise testing with a similar low incidence of only mild complications. In addition, dozens of children with anemia, heart disease, diabetes, and lung disease have been tested, and no major complications have been observed. Nonetheless, appropriate monitoring devices (pulse oximeters, electrocardiographs, blood pressure manometers) must be close at hand. Updated "crash carts" should be included in those laboratories in which children with diseases are to be tested. In addition, all laboratory personnel should be experienced in the fundamentals of cardiopulmonary resuscitation in children.

The American Heart Association Council on Cardiovascular Disease in the Young established a set of criteria for terminating exercise tests in the pediatric age group (1982). Included among the criteria are symptoms of severe chest pain and signs of hypovolemia. Moreover, exercise should be terminated if ventricular or supraventricular tachycardia is noted or if ST segmental depression exceeds 3 mm. Of course, evidence of either hypo- or hypertension should stop the exercise. Bar-Or (1983, p 337) has developed a set of contraindications for exercise testing in children with a variety of diseases. This list includes the presence of uncontrolled congestive heart failure, drug overdose, or asthma and severe bronchoconstriction at the time of testing.

NORMAL VALUES

In all aspects of pulmonary function testing and exercise assessment the clinician is faced with the problem of choosing normal values. As noted earlier, there are a number of large-series investigations of normal values for both pulmonary function testing and exercise results in children. But variations in methodology and in the racial and socioeconomic composition of population groups require the validation of normal values for any particular laboratory. For example, we compared the maximal $\dot{V}O_2$ obtained in our laboratory with values obtained by Åstrand in Sweden in 1950. Although the results for 6- to 18-year-old boys in our study were indistinguishable from the results for Swedish boys, the values for girls in our community were significantly lower than those for their Swedish counterparts (Åstrand, 1952). Apparently, cultural differences in patterns of physical activity resulted in marked reductions of fitness in the U.S. girls. Ideally, each laboratory should develop its own set of normal values. At the very least, a sample of local, healthy children can be tested to help choose an appropriate set of normal values.

THE CONCEPT OF FUNCTIONAL DISABILITY IN CHILDREN

In an adult, the concept of *disability* has both medical and economic significance. It can be assessed in the exercise laboratory by determining the extent to which cardiorespiratory impairment limits the performance of work-related tasks (Wasserman et al, 1987). The concept of *functional disability* can be applied in pediatrics as well by recognizing that the major tasks of children are running, jumping, and other activities associated with play. We believe that disability in children can be determined in part by measuring the cardiorespiratory response to exercise in the manners described previously. In addition, an assessment of the level of physical activity in the life of the child would clearly be useful, but precisely what constitutes a healthy or normal amount of physical activity is not yet known. Part of the problem

Table 8–4. CARDIORESPIRATORY RESPONSES TO EXERCISE—CASE 1

Age: 10 years	Weight: 31 kg	Height: 135 cm

Baseline (unloaded cycling) Values

$\dot{V}O_2$ .26 L/min $\dot{V}CO_2$ .21 L/min $\dot{V}_E$ 4.7 L/min   HR 85 beats/min

Progressive Cycle Ergometry (ramp-type protocol)

Peak $\dot{V}O_2$ 22 ml O_2/min/kg   :   Predicted (%)* 57

$\dot{V}O_2$ AT   Indeterminate due to hyperventilation for both $\dot{V}O_2$ and $\dot{V}CO_2$

$\Delta\dot{V}O_2/\Delta$WR (ml O_2/watt)	10	:	Predicted (%) 98
$\Delta\dot{V}O_2/\Delta$WR (ml O_2/beat)	7	:	Predicted (%) 95
$\Delta\dot{V}_E/\Delta\dot{V}CO_2$	26	:	Predicted (%) 101

O_2 saturation (ear oximeter) baseline 97%; peak exercise 96%

*Based on body height.

is that energy expenditure in physical activity has proved to be difficult to quantify under field conditions (i.e., in the environment of the *child,* not the investigator). Existing methodologies include a variety of questionnaires, interview techniques, and sensors of limb acceleration and body trunk motion (Wilson et al, 1986; La Porte, 1979; Dearwater et al, 1985). The data from these instruments must then be converted into units of metabolic energy metabolism (i.e., calories).

A number of techniques based on stable isotope chemistry (the stable isotopes are safe, nonradioactive substances) are likely to improve our ability to make noninvasive, precise measurements of energy expenditure in children under field conditions. In the 1950s Lifson and co-workers (1955) observed that following the ingestion of $^2H_2^{18}O$ (doubly labeled water) in animals, the washout kinetics of the ^{18}O differed from those of the ^2H. These investigators reasoned that the disparity between the two labeled atoms arose from the exchange of water oxygen with oxygen in CO_2; hence, the difference in the washout kinetics could be used to calculate the CO_2 production. This method was used to measure energy expenditure (as $\dot{V}CO_2$) in animal studies throughout the 1950s and 1960s. Attempts have been made to use the doubly labeled water technique in human subjects. A major limitation of this method is that it is accurate only for measuring energy expenditure over relatively long periods of time (several days to 2 weeks) (Schoeller et al, 1982; Saris, 1986), but activity in children is characterized by bursts over short periods of time (hours). Preliminary data using the stable isotope [^{13}C]bicarbonate (Cooper, Barstow, Sobel, and Epstein, 1988) suggest that a new method of measuring short bursts of activity under field conditions may soon be available.

The inappropriate diagnosis of disease as well as disease itself can result in impaired levels of physical activity in children. Bergman and Stamm (1967) introduced the concept of *cardiac nondisease* to characterize the disability and restrictions imposed on a group of healthy children who had been labeled as having heart disease. The participation of many of the children in physical activity was found to be severely restricted despite there being no physiologic

reason for these restrictions. In our experience, a major clinical task of the pediatrician interested in the physiology of physical activity will be to provide rational programs of exercise for healthy children and for those with chronic diseases. This task involves keeping precise measurements of the responses to exercise, assessing the child's level of physical activity, and being sensitive to the psychological needs of the family and child. No standards yet exist to perform such an evaluation in children, although a number of investigators are actively pursuing related areas (Orenstein, 1988; Nickerson, 1983). Two cases from our clinical experience are presented that might illustrate the problems and solutions involved in assessing the true functional disability of a child.

Case 1. A 10-year-old girl was referred to us for evaluation of cardiorespiratory response to physical activity. Three years earlier, the child had been involved in a motor vehicle accident, which resulted in severe trauma to the left chest wall with multiple rib fractures, pneumo- and hemothorax, and pulmonary contusion. The hospital course was complicated by pulmonary infections, multiple thoracenteses, ventilator dependence, and tracheostomy. By the time she was discharged, after four months, she was no longer ventilator dependent. Nighttime O_2 was prescribed, and the patient was advised not to participate in physical activities. On interviewing the child, it was clear that she wanted to increase her participation in physical activity substantially, but both she and her parents were wary of the consequences. It is noteworthy that the child was significantly overweight. The results of her exercise studies are shown in Table 8–4.

This case illustrates a number of points often encountered in the evaluation of functional disability of children. First, the peak or maximal $\dot{V}O_2$ is often of limited value in children who are deconditioned or who may have anxieties about the consequences of exercise. If we had relied only on the $\dot{V}O_{2max}$, then the abnormally low value found in this child might have led us to continue the severe restrictions imposed on her participation in physical activity. But by measuring the dynamic response to exercise, in this case the $\Delta\dot{V}_E/\Delta\dot{V}CO_2$, the $\Delta\dot{V}O_2/\Delta$HR, and changes in oxygen saturation (by ear oximetry), we established

Table 8–5. CARDIORESPIRATORY RESPONSES TO EXERCISE—CASE 2

Age: 12.2 years	Weight: 31 kg	Height: 154 cm

Baseline (unloaded cycling) Values

$\dot{V}O_2$ .22 L/min $\dot{V}CO_2$ .24 L/min $\dot{V}_E$ 4.7 L/min   HR 85 beats/min

Progressive Cycle Ergometry (ramp-type protocol)

Peak $\dot{V}O_2$	23 ml O_2/min/kg	:	Predicted (%)* 55
$\dot{V}O_2$-AT	15 ml O_2/min/kg	:	Predicted (%) 58
$\Delta\dot{V}O_2/\Delta$HR (ml O_2/watt)	8	:	Predicted (%) 76
$\Delta\dot{V}O_2/\Delta$HR (ml O_2/beat)	11	:	Predicted (%) 74
$\Delta\dot{V}_E/\Delta\dot{V}CO_2$	18	:	Predicted (%) 69

O_2 saturation (ear oximeter) baseline 94%; peak exercise 92%

*Based on body height.

an essentially normal response at the lower work rates. The low peak $\dot{V}O_2$ probably resulted from a combination of deconditioning and anxiety on the part of the child toward activities that she had been led to believe were dangerous and forbidden.

Second, by using a constant work rate test we were able to establish a level of exercise that was clearly below the child's AT. In reintroducing this child to physical activity, we felt that it would be important to determine what constituted high- and low-intensity exercise; in this way the child would not be suddenly exposed to work rates that would result in dyspnea, discomfort, and high levels of catecholamines. Using the constant work rate test, we demonstrated to ourselves and to the child that sustained exercise—even if only 6 min—could be performed. By finding the heart rate that correlated with the below-AT work rate, we established a starting point for a program designed to reintroduce this child to normal levels of physical activity.

Case 2. A 12-year-old boy suffered severe lung parenchymal and bronchial damage following a presumed viral pneumonia at age 3. He had been followed for several years in our pulmonary clinic, in which his lung volume was measured repeatedly and was always low (total lung capacity approximately 70 per cent of predicted). The parents were contemplating a vacation at a high-altitude resort (approximately 8500 feet above sea level) and were concerned about the possible effects on the patient. Progressive and constant work rate exercise testing was performed, and the results are shown in Table 8–5.

When the ability to match ventilation with CO_2 production is impaired by lung disease, exercise limitation may result from hypercapnea and its metabolic consequences. This limitation has been observed, for example, in some (but clearly not all) children with cystic fibrosis (Marcotte et al, 1986). In this patient, we found a low $\dot{V}O_{2max}$ and anaerobic threshold from the ramp test. Moreover, the slope of the $\dot{V}_E$ to $\dot{V}CO_2$ relationship was low, suggesting an elevated Pa_{CO_2}. In marked contrast to the normal finding of a constant end-tidal P_{CO_2} during progressive exercise with occasional decreases at very high work rates, the patient demonstrated a continual increase in the end-tidal CO_2 (Fig. 8–17). These data suggested a ventilatory impairment during exercise and an inability to normally excrete metabolically produced CO_2.

Hypoxia has a number of known effects on cardiorespiratory responses to exercise. Most notably, it stimulates ventilation (acutely) and impairs oxygen delivery, resulting in a reduced AT (Cooper et al, 1986; Dejours, 1963). In the case of this child, who had a marked ventilatory impairment, we wondered whether the high-altitude environment would create conditions in which almost any activity above resting would result in high-intensity (above AT) exercise. If so, the CO_2 load imposed during physical activity might be more than his ventilatory system could handle, Pa_{CO_2} would rise, and dyspnea and discomfort would ensue rapidly. By imposing hypoxic gas breathing equivalent to the Fi_{O_2} of the resort area (in this case, 15 per cent), we could determine at what level of exercise ventilation would become a limiting factor and desaturation of blood would occur. Using constant work rate exercise protocols, we then determined the heart rate above which the child might encounter difficulty. With this information, the family was able to monitor the child, appropriately limit his activity, and successfully complete the vacation.

ASTHMA AND EXERCISE

Often, the clinician is faced with the diagnostic dilemma of reported wheezing in a child who, by history, is normally active and participates in all

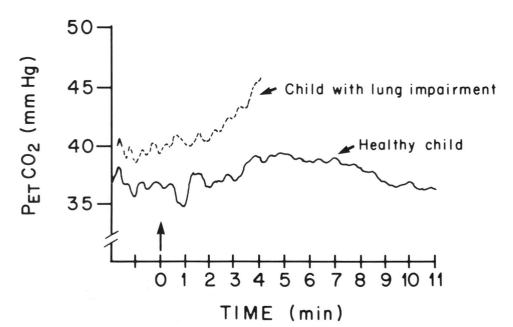

Figure 8–17. End-tidal P_{CO_2} during exercise in a child with a lung impairment *(dashed line)* and in a healthy 12-year-old child *(solid line)* during progressive exercise. Breath-by-breath values (y-axis) are plotted against time, where $t = 0$ is the onset of the ramp protocol. In the patient with lung disease, the end-tidal P_{CO_2} increases throughout exercise. This result suggests that the lungs are unable to adapt to the increasing CO_2 production due to exercise, and the concentration of CO_2 in the tissues is increasing.

Table 8–6. AN EXISTING PROTOCOL FOR EXERCISE CHALLENGE TEST FOR THE DIAGNOSIS OF
EXERCISE-INDUCED BRONCHOSPASM (EIB)

Pretest Preparation
1. Patient must avoid exertion for at least 2½ to 3 hours before testing.
2. Climatic conditions (temperature and humidity) should be standardized.
3. For a given patient, tests and retests should be at the same time of day.
4. Retesting, if necessary, should be performed between 1 day and 1 week of the original test.
5. A medical history should be obtained and a physical examination performed.
6. The child should be familiarized with the objectives of the test and the laboratory.
7. Baseline pulmonary function should be obtained.

Withdrawal of Medication
1. All β_2-sympathomimetics, methylxanthines, and anticholinergics should be discontinued at least 8 hours before testing.
2. Long-acting methylxanthines should be withdrawn 24 hours before testing.
3. Disodium cromoglycate should be withdrawn 24 hours before testing.

Exercise Protocol
1. Running up and down stairs in the office, hospital, or clinic is not sufficient.
2. Cycle ergometer or treadmill exercise is recommended.
3. Continuous monitoring of heart rate (HR) is necessary; monitoring of gas exchange is recommended.
4. Bar-Or recommends that a successful test consist of *at least* 5 min of constant work rate exercise at 80 to 90 per cent of the HR max. Thus the appropriate work rate must be estimated before testing by using normal values. The investigator may then have to adjust the work rate within the first several minutes.

Pulmonary Function Tests
1. Baseline (pre-exercise) testing (e.g., FVC and FEV_1) is done immediately before the exercise challenge.
2. Testing is repeated at 2, 5, and 10 min after the initial exercise and then repeated every 5 min until EIB subsides.
3. The most common calculation is the per cent value of the ratio:

$$\frac{\text{Pre-exercise pulmonary function value} - \text{Lowest postexercise value}}{\text{Pre-exercise value}}$$

4. A positive test is usually defined as a drop in pulmonary function of more than 15 per cent.

(Based on Bar-Or O: Pediatric Sports Medicine. New York, Springer Verlag, 1983, pp 102–104.)
FVC, forced vital capacity; FEV_1, forced expiratory volume in 1 sec.

aspects of sports and play. Because the incidence of exercise-induced bronchospasm (EIB) is high in children with asthma, using exercise to *uncover* wheezing has become a widely accepted means of diagnosing the condition (Bierman et al, 1975). The pathophysiology of EIB is not completely clear. Originally it seemed that airway cooling (dependent on water loss from the airways) was the responsible mechanism (McFadden et al, 1977). Consistent with this is the observation that swimming, in which the air breathed by the child is virtually 100 per cent saturated, results in far less EIB than does a comparable level of an exercise such as running, in which the air breathed is relatively dry (Bar-Or, 1983). But other investigators have suggested that the mechanism of EIB is not related to airway cooling. To support this contention, there are data that the bronchoconstriction following exercise occurs more slowly than does the bronchoconstriction following cold-air stimulation of the airways. Moreover, increased neutrophil chemotactic activity has been found during EIB (Lee et al, 1982).

There are a number of methodological problems concerning the exercise challenge test in the diagnosis of asthma. First, there is little standardization of the input of the exercise stimulus; there are no studies in which a "dose-response curve" has been adequately defined for children. Second, the criterion for a positive exercise challenge is not uniform among laboratories. Finally, there is a refractory period associated with the exercise challenge (Edmunds et al, 1978), which has been attributed to the depletion

of bronchoconstrictive mediators after repeated stimulation of mediator release by the exercise. This refractory period may explain the ability of many asthmatics to "break through" the wheezing at the onset of exercise simply by continuing to exercise. Alternatively, the breakthrough phenomenon and the refractoriness of EIB may be related to the bronchodilator effect of elevated levels of catecholamines associated with high-intensity exercise. Thus an exercise challenge test must require exercise of sufficient intensity to stimulate bronchoconstriction (Wilson et al, 1981)*; however, when the exercise input is sufficiently intense, catecholamine-induced bronchodilation may obscure the bronchoconstrictive effect. Bar-Or (1983) has suggested a standardized approach toward EIB, which is shown in Table 8–6.

Other types of challenge procedures to diagnose asthma have also been promoted by various investigators. The histamine and methacholine tests have been used widely in children, and standardized testing procedures are available (Chai et al, 1975). Cold-air testing (isocapnic hyperventilation with cold air [ICHA]) (Zach et al, 1984; McLaughlin and Dozor, 1983; Tal et al, 1984; Zach and Polgar, 1986) and ultrasonic nebulized distilled-water mist (USM) (Barker and Levison, 1972; Anderson et al, 1983) have also been proposed as relatively simple diagnostic challenge procedures. Differences in sensitivity and

---

*Interestingly, Wilson and co-workers (1981) found that the EIB for high-intensity exercise was disproportionately higher than the EIB observed for the lower-intensity exercise.

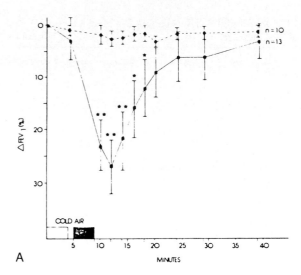

A

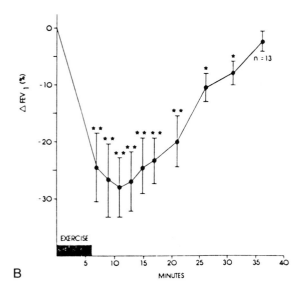

B

Figure 8–18. *A*, Change in FEV₁ (mean ± SE) in 13 asthmatic children *(solid squares)* and 10 healthy children *(solid circles)* after a cold-air challenge. Open box, lower left-hand corner, indicates 4 min of moderate hyperventilation; closed box indicates 4 min of maximal hyperventilation. *B*, Change in FEV₁ in 13 asthmatic children after an exercise test. *P<0.05; **P<0.01. (Data from Tal A, Pasterkamp H, Serrette C et al: Response to cold air hyperventilation in normal and in asthmatic children. J Pediatr 104:516, 1984.)

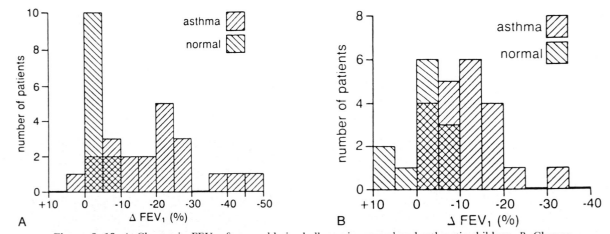

A   B

Figure 8–19. *A*, Change in FEV₁ after a cold-air challenge in normal and asthmatic children. *B*, Change in FEV₁ after an ultrasonic mist challenge in normal and asthmatic children.

specificity have been observed among the exercise, ICHA, USM, histamine, and methacholine challenge tests. For example, Tal and co-workers (1984) demonstrated that both cold-air and exercise induced bronchospasm to the same degree in a group of asthmatic children. However, they found that the response was faster for the cold-air test and the recovery longer for the exercise challenge (Fig. 8–18). Galdes-Sebaldt and co-investigators (1985) compared cold-air, methacholine, and ultrasonic nebulization. As shown in Figure 8–19, these challenges produced different patterns of responses among the asthmatic children and control subjects, suggesting different sensitivities and specificities for the procedures. The ideal role for exercise, histamine, methacholine, ICHA, and USM challenge testing in children has yet to be elucidated.

SUMMARY

In attempting to assess the health status of his or her patients, the pediatrician frequently asks the question, "How is the child doing?" With exercise testing, a precise answer to this question can often be obtained. We have attempted to demonstrate that the cardiorespiratory response to exercise is a measurement of metabolism and growth and development as well as an index of the functional capabilities of the heart and lungs. It is hoped that child health care professionals will avail themselves of this resource. Much more research has yet to be done before we understand fully the optimal role of physical activity in the lives of healthy children and in the lives of those suffering from chronic diseases.

REFERENCES

Alpert BS, Verrill DE, Flood NL et al: Complications of ergometer exercise in children. Pediatr Cardiol 4:91, 1983.

American Heart Association Council on Cardiovascular Disease in the Young: Standards for exercise testing in the pediatric age group. Circulation 66:1377A, 1982.

Anderson SD, Schoeffel RE, and Finney M: Evaluation of ultrasonically nebulised solutions for provocation testing in patients with asthma. Thorax 38:284, 1983.

Åstrand PO: Experimental Studies of Physical Working Capacity in Relation to Sex and Age. Copenhagan, Muskgaard, 1952.

Åstrand PO and Rodahl K: Textbook of Work Physiology. New York, McGraw-Hill Book Co, 1977.

Barker R and Levison H: Effects of ultrasonically nebulized distilled water on airway dynamics in children with cystic fibrosis and asthma. J Pediatr 80:396, 1972.

Bar-Or O: Pediatric Sports Medicine. New York, Springer Verlag, 1983.

Bergman AB and Stamm SJ: The morbidity of cardiac nondisease in school children. New Engl J Med 276:1008, 1967.

Bertrand JM, Beaudry PH, and Coates AL: Histamine inhalation challenge in children: a comparison of two methods. Ann Allergy 50:389, 1983.

Bierman CW and Pierson WE: Summary—symposium on exercise and asthma. Pediatrics 56:9500, 1975.

Casaburi R and Wasserman K: Exercise training in pulmonary rehabilitation. N Engl J Med 314:1509, 1986.

Chai H, Farr RS, Froehlich LA et al: Standardization of bronchial inhalation challenge procedures. J Allergy Clin Immunol 56:323, 1975.

Cooper DM: Development of the O_2 transport system in normal children. In Bar-Or O (ed): Pediatric Sports Sciences. Vol 3. Champaign, Ill, Human Kinetics Publishers, 1988.

Cooper DM, Barstow TL, Lee WNP, and Bergner A: Evidence for a threshold of glucose turnover during exercise in man. (Abstract). Physiologist 30:230, 1987.

Cooper DM, Barstow T, Sobel E, and Epstein E: Dynamics of exhaled $^{13}CO_2$ following oral administration of ^{13}C-bicarbonate. (Abstract). FASEB J 2:1302, 1988.

Cooper DM, Berry C, Lamarra N, and Wasserman K: Kinetics of O_2 uptake at the onset of exercise as a function of growth in children. J Appl Physiol 59:211, 1985.

Cooper DM, Hyman CB, Weiler-Ravell D et al: Gas exchange during exercise in children with thalassemia major and diamond-blackfan anemia. Pediatr Res 19:1215, 1985.

Cooper DM, Kaplan MR, Baumgarten L et al: Coupling of ventilation and CO_2 production during exercise in children. Pediatr Res 21:568, 1987.

Cooper DM, Wasserman DH, Vranic M, and Wasserman K: Glucose turnover in response to exercise during high- and low-Fi_{O2} breathing in man. Am J Physiol 251:E209, 1986.

Cooper DM, Weiler-Ravell D, Whipp BJ, and Wasserman K: Aerobic parameter of exercise as a function of body size during growth in children. J Appl Physiol 56:628, 1984a.

Cooper DM, Weiler-Ravell D, Whipp BJ, and Wasserman K: Oxygen uptake and heart rate during exercise as a function of growth in children. Ped Res 18:845, 1984b.

Cumming G: Gas mixing in disease. In Scadding JG and Cumming G (eds): Scientific Foundation of Respiratory Medicine. Philadelphia, WB Saunders Co, 1981.

Davis JA, Frank MM, Whipp BJ, and Wasserman K: Anaerobic threshold alteration caused by endurance training in middle-aged men. J Appl Physiol 46:1039, 1979.

Dearwater SR, LaPorte RE, Cauley JA, and Brenes G: Assessment of physical activity in inactive populations. Med Sci Sports Exerc 17:651, 1985.

Dejours P: Control of respiration by arterial chemoreceptors. Ann NY Acad Sci 109:682, 1963.

Driscoll DJ: Cardiovascular evaluation of the child and adolescent before participation in sports. Mayo Clin Proc 60:867, 1985.

Edmunds AT, Tooley M, and Godfrey S: The refractory period after EIA: its duration and relation to the severity of exercise. Am Rev Respir Dis 117:247, 1978.

Ekblom B, Kilbom A, and Soltysiack J: Physical training, bradycardia and autonomic nervous system. Scand J Clin Lab Invest 32:251, 1973.

Epstein LH, Wing RR, Penner BC, and Kress JM: Effect of diet and controlled exercise on weight loss in obese children. J Pediatr 107:358, 1985.

Escourrou P, Johnson DG, and Rowell LB: Hypoxemia increases plasma catecholamine concentrations in exercising humans. J Appl Physiol 57:1507, 1984.

Galdes-Sebaldt M, McLaughlin FJ, and Levison H: Comparison of cold air, ultrasonic mist, and methacholine inhalations as tests of bronchial reactivity in normal and asthmatic children. J Pediatr 107:526, 1985.

Godfrey S: Exercise Testing in Children. London, WB Saunders Co, Ltd, 1974.

Godfrey S, Silverman M, and Anderson SD: The use of the treadmill for assessing exercise-induced asthma and the effect of varying the severity and duration of exercise. Pediatrics 56:893, 1975.

Gray BF: On the surface law and basal metabolic rate. J Theor Biol 93:757, 1981.

Hagberg JM, Goldring D, Ehsani AA et al: Effect of exercise training on the blood pressure and hemodynamic features of hypertensive adolescents. Am J Cardiol 52:763, 1983.

Hansen JE, Casaburi R, Cooper DM, and Wasserman K: Oxygen uptake as related to work rate increment during cycle ergometer exercise. Eur J Appl Physiol 57:140, 1988.

Heusner AA: Energy metabolism and body size. I. Is the 0.75 mass exponent of Kleiber's equation a statistical artifact? Respir Physiol 48:1, 1982a.

Heusner AA: Energy metabolism and body size. II. Dimensional analysis and energetic non-similarity. Respir Physiol 48:13, 1982b.

Hunter WM, Fonseka CC, and Passmore R: Growth hormone: important role in muscular exercise in adults. Science 150:1051, 1965.

Idstrom J-P, Subramanian V, Chance B et al: Oxygen dependence of energy metabolism in contracting and recovering rat skeletal muscle. Am J Physiol 248:H40, 1985.

Jones NL, Robertson DG, and Kane JW: Difference between end-tidal and arterial P_{CO_2} in exercise. J Appl Physiol 47:954, 1979.

Katz A and Sahlin K: Regulation of lactic acid production during exercise. J Appl Physiol 65:509, 1988.

Kleiber M: The Fire of Life. New York, Robert E Krieger Publishing Co, 1975.

Klesges RC, Klesges LM, Swenson AM, and Pheley AM: A validation of two motion sensors in the prediction of child and adult physical activity levels. Am J Epidemiol 122:400, 1985.

La Porte RE: An objective measure of physical activity for epidemiologic research. Am J Epidemiol 109:158, 1979.

Lee TH, Nagy L, Nagakura T et al: Identification and partial characterization of an exercise-induced neutrophil chemotactic factor in bronchial asthma. J Clin Invest 69:889, 1982.

Lifson N, Forgon AB, and McClintock R: Measurement of total carbon dioxide production by means of D_2O^{18}. J Appl Physiol 7:704, 1955.

Lohman TG, Boileau RA, and Slaughter MH: Body composition in children and youth. In Boileau RA (ed): Advances in Pediatric Sports Sciences. Vol 1: Biological Issues. Champaign, Ill, Human Kinetics Publishers, Inc, 1984.

McFadden ER Jr, Ingram RH Jr, Haynes RL, and Wellman JJ: Predominant site of flow limitation and mechanisms of postexertional asthma. J Appl Physiol 42:746, 1977.

McLaughlin FJ and Dozor A: Cold air inhalation challenge in the diagnosis of asthma in children. Pediatrics 72:503, 1983.

McMahon TA: Muscles, Reflexes, and Locomotion. Princeton, NJ, Princeton University Press, 1984.

Marcotte JE, Grisdale RK, Levison H et al: Multiple factors limit exercise capacity in cystic fibrosis. Pediatr Pulmonol 2:274, 1986.

Nickerson BG, Baritista DB, Namey MA et al: Distance running improves fitness in asthmatic children without pulmonary complications or changes in exercise-induced bronchospasm. Pediatrics 71:147, 1983.

Orenstein DM: Exercise tolerance and exercise conditioning in children with chronic lung disease. J Pediatr 112:1043, 1988.

Phillipson EA, Bowes G, Townsend ER et al: Role of metabolic CO_2 production in ventilatory response to steady-state exercise. J Clin Invest 68:768, 1981.

Reybrouck T, Weymans M, Stijns H et al: Ventilatory anaerobic threshold in healthy children. Eur J Appl Physiol 54:278, 1985.

Reybrouck T, Weymans M, Vinckx J et al: Cardiorespiratory function during exercise in obese children. Acta Paediatr Scand 76:342, 1987.

Saris WH: Habitual physical activity in children: methodology and findings in health and disease. Med Sci Sports Exerc 18:253, 1986.

Schoeller DA and van Sante E: Measurement of energy expenditure in humans by doubly labeled water method. J Appl Physiol 53:955, 1982.

Shanis BS and Moshang T: Propranolol and exercise as a screening test for growth hormone deficiency. Pediatrics 57:712, 1976.

Sietsema KE, Cooper DM, Perloff JK et al: Dynamics of oxygen uptake during exercise in adults with cyanotic congenital heart disease. Circulation 73:1137, 1986.

Springer C, Barstow TJ, and Cooper DM: Effect of hypoxia on ventilatory control during exercise in children and adults. Pediat Res 25:285, 1989.

Springer C, Cooper DM, and Wasserman K: Evidence that maturation of the peripheral chemoreceptors is not complete in childhood. Respir Physiol 74:55, 1988.

Stratton R, Wilson DP, Endres RK, and Goldstein DE: Improved glycemic control after supervised 8-wk exercise program in insulin-dependent diabetic adolescents. Diabetes Care 10:589, 1987.

Tal A, Pasterkamp H, Serrette C et al: Response to cold air hyperventilation in normal and in asthmatic children. J Pediatr 104:516, 1984.

Taylor CR and Weibel ER: Design of the mammalian respiratory system. I. Problems and strategy. Respir Physiol 44:1, 1981.

Walsh ML and Banister EW: Possible mechanisms of the anaerobic threshold. A review. Sports Med 5:269, 1988.

Washington RL, VanGundy JC, Cohen C et al: Normal aerobic and anaerobic exercise data for North American school-age children. J Pediatr 112:223, 1988.

Wasserman K, Hansen JE, Sue DY, and Whipp BJ: Principles of exercise testing and interpretation. Philadelphia, Lea & Febiger, 1987.

Wasserman K, Van Kessel AL, and Burton GG: Interaction of physiological mechanisms during exercise. J Appl Physiol 22:71, 1967.

Wasserman K, Whipp BJ, and Davis JA: Respiratory physiology of exercise: metabolism, gas exchange, and ventilatory control. In Widdicombe JG (ed): Respiratory Physiology III. Baltimore, University Park Press, 1981.

Wasserman K, Whipp BJ, Koyal SN, and Beaver WL: Anaerobic threshold and respiratory gas exchange during exercise. J Appl Physiol 35:236, 1973.

Whipp BJ: Ventilatory control during exercise in humans. Ann Rev Physiol 45:393, 1983.

Whipp BJ and Mahler M: Dynamics of pulmonary gas exchange during exercise. In Pulmonary Gas Exchange. New York, Academic Press, 1980.

Whipp BJ and Wasserman K: Efficiency of muscular work. J Appl Physiol 26:646, 1969.

Whipp BJ, Davis JA, Torres F, and Wasserman K: A test to determine parameters of aerobic function during exercise. J Appl Physiol 50:217, 1981.

Whipp BJ, Lamarra N, Ward S et al: Estimating arterial P_{CO_2} from flow-weighted and time-averaged alveolar P_{CO_2} during exercise. In Swanson GD and Grodins FS (eds): Respiratory Control: Modelling Perspectives. New York, Plenum, (in press).

Wilson BA and Evans JN: Standardization of work intensity for evaluation of exercise-induced bronchoconstriction. Eur J Appl Physiol 47:289, 1981.

Wilson PWF, Pattenbarger RS Jr, Morris JN, and Havlik RJ: Assessment methods for physical activity and physical fitness in population studies: report of a NHLBI workshop. Am Heart J 111:1177, 1986.

Zach MS and Polgar G: Cold air challenge of airway hyperactivity in children: dose-response interrelation with a reaction plateau. J Allergy Clin Immunol 80:9, 1987.

Zach MS, Polgar G, Kump H et al: Cold air challenge of airway hyperactivity in children: practical application and theoretical aspects. Pediatr Res 18:469, 1984.

9

MARY ELLEN B. WOHL, M.D.,
and JERE MEAD, M.D.

AGE AS A FACTOR IN RESPIRATORY DISEASE

Respiratory diseases are among the leading causes of death in North America. Immaturity of the lung is a major contributing factor to the mortality associated with premature birth. Data taken from the Commonwealth of Massachusetts for 1979 show that in children less than 4 years of age, respiratory disease is the second most common cause of death (exceeded only by accidents). After early childhood, mortality rates are low, but respiratory diseases rank as at least the fifth most important cause of death. As mortality rates increase after age 60, respiratory diseases re-emerge as the third major cause of death.

Morbidity associated with respiratory infections is difficult to assess. Studies performed by Dingle and co-workers (1964) and Loda and co-workers (1972) suggest that on the average, every child experiences eight respiratory infections per year. There is a higher incidence in younger children. Estimates of the number of these infections that involve the lower respiratory tract range from 10 to 30 per cent. Although many factors, including sex, housing conditions, social class, the presence of older siblings, immunization, maternal smoking, and previous respiratory tract infections, contribute to the frequency of respiratory tract illness, age is a significant factor.

AGE SPECIFICITY OF RESPIRATORY PATHOGENS

Certain respiratory pathogens are age specific: they produce disease of consequence at certain ages and not at other ages. Some respiratory infections, such as cytomegalovirus pneumonia, depend on exposure in utero. With the exception of infections in the immunocompromised host, cytomegalovirus rarely causes disease beyond the perinatal period. Other infectious agents, such as chlamydia and group B streptococci, cause pneumonia after exposure of the host during birth. Respiratory syncytial virus produces a bronchiolitis in infants but usually only upper respiratory symptoms in school-age children and adults. Parainfluenza virus causes croup in the child between 2 and 3 years old. Acute epiglottitis is usually

but not always seen in children 2 to 7 years of age. Mycoplasma rarely produces disease in preschool children but is a common cause of bronchopneumonia in school-age children and young adults.

Part of the age specificity of respiratory pathogens is related to development of the immune system and to age-related exposure. The influence of age on respiratory structure and function, however, may contribute to this age specificity and is the subject of this chapter.

AGE AND ENERGY METABOLISM

The range of ventilatory demand for a newborn infant is much smaller than it is for adults. The weight-specific metabolic rate of infants at rest is about twice that of an adult, but their most strenuous activity, prolonged crying, only doubles the resting metabolic rate, whereas an adult increases metabolism by about 15 times during strenuous exercise. By the age of 5 years, children have roughly one half the metabolic scope of the adult, but because their basal metabolic rate is about twice the adult rate, the weight-specific ventilatory demand of a 5 year old during heavy exercise is comparable to that of an adult (Åstrand, 1952). It may well be that in health, only the preambulatory infant is spared from high ventilatory demand.

Low ventilatory demand connotes low respiratory reserve, which is compatible with immature lungs and chest wall. Accordingly, respiratory disease may be more life threatening in the very young, who have limited respiratory reserves.

AGE AND RESPIRATORY STRUCTURE

The respiratory system continues to develop throughout infancy and childhood and probably beyond adolescence. Its development is a subject of active investigation and review (Brody and Thurlbeck, 1986; Motoyama et al, 1988). A discussion of

175

some of the steps in the development of the lung that bear particularly on lung function during childhood and on the pattern of respiratory disease follows.

AIRWAYS

The airways are derived from an outpouching of the ventral groove of the embryo. During the embryonal period of lung development the proximal branches are formed. Further branching of the airways, which is more or less dichotomous, occurs during the pseudoglandular period, so named because of the appearance of the lung on microscopic section. By the seventeenth week of gestation the full number of generations of conducting airways has been established (Bucher and Reid, 1961). Thereafter no new conducting airways develop, but there is continuing growth (increase in size) of the existing airways, remodeling of the peripheral airways, and thinning of the epithelium.

The airway wall and the respiratory epithelium change during gestation and postnatal life. During fetal life the thick columnar glycogen-rich epithelium develops cilia and thins, particularly in the periphery of the airway. The thinning of the epithelium may continue postnatally in the human as it does in the rat. Although the epithelium of the infant's airway, like the adult's, is a ciliated pseudostratified columnar type in the trachea and gradually thins to a columnar type in the bronchioles, there are substantial differences. The infant's airway epithelium contains a higher ratio of mucous glands than the adult's, and the constituents of the secretions may change throughout childhood. The rate of tracheal mucociliary clearance, studied in animals, is greater in the young adult than in the infant (Whaley et al, 1987). Muscle is present in the airways of young children in the same proportion as that in adults, but more is distributed in central than in peripheral airways (Matsuba and Thurlbeck, 1972). Cartilage is present in bronchi at birth and does not extend farther toward the periphery until after about 25 weeks of gestation, when its distribution is similar to that of the adult (Bucher and Reid, 1961). Increased cartilage develops in the first years of life, probably contributing to the stiffening of the airways observed in the first months of postnatal life (Croteau and Cook, 1961; Burnard et al, 1965).

Postnatal growth of the airway has been investigated in only a limited number of anatomic studies. The data are conflicting. Hislop and associates (1972) show the infant's airway to be a miniature of the adult's. The limited anatomic and more extensive physiologic studies on excised human lung performed by Hogg and co-workers (1970) suggest that peripheral airways, those distal to the tenth or twelfth generation, increase in size relative to the central airways after the fifth year (Fig. 9–1).

Airway reactivity may be influenced by age. Although earlier investigations (Lenny and Milner, 1978) suggest that infants do not respond to bronchodilators, a number of studies have been done that suggest that normal infants can respond to both bronchoconstricting and bronchodilating stimuli (Tepper, 1987). Other studies demonstrate with considerable certainty that infants with bronchopulmonary dysplasia and cystic fibrosis respond to bronchodilators (Motoyama et al, 1987, Hiatt et al, 1988). Animal studies examining the ontogeny of airway reactivity show that in the lamb the bronchoconstricting response to histamine and carbachol increases with age (Sauder et al, 1986). The response to substance P may be the reverse (Grunstein et al, 1984). Taken together, it seems clear that young children and infants can respond to bronchoconstricting and bronchodilating stimuli and that the role of reversible obstruction needs to be evaluated clinically in the young as well as in the older child with airway disease.

ALVEOLI AND LUNG PARENCHYMA

Whereas the airways are established in early gestational life and grow by enlargement, the alveoli develop in late gestational life and grow in early childhood by forming new structures (i.e., alveolar ducts and alveoli) and only later by enlargement (Fig. 9–2). The development of alveoli is preceded by the formation of saccules at the end of the budding airway. These structures, larger and more irregular than alveoli, are probably capable of sustaining gas exchange. From 28 to 32 weeks of gestation, some of the subdivisions of the saccules have the cupped shape and single capillary layer characteristic of alveoli, but prematurely born infants may have virtually no alveoli.

Approximately 50 million alveoli are present at birth in the term infant. The number is likely to be extremely variable. Pulmonary hypoplasia is diagnosed when a baby has an associated abnormality, i.e., a congenital renal abnormality or a diaphragmatic hernia, and may be considered when a newborn develops a spontaneous pneumothorax. In all likelihood, considerable reduction in lung size as expressed by the number of terminal units may go undetected by the pediatrician but may influence the child's respiratory reserve. Dunhill (1962) carried out morphometric studies on lungs obtained at autopsy. His data suggest that most of the 300 million alveoli present in the adult lung are formed by the age of 2 years. Others report variable numbers of alveoli, from 200 to 600 million, in the adult and in the infant (Brody and Thurlbeck, 1986). This finding makes the age at which the increase in alveolar number ceases less certain. Nonetheless, a substantial fraction of the total number of alveoli is formed in the first few months and years of life. Thereafter, growth of alveoli takes place for the most part by enlargement.

It seems reasonable to assume that factors that

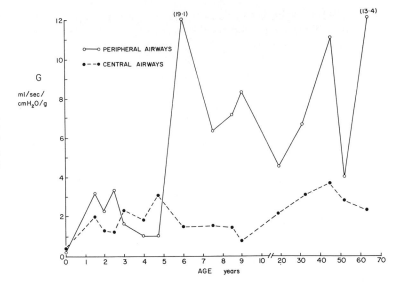

Figure 9–1. Comparison of peripheral and central airway conductance as a function of age in normal human lungs. The data are corrected for size by expressing the conductance as ml/sec/g of lung and for lung inflation by expressing all data at a transpulmonary pressure of 5 cm H₂O. (Replotted from Hogg JC, Williams J, Richardson JB et al: New Engl J Med 282:1283, 1970).

influence growth of the fetus during the last trimester and during the first year of life would be of particular importance to lung development. These factors are at present poorly understood; for example, there is little information available about lung growth in the 750-gram prematurely born neonate, in which the normal process of nutrition and growth is interrupted.

Maturation of the lung and in particular of the type II cell and the surfactant system can be assessed before birth. Delay in the maturation of the surfactant system is the principal cause of respiratory distress syndrome in the newborn. This subject is beyond the scope of this chapter; it has been reviewed in depth elsewhere (Post and van Golde, 1988).

Other structural changes within the lung parenchyma may relate to age as a factor in lung disease.

The interstitium of the lung contains little collagen and elastin during late gestation and at birth. This near absence of collagen and elastin may contribute to the relative ease of rupture of air spaces in the premature lung. Elastin, which appears to be closely related to the development of alveoli, increases during early postnatal life. Lung collagen also increases during postnatal life. The formation and changing ratio of elastin and collagen probably contribute to the change in volume-pressure relationships of the lung and to the increased stiffness of the lung with age.

PULMONARY VESSELS

The development of the vessels in the lung parallels the development of the airways and alveoli. The

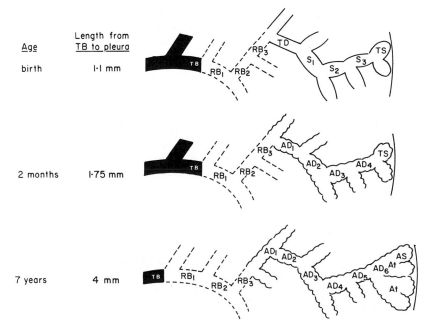

Figure 9–2. Diagram showing that the lung grows initially by increasing the number of alveoli by the ingrowth of septa and formation of the alveolar ducts. *TB*, terminal bronchiole; *RB*, respiratory bronchiole; *AD*, alveolar duct. (Modified from Hislop A and Reid L: Thorax 29:90, 1974.)

pulmonary arterial tree has two sets of vessels. "Conventional" arteries develop and branch in conjunction with the airways; most of the conventional arteries are established in early gestational life, but a few may develop as the respiratory bronchioles do. The "supernumerary" arteries branch from the conventional arterial tree and supply adjacent lung parenchyma; the supernumerary vessels, some of which form prenatally, serve adjacent respiratory parenchyma. Postnatally there is a marked increase in the number of arteries in the acinus. To some extent, this development parallels the postnatal development of alveoli.

In infants and adults, arteries of the same size have the same degree of muscularity. In infants and young children, an artery of a given size is located more proximally in the arterial tree than in adults. Thus muscular arteries extend only to the terminal bronchioles in the fetus and young child. During childhood, muscle extends out to the alveolar duct, and in the adult out to the alveoli (Reid, 1979). The extension of muscle out into the lung is consistent with increasing responsiveness to acute hypoxia with increasing age (Rendas et al, 1982).

A number of studies of the pulmonary vascular system relating structure to function have been carried out, and these reveal differences between infants and adults. The extension of muscle out into the acinus and the rise in the ratio of arteries to alveoli that occurs during childhood is consistent with an increasing responsiveness to acute hypoxia with increasing age (Rendas et al, 1982). However, the infant lung appears to be more responsive than the adult lung to chronic hypoxia (Lowen et al, 1987), with greater narrowing of large pulmonary arteries, increase in and extension of muscle into peripheral arteries, and decrease in the number of peripheral arteries, that is, decrease in the ratio of arteries to alveoli in the acinus (Rabinovitch et al, 1981).

Although structural features of the infant's pulmonary vasculature may influence the infant's response to a variety of vasoconstrictors and vasodilators, there may be substantial differences in response, perhaps governed at the cellular level and related to receptor density, between infants and adults. Little information is available on this subject.

CHEST WALL

In adults, lung volume at end-expiration or functional residual capacity (FRC) is mainly set passively by the balance between the recoils of the lung and chest wall. Newborns have compliant chest walls that would allow nearly complete collapse of lungs if it were not for the activity of muscles: expirations are braked by active glottic narrowing or interrupted by the onset of inspiration, or both. Indeed, the major function of the active Hering-Breuer reflex in infants may be to terminate expirations before lung volume gets too small. This response may disappear once the chest wall has become stiff enough to prevent collapse, but the passive characteristics of the young chest wall are not well enough known as yet to test this possibility. End-expiratory volume is actively maintained by infants until about 6 to 12 months of age, when the passive characteristics of the lung and chest wall appear to determine resting end-expiratory lung volumes.

The easy collapsibility of the rib cage is probably advantageous in utero, where it may help prevent pleural effusion (Agostoni and Mead, 1964), and during birth, when it allows for deformation of the chest as it passes through the birth canal and for easier expulsion of liquid from the lungs before the first breath. Thereafter the collapsibility is probably disadvantageous except during cardiopulmonary resuscitation (Dean et al, 1987) but affordable in a healthy infant because of relatively small metabolic demands. The parenchyma of the lungs matures largely postnatally, and the rib cage may be thought of as doing the same. The infant rib cage "caves in" during obstructed inspiration, whereas the adult rib cage does so to a much smaller extent. In one respect, however, the purely passive characteristics of the lungs and chest wall of infants may be suited to each other. As is mentioned later, the volume-pressure relationship of the lungs is more curvilinear in infants. Transpulmonary pressures are therefore smaller at end-expiration, and a smaller outward recoil is needed to maintain lung volume.

OTHER STRUCTURES

In the adult, collateral ventilation—the movement of gas from one acinus to another—occurs through holes in the alveoli, the pores of Kohn, and epithelial-lined channels between terminal bronchioles and adjacent alveoli called the canals of Lambert (Lambert, 1957). These structures may be present in the infant lung, but they are probably not of sufficient size to allow for air drift. Although collateral pathways in the adult are probably not of great significance for ventilation, they do prevent absorption of gas in regions distal to airway obstruction. The relative absence of collateral pathways probably contributes to the patchy atelectasis so common in airway disease of infants and young children.

The products of resistance and compliance, the time constants, of these collateral pathways have been investigated in maturing sheep (Terry et al, 1987) and in young adults (Inners et al, 1978). The time constants of pathways in the young lung and in the right middle lobe are longer than those in the older lung and in regions other than the right middle lobe, suggesting that atelectasis of the right middle lobe, so common with generalized airway diseases in infants and young children, may in part be related to comparatively little collateral ventilation and air drift into regions obstructed by secretions and cellular debris.

AGE AND RESPIRATORY FUNCTION

Respiratory structures change remarkably during growth. What are the functional implications of such changes? Lung volume and volume-pressure relationships (e.g., pulmonary compliance) should reflect parenchymal (air space) development, and airflows and pressure-flow relationships (resistances and conductances) should reflect airway development. But the relationships are not as direct as they might seem.

Pulmonary compliance depends on the number of air spaces expanded, the size and geometry of the air spaces, the characteristics of their surface lining layer, and probably the properties of the lung parenchyma that change with growth and maturation. Thus newborn lungs have low compliance in part because they are not completely aerated: unexpanded portions are extremely stiff. Compliance depends as well on the degree of lung expansion: fully aerated lungs are stiffer (less compliant) at higher expansion. The compliance of fully aerated lungs measured at equivalent degrees of expansion depends not only on lung size but also on structure. Lungs of a given size (degree of growth) may have very different volume-pressure characteristics depending on what they are made of. We already know that the air spaces of newborn lungs are immature. To what extent does the increase in compliance with age reflect changes in the air space wall brought about by maturation, and to what extent does it simply reflect an increase in lung size brought about by increasing numbers of alveoli? One might expect to obtain an answer by measuring excised lungs, which can be weighed. Structurally similar lungs would be expected to have similar weight-specific compliances. But lung weight includes more than simply lung parenchyma. The contribution of extraparenchymal structures, such as bronchi and blood vessels, to lung weight is greater in immature lungs. The low weight-specific compliance of young lungs must reflect the contribution of these extraparenchymal structures (Stigol et al, 1972). Morphometric measurement of the extraparenchymal fraction, which has not as yet been done, would permit correction of weight-specific compliances for this influence.

However, changes in the shape, magnitude or curvilinearity of volume-pressure curves do point to maturational changes in growing lungs. Volume-pressure curves are frequently normalized by expressing volumes as percentages of the maximal volume observed. At low distending pressures, such as 5 cm H_2O, differences in volume, expressed as percentage of maximal volume, must reflect characteristics of the lung other than its size. Volume-pressure curves from young lungs are more curvilinear than those from older lungs (Fig. 9–3). These differences may be explained by the fact that the young lungs have immature air sacs rather than mature alveoli, and they may reflect the differences in the ratio of elastin to collagen with age. It is interesting that the difference in the curves is similar to the difference between the curves of younger adult and older adult lungs: with increasing years, the volume-pressure relationship becomes more curvilinear once again. Although the morphologic basis for this is unknown, there are functional parallels between young and elderly lungs.

The lung volume at which airway closure occurs is higher in younger children (7 years) and in elderly adults than in older children and young adults (Mansell et al, 1972). The configuration of the relationship of maximal expiratory flow and lung volume—the maximal expiratory flow volume (MEFV) curve—is similar in the child and in the elderly; in both age groups the curves are alinear compared with curves from young adults. This alinearity is compatible with decreased elastic recoil (Mead, 1978).

Changes in pulmonary resistance with age are even more difficult to interpret. Whereas compliance measurements depend entirely on pulmonary properties, measurements of resistance or its inverse, conductance, depend in part on extrapulmonary structures—namely, the upper airways. Resistance decreases and conductance increases with age. Part of the increase reflects the fact that infants are obligate nose-breathers, and older children breathe through their mouths during measurements. But even when this difference is taken into account, interpretation of the increase in conductance is complicated because the contribution of the glottis is substantial and largely unknown. Measurements in excised lungs are, accordingly, of very great interest, and those of Hogg and associates (1970) remain the most comprehensive and provocative on this point. These researchers partitioned airway resistance by means of a retrograde catheter technique into central and peripheral components (see Fig. 9–1), and their results directly contradict the anatomic conclusion that the infant's tracheobronchial tree is simply a miniature of the adult one (Hislop et al, 1972). Such a conclusion implies that the airways increase in size equidimensionally, and if that were true the contribution of peripheral airways to the total would remain nearly the same. Hogg and associates found that up to the age of 5 years, peripheral airways accounted for a much larger fraction of the total resistance than they did in older lungs. This finding has important implications in disease and very much requires confirmation.

The specific bridges between structure and function in the growing lung appear few and shaky. Some less specific but nonetheless interesting insights are available from some unusual interpretations of relatively simple tests. Specific conductances express the ratio of airway conductance to the lung volume at which the conductance is measured. This sort of normalization has been useful in accounting for the influence of lung inflation on airway conductance. In regularly expanding structures at sufficiently low flow rates, conductance varies in direct proportion to airway volume, and hence to lung volume, if the

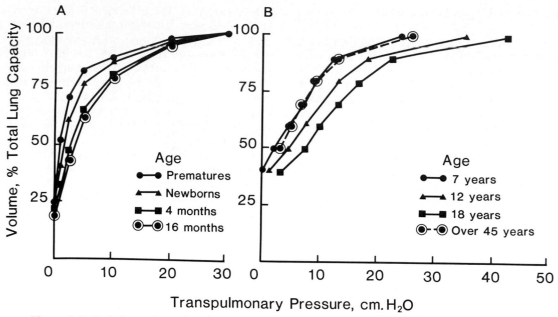

Figure 9–3. Deflation volume-pressure curves of the lung. *A,* Data plotted from curves on excised lungs obtained by Fagan (1976). The lung volume at a transpulmonary pressure of 30 cm H_2O is taken as 100 per cent of total lung capacity. *B,* Data taken from the work of Zapletal and co-workers (1976) are plotted in solid lines. Age is estimated from height. For comparison, the curve for subjects more than 45 years of age is shown with dashed lines (Turner et al, 1968). With increasing age up to young adulthood the curves become straighter, and at a given lung volume elastic recoil is greater. The curve from elderly subjects *(dashed line)* resembles that from a 7 year old.

regular expansion is shared by airways and parenchyma alike. Accordingly, specific conductance tends to be largely independent of the degree of lung expansion, which makes it a useful measurement, particularly when the degree of expansion may vary. A key point here is the use of lung volume as an indirect indicator of airway size. But lung volume is clearly a more direct indicator of parenchymal size (the volume of parenchyma and its degree of expansion). Conductance, on the other hand, does depend on airway size and on the degree of airway expansion. Therefore, specific conductance has both insensitivity to the degree of lung expansion and substantial sensitivity to the relative intrinsic size of the airways and lung parenchyma. We have seen that airways and parenchyma mature at different rates. The observation that specific conductance in infant lungs is greater than in older lungs is entirely consistent with the sequence of airway and parenchymal development (Stocks and Godfrey, 1977). The airways in the newborn lung are large compared with the relatively scanty parenchyma they serve.

Maximal expiratory flow (MEF), another measure of airway properties, depends entirely on pulmonary properties. The pertinent conductance governing MEF is entirely intrathoracic. Unfortunately, the anatomic extent of this conductance is variable, and it has no simple dependence on airway size. Nevertheless, MEFV curves can be interpreted in terms of the relative size of airways and parenchyma. The average slope of a flow-volume curve, i.e., the best straight line fit to the descending portion of the curve, ex-

presses the mean maximum rate of emptying. This rate depends mainly on the relative size of the airways and parenchyma. The smaller the lung, the more rapidly it empties through an airway of a given size and resistance. Similarly, the greater the size of the airways, and hence the lower their resistance, the more rapidly a lung of a given size empties. Estimates of the rate at which lungs empty can be made for infants, children, and adults. Infant lungs with rate constants of 7.8 empty some four times faster than adult lungs with rate constants of 1.7 (rate constant is flow/volume, which is 1/time) (Bryan and Wohl, 1986).

Dimensionally, the slope of a flow-volume curve is expressed as unit of volume/unit of time. It is no coincidence that specific conductance has the same dimension with the additional specification of pressure. Both the rate constant obtained from a flow-volume curve and the rate expressed by specific conductance reflect the "quickness" of lungs, which in turn depends on the size of airways in relation to the amount of lung being served.

CONCLUSIONS

The available measurements from infancy to adolescence reflect and parallel structural changes in the lungs. Compliance in absolute terms increases as new alveoli develop, but the changes in shape of the volume-pressure curve suggest that to some extent maturation makes the lung relatively stiffer. As the volume of the lung parenchyma enlarges relative to airway volume, specific conductance and indices of rates of emptying fall. However, these broad developmental changes may not be as important to the occurrence of lung disease as individual variability. In adults, considerable variability in indices of airway and lung size exists. Some individuals apparently have relatively large airways and small lungs, and vice versa. Some data (Dockery et al, 1983; Martin et al, 1988) indicate substantial tracking of lung volumes and of indices of airway size that have been documented from age 6 years through adolescence. These observations suggest that this dysanapsis between airway and lung parenchyma growth begins in early life and presumably is genetically determined. Whether it bears on disease susceptibility remains to be seen.

STRUCTURE AND FUNCTION AND THEIR RELATIONSHIP TO DISEASE

As pointed out in the beginning of this chapter, mortality from respiratory diseases is high in the first few years of life, falls, and then rises again with age. Similarities between the young and old lung that may be related to the pattern of incidence and severity of disease are as follows:

1. The young lung lacks elastic recoil. The aging lung loses elastic recoil.
2. As a consequence of this relative lack of lung recoil, the volume at which airways close is higher in the young and the old.
3. The high volume at which closure occurs may account for changes in arterial PO_2 with age. Arterial O_2 tensions increase throughout childhood (Gaultier et al, 1978) and decrease in the elderly.
4. The mucous gland "hypertrophy" of normal youngsters resembles changes produced by bronchitis in elderly adults.
5. Analysis of the forced expiratory maneuver—either the shape of the flow-volume curve or moment analysis of the volume-time trace (Neuberger et al, 1976)—suggests that inhomogeneity of emptying, particularly at low lung volumes, is more common in the very young and the elderly.

These similarities suggest that the immediate consequences of respiratory infections may be more severe in the young (e.g., bronchiolitis) and in the elderly (e.g., influenza).

However, the age at which a respiratory insult occurs makes a substantial difference in the lungs' regenerative response. One of the best examples may be the observation that correction of congenital diaphragmatic hernia does not result in complete development of the pulmonary vascular bed in later life (Wohl et al, 1977), presumably because the defect involves the branching of conducting pulmonary vessels, which occurs in early fetal life. In contrast, lobectomy in infancy for congenital lobar emphysema results in normal distribution of lung volumes and

pulmonary blood flow, suggesting that compensatory growth of vessels can take place after branching is complete (McBride et al, 1980). Children born prematurely appear to have impaired lung growth when examined in midchildhood (Mansell et al, 1987), perhaps because late fetal and early neonatal life is a time of alveolar multiplication. We do not know the long-term outcome with respect to lung function for very premature infants who are currently surviving into childhood. For some infants it is likely to be a complex interplay between airway and lung injury and nutritional deprivation at a time of alveolar multiplication on the one hand and the enormous regenerative capability of the infant lung on the other.

REFERENCES

Agostoni E and Mead J: Statics of the respiratory system. In Fenn WO and Rahn H (ed): Handbook of Physiology. Section 3: Respiration. Washington, DC, American Physiological Society, 1964.
Åstrand, PO: Experimental Studies of Physical Working Capacity in Relation to Sex and Age. Copenhagen, Ejnar Munksgaard, 1952.
Brody JS and Thurlbeck WM: Development, growth, and aging of the lung. In Fishman AP (ed): Handbook of Physiology. Section 3: The Respiratory System. Bethesda, Md, American Physiological Society, 1986.
Bryan AC and Wohl MEB: Respiratory mechanics in children. In Fishman AP (ed): Handbook of Physiology. Section 3: The Respiratory System. Bethesda, Md, American Physiological Society, 1986.
Bucher U and Reid L: Development of the intrasegmental bronchial tree: the pattern of branching and development of cartilage at various stages of intra-uterine life. Thorax 16:207, 1961.
Burnard ED, Grattan-Smith P, Picton-Warlow CG, and Grauaug A: Pulmonary insufficiency in prematurity. Aust Paediatr J 1:12, 1965.
Croteau JR and Cook CD: Volume-pressure and length-tension measurements in human tracheal and bronchial segments. J Appl Physiol 16:170, 1961.
Dean JM, Koehler RC, and Schleien CL: Age-related changes in chest geometry during cardiopulmonary resuscitation. J Appl Physiol 62:2212, 1987.
Dingle JG, Badger GF, and Jordan WS: Illness in the Home. Cleveland, The Press of Western Reserve University, 1964.
Dockery DW, Berkey CS, Ware JH et al: Distribution of forced vital capacity and forced expiratory volume in one second in children 6 to 11 years of age. Am Rev Respir Dis 128:405, 1983.
Dunhill MS: Postnatal growth of the lung. Thorax 17:329, 1962.
Fagan DG: Post-mortem studies of the semistatic volume-pressure characteristics of infants' lungs. Thorax 31:534, 1976.
Fagan DG: Shape changes in static V-P loops from children's lungs related to growth. Thorax 32:198, 1977.
Gaultier C, Boulé M, Allaire Y et al: Determination of capillary oxygen tension in infants and children. Assessment of methodology and normal values during growth. Bull Europ Physiopath Resp 14:287, 1978.
Grunstein MM, Tanaka DT, and Grunstein JS: Mechanism of substance P-induced bronchoconstriction in maturing rabbit. J Appl Physiol 57:1238, 1984.
Hiatt P, Eigen H, Yu P, and Tepper RS: Bronchodilator responsiveness in infants and young children with cystic fibrosis. Am Rev Respir Dis 137:119, 1988.
Hislop A, Muir DCF, Jacobsen M et al: Postnatal growth and function of the pre-acinar airways. Thorax 27:265, 1972.
Hogg JC, Williams J, Richardson JB et al: Age as a factor in the distribution of lower-airway conductance and in the pathologic

anatomy of obstructive lung disease. New Engl J Med 282:1283, 1970.

Inners CR, Terry PB, Traystman RJ, and Menkes HA: Collateral ventilation and the middle lobe syndrome. Am Rev Respir Dis 118:305, 1978.

Lenny W and Milner AD: At what age do bronchodilator drugs work? Arch Dis Child 58:532, 1978.

Loda FA, Glezen WP, and Clyde WA Jr: Respiratory disease in group day care. Pediatrics 49:428, 1972.

Lowen MA, Bergman MJ, Cutaia MV, and Porcelli RJ: Age-dependent effects of chronic hypoxia on pulmonary vascular reactivity. J Appl Physiol 63:1122, 1987.

McBride JT, Wohl MEB, Strieder DJ et al: Lung growth and airway function after lobectomy in infancy for congenital lobar emphysema. J Clin Invest 66:962, 1980.

Mansell AL, Bryan C, and Levison H: Airway closure in children. J Appl Physiol 33:711, 1972.

Mansell AL, Driscoll JM, and James LS: Pulmonary follow-up of moderately low birth weight infants with and without respiratory distress syndrome. J Pediatr 110:111, 1987.

Martin TR, Feldman HA, Fredberg JJ et al: Relationship between maximal expiratory flows and lung volumes in growing humans. J Appl Physiol 65:822, 1988.

Matsuba K and Thurlbeck WM: A morphometric study of bronchial and bronchiolar walls in children. Am Rev Respir Dis 105:908, 1972.

Mead J: Analysis of the configuration of maximum expiratory flow-volume curves. J Appl Physiol 44:156, 1978.

Motoyama EK, Brody JS, Colten HR, and Warshaw JB: Postnatal lung development in health and disease. Am Rev Respir Dis 137:742, 1988.

Motoyama EK, Fort MD, Klesh KW et al: Early onset of airway reactivity in premature infants with bronchopulmonary dysplasia. Am Rev Respir Dis 136:50, 1987.

Neuburger N, Levison H, Bryan AC, and Kruger K: Transit time analysis of the forced expiratory spirogram in growth. J Appl Physiol 40:329, 1976.

Post M and van Golde LMG: Metabolic and developmental aspects of the pulmonary surfactant system. Biochim Biophys Acta, 947:249, 1988.

Rabinovitch M, Gamble WJ, Miettinen OS, and Reid L: Age and sex influence on pulmonary hypertension of chronic hypoxia and on recovery. Am J Physiol 240:H62, 1981.

Reid LM: The pulmonary circulation: remodeling in growth and disease. Am Rev Respir Dis 119:531, 1979.

Rendas A, Branthwaite M, Lennox S, and Reid L: Response of the pulmonary circulation to acute hypoxia in the growing pig. J Appl Physiol 52:811, 1982.

Sauder RA, McNicol KJ, and Stecenko AA: Effect of age on lung mechanics and airway reactivity in lambs. J Appl Physiol 61:2074, 1986.

Stigol LA, Vawter GF, and Mead J: Studies on elastic recoil of the lung in a pediatric population. Am Rev Respir Dis 105:552, 1972.

Stocks J and Godfrey S: Specific airway conductance in relation to postconceptional age during infancy. J Appl Physiol 43:144, 1977.

Tepper RS: Airway reactivity in infants: a positive response to methacholine and metaproterenol. J Appl Physiol 62:1155, 1987.

Terry PB, Menkes JA, and Traystman RJ: Effects of maturation and aging on collateral ventilation in sheep. J Appl Physiol 62:1028, 1987.

Turner JM, Mead J, and Wohl MEB: Elasticity of human lungs in relation to age. J Appl Physiol 25:664, 1968.

Vital Statistics: Massachusetts 1979. Commonwealth of Massachusetts, Department of Public Health, 1980.

Whaley SL, Muggenburg BA, Seiler FA, and Wolff RK: Effect of aging on tracheal mucociliary clearance in beagle dogs. J Appl Physiol 62:1331, 1987.

Wohl MEB, Griscom NT, Strieder DJ et al: The lung following repair of congenital diaphragmatic hernia. J Pediatr 90:405, 1977.

Zapletal A, Paul T, and Samanek M: Pulmonary elasticity in children and adolescents. J Appl Physiol 40:953, 1976.

10

JOSEPH A. BELLANTI, M.D., and
JOSEF V. KADLEC, M.D., Ph.D.

HOST DEFENSE MECHANISMS

Significant advances have been made in our knowledge of the host defenses of the developing fetus, infant, and child that have had a profound impact on the study of pediatric pulmonary disease. This knowledge has led to a better understanding of the various mechanisms of tissue injury that occur at critical points of vulnerability of the developing lung. In the newborn period, for example, injury may result from immunologic immaturity and subsequent infection, e.g., group B streptococcal pneumonia, or from surfactant deficiency, e.g., respiratory distress of the newborn. In the older child, derangements of the immune system, both genetic and environmental in origin, may contribute to immune deficiency as well as to hypersensitivity and other forms of immunologically mediated pulmonary disease, e.g., asthma. The importance of this knowledge for those entrusted with the care of infants and children is seen not only in the form of better diagnostic and therapeutic measures for the child with pulmonary disease but also in the ultimate application in disease prevention through the identification and elimination of antecedent factors that contribute to end-stage lung disease in the adult.

This chapter focuses on (1) a unifying model for immunologic processes, (2) *nonspecific* and *specific* pulmonary defense mechanisms, (3) a unifying framework of immunologic mechanisms involved in pediatric pulmonary diseases, and (4) a summary of the clinical applications of this knowledge to specific pediatric pulmonary diseases.

A UNIFYING MODEL FOR IMMUNOLOGIC PROCESSES

In classic usage, host defense mechanisms have been traditionally divided into the *nonspecific* (e.g., phagocytosis and the inflammatory response) and the *specific* or *immunologic* (e.g., humoral [B cell] and cell-mediated [T cell]) responses (Bellanti, 1977). Although this is a convenient classification, it is generally recognized that the immunologic system is not so easily divisible into such components but rather represents an interrelated and interdependent network of cells and cell products responsive to a foreign stimulus. It is more appropriate to present a contemporary model of immunologic processes that takes into account not only the intrinsic interactive considerations within the immune system itself but also the modulating influences of other systems with which it is linked, e.g., neuroendocrine system (Bellanti, 1985).

For ease of discussion, consider six components of the immune response: (1) the environment, (2) the target cells, (3) the phagocytic cells, (4) the mediator cells and mediators, (5) the complement system and other biologic amplification systems, and (6) the specific antigen-recognition cells (B lymphocytes and T lymphocytes) and their products.

THE ENVIRONMENT

The basic requirement for induction of an immune response is contact with a foreign configuration, which usually arises from the external environment but which also may arise within the host as an alteration of a normal component of the internal environment (Fig. 10–1). These foreign substances within the external environment range from the simplest of low molecular weight chemicals to the most complex array of microbial agents; the foreign components that arise within the internal environ-

ment are exemplified by altered self-components (i.e., virally or chemically altered target cells) or transformed or malignant cells. Those substances that can evoke immunologic responses are commonly referred to as *immunogens* or *antigens,* and all of them are recognized as being *foreign* by the host. *Allergens* are a specialized class of immunogens and take part in hypersensitivity (i.e., allergic reactions).

Of particular importance in the development of pulmonary defense systems of the fetus and neonatal infant is the abrupt change from an aquatic environment in utero to an air-filled, gaseous environment at the moment of first breathing. Prominent in the internal environment associated with this event are large amounts of surfactant-related alveolar material produced by type II alveolar cells and residual debris in amniotic fluid, e.g., squamous epithelial cells (Bellanti et al, 1979). In the developing infant, alveolar macrophages play an important role in both the scavenging of inactive or excess intra-alveolar surfactant and the clearing of residual cellular debris. Moreover, as will be described later, the presence of intra-alveolar surfactant may also play an important modulatory role in the postnatal influx (i.e., chemotaxis) and the development of alveolar macrophages.

THE TARGET CELLS

The introduction of an environmental agent into the host may have an adverse effect on a wide variety of target cells (Fig. 10–2). These effects vary according to the type and location of the target cell as well as the portal of entry of the environmental agent (Table 10–1). The target cell may sustain a direct injury from the environmental agent or an indirect

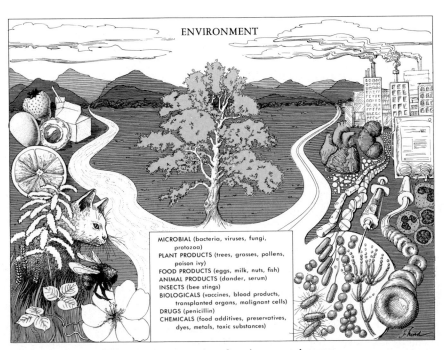

Figure 10–1. Examples of environmental agents.

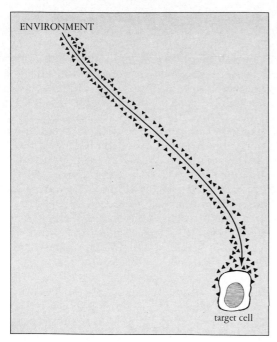

Figure 10–2. Effects of environmental agents on target cells.

injury through an immunologic attack on a target cell that has been altered by an environmental agent, e.g., a virus or a chemical. The net effect of these interactions is target cell dysfunction or cell death. Some of the more common target cells are shown in Table 10–1. Of importance in pulmonary defense are the epithelial, smooth muscle, and glandular cells of the respiratory tract. The impact of environmental agents or products of the inflammatory response on these target cells may be epithelial damage, bronchospasm, vasodilation, and increased secretion of mucus characteristic of such diseases as bronchial asthma.

THE PHAGOCYTIC CELLS

The phagocytic cells are those elements of the immunologic system that are involved in the process of engulfment and uptake of particles (i.e., phagocytosis) from the external environment. These cells are positioned strategically between the external en-

vironment and the target cells, thus providing a barrier protecting the target cells from subsequent injury (Fig. 10–3). In humans, phagocytosis is generally carried out primarily by mononuclear phagocytes (macrophages), neutrophils, and eosinophils. Shown in Table 10–2 are the phagocytic cells together with the agents responsible for their mobilization and their postulated function.

The pulmonary alveolar macrophage occupies a pivotal role as the primary cell of host defense linking both the nonspecific and specific immunologic systems. It is the only phagocytic cell that comes into direct contact with the external environment and is normally present in the alveolar space as a "resident cell"; neutrophils and eosinophils are called forth only under conditions of inflammation or hypersensitivity. As such, the alveolar macrophage functions in the detoxification of the inhaled particulate materials that reach the alveolus, and, as described earlier, in the scavenging of inactive or excess intraalveolar surfactant. The cell produces activated forms of oxygen that are important in microbicidal activity, e.g., superoxide and hydrogen peroxide, and is involved in the detoxification of these toxic oxygen metabolites by superoxide dismutase (SOD) (Bellanti et al, 1979).

The alveolar macrophage also plays an important role in the induction of specific immunologic responses and functions as an accessory cell facilitating antigen presentation and regulating lymphocyte function. Evidence suggests that the alveolar macrophage may serve a helper function in augmenting specific immune responses as well as a suppressor function in shielding the pulmonary lymphoid tissue from antigenic insult and subsequent immunologic injury (Herscowitz, 1985). As described later, there is a mobilization of inflammatory cells (neutrophils) into the lung tissue during conditions of chronic pulmonary infection or inflammation. Evidence suggests that the phagocytic cells that infiltrate as part of the inflammatory response—neutrophils, eosinophils and macrophages—may actually contribute to tissue injury by the release of intracellular products, such as lysosomal enzymes. Many of the pulmonary manifestations of diseases such as cystic fibrosis are thought to be caused by tissue injury resulting from these mechanisms; therapeutic approaches, such as

Table 10–1. EFFECTS OF THE ENVIRONMENT ON TARGET CELLS

Location of Target Cell	Example of Effect	Result
SKIN	Disruption of epidermal cells	Dermatitis
GASTROINTESTINAL TRACT		
Mucosal cell	Destruction	Gastrointestinal bleeding
Smooth muscle	Increased contractility	Diarrhea, vomiting
Glandular cell	Increased secretion	Increased mucus production
RESPIRATORY TRACT		
Smooth muscle	Increased contraction	Bronchospasm
Glandular cell	Increased secretion	Increased mucus production
CIRCULATORY SYSTEM		
Endothelial cell	Increased intercellular pore size	Edema
Formed elements	Destruction of erythrocytes	Anemia

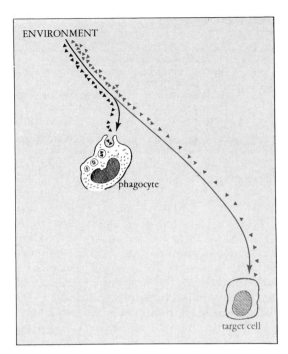

Figure 10–3. Phagocytic cells: mobilization factors and functions.

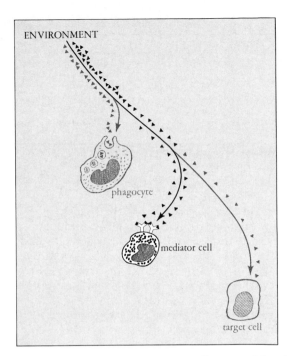

Figure 10–4. Mediator cells: products (mediators) and functions.

steroids, are being directed at the suppression of these responses.

THE MEDIATOR CELLS AND MEDIATORS

Certain cells of the body contain low molecular weight and macromolecular chemical substances with profound biologic properties that can amplify the effects of other cells of the immune system and that, at times, can have an adverse effect on target cells, contributing to dysfunction and disease (Fig. 10–4). These cells are referred to as the *mediator* cells and their products as the *mediator substances*. The mediator cells represent a heterogeneous collection of morphologic types that include mast cells, basophils, platelets, enterochromaffin cells, and phagocytic cells (Table 10–3). The best studied of these are the mast cells and basophils, which are important in certain immediate hypersensitivity diseases, including allergic rhinitis and asthma. Evidence suggests that there are at least two subsets of mast cells in the lung: (1) the *connective tissue mast cells,* which are found in the interstitial tissues surrounding bronchial mucosae, alveoli, and blood vessels; and (2) the *mucosal mast cells,* which are primarily located within the bronchial lumen and at the mucosal surface. Differences in mediator content have been observed between these two subpopulations, and, similarly, variations in response to specific pharmacologic agents, such as cromolyn, have been reported.

Following the interaction of the environmental agent with a mediator cell, the release of mediators occurs by one of two mechanisms: (1) *direct* or nonspecific release, which occurs following direct contact of the environmental agent with the cell membrane (e.g., radiocontrast material, codeine); and (2) *indirect* or specific release, which occurs after interaction of the environmental agent (e.g., allergen) with membrane-bound IgE specific antibody.

The mediator substances may be classified according to molecular size into (1) *low molecular weight mediators* (<1000), e.g., histamine, leukotrienes; and

Table 10–2. MOBILIZATION FACTORS AND FUNCTIONS OF PHAGOCYTIC CELLS

Phagocytic Cell	Agents Responsible for Mobilization of Cells	Cell Product or Function
Macrophages (monocytes)	Chemotactic factors, e.g., migration inhibitory factor (MIF), lymphokines	Processed immunogen, removal of environmental agent, prostaglandins
Neutrophils	Chemotactic factors (complement-associated and bacterial factors), lymphokines	Kallikreins (producing kinins), basic peptides, prostaglandins
Eosinophils	Identical with neutrophils, specific chemotactic factors, lymphokines	Ingestion of immune complexes, antagonize effects of mediators, e.g., leukotrienes

Table 10–3. PRODUCTS AND FUNCTIONS OF MEDIATOR CELLS

Mediator Cell	Mediator Product	Action
Mast cells	Histamine, leukotrienes C_4, D_4, E_4 (formerly SRS-A), prostaglandins, ECF-A	Increased vascular permeability, bronchoconstriction, eosinophilotaxis, increased mucus production
Basophils, platelets	Vasoactive amines (histamine, serotonin)	Increased vascular permeability, smooth muscle constriction, increased mucus production
Enterochromaffin cells	Serotonin	Vasodilation
Neutrophils	SRS, ECF	Contractility of smooth muscle, eosinophilotaxis

SRS-A, slow-reacting substance of anaphylaxis; ECF-A, eosinophil chemotactic factor of anaphylaxis; SRS, slow-reacting substance; ECF, extracellular fluid.

(2) *macromolecular mediators* (>1000), e.g., lysosomal enzymes (Table 10–4). Some of these mediators are synthesized and stored in the mast cells and are available for immediate release, for example, the preformed mediators, such as histamine; others are newly synthesized and require a period of time before being released, such as arachidonic acid metabolites. Once released or generated, the mediators have a twofold effect and can interact with either (1) a *target cell* with immediate sequelae, e.g., bronchospasm, edema, and mucus production—the immediate allergic response (IAR) characteristic of asthma; or (2) *cells of the immunologic system*, e.g., an influx of inflammatory cells with delayed manifestations—the *late allergic response (LAR)* (Fig. 10–5) (Nsouli et al, 1988).

THE COMPLEMENT SYSTEM AND OTHER BIOLOGIC AMPLIFICATION SYSTEMS

A number of other systems can amplify the immunologic responses, the most important of which is the complement system. This system involves at least 20 proteins that circulate in the plasma and that can be activated by two independent pathways termed the *classical* and the *alternative* pathways (Fig. 10–6). The complement system fulfills four major roles in host defense: (1) coating of pathogenic organisms or immune complexes with opsonins, which result in their removal by phagocytes (C3b); (2) activation of inflammatory cells, i.e., through stimulation of che-

motaxis (C5a and C567); (3) anaphylatoxin activity, which enhances the release of mediators from mediator cells (C3a, C4a and C5a); and (4) killing of target cells (activation of the entire sequence of activation through C9). In addition to the complement system, there are a number of other biologic amplification systems, including the clotting system and products of the neuroendocrine system, e.g., substance P, all of which can interact and enhance various components of the immune system.

THE SPECIFIC ANTIGEN-RECOGNITION CELLS (B LYMPHOCYTES AND T LYMPHOCYTES) AND THEIR PRODUCTS

The specific antigen-recognition cells include two universes of lymphocytes that interact with the environmental agent in an immunologically specific man-

Table 10–4. MEDIATORS RELEASED IN RESPONSE TO ENVIRONMENTAL AGENTS

Low molecular weight mediators (<1000)
  Histamine
  Serotonin
  Kinins
  Slow-reacting substance of anaphylaxis (SRS-A)
    (now leukotrienes C_4, D_4, E_4)
  Arachidonic acid metabolites
  Eosinophil chemotactic factors of anaphylaxis
    (i.e., prostaglandins, leukotrienes) (ECF-A)
  Platelet-activating factor (PAF)
Macromolecular mediators (>1000)
  Lysosomal enzymes
  Cationic proteins of polymorphonuclear leukocytes
  Complement and coagulation components; neuropeptides

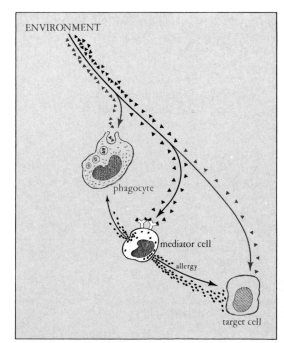

Figure 10–5. Mediator products and their effects on target cells (e.g., allergy) or phagocytic cells.

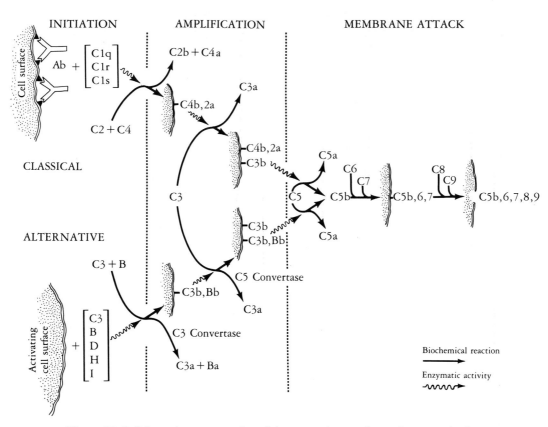

Figure 10–6. Schematic representation of the two pathways of complement activation.

ner. These include (1) the bone marrow, or bursa-dependent B lymphocytes, which provide humoral (antibody) immunity; and (2) thymus-dependent, or T lymphocytes, which participate in cell-mediated immunity.

B Lymphocytes and Their Products (Immunoglobulins)

The B lymphocytes are cells that respond to antigens by an exquisitely sensitive and specific receptor unit provided by intact immunoglobulin on the surface of these cells (Fig. 10–7). As a consequence of the binding of antigen with the surface receptor, the cell differentiates into clones of antibody-secreting plasma cells, each of which secretes a single class of immunoglobulin that is specific for the antigen. In humans there are five classes (isotypes) of immunoglobulins: IgG, IgM, IgA, IgD, and IgE. The physical, chemical, and biologic properties of these immunoglobulins are shown in Table 10–5.

Of importance in lung defense mechanisms is the discovery of an immunologic system unique to mucosal surfaces, the mucosa-associated lymphoid tissue (MALT), found in bodily tracts exposed to the external environment, e.g., respiratory and gastrointestinal tracts (Bellanti, 1971). In the lung, this system is referred to as the bronchus-associated lymphoid tissue (BALT) and is characterized by the presence of secretory immunoglobulin A (s-IgA), which is

structurally a dimer of serum IgA with an additional component—the secretory component—unique to this immunoglobulin (Bienenstock et al, 1983). Produced locally in B cells of the BALT, the s-IgA is an important immunoglobulin of local defense to microbial agents. Several clinical states have been described in which deficiency of s-IgA is associated with recurrent sinopulmonary infections, e.g., ataxiatelangiectasia.

From a developmental standpoint, the appearance of the immunoglobulins demonstrates a maturational sequence. The IgMs are the first to appear in infancy and can be demonstrated even in uterine life and in the neonate; the predominance of IgM-associated antibody responses during this period has been shown to be very helpful diagnostically. The IgGs attain maturation next, followed by IgA and IgE.

Once secreted by B lymphocytes, the primary effect of extracellular antibody is its binding with antigen. In addition, antibody may have secondary interactions with *phagocytic cells, mediator cells,* and *target cells.*

The effect of antibody on phagocytic cells is shown in Figure 10–8. Three types of interactions are seen: (1) the direct binding of antibody to the surface of the phagocytic cells (cytophilic antibody), (2) the uptake of antigen-antibody (complexes through the Fc receptor), and (3) the uptake of antigen-antibody-complement complexes through the C3b receptor of complement. The coating of certain encapsulated bacterial organisms by immunoglobulins (IgG, IgM)

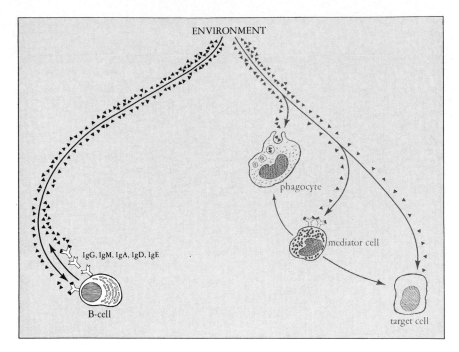

Figure 10-7. Reaction of B lymphocyte to environmental agent through its surface receptor, with resultant antibody production.

or by certain complement components (e.g., C3b) facilitates their uptake by phagocytic cells; collectively these substances are referred to as *opsonins*. The effect of antibody on mediator cells is shown in Figure 10-9. Certain classes of immunoglobulins, e.g., IgE, can attach to the mediator cells by virtue of their Fc fragments. Following the interaction of at least two of these membrane-bound molecules with antigen, the release of mediators occurs (see Fig. 10-9). Occasionally under abnormal circumstances, antibody may be directed against the target cells themselves (Fig. 10-10). This situation is totally anomalous, but it does occur in many of the immunologically mediated diseases, i.e., autoimmune diseases.

T Lymphocytes and Their Products

The T lymphocytes are those lymphocytes that come under the inductive influence of the thymus during maturation. These cells are responsible for cell-mediated immunity (delayed hypersensitivity)

and respond to the environmental agent through an interaction of antigen with another type of surface receptor (Fig. 10-11). The T antigen-specific receptor consists of certain domains of the immunoglobulin that allow the receptor to bind with its specific antigen.

Following the interaction of antigen with its receptor, the T cell undergoes a series of morphologic, biologic, and biochemical events. In this activated state, the T cell may function directly or through the elaboration of certain products, i.e., lymphokines. Shown in Table 10-6 is a partial list of these T cell products. The best studied of the classic lymphokines is migration inhibitory factor (MIF), which inhibits the migration of macrophages and activates these cells metabolically (Fig. 10-12). Many of these substances have been identified as molecules that are synthesized by one group of leukocytes and that stimulate another group, i.e., the interleukins (Table 10-7). A major investigative effort has been directed to the characterization of these molecules, particularly interleukin-2 (IL-2), which has been studied for

Text continued on page 193

Table 10-5. SOME PHYSICAL AND BIOLOGIC PROPERTIES OF HUMAN IMMUNOGLOBULIN CLASSES

Class	Mean Serum Concentration (mg/ 100 ml)	Molecular Weight	$S_{20,w}$	Mean Survival T/2 (days)	Biologic Function	Receptors On	Heavy Chain Designation	No. of Subclasses
IgG or γG	1240	150,000	7	23	Fix complement Cross placenta Heterocytotropic antibody	Polys, lymphocytes, monocytes	γ	4
IgA or γA	280	170,000	7, 10, 14	6	Secretory antibody Properdin pathway	Polys, lymphocytes, monocytes	α	2
IgM or γM	120	890,000	19	5	Fix complement	Lymphocytes	μ	1
IgD or γD	3	150,000	7	2.8	Lymphocyte surface receptor	—	δ	2
IgE or γE	0.03	196,000	8	1.5	Reaginic antibody Homocytotropic antibody	Mast cells Lymphocytes	ε	1

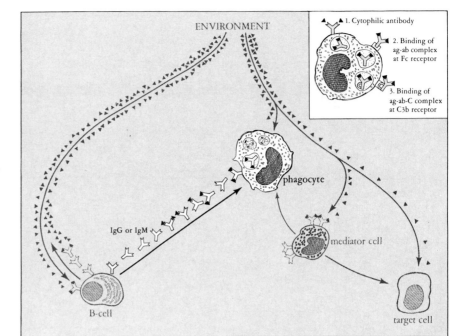

Figure 10–8. Responses of antibody with phagocytic cells.

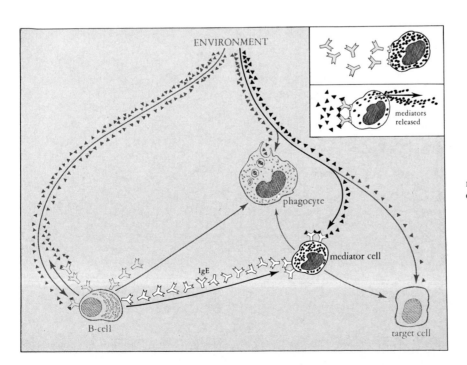

Figure 10–9. Responses of antibody with mediator cells with resultant release of mediators (inset).

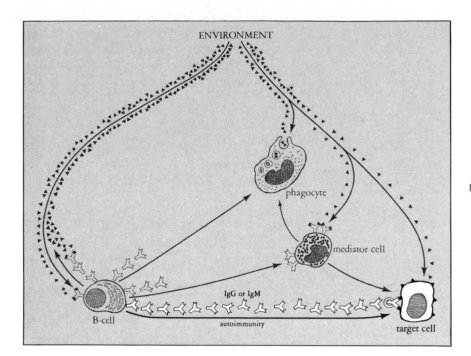

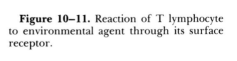

Figure 10–10. Effects of antibody on target cells with resultant autoimmunity.

Figure 10–11. Reaction of T lymphocyte to environmental agent through its surface receptor.

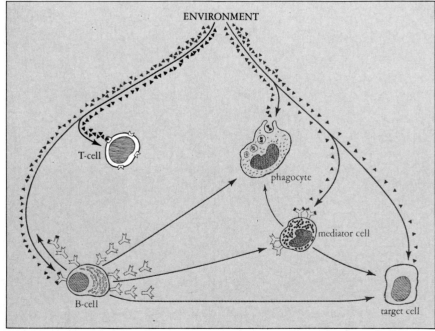

Table 10–6. PHYSICAL AND BIOLOGIC PROPERTIES OF EFFECTOR MOLECULES OF CELL-MEDIATED IMMUNITY

Lymphokine	Molecular Weight	Physical Properties	Activities	
			In vitro	In vivo
Transfer factors	<10,000 ?	Heat labile; (a) dialyzable polypeptide (b) nondialyzable	Mediator production Lymphocyte transformation	Transfer of reactivity to uncommitted lymphocytes
MIF (macrophage activating factor)	25,000–55,000	Heat stable; nondialyzable protein	Prevents random migration of macrophages; may activate macrophages	May lead to accumulation of macrophages; may increase phagocytosis and killing
Leukocyte inhibitory factor	68,000	Protein	Prevents migration of PMNs	Untested
Lymphotoxin(s)	25,000–150,000	Heat labile; nondialyzable protein	Target cell injury	May destroy target cells
Skin-reactive factor(s)	70,000			Localized cutaneous reaction
Chemotactic factors	12,000–60,000	Heat stable; nondialyzable protein	Attracts macrophages; attracts PMNs	Untested
Mitogenic factors	25,000	Heat stable; nondialyzable protein	Nonspecific lymphocyte transformation	Untested
Interferons (α, β, γ)	25,000–100,000	Heat stable; nondialyzable	Inhibits viral replication	Inhibits viral replication

PMN, polymorphonuclear neutrophils.

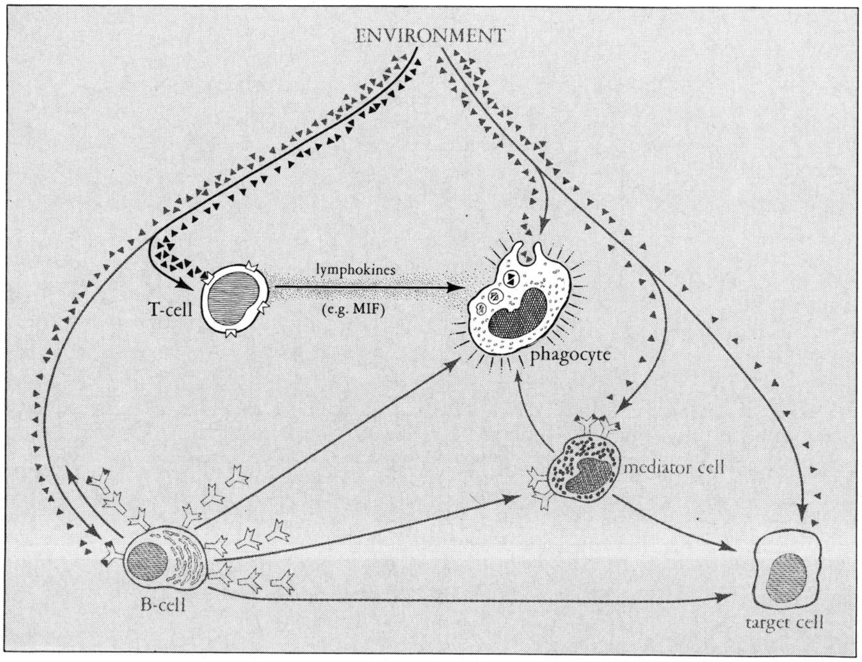

Figure 10–12. Responses of lymphokines (e.g., elaborated from T lymphocytes) on phagocytic cells (e.g., macrophages).

Table 10–7. CHARACTERISTICS OF INTERLEUKINS

	Form	Source	Targets
IL-1	Interleukin-1 alpha (15–17 KD, pI 5.0) Interleukin-1 beta (15–17 KD, pI 7.0)	Monocytes, macrophages Dendritic cells, fibroblasts Astrocytes, keritinocytes	T cells—stimulate lymphokine release B cells—stimulate activated B cells to proliferate with IL-4 and to differentiate with IL-6 NK cells—stimulate cytotoxicity Other—cell growth, catabolism, fever, chemotaxis
IL-2	Interleukin-2 (15 KD, pI 6.8, 7.1)	Activated T cells	T cells—stimulate growth of activated T cells and thymocytes, lymphokine production, and differentiation of activated B cells NK cells—stimulate cytotoxic activity Monocytes—stimulate cytotoxicity, metabolism Other—stimulate oligodendroglial cell maturation
IL-3	Interleukin-3 (14–28 KD)	Activated T cells	Multipotent stem cells—stimulate growth of progenitors including erythrocytes, neutrophils, eosinophils, basophils, macrophages, and megakaryocytes Mast cells—support growth
IL-4	Interleukin-4 (14 KD)	Activated T cells	T cells—proliferation of resting and activated T cells B cells—proliferation of activated B cells, increased expression of Fc episilon receptors and class II MHC molecules, and increased IgE and Fc episilon receptor secretion Mast cells—stimulation of growth Lymphoid precursors—stimulation of early (pre T and pre B) cells in bone marrow
IL-5	Interleukin-5 (12.3 KD)	Activated cells	T cells—induction of cytotoxic T cells and enhancement of IL-2 receptor expression B cells—stimulate the growth and differentiation of activated B cells, upregulate IL-2 receptor expression, increased synthesis of secretory IgA Eosinophils—differentiation
IL-6	Interleukin-6 (26 KD)	Activated monocytes HTLV-1 Transformed T cells, fibroblasts, and carcinoma cells	B cells/plasmacytomas—growth and differentiation Fibroblasts—increased class I MHC expression Hepatocytes—increased synthesis of acute phase proteins

KD, kathodol duration; HTLV-1, human T cell lymphotropic virus type I; NK, natural killer; MHC, major histocompatibility complex.

its therapeutic use, i.e., IL-2-stimulated or lympho-kine-activated killer cells (LAK) (Rosenberg et al, 1987).

In addition to its response to extracellular antigen, the T lymphocyte can also participate in the recognition of associated antigens in three major ways (Fig. 10–13): (1) direct lymphocyte-dependent cytotoxicity; (2) elaboration of lymphotoxin; and (3) antibody-dependent cytotoxicity (ADCC), in which certain T lymphocyte subsets, the killer (K) cells, linked by immunoglobulin, lead to target cell destruction. An additional pathway of direct target cell destruction is mediated by a group of cells that occur naturally, i.e., natural killer (NK) cells that do not require prior sensitization.

Because of the powerful approach of monoclonal antibody technology, the T lymphocytes have been characterized into several T cell subsets. Table 10–8 lists the more common T cell populations together with their postulated functions. Two of these T cell subsets that have received considerable significance in several clinical entities are the CD4 (cluster of diversity 4, formerly T4) and CD8 (cluster of diversity 8, formerly T8) subsets. The CD4 lymphocytes interact with B cells to facilitate the production of antibody, i.e., "helper cells"; the CD8 lymphocytes can inhibit the production of antibody by B cells, i.e., suppressor cells (Fig. 10–14). Normally the ratio of CD4 to CD8 is approximately 1.8:1, but in certain chronic disease states, i.e., chronic viral infections

such as acquired immune deficiency syndrome (AIDS), the CD4 to CD8 ratio is reversed owing to a destruction of the CD4 or an increase of the CD8 lymphocyte populations. There are similar controls exerted by T regulatory lymphocytes on T cell responses.

As described previously, the macrophage is a pivotal cell that interacts with T and B lymphocytes and is necessary for the induction of T cell responses as well as T cell-regulated B cell responses (Fig. 10–15). The cellular interactions of macrophages, T cells, and B cells appear to be genetically restricted by products of the major histocompatibility complex (MHC) locus. These products include class I molecules that are involved in T to T cellular interactions and class II molecules that are found on macrophages and other cells that present antigen to T cells, i.e., CD4 cells. A number of products of the macrophages, e.g., IL-1 and lymphocytes (IL-2), appear to play major roles in these intercellular communications. The total array of these responses is shown in Figure 10–16.

NONSPECIFIC AND SPECIFIC PULMONARY DEFENSE MECHANISMS

The respiratory mucous membrane is the most extensive tissue that forms a boundary between the

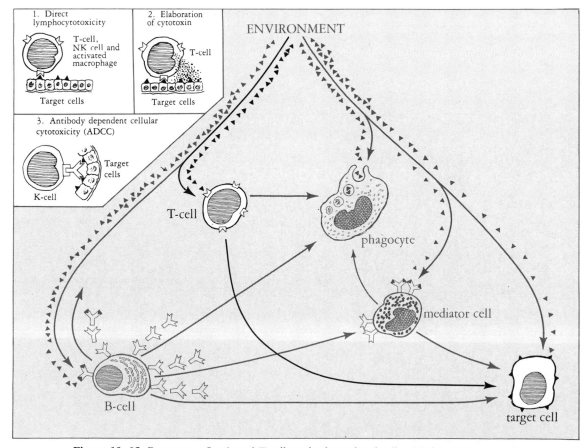

Figure 10–13. Responses of activated T cells and other related cells with foreign target cells.

Table 10–8. MONOCLONAL ANTIBODIES TO HUMAN T LYMPHOCYTE SURFACE ANTIGENS

Cluster Designation	Monoclonal Antibodies	Population Defined	Comments
CD5	Anti-T1	All mature T cells and medullary thymocytes express T1, T3, and T12. In addiction, T1 is expressed at low density on cortical thymocytes.	Modulates
CD3	Anti-T3	—	Modulates and is linked to antigen-specific T cell responses. Antibody is mitogenic for resting T cells.
	Anti-T12	—	Does not activate T cells or induce modulation.
CD4	Anti-T4	Majority of thymocytes and 50–65% of peripheral T cells	T4+—T cells contain all inducer functions and class II MHC specific CTL.
CD8	Anti-T5/8	Majority of thymocytes and 25–35% of peripheral T cells	T8+—T cells contain all suppressor function and class I MHC specific CTL.
CD1	Anti-T6	70–80% of thymocytes	Specific for cortical thymocytes. β_2M microglobulin associated.
	Anti-T10	All thymocytes, activated T cells, and plasma cells	Not T lineage specific
CD2	Anti-T11	All thymocytes, T cells, and plasma cells	E-rosette-associated protein. Greatest density on thymocytes and suppressor T cells.
	Anti 2H4	Present on 40% of total T cells. On T4 + cells, 40% are 2H4 + (suppressor/inducer). Also present on T8 + cells, subsets of B cells, null cells, and monocytes.	Does not activate T cells or induce modulation. T4+ 2H4+ defines the suppressor/inducer population.
	Anti-4B4	Present on 40% of total T cells. Of T4 + cells, 40% are 4B4 + (helper/inducer). Also present on T8 + cells, some B cells, null cells, and monocytes.	T4+ 4B4+ defines the helper/inducer population.
	Tal	Strongly expressed on activated T cells.	Specific for activated T cells.

CTL, cytotoxic lymphocytes; MHC, major histocompatibility complex.

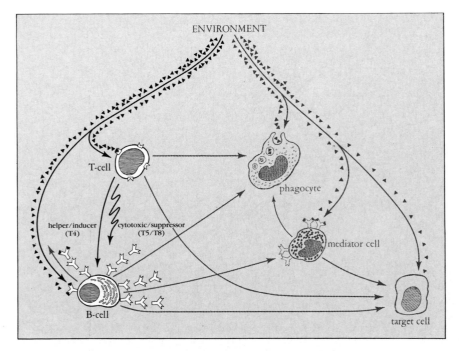

Figure 10–14. Helper and suppressor effects of T lymphocytes on B lymphocytes.

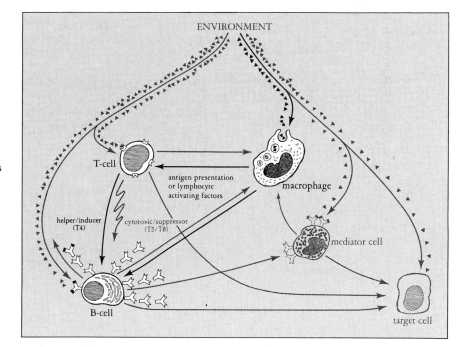

Figure 10–15. Responses of macrophages with T lymphocytes and B lymphocytes.

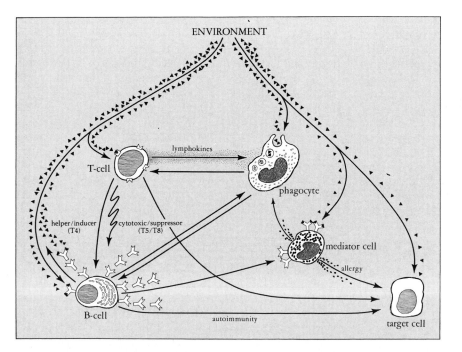

Figure 10–16. Total array of immunologic responses to the environment.

Table 10–9. NONSPECIFIC AND SPECIFIC
PULMONARY DEFENSE MECHANISMS

Nonspecific
Aerodynamic filtration
Movement of respiratory tract fluids, i.e., the mucociliary transport
  system
Detoxification systems
Chemotaxis, phagocytosis, and microbicidal activity of phagocytic
  cells
Specific
B cell (humoral)   } systemic and local
T cell (cell-mediated immunity)

host and the environment (Green et al, 1977). As such, it is exposed to the myriad of microorganisms, chemical toxins, inorganic and organic dusts, and other foreign substances that characterize the complex environment we live in. When an environmental agent enters the respiratory tract, it encounters a variety of pulmonary defense mechanisms. The degree to which these pulmonary defense mechanisms are effective determines whether the host will maintain a state of health or develop a respiratory disease. For ease of discussion, the pulmonary defense mechanisms are divided into nonspecific and specific mechanisms (Table 10–9) (Bellanti, 1977).

NONSPECIFIC DEFENSE MECHANISMS

Aerodynamic Factors

A number of anatomic and physiologic mechanisms in the lung provide a natural barrier to penetration of foreign materials beyond the respiratory epithelium. The lung has evolved as an effective organ of gas exchange. Its design is that of a bifurcating tubuloalveolar structure with multiple subdivisions capable of removing particulates by deposition in the proximal regions and by absorption of gas. Although the basic structure of the airways of the infant and those of the child share a common bronchopulmonary anatomy, significant anatomic and physiologic differences contribute to a greater vulnerability of the airways of the infant. As described in Chapter 1, the small airways make a greater contribution to airway resistance in the infant lung (50 per cent of small peripheral airways) than they do in the adult lung (20 percent). This contribution of the small airways not only affects aerodynamic flow of gases and particulates but also explains the greater propensity for occlusion of the airways of the infant and the young child in disease states characterized by edema fluid or inflammatory exudate, i.e., asthma or bronchiolitis.

Mucociliary Transport System

The airways are lined with an epithelial membrane that gradually changes to a ciliated pseudostratified columnar epithelium until it reaches the terminal bronchioles, after which it becomes a cuboidal epithelium at the gas exchanging units, i.e., the terminal respiratory units. Ciliary cells therefore predominate throughout the major portion of the airways and provide a rhythmic beating action, propelling mucus and attached particles in an upward motion to the pharynx (Sleigh et al, 1988). This mucociliary transport system is an important nonspecific defense mechanism of the lung and is responsible for removal of inhaled particles from the airways. A disruption of this mechanism is seen in a variety of clinical disorders, e.g., cystic fibrosis.

Detoxification Systems

The lung also functions as a detoxification system for all inhaled foreign substances, rendering them harmless (Green et al, 1977). The detoxification systems are complex and include both humoral mechanisms, i.e., fluids in the bronchi and alveoli, and cellular mechanisms provided by alveolar macrophages. The detoxification systems perform the following functions: (1) neutralization of inhaled gases, e.g., SO_2 and resultant acids; (2) detoxification of oxygen and oxygen metabolites; (3) solubilization of particles; (4) killing of bacteria; and (5) digestion of antigenic substances, rendering them nonantigenic. As described previously, the alveolar macrophage plays a major role in the uptake and digestion of inhaled particulate material that has evaded more proximal mechanisms and has reached the alveoli. The alveolar macrophage is capable of removing inert, nonreplicating material, such as carbon and silica, as well as replicating organisms, such as bacteria. The alveolar macrophages laden with these particles are expelled in an upward flow and represent the only phagocytes that are continually lost from the body—expectorated in sputum by the adult or swallowed (usually) by the infant and child. For those foreign substances capable of inducing specific immune responses, the alveolar macrophage is uniquely poised for processing and induction of humoral (B cell) and cell-mediated (T cell) responses.

The alveolar fluids contain phospholipids, the major portion of which is surfactant, i.e., phosphatidylcholine produced by type II cells. In addition to its primary function of reducing surface forces in alveoli at low lung volumes to prevent alveolar collapse, alveolar lining fluids also play several other roles in pulmonary defense. Evidence suggests that these fluids are important in the influx of alveolar macrophages into alveoli at the moment of birth. In addition, alveolar lining fluids play a modulating role in macrophage function.

Studies from several laboratories suggest that alveolar lining material also modulates bactericidal activity. Studies from our laboratory (Zeligs, 1984) have demonstrated an increased phagocytic uptake but decreased microbicidal activity and chemotaxis following incubation of alveolar macrophages of newborn rabbits with surfactant-related materials or di-palmityl lecithin (DPL) or both. Alveolar lining material may amplify phagocytic function through the spreading properties of surfactant, which may assist clearance of particulates by enhancing their transport or, alternatively, by a direct enhancing effect of the lipid active component on alveolar macrophage cell membranes.

SPECIFIC (IMMUNOLOGIC) DEFENSE MECHANISMS

General Characteristics

The respiratory tract has all the components of the immune system described previously (Kaltreider, 1976; Reynolds and Merrill, 1981). Some of the earlier literature appearing in the period between 1960 and 1970 described a two-compartment system: a *local immune* response and a *systemic immune* response (Table 10–10). The local immune response is characterized predominantly by a distinctly greater ratio of IgA to IgG in various external secretions of the upper airways and by the presence of a unique form of s-IgA. Factors that favor the production of s-IgA include the local application of antigen to the respiratory tract or the use of live agents given systemically; local cell-mediated immunity response is also influenced by similar factors. The systemic immune response displays a greater ratio of IgG that reflects the distribution found in serum. This system could be stimulated by systemic introduction of antigen.

It is generally accepted that this compartmentalization is not a rigid anatomic separation but rather a relative phenomenon. Further, there is good evidence to suggest a dynamic interaction between these two components and a recirculation of lymphocytes from one compartment to another (Bienenstock et al, 1983). For example, lymphocytes from the lamina propria of the gastrointestinal tract have been shown to recirculate in the lymphoid tissue of the breast that confers IgA into breast milk. Similar recirculation pathways have been demonstrated between the respiratory tract and the systemic sites. This pattern of recirculation is influenced by different types of immunizations, doses, and characteristics of antigen (e.g., particulate, soluble, living, killed) as well as by different routes of administration (e.g., intranasal, oral, or systemic).

Humoral (B Cell) Mechanisms

As described previously, the major immunoglobulins in respiratory tract secretions include both IgA and IgG; IgA predominates in the upper respiratory tract (nasopharynx), where it has been shown to be of critical importance in the defense of the upper airway. In contrast, bronchoalveolar lavage fluids have IgA and IgG contents that are intermediate between those of serum and upper airway passages, and IgG and alveolar macrophages play a greater role in the defense of the lower airways. Although both local synthesis and transudation from serum contribute to the immunoglobulin (IgA or IgG) present in the respiratory tract, IgA appears to be synthesized predominantly as a local response, whereas IgG enters the respiratory tract under conditions of inflammation and subsequent increased vascular permeability and transudation.

Of biologic interest is the finding that the IgA antibody in the respiratory tract neutralizes viruses and attaches to epithelial cells, providing a protective barrier, and does not fix complement through the classical pathway. In the respiratory tract, complement is present only in low concentrations. Thus the pulmonary defense system favors a protective mechanism that functions by direct antigen-antibody neutralization without the participation of complement activation and its potential for adverse inflammatory responses.

The IgG in the lower tract is found in relatively higher concentrations because it can activate complement. IgG participates in both protective mechanisms, i.e., opsinization and direct lysis of bacteria, but also in the immunopathogenesis of hypersensitivity lung disease. The IgM is found in relatively low concentrations in respiratory tract secretions, and a compensatory increase in this component is found in clinical states in which IgA is deficient (Bellanti, 1977).

IgE has been detected in respiratory tract secretions, and its participation in immediate hypersensitivity reactions is well known. On contact with a specific antigen, this immunoglobulin is responsible for symptoms of allergic rhinitis in the upper airways and immediate manifestations of asthma in the lower airways. A late asthmatic response has also been described that is caused by a slow accumulation of inflammatory cells that results from other mediators released by mast cells.

Table 10–10. COMPARISON OF LOCAL AND SYSTEMIC IMMUNE RESPONSES

	Local	Systemic
Immunoglobulin distribution	IgA IgG	IgG IgA
Type	s-IgA (11S dimer)	IgA (7S; aggregates)
Variables favoring stimulation	Local immunization; use of "living" or attenuated vaccines	Systemic immunization
Cell-mediated immunity	Local immunization	Systemic immunization

Cell-Mediated (T Cell) Immune Mechanisms

In contrast to humoral (B cell) mechanisms, relatively less is known about the expression of cell-mediated immunity. This lack of knowledge is due to both a technical problem of obtaining large numbers of lymphocytes from bronchoalveolar fluids and a dearth of investigative studies of this mechanism. Nonetheless, similar compartmentalization between local and systemic cell-mediated immune responses has been observed, and more recently the intercommunications between these two systems have been recognized. Cell-mediated immune responses are particularly prominent in states of chronic inflammation or chronic infection, such as tuberculosis.

A UNIFYING FRAMEWORK OF IMMUNOLOGIC MECHANISMS INVOLVED IN PEDIATRIC PULMONARY DISEASES

Having described the various components of the immunologic system and the nonspecific and specific pulmonary mechanisms, it is possible to construct a unifying framework as a basis for a presentation of the clinical applications of this knowledge to specific pediatric pulmonary diseases (Bellanti, 1985). The lung has a number of mechanisms for the recognition and elimination of foreign substances that it may encounter. For ease of discussion, these mechanisms may be divided into three categories of response based on a hierarchic scheme of efficiency of elimination of the foreign invader (Bellanti, 1985). These responses include (1) *primary* (nonspecific), (2) *secondary* (specific), and (3) *tertiary* (tissue-damaging) (Fig. 10–17).

PRIMARY (NONSPECIFIC) IMMUNE RESPONSES

These consist of phagocytosis and the inflammatory response. In the lung, these responses are carried out primarily by the resident alveolar macrophages; under conditions of inflammation, they are carried out by polymorphonuclear leukocytes and eosinophils. The degree to which these cellular types participate depends on the nature of the foreign substance (inert versus living) and its capacity to be eliminated. Some inert particles, e.g., carbon particles, are effectively cleared through unenhanced macrophage action without stimulation of the specific immune responses. Other more complex substances, e.g., bacteria, may stimulate the influx of other phagocytic cells, e.g., polymorphonuclear neutrophils, and are cleared through antibody and complement-mediated enhanced phagocytic and microbicidal responses. Still other microorganisms (e.g., *Mycobacterium tuberculosis*) can survive within macrophages and persist and evoke subsequent secondary immune responses and in certain situations tertiary responses. Thus the inflammatory response may be beneficial in the primary encounter with foreign substance, but if it persists, it may actually contribute to tissue injury and disease. If the foreign configuration can be eliminated by the primary immune responses, the host's encounter will be terminated. If antigen continues to persist, however, specific immune responses are stimulated.

SECONDARY (SPECIFIC) IMMUNE RESPONSES

The secondary or specific immune responses consist of two effector mechanisms: (1) the elaboration

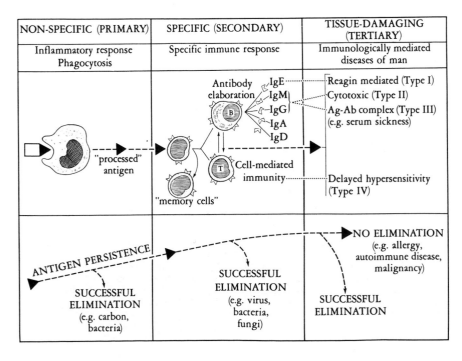

Figure 10–17. Schematic representation of the total immunologic capability of the host based on efficiency of elimination of foreign matter.

of specific antibody by B lymphocytes and (2) cell-mediated immunity that is carried out primarily by T lymphocytes (see Fig. 10–7).

Role of Antibody and Antibody-Mediated Reactions in Pulmonary Lung Defense Mechanisms

At least four (IgG, IgM, IgA, IgE) of the five known classes of human immunoglobulins participate in lung defense mechanisms. Although three classes (IgG, IgM, IgA) have been shown to exert antimicrobial (antiviral, antibacterial) activity, the IgG antibodies are the most thoroughly studied and are responsible for the major part of antimicrobial activity in serum (Bellanti, 1977). After immunization or infection with microbes, various classes of antibody appear sequentially, with IgM being stimulated initially, followed by IgG; the timing of IgA appears to be intermediate between IgM and IgG. Following reinfection, the antibodies in serum are predominantly IgG; relatively little IgM and IgA are found. The IgM responses characterize the fetal and neonatal responses.

As described earlier, the secretory IgA antibodies are produced locally at mucosal sites and appear to play an important role in localized types of infection of the upper airways. The IgG and to a lesser extent IgM play a greater role in the prevention of distal airway disease.

Some research suggests that certain viruses acting through the induction of IgE antibodies may also trigger immediate hypersensitivity responses through the release of vasoactive mediators, e.g., respiratory syncytial virus–induced bronchiolitis. Moreover, the studies of Ogra and colleagues have suggested a greater correlation between lower airway disease and the presence of IgE-associated antibody.

Role of Cell-Mediated Immune Responses in Pulmonary Defense Mechanisms

In contrast to the antibody responses that appear to function in the serum in systemic defense of immune responses to bacteria and viruses, cell-mediated immune responses are important in defense against chronic viral infections, e.g., cytomegalovirus, Epstein-Barr virus, fungal, e.g., and certain protozoal infections, e.g., *Pneumocystis carinii*. These T cell responses function by direct lysis of cells or by other mechanisms described previously. A failure of these responses is associated with a propensity to severe chronic pulmonary infections, e.g., *Pneumocystis carinii*. Local cell-mediated immune responses have been likewise demonstrated within the respiratory system and appear to be important in the defense of local infections. A characteristic pneumonitis particularly prominent in infants is lymphoid interstitial pneumonitis (LIP), which has been characteristically seen in pediatric AIDS. The precise basis for the lymphoid infiltration is not known, but several have suggested

it might be related to a chronic Epstein-Barr virus infection.

TERTIARY (TISSUE-DAMAGING) IMMUNE RESPONSES

If antigen continues to persist and cannot be eliminated by either primary or secondary immune responses, the tertiary, or tissue-damaging, responses are called into play (Bellanti, 1985). Antigen persistence may result from the nature of the antigen itself or from some genetic defect in antigen processing. If antigen persists, four types of immunologic interactions can be elicited: types I, II, III, and IV. These responses are no longer beneficial to the host and are manifested as disease phenomena. These phenomena may be either temporary or permanent, depending on the efficiency of antigen elimination. If antigen can be removed or eliminated, the tertiary response is terminated. However, if the tertiary response is ineffective and antigen still persists, the more harmful sequelae of the immune response are seen in the form of chronic inflammatory disease and pulmonary injury (Josephs, 1984).

Effector Mechanisms of Immunologic Injury

Basically, the mechanisms responsible for immune injury of the lung fall into four categories (Bellanti, 1985). The first of these, the anaphylactic or type I reaction, is mediated primarily by the IgE antibodies. Following the interaction of cell-membrane-bound IgE is a release of mediators that then leads to characteristic bronchospastic or inflammatory conditions characteristic of bronchial asthma. The type II or cytolytic response is usually mediated through complement-fixing properties of antibody. In the type III reaction, the mechanism of injury is mediated by antigen-antibody complexes that initiate a sequence of destructive inflammatory tissue reactions in the lung following the influx of phagocytic cells through chemotactic action. The fourth mechanism of immunologic injury is cell-mediated or type IV reaction. Unlike the previous three, this response does not involve antibody but is mediated directly by the action of sensitized T lymphocytes.

CLINICAL APPLICATIONS OF THIS KNOWLEDGE TO SPECIFIC PEDIATRIC PULMONARY DISEASES

The knowledge that has been generated concerning pulmonary defense mechanisms has had a direct application to a wide variety of clinical disorders. Shown in Table 10–11 are some illustrative examples of disorders of each of three compartments of the immune system presented earlier, together with their pathogenetic mechanisms and clinical manifestations. Some of these disorders are developmental in origin

Table 10–11. CLINICAL APPLICATIONS OF PULMONARY DEFENSE MECHANISMS

Type of Disorder	Example	Pathophysiologic Derangement	Clinical Manifestations
Primary (nonspecific) Immune Response			
Mucociliary transport	Cystic fibrosis	Abnormal viscid mucus	Bronchiolar obstruction, chronic infection
	Immotile cilia syndrome	Structural defect of cilia	Poor ciliary function; poor clearance; recurrent sinopulmonary infection
Alveolar macrophage	Respiratory distress syndrome	Surfactant deficiency; poor gas exchange; decreased numbers of alveolar macrophages	Respiratory failure; secondary infection
	Bronchopulmonary dysplasia	Accumulation of O_2 metabolites due to maturational deficiency of SOD in alveolar macrophages	Recurrent pneumonia, bronchiolitis, long-term sequelae
Secondary (specific) Immune Response			
Humoral	Agammaglobulinemia	Deficiency of opsonizing antibodies	Recurrent bacterial pneumonia, e.g., *Streptococcus pneumoniae*
Cell mediated	HIV infection	Deficiency of CMI	Chronic lymphoid interstitial pneumonia (LIP); opportunistic infections with CMV, EBV, *Pneumocystis carinii*
Tertiary (tissue injury) Response	Asthma	Type I; mediated by IgE; IgG4 (?)	Immediate asthmatic reaction (4–6 hours)
	Goodpasture syndrome	Type II; antibody to BM of lung and kidney—linear pattern of distribution	Pulmonary hemorrhage; hematuria
	Bronchopulmonary aspergillosis	Type I and type III; *Aspergillus fumigatus*	Pulmonary infiltration; obstructive pattern of disease; expectoration of golden mucus plugs; positive immediate skin tests and serum precipitins; can lead to chronic lung disease, e.g., emphysema
	Hypersensitivity lung disease	Type III and type IV; thermophilic actinomycetes	Pulmonary infiltrates; restrictive pattern; serum precipitins; positive delayed skin reactions; can lead to chronic lung disease, e.g., fibrosis
	Pulmonary hemosiderosis (Heiners syndrome)	Type III; antigen-antibody-complement complexes; idiopathic; some related to milk hypersensitivity; hemosiderin-laden alveolar cells; alveolar macrophages (BAL) or gastric lavage	Anemia; pulmonary infiltration; hematuria; gastrointestinal blood loss; guaiac positive stools
	Sarcoidosis	Type IV; noncaseating granuloma; alveolitis; increased T4/T8; lymphopenia	Fever; respiratory failure; chronic pulmonary infiltrates with mediastinal lymphadenopathy

HIV, human immunodeficiency virus; CMI, carbohydrate metabolism index; BAL, bronchoalveolar lavage; BM, basement membrane; CMV, cytomegalovirus; EBV, Epstein-Barr virus; SOD, superoxide dismutase.

and represent maturational delays in the appearance of immunologic cellular responses, e.g., alveolar macrophages; the inductive influences of surfactant; or critical enzymes, e.g., superoxide dismutase. Other entities are genetically determined (e.g., cystic fibrosis) and involve either defects of the primary immune system, e.g., the mucociliary transport system, or defects of the secondary immune system, e.g., the primary immune deficiency disorders. Some are disorders of tertiary function and are seen as manifestations of allergic reactions (e.g., asthma), hypersensitivity lung disease (e.g., bronchopulmonary aspergillosis), or pulmonary hemosiderosis or chronic inflammatory lung disease (e.g., sarcoidosis). These specific disease entities are described in greater detail in other chapters of this book but are represented here as examples that illustrate their clinical relevance to pediatric pulmonary disease.

REFERENCES

Bellanti JA: The biologic significance of the secretory IgA globulin system. Pediatrics 48:715, 1971.

Bellanti JA: Development of nonimmunologic, nonspecific mechanisms and specific mechanisms in resistance to airways and pulmonary infections in infants and children. Ped Res 11:224, 1977.

Bellanti JA (ed): Immunology III. Philadelphia, WB Saunders Co, 1985.

Bellanti JA, Nerurkar LS, and Zeligs BJ: Host defenses in the fetus and neonate: studies of the alveolar macrophage during maturation. Pediatrics 64:726, 1979.

Bienenstock J, Befus D, McDermott M et al: Regulation of lymphoblast traffic and localization in mucosal tissues with emphasis on IgA. Fed Proc 42:3213, 1983.

Green GM, Jakab GJ, Low RB, and Davis GS: Defense mechanisms of the respiratory membrane. Am Rev Respir Dis 115:479, 1977.

Herscowitz HB: In defense of the lung: paradoxical role of the alveolar macrophage. Ann Allergy 55:634, 1985.

Josephs SH: Immunologic mechanisms in pulmonary disease. Ped Clin N Am 31:919, 1984.

Kaltreider HB: Expression of immune mechanisms in the lung. Am Rev Respir Dis 113:347, 1976.

Newhouse M, Sanchis J, and Bienenstock J: Lung defense mechanisms. Parts I and II. New Engl J Med 295:990, 1045, 1976.

Nsouli TM, Nsouli SM, and Bellanti JA: Neuro-immuno-allergic inflammation: new pathogenetic concepts and future perspectives of immediate and late allergic reactions. Parts I and II. Ann Allergy 60:379, 483, 1988.

Reynolds HY and Merrill WW: Pulmonary immunology: Humoral and cellular immune responsiveness of the respiratory tract. In Simmons DH (ed): Current Pulmonology. Vol 3. New York, John Wiley and Sons, Inc, 1981.

Rosenberg SA, Lotze MT, Muul LM et al: A progress report on the treatment of 157 patients with advanced cancer using lymphokine-activated killer cells and interleukin-2 or high-dose interleukin-2 alone. New Engl J Med 316:889, 1987.

Sleigh MA, Blake JR, and Liron N: The propulsion of mucus by cilia. Am Rev Respir Dis 137:726, 1988.

Zeligs BJ, Nerurkar LS, and Bellanti, JA: Chemotactic and candidicidal responses of rabbit alveolar macrophages during postnatal development and the modulating roles of surfactant in these responses. Infect Immun 44:379, 1984.

INTENSIVE CARE FOR RESPIRATORY DISORDERS

11

REYNALDO D. PAGTAKHAN, M.D., and
HANS PASTERKAMP, M.D.

INTENSIVE CARE FOR RESPIRATORY DISORDERS

Disorders of respiratory structure and function with consequent ventilatory failure remain a significant cause of morbidity and mortality in infancy and childhood. This chapter considers the pediatric patient who is in imminent or frank respiratory failure, classifies the disorder according to the predominant functional abnormality, and discusses the principles of an intensive approach to therapy. Therapeutic advances have been made possible by the increased understanding of the pathophysiology of respiratory disorders, the growing availability of equipment that is appropriate for the pediatric patient for artificial ventilation and hemodynamic measurements, and the ability to monitor the results of respiratory therapy—in particular, the facility to measure arterial blood gas tensions easily by invasive as well as non-invasive techniques.

FUNCTIONAL CLASSIFICATION OF RESPIRATORY DISORDERS

Effective pulmonary exchange of oxygen and carbon dioxide requires clear airways, normal lungs and chest wall, and adequate pulmonary circulation. The integrity of the pulmonary system plus a normal respiratory control mechanism ensures adequate total alveolar ventilation and a proper relationship between ventilation and perfusion. The adequacy of gas exchange in the lungs is reflected in the tensions of oxygen and carbon dioxide in the arterial blood leaving the lung. This subject has been reviewed in great detail in Chapter 1.

Respiratory disorders may be classified according to the etiology and the dominant functional abnormality. The latter classification is utilized here because it forms the basis for a rational approach to intensive therapy of respiratory disorders. Three types of functional derangement may be delineated: (1) obstructive lung disease, (2) restrictive lung disease, and (3) primary inefficient gas transfer (Table 11–1). This approach is purposely oversimplified, and it is well recognized that in many disease processes all three types of functional derangement may be present. Inefficient gas transfer is most often

secondary to restrictive or obstructive lung disease, thus leading to a mismatching of ventilation and perfusion of the lung. Inefficient gas transfer may also appear as a primary disorder, such as a diffusion defect or an impaired ventilatory control mechanism, leading to alveolar hypoventilation.

It is possible to classify all pulmonary disease conditions into their dominant disturbance of function. Because most conditions affecting the respiratory system in the newborn period and early infancy are different from those in late infancy and childhood, it is useful to consider these separately. Tables 11–2, 11–3, and 11–4 contain illustrative causes of obstructive and restrictive lung disease and disorders of inefficient gas exchange in infancy and childhood. Any of these disorders may lead to failure of the respiratory system. The subsequent sections deal with the recognition of respiratory failure, the principles of emergency care, and the continued management of both acute and chronic respiratory disorders.

RECOGNITION OF RESPIRATORY FAILURE

Respiratory failure exists when the respiratory system is unable to deliver adequate oxygen to or to remove carbon dioxide from the pulmonary circulation, or both, thereby leading to arterial hypercapnia or hypoxemia or both. Thus respiratory failure is classified into two types to emphasize the underlying

Table 11–1. FUNCTIONAL CLASSIFICATION OF RESPIRATORY DISORDERS

Obstructive Lung Disease (Increased resistance to airflow)
  Upper respiratory tract
  Lower respiratory tract
Restrictive Lung Disease (Impaired lung expansion)
  Loss of lung volume
  Decreased distensibility
  Chest wall disturbance
Primary Inefficient Gas Transfer (Insufficient alveolar ventilation for carbon dioxide removal or impaired oxygenation of pulmonary capillary blood)
  Impaired respiratory control mechanism
  Diffusion defect

Table 11–2. CAUSES OF OBSTRUCTIVE RESPIRATORY DISEASE

	Specific Disease Conditions	
Site of Disturbance	NEWBORN AND EARLY INFANCY	LATE INFANCY AND CHILDHOOD
Upper Airway		
Anomalies	Choanal atresia, Pierre-Robin syndrome, flabby epiglottis, laryngeal web, tracheal stenosis, vocal cord paralysis, tracheomalacia, vascular ring	Tracheal stenosis, vocal cord paralysis, vascular ring, laryngotracheomalacia
Aspiration	Meconium, mucus, vomitus	Foreign body, vomitus
Infection		Laryngotracheitis, diphtheria, epiglottitis, peritonsillar or retropharyngeal abscess
Tumors	Hemangioma, cystic hygroma, teratoma	Papilloma, hemangioma, lymphangioma, teratoma, hypertrophy of tonsils and adenoids
Allergic or reflex	Laryngospasm from local irritation (intubation) or tetany	Laryngospasm from local irritation (aspiration, intubation, drowning) or tetany, allergy, smoke inhalation
Lower Airway		
Anomalies	Bronchostenosis, bronchomalacia, lobar emphysema, aberrant vessels	Bronchostenosis, lobar emphysema, aberrant vessels
Aspiration	Amniotic contents, tracheoesophageal fistula, pharyngeal incoordination, gastroesophageal reflux	Foreign body, vomitus, pharyngeal incoordination (Riley-Day syndrome), drowning, gastroesophageal reflux
Infection	Pneumonia, pertussis	Bronchiolitis, pneumonia, tuberculosis (endobronchial, hilar adenopathy), cystic fibrosis, bronchiectasis
Tumors		Bronchogenic cyst, teratoma
Allergic or reflex		Asthma, bronchospasm secondary to inhalation of noxious gases

pathogenetic mechanisms. Type I is characterized by a low arterial P_{O_2} (hypoxemia) with a normal or low arterial P_{CO_2} (eucapnia or hypocapnia). The major cause of Type I failure is a mismatching of ventilation and perfusion in the lungs. Hypoxemia may exist in the absence of respiratory failure if there is right-to-left cardiovascular shunt or low inspired P_{O_2}. Type II failure is characterized by an elevated arterial P_{CO_2} (hypercapnia) and concomitant hypoxemia (in the absence of an increased inspired O_2 concentration); thus the hallmark of Type II failure is alveolar hypoventilation.

Respiratory failure may also be classified as acute or chronic depending on its mode of development and the urgency of the need for medical attention. Chronic respiratory failure presupposes an underlying chronic respiratory disease associated with either Type I or Type II failure. The patient is often able to lead a relatively normal life but may present in acute failure as a result of a respiratory infection. The stability of chronic respiratory failure is due to the ability of the patient to adjust the work of breathing and to the adequacy of renal compensation for retained CO_2. Assessment of acid-base balance helps in the evaluation not only of CO_2 retention per se but also of whether the process is acute (before

Table 11–3. CAUSES OF RESTRICTIVE RESPIRATORY DISEASE

	Specific Disease Conditions	
Site of Disturbance	NEWBORN AND EARLY INFANCY	LATE INFANCY AND CHILDHOOD
Parenchymal		
Anomalies	Agenesis, hypoplasia, lobar emphysema, congenital cyst, pulmonary sequestration	Hypoplasia, congenital cyst, pulmonary sequestration
Atelectasis	Hyaline membrane disease	Thick secretions, foreign body
Infection	Pneumonia	Pneumonia, cystic fibrosis, bronchiectasis, pneumatocele
Alveolar rupture	Pneumothorax (spontaneous or iatrogenic), interstitial emphysema	Pneumothorax (trauma, asthma)
Others	Pulmonary hemorrhage, pulmonary edema, Wilson-Mikity syndrome	Pulmonary edema, lobectomy, chemical pneumonitis, pleural effusion, near-drowning
Chest Wall		
Muscular	Diaphragmatic hernia, eventration, edema	Amyotonia congenita, poliomyelitis, diphragmatic hernia, eventration, myasthenia gravis, muscular dystrophy, botulism
Skeletal malformations	Hemivertebrae, absence of ribs, thoracic dystrophy	Kyphoscoliosis, hemivertebrae, absence of ribs
Others	Abdominal distention	Obesity, flail chest

Table 11–4. CAUSES OF PRIMARY INEFFICIENT GAS TRANSFER

Site of Disturbance	Specific Disease Conditions
Pulmonary Diffusion Defect	
Increased diffusion path between alveoli and capillaries	Pulmonary edema, pulmonary fibrosis, collagen disorders, *Pneumocystis carinii* infection, sarcoidosis
Decreased alveolocapillary surface area	Pulmonary embolism, sarcoidosis, pulmonary hypertension, mitral stenosis, fibrosing alveolitis
Inadequate erythrocytes and hemoglobin	Anemia, hemorrhage
Respiratory Center Depression	
Increased cerebrospinal fluid pressure	Cerebral trauma (birth injuries, intracranial tumors, central nervous system infection (meningitis, encephalitis, sepsis)
Excess central nervous system depressant drugs	Maternal oversedation, overdosage with barbiturates, morphine, or diazepam
Excessive chemical changes in arterial blood	Severe asphyxia (hypercapnia, hypoxemia)
Toxic	Tetanus

any renal compensation has occurred) or chronic (after maximal renal compensation). Acid-base measurements also help delineate any concomitant or consequent metabolic problem. As a rough guide, a change in Pa_{CO_2} of 10 mm Hg is associated with a corresponding change in pH of 0.08 units, and a change in base bicarbonate of 10 mEq/L is associated with a corresponding change in pH of 0.15 units. Distinction of respiratory from nonrespiratory acidosis is crucial because the approaches to treatment differ.

Acute respiratory failure may also be of the Type I or Type II variety; it may be episodic, if caused by airway problems or poor ventilatory control, or complete, if caused by respiratory arrest. Either type may change to the other before the ultimate cure or demise of the patient. In general, a progression from Type I to Type II respiratory failure, particularly if associated with a sudden rise in arterial carbon dioxide tension, indicates that mechanical ventilation is required to avoid a clinical catastrophe.

Precise assessment of ventilatory adequacy must be based on both clinical and laboratory studies. Approximate normal values for commonly used indices of cardiopulmonary function are shown in Table 11–5. The clinical criteria for respiratory failure are determined by the adverse effects of disturbances in arterial blood gas tensions and pH on the function of susceptible organ systems, chiefly the lung, the heart, and the brain (Table 11–6). Hypoxemia interferes with brain metabolism, depresses the myocardium, and causes pulmonary hypertension. Hypercapnia depresses the central nervous system, and acidemia depresses myocardial function. The respiratory pump becomes fatigued either as a consequence of the disturbances in blood gases or as a result of the underlying respiratory disease. Thus the clinical manifestations may include restlessness, irritability, mood change, headache, mental confusion, convulsions, papilledema, and coma, which reflect cerebral dysfunction; bradycardia, tachycardia, blood pressure changes, and cardiac arrest, which reflect cardiovascular dysfunction; and cyanosis, absence or diminution of breath sounds, flaring of the alae nasi, intercostal retractions, wheezing, tachypnea, grunting, weakening of respiratory effort, and apnea, which reflect respiratory dysfunction. The adverse effects of hypoxemia, hypercapnia, and acidemia on any of these organ systems may be additive or synergistic. General fatigue and excessive sweating may also be useful clinical indices of acute respiratory failure.

Table 11–5. APPROXIMATE NORMAL VALUES

Parameter	Newborn Infant	Older Infant and Child
Respiratory frequency (breaths/min)	40–60	20–30 (to 6 years) 15–20 (above 6 years)
Tidal volume (ml/kg)	5–6	7–8
Arterial blood		
pH	7.30–7.40	7.30–7.40 (to 2 years) 7.35–7.45 (above 2 years)
P_{CO_2} (mm Hg)	30–35	30–35 (to 2 years) 35–45 (above 2 years)
Standard HCO_3^- (mEq/l)	20–22	20–22 (to 2 years) 22–24 (above 2 years)
P_{O_2} (mm Hg)	60–90	80–100
Heart rate (beats/min)	100–200	100–180 (to 3 years) 70–150 (above 3 years)
Blood pressure (mm Hg)		
Systolic	60–90	75–130 (to 3 years) 90–140 (above 3 years)
Diastolic	30–60	45–90 (to 3 years) 50–80 (above 3 years)

Table 11–6. CRITERIA OF RESPIRATORY FAILURE

Clinical Signs

RESPIRATORY
Tachypnea
Altered depth and pattern of
respiration (deep, shallow, apnea,
irregular)
Chest wall retractions
Flaring of alae nasi
Cyanosis
Decrease or absence of breath
sounds
Expiratory grunting
Wheezing and/or prolonged
expiration

CARDIAC
Tachycardia
Hypertension
Bradycardia
Hypotension
Cardiac arrest
CEREBRAL
Restlessness
Irritability
Headache
Mental confusion
Papilledema
Seizures
Coma

GENERAL
Fatigue
Excessive sweating

Laboratory Findings

Hypoxemia (acute or chronic)
Hypercapnia (acute or chronic)
Acidosis (metabolic and/or respiratory)

Two points cannot be overemphasized: (1) The manifestations of respiratory failure are not always clinically evident, and some of the symptoms, when present, may be due to nonrespiratory causes. (2) The strictly clinical assessment of arterial hypoxemia and hypercapnia is not reliable. Thus clinical judgment is required as to when arterial blood gas measurements should be taken. Close clinical observation of the patient over a period of time provides useful information; similarly, a longitudinal demonstration of a rising arterial P_{CO_2} or a falling arterial P_{O_2}, particularly if accompanied by clinical manifestations, is more important than a single determination of arterial blood gases. The degree of respiratory distress may not reflect the actual level of arterial oxygenation or of alveolar ventilation, so that significant changes in arterial gas tensions may well be present even in the absence of detectable clinical signs. For example, hypoxemia may be present in the complete absence of clinically detectable cyanosis. Depression of the respiratory center may cause hypoventilation without any respiratory distress, whereas an increase in dead space results in a marked compensatory increase in minute ventilation that may manifest as respiratory distress even though arterial P_{CO_2} is normal or only minimally elevated. Thus

precise assessment of oxygenation and ventilatory adequacy must be based on both clinical and laboratory status.

APPROACH TO MANAGEMENT

Table 11–7 outlines a systematic approach to the management of respiratory failure. Although estimation of arterial blood gases and pH is necessary for obtaining precise information about gas exchange in the lung, these studies obviously are unimportant in an emergency. Clinical judgment is paramount at this time, and the skilled physician or nurse must be able to assess the situation and initiate therapeutic measures within moments.

RESUSCITATION

Only minutes separate the onset of complete apnea from the ensuing ventricular fibrillation or asystole. No other clinical setting demands more immediate decision and more organized action, and both physicians and nurses must be skilled in emergency procedures. The sequential steps in resuscitation are outlined in Table 11–8. Resuscitation equipment should be readily accessible and should be checked daily. A list of suggested equipment is presented in Table 11–9.

Regardless of the cause of respiratory arrest and the age of the patient, the following basic approach not only should result in increased survival but also should prevent hypoxic brain damage. Appropriate modifications of this scheme may be made that reflect the presence and the number of other members of the resuscitation team. The cardinal rule is to use the simplest readily available procedure.

AIRWAY PATENCY

Rapid restoration of airway patency and institution of artificial ventilation are the first steps in resuscitation. In the absence of obstruction by secretions or foreign material, airway patency can be achieved by extending the neck and pulling the mandible forward, thereby lifting the tongue from the posterior

Table 11–7. SEQUENTIAL APPROACH TO MANAGEMENT OF RESPIRATORY FAILURE

Situation	Sequence	Action
Cardiorespiratory arrest	Recognize cardiorespiratory arrest	Initiate resuscitation measures within moments
Nonarrest	Suspect respiratory failure	Confirm diagnosis and define type through arterial blood gas analysis
	Define cause and severity of failure	Thoroughly evaluate clinical information and blood gas and other laboratory results
	Assess need for intensive clinical and laboratory monitoring	Transfer patient to intensive care unit if required
	Provide treatment modalities for specific functional disturbances and underlying etiology	Correct specific defects in oxygenation, ventilation, and acid-base equilibrium, and institute specific medical and/or surgical procedures as needed

Table 11–8. PRINCIPLES OF BASIC AND ADVANCED RESUSCITATION

Component	Basic Life Support*	Advanced Life Support†

Airway patency	Open the airway
	  Head lift–neck lift technique
	  Head lift–chin lift technique
	
	Confirm absence of breath
	  Observe for movement of chest and
	    abdomen
	  Feel for air from mouth and nose
	  Listen for air during expiration
		Adjuncts for airway
		  Pharyngeal airways (oral, nasal)
		  Tracheal intubation (oral, nasal)
		  Bronchoscopy
		Artificial surgical airway
		  Transtracheal catheterization
		  Cricothyrotomy
		  Tracheostomy

Breathing (oxygenation)	Mouth-to-mouth or mouth-to-mouth-and-
	  nose
	  For older child, 16 respirations per min
	  For infant, 20 respirations per min
	Manage airway obstruction
	  Blind removal (back blows and chest
	    thrusts)
	  Visualized removal (fingers)
		Adjuncts for breathing
		  Nasal cannulas
		  Face masks
		  Resuscitation bags
		Suctioning devices
		  Portable
		  Central-source

Circulation	Check pulse
	  For child, carotid
	  For infant, brachial
	External cardiac massage
	  For child, 80 compressions per min
	  For infant, 100 compressions per min
		External cardiac massage continued
		Electrocardiograph (ECG) monitoring and
		  recognition of dysrhythmia
		Defibrillation (electrical, pharmacologic)
		Intravenous lifeline
		Drug therapy

*Basic life support is continued until arrival of the advanced life support team.
†Adequate ventilation and circulation, intravenous lifeline, continuous ECG monitoring, and, in the very small infant, rewarming and stabilization of temperature are established before transfer to the intensive care unit.

pharyngeal wall. Overextension of the neck must be avoided in small infants. At this point one should check for the presence of air movement to and from the lungs, because absence of air movement may persist despite respiratory efforts in the presence of obstruction. Four breaths delivered in rapid succession (without allowing for full lung deflation) serve as a check for airway obstruction as well as a means of opening the peripheral airways. Manual relief of foreign body obstruction should not be undertaken as long as there is good air exchange. Blind finger sweep of the posterior oropharynx should be avoided so as not to push a foreign body farther back. Rather, it should be visualized before attempts are made to remove it with the finger. The proper maneuver for blind removal of a foreign body is a series of back blows and chest thrusts. Obstruction of the upper airway by a foreign body must be differentiated from that due to epiglottitis or croup, because back blows may precipitate a complete obstruction in these conditions.

If an airway cannot be established in such conditions as severe epiglottitis, laryngospasm, trismus, and laryngeal foreign body, an emergency tracheotomy must be performed. This procedure may be rapidly performed by percutaneous insertion of a 15-gauge needle into the trachea through the cricoid membrane. A single vertical slit made just below the cricoid through two or three tracheal rings without removing a segment of cartilage is the next procedure of choice. Often a bronchoscope may be inserted when tracheal intubation has failed, and this insertion may be followed by a less hurried tracheostomy. Emergency bronchoscopy is indicated for the removal of an aspirated foreign body when it is lodged in the trachea, but bronchoscopy is not an emergency procedure when the foreign body is lodged in a more distal airway. Bronchoscopic removal of thick mucopurulent secretions may be an emergency. Large volumes of secretions may be removed by direct laryngoscopy and endotracheal suction. Although speed should be exercised in initiating emergency treatment, the attending physician must always consider other causes of acute respiratory difficulty, such as tension pneumothorax, which is promptly relieved by needle thoracentesis.

ARTIFICIAL VENTILATION AND OXYGENATION

Mouth-to-mouth, mouth-to-nose, or bag-and-mask ventilation of the lung should be begun immediately after checking airway patency. A plastic oropharyngeal airway that prevents obstruction of the pharynx by the tongue should be inserted. Artificial respiration must be done cautiously with close observation of chest and abdominal wall expansion, because excessive pressure may produce pneumothorax, pneumomediastinum, and gastric distention. These complications are more apt to be encountered in newborn infants, who require no more than 15 to 20 ml tidal volume, an amount that is approximately the volume of the adult mouth with cheeks distended with air.

Several types of bag-and-mask arrangement are in common use. The conventional anesthesia bag requires an inflow of oxygen or air to reinflate the bag; the other type is a self-inflating bag. Either is satisfactory, but generally the concentration of oxygen by the latter type is limited. Whenever feasible, 100 per cent oxygen should be delivered. Bag-and-mask ven-

Table 11–9. CONTENTS OF A MOBILE PEDIATRIC RESUSCITATION CART

Category	Equipment	Specific Sizes or Types
Airway, ventilation, and oxygenation equipment	Oropharyngeal airways	Sizes 00, 1, 2, 3
	Face masks	Rendell-Baker sizes 0, 1, 2, 3 Everseal sizes 2, 3
	Breathing bags	Pediatric and adult Laerdal with reservoir Hope self-inflating type
	Suction apparatus	Bulb syringe Yankauer suction Suction catheters sizes 6, 8, 10, 12, 14 F Portable suction machine
	Endotracheal tubes and connectors	Sizes 3, 3.5, 4, 4.5, 5, 5.5, 6, 6.5, 7, 8, 9 mm
	Endotracheal adaptors	
	Laryngoscope	Straight blades: Miller sizes No. 1, 2 Curved blades: Macintosh No. 2, 3 Spare handles, batteries, and bulbs
	Introducers	
	Magil forceps	
	Tracheostomy tube and tray	
	Oxygen tank	
	Appropriate tubes and connectors for central O$_2$ source	
Cardiac equipment	Cardiac board	½-in thick plywood
	ECG monitor and DC defibrillator unit	
Intravenous and intraarterial administration set	Syringes	Sizes 2, 5, 10, 20, 50 ml
	Needles and cannulas	Regular type sizes 16, 18, 19, 20, 21, 22 Butterfly type sizes 21, 23, 25 Plastic over-the-needle or plastic through-the-needle catheters sizes 10, 12, 14, 16, 18, 20, 22 Umbilical artery catheters Intracardiac injection needle
	Tourniquets and alcohol swabs	
	Cutdown and umbilical catheterization trays	
	Local anesthetics	1% lidocaine
	Fluids and administration sets	Normal saline 50% and 5% dextrose in water 3.3% dextrose in saline
	Stopcocks	
Drugs	(see Table 11–22)	
Miscellaneous	Scissors	
	Stopwatch	
	Tape	
	Safety pins	
	Tincture of benzoin	

ECG, electrocardiograph; DC, direct current.

tilation must also be done cautiously to prevent lung rupture. Monitoring of inflation pressure with a manometer or providing a pressure relief valve to a bag-and-mask ventilation device will reduce the risk of lung rupture. It is worthwhile noting that aspirated vomitus and secretions will be driven down the tracheobronchial tree during positive pressure ventilation; suctioning is therefore a most important initial step. In the newborn period, diaphragmatic hernia should be ruled out as the cause of acute respiratory distress, because positive-pressure breathing may aggravate the situation by introducing air into the gastrointestinal tract. When an adequate upper airway cannot be established, tracheal intubation is required (Table 11–10).

EXTERNAL CARDIAC MASSAGE

As soon as airway patency is established and the initial breaths have been delivered, the third objective is to ascertain promptly the state of circulation. Cardiac standstill and absence of cerebral circulation can be tolerated for only a few minutes. Precordial palpation for the apical heart beats is not encouraged because precordial activity may represent an impulse rather than a true pulse and is therefore unreliable. In older children, absence of carotid pulsation is sufficient reason to commence external cardiac massage. In small infants, palpation of the brachial rather than the carotid pulse is preferred.

Two essentials of effective and safe cardiac massage must be fulfilled: (1) the patient's spine must be supported during compression of the sternum, and (2) sternal pressure must be forceful but not traumatic. Sternal compression applied too vigorously may result in rib and sternal fractures, hepatic tears, and stomach rupture. Effective cardiac massage may be achieved in very small infants by joining the fingers of both hands behind the patient's back with both thumbs on the middle sternum. In larger in-

Table 11–10. AVERAGE WEIGHTS AND ENDOTRACHEAL TUBE SIZES

Age	Average Wt Range (kg)	Endotracheal Tube Size (mm)
Premature and small newborn	1.0–2.5	2.5, 3.0
Newborn–3 mo	2.5–6.0	3.0, 3.5
4–18 mo	6.0–12.0	4.0, 4.5
1.5–3 yr	12.0–15.0	4.0, 4.5
3–5 yr	15.0–20.0	4.5, 5.0
5–7 yr	20.0–25.0	5.5, 6.0
8–10 yr	25.0–35.0	6.0 cuffed
11–12 yr	35.0–45.0	7.0 cuffed
>12 yr	—	7.5 cuffed

fants, one hand is placed under the infant's back and the heel of the other hand on the middle sternum. In an older child, a firm board (½-inch-thick plywood) is placed under the patient's spine, and both hands are used to compress the junction between the middle and lower thirds of the sternum. Cardiac massage should be started and maintained for 5 to 10 sec. Cardiac compression should be interspersed with ventilation at a ratio of one breath for every five compressions. Signs of recovery include palpable peripheral pulse, return of pupils to normal size, and disappearance of mottling and cyanosis.

At this stage, a fully equipped mobile resuscitation cart with an electrocardiographic (ECG) monitor-defibrillator should have arrived. The ECG monitor-defibrillator is hooked up to the patient, and, simultaneously, intravenous infusion is started to provide a direct route for administration of drugs, blood, or plasma expander.

DEFIBRILLATION

In contrast to asystole in adults, asystole in children is usually preceded by severe bradycardia or atrioventricular block of varying degrees or both. Ventricular fibrillation is a rare event. Thus defibrillation is usually undertaken only on definitive ECG demonstration of fibrillation. On occasion it may not be possible to distinguish between a fine fibrillation and a true asystole, and defibrillation is attempted.

Direct-current (DC) defibrillation is more effective than alternating-current (AC) defibrillation during periods of anoxia. Furthermore, direct current causes less myocardial damage, and therefore DC defibrillation is the method of choice. The initial dose of defibrillator energy varies with the size of the child, that is, 2 watt sec (joules) per kg of body weight for a child under 40 kg (Table 11–11). The subsequent energy dose is doubled if the initial dose does not reverse fibrillation. However, the dose for the patient who has been receiving digoxin should initially be the lowest that can be delivered by the defibrillator; it can be increased slowly if necessary to avoid irreversible myocardial arrest, a known complication of this combination of therapies. The initial dose for conversion of tachyarrhythmia is 1 watt sec (joule) per kg of body weight.

If defibrillation still does not occur in either situation, recheck that oxygenation is being maintained and metabolic acidosis is being corrected. Fibrillation of the fine type recalcitrant to countershock may be converted by epinephrine to a coarse type more susceptible to electrical treatment.

Proper placement of the two electrode paddles is important in determining the effectiveness of the defibrillation therapy. An anteroposterior placement with the heart in between delivers more current density to the heart. However, the anterior right-left placement (one paddle to the right of the sternum at the second rib level and the other at the left midclavicular line at the xiphoid level) is often utilized because it is less time consuming and interferes less with other resuscitation measures. To maximize current delivery a saline-soaked gauze pad is applied to the chest skin. Alcohol pads should not be used because they can burn the skin. Care must be taken that there is no saline contact between the paddles that would cause a short circuit. In small patients, a small set of paddles (4.5 cm in diameter) is crucial to maintain adequate separation of the electrode paddles. The 8.0-cm diameter paddles are suitable for older children who weigh more than 10 kg. It should be emphasized that the electrode paddles are charged only just before their actual application. Also, before delivery of the defibrillator shock, other members of the resuscitation team must be alerted to stand back for a moment.

The DC defibrillator may also be used, in a procedure known as synchronized cardioversion, to terminate dysrhythmias other than ventricular fibrillation. In emergency situations, rapid ventricular and supraventricular rhythms associated with inadequate cardiac output may be terminated by cardioversion. The procedures involve (1) activating the synchronizer circuit by placing the synchronizer switch in the "on" position and (2) holding the firing buttons depressed until the synchronizer causes discharge of the capacitor-stored energy approximately 10 ms after the peak of the R wave. The initial energy dose required for cardioversion is usually lower than that for defibrillation and is increased to levels recommended for the latter as desired. Delivery of an electrical discharge between the peak and the downward slope of the R wave is least likely to cause ventricular fibrillation. Should ventricular fibrillation be produced inadvertently, ensure that the synchronizer circuit is turned off and the defibrillator recharged before attempting defibrillation.

Table 11–11. INITIAL DOSE RANGE OF DEFIBRILLATOR SHOCK

Weight (kg)	Dose (watt sec or joules)*
<2.5	5
2.5–10	5–20
10–20	20–40
20–40	40–80
over 40	100

*Double this dose if unsuccessful.

Table 11–12A. PRIMARY RESUSCITATION DRUGS

Drug	Concentration Supplied	Dosage	Route* (Interval)	Indication(s)	Adverse Effect(s)
Oxygen	100%	Highest $F_{I_{O_2}}$	Face mask; ET (continuous)	All instances of acute need for resuscitation	Not of concern in these circumstances
Naloxone hydrochloride (Narcan)	0.02 mg/ml 0.40 mg/ml	0.01–0.10 mg/kg Minimum: 0.5 mg (newborn) 2.0 mg (older child)	IV; ET, ($\bar{q}$ 2–3 min)	Narcotic depression	None in the absence of narcotic depression Abrupt reversal symptoms (nausea, vomiting, tachycardia, hypertension, tremor)
Sodium bicarbonate†‡	0.9 mEq/ml (7.5%) 1.0 mEq/ml (8.4%)	1–2 mEq/kg	IV ($\bar{q}$ 5–10 min, according to pH)	Metabolic acidosis Ineffective countershock	Hyperosmolality Hypernatremia Metabolic alkalosis Fluid overload
Epinephrine†§ (Adrenalin)	0.1 mg/ml (1:10,000)**	0.01 mg/kg maximum: 0.5 mg	IV; ET ($\bar{q}$ 3–5 min)	Asystole Bradycardia Fine ventricular fibrillation	Hypertension Dysrhythmias Tachycardia
Atropine sulfate†	0.4 mg/ml 0.6 mg/ml 1.0 mg/ml	0.01–0.02 mg/kg maximum: 2 mg minimum: 0.1 mg	IV; ET ($\bar{q}$ 5–10 min)	Bradycardia plus hypotension AV block (2nd or 3rd degree) Slow idioventricular rates	Delirium Coma Ventricular and arterial tachyarrhythmias Paradoxical bradycardia
Calcium chloride‖ (27% Ca^{++}) Calcium gluconate‖ (9% Ca^{++})	100 mg/ml (10%) 100 mg/ml (10%)	20–50 mg/kg maximum: 1.0 g 100–200 mg/kg maximum: 2.0 g	IV slowly†† ($\bar{q}$ 10–20 min)	Cardiovascular collapse Electromechanical dissociation Ventricular standstill	Cardiac arrest Severe bradycardia Arrhythmias
Lidocaine† (Xylocaine)	10 mg/ml (1%) 20 mg/ml (2%)	0.5–1 mg/kg (bolus dose)	IV, ET ($\bar{q}$ 5–10 min) maximum: 5 mg/kg	Recurrent ventricular fibrillation Ventricular tachycardia Frequent premature ventricular contractions	Nausea, vomiting Lethargy Disorientation Convulsion Coma Bradycardia, hypotension

*ET, endotracheal; IV, intravenous; IM, intramuscular.
†These drugs are available in prefilled syringes; note their specific concentrations.
‡$NaHCO_3$ should not be mixed with epinephrine, atropine, calcium salts, or lidocaine.
§Epinephrine may precipitate with Ca^{++}.
‖Ca^{++} salts are used cautiously in a digitalized patient (0.01 ml/kg SC.)
**For anaphylaxis, the 1:1000 aqueous solution is used.
††IV dose administered at rate of less than 1 ml/min.

PHARMACOLOGIC AGENTS

Fundamentally, pharmacologic therapy during resuscitation is aimed at correcting specific disturbances—namely, hypoxia, narcosis, acidosis, asystole, bradycardia, dysrhythmia, and hypotension. The agents commonly used during the acute phase, along with their stock concentrations, doses, routes of administration, specific indications, and potential complications, are listed in Tables 11–12 and 11–13.

Oxygen is again considered in this section to reemphasize that its administration is indicated following all instances of cardiopulmonary arrest. It must be given promptly, continuously, and in the highest concentration available. Sources for oxygen include the rescuer's expired breath (16 to 17 per cent O_2),

bag-and-mask ventilation with room air (21 per cent O_2), and artificial ventilation with 100 per cent O_2 from a portable tank or a central outlet. Appropriately sized tubes and properly fitting connectors should be stored at all times in the resuscitation cart. In addition to the obvious benefit of correcting tissue hypoxia, oxygenation facilitates ventricular defibrillation by electrical countershock or drugs and, often, by itself converts arrhythmias accompanying hypoxia to normal rhythm.

Naloxone hydrochloride, a specific narcotic antagonist, is a competitive blocker of opiate receptor sites. It does not have agonist properties and therefore does not depress ventilation or aggravate respiratory depression. Maximal effect is seen 2 or 3 min after intravenous administration but is delayed to 15 min

Table 11–12B. ADDITIONAL EMERGENCY DRUGS

Drugs	Dose	Remarks
Diazepam (Valium)	IV— infuse 0.1–0.3 mg/kg q 2 min up to a total initial dose of 1.0 mg/kg	Be prepared to provide respiratory support if necessary.
Diphenhydramine (Benadryl)	IV 1–2 mg/kg slow infusion (5 min)	
Furosemide (Lasix)	IV, IM—1 mg/kg	Give slowly IV.
Glucose	IV—2–5 ml/kg (0.2–0.5 g/kg) of 10% dextrose in water and/or constant infusion of 10% dextrose in water at a rate of 100 ml/kg/24 h (8 mg of glucose/kg/min)	Blood glucose level should be determined following administration.
Morphine sulphate	IV (slowly) or IM— 0.1 mg/kg	Avoid IM if patient is hypotensive or in shock.
Pancuronium (Pavulon)	IV—0.1 mg/kg	Ventilatory support will be necessary.
Paraldehyde	Rectal—0.3 ml/kg of paraldehyde up to a maximum dose = 7 ml. Make up to 1:1 solution with mineral oil.	IM is contraindicated.
Phenobarbital	IV—10–20 mg/kg (loading dose). Maximum loading dose 30–40 mg/kg. Maintenance dose: 2–4 mg/kg/dose IV, IM, or PO q 12 h.	
Procainamide (Pronestyl)	IV—15 mg/kg per dose given during 30 min diluted in 5% dextrose IV infusion—20–80 μg/kg/min.	Be prepared for bradycardia and hypotension. Contraindicated in severe heart block. Widening of QRS interval by more than 0.02 sec or significant ventricular slowing suggests toxicity.

after intramuscular or subcutaneous administration. In the immediate neonatal period, naloxone is most often used to treat respiratory depression caused by placental transfer of narcotic analgesics administered to the mother. Failure to obtain improvement after two or three doses at 5 min intervals suggests that conditions other than narcotic depression may be responsible for the patient's condition.

Sodium bicarbonate is the agent of choice for the correction of metabolic acidosis and should be administered without waiting for blood pH measurement when severe hypoxia is suspected, for example,

Table 11–13. EMERGENCY DRUGS GIVEN BY CONTINUOUS INFUSION

Drug	Concentration Supplied	Dosage*	Indication(s)	Adverse Effect(s)
Epinephrine (Adrenalin)	1.0 mg/ml (1:1000)	0.01–1.0 μg/kg/min	Asystole Bradycardia Fine ventricular fibrillation	Hypertension Dysrhythmias Tachycardia
Isoproterenol (Isuprel)	0.2 mg/ml	0.05–1.0 μg/kg/min	Status asthmaticus	
Dopamine	40 mg/ml	2–30 μg/kg/min	Cardiogenic shock	Tachycardia Tachyarrhythmia Hypertension Excessive diuresis
Lidocaine (Xylocaine)	10 mg/ml (1%) 20 mg/ml (2%) 40 mg/ml (4%)	CHF†: 5–30 μg/kg/min§ No CHF: 35–50 μg/kg/min§	Recurrent ventricular fibrillation Ventricular tachycardia Frequent premature ventricular contractions	Nausea, vomiting Lethargy Disorientation Convulsion Coma Bradycarida, hypotension
Aminophylline	25 mg/ml 50 mg/ml	16–24 mg/kg/24 hours§	Severe bronchospasm	Transient hypotension Arrhythmia Nausea, vomiting Hyperreflexia Fasciculations Convulsion
Hydrocortisone hemisuccinate (Solu Cortef)	50 mg/ml 125 mg/ml	7 mg/kg/24 hours§	Acute asthma	None with short-term use
Methylprednisolone (Solu-Medrol)	40 mg/ml 62.5 mg/ml	2 mg/kg/24 hours§	Acute asthma	None with short-term use

*Infusion rate should start with the lower dose, and the rate should be increased gradually until the desired effect is achieved, usually at or before the higher dose is infused. Occasionally, a dose above the higher range is required; when applicable, drug blood level is measured.

†Congestive heart failure.

‡Infusion is decreased or stopped when toxicity occurs.

§The doses are preceded by a bolus dose (per kg of body weight); for lidocaine, 1 mg; for aminophylline 7 mg; for hydrocortisone, 7 mg; and for methylprednisolone, 5 mg.

after an unwitnessed cardiopulmonary arrest. Tris(hydroxymethyl)aminomethane (THAM) has also been used to correct metabolic acidosis. Dosage is calculated as follows:

$$mEq\ (0.3M\ THAM) = body\ weight\ (kg)$$
$$\times\ base\ excess\ \times\ 25\%$$

Half the dose is given over 4 hours. This drug has no advantage over sodium bicarbonate in terms of buffering capacity but does circumvent the administration of large quantities of sodium ion. Although such effects are of no significant concern during acute resuscitation, THAM may cause respiratory arrest and hypoglycemia. Correction of metabolic acidosis improves cardiac contractility and increases the efficacy of epinephrine.

Epinephrine increases myocardial contractility, stroke volume, and perfusion pressure and may convert fine ventricular fibrillation to a coarse type that is more amenable to electrical defibrillation. The preferred route of administration is by a central venous line, but a peripheral venous site or an endotracheal tube may be used. In patients younger than 3 years of age, rapid access to the vascular system may be effected through intraosseus administration of the drug. Intracardiac administration is done only as a last resort because of the dangers of cardiac tamponade, coronary artery laceration, intractable ventricular fibrillation, or pneumothorax in addition to the interruption of external cardiac massage. It must be emphasized that only the 1:10,000 dilution is used for cardiac resuscitation. The 1:1000 aqueous solution is the preparation of choice for anaphylactic shock and is given when a continuous infusion is later desired. Continuous drip requires close ECG and blood pressure monitoring of the patient.

Dopamine, a naturally occurring chemical precursor of epinephrine, is used in children to increase cardiac output and perfusion pressure. The drug is given as a continuous intravenous drip, and the patient is closely monitored to titrate the dose carefully to the desired effect. Low to moderate doses stimulate primarily the beta$_1$-adrenergic receptors, which increase cardiac output and renal blood flow, but high doses stimulate the alpha-adrenergic receptors, resulting in decreased renal perfusion. Dobutamine also stimulates beta receptors. In low doses, it produces mild peripheral vasoconstriction. In higher doses, peripheral vasodilation occurs. Thus it should not be used by itself in patients with hypotension. Additionally, this drug is more likely to reduce pulmonary vascular resistance, and therefore a combination of dopamine and dobutamine may be clinically indicated. In these circumstances, it is imperative that invasive hemodynamic monitoring be employed.

Calcium also improves myocardial contractility and is particularly helpful in profound cardiovascular collapse with electrical-mechanical dissociation of cardiac action. This condition can be recognized when electrical cardiac rhythm is orderly but there is hypotension, poor peripheral perfusion, and weak or undetectable peripheral pulse.

Atropine accelerates the arterial pacemaker and improves atrioventricular conduction. It is indicated for profound bradycardia only when there is associated hypotension or premature ventricular contractions. In the absence of these associated findings, bradycardia is treated with epinephrine or isoproterenol. Isoproterenol also causes peripheral arterial dilation, so that its use in the presence of hypovolemia increases the risk of hypotension. An insufficient dose of atropine stimulates the central medullary vagal nuclei and thereby causes paradoxical bradycardia; hence, the need for a minimum dose. Intravenous isoproterenol is also used for status asthmaticus but may cause cardiac arrhythmias; because the duration of action is short, this complication is easily treated by stopping the drug.

Lidocaine decreases myocardial excitability and slows electrical conduction in the heart. It is the drug of choice for recurrent ventricular fibrillation. Following a bolus dose, continuous intravenous administration is necessary because lidocaine has a short half-life. When lidocaine treatment fails, bretylium tosylate may be tried. This drug appears to be effective in some patients with life-threatening ventricular fibrillation or with tachycardia that is refractory to electrical countershock or lidocaine. The drug is a sympathetic blocker and therefore may cause hypotension. The mechanism by which bretylium tosylate affects ventricular fibrillation is not fully understood.

It cannot be overemphasized that familiarity with the stock concentrations, dosages, routes of administration, specific indications, and potential adverse effects of primary resuscitation and other emergency drugs is crucial to the delivery of intensive care to young infants and children with acute, serious respiratory disorders. For example, some drugs are supplied in different concentrations; prior planning and posting of a drug chart for the acutely ill patient can avoid delays and errors in calculation during an emergency. Awareness of the hazards of certain medications may prevent iatrogenic deaths. Personnel (pediatricians, anesthesiologists, resident-house staff, and nurses) should be familiar with the operation of resuscitation equipment (e.g., airways, laryngoscopes, defibrillator) and adept at starting a lifeline for drug administration. When a suitable number of personnel arrive at the scene, and in the absence of an organized resuscitation team, the most senior person knowledgeable about the principles and techniques of advanced life support should assume command and direct the entire maneuver. It is therefore advisable that personnel keep themselves up to date on the practice of basic and advanced life support by taking advantage of courses offered by various heart associations across the country.

RESUSCITATION OF THE NEWBORN INFANT

The newborn infant is able to tolerate asphyxia longer than the adult because of larger cardiac glycogen stores. In addition, it is likely that the brain of the neonate is more efficient at anaerobic metabolism than that of the older infant or child. Nonetheless, neurologic sequelae directly correlate with the duration of asphyxia, and resuscitation must therefore be as prompt as in older infants and children. Skilled personnel and special equipment are required because of the small size of the infant. The general approach to resuscitation is essentially the same in newborn infants as in older children, but asystole is rare, and an ineffective cardiac output is usually corrected by adequate oxygenation. It is unusual, then, for cardiac stimulants to be indicated in the newborn infant with respiratory failure, because such stimulants are rarely effective when bradycardia or a poor cardiac output fails to respond to artificial ventilation and oxygenation.

Because the newborn infant has a large surface area for heat loss, hypothermia is common unless the patient is immediately dried and an external heat source is supplied. Hypothermia increases the metabolic demand for oxygen, which may produce a critical situation in vital organs in the asphyxiated infant. An effective means of maintaining optimal body temperature of the infant in the delivery room is the use of infrared heat lamps. During resuscitation of the critically ill newborn infant, care must be taken to avoid excessive heat loss. The time taken to rewarm and stabilize a very small sick infant before transport to the intensive care nursery is well spent.

IMMEDIATE POSTRESUSCITATION PHASE

Recovery of adequate spontaneous ventilation following a period of respiratory arrest requires a minimum of 3 to 4 hours of continuous observation to recognize the development of posthypoxic complications, such as hyperexcitability, fever, visual disturbances, and seizures.

Patients must remain in the hospital following successful resuscitation and are usually admitted to an intensive care unit. Once the critical phase has passed, laboratory investigations are pursued as dictated by the history, a chest roentgenogram is obtained, and arterial blood gases and pH are determined. All of this information will aid in determining the need for further respiratory assistance, more laboratory investigations, and a specific treatment regimen.

CONTINUING RESPIRATORY CARE

The general principles underlying an intensive approach to the management of severe respiratory disorders involve continuing efforts at ensuring airway patency and adequate gas exchange in the lung and the institution of specific therapy (Table 11–14).

MAINTAINING AIRWAY PATENCY

In the intensive care unit, airway obstruction is most often caused by the retention of pulmonary secretions. An appreciation of this fact has resulted in the evolution of methods designed to aid the drainage of these secretions. In addition, airway obstruction may be caused by increased bronchomotor tone or mucosal edema, so therapy is also directed at increasing airway diameter.

Drainage of Secretions

It is generally accepted that adequate hydration by the administration of oral or parenteral fluids is the

Table 11–14. PRINCIPLES OF CONTINUING CARE OF RESPIRATORY DISORDERS

Maintenance of Airway Patency
DRAINAGE OF TRACHEOBRONCHIAL SECRETIONS
  Hydration of secretions
    Systemic fluid
    Humidification
    Aerosolized water (mist)
    Avoidance of drying agents
  Removal of secretions
    Coughing
    Suctioning (oropharyngeal, endotracheal)
    Chest pummeling and postural drainage
    Bronchoscopy
OPTIMAL AIRWAY DIAMETER
  Bronchodilator medication
    Aerosolized
    Systemic (oral, intravenous)
Oxygenation
METHODS OF ADMINISTRATION
  Face mask
  Tent
  Head box
  Incubator
INDICATION AND PRECAUTIONS
Tracheal Airway
INTUBATION
TRACHEOSTOMY
Mechanical Ventilatory Support
CRITERIA FOR SELECTION
TYPES OF MECHANICAL VENTILATORS
COMPLICATIONS AND THEIR MANAGEMENT
Additional Therapy
MEDICAL
  Bronchodilators
  Steroids
  Antimicrobials
  Diuretics
  Digitalis
  Analgesics and narcotics
  Chest wall strapping
  Oxygen
  Transfusion
SURGICAL
  Thoracentesis (air, fluid)
  Pleural drainage (air, fluid)
  Thoracotomy and direct repair
  Tonsillectomy and adenoidectomy

optimal way to ensure that tracheobronchial secretions are thinned and are able to move easily out of the respiratory tract. Overhydration, however, does not make secretions thinner. Increasing the water vapor content of inspired air (humidification) will reduce respiratory water loss, but full saturation at room temperature is only about 50 per cent saturation at body temperature. Under usual circumstances, the inspired air is fully humidified in the nose and upper airway. Dehydration of the lower respiratory tract is prone to occur during hyperventilation, during oxygen therapy, or in the patient with an artificial airway that bypasses the upper respiratory tract. Consequently, humidification is essential under these conditions to prevent drying of the lower respiratory tract mucosa and inspissation of mucus. Under these circumstances, the inspired air should be warmed and fully humidified.

Humidification is associated with the hazard of gram-negative infection, particularly *Pseudomonas*. Special precautions must be taken to ensure that the water reservoir remains sterile. In many intensive care units, it is recommended that the water reservoir and all tubing leading to the patient be changed every 24 hours. In the water reservoir of incubators, the addition of acetic acid has been shown to be effective in preventing the proliferation of gram-negative organisms.

Aerosolized water (mist) is commonly utilized to supply extra water to the respiratory tract, particularly in conditions such as croup, bronchitis, pneumonia, and cystic fibrosis. The rationale for the use of mist for lower respiratory tract diseases has been questioned, however, because of the evidence that most of the water droplets are filtered out of the nose and upper airway and are subsequently swallowed; only a minimal amount actually reaches the lung. Thus the effectiveness of mist therapy in thinning secretions is in considerable doubt and is most likely inefficient in comparison with adequate humidification and systemic hydration. Hazards associated with mist include infection, possible overhydration (particularly when ultrasonic nebulizers are used), and an unstable thermal environment.

In general, parasympatholytic drugs, such as atropine, and antihistamines must be avoided, because these agents dry respiratory mucus and interfere with proper drainage. For certain asthmatic children, atropine plays a beneficial role. It may act either by inhibiting production of cyclic guanosine monophosphate (GMP), thereby preventing smooth muscle contraction, or by abolishing the reflex increase in airway resistance induced by cold air, dust inhalation, and the like.

Cough is the most effective method of removing secretions. Deep inspiration augments the normal widening of thoracic airways and triggers an effective cough. When the cough mechanism is depressed or inadequate, as in the immediate postoperative period, oropharyngeal suction, which stimulates cough, must be done frequently. In the presence of endotracheal intubation or tracheostomy, the efficacy of cough can be seriously impaired, and direct suctioning is generally required. However, excessive suctioning may result in irritation of the tracheal mucosa and bleeding. Furthermore, suction catheters may damage respiratory mucosa unless there is a single end hole. The presence of side holes allows the respiratory mucosa to be sucked in and damaged if the end hole becomes occluded. The normal defense mechanisms of the upper airway have been bypassed, and bacteria are easily introduced unless special precautions are taken. It is generally recommended that sterile catheters be used once and then discarded and that personnel wear sterile disposable gloves when suctioning a patient.

Secretions may be mobilized by chest pummeling and postural drainage; this technique is widely employed in conditions associated with excessive secretions, such as pneumonia, bronchiectasis, and cystic fibrosis. Proper positioning for maximal drainage by gravity, which depends on the site of the involved lobe, is discussed in detail in Chapter 4. Therapeutic bronchoscopy is indicated for the removal of an aspirated foreign body and is used less commonly for the removal of thick secretions.

Optimal Airway Diameter

In normal subjects, bronchodilator agents have been shown to decrease airway resistance, indicating the presence of smooth muscle tone in small airways. Thus pharmacologic agents have been utilized extensively in respiratory disease to dilate small airways in the hope that secretions will be more effectively drained (see Table 11–13). Bronchodilators may act by decreasing smooth muscle tone (beta-adrenergic effect), by reducing mucosal congestion through vasoconstriction (alpha-adrenergic effect), or by exerting a direct relaxant action on smooth muscle. The commonly used bronchodilators include isoproterenol, salbutamol, terbutaline (all beta-adrenergic), epinephrine (alpha-adrenergic), ipratropium bromide (anticholinergic), and aminophylline (direct muscle relaxant). Salbutamol and terbutaline have more selective action on the beta$_2$-adrenergic receptors in the bronchial wall, thus avoiding significant cardiac stimulation. In the acutely ill patient, an adrenergic (sometimes in combination with an anticholinergic) drug is administered directly to the lungs as an aerosol; aminophylline is given intravenously. In addition to these treatment modalities, intravenous isoproterenol may be a useful adjunct to the therapy of children with severe bronchospasm and respiratory failure. Presumably, the drug increases effective pulmonary blood flow, which in turn allows an improvement in the metabolic function to the lung and an increase in perfusion with an associated lowering of the Pa_{CO_2}. It is mandatory that patients selected for this treatment be in the intensive care unit, where continuous cardiac monitoring is done.

Limitations of intravenous isoproterenol therapy include tachycardia above 200 beats/min and arrhythmia. Salbutamol given intravenously does not have these limitations.

Proper administration of aerosolized bronchodilator from metered-dose inhalers requires a deep, slow inspiration (lasting 5 or 6 sec) from functional residual capacity (FRC) and delivery of the aerosol at the beginning of inspiration. The breath should be held for approximately 10 sec at the end of inspiration. When the patient is unable to synchronize breaths, an aerochamber may be used. When the patient cannot take a deep inspiration, the drug may be administered by an intermittent positive-pressure device (IPPB). Aminophylline is a very effective bronchodilator when administered intravenously as a continuous infusion. It is mandatory to monitor blood levels of aminophylline for a more effective and safe therapy. Serum concentration should usually be 10 to 20 mg/ml. Aminophylline and caffeine have also been used in the treatment of apnea of prematurity. The premature infant may have insufficient hepatic enzymes to metabolize the drug, so measurement of these blood levels is mandatory. Steroids are employed early in the treatment of severe airflow obstruction due to asthma.

INCREASING OXYGEN TENSION IN INSPIRED GAS

Once the resuscitation phase has passed, the optimal method for determining the necessity for increasing the inspired oxygen concentration is by direct measurement of the arterial oxygen tension. Even in the absence of cyanosis, the presence of hypoxemia may be inferred by signs such as restlessness, confusion, and coma. Under these circumstances, oxygen should be administered immediately, and blood gas tension measurements should be obtained as soon as feasible. It must be emphasized that cyanosis is a poor indicator of hypoxemia, because this sign depends on the concentration of hemoglobin. Cyanosis will be apparent only when there is about 5 g/100 ml reduced hemoglobin in the capillaries. Thus in the presence of anemia, cyanosis may be difficult to detect; in the presence of polycythemia, cyanosis may be evident even though the blood oxygen content is adequate for tissue demands. Cyanosis requires the administration of oxygen until blood gas tensions are measured. In the presence of right-to-left cardiac shunt, oxygen will have little or no effect on arterial P_{O_2}.

There are several methods of oxygen administration (Table 11–15). Nasal catheters and cannulas are not usually tolerated by younger pediatric patients. Oxygen delivered via the oxygen inlet of an incubator is limited to a concentration of 40 per cent. When oxygen is delivered into a tent, the concentration varies, depending on leaks. Regardless of the tech-

Table 11–15. METHODS OF OXYGEN ADMINISTRATION

Method	Maximum Achievable F$_{I_{O_2}}$* (at 6–10 L/min of O$_2$) (%)
Nasopharyngeal catheter	50
Nasal prongs	50
Masks	
Without reservoir bag	50
With reservoir bag (partial rebreathing)	70
With reservoir bag (nonrebreathing)	95
Venturi	24,28,35,40
Incubator	40
Canopy tent	50
Head box	95

*Fractional concentration of inspired oxygen.

nique, it is essential that oxygen be heated and humidified by being bubbled through a heated nebulizer. To avoid damage to the lungs, oxygen administration should be discontinued as soon as possible (as indicated by serial blood gas tension measurements). Reduction of inspired oxygen concentration must be done stepwise and cautiously. Both concentration and duration of oxygen therapy must be recorded accurately. A well-calibrated oxygen analyzer must be used to check the inspired concentration at frequent intervals, at least every 2 hours. The necessity for closely monitoring arterial P_{O_2} in preterm newborn infants is related to both pulmonary oxygen toxicity and the danger of retrolental fibroplasia. In any patient, oxygen should be administered at the lowest concentration sufficient to maintain the arterial P_{O_2} above 50 mm Hg but not above 100 mm Hg. Continuous measurement of P_{O_2} by transcutaneous electrodes or oxygen saturation by oximetry has been used in addition to direct measurement of arterial blood gases for monitoring the adequacy of oxygenation.

The administration of oxygen may cause further respiratory depression if there has been chronic respiratory failure and a loss of sensitivity to carbon dioxide. This situation is uncommon in the pediatric patient but has been encountered in patients with cystic fibrosis.

NASOTRACHEAL INTUBATION AND TRACHEOSTOMY (TRACHEAL AIRWAY)

Although it is technically more difficult than orotracheal intubation, nasotracheal intubation is the preferred route when an adequate upper airway must be maintained for more than 12 hours. This route facilitates oral and pharyngeal hygiene and provides a more stable fixation, which reduces the chances of tracheal erosion and accidental extubation. Satisfactory placement of the tube should be confirmed by auscultation and roentgenogram. An ultrathin fiberoptic bronchoscope may also be used to check tube position. The tip of the tube should be at least 2 cm above the carina. This position places the tip of the tube at the level of T_3. Infants and children less than 10 years of age rarely require cuffed tubes. In older children, the cuff should be inflated to the minimum volume sufficient to provide an adequate tracheal seal and should be of the low-pressure type. The cuff should be deflated hourly for 2 to 5 min to minimize pressure necrosis.

In newborn infants, we have employed nasotracheal tubes for many weeks without complications. However, in older children, tracheostomy usually should be done if the tracheal airway is required beyond 1 week. Plastic polyvinylchloride tracheostomy tubes rather than metal ones are preferred by some physicians because they are simple to use and easily cleaned. However, the safety feature of an inner cannula in the metal tube is believed by some to be important. Cuffed tracheostomy tubes are seldom required.

MECHANICAL VENTILATORY SUPPORT

Selection of Patients

In general, patients in Type I or borderline Type II respiratory failure do not need mechanical ventilatory assistance and require only oxygen administration or adjunctive therapy or both to improve airway function. In contrast, Type II failure with a high level of hypercapnia, particularly with a rapidly rising P_{CO_2}, is a definitive indication for mechanical ventilation (Table 11–16). Also, mechanical support is necessary, even in the absence of Type II failure, when it is clinically evident on overall evaluation that the patient is likely to hypoventilate and develop more serious acidosis and critical hypoxemia. It must be emphasized that clinical signs and laboratory blood gas data should complement each other in the evaluation of all patients.

The crucial question is when to intubate a patient and commence mechanical ventilation in the absence of blood gas measurements and before the onset of apnea or cardiac arrest. Table 11–16 lists the generally accepted clinical selection criteria for a mechanical aid to breathing without which a patient's survival is unlikely, serious neurologic sequelae are anticipated, or respiratory crisis will occur. The clinical indices should include the state of cerebral, cardiac, and respiratory dysfunctions as well as the overall capacity of the patient to sustain further muscular activity. Clinical deterioration is ascertained when there is decreased breath sound, weakening of ventilatory effort, uncontrolled restlessness, anxious expression, lack of response to physical stimuli, severe changes in heart rate, peripheral cardiovascular collapse, loss of ability to cry, or limpness. Close clinical monitoring of the patient from the time of first observation should help tremendously in the assessment of increasing fatigue. Under these circumstances, mechanical ventilation may be initiated in an attempt to avoid crisis.

Types of Ventilators

A ventilator can substitute for or assist a patient's respiratory effort. When used as a substitute (controller), the ventilator cycles automatically at fixed settings and totally controls ventilation. When it is utilized to assist (assistor), the patient's inspiratory effort triggers the mechanical inspiratory phase of the ventilator. When provision is made for both machine control and patient's participation (controller-assistor), the ventilator controls respiration as long as the patient's respiratory frequency is below a preselected rate and assists breathing when the patient's respiratory frequency rises above the preselected rate. It must be noted that in small infants with weak respiratory efforts, the "assist" mode is usually unreliable.

Ventilators have also been classified as positive-pressure and negative-pressure machines depending on how lung inflation is artifically achieved. The positive-pressure machine inflates the lung by increasing airway pressure above atmospheric pressure; with a negative-pressure ventilator, a subatmospheric pressure is created around the chest wall while airway pressure remains atmospheric. Either class of ventilators produces an intermittent *positive* transpulmonary pressure (airway pressure greater than pleural pressure), which is essential for lung inflation.

Ventilators differ according to their primary control of cycling mechanism. The four main types are (1) volume-cycled—in which delivery of a fixed vol-

Table 11–16. SELECTION CRITERIA FOR MECHANICAL VENTILATION

Parameter*	Findings
Clinical†	
Respiratory	Apnea; decreased breath sounds despite rigorous chest wall movement; weakening ventilatory effort
Cardiac	Asystole; peripheral collapse; severe bradycardia or tachycardia
Cerebral	Coma; lack of response to physical stimuli; uncontrolled restlessness; anxious facial expression
General	Limpness; loss of ability to cry
Laboratory‡	
Pa_{CO_2}	Newborn infant: >60–65 mm Hg Older child: >55–60 mm Hg Rapidly rising (>5 mm Hg/hr)
Pa_{O_2} (FI_{O_2} = 100%)	Newborn infant: <40–50 mm Hg Older child: <50–60 mm Hg

*Clinical and/or laboratory data may dictate need for mechanical ventilation.

†More than one episode of apnea with bradycardia or an episode of cardiac arrest is adequate indication for initiating mechanical ventilation even in the absence of blood gas data.

‡Laboratory values less extreme than those indicated must be supplemented by clinical evidence of severity to warrant initiating mechanical ventilation.

ume of gas terminates the inspiratory phase; (2) pressure-cycled—in which attainment of a preselected pressure setting initiates the expiratory phase independent of the duration of inspiration; (3) time-cycled—in which inspiration and expiration are terminated by a preset cycle duration; and (4) flow-cycled—in which drop of flow to a present level initiates the changeover. Some ventilators cannot be assigned exclusively to any of these categories. Overriding time cycling is used as a safety feature in the first two types to ensure intermittent pulmonary inflation. The first three types have additional built-in safety features. Volume-cycled and time-cycled machines are pressure limited; pressure-cycled machines are flow rate limited.

Table 11–17 lists the commonly used ventilators. The efficacy of a particular ventilator depends on the skill and experience of the clinician and on the functional characteristics of the machine itself. One type may best suit a particular age group under certain conditions. The volume-cycled (pressure-limited) machine is effective when airway resistance is markedly increased and lung compliance is decreased, because even under these circumstances the appropriate tidal volume will continue to be delivered. However, a sudden increase in lung compliance may lead to lung rupture. Furthermore, it is difficult to detect leaks in the system unless inspiratory pressure is monitored. In contrast, use of the pressure-cycled (flow rate–limited) ventilator in the presence of leaks disturbs the attainment of the present pressure and thereby alters the cycling pattern; this situation should alert the intensive care unit staff. However, a decrease in lung compliance, such as that caused by accumulation of secretions, may be associated with a decrease in tidal volume. This situation

Table 11–17. EXAMPLES OF MECHANICAL VENTILATORS*

Volume-cycled (Pressure-limited)*
  Bennett MA-1
  Bourns LS-104
  Emerson Postoperative
  Engstrom
Pressure-cycled (Flow rate–limited)†
  Bennett PR-1 and PR-2
  Bird Mark VII and VIII
Time-cycled (Pressure-limited)
  Air Shields Isolette‡
  East-Radcliffe
  Air Shields
  Baby Bird§
  Sechrist Infant
  Biomed MVP-10
  Amsterdam Infant Mark 2
Flow-cycled
  Bennett PR-2

*Emerson postoperative and Engstrom ventilators are used as *controllers* only; all other types listed have provision for independent patient cycling *(assistor-controller)*.
†Has overriding time cycling in addition to the safety limit indicated.
‡Used as a negative pressure ventilator.
§Constant flow feature allows the use of intermittent mandatory ventilation (IMV).

may go unrecognized because the ventilator will continue to cycle at the preset pressure.

Overriding time cycling, a safety feature contained in most ventilators, ensures continued cycling should other mechanisms fail. Primary time-cycled (pressure-limited) machines deliver a tidal volume in the time allotted to inspiration. Because this type usually has a wide range of available flow rates, it can accommodate changes in airway resistance and lung compliance, but it functions most effectively when airways are relatively clear and lung compliance is stable. The constant-flow feature of the Baby Bird allows the infant to breath spontaneously even though a very slow rate is set on the machine (so-called intermittent mandatory ventilation or IMV). Many volume-cycled machines now incorporate a constant-flow feature to allow for IMV even in the older infant and the child.

A negative-pressure ventilator, available commercially as a purely time-cycled machine, has the advantage of not requiring tracheal intubation. However, the ventilator has not provided good control of alveolar ventilation in infants with hyaline membrane disease; that is, it has not been effective in lowering arterial P_{CO_2}. However, intermittent negative pressure ventilation with a portable device has been used in the treatment of chronic respiratory failure secondary to chronic obstructive lung disease.

In conditions associated with low lung volumes, such as hyaline membrane disease, atelectasis, and severe pneumonia (viral, *Pneumocystis*, meconium aspiration), alveolar collapse may be alleviated or prevented by the use of a positive end-expiratory pressure (PEEP). Alveolar pressure is not allowed to return to zero (atmospheric pressure) but is held at 3 to 5 cm H_2O above atmospheric pressure during expiration. This technique increases the efficiency of oxygen transfer in the lung (reduces the alveolar-arterial oxygen tension difference), thereby facilitating adequate tissue oxygenation at lower concentrations of inspired oxygen. The ability to oxygenate adequately at low inspired concentration of oxygen is important in preventing the toxic effect of oxygen on the lung. It is known that endotracheal intubation removes the normal laryngeal retardation of expiration (so-called physiologic PEEP). Thus a PEEP of 2 cm H_2O is used even in patients with normal lungs. PEEP has also been employed in patients with small airways disease, such as bronchiolitis, and is believed to prevent airway closure and air trapping. Hand-operated breathing bags with PEEP attachments are available, so PEEP can continue during manual inflation of the lungs shortly before and after suctioning of the patient on a mechanical ventilator.

In spontaneously breathing infants, constant positive transpulmonary pressure or continuous distending pressure (CDP) has been employed extensively in the treatment of hyaline membrane disease. Several methods have made this treatment possible in severely ill infants with adequate spontaneous alveolar ventilation (Type I failure) without having to resort to artificial ventilation. One method utilizes an endotracheal tube and bag system. The infant breathes into a rubber bag kept at a preset positive pressure. Carbon dioxide is washed out of the system by a high flow of gas, which leaks out at one end of the bag. The pressure in the bag is determined by the rate of gas inflow and by the screw clamp that controls the outflow. Later methods for the use of CDP have employed the principle of continuous application of positive airway pressure (CPAP) to the upper airways, using nasal prongs, a face mask, or a sealed head box. Another approach uses the negative-pressure ventilator in such a way as to provide a continuous subatmospheric chest wall pressure (CNP) while the infant breathes spontaneously. This method does not require endotracheal intubation and leaves the facial area clear for nursing care; however, access to the body is difficult, and significant leaks may cool the infant. CPAP has also been employed with varying success for the treatment of apnea of prematurity.

Mechanical ventilation at rates much higher than physiologic breathing frequencies has been tried in selected patients. So-called high-frequency jet or oscillatory ventilators use frequencies of up to 900 pulses/min. Theoretical advantages are a lower mean airway pressure and a reduced risk of lung rupture and chronic respirator lung damage. In preterm infants with hyaline membrane disease, results of high-frequency oscillation have been disappointing. Some infants with severe interstitial emphysema of the lung have been successfully treated with high-frequency ventilation, however.

Complications

Complications of ventilator therapy occur frequently, even with a highly skilled intensive care team, and personnel must be continually aware of the hazards associated with ventilatory support (Table 11–18). Aseptic technique is mandatory for tracheal airway care, because nosocomial infection constitutes a large and potentially preventable problem. *Pseudomonas* infection from contaminated water reservoirs can be prevented by careful attention to the source of water supply and by frequent changing of reservoirs and tubing.

Endotracheal intubation interferes with the drainage of pulmonary secretions, and special attention must be paid to maintaining effective drainage by means of suctioning and chest physiotherapy. Tubes may cause other problems, such as local necrosis, and cuffed tubes must be deflated every hour. Malposition of the tube is common; radiologic examination of the chest must be done to ensure proper placement.

A high concentration of inspired oxygen may be necessary to provide normal arterial oxygenation, but it must be accompanied by frequent analysis of arterial P_{O_2}. The premature infant is susceptible to retrolental fibroplasia, particularly if arterial P_{O_2} rises

Table 11–18. SOME COMPLICATIONS ASSOCIATED WITH MECHANICAL VENTILATION

Respiratory
Tracheal lesions (erosion, edema, stenosis, granuloma, obstruction, perforation)
Accidental endotracheal tube displacement (into main stem bronchus, esophagus, hypopharynx) or actual extubation
Infection (tracheitis, pneumonitis)
Air leaks (pneumothorax, pneumomediastinum, interstitial emphysema)
Trapping of gas (hyperinflation)
Excessive secretions (atelectasis)
O_2 hazards (depression of ventilation, bronchopulmonary dysplasia)
Pulmonary hemorrhage

Circulatory
Impairment of venous return (decreased cardiac output and systemic hypotension)
O_2 hazard (retrolental fibroplasia, cerebral vasoconstriction)
Septicemia
Intracranial hemorrhage (intraventricular, subarachnoid)
Hyperventilation (decreased cerebral blood flow)

Metabolic
Increased work of breathing ("fighting" the ventilator)
Alkalosis (potassium depletion, excessive bicarbonate therapy)

Renal and Fluid Balance
Antidiuresis
Excess water in inspired gas

Equipment Malfunction (Mechanical)
Power source failure
Ventilator malfunction (leaks, valve dysfunction)
Improper humidification (overheating of inspired gas, inspiratory line condensation)
Improper tubing connections (kinked line, disconnection)

above 150 to 200 mm Hg. Pulmonary fibrosis and necrosis of bronchiolar epithelium (bronchopulmonary dysplasia) are complications of the prolonged use of a high concentration of oxygen in association with mechanical ventilation and may reflect a direct toxic action of oxygen on the lung. It is likely that this complication can be reduced in frequency if inspired oxygen above 60 per cent is limited in application. Reduction of inspired oxygen concentration below 60 per cent should be made as rapidly as possible. Careful monitoring of both inspired oxygen concentration and arterial P_{O_2} is mandatory. In newborn infants with hyaline membrane disease, the use of CPAP, CNP, and artificial ventilation with PEEP has reduced the prevalence of bronchopulmonary dysplasia, but artificial ventilation with PEEP has doubled the prevalence of lung rupture, including interstitial emphysema of the lung, pneumomediastinum, and pneumothorax.

All ventilators increase pleural pressure relative to peripheral venous pressure; venous return to the heart may be impaired if excessive pressures are employed. The expiratory phase should be longer than the inspiratory phase, and a time ratio of 2:1 or higher is generally recommended. If the patient is not breathing in rhythm with the ventilator ("fighting" the ventilator), the work of breathing may be increased, thereby leading to increasing oxygen demand and carbon dioxide production. Under these circumstances, it is best to sedate the patient with morphine or diazepam or to paralyze the patient with curare or succinylcholine and to completely take over (control) respiration.

The use of ultrasonic nebulizers to humidify inspired gas may be associated with a positive water balance via the respiratory tract, and this effect must be taken into account in calculating fluid requirements. Proper function of the ventilator requires frequent checks on tubing connection, valve operation, humidifier apparatus, and the power source, whether pneumatic or electric. It should be emphasized that a clear understanding of the general principles of mechanical ventilation and the capabilities and limitations of the specific ventilator is crucial in reducing the incidence of complications or preventing fatalities.

ADDITIONAL THERAPY

Intensive management of respiratory disorders often requires additional treatment, depending on the etiologic or pathophysiologic features of the problem. The additional therapy may be either medical or surgical in nature (see Table 11–14).

Medical Therapy

The role of bronchodilator agents has been discussed earlier. Status asthmaticus may be refractory to such a drug until pH and blood gases are returned to normal. Steroids are effective, but there is often a delay of several hours. Steroids reduce the inflammatory response to inhaled or aspirated material and are particularly efficacious following the aspiration of gastric juice.

Appropriate antimicrobial treatment of infection requires culture and sensitivity studies of tracheal aspirate, sputum, blood, gastric aspirate, or loculated fluid in the chest. Pending the results of these studies, one is justified in beginning broad-spectrum antibiotic coverage in a patient who is acutely ill with an undetermined infection. Once the culture results are available, specific antibiotic coverage is begun.

Diuretics (e.g., furosemide, ethacrynic acid) and morphine are indicated in acute pulmonary edema. Morphine reduces venous return and thereby decreases pulmonary blood volume and pressures. Cardiac failure is treated with digoxin. Narcotic analgesics are also indicated in severe chest wall injury or severe chest pain, as in the immediate postoperative period. However, depression of ventilation and of the cough mechanism must be avoided; analgesics must, therefore, be given judiciously and discontinued as soon as possible. Pain associated with the movement of small flail segments of the chest wall may be reduced by compression strapping with a sandbag. Rib fracture, however, should not be strapped, because strapping interferes with expansion of the lung and leads to accumulation of secretions.

Severe hemoptysis or hemothorax may require blood transfusion. Not infrequently, the anemia may be so severe as to impair tissue oxygenation, and supplemental oxygen becomes essential until blood volume is restored. When a pneumothorax is small, nonprogressive, and mildly symptomatic, oxygen inhalation (100 per cent) is occasionally used to facilitate the absorption of air from the pleural cavity.

Surgical Therapy

Certain chest conditions can be properly and definitively managed only by surgical intervention. Thus a tension pneumothorax from any cause requires immediate aspiration of air. When air leakage continues, a chest tube is placed through the second intercostal space in the midclavicular line and is connected to an underwater seal. Suction may be required if the leak is large. The accumulation of liquid in the pleural space (e.g., blood) may also require tube drainage by placement of the tube in the dependent part of the pleural space. If the fluid is purulent and thick, open chest evacuation may be necessary; evacuation is followed by tube drainage. Control of persistent air leaks from the lung or of unrelenting hemorrhage requires thoracotomy for direct repair or emergency resection. Although never an emergency procedure, tonsillectomy with adenoidectomy provides a permanent cure of the pulmonary hypertension and respiratory failure occasionally associated with marked adenotonsillar hypertrophy and upper airway obstruction.

MONITORING

Close observation of the acutely ill child is mandatory but must be supplemented by other monitoring methods. The availability of modern blood gas equipment that allows the measurement of arterial pH, P_{CO_2}, and P_{O_2} on microsamples permits frequent assessment of these parameters. The need for continuous monitoring of the status of the patient and the operation of the equipment required for treatment has caused a remarkable growth in the availability of electronic devices. Associated with the use of such monitoring devices are certain hazards that are largely preventable.

MONITORING OF PATIENT STATUS

Close observation of the seriously ill child requires (1) visual inspection of skin color to estimate the level of arterial oxygen saturation, (2) observation of diaphragmatic movement and the use of accessory muscles to gauge respiratory difficulty, and (3) auscultation of the thorax to determine tube placement and the need for endotracheal suction. At the first sign of a change in status, arterial blood gas analysis must be done. Such measurements may be required as frequently as every 30 min if the patient's condition is unstable; if the clinical picture appears stable, blood gas studies need be done only two or three times a day. In the newborn infant, an indwelling umbilical arterial catheter is used for sampling and also for infusion of fluid. The tip of the catheter should be below the level of the renal arteries (L2) or at a high position above T_{10}. An arterialized capillary sample may suffice as an alternative, but P_{O_2} measurements are unreliable because they often do not reflect the arterial P_{O_2}. Continuous monitoring of arterial P_{O_2} and arterial P_{CO_2} is now feasible with the use of transcutaneous electrodes. Continuous monitoring of oxygen saturation is widely used with pulse oximeters. Temperature, heart rate, ECG, blood pressure, respiratory rate, and inspired oxygen concentration may be monitored continuously. It is beyond the scope of this chapter to comment in detail about precise methods of monitoring or the efficacy of or need for continuous monitoring of a patient or given parameter. Each intensive care facility should have its own specific guidelines, and these will vary with the age of the patient as well as with the personal preferences of the members of the intensive care team.

MONITORING OF EQUIPMENT FUNCTION

Constant surveillance of the equipment used for treatment and monitoring is essential to avoid complications. Not infrequently, equipment malfunction (see Table 11–18) may go unrecognized, compromising the patient's status beyond assistance. An audiovisual alarm is an appropriate method to signal any mechanical malfunction. Periodic checkup of the alarm system per se is essential. To ensure adequate monitoring of both patient and equipment, a flow sheet record of clinical observation, laboratory findings, and mechanical ventilatory adjustment is extremely useful.

ELECTRICAL HAZARDS AND SAFETY MEASURES

A potentially lethal hazard of using multiple monitoring devices is electrocution of patient or personnel. The hazard is introduced primarily because of stray electric currents or a faulty grounding system. Stray electric currents may be present because of a gross fault in the equipment. Frequent and regular inspection of all electrically operated devices in the intensive care unit, even when not in use, is most important in detecting obviously faulty equipment.

A more subtle source of stray electric current exists in all electronic monitoring devices because of leaks of small amounts of current to the metal case of the instrument. Every piece of equipment used in the intensive care area should be supplied with a three-pronged plug that contains a special third ground wire connected to the instrument case, by means of which current leaking to the case is carried to ground. Even though such current is small, it constitutes a hazard if it is allowed to flow close to the heart, for example, via the umbilical artery catheter. As little as 20 microamperes (20×10^{-6} amperes) may cause ventricular fibrillation when applied directly to the heart, whereas 5000 times this amount is required when the current is introduced externally.

Because of the subtle hazard of stray electrical currents, special attention must be paid to grounding, frequent testing, and personnel education. There should be a single effective ground consisting of a low-resistance wire that connects to all electric outlets in the unit. The use of the conduit for grounding is inadequate because the conduit is subject to mechanical damage or corrosion. Multiple pieces of equipment attached to the same patient must be grounded to a common point, such as a connection to a single bank of wall receptacles. This common grounding point is necessary to avoid small amounts of current flowing from one ground point to another (ground loops).

Despite the installation of a separate ground wire, breakage of ground connection frequently occurs inside the wall receptacle. Therefore, wall receptacles should be routinely tested for adequate ground connection. Equipment should also be routinely tested for leakage currents and other faults, because with the passage of time electrical components and insulating material gradually deteriorate. Tests for leakage current should be carried out at the instrument case as well as at the site of application to the patient (e.g., electrodes). Existing hospital safety codes are inadequate for medical equipment because they do not take into account the hazard of leakage current. Thus before purchasing equipment, one must obtain the manufacturer's specifications with regard to leakage current. Despite this precaution, each piece of equipment should be tested by the hospital engineer before actual use with a patient.

Each member of the intensive care team should be trained in the correct use of equipment and should also be aware of the potential hazard of electrical equipment. Consultation with a knowledgeable electrical engineer is advisable because the situation in a particular hospital is often complex and requires expert advice.

PSYCHOLOGICAL SUPPORT

Intensive respiratory care of children requires not only medical care of patients but also compassionate support for their siblings and parents. It is now clear that exposure to the intensive care setting is an emotionally traumatic experience for parents and siblings. Parents go through a series of severe psychological reactions, namely, shock and disbelief, self-blame, anticipatory waiting, and elation or mourning. To help families of patients cope, each member of the intensive care team must be aware of and able to recognize any of the psychosocial stresses associated with this experience. Specifically, all members of the team must know about the clinical events in the child's illness to avoid giving conflicting information to the families. Parents should be told of any therapeutic errors or iatrogenic complications that occur. The staff member who has overall responsibility for the care of the child should be made known to the parents, with whom this person must be prepared to communicate openly and frequently. Siblings should also be given equal attention and must be given information using language they can comprehend. Withdrawal of life support in the event of brain death must be presented to the parents as a staff decision; the parents should not believe that they are being asked to make the primary choice. Understanding of and dealing with these psychosocial issues are crucial components of pediatric intensive respiratory care.

SUMMARY

Intensive treatment of respiratory disease in infancy and childhood requires a clear understanding of the pathophysiology of disease processes in the younger age group and of the technological advances in respiratory care equipment. This chapter contains a classification of pediatric respiratory disorders according to the predominant functional derangement and a consideration of the recognition of imminent or frank respiratory failure. The principles of emergency and continuing intensive care of respiratory disorders have been discussed in depth. Details regarding intensive care unit organization, structural design, and equipment have been omitted. Therapeutic advances have been accelerated over the past decade because of the increasing skill of intensive care personnel as well as an improvement in equipment. In the final analysis, the success of such a unit depends on the availability of physicians, nurses, respiratory technologists, physiotherapists, and others organized into a team with special expertise and dedication.

REFERENCES

Avery ME, Fletcher BD, and Williams R: The Lung and Its Disorders in the Newborn Infant. 4th ed. Philadelphia, WB Saunders Co, 1981.

Ayers SM and Grace WJ: Inappropriate ventilation and hypoxemia as causes of cardiac arrhythmias. The control of arrhythmias without antiarrhythmic drugs. Am J Med 46:495, 1969.

Behrman RE, James LS, Klaus M et al: Treatment of the asphyxiated newborn infant. J Pediatr 74:981, 1969.

Berg T, Pagtakhan RD, Reed MH et al: Bronchopulmonary dysplasia and lung rupture in hyaline membrane disease: influence of continuous distending pressure. Pediatrics 55:51, 1975.

Bernstein JG and Koch-Weser J: Effectiveness of bretylium tosylate against refractory ventricular arrhythmias. Circulation 45:1024, 1972.

Bland RD: Special considerations in oxygen therapy for infants and children. Amer Rev Respir Dis 122:45, 1980.

Bohn D, Kalloghlian A, Jenkins J et al: Intravenous salbutamol in the treatment of status asthmaticus in children. Crit Care Med 12:892, 1984.

Chameides L, Brown GE, Raye JR et al: Guidelines for defibrillation in infants and children. Report of the American Heart Association target activity group: cardiopulmonary resuscitation in the young. Circulation 56:502A, 1977.

Chernick V and Raber M: Electrical hazards in the newborn nursery. J Pediatr 77:143, 1970.

Committee on Drugs of American Academy of Pediatrics: Emergency drug doses for infants and children. Pediatrics 81:462, 1988.

Daily WJR and Smith PC: Mechanical ventilation of the newborn infant. I and II. Curr Probl Pediatr 1:1 (June) and 1:1(July), 1971.

Dolovich M, Ruffin RE, Roberts R, and Newhouse MT: Optimal delivery of aerosols from metered dose inhaler. Chest 80(Suppl):911, 1981.

Downes JJ, Wood DW, Harwood I et al: Intravenous isoproterenol infusion in children with severe hypercapnia due to status asthmaticus. Crit Care Med 1:63, 1973.

Driscoll DJ: Use of inotropic and chronotropic agents in neonates. Clin Perinatol 14:931, 1987.

Driscoll DJ, Gillette PC, and McNamara DG: The use of dopamine in children. J Pediatr 92:309, 1978.

Egan DF: Fundamentals of Inhalation Therapy. 3rd ed. St. Louis, The CV Mosby Co, 1977.

Engle MA, Lewy JE, Lewy PR et al: The use of furosemide in the treatment of edema in infants and children. Pediatrics 62:811, 1978.

Goldring D, Hernandez A, and Hartmann AF: Cardiovascular emergencies in infants and children. Hosp Med 12:20, 1976.

Gutgesell HP, Tacker W, Geddes L et al: Energy dose for ventricular defibrillation in children. Pediatrics 58:898, 1976.

Jardin F, Farcot JC, Boisante L et al: Influence of positive end respiratory pressure on left ventricular performance. N Engl J Med 304:387, 1981.

Loughlin GM and Taussig LM: Upper airway obstruction. Semin Respir Med 1:131, 1979.

Martin L: Respiratory failure. Med Clin North Am 61:1369, 1977.

Mushin WW, Rendell-Baker L, Thompson PW, and Mapleson WW: Automatic Ventilation of the Lungs. 3rd ed. London, Blackwell Scientific Publications, 1980.

Newth CJL: Recognition and management of respiratory failure. Pediatr Clin North Am 26:617, 1979.

Orlowski JP: Cardiopulmonary resuscitation in children. Pediatr Clin North Am 27:495, 1980.

Pagtakhan RD, and Chernick V: Bronchiolitis. In Moss, AJ (ed): Pediatrics Update: Reviews for Physicians. New York, Elsevier North Holland, Inc, 1980.

Pagtakhan RD and Chernick V: Respiratory failure in the pediatric patient. Pediatr Rev 3:247, 1982.

Roberts JR, Greenberg MI, and Baskin SI: Endotracheal epinephrine in cardiorespiratory collapse. J Am Coll Emerg Phys 8:515, 1979.

Rothstein P: Psychological stress in families of children in a pediatric intensive care unit. Pediat Clin North Am 27:613, 1980.

Sackner MA, Brown LK, and Kim CS: Basis of an improved metered aerosol delivery system. Chest 80(Suppl):915, 1981.

Shoemaker W and Vidyasagar D (ed): Transcutaneous O_2 and CO_2 monitoring of the adult and neonate. Crit Care Med 9:689, 1981.

Sinclair JC (ed): Temperature Regulation and Energy Metabolism in the Newborn. New York, Grune and Stratton, Inc, 1978.

Smith RM: The critically ill child: respiratory arrest and its sequelae. Pediatrics 46:108, 1970.

Standards for Cardiopulmonary Resuscitation and Emergency Cardiac Care: Part III—Basic life support in infants and children. Part V—Advanced cardiac life support for neonates. JAMA 244:472, 1980.

Stephenson HE Jr (ed): Cardiac Arrest and Resuscitation. 4th ed. St. Louis, The CV Mosby Co, 1974.

Tabachnik E and Levison H: Clinical application of aerosols in pediatrics. Am Rev Respir Dis 122:97, 1980.

Taylor GJ, Tucker WM, Green HL et al: Importance of prolonged compression during cardiopulmonary resuscitation in man. N Engl J Med 296:1515, 1977.

Todres ID and Rogers MC: Methods of external cardiac massage in the newborn infant. J Pediatr 86:781, 1975.

Zaritsky A: Cardiopulmonary resuscitation in children. Clin Chest Med 8:561, 1987.

RESPIRATORY DISORDERS IN THE NEWBORN

ARNOLD M. SALZBERG, M.D., and
THOMAS M. KRUMMEL, M.D.

12

CONGENITAL MALFORMATIONS OF THE LOWER RESPIRATORY TRACT

THORACIC WALL DEFORMITIES

PECTUS CARINATUM (PIGEON BREAST)

Pectus carinatum is an uncommon structural deformity of the sternum in which sternal protrusion occurs with or without unilateral or bilateral costal cartilage recession. The excavatum abnormality is four to seven times more common than this variety (Fig. 12–1).

There are two basic types of deformity (Brodkin, 1953). The more common type involves a lower chondrogladiolar prominence (oblique form). The other type has an upper chondromanubrial prominence with a depressed gladiolus (arcuate form). Uncommonly, there may also be asymmetry with one-sided prominence. Males are much more often affected than females.

The surgical indications in the first 2 decades of life are mostly cosmetic and psychological.

The operative procedure consists of variously placed sternal osteotomies and chondrectomy of offending cartilages. Mortality and morbidity are very low, and the immediate and long-term results are satisfactory.

STERNAL CLEFTS (FISSURA STERNI CONGENITA)

A partial or total midline vertical split in the sternum represents a persistence of the embryonic separation of the two sternal cartilage bars, which have failed to unite (Hansen, 1919). Partial fissures are more common than total fissures. Furthermore, the partial split is more frequently seen in the cranial part of the sternum (Fig. 12–2). Isolated sternal clefts without other anomalies must clearly be differentiated from the sternal cleft that accompanies ectopia cordis, intrinsic congenital heart disease, and pathologic apertures in the abdominal wall, diaphragm, and pericardium (pentalogy of Cantrell).

The midline defect is appreciated on physical examination. The paradoxical movement of the anterior chest wall and the subcutaneous cardiac dance are specific findings; the opportunity for trauma as well as the cosmetic disfigurement is an indication for surgical intervention.

The unfused sternal bars of the flexible chest wall must be surgically apposed in the newborn before fixation and immobility take place. The lower or caudal bridge and xiphoid are divided, and appropriate chondrotomies are performed on the lateral sternal bars for surgical approximation of these two segments. This procedure is easily accomplished within the first 2 weeks of life. After this time, more complicated procedures are necessary, as suggested by Sabiston (1958), in which oblique mobilization of the costal cartilages is also included.

PECTUS EXCAVATUM (FUNNEL CHEST)

There are characteristic morphologic deformities in pectus excavatum that have been known since antiquity and that make the diagnosis fairly obvious on inspection. Physiologic implications and therapy are not quite so standardized.

The three anatomic segments of the sternum are not equally involved in pectus excavatum. The superior manubrium is normal. The sharp slope inward, toward the vertebral column, begins at the manubriogladiolar junction, and the depression is deepest at the gladiolar-xiphoid articulation. The depth of this concavity varies widely from a shallow excavation to near contact with the vertebral column. The xiphoid or ensiform may then proceed outward, deviate laterally, or become rotated. Deformities of the lower costal cartilages form an essential part of the malformation. From the costochondral junctions, the cartilages proceed away from the chest wall, then angulate sharply inward toward their sternal attachments, and thus become abnormal in length and

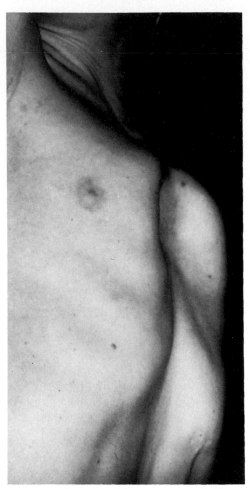

Figure 12–1. Pectus carinatum, or protrusion deformity of the anterior chest wall.

be minimal or extensive and may progress, regress, or remain stationary. With age, growth of the thorax in an anteroposterior direction is restricted but lateral development is uninhibited, and the disparity in the different diameters becomes obvious. Functionally, in the newborn and the infant, the labile breast bone may move paradoxically, but this movement subsides with fixation and rigidity, and a deeply concave pectus may move normally with respiration as the child grows older.

The depth of the gladiolar-ensiform excavation influences the position and volume of the intrathoracic viscera. There is cardiac compression between the sternum and vertebrae or dislocation of the heart into the left hemithorax with encroachment on the space occupied by the left lung. The basis for pulmonary and cardiac dysfunction exists, and the right side of the heart appears especially vulnerable, but it is difficult to document physiologic aberrations precisely. Bates and co-workers (1971) concluded that no consistent data have been accumulated that would incriminate pectus excavatum as an etiologic factor in the production of chronic pulmonary disease. Since their report, two highly sophisticated pulmonary function studies, performed under certain experimental circumstances, have incriminated the deformity as an etiologic factor in the production of cardiopulmonary disease (Bevegard, 1962; Beiser et al, 1972).

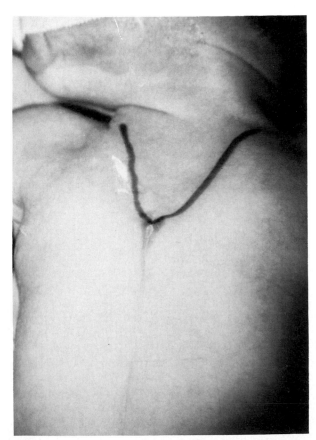

Figure 12–2. Partial sternal cleft in a newborn, outlined with marking pencil. Note typical raised fibrous cord between bottom of cleft and umbilicus.

direction. The deformity may be asymmetric, although the symmetric type is six times more common.

Theories about the causes of pectus excavatum are legion but can be distilled into a workable number. Both Brodkin (1953) and Chin (1957) have implicated a functional deficiency of the anterior diaphragm that, by default, allows the unopposed remaining diaphragm to distort a pliable sternum and the costal cartilages. Respiratory obstruction may not be a common cause but may aggravate an existing deformity by accentuating sternal retractions. Stanford and colleagues (1972) have emphasized defective pectoral muscles, whereas Brown (1939) described a short central tendon running between the diaphragm and the sternum. Neither factor is consistently present. An interesting possibility is that of a primary, misdirected, excessive growth of cartilage that eventually drives the lower part of the sternum backward. Of course, simultaneous or sequential diaphragmatic weakness with cartilage overgrowth is also a possibility. In addition, failure of osteogenesis and chondrogenesis, rather than diaphragmatic maldevelopment, has been emphasized by Mullard (1967).

The degree of structural deformity at birth may

Clinically, the deformity is apparent at or shortly after birth but is not associated with symptoms at this time, except for the occasional occurrence of paradoxical movement of the lower part of the sternum, which rarely produces respiratory distress. In the older infant or child, there may be decreased exercise tolerance, chest pain, palpitations, repeated upper respiratory tract infections, wheezing, stridor, and cough. The deformity at times is cosmetically objectionable and embarrassing to the child and the parents. The child is exposed to peer ridicule, will often not participate in outdoor activities, and may become reticent and introspective. The psychological impact may be the only or chief complaint, but in itself it can be crippling.

On physical examination, the inward angle of the gladiolar-xiphoid junction in the infant may be exaggerated with inspiration, documenting the paradoxical movement. Obliteration of the deformity should occur with expiration, and Chin (1957) believed that failure to do so was a sign of irreversibility. On further inspection, the anteroposterior diameter of the elongated chest is narrow compared with the lateral diameter. The round shoulders accentuate a dorsal kyphosis or kyphoscoliosis and protuberant abdomen (Fig. 12–3). The apical cardiac impulse is often shifted to the left and may be accompanied by a systolic murmur, which is usually innocent.

Examination by chest radiography quantitatively confirms the clinical diagnosis. The mediastinum and the heart are squeezed to the left of the vertebral column. The chest is wide on the posteroanterior view and narrow on the lateral view (Fig. 12–4). A radiopaque marker on the skin of the sternal depression nicely delineates the curvature and the restricted area between the posterior breast bone and the anterior vertebral column. Bronchograms have shown left lower lobe bronchiectasis, but correlation between this finding and the deformity remains poor.

The electrocardiogram may record a complex variety of changes, including right axis deviation, which probably represents displacement rather than intrinsic or concomitant heart disease. Increased venous pressure has been noted occasionally as a reflection of cor pulmonale and may be associated with a slight increase in right atrial pressure on cardiac catheterization. Pulmonary function studies have not demonstrated a consistent pattern. Often, vital capacity, maximal breathing capacity, and total lung capacity are within the normal range, although Orzalesi and Cook (1965) have reported lower than mean predicted values in 12 children with pectus excavatum. Only four of these, however, had an abnormally low vital or maximal breathing capacity. It is of some interest that in five of the 12 patients studied before and after surgical correction, there was no significant improvement in pulmonary function. Ravitch and Matzen (1968), however, have reported an 11-year-old girl with severe pectus excavatum and left lung agenesis whose pulmonary function improved after surgical repair. Welch (1958), too, has found a reduction in the vital and maximal breathing capacities in the lung volume in three of nine children so tested.

The clinical and laboratory information, then, in the majority of patients is likely to reflect a cosmetic deformity with variable psychological implications, vague cardiorespiratory symptoms, and minimal objective evidence of heart-lung dysfunction. Later in life a few patients with severe pectus excavatum and chronic pulmonary sepsis in whom the chest wall becomes rigidly fixed are said to have an insidious decrease in pulmonary function and perhaps emphysema. For this small group, operative correction has been advised as a prophylactic measure.

Additional indications for the surgical treatment of pectus excavatum might include seriously depressed funnel chest associated with measurable evidence of cardiopulmonary disease and a cosmetic deformity with poor posture that is psychologically oppressive and cannot be otherwise handled. This approach would exclude the newborn and the infant from surgery, except for the rare neonate with uncontrollable paradoxical movement whose diaphragm might be separated from the sternum, as suggested by Phillips (1960).

Figure 12–3. A moderate pectus excavatum in a 4-year-old boy with rounded shoulders, kyphosis, and protuberant abdomen. There is a reasonable cosmetic improvement 1 year after surgical correction.

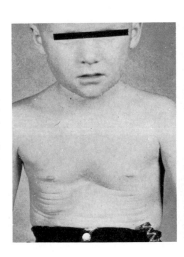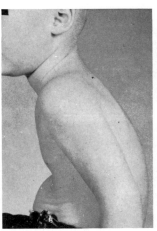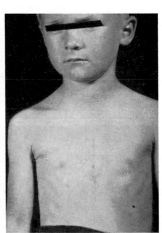

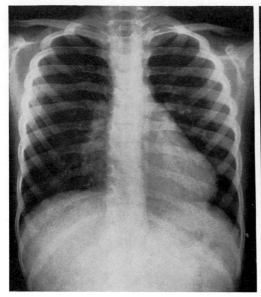
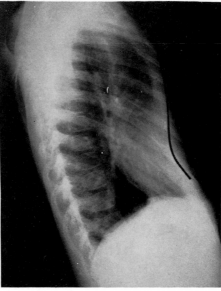

Figure 12–4. Typical roentgenographic findings in a 5-year-old boy with a pectus excavatum, demonstrating an absent right cardiac border and minimal deviation of the cardiac mass into the left hemithorax with angulation of the anterior ends of the middle and lower ribs. The chest is wide in the anteroposterior view and narrow in the lateral view. The lung fields are normal.

Meyer, in 1911, first attempted surgical correction of a pectus excavatum. The contemporary operative treatment for funnel chest was instigated by Brown (1939), who proposed the limited procedure of detaching or removing the xiphoid from the substernal ligament and diaphragm. Unfortunately, recurrence was frequent and stimulated the development of a host of more extensive thoracic wall operations. Basically, the deformity must be freed from all attachments, overcorrected, and splinted. The technique popularized by Ravitch (1949) is preferred by many because it fulfills the technical principles simply, without cumbersome external or internal appliances. Stanford and his group (1972) utilized a molded Silastic subcutaneous implant for correction of pectus defects in patients with cosmetic indications only. This technique is not applicable to patients in whom growth is still a significant consideration but may be useful in pectus excavatum complicated by unilateral absence of the pectoral muscles in adults.

Postoperatively, exercise tolerance may increase, and growth and development may accelerate. Other associated symptoms have been relieved. In a few instances, improvement in cardiac and pulmonary function has been noted. The immediate cosmetic results are usually acceptable and tend to remain so for the first 3 years, especially if the correction is performed between 3 and 8 years of age. Long-term follow-up studies are more divergent. Chin's clinic reported a 40 per cent recurrence after 10 years, although Wada and Ikeda's (1972) group had a 3 per cent recurrence rate. Younger patients corrected by Ravitch's technique have a low recurrence rate. The operative morbidity and mortality are acceptable.

CONGENITAL ABSENCE OF RIBS

This is an unusual bony deformity of the thoracic cage that is usually associated with other muscular and orthopedic anomalies (Fig. 12–5). The defect frequently involves the highest and lowest ribs, and clinical repercussions are minimal. Conversely, when ribs in the midthoracic region are absent, lung function may be altered.

In 1895, Thomson suggested that perhaps the hand of the fetus, applying pressure on the chest wall, produced the defect, which may be unilateral or bilateral and usually extends from the sternum anteriorly to the posterior axillary line. Involvement of the second, third, fourth, and fifth ribs would remove part of the origin of the pectoralis major muscle, and therefore absence of this muscle is a commonly associated defect; less common is breast

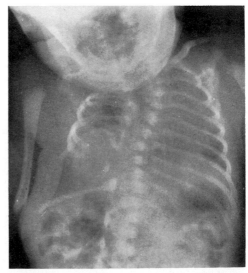

Figure 12–5. An anteroposterior radiograph of the thorax demonstrates deformed ribs and an absence of ribs on the right. Soft tissue changes consistent with the loss of supporting structures are also present. There is scoliosis with convexity to the left, and the heart is dislocated into the left hemithorax. Segmentation anomalies of the dorsal spine can also be seen.

agenesis on the same side. Hemivertebrae and kyphoscoliosis may be present.

The defect often produces no physiologic disturbance if the anomaly is single, small, and so localized that a lung hernia is not produced. If the second through the fifth ribs are absent anteriorly, a large lung hernia may occur, and lack of chest wall support here can lead to dramatic paradoxical respirations. Kyphoscoliotic heart disease, with cor pulmonale and congestive heart failure, may complicate congenital absence of ribs.

Symptoms may vary from none to severe dyspnea secondary to paradoxical respiratory movements and mediastinal flutter. Relatively few infants, however, present with advanced respiratory distress, and less serious difficulties will gradually disappear as the lung protrusion diminishes with growth.

Therapy is based on the contribution of the rib defect to the clinical picture and is seldom required. When symptoms are severe enough to produce respiratory embarrassment, local pressure may stabilize the chest, although Rickham (1959) believed that an inappropriate bandage may worsen the distress. Certainly, if critical symptoms persist in spite of conservative chest wall support, homologous rib grafting should be done. On occasion, adolescent girls may require cosmetic breast surgery for an ipsilateral rudimentary breast.

DIAPHRAGMATIC DEFORMITIES

CONGENITAL ANTERIOR DIAPHRAGMATIC HERNIA (MORGAGNI)

Morgagni hernias occur behind the sternum through defects in the diaphragm that are perhaps secondary to a developmental failure of the retrosternal segment of the septum transversum. The defect on the left is usually obliterated by pericardium; therefore, most of the hernias are on the right. Although these may be the most common tumors of the anterior inferior mediastinum in pediatric patients, they are the rarest type of congenital diaphragmatic hernia, accounting for one per 300 hernias. They are more common in females. More than half have a sac containing omentum or transverse colon. Hernias that do not contain bowel are the more difficult diagnostic problems.

In many infants and children, anterior diaphragmatic defects are asymptomatic, and the hernia is found incidentally on chest roentgenogram. Other patients may have abdominal complaints simulating those of gallbladder or peptic ulcer disease or constipation. A third group presents with chest symptoms of retroxiphoid pain, dyspnea, and cough. Finally, acute findings with strangulation are said to occur in 10 per cent of these patients. Here, succession sounds synchronous with the cardiac impulse may be diagnostic.

The diagnosis may be ultimately supported by roentgenograms showing a moderately dense tumor, usually at the right cardiophrenic angle in the posteroanterior film and in the anterior mediastinum on the lateral view (Fig. 12–6). A barium enema may delineate a thoracic transverse colon, which may also be elevated if omentum is incarcerated. An omental hernia may be suggested by changes in angulation of the transverse colon with inspiration and expiration. Liver scan and arteriography can be used to define those hernias containing liver.

Abdominal herniorrhaphy is advised for most Morgagni hernias because of the possibility of incarceration or strangulation, although the thoracic approach has been advocated by Boyd (1961). Results are consistently satisfactory.

CONGENITAL DIAPHRAGMATIC HERNIA OF BOCHDALEK

Posterolateral diaphragmatic hernia through the pleuroperitoneal sinus is perhaps the most urgent of all neonatal thoracoabdominal emergencies. If the diagnosis is not immediate in otherwise normal neonates who have symptoms in the first postnatal 24 hours, the mortality is excessive.

The maldevelopment has been catalogued as frequently as one in 2200 to 3500 births, or about 8 per cent of major congenital anomalies, and is left-sided in 85 to 90 per cent of the cases. It may be outnumbered by hiatal hernia but requires operative intervention as a lifesaving measure much more often. Concomitant defects that occur with some regularity are midgut malrotation, extralobar sequestration, and congenital heart disease.

Etiology. The hernia site between the chest and the abdomen results from a failure of closure of the pleuroperitoneal canal. The diaphragm is largely formed from the septum transversum and the dorsal mesentery, which at first separate the thoracic systems from the abdominal organs. The defect in the posterolateral areas of the diaphragm is the last to close and is eventually bridged at the sixth to eighth week (20-mm stage; 48 days) of fetal development by pleural and peritoneal membranes. Body wall mesoderm eventually insinuates between these membranes and becomes the diaphragmatic muscle. Early arrested development in the region of the foramen of Bochdalek, before the presence of pleura and peritoneum, produces a hernia without a sac, the most common anatomic situation. The left side is favored because diaphragmatic closure normally occurs here later than on the right. If the pleuroperitoneal membranes are formed without muscular development, a hernial sac for the Bochdalek defect has been created. Aborted muscle ingrowth between the properly fashioned pleura and the peritoneum may lead to a thin, fibrous tissue layer rather than substantial contractile muscle, and eventration results. Baffes (1962) has emphasized the role of an early return of the midgut

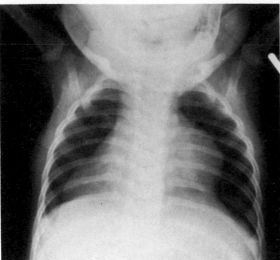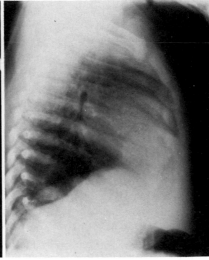

Figure 12–6. Anteroposterior and lateral films of the chest demonstrate a homogeneous shadow adjacent to the right heart border and diaphragm. The shadow is anterior in location with a smooth margin against the lung, as is seen with a Morgagni hernia. (Courtesy of Dr. MB Kodroff.)

(35-mm to 50-mm stage; 55 to 65 days) from its umbilical domicile to the peritoneal cavity in the creation and maintenance of Bochdalek hernias.

The aperture in the posterolateral leaf of the diaphragm may vary in size from a small defect to an absence or agenesis of the entire muscle, and may occur bilaterally. Small and large bowel, stomach, and spleen have been found in a pleural cavity on the left and the liver on the right. In less than 10 per cent of cases, a constricting hernia sac is present. Without this peritoneal or pleural investment, the herniated viscera may extend to the apex of the thorax. This migration of intraperitoneal structures is possible because of their insecure posterior peritoneal attachments and is reflected in the reported 20 per cent incidence of simultaneous malrotation. As in abdominal wall defects, the peritoneal cavity is small, lacking the growth stimulus of an expanding visceral volume.

Pathophysiology. Because the Bochdalek hernia has been present since early intrauterine life, compression of the ipsilateral lung may have occurred before the development of the lung buds (75 to 90 days); this process may also afflict the contralateral lung because of the severe mediastinal shift. The result of such compression is the development of bilateral pulmonary hypoplasia, more marked on the ipsilateral side; deLorimier and co-workers (1967) have produced a similar chain of events in fetal lambs with surgically produced Bochdalek hernias. This hypoplasia is a major factor in the excessive mortality in the early neonate with or without operation. The combined lung weights in nonsurvivors are distinctly below the average similar weights for other stillborns of the same range of body weight. Actually, lung expansion and growth occur in most survivors but may take days or weeks, depending on the degree of pulmonary differentiation.

The pathophysiologic features of the associated respiratory failure involve pulmonary hypoplasia as well as progressive pulmonary vascular hypertension.

The hypoplastic lungs cannot adequately ventilate or oxygenate, which leads to arterial oxygen desaturation, a mixed respiratory and metabolic acidosis, and, finally, pulmonary hypertension. This situation is compounded by the abnormal pulmonary arterial tree, which has more medial muscle and is thus more vasoreactive. Hypoxia, hypercarbia, and acidosis may all further stimulate vasoconstriction in the pulmonary arterial bed, raising pulmonary artery pressure and leading to right-to-left shunting through the foramen ovale or the ductus arteriosus. Such shunts increase venous admixture already produced by the ventilation-perfusion problem in the hypoplastic, collapsed lung. Oxygenation and ventilation are worsened, and the cycle is repeated.

Diagnosis. On examination of the newborn, immediate cardiorespiratory distress is striking and does not clear with pharyngotracheal cleaning. Cyanosis, dyspnea, tachypnea, and tachycardia are fairly constant. The involved hemithorax, usually the left, is relatively protuberant, and chest expansion is bilaterally uneven. Breath sounds are absent on the left, and percussion may be resonant. It is unusual to hear thoracic peristalsis. The apical cardiac impulse is dislocated to the right, and the abdomen is scaphoid.

The majority of patients with Bochdalek hernia have critical symptoms within the first 72 hours of life. After this, the patient is likely to have chronic respiratory and gastrointestinal ailments, and strangulation may occur.

Plain films of the chest in conventional views are almost always diagnostic, and the use of contrast material gives little aid to the work-up and introduces the danger of aspiration. The mediastinum is markedly displaced, and very little lung tissue on either side aerates properly. The diaphragmatic line on the affected side is difficult or impossible to visualize. Signet-ring radiolucencies in the thorax suggestive of air-filled loops of bowel are contrasted with a distinct loss of normal gastrointestinal pattern within the abdomen (Fig. 12–7). If the hernia is right sided, the liver alone may encroach on intrathoracic space, and liver scan may be necessary for diagnosis.

Differential Diagnosis. For differential diagnosis, Moore (1957) has emphasized the triad of dyspnea, cyanosis, and apparent dextrocardia. On radiography, the lesions simulate congenital cystic adenomatoid malformation, diffuse congenital pulmonary cysts, and pneumatoceles. Neither of the latter two is particularly frequent in the immediate neonatal period, and an infectious background is often lacking. Moreover, with all three, the abdominal gastrointestinal configuration is normal. Other entities that can be differentiated with minimal difficulty are laryngotracheal obstruction, atelectasis, pneumothorax, true dextrocardia, congenital heart and cerebral disease, and lobar emphysema. It may be impossible, but is unnecessary, to distinguish Bochdalek hernia, eventration, and phrenic nerve paralysis. The treatment in the presence of catastrophic symptoms is surgical in each instance.

Therapy. A number of neonates with congenital posterolateral diaphragmatic hernias expire shortly after birth even with a correct, prompt diagnosis, but proper emergency attention should enable most infants to survive. In this regard, effective, constant nasogastric suction may relieve or prevent the devastating intrathoracic gastrointestinal distention. Gentle positive-pressure resuscitation must be done through an endotracheal tube to avoid forcing oxygen down the esophagus and further distending the gastrointestinal tract. Overenthusiastic inflation of the lungs may produce unilateral or bilateral pneumothorax. The patient should be kept warm to reduce oxygen consumption. Serial blood gas and pH determinations, both pre- and postductal, must be obtained promptly, and vigorous treatment of the acidosis should be started in the preoperative period and continued throughout the operation.

Hedblom, in 1925, encouraged the emergency surgical approach for Bochdalek hernias by reporting a neonatal mortality rate of 75 per cent without operation. However, in recent years, Langer and colleagues (1988) have caused a critical reappraisal of this philosophy and have shown acceptable results with prolonged preoperative intensive medical management.

Thus the operation should be done following a period of preoperative resuscitation, stabilization, and correction of ventilatory and metabolic parameters. The surgical incision may be made transthoracically or transperitoneally, and there are advocates for each route (Fig. 12–8). A majority favors the abdominal route for neonates and the transpleural approach for infants older than 6 months. If reduction of the viscera in the abdomen and a layered abdominal wall closure create prohibitive intra-abdominal pressures, additional space may be obtained by creating a ventral abdominal Silastic pouch or by just approximating the skin. A further extension of this latter concept has been proposed by Meeker and Snyder (1962), who suggest the construction of a gastrostomy and an intentional ventral hernia when the operation is done in the newborn. Ventral herniorrhaphy may be accomplished after 1 year of age.

Closure of the posterolateral defect is usually uncomplicated, although the absence of a hemidiaphragm may pose serious technical problems, which have been ingeniously handled using Teflon, Marlex, and Ivalon grafts, pedicled abdominal or thoracic wall flaps, and the liver. Extreme care should be taken to avoid adrenal injury during the operation, because adrenal damage may contribute to mortality. An attempt should be made to visualize the lung on the involved side and the presence of a sac.

During the operation, the anesthesiologist cannot forcibly expand the atelectatic lung and, accordingly, must exert restraint in ventilating the patient in order to avoid pneumothorax, pneumomediastinum, and bronchopleural fistula. Postoperatively, the serial

Figure 12–7. *A,* The plain anteroposterior thoracoabdominal radiograph shows scoliosis of the spine and asymmetry of the chest, with the left side larger. The heart and trachea are dislocated to the left. The dome of the left diaphragm is intact; the right cannot be seen. Multiple signet ring radiolucencies and mottled densities are noted in the lower half of the right hemithorax. The right lung is confined to the upper half of the hemithorax, and the peripheral left lung is hyperaerated. The gastrointestinal air pattern normally seen within the abdomen is absent. *B,* Through the nasogastric tube, contrast material has been instilled that superfluously documents the finding of a Bochdalek hernia, which is apparent in the plain film.

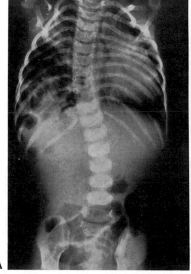
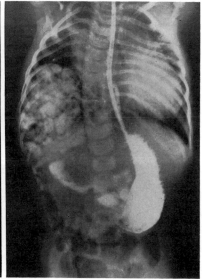

A   B

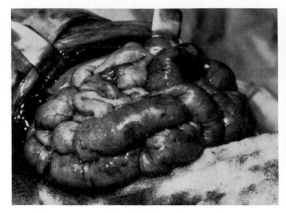
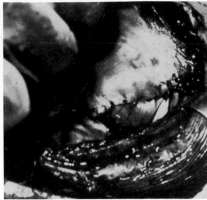

Figure 12–8. Small bowel extrudes through a low posterolateral right thoracotomy incision, relieving the pulmonary and mediastinal tamponade. After the hernial contents have been replaced within the abdomen, the diaphragmatic defect is closed in two layers.

monitoring of blood gases and pH is continued through an indwelling arterial line in both pre- and postductal positions, and ventilator support is managed accordingly. Pulse oximetry allows for continuous monitoring of oxygen saturation. Chest drainage is used without excessive negative pressure, and in the patient who survives, the lung will expand within a few days to several weeks. The insertion of a prophylactic chest tube on the contralateral side is gaining support, because the mortality of an unrecognized pneumothorax is so high.

Current investigative efforts are directed toward the pharmacologic control of pulmonary hypertension and the use of membrane oxygenators until pulmonary hypertension subsides. This research has been stimulated by the high mortality in newborns whose hernias are diagnosed within 8 hours of birth. Even though the defect is quickly repaired, persistent fetal circulation associated with relentless progressive acidosis, hypoxemia, and cardiovascular instability is followed by irreversible pulmonary failure and death. Early identification of these infants with severe but still reversible pulmonary failure would permit orderly application of conventional resuscitative measures, including antipulmonary hypertensives, such as tolazoline (Priscoline). If pulmonary failure persists in spite of maximal medical therapy, the mortality will be 100 per cent. Under these circumstances, extracorporeal membrane oxygenation (ECMO) using the internal jugular vein and common carotid artery for access to the right atrium and aortic arch seems justified. This type of extracorporeal support in patients with Bochdalek hernia may purchase the critical time necessary for the resolution of the underlying pulmonary hypertension. Numerous studies have documented its clinical effectiveness without serious untoward sequelae (Bartlett and Gazzaniga, 1977; Hardesty et al, 1981; Krummel et al, 1982).

The results of ECMO following repair of congenital diaphragmatic hernia were analyzed for 93 neonates reported to the neonatal ECMO registry (Langham et al, 1987). Although criteria for the initiation of ECMO support varied from institution to institution, most candidates for such support were judged moribund. Fifty-two infants (58 per cent) survived and were discharged. Mortality, despite ECMO support, was secondary to bleeding complications and renal insufficiency and was more common in small and premature infants. Survival rates as high as 90 per cent have been reported by other investigators (Stolar et al, 1988).

CONGENITAL HIATAL DIAPHRAGMATIC HERNIA

Some studies emphasize the frequency of hiatal hernias in the pediatric age group, especially during the first year. The extension of the stomach into the lower part of the chest occurs through an exaggerated crural defect that is usually congenital but may be acquired by gastric expansion in an upward direction during excessive vomiting. This may explain some of the hiatal hernias associated with pyloric stenosis.

The majority of hiatal protrusions in infancy and childhood are sliding hernias in which the esophagogastric junction is above the crural level of the diaphragm. This particular anatomic configuration abolishes the acute esophagogastric angle and, with a wide crural ring, allows free gastric reflux, which produces the symptoms of the disease. The rarer paraesophageal hiatal hernia has a normal esophagogastric junction and crural aperture, with the stomach herniating into the chest parallel to the esophagus but separated from it by strands of diaphragmatic muscle. Incarceration may occur with this arrangement, but reflux is less likely.

Persistent bile-free vomiting, projectile or regurgitant, is found consistently. This vomiting may begin soon after birth or at the third or fourth month and simulates vomiting seen in late pyloric stenosis. The incessant vomiting may occur at night with aspiration and repeated bouts of pneumonia. Slow growth and development are often systemic manifestations of malnutrition, dehydration, and chronic infection. Later, dysphagia from esophageal stricture and chronic pneumonitis with pulmonary fibrosis are seen. A peculiar contortion of the neck with hiatal hernia has been described.

Both hematemesis and melena can be confirmed by the clinical laboratory and are reflected in a blood loss anemia in about a third of the patients. The barium swallow with cinefluoroscopy corroborates the diagnosis and the stricture formation, and plain chest films document the aspiration pneumonia (Fig. 12–9). Burford and Lischer (1956) have emphasized the role of esophagoscopy in detailing the esophagitis and stenosis. Esophageal motility studies, continuous or intermittent monitoring of lower esophageal pH, and radioisotope scanning of the esophagogastric junction for reflux have all assumed significant diagnostic roles.

The differential diagnosis in the newborn and the infant involves other entities that produce rumination, chronic relentless vomiting with failure to thrive, actual malnutrition and depressed growth, repeated pneumonias, upper gastrointestinal tract bleeding, anemia, and dysphagia.

In the majority of patients, the hernia is small and symptoms are not critical, although there is no correlation between size and symptoms. In this sizable group, conservative therapy consisting of the continuous upright position (at least 60 degrees from horizontal), frequent, small, thickened feedings, and antispasmodics will suffice. Conservative therapy should be exhausted (continued for up to 10 weeks) before operative intervention is undertaken; 80 to 90 per cent of lesions respond to conservative measures, usually within 3 to 4 weeks. Surgical repair, either thoracic or abdominal, is reserved for patients who fail to grow and develop normally, continue to bleed, are developing a stricture, and accordingly are considered "medical failures." Hiatal herniorrhaphy can reverse this sequence of events by obliterating the hernial sac and reconstructing the normal esophagogastric junction and angle. The operation should occlude the patulous hiatus, anchor the esophagus below the diaphragm, and reinstate the acute gastroesophageal angle. Although many surgeons still favor anterior gastropexy, the operation of choice may be the Nissen fundoplication with crural suturing. This operation gives the lowest recurrence rate and an acceptable result. The morbidity and mortality following a technically satisfactory procedure are quite good, with relief of symptoms occurring in 90 per cent or more of the patients. The pylorus should always be evaluated for its role in the genesis of this problem. If any delay in gastric emptying is present or if the vagi are injured at surgery, pyloroplasty or pyloromyotomy should be done.

CONGENITAL EVENTRATION OF THE DIAPHRAGM

Eventration of all or part of one or both diaphragms follows maldevelopment of diaphragmatic muscle or, more commonly, phrenic nerve interruptions from birth or operative trauma. Thoracic operations for congenital heart disease with iatrogenic phrenic nerve injury have provoked a high incidence of unilateral postoperative eventration.

Embryologically, there is a complete or partial absence of muscular development in the septum transversum in the presence of normal pleura above and peritoneum below. These two membranes may be in direct juxtaposition or may be separated by only a thin fibrous sheath; usually, a small rim of muscle lies anteriorly between the pleuroperitoneal folds. Total eventration is said to be more frequent on the left, and a more localized or partial eventration is likely to be on the right side. The lesion has been found in the fetus, along with other local congenital anomalies, such as high renal ectopia and extralobar pulmonary sequestration.

Figure 12–9. A 7-month-old male infant with persistent bile-free vomiting, recurrent episodes of aspiration pneumonia, and poor weight gain. A, The lateral esophagogram reveals minimal dilation in the region of the middle third, with tapering and irritability of the distal portion of the esophagus. The presence of gastric mucosa above the diaphragm in a hiatal hernia is demonstrated. B, One month later, an air-fluid level is seen in the posterior mediastinum at the level of the carina with considerable dilation of the proximal part of the esophagus, documenting the progression of the stricture secondary to the hiatal hernia. A transthoracic approach to this sliding hiatal hernia with repair and dilation resulted in complete rehabilitation.

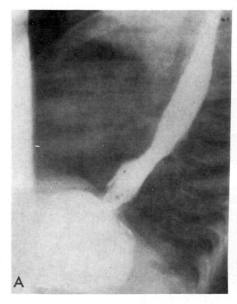
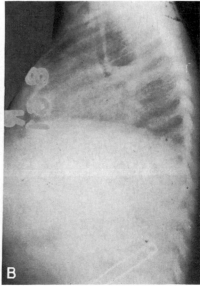

Gross pathologic analysis demonstrates an absence or diminution of the diaphragmatic muscle, which becomes fibrous, thin, and abnormally elevated. The phrenic nerve is smaller than normal; on microscopic examination, there is degeneration of the muscle but not of the nerve.

Symptoms are produced by an extremely elevated diaphragm with minimal or no function, but usually without paradoxical movements compressing the ipsilateral lung. The resultant mediastinal shift and rotation then encroach on the opposite lung. Respiratory findings are compounded by elevation and angulation of the stomach and are exaggerated after eating or in the Trendelenburg position.

The clinical picture may vary. It is not unusual to have respiratory distress of the order seen in a Bochdalek hernia—with dyspnea, tachypnea, and cyanosis. Physical examination may demonstrate tracheal and cardiac shift, with dullness and absence of breath sounds over the involved thorax as well as a scaphoid upper abdomen and fullness in the region of the lower chest on the involved side. Gastrointestinal complaints of vomiting, flatulence, and indigestion or cough with bronchitis and repeated pneumonia may predominate in the older child.

Fluoroscopy and chest roentgenograms are essential to the diagnosis. The degree of diaphragmatic elevation is precisely documented by visualization of a definite, thin, unbroken arc above the abdominal viscera (Fig. 12–10). At first, diaphragmatic excursions may be properly synchronous but minimal; later, perhaps, the diaphragm may move paradoxically and create mediastinal flutter. Atelectasis and mediastinal shift are seen.

The differential diagnosis includes congenital posterolateral diaphragmatic hernia and phrenic nerve paralysis. If the congenital eventration moves para-

doxically, it cannot be clinically separated from a hernia with a sac or a diaphragm elevated from nerve injury. In the usual Bochdalek hernia without a sac, however, the remaining diaphragm is difficult to see; when seen, it is located normally and is not elevated. Other diagnoses that should be considered are various tumors and cysts, Morgagni hernia, and, perhaps, pleural effusion. Barium studies and liver scan, separate or combined, can help in the differential diagnosis.

The course in congenital eventration is as unpredictable as are the symptoms. Deaths have been reported in the untreated patient, and survival may be complicated by chronic pulmonary suppuration, diaphragmatic rupture, and ulcer and volvulus of the stomach. Usually, however, supportive treatment suffices in the barely symptomatic infant. For dyspnea and cyanosis in the newborn, eventration should be handled by endotracheal intubation followed by surgical repair. With plication, which lowers the diaphragm, if the phrenic nerve is spared, mortality is low, respiratory distress is promptly abolished, and the immediate and long-term results are eminently satisfactory. The ipsilateral lung function may eventually approach normal. Goulston (1957) has demonstrated the efficacy of operation in older children with chronic gastric and respiratory complaints.

In the much more frequent, acquired, postthoracotomy phrenic nerve paralysis with eventration, removal of the endotracheal tube is associated with respiratory distress that is confirmed by arterial blood gas analysis. Fluoroscopy demonstrates the diaphragmatic elevation, but paradoxical respiration is consistent and dramatic and is the basis for the symptomatology. Conservative management with a nasotracheal tube and ventilation is indicated for 2 to 4 weeks. The key is postoperative end-expiratory pressures, which will control paradoxical movement. Persistent dyspnea without the airway is an indication for thoracotomy and plication. The results are predictably satisfactory.

CHYLOTHORAX

Pleural chylous effusion is a rare reason for neonatal respiratory distress but is important because the prognosis is fairly optimistic with conservative therapy.

Chylothorax, which occurs later in infancy or childhood, follows accident trauma, left thoracotomy (usually for congenital cardiovascular anomalies), mediastinal tumor, and infection. In the newborn, the causative factors are less precise. It has been reported after repair of a Bochdalek hernia. The basic noniatrogenic defect probably involves a malformation of the mediastinal and pulmonary lymphatics, with failure of orderly fusion and the production of multiple lymphatic fistulas. This defect may explain the generalized sources of chylous fluid found at postmortem examination.

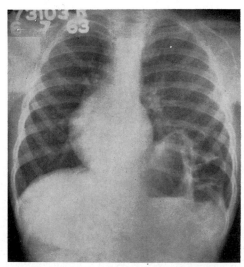

Figure 12–10. Radiograph of a 6-year-old boy with a modest, asymptomatic eventration of the diaphragm. The film was taken during an infrequent respiratory infection. The heart is shifted to the right, and the right diaphragm is intact and at the proper level. The arc of the left diaphragm is elevated two interspaces above the right and surrounds gas-containing abdominal viscera.

The remainder of the lymphatic system is usually normal, although widespread lymphangiomatous disease has been reported. Males are afflicted twice as often as females. Effusion occurs more commonly on the right.

A newborn may present with the usual stigmata of respiratory distress—dyspnea, tachypnea, and cyanosis without evidence of sepsis. On physical examination, the mediastinum is displaced, with unilateral dullness, and diminished breath sounds, although bilaterality has been reported at least once. Chest roentgenograms demonstrate opacification, usually on the right, with verification of the mediastinal shift.

The respiratory problem, which is secondary to compression atelectasis and mediastinal shift, is promptly relieved by aspiration of clear pleural fluid (the pleural fluid turns opalescent only after milk has been digested). The withdrawal of pleural chyle with a concentration of lipids greater than 400 mg/100 ml establishes the diagnosis, of course, and thoracenteses or intercostal chest tube drainage is continued until the pleural cavity remains dry. Varying numbers of thoracenteses have been used to control the effusion, which usually has a protein content of about 1 gm/100 ml. Ancillary help can be provided by a medium-chain-triglyceride, low-fat, high-protein, high-calorie diet. Parenteral hyperalimentation should be used if diet has failed to reduce chyle production.

In some instances, the chylothorax persisted in spite of multiple aspirations and intercostal tube drainage, and thoracotomy was performed. In one patient operated on by Randolph and Gross (1957), ligation of the thoracic duct controlled the lymphatic extravasation. Pleurodesis with iodized talc may also have a role in treatment. With diet and hyperalimentation, an operation should rarely be necessary.

Although the overall prognosis is favorable, death may occur from infection and malnutrition, and mortality rates have been reported as high as 25 per cent in some series.

TRACHEAL AND ESOPHAGEAL DEFORMITIES

TRACHEAL AGENESIS AND STENOSIS

Aplasia, atresia, or agenesis of the trachea is a rare congenital anomaly that to date seems incompatible with life. It would seem to occur because of a malformation in the development of the laryngotracheal groove.

Basically, the defect consists of partial or, more often, complete absence of the trachea below the larynx or cricoid; main stem bronchi that join in the midline; and a bronchoesophageal or tracheoesophageal fistula in 80 per cent of cases. The lungs may show lobulation abnormalities or intrapulmonary hemorrhage.

Clinically, these patients have respiratory problems at birth and die within a few hours. In at least one instance, the diagnosis was suspected and confirmed, and reconstructive surgery was ingeniously performed, with the patient surviving for 6 weeks. Intragastric oxygen at birth may prolong life if a fistula is present and thus may permit emergency surgical treatment. In a patient reported by Fonkalsrud and colleagues (1963), surgery consisted of division of the cervical esophagus with utilization of the proximal end as a salivary fistula and the distal stoma for the airway, division of the esophagus below the congenital esophagobronchial fistula, and gastrostomy. To date, there has been no satisfactory surgically treated case with long-term survival; this event may have to await further progress in transplantation or prosthetics.

Congenital stenosis of the trachea has been reported by Holinger and Johnston (1957) as a fibrous stricture in the form of webs; these webs are usually located in the subglottic area or just above the carina, although diffuse involvement has also been recorded. Respiratory difficulty is characterized by stridor. The diagnosis may be suspected on plain lateral radiographic films of the neck and chest and confirmed by contrast tracheogram or tracheoscopy. Dilation alone has not been particularly helpful, and tracheostomy may be necessary for acute respiratory problems. Successful transthoracic repair has been reported by Cantrell and Guild (1964). If possible, observation and conservative therapy should be exhausted, because growth at the stenotic area can eventuate in an adequate lumen. Othersen (1974) has reported the use of intraluminal stenting with a large-dose steroid injection into the stenotic area in a patient with congenital subglottic stenosis.

TRACHEOMALACIA

In infancy, the tracheal lumen is maintained largely by tracheal cartilages. If cartilaginous rings are congenitally absent, small, malformed, or too pliable, essential support is lacking, and such a lack may lead to functional tracheal stenosis and obstruction. This primary tracheomalacia is an unusual but most often benign form of respiratory distress in the newborn or infant and must be distinguished from the secondary type produced by extrinsic compression from a vascular ring or mediastinal tumor. The same pathologic process may be localized to a bronchus, with resultant congenital lobar emphysema.

Tracheal expansion and contraction occur with inspiration and expiration, respectively; these variations in airway size are minimized during sleep and shallow respiration and are exaggerated by forceful breathing, as with crying. With incomplete structural support of the trachea, the normal lumenal narrowing that occurs during expiration becomes exaggerated, and in severe instances the lumen may be small during inspiration.

Clinically, there may be wheezing, cough, stridor,

dyspnea, tachypnea, and cyanosis, all of which are made worse by pulmonary sepsis and secretions. On physical examination, expiration is prolonged, and there may be emphysema, but there is no localization by auscultation except with secondary infection. Opisthotonos has been reported. Neck, mouth, and pharynx are normal; ear cartilage may be absent. Chest roentgenograms are almost invariably done on inspiration, and the lungs may be exceptionally well aerated. Lateral films of the neck and chest taken during inspiration and, if possible, expiration may be helpful in the diagnosis.

The esophagogram is normal, but a contrast tracheogram done with cinefluorography in the lateral view may demonstrate the abnormal tracheal wall mobility. Laryngoscopy shows normal tissue down to the vocal cords, which, too, may be excessively soft; the combination of laryngotracheomalacia is not unusual. Careful bronchoscopy under local anesthesia may show close approximation of the anterior and posterior tracheal walls near the carina at any phase of respiration but most often at expiration. Passage of the bronchoscope to the carina is followed by less respiratory distress, because the flaccid area is being splinted by the instrument.

The differential diagnosis includes vascular ring, mediastinal tumor, tracheal web, foreign body, and obstructive lesions of the upper airway. Unfortunately, the ultimate diagnosis of tracheomalacia must often be established by exclusion. The findings of excessive tracheal wall mobility and airway relief with the passage of the bronchoscope are at times arbitrary and inconclusive.

Treatment involves the control of infection and secretions by specific antibiotics and humidification. Conservative therapy should be persistent, because cartilaginous development will eventually support the airway, and this improvement may be correlated with concomitant stiffening of the aural cartilages. Clinical improvement is definite in the majority of cases by 6 months of age, and spontaneous recovery in the remainder may be anticipated by 1 year. Tracheostomy has been used but is rarely indicated.

VASCULAR RING

In 1946, Gross and Ware inaugurated the current surgical management of vascular ring anomalies, more than 200 years after their morphologic description. Since then, documentation of this early contribution to cardiovascular surgery has been profuse.

Types. Although numerous variations from the normal aortic arch development have been reported, only a few distinct patterns can produce extrinsic tracheal obstruction, and even these may be incidental findings without clinical correlation. The most likely types that compromise the trachea and esophagus, singly or together, are (1) right aortic arch with left ligamentum arteriosum or patent ductus arteriosus, (2) double aortic arch, (3) anomalous innomi-

nate or left carotid artery, (4) aberrant right subclavian artery, and (5) pulmonary artery sling. Right aortic arch and double aortic arch account for the largest number.

A *right aortic arch* represents a persistent right fourth brachial vessel, which normally disappears. If the presence of this artery, in front of the trachea, is associated with a ductus or a ligamentum arteriosum that runs behind the esophagus, circular incarceration of the trachea and esophagus has taken place, and symptoms may follow. This anomaly has been reported to be more common in males, as opposed to the double aortic arch, which is allegedly more common in females.

With *double aortic arch*, the ascending aorta bifurcates and sends one branch to the right of the trachea and esophagus and then posteriorly to the esophagus to help form the descending aorta after joining the second branch of the arch, which proceeded in front and to the left of the trachea. Again, a ring is fashioned, and there may be respiratory distress.

Anomalous innominate or left carotid artery may produce direct anterior pressure on the tracheal wall because of delayed or premature origin from the arch. Thus the innominate origin from the arch is to the left of its normal source, whereas the left carotid arises to the right of its usual site. Both vessels must then run over the tracheal cartilages to reach their eventual destination and in so doing may produce a pressure phenomenon.

The *aberrant right subclavian artery* is most often asymptomatic but may constrict the posterior esophageal wall and produce dysphagia as it courses from the descending aorta toward the right and behind the esophagus. It is not likely to produce respiratory symptoms.

Pulmonary artery "sling" is perhaps the least common vascular cause of tracheal compression. In this congenital vascular anomaly, the left pulmonary artery originates from the proximal right pulmonary artery, traveling between the trachea and the esophagus to reach the left lung.

The common denominator in these arch anomalies is compression and narrowing of the tracheoesophageal complex. Air exchange is impeded, especially expiration. There is interference with deglutition, and esophageal distention near the area of obstruction may further constrict the narrowed trachea. Respiratory tract secretions are usually increased and poorly handled. Aspiration becomes almost inevitable.

Diagnosis. The clinical findings begin early, usually in the first year of life, and are most acute with a double aortic arch; they usually begin later and are less acute with a right aortic arch associated with an encircling ligamentum or ductus and are still less acute with anomalies that produce pressure only anteriorly, such as aberrant left carotid and innominate arteries.

Signs and symptoms (noisy respirations, intercostal retraction, dyspnea, and tachypnea) frequently are first observed while the newborn is still in the hospital's nursery. There is an invariable exacerbation of the respiratory problem with feedings, and cyanosis with coughing is likely at this time. On examination, the chest may be slightly emphysematous, expiration is prolonged, and stridor is apparent. Auscultation may demonstrate expiratory wheezing and rhonchi that are diffuse and sometimes transmitted. Opisthotonos is a common observation, and neck flexion is not tolerated.

Plain films in conventional views may show unusually well-aerated lungs, migratory atelectasis, pneumonia, and sometimes a right aortic arch. Chest roentgenograms may fail, however, to explain the respiratory difficulty. On good lateral films, the trachea may be seen to be narrowed just above the carina. Contrast material in the esophagus will document various combinations of posterior or lateral indentations at the same level as the tracheal constriction (Fig. 12–11). A normal esophagogram excludes a critically symptomatic vascular ring, so esophagography becomes the fundamental diagnostic study. Endoscopy will confirm these findings, and compression of the posterior esophageal pulsatile bulge by the scope with loss of right radial pulse is diagnostic of an aberrant right subclavian artery. If respiratory distress is not critical, contrast material in the trachea will delineate the anterior tracheal wall compression. In the infant, this can be done without general anesthesia by direct tracheal instillation or by overflow from the hypopharynx.

The presence of a vascular ring can be proved by angiocardiography (Fig. 12–12). This demonstration

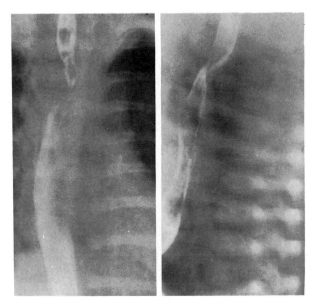

Figure 12–11. Posteroanterior and lateral views of a barium swallow demonstrate encirclement of the esophagus at the level of the aortic arch in a 2-month-old infant with dyspnea and noisy respirations. There is narrowing of the lumen from extrinsic pressure with forward displacement, noted best in the lateral projection. The posteroanterior film shows minimal deviation to the left, with tapering of the esophagus near a horizontal area of constriction.

in the presence of clinical symptoms and roentgenographic or endoscopic evidence of tracheoesophageal compression secures the diagnosis. In addition, contrast studies may facilitate the dissection and uncover other cardiovascular anomalies that were clinically unsuspected. Contrast studies can be of particular significance with a right aortic arch, because there is a high incidence of associated intracardiac anomalies.

Differential Diagnosis. The differential diagnosis involves the clinical picture of respiratory distress, stridor, and dysphagia. Cervical and hypopharyngeal obstruction can be ruled out by physical examination of the neck and the mouth and by laryngoscopy. Mediastinal tumors and most foreign bodies are excluded on the basis of radiographs. The diagnostic possibilities are thus restricted to a vascular ring, tracheal stenosis, tracheoesophageal fistula without atresia, and tracheomalacia. The esophagogram is the next step in the orderly establishment of the diagnosis and begins to limit the possibilities.

Treatment. After the diagnosis has been established, a short period of observation is useful, because only those patients with severe symptoms, recurrent respiratory infections, failure to thrive, dysphagia, and respiratory distress should be considered for surgery (Mustard, 1962). With prolonged hospitalization, however, a considerable mortality arises from the natural course of the disease, especially with a double aortic arch or right arch–left ligamentum arteriosum. Death may be sudden, due to compression or sepsis, and may be secondary to pneumonia. In the severely symptomatic infant, tube feeding, frequent pharyngeal suction, specific antibiotic therapy, high humidity, and control of oxygen and temperature are indispensable in the preoperative period. Careful, direct tracheal aspiration may be appropriate at this time.

The surgical treatment for an offensive vascular ring is now fairly standard. In all cases, careful attention should be paid to the anatomy of the recurrent laryngeal nerve. With right aortic arch and ligamentum arteriosum, division of the latter provides relief. A double aortic arch requires division of the smaller arch, usually the anterior one. The ligamentum or ductus should also be interrupted and the remnant of the anterior arch should be sutured to the undersurface of the sternum without separation from the trachea (Fig. 12–13). Inspection and palpation of the lateral tracheal walls may reveal a cartilaginous deformity, which might alter the postoperative course.

Surgical intervention for an aberrant left carotid artery is rarely required. When indicated, it consists in displacement of the vessel rather than division. An innominate artery, usually but not always aberrant (Mustard et al, 1969), may be a significant factor in producing varying degrees of tracheal obstruction by anterior tracheal compression. In severe cases, the diagnosis is suggested by a "reflex apneic" syndrome in the presence of other signs and symptoms of

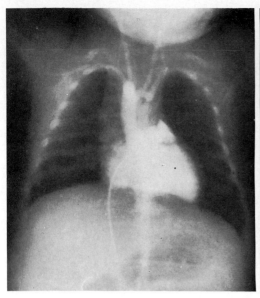

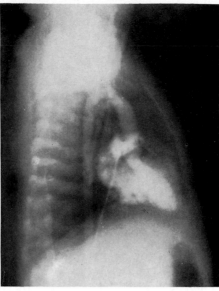

Figure 12–12. Selected posteroanterior and lateral films from a venous angiocardiogram through the right atrium, foramen ovale, and left atrium demonstrate two separate contrast-filled channels originating at the superior aspect of the ascending aorta. On the lateral view, the larger superior posterior arch and smaller inferior anterior limb fuse posteriorly at the origin of the descending aorta. In the two composite films, the innominate artery arises before the formation of the double arch, and the left-sided branches arise from the smaller anterior limb. In the frontal projection, the posterior arch has a short diagonal course to the left and downward before merging to form the descending aorta. (Courtesy of Dr. Page Mauck.)

vascular ring and is confirmed by contrast esophagogram, cinetracheography, endoscopy, and aortic angiography. The vast majority of patients can be treated medically, but about 10 per cent will need suspension of the innominate artery and base of the aorta to the sternum, which enlarges the tracheal lumen by drawing the anterior tracheal wall forward.

It appears that median sternotomy offers the best exposure for division of the aberrant left pulmonary artery with anastomosis to the main pulmonary artery with or without cardiopulmonary bypass. Simultaneous aortopexy and division of the ligamentum, or ductus arteriosus, will completely free the trachea.

In all vascular anomalies that encircle or compress the trachea, the esophagus, or both, it would appear that simultaneous bronchoscopy during open operation will ensure widest anatomic tracheal patency.

The period immediately after vascular ring surgery may be precarious because operative and anesthetic trauma may compromise the airway. Most complications occur in association with double aortic arch. Attention should be paid to the possibility of malacia of the trachea or a main stem bronchus and its effect on postoperative respirations. Fortunately, tracheostomy is rarely required. The stridor usually disappears, and feedings are taken without choking or aspiration. Respirations are not affected by flexion or extension of the head, but they continue to be loud for a few months.

Operative results are uniformly good, and relief from the respiratory distress is predictable. Surgical mortality and morbidity are low.

TRACHEOESOPHAGEAL FISTULA WITHOUT ESOPHAGEAL ATRESIA

Instances of communication between the trachea and the esophagus with an otherwise normal esophagus occur in about 3 per cent of tracheoesophageal fistulas, and according to Schneider and Becker (1962), approximately 28 infants so affected are born each year in the United States. Although symptoms from this congenital abnormality are fairly gross, the diagnosis is usually delayed, and a considerable amount of respiratory morbidity is likely to result (Fig. 12–14). The delay in diagnosis is unfortunate, because babies with an H-type fistula have a lower incidence of other anomalies and a higher birth

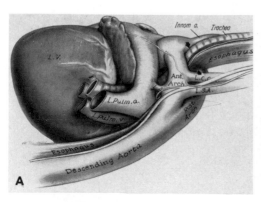

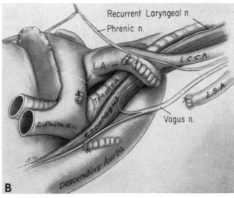

Figure 12–13. A, The operative findings through a left posterolateral fourth interspace incision confirm the presence of a double aortic arch. B, The left subclavian artery and ligamentum arteriosum were divided, and the smaller anterior arch was transected well to the left of the origin of the left common carotid artery. The remnant of the anterior arch may then be sutured to the undersurface of the sternum without being separated from the trachea.

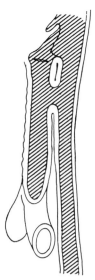

Figure 12–14. Diagram of tracheoesophageal fistula without esophageal atresia. The actual communication is much smaller than depicted.

weight than newborns with other types of tracheoesophageal fistula.

The tracheoesophageal connection is almost always small, and the majority are found in the neck, from below the larynx to the thoracic inlet. With this arrangement, the lungs become, in essence, a diverticulum of the esophagus, and continuous and relentless pulmonary soiling is the basis for extensive pulmonary infection.

The diagnosis should be considered in the presence of recurrent pneumonitis without clear cause or when bouts of coughing, choking, or cyanosis follow the ingestion of fluids. There is no dysphagia; solids may be swallowed and gavage feedings may be given without difficulty. On physical examination, gastric distention is prominent, especially after crying and coughing, as air is fed through the fistula into the esophagus and the stomach. The lung fields are noisy after liquid feedings but clear before such feedings. The severity of symptoms may parallel the size of the fistula.

Plain chest roentgenograms often demonstrate the stigma of chronic pulmonary sepsis, especially in the right upper lobe. In addition, attempts should be made to visualize the fistula by radiographic examination or endoscopy. Utilization of the Storz scope with the Hopkins telescopic lens system has made this approach extremely successful. Esophagograms in the various prone positions may be fruitful, especially if cinefluoroscopy is used. With continuous recording of the contrast-medium swallow, filling of the trachea through a fistula can be distinguished from overflow aspiration, and abnormal peristalsis of the esophagus distal to the fistula may sometimes be visualized. Several examinations may be necessary for radiographic diagnosis. Esophagoscopy and bronchoscopy are very likely to demonstrate the specific orifices, and dyes, such as methylene blue, inserted

into one lumen, may be recovered in the other lumen, especially if the esophagus distal to the fistula is occluded with a Foley catheter. This diagnosis may be difficult to substantiate, but studies should be repeated until it is confirmed. Surgery should not be done without a definitive diagnostic study.

The differential diagnosis of this variant of tracheoesophageal fistula should include chronic bacterial pulmonary disease, chalasia, achalasia, hiatal hernia, cystic fibrosis, neurogenic dysphagia, vascular ring, and agammaglobulinemia.

Operative division and suture of the fistula through a transcervical approach are very satisfactory in most instances. Very few fistulas must be handled transthoracically. The operative mortality is reasonable, and deaths are due largely to the crippling nature of the chronic pulmonary disease in patients whose diagnosis has not been prompt.

ESOPHAGEAL ATRESIA

The various types of esophageal atresia compose an important segment of those congenital abnormalities that produce respiratory distress in the newborn. The most common anatomic configuration of this primitive foregut anomaly, with an incidence of 85 per cent, is esophageal atresia with distal tracheoesophageal fistula. In perhaps 5 to 10 per cent of the cases of esophageal atresia, there is no fistula between the distal esophagus and the trachea (Fig. 12–15). Atresia with proximal tracheoesophageal fistula and tracheal fistula from both upper and lower esophageal pouches occur infrequently.

The incidence of this anomaly has been variously recorded, but one in 3500 births is a reasonable

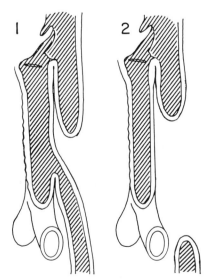

Figure 12–15. By far the most common morphologic variation of esophageal atresia is proximal atresia with distal tracheoesophageal fistula *(1)*. Much less frequent is proximal atresia without a tracheoesophageal fistula, in which the distal part of the esophagus, seen diagrammatically, actually ends blindly just above the crura of the diaphragm *(2)*.

consensus, and males predominate. At least 25 per cent of all patients are premature, and the same percentage have additional critical malformations, such as congenital heart disease, Down's syndrome, hydronephrosis, duodenal atresia, and tracheomalacia; 10 per cent of these babies have an imperforate anus, and one half have vertebral anomalies.

Aberrations in the development of the primary, common respiratory-digestive anlage form the basis for this anomaly. Separation into the anterior pulmonary and posterior gut components by fusion of internal septa is incomplete, perhaps explaining the presence of communications or fistulas. A complete lack of septal ingrowth is associated with the more serious, related deformity of laryngotracheoesophageal cleft. The intrauterine interruption of the vascular supply to the esophagus, the vascular anomalies with constriction, or the failure of intralumenal esophageal vacuolization may explain the atresia.

Pathology. Gross pathologic information is useful in the diagnosis and management of this lesion. With the usual proximal atresia and distal fistula arrangement, the upper blind pouch is large and substantial and usually ends about 8 cm from the superior alveolar ridge in the region of the azygos vein. The arterial supply from the inferior thyroid artery is rich, runs in a vertical manner, and is difficult to interrupt. Conversely, the lower segment is small and flimsy and originates from the region of the distal posterior membranous trachea, carina, or right main stem bronchus. Its arteries are distributed radially from the intercostals, and a small tracheal vessel may nourish the esophageal end of the tracheoesophageal fistula. Accordingly, ischemia and necrosis of the distal esophagus are constant hazards of the operative dissection. Congenital stenosis and a diaphragm-like atresia below the tracheoesophageal fistula in the distal esophagus have been reported. The attachment of the lower part of the esophagus to the region of the bifurcation of the trachea places this segment in somewhat of a juxtaposition to the upper pouch. Fortunately, in one fourth of such cases, the two muscle walls are in actual contact and anastomosis is relatively simple; in the remaining three fourths, the anastomosis is more difficult because the segments are separated by a gap varying from 1 mm to several centimeters.

In the 5 to 10 per cent of atresias without fistula, the proximal esophagus is similar to its counterpart in the more usual variance, but the distal esophagus is actually a small gastric diverticulum that barely extends above the diaphragmatic crura and, of course, ends blindly. The two segments are widely separated and cannot be joined surgically in the immediate postnatal period.

Pathophysiology. The respiratory distress sustained by newborns with proximal atresia and distal fistula is instigated by three factors. First, and obviously, secretions that collect in the upper pouch may overflow into the trachea. Second, gastric juice refluxes through the tracheoesophageal fistula and floods the lungs. Third, the fistula provides a convenient route for gastric distention, upward displacement of the diaphragm, and critical interference with pulmonary function.

Diagnosis. The clinical picture begins with a history of hydramnios in 25 per cent of the mothers. Profuse, bubbly, oral mucus appears early and almost continuously covers the baby's chin in spite of persistent oropharyngeal aspiration. Tachypnea and dyspnea soon follow, with intermittent episodes of choking and cyanosis. Regurgitation occurs promptly after the initial and subsequent feedings, and the aspiration explosively exacerbates the respiratory distress. This latter finding is exaggerated in the rare atresia with a proximal fistula, because the ingested liquid reaches the lungs directly through the fistula as well as by overflow of the proximal pouch. On further examination, the abdomen is protuberant, flatus is quickly and incessantly passed, and consolidation may be demonstrated in the region of the right upper lobe. If the abnormality is an atresia without a fistula, the incidence of maternal hydramnios may be higher, pulmonary consolidation may be lower, and the abdomen is scaphoid. Otherwise, the findings in these two types of atresia are similar.

Thoracoabdominal roentgenograms in conventional views may show consolidation of the right upper lobe or more diffuse pneumonitis. Air in the gastrointestinal tract is seen in the usual atresia with distal fistula, although it is said that small fistulas may prevent air from leaking into the stomach. Conversely, large amounts of gastric air may suggest a large fistula, and therapy becomes more urgent because of the exaggerated respiratory distress. An airless abdomen is presumptive evidence of atresia without a distal fistula. On lateral thoracic radiographic films, the proximal atretic pouch may be delineated by air, but this finding is made clearer by the insertion of a small radiopaque catheter. Coiling a fairly stiff catheter at a level between the second and fourth thoracic vertebrae concludes the regional diagnostic exercise. Contrast material should not be necessary. When used, it should be restricted to a small amount (0.5 ml) of water-soluble material. Gastrografin is especially irritating and should be avoided. The contrast material should be removed by aspiration at the conclusion of the examination (Fig. 12–16). Delays in diagnosis can be avoided if orogastric catheterization routinely follows pharyngeal suctioning in newborns, preferably with the same catheter.

These and other diagnostic studies are utilized to establish the presence of additional anomalies that may affect therapy. Thus the mediastinal dissection can be performed more readily if a right-sided aortic arch has been noted preoperatively. Congenital heart, cerebral, gastrointestinal, and neurologic anomalies must be considered and uncovered with some dispatch before the correct operative approach can be planned. Associated cardiovascular anomalies are particularly lethal.

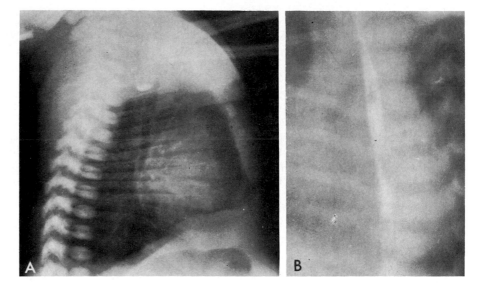

Figure 12–16. *A,* Lateral upright chest roentgenogram after instillation of 0.5 ml of contrast material into the esophagus has defined the atresia at the level of the fourth thoracic vertebra. There is gas in the stomach. *B,* A spot film 3 weeks after surgical repair demonstrates an adequate, undistorted lumen.

The diagnosis of atresia with fistula should be strongly suspected, then, on the basis of maternal hydramnios, excessive mucus, respiratory distress, and regurgitation. The suspicion is strengthened when passage of a catheter into the esophagus is stopped 6 to 8 cm from the gums. The final confirmation is obtained by fluoroscopic examination.

Treatment. Preoperatively, the upper pouch is aspirated through an indwelling catheter. A semi-upright position should be maintained during transportation or in the nursery Isolette to prevent or minimize gastric reflux through the fistula, although the Trendelenburg position has been advocated by some. High humidity and antibiotics are used to control pneumonia. Constant nursing care should be started on admission.

The operative management of isolated atresia without a fistula requires esophageal elongation and approximation of the blind ends by bougienage or an eventual reversed gastric tube or colon transplant, because the two ends of the esophagus are widely separated and cannot be anastomosed. The operation immediately after diagnosis is gastrostomy under local anesthesia. A contrast study through the stomach with the infant in sharp Trendelenburg position will outline the short, blind, distal esophageal stump. The proximal pouch is drained by a nasal sump-type catheter, and the gastrostomy tube is used for feeding. Both pouches are then elongated toward each other by bougienage until they are close enough for an anastomosis to be obtained. If this maneuver is not successful, a cervical esophagostomy is created to drain saliva, and esophageal replacement is anticipated at 18 months of age. The same steps have been followed when a large gap prevents anastomosis in the usual variety of atresia (Fig. 12–17). Proximal esophagomyotomy, in which a circular incision is made through the muscle layer down to the submucosa in the proximal thickened esophagus, has pro-

vided sufficient length for a satisfactory anastomosis even with large gaps between segments.

Several operative approaches are available for atresia with distal fistula. The ultimate decision is based on degree of prematurity, presence of other anomalies, time of diagnosis, presence or absence of pneumonia, exact anatomic configuration of the lesion, and preference of the surgeon. Transpleural or extrapleural ligation of the fistula and end-to-end or end-to-side esophagoesophagostomy with or without gastrostomy are ideal and constitute the accepted approach in the full-term newborn with no serious anomalies or pneumonia.

Varying degrees of prematurity, pneumonitis, and concomitant abnormalities drastically alter mortality, so that staged procedures have assumed some popularity in certain clinics. Gastrostomy alone may be chosen as the primary, emergency step to decompress the fistula and control the pneumonia. To this can be added parenteral hyperalimentation or a duo-

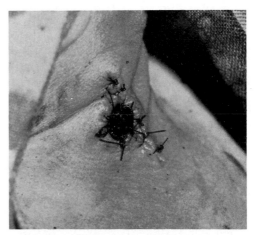

Figure 12–17. Proximal esophagostomy, or salivary fistula, in the right side of the neck of a newborn with esophageal atresia without fistula.

denal feeding tube along with suction of the proximal esophageal pouch. Meeker and Snyder (1962), Randolph and co-workers (1968), and Touloukian and co-workers (1974) have individually suggested transabdominal gastric division and double gastrostomy for the critically affected premature infant. Feedings are instilled into the distal tube, decompression of the tracheoesophageal fistula is accomplished through the proximal tube, and the thorax is not molested. Under ideal circumstances, these arrangements are commensurate with improvement in the size and health of the patient in preparation for definitive surgery. If these temporizing measures are inadequate, extrapleural ligation of the fistula and fixation of the oversewn distal esophagus to the endothoracic fascia permits feeding while the upper pouch remains on continuous or intermittent suction. With good nursing care, this arrangement is compatible with growth and development, and the esophageal anastomosis may be done electively, when the risk to the patient is lessened. If such nursing care cannot be provided, aspiration pneumonia from the upper pouch is almost inevitable, and in these circumstances, the very premature infant had best be treated by a salivary fistula and an esophageal substitute. This approach is less than ideal, but the mortality is improved distinctly over that of primary repair in this group.

The immediate postoperative period is critical and deserves maximum attention. The respiratory tract is especially vulnerable, and prophylaxis is the therapeutic goal. All the advantages of an Isolette are utilized. The pharynx must be aspirated carefully, without injury to the fresh anastomosis, to prevent aspiration and to stimulate coughing. Feedings should be started on the second to fourth postoperative day with homeopathic amounts of glucose water and formula, initially administered by slow drip through the gastrostomy tube. Oral feedings should be started after a barium swallow has verified a patent anastomosis without leaks.

Complications are legion, but the most catastrophic is disruption of the suture line and resultant empyema. The initial mortality from this disruption can be lessened by an extrapleural operative approach, which would confine the contamination to an extrapleural plane. Definitive treatment consists of effective naso-upper esophageal pouch and gastric catheter drainage along with duodenal feeding or parenteral hyperalimentation. The brassy postoperative cough is usually temporary and not related to a recurrence of the fistula, which does happen in about 10 per cent of cases and has a rather high mortality. This complication can be diagnosed nicely by esophagoscopy with the instillation of methylene blue through an endotracheal tube. Anastomotic strictures occur within 3 months in one fourth of the survivors and are heralded by dysphagia, regurgitation, cough, and recurrent pneumonia (Fig. 12–18). Treatment at first consists of dilation, started on the basis of dysphagia correlated with changes on the

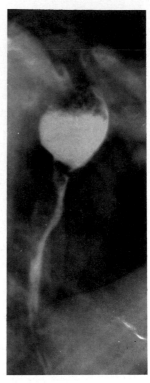

Figure 12–18. A barium swallow in a 1-year-old male infant with dysphagia, who was born with proximal esophageal atresia and distal tracheoesophageal fistula managed by ligation of the fistula and esophagoesophagostomy in one stage. This single film shows gross saccular dilation of the proximal esophagus above an area of stricture at the level of the anastomosis. Several dilations with a string provided an adequate lumen.

roentgenogram. Resection has been advised for recalcitrant strictures and perhaps should be combined with a gastric antireflux procedure. Gastroesophageal reflux is fairly common postoperatively and is treated in the usual medical, and occasionally surgical, fashion. Postoperative pneumonia can also be instigated by faulty motility of the distal esophagus with reflux following operative vagus nerve damage. Tracheal compression between a vascular structure anteriorly and a dilated upper esophagus posteriorly has been reported to cause recurrent respiratory problems with relief by anterior suspension of the aorta.

The overall rate of survivors with primary definitive operation, as derived from a sampling of children's and general hospitals, approaches 70 per cent; this rate has been elevated to 90 per cent in full-term newborns who are otherwise normal. Primary anastomosis in small babies with severe pneumonia or cardiac anomalies carries a 50 to 60 per cent mortality rate, which can be lowered with operative staging. However, primary repair should not be denied a marginally small baby because of size alone.

BRONCHIAL DEFORMITIES

CONGENITAL BRONCHIAL STENOSIS

Congenital stricture of the bronchus occurs predominantly in a main stem or middle lobe bronchus and can produce acute and chronic pulmonary infection (Swenson, 1962). Inflammatory scarring of the congenitally stenosed bronchus provides an ideal environment for distal suppuration, atelectasis, and bronchiectasis.

Chest roentgenograms demonstrate various stages of pneumonitis, atelectasis, and perhaps compensatory emphysema. Bronchoscopy and bronchography confirm the diagnosis.

Treatment consists of the resection of uncomplicated localized stenosis of main stem bronchi, with varying degrees of lung resection for more diffuse, complicated, and distal lesions.

FOREGUT CYSTS

A closed epithelial-lined sac developing abnormally in the thorax from the primitive anlage of both the upper gut and respiratory tract defines a foregut cyst. The actual congenital anomalies include bronchogenic, intramural esophageal, and posterior mediastinal cysts.

Embryologically, the respiratory system develops as a ventral diverticulum of the primitive foregut. During fetal growth, abnormal budding may lead to noncommunicating tracheal and bronchial cysts. Vacuolization of the cellular elements of the dorsal foregut—the eventual esophagus—creates its lumen. Persistent vacuolization, surrounded by cells of the esophageal wall, becomes an intramural esophageal cyst.

The notochord is the basis for the embryogenesis of posterior mediastinal cysts. In humans it may represent an early mesodermal cellular rod derived from the totipotent primitive streak around which the midline axial skeleton is formed. The notochord fuses with the juxtaposed embryonic endoderm, the precursor of the foregut. Normally the fusion degenerates, and vertebral and gut development occur autonomously. If fusion persists, endodermal cells are extracted from the foregut, and cyst formation that is separate from the esophagus can develop. Notochordal traction dorsally will often produce varying degrees of vertebral deformities, from a subtly widened vertebral body to anterior spina bifida. Descent of the foregut will dislocate the posterior mediastinal cysts to a level lower than the vertebral anomaly but will not disturb an attachment to the vertebral column.

The vast majority of foregut cysts in infancy are bronchogenic. Intramural esophageal cysts, although rare, occur more often than posterior mediastinal cysts.

Bronchogenic cysts are found in the posterior or middle mediastinum, most often in its mid third, close to the tracheobronchial tree (Fig. 12–19). These malformations are usually single and more common on the right; they may have a systemic blood supply. They are paratracheal, carinal, hilar, or paraesophageal in location, between 2 and 10 cm in diameter,

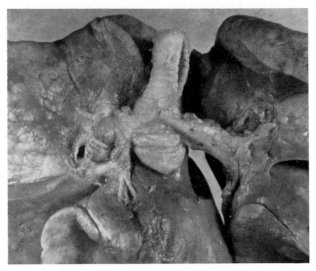

Figure 12–19. Autopsy specimen of a carinal bronchogenic cyst.

and unilocular (Maier, 1948). The clinical findings will include respiratory distress, pulmonary sepsis, and suppuration of the cyst. Some cysts are asymptomatic (Fig. 12–20).

The diagnosis may be suspected after chest roentgenograms, esophagogram, computed tomography (CT) scan, and magnetic resonance imaging. Occasionally endoscopy and bronchograms are helpful. Because bronchogenic cysts may rupture into a bronchus or pleura, bleed profusely, become badly infected, and produce sudden death, early diagnosis is imperative, and cystectomy with lung preservation should be utilized. A morbid location for a bronchogenic cyst is subcarinal. Here bronchial compression results in marked respiratory distress and should provoke urgent diagnostic and therapeutic steps (Fig. 12–21). Intraoperative airway manipulation must include preparation for one-lung anesthesia for possible resection and reconstruction.

Submucosal or intramural esophageal cysts are lined by esophageal, gastric, or respiratory epithelium, depending on site and time of development from the foregut. Like abdominal duplications, a common muscular wall is shared with the organ duplicated, and unlike posterior mediastinal cysts, vertebral anomalies are not concomitant.

As with other mediastinal cysts in infancy, respiratory distress and infection are more frequent than dysphagia, cough, and wheeze. Patients have been reported with hemoptysis from ulceration and perforation of a cyst lined with gastric mucous membrane into lung or bronchus as well as spontaneous drainage into the esophagus with hematemesis. Because the presence of gastric epithelium may alter therapy, the diagnostic work-up should include a 99m technetium pertechnetate scan. A chest radiograph in various projections may show a posterior or midmediastinal mass, and an esophagogram will demonstrate intramural narrowing of the lumen. Esophagoscopy and CT scans may be helpful.

Even though symptoms are minimal, complications

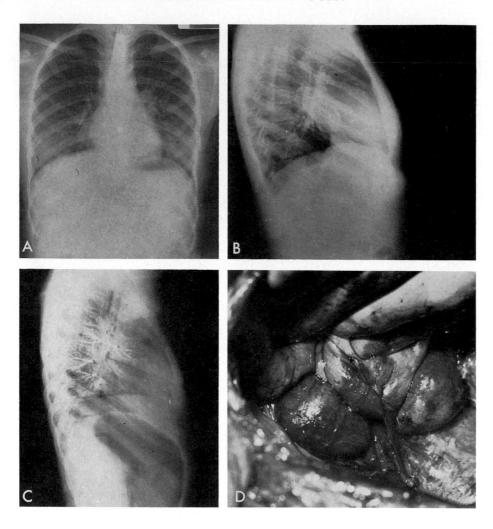

Figure 12-20. A 10-year-old girl exposed to tuberculosis, who had a markedly positive tuberculin skin test reaction. A mediastinal mass did not regress after 6 months of therapy in a sanatorium. A and B, The posteroanterior and lateral chest films show a normal cardiovascular silhouette. There is a mass posterior to the border of the right side of the heart with smooth margins, which covers almost two interspaces. The lateral film localizes the density to the area beneath the right hilus. The mass is denser than surrounding lung but more radiolucent than the heart. The lung fields are otherwise not remarkable. C, A lateral bronchogram shows no filling of the middle lobe but adequate filling elsewhere. D, At thoracotomy, a bilobed bronchogenic cyst in the region of the inferior pulmonary vein and ligament was resected.

are frequent, and the diagnosis is not secure without histologic confirmation. Accordingly, right thoracotomy with the inevitable nasogastric tube should be done for upper thoracic lesions, and left thoracotomy should be done for low-lying cysts. Because of the common esophageal muscle wall, resection would pose formidable reconstructive problems, and therapy lies between internal marsupialization and exci-

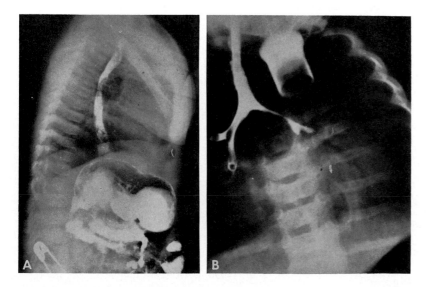

Figure 12-21. A 2-month-old infant with intermittent, severe respiratory distress. A, A lateral film with a barium-filled esophagus demonstrates an irregular, smoothly marginated radiolucency in the midmediastinum at the level of the carina with slight narrowing of the esophagus at this level. B, The anteroposterior tracheobronchogram reveals widening of the tracheal bifurcation and narrowing of the left main stem bronchus by extrinsic pressure. Within the limbs of the two main stem bronchi is an area of radiolucency with smooth borders, compatible with an air-filled cyst under tension. A bronchogenic cyst attached to the left main stem bronchus was removed.

sion of the mucous membrane. The former is acceptable for long tubular duplications if the epithelium is not gastric. A safer approach is partial excision of the extrinsic cyst wall and mucosectomy.

In the infant, the rare posterior mediastinal cyst is also heralded by respiratory distress from tracheobronchial compression with or without distal pneumonitis, usually right sided. Similarly, ulceration and bleeding induced by the gastric epithelium of the cyst may penetrate the esophagus, trachea, or bronchi, with alarming hemorrhage. Careful vertebral imaging will usually document some cervical-thoracic anomaly, and the diagnosis will become apparent. Additional embryologic repercussions of posterior mediastinal cysts are intra-abdominal intestinal duplications and neurologic deficits. Accordingly, these must be evaluated by appropriate radiologic studies. Finally, extension of an intrathoracic posterior mediastinal cyst through the diaphragm into the abdomen and origin of a cyst subdiaphragmatically with herniation into the thorax must be determined preoperatively.

The operative ideal is total excision of the entire mediastinal cyst and any extension without jeopardizing the integrity of vital structures above or below the diaphragm. It would be dangerous to terminate the operation and abandon a remnant of the cyst as a closed sac with gastric epithelium. Mucosectomy should be done if a cyst remnant must be left in order to remove gastric epithelium.

PULMONARY DEFORMITIES

PULMONARY AGENESIS, APLASIA, AND HYPOPLASIA

Varying degrees of absence of pulmonary tissue have been recorded in a number of instances. Bilateral pulmonary agenesis is a rare malformation that may occur in anencephalic monsters (Potter, 1952). Slightly more common is unilateral pulmonary agenesis, in which the trachea runs directly into the sole bronchus, with absence of the carina. Pulmonary aplasia, the most common variant, consists of a carina and main stem bronchial stump with absence of the distal lung. Functionally, unilateral lung agenesis and lung aplasia are similar. Lobar agenesis and aplasia are rarer than complete absence of one lung and usually affect the right upper and middle lobes together. Pulmonary hypoplasia has been described as a mass of poorly differentiated lung parenchyma connected to a malformed bronchus.

Embryologically, these malformations correspond to a failure of development of the respiratory system from the foregut. Arrest at the stage of the primitive lung bud produces bilateral pulmonary agenesis. The respiratory anlage at a later stage may develop only unilaterally and lead to lung agenesis. Lobar agenesis then becomes developmental arrest on one side in an older embryo. Pulmonary hypoplasia may occur during the last trimester of pregnancy with failure of final alveolar differentiation. The high incidence (greater than 50 per cent) of associated cardiac, gastrointestinal, genitourinary, and skeletal malformations, as well as frequent variations in the bronchopulmonary vasculature, lends support to generalized teratogenic factors.

Pathologically, the sole lung is larger than normal in pulmonary agenesis, and this enlargement is true hypertrophy and not emphysema. In addition, Lukas and co-workers (1953) have reported vascular changes secondary to hypertension in the residual lung, although others find no evidence that resting pulmonary artery hypertension or emphysema develops with a normal cardiovascular system.

The wide variation in clinical findings is explained only partially by the amount of involved pulmonary tissue, which is obviously an important factor. About 50 per cent of the patients with unilateral pulmonary agenesis survive. Death, however, is usually related to the associated serious anomalies.

The history may include harsh breathing, dyspnea, tachypnea, repeated upper respiratory tract infections, and respiratory distress, with cyanosis on exertion. Inspection of the chest does not suggest absence of a lung, because the external appearance is normal. Herniation of the sole lung and massive mediastinal shift and rotation fill the empty hemithorax. In addition, there is flat percussion over a dislocated heart, which may suggest dextrocardia in the presence of right-sided lung agenesis. Breath sounds from the herniated, hypertrophied lung are heard on the side of the agenesis except in the axilla and the base. With lobar agenesis, respiratory symptoms and mediastinal displacement are more subtle.

Radiographic films of the chest show a homogeneous density on the involved, agenetic side, with mediastinal rotation and shift. Lung herniation can be seen beneath the sternum on anterior films. Radiographic films of lobar agenesis may simply exhibit mediastinal shift. The electrocardiogram is useful in separating agenesis from dextrocardia, and pulmonary function studies demonstrate a reduction in vital capacity and exercise tolerance.

The diagnosis should be suspected when respiratory difficulty occurs with tracheal deviation in the presence of a symmetric chest and the chest roentgenogram is suggestive of massive atelectasis and mediastinal shift. Body section roentgenogram findings may strengthen the possibility of pulmonary agenesis. The diagnosis is confirmed by bronchoscopy and by bronchography with failure to demonstrate two major bronchi. With lobar aplasia, bronchograms are indispensable, because the pathologic changes may not be visible to the bronchoscopist. Angiography may demonstrate suspected cardiac anomalies and aberrant pulmonary vessels and has been used to diagnose the varying causes of unequal pulmonary aeration in children (Franken et al, 1973).

It is difficult to separate atelectasis from pulmonary or lobar agenesis on clinical grounds. In the differential diagnosis, Schaffer and Avery (1977) suggest that the finding of aeration in the peripheral lung on both sides rules out the diagnosis of unilateral pulmonary agenesis. Endoscopy and bronchography can settle the issue.

In reviewing the mortality from pulmonary agenesis, it is apparent that chronic dyspnea with cough and repeated respiratory infections are ominous prognostic signs; so indeed is right-sided agenesis, in which the mortality is twice that of left-sided agenesis. This higher mortality is probably related to a more severe mediastinal and cardiac displacement, with great vessel disturbances secondary to the greater mass of lung tissue on the right. A tracheobronchial foreign body may produce the initial symptoms, and at least three fatalities have been reported during attempts at endoscopic removal.

Pulmonary resection may be indicated in lobar agenesis if the lung parenchyma on the side of the agenesis is supplied by abnormal bronchi or arteries to which incapacitating symptoms can be ascribed (Adler et al, 1958). For pulmonary agenesis, acute infections are treated conventionally; repeated infections may require continuous antibiotic therapy and postural drainage. Borja and co-workers (1970) have emphasized the importance of conservative management, including the prevention of "spillage pneumonitis" from the agenetic stump in newborns.

CONGENITAL PNEUMATOCELE (PULMONARY HERNIA)

The presence of lung tissue outside the usual confines of an intact bony thorax is a most uncommon finding in the neonatal period. About 20 per cent of all lung hernias are congenital; the remainder follow trauma.

The usual site of a congenital pulmonary hernia is the cervical region, because of the absence of the endothoracic fascia in this area. Hernias in the region of the axilla have also been reported. Conversely, acquired posttraumatic hernias occur in the midthoracic region.

The infant with pneumatocele is usually asymptomatic, although local tenderness and slight dyspnea have been observed. Examination may demonstrate a supraclavicular mass that increases in size with crying. Treatment is usually superfluous.

CONGENITAL PULMONARY CYSTS

Cooke and Blades (1952) have classified congenital cystic disease of the lung into a bronchogenic type, an alveolar type, and a combination of these types. Altogether, the patients with these types are probably outnumbered by those with acquired cysts; nevertheless, the congenital group includes a substantial segment of salvageable infants and children with respiratory distress and suppuration. There is a relative absence of other anomalies; cystic disease elsewhere is rare, and pulmonary cysts, whether single or multiple, are usually limited to one lobe.

Because cysts have been recorded in late embryos and newborns, an anomalous development of the bronchopulmonary system at the stage of terminal bronchiolar or early alveolar formation has been postulated. This development may evolve by intrapulmonary alveolar dissociation or partial bronchiolar recanalization with stenosis. The distal alveolated pulmonary cyst is then formed on the basis of expiratory obstruction through an area of bronchiolar narrowing. These essential postuterine respiratory dynamics might explain the paucity of such cysts in embryos.

The usual gross pathologic specimen exhibits a single, multiloculated, unilobar, peripheral air-filled cyst with a tracheobronchial communication. Common variants include multiplicity of cysts, bilateral or segmental distribution, and absence of bronchial communication. Pus may be present. On microscopic examination, the thin wall of a congenital cyst contains bits of smooth muscle and perhaps cartilage and is lined by columnar epithelium. With the exception of acute staphylococcal pneumatocele, which has an obvious background of acute infection, most acquired cysts have an inner lining of squamous epithelium and can be separated histologically from congenital cysts. Unfortunately, contamination and inflammation may destroy these helpful criteria, so that infected congenital cyst, acquired cyst, and lung abscess may be indistinguishable pathologically and clinically.

The clinical pathogenesis derives from a cyst-airway connection, either direct or through the pores of Kohn, with free access on inspiration and obstruction during expiration. Under these circumstances, there is an acute or a chronic distention of the cyst leading to a progressive increase in intrathoracic tension, frequently in the neonatal period. Compression of the ipsilateral lung and of the diaphragm, mediastinal shift, and contralateral atelectasis are the usual sequence of events. If cyst drainage is poor, suppuration develops.

In the newborn and the infant, clinical findings are usually due to progressive tension as the congenital pulmonary cyst gradually distends with air. Tension pneumothorax can develop at this stage, either spontaneously or by needle aspiration. Respiratory and circulatory embarrassment is manifested by tachypnea, tachycardia, dyspnea, stridor, cyanosis, hyperresonance, absence of breath sounds, and displacement of the trachea and the heart without a history or signs of infection. By late infancy and childhood, infection is almost invariably present, and cough, fever, and hemoptysis with repeated, localized episodes of pulmonary sepsis become more prominent as the cyst evolves into a lung abscess.

Although at times there is a startling lack of correlation between symptoms and roentgenographic findings, plain roentgenograms of the chest usually corroborate the diagnosis or help in the differential diagnosis. The congenital pulmonary alveolar cyst may occupy the entire hemithorax and appear as a circular or oval, thin-walled, air-filled cavity containing faint strands of lung. Normally aerated or atelectatic lung may be present at the apex and the base but not at the hilus. There is a mediastinal shift, the diaphragm is depressed, pneumonia is absent, the pleura is not thickened, and other areas of translucency may be seen (Fig. 12–22). A fluid level within the cyst is unusual. Bronchography may be useful.

It is difficult, perhaps impossible, to separate pulmonary cysts from lobar emphysema. Emphysematous respiratory distress may be more explosive, but this difference is not a substantial factor in the face of common roentgenographic findings. The treatment is similar. The pulmonary cysts of cystic fibrosis and Letterer-Siwe disease should be excluded in the absence of other manifestations of the disease. Diaphragmatic hernia may simulate multiple lung cysts, but the immediate neonatal appearance of the hernia is very suggestive. Barium-contrast radiographic studies are useful in those cases in which clinical presentation occurs later in the neonatal period. A staphylococcal pneumatocele may complicate a virulent pneumonia, and the changes in size and configuration of this type of acquired cyst may be volatile. Spontaneous resolution here is expected, so it would be a great error to confuse pneumatoceles with congenital cysts. An infected congenital cyst and encapsulated empyema may look alike; in many patients with congenital cyst, chest drainage has been performed on the basis of a diagnosis of empyema, but characteristically, unlike empyema, obliteration of the infected cyst does not occur in the presence of adequate dependent drainage. Angiography may be useful in separating congenital from postinfectious cysts. The respiratory distress will suggest pneumothorax, but there are no linear strands in or around the area of translucency, and a hilar shadow representing compressed lung is likely with pneumothorax.

The fate of congenital pulmonary cystic disease is rarely spontaneous regression. If the cyst is left untreated, pleural rupture with tension pneumothorax, infection with abscess, recurrent disabling bronchopneumonia, bronchopleural fistula, hemorrhage, and cyst expansion with suffocation may be encountered. Accordingly, thoracotomy is advised to avoid these complications and the exceedingly poor prognosis associated with large, moderately symptomatic cysts. Elective lobectomy is the usual planned procedure, and every attempt should be made to conserve functioning pulmonary tissue (Fig. 12–23). Pneumonectomy for more generalized disease has been reported. At times, emergency resection must be done for the acute respiratory distress that threatens life. In this situation, needle aspiration and decompression of the tension cyst may be a worthwhile preparatory step on the way to the operative suite. Thoracentesis cannot be used definitively because pneumothorax and pleural soiling will follow.

The repeatedly infected lung cyst deserves systemic antibiotic therapy in the preoperative period, and resection should be done without prior drainage. At operation Clatworthy (1960) suggests aspiration of a fluid-filled cyst to provide exposure and to prevent bronchotracheal spillage. Aberrant systemic arteries must be considered, especially for lower lobe cysts. Postoperative nursing care should be done in an intensive care unit with appropriate equipment.

LOBAR EMPHYSEMA

Abnormal lobar distention can produce subtle or gross respiratory distress in an otherwise normal newborn or infant. Recognition of this entity is rewarding, because excisional therapy is fairly specific and the results are satisfactory.

The disease is usually unilobar and is often confined to either an upper or a middle lobe but may be segmental, bilobar, or bilateral or may involve an entire lung. The left upper lobe is the most common

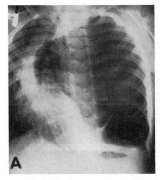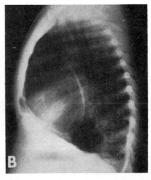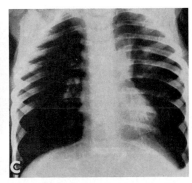

Figure 12–22. A 13-month-old infant with minimal respiratory distress. *A* and *B*, Posteroanterior and lateral chest films demonstrate gross hyperlucency of the left hemithorax. Frontal projection shows mediastinal displacement to the right. Pulmonary septal markings are noted within the area of hyperinflation. There is herniation of the left lung across the anterior mediastinum with flattening of the left diaphragm and widening of the left intercostal spaces. The right lung is compressed. *C*, After left upper lobe lobectomy, an overexposed radiograph reveals bilateral good aeration with return of the mediastinum toward the midline.

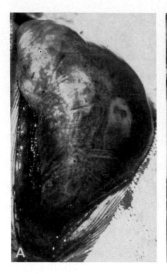
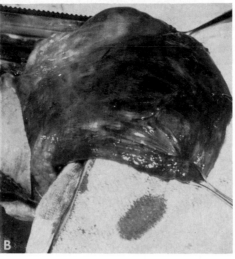

Figure 12–23. *A*, Extrusion of a left upper lobe pulmonary cyst, under tension, through an intercostal incision, with relief of respiratory distress that had become accentuated during the induction of anesthesia. *B*, The multiloculated cyst after deflation.

site, followed by middle and right upper lobes. At least 10 per cent of patients also have congenital heart disease, and a larger percentage have other anomalies.

Causative factors are profuse and, at times, specifically applicable; more often, the underlying mechanism is vague and escapes pathologic confirmation. Certainly, the emphysema secondary to a foreign body, tuberculosis, enteric cytopathogenic human orphan (ECHO) virus infection, mediastinal tumor, bronchial adenoma, and stenosis is well established, but these disorders do not often produce the distinctive pattern of infantile lobar emphysema. In only half the cases can a causative factor be found. The currently favored explanation for this form of lobar hyperaeration involves partial bronchial obstruction or intrinsic alveolar disease. The bronchial obstruction can be engendered by complete absence of cartilage, bronchomalacia, exuberant mucosal folds, extrinsic vascular and lymph node compression, bronchial distortion from an anterior mediastinal lung hernia, and retained secretions. The common denominator hinders expiration by organic bronchial narrowing compounded by functional expiratory bronchial collapse. This valvular arrangement leads to a hugely overdistended, noncollapsible lobe with widespread alveolar emphysema and rupture and small subpleural blebs. The pulmonary arteries are normal in lobar emphysema, unlike in unilateral pseudoemphysema, in which small pulmonary arteries supply a normal or small emphysematous lobe. The report of the surgical pathologist, although confirming the emphysematous nature of the parenchymatous disease, is often lacking in its specification of underlying causes. Perhaps the majority of surgical specimens are resected distal to intrinsic intrabronchial disease, or extrinsic causative factors, such as anomalous vessels, are left undisturbed. Lincoln and co-workers (1971), however, have reported hypoplasia or absence of bronchial cartilaginous plates in 22 of 28 resected patients. Bolande and colleagues (1956) have suggested that alveolar fibrosis cannot handle normal expiration with the development of emphysema. Others have suggested that alveolar elasticity is abnormal. Leape and Longino (1964), in a substantial clinical contribution, postulated the combination of alveolar disease and bronchial obstruction as causes.

The clinical profile is formed by a space-occupying emphysematous lobe producing ipsilateral lobar atelectasis and diaphragmatic compression, mediastinal shift, and contralateral lung atelectasis. Decompression of the overdistended lobe into the atelectic lobe is prevented by the immaturity and distortion of the pores of Kohn.

Progressive respiratory distress from birth to 6 months of age, but especially in the first month, parallels the degree of emphysema. Cough, wheezing, dyspnea, tachypnea, tachycardia, stridor, and intermittent cyanosis are aggravated with feeding. To this list may be added retraction and bulging of the thorax, tracheal and cardiac shift, hyperresonant percussion, and diminished breath sounds. There is no history of infection.

Thoracic roentgenograms in various positions, especially during expiration, must be obtained. On the lateral view, a translucent anterior mediastinum is suggestive of lung herniation. Anteroposterior films will show a large hyperlucent area containing vague lung and bronchovascular markings. The left upper lobe is most frequently involved. Adjacent lobes are compressed, the diaphragm is pushed downward, rib interspaces are wide, and the mediastinum is shifted into the opposite hemithorax with compression of the lung (Fig. 12–24). On fluoroscopy, the emphysematous segment remains constant in area, regardless of the phase of respiration. Air trapping can be confirmed by lateral decubitus films, because a normal dependent lung becomes relatively dense in this position, whereas the lucency persists with emphysema. Bronchograms demonstrate incomplete distal filling of the affected bronchi. A pulmonary scan will show reduced perfusion of the affected parenchyma and may be helpful.

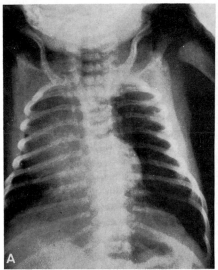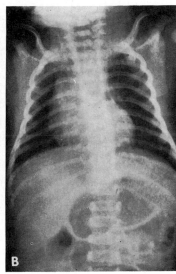

Figure 12–24. *A,* The anteroposterior chest roentgenogram of this newborn with respiratory distress demonstrates a shift of the mediastinum to the right with overinflation of the left lower lobe. There is depression of the left diaphragm, and the volume of the right lung is restricted. *B,* After left lower lobe lobectomy for lobar emphysema, the mediastinum has returned toward the midline, and the diaphragm is normally located. There is better aeration of the right lung and slight radiolucency of the upper lobe, which has expanded and filled the left hemithorax.

The differential diagnosis must exclude those lesions that produce respiratory distress but for which thoracotomy may not be indicated. Bronchoscopy can be utilized if a foreign body is a possibility and may be warranted in children whose first symptoms occur after 6 months of age. Postpneumonic pneumatocele and bronchiolitis both have a septic background. Pulmonary cystic disease may be similar but usually begins a little later in life. Fortunately, excision is proper for both. A tension pneumothorax will not have lung markings in the areas of radiolucency, and the nubbin of compressed lung in this condition is likely to be hilar rather than supradiaphragmatic or apical. Atelectasis with compensatory emphysema is not characterized by such pronounced respiratory distress. Pulmonary agenesis can be ruled out by bronchoscopy and bronchograms. Diaphragmatic hernia should not pose a problem but can be differentiated by the use of contrast material. The diagnosis of congenital lobar emphysema should be made with increasing hesitation in the infant with respiratory distress who is approaching 6 months of age. Asthma and bronchospasm can afflict an upper lobe to such an extent as to exactly mimic lobar emphysema; only at operation are the findings dissimilar.

Rarely, symptomatic infantile lobar emphysema will resolve spontaneously or with conservative therapy including bronchoscopy (Murray et al, 1967; Eigen et al, 1976). Such may be the case with obstruction secondary to a mucus plug. The usual course is relentlessly progressive toward tension emphysema. The prognosis without treatment, then, is exceedingly poor, and the mortality rate is high. Accordingly, excisional therapy, usually lobectomy but perhaps segmental resection (Lilly), should be done when the diagnosis is accompanied by symptoms. Only when the diagnosis is purely on a radiologic basis can thoracotomy be deferred.

Early age, concomitant congenital heart disease, or severe respiratory symptoms should not contraindicate operation. Lobectomy has been done successfully within the first day of life, and simultaneous pulmonary and cardiovascular surgery has been done on several occasions. If the newborn is in extremis, thoracentesis can provide time for thoracotomy at the expense of a tension pneumothorax. Buying time is its only role; aspiration should not be used definitively. During the induction of anesthesia, vigorous positive pressure may inflate the emphysematous lobe and produce an extension of the respiratory distress. The emergency is over when the distended lobe herniates through the posterolateral thoracotomy incision with decompression of the thorax. There is no peculiar postoperative morbidity, and relief is immediate.

The operative mortality rate is less than 5 per cent. Long-term follow-up shows normal growth and development, marred in rare instances by similar or less severe emphysema of other lobes and residual postoperative symptoms of pulmonary infection.

PULMONARY SEQUESTRATION

Pulmonary tissue that is embryonic and cystic, does not function, is isolated from normal functioning lung, and is nourished by systemic arteries has been aptly called *pulmonary sequestration.* The intrapulmonary variant is contained within otherwise normal lung parenchyma. The less common extralobar sequestration is divorced from and accessory to the ipsilateral lung.

Fundamentally, pulmonary sequestration represents a malformation of the primitive respiratory and vascular systems in which fetal lung tissue is segregated from the main tracheobronchial apparatus and ultimately has its own systemic artery. The sequence and time of these embryologic events have aroused a great deal of curiosity. Pryce (1946) believed that persistent aberrant fetal pulmonary blood vessels exerted traction on a segment of an equally primitive lung bud that then split off from the parent lung. The arterial trauma during and after the actual detachment is thought to lead to cystic degeneration. Others propose a primary pulmonary separation soon after the foregut stage, with subsequent acquisition of a blood supply from the nearest and most convenient source, which happens to be the aorta. Smith (1956) suggested that sequestration was secondary to pulmonary artery deficiency and that the cysts followed systemic blood pressure flow after birth. Boyden (1958) concluded from the available data that the respiratory and vascular anomalies were unexplained, could not be related as to cause, and occurred coincidentally. Halasz and associates (1961) postulated the presence of an additional low anterior foregut respiratory duplication with subsequent sequestration but retention of the original aortic blood supply. The occasional association of esophagobronchial fistula with sequestration supports this contention. Iwai and co-workers (1973) found independent occurrences of the malformed lung and aberrant artery. They support the theory of an accessory bronchopulmonary bud arising from the foregut.

Both types of sequestration have certain similar pathologic characteristics as well as clear-cut differences. The pathologic tissue is largely fetal and profusely cystic and contains disorganized, airless, and nonpigmented alveoli, bronchi, cartilage, respiratory epithelium, and a systemic artery. It is often secondarily infected, bronchiectatic, or atelectatic and is usually located in the region of the lower lobes (Figs. 12–25 and 12–26). The aberrant arteries may arise from the thoracic or abdominal aorta and, in the latter instance, may pierce the diaphragm and run through the pulmonary ligament before reaching the sequestration. The elastic vessel walls may become atherosclerotic, and the lumen varies considerably in size.

The intralobar sequestration is encircled by visceral pleura and has no pleural separation from the rest of the lobe; it usually occurs in the lower lobes, although Bruwer and co-workers (1950) have reported the lesion in the upper lobes. The remainder of the affected lobe and lung is normal, except that a small communication with the sequestration may have been maintained, may have reopened, or may have created infection. A communication with the gastrointestinal tract is rare, and so are other anomalies. The systemic arteries are likely to be large, and the veins drain into the pulmonary system. More than half the cases of intralobar sequestration are diagnosed after adolescence, and symptoms in neonates and infants are uncommon.

Extralobar sequestration can occur from the thoracic inlet to the upper part of the abdomen but characteristically is a left-sided (more than 90 per cent), ball-like, pliable mass between the diaphragm and the lower lobe and outside the visceral pleura. Communications with the trachea, bronchi, esophagus, stomach, and small bowel have been reported but are rare. The systemic arteries are small, the venous drainage is likewise systemic through the azygos system, and other anomalies, principally congenital pleuroperitoneal hernias, are frequently concurrent. More than half the cases of extralobar se-

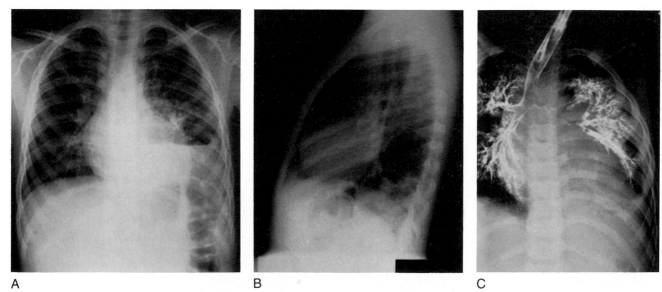

A   B   C

Figure 12–25. A 5-year-old child who has had repeated upper respiratory infections during the past 2 years. *A,* On the posteroanterior projection there is a cyst-like structure with an air-fluid level in the left lower lobe and minimal pleural fluid or thickening at the left base. Otherwise the lungs are clear except for minimal residual contrast from previous bronchography. The heart is slightly enlarged. *B,* The lateral view taken at a later date shows a cyst in the posterior aspect of the left lower lobe with a thin, well-defined rim. No air-fluid level is seen. The bronchi of the left lower lobe are compressed and displaced anteriorly. *C,* The bilateral bronchogram in the frontal projection demonstrates normal right bronchi and elevation of the left main stem bronchus. There is elevation and lateral displacement of the lower lobe bronchi, which are partially filled with fluid. (Courtesy of Dr. TR Howell.)

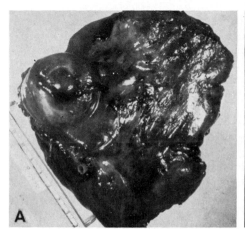 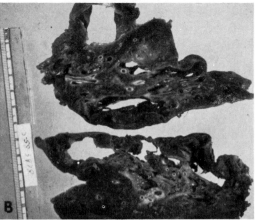

Figure 12–26. *A,* Gross external appearance of intralobar sequestration, left lower lobe, in an older child. Note the aberrant systemic artery in the lower left corner of the specimen. *B,* Cross section of an inflated, formalin-fixed specimen with multiple cysts, surrounded by compressed parenchyma. (Courtesy of Drs. James W Brooks and Saul Kay.)

questration are diagnosed before the patients are 1 year of age, and males are affected three to four times more often than females.

The basis for symptoms is infection through a fistula between the sequestration and either the airway or the digestive tract. The congenital, pathologic tissue may be contaminated by contiguous pneumonitis or hematogenous localization with the formation of the primary or additional fistulas. Accordingly, the arresting clinical feature, especially with intralobar sequestration, is recurrent or persistent pulmonary sepsis in the form of pneumonitis, lung abscess, or both, which is manifested by weight loss, chills, fever, cough, hemoptysis, and pyoptysis. Physical examination may elicit pathologic findings at the bases paravertebrally, and on several occasions a murmur has been noted. With extralobar sequestration, infection is less common, and the child may be asymptomatic except for an intrathoracic mass.

Plain chest films show a triangulated density in the region of the medial basal segment of a lower lobe, with displacement of the bronchovascular markings. Sometimes there is a dense linear projection toward the aorta. Body-section radiography may amplify these findings. With abscess, of course, a fluid level may be present along with surrounding pneumonitis. The diagnosis is suggested by the restriction and localization of roentgenographic findings to the same area that is associated with repeated clinical episodes.

Bronchography is extremely helpful, because the sequestration does not fill with dye but its periphery is outlined by bronchi that are filled. Aortography through the descending aorta delineates the anomalous arterial supply and thus confirms the nature of the pulmonary density. This evidence may also prove helpful at the time of surgery. At bronchoscopy, purulent secretions are absent from the main stem bronchi, even with pulmonary suppuration.

Extirpation is the only reasonable approach after the diagnosis has been established. Antibiotics must be given for the acute infection and should be given before and after the operation. Intralobar sequestration is handled by lobectomy; segmental resection will not suffice, because the sequestration is not clearly demarcated. An extralobar sequestration can be removed without disturbing the remaining lobes, and the Bochdalek hernia, if present, can be repaired. The only technical problem with either form of sequestration is the anomalous systemic artery and arteries, and exsanguination has followed their inadvertent division. The frequency of this vascular anomaly should always be kept in mind when performing thoracotomy for lower lobe lesions in infants and children.

Morbidity and mortality rates are exceedingly low if resection precedes repeated infections. Postoperative results are uniformly good.

CONGENITAL CYSTIC ADENOMATOID MALFORMATION OF THE LUNG

Cystic adenomatoid pulmonary hamartoma, first described by Chin and Tang in 1949, is a rare variant of congenital cystic disease and, similarly, can produce respiratory difficulty by tension and infection. Careful investigation of post-mortem material by Kwittken and Reiner (1962) would seem to implicate a developmental "adenomatoid" overgrowth of pulmonary tissue in the region of the end bronchioles, with suppression of alveolar growth. Examination reveals a massive and fleshy unilobar enlargement, although bilobar and bilateral involvements have been described. On microscopic examination, cystic degeneration, excessive terminal bronchiolar tissue, and areas of premature alveolar differentiation are interspersed with normal lung. Buntain and co-workers (1974) have suggested that the lesion is not a hamartoma but focal pulmonary dysplasia, because the cyst walls may contain skeletal muscle.

The basis for symptoms consists of pulmonary replacement by the malformation and compression of normal lung and mediastinum by the bulky size of the lesion and its enlarging cysts. Prematurity, hydramnios, and anasarca, possibly secondary to caval compression or torsion, are frequently associated findings, and respiratory distress soon after birth is the presenting sign. Examination demonstrates mediastinal shift toward the opposite side in a newborn with associated dyspnea, tachypnea, and perhaps cyanosis. Fairly specific radiologic findings, described by Craig and associates (1956), include pulmonary densities with radiolucent areas and mediastinal shift to the opposite side (Fig. 12–27).

The differential diagnosis is essentially a radiologic one and includes the more usual forms of congenital and acquired cystic disease, lobar emphysema, and Bochdalek hernia.

The urgency for operation in the newborn parallels that for obstructive emphysema, and indeed the tension phenomenon is remarkably similar. Lobectomy has been curative in a number of instances, some of which have been reported in small premature infants soon after birth. Segmental resections should not be done, because the complication rate is excessive. Later in life, secondary infection, which is almost inevitable, constitutes an indication for thoracotomy.

CONGENITAL PULMONARY LYMPHANGIECTASIS

This unusual congenital dilation of the pulmonary lymphatics produces severe respiratory distress in the newborn and is often associated with other crippling anomalies, such as congenital left heart disorders, especially anomalies producing obstruction to pulmonary venous flow. These anomalies may provide the basis for the persisting fetal pulmonary lymphatics.

Pathologically, according to Laurence (1955), there is diffuse overgrowth of the entire lymphatic system of both lungs, which become heavy, bulky, and inelastic, with grossly prominent subpleural cystic lymphatics. Lymphangiectasis is quite unlike a localized lymphangioma and is not associated with chylothorax.

Symptomatically, there is immediate respiratory distress with dyspnea and cyanosis, which may be aggravated by a pneumothorax. Radiographic films of the chest may show a diffuse, generalized mottling similar to that seen in hyaline membrane disease, along with emphysema in the remaining functioning lung (Carter and Vaughn, 1961). There may be some clinical resemblance to neonatal local hyperaeration (Wilson-Mikity syndrome), but differentiation can be accomplished.

Treatment is nonspecific, and the prognosis with diffuse involvement is hopeless.

PULMONARY ARTERIOVENOUS FISTULA

A congenital pulmonary arteriovenous fistula represents a direct intrapulmonary connection between pulmonary artery and vein without an intervening capillary bed. This cavernous arteriovenous aneurysm is the basis, then, for a right-to-left shunt and is an uncommon cause of symptoms, including cyanosis, in the pediatric age group. Accordingly, the

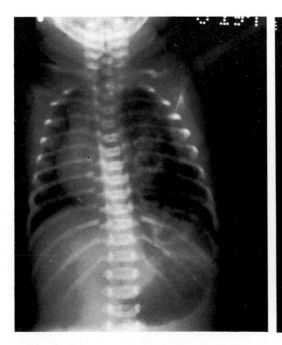
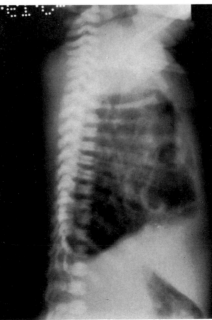

Figure 12–27. A 48-hour-old male infant with progressive respiratory distress since birth. Frontal and lateral projections demonstrate cardiac and mediastinal shifts to the right. The right lung is clear, as is the apex of the left lung. In the remainder of the left lung are multiple cyst-like areas interspersed with linear and nodular consolidations. There is no pleural fluid or pneumothorax. The gastric air bubble is normally located. Left lower lobe lobectomy was done promptly and confirmed the preoperative diagnosis of cystic adenomatoid malformation. (Courtesy of Dr. TR Howell.)

diagnosis is not often made in children in spite of its congenital nature. Bosher and colleagues, in an exhaustive review in 1959, reported 17 patients under 10 years of age, and Shumaker and Waldhausen, in 1963, reported 31 patients who were treated surgically between 5 months and 16 years of age. From this material it is apparent that the fistula occurs in the lower lobes in about 60 per cent of the instances, is single in 65 per cent, and is unilateral in 75 per cent. Bilateral multiplicity is found in the remainder.

The pulmonary vascular malformation represents a failure of maturation of the fetal splanchnic bed in which arteriovenous communications may normally exclude the pulmonary capillaries. There may, however, be a widespread basic blood vessel abnormality, because familial hemorrhagic telangiectasis of the Osler-Weber-Rendu variety often occurs simultaneously.

On gross pathologic examination, the actual arteriovenous fistula is subpleural or hilar and may simulate a saccular, cavernous hemangioma because of its aneurysmal swelling. The fistula is fed by at least one afferent artery, usually pulmonic and less often bronchial, and is drained by several veins, almost always pulmonary. There are numerous communications between artery and vein in this tortuous, dilated, worm-like vessel mass. On microscopic examination, the arteriovenous fistula is lined with vascular endothelium. Carcinomatous degeneration has been recorded by Hall (1935) and Wollstein (1931).

The clinical picture of this anomaly is created by an intrapulmonic right-to-left shunt in which unoxygenated pulmonary artery blood flows directly into the pulmonary veins and thence into the systemic circulation without gas exchange in the pulmonary capillaries. Although up to 50 per cent of the blood volume can be so rerouted in massive fistulization, a 25 per cent shunt will produce diagnostic clinical findings.

Generalized telangiectasis, noted especially on the skin and mucous membranes, has been described in half the patients with pulmonary arteriovenous fistula. Dyspnea, rubor, cyanosis, clubbing of the fingers and toes, hemoptysis, epistaxis, exercise intolerance, and hemorrhagic conjunctiva are common complaints. On physical examination, a thrill may be felt, and a systolic or continuous murmur and bruit may be heard over the shunt, especially during inspiration. The heart is normal to auscultation. The blood pressure, pulse, venous pressure, electrocardiogram, and cardiac output are within normal variations.

Clinical, pathologic, and radiologic studies are essential for the final diagnosis. Polycythemia with a red blood cell count in the range of 7 to 10 million/mm,[3] a hemoglobin concentration of 18 to 25 g/100 ml, and a hematocrit level of 60 to 80 per cent are fairly standard. The arterial oxygen saturation is consistently low, drops lower with exercise, and rises, but not to normal, with 100-per cent oxygen.

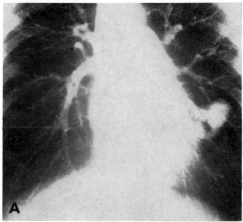

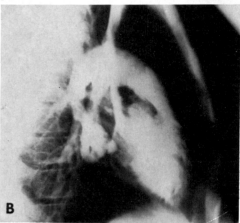

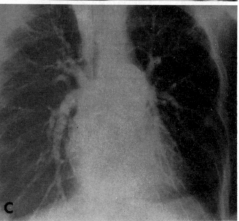

Figure 12–28. A virtually asymptomatic 15-year-old male with a family history of hereditary telangiectasia for 3 generations whose plain chest film showed a vague shadow in the left lower lung field. *A* and *B*, Preoperative posteroanterior and lateral angiocardiograms demonstrated a large pulmonary arteriovenous aneurysm in the anterior basal segment of the left lower lobe. A segmental resection was performed with total excision of the arteriovenous fistula. *C*, A postoperative posteroanterior angiocardiogram revealed no evidence of arteriovenous communication in either lung. (Courtesy of Dr. Thomas NP Johns.)

Routine chest films in various views demonstrate one or more homogeneous, noncalcified pulmonary densities with irregular, fairly sharp peripheral margins, confluent with the ipsilateral hilus. Body section roentgenograms may bring out the vascular nature of the tissue between the peripheral lesion and the hilus. The tumor may pulsate at fluoroscopy, decrease in size during the Valsalva maneuver, and become larger with the Müller test. Venous cineangiography with full chest films can delineate the offending fistula accurately and uncover smaller fistulas that were not hitherto suspected (Fig. 12–28). Pressure studies may record a normal systolic but a low diastolic pulmonary artery pressure.

Cyanotic cardiac anomalies are excluded in the differential diagnosis by the presence of a lung tumor and the absence of various murmurs and aberrations in pulse, blood pressure, venous pressure, cardiac output, heart size and configuration, and electrocardiogram, all of which are normal in pulmonary arteriovenous fistula.

Complications during the natural history of the untreated disease are formidable. Exsanguination from a massive spontaneous hemothorax or hemoptysis can occur. Any localized infection may initiate septicemia and brain abscess, and polycythemia can lead to embolic and thrombotic phenomena. The prognosis is obviously more serious and less manageable with widespread bilateral shunts or diffuse hereditary telangiectasis.

Excisional therapy should be done in symptomatic infants and children with localized disease, especially when accompanied by hereditary telangiectasis. In 31 pediatric patients there has been one operative death, and morbidity is equally low (Shumaker and Waldhausen, 1963). The results have been eminently satisfactory and have stimulated a more aggressive surgical approach toward the isolated pulmonary arteriovenous aneurysm with minimal or no symptoms and the more widely distributed fistulas with gross symptoms. Several experienced observers have commented on the clinical improvement following excision of the major dominant pulmonary fistula even though smaller diffuse fistulas remain untreated.

Lobectomy has been the procedure of choice in the majority of children. Unfortunately, normal pulmonary parenchyma was sacrificed because the dissection was not limited to the actual borders of the pathologic tissue. Because multiple shunts are often of paramount importance, postoperative results parallel the conservation of functioning lung. Accordingly, Bosher and associates (1959) and then Murdock (1962) and Björk (1967) have described the technique and practicality of local excision in a bloodless field in preference to segmental resection or lobectomy.

REFERENCES

General References

Arey LB: Developmental Anatomy: A Textbook and Laboratory Manual of Embryology. Rev. 7th ed. Philadelphia, WB Saunders Co, 1974.

Avery ME and Taeusch HW Jr (eds): Schaffer's Diseases of the Newborn. 5th ed. Philadelphia, WB Saunders Co, 1989.

Avery ME, Fletcher BD, and Williams R: The Lung and Its Disorders in the Newborn Infant. 4th ed. Philadelphia, WB Saunders Co, 1981.

Bates DV, Macklem PT, and Christie RV: Respiratory Function in Disease, an Introduction to the Integrated Study of the Lung. 2nd ed. Philadelphia, WB Saunders Co, 1971.

Brown JJM (ed): Surgery of Childhood. Baltimore, Williams & Wilkins Co, 1963.

Buntain WL, Isaacs H Jr, Payne VC Jr et al: Lobar emphysema, cystic adenomatoid malformation, pulmonary sequestration, and bronchogenic cyst in infancy and childhood: a clinical group. J Pediatr Surg 9:85, 1974.

Comroe JH Jr et al: The Lung, Clinical Physiology and Pulmonary Function Tests. 2nd ed. Chicago, Year Book Medical Publishers, Inc, 1962.

Demos NJ and Teresi A: Congenital lung malformations. A unified concept and a case report. J Thorac Cardiovasc Surg 70:260, 1975.

Flavell G: An Introduction to Chest Surgery. London, Oxford University Press, 1957.

Flavell G: The Oesophagus. London, Butterworth's, 1963.

Gross RE: Surgery of Infancy and Childhood: Its Principles and Techniques. Philadelphia, WB Saunders Co, 1953.

Gross RE: An Atlas of Children's Surgery. Philadelphia, WB Saunders Co, 1970.

Hamilton WJ, Boyd JD, and Mossman HW: Human Embryology (Prenatal Development of Form and Function). 2nd ed. Cambridge, W Heffer & Sons, Ltd, 1952.

Hutchin P: Congenital cystic disease of the lung. Rev Surg 28:79, 1971.

Landing BH and Wells TR: Tracheobronchial anomalies in children. Perspect Pediatr Pathol 1:1, 1973.

Leigh TF and Weens HS: The Mediastinum. Springfield, Ill, Charles C Thomas, 1959.

Lindskog GE, Liebow AA, and Glenn WWL: Thoracic and Cardiovascular Surgery, with Related Pathology. New York, Appleton-Century-Crofts, Inc, 1962.

Mustard WT et al (eds): Pediatric Surgery. 2nd ed. Vol 1. Chicago, Year Book Medical Publishers, Inc, 1969.

Nixon HH and O'Donnell B: The Essentials of Pediatric Surgery. London, William Heinemann, Ltd, 1961.

Patten BM: Human Embryology. 2nd ed. New York, McGraw-Hill Book Co, Inc, 1953.

Pierce WS, deParedes CG, Raphaely RC, and Waldhausen JA: Pulmonary resection in infants younger than one year of age. J Thorac Cardiovasc Surg 61:875, 1971.

Potts WJ: The Surgeon and the Child. Philadelphia, WB Saunders Co, 1959.

Rickham PP and Johnston JH: Neonatal Surgery. New York, Appleton-Century-Crofts, Inc, 1969.

Sabiston DC and Spencer FC (eds): Gibson's Surgery of the Chest. 4th ed. Philadelphia, WB Saunders Co, 1983.

Spencer H: Pathology of the Lung. New York, Macmillan Co, 1962.

Swenson O: Pediatric Surgery. 3rd ed. Vol 1. New York, Appleton-Century-Crofts, Inc, 1969.

Vaughan VC III, McKay RJ and Behrman RE (eds): Nelson Textbook of Pediatrics. 11th ed. Philadelphia, WB Saunders Co, 1981.

White M and Dennison WM: Surgery in Infancy and Childhood, a Handbook for Medical Students and General Practitioners. Edinburgh, E & S Livingstone, Ltd, 1958.

Thoracic Wall Deformities

Adkins PC: Pectus excavatum. Am Surg 24:571, 1958.

Adkins PC and Gwathmey O: Pectus excavatum: an appraisal of surgical treatment. J Thorac Surg 36:714, 1958.

Ashmore PG: Management of some deformities of the thoracic cage in children. Can J Surg 6:430, 1963.

Avery ME, Fletcher BD and Williams R: The Lung and Its Disorders in the Newborn Infant. 4th ed. Philadelphia, WB Saunders Co, 1981.

Bates DV, Macklem PT, and Christie RV: Respiratory Function in Disease: An Introduction to the Integrated Study of the Lung. 2nd ed. Philadelphia, WB Saunders Co, 1971.

Becker JM and Schneider KM: Indications for the surgical treatment of pectus excavatum. JAMA 180:22, 1962.

Beiser GD, Epstein SE, Stampfer M et al: Impairment of cardiac function in patients with pectus excavatum, with improvement after operative correction. N Engl J Med 287:267, 1972.

Bevegard S: Postural circulatory changes at rest and during exercise in patients with funnel chest, with special reference to factors affecting the stroke volume. Acta Med Scand 171:695, 1962.

Bevegard S, Holmgren A, and Jonsson B: The effect of body position on the circulation at rest and during exercise, with special reference to the influence on the stroke volume. Acta Phys Scand 49:279, 1960.

Bigger IA: The treatment of pectus excavatum or funnel chest. Am Surg 18:1071, 1952.

Billig DM and Immordino PA: Congenital upper sternal cleft: a case with successful surgical repair. J Pediatr Surg 5:257, 1970.

Brodkin AH Jr: Pectus excavatum: surgical indications and time of operation. Pediatrics 11:582, 1953.

Brodkin HA: Pigeon breast: congenital chondrosternal prominence. Arch Surg 77:261, 1958.

Brown AL: Pectus excavatum (funnel chest). J Thorac Surg 9:164, 1939.

Brown AL and Cook O: Cardiorespiratory studies in pre- and postoperative funnel chest (pectus excavatum). Dis Chest 20:378, 1951.

Brown JJM: The thoracic wall. In Brown HHM (ed): Surgery of Childhood. Baltimore, Williams & Wilkins Co, 1963.

Cantrell JR, Haller JA, and Ravitch MM: The syndrome of congenital defects involving the abdominal wall, sternum, diaphragm, pericardium, and heart. Surg Gynecol Obstet 107:602, 1958.

Chin EF: Surgery of funnel chest and congenital sternal prominence. Br J Surg 44:360, 1957.

Chin EF and Adler RH: Surgical treatment of pectus excavatum (funnel chest). Br Med J 1:1064, 1954.

Eijgelaar A and Butel JH: Congenital cleft sternum. Thorax 25:490, 1970.

Fink A, Rivin A, and Murray JF: Cardiopulmonary effects of funnel chest. Arch Intern Med 108:427, 1961.

Flavell G: An Introduction to Chest Surgery. London, Oxford University Press, 1957.

Gross RE: The Surgery of Infancy and Childhood: Its Principles and Techniques. Philadelphia, WB Saunders Co, 1953.

Groves LK: Deformities of the anterior chest wall. Cleveland Clin Q 30:55, 1963.

Haller JA Jr, Peters GN, Mazur D and White JJ: Pectus excavatum: a 20-year surgical experience. J Thorac Cardiovasc Surg 60:375, 1970.

Hanlon CR: Surgical treatment of funnel chest (pectus excavatum). Am Surg 22:408, 1956.

Hansen FN: The ontogeny and phylogeny of the sternum. Am J Anat 26:41, 1919.

Hansen JL and Jacoby O: Pulmonary function in pectus excavatum deformity. Acta Chir Scand 111:25, 1956.

Hay W and Dodsley J: Deformity. London, 1754.

Howard R: Funnel chest: its effect on cardiac function. Arch Dis Child 34:5, 1959.

Howard RN: Funnel chest: report of a series of one hundred cases. Med J Aust 2:1092, 1955.

Humphreys GH and Connolly JE: The surgical technique for the correction of pectus excavatum. J Thorac Cardiovasc Surg 40:194, 1960.

Jackson JL, George RE, Hewlett TH, and Bavers WF: Pectus excavatum: surgical experiences in thirty-four cases. Am J Surg 98:664, 1959.

Jensen NK, Schmidt WR and Garamella JJ: Funnel chest: a new corrective operation. J Thorac Cardiovasc Surg 43:731, 1962.

Jensen NK, Schmidt WR, Garamella JJ and Lynch MF: Pectus excavatum and carinatum: the how, when and why of surgical correction. J Pediatr Surg 5:4, 1970.

Jewett TC, Butsch WL, and Hug HR: Congenital bifid sternum. Pediatr Surg 52:932, 1962.

Keshishian JM and Cox PA: Management of recurrent pectus excavatum. J Thorac Cardiovasc Surg 54:740, 1967.

Kondrashin NI: Congenital funnel chest in children. Pediatriia 42:56, 1963.

Koop CE: The management of pectus excavatum. Surg Clin North Am 36:1627, 1956.

Lam CR and Brinkman GL: Indications and results in the surgical treatment of pectus excavatum. Arch Surg 78:322, 1959.

Lam CR and Taber RE: Surgical treatment of pectus carinatum. Arch Surg 103:191, 1971.

Lester CW: Funnel chest and allied deformities of thoracic cage. J Thorac Surg 19:507, 1950.

Lester CW: Funnel chest: its cause, effects, and treatment. J Pediatr 37:224, 1950.

Lester CW: Pigeon breast. Ann Surg 137:482, 1953.

Lester CW: Pigeon breast, funnel chest and other congenital deformities of chest. JAMA 156:1063, 1954.

Lester CW: The etiology and pathogenesis of funnel chest, pigeon breast, and related deformities of the anterior chest wall. J Thorac Surg 34:1, 1957.

Lester CW: Funnel chest, the status 360 years after its first description. Arch Pediatr 75:493, 1958.

Lester CW: Pectus carinatum, pigeon breast and related deformities of the sternum and costal cartilages. Arch Pediatr October 1960.

Lester CW: Surgical treatment of protrusion deformities of the sternum and costal cartilages (pectus carinatum, pigeon breast). Ann Surg 153:441, 1961.

Lindsey ES and Harris JA: Congenital and acquired chest deformities in children. South Med J 63:875, 1970.

Lindskog GE and Felton WL II: Considerations in the surgical treatment of pectus excavatum. Ann Surg 142:654, 1955.

Lindskog GE, Liebow AA, and Glenn WWL: Thoracic and Cardiovascular Surgery with Related Pathology. New York, Appleton-Century-Crofts, Inc, 1962.

Logan WD Jr, Crispin RH, Petterson JH et al: Ectopic cordis: report of a case and discussion of surgical management. Surgery 57:898, 1965.

Meyer L (1911): Cited in Ochsner A and DeBakey ME: Chonechondrosternon. Report of a case and review of the literature. J Thorac Surg 8:469, 1939.

Moghissi K: Long-term results of surgical correction of pectus excavatum and sternal prominence. Thorax 19:350, 1964.

Mullard K: Observations on the aetiology of pectus excavatum and other chest deformities, and a method of recording them. Br J Surg 54:115, 1967.

Orzalesi MM and Cook CD: Pulmonary function in children with pectus excavatum. J Pediatr 66:898, 1965.

Paltia V, Parkkulainen KV and Sulamaa M: Indications for surgery in funnel chest. Ann Pediatr Fenniae 5:183, 1959.

Peters RM and Johnson G Jr: Stabilization of pectus deformity with wire strut. J Thorac Cardiovasc Surg 47:814, 1964.

Phillips WL: Pectus excavatum. S Afr Med J 34:6, 1960.

Pilcher RS: Trachea, bronchi, lungs and pleura. In Brown JJM (ed): Surgery of Childhood. Baltimore, Williams & Wilkins Co, 1963.

Polgar G and Koop CE: Pulmonary function in pectus excavatum. Pediatrics 32:209, 1963.

Potts WJ: The Surgeon and the Child. Philadelphia, WB Saunders Co, 1959.

Ramsay BH: Transplantation of the rectus abdominis muscle in the surgical correction of a pectus carinatum deformity with associated parasternal depressions. Surg Gynecol Obstet 116:507, 1963.

Ravitch MM: Operative treatment of pectus excavatum. Ann Surg 129:429, 1949.

Ravitch MM: Pectus excavatum and heart failure. Surgery 30:178, 1951.

Ravitch MM: Operation for correction of pectus excavatum. Surg Gynecol Obstet 106:618, 1958.

Ravitch MM: Operative correction of pectus carinatum (pigeon breast). Ann Surg 151:705, 1960.

Ravitch MM: Operative treatment of congenital deformities of the chest. Am J Surg 101:588, 1961.

Ravitch MM: Congenital deformities of the chest wall. In Benson DD et al (eds): Pediatric Surgery. Vol 1. Chicago, Year Book Medical Publishers, Inc, 1962.

Ravitch MM: Technical problems in the operative correction of pectus excavatum. Ann Surg 162:29, 1965.

Ravitch MM: Congenital Deformities of the Chest Wall and Their Operative Correction. Philadelphia, WB Saunders Co, 1977.

Ravitch MM: Disorders of the sternum and the thoracic wall. In Sabiston DC Jr and Spencer FC (eds): Gibbon's Surgery of the Chest. 4th ed. Philadelphia, WB Saunders Co, 1983.

Ravitch MM and Matzen RN: Pulmonary insufficiency in pectus excavatum associated with left pulmonary agenesis, congenital clubbed feet and ectromelia. Dis Chest 54:58, 1968.

Rehbein F and Wernicke HH: The operative treatment of the funnel chest. Arch Dis Child 32:5, 1957.

Robicsek F, Daugherty HK, Mullen DC et al: Technical considerations in the surgical management of pectus excavatum and carinatum. Ann Thorac Surg 18:549, 1974.

Robicsek F, Sanger PW, Taylor FH, and Thomas MJ: The surgical treatment of chondrosternal prominence (pectus carinatum). J Thorac Cardiovasc Surg 45:691, 1963.

Roccaforte DS, Mehnert JJ and Peniche A: Repair of bifid sternum with autogenous cartilage. Ann Surg 149:448, 1959.

Sabiston DC: The surgical management of congenital bifid sternum with partial ectopia cordis. J Thorac Surg 23:118, 1958.

Sanger PW, Robicsek F, and Taylor FH: Surgical management of anterior chest deformities: a new technique and report of 153 operations without a death. Surgery 48:510, 1960.

Sanger PW, Taylor FH, and Robicsek F: Deformities of the anterior wall of the chest. Surg Gynecol Obstet 116:515, 1963.

Schaub F and Wegmann T: Elektrokardiographische Veranderungen bei Trichterbrust. Cardiologia 24:39, 1954.

Stanford W, Bowers DG, Lindberg EF et al: Silastic implants for correction of pectus excavatum. Ann Thorac Surg 13:529, 1972.

Swenson O: Pediatric Surgery. 2nd ed. New York. Appleton-Century-Crofts, Inc, 1962.

Van Buchem FSP and Nieveen J: Findings with funnel chest. Acta Med Scand 174:657, 1963.

Wachtel FW, Ravitch MM, and Grishman A: Relation of pectus excavatum to heart disease. Am Heart J 52:121, 1956.

Wada J and Ikeda K: Clinical experience with 306 funnel chest operations. Int Surg 57:707, 1972.

Welch KJ: Satisfactory surgical correction of pectus excavatum deformity in childhood. J Thorac Surg 36:697, 1958.

Welch KJ and Vos A: Surgical correction of pectus carinatum (pigeon breast). J Pediatr Surg 8:659, 1973.

Wichern WA Jr and Lester CW: Funnel chest. Arch Surg 84:170, 1962.

CONGENITAL ABSENCE OF RIBS

Aschner BB, Kaizer MN, and Small AR: Flaring of ribs associated with other skeletal anomalies. Conn Med J 19:383, 1955.

Brown JJM: The thoracic wall. In Brown JJM (ed): Surgery of Childhood. Baltimore, Williams & Wilkins Co, 1964.

Fishmann AP, Turino GM, and Bergofsky EH: Disorders of respiration and circulation in subjects with deformities of thorax. Mod Concepts Cardiovasc Dis 27:449, 1958.

Flavell G: An Introduction to Chest Surgery. London, Oxford University Press, 1957.

Goodman HI: Hernia of lung. J Thorac Surg 2:368, 1933.

Lindsey ES and Harris JA: Congenital and acquired chest deformities in children. S Med J 63:875, 1970.

Ravitch MM: The operative treatment of congenital deformities of the chest. Am J Surg 101:588, 1961.

Ravitch MM: The chest wall. In Benson CD et al (eds): Pediatric Surgery. Vol I. Chicago, Year Book Medical Publishers, Inc, 1962.

Ravitch MM: Disorders of the sternum and the thoracic wall. In Sabiston DC Jr and Spencer FC (eds): Gibbon's Surgery of the Chest. 4th ed. Philadelphia, WB Saunders Co, 1983.

Rickham PP: Lung hernia secondary to congenital absence of ribs. Arch Dis Child 34:14, 1959.

Swenson I: Pediatric Surgery. 2nd ed. New York, Appleton-Century-Crofts, Inc, 1962.

Thomson J: Teratologia. Vol 2. Edinburgh, W Green and Sons, 1895.

Diaphragmatic Deformities

CONGENITAL ANTERIOR DIAPHRAGMATIC HERNIA (MORGAGNI); CONGENITAL DIAPHRAGMATIC HERNIA OF BOCHDALEK

Avery ME, Fletcher BD, and Williams R: The Lung and Its Disorders in the Newborn Infant. 4th ed. Philadelphia, WB Saunders Co, 1981.

Baffes TG: Diaphragmatic hernia. In Benson CD et al (eds): Pediatric Surgery. Vol 1. Chicago, Year Book Medical Publishers, Inc, 1962.

Baran EM, Houston HE, Lynn HB and O'Connell EJ: Foramen of Morgagni hernias in children. Surgery 62:1076, 1967.

Bartlett RH and Gazzaniga AB: Extracorporeal membrane oxygenator (ECMO) support in neonatal respiratory failure. J Thorac Cardiovasc Surg 74:826, 1977.

Bartlett RH and Gazzaniga AB: Extracorporeal circulation for cardiopulmonary failure. Curr Probl Surg 15:1, 1978.

Bartlett RH, Gazzaniga AB, Fong SW et al: Extracorporeal membrane oxygenator (ECMO) support in neonatal respiratory failure. J Thorac Cardiovasc Surg 74:826, 1977.

Belsey R: The surgery of the diaphragm. In Brown JJM (ed): Surgery of Childhood. Baltimore, Williams & Wilkins Co, 1963.

Benjamin HB: Agenesis of the left hemidiaphragm. J Thorac Surg 46:265, 1963.

Bentley G and Lister J: Retrosternal hernia. Surgery 57:567, 1965.

Bloss RS, Turmen T, Beardmore HE, and Aranda JV: Tolazoline therapy for persistent pulmonary hypertension after congenital diaphragmatic hernia repair. J Pediatr 97:984, 1980.

Boix-Ochoa J, Peguero G, Seijo G et al: Acid-base balance and blood gases in prognosis and therapy of congenital diaphragmatic hernia. J Pediatr Surg 9:49, 1974.

Boles ET Jr, Schiller M and Weinberger M: Improved management of neonates with congenital diaphragmatic hernias. Arch Surg 103:344, 1971.

Bowers VM Jr, McElin TW and Dorsey MM: Diaphragmatic hernia in the newborn: diagnostic responsibility of the obstetrician. Obstet Gynecol 6:262, 1955.

Boyd DP: Diaphragmatic hernia of the foramen of Morgagni. Surg Clin North Am 41:839, 1961.

Butler N and Claireaux AE: Congenital diaphragmatic hernia as a cause of perinatal mortality. Lancet 1:659, 1962.

Campanale RP and Rowland RH: Hypoplasia of the lung associated with congenital diaphragmatic hernia. Ann Surg 142:176, 1955.

Carter REB, Waterson DJ and Aberdeen E: Diaphragmatic hernia in infancy. Lancet 1:656, 1962.

Cerilli GJ: Foramen of Bochdalek hernia. Ann Surg 159:385, 1964.

Chatrath RR, ElShafie M, and Jones RS: Fate of hypoplastic lungs after repair of congenital diaphragmatic hernia. Arch Dis Child 46:633, 1971.

Collins DL, Pomerance JJ, Travis KW et al: A new approach to congenital posterolateral diaphragmatic hernia. J Pediatr Surg 12:149, 1977.

Comer TP: Schmalhorst WR and Arbegast NR: Foramen of Morgagni hernia diagnosed by liver scan. Chest 63:1036, 1973.

Cook RCM and Beckwith JB: Adrenal injury during repair of diaphragmatic hernia in infants. Surgery 69:251, 1971.

deLorimier AA, Tierney DF and Parker HR: Hypoplastic lung in fetal lambs with surgically produced congenital diaphragmatic hernia. Surgery 62:12, 1967.

Dibbins AW and Weiner ES: Mortality from neonatal diaphragmatic hernia. J Pediatr Surg 9:653, 1974.

Farrel PM and Avery MR: Hyaline membrane disease: state of the art. Am Rev Resp Dis 111:657, 1975.

Filler RM, Randolph JG and Gross RE: Esophageal hiatus hernia in infants and children. J Thorac Surg 47:551, 1964.

Fitchett CW and Tavarex V: Bilateral congenital diaphragmatic herniation. Surgery 57:305, 1965.

Flavell G: An Introduction to Chest Surgery. London, Oxford University Press, 1957.

Gans SL and Hackworth LE: Respiratory obstructions of surgical import. Pediatr Clin North Am 6:1023, 1959.

Gross RE: The Surgery of Infancy and Childhood: Its Principles and Techniques. Philadelphia, WB Saunders Co, 1953.

Hajdu NH and Sidhva JN: Parasternal diaphragmatic hernia through the foramen of Morgagni. Br J Radiol 28:355, 1955.

Hardesty RL, Griffith BP, Debski RF et al: Extracorporeal membrane oxygenation. J Thorac Cardiovasc Surg 81:556, 1981.

Harrington SW: Various types of diaphragmatic hernia treated surgically: report of 430 cases. Surg Gynecol Obstet 86:735, 1948.

Haupt GL and Myers RN: Polyvinyl formalized (Ivalon) sponge in the repair of diaphragmatic hernia. Arch Surg 80:103; 613, 1960.

Hedblom CA: Diaphragmatic hernia. JAMA 85:947, 1925.

Hermann RE and Barber DH: Congenital diaphragmatic hernia in the child beyond infancy. Cleveland Clin Q 30:73, 1963.

Hill JD, O'Brien TG, Murray JJ et al: Prolonged extracorporeal oxygenation for acute post-traumatic respiratory failure (shock-lung syndrome). N Engl J Med 186:629, 1972.

Holcomb GW Jr: A new technique for repair of congenital diaphragmatic hernia with absence of the left hemidiaphragm. Surgery 51:534, 1962.

Hope JW and Koop CE: Differential diagnosis of mediastinal masses. Pediatr Clin North Am 6:379, 1959.

Jemerin EE: Diaphragmatic hernia through foramen of Morgagni. J Mount Sinai Hosp (NY) 30:415, 1963.

Johnson DG, Deaner RM and Koop CE: Diaphragmatic hernia in infancy: factors affecting the mortality rate. Surgery 62:1082, 1967.

Keith A: Human Embryology and Morphology. London, Edward Arnold, 1948.

Kelly KA and Bassett DL: An anatomic reappraisal of the hernia of Morgagni. Surgery 55:495, 1964.

Kenigsberg K and Gwinn JL: The retained sac in repair of posterolateral diaphragmatic hernia in the newborn. Surgery 57:894, 1965.

Kiesewetter WB, Gutierrez IZ, and Sieber WK: Diaphragmatic hernia in infants under one year of age. Arch Surg 83:561, 1961.

Kinsbourne M: Hiatus hernia with contortions of the neck. Lancet 1:1058, 1964.

Kitagawa M, Hislop A, Boyden EA, and Reid L: Lung hypoplasia in congenital diaphragmatic hernia. Br J Surg 58:342, 1971.

Krummel TM, Greenfield LJ, Kirkpatrick BV et al: Clinical use of an extracorporeal membrane oxygenator in neonatal pulmonary failure. J Pediatr Surg 1982.

Ladd WE and Gross ER: Abdominal Surgery of Infancy and Childhood. Philadelphia, WB Saunders Co, 1941.

Langer JC, Filler RM, Bohn DJ et al: Timing of surgery for congenital diaphragmatic hernia: is emergency operation necessary? J Pediatr Surg 23:731, 1988.

Langham MR Jr, Krummel TM, Bartlett RH et al: Mortality with extracorporeal membrane oxygenation following repair of congenital diaphragmatic hernia in 93 infants. J Pediatr Surg 22:1150, 1987.

Lewis MAH and Young DG: Ventilatory problems with congenital diaphragmatic hernia. Anaesthesia 24:571, 1969.

McNamara JJ, Eraklis AJ, and Gross RE: Congenital posterolateral diaphragmatic hernia in the newborn. J Thorac Cardiovasc Surg 55:55, 1968.

Meeker IA Jr and Snyder WH Jr: Surgical management of diaphragmatic defects in the newborn, a report of twenty infants each less than one week old. Am J Surg 104:196, 1962.

Moodie DS, Telander RL, Kleinberg F: Use of tolazoline in newborn infants with diaphragmatic hernia and severe cardiopulmonary disease. J Thorac Cardiovasc Surg 75:725, 1978.

Moore TC, Batterby JS, Rogenkamp MW, and Campbell JA: Congenital posterolateral diaphragmatic hernia in the newborn. Surg Gynecol Obstet 104:675, 1957.

Murdock AI, Burrington JB, and Swyer PR: Alveolar to arterial oxygen tension difference and venous admixture in newly born infants with congenital diaphragmatic herniation through the foramen of Bochdalek. Biol Neonate 17:161, 1971.

Murphy DR and Owen HF: Respiratory emergencies in the newborn. Am J Surg 101:58, 1961.

Neville WE and Clowes GHA Jr: Congenital absence of hemidiaphragm and use of a lobe of liver in its surgical correction. Arch Surg 69:282, 1954.

Nixon HH and O'Donnell B: The Essentials of Pediatric Surgery. London, William Heinemann, Ltd, 1961.

Ormazable M, Kirkpatrick B, and Mueller D: Alteration of alveolar-arterial O_2 gradient (A-a O_2) in response to tolazoline as a prediction of outcome in neonates with persistent pulmonary hypertension. Pediatr Res 14:607, 1980.

Osebold WR and Soper RT: Congenital posterolateral diaphragmatic hernia past infancy. Am Surg 131:748, 1976.

Polk HC and Burford TH: Hiatal hernia in infancy and childhood. Surgery 54:521, 1963.

Potts WJ: The Surgeon and the Child. Philadelphia, WB Saunders Co, 1959.

Raphaely RC and Downes JJ: Congenital diaphragmatic hernia: prediction of survival. J Pediatr Surg 8:815, 1973.

Richardson WR: Thoracic emergencies in the newborn infant. Am J Surg 105:524, 1963.

Riker WL: Congenital diaphragmatic hernia. Arch Surg 69:291, 1954.

Rosenkrantz JF and Cotton EK: Replacement of left hemidiaphragm by a pedicled abdominal muscular flap. J Thorac Cardiovasc Surg 48:912, 1964.

Sabga GA, Neville WE and Del Guercio LRM: Anomalies of the lung associated with congenital diaphragmatic hernia. Surgery 50:547, 1961.

Schuster SR: The recognition and management of diaphragmatic hernias in infancy and childhood. Q Rev Pediatr 15:171, 1960.

Shaffer JO: Prosthesis for agenesis of the diaphragm. JAMA 188:1060, 1964.

Simpson JS: Ventral silon pouch: method of repairing congenital diaphragmatic hernias in neonates without increasing intra-abdominal pressure. Surgery 66:798, 1969.

Snyder WH and Greany EM: Congenital diaphragmatic hernia: 77 consecutive cases. Surgery 57:576, 1965.

Starrett RW and deLorimier AA: Congenital diaphragmatic hernia in lambs: hemodynamic and ventilatory changes with breathing. J Pediatr Surg 10:575, 1975.

Stolar CJH, Dillon PW, and Reyes C: Selective use of extracorporeal membrane oxygenation in the management of congenital diaphragmatic hernia. J Pediatr Surg 23:207, 1988.

Sulamaa M and Viitamen I: Congenital diaphragmatic hernia and relaxation. Acta Chir Scand 124:288, 1962.

Thomsen G: Diaphragmatic hernia in the newborn: incidence of neonatal fatalities. Acta Chir Scand 283(Suppl):267, 1961.

White M and Dennison WM: Surgery in Infancy and Childhood. A Handbook for Medical Students and General Practitioners. Edinburgh, E & S Livingstone, Ltd, 1958.

Zapol WM, Snider MT, Hill JD et al: Extracorporeal membrane oxygenation in severe acute respiratory failure. JAMA 242:2193, 1979.

CONGENITAL HIATAL DIAPHRAGMATIC HERNIA

Avery ME, Fletcher BD, and Williams R: The Lung and Its Disorders in the Newborn Infant. 4th ed. Philadelphia, WB Saunders Co, 1981.

Blattner RJ: Hiatal hernia. J Pediatr 72:424, 1968.

Boles ET and Izant RJ Jr: Spontaneous chylothorax in the neonatal period. Am J Surg 99:870, 1960.

Burford TH and Lischer CE: Treatment of short esophageal hernia with esophagitis by Finney pyloroplasty. Ann Surg 144:647, 1956.

Cahill JL, Aberdeen E, and Waterston DJ: Results of surgical treatment of esophageal hiatal hernia in infancy and childhood. Surgery 66:597, 1969.

Euler AR, Byrne WJ, Amernt ME et al: Recurrent pulmonary disease in children: a complication of gastroesophageal reflux. Pediatrics 63:47, 1979.

Herbst J, Friedland GW, and Zboralske FF: Hiatal hernia and "rumination" in infants and children. J Pediatr 78:261, 1971.

Jewett TC Jr and Waterston DJ: Surgical management of hiatal hernia in children. J Pediatr Surg 10:757, 1975.

Jona JZ, Sty JR, and Glicklich M: Simplified radioisotope technique for assessing gastroesophageal reflux in children. J Pediatr Surg 16:114, 1981.

Kamal I and Guiney EJ: The treatment of hiatus hernia in children by anterior gastropexy. J Pediatr Surg 7:641, 1972.

Koch A and Gass R: Continuous 20–24 hr. esophageal pH monitoring in infancy. J Pediatr Surg 16:109, 1981.

Koch A and Ruggeberg J: Zur Funktion des unteren oesophagussphinkters im saulingsalter. Langenbeck's Arch Klin Chir Suppl 53–57, 1978.

Lilly JR and Randolph JG: Hiatal hernia and gastroesophageal reflux in infants and children. J Thorac Cardiovasc Surg 55:42, 1968.

Monereo J, Cortes L, and Blesa E: Peptic esophageal stenosis in children. J Pediatr Surg 8:475, 1973.

Prinsen JE: Hiatus hernia in infants and children: a long-term follow-up of medical therapy. J Pediatr Surg 10:97, 1975.

Rohatgi M, Shandling B, and Stephens CA: Hiatal hernia in infants and children: results of surgical treatment. Surgery 69:456, 1971.

Winans CS and Harris LD: Quantitation of lower esophageal sphincter competence. Gastroenterology 51:779, 1967.

CONGENITAL EVENTRATION OF THE DIAPHRAGM

Arnheim EE: Congenital eventration of the diaphragm in infancy. Surgery 35:809, 1954.

Avery ME and Taeusch HW Jr (eds): Schaffer's Diseases of the Newborn. 5th ed. Philadelphia, WB Saunders Co, 1989.

Avery ME, Fletcher BD, and Williams R: The Lung and Its Disorders in the Newborn Infant. 4th ed. Philadelphia, WB Saunders Co, 1981.

Baffes TC: Diaphragmatic hernia. In Benson CD et al (eds): Pediatric Surgery. Vol 1. Chicago, Year Book Medical Publishers, Inc, 1962.

Belsey R: The surgery of the diaphragm. In Brown JJM (ed): Surgery of Childhood. Baltimore, Williams & Wilkins Co, 1963.

Bisgard JD: Congenital eventration of diaphragm. J Thorac Surg 16:484, 1947.

Chin EF and Lynn RB: Surgery of eventration of the diaphragm. J Thorac Surg 32:6, 1956.

Firestone FN and Taybi H: Bilateral diaphragmatic eventration: demonstration by pneumoperitoneography. Surgery 62:954, 1967.

Flavell G: An Introduction to Chest Surgery. London, Oxford University Press, 1957.

Gans SL and Hackworth LE: Respiratory obstructions of surgical import. Pediatr Clin North Am 6:1023, 1959.

Goulston E: Eventration of the diaphragm. Arch Dis Child 32:9, 1957.

Haller JA, Pickard LR, Tepas JJ et al: Management of diaphragmatic paralysis in infants with special emphasis on selection of patients for operative plication. J Pediatr Surg 14:779, 1979.

Laxdal OE, McDougall H and Mellin GW: Congenital eventration of the diaphragm. N Engl J Med 250:401, 1954.

Lindskog GE, Liebow AA and Glenn WWL: Thoracic and Cardiovascular Surgery with Related Pathology. New York, Appleton-Century-Crofts, Inc, 1962.

Marcos JJ, Grover FL, and Trinkle JK: Paralyzed diaphragm—effect of plication on respiratory mechanics. J Surg Res 16:523, 1974.

Michelson E: Eventration of the diaphragm. Surgery 49:410, 1961.

Mickell JJ, Oh KS, Siewere RD et al: Clinical implications of postoperative unilateral phrenic nerve paralysis. J Thorac Cardiovasc Surg 76:297, 1978.

Othersen HB Jr and Lorenzo RL: Diaphragmatic paralysis and eventration: newer approaches to diagnosis and operative correction. J Pediatr Surg 12:309, 1977.

Pomerantz M: The diaphragm. In Sabiston DC Jr and Spencer FC (eds): Gibbon's Surgery of the Chest. 4th ed. Philadelphia, WB Saunders Co, 1983.

Robotham JL: A physiological approach to hemidiaphragm paralysis. Crit Care Med 12:563, 1979.

Schwartz MS and Filler RM: Plication of the diaphragm for symptomatic phrenic nerve paralysis. J Pediatr Surg 13:259, 1978.

Thomas TV: Nonparalytic eventration of the diaphragm. J Thorac Cardiovasc Surg 55:586, 1968.

Thomas TV: Eventration of the diaphragm. Ann Thorac Surg 10:180, 1970.

Chylothorax

Avery ME and Taeusch HW Jr (eds): Schaffer's Diseases of the Newborn. 5th ed. Philadelphia, WB Saunders Co, 1989.

Avery ME, Fletcher BD and Williams R: The Lung and Its Disorders in the Newborn Infant, 4th ed. Philadelphia, WB Saunders Co, 1981.

Boles ET and Izant RJ Jr: Spontaneous chylothorax in the neonatal period. Am J Surg 99:870, 1960.

Chernick V and Reed MH: Pneumothorax and chylothorax in the neonatal period. J Pediatr 76:624, 1970.

Eichenwald HF and McCracken GH Jr: Chylothorax. In Vaughan VC III and McKay RJ (eds): Nelson Textbook of Pediatrics. 11th ed. Philadelphia, WB Saunders Co, 1979.

Forbes GB: Chylothorax in infancy. J Pediatr 25:191, 1944.

Gingell JC: Treatment of chylothorax by producing pleurodesis using iodized talc. Thorax 20:261, 1965.

Higgins CB and Mulder DG: Chylothorax after surgery for congenital heart disease. J Thorac Cardiovasc Surg 61:411, 1971.

Maier HC: The pleura. In Sabiston DC Jr and Spencer FC (eds): Gibbon's Surgery of the Chest. 4th ed. Philadelphia, WB Saunders Co, 1983.

Morphis LG, Arcinue EL, and Krause JR: Generalized lymphangioma in infancy with chylothorax. Pediatrics 46:566, 1970.

Perry RE, Hodgman J and Cass AB: Pleural effusion in the neonatal period. J Pediatr 62:838, 1963.

Randolph JG and Gross RE: Congenital chylothorax. Arch Surg 74:405, 1957.

Ravitch MM: Chylothorax. In Benson CD et al (eds): Pediatric Surgery. Vol 1. Chicago, Year Book Medical Publishers, Inc, 1962.

Wiener ES, Owens L and Salzberg AM: Chylothorax after Bochdalek herniorrhaphy in a neonate. J Thorac Cardiovasc Surg 65:200, 1973.

Williams KR and Burford TH: The management of chylothorax. Ann Surg 160:131, 1964.

Tracheal and Esophageal Deformities

TRACHEAL AGENESIS AND STENOSIS

Bigler JA, Holinger PH, Johnston KC, and Schiller F: Tracheotomy in infancy. Pediatrics 13:476, 1954.

Cantrell JR and Guild HG: Congenital stenosis of the trachea. Am J Surg 108:297, 1964.

Fonkalsrud EW, Martell RR, and Maloney JV: Surgical treatment of tracheal agenesis. J Thorac Cardiovasc Surg 45:520, 1963.

Holinger PH: The infant with respiratory stridor. Pediatr Clin North Am 2:403, 1955.

Holinger PH and Johnston KC: Clinical aspects of congenital anomalies of the trachea and bronchi. Dis Chest 31:613, 1957.

Holinger PH, Johnston KC, Parchet VN et al: Congenital malformations of the trachea, bronchi and lung. Ann Otol 61:1159, 1952.

Hopkinson JM: Congenital absence of the trachea. J Pathol 107:63, 1972.

Joshi VV: Tracheal agenesis. Am J Dis Child 117:341, 1969.

Ochsner JL and Lejeune FE Jr: Tracheal and esophageal obstructions in infants. South Med J 57:1340, 1964.

Oliver P, Richardson JR, Clubb RW, and Flake CG: Tracheotomy in children. N Engl J Med 267:631, 1962.

Othersen HB Jr: The technique of intraluminal stenting and steroid administration in the treatment of tracheal stenosis in children. J Pediatr Surg 9:683, 1974.

Rubin LR et al: Elective tracheostomy in infants and children. Am J Surg 98:880, 1959.

Witzleben CL: Aplasia of the trachea. Pediatrics 32:31, 1963.

TRACHEOMALACIA

Cox WL and Shaw RR: Congenital chondromalacia of the trachea. J Thorac Cardiovasc Surg 49:1033, 1965.

Burford TH and Ferguson TB: Congenital lesions of the lungs and emphysema. In Sabiston DC Jr and Spencer FC (eds): Gibbon's Surgery of the Chest. 4th ed. Philadelphia, WB Saunders Co, 1983.

Holinger PH and Johnston KC: The infant with respiratory stridor. Pediatr Clin North Am 2:403, 1955.

Holinger PH et al: Congenital malformations of the trachea, bronchi, and lung. Ann Otol 61:1159, 1952.

Levin SJ, Scherer RA, and Adler P: Cause of wheezing in infancy. Ann Allergy 22:20, 1964.

Lynch JL: Bronchomalacia in children. Considerations governing medical vs. surgical treatment. Clin Pediatr 9:279, 1970.

Ochsner JL and LeJeune FE Jr: Tracheal and esophageal obstruction in infants. South Med J 57:1333, 1964.

VASCULAR RING

Abreu AL: Surgery of the heart and great vessels. In Brown JJM (ed): Surgery of Childhood. Baltimore, Williams & Wilkins Co, 1963.

Avery ME and Taeusch HW Jr (eds): Schaffer's Diseases of the Newborn. 5th ed. Philadelphia, WB Saunders Co, 1989.

Avery ME, Fletcher BD, and Williams R: The Lung and Its Disorders in the Newborn Infant. 4th ed. Philadelphia, WB Saunders Co, 1981.

Bahnson HT: The aorta. In Sabiston DC Jr and Spencer FC (eds): Gibbon's Surgery of the Chest. 4th ed. Philadelphia. WB Saunders Co, 1983.

Bernatz PE, Lewis DR, and Edwards JE: Division of the posterior arch of a double aortic arch for relief of tracheal and esophageal obstruction. Proc Staff Meet Mayo Clin 34:173, 1959.

Blumenthal S and Ravitch MM: Seminar on aortic vascular rings and other anomalies of the aortic arch. Pediatrics 20:896, 1957.

Boyle WF and Shaw CC: Right-sided aortic arch. N Engl J Med 256:392, 1957.

Campbell DN, Lilly JR, Heiser JC, and Clarke DR: Surgery of pulmonary artery "sling." J Pediatr Surg 18:855, 1983.

Cartwright RS and Bauersfield SR: Thoracic aortography in infants and children. Ann Surg 150:266, 1959.

De Bord RA: Double aortic arch in infancy. Ann Surg 161:479, 1965.

Eklof O, Ekstrom G, Eriksson BO et al: Arterial anomalies causing compression of the trachea and/or the oesophagus. Acta Paediatr Scand 60:81, 1971.

Fineberg C and Stofman HC: Tracheal compression caused by an anomalous innominate artery arising from a brachiocephalic trunk. J Thorac Surg 37:214, 1959.

Gans SL and Hackworth LE: Respiratory obstructions of surgical import. Pediatr Clin North Am 6:1023, 1959.

Griswold HE and Young MD: Double aortic arch: report of 2 cases and review of the literature. Pediatrics 4:751, 1949.

Gross RE: The Surgery of Infancy and Childhood: Its Principles and Techniques. Philadelphia, WB Saunders Co, 1953.

Gross RE: Thoracic surgery for infants. J Thorac Cardiovasc Surg 48:152, 1964.

Gross RE: An Atlas of Children's Surgery. Philadelphia, WB Saunders Co, 1970.

Gross RE and Neuhauser EBD: Compression of trachea or esophagus by vascular anomalies: surgical therapy in 40 cases. Pediatrics 7:69, 1951.

Gross RE and Ware PF: The surgical significance of aortic arch anomalies. Surg Gynecol Obstet 83:435, 1946.

Haller JA Jr, Peters GN, White JJ, and Dorst JP: Selection for operative correction of symptomatic tracheal compression from an aberrant innominate artery in infants. (Unpublished paper.)

Holinger PH and Johnston KC: The infant with respiratory stridor. Pediatr Clin North Am 2:403, 1955.

Holinger PH, Johnston KC, and Parchet VN: Congenital malformations of the trachea, bronchi and lung. Ann Otol 61:1159, 1952.

Lasher EP: Types of tracheal and esophageal constriction due to arterial anomalies of the aortic arch, with suggestions as to treatment. Am J Surg 96:228, 1958.

Lindskog GE, Liebow AA, and Glenn WWL: Thoracic and Cardiovascular Surgery, with Related Pathology. New York, Appleton-Century-Crofts, Inc, 1962.

Mahoney EB and Manning JA: Aortic arch: congenital abnormalities. Pediatr Digest March 1965.

Moes CAF, Izukawa T, and Trusler GA: Innominate artery compression of the trachea. Arch Otolaryngol 101:733, 1975.

Mustard WT: Vascular rings compressing the esophagus and trachea. In Benson CD et al (eds): Pediatric Surgery. Vol 1. Chicago, Year Book Medical Publishers, Inc, 1962.

Mustard WT, Bayliss CE, Fearon B et al: Tracheal compression by the innominate artery in children. Ann Thorac Surg 8:312, 1969.

Nikaidoh H, Riker WL, and Idriss FS: Surgical management of "vascular rings." Arch Surg 105:327, 1972.

Nixon HH and O'Donnell B: The Essentials of Paediatric Surgery. London, William Heinemann, Ltd, 1961.

Ochsner JL and LeJeune FE Jr: Tracheal and esophageal obstruction in infants. South Med J 57:1333, 1964.

Park CD, Waldhausen JA, Friedman S et al: Tracheal compression by the great arteries in the mediastinum. Arch Surg 103:626, 1971.

Richardson DW: Thoracic emergencies in the newborn infant. Am J Surg 105:524, 1963.

Riker WL and Potts WJ: Cardiac lesions amenable to surgery: current status. Pediatr Clin North Am 6:1055, 1959.

Swenson O: Pediatric Surgery. 2nd ed. New York, Appleton-Century-Crofts, Inc, 1962.

Vaughan VC III, McKay RJ, and Behrman RE (eds): Nelson Textbook of Pediatrics. 11th ed. Philadelphia, WB Saunders Co, 1979.

Wychulis AR, Kincaid OW, Weidman WH, and Danielson GK: Congenital vascular ring: surgical considerations and results of operation. Mayo Clin Proc 46:182, 1971.

TRACHEOESOPHAGEAL FISTULA WITHOUT ESOPHAGEAL ATRESIA; ESOPHAGEAL ATRESIA

Abrahamson J and Shandling B: Esophageal atresia in the underweight baby: a challenge. J Pediatr Surg 7:608, 1972.

Ashcraft KW and Holder TM: The story of esophageal atresia and tracheoesophageal fistula. Surgery 65:332, 1969.

Avery ME and Taeusch HW Jr (eds): Schaffer's Diseases of the Newborn. 5th ed. Philadelphia, WB Saunders Co, 1989.

Avery ME, Fletcher BD, and Williams R: The Lung and Its Disorders in the Newborn Infant. 4th ed. Philadelphia, WB Saunders Co, 1981.

Baker DC, Flood CA, and Ferrer JM Jr: Postoperative esophageal stenosis. Ann Otol 63:1082, 1954.

Battersby JS, Jolly WW, and Fess SW: Esophageal atresia: a comprehensive study of 210 patients. Bull Soc Int Chir No. 5/6, 1971.

Bedard P, Girvan DP and Shandling B: Congenital H-type tracheoesophageal fistula. J Pediatr Surg 9:663, 1974.

Blumberg JB: Laryngotracheoesophageal cleft, the embryologic implications: review of the literature. Surgery 57:559, 1965.

Burford TH and Ferguson TB: Congenital lesions of the lungs and emphysema. In Sabiston DC Jr and Spencer FC (eds): Gibbon's Surgery of the Chest. 4th ed. Philadelphia, WB Saunders Co, 1983.

Burgess JN, Carlson HC and Ellis FH Jr: Esophageal functions after successful repair of esophageal atresia and tracheoesophageal fistula. J Thorac Cardiovasc Surg 56:667, 1968.

Cohen SJ: Unusual types of esophageal atresia and tracheoesophageal fistula. Clin Pediatr 4:271, 1965.

Cohen SR: The diagnosis and surgical management of congenital tracheoesophageal fistula without atresia of the esophagus. Ann Otol Rhinol Laryngol 79:1101, 1970.

Comming WA: Esophageal atresia and tracheoesophageal fistula. Radiol Clin North Am 13:277, 1975.

DeBoar A and Potts WJ: Congenital atresia of the esophagus with tracheoesophageal fistula. Surg Gynecol Obstet 104:475, 1957.

DeLorimier AA and Harrison MR: Long gap esophageal atresia. Primary anastomosis after esophageal elongation by bougienage and esophagomyotomy. J Thorac Cardiovasc Surg 79:138, 1980.

Desjardins HG, Stephens CA, and Moes CAF: Results of surgical treatment of congenital tracheoesophageal fistula, with a note on cine-fluorographic findings. Ann Surg 100:14, 1964.

Dudgeon DL, Morrison CW, and Woolley MM: Congenital proximal tracheoesophageal fistula. J Pediatr Surg 7:614, 1972.

Eraklis AJ and Gross RE: Esophageal atresia—management following an anastomotic leak. Surgery 60:919, 1966.

Eraklis AJ, Rossello PJ, and Ballantine TVN: Circular esophago-myotomy of upper pouch in primary repair of long-segment esophageal atresia. J Pediatr Surg 11:709, 1976.

Falletta GP: Recommunication on repair of congenital tracheo-esophageal fistula. Arch Surg 88:779, 1964.

Ferguson CC: Management of infants with esophageal atresia and tracheoesophageal fistula. Ann Surg 172:750, 1970.

Filler RM, Rossello PJ, and Lebowitz RL: Life-threatening anoxic spells caused by tracheal compression after repair of esophageal atresia by surgery. J Pediatr Surg 11:739, 1976.

Flavell G: The Oesophagus. London, Butterworth's, 1963.

Franklin RH: The oesophagus. In Brown JJM (ed): Surgery of Childhood. Baltimore, Williams & Wilkins Co, 1963.

Gans SO and Hackworth LE: Respiratory obstructions of surgical import. Pediatr Clin North Am 6:1023, 1959.

Goldenberg IS: An unusual variation of congenital tracheoesoph-ageal fistula. J Thorac Cardiovasc Surg 40:114, 1960.

Gross RE: The Surgery of Infancy and Childhood: Its Principles and Techniques. Philadelphia, WB Saunders Co, 1953.

Groves LK: Surgical treatment of esophageal atresia and tracheo-esophageal fistula in the infant. Cleveland Clin Q 25:227, 1958.

Haight C: Congenital tracheoesophageal fistula without esopha-geal atresia. J Thorac Surg 17:600, 1948.

Haight C: The management of congenital esophageal atresia and tracheoesophageal fistula. Surg Clin North Am 41:1281, 1961.

Haight C: The esophagus. In Benson CD et al (eds): Pediatric Surgery. Vol 1. Chicago, Year Book Medical Publishers, Inc, 1962.

Hays DM: An analysis of the mortality in esophageal atresia. Am J Dis Child 103:765, 1962.

Hays DM: Esophageal atresia: current management. Pediatr Digest April 1965.

Hays DM and Snyder WH: Results of conventional operative procedures for esophageal atresia in premature infants. Am J Surg 106:19, 1963.

Heimlich HJ: Peptic esophagitis with stricture treated by recon-struction of the esophagus with a reversed gastric tube. Surg Gynecol Obstet 114:673, 1962.

Helmsworth JA and Pryles CV: Congenital tracheoesophageal fistula without esophageal atresia. J Pediatr 38:610, 1951.

Herwig J and Ogura J: Congenital tracheoesophageal fistula without esophageal atresia. J Pediatr 47:298, 1955.

Holder TM: Transpleural versus retropleural approach for repair of tracheoesophageal fistula. Surg Clin North Am 44:1433, 1964.

Holder TM: Thoracic surgery in infants. In Sabiston DC Jr and Spencer FC (eds): Gibbon's Surgery of the Chest. 4th ed. Philadelphia, WB Saunders Co, 1983.

Holder TM and Ashcraft KW: Esophageal atresia and tracheo-esophageal fistula. Ann Thorac Surg 9:445, 1970.

Holder TM and Gross RE: Temporary gastrostomy in pediatric surgery. Pediatrics 26:37, 1960.

Holder TM, Cloud DT, Lewis JE Jr et al: Esophageal atresia and tracheoesophageal fistula. A survey of its members by the Surgical Section of the American Academy of Pediatrics. Pedi-atrics 34:542, 1964.

Holder TM, McDonald VG, and Woolley MW: The premature or critically ill infant with esophageal atresia: increased success with a staged approach. J Thorac Cardiovasc Surg 44:344, 1962.

Holinger PH, Brown WT, and Maurizi DG: Endoscopic aspects of postsurgical management of congenital esophageal atresia and tracheoesophageal fistula. J Thorac Cardiovasc Surg 49:22, 1965.

Holinger PH, Johnston KC, and Parchet VN: Congenital malfor-mations of trachea, bronchi and lung. Ann Otol 61:1159, 1952.

Howard R and Meyers NA: Esophageal atresia—a technic for elongating the upper pouch. Surgery 58:725, 1965.

Humphreys GH, Hogg BM, and Ferrer J: Congenital atresia of esophagus. J Thorac Surg 32:332, 1956.

Johnson PW: Elongation of the upper segment in esophageal atresia. Report of a case. Surgery 58:741, 1965.

Kafrouni G, Baick CH, and Wooley MM: Recurrent tracheoesoph-ageal fistula: a diagnostic problem. Surgery 68:889, 1970.

Kappelman MM, Dorst J, Haller JA, and Stambler A: H-type tracheoesophageal fistula. Am J Dis Child 118:568, 1969.

Karlan M, Thompson J, and Clatworthy HW: Congenital atresia of the esophagus with tracheoesophageal fistula and duodenal atresia. Surgery 41:544, 1957.

Killen DA and Greenlee HB: Transcervical repair of H-type congenital tracheoesophageal fistula: review of the literature. Ann Surg 162:145, 1965.

Koop CE: Atresia of the esophagus: technical considerations in surgical management. Surg Clin North Am 42:1387, 1962.

Koop CE, Kiesewetter WB, and Johnson J: Treatment of atresia of the esophagus by the transpleural approach. Surg Gynecol Obstet 98:687, 1954.

Lafer DJ and Boley SJ: Primary repair in esophageal atresia with elongation of the lower segment. J Pediatr Surg 1:585, 1966.

Leix F and Schwab CE: End-to-side operative technic for esoph-ageal atresia with tracheoesophageal fistula. Am J Surg 118:225, 1969.

Lindskog GE, Liebow AA, and Glenn WWL: Thoracic and Car-diovascular Surgery with Related Pathology. New York, Apple-ton-Century-Crofts, Inc, 1962.

Livaditis A, Okmian L, Bjorek G et al: Esophageal suture anasto-mosis. Scand J Thorac Cardiovasc Surg 3:163, 1969.

Livaditis A, Radberg L, and Odensjo G: Esophageal end-to-end anastomosis. Scand J Thorac Cardiovasc Surg 6:206, 1972.

Lloyd JR and Clatworthy HW: Hydramnios as an aid to early diagnosis of congenital obstruction of the alimentary tract: a study of the maternal and fetal factors. Pediatrics 21:903, 1958.

Lynn HB and Divia LA: Tracheoesophageal fistula without atresia of the esophagus. Surg Clin North Am 41:871, 1961.

Mahour GH, Woolley MM, and Gwinn JL: Elongation of the upper pouch and delayed anatomic reconstruction in esophageal atresia. J Pediatr Surg 9:373, 1974.

Martin LW and Hogg SP: Esophageal atresia and tracheoesopha-geal fistula. Am J Dis Child 99:828, 1960.

Meeker IG and Snyder WH: Gastrostomy for the newborn surgical patient. Arch Dis Child 37:159, 1962.

Mellins RB and Blumenthal S: Cardiovascular anomalies and esophageal atresia. Am J Dis Child 107:160, 1964.

Moncrief JA and Randolph JG: Congenital tracheoesophageal fistula without atresia of the esophagus—a method for diagnosis and surgical correction. J Thorac Cardiovasc Surg 51:434, 1966.

Morse GW, Anderson EV, and Arenson N: Congenital tracheo-esophageal fistula without esophageal atresia: an improved method of demonstration. Am Surg 24:112, 1958.

Murphy DR and Owen HF: Respiratory emergencies in the newborn. Am J Surg 101:581, 1961.

Nixon HH and O'Donnell B: The Essentials of Pediatric Surgery. London, William Heinemann, Ltd, 1961.

Pieretti R, Shandling B, and Stephens CA: Resistant esophageal stenosis associated with reflux after repair of esophageal atresia: a therapeutic approach. J Pediatr Surg 9:355, 1974.

Randolph JG, Tunnell WP, and Lilly JR: Gastric division in the critically ill infant with esophageal atresia and tracheoesophageal fistula. Surgery 63:496, 1968.

Redo SF: Congenital esophageal atresia and tracheoesophageal fistula. Fifteen-year experience. NY State J Med November 1975.

Rehbein F and Yanagiswa F: Complications after operation for oesophageal atresia. Arch Dis Child 34:29, 1959.

Reploge RL: Esophageal atresia: plastic sump catheter for drain-age of the proximal pouch. Surgery 54:296, 1963.

Richardson WR: Thoracic emergencies in the newborn infant. Am J Surg 105:524, 1963.

Ricketts RR, Luck SR, and Raffensperger JG: Circular esophago-myotomy for primary repair of long-gap esophageal atresia. J Pediatr Surg 16:365, 1981.

Rigg W Jr: Congenital tracheoesophageal fistula without esopha-geal atresia. South Med J 62:135, 1969.

Sandegard E: The treatment of oesophageal atresia. Arch Dis Child 32:475, 1957.

Schneider KM and Becker JM: The "H-type" tracheoesophageal fistula in infants and children. Surgery 51:677, 1962.

Schultz LR and Clatworthy HW: Esophageal strictures after anas-tomosis in esophageal atresia. Arch Surg 87:136, 1963.

Schwartz SI and Dale WA: Unusual tracheoesophageal fistula with membranous obstruction of the esophagus and postoperative hypertrophic pyloric stenosis. Ann Surg 142:1002, 1955.

Shaw RR, Paulson DL, and Siebel EK: Congenital atresia of the esophagus with tracheoesophageal fistula, treatment of surgical complication. Ann Surg 142:204, 1955.

Stephens CA, Mustard WT and Simpson JS: Congenital atresia of the esophagus with tracheoesophageal fistula. Surg Clin North Am 36:1465, 1956.

Swenson O: Pediatric Surgery. 2nd ed. New York, Appleton-Century-Crofts, Inc, 1962.

Swenson O, Lipman R, Fisher JH, and DeLuca FG: Repair and complications of esophageal atresia and tracheoesophageal fistula. New Engl J Med 267:960, 1962.

Touloukian RH and Stinson KK: Temporary gastric partition: a mode for staged repair of esophageal atresia with fistula. Ann Surg 171:184, 1970.

Touloukian RJ, Pickett LK, Spackman T, and Biancani P: Repair of esophageal atresia by end-to-side anastomosis and ligation of the tracheoesophageal fistula: a critical review of 18 cases. J Pediatr Surg 9:305, 1974.

Tuqan NA: Annular stricture of the esophagus distal to congenital tracheoesophageal fistula. Surgery 52:394, 1962.

Waterston DJ, Bonham-Carter RE, and Aberdeen E: Oesophageal atresia: tracheo-oesophageal fistula. A study of survival in 218 infants. Lancet 1:819, 1962.

Waterston DJ, Bonham-Carter RE and Aberdeen E: Congenital tracheoesophageal atresia. Lancet 2:55, 1963.

Yahr WZ, Azzoni AA, and Santulli TV: Congenital atresia of the esophagus with tracheoesophageal fistula: an unusual variant. Surgery 52:937, 1962.

Young DG: Successful primary anastomosis in oesophageal atresia after reduction of a long gap between the blind ends by bouginage of the upper pouch. Br J Surg 54:321, 1967.

Zachary RB and Emery JL: Failure of separation of larynx and trachea from the esophagus: persistent esophagotrachea. Surgery 49:525, 1961.

Bronchial Deformities

CONGENITAL BRONCHIAL STENOSIS

Chang N, Hertzler JH, Gregg RH et al: Congenital stenosis of the right mainstem bronchus. Pediatrics 41:739, 1968.

Holinger PH, Johnston KC and Parchet VN: Congenital malformations of the trachea, bronchi and lung. Ann Otol 61:1159, 1952.

Swenson O: Pediatric Surgery. 2nd ed. New York, Appleton-Century-Crofts, Inc, 1962.

FOREGUT CYSTS

Ackerman LV: Personal communication. Cited in Gibbon JH Jr (ed): Surgery of the Chest. 2nd ed. Philadelphia, WB Saunders Co, 1969.

Alshabkhoun S, Starkey GW, and Asnes RA: Bronchogenic cysts of the mediastinum in infancy. Ann Thorac Surg 4:532, 1967.

Avery ME and Taeusch HW Jr (eds): Schaffer's Diseases of the Newborn. 5th ed. Philadelphia, WB Saunders Co, 1989.

Beardmore HE and Wigglesworth FW: Vertebral anomalies and alimentary duplications. Pediatr Clin North Am 5:457, 1958.

Bentley JFR and Smith JR: Developmental posterior enteric remnants and spinal malformations. Arch Dis Child 35:76, 1960.

Bressler S and Wiener D: Bronchogenic cyst associated with an anomalous pulmonary artery arising from the thoracic aorta. Surgery 35:815, 1954.

Bruwer A, Clagett OT and McDonald JR: Anomalous arteries to the lung associated with congenital pulmonary abnormality. J Thorac Surg 19:957, 1950.

Burford TH and Ferguson TB: Congenital lesions of the lungs and emphysema. In Sabiston DC Jr and Spencer FC (eds): Gibbon's Surgery of the Chest. 4th ed. Philadelphia, WB Saunders Co, 1983.

Culiner MM and Grimes OF: Localized emphysema in association with bronchial cysts or mucoceles. J Thorac Cardiovasc Surg 41:306, 1961.

Dabbs CH, Peirce EC and Rawson FL: Intrapericardial interatrial teratoma (bronchogenic cyst). N Engl J Med 256:541, 1957.

Desforges G: Primitive foregut cysts. Ann Thorac Surg 4:574, 1967.

Eraklis AJ, Griscom NT and McGovern JB: Bronchogenic cysts of the mediastinum in infancy. N Engl J Med 281:1150, 1969.

Fallon M, Gordon ARG, and Lendrum AC: Mediastinal cysts of foregut origin associated with vertebral anomalies. Br J Surg 41:520, 1954.

Flavell G: An Introduction to Chest Surgery. London, Oxford University Press, 1957.

Gans SL and Hackworth LR: Respiratory obstructions of surgical import. Pediatr Clin North Am 6:1023, 1959.

Gerami S, Richardson R, Harrington B, and Pate JW: Obstructive emphysema due to mediastinal bronchogenic cysts in infancy. J Thorac Cardiovasc Surg 58:432, 1969.

Greenfield LJ and Howe JS: Bronchial adenoma within the wall of a bronchogenic cyst. J Thorac Cardiovasc Surg 49:398, 1965.

Gross RE: The Surgery of Infancy and Childhood: Its Principles and Techniques. Philadelphia, WB Saunders Co, 1953.

Haller JA, Shermata DW, Donahoo JS et al: Life threatening respiratory distress from mediastinal masses in infants. Ann Thorac Surg 19:364, 1975.

Hope JW and Koop CE: Differential diagnosis of mediastinal masses. Pediatr Clin North Am 6:379, 1959.

Jones P: Developmental defects in lungs. Thorax 10:205, 1955.

Kirwan WO, Walbaum PR, and McCormack RJM: Cystic intrathoracic derivatives of the foregut and their complications. Thorax 28:424, 1973.

Leigh TF and Weens HS: The Mediastinum. Springfield, Ill, Charles C Thomas, 1959.

Lindskog GE, Liebow AA, and Glenn WWL: Thoracic and Cardiovascular Surgery, with Related Pathology. New York, Appleton-Century-Crofts, Inc, 1962.

Macpherson RI, Reed MH, and Ferguson CC: Intrathoracic gastrogenic cysts: a cause of lethal pulmonary hemorrhage in infants. J Assoc Can Radiol 24:362, 1973.

Maier HC: Bronchogenic cysts of the mediastinum. Ann Surg 127:476, 1948.

Moersch HJ and Clagett OT: Pulmonary cysts. J Thorac Surg 16:179, 1947.

Moore K: Development of the Notochord in the Developing Human. 3rd ed. Philadelphia, WB Saunders Co, 1982.

Opsahl T and Berman EJ: Bronchogenic mediastinal cysts in infants: case reports and review of literature. Pediatrics 30:372, 1962.

Pilcher RS: Trachea, bronchi, lungs and pleura. In Brown JJM (ed): Surgery of Childhood. Baltimore, Williams & Wilkins Co, 1963.

Pontius RG: Bronchial obstruction of congenital origin. Am J Surg 106:8, 1963.

Porkorny WJ and Goldstein IR: Enteric thoracoabdominal duplications in children. J Thorac Cardiovasc Surg 87:821, 1984.

Potts WJ: The Surgeon and the Child. Philadelphia, WB Saunders Co, 1959.

Raffensperger JG: Mediastinal masses. In Swenson O: Pediatric Surgery. 4th ed. New York, Appleton-Century-Crofts, Inc, 1980.

Schlumberger HG: Tumors of the mediastinum. In Atlas of Tumor Pathology. Fascicle 18. Washington, DC, Armed Forces Institute of Pathology, 1951.

Swenson O: Pediatric Surgery. 2nd ed. New York, Appleton-Century-Crofts, Inc, 1962.

Trossman CM: Push-up stridor caused by a bronchogenic cyst. Am J Dis Child 107:293, 1964.

Webb WR and Burford TH: Studies of the re-expanded lung after prolonged atelectasis. Arch Surg 66:801, 1953.

Weisel W, Claudon DB, and Darin JC: Tracheal adenoma in juxtaposition with a mediastinal bronchogenic cyst J Thorac Surg 37:687, 1959.

Pulmonary Deformities

PULMONARY AGENESIS, APLASIA, AND HYPOPLASIA

Adler RH, Herrmann JW, and Jewett TC: Lobar agenesis of the lung. Ann Surg 147:267, 1958.

Avery ME and Taeusch HW Jr (eds): Schaffer's Diseases of the Newborn. 5th ed. Philadelphia, WB Saunders Co, 1989.

Avery ME, Fletcher BD, and Williams R: The Lung and Its

Disorders in the Newborn Infant. 4th ed. Philadelphia, WB Saunders Co, 1981.

Booth JB and Berry CL: Unilateral pulmonary agenesis. Arch Dis Child 42:361, 1967.

Borja AR, Ransdell HT, and Villa S: Congenital development arrest of the lung. Ann Thorac Surg 10:317, 1970.

Brunner S and Nissen E: Agenesis of the lung. Am Rev Resp Dis 87:103, 1963.

Burford TH and Ferguson TB: Congenital lesions of the lungs and emphysema. In Sabiston DC Jr and Spencer FC (eds): Gibbon's Surgery of the Chest. 4th ed. Philadelphia, WB Saunders Co, 1983.

Claireaux AE and Ferreira HP: Bilateral pulmonary agenesis. Arch Dis Child 33:364, 1958.

Ferguson CF: Interesting bronchopulmonary problems of early life. Laryngoscope 80:1347, 1970.

Franken EA Jr, Hurwitz RA, and Battersby JS: Unequal aeration of the lungs in children. The use of pulmonary angiography. Radiology 109:401, 1973.

Harris GBC: The newborn with respiratory distress: some roentgenographic features. Radiol Clin North Am 1:499, 1963.

Holinger PH, Johnston KC and Parchet VN: Congenital malformations of the trachea, bronchi, and lung. Ann Otol 61:1159, 1952.

Landing BH: Anomalies of the respiratory tract. Pediatr Clin North Am 4:73, 1957.

Lindskog GE, Liebow AA, and Glenn WWL: Thoracic Cardiovascular Surgery, with Related Pathology. New York, Appleton-Century-Crofts, Inc, 1962.

Lukas DS, Dotter CT, and Steinberg I: Agenesis of the lung and patent ductus arteriosus with reversal of flow. N Engl J Med 249:107, 1953.

Maltz DL and Nadas AS: Agenesis of the lung. Pediatrics 42:175, 1968.

Martinez-Jimenez M, Pérez-Alvarez JJ, Pérez-Trevino C et al: Agenesis of the lung with patent ductus arteriosus treated surgically. J Thorac Cardiovasc Surg 50:59, 1965.

Minetto E, Galli E, and Boglione G: Agenesia, aplasia, hypoplasia pulmonare. Minerva Med 49:4635, 1958.

Morison JE: Foetal and Neonatal Pathology. London, Butterworth, 1952.

Morton DR, Klassen KP, and Baxter EH: Lobar agenesis of the lung. J Thorac Surg 20:665, 1950.

Oyamada A, Gasul BM, and Holinger PH: Agenesis of the lung. Report of a case with review of all previously reported cases. Am J Dis Child 85:182, 1953.

Pilcher RS: Trachea, bronchi, lungs, and pleura. In Brown JJM (ed): Surgery of Childhood. Baltimore, Williams & Wilkins Co, 1963.

Potter EL: Pathology of the Fetus and the Newborn. Chicago, Year Book Medical Publishers, Inc, 1952.

Ravitch MM: Agenesis of the lung. In Benson CD et al (eds): Pediatric Surgery. Vol 1. Chicago, Year Book Medical Publishers, Inc, 1962.

Spencer H: Pathology of the Lung. New York, Macmillan Co, 1962.

Tuynman PE and Gardner LW: Bilateral aplasia of lung. Arch Pathol 54:306, 1952.

Waddell JA, Simon G and Reid L: Bronchial atresia of the left upper lobe. Thorax 20:214, 1965.

CONGENITAL PNEUMATOCELE (PULMONARY HERNIA)

Goodman HI: Hernia of lung. J Thorac Surg 2:368, 1933.

Lindskog GE, Liebow AA, and Glenn WWL: Thoracic and Cardiovascular Surgery, with Related Pathology. New York, Appleton-Century-Crofts, Inc, 1962.

Ravitch MM: Disorders of the sternum and the thoracic wall. In Sabiston DC Jr and Spencer FC (eds): Gibbon's Surgery of the Chest. 4th ed. Philadelphia, WB Saunders Co, 1983.

Rickman PP: Lung hernia secondary to congenital absence of ribs. Arch Dis Child 34:14, 1959.

CONGENITAL PULMONARY CYSTS

Avery ME and Taeusch HW Jr (eds): Schaffer's Diseases of the Newborn. 5th ed. Philadelphia, WB Saunders Co, 1989.

Avery ME, Fletcher BD and Williams R: The Lung and Its Disorders in the Newborn Infant. 4th ed. Philadelphia, WB Saunders Co, 1981.

Bowden KM: Congenital cystic disease of lung. Med J Aust 2:311, 1948.

Boyden EA: Bronchogenic cysts and the theory of intralobar sequestration: new embryologic data. J Thorac Surg 35:604, 1958.

Burford TH and Ferguson TB: Congenital lesions of the lungs and emphysema. In Sabiston DC Jr and Spencer FC (eds): Gibbon's Surgery of the Chest. 4th ed. Philadelphia, WB Saunders Co, 1983.

Caffey J: On the natural regression of pulmonary cysts during early infancy. Pediatrics 11:48, 1953.

Clatworthy HW Jr: Intrathoracic tumors and cysts. In Ariel IM and Pack GT (eds): Cancer and Allied Diseases of Infancy and Childhood. Boston, Little, Brown & Co, 1960.

Cooke FN and Blades B: Cystic disease of the lungs. J Thorac Surg 23:546, 1952.

Crawford TJ and Cahill JL: The surgical treatment of pulmonary cystic disorders in infancy and childhood. J Pediatr Surg 6:251, 1971.

Dickson JA, Clagett OT, and McDonald JR: Cystic disease of the lung and its relation to bronchiectatic cavities: a study of 22 cases. J Thorac Surg 15:196, 1946.

Donald JG and Donald JW: Congenital cysts of the lung. Ann Surg 141:944, 1955.

Egan RW, Jewett TC, and Macmanus JE: Congenital lesions of the thorax in infancy demanding early surgical treatment. Arch Surg 77:584, 1958.

Gans SL and Hackworth LE: Respiratory obstructions of surgical import. Pediatr Clin North Am 6:1023, 1959.

Gilbert JW and Myers RT: Intrathoracic tension phenomena in the neonatal period and infancy. Arch Surg 76:402, 1958.

Grimes OF and Farber SM: Air cysts of the lung. Surg Gynecol Obstet 113:720, 1961.

Gross R: Congenital cystic disease: successful pneumonectomy in a three week old baby. Ann Surg 123:229, 1946.

Guest JL Jr, Yeh TJ, Ellison JT et al: Pulmonary parenchymal air space abnormalities. Ann Thorac Surg 1:102, 1965.

Herrmann JW, Jewett TC and Galletti G: Bronchogenic cysts in infants and children. J Thorac Surg 37:242, 1957.

Holinger PH, Johnston KC, and Parchet VN: Congenital malformations of trachea, bronchi, and lung. Ann Otol 61:1159, 1952.

Jones JC, Almond CH, Snyder HM, and Meyer BW: Congenital pulmonary cysts in infants and children. Ann Thorac Surg 3:297, 1967.

Landing BH: Anomalies of the respiratory tract. Pediatr Clin North Am 4:73, 1957.

Lichtenstein H: Congenital multiple cysts of the lung. Dis Chest 24:646, 1953.

Lindskog GE, Liebow AA, and Glenn WWL: Thoracic and Cardiovascular Surgery with Related Pathology. New York, Appleton-Century-Crofts, Inc, 1962.

Maier HC: The pleura. In Sabiston DC Jr and Spencer FC (eds): Gibbon's Surgery of the Chest. 4th ed. Philadelphia, WB Saunders Co, 1983.

Minnis JF Jr: Congenital cystic disease of the lung in infancy. J Thorac Cardiovasc Surg 43:262, 1962.

Murphy DR and Owen HF: Respiratory emergencies in the newborn. Am J Surg 101:581, 1961.

Nixon HH and O'Donnell B: The Essentials of Pediatric Surgery. London, William Heinemann, Ltd, 1961.

Opsahl T and Berman EJ: Bronchogenic mediastinal cysts in infants. Pediatrics 30:372, 1962.

Potts WJ: The Surgeon and the Child. Philadelphia, WB Saunders Co, 1959.

Potts WJ and Riker WL: Differentiation of congenital cysts of lung and those following staphylococcal pneumonia. Arch Surg 61:684, 1950.

Pryce DM: Lining of healed but persistent abscess cavities in lung with epithelium of ciliated columnar type. J Pathol Bacteriol 60:259, 1948.

Ravitch MM: Congenital cystic disease of the lung. In Benson CD et al (eds): Pediatric Surgery. Vol 1. Chicago, Year Book Medical Publishers, Inc, 1962.

Ravitch MM and Hardy JB: Congenital cystic disease of lung in infants and children. Arch Surg 59:1, 1949.

Riker WL: Lung cysts and pneumothorax in infants and children. Surg Clin North Am 36:1613, 1956.

Slim MS and Melhem RE: Congenital pulmonary air cysts. Arch Surg 88:923, 1964.

Spandler BP: Pathogenesis and treatment of pulmonary tension cavities. Am Rev Tuberc Pulmon Dis 76:370, 1957.

Spencer H: Pathology of the Lung. New York, Macmillan Co, 1962.

Swan H and Aragon GE: Surgical treatment of pulmonary cysts in infancy. Pediatrics 14:651, 1954.

Swenson O: Pediatric Surgery. 2nd ed. New York, Macmillan Co, 1962.

Szots I and Jakab T: Indications for urgent operation in pulmonary tension disorders in childhood. Arch Dis Child 39:172, 1964.

Vanhoutte JJ and Miller KE: Angiographic contribution to the determination of the etiology of some pulmonary cysts of infancy. Am J Roentgenol Radium Ther Nucl Med 108:569, 1970.

Woods FM: Cystic diseases of the lung. J Int Coll Surg 19:568, 1953.

LOBAR EMPHYSEMA

Avery ME and Taeusch HW Jr (eds): Schaffer's Diseases of the Newborn. 5th ed. Philadelphia, WB Saunders Co, 1989.

Avery ME, Fletcher BD, and Williams R: The Lung and Its Disorders in the Newborn Infant. 4th ed. Philadelphia, WB Saunders Co, 1981.

Backman A, Parkkulaimen KV, and Sulammaa M: Pulmonary tension emergencies in infants. Ann Pediatr Fenn 5:172, 1959.

Baker D: Chronic pulmonary disease in infants and children. Radiol Clin North Am 1:519, 1963.

Bates DV, Macklem PT, and Christie RV: Respiratory Function in Disease: An Introduction to the Integrated Study of the Lung. 2nd ed. Philadelphia, WB Saunders Co, 1971.

Binet JP, Nezelof C, and Fredet J: Five cases of lobar emphysema in infancy: importance of bronchial malformation and value of postoperative steroid therapy. Dis Chest 41:126, 1962.

Bolande RR, Schneider AF, and Boggs JD: Infantile lobar emphysema, an etiological concept. Arch Pathol 61:289, 1956.

Burford TH and Ferguson TB: Congenital lesions of the lung and emphysema. In Sabiston DC Jr and Spencer FC (eds): Gibbon's Surgery of the Chest. 4th ed. Philadelphia, WB Saunders Co, 1983.

Burman SO and Kent EM: Bronchiolar emphysema (cirrhosis of the lung). J Thorac Cardiovasc Surg 43:253, 1962.

Butterfield J, Moscovici C, Berry C, and Kempe CH: Cystic emphysema in premature infants, report of an outbreak with the isolation of type 19 ECHO virus in one case. N Engl J Med 268:18, 1963.

Campbell D, Bauer AJ, and Hewlett TH: Congenital localized emphysema. J Thorac Cardiovasc Surg 41:575, 1961.

Egan RW, Jewett TC, and Macmanus JE: Congenital lesions of the thorax in infancy demanding early surgical treatment. Arch Surg 77:584, 1968.

Ehrenhaft JL and Taber RE: Progressive infantile emphysema, a surgical emergency. Surgery 34:412, 1953.

Eigen H, Lemen RJ, and Waring WW: Congenital lobar emphysema: long-term evaluation of surgically and conservatively treated children. Am Rev Resp Dis 113:823, 1976.

Fischer HW, Lucido JL, and Lynxwiler CP: Lobar emphysema. JAMA 166:340, 1958.

Fischer HW, Potts WJ, and Holinger PH: Lobar emphysema in infants and children. J Pediatr 41:403, 1952.

Floyd FW, Repici AJ, Gibson ET, and McGeorge CK: Bilateral congenital lobar emphysema surgically corrected. Pediatrics 31:87, 1963.

Gans SL and Hackworth LE: Respiratory obstructions of surgical import. Pediatr Clin North Am 6:1023, 1959.

Hendren WH and McKee DM: Lobar emphysema of infancy. J Pediatr Surg 1:24, 1966.

Henry W: Localized pulmonary hypertrophic emphysema. J Thorac Surg 27:197, 1954.

Jewett TC Jr and Adler RH: Localized pulmonary emphysema of infancy. Surgery 43:1958.

Jones JC, Almond CH, Snyder HM et al: Lobar emphysema and congenital heart disease in infancy. J Thorac Cardiovasc Surg 49:1, 1965.

Kanphuys EHM: Congenital lobar emphysema. Arch Chir Neerl 14:93, 1962.

Kennedy JH and Rothman BF: The surgical treatment of congenital lobar emphysema. Surg Gynecol Obstet 121:253, 1965.

Korngold HW and Baker JM: Nonsurgical treatment of unilobar obstructive emphysema of the newborn. Pediatrics 14:296, 1954.

Kress MB and Finkelstein AH: Giant bulbous emphysema occurring in tuberculosis in childhood. Pediatrics 30:269, 1962.

Kruse RL and Lynn HB: Lobar emphysema in infants. Mayo Clinic Proc 44:525, 1969.

Landing BH: Anomalies of the respiratory tract. Pediatr Clin North Am 4:73, 1957.

Leape LL and Longino LA: Infantile lobar emphysema. Pediatrics 34:246, 1964.

Leape LL, Ching N, and Holder TM: Lobar emphysema and patent ductus arteriosus. Pediatrics 46:97, 1970.

Lewis JE and Potts WJ: Obstructive emphysema with a defect of the anterior mediastinum. J Thorac Surg 21:438, 1959.

Lincoln JCR, Stark J, Subramanian S et al: Congenital lobar emphysema. Ann Surg 173:55, 1971.

Lindskog GE, Liebow AA, and Glenn WWL: Thoracic and Cardiovascular Surgery with Related Pathology. New York, Appleton-Century-Crofts, Inc, 1962.

Mauney FM Jr and Sabiston DC Jr: The role of pulmonary scanning in the diagnosis of congenital lobar emphysema. Am Surg 36:20, 1970.

May RL, Meese EH, and Timmes JJ: Congenital lobar emphysema: case report of bilateral involvement. J Thorac Cardiovasc Surg 48:850, 1964.

Mercer RD, Hawk WA, and Karakjian G: Massive lobar emphysema in infants: diagnosis and treatment. Cleveland Clin Q 28:270, 1961.

Moore TC: Chondroectodermal dysplasia (Ellis–Van Creveld syndrome) with bronchial malformation and neonatal tension lobar emphysema. J Thorac Cardiovasc Surg 46:1, 1963.

Murphy DR and Owen HF: Respiratory emergencies in the newborn. Am J Surg 101:581, 1961.

Murray GF: Congenital lobar emphysema. Surg Gynecol Obstet 124:611, 1967.

Murray GF, Talbert JL, and Haller JA Jr: Obstructive lobar emphysema of the newborn infant—documentation of the "mucus plug syndrome" with successful treatment by bronchotomy. J Thorac Cardiovasc Surg 53:886, 1967.

Myers NA: Congenital lobar emphysema. Aust N Z J Surg 30:32, 1960.

Nelson TY: Tension emphysema in infants. Arch Dis Child 32:38, 1957.

Nelson TY and Reye D: Tension emphysema: a surgical emergency in infants. Med J Aust 2:342, 1954.

Nixon HH and O'Donnell B: The Essentials of Pediatric Surgery. London, William Heinemann, Ltd, 1961.

Overstreet RM: Emphysema of a portion of the lung in the early months of life. J Dis Child 57:861, 1939.

Pierce WS, deParedes CG, Friedman S, and Waldhausen JA: Concomitant congenital heart disease and lobar emphysema in infants: incidence, diagnosis, and operative management. Ann Surg 172:951, 1970.

Potts WJ: The Surgeon and the Child. Philadelphia, WB Saunders Co, 1959.

Raynor CC, Capp MP, and Sealy WC: Lobar emphysema of infancy. Ann Thorac Surg 4:374, 1967.

Riker WL: Neonatal respiratory distress. In Bendon CD et al (eds): Pediatric Surgery. Vol 1. Chicago, Year Book Medical Publishers, Inc, 1962.

Robertson R and James ES: Congenital lobar emphysema. Pediatrics 8:795, 1951.

Spencer H: Pathology of the Lung. New York, Macmillan Co, 1962.

Thomson J and Forfar JO: Regional obstructive emphysema in infancy. Arch Dis Child 33:97, 1958.

Urban AE, Stark J, and Waterston DJ: Congenital lobar emphysema. Thoraxchirurgie 22:255, 1975.

Vaughan VC III, McKay RJ, and Behrman RE (eds): Nelson Textbook of Pediatrics. 11th ed. Philadelphia, WB Saunders Co, 1979.

White M and Dennison WM: Surgery in Infancy and Childhood, a Handbook for Medical Students and General Practitioners. Edinburgh, E & S Livingstone, Ltd, 1958.

Williams H and Campbell P: Generalized bronchiectasis associated with deficiency of cartilage in the bronchial tree. Arch Dis Child 35:182, 1960.

Wiseman DH: Unilateral pseudoemphysema—a case report. Pediatrics 35:300, 1965.

Zatzkin HR, Cole PM, and Bronsther B: Congenital hypertrophic lobar emphysema. Surgery 52:505, 1962.

Pulmonary Sequestration

Asp K, Heikel PE, Pasila M et al: Pulmonary sequestration in children. Ann Paediatr Fenn 9:270, 1963.

Avery ME, Fletcher BD and Williams R: The Lung and Its Disorders in the Newborn Infant. 4th ed. Philadelphia, WB Saunders Co, 1981.

Boyden EA: Segmental Anatomy of the Lungs. New York, McGraw-Hill Book Co, Inc, 1955.

Boyden EA: Bronchogenic cysts and the theory of intralobar sequestration: new embryologic data. J Thorac Surg 35:604, 1958.

Breton A, Gaudier B, Caron J et al: Pulmonary sequestration: aortographic diagnosis: pathogenic discussion. Arch Franc Pediatr 16:751, 1959.

Britton RC, Weston JT, and Landing BH: Plastic injection techniques in pediatric pathology, with particular reference to roentgenographic analysis of injected specimens. Bull Int A M Mus 31:124, 1950.

Bruwer A, Clagett OT, and McDonald JR: Anomalous arteries to the lung associated with congenital pulmonary abnormality. J Thorac Surg 19:957, 1950.

Bryon ND, Campbell DC, and Hood RH: Lower accessory lung. J Thorac Cardiovasc Surg 47:605, 1964.

Buntain WL, Isaacs H Jr, Payne VC Jr et al: Lobar emphysema, cystic adenomatoid malformation, pulmonary sequestration, and bronchogenic cysts in infancy and childhood: a clinical group. J Pediatr Surg 9:85, 1974.

Burford TH and Ferguson TB: Congenital lesions of the lungs and emphysema. In Sabiston DC Jr and Spencer FC (eds): Gibbon's Surgery of the Chest. 4th ed. Philadelphia, WB Saunders Co, 1983.

Carter R: Pulmonary sequestration. Ann Thorac Surg 7:68, 1969.

Claman MA and Ehrenhaft JL: Bronchopulmonary sequestration. J Thorac Cardiovasc Surg 39:531, 1960.

DeBakey M, Arey JB, and Brunazzi R: Successful removal of lower accessory lung. J Thorac Surg 19:304, 1950.

Demos NJ and Teresi A: Congenital lung malformations. A unified concept and a case report. J Thorac Cardiovasc Surg 70:260, 1975.

Elliott GB, Miller GE, Walker RH, and Elliott KA: Thoracic sequestration cysts of fetal bronchogenic and esophageal origin. Can J Surg 4:522, 1961.

Ellis FH, McGoon DC, and Kincaid OW: Congenital vascular malformations of the lungs. Med Clin North Am 48:1069, 1964.

Flavell G: An Introduction to Chest Surgery. London, Oxford University Press, 1957.

Gallagher PG, Lynch JP and Christian HJ: Intralobar bronchopulmonary sequestration of the lung. N Engl J Med 257:643, 1957.

Gans SL and Potts WJ: Anomalous lobe of lung arising from the esophagus. J Thorac Surg 21:313, 1951.

Gerald FP and Lyons HA: Anomalous artery in intralobar bronchopulmonary sequestration. N Engl J Med 259:662, 1958.

Halasz NA, Lindskog GE, and Liebow AA: Esophagobronchial fistula and bronchopulmonary sequestration. Ann Surg 155:215, 1961.

Hutchin P: Congenital cystic disease of the lung. Rev Surg 28:79, 1971.

Iwai K, Shindo G, Hajikano H et al: Introlobar pulmonary sequestration with special reference to developmental pathology. Am Rev Resp Dis 107:911, 1973.

Kafka B and Becco T: Simultaneous intra- and extrapulmonary sequestration. Arch Dis Child 35:51, 1960.

Kergin FG: Congenital cystic disease of lung associated with anomalous arteries. J Thorac Surg 23:55, 1952.

Kilman JW, Battersby JS, Taybi H et al: Pulmonary sequestration. Arch Surg 90:648, 1965.

Landing BH: Anomalies of the respiratory tract. Pediatr Clin North Am 4:73, 1957.

Landing BH and Wells TR: Tracheobronchial anomalies in children. Perspect Pediatr Pathol 1:1, 1973.

Lindskog GE, Liebow AA, and Glenn WWL: Thoracic and Cardiovascular Surgery, with Related Pathology. New York, Appleton-Century-Crofts, Inc, 1962.

Mannix EP and Haight C: Anomalous pulmonary arteries and cystic disease of the lung. Medicine 34:193, 1955.

Muller H: Inaugural dissertation, University of Halle; quoted by Ramsey JN and Reiman DL: Bronchial adenomas arising in mucous glands. Am J Pathol 29:339, 1953.

Pierce WS, deParedes CG, Raphaely RC, and Waldhausen JA: Pulmonary resection in infants younger than one year of age. J Thorac Cardiovasc Surg 61:875, 1971.

Pryce DM: Lower accessory pulmonary artery with intralobar sequestration of lung. J Pathol Bacteriol 58:457, 1946.

Pryce DM, Sellors TH and Blair LG: Intralobar sequestration of lung associated with an abnormal pulmonary artery. Br J Surg 35:18, 1947.

Quinlan JJ, Shaffer VD, and Hiltz JE: Intralobar pulmonary sequestration. Can J Surg 6:418, 1963.

Ravitch MM: Congenital cystic disease of the lung. In Benson CD et al (eds): Pediatric Surgery. Vol 1. Chicago, Year Book Medical Publishers, Inc, 1962.

Simopoulos AP: Intralobar bronchopulmonary sequestration in children: diagnosis by intrathoracic aortography. Am J Dis Child 97:796, 1959.

Smith RA: A theory of the origin of intralobar sequestration of lung. Thorax 11:10, 1956.

Smith RA: Some controversial aspects of intralobar sequestration of the lung. Surg Gynecol Obstet 114:57, 1962.

Solit RW: The effect of intralobar pulmonary sequestration on cardiac output. J Thorac Cardiovasc Surg 49:844, 1965.

Song YS: Lower pulmonary aberrant lobe. South Med J 49:1137, 1956.

Spencer H: Pathology of the Lung. New York, Macmillan Co, 1962.

Sperling DR and Finck EJ: Intralobar bronchopulmonary sequestration. Association with a murmur over the back in a child. Am J Dis Child 115:362, 1968.

Symbas PN, Hatcher CR Jr, Abbott OA, and Logan WD Jr: An appraisal of pulmonary sequestration: special emphasis on unusual manifestations. Am Rev Resp Dis 99:406, 1969.

Talalak P: Pulmonary sequestration. Arch Dis Child 35:57, 1960.

Turk LN III and Lindskog GE: The importance of angiographic diagnosis in intralobar pulmonary sequestration. J Thorac Cardiovasc Surg 41:299, 1961.

Van Rens TJG: Intralobar sequestration of lung: review of its possible origin and report on five cases. Arch Chir Neerl 14:63, 1962.

Waddell WR: Organoid differentiation of fetal lung; histologic study of differentiation of mammalian fetal lung in utero and in transplants. Arch Pathol 47:277, 1949.

Witten DM, Clagett OT, and Hiltz JE: Intralobar pulmonary sequestration involving the upper lobes. J Thorac Cardiovasc Surg 43:523, 1962.

Congenital Cystic Adenomatoid Malformation of the Lung

Avery ME, Fletcher BD, and Williams R: The Lung and Its Disorders in the Newborn Infant. 4th ed. Philadelphia, WB Saunders Co, 1981.

Bain GO: Congenital adenomatoid malformation of the lung. Dis Chest 36:430, 1959.

Belanger R, Lefleche LR, and Picard JL: Congenital cystic adenomatoid malformation of the lung. Thorax 19:1, 1964.

Breckenridge RL, Rehermann RL, and Gibson ET: Congenital cystic adenomatoid malformation of the lung. J Pediatr 67:863, 1965.

Buntain WL, Isaacs H Jr, Payne VC Jr et al: Lobar emphysema, cystic adenomatoid malformation, pulmonary sequestration, and bronchogenic cysts in infancy and childhood: a clinical group. J Pediatr Surg 9:85, 1974.

Chin KY and Tang MY: Congenital adenomatoid malformation of one lobe of a lung with general anasarca. Arch Pathol 48:311, 1949.

Craig JM, Kirkpatrick J, and Neuhauser EBD: Congenital cystic adenomatoid malformation of the lung in infants. Am J Roentgenol 76:516, 1956.

Demos NJ and Teresi A: Congenital lung malformations. A unified concept and a case report. J Thorac Cardiovasc Surg 70:260, 1975.

Halloran LG, Silverberg SG, and Salzberg AM: Congenital cystic adenomatoid malformation of the lung: a surgical emergency. Arch Surg 104:715, 1972.

Holder TM and Christy MG: Cystic adenomatoid malformation of the lung. J Thorac Cardiovasc Surg 47:590, 1964.

Hutchin P: Congenital cystic disease of the lung. Rev Surg 28:79, 1971.

Kwittken J and Reiner L: Congenital cystic adenomatoid malformation of the lung. Pediatrics 30:759, 1962.

Landing BH: Anomalies of the respiratory tract. Pediatr Clin North Am 4:73, 1957.

Landing BH and Wells TR: Tracheobronchial anomalies in children. Perspect Pediatr Pathol 1:1, 1973.

Merenstein GB: Congenital cystic adenomatoid malformation of the lung. Report of a case and review of the literature. Am J Dis Child 118:772, 1969.

Pierce WS, deParedes CG, Raphaely RC, and Waldhausen JA: Pulmonary resection in infants younger than one year of age. Thorac Cardiovasc Surg 61:875, 1971.

CONGENITAL PULMONARY LYMPHANGIECTASIS

Avery ME, Fletcher BD, and Williams R: The Lung and Its Disorders in the Newborn Infant. 4th ed. Philadelphia, WB Saunders Co, 1981.

Brown MD and Reidbord HE: Congenital pulmonary lymphangiectasis. Am J Dis Child 114:654, 1967.

Carter RW and Vaughn HM: Congenital pulmonary lymphangiectasis. Am J Roentgenol 86:576, 1961.

Fronstein MH, Hooper GS, Besse BE, and Ferreri S: Congenital pulmonary cystic lymphangiectasis. Am J Dis Child 114:330, 1967.

Javett SN, Webster I, and Braundo JL: Congenital dilatation of the pulmonary lymphatics. Pediatrics 31:416, 1963.

Landing BH: Anomalies of the respiratory tract. Pediatr Clin North Am 4:73, 1957.

Laurence KM: Congenital pulmonary cystic lymphangiectasis. J Pathol Bacteriol 70:325, 1955.

Laurence KM: Congenital pulmonary lymphangiectasis. J Clin Pathol 12:62, 1959.

Laurence KM: Personal communication. Cited in Spencer H: Pathology of the Lung. New York, Macmillan Co, 1962.

Rywlin AM and Fojaco RM: Congenital pulmonary lymphangiectasis associated with a blind common pulmonary vein. Pediatrics 41:931, 1968.

Spencer H: Pathology of the Lung. New York, Macmillan Co, 1962.

PULMONARY ARTERIOVENOUS FISTULA

Björk VO: Local extirpation of multiple bilateral pulmonary arteriovenous aneurysms. J Thorac Cardiovasc Surg 53:293, 1967.

Bosher LH Jr, Blake DA and Byrd BR: An analysis of the pathologic anatomy of pulmonary arteriovenous aneurysms, with particular reference to the applicability of local excision. Surgery 45:91, 1959.

Burford TH and Ferguson TB: Congenital lesions of the lung and emphysema. In Sabiston DC Jr and Spencer FC (eds): Gibbon's Surgery of the Chest. 4th ed. Philadelphia, WB Saunders Co, 1983.

Charbon BC, Adams WF, and Carlson RF: Surgical treatment of multiple arteriovenous fistulas in the right lung in a patient having undergone a left pneumonectomy seven years earlier for the same disease. J Thorac Surg 23:188, 1952.

Clatworthy HW Jr: Intrathoracic tumors and cysts. In Ariel IM and Pack GT (eds): Cancer and Allied Diseases of Infancy and Childhood. Boston, Little, Brown & Co, 1960.

Dargeon HW: Tumors of Childhood, a Clinical Disease. New York, Paul B Hoeber, Inc, 1964.

Goldman A: Pulmonary arteriovenous fistula with secondary polycythemia occurring in two brothers. J Lab Clin Med 32:330, 1947.

Goldman A: Arteriovenous fistula of the lung: its hereditary and clinical aspects. Am Rev Tuberc 57:266, 1948.

Gomes MR, Bernatz PE, and Dines DE: Pulmonary arteriovenous fistulas. Ann Thorac Surg 7:582, 1969.

Hall EM: Malignant hemangioma of the lung with multiple metastasis. Am J Pathol 11:343, 1935.

Hodgson CH and Kaye RI: Pulmonary arteriovenous fistula and hereditary hemorrhagic telangiectasia. Dis Chest 43:449, 1963.

Hope JW and Koop CE: Differential diagnosis of mediastinal masses. Pediatr Clin North Am 6:379, 1959.

Husson GS and Wyatt TC: Primary pulmonary obliterative vascular disease in infants and young children. Pediatrics 23:493, 1959.

Klassen K: Personal communication to HW Clatworthy Jr. In Ariel IM and Pack GT (eds): Cancer and Allied Diseases of Infancy and Childhood. Boston, Little, Brown & Co, 1960.

Landing BH: Anomalies of the respiratory tract. Pediatr Clin North Am 4:73, 1957.

Lansdowne M: Discussion of paper by A Goldman. J Lab Clin Med 32:330, 1947.

Lindgren E: Roentgen diagnosis of arteriovenous aneurysm of the lung. Acta Radiol 27:586, 1946.

Lindskog GE, Liebow AA, and Glenn WWL: Thoracic and Cardiovascular Surgery, with Related Pathology. New York, Appleton-Century-Crofts, Inc, 1962.

Maier HC, Himmelstein A, Riley RL, and Bunim JJ: Arteriovenous fistula of the lung. J Thorac Surg 17:13, 1948.

Michael P: Tumors of Infancy and Childhood. Philadelphia, JB Lippincott Co, 1964.

Mitchell FN: Pulmonary arteriovenous telangiectasis. South Med J 47:1157, 1954.

Moyer JH and Ackerman AJ: Hereditary hemorrhagic telangiectasis associated with pulmonary arteriovenous fistula in two members of a family. Ann Intern Med 29:775, 1948.

Murdock CE: Pulmonary arteriovenous fistulectomy. Arch Surg 86:44, 1962.

Muri J: Arterio-venous aneurysm of the lung. Dis Chest 24:49, 1953.

Ravitch MM: Anomalies of the pulmonary vessels. In Benson CD et al (eds): Pediatric Surgery. Vol 1. Chicago, Year Book Medical Publishers, Inc, 1962.

Seaman WB and Goldman A: Roentgen aspects of pulmonary arteriovenous fistula. Arch Intern Med 89:70, 1952.

Shefts L: Discussion of paper by HC Maier et al (1948).

Shumaker HB Jr and Waldhausen JA: Pulmonary arteriovenous fistulas in children. Ann Surg 158:713, 1963.

Sweet RH: Discussion of paper by HC Maier et al (1948).

Taber RE and Ehrenhaft JL: Arteriovenous fistulae and arterial aneurysm of the pulmonary arterial tree. Arch Surg 73:567, 1965.

Vaughan VC, McKay RJ, and Behrman RE (eds): Nelson Textbook of Pediatrics. 11th ed. Philadelphia, WB Saunders Co, 1979.

Weiss DL and Czeredarczuk O: Rupture of an angiomatous malformation of the pleura in a newborn infant. Am J Dis Child 96:370, 1958.

Wollstein M: Malignant hemangioma of the lung with multiple visceral foci. Arch Pathol 12:562, 1931.

13

ANTHONY CORBET, M.D.

RESPIRATORY DISORDERS IN THE NEWBORN

The common respiratory problems of the newborn can be classified as (1) respiratory depression, or apnea; (2) respiratory distress, or rapid labored breathing; and (3) respiratory obstruction.

RESPIRATORY DEPRESSION (APNEA)

FETAL ASPHYXIA

Fetal asphyxia is an important cause of mortality and morbidity in newborn infants and is the usual cause of apnea at birth. Asphyxia is due to a reduction in respiratory gas exchange with excessive accumulation of carbon dioxide and oxygen deficiency, causing anaerobic metabolism and lactic acidosis. The fetus and the newborn survive asphyxia longer than the older child because they have higher glycogen stores, especially in the myocardium, which facilitate more sustained anaerobic metabolism and circulatory adaptation. This survival does not, however, reduce susceptibility to anoxic brain damage.

Placental Gas Exchange

Although the placenta is an adequate gas exchanger under normal circumstances, it does not have a large reserve. Intervillous oxygen tension, the placental equivalent of alveolar oxygen tension, is 45 to 60 mm Hg. The placenta itself has an oxygen consumption significantly greater than that of the lung. When fetal blood flow and maternal blood flow to the placenta are equal and are equally distributed in relation to each other, fetal villous capillary blood is not quite in equilibrium with intervillous blood. Umbilical venous blood, the most arterialized in the fetal circulation, has an oxygen tension of 30 to 35 mm Hg, much less than that of fetal villous capillary blood because fetal shunts circumvent the exchange surface. Fetal oxygen consumption is only half that of the neonate, because less is required to sustain thermal balance. Sufficient uptake of oxygen by the fetus depends on its having a higher hemoglobin concentration, a higher affinity of the hemoglobin

for oxygen, a more exaggerated Bohr effect, and especially a high blood flow through the fetal and maternal sides of the placenta. Impaired fetal or maternal circulation is very important in the disruption of fetal oxygen supplies. Placental reserve is low because maternal cardiac output and uterine blood flow are already high and cannot be increased to the same degree as alveolar ventilation in the lung.

Normal Delivery

Labor is accompanied by the development of mild fetal asphyxia during the second stage. Uterine blood flow is significantly restricted by normal uterine contractions and even more so with excessive uterine activity. At birth, umbilical arterial pH is 7.25 to 7.30 and P_{CO_2} 45 to 55 mm Hg. With normal cardiorespiratory function, newborn arterial blood gases are corrected rapidly in the first hour of postnatal life, but this correction occurs significantly more slowly in premature infants and in infants with pulmonary disorders.

Primary Apnea

Animal experiments that have included clamping the umbilical cord have demonstrated the sequence of events when the fetus is asphyxiated, and observations in the delivery room suggest that these experimental data can be applied in the human newborn infant. Although the fetus has frequent respiratory muscle contractions before the onset of labor, it is likely that no such activity occurs during labor. With the onset of asphyxia, transient respiratory activity occurs, a phenomenon partly responsible for the onset of breathing at birth. Progressive hypoxemia, however, depresses central respiratory neurons, and despite peripheral chemoreceptor activity, primary apnea supervenes.

The fetus, the mature newborn in the first few days, and the premature newborn in the first few weeks of life differ from the adult in that hypoxemia produces only transient respiratory stimulation followed by sustained depression. Most newborns who are apneic at birth are in a state of primary apnea.

Anesthesia and analgesic drugs given the mother during labor prolong primary apnea. The circulation remains intact, with increased cardiac output and mild peripheral vasoconstriction resulting in hypertension, which sometimes causes mild bradycardia through activation of the baroreceptors. The newborn infant is deeply cyanosed from arterial desaturation. Central respiratory neuron depression at this stage can be overcome by increasing the neuronal traffic through the brainstem reticular activating system, which is the purpose of vigorous cutaneous stimulation in the delivery room. An important point in the differentiation of primary apnea is that the stimulated infant resumes breathing first, and only after breathing is cyanosis relieved.

Terminal Apnea

If asphyxia is prolonged, the circulation deteriorates, with bradycardia from myocardial hypoxia and acidosis, severe peripheral vasoconstriction, and falling blood pressure. Primitive gasping due to severe cerebral hypoxia supervenes. After a variable period, gasping ceases, marking the onset of terminal apnea. Such infants have severe lactic acidosis and hypercarbia, very slow heart rate, low blood pressure, and intense vasoconstriction with shock. Brain and myocardial blood flow are preferentially preserved during this deterioration, but clearly there is significant deficiency. The time to last gasp can be prolonged by general anesthesia, barbiturates, or deep hypothermia. Delaying deterioration in the circulation by glucose or alkali administration also prolongs the time to last gasp. Previous episodes of asphyxia, which deplete glycogen stores, significantly shorten the period of gasping. Animal histologic evidence suggests that progressive brain damage results after the last gasp.

Once brain perfusion is impaired, central respiratory depression can be reversed only by improving the circulation. Until the circulation is improved, cutaneous stimulation will not revive the infant, as it will in primary apnea. Resuscitation is best accomplished by positive pressure ventilation of the lung with oxygen and by external cardiac massage to improve circulation to both the lungs and brain. Bicarbonate infusion and rapid correction of acidemia by hyperventilation improve cardiac output and reduce pulmonary vasoconstriction, thereby increasing oxygen uptake. Animal evidence suggests that the longer effective resuscitation is delayed after the last gasp, the longer it takes for the infant to respond and the more marked the brain damage. The initial response during resuscitation of terminal apnea is increased spontaneous heart rate, elevation of blood pressure, and relief of vasoconstriction, with color changing from the pale gray of desaturation and hypoperfusion to the healthy pink associated with adequate oxygenation and perfusion. Only after circulatory restoration does respiratory activity resume, an important point in the differentiation of terminal apnea. Effective resuscitation reduces brain damage even in infants asphyxiated to the point of extreme bradycardia.

Delivery Room Procedure

The infant is placed on a table head down to facilitate airway drainage. A radiant heat source is used to maintain skin temperature. The infant is dried rapidly with a towel to minimize evaporative heat losses, and the nasopharynx is gently suctioned. Both of these procedures may stimulate breathing. One hundred per cent oxygen is applied though a loose-fitting face mask and bag with a flow-through valve, and if breathing is not initiated by this stimulation, a slap on the soles may be effective. If response is not adequate, the infant should be ventilated by bag and close-fitting face mask at a pressure of about 30 cm H_2O, sufficient to move the upper chest visibly, with inflation sustained for 1 sec to promote diffusion into fluid-obstructed airways. If there is no spontaneous breathing after bag-and-mask ventilation, an endotracheal tube should be inserted and ventilation should be continued to correct hypoxemia and acidemia more rapidly.

When the heart rate is below 75 to 100 beats/min, external cardiac massage should be applied immediately. If spontaneous breathing is not initiated or the heart rate does not accelerate, an umbilical venous catheter should be inserted under sterile conditions, and after samples are obtained for blood gas measurements, sodium bicarbonate, 3 mEq/kg, should be injected over 3 min. Sinus bradycardia may respond to epinephrine, 1/10,000, 0.2 ml/kg. Continued bradycardia means an electrocardiogram (ECG) should be obtained. Bradycardia due to heart block from hyperkalemia may respond to cautious injection of 10 per cent calcium gluconate, 1 ml/kg. A problem such as pneumothorax, congenital diaphragmatic hernia, or hypoplastic lung must be considered. When vasoconstrictive shock persists after the heart rate has accelerated, blood loss should also be considered, but usually vasoconstriction is due to residual acidemia.

Persistent apnea may be due to narcotics administered to the mother, in which case repeated doses of naloxone hydrochloride are helpful. Persistent apnea may also indicate severe brain damage, and sustained mechanical ventilation may be undertaken or resuscitation may be abandoned. If resuscitation is abandoned, a period of 30 min of resuscitative effort appears justified.

MATERNAL DRUGS

The inhalation anesthetic agents, such as cyclopropane, enflurane, and halothane, all cross the placenta readily because they are of low molecular weight and are nonionized and highly lipid soluble. If given in sufficient concentration, inhalation anesthetics invariably depress respiration in the newborn. Fortunately, they are rapidly excreted by the lungs, so positive-pressure ventilation for about 5 min is usually all that is required. If the interval between induction and delivery is short (less than 20 min), maternal anesthetics have little effect in the newborn.

Because they are also lipid soluble and not highly ionized at physiologic pH, the barbiturates such as thiopental sodium readily cross the placenta, especially during cesarean section when uterine blood flow is not reduced by uterine contractions. Effects are not seen, however, if the interval between induction and delivery is less than 10 min. There is no correlation between depth of anesthesia in the mother and blood levels of the drug or respiratory depression in the newborn. Because the liver receives part of the umbilical venous flow, barbiturates may accumulate in the liver and be released slowly over a few hours. Uptake by the newborn brain may be limited because brain water content is high. The newborn's ability to metabolize barbiturates in the liver is poor, so respiratory depression due to high doses of maternal barbiturates may require prolonged mechanical ventilation for several hours.

Meperidine hydrochloride and other narcotic agents given to the mother for pain relief have all been associated in the neonate with delayed onset of breathing and excessive hypercarbia in the first 2 to 6 hours. They cross the placenta readily because of high lipid solubility. The risk is greatest if the interval between injection and delivery is 1 to 3 hours for intramuscular injection and 30 min to 1 hour for intravenous injection. There is no correlation between blood levels and respiratory depression, but a dose limited to 50 mg meperidine has not been associated with problems at any interval. The narcotic antagonist naloxone hydrochloride, 0.1 mg/kg given by peripheral vein or umbilical venous catheter, is effective in reversing respiratory depression. The dose may need to be repeated every hour until the effect of meperidine disappears. In the term newborn, the elimination half-life is approximately 24 hours, but the depressive effect on breathing should be much shorter in duration. Naloxone should not be given to infants of narcotic-addicted mothers, because it may precipitate an acute withdrawal reaction.

It is apparent that asphyxia and acidosis at birth make the newborn more susceptible to the effects of depressant drugs. The most likely explanation for this effect is that acidosis favors passage of the drug into the brain by altering protein binding and ionic dissociation, but there may also be an effect on the diffusion barrier, or asphyxia may divert more of the cardiac output to the brain. Asphyxia at birth should always be managed effectively before a diagnosis of respiratory depression by a drug is considered. In general, prolonged respiratory depression due to asphyxia is associated initially with peripheral vasoconstriction, whereas prolonged respiratory depression associated with a drug is accompanied by normal circulation.

Occasional instances of neonatal respiratory depression, peripheral rather than central in origin, have been reported in association with maternal administration of magnesium. Experience with adults suggests that this depression is unlikely to occur unless serum levels of magnesium exceed 10 mg/100 ml.

RECURRENT APNEA

This condition occurs commonly in newborns after the establishment of rhythmic breathing at birth. Although apneic spells are frequently brief, a significant or prolonged apneic spell may be described as cessation of respiratory gas exchange for more than 20 sec or for a shorter period if associated with cyanosis or bradycardia. In general, apnea is a common expression of many types of disorders in newborns, especially in premature infants, but it may occur without evidence of other abnormalities—so-called apnea of prematurity.

Control of Breathing

Breathing activity originates in a central pattern generator and is maintained by alternating discharges of inspiratory and expiratory neurons that are mutually inhibitory. These neurons are located diffusely in the medulla oblongata and are activated by the reticular activating system. The rhythm is initiated by a group of neurons called the *central inspiratory activator,* located near, but separate from, the central chemosensors on the ventral surface of the medulla.

Normally inspiration is active and expiration is passive. However, expiration is divided into two phases. In the first phase, a group of inspiratory neurons apply postinspiratory "braking" to slow exhalation. In the second phase, exhalation continues passively without braking, or it is accelerated by the contraction of expiratory muscles. The main inspiratory muscles are the diaphragm, intercostals, and upper airway abductors. The main expiratory muscles are intercostals, upper airway adductors, and abdominal groups.

Inspiration is terminated by an "off switch," which inhibits the central inspiratory activator and allows exhalation. The activity of the off switch and thus the rate and depth of breathing is regulated by inputs from the pulmonary stretch receptors and from the rostral pontine pneumotaxic center. The threshold of the off switch is modulated from multiple sources, including the central and peripheral chemosensors, the chest wall propriosensors, and the hypothalamus and cerebral cortex. A system so complex requires multiple neuronal connections and fast conduction times. These properties are insufficiently developed early in gestation and only develop to maturity by late infancy. During quiet sleep, modulation is chiefly chemical, but during active sleep and wakefulness, behavioral controls are much more important.

The activity of the pulmonary stretch receptors increases throughout gestation until term and then decreases, so that older children and adults do not have an active Hering-Breuer reflex. The net effect of the Hering-Breuer reflex in premature infants is more rapid, less deep breathing and a modest stimulation of ventilatory drive, factors that may be important for the maintenance of adequate lung volume.

The sensitivity of the central chemosensors to CO_2 is reduced in small premature infants and increases to adult levels at term. Hyperoxemia increases sensitivity and hypoxemia decreases sensitivity, the opposite interaction to that seen in adults. Regardless of gestation, adult levels of sensitivity are reached by 4 weeks postnatal age.

The newborn infant responds to hypoxia by transient hyperpnea, followed after a few minutes by relative ventilatory depression, suggesting rapid exhaustion and relative insufficiency of the peripheral chemosensor under circumstances of moderate central depression. The newborn's response contrasts with the adult's response in which there is sustained hyperpnea. In 100 per cent oxygen breathing, newborns demonstrate a transient depression of ventilation, as do adults, which is consistent with continued activity of the peripheral chemosensor under normal conditions. The hypoxic ventilatory depression disappears by a few days in mature newborns and in prematures by 2 to 3 weeks postnatal age, when the mature response of sustained hyperpnea becomes dominant. There is evidence in fetal lambs that the effect of hypoxia is not direct but mediated by primitive neurons in the rostral pons. Other evidence suggests a role for endorphins or adenosine, both of which are increased during hypoxia. It is not yet established whether maturation of the hypoxic response is due to disappearance of central depression or improvement in peripheral chemosensor function.

Periodic Breathing

This pattern consists of very brief apneas of 5- to 10- sec duration, followed by breathing for 10 to 15 sec before the next very brief apnea. Periodic breathing is uncommon during the first 3 to 4 days of life. There are no changes in the heart rate or color, but the net effect is mild hypoventilation. This pattern is very common in premature infants, especially at high altitudes, and it is relieved by supplemental oxygen and continuous distending airway pressure (CDAP). Although the prognosis is excellent, there is a clear relationship with apnea of prematurity.

Recurrent Apnea Secondary to an Underlying Disorder

All infants presenting with significant recurrent apnea should have a thorough clinical investigation before a diagnosis of apnea of prematurity is made. The diagnostic possibilities are as follows: (1) brain lesions, such as hemorrhage, ischemic damage, infection, kernicterus, and malformation; (2) lung disease producing severe hypoxemia or hypercarbia; (3) circulatory disorders, including septicemia, patent ductus arteriosus (PDA), dehydration, anemia, and polycythemia; (4) metabolic problems, such as hypoglycemia, hyperglycemia, hypernatremia, hyponatremia, hypocalcemia, hyperthermia, and malnutrition; and (5) hyperactive upper airway vagal reflexes initiated by gavage, suctioning, or pooling of secretions. Specific treatment is directed toward the underlying problem. In many centers, infection is the most frequent cause of secondary apnea.

Apnea of Prematurity

Incidence of apnea of prematurity increases as gestational age decreases. It is particularly high in neonates of 24 to 32 weeks' gestational age. Apneic spells occurring in the first few days of life are more likely to be secondary to an underlying disorder. Apnea of prematurity usually resolves by 38 weeks postconceptional age, but rarely it may persist until 42 weeks.

Pathogenesis. It is thought that 40 per cent of prolonged apnea episodes are central or diaphragmatic, 10 per cent are obstructive, and 50 per cent are mixed. Although this point is controversial, most mixed apneas begin as central and become obstructive. Although the cause is unknown, a number of theories have been proposed for the occurrence of central, diaphragmatic, and obstructive apnea.

1. The neurons of the central pattern generator are not connected by sufficient dendrites and synapses, causing inadequate amplification of the ventilatory drive signals originating from the central inspiratory activator. Infants with apnea have prolonged auditory brainstem conduction times when compared with control infants without apnea, which suggests that the nearby central pattern generator may be more disorganized.

2. The chest wall of premature infants is highly compliant, so more respiratory work is performed to generate a constant tidal volume. This extra work makes the diaphragm very susceptible to fatigue, in which case contractions will cease for a short period until a temporary recovery has occurred.

3. There is evidence that the upper airway abductors may activate insufficiently or late, so that diaphragmatic contraction induces upper airway closure. Load compensation to overcome this obstruction is reduced in premature infants, but increases with gestation. Small premature infants have a particular problem because of an active intercostal phrenic inhibitory reflex initiated by chest wall distortion, which shortens the inspiratory time and interferes with attempts at load compensation. This reflex predisposes to obstructive apnea, especially when in the supine position or when the neck is flexed.

Relationship to Sleep State. Apnea is more common during active sleep, when there is loss of intercostal muscle tone, diminished postinspiratory braking, reduced upper airway adductor activity, and decreased ventilatory drive. Secondary to these problems are a 30 per cent reduction in lung volume and a slight fall of arterial P_{O_2}. Both the ventilatory response to hypoxia and the sensitivity to CO_2 are depressed more in active sleep than in quiet sleep. The full-term newborn and premature infant spend 80 per cent of the time asleep; in the small infant, most of it is active sleep, thus increasing the susceptibility to apnea.

Treatment of Apnea. All infants considered to be at risk are monitored continuously for heart rate and sometimes for respiratory rate, using conventional electronic alarm systems. Those considered to be at risk are infants with a postconceptional age of less than 32 weeks or a body weight of less than 1500 g. Obstructive apnea may not be detected by thoracic impedence respiration monitors. A general increase in afferent stimulation may be obtained by using repeated body massage or flotation water beds. If apnea persists, mask-and-bag ventilation without a change in oxygen concentration should be applied. Some medical centers manage infants by maintaining continuous distending airway pressure, which prevents lung deflation and chest distortion. Others prefer a pharmacologic approach, utilizing caffeine or theophylline to increase central respiratory drive and improve CO_2 sensitivity. Caffeine is given as caffeine citrate, either intravenously or orally, at a loading dose of 20 mg/kg and a maintenance dose of 5 mg/kg once or twice daily. The half-life is about 4 days, and serum levels should be maintained between 10 and 20 mg/L. Theophylline may also be given intravenously or by mouth, at a loading dose of 6 mg/kg and a maintenance dose of 2 mg/kg two or three times daily. The half-life is 20 to 24 hours, and serum levels are maintained between 8 and 12 mg/L. Neither drug causes obvious toxicity, but tachycardia is more common with theophylline. The toxic to therapeutic ratio is higher for caffeine, and a significant fraction of theophylline is methylated to caffeine by premature infants. Caffeine gives much more stable plasma levels. The drugs may be used on a trial basis for 2 weeks and then stopped, or they may be continued until 32 weeks postconception when most cases should have resolved. It is uncommon for intubation and mechanical ventilation to be required for apnea of prematurity. Another drug sometimes prescribed for particularly troublesome apnea of prematurity is doxopram hydrochloride, which in low doses is said to stimulate the peripheral chemosensor and in higher doses directly stimulates respiratory neurons. Unfortunately, the U.S. preparation contains benzyl alcohol as a preservative, which limits its application. The usual starting dose is 0.5 mg/kg/hr, but doses as high as 2.5 mg/kg/hr have been prescribed. Hypertension is not uncommon at the higher dosage levels, and muscle twitching is frequently observed.

Feeding Hypoxemia

Feeding requires coordinated movements of sucking, swallowing, and breathing. Some term and large premature infants develop subventilation, apnea, cyanosis, and reflex bradycardia during feeding but not at other times. The problem usually resolves by 44 weeks postconception but may remain as late as 54 weeks. The treatment is frequent interruption and supplemental oxygen during feeding and in extreme cases gavage feeding. Atropine before feeding may be useful if bradycardia is a major problem.

Apnea Associated with Gastroesophageal Reflux

A few infants have frequent episodes of vomiting or regurgitation, sometimes accompanied by significant apnea, while they are awake. Accurate diagnosis of reflux-associated apnea depends on continuous recordings of esophageal pH and nasal air flow, with consistent demonstration of apnea preceded by episodes of pH less than 4.0. The final proof is resolution of the problem after gastric fundoplication, although some infants may respond to thickening of feeds and metoclopramide hydrochloride or bethanechol therapy.

Apnea of Infancy

Periodic breathing and brief apneas during sleep are not uncommon in normal term infants during the first few months of life. When prolonged apneas occur, especially if resuscitation is required, apnea of infancy may be diagnosed. Other possible causes of prolonged apneas are gastroesophageal reflux, pharyngeal incoordination, convulsions, infection, heart disease, breath-holding spells, central hypoventilation syndrome, and brain tumor. If a cause cannot be discovered and eliminated, the only possible treatment at present is hospital or home monitoring, with or without a respiratory stimulant, such as caffeine. There appears to be no relationship with sudden infant death syndrome (SIDS), which should be considered a separate disorder, because 90 to 95 per cent of SIDS infants do not have preceding apnea of infancy.

RESPIRATORY DISTRESS

TRANSIENT TACHYPNEA OF THE NEWBORN

The most common cause of respiratory distress in newborns, transient tachypnea of the newborn (TTN) has also been described as wet lung disease and type II respiratory distress syndrome. Affected infants have respiration rates of 60 to 120 breaths/min, often with early retractions and grunting. Onset is from birth, but signs are sometimes masked initially by central depression. Commonly the problem subsides within 12 to 24 hours, but in some infants the course extends over 3 to 7 days. There is an increased risk of pneumothorax.

Most patients are larger premature or term infants with a birth weight generally exceeding 1500 g. Incidence is higher in males and in association with prematurity, meperidine depression at birth, maternal diabetes, and cesarean section. Surfactant phospholipids in amniotic fluid and in tracheal aspirate after birth are normal. There may be hypercarbia in the first hours of life, reflecting fetal asphyxia or drug depression, but generally the arterial P_{CO_2} is normal by 8 hours. Cyanosis while breathing room air is common, but infants with TTN rarely require more than 40- to 50-per cent oxygen for adequate arterial saturation. There is no significant metabolic acidosis after the first few hours of life, and blood pressure, circulation, and urine output are normal. The oxygen requirement does not increase during the first 48 hours as it does in hyaline membrane disease or congenital pneumonia, and it soon improves. Occasionally, hyaline membrane disease (HMD) is masked by wet lung disease, which should be suspected if the oxygen requirement progresses or hypercarbia persists. In general, the prognosis in TTN is excellent with only supportive treatment, so distinction from HMD is important.

The chest may appear barrel shaped on physical examination. Lungs are clear to auscultation, although occasionally crackles suggest excessive alveolar fluid. Radiologically, the lungs may appear normal except for obvious hyperinflation (Fig. 13–1). Vascular markings are often increased, and a pattern of interstitial edema with small pleural effusions may be seen. Sometimes coarse, fluffy densities indicate alveolar edema, especially if radiographs are taken early. The pattern is sometimes more obvious on the right side on an anteroposterior (AP) view or posteriorly on a lateral view. Heart size is normal or slightly increased.

Although functional residual capacity measured by

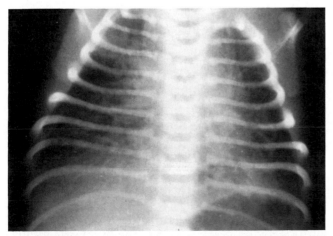

Figure 13–1. Transient tachypnea of the newborn with small bilateral pleural effusions. Note the hyperinflation and increased perihilar markings.

gas diffusion methods is normal in transient tachypnea of the newborn, chest radiographs suggest high lung volume and hence the presence of airway closure with excess trapped gas. Lung compliance is reduced. Hypoxemia is mainly from ventilation-perfusion inequality, rather than from right-to-left vascular shunts, which remain in the normal range.

Most clinical descriptions of TTN refer to larger infants, but many small premature infants placed immediately at birth on mechanical ventilation have a short-lived lung condition that is probably also wet lung disease. They may have high oxygen and ventilator requirements initially, but they wean to room air and low ventilator requirements by 24 hours of age. The chest radiograph is consistent with pulmonary edema and shows rapid clearing. The descriptive term *immature lung syndrome* has been used for this condition, but because these infants do not have HMD, this term does not seem appropriate.

Wet lung disease probably results from compression of peripheral conducting airways by excessive interstitial fluid. Before the onset of labor, the fetal lung contains about 25 ml/kg fetal lung liquid within the potential air spaces. Fetal lung fluid is rich in chloride but is nearly devoid of protein. During labor this fluid is transferred to the lung interstitial compartment and reabsorbed directly into the pulmonary capillary circulation. At birth only 6 ml/kg fluid remains in the airways, and with the onset of air breathing, this fluid too is rapidly transferred to the interstitial space, accumulating in sumps around peripheral airways rather than in gas exchange areas. After birth, lung lymph drainage and pulmonary blood flow increase, which are together responsible for clearing interstitial space fluid into the circulation. Normally this interstitial clearance is accomplished within 6 hours; the reason for its delay in TTN is not understood. The hypoproteinemia in TTN accounts for only a small amount of retained interstitial fluid. A few infants receive an excessive placental transfusion of blood, resulting in high vascular pressures that might delay clearance, but in most cases there is no evidence for pulmonary artery hypertension.

Some experimental work suggests that removal of lung liquid from the air spaces is under adrenergic hormone control. Plasma catecholamine levels in the fetus rise progressively during labor and reach extraordinarily high levels at birth, which accounts for the normal reduction in lung liquid occupying the air spaces. Possibly by a mechanism dependent on cyclic adenosine monophosphate (cyclic AMP), epinephrine inhibits the chloride pump responsible for lung liquid secretion and stimulates the amiloride-sensitive sodium channels responsible for lung liquid absorption. Once the chloride pump is inhibited, osmotic forces will also rapidly transfer fluid between the protein-poor air space and the protein-rich interstitial space. This situation suggests that infants with excessive alveolar fluid may be exposed to lower levels of plasma epinephrine during labor and delivery, especially if they are delivered by elective cesarean section without labor; alternatively, they may have a deficiency in lung adrenergic receptors. But it does not explain why there is such a delay in clearance of the interstitial compartment of the lung.

HYALINE MEMBRANE DISEASE

After TTN, HMD is the most common cause of newborn respiratory distress. It has been estimated that there are 40,000 cases annually in the United States, or about 1 per cent of deliveries. The incidence, about 50 per cent at 28 weeks, declines with gestational age to reach zero by 270 days; overall incidence is about 14 per cent in all infants weighing under 2500 g at birth. In the rare infant of more than 38.5 weeks gestational age who has HMD, physical criteria suggest that the patient is less mature. The disease is due to insufficient development of the pulmonary surfactant system and the lungs in general. There is evidence that body systems do not mature uniformly, so lung maturation may often be accelerated or decelerated in relation to gestational age. This uneven maturation rate explains why many immature infants are not affected by the disease, but some more mature infants die with severe HMD.

Risk Factors

Hyaline membrane disease is more common in male than in female infants, this difference not being apparent at 26 weeks but increasing toward term. Males with HMD have a higher mortality, suggesting slower lung development in the male. Premature infants are more likely to have HMD if in an earlier pregnancy the mother had a premature infant that was affected, which suggests some kind of maternal control over fetal lung development.

The role of cesarean section in HMD is controversial, but it appears that at any given gestational age the risk is higher in abdominal delivery than in vaginal delivery and that the indication for a cesarean section is a less important factor. The absence of labor increases the risk substantially, so it is elective cesarean section that is particularly incriminated. Determining the importance of cesarean section in HMD is compounded by the frequent uncertainty about maternal dates and the difficulty in defining lung maturity without laboratory investigation.

Occurrence of HMD is significantly increased in gestational diabetes and in insulin-dependent diabetic mothers without vascular disease. Most such infants are large for gestational age; similar infants whose mothers do not have diabetes are also at increased risk. On the other hand, the risk is decreased in diabetic or nondiabetic infants who are small for gestational age. Maternal conditions that decrease the incidence include chronic hypertension, subacute placental abruption, and narcotic addiction. Hyaline membrane disease is not seen in infants who pass meconium before delivery, nor is it common in infants of mothers with established amnionitis. The risk is significantly reduced in otherwise uncomplicated prolonged rupture of membranes, although the protective effect may not be seen for a variable period, 16 to 96 hours in different studies.

Although infants with HMD have lower Apgar scores and more abnormal fetal heart rate patterns, most are not more acidemic at birth than controls. The reason for the lower Apgar score is relative immaturity and defective lung function. The second-born of twins is more likely to have HMD but again is not more acidemic at birth despite a lower Apgar score. It is doubtful that fetal asphyxia could be a causative factor, but when present it probably increases the mortality.

Clinical Course

The infant with HMD is usually cyanotic in room air and has an edematous appearance. Most have rapid or labored breathing immediately after they have recovered from delivery. Persistent hypercarbia and mild metabolic acidosis are common. Usually, the infant requires 40 to 50 per cent oxygen after birth for relief of central cyanosis but then develops a progressive oxygen requirement over 24 to 48 hours that often reaches 100 per cent oxygen. In other infants, the oxygen requirement decreases as acidosis or hypothermia is corrected or fetal lung fluid is cleared and begins to progress only after 3 to 6 hours. More severely affected infants have an immediate high oxygen requirement, which rapidly progresses to 100 per cent, and they may die in 12 to 24 hours. Another group of larger, more mature infants needs little oxygen initially and manifests a slowly progressive course over 3 to 4 days that is often confused with congenital heart disease. If HMD is uncomplicated, recovery starts by 48 to 72 hours, the decline in oxygen requirement is relatively continuous, and oxygen can be discontinued by 7 days.

Radiology

There are diffuse, fine granular densities that sometimes are not present on initial films but that develop in the first 6 hours (Fig. 13–2). The appearance may be more marked at the base. Presence of an air bronchogram is consistent with HMD but not specific. Lung volume may appear normal early, especially if the infant is strong enough to overdistend less affected regions, but ultimately it decreases before recovery begins. Positive airway pressure frequently obliterates these diagnostic criteria.

Pathology

Gross findings include atelectasis, patent ductus arteriosus, and cerebral hemorrhage. Histologically, peripheral air spaces are collapsed, and alveolar ducts, lined with hyaline membranes and necrotic

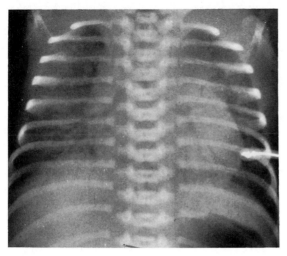

Figure 13–2. Hyaline membrane disease with typical reticulogranular appearance and air bronchogram.

epithelium, are distended. Pulmonary edema is prominent, with congested capillaries and distention of the interstitium and lymphatics with fluid.

Pathophysiology

Functional residual capacity of the lungs may be low from birth or may show a progressive decline over a few days. Dynamic compliance and specific compliance of the lung are significantly reduced. Nitrogen washout studies suggest that the distribution of ventilation in larger airways is remarkably even, but others consider the results to be consistent with a slow and a fast space model. Measurements of airway resistance have been normal, but these measurements reflect only the resistance in larger airways. Because the patency of small peripheral airways depends on the expansion of surrounding air spaces and the proximal spread of surfactant, peripheral resistance may be high in some regions of the lung and time constants may be prolonged. Indeed, airway closure with gas trapping has been observed experimentally. It has been observed that infants with more severe disease, destined to develop bronchopulmonary dysplasia, have significantly higher airway resistance than infants who make an uneventful recovery.

The $A-aD_{O_2}$ and right-to-left shunt while breathing 100 per cent oxygen are greatly increased, and it is commonly stated that large shunts at the foramen ovale and ductus arteriosus and in atelectatic lung constitute the major causes of severe hypoxemia. If true, increasing inspired oxygen would have little effect on arterial oxygen saturation, and oxygen therapy would be relatively ineffective. In fact, precipitous changes occur if inspired oxygen is reduced. These changes indicate the presence of an open, poorly ventilated compartment with extremely low Va/Q that produces variable hypoxic vasoconstriction and alterations in right-to-left shunt as the inspired oxygen changes. Because perfusion of this compartment makes only a small contribution to cardiac

output, measurements of $a-A_{DN_2}$ show only modest increase. On the other hand, measurements of $a-A_{DCO_2}$ and physiologic dead space are markedly increased. Minute ventilation is increased but alveolar ventilation is decreased, and because a large part of the lung is collapsed or poorly ventilated, most alveolar ventilation is directed to a relatively small compartment represented by the reduced functional residual capacity. Because this compartment cannot receive much perfusion, the $a-A_{DCO_2}$ is significantly increased. Measurements of pulmonary blood flow, utilizing the disappearance of gases that enter ventilated parts of the lung, confirm that perfusion is very low.

Surfactant

Analysis of purified lung lavage fluid with high surface activity gives an approximate estimate of surfactant composition. About 10 per cent is protein, and 90 per cent is lipid. Phospholipids represent 80 per cent of total surfactant lipid, and the remaining lipid is cholesterol or neutral fat. The major phospholipids are phosphatidylcholine (PC, 80 per cent) and phosphatidylglycerol (PG, 10 per cent), the rest being phosphatidylethanolamine, phosphatidylserine, lysolecithin, and sphingomyelin. Unlike surfactant in adults, surfactant in the newborn also contains significant phosphatidylinositol (PI). The level of saturation of fatty acids in PC, PG, and PI determines surface activity; at least 50 per cent of PC is desaturated (DSPC), and 30 to 60 per cent of PG and PI is desaturated, almost always with palmitic acid.

There are several types of surfactant protein: (1) SP-A, which has a relative molecular weight of 28,000; (2) SP-B, which is approximately 8000; and (3) SP-C, which is 5000. Much more is known about SP-A. Multiple isoforms are progressively larger than the basic molecule because of increasing glycosylation and may attain 30,000 to 40,000 relative molecular weight. The SP-A molecules are linked together by disulfide bonds to form large oligomers of greater than 300,000 relative molecular weight. SP-A has both hydrophilic and hydrophobic domains, whereas SP-B and SP-C are mainly hydrophobic. They all associate readily with lipids, but SP-A is water soluble and is removed in the process of lipid extraction.

Surfactant phospholipid molecules adsorb to the surface because they are hydrophilic at one end and hydrophobic at the other. The displacement of water molecules from the surface decreases the surface tension. When the surface is completely occupied by phospholipid molecules, the surface tension reaches so-called equilibrium. During exhalation, the surface is compressed. Less stable molecules, such as unsaturated PC and PG, are displaced from the surface, which therefore becomes enriched with DSPC. With continued exhalation, DSPC molecules tend to solidify and resist compression, so the surface tension becomes very low, approaching 0 dynes per cm. This decrease in surface tension prevents the lung saccules from collapsing at the end of expiration. During inhalation, unsaturated PC and PG return to the surface, the phospholipid mixture becomes more fluid, and it spreads rapidly over the surface as the interface tension returns to the equilibrium value of about 25 dynes per cm. Thus the function of unsaturated PC and PG is to increase the fluidity of DSPC and so accelerate spreading during inhalation. The function of surfactant protein is to increase the speed of adsorption to the surface, a function apparently shared by PG.

Etiology

Examination of pressure volume curves with air and saline in infants dying of HMD has established that there is surfactant insufficiency at the gas liquid interface of the lung. Minced lung tissue with unusually high surface tension, as measured by a Wilhelmy balance, is associated with reduced DSPC, but the amount of DSPC in lung mince far exceeds that theoretically required to form a stable alveolar surface. Infants with HMD may synthesize adequate DSPC, but they cannot make it function effectively as surfactant. There is controversy concerning the cause of this relative intracellular surfactant deficiency. One theory proposes acidosis and pulmonary vasoconstriction, as both have been shown to decrease surfactant. However, the occurrence of either phenomenon before the onset of HMD is poorly substantiated. The most widely accepted theory is that both cellular and alveolar surfactant deficiencies are developmental in origin and that birth occurs before the processes of surfactant synthesis, transport, secretion, and surface adsorption are adequately developed.

Synthesis of surfactant PC starts at 20 weeks in normal human gestation. By 24 weeks a large excess of surfactant as measured by the Wilhelmy balance technique is available in lung tissue; an even greater store is available by term. Surfactant phospholipids are synthesized in the microsomes of granular pneumocytes, transported through the Golgi apparatus where sorting and packaging occur, and stored as lamellar bodies. By a process of exocytosis, these lamellar bodies are later secreted along microtubules into the bulk phase of alveolar fluid, where they are transformed into tubular myelin structures, a process highly dependent on surfactant protein and calcium. These tubular myelin structures are ideally suited to rapid surface monolayer formation. Experimental evidence in fetal rabbits indicates that secretion of preformed lamellar bodies is rapid, but transport of surfactant phospholipid from microsomes takes longer.

Lamellar bodies are usually, but not always, difficult to find in infants dying of HMD, suggesting that intracellular packaging and transport may be the major problem. Others have suggested that lamellar bodies are plentiful, both intracellular and extracellular, but they can find no evidence for tubular myelin in infants dying of HMD, which might explain why lung mince surface tension was found to be high in the presence of seemingly adequate DSPC stores. The configuration of extracellular DSPC in HMD may not be appropriate for rapid surface adsorption.

After surface adsorption, surfactant is progressively desorbed from the surface and apparently is recycled by uptake into granular pneumocytes through a process of endocytosis, possibly mediated by surfactant proteins binding at specific receptor sites. The phospholipid is reincorporated in lamellar bodies and secreted again. It is not known if a disturbance of recycling may contribute to the etiology of HMD.

It has been suggested that surfactant function in infants with HMD may be inhibited by plasma proteins that leak into the airways, in particular a plasma protein of molecular weight 110,000 daltons. In experimental animals with surfactant insufficiency, considerable damage to the terminal airway epithelium occurs during spontaneous breathing or mechanical ventilation. Because the terminal air spaces cannot be adequately expanded, the conducting airways are overdistended. This distention tears off the epithelium, causing a considerable leakage of plasma. It may be of critical importance for the lungs to have adequate surfactant at the gas-liquid interface from the earliest possible moment after birth; otherwise acute lung injury may rapidly supervene.

Prenatal Prediction

The capacity to predict the occurrence of HMD before labor and delivery, utilizing measurement of secreted phospholipids in amniotic fluid, supports the notion that surfactant insufficiency has a developmental origin. Before birth, the surfactant system can be assessed in amniotic fluid, because some fetal lung fluid is not swallowed but enters the amniotic cavity. The most common material measured is lecithin (L), in particular DSPC, which is considered the major functional component of surfactant. The common procedure for isolating DSPC is precipitation in cold acetone and separation by thin-layer chromatography. Because changes in amniotic fluid volume may alter the concentration of DSPC, it is standardized to the concentration of sphingomyelin (S), which remains relatively constant throughout gestation and is expressed as the L/S ratio. There are problems in measuring this ratio if the amniotic fluid is stained with blood or meconium. In normal pregnancy, the L/S ratio follows a remarkably stable pattern, increasing slowly to 1.0 at 32 weeks (A 1 week), rising more rapidly to 2.0 at 35 weeks (A 1 week), and accelerating very rapidly thereafter, although exact values above 2.0 depend on whether the lecithin spot is measured by planimetry, densitometry, or phosphorus assay. In abnormal pregnancy, there is much wider scatter, reflecting conditions that accelerate or decelerate maturation. The ratio may reach 2.0 as early as 28 weeks or remain at 1.0 until term. The incidence of HMD is about 0.5 per cent for an L/S ratio of 2.0 or more and 100 per cent for an L/S ratio below 1.0; from 1.0 to 2.0 the incidence decreases until an acceptably low risk is achieved for an L/S ratio of 1.7. The L/S ratio represents the secretory activity of the lung, which is greatly accelerated at 35 weeks; however, because the appearance of secreted material in amniotic fluid is time dependent, the L/S ratio lags behind events in the fetal lung. A low L/S ratio near term may carry less risk because the lung is developing more rapidly.

Phosphatidylinositol (PI) in amniotic fluid increases progressively until 36 weeks and then decreases. At about this time, PG appears and increases until term. The appearance time of PG may be accelerated or delayed in the same way as lecithin. Absence of PG in the amniotic fluid of a diabetic mother with an L/S ratio between 2.0 and 3.0 suggests high risk. A test for surfactant function using amniotic fluid obtained from the mother or from the infant's stomach at birth (shake test) has proved a useful screen. Serial saline dilutions shaken with alcohol to exclude other surfactants from the surface are examined for bubble stability. A positive shake test result is associated with negligible risk, but a negative result is nonspecific, and an estimation of the L/S ratio should be performed.

After birth, the L/S measured in tracheal or pharyngeal aspirates increases further in infants without HMD but remains less than 2.0 in those with HMD until 48 to 72 hours after birth, when it does increase to above 2.0. Before birth or immediately after birth, PG is present in infants without HMD, but it does not appear in HMD infants until 48 to 72 hours of age. Recovery from HMD is also associated with an increase of PI in aspirated lung secretions.

Control of Lung Maturation

The rate of maturation of the surfactant system is influenced by many factors, and many researchers are interested in how it may be accelerated to prevent HMD. Thyroxine increases alveolar surfactant in fetal rabbits and adult rats, and the number of stored lamellar bodies is increased, but thyroxine does not increase tissue DSPC. Thyrotropin-releasing hormone stimulates secretion but not synthesis of surfactant. Infants with HMD have lower plasma thyroxine than control subjects, at birth and at 2 days of age. Estrogen in the form of estradiol-17b increases PC in both lung lavage fluid and lung tissue of fetal rabbits. Maternal administration of estrone accelerates the increase of L/S in amniotic fluid. Infants with HMD have lower cord levels and excrete less estriol in the first voided urine. Isoxsuprine and other beta-adrenergic agonists produce increased DSPC in lung tissue and lung lavage fluid of fetal rabbits. The evidence is inconclusive on whether infants of mothers treated with adrenergics for suppression of labor have a decreased incidence of HMD. Aminophylline increases the phospholipid

content of whole lung and alveolar lavage fluids. Cyclic AMP, probably increased by both isoxsuprine and aminophylline, has been shown to increase the production and secretion of lamellar bodies in adult rats. There is evidence that testosterone and insulin may delay surfactant maturation, possibly explaining the higher incidence of HMD in male and diabetic newborns.

Many experimental studies show that glucocorticoids increase lung tissue DSPC, lamellar body production, and surfactant secretion. Morphologic development of the lung is accelerated, and growth in cell number is reversibly reduced. Decreased amniotic fluid cortisol levels correlate well with the occurrence of HMD. Infants with HMD have lower cord cortisol levels, although the values are rapidly elevated with the onset of HMD, perhaps serving to accelerate postnatal maturation. In some animal species, a surge of cortisol secretion precedes the onset of labor, and infants born by cesarean section before labor have reduced cord cortisol levels and a high incidence of HMD. However, in the lamb, accelerated surfactant development significantly precedes increased cortisol secretion. In the human, maternal glucocorticoid administration increases the L/S ratio of amniotic fluid.

A number of clinical trials, most using maternal administration of betamethasone, 12 mg daily in two doses, have shown a significant reduction in the incidence and severity of HMD and in neonatal mortality, these effects being clearly demonstrated in both male and female newborns. Maternal glucocorticoid should probably not be given in severe hypertension of pregnancy, because the chance of late fetal death may be increased. The benefit of steroids may be seen as early as 26 weeks and can still be demonstrated as late as 34 weeks. At least 24 hours of steroid effect are necessary, and 48 hours are optimal. After 7 days, retreatment with betamethasone is required. The glucocorticoid levels in fetal blood are two or three times normal and are comparable to those seen during the course of HMD. Doubling the dose of maternal betamethasone produces no additional benefit. There has been no increased incidence of newborn infection with this therapy. Maternal glucocorticoids produce a further decrease in the incidence of HMD in infants of mothers with prolonged rupture of membranes, and the incidence of maternal infection is not significantly increased. The pituitary-adrenal axis has not been suppressed in newborn infants. Pharmacologic doses of glucocorticoid have been associated with cerebral dysfunction, retarded growth, and immune incompetence, but follow-up of infants given more physiologic doses of prenatal steroid for prevention of HMD has been very encouraging.

Conventional Treatment

It is important that fetal asphxia be avoided during delivery and that adequate resuscitation be performed at birth. Expansion of the lungs of small premature infants may be important in augmenting surfactant secretion. Because infants subjected to thermal stress have higher mortality, every effort should be made to maintain warmth in a neutral thermal environment to minimize metabolic activity. Enteral feeding and excessive manipulation should be avoided. Because urine output is initially low and infants are edematous, fluid is restricted during the first 2 days to 50 to 75 ml/kg/day, which may not prevent slight weight gain. Calories are provided in the form of 10 to 15 per cent glucose, which reduces excessive catabolism. Once fluids are liberalized, 100 ml/kg/day of 10 per cent glucose will further minimize catabolism, and 60 calories/kg/day with 2.5 per cent amino acids will produce a positive nitrogen balance. Oxygen transport is facilitated by a generous hemoglobin concentration, so the hematocrit is maintained above 40 per cent by infusions of packed red blood cells. Antibiotics are prescribed if the possibility of pneumonia cannot be excluded.

Warm humidified oxygen is initially administered by hood in concentrations sufficient to relieve central cyanosis. Arterial P_{O_2} measurements are made using samples collected from indwelling umbilical, radial, or tibial artery catheters, and the value is maintained between 50 and 70 mm Hg. It is important when sampling below a potential right-to-left ductal shunt to avoid exceeding this range, as retinal vasoconstriction may occur above 100 mm Hg. Routine use of transcutaneous P_{O_2} electrodes and pulse oximeters is immensely valuable in making fine adjustments to oxygen therapy. A single controlled trial has shown that mortality in neonates who weigh more than 1500 g is reduced by CDAP. The results of several trials show that early introduction of CDAP, at the stage when only 50-per cent oxygen is required, reduces the need for oxygen exposure and mechanical ventilation below that needed if one waits until 100-per cent oxygen is required. As breathing causes consumption of surfactant, the substance must be replaced continuously, but its consumption may be reduced by using CDAP, which prevents collapse and overdistention of the surface film. Because CDAP does not reduce the need for mechanical ventilation in neonates under 1500 g, it is often omitted. In infants over 2500 g at birth, the prognosis is usually good, especially if HMD is slowly progressive, and CDAP may be delayed until 75 to 100 per cent oxygen is required. The potential danger is overdistention, which may produce hypotension, hypercarbia, and pneumothorax. The usual practice is to initiate CDAP at 5 cm H_2O and increase the pressure toward 10 cm H_2O as compliance decreases and the oxygen requirement reaches 100 per cent. In larger infants, a pressure of 10 to 15 cm H_2O may be tried. During recovery, CDAP should be reduced as the oxygen requirement decreases.

Mechanical Ventilation

Mechanical ventilation is initiated for significant apnea, hypercarbia (45 mm Hg for infants with birth weight below 1500 g, 50 to 60 mm Hg for infants above 1500 g), and excessive oxygen requirement (50 per cent for infants with birth weight below 1500 g, 75 to 100 per cent for infants above 1500 g). Some institutions initiate mechanical ventilation in the delivery room for all infants whose birth weight is less than 1250 g, because such ventilation is thought to reduce the incidence of cerebral hemorrhage, a complication strongly associated with HMD. By ensuring adequate lung expansion, it may also favorably affect the development of HMD. The aim of mechanical ventilation is to relieve significant hypoxemia, hypercarbia, and acidosis without damaging the lungs and without embarrassing the circulation.

Most medical centers currently use time-cycled, positive pressure ventilators, generally limiting pressure to between 20 and 40 cm H_2O and positive end-expiratory pressure (PEEP) to between 4 and 8 cm H_2O. These ventilators incorporate a continuous gas flow, so spontaneous breaths are not loaded and infants may breathe spontaneously in the intermittent mandatory ventilation mode. There are several schools of thought on the use of mechanical ventilators. Many clinicians use a rate of 20 to 30 breaths per minute (bpm) and a 1.0 sec inspiration time, which allows considerable spontaneous breathing to contribute to the overall gas exchange. Others start with a rate of 60 bpm and a 0.2 sec inspiration time, and still others start with an intermediate rate of 40 bpm and an inspiration time of 0.5 sec. Arterial oxygenation is improved by increasing the mean airway pressure. The most efficient way to do this, in terms of arterial P_{O_2} and mean airway pressure, is by increasing the PEEP; increasing the inspiration time is clearly the least efficient method. Hypercarbia is controlled by the rate and tidal volume. In general, it follows that for constant alveolar ventilation, the tidal volume may be minimized at high r rates. The arterial P_{CO_2} is improved by increasing the peak pressure or decreasing PEEP. However, if the rate is initially slow, it is reasonable to first try a small increase.

There are no controlled trials demonstrating the superiority of any method. Those employing methods with long inspiration times have demonstrated improved oxygenation at lower peak pressures and claim that the incidence of bronchopulmonary dysplasia (BPD) is reduced. Those using methods with short inspiration times believe that the incidence of pulmonary air leaks is reduced, and the incidence of BPD is similar. In a single controlled trial, the use of an inspiration time of 0.5 sec and a rate of 60 bpm was associated with a reduced incidence of pulmonary air leaks when compared with an inspiration time of 1.0 sec and a rate of 30 bpm, but the incidence of death and BPD was unchanged.

The overall time constant in HMD is short, between 0.05 and 0.10 sec, which means that a long inspiration time is not necessary to achieve an adequate tidal volume. It also means that exhalation, at least initially, is readily accomplished in less than 0.5 sec without gas trapping. However, more diseased regions of the lung may have longer time constants because of destructive lesions of the terminal conducting airways. At higher rates, gas trapping may occur in more diseased parts of the lung, a selective recruitment that could be considered desirable, and may explain why oxygenation often improves at higher rates. However, as time passes and the larger airways are increasingly damaged, and as compliance improves, the general time constant may be more prolonged, and undesirable gas trapping may occur at higher rates of ventilation. The rate must be slowed after the acute phase of the disease has passed.

Many of the problems associated with mechanical ventilation are caused by general or regional overdistention, with resultant hypercarbia, circulatory depression, and pulmonary air leaks. Overdistention may be caused by excessive peak pressure, prolonged inspiration time, high PEEP, and gas trapping with high rates. At high volumes, lung compliance is significantly reduced, and ventilation is impaired. It is the more distensible airways that rupture and cause air leaks, not the atelectatic regions of the lung. Despite high recoil forces in HMD, approximately 40 to 60 per cent of airway pressure is transmitted to the circulation, especially during recovery, with the result that high pressures may impede the circulation and decrease oxygen transport. In small premature infants, there are no alveoli, so the terminal air sacs are tubular. According to the Laplace relationship, at any given radius and surface tension, recoil in a tube is only half that in a sphere. Surfactant insufficiency in small premature infants may allow considerable transmission of airway pressure to the circulation. Because of all these problems, it may sometimes be wise to allow only marginal blood gas levels, such as arterial P_{O_2} 35 to 40 mm Hg and hypercarbia with pH 7.20, rather than to raise the peak pressure or PEEP too high.

Muscle paralysis with pancuronium reduces the incidence of pneumothorax and smooths erratic fluctuation of blood gases and systemic blood pressure during mechanical ventilation. If a patient takes a breath at the same time as the ventilator, excessive lung distention may cause lung rupture. The fact that peak pressure must sometimes be raised does not mean overdistention of the lung, because pleural pressure is less negative under conditions of paralysis. Despite the rise in pleural pressure, it is claimed that paralysis may also reduce the incidence of brain hemorrhage. As a further most decided benefit, a controlled trial has shown that the use of paralysis reduces the incidence of bronchopulmonary dysplasia.

There is no agreement on how to wean the mechanical ventilator. Considering the increased risk of pulmonary air leaks, it seems reasonable to first reduce the peak pressure to 20 to 25 cm H_2O and then to adjust the PEEP to 3 cm H_2O. This approach places less emphasis on oxygen as a source of lung injury and suggests that oxygen should only be ad-justed when the mechanical ventilator settings have reached the safest possible settings consistent with the desired level of gas exchange. However, if reductions of peak pressure cause serious deterioration in the arterial P_{O_2}, it may prove safer to slowly wean the patient from oxygen for a few hours before trying again. After peak pressures have been obtained, and inspired oxygen reaches 40 per cent, it seems reasonable to adjust the rate, mindful that gradual lengthening of a short inspiration time to about 0.5 sec may be necessary as lung compliance improves and the time constant lengthens. There is reasonable evidence that theophylline, by stimulating respiratory drive or combating diaphragmatic fatigue, may significantly aid the weaning process. Because small endotracheal tubes have high resistance, it may be better to forgo a trial of endotracheal CDAP and change to hood oxygen or nasal CDAP when a slow rate of 10 bpm is tolerated.

Surfactant Replacement Therapy

Although early attempts at surfactant replacement met with failure, later results for small clinical trials are most encouraging. Two broad strategies are being investigated: (1) prophylaxis at birth in small premature infants at high risk for HMD and (2) treatment of infants with established HMD. Surfactant should be given by direct tracheal instillation under conditions of adequate PEEP to ensure appropriate distribution to surfactant-deficient regions of the lung. Although the lung surface requires only 3 mg/kg surfactant phospholipid, the dose should be 100 mg/kg to overcome the effects of destruction by macrophages and inhibition by plasma proteins.

Several different types of preparation are available, but none has obtained official approval. One approach is to lavage bovine lungs and extract lipid from the lavage fluid. Another is to mince bovine lungs and enrich the lipid extract with synthetic DSPC. A further preparation is derived from human amniotic fluid by sucrose gradient centrifugation. Finally, complete synthetic preparations have been made with DSPC and a fluidizing additive, PG, or hexadecanol. Preparations with surfactant protein added are under development.

The prophylactic approach under controlled conditions has shown a reduction in the incidence of HMD, but small premature infants have many other problems unrelated to surfactant insufficiency, and larger controlled trials have not yet established a reduction in the incidence of death or BPD. Controlled trials in established HMD have shown a significant improvement in oxygen requirements and to a lesser extent in ventilator requirements. Radiologic improvement has been apparent, and the incidence of pulmonary air leaks has been reduced. A few studies have shown a reduction in the incidence of BPD, but most have not, and it is very difficult to show a change of mortality when the mortality rate is already low. A large multicenter collaborative trial of Surfactant TA, using a single dose in the first 24 hours of life, showed a big improvement in the first 3 days, but no differences between treated and control infants could be discerned at 7 and 28 days of age. It is apparent that the effect is often short lived, presumably because of inhibition by plasma proteins, and that in some patients multiple doses are required. There are large trials under way that it is hoped will demonstrate a reduction in the incidence of BPD, which would have considerable long-term medical and economic benefits.

PATENT DUCTUS ARTERIOSUS

In the term infant, the ductus closes 1 to 3 days after birth, but in the preterm infant, especially one who is less mature, has HMD, or is on a mechanical ventilator, the ductus may remain open for weeks or months. The stimulus for closure is increased arterial P_{O_2}, but before birth and in premature infants for a few weeks after birth, patency may be maintained by local production of prostaglandin E, especially in the presence of episodic hypoxemia. After birth, in infants with high pulmonary vascular resistance, there is a small right-to-left shunt, but this shunt soon becomes bidirectional or left-to-right before ductal closure. Shunt size depends on the degree of ductal constriction, the cardiac output, and the balance between pulmonary and systemic vascular resistance.

Clinical Picture

There are two broad groups of patients with patent ductus arteriosus (PDA): (1) small premature infants without lung disease and (2) premature infants with lung disease who are on mechanical ventilation and in whom signs of PDA are superimposed. The shunt causes tachycardia, hyperdynamic precordium, accentuated pulse pressure, and, in many but not all cases, a late systolic or continuous murmur below the left clavicle. There is pulmonary congestion and later cardiomegaly consistent with left ventricular failure (Fig. 13–3). The respiration rate is increased, and rales are often heard. Because pulmonary compliance is reduced and airway resistance is increased by interstitial fluid, arterial P_{O_2} falls, hypercarbia develops, and the oxygen or ventilator requirement increases. There may be metabolic acidosis and reduced coronary, cerebral, mesenteric, renal, or peripheral perfusion, manifested by bradycardia, apnea, feeding intolerance, renal failure, or poor capillary filling. Liver enlargement suggests a progression to right heart failure, in which case specific signs disappear and confusion with septicemia or cerebral hemorrhage may occur. A direct relationship exists between closure of the ductus and the ability to wean patients off the ventilator; those with PDA require prolonged mechanical ventilation and incur a high risk for bronchopulmonary dysplasia.

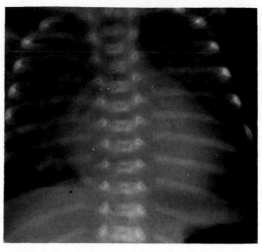

Figure 13–3. Patent ductus arteriosus without underlying lung disorder. Note cardiomegaly and increased pulmonary vascular markings.

Investigations

The left-to-right shunt may be semiquantitatively evaluated by radiopaque dye injection into the descending aorta through an indwelling umbilical arterial catheter, radionuclide scan after peripheral venous injection, aortic injection pulmonary artery echo contrast with aerated saline, two-dimensional echocardiography, pulsed Doppler ultrasonography, and other methods. Retrograde flow in the descending aorta normally occurs only early in diastole, so the finding on pulsed Doppler ultrasonography that retrograde flow extends throughout diastole may be very significant for the diagnosis of PDA. Similarly, diastolic forward flow in the main pulmonary artery may be recognized by this technique. Enlargement of the left atrium and ventricle standardized for weight, with the ratio of left atrial to aortic dimension greater than 1.2, as measured by M-mode echocardiography, is the most widely used method, but the sensitivity of this method in fluid-restricted infants leaves much to be desired.

Pulmonary Physiology

It can be argued that the magnitude of a left-to-right shunt is not as important as its effect on pulmonary function in small premature infants. Pulmonary vascular resistance increases with gestation, and small premature infants have a lower resistance and a larger physiologic decrease after birth, so a left-to-right ductal shunt is almost universal, and pulmonary edema is a frequent early complication.

There are many reasons for this complication. Surfactant insufficiency may cause lung interstitial pressure to be more negative. The colloid oncotic pressure of premature infants with HMD is reduced. Because resistance arterioles are poorly muscularized, pulmonary capillaries are exposed to greater hydrostatic pressure. Increased pulmonary blood flow may readily overload the left ventricle, which is less compliant and functions less efficiently in early gestation, thus increasing left atrial pressure. High blood flow also increases capillary hydrostatic pressure because in the newborn the capillary circulation is normally fully recruited, and capillary pressures cannot be protected by recruitment of additional vascular channels as in the adult. The net balance of these phenomena, according to the Starling relationship, would provide increased transcapillary filtration of fluid and may explain early pulmonary edema in the absence of a large shunt. There is evidence that infants given more than 125 ml/kg/day of fluid have a high incidence of symptomatic PDA.

Treatment

Conservative management consists of restricting fluids to between 75 and 125 ml/kg/day and administering furosemide, 1 mg/kg twice daily. Because myocardial contractility is increased in PDA, many physicians use digoxin only in advanced cases in which echocardiographic shortening fractions are clearly abnormal. Oxygen supplementation is given to maintain arterial P_{O_2} between 50 and 90 mm Hg; some physicians favor relative hyperoxemia to encourage ductal closure, but care is required to avoid exceeding 100 mm Hg. The use of CDAP (5 cm H_2O) is beneficial, and mechanical ventilation is indicated for recurrent apnea, hypercarbia, and inspired oxygen exceeding 50 per cent, particularly as prolonged exposure may predispose the patient to pulmonary oxygen toxicity.

If after 2 or 3 days of medical management, an infant cannot be weaned from the ventilator, it is reasonable to attempt pharmacologic closure of the ductus with indomethacin, 0.2 mg/kg intravenously every 12 to 24 hours for a total of three to five doses, if necessary. This drug presumably inhibits local synthesis of prostaglandin E. Before indomethacin is given, the serum creatinine and sodium levels and the platelet count should be evaluated; the drug commonly causes decreased renal perfusion and urine flow, fluid retention with hyponatremia, and decreased platelet function. Gastrointestinal bleeding has occurred, and a possible but unconfirmed danger is extension of a pre-existing cerebral hemorrhage.

In those weighing less than 1250 g and receiving mechanical ventilation, indomethacin in the first few days of life may produce an abrupt decrease in airway pressure and inspired oxygen requirement, suggesting an important role for PDA in primary lung disease. There is good evidence in small premature infants that if the ductus is not closed by the age of 3 days, it is not likely to close in the next few weeks, by which time considerable lung injury may occur. Early closure using indomethacin on the third or fourth day of life may reduce the incidence of bronchopulmonary dysplasia. This aggressive approach is favored for all infants under 1250 g on mechanical ventilation.

Indomethacin is most successful when used in the first 1 to 2 weeks, for which ductus closure rates of 50 to 90 per cent are reported. Unfortunately, closure is not always permanent, and second courses of the drug may be necessary. Many infants have an excellent constrictive response to indomethacin, but even after two courses the ductus does not close permanently. Permanent closure is a particular problem in infants under 750 g, presumably because of persistent production of prostaglandin E. The drug is not effective in infants beyond 36 weeks gestation, because by then prostaglandin E effects have greatly diminished. The half-life of indomethacin is prolonged, being 24 hours in the first week, but it decreases with time. Clinical failures have been attributed to peak serum levels under 1000 ng/ml or to rapid clearance with trough serum levels below 250 ng/ml. Because of these problems, many clinicians favor initial surgical closure, which reduces the time required for mechanical ventilation and length of hospital stay, but does not seem to influence the incidence of bronchopulmonary dysplasia, perhaps because surgery is undertaken too late. Early surgical closure appears to be relatively safe without predisposition to cerebral hemorrhage. A common complication of surgery is reversible paralysis of the left hemidiaphragm, which delays weaning from the ventilator.

CONGENITAL BACTERIAL PNEUMONIA

Congenital pneumonia may be acquired by the ascending route after production of chorioamnionitis, by aspiration of vaginal bacteria during delivery, or by transplacental spread. The incidence of congenital pneumonia is about five per thousand live births.

Postamnionitis Pneumonia

Inflammation begins at the os cervix in the amnion and spreads to the chorionic plate. The infiltrating white blood cells and those in amniotic fluid are of maternal origin, but later a fetal reaction occurs in the cord. Although chorioamnionitis is more frequent with increasing duration of membrane rupture, it is well established that chorioamnionitis may occur in the presence of intact fetal membranes. Amnionitis is much more frequent in premature gestations because of a developmental insufficiency of bacteriostatic factors in amniotic fluid. The longer the duration of labor, the greater the incidence of amnionitis. Frequent digital examinations are a predisposing factor. The condition appears to be more common in black, poor, and malnourished women and is also related to sexual activity. Amnionitis may be more common with incompetent cervix and in mothers with a urinary tract infection within 2 weeks of delivery.

Infants with postamnionitis pneumonia have histologic evidence of aspiration, namely, the presence of squamous cells in the terminal airways, and the clinical record commonly suggests fetal asphyxia. Although amnionitis has been ascribed to asphyxia, acidosis, and the presence of meconium without infection, this relationship has not been reproduced experimentally, whereas injected bacteria always cause an identical inflammatory response in the placenta and lungs of fetal rabbits. In most cases of amnionitis, bacteria can be isolated if appropriate cultures are made. However, not all the isolated organisms cause pneumonia in the fetus, e.g., mycoplasmas appear to be an important cause of amnionitis but not of intrauterine pneumonia. It has been suggested that some cases of pneumonia represent passive aspiration of amniotic fluid laden with maternal leukocytes, rather than true lung inflammation. The common organisms causing amnionitis and postamnionitis pneumonia are *Escherichia coli* and group B beta-hemolytic streptococci (GBS), but enterococcus, *Hemophilus influenzae*, pneumococcus, group D streptococci, *Listeria*, and anaerobes have also been implicated. There is a good correlation between bacteria causing amnionitis and vaginal bacterial flora. The mother may have abdominal tenderness, fever, leukocytosis, or foul-smelling cervical effluent, and there may be fetal tachycardia. Many infants with pneumonia are premature, often with birth weights of less than 1500 g, presumably because amnionitis is a very important cause of premature labor. The clinical picture is that of asphyxial depression at birth followed by immediate respiratory distress.

Transplacental Pneumonia

Transplacental pneumonia, which is comparatively rare, has been reported in *Listeria,* syphilis, tularemia, and others. The mother has evidence of a preceding systemic infection but no evidence of amnionitis.

Transnatal Pneumonia

In recent years, GBS has been an important cause of congenital pneumonia due to aspiration of vaginal bacteria. Between 5 and 25 per cent of GBS culture results from gravid women are positive. The newborns of these women are invariably colonized with GBS also. In transnatal pneumonia there is no evidence of preceding amnionitis or prolonged membrane rupture and no evidence of a relevant maternal systemic infection. Usually a latent interval of up to 24 hours occurs during which the infant appears normal, and then problems arise: sudden apnea, progressive respiratory distress, or the beginning of circulatory failure. Infants may have difficulty maintaining temperature, although fever sometimes appears in the more mature. Other infants are lethargic, have early jaundice, and feed poorly. A similar clinical picture and mode of infection may be seen with transnatal pneumonia due to listeriosis.

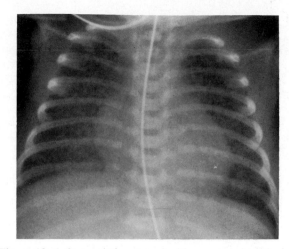

Figure 13–4. Congenital postamnionitis pneumonia with abnormal neutrophil count and group B streptococcus identified by blood culture. Radiograph demonstrates reticulogranular appearance.

Diagnosis

The diagnosis of congenital pneumonia depends on a high index of suspicion. Radiologically, there are coarse densities, and lung volume is normal or increased, or there may be a diffuse reticular nodular appearance, but frequently there is a reticular granular pattern resembling HMD (Figs. 13–4, 13–5, and 13–6). Small pleural effusions may be present, especially with GBS. The densities may not be evident at first but gradually evolve over a few hours or days. The presence of neutrophils (5 per high-power field) on smears of gastric aspirate suggests amnionitis but not necessarily pneumonia. Organisms in the gastric aspirate indicate vaginal colonization, which in the case of GBS may suggest a higher than usual risk of pneumonia. The peripheral white blood cell count is frequently useful, especially if repeated serially at intervals of 6 to 12 hours.

The infant with congenital pneumonia often has

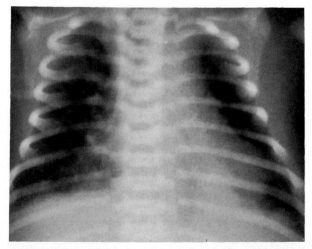

Figure 13–5. Congenital transnatal pneumonia with abnormal neutrophil count and group B streptococcus identified by blood culture. Radiograph shows coarse densities in the right lung field and probably behind the heart.

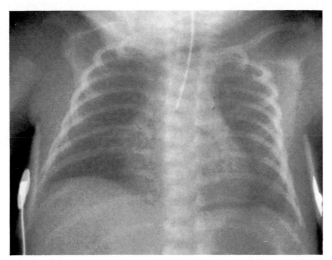

Figure 13–6. Congenital postamnionitis pneumonia due to *Escherichia coli*, which was growing in the infant's tracheal aspirate and blood and was present in the mother's urine and cervix. Radiograph demonstrates diffuse reticular nodular density.

an abnormally high or low neutrophil count in relation to age, and a ratio of immature neutrophils to total neutrophils that exceeds 0.2:1.0 should arouse suspicion. In the case of GBS, rapid test examinations for antigen with counterimmune electrophoresis or latex agglutination in urine or blood give excellent diagnostic results. If the infant must be mechanically ventilated, a requirement for only low peak pressures, especially in larger premature infants, has been suggested as evidence for pneumonia. Examination of tracheal aspirate samples for white blood cells and bacteria in the first 8 hours of life may be helpful, although bacterial contamination from the upper airway is common. The blood culture will be negative without systemic bacterial invasion, but because the premature newborn is known for an inability to localize serious infections, the blood culture is usually positive. In most cases, while awaiting the results of blood culture, the diagnosis must be presumptive and treatment must be started as soon as possible.

Treatment

Many cases respond to appropriate antibiotics, usually ampicillin and gentamicin or kanamycin for 10 to 14 days, and supportive measures. The more acute cases, despite antibiotic sensitivity, follow a rapid downhill course with endotoxic shock and persistent pulmonary hypertension. Because GBS are relatively resistant, the usual dosage of ampicillin should be increased; penicillin may be preferred, and gentamicin appears synergistic. The mortality rate in congenital pneumonia may exceed 50 per cent, which has focused attention on prevention, especially of GBS infection. Colonized mothers treated with penicillin are recolonized when antibiotics are stopped, especially if their partners, who may be urethral carriers, are not treated. Prescribing drugs for infants of all colonized mothers would represent an enormous expenditure, and the incidence of antibiotic resistant infection is known to be increased. Treatment of colonized mothers during labor seems to be a promising approach. It may not be necessary to treat infants whose mothers have GBS antibodies. Induction of maternal antibodies with vaccine may be possible in the future.

MECONIUM ASPIRATION PNEUMONIA

The fetus may pass meconium for several reasons. One theory is that during an episode of asphyxia, mesenteric vasoconstriction may cause hyperperistalsis, sphincter relaxation, and meconium passage, but the fetal acid-base disorder will be significant only if the episode is prolonged. Compression of the cord may initiate a vagal response leading to meconium passage, but only persistent or recurrent compression would cause significant acidemia.

Other researchers believe that a mature fetus may pass meconium spontaneously. During breech delivery, mechanical factors, as well as cord compression or asphyxia, may cause defecation. Thus although many meconium-stained infants have been asphyxiated in utero, many are not, the correlation with fetal acidemia is not always close, and many are not depressed at birth. The frequency of meconium staining is about 12 per cent of all deliveries, but only about 2 per cent of such infants develop meconium aspiration pneumonia (MAP). The condition is uncommon before 38 weeks, presumably because rectal maturation is important for its development. It is very common with acute fetal malnutrition, especially in postmature infants beyond 42 weeks, and it is also common among those with chronic fetal malnutrition who are small for gestational age.

Production of Pneumonia

An episode of asphyxia is very important in the production of MAP, because only deep gasping with severe hypoxemia before terminal apnea could be expected to move sufficient meconium into the trachea. The airways are filled with fetal lung fluid, and the constant flow up the trachea, the usual closed state of the glottis, and chest compression during vaginal delivery protect the lung from deeper aspiration before birth. In most cases, aspiration of meconium into the peripheral airways is a postnatal event. Release of chest compression at birth may move meconium deeper, and spontaneous breathing or mechanical ventilation would cause further peripheral dissemination. Suctioning the nasopharynx with perineal presentation of the face and suctioning the trachea immediately at delivery reduce the incidence of MAP. Absence of meconium in the larynx does not exclude the possibility of tracheal meconium, especially if the pharynx has been suctioned. Meconium that is well mixed with amniotic fluid to a uniform thin consistency does not cause a problem, and meconium passed late during breech delivery does not contact the newborn's upper airway.

Only if particulate meconium is mixed with amniotic fluid should tracheal suctioning be performed. Because standard suction catheters are too narrow for meconium removal, the usual technique is to pass an endotracheal tube and apply suction during withdrawal, repeating until meconium return is minimal. It is not beneficial to lavage the lungs, and this procedure may even cause deterioration. Sometimes bradycardia may seem to indicate immediate bag ventilation, but there is always time for one suctioning, which clears the airway and allows spontaneous inspiration or accelerates the response to bag ventilation. With relief of bradycardia, further suctioning should be performed. There is evidence that vigorous infants with normal Apgar scores and regular breathing do not require tracheal suctioning, because the trachea is unlikely to contain meconium, but pharyngeal suctioning during delivery is still advised. Infants from whom tracheal meconium was suctioned should be given a humidified oxygen mixture to breathe and chest physical therapy. Promotion of coughing by pharyngeal suction facilitates removal of residual meconium. The stomach should be emptied of meconium in case vomiting occurs.

Pathophysiology

Meconium aspiration into peripheral airways causes partial or complete obstruction with regional atelectasis and gas trapping. Radiologically, coarse densities are interspersed with areas of hyperinflation (Fig. 13–7). The functional residual capacity is usually normal and is only increased in those with less severe disease, but in severe cases with predominant atelectasis it is decreased. The dynamic compliance of the lung is decreased, and airway resistance is high. There may be lobar atelectasis or emphysema. Peripheral migration of meconium and a secondary irritant bronchopneumonia causes pulmonary func-

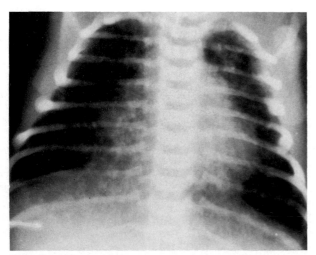

Figure 13–7. Meconium aspiration pneumonia with basal trapped gas.

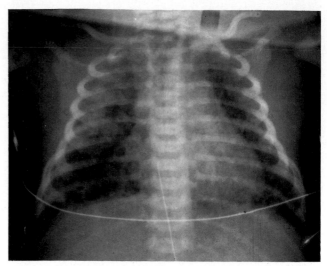

Figure 13–8. Meconium aspiration pneumonia with diffuse coarse densities, managed with continuous distending airway pressure alone. Radiologic clearing was delayed, and tachypnea lasted 3 weeks.

tion to deteriorate over the first 24 to 48 hours. Experimental evidence indicates that surfactant function may be impaired, contributing to the atelectasis. Because of regional overinflation, there is a substantial risk of pulmonary air leaks, which is even higher with mechanical ventilation. Many infants can achieve normal oxygen saturation with 100-per cent oxygen, suggesting that ventilation-perfusion inequality is the principal cause of hypoxemia in room air. Many infants have significant hypercarbia, and measurements of $a\text{-}AD_{CO_2}$ and $a\text{-}AD_{N_2}$ are increased, but less affected infants are able to lower arterial P_{CO_2} into the normal range. In severe cases, persistent pulmonary hypertension and large right-to-left shunts are found.

Clinical Course

Because infants with MAP have been asphyxiated, postasphyxial pulmonary edema plays a prominent role, and many have signs of postanoxic encephalopathy. Central respiratory depression may contribute to the blood gas disorder, and muscle hypertonicity and seizures may interfere with ventilation later. In many the cause of death is related more to cerebral damage than to lung disease. Meconium aspiration pneumonia is unlikely to resolve rapidly, so severe respiratory symptoms last 3 to 5 days, the findings on radiograph take 2 weeks or more to resolve, and tachypnea may last for a month. In those with a short course and rapid clearing on radiology it is likely that the symptoms are due to retained pulmonary fluid and not meconium.

Treatment

If the infant is severely asphyxiated at birth and is not subsequently vigorous in the delivery room, mechanical ventilation should be continued after initial resuscitation. Otherwise it is best to avoid mechanical ventilation. Infants should be treated with liberal amounts of oxygen, whether by hood or by ventilator. Because the risk of persistent pulmonary hypertension is high and the risk of retinopathy is low, arterial P_{O_2} may be tolerated at a level higher than that recommended for HMD, e.g., 90 to 100 mm Hg. Alkali infusions are often necessary to maintain the pH above 7.20. Hypotension in severely asphyxiated infants may require dopamine therapy. Fluid should be restricted to minimize the development of pulmonary and cerebral edema. Although many infants are treated with antibiotics, there is no evidence of benefit, despite observations that a mixture of meconium and amniotic fluid is a good culture medium. A controlled trial has shown that steroids are not efficacious. Nasal CDAP may be useful in maintaining the patency of peripheral airways, but caution should be exercised because excessive CDAP may readily produce overdistention, arterial oxygen desaturation, and hypercarbia. Mechanical ventilation is instituted if necessary for recurrent apnea, unacceptable hypercarbia (P_{CO_2} 70 mm Hg with pH below 7.2), and severe hypoxemia (P_{O_2} under 50 mm Hg) in 100 per cent oxygen. The PEEP may improve gas exchange by preventing airway closure, but the risk of overdistention is high.

PERSISTENT PULMONARY HYPERTENSION

After birth, the normal high fetal pulmonary vascular resistance falls with expansion and oxygenation of the lungs. Sometimes this reduction does not occur, or after initially falling the resistance increases subsequently. Because pulmonary blood flow is inadequate and the right-to-left shunt at the foramen ovale is large, infants with this condition cannot be well oxygenated; they appear cyanosed and usually have significant respiratory distress. The problem may occur transiently in hypothermia, hypoglycemia, hypovolemia, acidemia, or polycythemia, all of which are common in newborn infants. Transient pulmonary hypertension responds well to appropriate treatment of the underlying condition.

There is, however, a group of infants in whom the problem persists, some without obvious lung disease and others with postasphyxial pulmonary edema, congenital pneumonia, MAP, or pulmonary hypoplasia. Those without obvious lung disease are considered to have primary PPH, and the others mentioned are thought to have secondary PPH. In all these patients, arterial desaturation is more profound than can be explained by the lung disease. The second heart sound is accentuated, there is often a tricuspid insufficiency murmur, and the liver may enlarge. The systemic cardiac output is impaired in PPH for several reasons. Reduced pulmonary blood flow means that left ventricular preload is decreased. In addition, dilation of the right ventricle with shift of

the interventricular septum impinges on the left ventricle, further reducing the preload. Right ventricular hypertension also reduces diastolic coronary perfusion, and the resulting myocardial ischemia reduces cardiac output even more. If the infant has been severely asphyxiated, heart failure may supervene. The magnitude of the right-to-left shunt at the foramen ovale may depend more on the impairment of right ventricular function than on high pulmonary vascular resistance.

Radiographically, the lungs may appear undervascularized or hyperinflated, there may be changes consistent with pulmonary edema or pneumonia, and the heart may be enlarged (Fig. 13–9). The electrocardiogram (ECG) shows excessive right ventricular dominance. Structural heart disease should be excluded by echocardiography, which facilitates a simultaneous estimate of myocardial contractility. Systolic time intervals reflecting pulmonary vascular resistance should be evaluated, but these same intervals also reflect myocardial insufficiency. Two-dimensional echocardiography is particularly useful for demonstrating the large right-to-left shunt at the foramen ovale, with dilation of the right atrium and ventricle and deviation of the atrial septum into the left heart. If the ductus remains open, there may be a discrepancy between aortic blood oxygen saturation above and below the ductus, suggesting a right-to-left shunt. The absence of such a discrepancy does not exclude PPH, in which the most significant shunt occurs at the foramen ovale. Pulmonary venous blood obtained through an umbilical vein catheter is relatively well saturated, especially in the primary form of the condition without accompanying lung disease. In some cases cardiac catheterization must be performed to rule out total anomalous pulmonary venous return and other lesions, but echocardiography now makes this uncommon. In PPH systemic levels of pressure are measured in the pulmonary artery, which decline as the patient's condition improves. It has been observed that as systemic pressure exceeds

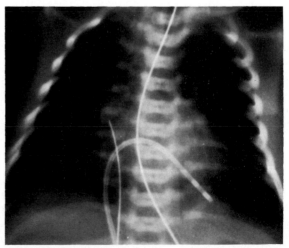

Figure 13–9. Persistent pulmonary hypertension with decreased vasculature.

pulmonary pressure there is a significant reduction of right-to-left shunt.

Pathogenesis

At least three major types have been recognized. In the first type, there is a functional persistent pulmonary vasoconstriction, but no structural changes in the pulmonary arteries are apparent. The cause is poorly understood, but fetal asphyxia may be a prominent feature of the recent clinical history. Hypoxia and acidosis both cause pulmonary vasoconstriction, and their effects are synergistic. An imbalance may exist between the effects of vasoconstrictors, such as thromboxane and leukotriene, and the effects of vasodilators, such as prostacyclin, prostaglandin, and bradykinin. The lung lavage fluid of patients with PPH is rich in leukotrienes. Thrombocytopenia is commonly reported and suggests that platelet-derived mediators, such as thromboxane, are important. In extreme cases of vasoconstriction, there is extensive microthrombosis of the pulmonary circulation, in which case a satisfactory response to treatment is unlikely. Infants with severe infection, commonly group B streptococcal disease, may have similar pulmonary vasoconstriction, probably caused by endotoxin and local mediators.

In the second type, PPH may result from an abnormal pulmonary artery medial muscle hypertrophy, with or without abnormal extension of medial muscle into acinar arteries, which are normally nonmuscular in the newborn infant. Animal models suggest that infants with chronic uteroplacental insufficiency over a period of 1 to 2 weeks may have this problem. Medial muscle hypertrophy and extension are commonly seen in infants dying of MAP, strongly suggesting the presence of chronic as well as acute fetal hypoxia. There is a high baseline pulmonary vascular resistance, and pulmonary vasoconstriction in response to acute stress may be exaggerated. Excessive muscle hypertrophy has also been described in infants of mothers with chronic salicylate ingestion. Closure of the fetal ductus arteriosus causes excessive perfusion of the fetal lungs at high vascular pressures, with resultant muscle hypertrophy.

In the third type of PPH associated with pulmonary hypoplasia, there is a reduction in the pulmonary vascular bed as the major cause of high pulmonary vascular resistance. This condition may be seen in infants with congenital diaphragmatic hernia and in infants with prolonged leakage of amniotic fluid. These infants may also have an element of medial muscle hypertrophy and complicating pulmonary vasoconstriction. Those with congenital diaphragmatic hernia who oxygenate poorly in the immediate postoperative period have severe muscle hypertrophy and extension, whereas those who oxygenate well during an initial "honeymoon" period and only deteriorate after 6 to 12 hours have predominant pulmonary vasoconstriction with less marked muscle hypertrophy.

Treatment

Most patients require mechanical ventilation with high concentrations of oxygen for correction of hypoxemia. Unless there is significant lung disease, PEEP is poorly tolerated and should be maintained at levels of 0 to 3 cm H_2O to avoid overdistending the lung and compromising the pulmonary circulation. Attempts to reduce inspired oxygen cause unexpectedly large reductions in oxygen saturation, presumably because of the exquisite sensitivity of pulmonary vessels to alveolar oxygen. Because most infants with PPH have a low risk of retinopathy, it is advisable to tolerate modest hyperoxemia (90 to 100 mm Hg) to avoid the problem of hyperreactivity.

Systemic hypotension and metabolic acidosis should be corrected with appropriate infusions of blood and alkali. Patients frequently oxygenate better when blood pressure is maintained in the high normal range. In newborn infants, dopamine at doses of 2 to 10 mg/kg/min augments the cardiac output by direct beta-adrenergic receptor stimulation and increases systemic blood pressure without change in systemic vascular resistance. It is possible that this treatment may improve pulmonary blood flow. At higher rates of infusion, up to 20 mg/kg/min, dopamine may increase the systemic vascular resistance because of its alpha-adrenergic agonist properties. Although this dose may redistribute blood flow to the lungs and improve coronary diastolic perfusion, it has not been established that the pulmonary vascular resistance is unchanged. Induction of respiratory alkalosis by mechanical hyperventilation, with rates up to 150 bpm and pressures up to 50 cm H_2O, is thought to improve oxygenation, often dramatically, at a critical pH of 7.55 to 7.65. However, other medical centers have obtained excellent results without resort to mechanical hyperventilation. It may be wiser to operate below the critical pH if peak pressures required are excessive. Because of the risks of gas trapping at high rates and because of the high incidence of pneumothorax with hyperventilation techniques, we have usually been satisfied with rates of 80 to 100 bpm. To avoid lung overdistention a short inspiration time (0.10 to 0.15 sec) is used. For this purpose patients are paralyzed with pancuronium and treated with liberal doses of morphine (0.1 mg/kg/3 hr) or fentanyl (5 mg/kg/hr). Infants in this condition become hypoxemic when handled, so disturbance should be minimal. Suctioning should be gentle and brief and only when indicated by secretions. Caution should be exercised in the administration of vasoactive agents, such as calcium, blood products, and hyperosmolar solutions.

After 5 days of high oxygen and vigorous mechanical ventilation, there is usually severe lung injury and pulmonary edema in all patients. The use of higher levels of PEEP to achieve adequate oxygenation is then appropriate, which means that peak pressures may be reduced to more reasonable levels and the ventilatory rate slowly reduced.

A number of other drugs have found a place in treatment of this disease, but no controlled trials have demonstrated efficacy. Tolazoline hydrochloride, 1 to 2 mg/kg over 1 to 2 min followed by 0.15 to 0.30 mg/kg/hour infused through a scalp vein, may sometimes be helpful, but systemic hypotension must be avoided by the use of volume loading and dopamine. Nitroprusside at infusion rates of 0.2 to 2.0 mg/kg/min has proved much easier to control and may be just as effective. Clinical trials have failed to establish the efficacy of prostacyclin and prostaglandins E and D.

It is customary to restrict fluids (50 ml/kg/day) with 25-per cent glucose in a central vein so that liberal colloid infusions may be given as necessary. There is value in monitoring central venous pressure to maintain adequate blood volume without overloading the heart. The use of pulmonary artery catheters has been abandoned because the results are no better, and the catheter may partially obstruct an already restricted pulmonary blood flow. It may be necessary to tolerate arterial P_{O_2} at a level of 35 mm Hg, in which case increasing the hematocrit to 50 per cent seems wise. Repeated measurements of serum lactate in the normal range may provide reassurance that significant hypoxia is not present. It is remarkable how many infants can recover from this difficult situation without clinicians running the risk of more vigorous mechanical ventilation. Noticeable improvement in the ability to oxygenate usually occurs around the age of 1 to 5 days. There has been significant improvement in the response to treatment in the last 5 years, with the result that mortality is now less than 20 per cent.

PULMONARY HYPOPLASIA

The definition of this condition is based on pathology, the combined lung weight being less than 1.2 per cent of body weight, less than 1.5 per cent in those newborns under 28 weeks of age. Otherwise, the standardized autopsy lung volume is less than 60 per cent of predicted, lung DNA is less than 100 mg/kg body weight, or the radial alveolar count is less than 4. Radiologically, the lungs are clear and small, but the latter characteristic may not be realized until multiple radiographs have been taken. These infants have hypercarbia that responds poorly to mechanical ventilation, and the risk of pneumothorax is very high. In addition, they frequently have PPH, because of a reduction in the vascular bed and secondary medial muscle hypertrophy of pulmonary arteries.

Normal fetal lung growth is dependent on lung distention, which in turn is dependent on space to occupy, expansion due to constant secretion of lung liquid against a usually closed glottis, and the muscular forces produced by fetal breathing. Conditions that are associated with oligohydramnios and fetal compression have resulted in pulmonary hypoplasia. These conditions include renal agenesis, renal dysplasia, obstructive uropathy, and chronic amnion rupture. Lung compression may also be due to congenital diaphragmatic hernia, membranous diaphragm, large abdominal or thoracic masses, ascites, and pleural effusion, all of which can cause pulmonary hypoplasia. Effective expansive forces caused by fetal breathing may be impaired by chest cage insufficiency, such as in the congenital thoracic dystrophy; by neuromuscular disease, such as motor neuron disease and myotonic dystrophy; and by central nervous system malformations, such as iniencephaly, that involve the brainstem. Patients with giant omphalocele may have pulmonary hypoplasia because the lower chest cage is not supported and expanded by normal abdominal contents. In a significant number of infants no cause for primary pulmonary hypoplasia can be found, although it is suspected that such infants might have chronic suppression of fetal breathing, possibly as the result of maternal smoking or barbiturate or ethanol ingestion.

In most cases, there is a reduction in the number of bronchial generations, suggesting an effect between 10 and 14 weeks gestation, as in congenital diaphragmatic hernia and renal dysplasia. Although the total number of acini is reduced, the number of alveoli per acinus may be relatively well preserved. In comparison, in many cases of chronic amnion rupture the onset is much later, the number of bronchial generations and acini is normal, and the main problem is a reduction in the number of alveoli in each acinus.

The possibilities for treatment are limited at the present time. Relief of conditions causing compression of the fetal lung has become a major objective

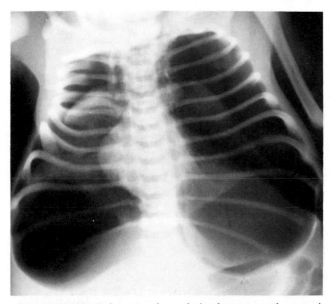

Figure 13–10. Pulmonary hypoplasia due to renal agenesis. Note the small chest cage and bilateral pneumothorax.

of the new discipline of fetal surgery. To avoid overdistention of the hypoplastic lung after birth, it is necessary to ventilate mechanically at rapid rates (80 to 100 bpm) using a short inspiration time (0.10 to 0.15 second) and the lowest pressures commensurate with adequate oxygenation and reasonable control of hypercarbia.

POSTASPHYXIAL PULMONARY EDEMA

The term postasphyxial pulmonary edema is used to describe severe respiratory distress with pulmonary edema, significant cardiomegaly, and postanoxic encephalopathy following an episode of severe fetal asphyxia without meconium aspiration. The affected infant often remains neurologically depressed after resuscitation and requires prolonged mechanical ventilation. Pulmonary edema following asphyxia is produced by increased transcapillary filtration, which results from high microvascular pressures rather than from putative capillary damage. It is not clear whether high microvascular pressures are due to pulmonary venous constriction or to transient heart failure, but left and right atrial pressures remain elevated for many hours after severe asphyxia, and in many infants pulmonary artery pressures are similar to systemic pressures. Both heart failure and PPH may result from severe anoxia and acidosis. In addition, the heart may suffer ischemic damage, especially to the papillary muscles of the mitral or tricuspid valve, resulting in valvular insufficiency. These infants may have pansystolic murmurs, hepatomegaly as well as pulmonary edema, gross cardiomegaly (Fig. 13–11), reduced systemic perfusion, intractable hypotension, and poor myocardial contractility assessed by echocardiography. Enzyme evidence of subendocardial infarction may evolve over a few days. The ECG may demonstrate ST depression in midchest leads and T-wave inversion in left chest leads.

Treatment

Unlike those with TTN, these infants with postasphyxial pulmonary edema require more than supportive treatment. Because of severe hypercarbia, metabolic acidosis, and hypoxemia, most require high concentrations of oxygen, infusions of base, and mechanical ventilation with PEEP. Seizures and hypertonicity must be adequately treated with phenobarbital to allow proper ventilation, and muscle paralysis is frequently necessary. Fluids are restricted because of pulmonary edema, oliguria, and cerebral swelling. When myocardial depression is prominent, correction of hypocalcemia is important. The cardiac output, systemic blood pressure, and urine flow may be augmented with dopamine, 2 to 10 mg/kg/min, occasionally supplemented with nitroprusside, 0.2 to 2.0 mg/kg/min, to reduce cardiac afterload. Despite

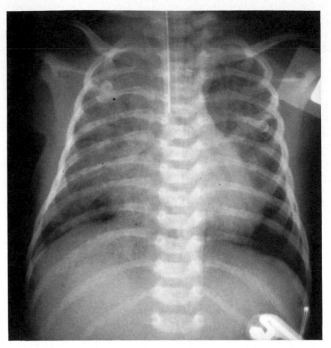

Figure 13–11. Postasphyxial pulmonary edema.

the need for fluid restriction, it is sometimes possible to improve pulmonary perfusion and oxygenate these infants only by expansion of blood volume with plasma or packed cells.

MASSIVE PULMONARY HEMORRHAGE

Mild interstitial pulmonary hemorrhage is a common autopsy finding, but sometimes massive pulmonary hemorrhage (MPH) with extension into airways is the principal cause of death. The airway fluid has a low hematocrit value, so the condition is really hemorrhagic pulmonary edema. There appear to be three important factors: high microvascular pressure causing increased fluid filtration, loss of capillary endothelial integrity, and pulmonary epithelial damage. High filtration pressures often occur in symptomatic PDA and in cardiac failure due to excessive fetal asphyxia or structural heart lesions. They are probably present in conditions of increased sympathetic discharge, such as cerebral edema or hemorrhage, in which pulmonary venous constriction may occur or massive systemic constriction may cause a shift of blood volume to the lungs. Capillary damage may result from oxygen toxicity, endotoxemia, or acute capillary distention. Epithelial damage has been reported in HMD, oxygen toxicity, infection, and mechanical ventilation, but may simply reflect overdistention of the interstitial space by liquid. Massive pulmonary hemorrhage is common in infants asphyxiated at birth, especially in those small for gestational age, and in small premature infants with HMD, PDA, and high inspired oxygen requirements. Most cases show no evidence of preceding coagulopathy.

The common presentation is an infant on mechanical ventilation for asphyxia or lung disease who suddenly deteriorates on the second or third day of life with frothy blood suctioned from the endotracheal tube. The chest radiograph shows the sudden appearance of coarse densities superimposed over HMD or postasphyxial pulmonary edema (Fig. 13–12). There is no established therapy, but treatment usually includes vigorous tracheal suctioning, mechanical ventilation, high PEEP (10 cm H_2O), oxygen, bicarbonate infusion, and correction of anemia and hypotension with transfusions. Specific treatment for PDA or congenital heart disease may also be necessary.

A second type of MPH is recognized. It occurs usually in older premature infants with nosocomial infection but sometimes in younger infants with congenital infection who have thrombocytopenia or a generalized disturbance of coagulation and who may bleed from other sites as well. These infants may respond to treatment of the infection; transfusion with blood, platelets, and fresh frozen plasma; and attempts to stem the lung hemorrhage by using mechanical ventilation at high levels of PEEP.

HYDROPIC PULMONARY EDEMA

Infants with hydrops fetalis have generalized edema, anemia, hepatosplenomegaly, ascites, and pleural effusions (Fig. 13–13). Many factors contribute to the lung disease, including surfactant insufficiency. In immune hydrops, the presence of hydrops correlates best with anemia rather than with hypoproteinemia, as was once thought. The most likely explanation is that anemia causes high output congestive cardiac failure, with elevated systemic venous pressure and impaired lymphatic drainage through the thoracic duct. Although blood volume is usually

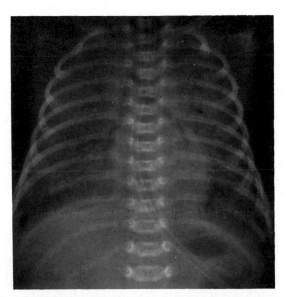

Figure 13–12. Massive pulmonary hemorrhage complicating hyaline membrane disease.

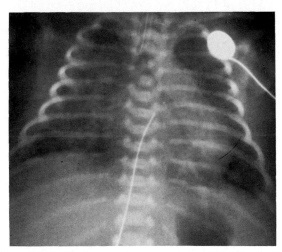

Figure 13–13. Hydropic pulmonary edema with pleural effusion on the right.

normal or decreased, vascular pressures tend initially to be high because of asphyxia and to decrease with correction of acidosis by mechanical ventilation and bicarbonate infusion. After resuscitation, the blood pressure may be low. The hemoglobin should then be corrected by a small transfusion of packed red blood cells (10 ml/kg) given slowly or by isovolemic exchange transfusion. Because this treatment may raise colloid osmotic pressure, there may be a shift of fluid from the extravascular to the vascular compartment, and pulmonary edema may be improved. Pleural effusions and ascitic fluid should be tapped if necessary to facilitate mechanical ventilation. Diuretics may deplete blood volume and impair renal function, so they should be used cautiously.

PULMONARY EDEMA WITH CONGENITAL CARDIAC DISEASE

Infants with cyanotic congenital heart disease due to uncomplicated pulmonary atresia or transposition of the great vessels may have respiratory symptoms in the form of deep breathing, but the chest radiograph shows normal or decreased pulmonary vasculature without pulmonary edema. Left-sided cardiac lesions, such as mitral atresia, critical aortic stenosis, preductal coactation, and aortic arch interruption, may present with pulmonary edema soon after the ductus arteriosus has closed during the first week of life. Newborns with severe cardiac arrhythmia, such as paroxysmal atrial tachycardia or heart block, those with a cerebral arteriovenous fistula, and those with viral myocarditis frequently develop left ventricular failure and pulmonary edema. Infants with ventricular septal defects complicated by such additional lesions as atrioventricular canal, double outlet right ventricle, truncus arteriosus, and aorticopulmonary transposition may present with signs of pulmonary edema but usually not until after the first week of life, when the pulmonary vascular resistance has

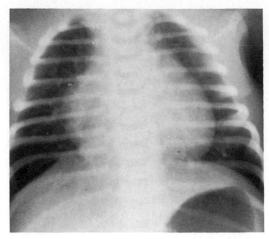

Figure 13–14. Mitral atresia with cardiomegaly and early congestion.

fallen sufficiently. Few cardiac malformations cause pulmonary edema in the newborn period and confusion with the usual causes of respiratory distress, but the two most common are mitral atresia and total anomalous pulmonary venous return (TAPVR) with obstruction.

Mitral Atresia

In mitral atresia, saturated pulmonary venous blood crosses the obstructed left atrium through an atrial septal defect to the right atrium, where it mixes with desaturated systemic venous blood and is pumped by the right ventricle into the pulmonary artery. While the ductus arteriosus remains patent, systemic flow is satisfactory and heart size is normal, but as the ductus closes, systemic blood flow is reduced and shock occurs. Increasing pulmonary perfusion causes pulmonary edema and cardiac enlargement (Fig. 13–14). Infants with these conditions develop respiratory symptoms and crepitant rales as early as the first day of life and are commonly thought to have lung disease. There is a soft pulmonary flow murmur, and the second heart sound is single. Liver enlargement signals right heart failure. Central cyanosis is mild, and with 100-per cent oxygen arterial saturation is normal. The ECG shows abnormal right ventricular hypertrophy with no R waves in the left chest leads. Neither mitral nor aortic valve motion can be demonstrated by echocardiography. These infants are often subjected to prostaglandin E treatment, cardiac catheterization, and experimental surgery, but the disease usually remains refractory to any treatment.

Total Anomalous Pulmonary Venous Return

Saturated pulmonary venous blood drains through abnormal veins into the right atrium to mix with desaturated systemic blood. The anomalous venous return is frequently into the portal venous system below the diaphragm, in which case severe obstruc-

tion with pulmonary venous congestion is usual because the portal system is not sufficiently large. There is a secondary reflex increased pulmonary vascular resistance with PPH, and the radiograph shows a diffuse granular density resembling HMD (Fig. 13–15). Because pulmonary perfusion is reduced, severe central cyanosis is unresponsive to 100 per cent oxygen. Peripheral pulses are normal early, but as the ductus closes the pulses become diminished, and there is reduced systemic circulation with right heart failure. These infants sometimes develop severe respiratory distress and crepitant rales within hours of birth and are commonly thought to have lung disease. There may be a tricuspid insufficiency murmur, and the second sound is single. The heart is quiet and enlarges late. The ECG shows abnormal right ventricular hypertrophy. Blood sampled from an umbilical catheter passed through the ductus venosus into the inferior vena cava is well saturated. The confluence of anomalous veins behind the heart may be detected by echocardiography, but a firm diagnosis requires cardiac catheterization. This disorder is refractory to medical treatment until the pulmonary venous confluence is freely anastomosed to the left atrium, after which mechanical ventilation, bicarbonate, digitalis, and diuretics may be effective.

CHRONIC PULMONARY INSUFFICIENCY OF PREMATURITY

A group of premature infants, weighing under 1250 g at birth, develop significant respiratory distress and recurrent apnea during the second week of life and generally recover during the second month of life. Lung volume is significantly reduced during the first month, and this reduction is reflected by the poorly defined diffuse density without cystic

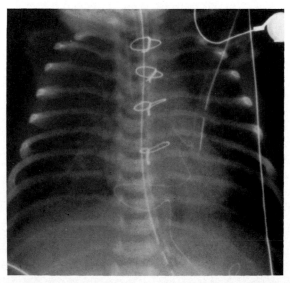

Figure 13–15. Total anomalous pulmonary venous return after recent surgical relief of obstruction. Diffuse granular densities are still present.

change seen on the chest radiograph (Fig. 13–16), an oxygen requirement of 25 to 40 per cent, and modest hypercarbia. The A-aD_{O_2}, a-AD_{CO_2}, and a-AD_{N_2} are increased. It has been suggested that chronic pulmonary insufficiency of prematurity (CPIP) is due to chronic surfactant insufficiency or to fluid overload, but the most likely explanation is chest cage insufficiency due to unusually high compliance. The problem responds well to prolonged nasal CDAP.

WILSON-MIKITY SYNDROME

The Wilson-Mikity syndrome describes a condition of prolonged respiratory distress in premature infants, who usually weigh under 1500 g at birth, that is accompanied by characteristic changes in the chest radiograph. The onset of slight tachypnea, chest retraction, and cyanosis occurs between 1 and 4 weeks of age. There is nothing characteristic in the obstetric history; exposure to oxygen and mechanical ventilation is minimal; HMD during the first week is usually absent; and there is no evidence for infection, excessive fluid administration, or PDA. The development of progressive distress occurs over a period of about 2 months, followed by a very slow improvement until most patients have recovered by 1 to 2 years of age. During development, the chest radiograph shows diffuse coarse streaky infiltrate with widespread cystic change, giving a "bubbly" appearance (Fig. 13–17); during the prolonged recovery phase, there is overinflation at the lung bases with flattening of the diaphragm and streaky atelectasis at the apices (Fig. 13–18).

Dynamic lung compliance is reduced, and airway resistance is increased. The measurements of lung volume appear normal initially, with a tendency to increase as the condition develops. Pathologically, the lung shows alternating areas of atelectasis and hyperinflation, accounting for the relatively normal measurements of lung volume. The A-aD_{O_2}, a-AD_{N_2},

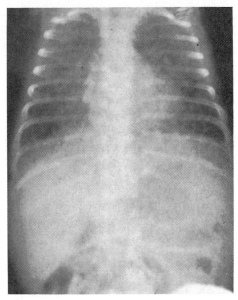

Figure 13–17. Wilson-Mikity syndrome during the development phase, showing diffuse density and cystic change.

and a-AD_{CO_2} are all increased, suggesting severe ventilation-perfusion imbalance, and most patients require only 30- to 50-per cent oxygen at the height of their disease. However, a significant number of infants die of chronic pulmonary artery hypertension and congestive cardiac failure.

The cause of this condition is unknown. The airways of very premature infants are extremely compliant, and if compliance values are unevenly distributed, this unevenness might cause airway closure during expiration, with gas trapping in certain regions and adjacent compression atelectasis in others. Although it was once quite common, this condition has became much less frequent since the advent of CDAP and mechanical ventilation. It is possible that

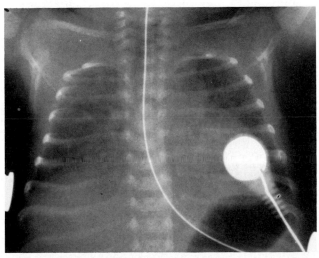

Figure 13–16. Chronic pulmonary insufficiency of prematurity.

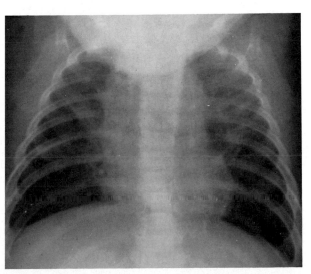

Figure 13–18. Wilson-Mikity syndrome during the recovery phase, showing hyperinflation at the bases and streaky density at the apices.

higher airway pressures stabilize the peripheral airways and prevent widespread closure.

PULMONARY AIR LEAKS

Excessive volume distention may cause rupture, usually at the base of a cluster of alveoli, into the periarterial sheath in the center of the pulmonary lobule. Alveolar pressures are more likely to be excessive when neighboring airways are closed by disease. Because its pores of Kohn are poorly developed, the newborn lung has little collateral ventilation and is therefore likely to rupture. When terminal air spaces are collapsed, as in HMD, rupture may occur in the highly distensible distal conducting airways. Proximal dissection through the periarterial interstitium toward the hilum occurs, but distal dissection through interlobular septae to the costal pleura also occurs. From the hilum there is dissection into the mediastinum, and because the mediastinum is easily ruptured, pneumothorax often results. In the mediastinum, air dissects around the thymus, producing the classic radiographic "sail sign," but it is unusual for air to dissect into the neck. More commonly, air dissects around or into the pericardium and into tracks between the parietal pleura and the diaphragm. It may even enter the retroperitoneal space and track forward in the mesentery and subserosa to give the appearance of necrotizing enterocolitis.

A rare but usually fatal complication is pulmonary venous air embolism. Pulmonary air leak (PAL) is common in HMD owing to inhomogeneity of surfactant development; in aspiration pneumonias, wet lung disease, and at birth owing to fluid-filled airways; in pulmonary hypoplasia owing to defective alveolar development; and in patients treated with mechanical ventilation or CDAP.

Pulmonary Interstitial Emphysema

Pulmonary interstitial emphysema (PIE) occurs mainly in small premature infants with abundant interstitial tissue but is nearly always associated with underlying lung disease and mechanical ventilation. The use of PEEP, inflation pressures over 20 cm H_2O, and especially prolonged inspiration time have all increased the incidence of this disorder. Radiologically, there are coarse elongated lucencies radiating from the hilum, sometimes reaching the pleura (Fig. 13–19). Lung volume is often increased, with bulging between the ribs and flattening of the diaphragm. The condition may be segmental, lobar, unilateral, or diffuse. With dissection and accumulation of air, interstitial blood vessels and airways are compressed. Pulmonary edema develops because pulmonary lymphatics are obstructed and lung compliance is greatly reduced. Hypercarbia is an early sign; later, pulmonary perfusion is impaired, and oxygenation becomes increasingly difficult. There may be systemic hypotension, metabolic acidosis, and tachycardia. De-

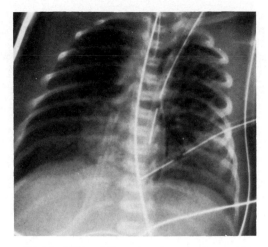

Figure 13–19. Diffuse bilateral pulmonary interstitial emphysema in hyaline membrane disease.

compression of PIE with the occurrence of pneumomediastinum or pneumothorax may cause temporary clinical improvement.

Treatment. In general this condition is managed by reducing the mean airway pressure, with attempted compensation by increased ventilator frequency and higher concentrations of inspired oxygen. If the interstitial gas has a high nitrogen content, breathing 100-per cent oxygen creates a large gradient between tissue and vascular nitrogen and thus promotes a more rapid resolution, but this approach cannot be recommended in small premature infants predisposed to retinopathy. In more malignant cases, the inspiration time should be short (0.10 to 0.15 sec), the peak pressure and PEEP should be reduced to the absolute minimum, and the ventilator rate should be 80 to 100 bpm. Serial chest radiographs should show that the lungs are relatively collapsed and that interstitial emphysema is improved. If not, then PEEP and peak pressures must be reduced further. If necessary, marginal blood gas values should be tolerated for a period of at least 3 days to accomplish healing of the lung rupture. Unilateral PIE may be managed by placing the index lung in the dependent position or by selective intubation of the main bronchus on the unaffected side, but clinical deterioration is not uncommon.

The most malignant forms of PIE are very difficult to manage. A few cases have been treated successfully by lobectomy. Multiple pleurotomies to promote pneumothorax have been suggested, but it is unlikely that uniform decompression would result. Reduction of peak pressure, PEEP, and inspiration time sometimes causes rapid deterioration, but the technique of high-frequency interruptor ventilation at 600 to 800 bpm appears promising. Because prolonged mechanical ventilation is required, survivors have a high incidence of bronchopulmonary dysplasia.

Pneumomediastinum and Pneumothorax

There is a high incidence (1 to 2 per cent) of air leak in normal term newborns because of the high transpulmonary pressures applied by the infant during the first breaths when airways are filled with lung fluid. It is rare for this air leak to occur in the preterm infant, whose compliant chest cage does not favor generation of high pressures. Another possibility, more common in premature infants, is that excessive pressures are applied to the lung during bag ventilation in the delivery room. Mediastinal air tends to collect anteriorly between the heart and the sternum, a condition well viewed on the lateral projection. Because tissue planes are loose and the mediastinum is easily ruptured, it is rare for pneumomediastinum to compress the venous return or to impinge significantly on the lung volume. Spontaneous pneumothorax in the term newborn likewise produces no increased tension and so resolves rapidly.

Infants with meconium aspiration have a high incidence of pneumothorax, both spontaneous and related to resuscitation or mechanical ventilation. Some pneumothoraces are asymptomatic, but often there is increased respiratory distress. Pneumothorax complicates wet lung disease in up to 10 per cent of patients, and the rate of spontaneous pneumothorax in HMD is 5 per cent. With CDAP the incidence of pneumothorax has increased in some reports up to 20 per cent, but in others there has been no change. Mechanical ventilation of patients with HMD, MAP, and pulmonary hypoplasia is associated with a high risk of pneumothorax, 10 to 40 per cent of HMD, up to 40 per cent in MAP, and as high as 100 per cent in pulmonary hypoplasia.

Clinical Picture. With respiratory distress, underlying lung disorder, or mechanical ventilation, one can assume that a pneumothorax is already under tension or will soon produce tension (Fig. 13–20). The lungs of premature newborns have so much

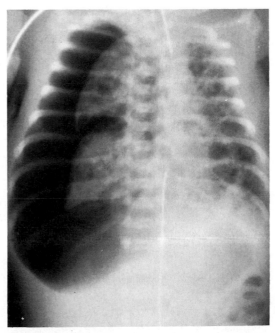

Figure 13–20. Tension pneumothorax on the right.

interstitium and fluid that they often do not collapse easily, and mediastinal shift is deceptively small. Pneumothoraces are usually larger than they appear, so if doubt persists it is best to take radiographs in frontal, lateral, and decubitus views. The decubitus view is invaluable for distinguishing pneumothorax from pneumomediastinum. Patients may have distention of the chest, tachycardia, bradycardia, increased respiratory distress, increased irritability, poor perfusion, hypotension, cyanosis, metabolic acidosis, and hypercarbia. In infants with a thin chest wall, transillumination with a fiberoptic light has been useful. When present, shift of the cardiac pulsation is suggestive, but differential air exchange detected with a stethoscope is an unreliable sign in small infants. Only in an emergency is needle aspiration a reasonable diagnostic procedure.

Treatment of Pneumothorax. Asymptomatic patients may be managed expectantly, or if mature, by 100-per cent oxygen breathing for 6 hours. Those with very mild symptoms may be managed by needle aspiration, but subsequent close observation is mandatory because the needle may damage the lung. In obviously symptomatic patients, a pneumothorax should be managed by insertion of a pleural catheter connected to an underwater seal. The catheter is placed through the second intercostal space in the midclavicular line or, less commonly, the fourth intercostal space in the midaxillary line. As gas rises, the catheter tip should be in the superior position (anterior in the supine infant). Rupture of the lung during catheter placement with a trocar may occur if the lung is first reinflated by needle aspiration, so many clinicians prefer to insert the catheter between the parted blades of blunt curved forceps. In newborns it is necessary to apply a negative pressure of 10 to 20 cm H_2O to the underwater seal. Pleural catheters may be left in place as long as the risk of pneumothorax remains; usually after 3 or 4 days, the suction may be discontinued for 12 to 24 hours of observation before removal of the tube.

RESPIRATORY OBSTRUCTION

CHOANAL ATRESIA

Choanal atresia is commonly associated with congenital heart disease, esophageal atresia, and colobomata and is more common in females. Atresia of the posterior nares at the posterior margin of the hard palate may be bony or membranous, but in some cases only stenosis is present. Unilateral involvement may cause few problems unless nasal secretions are increased. Because newborns are obligate nose breathers for 2 to 3 weeks, bilateral choanal atresia is associated with episodes of apnea and cyanosis and is relieved when crying is stimulated. During feeding the infant becomes cyanotic and may aspirate. When the mouth is held closed, movement of the alae nasi is not observed during attempted inspiration. Soft

No. 8 French plastic catheters cannot be passed through the nose, and radiopaque dye demonstrates obstruction by its failure to pass into the pharynx. Emergency prophylaxis consists of endotracheal intubation or taping a large oral airway in place, and the infant is fed by gavage. Surgical excision of the obstruction using a transnasal or transpalatal approach is performed, and both nares are intubated to prevent recurrence of the obstruction by swelling. The Silastic tubes are lavaged with saline and suctioned to maintain patency, and after 6 weeks they may be removed.

PIERRE-ROBIN SYNDROME

Infants with Pierre-Robin syndrome have severe mandibular hypoplasia with associated cleft or highly arched palate and develop intermittent airway obstruction because of posterior displacement of the tongue. Obstruction is maintained by negative pressures generated below the obstruction during inspiration and swallowing. It is more common in the supine position, during feeding, and in active sleep when pharyngeal muscle tone is absent. Chronic obstruction may result in pulmonary edema, pulmonary hypertension, and cor pulmonale. The infant should be kept in the prone position. A tube passed into the hypopharynx may prevent the development of negative pressures. It is helpful to stitch the tongue to the anterior gum, but in severe cases tracheostomy is necessary. Normal feeding is difficult because pharyngeal obstruction predisposes the infant to aspiration, and tube feeding or gastrostomy may be necessary. With adequate nutrition and growth of the mandible the problem resolves by 6 to 12 months of age.

LARYNGEAL OBSTRUCTION

The larynx may be partially or completely obstructed by a web, cyst, or papilloma that is seen directly at laryngoscopy. With partial obstruction the voice is weak or hoarse. An endotracheal tube can sometimes be passed beyond the obstruction; otherwise a large-bore needle is inserted percutaneously into the trachea below the larynx to maintain sufficient gas exchange until preparations for tracheostomy are made.

Bilateral vocal cord paralysis due to anoxic brainstem injury or congenital nuclear aplasia causes severe stridor. Swallowing difficulty, recurrent apnea, and aspiration are common because of associated pharyngeal paralysis. The anoxic injury may improve with time, but the prognosis is usually poor. Left-sided vocal cord paralysis from obstetric trauma to the recurrent laryngeal nerve causes mild stridor and hoarse voice. Left-sided vocal cord paralysis has also been reported after surgical ligation of the ductus arteriosus.

Laryngomalacia, which is relatively common, is due to the sucking of poorly supported aryepiglottic folds and the epiglottis into the airway during inspiration. Despite loud stridor and significant chest retraction the infant usually does not have cyanosis, hypercarbia, feeding difficulty, or growth failure, and the voice is normal. Congenital stridor is worse in the supine position with the neck flexed but better in the prone position with the neck hyperextended. Obstruction is worse during episodes of crying and upper respiratory infection. The condition improves over 6 to 12 months, as supporting cartilage matures.

SUBGLOTTIC OBSTRUCTION

Extubation after prolonged endotracheal intubation is sometimes followed by partial obstruction from subglottic edema. Pretreatment with dexamethasone is often suggested, but no controlled studies have been performed to determine its efficacy. Adequate humidification of inspired gas and nebulization of racemic epinephrine have proved useful. In cases with no response, reintubation with a smaller tube for a short period while growth occurs may be helpful. In some cases a cricoid split operation is successful, and in rare instances tracheostomy is necessary.

Subglottic hemangioma, often in the presence of cutaneous hemangiomata, may cause stridor that progresses with enlargement of the tumor. High-dose corticosteroid therapy may be successful, but prolonged intubation or tracheostomy is usually required during the interim.

OTHER CAUSES

The upper airway may be obstructed by tumors of the pharynx, such as teratoma, angiofibroma, and thyroglossal cyst. Thyroid goiter or cystic hygroma may sometimes be sufficiently large to compress the airway.

REFERENCES

Respiratory Depression

FETAL ASPHYXIA
Adamsons K: Transport of organic substances and oxygen across the placenta. Birth Def Orig Art Ser 1:27, 1965.
Behrman RE, James LS, Klaus M et al: Treatment of the asphyxiated newborn infant. J Pediatr 74:981, 1969.
Dawes GS: Birth asphyxia, resuscitation and brain damage. In Dawes GS (ed): Fetal and Neonatal Physiology. Chicago, Year Book Medical Publishers, Inc, 1968.
Scott H: Outcome of very severe birth asphyxia. Arch Dis Child 51:712, 1976.

MATERNAL DRUGS
American Academy of Pediatrics, Committee on Drugs: Naloxone use in newborns. Pediatrics 65:667, 1980.

Caldwell J, Wakile LA, Notarianni LJ et al: Maternal and neonatal disposition of pethidine in childbirth—a study using quantitative gas chromatography mass spectrometry. Life Sciences 22:589, 1978.

Cosmi EV: Drugs, anesthetics and the fetus. In Scarpelli EM and Ermelando VC (eds): Reviews in Perinatal Medicine. Baltimore, University Park Press, 1976.

James LS: The effect of pain relief for labor and delivery on the fetus and newborn. Anesthesiology 21:405, 1960.

James LS: Physiologic adjustments at birth. Effects of labor, delivery and anesthesia on the newborn. Anesthesiology 26:501, 1963.

Koch G and Wendel H: The effect of pethidine on the postnatal adjustment of respiration and acid base balance. Acta Obstet Gynecol Scand 47:27, 1968.

Lipsitz PJ: The clinical biochemical effects of excess magnesium in the newborn. Pediatrics 47:501, 1971.

RECURRENT APNEA

Aranda JV, Gorman W, Bergsteinsson H et al: Efficacy of caffeine in treatment of apnea in the low birth weight infant. J Pediatr 90:467, 1977.

Bairam A, Boutroy MJ, Badonnel Y et al: Theophylline versus caffeine: comparative effects in treatment of idiopathic apnea in the preterm infant. J Pediatr 110:636, 1987.

Barrington KJ, Finer NN, Torok-Both G et al: Dose-response relationship of doxapram in the therapy for refractory idiopathic apnea of prematurity. Pediatrics 80:22, 1987.

Bodegard G, Schweiler GH, Skoglund S et al: Control of respiration in newborn babies. Acta Paediatr Scand 58:567, 1969.

Brouillette RT and Thach BT: A neuromuscular mechanism maintaining extrathoracic airway patency. J Appl Physiol 46:772, 1979.

Bryan AC and England SJ: Maintenance of an elevated FRC in the newborn: paradox of REM sleep. Am Rev Resp Dis 129:209, 1984.

Dawes GS, Gardner WN, Johnston BM et al: Breathing in fetal lambs: the effect of brain stem section. J Physiol 335:535, 1983.

Euler Von C: On the central pattern generator for the basic breathing rhythmicity. J Appl Physiol 55:1647, 1983.

Gerhardt T and Bancalari E: Maturational changes of reflexes influencing inspiratory timing in newborns. J Appl Physiol 50:1282, 1981.

Gerhardt T and Bancalari E: Apnea of prematurity: I. Lung function and regulation of breathing. Pediatrics 74:58, 1984.

Gerhaardt T and Bancalari E: Apnea of prematurity: II. Respiratory reflexes. Pediatrics 74:63, 1984.

Gerhardt T, McCarthy J, and Bancalari E: Effects of aminophylline on respiratory center and reflex activity in premature infants with apnea. Pediatr Res 17:188, 1983.

Haddad GG and Mellins RB: The role of airway receptors in the control of respiration in infants: a review. J Pediatr 91:281, 1977.

Henderson-Smart DJ, Pettigrew AG, and Campbell DJ: Clinical apnea and brain-stem neural function in preterm infants. N Engl J Med 308:353, 1983.

Hoppenbrouwers T, Hodgman JE, Harper RM et al: Polygraphic studies of normal infants during the first six months of life: III. Incidence of apnea and periodic breathing. Pediatrics 60:418, 1977.

Jansen AH and Chernick V: Onset of breathing and control of respiration. Semin Perinatol 12:104, 1988.

Kattwinkel J: Neonatal apnea: pathogenesis and therapy. J Pediatr 90:342, 1977.

Kattwinkel J, Nearman HS, Fanaroff AA et al: Apnea of prematurity. J Pediatr 86:588, 1975.

Knill R and Bryan AC: An intercostal-phrenic inhibitory reflex in human newborn infants. J Appl Physiol 40:352, 1976.

Korner AF, Guilleminault C, Van den Hoed J et al: Reduction of sleep apnea and bradycardia in preterm infants on oscillating water beds: a controlled polygraphic study. Pediatrics 61:528, 1978.

Martin RJ, Miller MJ, and Carlo WA: Pathogenesis of apnea in preterm infants. J Pediatr 109:733, 1986.

Martin RJ, Nearman HS, Katona PG et al: The effect of a low continuous positive airway pressure on the reflex control of respiration in the preterm infant. J Pediatr 90:976, 1977.

Mathew OP, Roberts JL, and Thach BT: Pharyngeal airway obstruction in preterm infants during mixed and obstructive apnea. J Pediatr 100:964, 1982.

Miller MJ, Carlo WA, and Martin RJ: Continuous positive airway pressure selectively reduces obstructive apnea in preterm infants. J Pediatr 106:91, 1985.

National Institutes of Health Conference on Infantile Apnea and Home Monitoring: Consensus statement. Pediatrics 79:292, 1987.

Rigatto H: Respiratory control and apnea in the newborn infant. Crit Care Med 5:2, 1977.

Rigatto H: Ventilatory response to hypoxia. Semin Perinatol 1:357, 1977.

Rigatto H: Ventilatory response to hypercapnia. Semin Perinatol 1:363, 1977.

Rigatto H: Apnea. In Gregory GA and Thibeault DW (eds): Neonatal Pulmonary Care. Norwalk, Conn, Appleton-Century-Crofts, Inc, 1986.

Rigatto H and Brady JP: Periodic breathing and apnea in preterm infants. Evidence for hypoventilation possibly due to central respiratory depression. Pediatrics 50:202, 1972.

Rigatto H and Brady JP: Periodic breathing and apnea in preterm infants. Hypoxia as a primary event. Pediatrics 50:219, 1972.

Roberts JL, Mathew OP, and Thach BT: The efficacy of theophylline in premature infants with mixed and obstructive apnea and apnea associated with pulmonary and neurologic disease. J Pediatr 100:968, 1982.

Rosen CL, Glaze DG, and Frost JD: Hypoxemia associated with feeding in the preterm infant and full-term neonate. Am J Dis Child 138:623, 1984.

Spitzer AR, Boyle JT, Tuchman DN et al: Awake apnea associated with gastroesophageal reflux: a specific clinical syndrome. J Pediatr 104:200, 1984.

Stark AR and Thach BT: Mechanisms of airway obstruction leading to apnea in newborn infants. J Pediatr 89:982, 1976.

Respiratory Distress

TRANSIENT TACHYPNEA OF THE NEWBORN

Adams FH, Yanagisawa M, Kuzela D et al: The disappearance of fetal lung fluid following birth. J Pediatr 78:837, 1971.

Avery ME, Gatewood OB, and Brumley G: Transient tachypnea of the newborn. Am J Dis Child 111:380, 1966.

Bland RD: Lung liquid clearance and after birth. Semin Perinatol 12:124, 1988.

Bland RD, McMillan DD, Bressack MA et al: Clearance of liquid from lungs of newborn rabbits. J Appl Physiol 49:171, 1980.

Brice JEH and Walker CHM: Changing pattern of respiratory distress in newborn. Lancet 2:752, 1977.

Corbet AJS, Ross JA, Beaudy PH et al: Assessment of ventilation-perfusion inequality by aADN2 in newborn infants. Biol Neonate 36:10, 1979.

Edwards DK, Jacob J, and Gluck L: The immature lung: radiographic appearance, course and complications. AJR 135:659, 1980.

Fletcher BD, Sachs BF, and Kotas RV: Radiologic demonstration of postnatal liquid in the lungs of newborn lambs. Pediatrics 46:252, 1970.

Humphries PW, Normand ICS, Reynolds EOR et al: Pulmonary lymph flow and the uptake of liquid from the lungs of the lamb at the start of breathing. J Physiol 193:1, 1987.

Kitterman JA, Ballard PL, Clements JA et al: Tracheal fluid in fetal lambs: spontaneous decrease prior to birth. J Appl Physiol 47:985, 1979.

Lagercrantz H and Slotkin TA: The stress of being born. Scientific American 254:100, 1986.

Olver RE: Of labour and the lungs. Arch Dis Child 56:659, 1981.

Olver RE, Ramsden CA, Strang LB et al: The role of amiloride-blockable sodium transport in adrenaline-induced lung liquid reabsorption in the fetal lamb. J Physiol 376:321, 1986.

Rawlings CJ and Smith FR: Transient tachypnea of the newborn. Am J Dis Child 138:869, 1984.

Sundell H, Garrott J, Blankenship WJ et al: Studies on infants with type II respiratory distress syndrome. J Pediatr 78:754, 1971.

Taylor PM, Allen AC, and Stinson DA: Benign unexplained respiratory distress of the newborn infant. Pediatr Clin North Am 18:975, 1971.

Tudehope DI and Smyth MH: Is "transient tachypnea of the newborn" always a benign disease? Report of 6 babies requiring mechanical ventilation. Aust Paediatr J 15:160, 1979.

Walters DV and Olver RE: The role of catecholamines in lung liquid absorption at birth. Pediatr Res 12:239, 1978.

Walters DV and Ramsden CA: The secretion and absorption of fetal lung liquid. In Walters DV, Strang LB, and Geubelle F (eds): Physiology of the Fetal and Neonatal Lung. Boston, ATP Press Ltd, 1987.

HYALINE MEMBRANE DISEASE

Adams FH, Fujiwara T, Emmanouilides GC et al: Lung phospholipids of human fetuses and infants with and without hyaline membrane disease. J Pediatr 77:833, 1970.

Avery ME: Hyaline membrane disease. In Avery ME, Fletcher BD, and Williams RG (eds): The Lung and Its Disorders in the Newborn Infant. Philadelphia, WB Saunders Co, 1981.

Avery ME and Mead J: Surface properties in relation to atelectasis and hyaline membrane disease. Am J Dis Child 97:517, 1959.

Bland RD, Kim MH, Light MJ et al: High frequency mechanical ventilation in severe hyaline membrane disease. Crit Care Med 8:275, 1980.

Clements JA and Tooley WH: Kinetics of surface active material in the fetal lung. In Hodson WA (ed): Development of the Lung. New York, Marcel Dekker, Inc, 1977.

Collaborative group: Effect of antenatal dexamethasone administration on the prevention of respiratory distress syndrome. Am J Obstet Gynecol 141:276, 1981.

Corbet A: Surfactant secretion and turnover. In Stern, L (ed): Hyaline membrane disease. New York, Grune & Stratton, 1984.

Corbet A and Adams J: Current therapy in hyaline membrane disease. Clin Perinatol 5:299, 1978.

Corbet AJ and Soll RF: Surfactant replacement: what surfactant does, and recent advances. Neonatology Grand Rounds 3:1, 1986.

Corbet AJS, Ross JA, Beaudry PH et al: Ventilation-perfusion relationships as assessed by aADN$_2$ in hyaline membrane disease. J Appl Physiol 36:74, 1974.

Day R, Goodfellow AM, Apgar V et al: Pressure-time relations in the safe correction of atelactasis in animal lungs. Pediatrics 10:593, 1953.

DeMello DE, Chi EY, Doo E et al: Absence of tubular myelin in lungs of infants dying with hyaline membrane disease. Am J Pathol 127:131, 1987.

Drew JH: Immediate intubation at birth of the very low birth weight infant. Am J Dis Child 136:207, 1982.

Durand DJ, Goodman A, Ray P et al: Theophylline treatment in the extubation of infants weighing less than 1250 grams: controlled trial. Pediatrics 80:684, 1987.

Enhorning G, Sherman A, Possmayer F et al: Prevention of neonatal respiratory distress syndrome by tracheal instillation of surfactant: a randomized clinical trial. Pediatrics 76:145, 1985.

Farrell PM and Avery ME: State of the art: hyaline membrane disease. Am Rev Respir Dis 111:657, 1975.

Fedrick J and Butler NR: Certain causes of neonatal death: hyaline membranes. Biol Neonate 15:229, 1970.

Gandy G, Jacobson W, and Gairdner D: Hyaline membrane disease. I: cellular changes. Arch Dis Child 45:289, 1970.

Goldman SL, Gerhardt T, Sonni R et al: Early prediction of chronic lung disease by pulmonary function testing. J Pediatr 102:613, 1983.

Hallman M and Gluck L: Development of the fetal lung. J Perinat Med 5:3, 1977.

Hallman M, Merritt TA, Jarvenpaa AL et al: Exogenous human surfactant for treatment of severe respiratory distress syndrome: a randomized prospective clinical trial. J Pediatr 106:963, 1985.

Hansen TN, Corbet AJS, Kenny JD et al: Effects of oxygen and constant positive pressure breathing on aADCO$_2$ in hyaline membrane disease. Pediatr Res 13:1167, 1979.

Heicher DA, Kasting DS, and Harrod JR: Prospective clinical comparison of two methods for mechanical ventilation of neonates: rapid rate and short inspiratory time versus slow rate and long inspiratory time. J Pediatr 98:957, 1981.

Howie RN: Pharmacological acceleration of lung maturation. In Raivio KO et al (eds): Respiratory Distress Syndrome. New York, Academic Press, 1984.

Ikegami M, Jacobs H, and Jobe A: Surfactant function in respiratory distress syndrome. J Pediatr 102:443, 1983.

Ikegami M, Jobe A, and Berry D: A protein which inhibits surfactant in respiratory distress syndrome. Biol Neonate 50:121, 1986.

Jefferies AL, Coates G, and O'Brodovich H: Pulmonary epithelial permeability in hyaline membrane disease. N Engl J Med 311:1075, 1984.

Jobe A, Kirkpatrick E, and Gluck L: Lecithin appearance and apparent biologic half-life in term newborn rabbit lung. Pediatr Res 12:669, 1978.

Kanto WP, Borer RC, Barr M et al: Tracheal aspirate lecithin-sphingomyelin ratios as predictors of recovery from respiratory distress syndrome. J Pediatr 89:612, 1976.

Kenny JD, Adams JM, Corbet AJS et al: The role of acidosis at birth in the development of hyaline membrane disease. Pediatrics 58:184, 1976.

Kenny JD, Corbet AJ, Adams JM et al: Hyaline membrane disease and acidosis at birth in twins. Obstet Gynecol 50:710, 1977.

Kim EH and Bontwell WC: Successful direct extubation of very low birth weight infants from low intermittent mandatory ventilation rate. Pediatrics 80:409, 1987.

Landers S, Hansen TN, Corbet AJS, et al: Optimal constant positive airway pressure assessed by arterial alveolar difference for CO$_2$ in hyaline membrane disease. Pediatr Res 20:884, 1986.

Liggins GC and Howie RN: A controlled trial of ante-partum glucocorticoid treatment for prevention of respiratory distress syndrome in premature infants. Pediatrics 50:515, 1972.

Long WA and Sanders RL: New treatment methods in neonatal respiratory distress syndrome: replacement of surface active material. In Guthrie RD (ed): Neonatal Intensive Care. New York, Churchill Livingstone, Inc, 1988.

MacArthur BA, Howie RN, Dezoete JA et al: School progress and cognitive development of 6 year old children whose mothers were treated antenatally with betamethasone. Pediatrics 70:99, 1982.

Naeye RL, Freeman RK, and Blanc WA: Nutrition, sex and fetal lung maturation. Pediatr Res 8:200, 1974.

Nilsson R, Grossman G, and Robertson B: Pathogenesis of neonatal lung lesions induced by artificial ventilation: evidence against the role of barotrauma. Respiration 40:218, 1980.

Notter RH and Shapiro DL: Lung surfactant in an era of replacement therapy. Pediatrics 68:781, 1981.

Pollitzer MJ, Reynolds EOR, Shaw DG et al: Pancuronium during mechanical ventilation speeds recovery of lungs of infants with hyaline membrane disease. Lancet 1:346, 1981.

Primhak RA: Factors associated with pulmonary air leak in premature infants receiving mechanical ventilation. J Pediatr 102:764, 1983.

Rhodes PG, Graves GR, Patel DM et al: Minimizing pneumothorax and bronchopulmonary dysplasia in ventilated infants with hyaline membrane disease. J Pediatr 103:634, 1983.

Richardson CP and Jung AJ: Effects of continuous positive airway pressure on pulmonary function and blood gases of infants with respiratory distress syndrome. Pediatr Res 12:771, 1978.

Robert MF, Neff RK, Hubbell JP et al: Association between maternal diabetes and the respiratory distress syndrome in the newborn. N Engl J Med 294:357, 1976.

Robertson B: Lung surfactant for replacement therapy. Clin Physiol 3:97, 1983.

Ross Collaborative Group: Multicenter trial of single dose Surfactant TA for prevention of respiratory distress syndrome. Pediatr Res 23:425A, 1988.

Ross Collaborative Group: Multicenter trial of single dose Surfactant TA for treatment of respiratory distress syndrome. Pediatr Res 23:410A, 1988.

Simbruner G: Inadvertent positive end-expiratory pressure in mechanically ventilated newborn infants: detection and effect on lung mechanics and gas exchange. J Pediatr 108:589, 1986.

Stark AR, Baccom R, and Frantz ID: Muscle relaxation in mechanically ventilated infants. J Pediatr 94:439, 1979.

Stewart AR, Finer NN, and Peters KL: Effects of alterations of inspiratory and expiratory pressures and inspiratory-expiratory ratios on mean airway pressure, blood gases and intracranial pressure. Pediatrics 67:474, 1981.

Symposium on Perinatal and Developmental Medicine, Bloom RS, Sinclair JC, and Warshaw JB (advisory board): The surfactant system and the neonatal lung. Evansville, Ill, Mead Johnson and Co, 1979.

Tooley WH: Hyaline membrane disease. In Rudolph AM (ed): Pediatrics. New York, Appleton & Lange, 1987.

Weller PH, Jenkins PA, Gupta J et al: Pharyngeal lecithin-sphingomyelin ratios in newborn infants. Lancet 1:12, 1976.

Whitsett JA, Hull W, Ross G et al: Characteristics of human surfactant-associated glycoproteins A. Pediatr Res 19:501, 1985.

Zachman RD: The NIH multicenter study and miscellaneous clinical trials of antenatal corticosteroid administration. In Farrell PM (ed): Lung Development: Biological and Clinical Perspectives. Vol II: Neonatal Respiratory Distress. New York, Academic Press, 1982.

PATENT DUCTUS ARTERIOSUS

Bell EF, Warburton D, Stonestreet BS et al: Effect of fluid administration on the development of symptomatic patent ductus arteriosus and congestive heart failure in premature infants. N Engl J Med 302:598, 1980.

Brash AR, Hickey DE, Graham TP et al: Pharmacokinetics of indomethacin in the neonate: relation of plasma indomethacin levels to response of the ductus arteriosus. N Engl J Med 305:67, 1981.

Cifuentes RF, Olley PM, Balfe JW et al: Indomethacin and renal function in premature infants with persistent patent ductus arteriosus. J Pediatr 95:583, 1979.

Cooke RWI and Pickering D: Poor response to oral indomethacin therapy for persistent ductus arteriosus in very low birthweight infants. Br Heart J 41:301, 1979.

Cotton RB, Stahlman MT, Bender HW et al: Randomized trial of early closure of symptomatic patent ductus arteriosus in small pre-term infants. J Pediatr 93:647, 1978.

Danilowitz D, Rudolph AM, and Hoffman JIE: Delayed closure of the ductus arteriosus in premature infants. Pediatrics 37:74, 1966.

Dudell GG and Gersony WM: Patent ductus arteriosus in neonates with severe respiratory disease. J Pediatr 104:915, 1984.

Friedman WF, Fitzpatrick KM, Merritt TA et al: The patent ductus arteriosus. Clin Perinatol 5:411, 1978.

Fujiwara T, Chida S, Watahe Y et al: Artificial surfactant therapy in hyaline membrane disease. Lancet 1:55, 1980.

Gentile R, Stevenson G, Dooley T et al: Pulsed doppler echocardiographic determination of time of ductal closure in normal newborn infants. J Pediatr 98:443, 1981.

Gersony WM, Peckham GJ, Ellison RC et al: Effects of indomethacin in premature infants with patent ductus arteriosus: results of a national collaborative study. J Pediatr 102:895, 1983.

Hammerman C, Strates E, and Valaitis S: The silent ductus: its precursors and its aftermath. Pediatr Cardiol 7:121, 1986.

Heymann MA, Rudolph AM, and Silverman NH: Closure of the ductus arteriosus in premature infants by inhibition of prostaglandin synthesis. N Engl J Med 295:540, 1976.

Jacob J, Gluck J, DiSessa TG et al: The contribution of PDA in the neonate with severe RDS. J Pediatr 96:79, 1980.

McCarthy JS, Zies LG, and Gelband H: Age-dependent closure of the patent ductus arteriosus by indomethacin. Pediatrics 62:706, 1978.

Mellander M, Leheup B, Lindstrom DP et al: Recurrence of symptomatic patent ductus arteriosus in extremely premature infants, treated with indomethacin. J Pediatr 105:138, 1984.

Merritt TA, Harris JP, Roghmann K et al: Early closure of the patent ductus arteriosus in very low birth weight infants: a controlled trial. J Pediatr 99:281, 1981.

Peckham GJ, Miettinen OS, Ellison RC et al: Clinical course to 1 year of age in premature infants with patent ductus arteriosus: results of a multi-center randomized trial of indomethacin. J Pediatr 105:285, 1984.

Ramsay JM, Murphy DJ, Vick W et al: Response of the patent ductus arteriosus to indomethacin treatment. Am J Dis Child 141:294, 1987.

Record RG and McKeown T: Observations relating to the aetiology of patent ductus arteriosus. Br Heart J 15:376, 1953.

Seyberth HW, Knapp G, Wolf D et al: Introduction of plasma indomethacin level monitoring and evaluation of an effective threshold level in very low birthweight infants with symptomatic patent ductus arteriosus. Eur J Pediatr 141:71, 1983.

Siassi B, Blanco C, Cabal LA et al: Incidence and clinical features of patent ductus arteriosus in low birthweight infants: a prospective analysis of 150 consecutively born infants. Pediatrics 57:347, 1976.

CONGENITAL BACTERIAL PNEUMONIA

Ablow RC, Driscoll SG, Effmann EL et al: A comparison of early-onset group B streptococcal neonatal infection and the respiratory distress syndrome of the newborn. N Engl J Med 294:65, 1976.

Baker CJ: Summary of NIH workshop on perinatal infections due to Group B streptococcus. J Infect Dis 135:137, 1977.

Baker CJ: Group B streptococcal infections in neonates. Pediatrics in Review 1:5, 1979.

Blanc WA: Pathways of fetal and early neonatal infection. J Pediatr 59:473, 1961.

Brook I, Martin WJ, and Finegold SM: Bacteriology of tracheal aspirates in intubated newborn. Chest 78:875, 1980.

Burchell RC: Premature spontaneous rupture of the membranes. Am J Obstet Gynecol 88:251, 1964.

Hamoudi AC, Marcon MJ, Cannon HJ et al: Comparison of three major antigen detection methods for the diagnosis of group B streptococcal sepsis in neonates. Pediatr Infect Dis J 2:432, 1983.

Lauweryns J, Bernat R, Lerut A et al: Intrauterine pneumonia: an experimental study. Biol Neonate 22:301, 1973.

Manroe BL, Rosenfeld CR, Weinberg AG et al: The differential leucocyte count in the assessment and outcome of early-onset neonatal group B streptococcal disease. J Pediatr 91:632, 1977.

Naeye RL: Coitus and associated amniotic-fluid infections. N Engl J Med 29:1198, 1979.

Naeye RL and Blanc WA: Relation of poverty and race to antenatal infection. N Engl J Med 283:555, 1970.

Naeye RL and Peters EC: Amniotic fluid infections with intact membranes leading to perinatal death: a prospective study. Pediatrics 61:171, 1978.

Philip AGS and Hewitt JR: Early diagnosis of neonatal sepsis. Pediatrics 65:1036, 1980.

Ramos A and Stern L: Relationship of premature rupture of the membranes to gastric fluid aspirate in the newborn. Am J Obstet Gynecol 105:1247, 1969.

Schlievert P, Larsen B, Johnson W et al: Bacterial growth inhibition by amniotic fluid. Am J Obstet Gynecol 122:809, 1975.

Schutte MF, Treffers PE, Kloosterman GJ et al: Management of premature rupture of membranes: the risk of vaginal examination to the infant. Am J Obstet Gynecol 146:395, 1983.

Sherman MP, Chance KH, and Goetzman BW: Gram's stains of tracheal secretions predict neonatal bacteremia. Am J Dis Child 138:848, 1984.

Sherman MP, Goetzman BW, Ahlfors CE et al: Tracheal aspiration and its clinical correlates in the diagnosis of congenital pneumonia. Pediatrics 65:258, 1980.

Yoder PR, Gibbs RS, Blanco JD et al: A prospective, controlled study of maternal and perinatal outcome after intraamniotic infection at term. Am J Obstet Gynecol 145:695, 1983.

MECONIUM ASPIRATION PNEUMONIA

Bancalari E and Berlin JA: Meconium aspiration and other asphyxial disorders. Clin Perinatol 5:317, 1978.

Carson BS, Losey RW, Bowes WA et al: Combined obstetric and pediatric approach to prevent meconium aspiration syndrome. Am J Obstet Gynecol 126:712, 1976.

Clark DA, Nieman GF, Thompson JE et al: Surfactant displacement by meconium free fatty acids: an alternative explanation for atelectasis in meconium aspiration syndrome. J Pediatr 110:765, 1987.

Fox WW, Berman LS, Downes JJ et al: The therapeutic application of end-expiratory pressure in the meconium aspiration syndrome. Pediatrics 56:214, 1975.

Gregory GA, Gooding CA, Phibbs RH et al: Meconium aspiration in infants—a prospective study. J Pediatr 85:848, 1974.

Linder N, Aranda JV, Tsur M et al: Need for endotracheal intubation and suction in meconium-stained neonates. J Pediatr 112:613, 1988.

Philips JB: Management of the meconium-stained infant. Neonatology Grand Rounds 3:1, 1986.

Ting P and Brady JP: Tracheal suction in meconium aspiration. Am J Obstet Gynecol 122:767, 1975.

Tran N, Lowe C, Sivieri EM et al: Sequential effects of acute meconium obstruction on pulmonary function. Pediatr Res 14:34, 1980.

Truog WE, Lyrene RK, Standaert TA et al: Effects of PEEP and tolazoline infusion on respiratory and inert gas exchange in experimental meconium aspiration. J Pediatr 100:284, 1982.

Tyler DC, Murphy J, and Cheney FW: Mechanical and chemical damage to lung tissue caused by meconium aspiration. Pediatrics 62:454, 1978.

Vidyasagar D, Yeh TF, Harris V et al: Assisted ventilation in infants with meconium aspiration syndrome. Pediatrics 56:213, 1975.

Yeh T, Lilien LD, Barathi A et al: Lung volume, dynamic lung compliance, and blood gases during the first 3 days of postnatal life in infants with meconium aspiration syndrome. Crit Care Med 10:588, 1982.

Yeh TF, Srinivasan G, Harris V et al: Hydrocortisone therapy in meconium aspiration syndrome: a controlled study. J Pediatr 90:140, 1977.

PERSISTENT PULMONARY HYPERTENSION

Benitz WE, Malachowski N, Cohen RS et al: Use of sodium nitroprusside in neonates: efficacy and safety. J Pediatr 106:102, 1985.

Crouse DT and Philips JB: Persistent pulmonary hypertension of the newborn. Perinatology-Neonatology 8:10, 1987.

Drummond WH, Gregory GA, Heymann MA et al: The independent effects of hyperventilation, tolazoline, and dopamine on infants with persistent pulmonary hypertension. J Pediatr 98:603, 1981.

Fox WW and Duara S: Persistent pulmonary hypertension in the neonate: diagnosis and management. J Pediatr 103:505, 1983.

Fox WW, Gewitz MH, Dinwiddie R et al: Pulmonary hypertension in the perinatal aspiration syndromes. Pediatrics 59:205, 1977.

Geggel RL, Murphy JD, Langleben D et al: Congenital diaphragmatic hernia: arterial structural changes and persistent pulmonary hypertension after surgical repair. J Pediatr 107:457, 1985.

Goetzman BW and Riemenschneider TA: Persistence of the fetal circulation. Pediatrics in Review 2:37, 1980.

Goetzman BW, Sunshine P, Johnson JD et al: Neonatal hypoxia and pulmonary vasospasm: response to tolazoline. J Pediatr 89:617, 1976.

Hammerman C, Komar K, and Abu-Khudair H: Hypoxic vs. septic pulmonary hypertension. Am J Dis Child 142:319, 1988.

Hansen TN and Gest AL: Oxygen toxicity and other ventilatory complications of treatment of infant with persistent pulmonary hypertension. Clin Perinatol 11:653, 1984.

Levin DL, Heymann MA, Kitterman JA et al: Persistent pulmonary hypertension of the newborn infant. J Pediatr 89:626, 1976.

Levin DL, Weinberg AG, and Perkin RM: Pulmonary microthrombi syndrome in newborn infants with unresponsive persistent pulmonary hypertension. J Pediatr 102:299, 1983.

Manchester D, Margolis HS, and Sheldon RE: Possible association between maternal indomethacin therapy and primary pulmonary hypertension of the newborn. Am J Obstet Gynecol 126:467, 1976.

Murphy JD, Vawter GF, and Reid LM: Pulmonary vascular disease in fatal meconium aspiration. J Pediatr 104:758, 1984.

Padbury JF, Agata Y, Baylen BG et al: Dopamine pharmacokinetics in critically ill newborn infants. J Pediatr 110:293, 1987.

Peckham GJ and Fox WW: Physiologic factors affecting pulmonary artery pressure in infants with persistent pulmonary hypertension. J Pediatr 93:1005, 1978.

Perkin RM and Anas NG: Pulmonary hypertension in pediatric patients. J Pediatr 105:511, 1984.

Segall ML, Goetzman BW, and Schick JB: Thrombocytopenia and pulmonary hypertension in the perinatal aspiration syndromes. J Pediatr 96:727, 1980.

Soifer SJ, Clyman RI, and Heymann MA: Effects of prostaglandin D_2 on pulmonary arterial pressure and oxygenation in newborn infants with persistent pulmonary hypertension. J Pediatr 112:774, 1988.

Spear ML, Spitzer AR, and Fox WW: Hyperventilation therapy for persistent pulmonary hypertension of the newborn. Perinatology-Neonatology 8:27, 1985.

Stenmark KR, James SL, Voelkel NF et al: Leukotriene C_4 and D_4 in neonates with hypoxemia and pulmonary hypertension. N Engl J Med 309:77, 1983.

Vacanti JP, Crone RK, Murphy JD et al: The pulmonary hemodynamic response to perioperative anesthesia in the treatment of high-risk infants with congenital diaphragmatic hernia. J Pediatr Surg 19:672, 1984.

Ward RM, Daniel CH, Kendig JW et al: Oliguria and tolazoline pharmacokinetics in the newborn. Pediatrics 77:307, 1986.

Wung JT, James LS, Kilchevsky E et al: Management of infants with severe respiratory failure and persistence of the fetal circulation, without hyperventilation. Pediatrics 76:488, 1985.

PULMONARY HYPOPLASIA

Alcorn D, Adamson TM, Lambert TF et al: Morphological effects of chronic tracheal ligation and drainage in the fetal lamb lung. J Anat 123:649, 1977.

Collins MH, Moessinger AC, Kleinerman J et al: Fetal lung hypoplasia associated with maternal smoking: a morphometric analysis. Pediatr Res 19:408, 1985.

Goldstein JD and Reid LM: Pulmonary hypoplasia resulting from phrenic nerve agenesis and diaphragmatic amyoplasia. J Pediatr 97:282, 1980.

Hershenson MB, Brouillette RT, Klemka L et al: Respiratory insufficiency in newborns with abdominal wall defects. J Pediatr Surg 20:348, 1985.

Hislop A, Hey E, and Reid L: The lungs in congenital bilateral renal agenesis and dysplasia. Arch Dis Child 54:32, 1979.

Langston C and Thurlbeck WM: Conditions altering normal lung growth and development. In Thibeault DW and Gregory GA (eds): Neonatal Pulmonary Care. Norwalk, Conn, Appleton-Century-Crofts, Inc, 1986.

Nimrod C, Varela-Gittings F, Machin G et al: The effect of very prolonged membrane rupture on fetal development. Am J Obstet Gynecol 148:540, 1984.

Perlman M, Williams J, and Hirsch M: Neonatal pulmonary hypoplasia after prolonged leakage of amniotic fluid. Arch Dis Child 51:349, 1976.

Thibeault DW, Beatty EC, Hall RT et al: Neonatal pulmonary hypoplasia with premature rupture of fetal membranes and oligohydramnios. J Pediatr 107:273, 1985.

Swischuk LE, Richardson CJ, Nichols MM et al: Primary pulmonary hypoplasia in the neonate. J Pediatr 95:573, 1979.

Thomas IT and Smith DW: Oligohydramnios, cause of the nonrenal features of Potter's syndrome, including pulmonary hypoplasia. J Pediatr 84:811, 1974.

Wigglesworth JS and Desai R: Is fetal respiratory function a major determinant of perinatal survival? Lancet 1:264, 1982.

POSTASPHYXIAL PULMONARY EDEMA

Adamson TM, Boyd RDH, Hill JR et al: Effect of asphyxia due to umbilical cord occlusion in the foetal lamb on leakage of liquid from the circulation and on permeability of lung capillaries to albumin. J Physiol 207:493, 1970.

Bucciarelli RL, Nelson RM, Egan EA et al: Transient tricuspid insufficiency of the newborn: a form of myocardial dysfunction in stressed newborns. Pediatrics 59:330, 1977.

Burnard ED and James LS: Failure of the heart after undue asphyxia at birth. Pediatrics 28:545, 1961.

Cabal LA, Devaskar U, Siassi B et al: Cardiogenic shock associated with perinatal asphyxia in preterm infants. J Pediatr 96:705, 1980.

DiSessa TG, Leitner M, Ti CC et al: The cardiovascular effects of dopamine in the severely asphyxiated neonate. J Pediatr 99:772, 1981.

Donnelly WH, Bucciarelli RL, and Nelson RM: Ischemic papillary muscle necrosis in stressed newborn infants. J Pediatr 96:295, 1980.

Finley JP, Howman-Giles RB, Gilday DL et al: Transient myocardial ischemia of the newborn infant demonstrated by thallium myocardial imaging. J Pediatr 94:263, 1979.

Hansen TN, Hazinski TA, and Bland RD: Effects of asphyxia on lung fluid balance in baby lambs. J Clin Invest 74:370, 1984.

Riemenschneider TA, Nielsen HC, Ruttenberg HD et al: Disturbances of the transitional circulation: spectrum of pulmonary hypertension and myocardial dysfunction. J Pediatr 89:622, 1976.

Rowe RD and Hoffman T: Transient myocardial ischemia of the newborn infant: a form of severe cardiorespiratory distress in full-term infants. J Pediatr 81:243, 1972.

Strang LB: Neonatal lung oedema. In Strang LB (ed): Neonatal Respiration. Oxford, Blackwell Scientific Publications, 1977.

Walther FJ, Siassi B, Ramadan NA et al: Cardiac output in newborn infants with transient myocardial dysfunction. J Pediatr 107:781, 1985.

HYDROPIC PULMONARY EDEMA

Nicolaides KH, Clewell WH, and Rodeck CH: Measurement of human fetoplacental blood volume in erythoblastosis fetalis. Am J Obstet Gynecol 157:50, 1987.

Nicolaides KH, Warenski JC, and Rodeck CH: The relationship of fetal plasma protein concentration and hemoglobin level to the development of hydrops in iso-immunization. Am J Obstet Gynecol 152:341, 1985.

Phibbs RH, Johnson P, Kitterman JA et al: Cardiorespiratory status of erythroblastotic newborn infants. III: Intravascular pressures during the first hours of life. Pediatrics 58:484, 1976.

WILSON-MIKITY SYNDROME

Burnard ED: The pulmonary syndrome of Wilson and Mikity, and respiratory function in very small premature infants. Pediatr Clin North Am 13:999, 1966.

Hodgman JE, Mikity VG, Tatter D et al: Chronic respiratory distress in the premature infant: Wilson-Mikity syndrome. Pediatrics 44:179, 1969.

Krauss AN, Levin AR, Grossman H et al: Physiologic studies on infants with Wilson-Mikity syndrome. J Pediatr 77:27, 1970.

PULMONARY AIR LEAKS

Allen RW, Jung AL, and Lester PD: Effectiveness of chest tube evacuation of pneumothorax in neonates. J Pediatr 99:629, 1981.

Banagale RC, Outerbridge EW, and Aranda JV: Lung perforation: a complication of chest tube insertion in neonatal pneumothorax. J Pediatr 94:973, 1979.

Brazy JE and Blackmon LR: Hypotension and bradycardia associated with airblock in the neonate J Pediatr 5:796, 1977.

Brooks JG, Bustamante SA, Koops BL, et al: Selective bronchial intubation for the treatment of severe localized pulmonary interstitial emphysema in newborn infants. J Pediatr 91:648, 1977.

Caldwell EJ, Powell RD, and Mullooly JP: Interstitial emphysema: a study of physiologic factors involved in experimental induction of the lesion. Am Rev Respir Dis 102:516, 1970.

Frantz ID, Werthammer J, and Stark AR: High frequency ventilation in premature infants with lung disease: adequate gas exchange at low tracheal pressure. Pediatrics 71:483, 1983.

Hall RT and Rhodes PG: Pneumothorax and pneumomediastinum in infants with idiopathic respiratory distress syndrome receiving continuous positive airway pressure. Pediatrics 55:493, 1975.

Madansky DL, Lawson EE, Chernick V et al: Pneumothorax and other forms of pulmonary air leak in newborns. Am Rev Respir Dis 120:729, 1979.

Ng KPK and Easa D: Management of interstitial emphysema by high-frequency low positive-pressure hand ventilation in the neonate. J Pediatr 95:117, 1979.

Ogata ES, Gregory GA, Kitterman JA et al: Pneumothorax in the respiratory distress syndrome: incidence and effect on vital signs, blood gases, and pH. Pediatrics 58:177, 1976.

Plenat F, Vert P, Didier F, and Andre M: Pulmonary interstitial emphysema. Clin Perinatol 5:351, 1978.

Swingle HM, Eggert LD, and Bucciarelli RL: New approach to management of unilateral tension pulmonary interstitial emphysema in premature infants. Pediatrics 74:354, 1984.

Thibeault DW: Pulmonary barotrauma: interstitial emphysema, pneumomediastinum and pneumothorax. In Thibeault DW and Gregory GA (eds): Neonatal Pulmonary Care. Norwalk, Conn, Appleton-Century-Crofts, Inc, 1986.

Webb WR, Johnston JH, and Geisler JW: Pneumomediastinum: physiologic observations. J Thorac Surg 35:309, 1958.

Weiner JH, Kliegman RM, Fanaroff AA et al: Pulmonary venous air embolism in the neonate. Crit Care Med 14:67, 1986.

OTHER TYPES OF RESPIRATORY DISTRESS

Adamson TM, Boyd RDH, Normand ICS et al: Haemorrhagic pulmonary oedema (massive pulmonary haemorrhage) in the newborn. Lancet 1:494, 1969.

Krauss AN, Klain DB, and Auld PAM: Chronic pulmonary insufficiency of prematurity (CPIP). Pediatrics 55:55, 1975.

Rudolph AM: Congenital Diseases of the Heart. Chicago, Year Book Medical Publishers, Inc, 1974.

Respiratory Obstruction

Avery ME, Fletcher BD, and Williams RG: Normal and abnormal airways. In Avery ME, Fletcher BD, and Williams RG (eds): The Lung and Its Disorders in the Newborn Infant. Philadelphia, WB Saunders Co, 1981.

Krauss AN and Schley WS: Diseases of the upper airways. In Scarpelli EM et al (eds): Pulmonary Disease of the Fetus, Newborn and Child. Philadelphia, Lea & Febiger, 1978.

14

BRONCHOPULMONARY DYSPLASIA

Bronchopulmonary dysplasia (BPD) is a syndrome characterized by the triad of oxygen dependence, radiographic abnormalities, and respiratory symptoms that persist beyond 28 days of life in infants with respiratory failure at birth. It is now the most common chronic lung disease of infants. In Tennessee, for example, the incidence of BPD is at least sevenfold higher than cystic fibrosis and fifteenfold higher than chronic interstitial lung disease. The pathophysiology of BPD is complex and is not yet well understood; its treatment has been derived largely by analogy to other chronic lung disorders, such as asthma, congestive heart failure, and chronic obstructive pulmonary disease (COPD). As a result, the treatment of BPD does not yet have a firm scientific rationale.

Several reviews discuss in detail the etiology and pathogenesis of BPD (O'Brodovich and Mellins, 1987; Nickerson, 1985; Stahlman, 1987; Koops et al, 1984; Bronchopulmonary dysplasia, 1986). This chapter discusses these topics briefly but focuses mainly on inpatient and outpatient management, because 40 to 50 per cent of infants who develop BPD will require ongoing therapy at home, and some of these will develop chronic respiratory disease that may persist into adulthood.

EPIDEMIOLOGY

The epidemiology of BPD has changed dramatically in the last 2 decades. In the early 1960s, premature infants with respiratory failure, usually due to hyaline membrane disease (HMD), began to receive oxygen therapy and mechanical ventilation. At that time, most infants who survived for 72 hours went home in 7 to 10 days without evidence of lingering lung disease. However, as these therapies were applied more widely, several medical centers reported infants who did not recover rapidly but instead developed chronic pulmonary symptoms, hypoxemia, and chest radiographic abnormalities. For example, Shephard and colleagues (1964) reported that 50 per cent of the premature neonates who

received one or both therapies developed persistent symptomatic pulmonary infiltrates beyond the age of 6 months.

Northway and co-workers (1967), following up their earlier study (Rosan et al, 1966), reported on 32 mechanically ventilated infants who also had received high concentrations of oxygen. The infants averaged 2.2 kg and 34 weeks of gestation at birth. In their study, 19 infants died, and the lungs of these infants were examined for pathologies. All of the surviving infants had respiratory symptoms and abnormal chest radiographs beyond the first 4 weeks of life. The investigators compiled their clinical and pathologic findings and defined a new respiratory syndrome, which they termed *bronchopulmonary dysplasia*, ". . . to emphasize the involvement of all the tissues of the lung in the pathologic process." The researchers correctly conceptualized BPD as resulting from three interacting factors: (1) lung immaturity; (2) initial lung injury caused by oxygen, mechanical ventilation, and other factors; and (3) inadequate repair of the initial lung injury. Advances in neonatal-perinatal medicine, such as improved delivery room care and the development of regional perinatal units, have made it possible to eliminate each of these three factors to some extent. Indeed, the success of neonatal care is evidenced by the fact that BPD has virtually disappeared in moderately premature infants who were the subjects of initial reports (Shepard et al, 1968).

BPD is now rare in infants who are older than 32 weeks of gestation and is uncommon beyond 30 weeks. However, at least in North America and Europe, there has been an increase in the number and survival rates of premature infants of 25 to 28 weeks of gestation, so that more than 75 per cent of infants with BPD are from this very low birth weight group (Fig. 14–1). In these immature infants, even minimal exposure to oxygen and mechanical ventilation can lead to BPD. Thus as survival rates of extremely premature infants increase, the number of infants with BPD will also increase (Fig. 14–2).

The epidemiology of BPD is difficult to determine because the current definition of BPD lacks precision and sensitivity. This lack of precision exists for three reasons. First, the definition does not include severity criteria. For example, consider two infants born at 27 weeks of gestation: at 28 days of age, one is

This work was supported by grants from the Department of Health and Human Services (HL 14214) and by a Career Investigator Award from the American Lung Association.

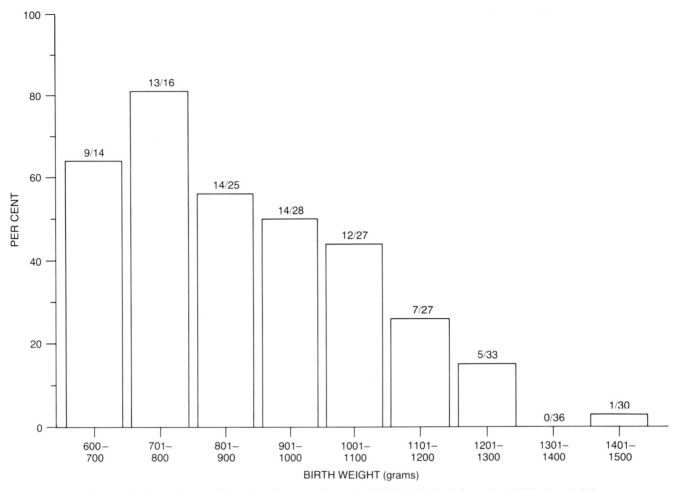

Figure 14–1. Incidence of bronchopulmonary dysplasia (BPD) by birthweight at Vanderbilt Hospital for the 18 months before July 1, 1989. The incidence of BPD is depicted as the percentage of infants who survived more than 28 days.

receiving 23 per cent oxygen via nasal cannula and the other is receiving 100 per cent oxygen and mechanical ventilation. Both of these infants have BPD, but the treatment for and prognosis of each of them are very different.

Second, the definition considers only postnatal age and not gestational age; it is not surprising that infants born at less than 28 weeks of gestation with severe HMD will still require oxygen therapy after 28 days when they are not yet 32 weeks of postconceptional age. Indeed, in this group, as shown in Figure 14–3, BPD is the cost of successful treatment of respiratory failure (Cotton and Parker, 1988; Tooley, 1979).

Third, because the definition of BPD includes oxygen dependence, a nursery that administers oxygen until the infant's room air saturation is always greater than 94 per cent will have more infants in oxygen than a nursery that discontinues oxygen therapy when room air saturation is greater than 90 per cent. In addition, nurseries in cities high above sea level, such as Denver, Albuquerque, and Reno, might be expected to use oxygen therapy for longer periods. Thus the broad definition of BPD has made interpretation of BPD incidence figures from different medical centers very difficult. Table 14–1 depicts the incidence of BPD *in the same center* using different denominators. Regardless of the definition used, however, advances in neonatal care will inevitably result in an increase in the number of infants with BPD who will require ongoing care in the first years of life.

RISK FACTORS

Although it is simple to list the risk factors for the development of BPD, the importance of any single factor in any individual infant is impossible to determine. The key risk factor for the development of BPD is respiratory failure in an infant with an immature lung. Respiratory failure can be caused by various factors that are described in what follows.

Lung Immaturity. It has long been recognized that some extremely premature infants do not develop BPD, but some near-term infants do (Wilson and Mikity, 1960; Krauss et al, 1975; Truog et al, 1985). These observations have led to the notion that it is not prematurity per se but lung immaturity that is the primary risk factor for BPD. However, because most infants with immature lungs have very low birth

BPD AT CHILDREN'S HOSPITAL, VANDERBILT

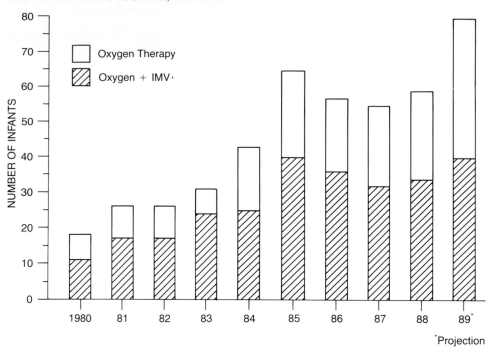

Figure 14–2. Number of infants diagnosed with bronchopulmonary dysplasia (BPD) at 28 days of life at Children's Hospital, Vanderbilt, from 1980 to 1989. The height of each bar represents the number of 28-day-old oxygen-dependent infants, and the hatched area represents the number of such infants who also required mechanical ventilation. The projection for 1989 is based on data from the first 6 months of that year.

weights, the most important single predictive factor for the development of BPD is birth weight (see Fig. 14–2).

Although discussions of lung immaturity usually focus on alveolar development and on the functional immaturity of the surfactant system in type II cells, all of the components of the immature respiratory system can be underdeveloped at birth, which can lead to respiratory failure. Lung development is

discussed in detail in Chapter 1, but it should be evident that normal lung development depends on the orderly differentiation of more than 30 other cell types, the function of many of which is not yet understood.

The anatomic features of the immature but rapidly developing respiratory system easily explain the pathogenesis of respiratory failure in immature infants. For example, in the fetal lung at 22 to 26

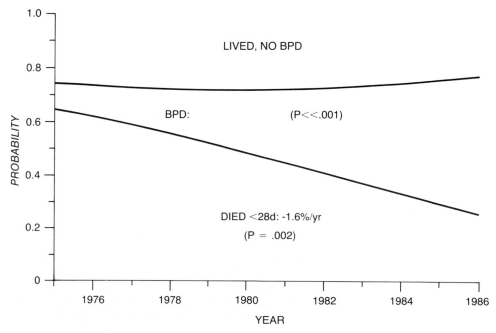

Figure 14–3. Logistic regression analysis of the changing outcomes for premature male infants from 1975 to 1986. Note that the fall in mortality is almost exactly balanced by the increased probability of developing bronchopulmonary dysplasia (BPD), but the chances of survival without BPD have remained essentially unchanged. (Data from Cotton RB and Parker RA: Pediatr Res 23:445A, 1988.)

[BW: 1000 g, HMD, NO PTX, MALE, WHITE, INBORN]

Table 14–1. INCIDENCE OF BRONCHOPULMONARY DYSPLASIA AT VANDERBILT NEONATAL INTENSIVE CARE UNIT, JAN 1 THROUGH JUNE 30, 1989

2% of all ventilated surviving infants between 1500 and 3000 g
8% of all infants ventilated at birth
10% of all nursery admissions
19% of all ventilated surviving infants
42% of all admissions ¢1000 g
55% of all surviving infants ¢1000 g
62% of all inborn infants ¢1250 g
75% of all inborn surviving infants ¢1250 g
70% of all survivors ¢750 g
100% of all surviving infants with hyaline membrane disease ¢750 g

weeks of gestation and in more mature infants in whom lung maturation has been delayed (e.g., in infants of diabetic mothers), most of the capillaries are still embedded in mesenchyme, and capillary-airway interfaces are infrequent (Stahlman and Gray, 1987). Moreover, these lung capillaries have increased permeability to water and protein that can lead to pulmonary edema after birth as pulmonary blood flow increases. As a result, even though type II cell number and function may be adequate and airway anatomy well developed, ventilation-perfusion mismatch is an anatomic inevitability and respiratory failure will occur. A flail chest wall; immature respiratory control system; and underdeveloped tone, power, and coordination of respiratory muscles all contribute to the development of respiratory failure. These features explain why BPD will continue to occur even in infants whose type II cell development has been accelerated by maternal corticosteroid treatment or augmented by surfactant replacement therapy.

There has been an increase in the number of near-term infants who develop severe hypoxemic respiratory failure in association with perinatal asphyxia and persistent pulmonary hypertension or persistent fetal circulation (PFC). The morbidity and mortality of severe hypoxemic respiratory failure is substantial, and a number of these infants develop BPD that may be particularly severe. The early identification and treatment of these infants along with the introduction of extracorporeal membrane oxygenation (ECMO) may reduce the incidence of BPD in this new group at risk.

Genetic Factors. Several studies have suggested that there may be a genetic predisposition to the development of BPD. In most medical centers, race (white) and gender (male) are independent risk factors for the development of BPD (Avery et al, 1987), probably because HMD is more severe in these groups. Others have reported a higher than expected incidence of atopic disorders in families of BPD infants, which has led to the speculation that bronchial hyperreactivity may be a key risk factor for BPD (Nickerson and Taussig, 1980). Other studies indicate that premature infants without BPD also have bronchial hyperreactivity so that its association with BPD may be secondary to preterm birth.

Oxygen Toxicity. Oxygen therapy is a two-edged sword for the immature infant with respiratory failure. On the one hand, oxygen is necessary to maintain systemic oxygen delivery. On the other hand, the detrimental effects of acute and long-term oxygen exposure on lung function and lung development have been known for decades. Most clinicians agree that the mechanism by which oxygen injures the lung is related to the accelerated production of a toxic oxygen species that cannot be detoxified by antioxidant defenses (Frank and Massaro, 1980; Deneke and Fanburg, 1980). Past research has focused mainly on the key role of lung antioxidant enzymes in the defense against oxygen injury. However, later research has focused on enzymatic sources of oxidant production and on the key role of nonenzymatic antioxidants, such as glutathione and alpha$_1$-protease inhibitor (Hazinski et al, 1988; Hazinski et al, 1989).

Although high concentrations of oxygen affect all lung cells, the endothelial cell is particularly vulnerable to injury because antioxidant defenses are inadequate, oxidant production is markedly accelerated in these cells, or both. Thus acute oxygen toxicity is marked by the increase in lung microvascular permeability, the development of acute pulmonary edema, and the development of acute necrotizing tracheobronchitis (van Asbeck et al, 1985). Alveolar permeability is also increased by oxygen exposure. In addition, the oxidant stress of acute oxygen exposure can disrupt normal lung development, interfere with surfactant production and ciliary motility, and cause oxidative inactivation of cellular antioxidants (Nash et al, 1967; Pratt et al, 1979; Kapanci et al, 1969).

Long-term exposure to high concentrations of oxygen also has detrimental effects: recruitment and activation of lung neutrophils and macrophages, necrosis of bronchiolar epithelium, necrosis of type I cells, hyperplasia of type II cells, and a marked proliferation of fibroblasts and macrophages in lung interstitium. All of these pathologic features are present in infants with BPD.

It is impossible to define a safe level or duration of oxygen exposure for infants with immature lungs. Indeed, even 21 per cent oxygen (PA$_{O_2}$ ¯ 110 mm Hg) is relatively hyperoxic for the premature infant whose in utero alveolar oxygen tension is less than 40 mm Hg. Moreover, oxygen-induced lung injury depends not only on FI$_{O_2}$ but also on an imbalance between oxidant production and oxidant destruction within specific lung cells. In animal studies, lung levels of antioxidant enzymes have been found to increase throughout gestation, but so do enzyme systems that increase oxidant production. As a result, the oxidant/antioxidant balance may remain relatively constant throughout gestation so that the immature infant's susceptibility to oxygen injury may reside in part on an inability to respond rapidly to oxygen exposure by inducing antioxidant production and by inhibiting oxidant production. Future strategies to reduce oxidant-mediated lung injury will likely be based on a better understanding of the regulation of these oxidant- and antioxidant-producing pathways.

Despite these observations, the role of oxygen toxicity in the pathogenesis of BPD has always been speculative, in part because BPD was rare in premature infants treated with oxygen alone. However, studies of a primate model of premature respiratory failure demonstrated that breathing 100 per cent oxygen for 6 to 8 days increases the risk of BPD even when the effect of mechanical ventilation is taken into account (deLemos, Coalson, Gerstmann et al, 1987; Coalson et al, 1988).

Positive-Pressure Ventilation with Lung Stretch. Positive airway pressure of even mild degree can augment oxygen toxicity by stinting previously unventilated alveolar units with low compliance, thereby increasing PA_{O_2} in these lung units. The immature lung can also be injured by the mechanical effects of positive-pressure ventilation. Pathologic studies of premature infants and experimental animals have demonstrated marked distortion of the lung, especially terminal bronchioles, during mechanical ventilation. In the surfactant-deficient lung with low compliance, the increase in alveolar volume during positive pressure-driven inspiration is *less* than the increase in terminal airway volume, indicating that bronchiolar compliance is higher than alveolar compliance (Meredith et al, in press). Conversely, spontaneously breathing premature infants may collapse these compliant terminal airways during exhalation. As a result of this cyclic bronchiolar stretching, terminal airway ischemia and necrosis develop, which eventually lead to interstitial air dissection, interstitial emphysema, pneumothorax, and further lung injury (deLemos, Coalson, Null et al, 1987; Stahlman et al, 1979). Data indicate that high tidal volume ventilation can also increase lung microvascular permeability, which may augment edema formation and result in the need for more aggressive mechanical ventilation (Carlton et al, 1989).

Although this injury mechanism has been termed *barotrauma,* studies indicate that lung stretch is the real culprit and that high levels of positive pressure alone are well tolerated by the newborn lung if lung stretch is prevented. These findings have spurred the search, thus far unsuccessful, for less damaging ways to apply conventional ventilation and to the development of unconventional ventilation techniques, including high-frequency ventilation (HIFI study group, 1989). There is no conclusive evidence yet that one ventilator or ventilation technique is superior to another.

Inflammation. Neonatal pneumonia can lead to respiratory failure. The intubated infant with respiratory failure is exposed to various airway irritants and is at high risk for repeated bouts of airway infection; any of these events can trigger the inflammation pathway and upset the balance between inflammatory and anti-inflammatory mechanisms in the lung. Thus neutrophil-, macrophage-, and lymphocyte-derived inflammatory mediators have been proposed as prominent risk factors for the development of BPD. Neutrophils can produce and release

toxic oxygen species, and neutrophil accumulation has been observed near edematous endothelial cells in some models of acute lung injury. Lung lavage fluid from infants who ultimately develop BPD contains elevated levels of neutrophil-derived protease activity and reduced or inactivated antiprotease defenses (Burnett et al, 1987; Clement et al, 1988; Jackson et al, 1987; Merritt et al, 1983; Ogden et al, 1983; Merritt et al, 1981). Studies of lavage fluid from other newborn infants with respiratory failure have also demonstrated high concentrations of vasoactive and bronchoactive metabolites of arachidonic acid, indicating that these inflammatory mediators may play a role in the functional abnormalities of infants with BPD. It has also been shown that both growth factors and cytokines are produced at sites of inflammation and that these agents can have potent vasoactive and mitogenic effects (Johnson et al, 1989; Johnson et al, 1982); these effects are likely to have unique consequences in the immature lung.

Abnormal Nutrition. The amount, route, and composition of nutrients provided to the extremely premature neonate are inadequate when compared with the infant in utero. The early administration of intravenous dextrose, amino acid and lipid emulsions, and improved enteral formulas have played an important role in the immediate and long-term care of the immature neonate, but evidence indicates that these solutions may lack factors important for lung growth, repair, and defense against injury. For example, based on data that suggested that the antioxidant vitamin E was deficient in premature infants, an early study indicated that vitamin E supplementation reduced the incidence of BPD (Ehrenkranz et al, 1978). Subsequent studies could not confirm this finding (Ehrenkranz et al, 1979; Saldanha et al, 1982), probably because by the time these later studies were done, parenteral nutrition solutions and infant formulas were enriched in this nutrient, so that even the control groups in subsequent studies were vitamin E sufficient.

Vitamin A has been identified as a key nutrient for the premature infants at risk to develop BPD. Based on the observations that squamous metaplasia was a pathologic feature of both vitamin A deficiency and BPD and that premature infants have low plasma levels of vitamin A, Shenai and colleagues conducted a double-blind, placebo-controlled study of vitamin A supplementation in premature infants (1987). They found that the incidence and severity of BPD were significantly reduced by the administration of parenteral vitamin A in doses designed to result in levels in plasma that were in the normal range for term infants. This finding has been confirmed in another small study (Papagaroufalis et al, 1988), and if it is shown to be true in larger trials, it may be an important step in the understanding of the role of specific nutrient deficiencies in the pathogenesis of BPD. In addition, because vitamin A is known to play a key role in lung repair and differentiation, these studies lend substantial support to Northway's original hypothesis that BPD represented ". . . the prolongation of the healing phase of the (respiratory distress) syndrome."

Growth Factor Imbalance. More than 200 growth factors or signaling factors have been described, and a few of these have been identified in the developing and healing lung. For example, as the name implies, epidermal growth factor (EGF) is present in the fetal lung epithelium and stimulates proliferation of undifferentiated stem cells that are present in those portions of the airways that are undergoing the most rapid growth. Neither EGF nor its receptor is present in well-differentiated terminal airways of near-term infants with normal lungs, but it is abundant in sites of airway injury that are undergoing repair in BPD infants (Stahlman et al, 1989). This finding of EGF in the regenerating dysplastic epithelium of BPD infants suggests that abnormal EGF-stimulated airway growth without concomitant differentiation may contribute to the morphologic and functional abnormalities of terminal airways in infants with BPD. It is likely that further understanding of BPD will depend largely on the understanding of the factors that control normal lung growth and injury repair, because there is increasing evidence that these two mechanisms may be quite similar.

PATHOLOGY

In the years following the initial description of BPD, the treatment of neonatal respiratory failure and its consequences has changed dramatically. In addition, the impact of extremely premature birth on lung injury and repair mechanisms has rendered the original pathologic descriptions of BPD in near-term infants difficult to apply. Moreover, in vivo lung biopsy studies of infants with mild BPD are scarce, and most infants who die with BPD die of an acute pulmonary infection. As a result of these factors, the precise pathologic features of BPD, their time of onset, and their implications have been difficult to determine. The most comprehensive studies have been performed by Stocker (1986) and Stahlman (1987; Stahlman and Gray, 1987), who have divided the pathologic findings into early, reparative, and chronic categories. A summary of pathologic findings is presented in Table 14–2.

In the early stages of BPD (i.e., infants who die within 3 to 5 days of age), the gross appearance of the lungs is similar to that of HMD. Lung weight is 25 to 150 per cent of predicted, and the lungs are consolidated with focal hemorrhage and diffuse interstitial emphysema. The trachea and large bronchi may have diffuse or focal areas of epithelial ulceration. On microscopic examination, bronchial epithelium is devoid of ciliated cells, and hyaline membranes are present within alveoli. There is airway and alveolar necrosis with interstitial edema. Pulmonary arterioles and veins are usually normal.

In the reparative or subacute phase, there is a suggestion of a cobblestone appearance to the pleural surface that reflects the underlying uneven distribution of alveolar inflation. Large, air-filled, subpleural cysts lined by lymphatic endothelium are present, whose lumens can be traced to the hilum along septal planes. At this stage, some parts of the lung appear relatively normal, and there are often obvious demarcation lines between normal and abnormal areas. The trachea and large bronchi appear relatively normal, but tracheomalacia may be present in some infants. Microscopic examination reveals a spectrum of bronchial abnormalities, ranging from mild metaplastic changes in patent bronchioles to complete obliteration of others. Some bronchial lumens are narrowed by hyperplastic squamous metaplasia, and some ciliated epithelial cells begin to reappear. Small and medium-sized bronchi are surrounded by thick bands of smooth muscle, and muscular hypertrophy may extend beyond respiratory bronchioles. The focal nature of the injury is apparent in lung sections, as completely occluded and edematous bronchi are surrounded by relatively normal alveoli. In other areas, dysplastic alveoli seem to be compressed by fibroblast proliferation. Pulmonary arterioles display medial hypertrophy and intimal hyperplasia. Thus the major features of this phase of BPD are the focal nature and the dysplastic changes at the level of the bronchi, terminal airways, and respiratory bronchioles.

The focal nature of this phase of BPD, which has also been seen in the primate model of BPD (Coalson et al, 1988; Meredith et al, in press), has led Stocker and others to suggest that alveolar units distal to completely obstructed airways are protected from both high oxygen tensions and stretch injury; in these units, lung repair might be more effective because ongoing lung injury was diminished (Fig. 14–4). Although it would be desirable to permit lung repair to occur, this unventilated region, if normally perfused, would also function as an anatomic shunt, which in turn might lead to the use of increased oxygen concentrations. In addition, those airways that remained partially open would be subjected to high oxygen tensions and be even more susceptible to stretch injury if these units inflate rapidly but deflate slowly. Thus the focal and dynamic nature of the anatomic features of this phase of BPD makes the design of general treatment strategies difficult.

Cardiac involvement has also been demonstrated in infants with BPD. There may be evidence of myocardial ischemia or myocardial infarction, and left-sided, right-sided, and biventricular hypertrophy have been described (Tomashefski et al, 1984).

In the chronic phase of BPD (usually infants older than 2 months of age), the cobblestone appearance of the lung's surface is much more pronounced, as hyperexpanded units are present alongside atretic and fibrotic units to impart a "pseudofissuring" to the surface of the lung. With time and growth of relatively normal areas of the lung, the cobblestone effect disappears, but large pseudofissures remain,

Table 14–2. PATHOLOGIC FEATURES OF BRONCHOPULMONARY DYSPLASIA

	Acute	Reparative	LSHBPD*
TRACHEA			
Mucosa	Dysplasia	Metaplasia	Normal or metaplasia
	Necrosis	Metaplasia	Metaplasia
Submucosa	Inflammation acute or chronic	Inflammation chronic	
	Necrosis and/or edema	Fibroplasia	Fibrosis (pseudopolyp)
Glands	Hypertrophy	Hyperplasia	Hyperplasia or normal
BRONCHI			
Mucosa	Dysplasia	Metaplasia	Normal or metaplasia
Submucosa	Inflammation acute or chronic	Inflammation chronic	Normal
	Edema	Muscular hyperplasia	
BRONCHIOLES			
Mucosa	Luminal occlusion by hyaline membrane	Organization	Normal
	Dysplasia	Metaplasia	Normal
	Necrosis	Metaplasia	Normal
	Necrosis	Organization	Normal
Submucosa	Necrotizing "obstructive" bronchiolitis	Intrinsic fibroplasia	Partial or complete obliteration
	Edema	Muscular hyperplasia	Muscular hyperplasia
	Inflammation acute and chronic	Extrinsic fibroplasia	Fibrosis
ALVEOLAR DUCT			
Mucosa	Hyaline membranes	Organization	Normal
	Dysplasia	Metaplasia	Normal
	Necrosis	Intrinsic fibroplasia	Fibrosis or obliteration
Submucosa	Necrosis and edema	Extrinsic fibroplasia	Fibrosis or obliteration
ALVEOLUS			
Lining cells	Hyaline membranes	Organization	Normal
	Necrosis	Fibroplasia	Fibrosis with obliteration
Interstitium	Edema	Edema	Normal
	Necrosis	Fibroplasia	Fibrosis or obliteration
INTERLOBULAR SEPTA			
	Edema	Edema	Normal
	Interstitial emphysema, acute	Organization	Normal
	Interstitial emphysema, persistent	Giant-cell reaction	Fibrosis
PULMONARY ARTERIES			
	Adventitial edema	Medial hyperplasia and adventitial edema	Medial hyperplasia and/or adventitial fibrosis

*Long-standing healed bronchopulmonary dysplasia.
(From Stocker JT and Dehner LP: Acquired pulmonary disease in the pediatric age group. In Dail D and Hammer S: Pulmonary Pathology. New York, Springer Verlag, 1987.)

and normal lobes are impossible to identify. Tracheomegaly, tracheomalacia, and ciliary dysfunction may be present as either focal or diffuse abnormalities (Bhutani et al, 1986; O'Brodovich et al, 1984). Granulomatous nodules, concentric fibrosis, and polyps may also be present and may cause tracheal or bronchial obstruction. On microscopic examination, the hallmark of this phase of BPD is alveolar septal fibrosis such that the width of the alveolar septa are ten times greater than normal. The focal nature of BPD is still present with fibrotic, hyperexpanded, and normal lung units adjacent to one another. There is mucous gland hypertrophy in the bronchial mucosa, and squamous metaplasia is more pronounced. In addition, muscular hyperplasia around pulmonary arteries and especially around bronchioles can now be identified in more than 80 per cent of infants who die during this phase of the disease; however, even these abnormalities may be focal, and normal bronchovascular anatomy may be seen in many lung regions.

Ventricular hypertrophy occurs in most infants who die with BPD at this stage. Right ventricular hypertrophy has been seen in 73 per cent of these infants, whereas left ventricular hypertrophy (17 per cent) and biventricular hypertrophy (10 per cent) are less frequent. Myocardial fibrosis is also present.

RADIOLOGIC FINDINGS

Although persistent radiologic abnormalities form part of the triad of the diagnosis of BPD and were once used to stage the progression of disease, these changes have proved to be less useful than they once were. It is now possible to measure the clinical and functional consequences of BPD, such as the FI_{O_2} needed to maintain a certain saturation, and to measure compliance and resistance directly; these findings often are little correlated with chest radiographic assessment. In general, however, two radiographic abnormalities predominate (Heneghan et al, 1986). The most common radiologic manifestation of BPD is the presence of diffuse, fine infiltrates without

Figure 14–4. *Top:* Schematic drawing of normally expanded and aerated pulmonary lobules. *Middle:* Acute bronchopulmonary dysplasia. *A,* Necrotizing bronchiolitis occludes the bronchiolar lumen "protecting" the parenchyma distal to it from the high oxygen tension and pressure needed to maintain adequate oxygenation. *B,* The bronchiole is narrowed by mucosal necrosis, hyperplasia, or both, and submucosal edema, fibroplasia, or both, thereby reducing the amount of pressure and oxygen tension in the lobule distal to it. Alveolar cell hyperplasia, septal fibroplasia, and alveolar macrophage dysplasia, however, occur to a mild to moderate degree. *C,* The bronchiole is widely patent, exposing the distal sublobule to the full ventilatory pressure and high oxygen tension. The alveolar lumens are largely obliterated by alveolar macrophages, alveolar cell hyperplasia, and marked septal fibroplasia. *Bottom:* Longstanding "healed" bronchopulmonary dysplasia (LSHBPD). *A,* With resolution of the necrotizing bronchiolitis that occluded the lumen of the bronchiole, the uninjured sublobule overexpands to compensate for the less expansile injured portions of lung *(B* and *C). B,* With resolution of the mild to moderate injury incurred by the parenchyma during the acute stages of bronchopulmonary dysplasia, the sublobule displays the hallmark of LSHBPD—septal fibrosis. *C,* The sublobule is virtually obliterated by organization of the severe acute bronchopulmonary dysplasia. (From Stocker JT: Hum Pathol 17:943, 1986.)

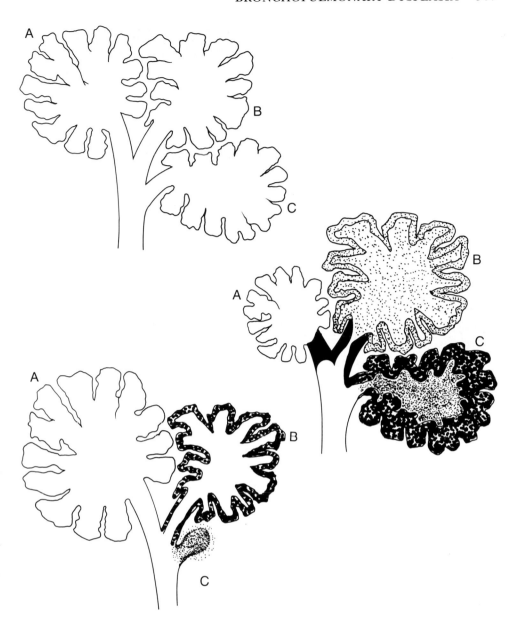

appreciable emphysema (Fig. 14–5*A*). Infants with these infiltrates may have no oxygen requirement and be asymptomatic, or they may still require mechanical ventilation for severe hypercarbia. Infants with severe respiratory impairment usually have coarse infiltrates with emphysema, but even some infants with this radiographic picture may have mild disease (Fig. 14–5*B*). A system for scoring the radiographic severity of BPD has been proposed (Toce et al, 1984) but has not gained widespread use because of the subjective and qualitative nature of the variables employed to compute a final score.

A peculiar feature of some infants with BPD who are older than 6 months is the presence of a flat chest, seen on lateral chest radiographs (Edwards and Hilston, 1987). This abnormality is apparently unrelated to the extent of BPD severity at the time the radiographs were taken but may reflect the resid-

ual effects of abnormal lung mechanics on chest growth.

CARDIOPULMONARY FUNCTION

The functional consequences of the pathologic abnormalities in the early stages of BPD have been well documented in many studies, in part because of the availability of computer-assisted devices that measure the active and passive characteristics of the respiratory system (England, 1988; Guslits et al, 1987; Gerhardt et al, 1989). All of these devices, however, have as their major limitation the inability to measure multiple compartments of the lung affected by BPD; instead they measure only an average value for the lung or respiratory system as a whole. As predicted from the pathologic description of BPD,

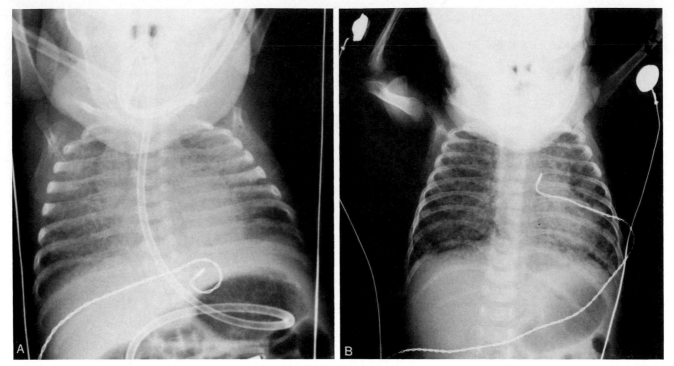

Figure 14–5. Two typical radiographic appearances of chronic bronchopulmonary dysplasia. *A* demonstrates the diffuse haziness pattern seen in some infants. *B* illustrates the bilateral cystic appearance of the lungs with hyperinflation. Both of these 3-month-old infants required more than 80 per cent oxygen to maintain normal oxygen saturation.

the major physiologic abnormalities should be related to focal small airway narrowing due to edema, fibrosis, and muscle hypertrophy. Thus infants with BPD at 28 days of age have an increased total respiratory resistance, expiratory resistance, and severe flow limitation, especially at low lung volumes (Loeber et al, 1980; Tepper et al, 1986; Wolfson et al, 1984; Lindroth et al, 1980) (Fig. 14–6). Indeed, in some studies, an elevated pulmonary resistance in infants less than a week old accurately predicts those infants who will go on to develop chronic BPD (Goldman et al, 1983). Dynamic lung compliance is also markedly reduced in infants with BPD (Wolfson et al, 1984; Lindroth et al, 1980), even in those who no longer require oxygen therapy (Kao, Warburton, Cheng et al, 1984). The reduction in compliance is due not only to small airway narrowing but also to interstitial fibrosis, edema, and atelectasis. Functional residual capacity (FRC) is usually decreased but may be increased or normal. These dynamic abnormalities lead to an increase in the work of breathing and to ventilation-perfusion mismatching. Highly unusual ventilation-perfusion patterns have been observed during ventilation-perfusion scanning studies (Slavin et al, 1986). Nitrogen washout is prolonged, particularly in hyperexpanded regions.

Pulmonary vascular hypertension may also be present in infants with BPD and is characterized pathologically by structural remodeling of pulmonary arterioles and by altered vasoreactivity (Tomashefski et al, 1984; Melnick et al, 1980). Before the use of

continuous oxygen therapy in infants with severe BPD became widespread, these commonly succumbed to cor pulmonale; this complication is now seen only in the most severe ventilator-dependent infants who have never been discharged from the hospital.

Systemic hypertension and left-ventricular dysfunction may also be present in infants with BPD; their causes are poorly understood (Abman, Warady, Lum, and Koops, 1984; Goodman et al, 1988). Infants with BPD have been shown to have abnormal pulmonary clearance of norepinephrine (Abman et al, 1987) and to have elevated vasopressin levels (Hazinski et al, 1988), but the relationship between these two observations and the development of systemic hypertension is unclear. Systemic hypertension usually does not require long-term treatment and disappears as lung function improves.

As a result of these abnormalities, hypoxia with or without hypercarbia is present. However, the degree of gas exchange impairment correlates poorly with resistance and compliance measurements. Oxygen consumption at rest is also 30 to 50 per cent higher (Fig. 14–7), but this value cannot be accounted for entirely by the increased work of breathing (Kurzner et al, 1988; Weinstein and Oh, 1981).

A few studies have assessed the changes in pulmonary function of BPD infants beyond the first few months of life (Gerhardt et al, 1987). Most infants with BPD show improvement of pulmonary function with time, so that lung function is usually in the

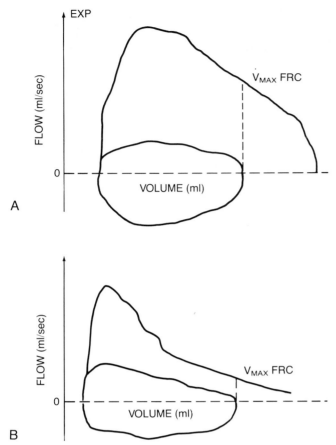

Figure 14–6. Partial expiratory flow-volume curves. The smaller inner curve represents tidal breathing, and the larger curve represents maximal expiratory flow generated by the rapid compression technique. The maximal expiratory flow at functional residual capacity $(V_{max}FRC)$ is indicated by a *dashed line*. The difference between tidal breathing and maximal expiratory flow represents the expiratory flow reserve. *A*, The normal control infant has a convex to linear maximal expiratory flow volume curve, with a large expiratory flow reserve. *B*, The infant with bronchopulmonary dysplasia has a concave flow volume curve, with a decreased expiratory flow reserve and $V_{max}FRC$, compared with the infant in *A*. (Data from Tepper et al: J Pediatr 109:1040, 1986.)

normal range by 2 to 3 years of age. Whether this improvement represents repair of damaged lung or growth of new lung (or both) has not been determined. Infants whose lung function remains unchanged or worsens are usually those whose somatic growth is markedly delayed, but the relationship between abnormal lung repair and delayed somatic growth is unclear. Some neonatologists have used this latter observation to justify aggressive nutritional supplementation for infants with BPD, with unproven success. Indeed, it may be equally likely that the delay in somatic growth in these severely affected infants is the result of chronic hypoxemia or an adaptive response to delayed lung repair.

Studies of pulmonary function in older children who were born prematurely have indicated that although subtle defects of small airway function may be present in childhood, these abnormalities are not more frequent in infants with BPD than in premature

infants without BPD (Bertrand et al, 1985). These studies suggest that prematurity per se may have a small but measurable impact on lung growth, which may predispose an individual to the development of lung disease later in life.

CLINICAL MANIFESTATIONS

The pulmonary signs and symptoms of BPD should be apparent from the previous discussions of the pathology and physiology of the syndrome. Tachypnea, dyspnea, and wheezing may be intermittently or chronically present. The chest wall may appear hyperinflated, or a flat chest may be seen (Edwards and Hilston, 1987). Inguinal hernias may also be present, which may reflect the continual increase in abdominal pressure caused by high airway resistance and the use of accessory respiratory muscles. Infants with BPD who have been intubated for long periods may develop subglottic stenosis or intratracheal scars or polyps, which may cause stridor or prohibit extubation. Infants with moderate to severe BPD are frequently described as irritable and difficult to feed and comfort; they may develop irregular sleep patterns or have such disrupted patterns imposed on them. These symptoms may indicate hypoxia or underlying neurologic dysfunction. Pallor and severe growth failure usually indicate chronic hypoxia despite oxygen therapy or myocardial dysfunction due either to underlying pulmonary vascular disease or to the pulmonary vascular effects of

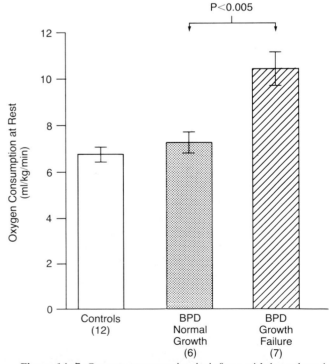

Figure 14–7. Oxygen consumption in infants with bronchopulmonary dysplasia with and without growth failure. (From Kurzner SI, Garg M, Bautista DB et al: Growth failure in bronchopulmonary dysplasia: elevated metabolic rates and pulmonary mechanics. J Pediatr 112:76, 1988.)

mechanical ventilation. Digital clubbing is seen in the most severe cases; in my experience, the presence of digital clubbing signals a bleak prognosis.

Infants with severe BPD often have episodic disorders that are difficult to explain and to treat. Perhaps the worst complication of infants with severe BPD is the development of *recurrent cyanotic episodes.* These episodes may be caused by agitation with tracheal obstruction due to tracheal distortion or by idiopathic *necrotizing tracheobronchitis.* This latter problem is heralded radiographically by the appearance of migratory focal consolidations and clinically by the sudden development of partial or complete airway obstruction, for which emergency bronchoscopy may be the only treatment. These infants also may develop *intermittent systemic edema,* which may be iatrogenic due to volume overload (blood transfusion, excess fluid intake from diluted oral drugs, frequent tracheal lavage with saline, etc.) or may be related to vasopressin excess or to transient myocardial dysfunction. Also, like many patients with chronic obstructive lung disease, they may develop intermittent high *fever* without documented infection. *Supraventricular tachycardia* may also occur in these infants spontaneously, in association with diuretic-induced electrolyte imbalance or during bronchodilator therapy. Recently, a generalized disorder of movement has been described in infants with severe BPD (Perlman and Volpe, 1989).

RESPIRATORY MANAGEMENT

The goals of respiratory management of infants with BPD are to maintain normal oxygenation while at the same time avoiding those interventions that increase the risk of further pulmonary damage or delay lung repair. The clinician must recognize that these goals are often in conflict with one another and in some cases are in conflict with the principles of optimal pediatric care. As with any chronic disease, tradeoffs must inevitably be made with a view toward the best interests of the child and the child's caretakers.

Mechanical Ventilation. Positive-pressure ventilation via endotracheal tube should be discontinued as soon as possible. If mechanical ventilation is necessary, the lowest inflation pressures should be used, and expiratory time should be long enough (i.e., $\geq$ 400 ms) to allow hyperinflated and highly compliant lung units to empty completely. The oft-quoted assertion that mechanical ventilation decreases the work of breathing and spares calories for growth and repair is unproved for infants and has been shown to be absolutely wrong for adults with COPD; in fact, mechanical ventilation actually increases the work of breathing in adult patients (Marini et al, 1988). The value of chest physiotherapy in either ventilated or spontaneously breathing infants is unproved but is probably useful in the ventilated infant prone to atelectasis. Gentle technique and adequate oxygena-

tion during the procedure are mandatory. A very useful weaning strategy for ventilated infants with BPD has been recently described by Goldberg and Bancalari (1988).

The three most common mistakes made in weaning infants with BPD from mechanical ventilation are (1) the failure to distinguish between the need for ventilation (i.e., carbon dioxide removal) and the need for oxygenation (i.e., Fi_{O_2}); (2) the belief that arterial pH and P_{CO_2} must be in the normal range before and immediately after making a reduction in ventilator support; and (3) the realization that postextubation symptoms must develop before the administration of antiedema aerosol therapy with racemic epinephrine, proper positioning, and additional oxygen therapy.

To avoid the first two mistakes during weaning, the clinician should use whatever Fi_{O_2} that results in oxygen saturations that are greater than 92 per cent at all times by accurate oximetry. In chronic BPD, arterial blood gas values may be less helpful, and the clinician should instead conclude that a reduction in ventilatory support is successful if the patient's general appearance is unchanged and a venous or arterial pH is greater than 7.25. In addition, the physician must recognize that a diuretic-induced metabolic alkalosis can cause hypoventilation and hypercarbia; the treatment for this condition is to correct the electrolyte imbalance, *not* to increase mechanical ventilatory support. Some infants with BPD and tracheomegaly and tracheobronchomalacia may require long-term continuous positive airway pressure (CPAP) therapy to maintain large airway patency; these infants are particularly prone to acute cyanotic episodes that may be both caused and worsened by agitation. In these infants, sedation may improve gas exchange so that an increase in mechanical ventilation is unnecessary.

To avoid the third mistake, the clinician should anticipate the occurrence of postextubation edema and begin aerosol therapy immediately after extubation and as often as necessary for at least 24 hours thereafter to prevent stridor and wheezing. Infants who cannot be extubated successfully after two or three attempts should be evaluated thoroughly for airway obstructive lesions; flow-volume curves and flexible or rigid bronchoscopy may be quite valuable in this regard (Cohn et al, 1988).

Although almost routine in some medical centers, the decision to perform a tracheostomy in infants with severe BPD should not be undertaken lightly. It should be performed only for clear-cut indications, such as untreatable upper airway obstruction or, very occasionally, patient comfort. Tracheostomy care in a patient with lower airway and parenchymal disease is very difficult, especially at home, and the risks of recurrent infection, accidental decannulation, and airway obstruction due to tracheal distortion are always present.

The long-term medical care of these infants is expensive, and families must be assisted in securing financial resources from all relevant agencies. Although mechanical ventilation of infants with BPD has been performed at home and can be justified on psychological and economic grounds, it is the exceptional family that can undertake such a responsibility.

Despite meticulous care of long-term ventilator-dependent infants, approximately 10 to 30 per cent of those with BPD at 28 days of life die before being discharged. The cause of death may be an intercurrent respiratory illness or necrotizing tracheobronchitis, but often death is sudden and unexpected. A unique feature of sudden unexpected death is the refractory nature of the bradycardia that occurs. Post-mortem studies of these infants are infrequent, and physicians have questioned whether a neurologic event or a cardiac arrhythmia may be responsible, perhaps related to multiple-drug therapy.

Oxygen Therapy. The most important feature of BPD therapy is to maintain adequate oxygenation to promote normal somatic growth and neurologic development and to prevent the development of pulmonary vascular disease and right ventricular hypertrophy. A multicenter trial on adults with COPD has shown that oxygen therapy is beneficial (Nocturnal Oxygen Therapy, 1980; Levine et al, 1967), but no such trials have been performed on infants. In the past, aggressive weaning from oxygen has been favored because of the unavailability of suitable delivery systems for infants, the need to discharge older infants, and the psychological needs of physicians who viewed oxygen-dependent infants as sicker than those who were breathing room air. However, evidence continues to mount that chronic alveolar hypoxia and hypoxemia are detrimental. For example, alveolar hypoxia can cause pulmonary vasoconstriction and bronchoconstriction (Teague et al, 1988), which can further aggravate chronic respiratory distress. Hypoxemia may also interfere with nutrient absorption in the gastrointestinal tract (Askanazi et al, 1982). Indeed, slow somatic growth frequently can be improved by optimizing oxygen therapy, not by increasing caloric intake, suggesting that hypoxia and not malnutrition is the factor that is limiting growth (Groothuis et al, 1986). However, in severely affected infants with severe ventilation-perfusion defects, even the breathing of 100 per cent oxygen will not prevent alveolar hypoxia in some lung units, and pulmonary hypertension can develop even with maximal oxygen therapy. Moreover, myocardial dysfunction and anatomic right-to-left shunts in the heart or lungs may result in inadequate systemic oxygen delivery even when arterial oxygen tensions are in the normal range.

Oxygen can be administered through a hood, tent, face mask, or nasal catheter. A nasal catheter is preferred because it interferes minimally with other aspects of infant care and it allows low flow rates to be used so that various oxygen sources can be attached to it. Its disadvantages are that it may become dislodged during sleep, that FI_{O_2}s greater than 35 to 40 per cent cannot be achieved, and that oxygen delivery is reduced in the crying or agitated infant who breathes orally.

Although it would be most accurate to adjust oxygen therapy based on an analysis of gas tensions in arterial blood, repeated arterial punctures are difficult and hazardous and probably do not reflect steady-state gas exchange in chronically ill infants. Fortunately, the accuracy and increased availability of oximeters has greatly facilitated the monitoring of oxygen therapy in both hospitalized infants and infants at home (Ramanathan et al, 1987; Solimano et al, 1986). Transcutaneous oxygen and carbon dioxide monitoring, which have proved so useful in acute neonatal care, have proved less useful in long-term oxygen management because of calibration difficulties, long warm-up times, thermal skin effects, and possible inaccurate readings in older infants with BPD.

Available evidence indicates that there is substantial variability among individuals in the level of hypoxia that results in heart strain and the level of hyperoxia that results in ongoing injury. It is the view in our clinic that oxygen should be used and monitored as a medication, following strict guidelines. Our practice is to maintain oxygen saturation between 92 and 95 per cent while the infant is both awake and asleep. In infants with BPD, the sleep state does not appear to affect oxygenation, but sleep-associated desaturation does occur (Rome et al, 1987). In our experience, the more severely affected infants will improve their oxygenation during sleep, perhaps because oxygen consumption is reduced; infants with mild to moderate BPD will desaturate during sleep. If saturation is adequate when infants are awake, they can be weaned from continuous oxygen therapy to night and nap oxygen therapy for an additional 4 to 6 weeks. During this time, any ancillary medications are discontinued, if possible. If the infant's growth rate remains the same and respiratory symptoms are not increased, oxygen therapy can be discontinued. The oxygen delivery apparatus is kept available in the home for another month or so in case an intercurrent respiratory infection develops and respiratory symptoms return. The physician should remember that even when oxygen therapy is discontinued, pathologic abnormalities and ventilation-perfusion defects may be present for some time. These infants should be carefully evaluated when respiratory infections appear. Some infants will reacquire the need for oxygen following infectious episodes, after which the weaning process should begin again.

Family members and primary care physicians frequently ask when oxygen therapy can be discontinued, because continuous oxygen therapy is often cumbersome and limits the family's activity. Currently, there is no way to predict the duration of oxygen therapy for individual infants. At Vanderbilt, at least 60 per cent of those discharged receiving oxygen therapy will be weaned from oxygen within 3 months; two thirds of the remainder will no longer require oxygen after 6 months of therapy, and the remainder will require oxygen therapy for at least 9 to 12 months. Overall, approximately 10 per cent will require oxygen therapy for longer than a year.

Environmental Control. The environment is an often neglected aspect of the outpatient care of infants with resolving or resolved BPD and of premature infants in general. The infant's environment, both at home and at the day-care center, should be free of dander-producing pets, smokers, and wood-burning or kerosene stoves (Honicky et al, 1985; Greenberg et al, 1989). The filters in heating and air-conditioning units should be changed frequently. In addition, large crowds and individuals with active respiratory infections should be avoided, if possible. Caretakers and siblings should be told to wash their hands with soap before and after they handle the baby.

Coexisting Pulmonary Disease. Although not yet reported, it seems only a matter of time before an infant with severe chronic BPD is found to have cystic fibrosis or an immunodeficiency syndrome. In selected infants, a sweat test and a human immuno-deficiency virus (HIV) antibody test may be indicated to rule out these disorders.

DRUG THERAPY

Pharmacotherapy in infants with BPD is still evolving, and current therapeutic strategies are derived by analogy with other chronic lung diseases. There is not a drug regimen that is likely to be effective in all infants because of the complex nature of the disease in these infants. In addition, there is no simple relationship between improvement in lung mechanics and improvement in gas exchange in these infants. Indeed, as predicted by Stocker (1986) and occasionally observed clinically, the administration of a diuretic or bronchodilator may either have no effect or else actually cause further deterioration in gas exchange even when lung mechanics are improved. An improvement in compliance of a fibrotic, unventilated lung unit or a reduction in resistance in an airway that serves a poorly perfused lung unit will not result in improved gas exchange. It should be recognized also that in clinical trials of drug therapy, transient improvements in lung function that are statistically significant may be physiologically unimportant for the infant with severe disease.

DIURETIC THERAPY

The rationale for diuretic therapy in infants with BPD is based on four observations. First, infants with uncomplicated HMD have oliguria when their pulmonary function is most abnormal, and a diuresis signals the return of normal lung function after 3 to 5 days of therapy (Spitzer et al, 1981). Second, infants with BPD have histologic, clinical, and radiographic evidence of peribronchiolar pulmonary edema; their endogenous regulation of fluid balance may be intrinsically abnormal (Hazinski et al, 1988) and may lead to intermittent or chronic hypervolemia. Third, drugs with diuretic properties have been shown to reduce pulmonary edema and to improve gas exchange in patients whose pulmonary edema is due to congestive heart failure. Fourth, anecdotal reports and controlled clinical trials (Engelhardt et al, 1986; Kao et al, 1983, 1987; McCann et al, 1985; Patel et al, 1985) documented that some but not all diuretic agents improve lung function in infants with BPD. Despite these demonstrations of efficacy, the mechanisms by which drugs with diuretic properties improve lung function (and occasionally gas exchange) are unknown. These drugs were originally chosen for their diuretic properties, and clinicians have always hoped (without evidence) that diuresis will permit a higher caloric intake and that improved lung mechanics will spare ingested calories for somatic growth and lung repair. However, diuresis alone is insufficient to cause improvement in lung mechanics and gas exchange (Engelhardt et al, 1989). Drugs termed *diuretics* have nondiuretic properties, which may also explain their beneficial effects on lung function. For example, furosemide and some thiazide drugs exert a nitrate-like effect on vascular smooth muscle (Mironneau et al, 1981; Davila and Davila, 1981), and furosemide has been shown to affect chloride transport in tracheal epithelium (Widdicombe et al, 1983), to dilate constricted airways when given by inhalation (Bianco et al, 1988), and to reduce lung edema formation even in anephric animals (Bland et al, 1978).

Although furosemide is effective, it can cause severe side effects. For example, long-term furosemide therapy causes chloride and potassium depletion that leads to alkalosis and hypoventilation (Hazinski, 1985; Perlman et al, 1986), hypercalcuria and nephrocalcinosis due to secondary hyperparathyroidism (Hufnagle et al, 1982), possible hearing deficits, glucosuria, and stimulation of renal prostaglandin synthesis. Other evidence indicates that infants may accumulate furosemide and have progressively elevated plasma levels when given standard doses of the drug (Mirochnick et al, 1988).

Other diuretic agents, such as thiazides, spironolactone, and acetazolamide, have fewer side effects than furosemide but may be less effective. In addition, high doses of these agents can lead to electrolyte imbalance, especially when used in combination with other drugs. Initial reports that low doses of thiazides can prevent furosemide-induced hypercalciuria have not been confirmed.

Intermittent Furosemide Therapy. During the acute phase of BPD in hospitalized infants, diuretic therapy is used intermittently when symptoms of acute fluid intolerance occur, such as rapid weight gain, systemic edema, and increased respiratory symptoms or oxygen requirements that cannot be explained by infection. Doses of 1 mg/kg are given intramuscularly or intravenously every 12 hours (or

2 mg/kg/dose every 12 hours by mouth) for 2 to 3 days, then discontinued, and the patient is reassessed. If the infant responds favorably to furosemide, the aforementioned doses are continued and potassium chloride (2 mEq/kg/dose) is added to prevent metabolic alkalosis.

Long-Term Furosemide Therapy. Two types of infants with BPD should be considered for long-term furosemide therapy with close monitoring of serum electrolyte, pH, and clinical response: the continously hospitalized, ventilator-dependent infant with severe BPD, and the unventilated infant whose oxygen requirement exceeds 35 to 40 per cent, who thus cannot go home safely. The role for continuous diuretic therapy in infants with mild to moderate BPD is unclear, especially in view of the risks of diuretic therapy and the lack of long-term studies. Supplementation with potassium chloride and occasionally sodium chloride (in fluid-restricted infants receiving dilute formulas) is required to prevent metabolic alkalosis. The physician should remember that in these hypercarbic infants the primary acid-base abnormality is a chronic respiratory acidosis with secondary renal conservation of bicarbonate. Renal compensation can never restore arterial pH to normal if hypercarbia is present. Thus if a hypercarbic infant who is receiving diuretic therapy develops a normal or elevated pH, it is likely that a diuretic-induced metabolic alkalosis is present that is due to excessive urinary losses or intake of potassium and chloride.

It has been reported that alternate-day furosemide therapy can improve lung function and that some metabolic side effects can be avoided (Rush et al, 1989). This alternate-day regimen may be useful either as initial therapy for infants with moderate disease or as a way to wean infants from daily diuretic therapy.

BRONCHODILATOR THERAPY

The rationale for bronchodilator therapy is based on three observations. First, despite earlier evidence to the contrary, premature infants have enough bronchial smooth muscle to constrict in response to inhaled substances, such as cold air and histamine (Lesouef et al, 1989; Motoyama et al, 1987). Second, infants with BPD have hyperplasia of bronchial and bronchiolar smooth muscle, and their tendency to be offspring of atopic individuals has already been noted. Third, short-term clinical trials of inhaled or parenteral beta-agonist and methylxanthine therapy have demonstrated improvement in both lung mechanics and gas exchange. Unfortunately, most of these studies to date have examined only the acute response to single doses of a drug. However, many physicians rely on these agents for long-term therapy, believing that the lessening in airway resistance, particularly in infants with severe disease, can reduce

the incidence and severity of subsequent lung damage.

Theophylline and Caffeine. The drugs theophylline and caffeine appear to offer a number of benefits to the infant with BPD, but their erratic pharmacokinetics make them difficult to use on a long-term basis (Loisel et al, 1987). These agents may have a bronchodilator effect, but the effect has been difficult to measure directly (Davis et al, 1989). Theophylline, for example, does not reliably relax bronchial smooth muscle in vitro until concentrations three- to sixfold higher than those achieved clinically are used (JR Sheller, M.D., personal communication). These drugs may also have diuretic properties and improve respiratory muscle efficiency. They are well-known respiratory stimulants and may hasten extubation of some neonates whose ventilator dependence is due to inadequate respiratory drive (Harris et al, 1983). Dose recommendations are difficult to make, and various nomograms have been published to guide long-term therapy. None of these formulas is foolproof, however, and frequent monitoring of steady-state serum concentrations is mandatory when these agents are used at doses that are supposed to produce bronchodilation (e.g., 10 to 20 mg/dL).

Beta-Agonist Therapy. Isoproterenol, terbutaline, salbutamol, and metaproterenol have been shown to reduce airway resistance immediately and to improve gas exchange, presumably because of their bronchodilator effects (Solulski et al, 1986; Kao, Warburton, Platzker, and Keen, 1984; Cabal et al, 1987; Kao et al, 1989; Gomez-Del Rio et al, 1986). However, these drugs may also reduce lung edema (Niermeyer, 1988), enhance mucociliary transport, and improve pulmonary blood flow. Most published studies have examined the effect of aerosol therapy because of its rapid onset of action and ease of delivery via endotracheal tube or face mask. However, resistance of infants to this therapy, the linkage of drug absorption to the infant's ability to breathe deeply, and the inability to determine precisely the administered dose may substantially reduce the efficacy of this route. Improved aerosol delivery systems are being developed (Conner et al, 1989). Oral therapy would appear to be more effective for long-term management. Unfortunately, no studies of oral therapy have been reported, and it cannot be recommended for routine care of infants with BPD. Bronchodilators that can be used to treat BPD are listed in Table 14–3.

Short-term beta-agonist therapy is effective when acute bronchospasm is present. Any infant with BPD and acute wheezing or hypercarbia deserves a therapeutic trial of these agents. However, the physician should be mindful of their short duration of action, their cardiac side effects, and the possibility of rebound bronchospasm.

OTHER DRUGS

Corticosteroids. Corticosteroid therapy is perhaps the most controversial area of BPD care. Early re-

Table 14–3. AVAILABLE DOSES OF BRONCHODILATORS USED IN THE TREATMENT OF
BRONCHOPULMONARY DYSPLASIA (BPD)

Drug	Dose	Route
Salbutamol (Albuterol)	0.04 ml/kg in 1.5 ml NS*	Aerosol
Isoproterenol	0.2 ml of 1:200 solution in 2 ml of 0.45 NS	Aerosol
Metaproterenol	2.0 ml of 0.3% solution	Aerosol
Atropine	0.05 mg/kg in 2 ml of 0.45 NS	Aerosol
Theophylline	8 w postnatal age (months) z total daily dose in mg/kg†	PO—IV
Caffeine‡	10 mg/kg load; 2.5 mg/kg/day maintenance	PO—IV

*Respirator solution 5 mg of salbutamol base/ml.
†Dose modified for BPD by Nickerson BG: Chest 87:528, 1985, from Nassif EG, Weinberger MM, Shannon D et al: J Pediatr 98:158, 1981.
‡Caffeine base.
NS, normal saline; PO, orally; IV, intravenously.
(For documentation of dosages listed and for recommendations on the frequency of administration, see Blanchard et al: Clin Perinatol 14:881, 1987.)

ports suggested that improved pulmonary function and weaning from mechanical ventilation could be achieved after 3 to 7 days of steroid therapy but that incidence of bacterial sepsis and hypertension was higher than expected and long-term benefits could not be demonstrated (Mammel et al, 1983; Mammel et al, 1987; Avery et al, 1985; Gerdes et al, 1988; Mohsini et al, 1987). In these studies, there were substantial differences in terms of patient selection, drug dosage, and duration of therapy. None of these studies explored possible mechanisms of action, although subsequent researchers have postulated that steroid therapy enhances the diuretic and other effects of furosemide and thus improves fluid balance abnormalities in infants with BPD (Donn et al, 1983). However, steroid treatment in some animal models of lung injury has aggravated the injury (Kehrer et al, 1984). As a result, most physicians have been wary of corticosteroid therapy and have used it only rarely in infants, with equivocal results. However, a randomized clinical trial by Cummings and colleagues (1989) demonstrated that if 2-week-old ventilator-dependent infants were given 42 days of dexamethasone in progressively lower doses, the duration of mechanical ventilation and oxygen dependence was reduced by more than 50 per cent. The incidence of sepsis was no higher in the steroid-treated group, and neurodevelopmental outcome (at 1 year of age) was better in the steroid-treated infants. Unfortunately, 13 of the 36 enrolled infants (and 45 per cent of the placebo-treated infants) died before discharge, and the mechanism by which steroid treatment improved outcome was not addressed. Despite this small sample size and high mortality rate beyond the second week of life, this provocative study indicates that the benefit of steroid therapy is likely to be early rather than late in the clinical course of these infants. A multicenter trial of this therapy is the logical next step in evaluating the role of corticosteroids in BPD. The role for inhaled corticosteroid therapy, which seems promising for patients with asthma, has not yet been evaluated.

Vasoactive Drugs. There has been an increased interest in the role of nondiuretic vasoactive drugs for the treatment of abnormal circulatory dynamics and gas exchange in infants with BPD. Nifedipine (Kochanek and Zaritsky, 1986; Brownlee et al, 1988), hydralazine (Thompson et al, 1986), and almitrine (Magny et al, 1987) have been reported to be effective occasionally, but these drugs should still be considered experimental. Systemic hypertension does not usually require therapy, but when therapy is indicated, these infants respond to either diuretics, captopril, or hydralazine (Blanchard et al, 1987).

Vitamin A. As mentioned previously, the role of the deficiency of specific nutrients is a relatively unexplored area of neonatal lung research. Shenai and colleagues (1987) have studied the role of vitamin A metabolism on lung growth and development and demonstrated that correction of vitamin A deficiency substantially reduced the incidence of BPD in high-risk infants. In most of these infants, a daily vitamin A intake higher than currently recommended for premature infants was necessary to achieve plasma vitamin A levels in the normal range. Moreover, some infants could not achieve normal levels even at very high daily doses. Levels of vitamin A associated with toxicity did not occur in this study because serum levels were monitored frequently and dose adjustments made as necessary. As with steroid therapy, the applicability of the results of this exciting study will have to be confirmed by other medical centers before vitamin A can be adopted as routine therapy. It might also be possible to improve the premature infant's vitamin A stores prenatally by supplementing the supply in mothers at risk for premature labor, but this possibility has not yet been tested for safety and efficacy.

NUTRITION

All investigators agree that optimal nutrition is important for the treatment of BPD, but no agreement exists about how this goal should be met. Several studies have linked growth failure to poor neurodevelopmental outcome, but a cause-and-effect relationship between these two events may be inappropriate (Markestad and Fitzhardinge, 1981; Hack et al, 1982). The most extremely afflicted infants are inevitably malnourished and malnurtured, and it is not surprising that growth retardation occurs in infants with severe BPD who are long-term residents of intensive care nurseries. An elevated resting metabolic rate, frequent respiratory exacerbations, neurologic damage with subsequent feeding problems, fluid restriction protocols, and aggressive weaning from oxygen all contribute to growth failure in these infants. For these infants, gentle nursing care, pleasant oral stimulation, and a quiet environment are crucial elements for a successful nutritional program and may be more important than type of formula or total caloric intake. However, even with an optimal environment, some infants with BPD will not begin to grow well until lung repair is well under way, as evidenced by a fall in F_{IO_2} and a reduction of symptoms.

A realistic goal in nutrition therapy for infants with moderate BPD would be to provide a caloric intake of 110 to 150 kcal/kg/day to produce a weight gain of 15 to 20 g/day. Newer formulas designed for premature infants with a caloric density of 24 kcal/oz are usually satisfactory. The additional calcium and phosphorus in these formulas may provide an extra safeguard against developing a deficiency of these substances during diuretic therapy. However, the sodium content of these formulas may be inadequate for the growing infant with BPD, the infant receiving dilute formulas in restricted amounts, or the infant receiving concomitant diuretic therapy.

Although commonly done, increasing the caloric density of infant formulas to greater than or equal to 30 kcal/oz with glucose polymers, corn syrup, or fats should be regarded as unproven and potentially hazardous therapy. The additional fluid and carbohydrate load may cause fluid overload or osmotic diarrhea. High carbohydrate diets may also result in an increased CO_2 load on the respiratory system and thus may worsen respiratory distress. Some fat supplements, such as medium-chain triglycerides, are costly and offer no advantage over less expensive fat sources, such as corn oil. In some infants in whom somatic growth has occurred in the absence of lung repair, the need for oxygen therapy has increased. Conversely, some infants have rapid resolution of BPD while receiving less than 100 kcal/kg/day. Moreover, excessive dietary manipulations complicate care and are rarely effective in accelerating growth. These findings suggest that regulation of somatic growth may be linked to the rate of lung repair, which is not particularly responsive to caloric intake.

SPECIAL PROBLEMS OF THE INFANT

Nursery Discharge. An important advance in the treatment of infants with BPD has been the recognition of the importance of complete discharge planning, which should begin 10 to 14 days before the anticipated discharge date. In the Vanderbilt nursery, an infant with BPD is considered ready for discharge if the F_{IO_2} is less than 0.40 *and* the infant's saturation in room air is greater than 85 per cent. In our experience, failure to meet this latter criterion is invariably associated with rehospitalization within a month. If medications are thought to be no longer necessary, they should be discontinued far enough in advance of discharge so that the effects of complete weaning can be evaluated in the hospital. A single individual, often an experienced nurse or social worker, reviews the infant's pulmonary and nonpulmonary needs, arranges for home nursing care if necessary, contacts the oxygen delivery service, assesses the home environment, and notifies the infant's private physician that discharge is imminent. The infant's caretakers are taught heart rate monitoring, if it is prescribed (see subsequent discussion), and are also taught cardiopulmonary resuscitation (CPR). The purpose and side effects of each prescribed medication, including oxygen therapy, are explained. In addition, the signs and symptoms of respiratory distress are reviewed. During the final week of hospitalization, routine aspects of newborn care should be emphasized and demonstrated. In the past, parents were sent home with exemplary respiratory therapy skills but were not taught how to bathe their baby! When home nursing care is deemed necessary, we emphasize that the infant's parents or primary caretaker will be the best teacher and manager of these individuals.

Immunizations given before discharge should be noted and conveyed to the primary care physician along with a brief but relevant discharge summary. Our practice is to discharge the infant with a recent chest radiograph taken at a time when the baby is free of acute respiratory problems; the primary care physician can use this radiograph for comparison with subsequent films if respiratory problems develop. A 12-lead electrocardiogram (ECG) is also obtained and retained in the infant's record. A follow-up appointment should be made with the primary care physician as soon as possible so that the child can be examined when stable.

In addition, the parents should be encouraged to discuss their child's current and future needs with knowledgeable individuals in the days before discharge. The nursery staff must realize that this is a stressful time for families and should express confidence in the family's ability to care for the baby. A well-written pamphlet is available from the American Lung Association that may be helpful in preparing the family for discharge.*

Apnea and Heart Rate Monitoring. The incidence of sudden infant death syndrome (SIDS) in infants with BPD is the same as the incidence for all premature infants; i.e., 0.5 to 1.5 per cent (Hack et al, 1982). Regional differences exist regarding the prac-

*This pamphlet may be obtained from the American Lung Association of New Mexico at the following address: 216 Truman Avenue N.E., Albuquerque, NM 87108.

tice of monitoring premature infants, but in our region, monitoring is infrequent unless other risk factors exist or parental concerns are expressed. However, some physicians and many parents may elect to monitor infants with BPD in the hope that the monitor will provide early warning of an impending respiratory exacerbation. The advantages and disadvantages of monitoring must be discussed with each family; heart rate monitoring itself is stressful for the family and has not been shown to reduce the incidence of SIDS.

Upper Airway Obstruction. Upper airway obstruction due to subglottic stenosis, tracheal scarring, or granuloma or polyp formation should be suspected in infants who cannot be permanently extubated and whose respiratory distress is out of proportion to their oxygen requirements. The airways of these infants should be examined by experienced individuals, using flexible or rigid bronchoscopy (Saigal et al, 1984). Tracheostomy, cricoid or tracheal surgery, or laser therapy may be useful in selected infants (Fan and Flynn, 1981; Pashley, 1984; Pashley et al, 1984).

Unsuspected Cardiac Disease. Infants with BPD who have severe refractory disease, those who do not show steady improvement, and those whose right ventricular hypertrophy is out of proportion to the degree of pulmonary disease should be evaluated for the presence of structural cardiac defects. Small septal defects and patent ductus arteriosus (PDA), which might be of little consequence to an infant without chronic lung disease, may cause chronic congestive heart failure and pulmonary hypertension (Abman, Accurso, and Bowman, 1984).

Gastroesophageal Reflux and Chronic Aspiration. Because abnormal lung mechanics lead to abnormal pressure gradients between the chest and abdomen, it is not surprising that gastroesophageal reflux (GER) and BPD have been associated. However, the contribution of GER to ongoing lung injury is difficult to ascertain in individual infants who may suffer reflux into the esophagus without pulmonary effects (Guiffre et al, 1987). If GER is suspected, a barium esophagogram is performed first to examine oropharyngeal function and esophageal motility and to search for unsuspected tracheoesophageal malformations. Esophagograms are *not* useful in diagnosing GER because reflux will occur in many infants without GER during the study. If the esophagogram is nondiagnostic, lung scans following a technetium meal are performed. If this test finding is positive, positional therapy (prone) and antacids are given, with bethanecol and metoclopramide therapy reserved for more severely affected infants. Surgery is rarely required; even when attempted, it may yield unfavorable results in infants with coexisting neurologic impairment.

It is also important to differentiate between infants who aspirate and those who have GER (some infants have both). Aspiration due to neurologic dysfunction may be transient, and tube feedings can be performed until improvement occurs.

Acute Respiratory Exacerbations. More than 80 per cent of BPD infants will develop a lower respiratory infection within a year after discharge, and more than one half of these infants will require hospitalization (Markestad and Fitzhardinge, 1981). Infants with chronic BPD may suddenly develop severe respiratory failure in the midst of a seemingly innocuous upper respiratory infection. Therefore, these infants should be evaluated early in the course of respiratory illnesses, and close contact should be maintained with the infant's family. When treating such an infant, the physician should assume that any of *four treatable and synergistically acting lung conditions* may be present: hypoxia, edema, bronchoconstriction, and bacterial infection. Unlike adults with COPD, infants with BPD do not ordinarily hypoventilate when given high concentrations of oxygen (Hazinski et al, 1984), and oxygen should be given liberally to these infants until oxygen therapy can be adjusted by oximetry or by blood gas measurements. If the infant exhibits signs of fluid overload or wheezing, a parenteral dose of furosemide (1 mg/kg) is used. Because this therapy may not have any effect for 20 to 30 min, an immediate trial of beta-agonist by aerosol or subcutaneous route should also be considered. Although bacterial pneumonia is rare in these infants, a febrile infant should be given a broad-spectrum antibiotic, such as ampicillin or a cephalosporin, and blood cultures and cerebrospinal fluid cultures should be obtained if indicated. Chest radiographs are rarely helpful, but serial films can confirm the presence of edema or acute hyperinflation. Intubation and mechanical ventilation can and should be avoided by the judicious use of the previously mentioned therapies. The indication for intubation should be apnea, an unfavorable general appearance, or both; a single blood gas determination, even if its results are alarming, should not be used *alone* as an indication to intubate if the infant is stable and appears to be responding to medical treatment.

Because bronchial and bronchiolar damage is already present in infants with active or resolved BPD, these infants are particularly vulnerable to respiratory viruses that are tropic for bronchial epithelium, such as adenovirus, cytomegalovirus (CMV), and respiratory syncytial virus (RSV) (Sawyer et al, 1987; Groothuis et al, 1988; Toms and Scott, 1987). Although rapid diagnostic methods are available for RSV infection, some investigators recommend the institution of antiviral therapy with ribavirin while waiting for the definitive diagnosis. The drug must be given by continuous inhalation, and the appropriate delivery system must be available if the infant is being mechanically ventilated.

Elective Surgery. Because of the risk of acquiring a nosocomial infection from other hospitalized children, elective surgery should not be performed during local outbreaks of viral infections. If hospitalizations are necessary, respiratory precautions should be taken, and the infant should be discharged as soon as possible.

LONG-TERM PROGNOSIS

With time, nutrition, growth, adequate oxygenation, and access to attentive medical care, the majority of infants with BPD will improve. For those severely affected infants, lung or heart-lung transplantation can now be considered because technical barriers to its implementation may have been overcome already in some medical centers. However, donor availability, lifelong dependence on immunosuppressive drugs, rejection-induced respiratory failure, and expensive follow-up care are unsolved problems, so transplantation may not be in the best interests of the infant or family.

Infants with resolved or resolving BPD (and perhaps most extremely premature infants) may have chronic bronchial hyperreactivity, which may develop into typical bronchial asthma. In up to 50 per cent of children with a history of BPD, exercise-associated desaturation can occur, but overall exercise ability is not impaired (Bader et al, 1987; Gibson et al, 1988). As mentioned previously, the families of these infants must be cautioned about the risks of passive and active smoking.

The impact of this chronic disease on long-term neurologic development has raised considerable concern. Most studies indicate that infants with BPD have developmental delay for the first 24 to 36 months of life, even in the absence of such coexisting conditions as posthemorrhagic hydrocephalus and hearing or visual impairment (Meisels et al, 1986). All aspects of development are affected: physical growth as well as cognitive, language, and sensorimotor skills. This developmental delay is usually transient in infants without such coexisting problems, suggesting that it is due to chronic disease with lengthy and repeated hospitalizations and often to a disruptive and stressful postnatal environment (Sauve and Singhal, 1985). Some experts have attributed more severe forms of developmental delay in BPD infants to perinatal events, such as perinatal asphyxia and initial severity of respiratory failure (Markestad and Fitzhardinge, 1981; Horbar et al, 1988). For all premature infants, a crucial determinant of long-term neurodevelopmental outcome is the overall quality of the postnatal environment, which may be quite limited in some populations at high risk to develop BPD.

FUTURE TRENDS AND RESEARCH DIRECTIONS

Because the best way to treat a disease is to prevent it, a glance at Figure 14–1 illustrates that the single most effective way to reduce the incidence of BPD (and most other chronic disorders of premature infants) is to delay or prevent the onset of premature labor before 28 weeks of gestation, i.e., to prevent extreme prematurity.

Caring for infants with BPD is costly, and parents and hospitals often lack the necessary economic resources to provide long-term care for severely affected infants. These goals are attainable but require a substantial commitment of resources, which many countries have been willing to make. Commentaries on the situation in the United States indicate that these resources are not likely to be available soon (Stahlman, 1989; Koops, 1988).

Improvements in BPD care will also require a better understanding of lung development and lung repair mechanisms, including the role of growth factors, inflammatory cells and mediators, and specific nutrients in these processes. Animal models of this disease and its relevant features need to be developed and studied. The exciting possibilities of powerful molecular biology techniques, genetically engineered drugs, and human gene therapy await the successful demonstration of their therapeutic value. Clinical trials of the efficacy of long-term therapy with drugs currently used with little firm scientific rationale should be performed.

REFERENCES

Abman SH, Accurso FJ, and Bowman CM: Unsuspected cardio-pulmonary abnormalities complicating bronchopulmonary dysplasia. Arch Dis Child 59:966, 1984.

Abman SH, Schaffer MS, Wiggins J et al: Pulmonary vascular extraction of circulating norepinephrine in infants with bronchopulmonary dysplasia. Pediatr Pulmonol 3:386, 1987.

Abman SH, Warady BA, Lum GM, and Koops BL: Systemic hypertension in infants with bronchopulmonary dysplasia. J Pediatr 104:929, 1984.

Askanazi J, Weissman C, Rosenbaum SH et al: Nutrition and the respiratory system. Crit Care Med 10:163, 1982.

Avery GB, Fletcher AB, Kaplan M, and Brudno DS: Controlled trial of dexamethasone in respirator-dependent infants with bronchopulmonary dysplasia. Pediatrics 75(1):106, 1985.

Avery ME, Tooley WH, Keller MPH et al: Is chronic lung disease in low birth weight infants preventable? A survey of eight centers. Pediatrics 79(1):26, 1987.

Bader D, Ramos AD, Lew CD et al: Childhood sequelae of infant lung disease: exercise and pulmonary function abnormalities after bronchopulmonary dysplasia. J Pediatr 110:693, 1987.

Bertrand J-M, Riley SP, Popkin J, and Coates AL: The long-term pulmonary sequelae of prematurity: the role of familial airway hyperreactivity and the respiratory distress syndrome. N Engl J Med 312:742, 1985.

Bhutani VK, Ritchie WG, and Shaffer TH: Acquired tracheomegaly in very preterm neonates. Am J Dis Child 140:449, 1986.

Bianco S, Vaghi A, Robuschi M, and Pasargiklian M: Prevention of exercise-induced bronchoconstriction by inhaled furosemide. Lancet 7:252, 1988.

Blanchard PW, Brown TM, and Coates AL: Pharmacotherapy in bronchopulmonary dysplasia. Clin Perinatol 14:881, 1987.

Bland RD, McMillan DD, and Bressack MA: Decreased pulmonary transvascular fluid filtration in awake newborn lambs after intravenous furosemide. J Clin Invest 62:601, 1978.

Bronchopulmonary dysplasia and related chronic respiratory disorders. In Farrell PM and Taussig LM (eds): Report of the Ninetieth Ross Conference on Pediatric Research Columbus, Ohio, Ross Laboratories, 1986.

Brownlee JR, Beekman RH, and Rosenthal A: Acute hemodynamic effects of nifedipine in infants with bronchopulmonary dysplasia and pulmonary hypertension. Pediatr Res 24:186, 1988.

Burnett D, Chamba A, Hill SL, and Stockley RA: Neutrophils from subjects with chronic obstructive lung disease show enhanced chemotaxis and extracellular proteolysis. Lancet 11:1043, 1987.

Cabal LA, Larrazabal C, Ramanathan R et al: Effects of metaproterenol on pulmonary mechanics, oxygenation, and ventilation in infants with chronic lung disease. J Pediatr 110:116, 1987.

Carlton DP, Cummings JJ, Poulain FR, and Bland RD: Threshold effect of lung overinflation on pulmonary vascular protein permeability in lambs. Pediatr Res 25(4):34A, 1989.

Clement A, Chadelat K, Sardet A et al: Alveolar machrophage status in bronchopulmonary dysplasia. Pediatr Res 23:470, 1988.

Coalson JJ, Kuehl TJ, Prihoda TJ, and deLemos RA: The role of diffuse alveolar damage in the evolution of bronchopulmonary dysplasia in the baboon. Pediatr Res 34:357, 1988.

Cohn RC, Keresmar C, and Dearborn D: Safety and efficacy of flexible endoscopy in children with bronchopulmonary dysplasia. Am J Dis Child 142:1225, 1988.

Conner WT, Dolovich MB, Frame RA, and Newhouse MT: Reliable salbutamol administration in 6- to 36-month-old children by means of a metered dose inhaler and aerochamber with mask. Pediatr Pulmonol 6:263, 1989.

Cotton RB and Parker RA: Bronchopulmonary dysplasia (BPD): an effect of newborn intensive care efficacy. Pediatr Res 23(4):445A, 1988.

Cummings JJ, D'Eugenio DB, and Gross SJ: A controlled trial of dexamethasone in preterm infants at high risk for bronchopulmonary dysplasia. N Engl J Med 320:1505, 1989.

Davila D and Davila T: Thiazide diuretics inhibit contractions of isolated smooth muscles. Pharmacology 22:108, 1981.

Davis JM, Bhutani VK, Stefano JL et al: Changes in pulmonary mechanics following caffeine administration in infants with bronchopulmonary dysplasia. Pediatr Pulmonol 6:49, 1989.

deLemos RA, Coalson JJ, Gerstmann DR et al: Oxygen toxicity in the premature baboon with hyaline membrane disease. Am Rev Respir Dis 136:677, 1987.

deLemos RA, Coalson JJ, Null DM Jr et al: Ventilatory management of infant baboons with hyaline membrane disease: the use of high frequency ventilation. Pediatr Res 21:594, 1987.

Deneke SM and Fanburg BL: Normobaric oxygen toxicity of the lung. N Engl J Med 303:76, 1980.

Donn SM, Faix RG, and Banagale RC: Dexamethasone for bronchopulmonary dysplasia. Lancet 8:460, 1983.

Edwards DK and Hilston SVW: Flat chest in chronic bronchopulmonary dysplasia. AJR 149:1213, 1987.

Ehrenkranz RA, Ablow RC, and Warshaw JB: Prevention of bronchopulmonary dysplasia with vitamin E administration during the acute stage of respiratory distress syndrome. J Pediatr 95:873, 1979.

Ehrenkranz RA, Bonta BW, Ablow RC, and Warshaw JB: Amelioration of bronchopulmonary dysplasia after vitamin E administration. N Engl J Med 299:564, 1978.

Engelhardt BE, Blalock WA, Donlevy S et al: Effect of spironolactone-hydrochlorothiazide on lung function in infants with chronic bronchopulmonary dysplasia. J Pediatr 114(4):619, 1989.

Engelhardt BE, Elliott S, and Hazinski TA: Short- and long-term effects of furosemide on lung function in infants with bronchopulmonary dysplasia. J Pediatr 109:1034, 1986.

England SJ: Current technologies for assessing pulmonary function in the newborn and infant: advantages and limitations. Pediatr Pulmonol 4:48, 1988.

Fan LL and Flynn JW: Laryngoscopy in neonates and infants: experience with the flexible fiberoptic bronchoscope. Laryngoscope 91:451, 1981.

Frank L and Massaro D: Oxygen toxicity. Am J Med 69:117, 1980.

Gerdes JS, Harris MC, and Polin RA: Effects of dexamethasone and indomethacin on elastase, beta₁-proteinase inhibitor, and fibronectin in bronchoalveolar lavage fluid from neonates. J Pediatr 113:727, 1988.

Gerhardt T, Hehre D, Feller R et al: Serial determination of pulmonary function in infants with chronic lung disease. J Pediatr 10:448, 1987.

Gerhardt T, Reifenberg L, Duara S, and Bancalari E: Comparison of dynamic and static measurements of respiratory mechanics in infants. J Pediatr 114:120, 1989.

Gibson RL, Jackson JC, Twiggs GA et al: Bronchopulmonary

dysplasia. Survival after prolonged mechanical ventilation. Am J Dis Child 142:721, 1988.

Giuffre RM, Rubin S, and Mitchell I: Antireflux surgery in infants with bronchopulmonary dysplasia. Am J Dis Child 141:648, 1987.

Goldberg RN and Bancalari E: Respiratory management of infants with bronchopulmonary dysplasia. In Bancalari E and Stocker JT (eds): Bronchopulmonary Dysplasia. Washington, DC, Hemisphere Publishing Corp, 1988.

Goldman SL, Gerhardt T, Sonni R et al: Early prediction of chronic lung disease by pulmonary function testing. J Pediatr 102:613, 1983.

Gomez-Del Rio M, Gerhardt T, Hehre D et al: Effect of a beta-agonist nebulization on lung function in neonates with increased pulmonary resistance. Pediatr Pulmonol 2:287, 1986.

Goodman G, Perkin RM, Anas NG et al: Pulmonary hypertension in infants with bronchopulmonary dysplasia. J Pediatr 112:67, 1988.

Greenberg RA, Bauman KE, Loda FA et al: Ecology of passive smoking by young infants. J Pediatr 114:774, 1989.

Groothuis JR, Gutierrez KM, and Lauer BA: Respiratory syncytial virus infection in children with bronchopulmonary dysplasia. Pediatrics 82:199, 1988.

Groothuis JR, Rosenberg AA, and Zerle GO: Home oxygen promotes weight gain in infants with bronchopulmonary dysplasia. Pediatr Res 20:227A, 1986.

Guslits BG, Wilkie RA, England SJ, and Bryan AC: Comparison of methods of measurement of compliance of the respiratory system in children. Am Rev Respir Dis 136:727, 1987.

Hack M, Merkatz IR, Gordon D et al: The prognostic significance of postnatal growth in very low-birth-weight infants. Am J Obstet Gynecol 143:693, 1982.

Harris MC, Baumgart S, Rooklin AR et al: Successful extubation of infants with respiratory distress syndrome using aminophylline. J Pediatr 103:303, 1983.

Hazinski TA: Furosemide decreases ventilation in young rabbits. J Pediatr 106:81, 1985.

Hazinski TA, Blalock WA, and Engelhardt BE: Vasopressin excess in infants with bronchopulmonary dysplasia. Pediatr Res 23:86, 1988.

Hazinski TA, Severinghaus JW, Marin MS, and Tooley WH: Estimation of the ventilatory response to carbon dioxide in patients with chronic lung disease. J Pediatr 105:389, 1984.

Hazinski TA, France ML, Kennedy KA, and Hansen TN: Cimetidine reduces hyperoxic lung injury in lambs. J Appl Physiol, December 1989.

Hazinski TA, Kennedy KA, France ML, and Hansen TN: Pulmonary oxygen toxicity in lambs: physiological and biochemical effects of endotoxin infusion. J Appl Physiol 65(4):1579, 1988.

Heneghan MA, Sosulski R, and Baquero JM: Persistent pulmonary abnormalities in newborns: the changing picture of bronchopulmonary dysplasia. Pediatr Radiol 16:180, 1986.

HIFI Study Group: High-frequency oscillatory ventilation compared with conventional mechanical ventilation in the treatment of respiratory failure in preterm infants. N Engl J Med 320:88, 1989.

Honicky R, Osborne J, and Akpom C: Symptoms of respiratory illness in young children and the use of wood-burning stoves for indoor heating. Pediatrics 75:587, 1985.

Horbar JD, McAuliffe TL, Adler SM et al: Variability in 28-day outcomes for very low birth weight infants: an analysis of 11 neonatal intensive care units. Pediatrics 82:554, 1988.

Hufnagle KG, Khan SN, Pen D et al: Renal calcifications: a complication of long-term furosemide therapy in preterm infants. Pediatrics 70:360, 1982.

Jackson JC, Chi EY, Wilson CB et al: Sequence of inflammatory cell migration into lung during recovery from hyaline membrane disease in premature newborn monkeys. Am Rev Respir Dis 135:937, 1987.

Johnson DE, Lock JE, Elde RP, and Thompson TR: Pulmonary neuroendocrine cells in hyaline membrane disease and bronchopulmonary dysplasia. Pediatr Res 16:446, 1982.

Johnson MD, Gray ME, Carpenter GR et al: Ontogeny of epidermal growth factor receptor/kinase and of lipocortin-1 in the ovine lung. Pediatr Res 25:535, 1989.

Kao LC, Durand DJ, and Nickerson BG: Effects of inhaled metaproterenol and atropine on the pulmonary mechanics of infants with bronchopulmonary dysplasia. Pediatr Pulmonol 6:74, 1989.

Kao LC, Durand DJ, Phillips BL, and Nickerson BG: Oral theophylline and diuretics improve pulmonary mechanics in infants with bronchopulmonary dysplasia. J Pediatr 111:439, 1987.

Kao LC, Warburton D, Cheng MH et al: Effect of oral diuretics on pulmonary mechanics in infants with chronic bronchopulmonary dysplasia: results of a double-blind crossover sequential trial. Pediatrics 74:37, 1984.

Kao LC, Warburton D, Platzker ACG, and Keens TG: Effect of isoproterenol inhalation on airway resistance in chronic bronchopulmonary dysplasia. Pediatrics 73(4):509, 1984.

Kao LC, Warburton D, Sargent CW et al: Furosemide acutely decreases airway resistance in chronic bronchopulmonary dysplasia. J Pediatr 103:624, 1983.

Kapanci Y, Weibel ER, Kaplan HP et al: Pathogenesis and reversibility of the pulmonary lesions of oxygen toxicity in monkeys. II. Ultrastructural and morphometric studies. Lab Invest 20:101, 1969.

Kehrer JP, Klein-Szanto JP, Sorenson EMB et al: Enhanced acute lung damage following corticosteroid treatment. Am Rev Respir Dis 130:256, 1984.

Kochanek PM and Zaritsky A: Nifedipine in the treatment of a child with pulmonary hypertension associated with severe bronchopulmonary dysplasia. Clin Pediatr 25:214, 1986.

Koops BL: Commitment to long-term support: clinical, economic, and ethical issues. In Bancalari E and Stocker JT (eds): Bronchopulmonary Dysplasia. Washington, DC, Hemisphere Publishing Corp, 1988.

Koops BL, Abman SH, and Accurso FJ: Outpatient management and follow-up of bronchopulmonary dysplasia. Clin Perinatol 11(1):101, 1984.

Krauss A, Klain D, and Auld P: Chronic pulmonary insufficiency of prematurity. Pediatrics 55:55, 1975.

Kurzner SI, Garg M, Bautista DB et al: Growth failure in bronchopulmonary dysplasia: elevated metabolic rates and pulmonary mechanics. J Pediatr 112:73, 1988.

Lesouef PN, Geelhoed GC, Turner DJ et al: Response of normal infants to inhaled histamine. Am Rev Respir Dis 139:62, 1989.

Levine BE, Bigelow DB, Hamstra RD et al: The role of long-term continuous oxygen administration in patients with chronic airway obstruction and hypoxemia. Ann Intern Med 66:639, 1967.

Lindroth M, Jonson B, Svenningsen NW, and Mortensson W: Pulmonary mechanics, chest x-ray and lung disease after mechanical ventilation in low birth weight infants. Acta Paediatr Scand 69:761, 1980.

Loeber NV, Morray JP, Kettrick RG, and Downes JJ: Pulmonary function in chronic respiratory failure of infancy. Crit Care Med 8(10):596, 1980.

Loisel DB, Smith MM, and MacDonald MG: Plasma theophylline levels as related to toxicity in infants with severe chronic lung disease. Neonatal Network 10:15, 1987.

McCann EM, Lewis K, Deming DD et al: Controlled trial of furosemide therapy in infants with chronic lung disease. J Pediatr 107:957, 1985.

Magny JF, Bromet N, Bonmarchand M, and Dehan M: Study of the pharmacokinetics and pharmacodynamic activity of almitrine bismesylate in infants during the recovery phase following bronchopulmonary dysplasia. Dev Pharmacol Ther 10:369, 1987.

Mammel MC, Fiterman C, Coleman M, and Boros SJ: Short-term dexamethasone therapy for bronchopulmonary dysplasia: acute effects and 1-year follow-up. Dev Pharmacol Ther 10:1, 1987.

Mammel MC, Green TP, Johnson DE, and Thompson TR: Controlled trial of dexamethasone therapy in infants with bronchopulmonary dysplasia. Lancet 6:1356, 1983.

Marini JJ, Smith TC, and Lamb VJ: External work output and force generation during synchronized intermittent mechanical ventilation. Am Rev Respir Dis 138(5):1169, 1988.

Markestad T and Fitzhardinge PM: Growth and development in children recovering from bronchopulmonary dysplasia. J Pediatr 98:597, 1981.

Meisels SJ, Plunkett JW, Roloff DW et al: Growth and development of preterm infants with respiratory distress syndrome and bronchopulmonary dysplasia. Pediatrics 77:345, 1986.

Melnick G, Pickoff AS, Ferrer PL et al: Normal pulmonary vascular resistance and left ventricular hypertrophy in young infants with bronchopulmonary dysplasia: an echocardiographic and pathologic study. Pediatrics 66(4):589, 1980.

Meredith KS, deLemos RA, Coalson JJ et al: The role of lung injury in the pathogenesis of hyaline membrane disease in the premature baboon. J Appl Physiol (in press).

Merritt TA, Cochrane CG, Holcomb K et al: Elastase and alpha$_1$-proteinase inhibitor activity in tracheal aspirates during respiratory distress syndrome. J Clin Invest 72:656, 1983.

Merritt TA, Stuard ID, Puccia J et al: Newborn tracheal aspirate cytology: classification during respiratory distress syndrome and bronchopulmonary dysplasia. J Pediatr 98(6):949, 1981.

Mirochnick MH, Miceli JJ, Kramer PA et al: Furosemide pharmacokinetics in very low birth weight infants. J Pediatr 112:653, 1988.

Mironneau J, Savineau J-P, and Mironneau C: Compared effects of indapamide, hydrochlorothiazide and chlorthalidone on electrical and mechanical activities in vascular smooth muscle. Eur J Pharmacol 75:109, 1981.

Mohsini K, Reid D, and Tanswell K: Resolution of acquired lobar emphysema with dexamethasone therapy. J Pediatr 111:901, 1987.

Motoyama EK, Fort MD, Klesh KW et al: Early onset of airway reactivity in premature infants with bronchopulmonary dysplasia. Am Rev Respir Dis 136:50, 1987.

Nash G, Blennerhassett JB, and Pontoppidan H: Pulmonary lesions associated with oxygen therapy and artificial ventilation. N Engl J Med 276:368, 1967.

Nickerson BG: Bronchopulmonary dysplasia. Chronic pulmonary disease following neonatal respiratory failure. Chest 87(4):528, 1985.

Nickerson BF and Taussig LM: Family history of asthma in infants with bronchopulmonary dysplasia. Pediatrics 65:1140, 1980.

Niermeyer S: Nutritional and metabolic problems in infants with bronchopulmonary dysplasia. In Bancalari E and Stocker JT (eds): Bronchopulmonary Dysplasia. Washington, DC, Hemisphere Publishing Corp, 1988.

Nocturnal Oxygen Therapy Trial Group: Continuous or nocturnal oxygen therapy in hypoxemic chronic obstructive lung disease. Ann Intern Med 93:391, 1980.

Northway WH, Rosan RC, and Porter DY: Pulmonary disease following respirator therapy of hyaline-membrane disease. N Engl J Med 276(7):357, 1967.

O'Brodovich HM and Mellins RB: Bronchopulmonary dysplasia. Unresolved neonatal acute lung injury. In Cherniack RM (ed): Lung Disease. State of the Art. New York, American Lung Association, 1987.

O'Brodovich H, Forrest JB, and Newhouse MT: Ciliary defects associated with the development of bronchopulmonary dysplasia. Am Rev Respir Dis 129:190, 1984.

Ogden BE, Murphy S, Saunders GC, and Johnson JD: Lung lavage of newborns with respiratory distress syndrome. Chest 83S:31, 1983.

Papagaroufalis C, Cairis M, Pantazatou E et al: A trial of vitamin A supplementation for the prevention of bronchopulmonary dysplasia (BPD) in very-low-birth-weight (VLBW) infants. Pediatr Res 23:518A, 1988.

Pashley NRT: Anterior cricoidotomy for congenital and acquired subglottic stenosis in infants and children. J Otolaryngol 13:187, 1984.

Pashley NRT, Jaskunas JM, and Waldstien G: Laryngotracheoplasty with costochondral grafts: clinical correlate of graft survival. Laryngoscopy 94:1493, 1984.

Patel H, Yeh T-F, Jain R, and Pildes R: Pulmonary and renal responses to furosemide in infants with stage III–IV bronchopulmonary dysplasia. Am J Dis Child 139:917, 1985.

Perlman JM and Volpe JJ: Movement disorder of premature infants with severe BPD: a new syndrome. Pediatrics 84:215, 1989.

Perlman JM, Moore V, Siegel MJ, and Dawson J: Is chloride depletion an important contributing cause of death in infants with bronchopulmonary dysplasia? Pediatrics 77:212, 1986.

Pratt PC, Vollmer RT, Shelburne JD et al: Pulmonary morphology in a multihospital collaborative extracorporeal membrane oxygenation project. I. Light microscopy. Am J Pathol 95:191, 1979.

Ramanathan R, Durand M, and Larrazabal C: Pulse oximetry in very low birth weight infants with acute and chronic lung disease. Pediatrics 79(4):612, 1987.

Rome ES, Miller MJ, Goldthwait DA et al: Effect of sleep state on chest wall movements and gas exchange in infants with resolving bronchopulmonary dysplasia. Pediatr Pulmonol 3:359, 1987.

Rosan RC, Porter DY, and Northway WH Jr: Pulmonary dysplasia following survival from severe respiratory distress syndrome (RDS) of newborn: new disease? Federation Proc 25:603, 1966.

Rush MG, Engelhardt BE, DonLevy S, and Hazinski TA: Double-blind placebo-controlled trial of alternate day furosemide therapy in infants with chronic BPD. Pediatr Res 25:308A, 1989.

Saigal S, Rosenbaum P, Stoskopf B, and Sinclair JC: Outcome in infants 501–1000 gm birth weight delivered to residents of the McMaster Health Region. J Pediatr 105:969, 1984.

Saldanha RL, Cepeda EE, and Poland RL: The effect of vitamin E prophylaxis on the incidence and severity of bronchopulmonary dysplasia. J Pediatr 101:89, 1982.

Sauve RS and Singhal N: Long-term morbidity of infants with bronchopulmonary dysplasia. Pediatrics 76:725, 1985.

Sawyer MH, Edwards DK, and Spector SA: Cytomegalovirus infection and bronchopulmonary dysplasia in premature infants. Am J Dis Child 141:303, 1987.

Shenai JP, Kennedy KA, Chytil F, and Stahlman MT: Clinical trial of vitamin A supplementation in infants susceptible to bronchopulmonary dysplasia. J Pediatr 111(2):269, 1987.

Shephard F, Gray J, and Stahlman MT: Occurrence of pulmonary fibrosis in children who had idiopathic respiratory distress syndrome. J Pediatr 65:1078, 1964.

Shepard FM, Johnston RB, Klatte EC et al: Residual pulmonary findings in clinical hyaline membrane disease. N Engl J Med 279:1063, 1968.

Slavin JD, Mathews J, and Spencer RP: Pulmonary ventilation/perfusion and reverse mismatches in an infant. Acta Radiologica Diagn 27:708, 1986.

Sobonya RE, Logvinogg MM, Taussig LM, and Theriault A: Morphometric analysis of the lung in prolonged bronchopulmonary dysplasia. Pediatr Res 16:969, 1982.

Solimano AJ, Smyth JA, Mann TK et al: Pulse oximetry advantages in infants with bronchopulmonary dysplasia. Pediatrics 78(5):844, 1986.

Sosulski R, Abbasi S, Bhutani BK, and Fox WW: Physiologic effects of terbutaline on pulmonary function of infants with bronchopulmonary dysplasia. Pediatr Pulmonol 2:269, 1986.

Spitzer AR, Fox WW, and Delivoria-Papadopoulos M: Maximum diuresis—a factor in predicting recovery from respiratory distress syndrome and the development of bronchopulmonary dysplasia. J Pediatr 98:476, 1981.

Stahlman MT: Chronic lung disease in the newborn infant. In Stern L and Vert P (eds): Neonatal Medicine. New York, Masson Publishing Co, 1987.

Stahlman MT: Medical complications in premature infants. N Engl J Med 320:1551, 1989.

Stahlman MT and Gray ME: The fetus and neonate overview. The lung. In Kretchmer N, Quilligan EJ, and Johnson JD (eds): Prenatal and Perinatal Biology and Medicine. Vol 1. New York, Harwood Academic Publishers, 1987.

Stahlman MT, Cheatham W, and Gray ME: The role of air dissection in bronchopulmonary dysplasia. J Pediatr 95(5):878, 1979.

Stahlman MT, Orth DN, and Gray ME: Immunocytochemical localization of epidermal growth factor in the developing human respiratory system and in acute and chronic lung disease in the neonate. Lab Invest 60:579, 1989.

Stocker JT: Pathologic features of long-standing "healed" bronchopulmonary dysplasia: a study of 28 3- to 40-month-old infants. Hum Pathol 17:943, 1986.

Teague WG, Pian MS, Heldt GP, and Tooley WH: An acute reduction in the fraction of inspired oxygen increases airway constriction in infants with chronic lung disease. Am Rev Respir Dis 137:861, 1988.

Tepper RS, Morgan WJ, Cota K, and Taussig LM: Expiratory flow limitation in infants with bronchopulmonary dysplasia. J Pediatr 109:1040, 1986.

Thompson D, McCann F, and Lewis K: A controlled trial of hydralazine in infants with bronchopulmonary dysplasia. Pediatr Res 20:443A, 1986.

Toce SS, Farrell PM, Leavitt LA et al: Clinical and roentgenographic scoring systems for assessing bronchopulmonary dysplasia. Am J Dis Child 138:581, 1984.

Tomashefski JF, Oppermann HC, Vawter GF, and Reid LM: Bronchopulmonary dysplasia: a morphometric study with emphasis on the pulmonary vasculature. Pediatr Pathol 2:469, 1984.

Toms JL and Scott R: Respiratory syncytial virus and the infant immune response. Arch Dis Child 62:544, 1987.

Tooley WH: Epidemiology of bronchopulmonary dysplasia. J Pediatr 95(5):851, 1979.

Truog WE, Jackson JC, Badura RJ et al: Bronchopulmonary dysplasia and pulmonary insufficiency of prematurity. Am J Dis Child 139:351, 1985.

van Asbeck BS, Hoidal J, Vercellotti GM et al: Protection against lethal hyperoxia by tracheal insufflation of erythrocytes: role of red cell gluatathione. Science 227:756, 1985.

Weinstein MR and Oh W: Oxygen consumption in infants with bronchopulmonary dysplasia. J Pediatr 99(6):958, 1981.

Widdicombe JH, Nathanson IT, and Highland E: Effects of "loop" diuretics on ion transport by dog tracheal epithelium. Am J Physiol 245(5):C388, 1983.

Wilson M and Mikity V: A new form of respiratory disease in premature infants. Am J Dis Child 99:489, 1960.

Wolfson MR, Bhutani BK, Shaffer TH, and Bowen FW: Mechanics and energetics of breathing helium in infants with bronchopulmonary dysplasia. J Pediatr 104:752, 1984.

INFECTIONS OF THE RESPIRATORY TRACT

15

JEROME O. KLEIN, M.D.

ANTIMICROBIAL THERAPY

Effective antimicrobial agents are now available for eradication of most microorganisms (with the exception of viruses) responsible for pulmonary infections in children. These drugs can be classified into four groups:

1. Beta-lactam drugs—penicillins and cephalosporins.
2. Broad-spectrum drugs—erythromycins, lincomycin and clindamycin, tetracyclines, and sulfonamides and trimethoprim-sulfamethoxazole.
3. Drugs used primarily for infections due to gram-negative bacteria—aminoglycosides, chloramphenicol, and polymyxins.
4. Drugs used primarily for infections due to gram-positive bacteria—vancomycin.

In this section, consideration is given to the properties that govern use of these drugs: in vitro efficacy, absorption and excretion, adverse side effects and toxicity, and selected aspects of administration. Antibiotics of value in treating diseases due to fungi and mycobacteria are discussed in the chapters dealing with those pathogens.

Some drugs that are of value for treating respiratory infections in adults but that have not yet been approved for use in infants and children include piperacillin, cefoperazone, cefotetan, imipenem, ampicillin in combination with sulbactam, and the quinolones. The quinolones are oral antibiotics that merit special attention because of their broad spectrum of activity, including efficacy against *Pseudomonas aeruginosa;* use in children is now prohibited because of the findings of destruction of cartilage in juvenile small animals during studies of safety. Use of the quinolones in children is now restricted to therapy provided within investigational protocols. In this chapter, only antibiotics approved for use in infants and children in January of 1989 are discussed.

BETA-LACTAM DRUGS

THE PENICILLINS

Penicillin G

Penicillin G approaches the ideal antibiotic in combining maximal bactericidal activity with absence of toxicity. It is the drug of choice for treatment of respiratory infections caused by *Streptococcus pneumoniae,* non–penicillinase-producing strains of *Staphylococcus aureus,* groups A and B beta-hemolytic streptococci, anaerobic streptococci, oropharyngeal strains of *Bacteroides* species, and organisms less commonly associated with disease of the respiratory tract such as *Corynebacterium diphtheriae, Neisseria meningitidis, Bacillus anthracis,* and *Pasteurella multocida.* It is remarkable that no strains of group A or B beta-hemolytic streptococci resistant to penicillin G have emerged during the more than 40 years since this antibiotic has been in use. In contrast, many strains of *S. aureus* are resistant to penicillin G, and initial therapy for significant respiratory disease believed to be due to this organism must include a penicillinase-resistant penicillin.

Strains of *S. pneumoniae* resistant to penicillin G and also to other antibiotics that might be used as alternatives to penicillin G, i.e., cephalosporins, erythromycin, clindamycin, and tetracyclines, were first reported from South Africa in 1977. Few multiresistant strains have appeared in the United States. The minimal inhibitory concentration (MIC) of highly resistant strains is 4 mg/ml, whereas the median MIC for most strains of *S. pneumoniae* is 0.02 mg/ml. Of equal concern are reports of moderate resistance (MIC 0.1 to 1.0 mg/ml) from different areas of the United States. Treatment of patients who have mild to moderate disease caused by these strains may require an increase in the usual dosage of penicillin G.

Several oral and parenteral forms of penicillin G are available. The choice of parenteral preparation of this antibiotic is based on the pattern of absorption.

Aqueous (soluble) penicillin G produces high peak levels of antibacterial activity in serum within 30 min after intramuscular (IM) administration but is rapidly excreted, and most activity is dissipated within 2 to 4 hours. If this agent is given by the intravenous (IV) route, the peak is higher and earlier, and the duration of antibacterial activity in serum is shorter (approximately 2 hours).

Procaine penicillin G (IM) produces lower levels of serum antibacterial activity (approximately 10 to 30 per cent of the level achieved by the same dose of the aqueous form); however, the activity remains in the serum for 6 to 12 hours.

Benzathine penicillin G (IM) is a repository preparation providing low (approximately 1 to 2 per cent of the level achieved by the same dose of the aqueous form) but prolonged levels of antibacterial activity, measurable in serum for 14 days or more.

Oral (PO) preparations of buffered penicillin G and phenoxymethyl penicillin (penicillin V) are absorbed well from the gastrointestinal tract; the peak level of serum activity of penicillin V (PO) is approximately 40 per cent, and that of buffered penicillin G (PO) is approximately 20 per cent of the level achieved by the same dose of aqueous penicillin G administered IM.

The PO preparations can be used for patients with minor respiratory infections or during convalescence from severe disease when parenteral therapy is no longer required. Children who appear severely ill initially, who have significant underlying disease, or who have complications (empyema, abscess) require the higher serum and tissue antibacterial activity provided by a parenteral form of penicillin G.

Aqueous penicillin G (IM or IV) is used for severe or complicated pneumonia. The doses in such cases should be given at frequent intervals, usually every 4 hours, until the infection has been brought under control. The peak level of serum activity of procaine penicillin (IM) is lower than the level provided by a comparable PO dose of penicillin V. Therefore, IM administration of procaine penicillin should be reserved for patients who cannot tolerate oral penicillins because of vomiting or diarrhea, who are comatose, or who require the consistency and reliability of a parenteral preparation even though the disease is not severe enough to warrant frequent doses of aqueous penicillin G (IM or IV).* Benzathine penicillin G (IM) is appropriate only for highly sensitive organisms in tissues that are well vascularized so that the drug can diffuse readily to the site of infection. Although this preparation has been effective in some cases of uncomplicated pneumonia due to *S. pneumoniae*, the level of antibacterial activity in serum and tissues is low, and clinical and bacteriologic failure is frequent when benzathine penicillin G is used.

Penicillinase-Resistant Penicillins

The vast majority of strains of *S. aureus* that cause disease in hospitalized patients are resistant to penicillin G, and the number of strains of resistant staphylococci in patients who have community-acquired disease is increasing rapidly. Thus, at present, the penicillinase-resistant penicillins are the drugs of choice for initial management of patients with staphylococcal disease.

Methicillin was the first penicillinase-resistant penicillin to be introduced, and it proved effective for severe staphylococcal disease. However, it is available only in parenteral form. Oxacillin and nafcillin, which were introduced later, are available in both parenteral and oral preparations and have greater in

---

*See Chapter 19 for a somewhat different approach.

vitro activity against gram-positive cocci. Cloxacillin and dicloxacillin are available only in PO forms and are absorbed more efficiently from the gastrointestinal tract than are the other PO drugs. Although differences exist among these five penicillins in protein-binding properties, degradation by penicillinase, and in vitro antistaphylococcal activity, all five drugs are effective in treatment of staphylococcal disease, and clinical studies have shown them to be comparable when used in appropriate dosage schedules. In addition, all but methicillin have proved effective against infections due to *S. pneumoniae* and beta-hemolytic streptococci, although penicillin G should still be considered the drug of choice for these infections.

Staphylococci resistant to methicillin and other penicillinase-resistant penicillins and cephalosporins were identified soon after the introduction of these drugs. The incidence of such strains in the United States remains low (approximately 1 per cent in recent reports), but outbreaks of disease have occurred in newborn nurseries and surgical units. Bacterial resistance must be considered a possible cause of therapeutic failure whenever staphylococcal disease in a patient who is receiving an adequate amount of penicillinase-resistant penicillin does not respond appropriately. Gentamicin or vancomycin is usually effective against these methicillin-resistant strains of staphylococci.

Ampicillin, Amoxicillin, and Amoxicillin-Clavulanate

Ampicillin and amoxicillin are effective in vitro against a wide spectrum of bacteria: *S. pneumoniae*, beta-hemolytic streptococci, non–penicillinase-producing strains of *S. aureus*, oropharyngeal strains of anaerobic bacteria, *N. meningitidis*, non–penicillinase-producing strains of *Hemophilus influenzae*, and some gram-negative enteric bacilli, including strains of *Escherichia coli* and *Proteus mirabilis*.

Ampicillin is available for oral or parenteral administration; amoxicillin is available in PO form only. For PO use, amoxicillin is preferred because it provides levels of activity in serum that are higher and more prolonged than those achieved with equivalent doses of ampicillin. An additional advantage of amoxicillin is that absorption is not altered when the antibiotic is administered with food, whereas absorption of penicillin is decreased significantly when it is given with food.

Because it is effective against both *S. pneumoniae* and *H. influenzae*, the major pathogens in pulmonary infections in pre–school-age children, amoxicillin has been widely used for respiratory infections in this age group. However, resistant strains of both nontypeable and type B *H. influenzae* have been reported throughout the United States and Western Europe. This resistance appears to be a recent phenomenon; few resistant strains were detected before 1972. Resistance to ampicillin is attributable to production of a penicillinase that hydrolyzes ampicillin, amoxicillin, penicillin G and V, and carbenicillin. Ampicillin or amoxicillin continues to be the antibiotic of choice for children with mild to moderately severe pneumonia that may be due to *H. influenzae;* however, the physician must obtain results of antibiotic susceptibility tests when *H. influenzae* is isolated from the sputum, blood, or other significant body fluid or secretion and must follow the patient's clinical course to be certain that the response to the antibiotic is satisfactory.

Amoxicillin in combination with a beta-lactamase inhibitor clavulanic acid (amoxicillin-clavulanate) is a PO preparation that extends the spectrum of amoxicillin to include beta-lactamase-producing strains of *S. aureus, H. influenzae, Branhamellla catarrhalis,* and gram-negative enteric bacteria. Clavulanate potassium, the salt of clavulanic acid, is a beta-lactam antibiotic with poor in vitro activity against pathogenic bacteria but potent activity as an inhibitor of beta-lactamase enzymes. The activity of amoxicillin-clavulanate against beta-lactamase-producing strains is equivalent to amoxicillin alone against susceptible organisms. The combination drug may be considered if a beta-lactamase-producing organism is known or suspected to be the cause of the respiratory infection. A parenteral drug that combines ampicillin with a different beta-lactamase inhibitor, sulbactam, is available for use in adults but has not yet been approved for use in infants and children.

Carbenicillin and Ticarcillin

These semisynthetic penicillins are efficacious against gram positive cocci, *H. influenzae,* anaerobic bacteria including *Bacteroides fragilis,* and some gram-negative enteric bacilli resistant to other penicillins. The last group includes Enterobacter species, *P. aeruginosa,* and most strains of *Proteus* (including *P. mirabilis* and indole-positive species). Ticarcillin is similar to carbenicillin but is more active against some strains of *P. aeruginosa* and less active against gram-positive cocci. Because of the increased activity, smaller doses of ticarcillin may be used for treatment of disease due to gram-negative organisms.

The value of carbenicillin and ticarcillin in systemic infection appears to be limited by the relatively high serum concentrations of drug required for inhibition of sensitive organisms, but this deficiency is overcome, in part, by the low toxicity of the drug even when it is given in large IV doses. Combination of either of these penicillins with gentamicin or tobramycin provides broad coverage and synergistic activity against some gram-negative enteric bacilli. Such combinations have been effectively used in treatment of serious infections due to *P. aeruginosa* in patients with compromised defense mechanisms.

Ticarcillin and carbenicillin have no dose-related toxicity, but both drugs are disodium salts, and large amounts of either include significant quantities of sodium. One gram of carbenicillin contains 4.7 mEq, or 108 mg, of sodium; 1 g of ticarcillin contains 5.2 mEq, or 120 mg, of sodium. The amount of sodium administered may be of concern in treatment of certain patients with renal or cardiac disease.

Azlocillin and Mezlocillin

Azlocillin and mezlocillin are parenteral penicillins with a spectrum of activity similar to that of carbenicillin and ticarcillin but greater activity in vitro against some gram-negative bacilli and anaerobic bacteria including most strains of *Klebsiella pneumoniae* and many strains of *Serratia marcescens.* Azlocillin is more potent than ticarcillin for strains of *P. aeruginosa.* Combinations of azlocillin or mezlocillin and an aminoglycoside are synergistic against some gram-negative bacteria and have more killing activity than either drug alone. Azlocillin and mezlocillin have less than half the sodium content (1.8 to 2.0 mEq/g) of carbenicillin or ticarcillin.

Toxicity and Sensitization of the Penicillins

The penicillins have no dose-related toxicity unless excessively large doses are used. They do have an epileptogenic potential; a regimen of 60 million or more units per day or very rapid IV injection of 5 million or more units in adults has resulted in seizures. This reaction does not occur with smaller dosage schedules in adults except in patients who are in renal failure or have underlying focal brain lesions. Nephritis and bone marrow depression have been reported in a few cases after methicillin therapy, but this finding is uncommon and does not warrant any change in consideration of the drug for the patient with serious staphylococcal disease. Thrombocytopenia with purpura due to drug-induced platelet aggregation has been noted after use of carbenicillin and penicillin G.

The major concern with use of penicillin is not toxicity but sensitization. Acute anaphylactic reactions are infrequent (approximately one per 20 thousand courses), but a significant number of fatalities occur each year because such a large number of individuals are treated with this antibiotic. The physician must identify the patient who will react to penicillin to avoid use of the drug in that patient. Serologic assays for detection of antibodies to penicillin are not of proven value in identification of patients who will have an immediate life-threatening reaction. Antigens used for skin testing have not received broad acceptance because of false-negative reactions (inability to detect the patient who subsequently reacts to penicillin). In addition, some patients have had an anaphylactic reaction from the small amount of antigen administered. New skin-test antigens, including penicilloyl polylysine and the minor determinant mixture (containing benzyl penicillin and its metabolic breakdown products), have been investigated by Levine (1966). Penicilloyl polylysine is available for skin testing,* but there is no standard material available for the minor determinant mixture. At present, the physicians must rely on the patient's history of an adverse reaction after administration of a penicillin. If the reaction appears to be related to the penicillin, the drug should be avoided for minor infections. If a life-threatening infection should occur and penicillin is clearly the optimal drug, as in the case of overwhelming pneumonia due to *S. pneumoniae*, the physician may choose to administer the drug under carefully controlled conditions; a small dose may be injected initially in an extremity, followed by increasing doses given every 30 min. Epinephrine, a tourniquet, and a tracheotomy set should be available in case of a severe reaction during the testing period. All penicillins are cross-reactive in regard to sensitization, and allergy to any one implies sensitization to all.

THE CEPHALOSPORINS

The cephalosporins are among the antimicrobial agents that may be used as alternatives to penicillins for therapy of patients allergic to penicillin. The cephalosporins have a broad range of activity that encompasses gram-positive cocci (including penicillinase-producing *S. aureus*), some gram-negative enteric bacilli, and anaerobic bacteria. At present, 19 cephalosporins are available in the United States, and several are undergoing clinical trials. The cephalosporins have been categorized as first, second, and third generation based on time of introduction and, in general, similar in vitro activity.

First-Generation Cephalosporins

First-generation cephalosporins are effective against gram-positive cocci, including beta-lactamase-producing *S. aureus*, and have variable activity against gram-negative enteric bacilli. Six first-generation cephalospirns are currently available for use in infants and children: the parenteral drugs cephalothin, cefazolin, and cephaparin; the oral drugs cephalexin and cefadroxil; and cephradine, which is available in both oral and parenteral forms. The first-generation cephalosporins may be considered alternatives to penicillin for disease caused by *S. aureus*, *Streptococcus pyogenes*, *S. pneumoniae*, and susceptible gram-negative enteric bacilli. Activity against *H. influenzae* is limited. First-generation cephalosporins are not the drugs of choice for any pediatric respiratory infection but may be of value for children who have disease due to susceptible organisms and who are known or suspected to be allergic to penicillin. Because of the ambiguity about cross-allergenicity of penicillins and cephalosporins, cephalosporins should not be used if the patient has had an immediate or accelerated reaction to penicillin.

*Pre-pen, Kremers-Urban Company, Milwaukee, Wis.

Second-Generation Cephalosporins

The second-generation cephalosporins approved for use in children consist of three parenteral drugs—cefamandole, cefoxitin, and cefuroxime—and one PO preparation, cefaclor.

Cefoxitin has excellent activity against anaerobic organisms, particularly *B. fragilis*, and selective activity against gram-negative enteric bacilli. The indications include infections in which anaerobic bacteria are known or suspected to be causes of the respiratory tract infection.

Cefamandole is active against gram-negative cocci and was the first cephalosporin to be effective for *H. influenzae*, including beta-lactamase-producing strains. Activity against *S. pneumoniae*, *S. aureus*, and *H. influenzae* prompted use of cefamandole for presumptive therapy of acute sinusitis, periorbital cellulitis, and severe pneumonia. Because of erratic diffusion of the drug into cerebrospinal fluid and reports of its failure to cure meningitis due to *H. influenzae*, cefamandole should not be used if sepsis and potential spread to the central nervous system are possible.

Cefuroxime has an in vitro spectrum of activity similar to that of cefamandole but appears to diffuse better across biologic membranes, as exemplified by success in treatment of bacterial meningitis. Cefuroxime is now preferred to cefamandole for treatment of acute sinusitis, periorbital cellulitis, and severe pneumonia.

Cefaclor is the only oral cephalosporin with significant activity in vitro against *H. influenzae*, including beta-lactamase-producing strains. The major use has been in treatment of otitis media, but cefaclor may also be useful in therapy of mild to moderately severe pneumonia and to complete a course of treatment initiated with a parenteral antibiotic.

Third-Generation Cephalosporins

Cefotaxime, ceftriaxone, and ceftazidime are the most effective of the new cephalosporins and have found important uses for selected infectious problems of infants and children. Each of the three drugs is very effective against gram-negative enteric bacilli and *H. influenzae*. Activity against gram-positive organisms is variable; strains of *S. pneumoniae* are consistently sensitive, but some strains of *S. aureus* require high concentrations of drug for inhibition. Although effective in vitro and with clinical success, a third-generation cephalosporin, moxalactam, is now limited in use because of bleeding problems associated with its administration.

Ceftriaxone is unique among cephalosporins in possessing a long half-life of 6.5 to 8 hours, allowing a dosage schedule of once or twice a day (the once-a-day schedule is approved for use in adults, but only administration every 12 hours is approved for use in children). Because of its long half-life and reduced number of daily doses, ceftriaxone may be of value when the patient may be treated outside the hospital.

Uses outside the hospital include treatment of mild to moderate pneumonia that does not require intensive nursing or for continued therapy of diseases requiring prolonged courses of drug after other needs for hospitalization have ended (see "Home Intravenous Antibiotic Therapy," later).

Ceftazidime has in vitro activity similar to that of cefotaxime and ceftriaxone but has better in vitro activity against *P. aeruginosa,* including strains resistant to antipseudomonal penicillins. Ceftazidime is the most effective of all antimicrobial agents against *P. aeruginosa* and should be considered for acute exacerbations of respiratory infections in children with cystic fibrosis or for management of chronic suppurative otitis media.

Toxicity and Sensitization of the Cephalosporins

The cephalosporins, like the penicillins, are safe for infants and children and have no dose-related toxicity. Uncommon reactions include nephrotoxicity, biliary concretions, alcohol intolerance, and bleeding. A serum sickness–like reaction has occurred in children who received cefaclor. Nephrotoxicity has been reported in adults who received cephalothin in combination with gentamicin. A reversible precipitation of biliary and calcium salts has been associated with administration of ceftriaxone; patients who receive ceftriaxone and experience colicky abdominal pain should have abdominal ultrasonography and appropriate biochemical tests to determine this possibility. A disulfiram-like response occurred in patients consuming alcoholic beverages after administration of cefamandole and moxalactam. Bleeding problems due to hypothrombinemia, thrombocytopenia, or platelet dysfunction have been reported in infants after use of moxalactam.

BROAD-SPECTRUM DRUGS

ERYTHROMYCIN

Erythromycin is effective in vitro against gram-positive cocci of importance in respiratory infections, i.e., *S. pneumoniae,* beta-hemolytic streptococci, and penicillinase-producing and non–penicillinase-producing *S. aureus.* In addition, the drug is highly active against *Mycoplasma pneumoniae, C. diphtheriae, Bordetella pertussis,* and *Legionella pneumophila.* Erythromycin is active against some anaerobic bacteria of the respiratory tract but is not uniformly active against *H. influenzae.* Reports of erythromycin-resistant strains of group A streptococci and *S. pneumoniae* suggest vigilance in patients who have these infections but who do not have appropriate clinical responses to therapy with erythromycin.

Several preparations are available for PO administration. These include erythromycin base, erythromycin stearate (a salt), erythromycin ethylsuccinate (an ester), and erythromycin estolate (the salt of an ester). Erythromycin base is unstable at the low pH of the stomach; thus, absorption of this compound taken PO is incomplete. The other forms are absorbed better from the gastrointestinal tract, but because the base is the only compound with antibacterial activity, the other preparations must be hydrolyzed to the base in the body. The estolate provides the highest serum concentrations, but there is still controversy about which of the preparations provides the highest amount of biologically active drug at the site of infection.

Two preparations are available for IV administration, the glucoheptonate and the lactobionate. IM administration of these forms is painful and should be avoided.

With the exception of the estolate, the available preparations of erythromycin are well tolerated and are not toxic. The estolate may give rise to a cholestatic jaundice that is believed to be a hypersensitivity reaction. This syndrome has also been observed with other forms of erythromycin, but the majority of reported cases have been associated with administration of the estolate. The ester is thought to be responsible for the hepatotoxicity. The jaundice has been noticed in patients who receive the drug for more than 14 days. Jaundice disappears when administration of the drug is stopped. Few cases have been reported in children. At present, potential hepatotoxicity does not appear to be a contraindication to use of the estolate in children. Nevertheless, physicians using this preparation should limit duration of therapy to 10 days and should be alert for signs of liver toxicity.

In some patients, erythromycin has a significant inhibitory effect on clearance of theophylline. Patients who receive both erythromycin and theophylline may develop theophylline toxicity owing to elevated serum concentrations. Patients receiving both drugs should have frequent measurements of serum theophylline.

Erythromycin is an effective alternative to penicillin for treatment of pulmonary infections due to *S. pneumoniae* or beta-hemolytic streptococci. The drug is also effective for mild to moderate infections due to *S. aureus.* For patients with severe disease due to *S. aureus,* erythromycin should be combined with another effective agent, such as chloramphenicol, because of the rapid development of resistance to erythromycin with prolonged use. If *H. influenzae* is believed to be the cause of the respiratory infection, erythromycin is inadequate for initial therapy. This agent is effective in alleviating the signs and symptoms of respiratory disease due to *M. pneumoniae,* although the organism usually is not cleared from the upper respiratory tract. Erythromycin eradicates *B. pertussis* from the nasopharynx and is used to reduce the period of infectivity of patients with *B. pertussis* infection. The drug is also used as prophylaxis for persons in intimate contact with such patients. It is less certain that erythromycin alters the clinical course of pertussis. Erythromycin appears to be of value in treating respiratory disease due to *L. pneumophila*, but to date, few cases have been reported in children.

LINCOMYCIN AND CLINDAMYCIN

Both lincomycin and clindamycin are effective in vitro against gram-positive cocci but are inactive against *H. influenzae*, *N. meningitidis*, and gram-negative enteric bacilli. Clindamycin is also active against some anaerobic bacteria, including penicillin-resistant *Bacteroides* species. Clindamycin provides higher levels of activity in serum than does lincomycin, and in contrast to lincomycin, its absorption through the intestines is not decreased when the drug is taken in close temporal relation to meals. Because of these advantages, clindamycin has largely replaced lincomycin for therapy of appropriate infectious diseases.

Diarrhea and pseudomembranous enterocolitis may follow use of clindamycin; however, most cases of such adverse reactions have been in patients who are elderly, have severe illness, or are receiving several antibiotics. Recent studies indicate that overgrowth of toxin-producing strains of *Clostridium difficile* is probably responsible for most cases of antibiotic-associated colitis. The antibiotic suppresses the normal flora in the colon, and the *C. difficile* organisms proliferate and produce an enterotoxin that is responsible for the disease. The drug has been well tolerated in children; diarrhea has not been a common side effect, and there are few reports of enterocolitis. Clindamycin and lincomycin may be considered as alternatives to penicillin for allergic patients with streptococcal, pneumococcal, or sensitive staphylococcal infections. Most pulmonary infections due to anaerobic organisms in the respiratory tract are sensitive to penicillin G, but some strains may be sensitive only to clindamycin.

THE TETRACYCLINES

The tetracyclines are effective against a broad range of microorganisms, including gram-positive cocci, some gram-negative enteric bacilli, *M. pneumoniae*, rickettsiae, chlamydiae, and *B. pertussis*. Caution must be used in consideration of the tetracyclines as alternatives to penicillin for allergic patients; a significant proportion of group A streptococci and some strains of *S. pneumoniae* are resistant to tetracycline.

Seven tetracycline compounds are available for PO administration in the United States: tetracycline, chlortetracycline, oxytetracycline, demethylchlortetracycline, methacycline, doxycycline, and minocycline. Tetracycline, chlortetracycline, doxycycline, and minocycline are also available for IV administration. With few exceptions, there are only minor differences in the in vitro activity of the different preparations, although minocycline may be effective for some strains of *S. aureus* resistant to other tetracyclines, and doxycycline may inhibit strains of *B. fragilis*.

Tetracyclines are deposited in teeth during the early stages of calcification, and dental staining occurs. A relationship between total dose and visible staining has been established. Discoloration of the teeth has been seen in babies of mothers who received tetracycline after the sixth month of pregnancy. The permanent teeth are stained if the drug is administered between 6 months and 6 years of age.

There are few indications for tetracycline in young children with respiratory infection; other effective antimicrobial agents are available for almost all infections against which tetracycline might be used. Therefore, the use of tetracycline in children should be avoided unless there is a specific indication. Tetracyclines may be considered for children 8 years of age and older for treatment of Q fever, psittacosis, and *M. pneumoniae* infection. The committee of the Food and Drug Administration that oversees use of antibiotics has advised against tetracycline drops for use in children and also recommended stronger label warnings on pediatric uses of the syrup.

THE SULFONAMIDES

Sulfapyridine, discovered in 1938, was the first antimicrobial agent to be effective for therapy of pneumococcal pneumonia. Prontosil, described in 1935 by Domagk, had earlier been demonstrated to be effective against infections due to hemolytic streptococci. Soon after, however, resistance to the sulfonamides appeared in both streptococci and pneumococci. Today, applicability of sulfonamides for respiratory infection is limited; they are the drugs of choice only for treatment of pulmonary infection due to *Nocardia*. The sulfonamides are effective for upper respiratory infections (such as otitis media) due to *H. influenzae*, for treatment of pneumonitis caused by *Chlamydia trachomatis*, and for bacteremia and focal disease (including pneumonia) due to susceptible strains of the meningococcus (*N. meningitidis*). These drugs should not be considered as alternatives to penicillin for treatment of infections due to *S. pneumoniae*, beta-hemolytic streptococci, or *S. aureus*.

TRIMETHOPRIM-SULFAMETHOXAZOLE

Trimethoprim-sulfamethoxazole (TMP-SMZ) is an antimicrobial combination with significant activity against a broad spectrum of gram-positive and gram-negative pathogens. Trimethoprim is more active than sulfonamide, but the combination is frequently more effective than either drug alone. Sulfamethoxazole was the sulfonamide chosen to be used in combination with trimethoprim because it has similar patterns of absorption and excretion. Both agents are well absorbed from the gastrointestinal tract, and food does not affect absorption. An IV form is available for treatment of sepsis or severe pneumonia due to susceptible organisms such as *Pneumocystis carinii*. The same dosage is used for tablets, suspension, and IV formulations.

Adverse reactions to the combination include rashes similar to those previously associated with sulfonamides (maculopapular or urticarial rashes, purpura, photosensitivity reactions, and erythema multiforme bullosum) and gastrointestinal symptoms, primarily nausea and vomiting. Hematologic indices have been carefully evaluated because of the antifolate activity of trimethoprim. Leukopenia, neutropenia, thrombocytopenia, agranulocytosis, and aplastic anemia have been associated with administration of TMP-SMZ, but the incidences of these adverse reactions appear to be low.

Use of TMP-SMZ for respiratory infections includes treatment of disease due to *P. carinii, S. pneumoniae, H. influenzae,* and gram-negative enteric bacilli that are uniquely susceptible to the combination. Disease due to beta-hemolytic streptococci does not respond to treatment with sulfonamides or TMP-SMZ.

DRUGS USED PRIMARILY AGAINST INFECTIONS DUE TO GRAM-NEGATIVE BACILLI

THE AMINOGLYCOSIDES

The aminoglycosides of current therapeutic importance include streptomycin, kanamycin, gentamicin, tobramycin, netilmicin, and amikacin. The in vitro activity of these antibiotics against gram-negative enteric bacilli varies and must be defined for each institution on the basis of current results of sensitivity tests. Streptomycin is ineffective against a significant proportion of infections caused by this group of bacteria, whereas kanamycin, gentamicin, and tobramycin are active against most isolates of *E. coli, Enterobacter, Klebsiella, and Proteus.* At present, gentamicin, tobramycin, netilmicin, and amikacin are the most active of the aminoglycosides against these organisms and also the only drugs active against *P. aeruginosa.*

The spectra of activity for gentamicin, tobramycin, and netilmicin are similar, and strains resistant to one are usually resistant to the others. The major advantage of tobramycin is its activity against some strains of *P. aeruginosa* that are resistant to gentamicin. The spectrum of activity of amikacin is similar to that of gentamicin and tobramycin, but there is little cross-resistance, and some gram-negative organisms resistant to gentamicin and tobramycin are sensitive to amikacin.

The aminoglycosides have significant in vitro activity against *S. aureus* but are ineffective for groups A and B beta-hemolytic streptococci and *S. pneumoniae.* A combination of a penicillin and an aminoglycoside commonly results in more rapid killing and a lower concentration of aminoglycoside required to inhibit strains of gram-negative enteric bacilli.

After parenteral administration, the aminoglycosides distribute rapidly in extracellular body water. The drugs are excreted unchanged in urine and are filtered almost exclusively by the glomeruli, with limited tubular reabsorption.

All of the aminoglycosides may produce renal injury and damage to the eighth nerve in the form of impaired hearing or diminished vestibular function. Eighth nerve damage appears to be dose related, although it has followed the use of relatively small doses, especially in patients with renal failure. Toxicity has not been a problem in children who have normal kidney function and who were treated with aminoglycosides in currently recommended dosage schedules.

The concentrations of aminoglycosides in serum are variable and unpredictable; infants and children who receive aminoglycosides require monitoring of serum concentrations of drug to determine the safety as well as the efficacy of the agent. Blood should be obtained at the expected peak (1 to 2 hours after administration) or trough (just before the next dose). Specimens should be obtained early in the course of therapy (within the first 3 days) to be certain that effective levels in serum are achieved and at subsequent intervals (every 3 to 4 days) to determine that the concentration of aminoglycoside in the serum is not in the toxic range. The desired peaks for aminoglycosides are as follows: for gentamicin and tobramycin 5 to 10 mg/ml, and for kanamycin and amikacin 15 to 25 mg/ml. The trough should not exceed 2 mg/ml for gentamicin and tobramycin or 10 mg/ml for kanamycin and amikacin. The toxic ranges are considered to be more than 14 mg/ml for gentamicin and tobramycin and more than 40 mg/ml for kanamycin and amikacin. Dosage schedules should be modified if concentrations in serum are either too low and therefore inadequate for optimal therapy or too high and therefore potentially toxic.

If there is reason to suspect pulmonary infection due to gram-negative enteric bacteria (as in immunocompromised patients and in the case of pneumonia in newborns), the most effective aminoglycoside should be used. The physician must inspect, on a regular basis, the data provided by the hospital laboratory for current antibiotic susceptibility patterns. At present, gentamicin is used at the Boston City Hospital for initial therapy of patients with respiratory infection that may be due to gram-negative enteric bacilli. Tobramycin and amikacin are reserved for use in infections that would be uniquely sensitive to these drugs. The initial regimen is reevaluated when the results of cultures and susceptibility tests are available.

CHLORAMPHENICOL

Chloramphenicol is active against a broad range of gram-positive and gram-negative bacteria, chlamydiae, and rickettsiae. The oral preparations are absorbed well. Chloramphenicol palmitate, an ester of chloramphenicol, is a liquid preparation that lacks the bitter taste of chloramphenicol in solution or suspension. The palmitate ester is hydrolyzed by enzymes in the gastrointestinal tract to free chloramphenicol, which is well absorbed and biologically active. The encapsulated forms of chloramphenicol also have excellent bioavailability. Recent reports indicate that the bioavailability of PO administered chloramphenicol palmitate is superior to that of chloramphenicol succinate given IV. Hydrolysis of chloramphenicol succinate to free chloramphenicol occurs in the liver, and the rate of hydrolysis appears to vary among individual patients. Only the IV route should be used for parenteral administration, because lower levels of serum activity follow IM use.

Concern for the infrequent but severe effect of chloramphenicol on bone marrow has limited the role of this antibiotic. Aplastic anemia is an idiosyncratic reaction that occurs in approximately 1 in 20,000 to 40,000 courses of the drug. With few exceptions, aplastic anemia has followed use of the PO preparation. A dose-related anemia characterized by decreased reticulocyte count, increased concentrations of iron in serum, and vacuolization of erythroid and myeloid precursors in bone marrow may also occur but ceases when the drug is discontinued.

Chloramphenicol should be used for initial treatment of severe respiratory infections that are or are suspected to be due to ampicillin-resistant *H. influenzae* and in the treatment of pneumonia due to gram-negative enteric bacilli in the rare cases in which chloramphenicol is the only effective agent.

THE POLYMYXINS

Polymyxin and colistin are effective in vitro against a broad spectrum of gram-negative enteric bacilli, including *P. aeruginosa*. These drugs do not diffuse well across biologic membranes and are most effective when they come into direct contact with the causative agent, as in urinary tract infections or when applied topically. The polymyxins are less effective in pneumonia and usually fail to eradicate suppurative foci or other tissue infections.

DRUGS USED PRIMARILY FOR INFECTIONS DUE TO GRAM-POSITIVE ORGANISMS

VANCOMYCIN

Vancomycin is a parenterally administered antibiotic whose spectrum of activity is limited to gram-positive organisms. It is administered only by the IV route because IM injection causes pain and tissue necrosis. Ototoxicity may result from high concentrations of vancomycin in serum. The principal use of this agent is treatment of serious staphylococcal disease in which the organism is resistant to the penicillinase-resistant penicillins and cephalosporins. Vancomycin is one of the few drugs (rifampin, fusidic acid, and bacitracin are others) effective in vitro against the highly resistant strains of *S. pneumoniae* isolated recently in South Africa and may be an important therapeutic agent if this strain becomes more widespread.

IMPORTANT ASPECTS OF ADMINISTRATION OF ANTIBIOTICS

DOSAGE SCHEDULES IN NEWBORN INFANTS

Dosage schedules for parenteral antibiotics used in treatment of serious infections (including pneumonia) in newborn infants (up to 28 days of age) are given in Table 15–1. Gestational age and postnatal age are important factors in the clinical pharmacology of antibiotics during the first month of life; enzyme systems involved in the detoxification of drugs such as chloramphenicol may be deficient in premature infants. Rapidly maturing renal function requires alteration of dosage schedules after the first week of life so that antimicrobial activity of drugs excreted mainly by the kidneys will be maintained in serum and tissues. Thus, different dosage schedules for the penicillins and some aminoglycosides are recommended for infants with birth weight 2000 g or less or greater than 2000 g and 6 days of age or younger and for infants 1 to 4 weeks of age.

DOSAGE SCHEDULES IN INFANTS AND CHILDREN

The dosage schedules listed in Table 15–2 are classified according to whether the disease is mild to moderate or severe. In general, the higher dosage schedules are used for infections that are more severe, due to less susceptible organisms, or located in areas of the body where diffusion of the antimicrobial agent is limited.

DOSAGE SCHEDULES IN CHILDREN WITH RENAL INSUFFICIENCY

The kidneys are the major organs of excretion for most antimicrobial agents, including the penicillins, aminoglycosides, polymyxins, and tetracyclines (with the exception of doxycycline). Impaired excretion may result in high and possibly toxic concentrations

Table 15–1. DAILY DOSAGE SCHEDULES FOR ANTIBIOTICS OF VALUE IN TREATING
BACTERIAL PNEUMONIA IN NEONATES*

Drug	Route	¢ 7 Days of Age		· 7 Days of Age	
		BW [2000 G	BW $ 2000 G	BW [2000 G	BW $ 2000 G
Penicillins					
Penicillin G, crystalline	IV, IM	25,000 U q 12 hr	25,000 U q 8 hr	25,000 U q 8 hr	25,000 U q 6 hr
Ampicillin	IV, IM	25 U q 12 hr	25 U q 8 hr	25 U q 8 hr	25 U q 6 hr
Oxacillin	IV, IM	25 U q 12 hr	25 U q 8 hr	25 U q 8 hr	25 U q 6 hr
Nafcillin	IV	25 U q 12 hr	25 U q 8 hr	25 U q 8 hr	25 U q 6 hr
Carbenicillin	IV, IM	100 U q 12 hr	100 U q 8 hr	100 U q 8 hr	100 U q 6 hr
Ticarcillin	IV, IM	75 U q 12 hr	75 U q 8 hr	75 U q 8 hr	75 U q 6 hr
Cephalosporins					
Cefotaxime	IV, IM	50 U q 12 hr	50 U q 8 hr	50 U q 8 hr	50 U q 6 hr
Ceftazidime	IV, IM	50 U q 12 hr	30 U q 8 hr	30 U q 8 hr	30 U q 8 hr
Ceftriaxone	IV, IM	50 U q 24 hr	50 U q 24 hr	50 U q 24 hr	50 U q 24 hr
Aminoglycosidest					
Amikacin	IV†, IM	7.5 U q 12 hr	7.5 U q 12 hr	75. U q 8 hr	10 U q 8 hr
Gentamicin	IV†, IM	2.5 U q 12 hr	2.5 U q 12 hr	2.5 U q 8 hr	2.5 U q 8 hr
Kanamycin	IV†, IM	7.5 U q 12 hr	7.5 U q 12 hr	7.5 U q 8 hr	10 U q 8 hr
Tobramycin	IV†, IM	2 U q 12 hr	2 U q 12 hr	2 U q 8 hr	2 U q 8 hr
Chloramphenicol†	IV	25 U q 24 hr	25 U q 24 hr	25 U q 24 hr	25 U q 12 hr
Clindamycin	IV, IM	5 U q 12 hr	5 U q 8 hr	5 U q 8 hr	5 U q 6 hr
Vancomycin†	IV‡	10 U q 12 hr	10 U q 12 hr	10 U q 8 hr	10 U q 8 hr

*Dose in mg/kg or units/kg and frequency of administration in hours.
†Serum concentrations needed to determine optimal schedule.
‡IV administration over 30 to 60 min.

of the drug in the blood and tissues if alterations in the dosage schedule are not considered.

Agents requiring adjustment of dosage include the aminoglycosides, tetracyclines (with the exception of doxycycline), vancomycin, and polymyxins.

Agents requiring adjustment of dosage only when renal failure is severe include the penicillins, the cephalosporins, and clindamycin.

Agents that do not require adjustment of the dosage schedule in renal impairment include erythromycin, chloramphenicol, and doxycycline.

The dosage schedules may be altered by increasing the interval between doses or by decreasing individual doses. In most cases, the first dose can be given in the usual amount and the intervals between subsequent doses can be lengthened. Bioassays of antimicrobial activity in serum are now available in many hospital laboratories and should be used when aminoglycosides are administered to children with renal insufficiency. Serum specimens should be obtained at the time of the anticipated peak level (approximately 1 hour for aminoglycosides) and of the trough level (just before administration of the next dose) on the first day. Samples should be obtained again on subsequent days to ensure that a safe and effective dosage schedule is being used.

FOOD INTERFERENCE WITH THE ABSORPTION OF SOME ORAL ANTIBIOTICS

The intestinal absorption of some antibiotics is significantly decreased when the drugs are ingested with food (Table 15–3). Absorption of other antibiotics is only slightly affected by food. Antibiotics whose absorption is hindered by concurrent ingestion of food should be taken at least 1 hour before or 2 hours after meals.

SOME CONSIDERATIONS IN ADMINISTRATION OF PARENTERAL PREPARATIONS

The availability of PO antimicrobial agents is of value in treatment of mild pulmonary disease. Most PO antibiotics vary in their absorption, however, and because higher serum levels of antibacterial activity are achieved by parenteral routes, the latter are preferable for moderately severe and severe infections. Only parenteral antibiotics should be used in newborn infants with systemic infection.

Unless a patient is in shock or suffers from a bleeding diathesis, there is little or no therapeutic advantage of IV over IM administration of the antibiotic. If prolonged parenteral therapy is anticipated, however, the pain on injection and the small muscle mass of a young child preclude the IM route and make IV therapy preferable. Chloramphenicol, the tetracyclines, and erythromycin should be given by the IV rather than the IM route. Chloramphenicol is poorly absorbed from IM sites. IM injection of tetracyclines and erythromycin causes local irritation and pain.

Penicillins may be administered by the "push"

Table 15–2. DAILY DOSAGE SCHEDULES FOR ANTIBIOTICS OF VALUE IN TREATING BACTERIAL PNEUMONIA IN PEDIATRIC PATIENTS BEYOND THE NEWBORN PERIOD

Drug (Trade Name)	Route	Dosage/kg/24 Hours	
		Mild to Moderate Infections	*Severe Infections*
Penicillin G, crystalline (numerous)	IV, IM	25,000–50,000 units in 4 doses	100,000–300,000 units in 4–6 doses
Penicillin G, procaine	IM	25,000–50,000 units in 1–2 doses	Inappropriate
Penicillin G, benzathine	IM	¢60 lbs: 600,000 u ·60 lbs: 1,200,000 u	Inappropriate
Penicillin G, potassium (numerous)	PO	25,000–50,000 units in 4 doses	Inappropriate
Phenoxymethyl penicillin, penicillin V (numerous)	PO	25,000–50,000 units in 4 doses	Inappropriate
Penicillinase-resistant penicillins:			
Methicillin (Staphcillin, Celbenin)	IV, IM	100–200 mg in 4 doses	200–300 mg in 4–6 doses
Oxacillin (Prostaphlin, Bactocil)	IV, IM	50–100 mg in 4 doses	100–200 mg in 4–6 doses
	PO	50–100 mg in 4 doses	Inappropriate
Nafcillin (Unipen)	IV, IM	50–100 mg in 4 doses	100–200 mg in 4–6 doses
	PO	50–100 mg in 4 doses	Inappropriate
Cloxacillin (Tegopen)	PO	50–100 mg in 4 doses	Inappropriate
Dicloxacillin (Dynapen, Pathocil, Veracillin)	PO	25–50 mg in 4 doses	Inappropriate
Broad-spectrum penicillins:			
Ampicillin (numerous)	IV, IM	50–100 mg in 4 doses	200–300 mg in 4 doses
	PO	50–100 mg in 4 doses	Inappropriate
Amoxicillin (Amoxil, Larotid, Polymox)	PO	20–40 mg in 3 doses	Inappropriate
Amoxicillin-clavulanate (Augmentin)	PO	20–40 mg in 3 doses	Inappropriate
Carbenicillin (Geopen, Pyopen)	IV, IM	100–200 mg in 4 doses	400–600 mg in 4–6 doses
Ticarcillin (Ticar)	IV, IM	50–100 mg in 4 doses	200–300 mg in 4–6 doses
Cephalosporins:			
Cephalexin (Keflex)	PO	25–100 mg in 4 doses	Inappropriate
Cephradine (Anspor, Velosef)	PO	25–100 mg in 2–4 doses	Inappropriate
	IV, IM	50 mg in 4 doses	50–100 mg in 4 doses
Cefadroxil (Duricef)	PO	30 mg in 1 dose*	
Cefaclor (Ceclor)	PO	20–40 mg in 3 doses	Inappropriate
Cephalothin (Keflin)	IV, IM	80–100 mg in 4 doses	100–150 mg in 4–6 doses
Cefazolin (Kefzol, Ancef)	IV, IM	25–50 mg in 2–4 doses	50–100 mg in 4 doses
Cephapirin (Cefadyl)	IV, IM	40 mg in 4 doses	40–80 mg in 4 doses
Cefamandole (Mandol)	IV, IM	50–100 mg in 3–4 doses	100–150 mg in 4–6 doses
Cefoxitin (Mefoxin)	IV, IM	80–100 mg in 3–4 doses	80–160 mg in 4–6 doses
Cefuroxime (Zinacef)	IV, IM	75–100 mg in 3 doses	175–240 mg in 3 doses
Cefotaxime (Claforan)	IV, IM	75–100 mg in 4 doses	150–200 mg in 4 doses
Ceftriaxone (Rocephin)	IV, IM	50–75 mg in 2 doses	80–100 mg in 2 doses
Ceftazidime (Fortaz)	IV, IM	75–100 mg in 3 doses	125–150 mg in 3 doses
Erythromycin:			
Erythromycin glucoheptonate (Ilotycin, IV)	IV	Inappropriate	20–50 mg in 4 doses
Erythromycin lactobionate (Erythrocin, IV)			
Erythromycin base (Ilotycin, E-mycin)	PO	20–50 mg in 3–4 doses	Inappropriate
Erythromycin ethylsuccinate (Pediamycin, Erythrocin)			
Erythromycin stearate (Erythrocin)			
Erythromycin estolate (Ilosone)			
Clindamycin (Cleocin)	IV, IM	15–25 mg in 3–4 doses	25–40 mg in 3–4 doses
	PO	10–20 mg in 4 doses	Inappropriate
Aminoglycosides:‡			
Streptomycin (numerous)	IM	Inappropriate	20–40 mg in 3 doses
Kanamycin (Kantrex)	IV, IM	Inappropriate	15–30 mg in 2–3 doses
Gentamicin (Garamycin)	IV, IM	Inappropriate	3–7.5 mg in 3 doses
Tobramycin (Nebcin)	IV, IM	Inappropriate	3–7.5 mg in 3 doses
Amikacin (Amikin)	IV, IM	Inappropriate	15–30 mg in 2–3 doses
Netilmicin (Netromycin)	IV, IM	Inappropriate	3–7.5 mg in 3 doses
Tetracycline (numerous)	IV	Inappropriate	10–20 mg in 2 doses
	PO	20–40 mg in 4 doses	Inappropriate
Chloramphenicol‡ (Chloromycetin)	IV	Inappropriate	50–100 mg in 3–4 doses
	PO	Inappropriate	50–100 mg in 3–4 doses
Vancomycin (Vancocin)‡	IV	40 mg in 4 doses	40–60 mg in 4 doses
Sulfonamides:			
Sulfadiazine	IV, SC	Inappropriate	100–150 mg in 4 doses
Sulfisoxazole (Gantrisin)	IV, SC	Inappropriate	100–150 mg in 4 doses
	PO	100–150 mg in 4 doses	Inappropriate
Triple sulfas (numerous)	PO	120–150 mg in 4 doses	120–150 mg in 4 doses
Trimethoprim/sulfamethoxazole (Bactrim, Septra)	PO	8 mg trimethoprim/40 mg sulfamethoxazole in 2 doses	20 mg trimethoprim/100 mg sulfamethoxazole in 4 doses§
	IV	Inappropriate	20 mg trimethoprim/100 mg sulfamethoxazole in 4 doses†

*For streptococcal pharyngitis.
†For use only in *Pneumocystis carinii* pneumonia or when microorganism is uniquely susceptible and oral form cannot be administered.
‡Serum concentrations needed to determine optimal schedule.
§For use only in *Pneumocystis carinii* pneumonia.

Table 15–3. EFFECT OF FOOD ON ABSORPTION OF SELECTED ORAL ANTIBIOTICS

Major Decrease	Minimal or No Decrease
Unbuffered penicillin G	Buffered penicillin G
Ampicillin	Penicillin V
	Amoxicillin, amoxicillin-clavulanate
Penicillinase-resistant penicillins: oxacillin, nafcillin, cloxacillin, dicloxacillin	Cephalosporins: cephalexin, cephradine, cefaclor
	Clindamycin
Lincomycin	Chloramphenicol
Tetracyclines	Erythromycin

(intermittent) method of IV therapy, in which the drug is administered in 5 to 15 min and produces high serum levels of antibacterial activity of short duration. The "steady drip" method produces a sustained low level of activity. There are no data to indicate a clinical advantage of one method over the other. Rapid administration (less than 5 min) of large IV doses of penicillins should be avoided because of possible central nervous system effects.

The antibacterial activity of some penicillins deteriorates if they are kept in solution at room temperature for a long period. Therefore, it is good practice to administer fresh solutions of the penicillin every 6 to 8 hours when the steady drip method is used.

The aminoglycosides (kanamycin, gentamicin, tobramycin, and amikacin) may be administered IV over 30 to 60 min. Because of possible eighth nerve toxicity at very high blood or tissue levels, these drugs should not be given by the push method.

HOME INTRAVENOUS ANTIBIOTIC THERAPY

Patients who remain hospitalized only for prolonged courses of IV antimicrobial agents may now be treated at home. The criteria for home use include the following: the patient's condition is stable; the patient or parent can monitor the therapy; the home environment is suitable, including a phone for emergency communication and a refrigerator for storage of the drug. Antibiotics used in outpatient care should have low toxicity and long half-life, allowing for less frequent dosing. Visiting nurse associations or hospital pharmacy or community programs are usually capable of implementing programs based on the physician's plan. Advantages include patient comfort, decreased cost, decrease in nosocomial infection, and involvement of the patient and family in the patient's care and progress to recovery.

USE OF PROBENECID WITH PENICILLINS

Probenecid increases the peak and duration of penicillin activity in the serum. The drug is used as an adjunct to penicillin therapy when high levels are necessary. Although this combination is not usually appropriate when parenteral penicillin is given to a child with pulmonary disease, probenecid may be of value in increasing levels of penicillin in serum and pleural effusions when PO treatment with penicillin is necessary. Probenecid is used most commonly when a prolonged course of therapy is necessary and there are no more sites to insert needles for IV administration. PO penicillin alone or a combination of PO penicillin and one or two IM doses each day plus one dose of probenecid may provide adequate levels to complete a course of therapy. The dosage of probenecid is 10 mg/kg every 6 hours (adult dose, 500 mg every 6 hours).

DIRECT INSTILLATION OF ANTIMICROBIAL AGENTS

Direct instillation of antimicrobial agents into various body fluids may be of value when diffusion of the drug to the site of infection is inadequate. Antibiotics diffuse well into the pleural space after parenteral administration, but intrapleural instillation should be considered when the empyema fluid is loculated by fibrous bands. If a chest tube is in place, antibiotics are instilled through the tube after irrigation. In susceptible infection, aqueous crystalline penicillin G (10,000 to 60,000 units), ampicillin (10 to 50 mg), or a penicillinase-resistant penicillin or cephalosporin (10 to 50 mg) may be injected into the chest tube in 10 ml of 0.85 per cent sodium chloride or sterile water. The clamp is maintained for 1 hour and then released for drainage. The instillations should be repeated three to four times during each day that the tube remains in place. If thoracenteses are done, antibiotic is introduced after the pleural fluid is aspirated.

USE OF ANTIMICROBIAL AGENTS FOR PROPHYLAXIS

Chemoprophylaxis refers to use of drugs to prevent infections and thus use of the drug before onset of infection. Prophylaxis is of most value when the following criteria are met: use of a single drug with a narrow spectrum of activity; use of a drug with minimal side effects and no important toxicity; prevention of colonization with an organism of known sensitivity that is unlikely to become resistant to the drug used.

Use of antimicrobial agents for prophylaxis in children has proved to be of value in many circumstances, including selected use for prevention of infections of the respiratory tract. These uses include isoniazid for prevention of tuberculous infection in household contacts; TMP-SMZ for prevention of pneumonia due to *P. carinii* in children who have malignancy and who are receiving immunosuppressive therapy or children with acquired immune deficiency syndrome; amoxicillin or sulfisoxazole for prevention of recurrent episodes of acute otitis media; amantadine for influenza A virus infection; and rifampin for contacts of patients with invasive disease due to *H. influenzae* or *N. meningitidis*. Other uses should await the results of appropriate investigations.

USE OF ANTIMICROBIAL AGENTS FOR CHILDREN IN SCHOOL OR GROUP DAY-CARE

Infants and children may return to school or day-care during a course of antimicrobial therapy. Physicians should recognize the problems of administration of drug by caretakers outside of the home and should consider medications that are given infrequently and need only simple directions for administration. Drugs administered two or three times a day are preferred. Chewable tables when available are of value in reducing the need to measure specific amounts of suspension. Once-a-day dosage schedules are an important administrative advantage to obtain maximum compliance with the prescribed schedule: cefadroxil is available for therapy of streptococcal pharyngitis; cefixime was approved by the Food and Drug Administration in the spring of 1989 for therapy of acute otitis media. Single-dose regimens, such as IM benzathine penicillin G for group A streptococcal infections, may be advantageous. Guidelines for administration of medications in school have recently been published by the Committee of School Health of the American Academy of Pediatrics and may also serve as a model for the physician who is prescribing drugs to be administered in day-care (Zanga et al, 1984).

WHAT TO LOOK FOR WHEN ANTIMICROBIAL THERAPY FAILS

If a patient does not respond appropriately to therapy with antimicrobial agents or subsequently has a relapse or recurrence of infection, the physician must review the illness to determine the reasons for failure. Variables affecting the outcome of antimicrobial therapy, including characteristics of the disease, the host, the drug, and the microorganism, should be reevaluated. A list of factors responsible for or contributing to failure of antimicrobial agents is given in Table 15–4.

Table 15–4. FACTORS CONTRIBUTING TO FAILURE OF ANTIMICROBIAL AGENTS IN PULMONARY INFECTION

Disease-related
  Antibiotic inappropriate for disease
  Ancillary therapy not instituted
  Sequestered focus of infection (undetected or inaccessible)
Host-related
  Defect in immune response to infection
  Anatomic defect
  Foreign body
Drug-related
  Inadequate compliance
  Improper dosage schedule—route, dose, or duration
  Inadequate diffusion to site of infection
  Incompatibility of mixed drugs for oral or parenteral route
  Deterioration of drug on storage
Organism-related
  Protoplast formation
  "Persisters"
  Acquired resistance to antimicrobial agent
  Superinfection with resistant bacteria

DISEASE FACTORS

The use of antibiotics for viral infection and incorrect choice of drugs for bacterial disease are major factors in apparent lack of response.

Failure to consider the role of drainage of a suppurative focus, such as empyema fluid, may result in persistent fever and toxicity. Organisms may remain sequestered in undetected or inaccessible loci and cause a recurrence of disease after therapy is discontinued. Patients with pulmonary disease may have infections at other sites that require special management. Identification of the focus and drainage or more prolonged or different therapy may be necessary to effect a cure.

HOST FACTORS

Patients whose normal humoral or cellular defense mechanisms are compromised by congenital or acquired disease or immunosuppressive medication suffer from frequent infections, often of the respiratory tract. Bactericidal antibiotics are usually necessary in treating infection in these patients, because bacteriostatic agents depend on normal phagocytic and immunologic mechanisms to eradicate the infection.

Anatomic defects, congenital or traumatic, often result in infections and recurrence or relapse after apparently successful antimicrobial therapy. Thus, patients with tracheoesophageal fistula or sequestration of segments of lung may pose a difficult problem in eradication of local infection.

A foreign body, such as an aspirated particle, may serve as a nidus for a persisting pulmonary infection.

DRUG FACTORS

The most common drug-related factor in failure of antibiotic therapy is inadequate compliance—the patient did not take the medicine as prescribed. Before embarking on expensive and time-consuming tests to determine the basis for failure, the physician must be assured that the patient took the medication as instructed.

Other drug-related factors include poor choice of route of administration, inappropriate dosage schedule, and inadequate duration of therapy. For the most part, physicians must rely on empirically derived dosage schedules to provide assured results with minimal risk in terms of clinical failure and toxicity of the drug. Because recommendations change as new information is presented, physicians must be alert to the need to modify dosage schedules.

Incompatibility of IV administered drugs may result in physical or chemical changes and possible alteration of antibacterial activity. Whenever possible, each IV drug should be administered separately.

Some antimicrobial agents deteriorate on prolonged storage. Adherence to expiration dates recommended by the manufacturer safeguards against inadequate potency of the drug.

Diffusion of the drug to the site of infection may be inadequate. Some drugs, such as polymyxin, diffuse poorly across biologic membranes and would be expected to be ineffective for treatment of pulmonary abscesses and other suppurative foci.

BACTERIAL FACTORS

Factors directly related to the interaction of drugs and infecting organism include persistence of infection due to the formation of protoplasts or ill-defined "persisters" at the site of infection.

Development of resistance may be important in infection due to gram-negative enteric bacilli and in tuberculosis but does not appear to be of clinical concern in staphylococcal disease treated with penicillinase-resistant penicillins (although resistance may develop if erythromycin alone is used).

Superinfection with new organisms resistant to previously administered antibiotics is a particular problem in patients with defective immune mechanisms or chronic respiratory infection.

Selected reviews are listed in the references for readers who are interested in further information about the use of antimicrobial agents for treatment of pulmonary infections in children.

REFERENCES

Beta-Lactam Drugs

Acar JF and Neu HC (eds): Gram-negative aerobic bacterial infections: a focus on directed therapy, with special reference to aztreonam. Rev Infect Dis 4:537, 1985.

Frenkel LD and the Multicenter Ceftriaxone Pediatric Study Group: Once-daily administration of ceftriaxone for the treatment of selected serious bacterial infections in children. Pediatrics 82:486, 1988.

Jacobs MR, Koornhof HJ, Robins-Browne RM et al: Emergency of multiply resistant pneumococci. N Engl J Med 299:735, 1978.

Kirby WMM (chairman of symposium): Symposium on carbenicillin. A clinical profile. J Infect Dis 122(Suppl):S1, 1970.

Klein JO: Symposium on long-acting penicillins. Pediatr Infect Dis 5:569, 1985.

Klein JO and Finland M: The new penicillins. N Engl Med 269:1019, 1963.

Levin S and Harris AA: Principles of combination therapy. Bull NY Acad Med 51:1020, 1975.

Levine BB: Immunologic mechanisms of penicillin allergy. A haptenic model system for the study of allergic diseases of man. N Engl J Med 275:1115, 1966.

Marques JC, Tornell SG, and Tahull JMG: Invasive infections caused by multiply resistant Haemophilus influenzae type b. J Pediatr 104:164, 1984.

Neu HC (ed): Beta-lactamase inhibition: therapeutic advances. Am J Med 79(5B):1, 1985.

Word BW and Klein JO: Current therapy of bacterial sepsis and meningitis in infants and children: a poll of directors of programs in pediatric infectious diseases. Pediatr Infect Dis 7:267, 1988.

Broad-Spectrum Drugs

Braun P: Hepatotoxicity of erythromycin. J Infect Dis 119:300, 1969.

Cook FV and Farrar WE Jr: Vancomycin revisited. Ann Intern Med 88:313, 1978.

Dillon HC and Derrick CW: Clinical experience with clindamycin hydrochloride. I. Treatment of streptococcal and mixed streptococcal-staphylococcal skin infections. Pediatrics 55:205, 1975.

Finland M, Kass EH, and Platt R (guest ed): Trimethoprim-sulfamethoxazole revisited. Rev Infect Dis 4:185, 1982.

Genot MT, Golan HP, Porter PJ et al: Effect of administration of tetracycline in pregnancy on the primary dentition of the offspring J Oral Med 25:75, 1970.

Grossman ER, Walchek A, Freedman H et al: Tetracyclines and permanent teeth. The relation between dose and tooth color. Pediatrics 47:567, 1971.

Kass EH and Evans DA: Future prospects and past problems in antimicrobial therapy: the role of cefoxitin. Rev Infect Dis 1:1, 1979.

Keusch GT and Present DH: Summary of workshop on clindamycin colitis. J Infect Dis 133:578, 1976.

LaForce CF, Miller MF, and Chai H: Effect of erythromycin on theophylline clearance in asthmatic children. J Pediatr 99:153, 1981.

Moellering RC Jr: Symposium on cefamandole. J Infect Dis 137:151, 1978.

Moellering RC Jr and Swartz MN: The newer cephalosporins. N Engl J Med 294:24, 1976.

Nelson JD: The evolving role of erythromycin in medicine. Pediatr Infect Dis 5:118, 1986.

Raeburn JA, Govan JRW, McCrae WM et al: Ciprofloxacin therapy in cystic fibrosis. J Antimicrob Chemother 20:295, 1987.

Yaffe SJ: Chairman for the Committee on Drugs. Requiem for tetracyclines. Pediatr 55:142, 1975.

Drugs Used Primarily for Infections Due to Gram-Negative Bacilli

Evans WE, Feldman S, Barker LF et al: Use of gentamicin serum levels to individualize therapy in children. J Pediatr 93:133, 1978.

Finland M and Hewitt WL (guest eds): Second international symposium on gentamicin, an aminoglycoside antibiotic. J Infect Dis 124(Suppl):S1, 1971.

Finland M and Neu HC (guest eds): Symposium of the Ninth International Congress of Chemotherapy in London, England: Tobramycin. J Infect Dis 134(Suppl):S1, 1976.

Finland M, Brumfitt W, and Kass EH (guest eds): Advances in aminoglycoside therapy: amikacin. J Infect Dis 134(Suppl):S235, 1976.

Kauffman RE, Thirumoorthi MB, Buckley JA et al: Relative bioavailability of intravenous chloramphenicol succinate and oral chloramphenicol palmitate in infants and children. J Pediatr 99:963, 1981.

Moellering RC Jr and Siegenthaler WE: Aminoglycoside therapy—the new decade: a world-wide perspective. Am J Med 80(6B):1, 1986.

Scott JL, Finegold SM, Belkin GA, et al: A controlled double-blind study of the hematologic toxicity of chloramphenicol. N Engl J Med 272:1137, 1965.

Whitelock O-V St (ed-in-chief): The basic and clinical research of the new antibiotic, kanamycin. Ann NY Acad Sci 76:17, 1958.

Important Aspects of Administration of Antibiotics

Klein JO: Antimicrobial prophylaxis for recurrent acute otitis media. Pediatr Ann 5:398, 1984.

Kunin CM: Antibiotic usage in patients with renal impairment. Hosp Pract, January 1972, p. 141.

McCracken GH: Clinical pharmacology of antibacterial agents. In Remington JS and Klein JO (eds): Infectious Diseases of the Fetus and Newborn Infants.3rd ed. Philadelphia, WB Saunders Co, 1990.

Peter G (ed): *Hemophilus influenzae* Infections: Control Measures. Report of the Committee of Infectious Diseases. 20th ed. Elk Grove Village, Ill, American Academy of Pediatrics, 1988.

Wallerstein RO, Condit PK, Kasper CK et al: Statewide study of chloramphenicol therapy and fatal aplastic anemia. JAMA 208:2045, 1969.

Weinstein L and Dalton AC: Host determinants of response to antimicrobial agents. N Engl J Med 279:467, 1968.

Zanga J, Douland MA, Newton J, et al: Administration of medication in school. Pediatrics 74:433, 1984.

16

RONI GRAD, M.D., and
LYNN M. TAUSSIG, M.D.

ACUTE INFECTIONS PRODUCING UPPER AIRWAY OBSTRUCTION

Infections of the supraglottis, glottis, subglottis, and trachea are relatively common in infants and children. Collectively they are often referred to as the *croup syndrome* (Nelson, 1984). Although these disease processes primarily produce symptoms in infants and young children because of the small airway diameter in these patients, older children and adults may be affected as well.

Before 1900, the term *croup* was used to refer almost exclusively to diphtheria; however, attempts to classify different patterns of laryngeal infections date to 1812 (Stool, 1988). Epiglottitis was first recognized as a separate entity in 1900, although George Washington may have died of this disorder in 1799 (Scheidemandel, 1976). *Hemophilus influenzae* was first isolated from patients with epiglottitis in 1936. Laryngotracheobronchitis was initially described as a separate entity in 1928, and parainfluenza virus was first isolated from afflicted patients in 1956. Bacterial tracheitis was "rediscovered" as a separate entity in 1979 (Jones et al, 1979); however, this disease process was well described in literature from the early part of the twentieth century (Nelson, 1984). Laryngeal diphtheria is now rare in industrialized countries, with the advent of immunization programs.

Treatment of laryngeal infections in the early nineteenth century consisted of phlebotomy and the application of leeches. Tracheotomy was rarely performed because of the high risk of secondary neck damage and death due to bacterial toxemia (Stool, 1988). In the late nineteenth century, a series of endotracheal tubes was introduced by Joseph O'Dwyer. These tubes were inserted orally, resulting in a patent airway and decreased mortality; however, complications developed subsequent to their use, including laryngeal stenosis. In the early twentieth century, advances by Chevalier Jackson improved the tracheotomy procedure, reducing mortality and the complication of laryngeal stenosis. With the advent of polypropylene plastic endotracheal tubes, complications have been further reduced, and endotracheal intubation is usually advocated instead of tracheostomy for airway maintenance. The introduction of antibiotics and corticosteroids in the midtwentieth century and the recent use of racemic epinephrine have further improved the standard of care of patients with laryngeal infections.

Considerable confusion exists regarding nomenclature of these disorders, with some using the term *croup* to refer to any inflammatory disorder of the upper airway and others restricting the use of the term to refer specifically to subglottic disease, usually of viral origin. This chapter describes infectious processes causing inflammation of the paraglottic structures, focusing primarily on laryngotracheobronchitis, epiglottitis, and bacterial tracheitis. The term *croup* will be largely avoided to minimize confusion.

LARYNGEAL ANATOMY

To understand the pathogenesis of symptoms due to acute upper airway infections, it is necessary to

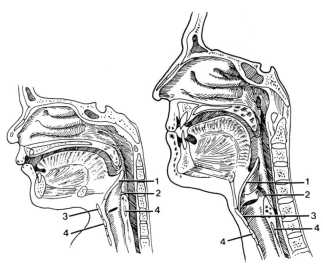

Figure 16–1. Anatomy of the larynx in an infant and an adult. Specific landmarks: *1*, epiglottis; *2*, arytenoid cartilages; *3*, thyroid cartilage; *4*, cricoid cartilage. The infant larynx is situated relatively high in the cervical region. Additionally, the base of the infant's tongue is close to the larynx, and the epiglottis is located near the palate. These anatomic differences partially explain the obligate nose breathing of the young infant, as well as the relative ease with which infants develop upper airway obstructions.

consider the anatomy of the larynx (Figs. 16–1 to 16–3). The larynx consists of four major cartilages—the thyroid, cricoid, arytenoid, and epiglottic cartilages—joined by muscles, ligaments, and fibroelastic and mucous membranes.

The thyroid cartilage is the largest of the laryngeal cartilages and surrounds the larynx anteriorly and laterally. The cricoid cartilage completely surrounds the larynx inferior to the vocal cords, thus providing a critical airway orifice. The arytenoid cartilages articulate at a synovial surface with the upper lateral

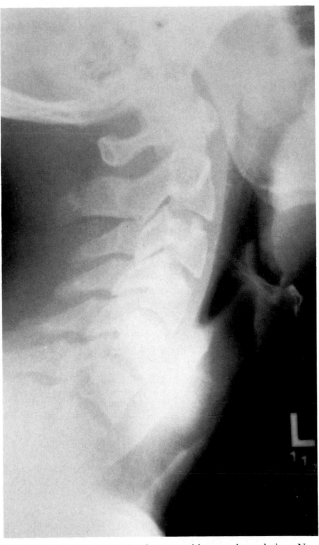

Figure 16–3. Radiograph of a normal larynx: lateral view. Note the sharp epiglottis, the nondistended hypopharynx, and the patent subglottic space. (Courtesy of Dr. George Barnes.)

borders of the cricoid lamina, allowing them to move anteriorly, posteriorly, laterally, and medially, as well as to rotate. The vocal cords are attached to the arytenoid cartilages. The epiglottic cartilage provides support for the supraglottic area and projects superiorly in the pharynx posterior to the tongue. This cartilage is covered with a mucous membrane and separates the vallecula posteriorly from the laryngeal vestibule anteriorly. The arytenoepiglottic folds are folds of mucous membranes extending from the arytenoids superiorly, laterally, and anteriorly to the lateral border of the epiglottic cartilage, separating the piriform sinuses from the laryngeal orifice.

The laryngeal cavity consists of three areas divided by two sets of mucous membrane folds. The bulky vestibular folds separate the vestibule superiorly from the ventricle inferiorly, and the vocal cords separate the ventricle from the subglottic cavity inferiorly. The vocal cords are formed by the conus elasticus, a fibroelastic membrane arising from the arch of the cricoid cartilage.

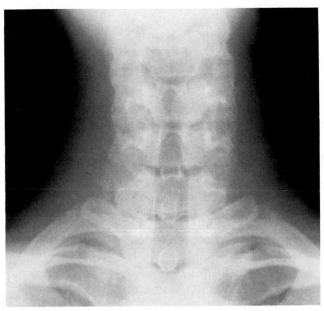

Figure 16–2. Radiograph of a normal larynx: anteroposterior view. (Courtesy of Dr. George Barnes.)

The mucous membrane of the larynx consists of stratified squamous epithelium along the wall of the vestibule and on the vocal ligaments and ciliated columnar epithelium in the ventricle and subglottic cavity. The mucous membrane is tightly adherent along the laryngeal surface of the epiglottis and the vocal folds and loosely adherent along the other surfaces above the vocal folds.

The anatomy of the larynx in infants differs from that of adults, and these differences render the infant at special risk for the development of certain symptoms with upper airway infections (see Fig. 16–1). The larynx of a neonate is situated high in the neck. The epiglottis is narrow, omega shaped, and vertically positioned. The submucosa in the subglottic area, the narrowest segment of the larynx, is nonfibrous, resulting in a looser attachment of the mucous membrane than in adults, facilitating the accumulation of edema (Kushner and Harris, 1978). Additionally, the cartilaginous support of the airways in infants is soft, easily allowing for dynamic collapse of the airways during inspiration.

The airway of a neonate measures 5 to 6 mm in diameter at its narrowest point, the cricoid ring. Infants are thus at very high risk for respiratory failure with any compromise to the patency of the small airway, as they are easily fatigued by the work of breathing necessary to generate the pressures needed to maintain airflow.

During inspiration, airflow is generated by a drop in intrathoracic and intratracheal pressure to levels below extrathoracic atmospheric pressure. The difference between intrathoracic and extrathoracic pressures necessary to maintain a given flow through the upper airway is inversely proportional to the fourth or fifth power of the radius of the airway (Badgwell et al, 1987). A 50 per cent decrease in the radius may increase the necessary pressure by a factor of 32. Thus, greater negative intrathoracic pressures must be generated by patients with airway obstruction. To achieve this, patients use accessory muscles of respiration, which will be prominent on physical examination. As a result of high negative intrathoracic pressures, patients exhibit retractions of the soft tissues of the chest wall. An elevation of the pulsus paradoxus develops, as an increased pressure differential between the abdominal and thoracic aorta presents the left ventricle with an increased afterload. Finally, dynamic collapse of the soft extrathoracic airways results, further worsening the airway obstruction and feeding a vicious cycle (Figs. 16–4 and 16–5).

Airflow across the upper airway is turbulent. Obstruction of the glottis and the subglottic area results in airflow of increased turbulence and velocity. As high-velocity airflow passes across the vocal cords and arytenoepiglottic folds, these structures vibrate, resulting in stridor. Initially, the stridor is low pitched, loud, and inspiratory; however, as obstruction worsens, the stridor becomes softer and higher pitched and extends into exhalation. With severe obstruction,

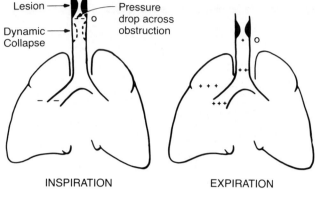

A. EXTRATHORACIC OBSTRUCTION

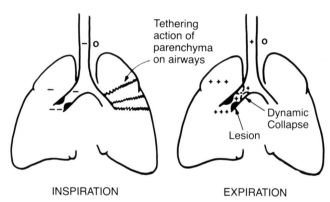

B. INTRATHORACIC OBSTRUCTION

Figure 16–4. Differential effects of the respiratory phase on extrathoracic and intrathoracic obstructions. During inspiration, negative intratracheal pressures relative to atmospheric pressure lead to dynamic collapse of the extrathoracic airway, thus worsening the effects of any extrathoracic obstructive lesion. In contrast, intrathoracic obstruction improves during inspiration because of the tethering effect of the lung parenchyma opening the intrathoracic airways. During expiration, intratracheal pressure is positive relative to atmospheric pressure, opening the extrathoracic trachea and lessening the obstructive effect of any lesions. In contrast, intrathoracic obstruction worsens because of lower pressure in the airways relative to the surrounding parenchyma, collapsing the airways. (From Loughlin GM and Taussig LM: Upper airway obstruction. Semin Resp Med 1[2]:131–46, 1979, Thieme Medical Publishers, Inc. Reprinted by permission.)

soft expiratory crowing (or wheezing) may be heard, and sudden cessation of airflow may eventually develop.

EPIDEMIOLOGY

Very little information exists regarding the true incidence of croup syndromes in the general population. The attack rates for viral laryngotracheobronchitis among preschool-age children in a prepaid group practice in Seattle were 5.2:1000 children per year in the 0- to 5-month-old age group, 11 in the

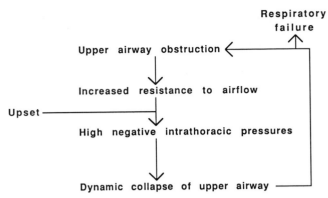

Figure 16–5. Dynamic demonstration of the vicious cycle in acute upper airway obstructive diseases.

6- to 12-month group, 14.9 in the 1-year-old group, 7.5 in the 2- to 3-year-old group, and 3.1 in the 4- to 5-year-old group (Foy et al, 1973). Comparable figures from a large pediatric practice in Chapel Hill, N.C., were 24.3, 39.7, 47, 31.2, and 14.5 (Denny et al, 1983). Of these, 1.26 per cent required hospitalization. In Tucson, Ariz., the attack rate during the first year of life was 107 cases in 961 children in a prepaid group practice (Wright et al, 1989). Despite the discrepancies in incidence rates, a common finding is a peak incidence in the 1- to 2-year-old age group for viral laryngotracheobronchitis. Before age 6, males are affected more commonly than females, with a male-to-female incidence ratio of 1.43:1 (Denny et al, 1983). In older children, males and females are affected equally. Most cases occur in the fall as a result of the preponderance of parainfluenza virus in this syndrome.

The incidence of acute epiglottitis has been studied in a population of children age 0 to 15 years in Gothenburg, Sweden (Claesson et al, 1984). In that population, during a 10-year period, the age-specific incidence of acute epiglottitis was 14:100,000 per year. Further population studies in other areas are needed, however, before this finding can be generalized. Globally, epiglottitis accounts for 1 in every 400 to 1000 pediatric admissions to the hospital (Blanc et al, 1986; Lazoritz et al, 1979). Peak incidence for epiglottitis occurs in the 2- to 6-year-old age group, and most cases occur in the fall and winter months.

Bacterial tracheitis affects from 2 (Sofer et al, 1983) to 5 per cent (Mahajan et al, 1985) of patients hospitalized with acute infectious upper airway obstruction. Information about its incidence in the general community is lacking; however, it appears to be uncommon. No obvious seasonal pattern has been described.

ETIOLOGY

Table 16–1 summarizes the etiologic agents responsible for acute upper airway infections. Parainfluenza virus type 1 is responsible for most cases of viral laryngotracheobronchitis, followed closely by types 2 and 3. Other agents—most notably influenza A and B, adenovirus, and respiratory syncytial virus—may also be responsible for outbreaks. *H. influenzae* type B is responsible for almost all cases of epiglottitis in otherwise healthy patients. Immunocompromised patients may be at risk for epiglottitis due to infection with *Candida albicans* (Colman, 1986). Bacterial tracheitis is most commonly due to *Staphylococcus aureus;* however, other organisms including *H. influenzae*, streptococci, *Neisseria, Escherichia coli, Klebsiella, Pseudomonas,* and *Chlamydia trachomatis* have been isolated from these patients. Bacterial tracheitis may, in some instances, reflect a bacterial superinfection of a primary viral tracheitis or a co-infection. *Corynebacterium diphtheriae* is now rare but should be considered in nonimmunized patients.

PATHOGENESIS AND PATHOPHYSIOLOGY

Parainfluenza viruses primarily infect ciliated respiratory epithelium; thus, the ventricular and subglottic regions are the chief sites involved in viral laryngotracheobronchitis. Some parainfluenza virus strains, particularly types 2 and 3, are cytopathic, causing cell fusion, multinucleated syncytial giant cells, and cell death, whereas other strains are not cytopathic. Viral particles are found in the cytoplasm of infected cells, and cell-to-cell transmission of the virus is mediated by the viral F protein, which inserts into the membrane of epithelial cells (Winn and Walker, 1988).

After infection of respiratory epithelium, an inflammatory response to the virus develops, resulting in an influx of polymorphonuclear leukocytes (Rabe, 1948a) and mononuclear cells. Vascular congestion and edema then develop, and this accounts, in part, for the obstructive airway symptoms in this disorder. As the process continues, surface ulcerations may

Table 16–1. ETIOLOGIC AGENTS IN ACUTE UPPER AIRWAY INFECTIONS

Bacterial
Haemophilus influenzae type B
Staphylococcus aureus
Corynebacterium diphtheriae
Group A streptococcus
Neisseria sp.
Escherichia coli
Klebsiella sp.
Pseudomonas sp.
Chlamydia trachomatis
Fungal
Candida albicans
Viral
Parainfluenza types 1,2,3
Influenza A, B
Adenovirus
Respiratory syncytial virus
Enterovirus sp.
Measles

develop as virus-infected epithelium is destroyed (Rabe, 1948a).

Despite the tropism of the parainfluenza virus for the ciliated epithelium, only 27 per cent of patients from birth to 2.5 years of age develop evidence of disease with primary parainfluenza infection (Welliver, Wong, Choi, and Ogra, 1982). It is thus likely that additional factors other than mere infection contribute to the development of laryngotracheobronchitis.

In addition to edema, laryngeal muscle spasm may form an important component in the airway obstruction of viral laryngotracheobronchitis. This concept was expounded by Cramblett (1960) and is supported by the prompt temporary relief experienced by these patients on administration of racemic epinephrine (Taussig et al, 1975). Spasm may play a relatively greater role in patients with recurrent (spasmodic) croup. Patients with a history of laryngotracheobronchitis may later demonstrate hyperreactivity of the airways (Loughlin and Taussig, 1979; Gurwitz et al, 1980; Zach et al, 1980), and those with recurrent laryngotracheobronchitis demonstrate hyperreactivity of the extrathoracic as well as intrathoracic airways (Zach et al, 1980). Patients with sudden-onset parainfluenza type 1 laryngotracheobronchitis may show serologic evidence of prior infection with parainfluenza type 3 (Uruquhart et al, 1979). Furthermore, patients with laryngotracheobronchitis have been shown to exhibit high concentrations of parainfluenza virus-specific IgE and histamine concentrations in nasopharyngeal secretions, as opposed to parainfluenza virus-infected individuals with mild cold-like symptoms only (Welliver, Wong, Middleton et al, 1982). Spasm may thus result from a type I hypersensitivity response to parainfluenza virus with release of spasmogenic mediators. In addition, patients with laryngotracheobronchitis demonstrate increased lymphoproliferative responses to parainfluenza virus antigen and decreased histamine-induced suppression of these responses (Welliver et al, 1985), suggestive of a defect of suppressor cell function as a major factor in the pathogenesis of laryngotracheobronchitis.

H. influenzae type B is carried in the nasopharynx by 5 per cent of asymptomatic children. Invasive disease, however, occurs in only 1 per cent of these carriers (Mendelman and Smith, 1987). Nasal inoculation of *H. influenzae* type B results in formation of colonies of these organisms in the nasal mucosal epithelium and in the submucosa. The organism is then believed to spread to the blood stream via the lymphatics and, once in the blood stream, may seed any serosal surface (Mendelman and Smith, 1987). Thus, although situated in close proximity to the nose, the supraglottic area is likely seeded via the blood stream rather than by spread along mucosal surfaces, as reflected by the high yield of positive blood cultures in epiglottitis and relatively low incidence of epiglottitis among carriers of *H. influenzae*.

Infection of the epiglottis causes a local inflammatory response resulting in a cherry-red edematous epiglottis (Fig. 16–6). The arytenoids, arytenoepiglottic folds, and ventricle are involved as well (Rabe, 1948b). Destruction of infected epithelial tissue results in mucosal ulcerations, which may appear on the epiglottis, larynx, and trachea (Rabe, 1948b). Submucosal glands are involved as well, with the formation of abscesses (Rabe, 1948b).

The factors governing the specific seeding of the epiglottis in invasive *H. influenzae* disease are unknown. The incidence of *H. influenzae* epiglottis relative to meningitis varies according to geographic region, with a higher incidence of epiglottitis in Gothenburg, Sweden (Claesson et al, 1984), and a lower incidence in the United States. Epiglottitis affects older children than does meningitis. In addition to age and environment, immunogenetic factors may play a role in the predisposition to epiglottitis. Whites are affected more commonly than blacks (Granoff et al, 1984). Increased risk of epiglottitis may be associated with certain erythrocyte genotypes (Whisnant et al, 1976; Granoff et al, 1984). Although

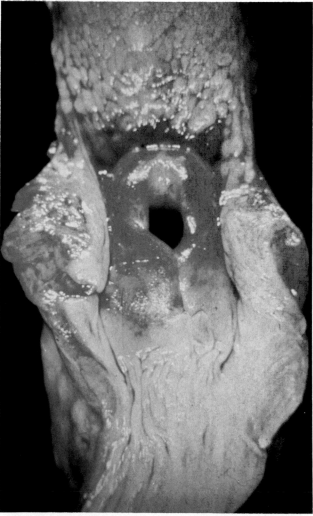

Figure 16–6. Post-mortem larynx from a patient who died of epiglottitis. Note epiglottic edema and surface mucosal ulcerations. (Courtesy of Dr. Robert Berg.)

several studies have examined the frequencies of HLA specificities in patients with epiglottitis (Granoff et al, 1984), there is no conclusive evidence linking these genetic foci with increased frequency of this disease.

Bacterial tracheitis may represent a primary bacterial infection (Jones et al, 1979), a bacterial superinfection of a primary viral disease, or dual infection (Edwards et al, 1983; Henry et al, 1983a; Liston et al, 1983). Influenza, parainfluenza, and enteroviruses have been isolated from patients with bacterial tracheitis. In addition, one case of staphylococcal tracheitis complicating *H. influenzae* epiglottitis has been reported (Liston et al, 1983).

The pathologic findings from a 3-year-old girl dying of staphylococcal tracheitis have been reviewed, shedding some light on the pathogenesis of this disorder (McKenzie et al, 1984). Staphylococcal organisms infect tracheal mucosal epithelium, resulting in an influx of polymorphonuclear leukocytes. Mucosal cells are destroyed and the resulting collection of necrotic cells, bacterial organisms, and fibrin form a pseudomembrane along the surface of the trachea (hence, some refer to this entity as pseudomembranous croup). Submucosal vessels become dilated and engorged, and submucosal glands are dilated. This process may extend peripherally to the bronchioles. Airway obstruction is caused by the purulent exudate in the trachea and the sloughing tracheal pseudomembrane.

CLINICAL PRESENTATION, DIAGNOSIS, AND MANAGEMENT

VIRAL AND SPASMODIC LARYNGOTRACHEOBRONCHITIS

Viral disease may involve the larynx (laryngitis), the larynx and trachea (laryngotracheitis), or the larynx, trachea, bronchi, and bronchioles (laryngotracheobronchitis). For simplicity, the term *laryngotracheobronchitis* will be used to refer to the spectrum of virus-induced subglottic disease. Typically, the child has an antecedent mild febrile upper respiratory infection for several days. The patient then develops a barking cough, hoarseness, and inspiratory stridor, with or without fever (Table 16–2). Patients with spasmodic croup typically are well and awaken suddenly at night with symptoms similar to those of viral laryngotracheobronchitis. The course of viral laryngotracheobronchitis tends to be insidious, peaking at 3 to 4 days, with symptoms tending to worsen at night. The disease gradually resolves over a 1-week period. In patients with severe obstruction, tachypnea and suprasternal and supraclavicular retractions are present, along with an elevation of the pulsus paradoxus due to high negative intrathoracic pressures. The child is apprehensive, and agitation and crying worsen the stridor as a result of dynamic compression of the obstructed upper airway.

Late findings may include decreased stridor due to fatigue or lack of airflow from severe obstruction, together with cyanosis.

Laryngoscopic examination in viral laryngotracheobronchitis reveals a deep red laryngeal mucosa with swelling of the subglottic tissues. Occasional patches of secretions are noted. The appearance of the mucosa in spasmodic croup is somewhat paler (Baugh and Gilmore, 1986).

The diagnosis of laryngotracheobronchitis is suggested by the clinical history and physical examination. Viral cultures are positive in most patients (Wagener et al, 1986). Blood counts may demonstrate a mild leukocytosis and lymphocytosis (Wagener et al, 1986). Lateral neck radiographs demonstrate subglottic narrowing, usually extending a centimeter below the glottis (Capitanio and Kirkpatrick, 1968). Anteroposterior neck radiographs demonstrate tapering of the upper trachea in the subglottic area, known as the "steeple sign" (Fig. 16–7). Inspiratory distention of the hypopharynx may be present on the lateral neck radiograph as a result of airway obstruction (Capitanio and Kirkpatrick, 1968) (Fig. 16–8). Although radiographs may be useful in differentiating laryngotracheobronchitis from other causes of laryngeal obstruction, they are generally not helpful in the management of patients with laryngotracheobronchitis (Wagener et al, 1986). Radiographic changes do not relate to the severity of the disease and depend heavily on the stage of the respiratory cycle during which the radiographs are taken.

The management of laryngotracheobronchitis must be preceded by a determination of the severity of respiratory distress in the patient. Before the initiation of therapy, a decision regarding the need for hospitalization must be made. Older, previously healthy patients presenting with a barking cough but good air entry without stridor, tachypnea, chest wall retractions, and elevation of the pulsus paradoxus may be managed at home with clear instructions to return if respiratory distress should develop. A decision to hospitalize is based on the need for therapy and the risk of respiratory failure if left untreated. Children presenting with respiratory distress in the morning probably should be hospitalized, as the symptoms are likely to worsen during the following night. Additionally, it is reasonable to hospitalize children with underlying lesions narrowing the upper airway and any infant with signs and symptoms of relatively severe airway obstruction.

Patients with laryngotracheobronchitis should be approached in a calm and reassuring manner, as emotional upset will worsen the child's respiratory distress as a result of dynamic compression of the edematous upper airway. Most patients with laryngotracheobronchitis are hypoxemic (Newth et al, 1972); hence, oxygenation should be assessed and humidified oxygen delivered. Oxygenation may be assessed initially by noninvasive pulse oximetry to minimize patient discomfort and maximize calm;

Table 16–2. COMPARISON OF UPPER AIRWAY INFECTIONS

	Spasmodic Croup	Laryngotracheo-bronchitis	Bacterial Tracheitis	Epiglottitis
Age range	6 mo–3 yr	0–5 yr (peak 1–2 yr)	1 mo–6 yr	2–6 yr
Etiology	? Viral ? Airway reactivity	Parainfluenza Influenza Adenovrus Respiratory syncytial virus	S. aureus H. influenzae	H. influenzae
Onset	Sudden	Insidious	Slow/sudden deterioration	Sudden
Clinical manifestations	Afebrile Nontoxic Barking cough Stridor Hoarse	Low-grade fever Nontoxic Barking cough Stridor Hoarse	High fever Toxic Barking cough Stridor Hoarse	High fever Toxic Nonbarking cough Muffled voice Drooling Dysphagia Sitting, leaning forward
Endoscopic findings	Pale mucosa Subglottic swelling	Deep red mucosa Subglottic swelling	Deep-red mucosa Copious tracheal secretions	Cherry-red epiglottis Arytenoepiglottic swelling
Complete blood count, differential	Normal	Mild leukocytosis Lymphocytosis	Normal-mild leukocytosis; marked bandemia	Marked leukocytosis Bandemia
Radiographic findings	Subglottic narrowing	Subglottic narrowing	Subglottic narrowing Irregular tracheal border	Large epiglottis Thick arytenoepiglottic folds
Therapy	Mist Calm (occasionally) Racemic epinephrine (occasionally) Steroids	Mist Calm Racemic epinephrine ?Steroids Intubation (if necessary)	Intubation Antibiotics	Intubation Antibiotics
Response	Rapid	Transient	Slow (1–2 wk)	Rapid (40 hr)
Intubation	Rare	Occasional	Usual	Usual

however, if respiratory distress is severe and unresponsive to initial treatment, arterial blood gas tensions should be measured to assess for hypercapnia and respiratory acidosis. It should be noted that a normal Pa_{CO_2} may not reflect a lack of severity, as obstruction may occur suddenly. By the time hypercapnia is present, most patients require an artificial airway.

The use of mist therapy has been based on empiricism. Data in kittens suggest that inhalation of saline mist results in a mechanoreceptor-mediated reflex slowing of the inspiratory flow rate and respiratory rate, resulting in improved air exchange most likely secondary to less dynamic collapse of the trachea; this effect is mediated by the trigeminal and superior laryngeal nerves (Sasaki and Suzuki, 1977). Evidence that this mechanism is indeed operative in children with laryngotracheobronchitis is lacking; the response often noted in the home to the steam from hot water in the bathroom may relate more to a calming effect on the child than to a physiologic benefit of the steam (Henry, 1983). The placement of a child in a mist tent may increase anxiety and worsen respiratory distress (Henry, 1983). In view of the potential benefit of inhaled aerosol mist, it seems reasonable to place a sleeping infant in a mist tent, although an awake, anxious child may fare better in the arms of a parent.

The decision on feeding must relate to the severity of the respiratory distress. Patients who are severely distressed should not be fed and should receive intravenous fluids. Fluids should be restricted to 80 to 90 per cent of maintenance requirements (in a nondehydrated patient), to decrease the pulmonary artery fluid load.

Nebulized racemic epinephrine transiently improves respiratory distress in patients with laryngotracheobronchitis, an effect noted within one-half hour of aerosol treatment and usually gone by 2 hours (Taussig et al, 1975; Westley et al, 1978). There is no evidence that the use of racemic epinephrine alters the natural history of laryngotracheobronchitis; however, its use has led to a decreased need for artificial airways (Adair et al, 1971; Singer and Wilson, 1976; Shaw and Mansmann, 1977) (Table 16–3). Because of the transient effects of this treatment modality, racemic epinephrine should not be used on an outpatient basis. In the past, racemic epinephrine was nebulized with intermittent positive pressure breathing (IPPB) (Taussig et al, 1975; Westley et al, 1978); however, nebulization without IPPB is as effective as nebulization with IPPB (Fogel et al, 1982). Racemic epinephrine may be given as frequently as every half hour if needed to relieve respiratory distress. The agent is administered in doses of 0.25 ml of a 2.25 per cent solution for every 5 kg of body weight to a maximum dose of 1.5 ml. Racemic epinephrine should be nebulized in oxygen, as the agent

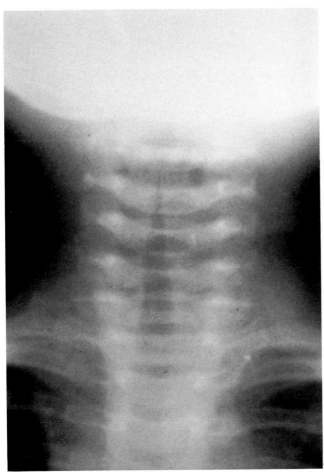

Figure 16–7. "Steeple sign." Note subglottic narrowing. (Courtesy of Dr. Robert Berg.)

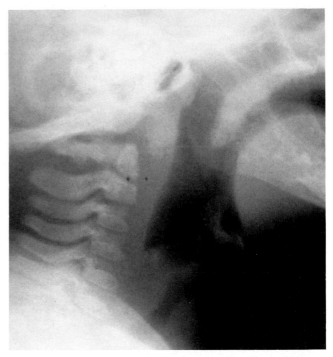

Figure 16–8. Lateral neck radiograph of a patient with laryngotracheobronchitis demonstrating hypopharyngeal distention. (Courtesy of Dr. Robert Berg.)

causes transient worsening of intrapulmonary ventilation-perfusion mismatching. Pulse and cardiac rhythm should be monitored, and the drug discontinued should an arrhythmia develop.

Considerable controversy exists regarding the use of corticosteroids in the treatment of laryngotracheobronchitis. Studies evaluating the efficacy of steroids are plagued by methodologic flaws and the use of low doses (Tunnessen and Feinstein, 1980). There is evidence that steroid doses equivalent to 100 mg cortisol may be effective in attenuating the severity of laryngotracheobronchitis (Tunnessen and Feinstein, 1980). A recent prospective, randomized, double-blind study has demonstrated the efficacy of a single dose of 0.6 mg/kg dexamethasone in attenuating the symptoms and quickening the recovery in patients hospitalized with severe spasmodic croup (Kuusela and Vesikari, 1988). The same dose of dexamethasone may be beneficial in attenuating the severity of viral laryngotracheobronchitis as well (Super et al, 1989). It must be remembered that dosing regimens vary, and no specific guidelines yet exist. In patients with severe respiratory distress, a therapeutic trial of steroids may be beneficial in preventing the need for an artificial airway. However, before steroids can be unequivocally recommended, further studies are needed.

Syrup of ipecac has been used to alleviate laryngeal muscle spasm in patients with laryngotracheobronchitis (Cramblett, 1960). Although given in subemetic doses, the drug may not demonstrate full therapeutic effect until vomiting is induced (Cramblett, 1960). No careful studies have been performed to document the efficacy of this agent, and the use of ipecac should be avoided in children with respiratory distress because of the risk of aspiration of vomitus.

Helium-oxygen has been used successfully to improve airflow in patients with upper airway obstruction (Lu et al, 1976). The low density of helium theoretically enhances turbulent airflow. A controlled study of this treatment modality in laryngotracheobronchitis is warranted, as it may further decrease the need for endotracheal intubation.

Despite optimal medical management, patients with laryngotracheobronchitis occasionally require endotracheal intubation. Intubation should be performed with great care, so as to minimize further

Table 16–3. IMPACT OF RACEMIC EPINEPHRINE (RE) ON NEED FOR ARTIFICIAL AIRWAYS IN LARYNGOTRACHEOBRONCHITIS

Series	% Requiring Tracheostomy/Intubation	
	BEFORE RE	AFTER RE
Adair et al (1971)	7% of 205 (1961–1963)	0% of 351 (1964–1970)
Singer and Wilson (1976)	2.5% of 509 (1970–1972)	0.3% of 359 (1973–1974)
Shaw and Mansmann (1977)	2 of 2195 (1969–1973)	0.5% of 413 (1975)
	4.8% of 588 (971–1975)	

airway injury and inflammation. Endotracheal tubes one half to one full size smaller than indicated by the age of the patient (or by the size of the small finger of the patient) should be used, and the tube cut to shorten its length and the resistance to airflow. There is no distinct advantage to nasotracheal over oral intubation, and patients should not be reintubated electively, as this may increase the airway injury and further worsen airway obstruction. Once intubated, patients rarely require mechanical ventilation or positive end-expiratory pressure. In fact, tethering of the endotracheal tube to a ventilator may further aggravate airway injury and edema when the patient moves. Patients should thus be placed in a tent with humidified, oxygenated air while intubated, with close attention paid to mucociliary clearance. Suctioning should be minimized, again to minimize airway injury. Adequate restraint is mandatory to prevent self-extubation. Extubation may be attempted after the development of an air leak around the endotracheal tube. The recent development of thin flexible fiberoptic bronchoscopes may facilitate the decision to extubate. The presence of pallor around the endotracheal tube indicates that the airway mucosa remains sufficiently swollen to necessitate ongoing intubation, whereas absence of this finding suggests that extubation may be attempted. Tracheostomy is rarely necessary in otherwise healthy children with laryngotracheobronchitis; however, the facility to perform this procedure emergently must be available.

Children with laryngotracheobronchitis may require hospitalization for as little as 24 hours or for as long as 1 week or more. Criteria for discharge should include resolution of the respiratory distress and a 24-hour lack of need for specific therapies.

EPIGLOTTITIS

Epiglottitis is a rapidly progressive medical emergency that is often fatal if not properly recognized and treated. Although most common in the 2- to 6-year-old age group, epiglottitis is increasing in incidence in older children and adults (MayoSmith et al, 1986) and must be considered in these groups as well. The onset of epiglottitis is abrupt, with high fever, sore throat, and cough progressing within 12 hours to the development of stridor, dysphagia, air hunger, and a toxic appearance. There is usually no history of a prior upper respiratory tract infection. Characteristically, the patient is anxious, drooling, and sitting forward with the neck hyperextended (Lazoritz et al, 1979), occasionally in a tripod position (Fig. 16–9). Complete, fatal airway obstruction may occur suddenly and without warning regardless of the patient's age (MayoSmith et al, 1986).

The diagnosis of epiglottitis must be assumed in patients with a classic presentation. The first priority in the management of these patients must be the establishment of a stable artificial airway. Physical

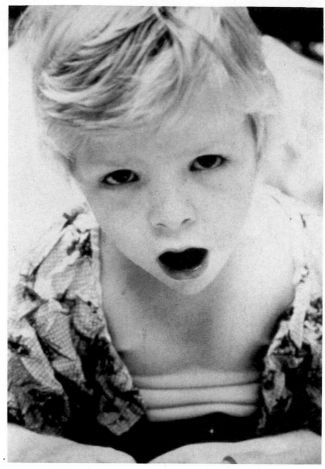

Figure 16–9. Characteristic posture in a patient with epiglottitis. Note that the child is leaning forward and drooling, and the neck is hyperextended. (Courtesy of Dr. Robert Berg.)

examination of the child and painful diagnostic tests should be deferred, as emotional upset may precipitate complete airway obstruction. When epiglottitis is clinically suspected, the child should be approached in a calm and reassuring manner. The child should be taken to the operating room or the intensive care unit, held by a parent, and accompanied by a physician carrying a laryngoscope, an endotracheal tube, and a percutaneous tracheostomy tray. Should the child suddenly develop complete airway obstruction, performance of a Heimlich maneuver may temporarily relieve the obstruction. Alternatively, forward traction may be applied to the mandible to relieve the obstruction. In the operating room or the intensive care unit, a lateral neck radiograph may be taken; classic findings include loss of distinctive anatomy with enlargement of the epiglottis, thickening of the arytenoepiglottic folds, and distention of the hypopharynx (Capitanio and Kirkpatrick, 1968) (Fig. 16–10). Laryngoscopy and endotracheal intubation should then be performed by an individual skilled in airway management. Laryngoscopic findings include a cherry-red epiglottis and edema of the arytenoepiglottic folds (Fig. 16–11). Although tracheostomy is rarely necessary, the medical team should be pre-

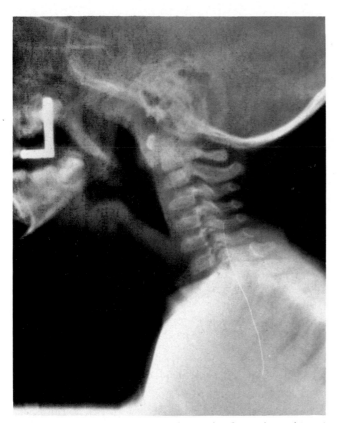

Figure 16–10. Lateral neck radiograph of a patient with epiglottitis. Note the enlargement of the epiglottis and the distention of the hypopharynx. (Courtesy of Dr. Robert Berg.)

pared to perform this emergently should the need arise.

After an artificial airway is established, the child should be managed in the intensive care unit. Considerations of airway management and oxygen delivery are similar to those described for laryngotracheobronchitis, and mechanical ventilation should be used only if absolutely necessary. Restraint of the child is of utmost importance to prevent self-extubation and death; the upper extremities should be taped to arm boards to prevent reaching for the endotracheal tube. Light sedation may be helpful in calming the patient and reducing the risk of self-extubation.

Once the patient is intubated, blood counts should be done and cultures should be drawn, an intravenous catheter inserted, and antibiotics begun. Prime consideration must be given to coverage for penicillinase-producing *H. influenzae*. Thus, chloramphenicol (75 mg/kg/day) or a cephalosporin (cefotaxime [100 to 200 mg/kg/day] or cefuroxime [75 to 150 mg/kg/day]) should be started; however, other organisms including fungi should be given consideration, particularly in immunocompromised patients. Cultures of the epiglottis obtained during endotracheal intubation may be helpful. Urine antigen studies may be of help in children already on antibiotic therapy at the time of presentation. Blood counts typically dem-

onstrate a marked leukocytosis with a left shift. C-reactive protein is universally elevated in epiglottitis and may occasionally prove useful in differentiating this bacterial disease from severe viral laryngotracheobronchitis (Peltola, 1983).

There is some empiric evidence that corticosteroids may improve the course of epiglottitis (Strome and Jaffe, 1974). Racemic epinephrine is of no benefit in epiglottitis (Adair and Ring, 1975).

Duration of intubation for epiglottitis averages about 40 hours, but there is great individual variability. A decision to extubate may be made when an air leak develops around the endotracheal tube; however, extubation is best performed under direct visualization. Again, facilities for performance of emergency tracheostomy must be available. Patients should be examined daily for signs of metastatic *H. influenzae* disease to the joints or other serosal surfaces. Before discharge, patients should be free of respiratory distress for 24 hours and should be non-toxic. Antibiotics should be continued for a full 10-day course, and contacts should be given appropriate prophylaxis against *H. influenzae*.

A syndrome of supraglottitis due to group A streptococci has recently been described (Lacroix et al, 1986). Affected patients typically present with acute, severe respiratory distress, as do patients with *H. influenzae* epiglottitis; however, the streptococcal variant tends to affect older children, is associated with a longer prodrome which may last more than 24 hours, primarily involves the arytenoepiglottic folds while sparing the epiglottis, and has a protracted

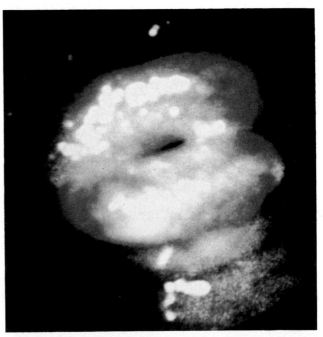

Figure 16–11. Laryngoscopic view of the edematous epiglottis in a patient with epiglottitis. (Courtesy of Dr. Robert Berg.)

course. The principles of management are similar to those for epiglottitis.

BACTERIAL TRACHEITIS

Bacterial tracheitis is a medical emergency that, like epiglottitis, may result in sudden, complete airway obstruction and death. Patients with bacterial tracheitis may experience an antecedent mild upper respiratory infection or laryngotracheobronchitis, which may be present for 1 hour to 6 days before presentation for severe airway obstruction (Jones et al, 1979; Liston et al, 1983; Sofer et al, 1983; Edwards et al, 1983; Mahajan et al, 1985). Patients then develop inspiratory stridor, barking cough, high fever, and a toxic appearance. Although the initial pattern of respiratory distress closely resembles that of laryngotracheobronchitis, the degree of fever and toxic appearance should alert the clinician to a high probability of a bacterial disease. Patients may present with a picture highly suggestive of epiglottitis (Edwards et al, 1983), and epiglottitis and bacterial tracheitis may coexist in the same patient (Liston et al, 1983).

Despite a clinical appearance similar to laryngotracheobronchitis, patients with bacterial tracheitis usually fail to respond to racemic epinephrine (Jones et al, 1979; Liston et al, 1983; Mahajan et al, 1985). Because of the copious amount of secretions in the trachea, it is not surprising that almost all patients with bacterial tracheitis require the establishment of an artificial airway. The diagnosis of bacterial tracheitis is confirmed by the presence of large amounts of thick secretions visualized and aspirated on intubation of the trachea.

Radiography of the neck may reveal subglottic narrowing on posteroanterior and lateral projections (Jones et al, 1979; Liston et al, 1983; Mahajan et al, 1985). The epiglottis and arytenoepiglottic folds are normal, unless epiglottitis coexists. The tracheal mucosa may appear irregular as a result of the formation of a pseudomembrane or mucosal sloughing (Fig. 16–12). There is often a suggestion of radiopaque foreign material in the lumen of the airway, which represents a tracheal pseudomembrane (Henry et al, 1983).

Blood counts often reveal a bandemia in the presence of normal to mildly elevated total leukocyte counts. Blood cultures are typically negative; however, Gram stains and cultures of the tracheal secretions characteristically yield pure growth of the offending organism.

Patients with suspected bacterial tracheitis should be admitted to an intensive care unit. Endotracheal intubation should be performed early in toxic, febrile patients with a laryngotracheobronchitis-like illness and severe airway obstruction unresponsive to racemic epinephrine. Once an artificial airway is established, principles of airway management are similar to those described for laryngotracheobronchitis and

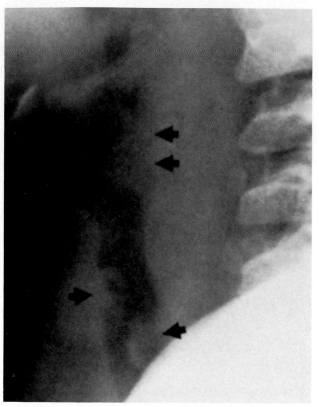

Figure 16–12. Lateral neck radiograph demonstrating an irregular tracheal mucosa in a patient with bacterial tracheitis. (Reproduced with permission from Han BK, Dunbar JS, and Striker TW: Membranous laryngotracheobronchitis. AJR 133:53–58, 1979. © American Roentgen Ray Society.)

epiglottitis. Tracheal toilet is a major problem in these patients, and frequent suctioning is often necessary to prevent blockage of the endotracheal tube.

Patients with bacterial tracheitis should receive broad-spectrum antibiotic coverage initially, covering for the possibilities of S. aureus, H. influenzae, and Streptococcus pneumoniae. The combination of nafcillin (100 mg/kg/day) and chloramphenicol (75 mg/kg/day) or alternatively a third-generation cephalosporin alone may be used. Antibiotic therapy can be adjusted according to the results of the cultures.

Duration of intubation varies widely in patients with bacterial tracheitis; typically, the disease is more protracted than epiglottitis, lasting about 1 week (Sofer et al, 1983). Although death may occur from sepsis (McKenzie et al, 1984), deaths are more likely to occur from acute airway obstruction with respiratory arrest and its neurologic sequelae (Liston et al, 1983; Sofer et al, 1983). Restraint of the child is mandatory to avoid premature extubation. Considerations for extubation and hospital discharge are similar to those for epiglottitis.

DIFFERENTIAL DIAGNOSIS

Table 16–4 summarizes the other infectious and noninfectious causes of acute upper airway obstruc-

Table 16–4. INFECTIOUS AND NONINFECTIOUS CAUSES OF ACUTE UPPER AIRWAY OBSTRUCTION

Infectious
Laryngotracheobronchitis
Epiglottitis
Bacterial tracheitis
Diphtheria
Retropharyngeal abscess
Peritonsillar abscess

Noninfectious
Foreign body
Trauma
Angioneurotic edema
Hypocalcemic tetany
Caustic burns

tive syndromes. Several of these deserve further mention.

Laryngitis secondary to *C. diphtheriae*, once the most common infectious cause of acute upper airway obstruction, is now uncommon because of the widespread success of immunization programs but must be considered in unimmunized patients and populations. Patients typically present with a 3- to 4-day history of upper respiratory infection and exhibit a serosanguineous nasal discharge and a posterior pharyngeal membrane. The patient appears toxic with symptoms of laryngotracheobronchitis and may quickly develop signs of severe airway obstruction if the pharyngeal membrane dislodges and obstructs the airway.

Retropharyngeal abscess may follow a nasopharyngeal infection or a penetrating pharyngeal injury. Patients present with acute onset of dysphagia, hoarseness, dyspnea, and fever. Although now rare since the advent of antibiotics, this condition is a medical emergency and must be recognized and treated immediately. These abscesses usually occur in children under 2 years of age.

Airway foreign bodies represent the most common noninfectious cause of acute upper airway obstruc-

tion in children. Symptoms depend largely on the specific airway location of the foreign body, the nature of the foreign body, and the degree of airway obstruction. Laryngeal foreign bodies typically produce pain, laryngeal spasm, dyspnea, inspiratory stridor, and hoarseness (Rowe, 1988). Tracheal foreign bodies tend to produce inspiratory and expiratory wheezing (Rowe, 1988). Foreign bodies lodged in the region of the cricopharyngeus muscle produce dysphagia and drooling rather than stridor, unless tissue edema is present, obstructing the airway (Capitanio and Kirkpatrick, 1968). Onset of symptoms may be acute, in the case of a relatively large foreign body causing severe obstruction, or insidious, in the case of a small foreign body that is not large enough to be obstructive per se but is irritating to laryngeal and tracheal mucosa, causing airway narrowing secondary to edema. In cases of severe airway obstruction, the voice may be aphonic and the breath sounds quiet. This condition represents a medical emergency, requiring immediate visualization of the larynx and trachea and removal of the foreign body by a physician experienced in this procedure.

Acute upper airway obstruction may result from the ingestion of caustic substances, with resulting pharyngeal burns, edema, and inflammation of the epiglottis, arytenoepiglottic folds, larynx, and trachea (Capitanio and Kirkpatrick, 1968).

Angioneurotic edema may cause acute laryngeal swelling and airway obstruction. Patients appear nontoxic and may exhibit other signs of allergic disease, such as urticaria and abdominal pain. In hereditary angioneurotic edema, the family history may be positive for others afflicted with recurrent episodes of this disorder.

COMPLICATIONS

Involvement of the lung parenchyma is common in patients with laryngotracheobronchitis, epiglottitis,

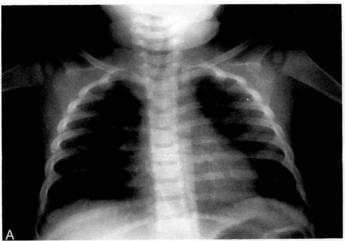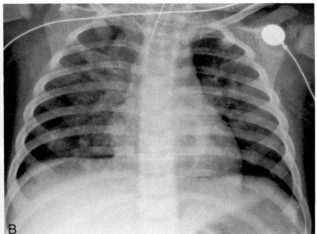

Figure 16–13. Chest radiograph before *(A)* and after *(B)* intubation in a patient with epiglottitis, demonstrating the development of postintubation pulmonary edema.

and bacterial tracheitis. Radiographic manifestations often include focal atelectasis, pneumonitis, and edema. Blood gas changes in laryngotracheobronchitis are not fully explained by alveolar hypoventilation resulting from upper airway obstruction (Newth et al, 1972; Taussig et al, 1975). Similar observations were made in patients with epiglottitis (Costigan and Newth, 1983), suggesting involvement of the lower respiratory tract in these disease processes with resultant ventilation-perfusion abnormalities.

The appearance of florid pulmonary edema following relief of upper airway obstruction is well described (Travis et al, 1977; Galvis et al, 1980; Sofer et al, 1984) (Fig. 16–13), although the edema may actually develop during the obstructive event because of increased pulmonary vascular volumes and high negative pleural and interstitial pressures (Sofer et al, 1984). The pulmonary edema tends to resolve quickly, but short-term mechanical ventilation may be necessary in some instances.

Pneumothorax has been reported in two children with bacterial tracheitis undergoing tracheostomy (Liston et al, 1983). Granulation tissue resulting in granulomas, subglottic stenosis, and webs may develop on affected laryngeal structures after the use of artificial airways (Cunningham and Taussig, 1986), but this appears to be a rare complication. Toxic shock syndrome occasionally develops in patients with bacterial tracheitis due to S. aureus (Chenaud et al, 1986). Evidence linking laryngotracheobronchitis to the presence of airway reactivity later in life was discussed previously.

Perhaps the most important complication of all of these disease processes is hypoxic ischemic encephalopathy resulting from respiratory arrest due to severe airway obstruction. This tragic complication is completely preventable with suspicion, prompt diagnosis, and management of the child with infectious compromise of the glottic, supraglottic, and subglottic structures.

REFERENCES

Adair JC and Ring WH: Management of epiglottitis in children. Anesth Analg 54:622, 1975.
Adair JC, Ring WH, Jordan WS, and Elwyn RA: Ten-year experience with IPPB in the treatment of acute laryngotracheobronchitis. Anesth Analg 50:649, 1971.
Badgwell JM, McLeod ME, and Friedberg J: Airway obstruction in infants and children. Can J Anaesth 34:90, 1987.
Baugh R and Gilmore BB. Infectious croup: a critical review. Otolaryngol Head Neck Surg 95:40, 1986.
Blanc VF, Duquenne P, and Charest J: Acute epiglottitis: an overview. Acta Anaesthesiol Belg 37:171, 1986.
Capitanio MA and Kirkpatrick JA: Upper respiratory tract obstruction in infants and children. Radiol Clin North Am 6:265, 1968.
Chenaud M, Leclerc F, and Martinot A: Bacterial croup and toxic shock syndrome. Eur J Pediatr 145:306, 1986.
Claesson B, Trollfors B, Ekstrom-Jodal B et al: Incidence and prognosis of acute epiglottitis in children in a Swedish region. Pediatr Infect Dis 3:534, 1984.

Colman MF: Epiglottitis in immunocompromised patients. Head Neck Surg 8:466, 1986.
Costigan DC and Newth CJL: Respiratory status of children with epiglottitis with and without an artificial airway. Am J Dis Child 137:139, 1983.
Cramblett HG: Croup—present day concept. Pediatrics 25:1071, 1960.
Cunningham JC and Taussig LM: Infection of the larynx and trachea. In Nelson JD (ed). Current Therapy in Pediatric Infectious Disease. St. Louis, CV Mosby Co, 1986.
Denny FW, Murphy TF, Clyde WA et al: Croup: an 11-year study in a pediatric practice. Pediatrics 71:871, 1983.
Edwards KM, Dundon C, and Altemeier WA: Bacterial tracheitis as a complication of viral croup. Pediatr Infect Dis 2:390, 1983.
Fogel JM, Berg IJ, Gerber MA, and Sherter CB: Racemic epinephrine in the treatment of croup: nebulization alone versus nebulization with intermittent positive pressure breathing. J Pediatr 101:1028, 1982.
Foy HM, Cooney MK, Maletzky AJ, and Grayston JT: Incidence and etiology of pneumonia, croup and bronchiolitis in preschool children belonging to a prepaid medical care group over a four year period. Am J Epidemiol 97:80, 1973.
Galvis AG, Stool S, and Bluestone CD: Pulmonary edema following relief of acute upper airway obstruction. Ann Otol 89:124, 1980.
Granoff DM, Boies EG, Squires JE et al: Histocompatibility leukocyte antigen and erythrocyte MNSs specificities in patients with meningitis or epiglottitis due to Haemophilus influenzae type B. J Infect Dis 149:373, 1984.
Gurwitz D, Corey M, and Levison H: Pulmonary function and bronchial reactivity in children after croup. Am Rev Respir Dis 122:95, 1980.
Henry R: Moist air in the treatment of laryngotracheitis. Arch Dis Child 58:577, 1983.
Henry RL, Mellis CM, and Benjamin B: Pseudomembranous croup. Arch Dis Child 58:180, 1983.
Jones R, Santos JI, and Overall JC: Bacterial tracheitis. JAMA 242:721, 1979.
Kushner DC and Harris GB: Obstructing lesions of the larynx and trachea in infants and children. Radiol Clin North Am 16:181, 1978.
Kuusela AL and Vesikari T: A randomized double-blind placebo controlled trial of dexamethasone and racemic epinephrine in the treatment of croup. Acta Paediatr Scand 77:99, 1988.
Lacroix J, Ahronheim G, Arcand P et al: Group A streptococcal supraglottitis. J Pediatr 109:20, 1986.
Lazoritz S, Saunders BS, and Bason WM: Management of acute epiglottitis. Crit Care Med 7:285, 1979.
Liston SL, Gehrz RC, Siegel LG, and Tilelli J: Bacterial tracheitis. Am J Dis Child 137:764, 1983.
Loughlin GM and Taussig LM: Pulmonary function in children with a history of laryngotracheobronchitis. J Pediatr 94:365, 1979.
Lu TS, Ohmura A, Wong KC, and Hodges MR. Helium-oxygen in treatment of upper airway obstruction. Anesthesiology 45:678, 1976.
McKenzie M, Norman MG, Anderson JD, and Thiessen PN. Upper respiratory tract infection in a 3-year-old girl. J Pediatr 105:129, 1984.
Mahajan A, Alvear D, Chang C et al: Bacterial tracheitis, diagnosis and treatment. Int J Pediatr Otorhinolaryngol 10:271, 1985.
MayoSmith MF, Hirsch PJ, Wodzinski SF, and Schiffman FJ. Acute epiglottitis in adults. N Engl J Med 314:1133, 1986.
Mendelman PM and Smith AL: Hemophilus influenzae. In Feigin RD and Cherry JD (eds): Textbook of Pediatric Infectious Diseases. 2nd ed. Philadelphia, WB Saunders Co, 1987.
Nelson WE: Bacterial croup: a historical perspective. J Pediatr 105:52, 1984.
Newth CJL, Levison H, and Bryan AC. The respiratory status of children with croup. J Pediatr 81:1068, 1972.
Peltola H: C-reactive protein in rapid differentiation of acute epiglottitis from spasmodic croup and acute laryngotracheitis: a preliminary report. J Pediatr 102:713, 1983.
Rabe EF: Infectious croup. II. "Virus" croup. Pediatrics 2:415, 1948a.
Rabe EF: Infectious croup. III. Hemophilus influenzae type B croup. Pediatrics 2:559, 1948b.

Rowe LD: Airway obstruction in the pediatric patient. In Crumley RL (ed): Common Problems of the Head and Neck Region. Philadelphia, WB Saunders Co, 1988.

Sasaki CT and Suzuki M: The respiratory mechanism of aerosol inhalation in the treatment of partial airway obstruction. Pediatrics 59:689, 1977.

Scheidemandel HHE: Did George Washington die of quinsy? Arch Otolaryngol 102:519, 1976.

Shaw LL and Mansmann HC: Decisions in the evaluation and treatment of acute viral croup. Pediatr Ann 6:476, 1977.

Singer OP and Wilson WJ: Laryngotracheobronchitis: 2 years' experience with racemic epinephrine. CMA Journal 115:132, 1976.

Sofer S, Duncan P, and Chernick V: Bacterial tracheitis—an old disease rediscovered. Clin Pediatr 22:407, 1983.

Sofer S, Bar-Ziv J, and Scharf SM: Pulmonary edema following relief of upper airway obstruction. Chest 86:401, 1984.

Stool SE: Croup syndrome: historical perspective. Pediatr Infect Dis 7:S157, 1988.

Strome M and Jaffe B: Epiglottitis—individualized management with steroids. Laryngoscope 84:921, 1974.

Super DM, Cartelli NA, Brooks LJ et al: A prospective randomized double-blind study to evaluate the effect of dexamethasone in acute laryngotracheitis. J Pediatr 115:323, 1989.

Taussig LM, Castro O, Beaudry PH et al: Treatment of laryngotracheobronchitis (croup). Am J Dis Child 129:790, 1975.

Travis KW, Todres ID, and Shannon DC: Pulmonary edema associated with croup and epiglottitis. Pediatrics 59:695, 1977.

Tunnessen WW, and Feinstein AR: The steroid-croup controversy: an analytic review of methodologic problems. J Pediatr 96:751, 1980.

Uruquhart GED, Kennedy DH, and Ariyawansa JP: Croup associated with parainfluenza type 1 virus: two subpopulations. Br Med J 1:1604, 1979.

Wagener JS, Landau LI, Olinsky A, and Phelan PD: Management of children hospitalized for laryngotracheobronchitis. Pediatr Pulmonol 2:159, 1986.

Welliver RC, Sun M, and Rinaldo D: Defective regulation of immune responses in croup due to parainfluenza virus. Pediatr Res 19:716, 1985.

Welliver R, Wong DT, Choi TS, and Ogra PL: Natural history of parainfluenza virus infection in childhood. J Pediatr 101:180, 1982.

Welliver RC, Wong DT, Middleton E et al: Role of parainfluenza virus-specific IgE in pathogenesis of croup and wheezing subsequent to infection. J Pediatr 101:889, 1982.

Westley CR, Cotton EK, and Brooks JG: Nebulized racemic epinephrine by IPPB for the treatment of croup. Am J Dis Child 132:484, 1978.

Whisnant JK, Rogentine GN, Gralnick MA et al: Host factors and antibody response in Haemophilus influenzae type B meningitis and epiglottitis. J Infect Dis 133:448, 1976.

Winn WC and Walker DH: Viral infection. In Dail DH and Hammar SP (eds): Pulmonary Pathology. New York, Springer Verlag, 1988.

Wright AL, Taussig LM, Ray CG et al: The Tucson children's respiratory study. II. Lower respiratory tract illnesses in the first year of life. Am J Epidemiol 129:1232, 1989.

Zach MS, Schnall RP, and Landau LI: Upper and lower airway reactivity in recurrent croup. Am Rev Respir Dis 121:979, 1980.

17

GERALD M. LOUGHLIN, M.D.

BRONCHITIS

Bronchitis in children is encountered in various clinical settings. It occurs as a major component of the illness associated with asthma or cystic fibrosis, as well as an acute illness generally secondary to a viral upper respiratory infection. Between these extremes, bronchitis also occurs as a complication of inhalation of noxious substances, as a bacterial infection superimposed on a relatively minor airway injury, and finally as a complication of inadequate airway or immune defenses.

On the surface, it would seem that bronchitis should be relatively simple to define and characterize. Unfortunately, this is not the case, largely because the primary and at times exclusive respiratory manifestation of disease is cough—a symptom that has little diagnostic specificity. The diagnostic label is also inadequate because inflammation of the bronchi rarely occurs in an isolated manner. The nasal mucosa, sinuses, trachea, and bronchioles frequently are also involved, yet the focus is on bronchitis. The picture is further clouded by the overlap between asthma and bronchitis in children. Both conditions are marked by inflammation of the airways, and the clinical presentation of asthma exacerbations is often similar to that in a child with presumed chronic recurrent bronchitis.

Despite these limitations, it is important to try to understand bronchitis, because in its many forms it is a common clinical childhood respiratory problem that may play an important role in the development of bronchitis in adults (Barker and Osmond, 1986). This chapter attempts to provide this perspective by focusing on acute bronchitis, the relationship between airway epithelial injury and chronic/recurrent bronchitis, the relationship between asthma and bronchitis, and finally the long-term consequences of bronchitis in children. Certain conditions in which bronchitis occurs as a component of a distinct clinical problem, such as cystic fibrosis or immotile cilia syndrome, are included in the differential diagnosis but are discussed in separate chapters.

DEFINITIONS

The literature and clinical experience would suggest that bronchitis exists in acute, chronic, and recurrent forms. Unfortunately, the distinction among these forms is frequently ambiguous, and it is often difficult to determine where one type ends and another begins. The implications of chronic disease in children justify some attempt at distinguishing acute from chronic/recurrent disease. The chronic/recurrent symptoms suggest that the stimulus of the inflammation is still present, a complication of acute bronchitis has developed, significant and perhaps permanent airway damage has occurred, or conditions of an underlying disease, such as cystic fibrosis or immotile cilia syndrome, may be present.

For purposes of this chapter, the following broad definitions have been developed from the literature. Acute bronchitis is defined as a transient inflammatory process involving the trachea and major bronchi manifested primarily, and at times exclusively, by cough. It usually resolves without therapy within 2 weeks (Edwards, 1966; Parks, 1979). The definition of chronic bronchitis, on the other hand, is less clear. The American Thoracic Society (1962) defines chronic bronchitis as productive cough occurring for 3 months a year for 2 consecutive years without evidence of other respiratory disease. This definition, although possibly useful for adults, is probably not relevant to children. It also seems to have little impact on the diagnostic practices of pediatricians (Taussig et al, 1981).

Because symptoms from an isolated episode of bronchitis following an acute insult infrequently last for more than 2 to 3 weeks, it would seem that the persistence of symptoms beyond this period should be considered unusual and as such suggest that a chronic condition exists. Critics may argue that this definition is too inclusive and encourages overdiagnosis, but data from Taussig and associates (1981), although limited, suggest that this is not the case.

The definition of recurrent bronchitis is perhaps more ambiguous than chronic bronchitis because it is difficult to determine where isolated, recurrent, acute episodes end and a chronic state begins (Kubo et al, 1978). On the basis of clinical experience, it seems that four or more episodes of bronchitis per year constitute a recurrent condition (Williams and Phelan, 1975; Kubo et al, 1978). There currently is no consensus on the significance of recurrent attacks of acute bronchitis. At what point should acute episodes be considered no longer isolated, unrelated events but instead indicative of underlying airway damage? How many episodes are "too many"? Is the interval between episodes as significant as the number of attacks? What is the relationship between recurrent

bronchitis and asthma? All of these questions are unanswered. Regardless, it is prudent to approach a child with recurrent episodes of bronchitis as one would a child whose symptoms persist unabated. An approach to the child with bronchitis is presented in Table 17–1.

ACUTE BRONCHITIS

BRONCHITIS CAUSED BY VIRUS

Multiple epidemiologic studies have demonstrated that viruses produce most attacks of acute bronchitis (Glezen and Denny, 1973; Horn et al, 1975). Attacks can occur at any time but are most common in the winter months, paralleling the peak of the respiratory virus season (Ayres, 1986). This disorder appears to be more common in younger children and males. *Rhinovirus* is the organism most frequently recovered from children with acute bronchitis, particularly those whose disease is associated with wheezing. Respiratory syncytial virus, influenza, parainfluenza, adenovirus, and the paramyxoviruses have also been identified. Rubeola is almost universally associated with acute bronchitis, the respiratory symptoms often preceding the more classic manifestations of this infection.

Onset of viral bronchitis is usually gradual, with cough appearing 3 to 4 days after the rhinitis. The presence of cough denotes extension of the infection to the trachea and bronchi. The cough, which may be the primary clinical manifestation, is initially nonproductive, but several days into the illness it may evolve into a loose, gurgly cough with sputum production. Young children generally swallow the mucus. Vomiting associated with coughing paroxysms can occur. The vomitus frequently contains mucus, confirming the productive nature of the cough. In

Table 17–1. APPROACH TO THE PATIENT WITH CHRONIC BRONCHITIS

History: Age, onset of symptoms, relationship to feeding, previous episodes, exposures, associated symptoms, characteristics of the cough, timing productivity, factors that relieve or exacerbate symptoms, family history, environmental triggers.
Physical examination: Growth and development, respiratory signs—rales, rhonchi, wheezes, clubbing, sinus tenderness, or swelling.
Laboratory:
  Initial—should be obtained in all patients.
    Chest radiograph
    Complete blood count, differential
    Sputum culture, Gram and Wright stain
    Purified protein derivative
  As indicated by above data
    Sweat chloride
    Immunoglobulins including IgE and IgG subclasses
    Barium swallow
    Bronchoscopy
    Cilia biopsy
    Sinus radiographs and/or computed tomography
    Pulmonary function tests, before and after bronchodilators
    Serology

general, there are few constitutional symptoms unless the bronchitis is secondary to a more severe systemic illness such as rubeola or typhoid fever.

Auscultation of the chest is frequently unremarkable in the early stages. Rhonchi may be heard as the cough progresses. Crackles are infrequent. Wheezing is common, and its presence has been considered to be indicative of an asthmatic state (asthmatic or wheezy bronchitis) (Kubo et al, 1978); this association is discussed later. Symptoms usually resolve within 10 to 14 days. If the cough persists beyond this period, one should suspect secondary infection, a complication such as pneumonia or atelectasis, or the possibility of a previously unrecognized asthmatic condition.

Material for pathologic investigation of acute bronchitis is limited because the disease is usually mild and self-limited. Congestion of the mucosa develops initially. Secretions are usually sparse, but mucous gland activity increases as the inflammatory process continues, resulting in sputum production. Infiltration of polymorphonuclear leukocytes into the airway walls and lumen contributes to the purulent appearance of the secretions. Because this leukocytic migration is a nonspecific response, the mere presence of purulent sputum is not tantamount to bacterial infection. Desquamation of the ciliated epithelium occurs as well (Spencer, 1977) and may represent an important contributing factor to the proposed predisposition to secondary bacterial infections following viral tracheobronchitis (Smith et al, 1976).

The diagnosis of acute viral bronchitis is a clinical one. Chest roentgenograms are usually normal, but peribronchial thickening may occasionally be present. Hyperinflation suggests involvement of more peripheral airways. As noted, pneumonia or atelectasis may complicate bronchitis; a radiograph is often required for confirmation. A sputum culture as well as Gram and Wright staining of the sputum may be useful in cases in which a secondary infection or unusual etiology is suspected (Epstein, 1972).

Treatment of acute viral bronchitis is largely palliative. Adequate rest and proper humidification of the ambient air are usually sufficient. Exposure to noxious agents such as cigarette smoke should be avoided. The usual mild case does not require antibiotics or other pharmacologic agents. The mere presence of purulent-appearing sputum does not necessarily indicate bacterial infection. Thus, antibiotics should be reserved for conditions in which a bacterial infection has been proved by culture if possible or is highly suspected from the clinical course. A productive cough is common, so the use of cough suppressants should be discouraged and in fact is contraindicated. Bronchodilators, particularly theophylline, may be useful in patients with viral bronchitis because many of these children actually have asthma (see the later discussion of the association between asthma and bronchitis). Persistent cough after the acute infection has cleared may be the only manifestation of an asthma exacerbation (McFadden, 1975). Although most cases of acute bronchitis do not require treatment, a child with marked symptoms that disturb sleep or disrupt classroom activities or the child's performance in school may benefit from a trial of theophylline, particularly in the presence of exercise intolerance or a family history of asthma or atopy. There currently are no data on the use of inhaled or oral sympathomimetics or prednisone in the treatment of bronchitis in children. Clinical experience suggests that, as with children who wheeze, combination therapy with β_2 agonists and/or steroids is occasionally indicated.

BRONCHITIS CAUSED BY BACTERIA

Most episodes of acute tracheobronchitis caused by bacteria occur as secondary infections during a period of vulnerability of the mucosal surface caused by a prior viral infection or other airway insult. Work by Ramphal and co-workers (1980) in mice and ferrets demonstrates that influenza infection induces a widespread desquamation of the ciliated epithelium of the trachea. In this state, *Pseudomonas aeruginosa* organisms, which were previously swept out by cilial movement, adhere to the injured cells and exposed basement membrane. Penetration of the mucosal barrier by bacteria can occur and may contribute to secondary bacterial bronchitis. Recovery of the ciliated epithelium occurs over 5 to 7 days in uncomplicated bronchitis.

Streptococcus pneumoniae, Staphylococcus aureus, and *Hemophilus influenzae,* both type B and nontypeable species, have been implicated as causative agents. In addition, recent work has also suggested an expanding role for *Branhamella catarrhalis* (Christensen et al, 1986) in producing acute bacterial bronchitis. Because many of these bacteria can be found in the nasopharynx of healthy children, it is not always possible to link a positive nasopharyngeal culture with the cause of a lower respiratory tract illness. Quantitative sputum cultures may be useful in identifying a significant pathogen (Guckian and Christensen, 1978). In a younger child, who frequently does not expectorate sputum, a deep nasopharyngeal culture obtained while the child is coughing may identify a dominant organism (Huang et al, 1961). Application of recently developed rapid noninvasive diagnostic techniques such as measurement of C-reactive protein, microbial antigen detection, and both labeled and unlabeled antibody detection may be helpful not only in separating viral from bacterial infections but also in identifying the causative agent (Florman et al, 1987). Treatment of these infections is generally empiric, based largely on the organisms commonly encountered and the age of the patient.

Mycoplasma pneumoniae generally produces an indolent, protracted pneumonitis. However, it has also been infrequently identified as the pathogen producing bronchitis (Denny et al, 1971). As with pneumonia, there are no characteristic clinical findings of bronchitis caused by *Mycoplasma*. It should be considered in an older child or adolescent in whom other causes of prolonged bronchitis have been ruled out. Positive cold hemagglutination titers supported by a rise in specific *Mycoplasma* titers confirm the diagnosis. Erythromycin therapy can be effective, but the response to therapy may be variable (Stevens et al, 1978).

Bordetella pertussis and *Corynebacterium diphtheriae* produce a characteristic tracheobronchitis in unimmunized children (Krugman et al, 1977). The early catarrhal stage of *B. pertussis* infection is marked by symptoms of upper respiratory tract infection. A dry, hacking cough is present and progresses during the week to become paroxysmal. As the paroxysmal stage develops, the cough takes on a more classic nature: multiple bursts of coughing interrupted by a deep inspiratory whoop. This cough eventually produces thick, tenacious mucus. The number of paroxysms varies considerably, depending on the severity of the illness. This stage lasts 4 to 6 weeks, followed by a period of prolonged convalescence.

Inflammatory changes in the respiratory tract extend from the nasopharynx to the bronchi. Congestion of the mucosa with infiltration of leukocytes is seen. Clumps of organisms can be found enmeshed in the cilia. Necrosis of the midzonal and basilar layers of the mucosal lining beneath these clumps is thought to be a characteristic pathologic finding of pertussis bronchitis. Clinical manifestations should suggest the diagnosis. Culture and fluorescent antibody tests of secretions can provide laboratory confirmation. Cultures are commonly positive in the first 2 weeks, before the onset of the paroxysmal phase. The fluorescent antibody test is a more useful diagnostic technique, because often, by the time one suspects the disease clinically, the infection has reached a point at which cultures are negative. Adenovirus and parapertussis can produce an illness that mimics classic pertussis syndrome.

Treatment of pertussis is largely supportive. Factors that may trigger paroxysms, such as smoke and dry ambient air, should be avoided. Erythromycin or ampicillin can be used to decrease spread of disease; however, these drugs have little effect on the course of the illness. Patience is required on the part of parents and physicians.

Chlamydia infections can also produce an acute tracheobronchitis and pneumonitis in young infants beginning at several weeks of age (Beem and Saxon, 1977). Respiratory symptoms that include a characteristic staccato cough may be preceded by blepharitis or conjunctivitis. Infection is acquired at birth. The diagnosis can be confirmed by culture or serology. Interestingly, the clinical symptoms of *Chlamydia* infection frequently are indistinguishable from infections due to cytomegalovirus, *Pneumocystis*, and *Ureaplasma* in the same population (Stagno et al, 1981). Treatment is largely supportive but also includes a trial of erythromycin.

Infection with *Mycobacterium tuberculosis* and certain fungi, particularly *Histoplasma capsulatum*, should also be considered as possible causes of acute and chronic bronchitis, especially if afflicted children come from endemic areas (Goodwin et al, 1981). Tuberculosis is discussed in Chapter 48. Cough associated with other constitutional symptoms can be encountered with fungal infections. Cough is generally nonproductive and may be related to airway compression from lymph node enlargement. Fungal serology, delayed hypersensitivity skin testing, and cultures when available may be helpful in establishing a diagnosis. Frequently, an important clue to the diagnosis is a history of a significant exposure to the fungus or residence in an endemic area.

With a few exceptions, most episodes of acute bronchitis are caused by infection. Although massive exposure to irritants such as gastric acid or environmental pollutants can produce acute symptoms, these insults generally are more subtle and produce or contribute to chronic indolent symptoms.

CHRONIC AND RECURRENT BRONCHITIS

Persistence of signs and symptoms of acute tracheobronchitis after 2 to 3 weeks or frequent recurrences (more than four per year) should not be treated lightly but should initiate an attempt to identify an underlying disorder. As suggested by Morgan and Taussig (1984), chronic/recurrent bronchitis is best viewed as an interaction between intrinsic (host) and extrinsic factors that in combination result in chronic inflammation and damage to the airways. As a general rule, chronic/recurrent bronchitis denotes either the presence of airway damage after an acute injury, the continued exposure of the airways to a noxious agent triggering chronic inflammation, the presence of a condition such as asthma or cystic fibrosis that predisposes to airway inflammation, or a defect in host defenses as in IgA deficiency or immotile cilia syndrome (Table 17–2). The remainder of this chapter focuses on the interaction of those factors contributing to chronic/recurrent disease.

The one notable exception to the rule is a chronic cough that has a psychogenic or functional basis. This cough occurs in a healthy child without evidence of underlying lung disease. It is generally a loud, honking cough that usually attracts considerable attention. Characteristically, the cough stops during sleep or when the child believes he or she is unobserved. The child frequently appears quite unconcerned, whereas the parents are usually very anxious about the persistence of the cough. When a functional cough is suspected, initial efforts should focus on defining a treatable condition. However, once a reasonably comprehensive evaluation has been completed, attention should be turned to identifying the secondary gain accruing to the child by persistence of the cough.

Table 17–2. DIFFERENTIAL DIAGNOSIS OF BRONCHITIS IN CHILDREN

Acute	
Viral	Parainfluenza, influenza, adenovirus, rhinovirus
Infection—viral, bacterial	*S. pneumoniae, S. aureus, H. influenzae* (type B, nontypeable), *Mycoplasma, Chlamydia,* pertussis, tuberculosis, diphtheria
Chemical reaction, acute aspiration, smoke inhalation	
Chronic/recurrent	
Cystic fibrosis	
Asthma	
Immotile cilia syndrome	
Tuberculosis	
Retained foreign body (airway, esophageal)	
Aspiration	Anatomic abnormalities (tracheoesophageal fistula, laryngeal cleft); dysfunctional swallowing with and without gastroesophageal reflux, gastroesophageal reflux
Immunodeficiency	IgA, IgG; IgG subclass; Combination IgA and IgG subclass
Inhalation injury	Smoking—active or passive; Indoor pollution; Outdoor pollution
Chronic airway damage	Postinfection or traumatic airway injury with delayed or incomplete healing
Large airway compression	Dynamic—tracheomalacia, bronchomalacia; Extrinsic—vascular or nodal compression

INCIDENCE OF CHRONIC BRONCHITIS IN CHILDREN

As with the definition of chronic bronchitis, it is difficult to determine the incidence of chronic bronchitis in children. Overlap with asthma and the lack of an accepted definition contribute to the confusion (Williams and McNicol, 1969; Hamman et al, 1975). Data from Peat and associates (1980), using a definition similar to the one used in this chapter, revealed that a cumulative incidence of chronic bronchitis in a group of Australian children 9 to 18 years of age ranged between 14 and 24 per cent. It was three times higher than the incidence of asthma in the same population. The incidence was also higher in boys. Similarly, Hall and associates (1972) reported the occurrence of productive cough alone in 32 per cent of 7-year-old Tasmanian children. In the United States, a National Health Survey conducted in 1970 using parental questionnaires revealed 2.5 million children with chronic bronchitis (Wilder, 1970). However, the study by Taussig and associates (1981) suggests that chronic bronchitis is diagnosed infrequently by both pediatricians and family practitioners. It seems that without a better definition and further epidemiologic studies, it is impossible at this point to determine accurately the actual incidence and prevalence of chronic bronchitis in children.

PATHOLOGIC AND RADIOGRAPHIC FINDINGS IN NONSPECIFIC CHRONIC BRONCHITIS

The pathology of chronic bronchitis in adults is fairly well established (Table 17–3), but data on the pathology of chronic bronchitis in childhood are limited (Heard et al, 1979). Again, problems with definition and overlap with other diseases cloud the picture. The radiographic signs of peribronchial thickening and the clinical finding of productive cough suggest that the pathology of chronic bronchitis in children may be similar to that in adults. Székely and Farkas (1978) compared biopsy material from 59 children who did not have asthma but who had signs of chronic bronchial inflammation with that from children with bronchial asthma; their histologic findings are summarized in Table 17–4. Smith

Table 17–3. PATHOLOGIC CHARACTERISTICS OF CHRONIC BRONCHITIS IN ADULTS

Thickened bronchial walls
Mucous gland hypertrophy
Goblet cell hypertrophy
Squamous metaplasia of epithelium
Chronic inflammation

Table 17–4. PATHOLOGIC CHARACTERISTICS OF CHRONIC BRONCHITIS AND ASTHMA IN CHILDREN

	Percentage of Cases	
Characteristic	Chronic Bronchitis	Asthma
Round cell infiltration	100	100
Eosinophils	14	49
Hypertrophied submucosal glands	39	20
Increased mucus	20	12
Metaplasia of epithelium	0	6
Intact epithelium	86	86

(Data from Székely E and Farkas E: Pediatric Bronchology. Baltimore, University Park Press, 1978.)

and colleagues (1985) demonstrated similar findings in a group of children whose chronic bronchitis was diagnosed by bronchoscopic observations. Increased numbers of neutrophils in bronchial secretions were also present in almost all children evaluated. Mucosal gland hypertrophy, which is believed to be a highly typical feature in adults, was present in only 39 per cent of the children studied. Also, metaplasia of the epithelium, which is common in adults, is rare in children. Further studies are needed to clarify these differences and to determine the relationship between these changes in children and those found in adults.

RELATIONSHIP BETWEEN CHRONIC/ RECURRENT BRONCHITIS AND ASTHMA

Burrows and associates (1976) have demonstrated a relationship between symptoms of bronchitis and allergy skin test reactivity in children younger than 15 years. In addition, in 74 per cent of the children with the diagnosis of chronic bronchitis, wheezing was also present (Burrows and Lebowitz, 1975). Like cough, wheezing is a nonspecific symptom. It reflects airway narrowing without regard to mechanism. In bronchitis, airway narrowing can result from excessive mucus production, associated with mucosal edema, as well as from smooth muscle constriction. This overlap of the clinical presentations of asthma (reversible obstructive airways disease) and bronchitis has made it difficult to distinguish between these conditions. Consequently, the terms *asthmatic* and *wheezy bronchitis* have been applied to the diseases of patients with predominant cough and mild or variable wheezing (Williams and McNicol, 1969). Although these are descriptive terms, they are also quite useful in that they reflect the fact that asthma and certain forms of bronchitis are merely different parts of the clinical spectrum of a single disease rather than separate conditions.

Multiple clinical studies have documented an association between attacks of wheezy bronchitis and viral infections (Horn, Brain, Gregg et al, 1979; Horn, Reed, and Taylor, 1979) and cigarette smoke (Ferguson et al, 1980). Both of these factors are also known to exacerbate symptoms of asthma as well. As with asthma, an increased incidence of airway hyperreactivity has also been observed in patients with wheezy bronchitis and their first-degree relatives (König et al, 1972; König and Godfrey, 1973). On the basis of this evidence, it has been postulated that a child who has bronchitis and wheezes actually has asthma (Williams and McNicol, 1969; Kubo et al, 1978). Recent work has suggested that this relationship between bronchitis and asthma may also extend to some patients without wheezing. Bronchitis without wheezing was previously considered by many researchers to be unrelated to asthma. However, the absence of wheezing in adults and children with chronic cough does not preclude a variant presentation of asthma. McFadden (1975) has demonstrated that cough without wheezing can be a manifestation of an asthma attack in adults with known asthma. Similarly, Corrao and associates (1979) have demonstrated, again in adults, that cough may be equivalent to wheezing and, as such, a marker of underlying asthma. In a group of 15 children who had isolated cough without wheezing, Cloutier and Loughlin (1981) have shown exercise-induced airway hyperreactivity similar to that in children with asthma. Both the cough and airway hyperreactivity were relieved by oral theophylline therapy.

The implications of these observations may be quite important for clinicians managing children with chronic bronchitis. Inhalation or exercise challenges can be used to identify these patients. Analysis of sputum for eosinophils may also be useful in this setting, because the presence of more than 20 per cent eosinophils in the sputum is highly correlated with asthma (Chodosh, 1970). Theophylline is effective in controlling the cough. Interestingly, theophylline has been found to block the cough without altering baseline lung function, suggesting that bronchodilation is not involved in the drug's mechanism of action. The role of other bronchodilators and steroids is most likely similar to that encountered in dealing with conventional asthma. Because inflammation rather than bronchospasm is a major factor in producing symptoms, steroids should be an important component of any therapeutic approach, but further study is needed.

RELATIONSHIP BETWEEN IMMUNE DEFICIENCY AND CHRONIC/ RECURRENT BRONCHITIS

Although tracheobronchitis is not indicated specifically, there have been a number of recent reports of children with selective immune system deficiencies that suggest that these children have increased susceptibility to respiratory infections, in particular those associated with encapsulated organisms. Deficiencies encountered include selective IgA deficiency (Bretza and Novey, 1985); IgA deficiency associated with IgG subclass deficiency; especially IgG2 (Oxelius et al, 1981); and combined deficiency of IgG2 and IgG4 in the presence of normal total IgG and IgA (Oxelius, 1974). Selective IgA and IgG2 deficiency has also been reported to increase respiratory symptoms in patients with nonallergic asthma (Smith et al, 1984).

Recognition of these deficiencies, particularly of the IgG subclasses, can be have important therapeutic implications, because more aggressive antibiotic therapy coupled with antibody replacement therapy is indicated (Berger, 1987).

BRONCHITIS RELATED TO FOCAL AIRWAY INJURY OR COMPRESSION

Although limited information is available, recent experience with fiberoptic bronchoscopy has identified a group of children with chronic/recurrent cough whose symptoms arise as a consequence of injury to a bronchial segment. The injury results in compromised airway function and defenses, leading to an apparent increased susceptibility to infection as well as a delay in the recovery from an individual infection. The right middle lobe appears to be involved most commonly (see Chapter 37), but no one area appears to be immune to injury. These children present with chronic/recurrent productive cough, associated with fever and a focal infiltrate (atelectasis or pneumonia). At bronchoscopy, one finds a localized inflammatory process involving a segmental or subsegmental bronchus. Malacia of the bronchial wall is often seen. Secretions are increased and frequently contain many neutrophils. Cultures are positive for organisms such as *H. influenzae,* both type B and nontypeables, and *B. catarrhalis.* Exacerbations are usually triggered by viruses, followed by secondary bacterial infection. Extended antibiotic coverage is frequently required for effective therapy. The natural history of this disorder is not known. Most patients improve with therapy, but an occasional patient suffers permanent injury and requires resection of the damaged segment in order to control symptoms and prevent recurrences.

Tracheobronchial malacia and compression of airway caliber by lymph nodes or vascular structures including the left atrium are associated with a predisposition to chronic/recurrent bronchitis most likely secondary to the effects of deformation of the airway on clearance mechanisms.

RELATIONSHIP BETWEEN IRRITANTS AND CHRONIC/RECURRENT BRONCHITIS

In adults, the association between chronic exposure to irritants and bronchitis is fairly well established. Recent studies have suggested that children have their own unique "occupational" hazards that increase the risk of developing inflammatory disease of the major airways. The major sources of chemical irritation of the child's airways include (1) aspiration of food or gastric contents or other foreign substances and (2) inhalation of polluted air.

Aspiration

Aspiration in children occurs secondary to anatomic defects of the trachea and esophagus, swallowing dysfunction, gastroesophageal reflux, and accidents. The presence of a retained foreign body must always be considered in evaluating children with chronic cough. This condition is discussed in more detail in Chapter 31.

Tracheoesophageal fistula and esophageal atresia are discussed in Chapter 12. The H-type fistula, although one of the least common, deserves comment here because it is the most common type of fistula diagnosed after the newborn period and must be considered in the differential diagnosis of a young child with chronic cough (Sundar et al, 1975). Symptoms may occur immediately after ingestion of food, especially liquids. Occasionally, this important clinical observation is not present, because recurrent aspiration may attenuate the immediate cough response. Thus the aspiration event may produce only minimal acute symptoms, yet the child may present with chronic, recurrent cough or wheezing. As with other forms of bronchitis, auscultation of the chest may be unremarkable until immediately after a liquid meal, when wheezes or rhonchi may be heard. Chest radiographs may demonstrate perihilar infiltrates and peribronchial thickening.

The diagnosis of an H-type tracheoesophageal fistula can be established with a barium swallow. Using a catheter to increase intraesophageal pressure and positioning the patient in the prone, head-down position improves the yield from this study. However, despite the best radiographic techniques, bronchoscopy is occasionally necessary to establish the diagnosis. Introduction of a color dye may aid the bronchoscopist in identifying a small fistula.

Treatment is surgical, but patients may have persistent symptoms despite surgical correction (Dudley and Phelan, 1976), perhaps because of permanent airway damage from prior aspiration or because of an induced airway hyperreactive state secondary to chronic aspiration (Milligan and Levison, 1979).

Several authors have suggested a relationship between gastroesophageal reflux and pulmonary disease such as bronchitis, asthma, and pneumonia (Danus et al, 1976; Herbst, 1981; Orenstein and Orenstein, 1988). Although the evidence is not conclusive, the amelioration of respiratory symptoms with control of gastroesophageal reflux lends support to this relationship. Barium swallow, radionuclide scan, and continuous esophageal pH probe monitoring can be used to diagnose reflux. Correlation of cough with a preceding drop in esophageal pH or the finding of aspirated radionuclide confirms the association (McVeagh et al, 1987). However, this solid association is frequently lacking and the diagnosis must be made on clinical grounds. Bronchoscopy may be useful to document evidence of tracheobronchitis and to collect secretions that can be stained to detect the presence of fat-laden macrophages indicative of aspiration. Initial treatment of reflux is medical, including upright position, thickened feedings, and drugs such as metoclopramide or bethanechol. Surgery should be reserved for documented severe cases that are life threatening or unresponsive to medical management.

In children without gastroesophageal reflux, accidental aspiration of large amounts of gastric contents is usually an isolated event generally occurring in association with another condition such as endotracheal intubation or a seizure. The resulting bronchitis is usually an acute self-limited process, which may be followed by a secondary bacterial infection.

Aspiration can also result from swallowing dysfunction (Fisher et al, 1981). This problem can be encountered in neurologically and developmentally normal children but is certainly an important cause of bronchitis in children with mental retardation and cerebral palsy, particularly in an institutionalized population (unpublished observations).

Fluoroscopic evaluation of swallowing using a barium meal of varying consistencies (Kramer, 1985) is useful in detecting both an abnormal swallowing pattern as well as associated aspiration. Even if aspiration is not noted, the finding of a dysfunctional swallow is highly suggestive that respiratory symptoms are related to aspiration during swallowing. Clinical observation of feeding is essential in establishing a diagnosis, because these patients frequently have more difficulty with thinner liquids and thicker barium may minimize symptoms during the study. Treatment of this disorder generally involves thickening feedings in otherwise normal children. However, in neurologically impaired children, nasogastric feedings on a temporary basis and gastrostomy as a more permanent solution are required.

Aspiration of a foreign substance produces an inflammatory response in the airways similar to that in viral tracheobronchitis. The intensity of this response is related to the composition of the aspirated substance. Inert materials frequently produce less inflammation. Work by Wynne and co-workers (1981) has shed light on the relationship between aspiration and chronic and recurrent bronchitis. Scanning electron microscopic studies have demonstrated that following aspiration of gastric contents there is a loss of ciliated epithelium. As previously noted, this situation reduces the defenses of the respiratory epithelium and may predispose to infection. If the insult is recurrent, as it can be in several of these situations, there may not be sufficient time for healing to occur, and the patient may become predisposed to chronic disease.

Effects of Air Pollution

Air pollution is the other major airway irritant thought to produce either chemical bronchitis or a predisposition to recurrences of infectious bronchitis. Variability in the types of pollutants and lengths of exposure, and an inability to separate the effects of pollution alone from interactions between pollution and other provocative factors have contributed to some confusion in the literature regarding the relationship between pollution and bronchitis (Kerrebijn et al, 1977). In general, atmospheric pollution has two major components: *reducing substances*—smoke, soot, and sulfur compounds (sulfur dioxide, sulfuric acid, and sulfates)—and *oxidizing substances*—hydrocarbons, nitrous oxide, and reaction products catalyzed by sunlight (ozone, aldehydes, and ketones). The relationship between pollution and a particular case of bronchitis becomes clearer if the type of pollutant is known.

Although outdoor air pollution does not appear to be a factor in acute bronchitis, long-term exposure to high levels of atmospheric pollution composed of reducing substances increases the incidence of chronic and recurrent lower respiratory tract disease, including bronchitis (Pearlman et al, 1971). Reducing substances have also been shown to produce chronic pulmonary function abnormalities unassociated with increased incidence of respiratory infections or symptoms (Ferris, 1970; Zapletal et al, 1973). Lunn and co-workers (1967) showed that both upper and lower respiratory tract illnesses occurred more frequently in children who lived in highly polluted areas. Interestingly, in a follow-up study 4 years later, there was a reduction in the incidence of bronchitis concomitant with a reduction in pollution (Lunn et al, 1970). Similarly, Colley and associates (1973) as well as Chiaramonte and co-workers (1970) found an association between bronchitis and chronic cough and pollution. These data suggest that long-term exposure to pollution composed of reducing substances produces a dysfunction of the airways, which then predisposes these children to develop chronic or recurrent lower respiratory tract illness. As in other forms of bronchitis, viral respiratory infections certainly play a role in these exacerbations. The available data suggest that in contrast to the effects of reducing substances, neither acute severe nor more subtle chronic exposure to oxidizing air pollutants increases the incidence of bronchitis or the predisposition to lower respiratory tract illness in children (McMillan et al, 1969; Shy et al, 1973).

Indoor air pollution also plays a part in predisposing children to chronic respiratory symptoms, including increased susceptibility to recurrent viral upper respiratory infections. An extensive review of the current status of the health effects of indoor air pollution is provided by Samet and co-workers (1987). Table 17–5, adapted from this review, summarizes common sources of indoor air pollution commonly encountered by children.

Although the relationship between respiratory symptoms and a number of these agents is not clearly established, the data on the effects of two common pollutants, emissions from wood-burning stoves and especially cigarette smoke, is worthy of discussion.

Work by Honicky and co-workers (1985) has dem-

Table 17–5. COMMON SOURCES OF AIR POLLUTION IN THE HOME

Cigarette smoke	Respirable particles, carbon monoxide, volatile organic substances
Gas stoves	Nitrous oxide, carbon monoxide
Wood-burning stoves, fireplaces	Respirable particles, carbon monoxide, polycyclic aromatic hydrocarbons
Kerosene heaters	Nitrous oxide, carbon monoxide, sulfur dioxide
Building materials	
Dust, inhaled allergens	Formaldehyde

(Adapted from Samet JM, Marbury MC, and Spengler JD: Health effects of indoor air pollution. Am Rev Respir Dis 136:1486, 1987.)

onstrated an increased occurrence of bronchitis and asthma in children living in homes heated by wood-burning stoves as compared with a control group. The increased use of these stoves in conjunction with improvement in home insulation has increased children's exposure to the by-products of combustion.

Effects of Cigarette Smoke

Cigarette smoke appears to be a major etiologic agent and an important predisposing factor in bronchitis in children. Exposure to cigarette smoke occurs in either an active or a passive manner. The latter occurs when children inhale air polluted by smokers, usually their parents or relatives.

The case for active smoking as a factor in producing tracheobronchitis is quite clear. Cigarette smoking among children and adolescents has been shown to be related not only to the etiology of chronic cough but also to an increased incidence and frequency of bronchitis produced by respiratory viruses (Kiernan et al, 1976; Bland et al, 1978). The effects of involuntary (passive) smoking on the lungs are more subtle but just as real. Work by several investigators has documented an association between bronchitis and pneumonia and parental, especially maternal, smoking (Cameron et al, 1969; Yarnell and St. Leger, 1979; Taylor and Wadsworth, 1987). This effect appears to be age dependent and is more apparent in the first year of life (Harlap and Davies, 1974). In addition, several investigators have reported an association between respiratory cough with phlegm in children and parental smoking. However, the presence of parental symptoms must be taken into account in analyzing these data, because adjusting for the presence of similar respiratory symptoms in the parents weakens but does not eliminate this association between passive smoking and bronchitis in children (Colley, 1974; Lebowitz and Burrows, 1976). Cessation of parental smoking may produce dramatic relief of symptoms in certain children. Consequently, it is vital to include a smoking history of both the adults and the child in the household when evaluating the cause of unexplained bronchitis and cough. Furthermore, it must be remembered that a smoking history obtained from an older child or adolescent with parents present is frequently unreliable.

LUNG FUNCTION IN CHILDREN WITH BRONCHITIS

To date, there are limited data on the effects of bronchitis on pulmonary function. Lung function changes that may occur during and immediately after acute viral bronchitis have not been studied. However, information on the effects of bronchitis on lung function can be gleaned from studies of viral upper respiratory tract infection in children. In one such study, these illnesses were associated with decreases in many spirometric values, reflecting a reduction in

caliber of large and small airways alike (Collier et al, 1978). Cough was a clinical manifestation of the illness in many of these children, so it is likely that there was also a component of tracheobronchitis. Thus, these changes may be indicative of the lung function abnormalities associated with bronchitis. Studies of children with wheezy bronchitis have demonstrated evidence of increases in airway resistance and airway hyperreactivity; airway obstruction was reversible in the older children but not in the infants (Rutter et al, 1975; Lenney and Milner, 1978).

Boule and co-workers (1979) investigated the effects of recurrent bronchitis on subsequent lung function in children. They observed evidence of airway obstruction and airway hyperreactivity in a significant number of these children. These abnormalities were present in subjects with and without wheezing during the episode. All children were studied at least 6 weeks after the last attack of bronchitis. Moreover, Woolcock and co-workers (1979) have demonstrated that these lung function abnormalities may persist for years after the attacks have resolved. Additional clinical and epidemiologic studies are needed to clarify the effects of acute and chronic bronchitis on lung growth, development, and function in children.

LONG-TERM CONSEQUENCES OF CHILDHOOD BRONCHITIS

Multiple clinical studies have implicated chronic bronchitis in children as a factor in the persistence of lung dysfunction and chronic respiratory symptoms. Bland and associates (1974) have shown that children with a history of bronchitis before age 5 have an increased risk of bronchitis, colds, wheezy chest, coughing, and phlegm production at age 11. Lung function was also adversely affected. Work by Colley and others has demonstrated an association between cough prevalence at age 20 and 25 and a history of bronchitis before age 2 (Colley et al, 1973; Kiernan et al, 1976). Current smoking habits increased the tendency for chronic symptoms in those with a history of bronchitis. Woolcock and associates (1979) confirmed this association between bronchitis in infancy and chronic symptoms later in life. Subtle pulmonary function abnormalities similar to those in younger children with recurrent bronchitis were found in this population. Burrows and co-workers (1977), in a large epidemiologic study, demonstrated an association between childhood respiratory illness and impairment of ventilatory function in adults over age 20. They also observed that the decline in lung function with aging is accelerated with cigarette use in persons who had childhood respiratory illness.

These studies support the notion that chronic and recurrent bronchitis in children should not be taken lightly. It appears to be a significant factor in predisposing adults not only to chronic respiratory symptoms but also to lung dysfunction (Burrows and

Taussig, 1980). Smoking appears to aggravate the situation. Thus it is imperative that children with chronic bronchitis and their parents be advised of the significant risks of smoking, because it may well contribute not only to current symptoms but also to lasting lung injury.

REFERENCES

American Thoracic Society, Committee on Diagnostic Standards for Nontuberculous Respiratory Diseases: definitions and classification of chronic bronchitis, asthma, and pulmonary emphysema. Am Rev Respir Dis 85:762, 1962.

Ayres JG: Seasonal pattern of acute bronchitis in general practice in the United Kingdom 1976–83. Thorax 41:106, 1986.

Barker DJ and Osmond C: Childhood respiratory infection and adult chronic bronchitis in England and Wales. Br Med J 293:1271, 1986.

Beem MO and Saxon EM: Respiratory tract colonization and a distinctive pneumonia syndrome in infants infected with *Chlamydia trachomatis*. N Engl J Med 296:306, 1977.

Berger M: Immunoglobulin G subclass determination in diagnosis and management of antibody deficiency syndromes. J Pediatr 110:325, 1987.

Bland JM, Holland WW, and Elliott A: The development of respiratory symptoms in a cohort of Kent schoolchildren. Bull Physiopathol Resp 10:699, 1974.

Bland M, Bewley BR, Pollard V et al: Effects of children's and parent's smoking on respiratory symptoms. Arch Dis Child 53:100, 1978.

Boule M, Gaultier C, Tournier G et al: Lung function in children with recurrent bronchitis. Respiration 38:127, 1979.

Bretza JA and Novey HS: IgA: Biologic function in health and disease. Immunol Allergy Prac 308:15, 1985.

Burrows B and Lebowitz MD: Characteristics of chronic bronchitis in a warm, dry region. Am Rev Respir Dis 112:365, 1975.

Burrows B and Taussig LM: "As the twig is bent, the tree inclines" (perhaps). Am Rev Respir Dis 122:813, 1980.

Burrows B, Knudson RJ, and Lebowitz MD: The relationship of childhood respiratory illness to adult obstructive airway disease. Am Rev Respir Dis 115:751, 1977.

Burrows B, Lebowitz MD, and Barbee RA: Respiratory disorders and allergy skin test reactions. Ann Intern Med 84:134, 1976.

Cameron P, Kostin JS, Zaks JM et al: The health of smokers' and non-smokers' children. J Allergy 43:336, 1969.

Chiaramonte LT, Bongiorno JR, Brown R et al: Air pollution and obstructive respiratory disease in children. NY State J Med 70:394, 1970.

Chodosh S: Examination of sputum cells. N Engl J Med 282:854, 1970.

Christensen JJ, Gadeberg O, and Bruun B: *Branhammella catarrhalis*: significance in pulmonary infections and bacteriological features. Acta Pathol Microbiol Immunol Scand [B] 94:98, 1986.

Cloutier MM and Loughlin GM: Chronic cough in children: a manifestation of airway hyperreactivity. Pediatrics 67:6, 1981.

Colley JRT: Respiratory disease in childhood. Br Med Bull 27:9, 1971.

Colley JRT: Respiratory symptoms in children and parental smoking and phlegm production. Br Med J 2:201, 1974.

Colley JRT, Douglas JWB, and Reid DD: Respiratory disease in young adults: influence of early childhood lower respiratory tract illness, social class, air pollution and smoking. Br Med J 3:195, 1973.

Collier AM, Pimmel RL, Hasselbad V et al: Spirometric changes in normal children with upper respiratory infections. Am Rev Respir Dis 117:47, 1978.

Corrao WN, Braman SS, and Irvin RS: Chronic cough as the sole presenting manifestation of bronchial asthma. N Engl J Med 300:633, 1979.

Corwin RW and Irwin RS: The lipid-laden alveolar macrophage as a marker of aspiration in parenchymal lung disease. Am Rev Respir Dis 132:576, 1985.

Danus O, Casar C, Larrain A et al: Esophageal reflux—an unrecognized cause of recurrent obstructive bronchitis in children. J Pediatr 89:220, 1976.

Denny FW and Clyde WA Jr: Acute lower respiratory tract infections in non-hospitalized children. J Pediatr 108:635, 1986.

Denny FW, Clyde WA, and Glezen WP: *Mycoplasma pneumoniae* disease: clinical spectrum, pathophysiology, epidemiology and control. J Infect Dis 123:74, 1971.

Dudley NE and Phelan PD: Respiratory complications in long-term survivors of oesophageal atresia. Arch Dis Child 51:279, 1976.

Edwards G: Acute bronchitis—aetiology, diagnosis and management. Br Med J 1:963, 1966.

Epstein RL: Constituents of sputum: a simple method. Ann Intern Med 77:257, 1972.

Fergusson DM, Horwood LJ, and Shannon FT: Parental smoking and respiratory illness in infancy. Arch Dis Child 55:358, 1980.

Ferris BG: Effects of air pollution on school absences and differences in lung function in first and second graders in Berlin, New Hampshire, January 1966 to June 1967. Am Rev Respir Dis 102:591, 1970.

Fisher SE, Painter M, and Milmoe G: Swallowing disorders in infancy. Pediatr Clin North Am 28:845, 1981.

Florman AL, Cushing AH, and Umland ET: Rapid non-invasive techniques for determining etiology of bronchitis and pneumonia in infants and children. Clin Chest Med 8:669, 1987.

Glezen WP and Denny FW: Epidemiology of acute lower respiratory disease in children. N Engl J Med 288:498, 1973.

Goodwin RA, Loyd JE, and Des Prez RM: Histoplasmosis in normal hosts. Medicine 60:231, 1981.

Guckian JC and Christensen WD: Quantitative culture and gram stain of sputum in pneumonia. Am Rev Respir Dis 118:997, 1978.

Hall GLJ, Gandevia B, Silverstone H et al: The interrelationships of upper and lower respiratory tract symptoms and signs in seven-year-old children. Int J Epidemiol 1:389, 1972.

Hamman RF, Halil T, and Holland WW: Asthma in schoolchildren. Br J Prev Soc Med 29:228, 1975.

Harlap S and Davies AM: Infant admissions to hospital and maternal smoking. Lancet 1:529, 1974.

Heard BE, Khatchatourov V, Otto H et al: The morphology of emphysema, chronic bronchitis and bronchiectasis: definition, nomenclature and classification. J Clin Pathol 32:882, 1979.

Herbst JJ: Gastroesophageal reflux. J Pediatr 98:859, 1981.

Honicky RE, Osborne JS III, and Akpom CA: Symptoms of respiratory illness in young children and the use of wood-burning stoves for indoor heating. Pediatrics 75:587, 1985.

Horn MEC, Brain E, Gregg I et al: Respiratory viral infection in childhood: a survey in general practice, Roehampton 1967–1972. J Hyg (Camb.), 74:157, 1975.

Horn MEC, Brain EA, Gregg I et al: Respiratory viral infection and wheezy bronchitis in childhood. Thorax 34:23, 1979.

Horn MEC, Reed SE, and Taylor P: Role of viruses and bacteria in acute wheezy bronchitis in childhood: a study of sputum. Arch Dis Child 54:587, 1979.

Huang NN, Van Loon EL, and Sheng KT: The flora of the respiratory tract of patients with cystic fibrosis of the pancreas. J Pediatr 59:512, 1961.

Kerrebijn KF, Hoogeveen-Schroot HCA, and Van Der Wal MC: Chronic nonspecific respiratory disease in children: a five-year follow-up study. Acta Paediatr Scand (Suppl) 261:3, 1977.

Kiernan KE, Colley JRT, Douglas JWB et al: Chronic cough in young adults in relation to smoking habits, childhood environment, and chest illness. Respiration 33:236, 1976.

König P and Godfrey S: Exercise-induced bronchial lability and atopic status of families of infants with wheezy bronchitis. Arch Dis Child 48:942, 1973.

König P, Godfrey S, and Abrahamov A: Exercise-induced bronchial lability in children with a history of wheezy bronchitis. Arch Dis Child 47:578, 1972.

Kramer SS: Special swallowing problems in children. Gastrointest Radiol 10:241, 1985.

Krugman S, Ward R, and Katz SL: Infectious Diseases of Children. St. Louis, CV Mosby Co, 1977.

Kubo S, Funabashi S, Uehara S et al: Clinical aspects of "asthmatic bronchitis" and chronic bronchitis in infants and children. J Asthma Res 15:99, 1978.

Lebowitz MD and Burrows B: Respiratory symptoms related to smoking habits of family adults. Chest 69:48, 1976.

Lenney W and Milner AD: Recurrent wheezing in the preschool child. Arch Dis Child 53:468, 1978.

Lunn JE, Knowelden J, and Handyside AJ: Patterns of respiratory illness in Sheffield infant school children. Br J Prev Soc Med 21:7, 1967.

Lunn JE, Knowelden J, and Roe JW: Patterns of respiratory disease in Sheffield junior school children. Br J Prev Soc Med 24:223, 1970.

McFadden ER: Exertional dyspnea and cough as preludes to acute attacks of bronchial asthma. N Engl J Med 292:555, 1975.

McMillan RS, Wiseman DH, Hanes B et al: Effects of oxidant air pollution on peak expiratory flow rates in Los Angeles school children. Arch Environ Health 18:941, 1969.

McVeagh P, Howman-Giles R, and Kemp A: Pulmonary aspiration studied by radionuclide milk scanning and barium swallow roentgenography. Am J Dis Child 141:917, 1987.

Milligan DWA and Levison H: Lung function in children following repair of tracheoesophageal fistula. J Pediatr 95:24, 1979.

Morgan WJ and Taussig LM: The chronic bronchitis complex in children. Pediatr Clin North Am 31:851, 1984.

Orenstein SR and Orenstein DM: Gastroesophageal reflux and respiratory disease in children. J Pediatr 112:847, 1988.

Oxelius V-A: Chronic infections in a family with hereditary deficiency of IgG2 and IgG4. Clin Exp Immunol 17:19, 1974.

Oxelius V-A, Laurell A-B, Lindquist B et al: IgG subclasses in selective IgA deficiency. N Engl J Med 304:1476, 1981.

Parks CR: Bronchitis, bronchiolitis and asthma. In Kelly VC (ed): Practice of Pediatrics. Vol. IV. Hagerstown, Maryland, WF Pryor Co, 1979.

Pearlman ME, Finklea JF, Creason JP et al: Nitrogen dioxide and lower respiratory illness. Pediatrics 47:391, 1971.

Peat JK, Woolcock AJ, Leeder SR et al: Asthma and bronchitis in Sydney schoolchildren. I. Prevalence during a six-year study. Am J Epidemiol 111:721, 1980.

Ramphal R, Small PM, Shands JW Jr et al: Adherence of *Pseudomonas aeruginosa* to tracheal cells injured by influenza infection or by endotracheal intubation. Infect Immun 27:614, 1980.

Rutter N, Milner AD, and Hiller EJ: Effect of bronchodilators on respiratory resistance in infants and young children with bronchiolitis and wheezy bronchitis. Arch Dis Child 50:719, 1975.

Samet JM, Marbury MC, and Spengler JD: Health effects of indoor air pollution. Parts I and II. Am Rev Respir Dis 136:1486, 1987; 137:221, 1988.

Shy CM, Hasselblad V, Burton RM et al: Air pollution effects on ventilatory function of U.S. school children. Arch Environ Health 27:124, 1973.

Smith CB, Golden C, Klauber MR et al: Interactions between viruses and bacteria in patients with chronic bronchitis. J Infect Dis 134:552, 1976.

Smith TF, Ireland TA, Zaatari GS et al: Characteristics of children with endoscopically proven chronic bronchitis. Am J Dis Child 139:1039, 1985.

Smith TF, Morris EC, and Bain RP: IgG subclasses in non-allergic children with chronic chest symptoms. J Pediatr 105:896, 1984.

Spencer H: Pathology of the Lung. Vol. 1. Oxford, Pergamon Press, 1977.

Stagno S, Brasfield DM, Brown MB et al: Infant pneumonitis associated with cytomegalovirus, chlamydia, pneumocystis and ureaplasma: a prospective study. Pediatrics 68:322, 1981.

Stevens D, Swift PGF, Johnston PGB et al: *Mycoplasma pneumoniae* infections in children. Arch Dis Child 53:38, 1978.

Sundar B, Guiney EJ and O'Donnell B: Congenital H-type tracheo-oesophageal fistula. Arch Dis Child 50:862, 1975.

Székely E and Farkas E: Pediatric Bronchology. Baltimore, University Park Press, 1978.

Taussig LM, Smith SM, and Blumenfeld R: Chronic bronchitis in childhood: what is it? Pediatrics 67:1, 1981.

Taylor B and Wadsworth J: Maternal smoking during pregnancy and lower respiratory tract illness in early life. Arch Dis Child 62:786, 1987.

Wilder CS: Prevalence of Selected Chronic Respiratory Conditions. (Vital and Health Statistics, Series 10, No. 84.) Rockville, Md, U.S. Department of Health, Education and Welfare, 1970.

Williams H and McNicol KN: Prevalence, natural history and relationship of wheezy bronchitis and asthma in children: an epidemiologic study. Br Med J 4:321, 1969.

Williams HE, and Phelan PD: Respiratory Illness in Children. Oxford, Blackwell Scientific Publications, 1975.

Woolcock AJ, Leeder SR, Peat JK, et al: The influence of lower respiratory illness in infancy and childhood and subsequent cigarette smoking on lung function in Sydney schoolchildren. Am Rev Respir Dis 120:5, 1979.

Wynne JW, Ramphal R, and Hood CI: Tracheal mucosal damage after aspiration: a scanning electron microscopic study. Am Rev Respir Dis 124:728, 1981.

Yarnell JWG and St. Leger AS: Respiratory illness, maternal smoking habit, and lung function in children. Br J Dis Chest 73:230, 1979.

Zapletal A, Jech J, Paul T et al: Pulmonary function studies in children living in an air-polluted area. Am Rev Respir Dis 107:400, 1973.

MARY ELLEN B. WOHL, M.D.

18

BRONCHIOLITIS

Bronchiolitis means inflammation of the bronchioles. In a child less than 2 years of age, the term is usually applied to a clinical syndrome characterized by rapid respiration, chest retractions, and wheezing.

CLINICAL PRESENTATION

Bronchiolitis is one of the major causes of hospital admission in infants under the age of 1 year; most commonly, it affects infants between the ages of 2 and 6 months (Henderson, Clyde, Collier et al, 1979). The infant characteristically has symptoms of a viral infection such as mild rhinorrhea, cough, and sometimes a low-grade fever. Within 1 or 2 days, these symptoms are followed by the onset of rapid respiration, chest retractions, and wheezing. The infant may be irritable, may feed poorly, and may vomit (Reilly et al, 1961; Heycock and Noble, 1962; Gardner, 1973; Hall et al, 1976; McConnochie, 1983).

On physical examination, the respiratory rate is increased, often to rates above 50 or 60 breaths/min. The pulse rate is usually increased, and body temperature may be normal or elevated as high as 41°C. Mild conjunctivitis or otitis is observed in some patients and pharyngitis in about one half (Reilly et al, 1961; Gardner, 1973). Chest retractions are present. Prolonged expirations are frequently found, but breath sounds may be normal. Rhonchi and wheezes or rales are usually heard throughout the lungs. Respiratory distress may prevent adequate oral fluid intake and cause dehydration. Although severe abnormalities in gas exchange can develop, cyanosis is detectable in only a minority of the infants. Increased respiratory rate is a more sensitive indicator of impaired gas exchange, and rates of 60 breaths/min or higher are associated with reduction of arterial oxygen tension and elevation of carbon dioxide tension (Reynolds, 1963a, b; Hall, Hall, and Speers, 1979).

The radiographic manifestations of bronchiolitis are nonspecific and include diffuse hyperinflation of the lungs with flattening of the diaphragms, prominence of the retrosternal space, and bulging of the intercostal spaces (Rice and Loda, 1966; W Simpson et al, 1974) (Fig. 18–1). Patchy or peribronchial infiltrates suggestive of interstitial pneumonia occur in the majority of infants. Pleural thickening and fluid are rarely observed and, when present, are minimal. Some infants with illness severe enough to require hospitalization have normal chest roentgenograms.

ETIOLOGY

In 1957, Chanock and Finberg isolated respiratory syncytial virus (RSV) from two infants with lower respiratory tract disease. Beem and co-workers in 1960 identified this virus, originally isolated from the chimpanzee and termed the *chimpanzee coryza agent*, in 31 of 95 infants less than 2 years of age with acute lower respiratory tract disease. Subsequently, RSV has been found to be the etiologic agent in the majority of infants with bronchiolitis. (See Cradock-Watson et al, 1971; Brandt et al, 1973; Gardner, 1973; Kim et al, 1973; Parrott et al, 1973; Henderson, Clyde, Collier et al, 1979.) Infection with other viruses, primarily adenovirus, parainfluenza virus types 1 and 3, enterovirus, and influenza virus, has been associated with bronchiolitis in smaller numbers of cases (Becroft, 1971; Cradock-Watson et al, 1971; Glezen and Denny, 1973; Zollar et al, 1973; Henderson, Clyde, Collier et al, 1979; Welliver, Wong, Sun, and McCarthy, 1986). Particularly severe bronchiolitis associated with adenovirus infections has been observed in native (Indian, Eskimo, Métis) Canadian children (Morrell et al, 1975) and in native (Maori) New Zealand and Pacific Island children (Lang et al, 1969; James et al, 1979).

Epidemics of RSV disease occur between October and June, last approximately 5 months, and follow a characteristic pattern of alternating short (7 to 12 months) and long (13 to 16 months) intervals between epidemic peaks (Brandt et al, 1973; Glezen and Denny, 1973; Kim et al, 1973). Adults as well as children are infected, and epidemics have been reported in newborns' nurseries (Hall, Kopelman, Douglas et al, 1979). In very young or premature infants, however, the disease is atypical. In general only infants older than 1 month develop the clinical syndrome of bronchiolitis (Parrott et al, 1973; Hall et al, 1976). In large urban populations, the peak age incidence of RSV bronchiolitis is at 2 months (Parrott et al, 1973); in more rural settings, RSV-

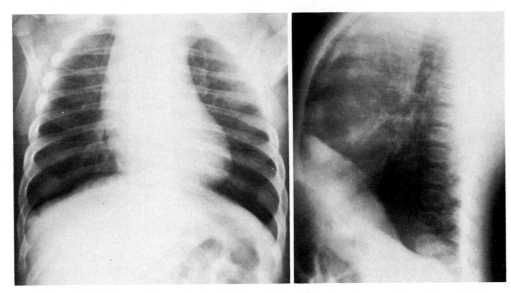

Figure 18–1. Chest radiograph of an infant with the clinical syndrome of acute bronchiolitis.

associated bronchiolitis is observed up to the age of 2 years (Glezen and Denny, 1973). Although the incidence of RSV infections appears to be the same in males and females, severe bronchiolitis is more likely to occur in male infants.

Epidemiologic studies of RSV indicate that during an epidemic all age groups have appreciable attack rates. The lowest attack rate, 17 per cent, is in adults (Hall et al, 1976). The highest, 98 per cent, is reported in previously uninfected infants in a day-care setting (Henderson, Collier, Clyde, and Denny, 1979). Virtually all children in intensively populated urban settings acquire infection by 2 years of age (Kim et al, 1973; Glezen et al, 1981). In a study of transmission of RSV within families, 45 per cent of family members acquired infection once the virus was introduced, usually by a school-age child (Hall et al, 1976). Groups at particular risk for infection are infants hospitalized for other reasons during an RSV epidemic, and hospital staff caring for infants. Forty-five per cent of infants hospitalized for 1 week and 100 per cent of those hospitalized for 1 month acquired infection (Hall, Douglas, Geiman, and Messner, 1975). About one-half of hospital personnel working with infants acquire infection during an epidemic (Hall, Douglas, Geiman, and Messner, 1975), and the major mode of transmission appears to be by large particles and by self-inoculation after touching contaminated surfaces (Hall and Douglas, 1981). Observing strict hand-washing practice and cohorting infants and staff (making sure the same staff members care for the same infants during an epidemic) can reduce the rate of infection among infants but not among staff (Hall et al, 1978). Gown and glove precautions reduce nosocomial spread dramatically (LeClair et al, 1987). Almost all infected individuals, including adults, develop symptoms, particularly nasal congestion and cough. Severe and fatal disease can occur in hospitalized infants who acquire RSV infection.

RSV continues to be shed from the respiratory tract for an average of 9 days in children less than 1 year of age. High titers of virus may remain in nasal washings despite clinical improvement (Hall, Hall, and Speers, 1979). Some infants, particularly those with immunodeficiency syndromes, shed virus for months after infection (Fishaut et al, 1980). These and other observations indicate that factors other than the cytolytic effect of viral replication in the airways may be responsible for bronchiolitis in young infants.

Immunopathologic mechanisms appear to contribute to the manifestations of RSV infections in infants (McIntosh and Fishaut, 1980). Infants who had received a killed RSV vaccine developed high levels of complement-fixing and neutralizing antibody to RSV (Chanock et al, 1970). Yet in an epidemic of RSV infection, their disease was more severe than that in control infants. Severe bronchiolitis occurs in young infants in whom maternally acquired antibody might be highest. These observations suggest that the presence of antibody contributes to the production of disease. The hypothesis has been put forth that antigen-antibody complexes toxic to cells are formed. The observation that older infants with no evidence of antibody acquire typical RSV bronchiolitis does not support this hypothesis (Parrott et al, 1973). Work by Glezen and co-workers (1981) shows that infants with lower levels of antibody have more severe illness and suggests that maternal antibody is associated with protection.

The vaccinated infants also had evidence of specific cell-mediated immunity (delayed hypersensitivity) to RSV (Kim et al, 1976), and this finding, coupled with the observation that there are accumulations of lymphocytes around peripheral airways in infants with bronchiolitis, has led to the speculation that a type IV or cell-mediated immune response contributes to the production of disease. Although some investigators (Welliver et al, 1979) have found evidence of increased lymphocyte proliferative responses developing earlier in infants with bronchiolitis than in infants with RSV disease pneumonia, others (Mito et al, 1984) have not confirmed these results, and the exact role of cell-mediated immune responses in determining the manifestations of infection is not clear.

The relative paucity of virus in the airways of infants with bronchiolitis examined at autopsy contrasted with the large quantities of virus present in the lungs of infants dying of RSV pneumonia has led to the suggestion that a small amount of virus might trigger a type I immune response with the subsequent release of mediator substances (Gardner et al, 1970). RSV-specific IgE and elevated levels of histamine have been demonstrated in nasopharyngeal secretions during RSV infection, particularly bronchiolitis with hypoxia (Welliver et al, 1981), and virus-specific IgE and IgG4 antibodies have been detected in serum of children with RSV bronchiolitis (Bui et al, 1987). Leukotriene C4 has been found in secretions during viral infections accompanied by wheezing (Volovitz et al, 1988). It appears that histamine and other mediators of inflammation are released locally in children with viral bronchiolitis, but why this occurs in some infected infants and not in all remains unknown.

The relative rate of maturation of various components of the immune system may influence the type of disease produced by RSV. The presence of secretory IgA antibody to RSV on the nasal mucosa conveys some degree of protection, and the relative delay in the development of this system may be related to the occurrence of disease. The development of specific IgA antibody in respiratory secretions is related temporally to the termination of viral shedding (McIntosh et al, 1979).

Anatomic differences between the lungs of young infants and older children may contribute to the severity of bronchiolitis in infants. Resistance of peripheral airways is a larger part of overall airway resistance in infants than in adults. In normal adults, the resistance of peripheral airways has little influence on the distribution of ventilation. This may not be true in infants. One may further speculate that a given amount of cellular debris and edema produces a greater degree of obstruction in an infant's small peripheral airways than in an older child's larger peripheral airways. The absence of effective collateral ventilation in infants may contribute to the development of patchy atelectasis and the abnormalities of gas exchange. Smooth muscle exists in the periphery of an infant's lung as it does in the lung of the older child, so the infant's airways may respond to mediator substances if these are released. Finally, there are changes in the cell composition of the lung and in the composition of mucus that may contribute, in yet undefined ways, to the reduction in the incidence and severity of bronchiolitis with increasing age (Reid, 1977).

Concurrent pulmonary pathology may also influence the severity of RSV infection. Infants who are premature and develop bronchopulmonary dysplasia appear to be at particular risk (Groothuis et al, 1988). Injury to respiratory epithelium, distortion of the pulmonary architecture, increased bronchial reactivity, and low levels of maternally acquired protective antibody are likely factors contributing to the severity of disease in the former premature infant. Other populations considered to be at increased risk of severe disease include infants with trisomy 21 and with congenital heart disease with pulmonary hypertension (MacDonald et al, 1982).

PATHOLOGY

The initial abnormalities of the lower respiratory tract in RSV bronchiolitis are necrosis of the respiratory epithelium and destruction of ciliated epithelial cells, followed by peribronchiolar infiltration with lymphocytes. The submucosa becomes edematous, but there is no destruction of collagen or elastic tissue Fig. 18–2. Cellular debris and fibrin form plugs within the bronchioles. The alveoli usually are normal, except those immediately adjacent to the inflamed bronchioles. Occasionally there is more extensive alveolar involvement, and the increased cellularity of the subepithelial tissue of the bronchi and bronchioles extends to distant intra-alveolar walls. In such cases, edema fluid may accumulate within alveoli (McLean, 1956; Aherne et al, 1970).

In addition to these changes, RSV may cause severe

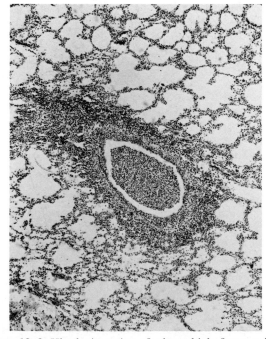

Figure 18–2. Histologic section of a bronchiole from an infant who later died of acute bronchiolitis. The respiratory syncytial virus was grown from necropsy specimens. Peribronchiolar lymphoid infiltration and plugging of the lumen with exudate and cell debris can be seen. The surrounding alveoli are little affected. (Courtesy of Dr. W Aherne.)

pneumonia with extensive destruction of respiratory epithelium, necrosis of lung parenchyma, and formation of hyaline membranes, similar to the pneumonia that occurs in adenovirus and parainfluenza type 3 infections (Aherne et al, 1970).

Recovery from acute bronchiolitis begins with regeneration of the bronchiolar epithelium after 3 or 4 days, but cilia do not appear until much later, probably about 15 days. Mucus plugs are removed by macrophages (Aherne et al, 1970).

PATHOPHYSIOLOGY

As a result of the edema of the airway wall and the accumulation of mucus and cellular debris, and perhaps even as a result of muscle spasm, many peripheral airways are narrowed, and some are partially and others totally occluded. The patchy distribution and variable degree of obstruction produce atelectasis in some areas of the lung and overdistention in others.

The mechanics of respiration are abnormal (Krieger, 1964; Phelan, Williams, and Freeman, 1968; Wohl et al, 1969). The infant breathes at a high lung volume, and resting end-expiratory lung volume (functional residual capacity) is approximately twice normal. Dynamic compliance is decreased, in part because the infant is breathing at a higher lung volume and hence on a stiffer portion of the volume-pressure curve of the lung, and in part because of the uneven distribution of resistances within the lung. Airway resistance is increased, although to a variable extent. Most studies have shown the greater increase to be on expiration, which is compatible with lower airway obstruction; the data of Krieger (1964), however, suggest a substantial upper airway (above the level of the carina) component to the obstruction. The decrease in compliance and increase in resistance result in a substantial increase in the work of breathing.

Serious alterations in gas exchange occur as a result of the airway obstruction and patchy distribution of atelectasis (Reynolds, 1963a; Downes et al, 1968; H Simpson et al, 1974; Hall, Hall, and Speers, 1979). Arterial hypoxemia develops as the result of mismatching of pulmonary ventilation and perfusion ($\dot{V}/\dot{Q}$ abnormality), with continued perfusion of underventilated units and overventilation of poorly perfused units. The evidence that $\dot{V}/\dot{Q}$ abnormalities usually account for the hypoxemia comes from the observation that the hypoxemia can be corrected by the administration of 40 per cent oxygen (Reynolds, 1963a). The tension of carbon dioxide in arterial blood is variable. In young infants in particular, some degree of carbon dioxide retention is noted sometime in the course of the disease. The likely mechanisms are severe $\dot{V}/\dot{Q}$ and hypoventilation secondary to the markedly increased work of breathing. Blood pH is variable. Some infants exhibit a mild respiratory alkalosis. More commonly, metabolic acidosis is ob-

served. Poor caloric and fluid intake and the administration of salicylate may contribute to the ketoacidosis in such infants. Finally, carbon dioxide retention can produce acute respiratory acidosis.

DIAGNOSIS

The diagnosis of acute viral bronchiolitis is suggested by the clinical presentation, the age of the child, and the presence of an epidemic of RSV in the community. Viral identification can be performed rapidly on nasal secretions using immunofluorescent techniques now available for RSV and most other respiratory viruses. Routine laboratory tests are not specific. Chest roentgenograms, as noted previously, may be normal or may show peribronchial thickening, patchy atelectasis, segmental collapse, or hyperinflation. The white blood cell count ranges from 5000 to 24,000 cells/mm.[3] In patients with elevated white blood cell counts, there is a preponderance of polymorphonuclear leukocytes and band forms. A determination of hemoglobin level is not useful diagnostically but is helpful in assessing the effects of a decrease in arterial oxygen tension.

Other causes of chest retraction and airway obstruction need to be ruled out by careful physical and radiographic examination. These include obstruction of the nasopharynx by hypertrophied adenoids or a retropharyngeal abscess; laryngeal obstruction caused by abnormalities of the larynx, croup, or a foreign body; and lobar emphysema. Occasionally, the hyperpnea of metabolic disorders such as salicylate poisoning may mimic bronchiolitis. Measurements of arterial blood gas tensions, pII, salicylate level (if salicylates have been given), and serum electrolytes aid in making the proper diagnosis. Congestive heart failure secondary to a congenital malformation or viral myocarditis may manifest clinical findings very similar to those of bronchiolitis, and the palpable liver and spleen found frequently in infants with bronchiolitis may contribute to the confusion. A history of normal growth and development and the absence of a cardiac murmur assist in the diagnosis. Cardiac size should be evaluated on chest roentgenogram, and in case of doubt, an electrocardiogram should be obtained. However, infants with cardiac disease often develop congestive heart failure during viral infections, and the two conditions may coexist. The lung disease of cystic fibrosis may present as acute bronchiolitis. Certainty of diagnosis requires the identification of the virus or the viral antigen in nasopharyngeal secretions. Detection of antigen is now done by enzyme-linked immunosorbent assay (ELISA) or immunofluorescence, and results can be available within hours. If samples are properly obtained by aspiration or gentle washing, are inoculated at the bedside (Hall and Douglass, 1975), or are transported promptly on wet ice, not frozen, to a culture laboratory and are inoculated onto sensitive tissue culture cell lines, results can be available within a few days for RSV and some other common viruses.

TREATMENT

Mild bronchiolitis is often treated at home. For infants with mild respiratory distress, careful observation and adequate fluid administration are appropriate. Infants with moderate or severe respiratory distress should usually be hospitalized. The aims of treatment in hospital are (1) to support the infant, (2) to detect and treat possible complications, and (3) to treat with specific antiviral agents if indicated. Controversies in the treatment of bronchiolitis center around the use of specific antiviral agents and the use of bronchodilators.

Supportive care for hospitalized infants with bronchiolitis includes administration of oxygen; careful monitoring to detect hypoxemia, apnea, and respiratory failure; attention to temperature regulation; and appropriate fluid administration.

The major consequence of the airway obstruction and concomitant maldistribution of ventilation and perfusion is hypoxemia. Oxygen should be administered to infants with all but the mildest illnesses. Any techniques familiar to nursing personnel may be used, provided that the oxygen is humidified and the flow rate of gas through the device is sufficient to prevent accumulation of carbon dioxide. The inspired oxygen concentration must be monitored frequently. Concentrations of 35 to 40 per cent have been found to correct the arterial hypoxemia in most, but not all, infants (Reynolds, 1963a; H Simpson et al, 1974). In infants with no history of chronic obstructive pulmonary disease, oxygen can be safely administered without fear of significantly depressing respiration by blunting the hypoxic drive. However, a growing number of infants of very low birth weight are surviving respiratory distress syndrome of the newborn to be left with bronchopulmonary dysplasia of variable severity. Acute viral bronchiolitis presents special problems in such infants. Some of them have chronic compensated carbon dioxide retention. Further impairment of gas exchange may make them severely hypoxemic. The administration of increased concentrations of inspired oxygen may be associated with further carbon dioxide retention because hypoxemia may be their major respiratory stimulus. Frequent measurement of oxygen saturation by pulse oximeter is required in these patients, and the minimum inspired concentrations consistent with an arterial saturation of 94 to 96 per cent should be delivered. Care should be taken to measure saturations while the infant is quiet, because decreases in oxygen saturations can occur when an infant cries, for example. Unnecessarily high inspired oxygen tensions will be delivered if the goal is the prevention of any episode of desaturation, however brief. Carbon dioxide retention should be monitored by periodic assessment of arterial blood gas tensions. It should be noted that in patients with chronic carbon dioxide and bicarbonate retention, a decrease in the hypoxic drive associated with administration of oxygen usually produces additional carbon dioxide retention. This retention is to be expected and need not reflect worsening of the underlying disease.

Mist has not proved beneficial to any appreciable degree, because little water reaches the lower respiratory tract to liquefy secretions.

With fever, chilling, or shivering, oxygen consumption is increased. Small infants should be nursed in incubators or under radiant warmers; care should be taken that temperature is controlled in oxygen tents or other devices used for the administration of oxygen.

Because RSV is shed in high titers for days after the onset of illness and hospital-acquired infections are common (Hall, Douglas, and Geiman, 1975; Hall, Douglas, Geiman, and Messner, 1975; Hall et al, 1978), careful attention must be paid to the prevention of transmission of infection to staff and other patients. Limitation of child-to-child contact, cohorting of patients, and careful hand washing are useful methods of limiting nosocomial infections with RSV, but the most practical measure may be glove and gown precautions applied to all infants with suspected viral bronchiolitis (Leclair et al, 1987).

On admission to hospital, some infants are dehydrated because of poor fluid intake and have mild metabolic acidosis. Intravenous fluids should be given with care. It may be speculated that in the presence of the large negative intrapleural pressures required to overcome the airway obstruction, added demands are made on the left ventricle. Furthermore, the negative intrathoracic pressures are probably transmitted to the interstitium surrounding the fluid-exchanging vessels, enhancing fluid accumulation in the lung. The uneven distribution of the airway obstruction may result in amplification of these negative pressures, further enhancing fluid accumulation. The details of these mechanisms are discussed in Chapter 38.

The routine administration of antibiotics has not been shown to influence the course of bronchiolitis (Field et al, 1966; Friis et al, 1984), and there is little rationale for their use. Lack of rapid diagnostic techniques to identify RSV or other viruses, the uncertainty about the cause of the disease in small, acutely ill infants, and the concern that viral infection may predispose to secondary bacterial invasion are arguments used to justify the administration of antibiotics. In children in whom a viral cause can be established, who present with clinical features consistent with viral infection, including otitis media and segmental atelectasis, both common features of RSV infection, treatment with antibiotics is not recommended. A recent study (Hall et al, 1988) of children under 2 years of age who were hospitalized with RSV lower respiratory infection reports that those children given parenteral antibiotics for 5 days or longer had a 9 per cent incidence of secondary bacterial infection in contrast to the overall incidence of 1.2 per cent. The diversity of bacterial organisms reported in association with viral lower respiratory tract disease (Zoller et al, 1973; Hall et al, 1988) mandates that tracheal secretions be examined by Gram stain and cultured if clinical deterioration takes place, and infants who present with or develop fever, elevated or shifted peripheral white blood cell counts, or clinical features suggesting sepsis should have bacterial cultures of blood, urine, and cerebrospinal fluid.

The role of bronchodilators is controversial. The relative importance of mechanical obstruction secondary to edema, accumulated secretions, and cellular debris and of potentially reversible smooth muscle contraction is unknown. Revival of interest in measurements of mechanics of respiration in infants has led to a number of studies evaluating the use of nebulized and inhaled sympathomimetic agents such as albuterol and of atropine derivatives such as ipratropium bromide (Hughes et al, 1987). The results are inconclusive, in part because of the large variability in measurements and the relative insensitivity of the test used. The aim of therapy should be improvement in gas exchange, and as yet there are no well-designed control studies evaluating treatment with bronchodilators on parameters of gas exchange or outcome variables such as duration of hospitalization. Ipratropium bromide, sympathomimetic agents, and theophylline may yet prove to benefit selected patients.

Initial studies of the treatment of bronchiolitis with corticosteroids suggested that these drugs might favorably influence mortality and morbidity. However, large controlled studies have failed to demonstrate any significant clinical effect (Leer et al, 1969). In particular, the response to corticosteroids in infants with a family history of allergy differed not at all from the response in infants without such a history. A small but well-designed study (Tal et al, 1983) has demonstrated clinical improvement in infants treated with inhaled salbutamol and intramuscular dexamethasone, but no alteration in parameters of gas exchange.

Ribavirin, a synthetic nucleoside analog resembling guanosine, has been shown to have a wide antiviral effect, probably by inhibiting viral protein synthesis. Delivered as a small-particle aerosol for 18 to 20 hours per day, it has led to improvement in oxygenation and clinical state (Hall et al, 1983; Taber et al, 1983; Hall et al, 1985). Candidates for treatment currently include infants at high risk; those with bronchopulmonary dysplasia, chronic pulmonary infection such as cystic fibrosis, immunodeficiencies, and congenital heart disease; infants who are severely ill (hypoxemic with increasing levels of carbon dioxide); and infants in whom respiratory disease might be particularly "detrimental to an underlying condition" (Committee on Infectious Diseases, 1987). Despite initial concerns, the drug can be effectively given to patients on ventilators (Outwater et al, 1988). The somewhat modest improvement demonstrated

in studies carefully evaluating the benefits, the overall low mortality rates associated with bronchiolitis caused by RSV in developed countries, the somewhat difficult and cumbersome methods of delivery, and concerns about the long-term teratogenicity are reasons most clinicians restrict the administration of ribavirin to high-risk infants.

Immunotherapeutic approaches to bronchiolitis are under investigation. A preliminary trial of human intravenous immunoglobulin containing high titers of RSV-neutralizing antibody demonstrated a reduction in titers of RSV shed and an improvement in oxygenation although no overall influence on morbidity in the treated group (Hemming et al, 1987).

COURSE AND COMPLICATIONS

Although they may appear extremely ill on admission to the hospital, most infants with bronchiolitis, given adequate supportive care, are clinically improved within 3 to 4 days (Heycock and Noble, 1962). By 2 weeks after the height of the illness, the respiratory rate is normal, and arterial oxygen and carbon dioxide tensions are within the normal range in most infants (Reynolds, 1963b). Radiographic abnormalities have generally cleared by 9 days from admission (Rice and Loda, 1966).

However, the clinical course may be prolonged (Heycock and Noble, 1962). Approximately 20 per cent of infants have a protracted course, with persistent wheezing and hyperinflation of chest, evidence of continued airway obstruction on physiologic studies (Phelan, Williams, and Freeman, 1968; Wohl et al, 1969), and persistent abnormalities of gas exchange (Reynolds, 1963b). These abnormalities may persist for many months. In addition, some infants with proven RSV bronchiolitis go on to develop lobar collapse (Rice and Loda, 1966); the cause is unknown, but the radiographic abnormality may persist for several weeks or longer.

Sudden clinical deterioration followed by apnea can occur (Bruhn et al, 1977; Hall, Hall, and Speers, 1979), even in infants in whom frequent monitoring of arterial gases did not indicate progressive carbon dioxide retention. At present, the cause of apnea remains unexplained, but upper airway obstruction and hypoxia may be contributing factors.

Estimates of the number of hospitalized infants requiring mechanical ventilation vary but can be as high as 7 per cent in a retrospective study of bronchiolitis admissions in 1982–1983 (Outwater and Crone, 1984). The major indications for intubation and mechanical ventilation were clinical deterioration (worsening respiratory distress, heart rates over 200 beats/min, listlessness, and poor peripheral perfusion), apnea and/or bradycardia, and hypercarbia. No infant required intubation for oxygenation alone. The median duration of mechanical ventilation was 5 days, but 4 of 15 infants were ventilated for periods ranging from 9 to 18 days.

RELATIONSHIP TO ASTHMA

Numerous observations have been made of the high incidence (30 to 50 per cent) of asthma developing subsequently in children who had bronchiolitis during infancy (Wittig et al, 1959; Eisen and Bacal, 1963; Simon and Jordan, 1967). There is a strong association between proven RSV bronchiolitis and the subsequent development of asthma. More than half of the children studied 2 to 7 years after proven RSV bronchiolitis have recurrent episodes of wheezing characteristic of asthma (Rooney and Williams, 1971). The clinical continuum between the infant with bronchiolitis and the older child with virus-related wheezing (McIntosh, 1976; McIntosh and Fishaut, 1980) suggests shared pathogenic mechanisms as well as shared pathologic changes. Antigen can coexist with antibody of the IgA, IgM, and IgG classes in the upper respiratory tract (McIntosh et al, 1979). Virus-specific IgE antibody has been detected in nasopharyngeal secretions of infants with bronchiolitis caused by RSV and by parainfluenza virus (Welliver, Sun, Rinaldo, and Ogra, 1986; Welliver, Wong, Sun, and McCarthy, 1986). The titers of anti-RSV IgE antibody during an episode of bronchiolitis are good predictors of further episodes of wheezing. Elevated levels of histamine and arachidonic acid metabolites, isolated from secretions of infants with bronchiolitis and from blood of children with asthma (Skoner et al, 1988), further support shared pathologic mechanisms in bronchiolitis and asthma.

LONG-TERM SEQUELAE

In some infants, lung function studies remain abnormal for months after bronchiolitis. However, until recently it was believed that no residual effects of the disease persist into late childhood except for a greater than expected incidence of asthma. A number of studies (Katten et al, 1977; Sims et al, 1978; Gurwitz et al, 1981; Pullen and Hey, 1982) now document that infants hospitalized with bronchiolitis or RSV infection or both continue to demonstrate abnormalities in lung function. As a group, these children, when seen at ages 8 to 11 years and compared with control children, have experienced more frequent episodes of wheezing, demonstrate increased bronchial hyperreactivity, and have small but significant alterations in measurements of lung function. Lung function abnormalities are present even in those children who had no further episodes of wheezing. These abnormalities are not accompanied by skin test evidence of atopy. These studies have not been able to determine whether the bronchiolitis or RSV infection was responsible for the subsequent abnormalities. It may be that both hospitalizations for bronchiolitis and the subsequent abnormalities in lung function are manifestations of individual differences in airway reactivity, function, or size.

BRONCHIOLITIS OBLITERANS

Bronchiolitis obliterans, a chronic form of bronchiolitis first described by Lange in 1901, has been reported following inhalation of hydrochloric and nitric acids and sulfur dioxide (Blumgart and MacMahon, 1929; Azizirad et al, 1975; Charan et al, 1979). It has been described in adults, in association with rheumatoid arthritis (Geddes et al, 1977) and in association with childhood onset of lupus erythematosus (Nadorra and Landing, 1987). Attention has been focused on its occurrence as a component, often severe, of graft-versus-host disease in bone marrow transplantation (Ralph et al, 1984; Chan et al, 1987) and its occurrence after heart-lung transplantation in young adults (McGregor et al, 1986).

In infants and young children, bronchiolitis obliterans following infections with adenovirus has been well described (Lang et al, 1969; Gold et al, 1969; Cumming et al, 1971; Strieder and Nash, 1975). The initial clinical presentation does not differ from that of acute bronchiolitis caused by the RSV, except for the fact that rhinorrhea is not a prominent feature and evidence for bronchopneumonia is more common. The infant becomes ill with cough and fever and goes on to develop dyspnea and wheezing. On physical examination, wheezes and rales are heard. The radiographic features are initially nonspecific and consist of peribronchial thickening and increased interstitial markings with areas of patchy bronchopneumonia. Collapse and consolidation of segments or lobes are common.

Characteristically, the clinical and radiographic features of the disease wax and wane for several weeks or months, with recurrent episodes of atelectasis, pneumonia, and wheezing. Recovery assessed clinically may be complete, but approximately 60 per cent of children with documented adenovirus pneumonia or bronchiolitis go on to develop evidence of chronic pulmonary disease. Persistent atelectasis (particularly of the right upper lobe in young children and of the left lower lobe in older children), bronchiectasis, recurrent pneumonias, generalized hyperinflation, increased pulmonary markings on chest radiographs, and the development of the unilateral hyperlucent lung syndrome are among the reported long-term complications of adenovirus infection, particularly types 7 and 21. At least half of children admitted with adenovirus type 7 pneumonia had evidence of substantial airways obstruction when studied about 12 years later (Sly et al, 1984).

Little is known about host factors that predispose to this unusual form of bronchiolitis. Maternal antibody may be protective, because the disease characteristically occurs in infants older than 6 months. In Canada it is seen more frequently in the Indian population, and in New Zealand in Polynesian children, suggesting that racial or socioeconomic factors may be important (Wohl and Chernick, 1978). No infectious agent has been clearly implicated in the bronchiolitis obliterans associated with bone marrow transplantation and graft-versus-host disease.

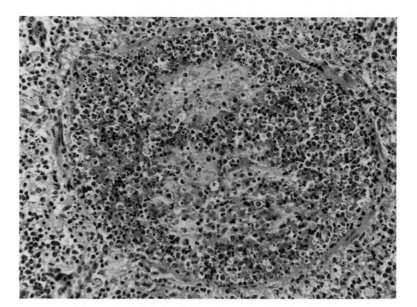

Figure 18–3. Necrotizing adenovirus bronchiolitis. The epithelial lining has been completely destroyed, and the lumen is filled with cellular debris. The smooth muscle is still largely intact. Adenovirus type 3 was recovered in tissue culture. (Original magnification ×240; courtesy of Dr. J Hoogstraten.) (Reproduced with permission from Wohl ME and Chernick V: Bronchiolitis. Am Rev Respir Dis 118:759, 1978.)

In lungs examined histologically, abnormalities of large and medium-sized bronchi range from hypertrophy and piling up of the bronchial epithelium to cellular infiltration of the wall extending to the peribronchial space, with destruction and disorganization of the muscle and elastic tissue of the wall. Fibrosis of the wall and surrounding areas occurs. The most striking changes occur in the small bronchi and bronchioles. Here the mucosa is destroyed and the lumen is filled with fibrous tissue (Figs. 18–3 and 18–4). Typically, the terminal bronchioles are occluded and the distal respiratory bronchioles are dilated. The vessels are narrowed, and areas of overdistention, atelectasis, and fibrosis occur within the alveolar region of the lung.

Bronchograms reveal marked pruning of the bronchial tree, and pulmonary angiograms reveal decreased vasculature in the involved lung (Fig. 18–5). These findings may be localized, as in those children who develop unilateral hyperlucent lung syndrome, or may be more diffuse. Similar sequelae, either diffuse or localized as described by Swyer and James (1953) and Macleod (1954), have also been observed after other infections, including influenza and *Mycoplasma* infections (Laraya-Cuasay et al, 1977; Stokes et al, 1978). These sequelae should be considered in the diagnostic evaluation of children who develop recurrent infections and fixed airway obstruction after what may be presumed to be severe viral bronchiolitis and pneumonia. However, there are few data to support the association of bronchiolitis obliterans with RSV infections, and bronchiolitis obliterans should not be considered a complication of RSV bronchiolitis.

The incidence of bronchiolitis obliterans in the pediatric population is not known. Between 1960 and 1985, 19 cases were identified at a large urban teaching hospital (Hardy et al, 1988). In some of these patients, aspiration and gastroesophageal reflux appeared to contribute to the development of the

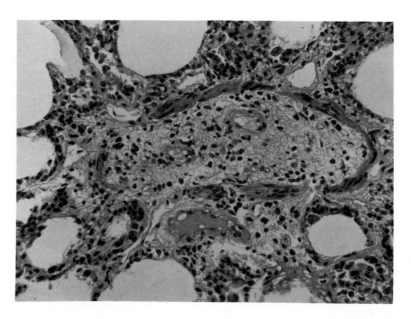

Figure 18–4. Obliterative bronchiolitis in a 1.5-year-old child who had had severe adenovirus bronchiolitis and pneumonia 1 year previously. The obliterated lumen of the bronchiole is filled with vascularized connective tissue. (Original magnification ×240; courtesy of Dr. J Hoogstraten.) (Reproduced with permission from Wohl ME and Chernick V: Bronchiolitis. Am Rev Respir Dis 118:759, 1978.)

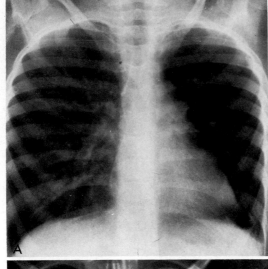

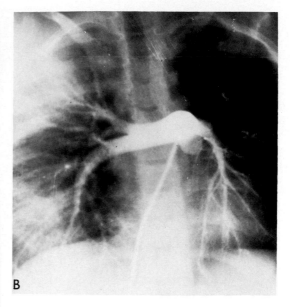

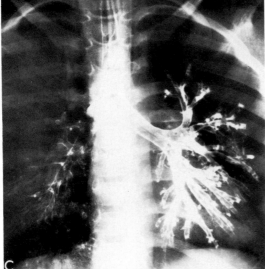

Figure 18–5. Left unilateral hyperlucent lung in a 4-year-old child secondary to adenovirus infection in early infancy. *A*, Plain chest film shows increased radiolucency of the left lung due to decreased bronchovascular markings. *B*, Decreased blood flow to the left lung is evident on the pulmonary angiogram. *C*, Bronchogram demonstrates a typical "pruned-tree" appearance. (Reproduced with permission from Wohl ME and Chernick V: Bronchiolitis. Am Rev Respir Dis 118:759, 1978.)

disease. Patients who have persistent wheezing and cough following viral or *Mycoplasma* pneumonia, who have persistent localized physical findings after a respiratory insult, who develop progressive airways obstruction poorly responsive to bronchodilators after bone marrow transplantation, or who develop or are found to have unilateral or patchy regions of hyperlucency on chest radiographs should be considered for further investigation including ventilation-perfusion scans, bronchoscopy, bronchography, and lung biopsy. As this process is better understood and the clinical features better defined, therapeutic interventions may develop.

Some pathologic studies of bronchopulmonary dysplasia in infants have focused on the importance of the damage to the ciliary apparatus, the severe necrotizing bronchiolitis, and the obliterative bronchiolar fibrosis that occur in this disease (Bonikos, 1976). Thus in adults and in children, a chronic, necrotizing, and ultimately fibrosing process may occur in response to epithelial injury associated with chemicals, oxygen, barotrauma, and infection.

REFERENCES

Aherne W, Bird T, Court SDM et al: Pathological changes in virus infections of the lower respiratory tract in children. J Clin Pathol 23:7, 1970.

Anas N, Boettrich C, Hall CB, and Brooks JG: The association of apnea and respiratory syncytial virus infection in infants. J Pediatr 101:65, 1982.

Azizirad H, Polgar G, Borns PF, and Chatten J: Bronchiolitis obliterans. Clin Pediatr 14:572, 1975.

Becroft DMO: Bronchiolitis obliterans, bronchiectasis, and other sequelae of adenovirus type 21 infection in young children. J Clin Pathol 24:72, 1971.

Beem W, Wright FH, Hamre D et al: Association of the chimpanzee coryza agent with acute respiratory disease in children. N Engl J Med 263:523, 1960.

Blumgart HL and MacMahon HE: Bronchiolitis fibrosa obliterans: a clinical and pathologic study. Med Clin North Am 13:197, 1929.

Bonikos DS, Bensch KG, Northway WH Jr, and Edwards DK: Bronchopulmonary dysplasia: the pulmonary pathologic sequel of necrotizing bronchiolitis and pulmonary fibrosis. Hum Pathol 7:643, 1976.

Brandt CD, Kim HW, Arrobio JO et al: Epidemiology of respiratory syncytial virus infection in Washington, D.C. III. Composite analysis of eleven consecutive yearly epidemics. Am J Epidemiol 98:355, 1973.

Bruhn FW, Mokrohisky ST, and McIntosh K: Apnea associated with respiratory syncytial virus infection in young infants. Pediatrics 90:382, 1977.

Bui RH, Molinaro GA, Kettering JD, et al: Virus-specific IgE and IgG4 antibodies in serum of children infected with respiratory syncytial virus. J Pediatr 110:87, 1987.

Chan CK, Hyland RH, Hutcheon MA et al: Small-airways disease in recipients of allogeneic bone marrow transplants. Medicine 66:327, 1987.

Chanock R and Finberg L: Recovery from infants with respiratory illness of a virus related to chimpanzee coryza agent (CCA). II. Epidemiologic aspects of infection in infants and young children. Am J Hyg 66:291, 1957.

Chanock RM, Kapikian AZ, Mills J et al: Influence of immunological factors in respiratory tract. Arch Environ Health 21:347, 1970.

Charan NB, Myers CG, Lakshminarayan S, and Spencer, TM: Pulmonary injuries associated with acute sulfur dioxide inhalation. Am Rev Resp Dis 119:555, 1979.

Committee on Infectious Diseases: Ribavirin therapy of respiratory syncytial virus. Pediatrics 79:475, 1987.

Cradock-Watson JE, McQuillin J, and Gardner PS: Rapid diagnosis of respiratory syncytial virus infection in children by the immunofluorescent technique. J Clin Pathol 24:308, 1971.

Cumming GR, Macpherson RI, and Chernick V: Unilateral hyperlucent lung syndrome in children. J Pediatr 78:250, 1971.

Downes JJ, Wood DW, Striker TW, and Haddad C: Acute respiratory failure in infants with bronchiolitis. Anesthesiology 29:426, 1968.

Eisen AH and Bacal HL: The relationship of acute bronchiolitis to bronchial asthma—a 4- to 14-year follow-up. Pediatrics 31:859, 1963.

Epler GR, Snider GL, Gaensler EA et al: Bronchiolitis and bronchitis in connective tissue disease. JAMA 242:528, 1979.

Field CMB, Connally JH, Murtagh G et al: Antibiotic treatment of epidemic bronchiolitis—a double-blind trial. Br Med J 1:83, 1966.

Fishaut M, Tubergen D, and McIntosh K: Cellular response to respiratory viruses with particular reference to children with disorders of cell-mediated immunity. J Pediatr 96:179, 1980.

Friis B, Anderson P, Brenoe E et al: Antibiotic treatment of pneumonia and bronchiolitis a prospective randomised study. Arch Dis Child 59:1038, 1984.

Gardner PS: Respiratory syncytial virus infections. Postgrad Med J 49:788, 1973.

Gardner PS, McQuillin J, and Court SDM: Speculation on pathogenesis in death from respiratory syncytial virus infection. Br Med J 1:327, 1970.

Geddes DN, Corrin B, Brewerton DA et al: Progressive airway obliteration in adults and its association with rheumatoid disease. Q J Med 46:427, 1977.

Glezen WP and Denny FW: Epidemiology of acute lower respiratory disease in children. N Engl J Med 288:498, 1973.

Glezen WP, Paredes A, Allison JE et al: Risk of respiratory syncytial virus infection for infants from low-income families in relationship to age, sex, ethnic group, and maternal antibody level. J Pediatr 98:708, 1981.

Groothuis JR, Gutierrez KM, and Lauer BA: Respiratory syncytial virus infection in children with bronchopulmonary dysplasia. Pediatrics 82:199, 1988.

Gold R, Wilt JC, Adhikari PK, and Macpherson RI: Adenoviral pneumonia and its complications in infancy and childhood. J Can Assoc Radiol 20:218, 1969.

Gurwitz D, Mindorff C, and Levison H: Increased incidence of bronchial reactivity in children with a history of bronchiolitis. J Pediatr 98:551, 1981.

Hall CB and Douglas RG: Clinically useful method for the isolation of respiratory syncytial virus. J Infect Dis 131:1, 1975.

Hall CB and Douglas RG: Modes of transmission of respiratory syncytial virus. J Pediatr 99:100, 1981.

Hall CB, Douglas RG, and Geiman JM: Quantitative shedding patterns of respiratory syncytial virus in infants. J Infect Dis 132:151, 1975.

Hall CB, Douglas RG, Geiman JM, and Messner MK: Nosocomial respiratory syncytial virus infections. N Engl J Med 293:1343, 1975.

Hall CB, Geiman JM, Biggar R et al: Respiratory syncytial virus infections within families. N Engl J Med 294:414, 1976.

Hall CB, Geiman JM, Douglas RG Jr, and Meager MP: Control of nosocomial respiratory syncytial viral infections. Pediatrics 62:728, 1978.

Hall CB, Hall WJ, and Speers DM: Clinical and physiological manifestations of bronchiolitis and pneumonia. Am J Dis Child 133:798, 1979.

Hall CB, Kopelman AE, Douglas RG et al: Neonatal respiratory syncytial virus infection. N Engl J Med 300:393, 1979.

Hall CB, McBride JT, Gala CL et al: Ribavirin treatment of respiratory syncytial viral infection in infants with underlying cardiopulmonary disease. JAMA 254:3047, 1985.

Hall CB, McBride JT, Walsh EE et al: Aerosolized ribavirin treatment of infants with respiratory syncytial viral infection. N Engl J Med 308:1443, 1983.

Hall CB, Powell KR, Schnabel KC et al: Risk of secondary bacterial infection in infants hospitalized with respiratory syncytial viral infection. J Pediatr 113:266, 1988.

Hardy KA, Schidlow DV, and Zaeri N: Obliterative bronchiolitis in children. Chest 93:460, 1988.

Hemming VG, Rodriguez W, Kim HW et al: Intravenous immunoglobulin treatment of respiratory syncytial virus infections in infants and young children. Antimicrob Agents Chemother 31:1882, 1987.

Henderson FW, Clyde WA, Collier AM et al: The etiologic and epidemiologic spectrum of bronchiolitis in pediatric practice. J Pediatr 95:183, 1979.

Henderson FW, Collier AM, Clyde WA Jr, and Denny FW: Respiratory-syncytial-virus infections, reinfections and immunity. N Engl J Med 300:530, 1979.

Heycock JB and Noble TC: 1,230 cases of acute bronchiolitis in infancy. Br Med J 2:879, 1962.

Hughes DM, Lesouef PN, and Landau LI: Effect of salbutamol on respiratory mechanics in bronchiolitis. Pediatr Res 22:83, 1987.

James AG, Lang WR, Liang AY et al: Adenovirus type 21 bronchopneumonia in infants and young children. J Pediatr 95:530, 1979.

Kattan M, Keens TG, Lapierre J et al: Pulmonary function abnormalities in symptom-free children after bronchiolitis. Pediatrics 59:683, 1977.

Kim HW, Arrobio JO, Brandt CD et al: Epidemiology of respiratory syncytial virus infection in Washington, D.C. I. Importance of the virus in different respiratory tract disease syndromes and temporal distribution of infection. Am J Epidemiol 98:216, 1973.

Kim HW, Leikin SL, Arrobio J et al: Cell-mediated immunity to respiratory syncytial virus induced by inactivated vaccine or by infection. Pediatr Res 10:75, 1976.

Krieger I: Mechanics of respiration in bronchiolitis. Pediatrics 33:45, 1964.

Lang WR, Howden CW, Laws J, and Burton JF: Bronchopneumonia with serious sequelae in children with evidence of adenovirus type 21 infection. Br Med J 1:73, 1969.

Lange W: Über eine eigentumliche Erkrankung der klemen: Branchen and Branchiolen (Bronchitis et Bronchiolitis obliterans). Deutsch Arch Klin Med 70:342, 1901.

Laraya-Cuasay LR, DeForest A, Huff D et al: Chronic pulmonary complications of early influenza virus infection in children. Am Rev Respir Dis 116:617, 1977.

Leclair JM, Freeman J, Sullivan BF, et al: Prevention of nosocomial respiratory syncytial virus infections through compliance with glove and gown isolation precautions. N Engl J Med 317:330, 1987.

Leer JA, Green JL, Heimlick EM et al: Corticosteroid treatment in bronchiolitis. A controlled, collaborative study in 297 infants and children. Am J Dis Child 117:495, 1969.

McConnochie KM: Bronchiolitis. Am J Dis Child 137:11, 1983.

MacDonald NE, Hall CB, Suffin SC et al: Respiratory syncytial viral infection in infants with congenital heart disease. N Engl J Med 307:397, 1982.

McGregor CGA, Jamieson SW, Baldwin JC et al: Combined heart-lung transplantation for end-stage Eisenmenger's syndrome. J Thorac Cardiovasc Surg 91:443, 1986.

McIntosh K: Bronchiolitis and asthma: possible common pathogenetic pathways. J Allergy Clin Immunol 57:595, 1976.

McIntosh K and Chanock RM: Respiratory synctial virus. In Fields BN, Knipe DM, Chanock RM et al (eds): Virology. 2nd ed. New York, Raven Press, 1990.

McIntosh K and Fishaut JM: Immunopathologic mechanisms in lower respiratory tract disease of infants due to respiratory syncytial virus. In Melnick JL (ed): Progress in Medical Virology. New York, S Karger, 1980.

McIntosh K, McQuillin J, and Gardner PS: Cell-free and cell-bound antibody in nasal secretions from infants with respiratory syncytial virus infection. Infect Immun 23:276, 1979.

McLean KH: The pathology of acute bronchiolitis—a study of its evolution. I. The exudative phase. Australas Ann Med 5:254, 1956.

Macleod WM: Abnormal transradiancy of one lung. Thorax 9:147, 1954.

Mito K, Chiba Y, Suga K, and Nakao T: Cellular immune response to infection with respiratory syncytial virus and influence of breast-feeding on the response. J Med Virol 14:323, 1984.

Morrell RE, Marks MI, Champlin R, and Spence L: An outbreak of severe pneumonia due to respiratory syncytial virus in isolated arctic populations. Am J Epidemiol 101:231, 1975.

Nadorra RL and Landing BH: Pulmonary lesions in childhood onset systemic lupus erthematosus: analysis of 26 cases, and summary of literature. Pediatr Pathol 7:1, 1987.

Outwater KM and Crone RK: Management of respiratory failure in infants with acute viral bronchiolitis. Am J Dis Child 138:1071, 1984.

Outwater KM, Meissner HC, and Peterson MB: Ribavirin administration to infants receiving mechanical ventilation. Am J Dis Child 142:512, 1988.

Parrott RH, Kim HW, Arrobio JO et al: Epidemiology of respiratory syncytial virus infection in Washington, D.C. II. Infection and disease with respect to age, immunologic status, race and sex. Am J Epidemiol 98:289, 1973.

Phelan PD and Williams HE: Sympathomimetic drugs in acute viral bronchiolitis. Their effect on pulmonary resistance. Pediatrics 44:493, 1969.

Phelan PD, Williams HE, and Freeman M: The disturbances of ventilation in acute viral bronchiolitis. Aust Paediatr J 4:96, 1968.

Pullan CR and Hey EN: Wheezing, asthma, and pulmonary dysfunction 10 years after infection with respiratory syncytial virus in infancy. Br Med J 284:1665, 1982.

Ralph DD, Springmeyer SC, Sullivan KM et al: Rapidly progressive air-flow obstruction in marrow transplant recipients. Am Rev Respir Dis 129:641, 1984.

Reid L: Influence of the pattern of structural growth of lung on susceptibility to specific infectious diseases in infants and children. Pediatr Res 11:210, 1977.

Reilly CM, Stokes J, McClelland L et al: Studies of acute respiratory illnesses caused by respiratory syncytial virus. 3. Clinical and laboratory findings. N Engl J Med 264:1176, 1961.

Reynolds EOR: The effect of breathing 40 per cent oxygen on the arterial blood gas tensions of babies with bronchiolitis. J Pediatr 63:1135, 1963a.

Reynolds EOR: Recovery from bronchiolitis as judged by arterial blood gas tension measurements. J Pediatr 63:1182, 1963b.

Rice RP and Loda F: A roentgenographic analysis of respiratory syncytial virus pneumonia in infants. Radiology 87:1021, 1966.

Rooney JC and Williams HE: The relationship between proved viral bronchiolitis and subsequent wheezing. J Pediatr 79:744, 1971.

Simon G and Jordan WS: Infections and allergic aspects of bronchiolitis. J Pediatr 70:533, 1967.

Simpson H, Matthew DJ, Inglis JM, and George EL: Virological findings and blood gas tensions in acute lower respiratory tract infections in children. Br Med J 2:629, 1974.

Simpson W, Hacking PM, Court SDM, and Gardner PS: The radiological findings in respiratory syncytial virus infection in children II. The correlation of radiological categories with clinical and virological findings. Pediatr Radiol 2:155, 1974.

Sims DG, Downham MAPS, Gardner PS et al: Study of 8-year-old children with a history of respiratory syncytial virus bronchiolitis in infancy. Br Med J 1:11, 1978.

Skoner DP, Page R, Asman B et al: Plasma elevation of histamine and a prostoglandin metabolite in acute asthma. Am Rev Respir Dis 137:1009, 1988.

Sly PD, Soto-Quiros ME, Landau LI et al: Factors predisposing to abnormal pulmonary function after adenovirus type 7 pneumonia. Arch Dis Child 59:935, 1984.

Stokes D, Sigler A, Khouri N, and Talamo RC: Unilateral hyperlucent lung (Swyer-James syndrome) after severe Mycoplasma pneumoniae infection. Am Rev Respir Dis 117:145, 1978.

Strieder DJ and Nash G: Case records of the Massachusetts General Hospital. N Engl J Med 292:634, 1975.

Swyer P and James G: Case of unilateral pulmonary emphysema. Thorax 8:133, 1953.

Taber LH, Knight V, Gilbert BE et al: Ribavirin aerosol treatment of bronchiolitis associated with respiratory syncytial virus infection in infants. Pediatrics 72:613, 1983.

Tal A, Bavilski C, Yohai D et al: Dexamethasone and salbutamol in the treatment of acute wheezing in infants. Pediatrics 71:13, 1983.

Volovitz B, Faden H and Ogra PL: Release of leukotriene C4 in respiratory tract during acute viral infection. J Pediatr 112:218, 1988.

Welliver RC, Kaul A, and Ogra PL: Cell-mediated immune response to respiratory syncytial virus infection: relationship to the development of reactive airway disease. J Pediatr 94:370, 1979.

Welliver RC, Sun M, Rinaldo D, and Ogra PL: Predictive value of respiratory syncytial virus-specific IgE responses for recurrent wheezing following bronchiolitis. J Pediatr 109:776, 1986.

Welliver RC, Wong DT, Sun M, and McCarthy N: Parainfluenza virus bronchiolitis epidemiology and pathogenesis. Am J Dis Child 140:34, 1986.

Welliver RC, Wong DT, Sun M et al: The development of respiratory syncytial virus–specific IgE and the release of histamine in nasopharyngeal secretions after infection. N Engl J Med 305:841, 1981.

Wittig HJ, Cranford NJ, and Glaser J: The relationship between bronchiolitis and childhood asthma. J Allergy 30:20, 1959.

Wohl MEB and Chernick V: Bronchiolitis. Am Rev Respir Dis 118:759, 1978.

Wohl MEB, Stigol LC, and Mead J: Resistance of the total respiratory system in healthy infants and infants with bronchiolitis. Pediatrics 43:495, 1969.

Zollar LM, Krause HE, and Mufson MA: Microbiologic studies on young infants with lower respiratory tract disease. Am J Dis Child 126:56, 1973.

ADRIANO G. ARGUEDAS, M.D., HARRIS R. STUTMAN, M.D.,
and MELVIN I. MARKS, M.D.

19

BACTERIAL PNEUMONIAS

Pneumonia remains a major cause of acute morbidity in the United States. Annual attack rates in preschool children average 40 per thousand and decrease gradually to 9 per thousand by 9 to 15 years of age. Predisposing factors include poor socioeconomic status, increased number of siblings, parental smoking, preterm delivery, and urban residence.

Hospitalization is also an important predisposing factor. Clustering of very ill infants and children receiving respiratory support in intensive care units, the increasing use of immunosuppressive therapies, and various medical and surgical illnesses enhance nosocomial colonization and infection as a result of an increasing diversity of respiratory pathogens.

Certain additional factors increase susceptibility to pneumonia: (1) congenital anatomic defects; (2) pulmonary sequestration and tracheoesophageal fistula; (3) foreign body; (4) defects in immune function, congenital or acquired (including acquired immune deficiency syndrome [AIDS] and sickle cell disease); (5) cystic fibrosis; and (6) congestive heart failure.

New diagnostic techniques (e.g., bacterial antigen detection, fiberoptic bronchoscopy, bronchoalveolar lavage, and lung biopsy) have led to a better understanding of the etiology of acute pneumonias and, therefore, to improvements in specific therapeutic regimens.

ETIOLOGY OF ACUTE PNEUMONIA

The pathogens causing pneumonia vary with the age of the patient, the patient's immune status, and environmental conditions. However, viruses account for the majority of cases of pneumonia at all ages, with respiratory syncytial, parainfluenza, influenza, and adenovirus the most prevalent etiologic agents.

The most common bacterial causes of pneumonia in *newborns* in North America are group B streptococci, mainly serotypes I and II, followed by gramnegative enteric bacilli and *Chlamydia*, the latter occurring between birth and 6 months of age. Syphilis may produce pulmonary disease (pneumonia alba) and must be suspected given appropriate epidemiologic circumstances. In children 1 month through 6 years of age, *Streptococcus pneumoniae* and *Haemophilus influenzae* serotype B are the most common pathogens. The latter is especially likely in children between 4 months and 2 years of age and is often associated (60 to 70 per cent) with bacteremia. In adolescents, *Mycoplasma pneumoniae* and *S. pneumoniae* are the most common etiologic agents.

Legionnaires' disease in children is rare but has been reported, especially in immunocompromised hospitalized children. It should be suspected in patients who present with high fever, slow pulse, nonproductive cough, pleuritic pain, and gastrointestinal problems (diarrhea, vomiting or abdominal pain), especially if exposed to water-cooled air-conditioners.

Under certain circumstances, other organisms, well discussed in other sections of this book, may cause pneumonia. *Branhamella (Moraxella) catarrhalis* and group A streptococci are occasional pathogens in infants and older children. Other causes of pneumonia include *Francisella tularensis* (tularemia after exposure to rabbits), *Chlamydia psittaci* (psittacosis after exposure to parrots and other birds), *Coxiella burnetii* (Q fever after contact with sheep), and *Salmonella choleraesuis* after exposure to pigs.

Specific geographic locations and exposures must also be considered. Coccidioidomycosis is occasionally encountered in children from the southwestern United States, Mexico, and some areas of Central and South America, melioidosis (*Pseudomonas pseudomallei*) in individuals from Southeast Asia, and tuberculosis in immigrant populations. Tuberculosis remains endemic in the United States, especially in urban populations. Cryptococcosis and histoplasmosis occur most commonly among pigeon breeders, and histoplasmosis may be suspected in children having contact with chickens or bats.

Hospital-associated pneumonia almost always follows aspiration of oropharyngeal flora. In ill, immunosuppressed patients, as well as in children receiving broad-spectrum antibiotics, the oropharynx is colonized with gram-negative rods derived from intestinal flora or from the hospital environment, and these bacteria may assume a pathogenic role. Hence, in addition to the bacterial pathogens mentioned above, one must consider gram-negative rods such as *Pseudomonas* sp., *Klebsiella* sp., *Escherichia coli*, and *Serratia marcescens*, and fungi, especially *Candida al-*

The authors thank Michael Weller, M.D., for radiographic consultation, and Joyce Bagan for editorial assistance.

bicans. These latter possibilities are especially likely in children under ventilatory support; in patients receiving broad-spectrum antibiotics, steroids, or intravenous-parenteral nutrition; as well as in immunosuppressed patients.

PATHOLOGY AND PATHOGENESIS

The airways are normally sterile from the sublaryngeal area to the terminal lung units. Under normal circumstances, the lungs are protected from bacterial infection by a number of mechanisms, including (1) filtration of particles in the nares, (2) prevention of aspiration by the epiglottal reflex, (3) expulsion of aspirated material by the cough reflex, (4) entrapment and expulsion of organisms by mucus-secreting and ciliated cells, (5) ingestion and killing of bacteria by alveolar macrophages, (6) neutralization of bacteria by local immune substances, and (7) transport of particles from the lungs by lymphatic drainage. Pulmonary infection may occur when one or more of these defense mechanisms are altered and organisms reach the lower respiratory tract either by aspiration or by the hematogenous route. Aspiration is the more common route, and evidence is increasing that viruses may enhance the susceptibility of the lower respiratory tract to infection in several different ways: (1) increased secretions promoting the aspiration of bacteria-laden fluid into the lung, (2) decreased ciliary activity diminishing bacterial clearance, and (3) impairment of local immune responses and bactericidal activity of alveolar macrophages.

When respiratory pathogens reach the terminal bronchioles and beyond, there is an outpouring of edema fluid into the alveoli, followed by large numbers of leukocytes. Later, macrophages remove cellular and bacterial debris. The process may extend farther within the same segment or lobe or may spread by infected bronchial fluid to other parts of the lung. Pulmonary lymphatics enable bacteria to reach the blood stream or the visceral pleura.

As lung tissue becomes consolidated, the vital capacity and lung compliance decrease and blood flow through consolidated, nonventilated areas creates a physiologic right-to-left shunt with ventilation-perfusion mismatching and resultant hypoxia. Cardiac work may be increased because of oxygen desaturation and hypercapnia.

CLINICAL FEATURES

The signs and symptoms of bacterial pneumonia vary with the bacterial pathogen, the age and immunologic condition of the patient, and the severity of disease. Clinical manifestations are extremely diverse and, especially in newborns, may occasionally be absent. Symptoms and signs of pneumonia in children can be classified as general or nonspecific, pulmonary, pleural, and extrapulmonary. Nonspecific complaints include fever, chills, headache, irritability, restlessness, and apprehension. Some patients may have gastrointestinal problems, such as vomiting, abdominal distention, diarrhea, and abdominal pain.

Although pulmonary signs are most helpful, they may not be present from onset: these include nasal flaring (most prominent in newborns), tachypnea, dyspnea, and apnea. Accessory intercostal and abdominal muscles may be used. Cough is usually absent in infants but is common in older children; the cough may initially be dry but later becomes productive of purulent or even bloody sputum. The respiratory rate is the most sensitive index of disease severity and is used both to suggest the diagnosis and, when measured during sleep or at rest, to guide management. Percussion is of no diagnostic value in the presence of a patchy pneumonia; dullness to percussion in children is more often associated with pleural effusion than with involvement of the lung parenchyma. Decreased breath sounds are frequently noted by auscultation, but the presence of fine crackles, characteristic of pneumonia in older patients, may be absent in infants. Breath sounds are often exaggerated on the noninvolved side. In an infant with empyema, the breath sounds are not always reduced even over the area of dullness, because of the relatively small size of the chest, the thinness of the layer of fluid, and the short path of transmission for breath sounds.

Pleural inflammation, not an uncommon finding in *S. pneumoniae* and *Staphylococcus aureus* pneumonia, may be accompanied by chest pain at the site of inflammation. Pain may be severe, limiting chest movement during inspiration, and sometimes may radiate to the neck or abdomen.

Extrapulmonary infection may be present in some cases (Table 19–1). Abscesses of the skin or soft tissue are often present in *S. aureus* pneumonia. Otitis media, sinusitis, and conjunctivitis can be found in the presence of *S. pneumoniae* or *H. influenzae*, and epiglottitis and meningitis are particularly likely to be associated with *H. influenzae* pneumonia.

Table 19–1. CLINICAL CLUES TO THE ETIOLOGY OF PNEUMONIA

Skin or extrapulmonary abscesses	*Staphylococcus aureus*
Skin petechiae	*Neisseria meningitidis*
Palatal petechiae	Streptococcus group A
Perianal purpuric lesion (immunosuppressed patients)	*Pseudomonas* sp.
Otitis media	*Streptococcus pneumoniae*
	Haemophilus influenzae
Cystic fibrosis	*S. aureus*
	H. influenzae
	Pseudomonas sp.
Sickle cell disease	*S. pneumoniae*
	H. influenzae

(Reproduced with permission from Marks MI: Pediatric Infectious Diseases for the Practitioner. New York, Springer-Verlag, 1984.)

RADIOLOGY

Although the diagnosis of pneumonia is suggested by clinical signs, a chest radiograph should be obtained to support the clinical impression and to define the extent of the pathology more accurately.

Lateral and frontal projections are essential in order to determine the anatomic location of the pneumonic process. Patchy infiltrates are most common during infancy; however, lobar consolidation is the more widely recognized finding, especially when *S. pneumoniae* or *H. influenzae* is the etiologic agent (Fig. 19–1). Hilar lymph nodes are often enlarged in pneumonia due to *H. influenzae* or *S. aureus* but less commonly in that caused by *S. pneumoniae*. Other diseases associated with hilar adenopathy are tuberculosis, histoplasmosis, and lymphoma. The presence of pneumatocele on a film should suggest *S. aureus*, especially during the convalescent phase of disease (Fig. 19–2). Gram-negative bacteria, especially *Klebsiella*, can also produce this radiologic finding. The chest roentgenogram clears within 3 to 4 weeks in 80 per cent of the cases and most of the remainder within 3 to 4 months. Radiographs do not need to be repeated during the convalescent period unless pneumatocele, abscess, pneumothorax, or other complications have developed or unless the child has an underlying immunosuppression or sickle cell disease.

LABORATORY EVALUATION

In the majority of cases, an extensive work-up is not required, but laboratory results may help the physician to focus on likely etiologic organisms.

An elevated white blood cell count (>15,000/mm³) is frequently but not invariably found. A count greater than 30,000 with a predominance of neutrophils suggests pneumococcal pneumonia, although other organisms including *H. influenzae* and *S. aureus* may produce this. The erythrocyte sedimentation

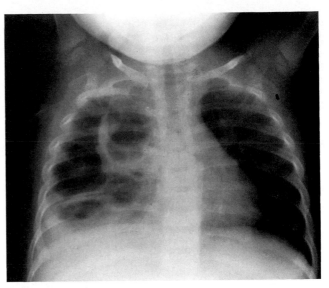

Figure 19–2. Patient with right-sided pneumatoceles due to *Staphylococcus aureus* pneumonia. (Courtesy of Dr. M Weller.)

rate and C-reactive protein concentrations are nonspecific indicators of inflammation and provide little direct help in patient management. When pneumonia is chronic (e.g., tuberculosis, cystic fibrosis) or associated with complications, however, these tests can be helpful in distinguishing acute exacerbations from chronic disease.

Although the blood culture is a specific method for establishing an etiologic diagnosis, it is positive only in 10 to 15 per cent of cases, mainly in younger children with pneumonia caused by *H. influenzae*, *S. aureus*, or *S. pneumoniae*. Because of the associated risks of bacteremia, cultures should be drawn in any child with suspected bacterial pneumonia before starting antibiotic therapy.

Cultures and Gram stain of secretions from the sputum should be obtained in all patients with productive cough and expectoration. The sputum evaluation can provide significant clues to the pathogens causing lower respiratory tract disease. An interpretable specimen must, however, have more than 25 polymorphonuclear and fewer than 25 epithelial cells per high-power field. Otherwise the material obtained is unlikely to be helpful and should not be processed. In neutropenic hosts, tuberculosis, and viral or mycoplasma infection, knowledge of upper respiratory flora may of course be useful information, regardless of the presence or absence of leukocytes.

Diagnostic tests based on detection of bacterial antigen have been developed and include counterimmunoelectrophoresis and latex particle agglutination. These tests permit detection of specific bacterial polysaccharide antigens in body fluids such as serum, urine, and pleural and spinal fluid. Either procedure can be carried out expeditiously, and antiserum is available for *S. pneumoniae*, *H. influenzae* type B, *Neisseria meningitidis* serotypes A, B, C, Y, W 135, and group B streptococci. Antigen is not usually detectable in individuals who are merely carriers of respi-

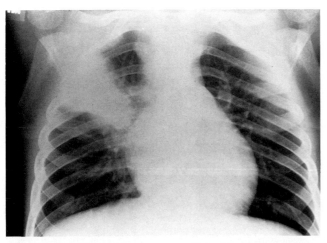

Figure 19–1. Chest roentgenogram of a patient with right lobar consolidation due to *Streptococcus pneumoniae*. (Courtesy of Dr. M Weller.)

ratory pathogens. In bacteremic pneumonias, the antigen screening is positive in serum in more than 90 per cent of documented *H. influenzae* pneumonias (100 per cent specificity), but in only 30 to 35 per cent of cases caused by *S. pneumoniae, N. meningitidis,* or group B streptococci (100 per cent specificity); in the urine, the sensitivity and specificity for *H. influenzae* and group B streptococci are more than 90 per cent, but the sensitivity for *S. pneumoniae* is less than 4 per cent. Urinary antigen screening for *N. meningitidis* is not recommended because of frequent false-positive results (5 per cent). Although negative results may not be predictive, positive results may guide specific antimicrobial therapy.

Percutaneous transtracheal aspiration has yielded reliable information on the cause of pulmonary infection in adults but is not recommended in children because of the high risk of complications (hemoptysis, cardiac arrhythmia, and hematoma formation). Diagnostic lung aspiration or biopsy should be considered in a severely ill child in whom a prompt diagnosis is essential, such as one with progressive disease who has responded poorly to therapy, or in a child with underlying immunodeficiency in whom empiric broad-spectrum treatment is hazardous because of the risk of superinfection and other adverse effects. Material may be obtained by open-lung biopsy, closed needle biopsy, or percutaneous needle aspiration; positive results for open biopsy vary between 70 and 75 per cent.

The presence of pleural fluid in a patient with pneumonia strongly suggests a bacterial cause of pneumonia (Tables 19–2 and 19–3). Bacterial empyema appears more frequently in infants less than 2 years of age and in males. The specific bacterial etiology depends on the age of the patient, *S. aureus* being most common in infants less than 6 months of age, *H. influenzae* and *S. aureus* between 7 and 24 months of age, and *S. pneumoniae* and *S. aureus* in infants older than 2 years. Anaerobes, the most common cause of empyema in adults (76 per cent), are rarely isolated from pleural fluid in children, except in those with impaired consciousness or poor oral hygiene. Other gram-negative organisms, excluding *H. influenzae,* are rare causes of empyema but may be the cause of pleural fluid superinfection in patients undergoing closed chest-tube drainage. Establishing the precise cause of the pleural effusion is very important, because the choice of antimicrobial therapy and the complications vary with the infecting organism.

Once the radiographic diagnosis of pleural effusion is made, diagnostic thoracentesis should be performed as the most direct method of identifying the responsible pathogen. Macroscopic appearance of the pleural fluid may be helpful; in the case of purulent fluid, an infectious cause is assumed and Gram stain with appropriate cultures is the first examination required. If the fluid is nonpurulent (turbid, serosanguineous, bloody), the first step is to differentiate between exudate (>3.0 g/dL of protein) and transu-

date (<3.0 g/dL of protein). A transudate occurs in patients with nephrotic syndrome, congestive heart failure, or hypoalbuminemia. Glucose concentration should also be measured; levels below 40 mg/dL are suggestive of bacterial infection, as are lactic dehydrogenase determinations greater than 1000 IU/L. Measurements of pH are sometimes helpful in the

Table 19–2. ETIOLOGY OF PLEURAL EMPYEMA

Bacteria
Staphylococcus aureus
Streptococcus pneumoniae
Streptococcus pyogenes
Haemophilus influenzae
Group B streptococcus
Haemophilus parainfluenzae
Anaerobes (streptococci, bacteroides, clostridia)
Mycobacterium tuberculosis
Pasteurella multocida
Yersinia enterocolitica

Viruses
Adenovirus
Coxsackievirus
Influenza
Epstein-Barr virus

Combined
Staphylococcus aureus (+) influenza A virus

Fungi
Histoplasma capsulatum
Candida albicans
Aspergillus

Others
Mycoplasma pneumoniae
Chlamydia
Parasites

(Reproduced with permission from Marks MI: Pediatric Infectious Diseases for the Practitioner. New York, Springer-Verlag, 1984.)

Table 19–3. NONINFECTIOUS PLEURAL EFFUSION

Neonatal
Chylothorax
Congenital pleural effusion (usually bilateral)

Others
Congestive heart failure
Myxedema
Pancreatitis
Nephrosis
Cirrhosis
Constrictive pericarditis
Rheumatoid arthritis
Polyarteritis nodosa
Systemic lupus erythematosus
Sarcoidosis
Hemothorax
Pulmonary infarction
Lymphoma
Mediastinal irradiation
Foreign body
Ovarian cyst
Tumor
Hypersensitivity (drug, parasite)
Subdiaphragmatic abscess

(Reproduced with permission from Marks, MI: Pediatric Infectious Diseases for the Practitioner. New York, Springer-Verlag, 1984.)

diagnosis and prognosis of pleural empyema. If pleural fluid is collected anaerobically in a heparinized syringe and transported to the laboratory on ice, values below 7.20 are usually associated with the presence of bacteria. Most of these patients require chest-tube drainage, especially if low pH is associated with a pleural fluid glucose level of less than 40 mg/dL. In the presence of grossly purulent pleural fluid, pH measurements are not necessary and do not provide any useful information.

Gram stain should be carried out on every pleural fluid. Acid-fast (mycobacterial pathogens) or India ink stains (*Cryptococcus*) are indicated when based on epidemiologic and clinical suspicions. Antigen screening (*H. influenzae, S. pneumoniae, N. meningitidis* and group B streptococci) in pleural fluid is helpful, especially in those patients in whom Gram stain and cultures may be negative because of previous antibiotic therapy. In these situations, antigen can often be detected in pleural fluid for several days up to 6 weeks after initiation of therapy. Anaerobic, fungal, viral, and aerobic cultures from pleural fluid should also be considered. In the case of purulent exudates, the etiologic microorganism is cultured in 82 per cent of the cases.

COMPLICATIONS

In most uncomplicated cases of bacterial pneumonia in children, mortality is very low (less than 1 per cent) and pulmonary function quickly returns to normal. Death is more common in patients with an underlying disease or with a complicated course. Children who do not have an underlying problem and in whom therapy is restored promptly and adequately have the best prognosis for recovery, with normal growth and development, normal pulmonary function test results, and no increase in susceptibility to infections.

S. aureus pneumonia is more likely to have a complicated course if not treated promptly or if it afflicts children less than 2 years of age. Empyema, pneumothorax, or lung abscess may complicate the acute phase of the disease. Cystic fibrosis should be suspected in children with failure to thrive and *S. aureus* pneumonia; therefore, a sweat test and immunologic studies are indicated with this clinical syndrome.

H. influenzae pneumonia, when treated properly, usually has a benign course. Pleural effusion may occur with a propensity to produce loculated fluid. One quarter of patients may have meningeal, epiglottal, or articular involvement.

S. pneumoniae pneumonia has a low mortality (1 per cent) and low long-term morbidity rate. Concomitant infection in other locations such as the middle ear may precede respiratory symptoms but rarely occurs after appropriate antibiotic therapy is begun. Local complications such as lung abscess and em-

pyema are uncommon if children have received early medical therapy with appropriate agents.

It is important to monitor the patient's cardiovascular status because of the possibility of pericardial effusion secondary to pulmonary infection. This condition must be suspected with the appearance of a murmur, a decrease in heart sounds, or signs of congestion. An electrocardiogram and an echocardiogram are indicated under those circumstances.

SPECIFIC PATHOGENS

GROUP B STREPTOCOCCI

Group B streptococci can be subdivided into five serotypes (Ia, Ib, Ic, II, and III) based on specific polysaccharide antigens. Serotypes I and II are usually associated with lung disease (early onset disease) and serotype III with meningeal involvement (late-onset disease).

Epidemiology

Group B streptococci are associated with infections at any age; however, these organisms are more common in infants less than 3 months of age. Acquisition of group B streptococci by newborns is usually vertical, from the maternal genital tract in utero, or during passage through the birth canal. Serotypes in the maternal genital tract are identical with those in the newborn. Colonization rates of the birth canal, at delivery, in the United States vary between 25 and 30 per cent. The rate of early onset infection in most parts of the United States varies from 3.0 to 4.2 per 1000 live births.

Early onset illness is usually associated with maternal fever at the time of delivery, prolonged rupture of membranes, amnionitis, prematurity (< 37 weeks gestation), and low birth weight.

Clinical Features

Neonates with early onset infection usually manifest clinical symptoms within the first 6 to 12 hours of life. These include fever, respiratory distress, apnea or tachypnea, and signs of hypoxemia; by 12 to 24 hours, signs of cardiovascular collapse usually appear. The syndrome of persistent fetal circulation, secondary to pulmonary hypertension, is frequent, and pulmonary or intracranial hemorrhage is a common terminal event.

The differentiation between group B streptococcal pneumonia and respiratory distress syndrome (RDS) is often difficult. The history of obstetric complications at the time of delivery, cardiovascular collapse during the first 24 hours of life, and the presence of leukopenia or leukocytosis with increased numbers of immature forms may suggest this infection. Peak inspiratory pressures are said to be lower in patients with group B streptococcal infection than in patients with RDS.

Laboratory

Isolation of the organism establishes the diagnosis of group B streptococcal infection. Cultures from the blood and cerebrospinal fluid must be obtained in all neonates with suspected group B streptococcal pneumonia. The organism can also be cultured from gastric fluid, the ear canal, the umbilical cord, and skin surfaces, although positive cultures from any of these sites is only suggestive evidence. Several techniques for the detection of group B streptococcal antigen in body fluids have shown to be helpful in providing a rapid etiologic diagnosis; these include latex agglutination, countercurrent immunoelectrophoresis, slide coagglutination tests, and enzyme immunoassays. Among these, latex agglutination is the fastest, simplest, and most sensitive. Concentrated urine is more sensitive (90 to 95 per cent) than serum (25 to 30 per cent) or spinal fluid (80 to 85 per cent). False-positive results are rare (0 to 3 per cent) if concentrated urine is used.

Leukopenia or leukocytosis with an increase in immature granulocytes and elevation in the C-reactive protein concentration and sedimentation rate are common but not specific to this infection.

Radiology

The radiographic findings of neonates with group B streptococcal pneumonia can be divided into those (40 per cent) in whom lobar consolidation is characteristic and those in whom the radiologic findings (diffuse reticulonodular pattern with air bronchogram) are indistinguishable from the findings in RDS (Fig. 19–3).

Treatment

Aggressive cardiovascular and ventilatory support is required, especially during the first 24 to 48 hours

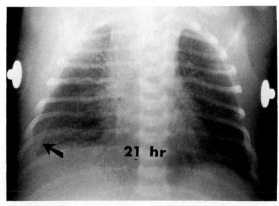

Figure 19–3. Chest roentgenogram of a 21-hour-old infant with group B streptococcal pneumonia, showing a typical air bronchogram, a diffuse reticulonodular infiltrate, and a right pleural effusion *(arrow)*. (Courtesy of Dr. M Weller.)

of life, when shock is a common complication. Antibiotic therapy should include a combination of ampicillin or penicillin and gentamicin. The initial use of an aminoglycoside is recommended because gram-negative organisms are part of the differential diagnosis and the rate of killing of group B streptococci by penicillin alone is enhanced by its association with an aminoglycoside. If the minimum bactericidal concentration for penicillin is adequate, gentamicin can be discontinued and penicillin given alone. If not, both drugs are continued for a duration of therapy of 10 to 14 days.

Prognosis

Although the mortality of group B streptococcal pneumonia has been high (50 to 60 per cent), studies suggest an improvement with prompt initiation of therapy. A number of infants have experienced a second episode of infection 1 week or more after cessation of antibiotic therapy. This recurrence could be the result of exogenous recolonization or reinvasion by the streptococci, which persist on mucous membranes after penicillin therapy. Those neonates in whom meningeal involvement is present in conjunction with group B streptococcal pneumonia (30 per cent) may have neurologic sequelae (20 to 50 per cent).

PNEUMOCOCCAL PNEUMONIA

The pneumococcus (*S. pneumoniae*) is a gram-positive diplococcus. Although immunologic classification of pneumococci into some 84 serotypes has been recognized, approximately 80 per cent of serious infections are caused by only 12 serotypes (1, 4, 6, 8, 9, 12, 14, 19, 23, 25, 51, and 56). In children, types 1, 3, 6A, 14, 18C, 19F, and 23F account for 60 to 70 per cent of pneumococcal infections.

Epidemiology

Pneumococci are a major cause of pneumonia, meningitis, and acute otitis media in infants and children and in the elderly. It is estimated that there are between two and five cases of pneumococcal pneumonia per 1000 persons each year in the United States. This figure represents 200,000 to 1 million cases annually, with an annual cost in hospitalization and days lost from work of approximately $420 million.

The incidence is highest in infants younger than 2 years of age, with a peak between 3 and 5 months of age. Males are affected more frequently than females, in a ratio of 3:2. Pneumococcal disease is more common in the black population; socioeconomic factors and sickle cell anemia may be important reasons. The seasonal incidence of pneumococcal disease parallels the seasonal variations of other respiratory tract infections, with the greatest incidence in winter and spring. Patients with asplenia or functional hyposplenia, as well as those with malignancy (such as Hodgkin's disease) or those receiving immunosuppressive drugs, are at special risk of developing invasive pneumococcal disease, including pneumonia.

Radiologic Features

Patchy bronchopneumonia is the most common radiologic finding, particularly in infants. Lobar or segmental consolidation is not uncommon, especially in moderate or severe cases. Less commonly, pleural effusion or pneumatocele may appear.

Therapy

Penicillin is the drug of choice in the treatment of pneumococcal pneumonia. Once a positive culture for *S. pneumoniae* is obtained, an oxacillin disk test should be performed, to detect penicillin–relatively-resistant pneumococci (3 to 16 per cent in some parts of the United States). Depending on the severity of the clinical picture, the patient with a penicillin-sensitive pneumococcal infection may be treated with oral penicillin (50 to 250 mg/kg/day every 4 to 6 hours) or oral erythromycin estolate (30 to 50 mg/kg/day every 6 hours). If the patient appears toxic, respiratory distress is moderate, or there are complications such as abscess or empyema, hospitalization and parenteral therapy should be initiated with aqueous penicillin G administered intravenously (100,000 to 200,000 U/kg/day every 4 to 6 hours). Infections due to penicillin–relatively-resistant *S. pneumoniae* are effectively treated with vancomycin, chloramphenicol, or beta-lactam antibiotics such as cefuroxime, ceftriaxone, and cefotaxime. Ampicillin or amoxicillin can also be used if meningitis and immunodeficiency are not present. Disease due to penicillin–relatively-resistant pneumococci should be considered in patients who have received prior therapy with beta-lactam antibiotics.

In penicillin-allergic patients, erythromycin (oral estolate 30 to 50 mg/kg/day every 6 hours) is the best alternative. Other drugs that can be used in these patients are cephalosporins (5 to 16 per cent cross-reactions in patients allergic to penicillin), chloramphenicol, and clindamycin.

Antimicrobial therapy should be continued for at least 48 to 72 hours after defervescence (usually a total of 5 to 7 days).

Prevention

Children who are at high risk of developing pneumococcal infections may benefit by receiving the 23-valent pneumococcal vaccine, licensed in the United States in 1983. This vaccine includes the capsular antigens representing nearly all serotypes causing invasive disease in childhood. Children in high-risk groups, age 2 years or older, should be vaccinated with 0.5 ml of the 23-valent pneumococcal vaccine, administered subcutaneously or intramuscularly. The vaccine is usually well tolerated, with local soreness or induration observed in 29 to 44 per cent of vaccinated children and fever greater than 37.7°C (99.9°F) in 3 to 19 per cent. Anaphylactoid reactions have been reported very rarely.

HAEMOPHILUS INFLUENZAE

Organisms of the genus *Haemophilus* are small, nonmotile, gram-negative rods that occur in encapsulated and nonencapsulated forms. The encapsulated forms are divided into six capsular types based on their polysaccharide (types A to F). Approximately 90 to 95 per cent of invasive disease (including pneumonia) is caused by serotype B. The nonencapsulated forms are normal habitants of the nasopharynx and, although a major cause of otitis media, sinusitis, and upper respiratory mucosal infections, are rare causes of bacteremic disease or pneumonia in children.

Epidemiology

H. influenzae causes about 20,000 cases of invasive diseases annually, including bacteremia, meningitis, and pneumonia. The incidence of pneumonia is higher in infants younger than 5 years of age, with a peak between 4 and 7 months of age. Most studies show equal rates of disease in males and females. High incidence has been observed in blacks, Hispanics, and native Americans, as well as in families with low income and substandard educational levels. Chronic diseases known to be associated with increased risk include sickle cell anemia, antibody deficiency syndromes, and malignancies, especially during chemotherapy.

Radiologic Features

The radiologic findings in *H. influenzae* pneumonia show no characteristic or consistent pattern. Segmental infiltrates involving a single lobe, without predilection for a specific anatomic location, are a common finding, but involvement of two or more lobes may occur. Hilar adenopathy may be present early in the course of the disease. Pleural effusion, when present, is usually adjacent to the pneumonic process.

Therapy

Once the diagnosis of *H. influenzae* pneumonia is made, based on a positive culture, identification of beta-lactamase–positive strains (40 to 60 per cent in certain parts of the United States) and susceptibility testing must be done (a few strains are beta-lactamase negative but still ampicillin resistant).

In a hospitalized patient, a combination of ampicillin plus chloramphenicol or a cephalosporin such as cefuroxime, cefotaxime, or ceftriaxone is effective. If the isolate is ampicillin sensitive and ampicillin and chloramphenicol were initially selected, chloramphenicol can be discontinued and ampicillin given alone. If the pathogen is beta-lactamase positive, ampicillin should be discontinued and chloramphenicol given to maintain blood concentrations of 15 to 25 μg/ml. If chloramphenicol blood concentrations are not available or there are any contraindications to its use (blood dyscrasias, newborn, hepatotoxicity, shock), one of the cephalosporins should be selected. Oral therapeutic regimens include amoxicillin, erythromycin-sulfamethoxazole, cefaclor, and cefuroxime axetil.

Although a course of 7 days of therapy is sufficient for most uncomplicated cases, complicated processes may require therapy extended to 10 or 14 days.

Prevention

Immunization against *H. influenzae* type B infection with a capsular polysaccharide vaccine (PRP) has been available in the United States since April of 1985. In December of 1987, a conjugate vaccine against *H. influenzae* type B was licensed containing *H. influenzae* polysaccharide and diphtheria toxoid (PRP-D). PRP-D is recommended, as a single dose, for all children at 18 months of age or for those children who received a dose of PRP between 18 and 23 months of age. PRP-D is not recommended for children vaccinated with PRP at the age of 24 months or older, for children who have had invasive *H. influenzae* infection at 24 months of age or older, or for children less than 18 months of age. Local reactions (tenderness, swelling and redness) occur in 10 to 12 per cent of recipients and fever (rectal temperature > 39°C) in 1 per cent. Convulsions and thrombocytopenia have been reported rarely.

Children who are household contacts of an index patient with *H. influenzae* type B infection and who are under 4 years of age are approximately 500 times more susceptible than the general population to acquire an *H. influenzae* infection. According to the American Academy of Pediatrics, rifampin prophylaxis should be given to (1) all members of a household when there are susceptible contacts less than 4 years of age; (2) nursery school and day-care center contacts (but not their families) and adult staff when they have spent 4 hours or more per day with the index patient for 5 of the 7 days preceding hospital admission; and (3) the index patient if, after being discharged from the hospital, he or she will be in contact with susceptible children (less than 4 years of age). Rifampin is given at 20 mg/kg once daily (maximum dose 600 mg/daily) for 4 days, resulting in carriage eradication rates of greater than 90 per cent. Side effects, mainly nausea and diarrhea, occur in less than 5 per cent of individuals.

STAPHYLOCOCCAL PNEUMONIA

Staphylococci are gram-positive bacteria frequently found on the skin, on nasal and other mucous membranes. Three major species are recognized: *S. aureus*, *S. epidermidis*, and *S. saprophyticus*. Coagulase formation characterizes most of the *S. aureus* strains. Extracellular products of staphylococci include hemolysins, enterotoxins, hyaluronidase, leukocytotoxic substances, and in some strains, penicillinase, an enzyme that opens the beta-lactam ring of the penicillin molecule.

Epidemiology

S. aureus is ubiquitous and grows over a wide temperature range. A person colonized in the nose and throat or perineal region is the major source of the organism. Twenty to 30 per cent of normal individuals carry *S. aureus* in the anterior nares.

Transmission of *S. aureus* generally occurs by direct contact or by spread of heavy particles. Infection may follow colonization and depends on the quantity of bacteria transmitted and the susceptibility of the host. Conditions that enhance the likelihood of infection include wounds, skin disease, intravenous drug abuse, use of corticosteroids, and diabetes mellitus.

Radiologic Features

The radiologic findings in a patient with *S. aureus* pneumonia vary according to the stage of the disease; during the acute phase, consolidation is the most common finding, often associated with pleural effusion (55 per cent) or pneumothorax (21 per cent). Characteristically, the radiologic picture changes rapidly, from minimal changes at disease onset, to patchy consolidated lesions with empyema (Fig. 19–4) or pneumothorax a few hours later. Pneumatoceles usually appear during the convalescent phase and may persist for months to years in asymptomatic children, without clinical implications.

Therapy

Because the clinical course of staphylococcal pneumonia may be fulminant, every patient in whom this

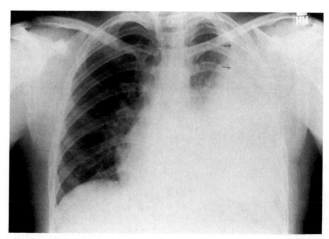

Figure 19–4. Patient with a large left pulmonary empyema due to *Staphylococcus aureus*.

condition is suspected should be hospitalized and therapy promptly begun after cultures of blood and suspicious sites (e.g., skin abscess) are obtained.

The initial therapeutic approach should include a drug resistant to inactivation by penicillinase: nafcillin (100 to 150 mg/kg/day divided every 6 hours IV), oxacillin (100 to 150 mg/kg/day divided every 6 hours IV), cefazolin (100 mg/kg/day divided every 8 hours IV), or clindamycin (10 to 40 mg/kg/day divided every 6 to 8 hours IV). Methicillin-resistant *S. aureus* accounts for up to 11.5 per cent of isolates in the United States, and vancomycin (40 mg/kg/day divided every 6 hours IV) should be given when these organisms are isolated. Duration of therapy is usually 21 days; during therapy, one should carefully watch for signs of extrapulmonary infection (pericardium, bone, kidneys).

REFERENCES

Akierman AR and Mayock DE: Group B streptococcal septicemia and delayed-onset congenital right-sided diaphragmatic hernia. Can Med Assoc J 129:1289, 1983.

Alario AJ, McCarthy PL, Markowitz R et al: Usefulness of chest radiographs in children with acute lower respiratory tract disease. J Pediatr 111:187, 1987.

Anderson KC, Maurer MJ, and Dajani AS: Pneumococci relatively resistant to penicillin: a prevalence survey in children. J Pediatr 97:939, 1980.

Asmar BI, Slovis TL, Reed JO et al: *Haemophilus influenzae* type b pneumonia in 43 children. J Pediatr 93:389, 1978.

Baigelman W and Chodosh S: Sputum "wet preps": window on the airways. J Respir Dis 5:59, 1984.

Baker CJ: Summary of the workshop on perinatal infections due to group B streptococcus. J infect Dis 136:137, 1977.

Baker CJ and Kasper DL: Group B streptococcal vaccines. Rev Infect Dis 7:458, 1985.

Baker CJ and Rench MA: Commercial latex agglutination for detection of group B streptococcal antigen in body fluids. J Pediatr 102:393, 1983.

Baker CJ, Webb BJ, Jackson CV et al: Countercurrent immunoelectrophoresis in the evaluation of infants with group B streptococcal disease. Pediatrics 65:1110, 1980.

Barrett DJ, Lee OG, Ammann AJ et al: IgG and IgM pneumococcal polysaccharide antibody responses in infants. Pediatr Res 18:1067, 1984.

Black SB, Shinefield HR, Hiatt RA et al: Efficacy of *Haemophilus influenzae* type b capsular polysaccharide vaccine. Pediatr Infect Dis 7:149, 1988.

Bolan G, Ajello GW, Hayes PS et al: The utility of commercial latex agglutination tests for detection of *H. influenzae* type b and *S. pneumoniae* antigens in bacteremic pneumonia patients. Interscience Conference on Antimicrobial Agents and Chemotherapy, Abstract 73:110, New Orleans, 1986.

Bolan G, Broome V, Facklam RR et al: Pneumococcal vaccine efficacy in selected populations in the United States. Ann Intern Med 104:1, 1986.

Boyer KM and Gotoff SP: Prevention of early-onset neonatal group B streptococcal disease with selective intrapartum chemoprophylaxis. N Engl J Med 314:1665, 1986.

Boyer KM, Gadzala CA, Burd LI et al: Selective intrapartum chemoprophylaxis of neonatal group B streptococcal early-onset disease. I. Epidemiologic rationale. J Infect Dis 148:795, 1983.

Bromberger PI, Chandler B, Gezon H et al: Rapid detection of neonatal group B streptococcal infections by latex agglutination. J Pediatr 96:104, 1980.

Brunell PA, Bass JW, Daum RS et al: Recommendations for using pneumococcal vaccine in children. Pediatrics 75:1153, 1985.

Cates KL, Krause PJ, Murphy TV et al: Second episodes of

Haemophilus influenzae type b disease following rifampin prophylaxis of the index patients. Pediatr Infect Dis 6:512, 1987.

Chitayat D, Diamant SH, Lazevnick R et al: *Haemophilus influenzae* type b pneumonia with pneumatocele formation. Clin Pediatr 19:151, 1979.

Christensen KK, Christensen P, Bucher HU et al: Intravenous administration of human IgG to newborn infants: changes in serum antibody levels to group B streptococci. Eur J Pediatr 143:123, 1984.

Cochi SL and Broome CV: Vaccine prevention of *Haemophilus influenzae* type b disease: past, present and future. Pediatr Infect Dis 5:12, 1986.

Cochi SL, Fleming DW, Hightower AW et al: Primary invasive *Haemophilus influenzae* type b disease: a population-based assessment of risk factors. J Pediatr 108:887, 1986.

Cole FS, Saryan JA, and Smith AL: The risk of additional systemic bacterial illness in infants with systemic *Streptococcus pneumoniae* disease. J Pediatr 99:91, 1981.

Congeni BL, Igel HJ, and Platt MS: Evaluation of a latex particle agglutination kit in pneumococcal disease. Pediatr Infect Dis 3:417, 1984.

Davis C and Millard D: How useful is urine latex agglutination to diagnose group B streptococcal disease in term newborns at risk for infection? Proceedings of the American Pediatric Society, Abstract 993, Washington, DC, 1988.

Denny FW and Clyde WA Jr: Acute lower respiratory tract infections in nonhospitalized children. J Pediatr 108:635, 1986.

Early GL, Williams TE, and Kilman JW: Open lung biopsy. Its effects on therapy in the pediatric patient. Chest 87:467, 1985.

Editorial: Pneumonia in childhood. Lancet 1:741, 1988.

Eskola J, Peltola H, Takala AK et al: Efficacy of *Haemophilus influenzae* type b polysaccharide-diphtheria toxoid conjugate vaccine in infancy. N Engl J Med 317:717, 1987.

Faix RG and Donn SM: Association of septic shock caused by early-onset group B streptococcal sepsis and periventricular leukomalacia in the preterm infant. Pediatrics 76:415, 1985.

Feld LG, Springate JE, Darragh R et al: Pneumococcal pneumonia and hemolytic uremic syndrome. Pediatr Infect Dis 6:693, 1987.

Fischer GW, Weisman LB, Hemming VG et al: Intravenous immunoglobulin in neonatal group B streptococcal disease. Am J Med 76:117, 1984.

Freij BJ, Kusmiesz H, Nelson JD et al: Parapneumonic effusions and empyema in hospitalized children: a retrospective review of 227 cases. Pediatr Infect Dis 3:578, 1984.

Friedman CA, Wender DF, and Rawson JE: Rapid diagnosis of group B streptococcal infection utilizing a commercially available latex agglutination assay. Pediatrics 73:27, 1984.

Fuchs GJ, LaRocco M, Robinson A et al: Fatal legionnaires' disease in an infant. Pediatr Infect Dis 5:377, 1986.

Gilsdorf JR: Dynamics of nasopharyngeal colonization with *Haemophilus influenzae* b during antibiotic therapy. Pediatrics 77:242, 1986.

Gilsdorf JR and Herring G: Recovery of *Haemophilus influenzae* type b from hospital environmental surfaces. Am J Infect Control 15:33, 1987.

Ginsburg CM, Howard JB, and Nelson JD: Report of 65 cases of *Haemophilus influenzae* b pneumonia. Pediatrics 64:283, 1979.

Glode MP, Daum RS, Boies EG et al: Effect of rifampin chemoprophylaxis on carriage eradication and new acquisition of *Haemophilus influenzae* type b in contacts. Pediatrics 76:537, 1985.

Gloser H, Bachmayer H, and Helm A: Intravenous immunoglobulin with high activity against group b streptococci. Pediatr Infect Dis 5:S176, 1986.

Gotoff SP: Chemoprophylaxis of early onset group B streptococcal disease. Pediatr Infect Dis 3:401, 1984.

Granoff DM, Gilsdorf J, Gessert C et al: *Haemophilus influenzae* type B disease in a day care center: eradication of carrier state by rifampin. Pediatrics 63:397, 1979.

Grossman LK, Wald ER, Nair P et al: Roentgenographic follow-up of acute pneumonia in children. Pediatrics 63:30, 1979.

Jackson MA, Shelton S, Nelson JD et al: Relatively penicillin-resistant pneumococcal infections in pediatric patients. Pediatr Infect Dis 3:129, 1984.

Jacobs NM and Harris VJ: Acute *Haemophilus* pneumonia in childhood. Am J Dis Child 133:603, 1979.

Jones DE, Kanarek KS, Lim DV: Group B streptococcal colonization patterns in mothers and their infants. J Clin Microbiol 20:438, 1984.

Klein JO: The epidemiology of pneumococcal disease in infants and children. Rev Infect Dis 3:246, 1981.

Kohler RB, Winn WC Jr, and Wheat LJ: Onset and duration of urinary antigen excretion in legionnaires' disease. J Clin Microbiol 20:605, 1984.

Koskela M, Leinonen M, Haiva VM et al: First and second dose antibody responses to pneumococcal polysaccharide vaccine in infants. Pediatr Infect Dis 5:45, 1986.

Kumar A and Nankervis GA: Latex agglutination test and countercurrent immunoelectrophoresis for detection of group B streptococcal antigen. Pediatrics 97:328, 1980.

Leinonen M, Sakkinen A, Kalliokoski R et al: Antibody response to 14-valent pneumococcal capsular polysaccharide vaccine in pre-school age children. Pediatr Infect Dis 5:39, 1986.

Li KI, Dashefsky B, and Wald ER: *Haemophilus influenzae* type B colonization in household contacts of infected and colonized children enrolled in day care. Pediatrics 78:15, 1986.

Lim DV, Morales WJ, Walsh AF et al: Reduction of morbidity and mortality rates for neonatal group B streptococcal disease through early diagnosis and chemoprophylaxis. J Clin Microbiol 23:489, 1986.

Long SS: Treatment of acute pneumonia in infants and children. Pediatr Clin North Am 30:297, 1983.

McCarthy PL, Spiesel SZ, Stashwick CA et al: Radiographic findings and etiologic diagnosis in ambulatory childhood pneumonias. Clin Pediatr 20:686, 1981.

McHenry MC: The infectious pneumonias. Hosp Practice 15:41, 1980.

Makintubee S, Istre GR, and Ward JI: Transmission of invasive *Haemophilus influenzae* type b disease in day care settings. J Pediatr 111:180, 1987.

Marks MI: Pediatric pneumonia: viral or bacterial? J Respir Dis 3:108, 1982.

Marks MI: Pneumonia. In Pediatric Infectious Diseases for the Practitioner. New York, Springer-Verlag, 1984.

Marks MI and Dorchester WL: Secondary rates of *Haemophilus influenzae* type b disease among day care contacts. J Pediatr 111:305, 1987.

Masur H, Shelhamer J, and Parrillo JE: The management of pneumonias in immunocompromised patients. JAMA 253:1769, 1985.

Mufson MA: Pneumococcal infections. JAMA 246:1942, 1981.

Murphy D, Lockhart CH, and Todd JK: Pneumococcal empyema. Am J Dis Child 134:659, 1980.

Murphy TV: *Haemophilus* B polysaccharide vaccine: need for continuing assessment. Pediatr Infect Dis 6:701, 1987.

Murphy TV, McCracken GH Jr, Moore BS et al: *Haemophilus influenzae* type B disease after rifampin prophylaxis in a day care center: possible reasons for its failure. Pediatr Infect Dis 2:193, 1983.

Murphy TV, McCracken GH Jr, Zweighaft TC et al: Emergence of rifampin-resistant *Haemophilus influenzae* after prophylaxis. J Pediatr 99:406, 1981.

Novak RW and Platt MS: Significance of placental findings in early-onset group B streptococcal neonatal sepsis. Clin Pediatr 24:256, 1985.

Peter G: The child with pneumonia: diagnostic and therapeutic considerations. Pediatr Infect Dis 7:453, 1988.

Philip AG: Response of C-reactive protein in neonatal group B streptococcal infection. Pediatr Infect Dis 4:145, 1985.

Plotkin SA, Daum RS, Giebink GS et al: *Haemophilus influenzae* type B conjugate vaccine. Pediatrics 81:908, 1988.

Prober CG, Whyte H, and Smith CR: Open lung biopsy in immunocompromised children with pulmonary infiltrates. Am J Dis Child 138:60, 1984.

Pyati SP, Pildes RS, Jacobs NM et al: Penicillin in infants weighing two kilograms or less with early-onset group B streptococcal disease. N Engl J Med 308:1383, 1983.

Ramsey BW, Marcuse EK, Foy HM et al: Use of bacterial antigen detection in the diagnosis of pediatric lower respiratory tract infections. Pediatrics 78:1, 1986.

Rancilio L, Rusconi F, Arizzi AF et al: Counterimmunoelectrophoresis and latex agglutination in the etiologic diagnosis of severe presumptive bacterial pneumonia in childhood. Interscience Conference on Antimicrobial Agents and Chemotherapy, Abstract 362:160, New York, 1987.

Riley ID, Alpers MP, Gratten M et al: Pneumococcal vaccine prevents death from acute lower respiratory tract infections in Papua New Guinean children. Lancet 2:878, 1986.

Rubin LG, Carmody L, Frogel M et al: Pneumococcal & *Haemophilus influenzae* B antigen detection in children at risk for occult bacteremia. Interscience Conference on Antimicrobial Agents and Chemotherapy, Abstract 75:110, New Orleans, 1986.

Rytel MW: Pneumococcal pneumonia: diagnosis and management. J Respir Dis 58:80, 1983.

Saubolle MA and Wright RE: Comparative value of urine latex agglutination for detection of four bacterial antigens. Interscience Conference on Antimicrobial Agents and Chemotherapy, Abstract 74:110, New Orleans, 1986.

Shann F: Etiology of severe pneumonia in children in developing countries. Pediatr Infect Dis 5:247, 1986.

Shann F and Germer S: Hyponatraemia associated with pneumonia or bacterial meningitis. Arch Dis Child 60:963, 1985.

Shapiro ED and Wald ER: Efficacy of rifampin in eliminating pharyngeal carriage of *Haemophilus influenzae* type B. Pediatrics 66:5, 1980.

Sherman MP, Goetzman BW, Ahlfors CE et al: Tracheal aspiration and its clinical correlates in the diagnosis of congenital pneumonia. Pediatrics 65:258, 1980.

Swingle HM, Bucciarelli RL, Ayoub EM: Synergy between penicillins and low concentrations of gentamicin in the killing of group B streptococci. J Infect Dis 152:515, 1985.

Teele DW, Dorion ME, and Nanan C: Pneumococcuria: clue to the diagnosis of systemic pneumococcal infections? J Pediatr 98:70, 1981.

Turner RB, Hayden FG, and Hendley JO: Counterimmunoelectrophoresis of urine for diagnosis of bacterial pneumonia in pediatric outpatients. Pediatrics 71:780, 1983.

Turner RB, Lande AE, Chase P et al: Pneumonia in pediatric outpatients: cause and clinical manifestations. J Pediatr 111:194, 1987.

Wald ER and Levine MM: Frequency of detection of *Hemophilus influenzae* type B capsular polysaccharide in infants and children with pneumonia. Pediatrics 57:266, 1976.

Young LS: Respiratory infections in the patient at risk: an overview. Am J Med 76:78, 1984.

20

WALTER T. HUGHES, M.D.

PNEUMOCYSTIS CARINII PNEUMONITIS

Pneumocystis carinii pneumonitis is a unique infection of humans and lower animals with an unyielding penchant for the debilitated and immunodeficient host. Unlike other opportunistic infections of the compromised patient, this disease process and the causative agent with rare exception remain confined to the lungs even in fatal cases. *P. carinii* was recognized as a cause of interstitial plasma cell pneumonitis of premature and marasmic infants in Europe during and following World War II, when the disease occurred in epidemic form. The first case of *P. carinii* pneumonitis in the United States was reported only 30 years ago. In contrast to the epidemic, infantile form in Europe, the American cases have been sporadic and have occurred in children and adults with some underlying disease. Although the infantile form has become less prevalent over the past 25 years, the sporadic form in the United States has progressively increased in frequency. More extensive use of immunosuppressive therapy and advances in medicine that have extended the longevity of patients with impaired resistance to infection account in part for the increasing prevalence of the infection, but the epidemic of acquired immune deficiency syndrome (AIDS) has accounted for the vast majority of cases since 1981.

PREDISPOSING FACTORS

In addition to AIDS, underlying diseases or conditions related to the provocation of *P. carinii* pneumonitis have included lymphoproliferative malignancies, solid tumors, congenital immune deficiency disorders, organ transplantation, Kaposi's sarcoma, Waldenström macroglobulinemia, rheumatoid arthritis, rheumatic fever, Henoch-Schönlein purpura, thrombotic thrombocytopenic purpura, hemophilia, aplastic anemia, hemolytic anemia, Wiskott-Aldrich syndrome, nephrosis, hypoproteinemia, and protein-calorie malnutrition. It has also occurred with some chronic infectious disease, such as tuberculosis, cryptococcosis, and congenital rubella. *P. carinii* infection has been encountered in Vietnamese refugee children and in certain homosexual men. Studies suggest that *P. carinii* may be a more common cause of pneumonitis in presumably normal infants than previously recognized; in one series of infants between 1 and 3 months of age with pneumonitis, *P. carinii* was implicated in 14 to 22 per cent of cases (Stagno et al, 1980; Stagno et al, 1981; Rowecka-Trzebicka et al, 1988).

The incidence of *P. carinii* pneumonitis has been related directly to the intensity of immunosuppressive therapy. Careful surveillance for 2.5 years of a group of children with acute lymphocytic leukemia randomized in a prospective study to receive gradations of chemotherapy agents showed the incidence of this infection to be 5 per cent in those receiving only one drug for maintenance therapy; in those receiving four anticancer drugs, however, 22 per cent had *P. carinii* pneumonia. When mediastinal irradiation was added to intensive chemotherapy, the incidence of the pneumonitis was 36 per cent (Hughes, Feldman, Aur et al, 1975). At least 43 per cent of infants with severe combined immunodeficiency syndrome acquire *P. carinii* pneumonitis, and between 50 and 75 per cent of those with AIDS will have the pneumonitis. Furthermore, in the AIDS patients about one third of those successfully treated for *P. carinii* pneumonia will have a recurrence of the infection.

CLINICAL FEATURES

SIGNS AND SYMPTOMS

Two somewhat different clinical patterns may be recognized with *P. carinii* pneumonitis. Because one pattern has been predominant in premature and debilitated infants, it will be referred to as the *infantile type*.

In the infantile type the onset is usually slow, with nonspecific signs, such as poor feeding and restlessness. Tachypnea and a peculiar cyanosis about the mouth and under the eyes may be the first signs of pulmonary involvement. Coryza, cough, and fever are usually not present, and crackles are often heard. Within 1 to 2 weeks, the respiratory distress has become severe, with marked tachypnea, flaring of nasal alae, sternal retraction, and cyanosis. Sudden attacks of coughing may occur. Usually the duration of the illness is 4 to 6 weeks, and 25 to 50 per cent of the cases will end fatally if untreated (Gajdusek, 1957). Infants between 3 and 6 months of age are most frequently affected.

The second type is encountered primarily in the immunosuppressed child and adult. Abrupt onset and fever are characteristic features here, in contrast to the infantile type. Other signs and symptoms are listed in Figure 20–1. The absence of crackles is a usual feature. The natural course of the disease is one of a rapidly progressive course ending fatally in almost all the cases.

It should be kept in mind that either of the clinical types may occur in infants, children, and adults and that patterns described have only general application. A fulminating, rapidly fatal course may occur in infants, and a subtle but progressive course may sometimes be encountered in adults and children. Infants and children with AIDS may have signs and symptoms of either of the clinical types or the pneumonitis may be of intermediate magnitude.

ROENTGENOGRAM

The chest roentgenogram, with rare exception, depicts bilateral diffuse alveolar disease. The hilar areas are involved initially, with spread to the periphery. The infantile form shows interstitial infiltrate with hyperexpanded lung fields, whereas the other type is characterized by alveolar disease (Fig. 20–2). Rarely the pulmonary infiltrate manifests as a lobar pneumonitis resembling that of bacterial origin, a solitary nodular lesion suggesting malignancy, a unilateral hyperinflation suggesting airway obstruction, or a pneumonitis in areas of previous therapeutic irradiation suggesting radiation pneumonitis.

ACID-BASE AND BLOOD GAS PROFILES

Hypoxia with quite low arterial oxygen tension (Pa_{O_2}) almost always occurs once the disease is clinically or radiographically discernible. Carbon dioxide retention is rarely present, and the arterial pH is usually increased. Concomitant with a decrease in Pa_{O_2} is an increase in alveolar-arterial gradient and intrapulmonary right-to-left shunt.

NONSPECIFIC LABORATORY TESTS

The white blood cell count is usually unaffected by the infection. Although eosinophilia has been reported with P. carinii pneumonitis in sex-linked agammaglobulinemia, this response is the exception rather than the rule.

The serum immunoglobulin levels may be normal or decreased, depending on the type of primary disease. In the infantile form of the infection, the low immunoglobulin levels usually reached at the third to fourth month of age are believed to precondition the infant to intra-alveolar proliferation of P. carinii. When severe protein-calorie malnutrition is the predisposing condition, serum albumin values may be low. (See Hughes, Feldman, and Sanyal, 1975; Hughes, Feldman, Aur et al, 1975.)

PATHOLOGY

In fatal cases of P. carinii pneumonitis, the lungs are diffusely involved, heavy, noncompliant, and have the consistency and coloration of liver.

The histopathologic features of the infantile epidemic type differ from those in pneumonia that occur as a result of immunosuppression in children and adults (Dutz et al, 1973). In the infantile form, there is extensive involvement of the alveolar septa with plasma cell and lymphocyte infiltration. The septa may be five to 20 times the normal thickness.

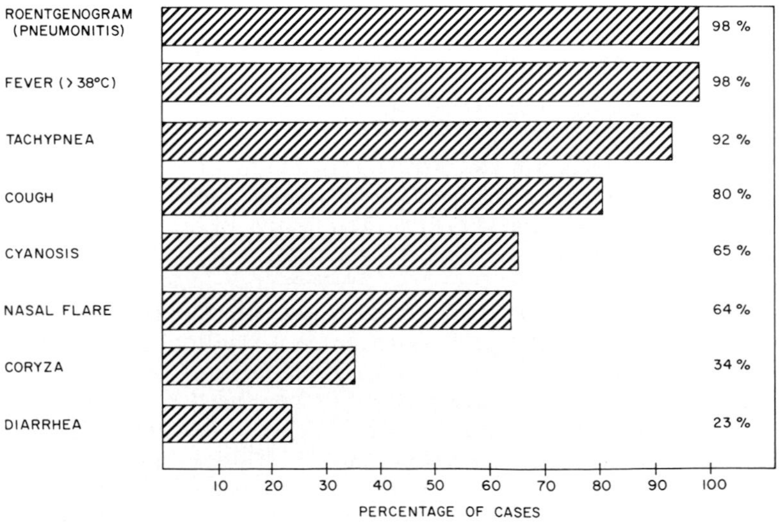

Figure 20–1. Clinical profile of 100 children with Pneumocystis carinii pneumonitis and childhood malignancies admitted to St. Jude Children's Research Hospital, Memphis, Tenn. The diagnosis was made by lung aspirate, biopsy, or autopsy studies. Bars indicate the percentage of patients with the respective abnormality at the time of admission.

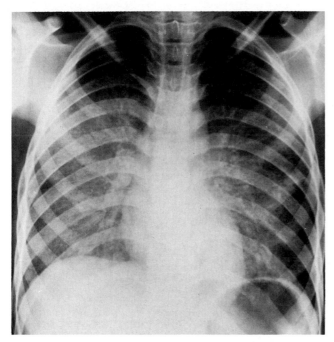

Figure 20–2. Chest roentgenogram showing evidence of moderately severe *Pneumocystis carinii* pneumonitis. The pattern is one of diffuse alveolar disease with bilateral distribution. The superior portions of the upper lobes are usually the least involved, and the perihilar areas are the most commonly affected sites. Air bronchograms are discernible.

Up to three fourths of the entire lung space is occupied by the distended septa. The alveolar spaces are also heavily infiltrated with organisms. In milder cases, often clinically undetected, *P. carinii* organisms are found in subpleural posterior alveoli with minimal focal interstitial plasma cell response.

In the immunodeficient child and adult, the disease process is predominantly in the alveolar spaces with considerably less involvement of the alveolar septa than that seen in infants. The histopathologic features have been correlated with the extent of clinical disease (Price and Hughes, 1974). In Stage I, isolated organisms are found adjacent to the alveolar wall or in the cytoplasm of the macrophage with no inflammatory response; there is no clinical evidence of the disease. In Stage II there is desquamation of alveolar cells containing organisms into the alveolar lumen with increasing numbers of organisms and minimal or no inflammatory response in alveolar septa; there may or may not be clinical evidence of pneumonitis. With Stage III, extensive reactive and desquamative alveolopathy is found with large numbers of organisms within the alveolar cellular desquamate, and there is also extensive alveolar septal thickening with mononuclear inflammatory cells (Fig. 20–3). All patients with Stage III disease have clinical manifestations of pneumonitis.

CHARACTERISTICS OF THE ORGANISM

The taxonomy of *P. carinii* has not been established. Recent studies of *P. carinii* ribosomal RNA suggest greater similarity to ascosporous yeasts than to certain protozoa (Edman et al, 1988). The organism exists in three developmental forms, which represent stages in the life cycle. The largest form is at least 4 to 6 microns in diameter. This *cyst* form is rounded or crescent shaped and possesses a thick cell wall. The cyst wall is readily impregnated with Gomori methenamine–silver nitrate stain or toluidine blue O stain (Fig. 20–4*A* and *B*) but does not take up polychrome stains, such as Giemsa, Wright, or polychrome methylene blue reagents. However, these latter stains identify the intracystic structures referred to as *sporozoites* (Fig. 20–4*C*). Up to eight sporozoites are found in mature cysts. These round, sickle-shaped, or pleomorphic intracystic forms measure 1 to 2 microns in diameter. The extracystic forms are termed *trophozoites*. These cells vary greatly in size and measure from 2 to 4 microns in diameter. The cytoplasm is bluish and bounded by an indefinite cell membrane. The nuclei are small and usually located eccentrically.

Little is known about the macromolecular structure of *P. carinii;* however, some histochemical studies have shown the cyst wall to consist of mucopolysaccharides, lipoproteins, and chitinic acid.

P. carinii has been propagated for limited periods in vitro in embryonic chick epithelial lung cell cultures (Pifer and Hughes, 1975) and Vero cells (Latorre et al, 1977). Here something has been learned of the reproductive cycle. The trophozoite attaches to but does not penetrate the host cell. While joined by microtubules, the parasite enlarges; then it detaches and develops into a mature cyst. The method of cell replication has not been determined. Excystment occurs through breaks in the cyst wall through which the sporozoites are expelled to become trophozoites (Fig. 20–4*D*). Chromatofocusing and lectin-binding studies have shown that the surface antigen of a 115- to 120-kDa cyst is an acidic glycoprotein that contains mannose, glucose, or both, and *N*-acetylglucosamine sugar residues (Gigliotti et al, 1988).

DIAGNOSIS

For a definitive diagnosis, *P. carinii* must be demonstrated in lung tissue or in fluid derived from the lung or lower respiratory tract. Several approaches have been taken to obtain specimens for diagnosis. Tracheal aspirates have been a reliable source of *P. carinii* organisms in infants with interstitial plasma cell pneumonia. This procedure has been less reliable for older children and adults.

Sputum, pharyngeal smears, and gastric aspirates may only occasionally contain the organisms, and culture of such specimens cannot be depended on to exclude the diagnosis. Induced sputum specimens properly collected have been especially useful in adults with AIDS.

Fiberoptic bronchoscopy with bronchoalveolar lavage is a useful method to obtain specimens of

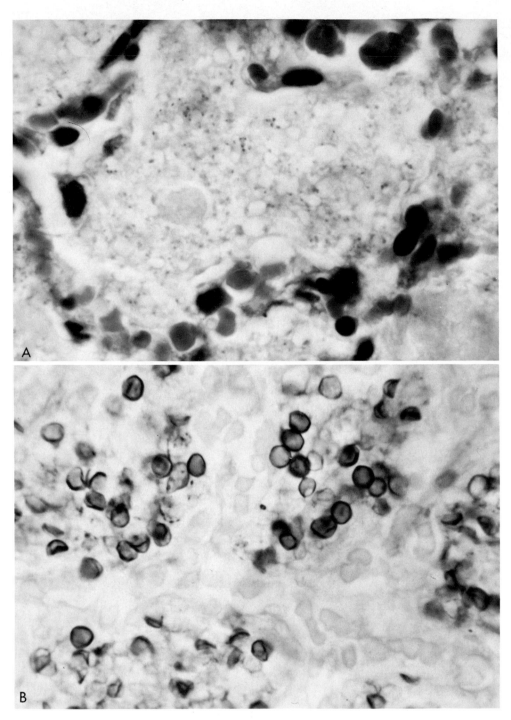

Figure 20–3. Histopathologic features of *Pneumocystis carinii* pneumonitis. *A*, Hematoxylin and eosin (H and E) stain of extensively infected (Stage III) lung. *P. carinii* organisms do not stain with H and E; therefore, the alveolar spaces appear to be filled with a pinkish "foamy proteinaceous" material. The alveolar septa are widened because of interstitial edema and lymphocytic infiltration (original magnification ×1180). *B*, Gomori methenamine–silver nitrate stain of the same lung section. *P. carinii* organisms fill the alveolar spaces. Only the cyst forms are stained. Cysts are 4 to 6 microns in diameter, brownish black, round, oval, and cup shaped; two "nucleoid" bodies shaped like parentheses may be seen in some of the organisms (original magnification ×1180).

diagnostic value. Endobronchial brush biopsy has been used successfully in adults, but its use has been limited in children with *P. carinii* pneumonitis. Although adequate specimens may be obtained by percutaneous needle biopsy of the lung, this procedure is frequently followed by complications of pneumothorax and hemoptysis. Transbronchial lung biopsy may be utilized by the skillful operator. The standard surgical open-lung biopsy is the most dependable method for the diagnosis of this infection. It has the advantage of providing a specimen that reveals the histologic characteristics of the disease process, and

the presence of a concomitant infection of another cause may be recognized. General anesthesia and endotracheal intubation are disadvantages.

Percutaneous needle aspiration of the lung provides a specimen that contains identifiable organisms in 85 per cent of the cases. When this procedure is repeated in suspicious cases with nondiagnostic initial aspirates, the diagnosis can be made in more than 90 per cent of the cases. However, pneumothorax is a complication that frequently follows this procedure as well as that of the other invasive techniques.

Several staining techniques have been employed to

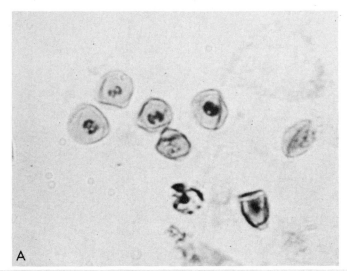

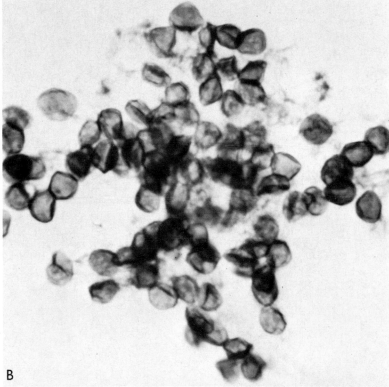

Figure 20–4. Specimens obtained by percutaneous transthoracic needle aspiration of the lung showing *Pneumocystis carinii* stained by different methods. *A,* Gomori methenamine–silver nitrate stain reveals the cysts as brownish black, rounded, and sometimes folded structures. The parenthesis-like "nucleoid" bodies are seen in some cysts and represent components of the cell wall. The intracystic sporozoites and extracystic trophozoite are not stained (original magnification × 1180). *B,* Toluidine blue O stain depicts the same features as the Gomori stain, except that the cysts stain violet to lavender (original magnification × 1180).

Illustration continued on following page.

identify *P. carinii.* The Gomori methenamine–silver nitrate stain and toluidine blue O stain are most useful for localizing organisms in specimens. These stains clearly outline the cyst forms but not the trophozoites. The Gomori stain is more complex and requires some 4 hours to complete, whereas the toluidine blue O method requires only 10 to 20 min. These methods also stain fungi and nonbudding yeasts, which may resemble *P. carinii* cysts. The Giemsa, polychrome methylene blue, Wright, and Gram-Weigert stains are most informative for detailed study of the organisms, because the cyst with sporozoites as well as trophozoites is identifiable. The cyst wall does not stain with these reagents. Fluorescein-labeled antibody methods using specific mono-clonal antibodies have been applied to clinical specimens but offer no significant advantages over the other staining procedures.

SEROLOGY

In the epidemic-infantile type, antibodies to *P. carinii* may be detected by the complement fixation test in 75 to 95 per cent of the cases. Seroconversion usually occurs during the second week of the illness; however, this test has not been sufficiently sensitive for diagnostic purposes in the immunodeficient child and adult with the infection. Furthermore, it is not available in the United States.

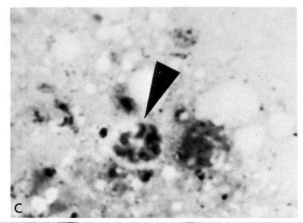

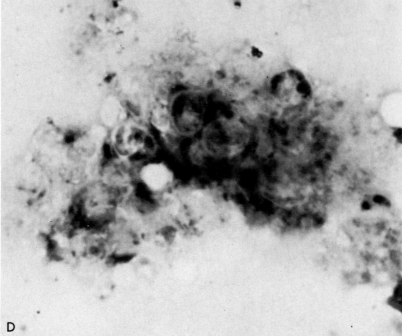

Figure 20–4 *Continued C,* Polychrome methylene blue stain showing cysts with crescent-shaped sporozoites. The cyst wall does not stain, resulting in a clear zone or "halo" around the intracystic sporozoites *(arrow).* The cytoplasm of the sporozoites stains light blue with a dark-staining nucleus. As many as eight sporozoites may be seen in one cyst (original magnification ×1440). *D,* Polychrome methylene blue stain showing a massive cluster of cysts and trophozoites. The trophozoites are 2 to 4 microns in diameter with light blue cytoplasm and small, punctate, sometimes eccentrically located nuclei. They are pleomorphic, with a marked affinity for clustering in masses. The trophozoite is not sufficiently unique for identification as *P. carinii,* because platelet and cell remnants may mimic this stage of the organism (original magnification ×1440).

An immunofluorescence method developed at the Centers for Disease Control (CDC) in Atlanta detected antibody in the serums of 35 per cent of suspected or confirmed cases of *P. carinii* pneumonitis of the child-adult type and was more sensitive than the complement fixation test. Unfortunately, antibody was also detected in patients without *P. carinii* infection, thus limiting the reliability of this technique in the diagnosis of active infection.

P. carinii antigenemia has been detected by counterimmunoelectrophoresis using rabbit antiserums (Pifer et al, 1978). Because the antigen can be detected in at least 15 per cent of cancer patients without pneumonitis and neither the antiserums nor the control antigen has been standardized, this technique cannot be relied on for diagnosis in general hospital laboratories.

TREATMENT

SPECIFIC DRUGS

Various drugs have been evaluated in the treatment of *P. carinii* pneumonitis.

Pentamidine isethionate, a diamidine with antifungal and antiprotozoan activity, was the first drug used successfully. With the infantile interstitial plasma cell pneumonitis, the mortality rate was reduced from 50 per cent to about 3 per cent with pentamidine therapy. This drug became available in the United States in 1967 solely through the CDC. The mortality rate in untreated cases of *P. carinii* pneumonitis in the United States is about 100 per cent. Data from the CDC have shown that 43 per cent of 163 pentamidine-treated patients recovered (Walzer et al, 1974).

More favorable results have come from specific medical centers, reporting recovery rates of up to 75 per cent. Pentamidine is administered as a single daily dose of 4 mg/kg intravenously over a 2-hr period for 10 to 14 days. The total dose should not exceed 56 mg/kg. Unfortunately, an inordinate number of toxic and adverse side effects are associated with pentamidine therapy. Adverse effects, which can be expected in half the patients, include impaired renal or liver function, hypoglycemia, injection site reactions, anemia, thrombocytopenia, neutropenia, hypotension, skin rashes, and hypocalcemia.

The drug combination trimethoprim-sulfamethoxazole has been evaluated for the treatment of this infection. The dosage of 20 mg trimethoprim–100 mg sulfamethoxazole/kg/day, orally, in four divided doses for 2 weeks has been shown to be the preferred one for the treatment of humans (Hughes, Feldman, and Sanyal, 1975; Lau and Young, 1976).

One study has compared the therapeutic efficacies of pentamidine isethionate and trimethoprim-sulfamethoxazole (Hughes et al, 1978). Of 50 patients with cancer and *P. carinii* pneumonitis, 77 per cent of the 26 children treated initially with trimethoprim-sulfamethoxazole and 75 per cent of the 24 children treated with pentamidine recovered. No significant adverse effects occurred in the drug combination group; however, the high incidence of reactions as found in other studies occurred with the pentamidine group. Thus trimethoprim-sulfamethoxazole is as effective as pentamidine but has the advantage of fewer adverse side effects. Patients with AIDS, however, have an exaggerated rate of adverse reactions to this drug combination to the extent that 50 per cent of them will have a rash, neutropenia, fever, or other unwanted reactions. The combination is available in oral tablet and suspension forms as well as in a solution for intravenous (IV) infusion. The IV preparation is administered in a dosage of 15 mg trimethoprim–75 mg sulfamethoxazole/kg/day in four divided doses. The oral dose is 20 mg trimethoprim–100 mg sulfamethoxazole/kg/day in four divided doses. If either the oral or the IV form is used, serum levels of the drugs should be measured and the dosages should be adjusted to achieve 2-hr postdose levels of 3 to 5 μg/ml trimethoprim–100 to 150 μg/ml sulfamethoxazole. Other drugs under clinical investigation include pyrimethamine-sulfadoxine (Fansidar), dapsone, dapsone-trimethoprim, trimetrexate with leucovorin, and aerosolized pentamidine (Kovacs and Masur, 1988). Each has been demonstrated to have some degree of efficacy for *P. carinii* pneumonitis therapy, but priority of choices for therapy has not been established.

SUPPORTIVE MEASURES

Oxygen should be administered as required to keep the arterial oxygen tension (Pa_{O_2}) above 70 mm Hg. The fraction of inspired oxygen (Fi_{O_2}) should be kept below 50 volumes per cent, if possible, to prevent oxygen toxicity. Assisted or controlled ventilation is indicated when the Pa_{O_2} is less than 60 mm Hg at Fi_{O_2} of 50 volumes per cent or greater. A continuous negative pressure system has been useful in the management of patients requiring assisted ventilation (Sanyal et al, 1975).

Because the mode of transmission of *P. carinii* is not known, and because some instances of possible person-to-person transmission have been reported, it is probably wise to admit patients to contagion isolation rooms.

Our policy has been to withhold immunosuppressive drugs during the acute phase of the infection if the status of the primary disease permits.

PREVENTIVE MEASURES

P. carinii pneumonitis can be effectively prevented by the prophylactic administration of 5 mg trimethoprim–25 mg sulfamethoxazole/kg daily (Hughes et al, 1977) or even 3 days a week (Hughes et al, 1987). Protection is afforded only as long as the drugs are administered, because *P. carinii* is not eradicated by them. This approach should be considered for individuals who are at unusually high risk for this type of pneumonitis. Aerosolized pentamide has been used successfully in adults, but studies have not been done in infants and children.

ATYPICAL CASES

Rare cases of disseminated *P. carinii* infection involving hematopoietic tissues, liver, spleen, thymus, lymph node, thyroid, ear, eye, intestine, and bone marrow have been reported. A few descriptions of *P. carinii* pneumonitis in neonates have strongly suggested the possibility of intrauterine infection.

Recurrent infection or reinfection has occurred several months to a year after recovery from an initial episode of *P. carinii* pneumonitis. The clinical manifestations and response to treatment are similar to those in the primary infection.

REFERENCES

Dutz W, Post C, Kohout E, and Aghamohammadi A: Cellular reaction to *Pneumocystis carinii*. Z Kinderheilkd 114:1, 1973.

Edman J, Kovacs J, Masur H et al: Ribosomal RNA sequence shows *Pneumocystis carinii* to be a member of the fungi. Nature 334:519, 1988.

Gajdusek DC: *Pneumocystis carinii*—etiologic agent of interstitial plasma cell pneumonia of premature and young infants. Pediatrics 19:543, 1957.

Gigliotti F, Ballou LR, Hughes WT, and Mosley B: Purification and initial characterization of a *Pneumocystis carinii* surface antigen capable of inducing protective antibody (abstract). Pediatr Res 23:369A, 1988.

Hughes WT, Feldman S, and Sanyal SK: Treatment of *Pneumocystis carinii* pneumonitis and trimethoprim-sulfamethoxazole. Can Med J 112(Suppl.):47, 1975.

Hughes WT, Feldman S, Aur RJA et al: Intensity of immunosuppressive therapy and incidence of *Pneumocystis carinii* pneumonitis. Cancer 36:2004, 1975.

Hughes WT, Feldman S, Chaudhary S et al: Comparison of trimethoprim-sulfamethoxazole and pentamidine in the treatment of *Pneumocystis carinii* pneumonitis. J Pediatr 92:285, 1978.

Hughes W, Kuhn S, Chaudhary S et al: Successful chemoprophylaxis for *Pneumocystis carinii* pneumonitis. N Engl J Med 297:1419, 1977.

Hughes WT, Rivera GK, Schell MJ, Thornton D, and Lott L: Successful intermittent chemoprophylaxis for *Pneumocystis carinii* pneumonitis. N Engl J Med 316:1627, 1987.

Kovacs JA and Masur H: *Pneumocystis carinii* pneumonia: therapy and prophylaxis. J Infect Dis 158:254, 1988.

Latorre CR, Sulzer AT, and Norman LG: Serial propagation of *Pneumocystis carinii* in cell line cultures. Appl Environ Microbiol 33:1204, 1977.

Lau WK and Young LS: Co-trimoxazole treatment of *Pneumocystis carinii* pneumonia in adults. N Engl J Med 295:716, 1976.

Pifer LL and Hughes WT: Cultivation of *Pneumocystis carinii* in vitro (abstract). Pediatr Res 9:344, 1975.

Pifer LL, Hughes WT, Stagno S, and Woods D: *Pneumocystis carinii* infection: evidence for high prevalence in normal and immunosuppressed children. Pediatrics 61:35, 1978.

Price R and Hughes W: Histopathology of *Pneumocystis carinii* infestation and infection of malignant disease of childhood. Hum Pathol 5:737, 1974.

Rowecka-Trzebicka K, Kassur-Siemienska B, Dobryanska A, and Milewska-Bobula B: *Pneumocystis carinii* pneumonia in neonates (abstract). Pediatr Res 24:271, 1988.

Sanyal SK, Mitchell C, Hughes WT et al: Continuous negative chest wall pressure as therapy for severe respiratory distress in older children. Chest 68:143, 1975.

Stagno S, Brasfield DM, Brown MB et al: Infant pneumonitis associated with cytomegalovirus, chlamydia, pneumocystis, and ureaplasma: a prospective study. Pediatrics 68:322, 1981.

Stagno S, Pifer L, Hughes W et al: *Pneumocystis carinii* pneumonitis in young immunocompetent infants. Pediatrics 66:56, 1980.

Walzer PD, Perl DP, Krogstad DJ et al: *Pneumocystis carinii* pneumonia in the United States. Ann Intern Med 80:83, 1974.

21

W. PAUL GLEZEN, M.D.

DIAGNOSIS OF VIRAL RESPIRATORY ILLNESS

The National Health Survey estimates that every year U.S. citizens experience about 250 million acute respiratory illnesses that cause them to alter their activities or to seek medical care. Almost 40 per cent of these illnesses are medically treated, which translates into about 100 million clinic visits per year. More than 60 per cent of acute respiratory illnesses of preschool children generate a health care visit; the rate for school children is about 30 per cent. It is, therefore, important for clinicians to understand the pathogenesis of these infections and to treat them appropriately. Most (about 80 per cent) of these illnesses are caused by viruses.

More than 200 different viruses infect the human respiratory tract (Table 21–1); most have on occasion been associated with all of the clinical syndromes of acute respiratory disease ranging from rhinitis to pneumonia. Table 21–2 provides an approximation of the frequency of association of specific virus infections with the various clinical syndromes. Some viruses have typical clinical presentations, which may be helpful in assessing the etiology of illnesses when

considered in conjunction with epidemiologic factors, such as seasonality and age of the patient. For the most part, specific virologic studies are necessary to specify the etiology. New technologies are being brought to bear on this problem, which make viral diagnosis increasingly available and clinically useful. This chapter summarizes general aspects of the laboratory diagnosis of respiratory virus infections, addresses some of the distinguishing features of the major virus families, and presents the clinical and epidemiologic patterns of occurrence of the viruses associated with acute lower respiratory tract infections in children.

Rationale for Viral Diagnosis. Determination of the etiology of virus infections becomes increasingly

Table 21–1. HUMAN RESPIRATORY VIRUSES

Type	Number of Serotypes
Influenza viruses	3 (3 subtypes of type A)
Respiratory syncytial virus	1 (2 subtypes)
Parainfluenza	4
Adenoviruses	33
Rhinoviruses	~100
Enteroviruses	63
Coronaviruses	4
Herpesvirus	1 (2 subtypes)
Cytomegalovirus	1

This work was supported in part by contracts AI62517 and AI 22672 from the Development and Applications Branch, National Institute for Allergy and Infectious Diseases, NIH. The author is grateful to Sherry Watson for manuscript preparation.

Table 21–2. ASSOCIATION OF RESPIRATORY VIRUSES WITH CLINICAL SYNDROMES

Viruses	Upper Respiratory Illness (URI)	Pharyngitis	Febrile URI or Flu-like Illness	Tracheo-bronchitis	Croup	Bronchiolitis	Pneumonia
Influenza A	+	+	+ + +	+ +	+	+	+ +
Influenza B	+	+	+ + +	+ +	+	±	+ +
Respiratory syncytial	+	±	+	+ +	+	+ + +*	+ + +
Parainfluenza type 1	+	+	+	+ +	+ + +*	+	+ +
Parainfluenza type 2	+	+	+	+	+	±	+ +
Parainfluenza type 3	+	+	+	+ +	+ +	+	+ +
Adenoviruses	+	+ +	+ +	+	±	±	+
Rhinoviruses	+ + +	+	+	+	±	+	±
Influenza C	+ +	±	±	±	±	±	±
Coronaviruses	+ +	+	+	±	±	+	±
Herpesvirus hominis	+	+ + +	+	+	±	±	+
Enteroviruses	+	+	+	±	±	±	+
Cytomegalovirus	–	–	–	–	–	–	+

*Signal illness

important with the introduction of specific viral chemotherapy. Some therapies are commenced on the basis of a presumptive diagnosis; a specific diagnosis may be important to confirm the initial impression and to determine the length of time for treatment. Conversely, viral diagnosis is important to curtail the unnecessary use of antibiotics.

Viral diagnosis is also important for the surveillance of nosocomial infections. Several respiratory viruses have been implicated in nosocomial outbreaks. Control measures have been recommended that are dependent on etiologic studies for implementation and evaluation. Viral diagnosis is necessary for the evaluation of vaccine efficacy. For instance, many respiratory viruses may cause influenza-like illnesses, and influenza viruses may be responsible for other respiratory syndromes; therefore, influenza vaccine efficacy can best be determined by virologic methods.

LABORATORY DIAGNOSIS

Virus Identification. Isolation of viruses in tissue culture is the standard method of virus diagnosis. Although some rapid antigen detection systems are used routinely, they do not yet have the flexibility or sensitivity to replace tissue culture isolation. The tissue cultures commonly used to isolate and identify respiratory viruses are primary monkey kidney, human fetal lung fibroblasts (or some other human diploid line), and a continuous cell line, such as HEp-2 cells, known to be sensitive to respiratory syncytial virus (RSV). Primary monkey kidney cells will support the growth of influenza viruses, parainfluenza viruses, and enteroviruses. Primary monkey kidney cultures are relatively expensive, and certain less expensive continuous cell lines maintained in media containing active trypsin can be used. MDCK cells are sensitive to influenza viruses, and LLC-MK2 cells can be used to isolate parainfluenza viruses. These cell lines are not satisfactory for enteroviruses. Human fetal lung fibroblast cultures are best for

growing rhinoviruses and herpesviruses, including Herpesvirus hominis, varicella-zoster, and cytomegalovirus (CMV). Most enteroviruses can also be cultivated on these cells. Of the continuous cell lines, HEp-2 cells are usually favored for the isolation of RSV and adenoviruses. After many generations, HEp-2 cells may lose their ability to support the growth of RSV; therefore, it is important to monitor the cell line with positive controls and to replace the line when it appears to be losing sensitivity.

Several antigen detection methods are useful for virus diagnosis, and some are used routinely in virus diagnostic laboratories. The major advantage of these tests is that they can be performed rapidly and can provide results within 24 hours of receiving the specimen in the laboratory. The disadvantages are that they are usually less sensitive and that they have limited scope; that is, reagents are available for a limited number of agents. This limited scope means that rapid diagnosis is available currently for only a small number of viruses—but usually the most important ones—such as RSV, parainfluenza, and influenza viruses. The same techniques can be applied to viruses grown in tissue culture to speed up identification. For clinical specimens that do not contain enough viral antigen for immediate, direct identification, the virus content can be amplified by short periods (24 to 72 hours) of incubation in tissue culture. After a few cycles of virus replication, sufficient antigen may be present for typing.

Several methods for the rapid detection of viral antigens have been tested. These include immune electron microscopy, immunofluorescence (fluorescent antibody technique [FA]), enzyme-linked immunosorbent assay (ELISA), enzyme-linked fluorescent assay, and tissue culture amplification (TCA). Several modifications of these tests have been proposed for use with different virus groups. The tests that have found practical application for respiratory viruses are FA, ELISA, and TCA. From the standpoint of both the number of viruses to which it has been applied and the number of laboratories that employ it, FA has the broadest application. The

ELISA kits are available for identification of several viruses, and the kits for RSV identification are widely used. For influenza virus identification, TCA has been employed successfully. Efficient use of these methods requires that the clinicians and the laboratory directors have a good understanding of the clinical and epidemiologic features of the viruses for which the reagents are available. Knowledge of the seasonality, age incidence, and major clinical manifestations of the viruses is essential.

A new method for virus recognition in clinical specimens is nucleic acid hybridization. The unknown DNA or RNA is fixed to nitrocellulose to be reacted with a radio-labeled probe. The test should have great sensitivity and specificity. The problem will be the development of a battery of appropriate radio-labeled probes and strategies for their efficient use.

Specimen collection and transportation of specimens to the laboratory can be critical for the diagnosis of respiratory virus infection. Specimens should be obtained as early as possible after the onset of symptoms. Nasal aspiration or a small nasal washing combined with a throat swab is probably the optimal specimen. The nasal washing should be performed with a balanced (neutral pH) salt solution. Tracheal aspirate or percutaneous lung aspirate can be cultured, if available. The virus-holding medium should contain antibiotics and a protein stabilizer, such as 0.5 per cent bovine serum albumin or gelatin. The specimen should be transported to a laboratory on wet ice as soon as possible.

Antibody Detection. In usual clinical practice, serologic tests are less helpful but may be important under certain circumstances. For most respiratory virus infections, antibodies in serum and secretions do not develop until the patient is recovering. An important exception is CMV, which may produce an indolent pneumonia in the neonatal period; measurement of specific IgM antibodies to CMV can be diagnostic in such cases. Detection of IgM antibodies to other respiratory viruses also could be helpful, but specificity has been a problem in the detection of some IgM antibodies.

Testing of paired serum specimens to measure a rise in antibodies to respiratory viruses may be important for severe infections that produce complications, such as obliterative bronchiolitis, myocarditis, pericarditis, or encephalitis. The diagnosis may help determine a prognosis in such cases. Testing also may be important for determining the susceptibility to certain viruses of pregnant women, nursing staff, and medical staff. Antibody testing is obviously important for clinical investigations and for vaccine evaluation.

A battery of serologic tests are available and can be useful, depending on the purpose of the investigation. Complement fixation (CF) tests are available for most of the respiratory viruses and have special applications for some of them. For instance, adenoviruses have a common internal antigen, and the CF test is useful as a screen for a recent adenovirus infection, but it does not indicate type. The CF test for influenza viruses utilizing the internal or nucleoprotein antigen is type specific for types A, B, and C. It can be employed for the detection of serum antibodies; high titers may indicate a recent infection because CF titers usually wane after a few months. Disadvantages include the fact that the CF test is not very sensitive and shows cross reactions among the paramyxoviruses (including mumps). The CF test may also be used—with monospecific serum—to classify viruses by type.

Many respiratory viruses will absorb red blood cells to infected tissue culture cells. This property is useful for detecting growth of the virus in culture systems, for identifying the viruses, and for testing serum specimens for antibody. Testing for hemadsorption may be the only indication of infection of culture systems. Inhibition of hemadsorption by specific antiserums is one method for identifying the same viruses. Inhibition of hemagglutination of a known virus with dilutions of the patient's serum is a practical and useful antibody test for many of these viruses. Most serum specimens must be pretreated to eliminate nonspecific inhibitors before combining them with the hemagglutinating antigen and the red blood cells. The animal source of red blood cells may be specific for certain viruses; this property can be employed to classify viruses. For instance, adenoviruses can be grouped by hemadsorption of either rhesus or rat red blood cells.

Neutralization of virus growth in tissue culture with dilutions of serum is a particularly informative test for determining immunity. In general, the neutralization test is considered the best correlate of immunity and is frequently used to evaluate vaccines. Neutralization tests take several days to complete and are relatively expensive to perform.

The ELISA tests have been adapted to measure specific antibody by immunoglobulin class and subclass. Because commercial kits can be prepared for hospital laboratories, it is likely that many will become available in the future. The IgM-capture ELISA would be particularly useful for clinical virology. In general, ELISA antibody tests are very sensitive and may detect nonneutralizing antibodies. The problem is, of course, to preserve the specificity of these tests.

MAJOR RESPIRATORY VIRUS GROUPS

Influenza Viruses. The influenza viruses belong to the Orthomyxoviridae family. Under the genus influenza virus are three serotypes: A, B, and C. Three subtypes of influenza A have been known to infect humans (Table 21–3). The subtypes are classified by the surface antigens: hemagglutinin (H) and neuraminidase (N). In addition to the three subtypes that infect humans, ten other subtypes are known to infect avian species. These animal reservoirs are thought to

Table 21–3. INFLUENZA VIRUSES

Type	Subtype	Prototype	Common Designation
A	H_1N_1	A/Puerto Rico/8/34	PR8
		A/New Jersey/1/76	Swine flu
		A/USSR/90/77	Russian flu
	H_2N_2	A/Japan/305/57	Asian flu
	H_3N_2	A/Hong Kong/1/68	Hong Kong flu
B	None	B/Lee/40	B/Lee
C	None	C/Taylor/1233/47	Taylor

be the source of subtypes that cause pandemics, such as the Hong Kong influenza pandemic of 1968–1969. Multiple variants resulting from antigenic "drift" have been described for each of the A subtypes and for influenza B. Table 21–4 shows the most important variants that have circulated between 1978 and 1988.

Influenza viruses are the most important causes of acute respiratory illnesses that receive medical attention. They regularly cause serious infections that result in hospitalization. The surface antigens of the viruses—hemagglutinin and neuraminidase—are constantly changing so that previously acquired immunity from natural infection or vaccination may not protect against a new variant. Antiviral therapy is available; amantadine is effective against influenza A viruses, and a broader spectrum antiviral, ribavirin, is licensed for treatment of infants with RSV disease. Ribavirin has been shown to shorten the course of illness caused by both influenza B and influenza A. The need for rapid diagnosis of these potentially life-threatening infections is obvious. Immunofluorescence can be used for identification of virus in cells shed from the upper respiratory tract. In addition, ELISA and tissue culture amplification have been tested and should be commercially available in the near future.

Besides tissue cultures, embryonated eggs have long been used to isolate influenza viruses and have been the standard for many years. Eggs, 11 to 13 days old, are generally inoculated and incubated for 3 days before harvesting and testing the fluid for hemagglutination. Influenza C viruses can be isolated only in eggs; the problem is that type C takes longer to grow than types A or B. For detecting influenza C, it is generally necessary to inoculate 6- to 8-day-old eggs and then incubate them for 5 days. Only chick red blood cells can be used to detect the virus.

Table 21–4. VARIANTS OF INFLUENZA VIRUSES PREVALENT IN THE UNITED STATES, 1978–1988, BY TYPE AND SUBTYPE

Type A		Type B
H_1N_1	H_3N_2	
A/USSR/90/77	A/Texas/1/77	B/Singapore/222/79
A/Brazil/11/78	A/Bangkok/1/79	B/USSR/100/82
A/England/333/80	A/Philippines/2/82	B/Ann Arbor/1/86
A/Chile/1/83	A/Mississippi/1/85	B/Victoria/2/87
A/Taiwan/1/86	A/Leningrad/360/86	
	A/Sichuan/2/87	

Because of these differences in procedure, influenza C virus is rarely detected by routine virus diagnostic methods. Available evidence suggests that infection is common because serologic surveys have shown that most children have been infected by the age of 5 years. Limited clinical studies suggest that the virus infection usually involves the upper respiratory tract without complications.

Respiratory Syncytial Virus. Respiratory syncytial virus is a member of the Paramyxoviridae family, genus *pneumovirus*. It is an enveloped RNA-containing virus that has two surface glycoproteins, as do other viruses of this family. The major difference is that RSV does not hemagglutinate red blood cells like the others do. The virus does have an active fusion protein that acts to fuse cell membranes of contiguous cells in culture, which produces large syncytia. The RSV is labile, with a lipid envelope; it is inactivated by lipid solvents as well as by acid pH. Infectivity is usually lost below pH 3.0. Freezing of clinical specimens will inactivate the virus unless the freezing is accomplished under special conditions (snap freezing at $-70°C$ with the specimen in a holding medium containing a protein stabilizer).

The most important cause of acute lower respiratory disease in infants is RSV. Epidemics occur each winter and result in the hospitalization of approximately 1 per cent of children younger than 1 year of age. Most children are infected at least once by 2 years of age; reinfection is common in older children and adults. Specific therapy, ribavirin aerosol, is available for hospitalized infants. The major distinguishing clinical manifestation of RSV infection is bronchiolitis. During epidemics, it is not necessary to obtain specific virologic diagnosis before instituting ribavirin aerosol therapy of severely involved wheezing infants. Rapid diagnosis is available routinely in many hospitals; laboratories utilize FA or ELISA kits. The best specimen for detection of RSV antigen is a nasal aspirate or small nasal washing. Because RSV is labile, the clinical specimen should be transported to the laboratory on wet ice as soon as possible.

Parainfluenza Viruses. Parainfluenza viruses belong to the Paramyxoviridae family along with mumps virus. After RSV, parainfluenza viruses are the next most common causes of acute lower respiratory tract disease in children. As a group they account for almost as many hospitalizations each year as RSV. The surface glycoproteins of the parainfluenza viruses include one with hemagglutinin activity. Hemadsorption of guinea pig red blood cells allows early recognition of the growth of the viruses in tissue culture; therefore, parainfluenza antiserums are usually incorporated into the battery used for identification of hemadsorbing viruses by immunofluorescence. Parainfluenza viruses are relatively stable at 4°C in a protein-stabilized holding medium.

Hemagglutination inhibition can be employed to measure antibodies in serum, but it should be remembered that cross reactions may occur among the group, including mumps virus. The first three types have closely related viruses in nature. Sendai virus of rodents is antigenically similar to parainfluenza virus type 1. A simian virus, SV5, is related to parainfluenza type 2; this virus may arise as a contaminant when primary monkey kidney tissue cultures are being utilized for virus isolation in the clinical laboratory. The shipping fever virus of cattle is similar to parainfluenza virus type 3.

Adenoviruses. Adenoviruses are stable viruses consisting of a single-stranded DNA core surrounded by a protein coat that exhibits icosahedral symmetry. Adenoviruses are present throughout the year and can cause acute respiratory tract illnesses ranging from conjunctivitis to life-threatening obliterative bronchiolitis. Infections with types 1, 2, 5, and 6 are common in children younger than 2 years of age. Primary infection usually results in a febrile upper respiratory illness. Exudative pharyngitis in an infant younger than 2 years of age is likely to be due to one of these adenoviruses. Otitis media is a common complication of adenovirus infection in this age group.

Types 3 and 7 are common causes of pharyngo-conjuctival fever in older children and young adults. Rarely, these viruses, along with types 11 and 21, cause a severe necrotizing pneumonia in infants. This pneumonia is often fatal, and survivors may have permanent damage from obliterative bronchiolitis. These infections appear to be more common in native Americans and in infants from the Far East.

Adenovirus types 4, 7, and 21 have been frequent causes of acute respiratory disease and pneumonia in military recruits. A successful vaccine for types 4 and 7 is currently in use in the United States. The viruses are enclosed in an enteric-coated capsule for administration, which results in asymptomatic infection of the gastrointestinal tract and solid immunity against respiratory tract infection.

Adenoviruses are relatively stable, and virus recovery is easily accomplished. The viruses produce a typical cytopathic effect in tissue culture that results

in clumping of rounded and swollen cells. Human fetal kidney cells are the most sensitive tissue culture but are not routinely available. Identification of specific serotypes is usually accomplished by neutralization with specific antiserums. The less common types may be grouped by their hemadsorption with rhesus and rat red blood cells.

Coronaviruses. Coronaviruses were so named because of the crown-like projections visible on the surface. The virus has a single-stranded RNA core and is labile at low pH and in lipid solvents. This group of viruses has not been well studied because of the difficulties in viral diagnosis. Coronaviruses do not grow in usual tissue cultures, a fact that has hampered investigations, but ELISA methods have been applied both to antigen detection in respiratory secretions and to antibody measurements in serum. Most studies attribute upper respiratory tract infections to these viruses, but a study from the United Kingdom reported that coronavirus infections frequently trigger wheezing episodes in children with reactive airway disease. Further technologic advances should increase our understanding of these viruses in the future.

Rhinoviruses. Rhinoviruses belong to the Picornaviridae family and are small RNA viruses with a stable protein coat. Unlike the enteroviruses, rhinoviruses are not found in the gastrointestinal tract, probably because of their instability in acid pH. Presumably they are inactivated in the stomach. Rhinoviruses are responsible for about 30 per cent of upper respiratory illnesses in adults. (Adults average about one acute respiratory illness per year that alters their activity or causes them to seek medical care.) These viruses are also frequent causes of acute respiratory illnesses in children, but they are overshadowed by RSV, parainfluenza, and influenza viruses, which are more likely causes of lower respiratory tract infections.

Rhinoviruses can be isolated on human diploid fibroblasts, but identification beyond demonstrating

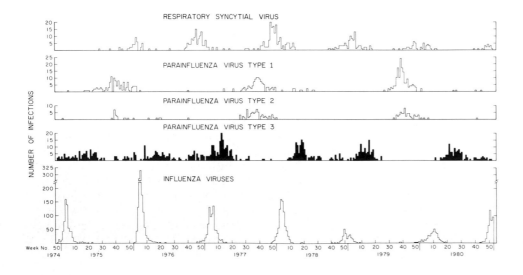

Figure 21–1. Number of respiratory viruses isolated from patients with acute respiratory illnesses who attended sentinel clinics, and from persons observed in the Houston Family Study, Houston, Texas, 1974–1980. The parainfluenza virus type 3 isolates are shaded to emphasize the change from endemic to seasonal occurrence. (Reproduced with permission from Glezen WP, Frank AL, Taber LH, and Kasel JA: J Infect Dis 150:852, 1984. © by the University of Chicago. All rights reserved.)

Table 21–5. CLINICAL AND EPIDEMIOLOGIC FEATURES RELATED TO ETIOLOGY OF LOWER RESPIRATORY TRACT DISEASE IN CHILDREN

Virus	Age	Season	Signal Illness
Parainfluenza type 1	6–24 mo	Autumn (biannual)	Croup
Respiratory syncytial	2–6 mo	Midwinter	Bronchiolitis
Influenza	2–18 yr	Midwinter	Flu-like, tracheobronchitis
Parainfluenza type 3	3–8 mo	Spring	Bronchiolitis, pneumonia

acid lability is not practical except for clinical and epidemiologic investigations. Replication of rhinoviruses is inhibited below pH 3.0, whereas enteroviruses are acid stable; this property of acid stability is commonly used to separate the two groups of viruses, because the cytopathic effects in tissue culture may be similar. More than 100 rhinovirus serotypes have been described, and other putative serotypes have been reported. Serotyping has no clinical significance, because the manifestations of infection are the same. Because of the multiplicity of types, serologic testing is not practical.

CLINICAL AND EPIDEMIOLOGIC ASSESSMENT OF ACUTE LOWER RESPIRATORY ILLNESSES IN CHILDREN

Some consistent clinical features and epidemiologic patterns of occurrence of the major respiratory viruses associated with lower respiratory disease have emerged to assist clinicians in their assessment of causes. These features may be important for those who do not have access to clinical virology laboratories. They also allow initiation of antiviral therapy for children with life-threatening infections before laboratory results are available. The major respiratory viruses—RSV, parainfluenza, and influenza viruses—occur in predictable seasonal patterns as relatively discrete outbreaks, as shown in Figure 21–1. When the activity of one virus is at its peak, the others tend to be relatively inactive. For example, epidemics of parainfluenza type 1 virus occur biannually during the autumn of odd-numbered years. In Houston, Texas, these epidemics have been documented in 1975, 1977, 1979, 1981, 1983, and 1987, with the peak in late September to mid-October. Epidemics of RSV occur every year during the winter and usually peak in December or January. These RSV epidemics usually have preceded the yearly influenza epidemic, which typically peaks in February; however, in 3 of the last 14 years, influenza activity has had an early peak in December, and most RSV activity has occurred later, as is shown for the 1978–1979 respiratory disease season in Figure 21–1. Parainfluenza virus type 3 may appear at any time during the year, but since 1977, most of the infections with this virus have been in late winter or early spring after influenza activity has subsided.

The major clinical manifestations of these virus infections may alert clinicians to their presence in the community. Although all of these viruses can produce any clinical syndrome in the spectrum of severity from rhinitis to fulminating pneumonia, some have characteristic clinical presentations that signal their presence. The signal illness for parainfluenza virus type 1 is croup or laryngotracheobronchitis; therefore, when a number of children with croup are observed at the expected season (autumn of odd-numbered years), clinicians can assume that most of the viral infections seen concurrently are caused by parainfluenza virus 1 (or type 2, which usually accompanies it, although with less serious consequences). Similarly, when infants with wheezing and bronchiolitis appear, it may be assumed that the bulk of the acute respiratory illness may be related to RSV. Bulletins from the Centers for Disease Control in Atlanta and increasing numbers of schoolchildren with febrile illnesses—particularly tracheobronchitis—usually signal the yearly influenza epidemic.

Table 21–5 summarizes the clinical and epidemiologic features of infections with the major respiratory viruses. Wherever possible this information should be reinforced by virologic studies of a systematic sample of children presenting for medical care with acute respiratory illnesses. The information so gained should be published as bulletins for clinicians in the same geographic regions so that they can estimate the etiology of the illnesses with which they are confronted during the same period of time. This information should allow them to administer antiviral therapy judiciously and to limit the unnecessary use of antibiotics.

REFERENCES

Ahluwalia G, Embree J, McNicol P et al: Comparison of nasopharyngeal aspirate and nasopharyngeal swab specimens for respiratory syncytial virus diagnosis by cell culture, indirect immunofluorescence assay, and enzyme-linked immunosorbent assay. J Clin Microbiol 25:763, 1987.

Baxter BO, Couch RB, Greenberg SB, and Kasel JA: Maintenance of viability and comparison of identification methods for influenza and other respiratory viruses of humans. J Clin Microbiol 6:19, 1977.

Couch RB, Kasel JA, Glezen WP et al: Influenza: its control in persons and populations. J Infect Dis 153:431, 1986.

Current estimates from the national health interview survey, United States, 1986. DHHS Publication No (PHS) 87-1592, October 1987.

Evans AS and Olson B: Rapid diagnostic methods for influenza virus in clinical specimens: a comparative study. Yale J Biol Med 55:391, 1982.

Frank AL, Couch RB, Griffis CA, and Baxter BD: Comparison of different tissue cultures for isolation and quantitation of influenza and parainfluenza viruses. J Clin Microbiol 10:32, 1979.

Frank AL, Puck J, Hughes BJ, and Cate TR: Microneutralization test for influenza A and B and parainfluenza 1 and 2 viruses that uses continuous cell lines and fresh serum enhancement. J Clin Microbiol 12:426, 1980.

Glezen WP and Denny FW: Epidemiology of acute lower respiratory tract disease in children. N Engl J Med 288:498, 1973.

Glezen WP, Frank AL, Taber LH, and Kasel JA: Parainfluenza virus type 3: seasonality and risk of infection and reinfection in young children. J Infect Dis 150:851, 1984.

Glezen WP, Taber LH, Frank AL, and Kasel JA: Risk of primary infection and reinfection with respiratory syncytial virus. Am J Dis Child 140:543, 1986.

Khamapirad T and Glezen WP: Clinical and radiographic assessment of acute lower respiratory tract disease in infants and children. Semin Respir Infect 2:130, 1987.

Krilov LR, Marcoux L, and Isenberg HD: Comparison of three enzyme-linked immunosorbent assays and a direct fluorescent-antibody test for detection of respiratory syncytial virus antigen. J Clin Microbiol 26:377, 1988.

Lennette EH and Schmidt NJ (eds): Diagnostic procedures for viral, rickettsial and chlamydial infections. 5th ed. New York, American Public Health Association, Inc, 1979.

MacNaughton MR, Flowers D, and Isaacs D: Diagnosis of human coronavirus infections in children using enzyme-linked immunosorbent assay. J Med Virol 11:319, 1983.

Masters HD, Weber KO, Groothuis JR et al: Comparison of nasopharyngeal washings and swab specimens for diagnosis of respiratory syncytial virus by EIA, FAT and cell culture. Diagn Microbiol Infect Dis 8:101, 1987.

Richman D, Cleveland PH, Redfield DC et al: Rapid viral diagnosis. J Infect Dis 149:298, 1984.

Richman D, Schmidt N, Plotkin S et al: Summary of a workshop on new and useful methods in rapid viral diagnosis. J Infect Dis 150:941, 1984.

Schmidt OW: Antigenic characterization of human coronaviruses 229E and OC43 by enzyme-linked immunosorbent assay. J Clin Microbiol 20:175, 1984.

Yolken RH: Enzyme immunoassays for the detection of infectious antigens in body fluids: current limitations and future prospects. Rev Infect Dis 4:35, 1982.

Zahradnik JM: Adenovirus pneumonia. Sem Respir Infect 2:104, 1987.

22

W. PAUL GLEZEN, M.D.

VIRAL PNEUMONIA

The National Health Survey for 1986 reports that more than 1 million episodes of pneumonia occurred among children in the United States. Virtually all were medically attended; the proportion of children hospitalized is unknown, but it is likely that many were because about 75 per cent of the pneumonia episodes occurred in children less than 5 years of age. In Houston and in Harris County, Texas, the rate of hospitalization for children with acute respiratory illnesses was 87 per 10,000 between 1977 and 1978. The rate was highest in infants and ranged from 460 per 10,000 for those less than 1 year of age to only 16 per 10,000 for those between 10 and 14 years of age. The discharge diagnosis for the majority of these hospitalized children was pneumonia; tracheobronchitis, bronchiolitis, and croup were less common. Because most children with bronchiolitis and many with croup have some pneumonic involvement, the proportion with some pneumonitis was high. For preschool children seen in primary care facilities serving middle- and upper-income pop-

ulations, the pneumonia rate has been about 40 per 1000. It is likely that the rate is higher for infants from low-income families.

Respiratory viruses are responsible for most pediatric lower respiratory tract infections, including pneumonia. Virologic studies in many geographic sites have documented this finding, and epidemiologic studies have shown that the occurrence of most lower respiratory tract illnesses coincides with epidemics of infections with the major respiratory viruses—respiratory syncytial virus (RSV), parainfluenza viruses, and influenza viruses. Adenoviruses and picornaviruses also have been associated with lower respiratory tract illnesses in nonepidemic periods. Overall, it is estimated that about 80 to 85 per cent of pediatric pneumonias are caused by viruses through a direct invasion of the lower respiratory tract or an indirect facilitation of access of bacterial pathogens. Table 22–1 lists the common virus groups associated with pneumonia in children with an approximation of the frequency of association in three age groups: infancy, preschool, and school age.

This chapter summarizes the pathogenesis of viral pneumonia, examines the unique features of lower respiratory tract infections caused by the major respiratory viruses, and describes specific therapies that are available. The last section is devoted to differ-

The author is grateful to Dr. Tuenchit Khamapirad, pediatric radiologist, for interpretation of chest radiographs and development of the scoring system, and to Sherry Watson for manuscript preparation. This work was supported by contracts AI62517 and AI22672 from the Development and Applications Branch, National Institute for Allergy and Infectious Diseases, NIH.

Table 22–1. VIRUSES ASSOCIATED WITH PNEUMONIA IN CHILDREN

Viruses	Age Group		
	Infants	Preschool	School Age
Respiratory syncytial	+++	++	±
Parainfluenza type 3	++	+	+
Parainfluenza type 1	++	++	+
Influenza A	+	++	++
Influenza B	±	+	++
Parainfluenza type 2	+	+	±
Adenovirus	+	±	±
Measles	+*	+*	±
Cytomegalovirus	+	±	±
Picornaviruses	±	±	±

*Important cause in developing countries.

ential diagnosis of viral infections and other treatable causes of pneumonia in both hospital and ambulatory settings.

PATHOGENESIS

Inoculation of viruses may take place by direct contact, droplet nuclei, or aerosol. There is epidemiologic and experimental evidence, although not conclusive, for all three routes. Whether by extension down the airways from upper tract infection or by direct implantation, the virus invades the terminal airways and the alveoli. The smallest airways ranging in diameter from 75 to 300 μ are probably the primary target. The involvement is usually patchy, affecting multiple lobes. At any given time of observation—either at autopsy or surgical biopsy—the stage of infection will vary at different sites. Some sites will demonstrate early changes, some will be advanced, and some will have evidence of regeneration.

The earliest lesion is probably destruction of ciliated epithelium with sloughing of cellular debris into the lumen. The inflammatory response initially involves infiltration of mononuclear cells into the submucosa and into contiguous perivascular areas. A few polymorphonuclear cells will be found in the lumen of small airways. As the process advances, the amount of debris accompanied by mucus and inflammatory cells increases in the small airways, leading to complete or partial obstruction. Complete obstruction results in the collapse of the contiguous alveoli; infants lack collateral ventilation that in older children and adults may delay or prevent atelectasis. Partial obstruction may cause air trapping, because the airways tend to collapse with expiration. The inflammatory response will also be accompanied by edema of the submucosa, which may extend into the alveolar walls. The inflammatory response within the alveoli as well as in the interstitial space will consist of mononuclear cells. The pathologic changes that occur early in the course of infection are mimicked by those produced in the hamster by intranasal inoculation with parainfluenza virus type 3 (Fig. 22–1).

Severe infections progress with further denudation of the epithelium and development of a hemorrhagic exudate. Rarely, the interstitial infiltration will progress with the development of fibrosis. Either of these developments may cause permanent disability if the patient survives.

Even as some areas of the lung show evidence of advanced involvement, other areas show exuberant proliferation of the epithelium, with piling up of the cells and evagination into the lumen. This proliferation is assumed to occur with regeneration, but it may prolong respiratory difficulties. Usually the host immune response consisting of interferon, cytotoxic cells, and specific antibody limits the progression of the infection and helps promote a recovery. The sequence of these events is illustrated diagramatically in the hamster–parainfluenza type 3 pneumonia model (Fig. 22–2).

Welliver and associates have presented data to suggest that other mechanisms may contribute to the pathologic process. They have detected IgE antibody specific for RSV or parainfluenza viruses in the respiratory secretions of children with these viruses who have severe lower respiratory tract infections. High levels of IgE antibody were accompanied by detectable histamine release. The frequency and quantity of IgE antibody were directly related to the severity of the illness. Therefore, the inflammatory response to infection may be enhanced by release of chemical mediators of atopy; the resulting increase in edema and mucus production as well as in bronchospasm may contribute to the development of pneumonia.

Considerable evidence suggests that virus infections may precede the development of bacterial pneumonia in children. Studies of the bacterial flora of the nasopharynx of children with pneumonia compared with age-matched controls and of children followed longitudinally with and without acute respiratory illness have shown that the potential pathogens usually associated with bacterial pneumonia frequently reside in the nasopharynx of healthy children and are present in the nasopharynx of ill children with only slightly increased frequency. Because these potential bacterial pathogens appear to be normal flora of the upper respiratory tract, an injury must occur to allow them access to the lower tract. For children who have no underlying condition, such as asthma or cystic fibrosis, the injury that makes them more vulnerable to the development of pneumonia is in most instances probably a virus infection. At any one time, pneumococci can be found in the nasopharynx of about 45 per cent of healthy children. For ill children, the frequency is increased to about 50 per cent. *Haemophilus influenzae* organisms (including typable and nontypable strains) are found in about 25 per cent of children under 4 years of age, and staphylococci are carried by about 10 per cent of them. Group A streptococci are unusual in the nasopharynx of infants but occur with increasing frequency as children approach school age.

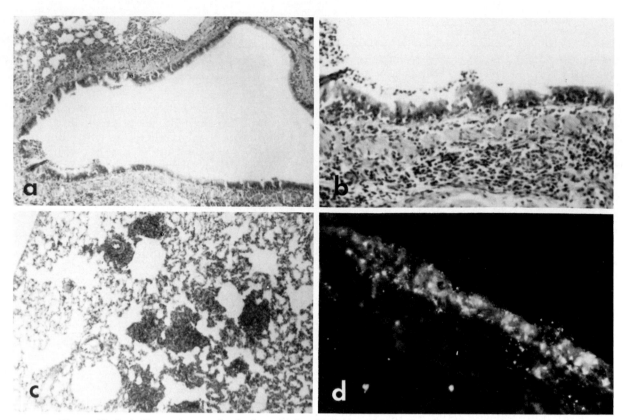

Figure 22–1. *A,* Photomicrograph of a bronchiole with peribronchiolar lymphocytic infiltration and scant intralumenal exudate in the lung of a hamster infected with parainfluenza virus type 3. *B,* High magnification of the intralumenal exudate, showing both mononuclear and polymorphonuclear cells. *C,* Perivascular mononuclear cell infiltration and scattered areas of interstitial infiltration. *D,* Parainfluenza virus type 3 antigen stained by direct immunofluorescence in the respiratory epithelial cells of a hamster bronchus. (Reproduced with permission from Glezen WP and Fernald GW: Infect Immun 14:212–216, 1976.)

Bacteria may invade the lower respiratory tract by two routes, facilitated by infection by respiratory viruses. The first route is via the blood stream; inflammation of the nasal mucosa may allow direct seeding into the blood stream, or it may trap bacteria in the middle ear or paranasal sinuses, which leads to a purulent infection and the additional possibility of bacteremia. The blood-borne bacteria may be filtered out in the lungs or pleura and may result in pneumonia, with or without empyema.

If the viral infection involves the lower respiratory tract, a breakdown of the normal pulmonary clearance mechanisms may allow bacteria from the nasopharynx to invade the lower tract and produce bacterial pneumonia. An understanding of the possible pathogenetic mechanisms is important because the

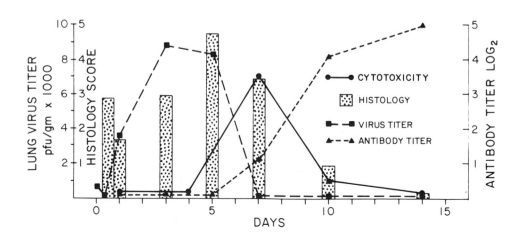

Figure 22–2. Sequence of detection of cell-mediated cytotoxicity, lung histopathology, lung virus, and serum neutralizing antibodies in hamsters infected intranasally with parainfluenza virus type 3. Interferon activity paralleled the curve for lung virus titers. (Reproduced with permission from Kimmel KA, Wyde PR, and Glezen WP: J Reticuloendothel Soc 31:71–83, 1982.)

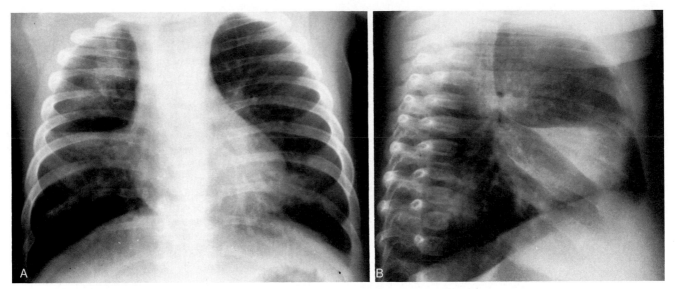

Figure 22–3. Chest radiograph of an infant with respiratory syncytial virus bronchiolitis. Bilateral perihilar and peribronchial infiltrations are evident as well as partial atelectasis of the right middle and right upper lobes. *A,* Posteroanterior view; *B,* lateral view. (Reproduced with permission from Khamapirad T and Glezen WP: Semin Respir Infect 2:130–144, 1987.)

two etiologic classifications—viral and bacterial—are not mutually exclusive. Pneumonia may result from a viral infection alone, or it may result from sequential invasion of the lower tract by a virus followed by a bacterial pathogen. In the latter instance, the patient may seek medical attention at any stage of the evolution from the predominantly viral to the predominantly bacterial. Therefore, continuing evaluation and clinical reassessment of the patient are important in medical management.

MAJOR VIRUS GROUPS

Respiratory Syncytial Virus. Respiratory syncytial virus is the most important cause of pneumonia in infants. Although bronchiolitis is the signal illness of infants infected with RSV, most have accompanying evidence of pneumonitis on chest radiographs. Even though lower tract involvement is common, many infants will have only upper respiratory tract involvement with the first infection. About one third will have evidence of lower respiratory tract involvement. The usual illness begins with low-grade fever—usually less than 102°F— and signs of upper respiratory infection. Coughing increases over the first 3 days, and wheezing may ensue. It is not unusual to find both inspiratory rales and expiratory wheezing on auscultation of the lungs. If infants are examined daily during the course of illness, wheezing may predominate during one examination and rales will be the major finding at the next. The usual course of illness is 5 to 7 days, although cough may persist for a longer period of time. More severe involvement develops for about 1 per cent of infants during the first year of life, evidenced by intercostal retractions and hyperpnea. Mild to moderate hypoxia can be

demonstrated, in which case hospitalization is indicated. The risk of lower respiratory tract involvement decreases both with age and with number of reinfections; the latter are very common with this virus. Two antigenic subtypes of the virus have been described. One of the surface glycoproteins, the fusion protein, is antigenically constant, but the large, heavily glycosylated G protein has differing epitopes for the two subtypes, A and B. Some investigators have suggested that sequential infections with RSV are more likely to alternate between the two subtypes, but the data are inconclusive.

From the foregoing, it is evident that there is no sharp demarcation between the clinical classifications of pneumonia and bronchiolitis; the lower tract involvement of most children will overlap these two categories. In most reported series, the presence of wheezing results in the classification of the illness as bronchiolitis, whether or not pneumonitis is present also. In our series of chest radiographs of hospitalized infants with lower tract disease, almost all (96 per cent) had infiltrations involving multiple lobes. The infiltrations ranged from mild peribronchial thickening to mild interstitial infiltrations. Only about 4 per cent had moderate interstitial involvement. About 21 per cent had radiographic signs of air trapping; only two, or 4 per cent, had air trapping as the only radiographic abnormality. Atelectasis was common, as illustrated by the radiograph of a typical case (Fig. 22–3). This 3-month-old infant had scattered infiltrates and partial atelectasis of the right middle and upper lobes. Atelectasis of the right middle or upper lobe was a common accompaniment of RSV lower respiratory tract disease. Atelectasis was usually present in multiple areas and was segmental, subsegmental, or lobular. Figure 22–4 illustrates the occurrence of bacterial superinfection of

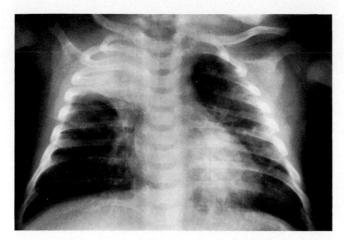

Figure 22–4. Chest radiograph of a child infected with respiratory syncytial virus; pneumococcus was also recovered from the blood culture. Scattered, streaky perihilar and peribronchial infiltrations are present in multiple lobes. The volume of the right upper lobe is reduced, but it also contains a dense infiltrate suggesting bacterial infection. (Reproduced with permission from Khamapirad T and Glezen WP: Semin Respir Infect 2:130–144, 1987.)

RSV disease. This 1-month-old infant had atelectasis of the right upper lobe with a dense infiltrate, which was probably evidence of a pneumococcal infection; this bacterium was recovered from the blood stream at the time of admission, when RSV also was isolated from nasopharyngeal secretions. Despite this finding and the presence of otitis media, the admission temperature was only 100.5°F. In our series, the right upper lobe was the most common site (36 per cent) of atelectasis, but complete collapse was seen only once, or in 2 per cent of the cases. The right middle lobe was the next most common site at 22 per cent followed by the lingula at 16 per cent. Atelectasis involving the lower lobes or the left upper lobe was less frequent, occurring in only about 5 per cent of the cases for each site. In most instances, the atelectasis involved multiple lobes and was segmental, subsegmental, or lobular, so the frequencies cited are cumulative and not mutually exclusive.

In the past, mortality was relatively common with RSV lower tract disease; deaths were reported for about 5 per cent of hospitalized children. Most fatalities occurred among infants with underlying conditions, such as congenital heart disease, bronchopulmonary dysplasia, or immunodeficiency. Advances in methods of ventilatory support and the development of specific therapy have changed the fatality rate. The specific therapy is ribavirin aerosol, which has been shown to shorten the course of the illness and to improve oxygenation. Survival of infants in high-risk conditions who have been treated with ribavirin aerosol has been remarkable. Therapy should be considered for all infants admitted with arterial P_{O_2} less than 60 mm Hg. If the P_{O_2} does not respond to oxygen therapy by hood within the first few hours after admission, ribavirin aerosol therapy should be instituted. The goal should be to keep these infants off ventilators and out of intensive care units. Delay in initiation of therapy can lead to the advanced pathologic changes described previously, after which antiviral therapy can have little effect.

Parainfluenza Viruses. As a group, the parainfluenza viruses account for about the same total morbidity as does RSV. There are sharp differences in the seasonal patterns. RSV produces annual midwinter epidemics. Parainfluenza virus types 1 and 2 occur biannually in autumn, and parainfluenza type 3 is endemic, with a tendency to occur in the late winter or early spring. Parainfluenza virus type 3, like RSV, may produce serious lower respiratory tract infections in infants. Although infections with RSV and parainfluenza type 3 virus occur with about the same frequency in the first year of life, infection with parainfluenza type 3 is much less likely to produce lower tract involvement. Parainfluenza types 1 and 2 usually do not cause serious infections before 6 months of age. Croup is the signal illness for these viruses, but pneumonia is a common manifestation.

The clinical course and radiographic findings for patients with parainfluenza pneumonia are similar to those for RSV. Figure 22–5 is a typical radiograph of an infant with pneumonia caused by parainfluenza virus type 3. This 11-month-old boy was admitted to the hospital with a temperature of 103°F. The chest radiograph was interpreted to show scattered infiltrates of the left lung, especially involving the lower lobe. Figure 22–6 illustrates the type of involvement that may be life threatening for infants in high-risk conditions. This 3-month-old infant with a ventricular septal defect was admitted to the hospital with extensive pneumonitis and atelectasis of the right upper lobe. A percutaneous aspirate of the partially collapsed lobe was cultured for viruses and bacteria, and the cultures revealed only parainfluenza virus type 3. On other occasions, only RSV has been recovered from atelectatic right upper lobes. This finding illustrates the fact that the presence of a densely atelectatic right upper lobe is not necessarily evidence of bacterial infection.

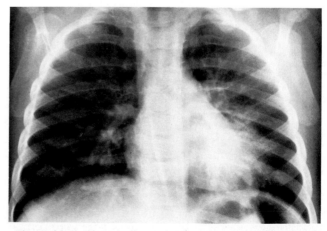

Figure 22–5. Chest radiograph of an 11-month-old infant infected with parainfluenza virus type 3. Scattered infiltrates are concentrated on the left side, with a dense infiltrate located posteriorly in the left lower lobe.

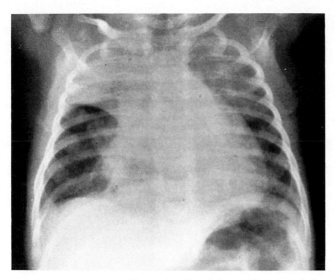

Figure 22–6. Chest radiograph of an infant with a ventricular septal defect and a parainfluenza virus type 3 infection. Multiple scattered infiltrates are present, with partial atelectasis of the right upper lobe. Parainfluenza virus type 3 was isolated from percutaneous aspirate of the right upper lobe.

No specific therapy is available for parainfluenza viruses; however, in vitro tests have shown that the growth of these viruses is inhibited by ribarivin. A few children with severe combined immunodeficiency have been treated with ribavirin, with a resulting clinical improvement and decrease in virus shedding. Controlled clinical trials are needed, but it is likely that parainfluenza viruses also can be treated with ribavirin aerosol.

Influenza Viruses. Influenza viruses are the most important causes of pneumonia that lead to the hospitalization of school-age children. The morbidity rate for infants and preschool children with influenza viruses is also considerable and ranks just behind that for RSV and parainfluenza viruses. Currently, two subtypes of influenza A and influenza B are prevalent. The problem is compounded by the fact that the genes for the surface glycoproteins of these viruses are unstable, so that mutations occur regularly. New variants emerge for which immunity acquired from previous infection or vaccination may not be protective. Fifteen major variants of these three viruses have produced epidemics during the past 10 years. Midwinter epidemics are the rule, and the peak of visits to health care facilities for acute respiratory illness each year coincides with the peak of influenza virus activity.

Influenza virus infection is particularly destructive for the ciliated respiratory epithelium. Spread is often by aerosol, so that tracheitis is a common occurrence. If the lesions extend to the distal airways, a severe fulminating pneumonia may result with a hemorrhagic exudate that contains both polymorphonuclear and mononuclear cells. Death may result unless timely intervention with ventilatory assistance and specific therapy is provided. Destruction of the respiratory epithelium also may lead to secondary bacterial pneumonia; infections with staphylococci, pneumococci, and *H. influenzae* are frequent complications of influenza virus infection.

The clinical course of influenza virus infection is usually more abrupt and intense than the course of other respiratory viruses. A fever of 103°F or higher is common; older children will complain of myalgia and headache. A scratchy sore throat and a dry hacking cough usually precede the development of pneumonitis. A common clinical feature is a white blood cell count of less than 5000. Figure 22–7 illustrates the chest radiograph of a 2-year-old child who was admitted to the hospital with a temperature of 103°F and a peripheral white blood cell count of 6800. Wide bands of atelectasis are often evident with influenza virus infections. This radiograph is fairly typical, showing infiltrates involving multiple lobes and partial atelectasis of the right upper lobe.

Influenza A virus infections can be treated with amantadine hydrochloride. Numerous studies have demonstrated that amantadine will shorten the course of illness of uncomplicated influenza infections in otherwise healthy young adults and children if it is instituted within the first 48 hours. Amantadine is not effective for influenza B. About 5 per cent of persons treated with amantadine will complain of some central nervous system–related symptoms, such as anorexia, insomnia, dizziness, light-headedness, or nausea. These symptoms resolve when the drug is stopped and even when the drug is continued for patients being treated for parkinsonism. The drug may lower the seizure threshold for children with underlying seizure disorders but, conversely, the drug has been used to treat children with seizures refractory to other medications. Rimantadine hydrochloride, an analogue of amantadine, is just as effective without having the side effects of amantadine. Ribavirin aerosol has been demonstrated to be effective in shortening the course of both influenza A and B infections in college students. Case reports of treatment of seriously ill adults with complicated infections suggest that the drug is also effective for moderating infection under these circumstances. Further studies of all three drugs for treatment of hospitalized patients are needed to determine the role of antiviral therapy. It is also possible that combined treatment with amantadine or rimantadine and ribavirin will be the optimal therapy for children with severe pneumonias caused by the influenza A virus. In the meantime, ribavirin aerosol should be considered for children with life-threatening infections with influenza B virus.

Adenoviruses. Adenoviruses vary considerably in their potential for causing pneumonia in children. The serotypes that infect children most commonly (types 1, 2, 5, and 6) usually involve the upper respiratory tract only. These viruses are present throughout the year and cause febrile upper respiratory tract illnesses; in children under 2 years of age they are the most common cause of exudative pharyngitis. Adenovirus infections also are frequently complicated by the development of otitis

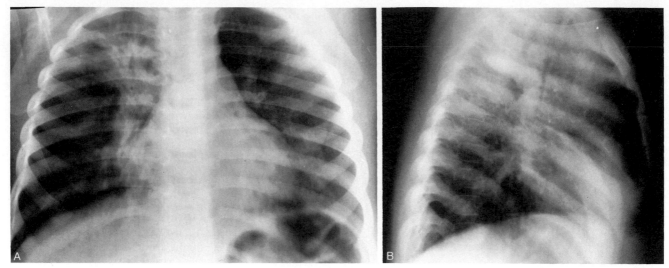

Figure 22–7. Chest radiograph of a 2-year-old child with an influenza A virus infection. Multiple perihilar infiltrates are evident as well as partial atelectasis of the right middle lobe. *A*, Posterior view; *B*, lateral view. (Reproduced with permission from Khamapirad T and Glezen WP: Semin Respir Infect 2:130–144, 1987.)

media. Adenoviruses were first isolated from fresh adenoidal tissue maintained in culture after having been surgically removed from young children. Edema and inflammation of adenoids and surrounding respiratory epithelium would most certainly affect eustachian tube function and promote the development of otitis media with effusion.

Another group of adenoviruses—types 3, 7, 11, and 21—may produce severe, necrotizing pneumonia in infants. Only sporadic reports of outbreaks have originated from the United States, but outbreaks have been reported in aboriginal children from Canada and New Zealand as well as from mainland China. The mortality rate is high, and the pathologic findings include obliterative bronchiolitis. Survivors are likely to have permanent lung disability, and the radiographic picture of "unilateral hyperlucent lung syndrome" has been described for some of these children. In Europe, outbreaks have been reported in hospitalized children and in day-care centers. Measles virus infection of the lung in infants can produce the same clinical and pathologic findings and is the most important cause of fatal pneumonia in many developing countries.

Fortunately, the disease caused by adenovirus types 3 and 7 in older children and adults is usually mild and self-limited. The usual picture is pharyngitis or pharyngoconjunctival fever. In one special environment, namely, military recruit training, more severe disease may be seen. Adenovirus types 4, 7, and 21 frequently cause influenza-like illnesses and pneumonia in unimmunized recruits. A vaccine consisting of live adenovirus types 4 and 7 in an enteric-coated capsule is routinely given to recruits in the United States. The vaccine viruses establish asymptomatic infection in the gastrointestinal tract that provides solid protection against respiratory tract infection. Adenovirus types 11 and 21 also have been associated with benign hemorrhagic cystitis. There is no specific treatment for adenoviral infections, although Chinese investigators have reported using ribavirin aerosol for severe pneumonias. In vitro studies are not encouraging for this application of the drug.

DIFFERENTIAL DIAGNOSIS

Hospitalized Children. In Chapter 21 some consistent seasonal patterns, clinical manifestations, and age-specific infection rates were presented for estimating the causes of viral infections of the lower respiratory tract. These epidemiologic factors, however, do not provide much help in differentiating the sporadic bacterial infections that occur throughout the respiratory disease season. A scoring system has been developed to provide guidelines for recognizing pneumonias that probably have a bacterial source. For this purpose, only the clinical data available at the time of the admission work-up are used. The scoring system was tested retrospectively by reviewing blindly cases with proven viral or bacterial causes, recognizing that the two conditions often occur sequentially.

The most important feature of the clinical scoring system is the evaluation of the chest radiograph. The characteristics of the chest radiographs to be considered are shown in Table 22–2. Positive scores are assigned to characteristics associated with bacterial infections and negative scores to those associated with viral infections. In general, bacterial infections are judged to produce infiltrates that are well defined, involve only one lobe, and are more likely to be located in the mid or peripheral lung field. Fluid in the pleural space and abscess or pneumatocele formation are considered characteristic of bacterial infection. In contrast, infiltrates resulting from viral infections are likely to be poorly defined, involve more than one lobe, and located in the perihilar

Table 22–2. SCORING FOR FEATURES OF PNEUMONIA ON CHEST RADIOGRAPH

Characteristic	Score Bacterial	Viral
INFILTRATE		
Well-defined lobar, lobular, segmental, subsegmental (rounded)	+2	
Less well defined, patchy	+1	
Poorly defined, interstitial, or peribronchial		−1
LOCATION		
Single lobe	+1	
Multiple lobes but well defined	+1	
Multiple sites, perihilar, poorly defined		−1
FLUID IN PLEURAL SPACE		
Minimal blunting of angle	+1	
Obvious fluid	+2	
ABSCESS, PNEUMATOCELE, OR BULLAE		
Equivocal	+1	
Obvious	+2	
ATELECTASIS		
Subsegmental (usually multiple site)		−1
Lobar involving right middle or upper lobes		−1

(Adapted from Khamapirad T and Glezen WP: Semin Respir Infect 2:130, 1987.)

areas. Scattered areas of atelectasis or atelectasis involving the right upper or middle lobes is considered to be associated with viral infections. The retrospective evaluation of the scoring system, with the radiologist uninformed as to the etiology, gave an average score of +4.5 for bacterial pneumonias and −1.9 for viral pneumonias.

A supplementary score for clinical features considered to be characteristic of bacterial infections is added to that for the chest radiograph. The average values for these clinical features for our series is shown in Table 22–3. Therefore, +1 is added if the admission fever is 103°F or greater, if the total white blood cell count is 20,000 or higher, if the absolute polymorphonuclear cell count is higher than 10,000, and if the immature polymorphonuclear cell count is greater than 500. In addition, we found that a very small proportion of infants younger than 6 months of age had bacterial infections, but almost 20 per cent of older infants and children proved to have such infections. Therefore, a child 7 months of age or older admitted to the hospital with pneumonia is given an additional +1.

In the retrospective analysis, the total score for each child was examined for ability to select children

Table 22–3. AVERAGE TEMPERATURE AND WHITE BLOOD COUNT OF CHILDREN WITH PNEUMONIA BY ETIOLOGY, BEN TAUB HOSPITAL, 1975–1977

Agent	Average Values Age (mo.)	Temp. (F)	WBC*	PMN	Immature PMN
Viral	9	101.4°	11.4	4458	350
Bacterial	20	103.3°	21.5	11049	1957

*Total white blood count × 1000.

with bacterial or viral infection. A score of zero or less indicated a probable viral cause, and a score of one or greater indicated a probable bacterial cause. A score of zero or less correctly predicted a viral origin in 37 of 39 cases, for a positive predictive power of 95 per cent. The sensitivity was 84 per cent, and the specificity was 87 per cent. The positive predictive power of a positive score of one or greater, indicating a probable bacterial origin, was 70 per cent. Seven cases without a proven bacterial infection had positive scores and therefore would have been treated under this scoring system. This result might be considered "unnecessary" treatment of 11 per cent which in itself is acceptable; however, it is also possible that most of these children in fact had undetected secondary bacterial infections and would be correctly treated with antibiotics. Two children with negative scores had pneumococci recovered from their blood streams. One of these children had an acute otitis media, which may have been the site from which the blood stream was seeded with the pneumococci; the child was treated for the otitis media, but the lung involvement was typical for RSV, which was recovered from nasopharyngeal secretions. The other child had bronchopulmonary dysplasia and occult bacteremia. This child is the only one with a bacterial infection who may not have received antibiotics on admission under these guidelines. The retrospective analysis suggests that the scoring system may serve as a reasonable guide for initiating antibiotic therapy before the results of cultures are available.

Another treatable cause of pneumonitis of infants is *Chlamydia trachomatis*. Typically, chlamydial pneumonitis is an indolent, progressive infection that becomes evident during the first weeks of life; the infection is presumably acquired intrapartum from the mother's genital tract. Some children will have a history of conjunctivitis during the first 10 days of life; a progressively worsening cough will develop between 3 and 6 weeks of age. The infants are typically afebrile, but the cough may attain sufficient severity to interfere with feeding so that the child may appear to be poorly nourished. The chest radiograph usually shows diffuse infiltrates radiating from the hilar area. The clinical picture is similar to that described for cytomegalovirus pneumonitis in early infancy. In fact, many infants with chlamydial infection are coinfected with cytomegalovirus. Other infants have been reported to be coinfected with RSV or other respiratory viruses, but these infants do not have the indolent, afebrile course of typical chlamydial pneumonitis. These infants probably have lower respiratory tract disease caused by the virus and are coincidentally carrying the chlamydia in their nasopharynx. Chlamydial infection is treated with erythromycin.

Ambulatory Setting. The most important cause of pneumonia in school children without underlying chronic conditions is *Mycoplasma pneumoniae*. *M. pneumoniae* pneumonia is unusual in infants and is relatively uncommon in preschool children. *M. pneumoniae* infection has a relatively indolent course and develops over 5 to 7 days. The first signs are usually a low-grade fever and a scratchy sore throat. Systemic symptoms, such as aching and headache, will increase as a dry, hacking cough begins. After a few days, crackling rales will be present on auscultation of the lungs, particularly in the lower lung fields where infiltrates are usually present. Although not necessarily specific for *M. pneumoniae,* a cold agglutinin titer of 1:64 or greater is evidence for this origin. This type of pneumonia has been correctly designated as "walking pneumonia" because it is rarely necessary to hospitalize a child who has no underlying condition. Children with sickle cell disease may develop a severe pneumonia with this agent and may require many days of treatment in the hospital. Erythromycin is the treatment of choice for children.

Recognition of bacterial pneumonia in the ambulatory setting is difficult because it often must be accomplished without a chest radiograph or a complete white blood cell count. The clinical manifestations, including high fever and "toxicity," may be helpful in recognizing bacterial infections, and a high proportion will require hospitalization so that the clinical tests will be available. Knowledge of the seasonal occurrence of the major respiratory viruses along with their characteristic clinical manifestations and age-specific infection rates will be helpful in assessing the disease's origin.

REFERENCES

Aherne W, Bird T, Court SDM et al: Pathological changes in virus infections of the lower respiratory tract in children. J Clin Path 23:7, 1970.

Becroft DMO: Histopathology of fatal adenovirus infection of the respiratory tract in young children. J Clin Path 20:561, 1967.

Becroft DMO: Bronchiolitis obliterans, bronchiectasis, and other sequelae of adenovirus type 21 infection in young children. J Clin Path 24:72, 1971.

Beem MO and Saxon BS: Respiratory-tract colonization and a distinctive pneumonia syndrome in infants infected with *Chlamydia trachomatis.* N Engl J Med 296:306, 1977.

Couch RB, Kasel JA, Glezen WP et al: Influenza: its control in persons and populations. J Infect Dis 153:431, 1986.

Current estimates from the national health interview survey, United States, 1986. DHHS Publication No (PHS) 87-1592, October 1987.

Denny FW, Clyde WA Jr, and Glezen WP: *Mycoplasma pneumoniae* disease: clinical spectrum, pathophysiology, epidemiology and control. J Infect Dis 123:74, 1971.

Downham MAPS, Gardner PS, McQuillin J, and Ferris JAJ: Role of respiratory viruses in childhood mortality. Brit Med J 1:235, 1975.

Foy HM, Cooney MK, McMahan R, and Grayston JT: Viral and mycoplasmal pneumonia in a prepaid medical care group during an eight-year period. Am J Epidemiol 97:93, 1973.

Glezen WP: Viral pneumonia as a cause and result of hospitalization. J Infect Dis 147:765, 1983.

Glezen WP, Collier AM, and Loda FA: Significance of *Diplococcus pneumoniae* and *Haemophilus influenzae* cultured from the nasopharynx of children. Pediatr Res 8:425, 1974.

Glezen WP, Decker M, Joseph SW et al: Acute respiratory disease associated with influenza epidemics in Houston, 1981–1983. J Infect Dis 115:1119, 1987.

Glezen WP and Fernald GW: Effect of passive antibody on parainfluenza virus type 3 pneumonia in hamsters. Infect Immun 14:212, 1976.

Glezen WP, Paredes A, and Taber LH: Influenza in children. Relationship to other respiratory agents. JAMA 243:1345, 1980.

Harmon AT, Harmon MW, and Glezen WP: Evidence of interferon production in the hamster lung after primary or secondary exposure to parainfluenza virus type 3. Am Rev Respir Dis 125:706, 1982.

Khamapirad T and Glezen WP: Clinical and radiographic assessment of acute lower respiratory tract disease in infants and children. Semin Respir Infect 2:130, 1987.

Kimmel KA, Wyde PR, and Glezen WP: Evidence of a T-cell-mediated cytotoxic response to parainfluenza virus 3 pneumonia in hamsters. J Reticuloendothelial Soc 31:71, 1982.

Knight V and Gilbert BE: Ribavirin aerosol treatment of influenza. Infect Dis Clinics North Am 1:441, 1987.

Loda FA, Collier AM, Glezen WP et al: Occurrence of *Diplococcus pneumoniae* in the upper respiratory tract of children. J Pediatr 87:1087, 1975.

Murphy TF, Henderson FW, Clyde WA Jr et al: An eleven-year study in a pediatric practice. Am J Epidemiol 113:12, 1981.

Rodriguez WJ and Parrott RH: Ribavirin aerosol treatment of serious respiratory syncytial virus infections in infants. Infect Dis Clinics North Am 1:425, 1987.

Tominack RL and Hayden FG: Rimantadine hydrochloride and amantadine hydrochloride use in influenza A virus infections. Infect Dis Clinics North Am 1:459, 1987.

Welliver RC, Wong DT, Middleton E Jr et al: Role of parainfluenza virus—specific IGE in pathogenesis of croup and wheezing subsequent to infections. J Pediatr 101:889, 1982.

Welliver RC, Wong DT, Sun M et al: The development of respiratory syncytial virus—specific IgE and the release of histamine in nasopharyngeal secretions after infection. N Engl J Med 305:841, 1981.

Zahradnik JM: Adenovirus pneumonia. Semin Respir Infect 2:104, 1987.

23

WALLACE A. CLYDE, JR., M.D.

INFECTIONS OF THE RESPIRATORY TRACT DUE TO *MYCOPLASMA PNEUMONIAE*

Mycoplasma species are the cause of a wide variety of diseases among all higher life forms. The prototype species, *M. mycoides,* produces pleuropneumonia of cattle, a chronic, progressive destructive process involving the lungs and pleura. In humans, the most important mycoplasmal disease is caused by *M. pneumoniae,* although pathologic associations have been made with other species, including *M. hominis, M. genitalium,* and *Ureaplasma urealyticum.* Biologic properties shared by all species are small size (average dimension 0.250 m) and lack of a rigid cell wall structure comparable to that of classic bacterial species. These properties make mycoplasmas invisible by light microscopy, nonstainable by the Gram method, and resistant to antibiotics whose mode of action interferes with cell wall synthesis.

Mycoplasma pneumoniae was isolated initially by Monroe Eaton in 1940, through production of pneumonic lesions in cotton rats and hamsters following inoculations of sputa from patients with the atypical pneumonia syndrome. However, this work was not accepted for many years because it was not confirmed by other investigators. *M. pneumoniae* is recognized now as the most common single cause of atypical pneumonia, although nonpneumonic syndromes of tracheobronchitis and asymptomatic infections are at least thirtyfold more common.

MICROBIOLOGY

The atypical pneumonia agent of Eaton was thought to be a large virus or psittacosis-like agent until 1960, when it was visualized as an extracellular parasite through the use of special staining techniques, first in infected chick embryo lungs and then in cell cultures. In 1961, the organism was first grown in synthetic media and was shown to have properties of the *Mycoplasmataceae.* The binomial nomenclature *Mycoplasma pneumoniae* was proposed in 1962, providing a counterpart to the common classic bacterial agent of pneumonia, *Streptococcus pneumoniae.*

Although *M. pneumoniae* lacks cell wall structures

and is contained by a trilaminar unit membrane, it exists as a slender filament measuring roughly 0.1 x 2.0 m. At one end is a differentiated organelle that mediates attachment to the membranes of respiratory epithelial cells (Fig. 23–1). In solid media made of beef heart infusion agar with horse serum and yeast extract, the organisms form microscopic colonies (10 to 100 m in diameter) after 7 to 10 days' incubation. In liquid media, no turbidity is produced by growth; metabolism of the organisms is shown by fermentation of dextrose and other carbohydrates. Like many other mycoplasmas, *M. pneumoniae* is sensitive to the tetracycline antibiotics and totally insensitive to the penicillins and cephalosporins. Unlike other species, *M. pneumoniae* also is very sensitive to erythromycins.

EPIDEMIOLOGY

Infections with *M. pneumoniae* are among the most frequent respiratory diseases of children, adolescents, and young adults. In U.S. urban areas, the overall

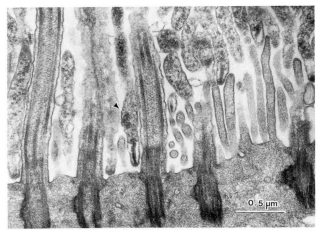

Figure 23–1. Electron micrograph of a tracheal organ culture infected with *Mycoplasma pneumoniae.* An attached organism is seen between two adjacent cilia (*arrow*). Tips of other organisms are seen in the upper right portion of the micrograph, attached to microvilli.

403

incidence of pneumonia caused by this organism is 1 to 3 per 1000 population per year, but in the age group of highest incidence (10 to 15 years) the rate is two to three times greater. Based on these figures, an estimated 500,000 cases per year occur in the United States. However, annual prevalence varies in roughly 4-year cycles in parts of the world where adequate surveillance has been undertaken. It is popularly held that *M. pneumoniae* infections are uncommon during the preschool years, but in fact numerically they are as common then as they are in older children; below the age of 4 years, the frequency of pneumonias is 45 per 1000 population per year, of which 5 per cent are caused by this organism.

The spread of mycoplasmal respiratory infections is via the droplet route and is facilitated by close contact, such as in family units and dormitory settings. The infections are highly communicable under such conditions, affecting 75 per cent of susceptible individuals within households. The incubation period is about 3 weeks, and thus family outbreaks may take several months to run their course. Other groups at high risk for infection include college students, in whom the mycoplasma causes 50 per cent of all pneumonias, and military recruits, in whom the organism is responsible for about 25 per cent of cases (adenoviral atypical pneumonia being at least twice as common).

Outbreaks of mycoplasmal pneumonia can occur in any season, but have been noted frequently during the fall months, when other types of respiratory infections are less common. The disease also occurs in all geographic areas where it has been investigated, generally during the rainy season in tropical climates.

PATHOLOGY

An understanding of the lung tissue pathology that occurs in *M. pneumoniae* disease is useful in interpreting the roentgenographic changes that can be seen, as well as the basis of the pathophysiologic disturbances. Because the disease is only rarely fatal, this information is based on rare autopsy studies that have been published. The lungs appear irregularly mottled, most prominently in the lower lobes. Small amounts of straw-colored pleural fluid are common. On cut surfaces, bronchial branches appear thickened, and mucopurulent exudate may be noted.

Microscopic sections reveal cuffing of smaller bronchial branches by thick infiltrations of small lymphocytes and plasma cells (Fig. 23–2); such infiltrates also may be found in perivascular locations and in the interstitial spaces (Fig. 23–3). The bronchial lumens contain a variable amount of exudate consisting of macrophages, polymorphonuclear leukocytes, fibrin, and sheets of desquamated bronchial epithelial cells (Fig. 23–4). These exudates may occlude the airway, leading to areas of segmental or subsegmental atelectasis.

With the electron microscope, the nature of the

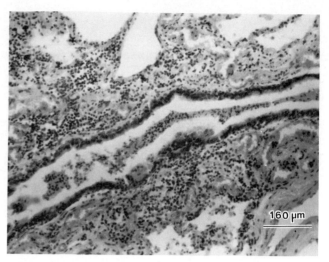

Figure 23–2. Section of a human lung with mycoplasmal pneumonia (hematoxylin and eosin stain). A bronchial branch shows dense peribronchial infiltration with lymphocytes and plasma cells. An exudate partially obstructs the lumen.

host cell parasite interaction is revealed (see Fig. 23–1). The organisms appear as slender filaments among cilia or on nonciliated epithelia, and they adhere to these cell membranes using a differentiated organelle. This adherence is not reversible, and parasitized cells ultimately are lost from the mucosal border. It is from this extracellular location that the organisms direct cell injury and leukocyte recruitment and proliferation. In addition to peroxide secretion, which is injurious to the host-cell membrane, the organisms produce a factor that inhibits the endogenous host-cell catalase. This factor leads to suppression of the epithelial cell protein synthesis, nucleic acid replication, macromolecular transport, and oxygen utilization. Histologically, these biochemical changes are reflected as cytoplasmic vacuolization, nuclear swelling, chromatin margination, and disruption of the cell membrane integrity.

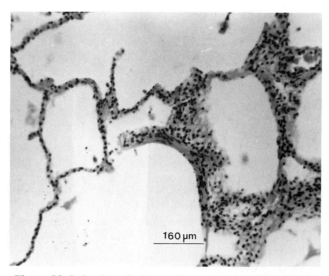

Figure 23–3. Section of a human lung with mycoplasmal pneumonia (hematoxylin and eosin stain). An area of interstitial lymphocytic infiltration.

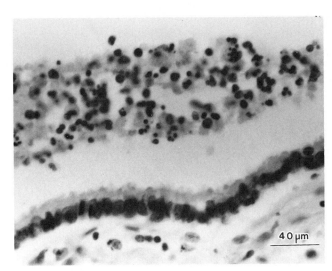

Figure 23–4. Section of a human lung with mycoplasmal pneumonia (hematoxylin and eosin stain). The intralumenal exudate (see Fig. 23–2) consists mainly of polymorphonuclear leukocytes and macrophages.

Ultrastructural changes that are seen in parasitized cells include disappearance of ciliary necklace structures (large integral membrane proteins) and dissolution of gap and tight junctions between adjacent cells. These changes would be expected to cause disruption in ciliary beat frequency and synchrony, which in fact has been demonstrated in tracheal organ culture models. The injury to junctional complexes would affect cell nutrition and the integrity of the bronchial epithelial layer.

IMMUNOLOGY

The membranes of *M. pneumoniae* contain glyceroglycolipid moieties that resemble lipids found in skeletal and heart muscles, the lung itself, erythrocyte membranes, and brain tissues. This property may allow "biologic mimicry," which initially could protect the organisms from host immune recognition, but these antigenic similarities also may be the basis for the antibodies to host tissues that many patients later develop, including the cold hemagglutinin response. As yet uncharacterized factors of *M. pneumoniae* cause polyclonal B lymphocyte activation, T lymphocyte suppression, and macrophage inhibition. The organisms also trigger the properdin pathway. These factors in concert likely are responsible for inflammatory cell recruitment and lymphocyte proliferation within the lung tissue.

Despite the similarities between organism and host-cell membranes, all arms of the immune response eventually are stimulated. The first humoral antibody to be produced, the cold hemagglutinin, has specificity for the I antigen of erythrocyte membranes and is an IgM molecule. This response occurs during the end of the first week of illness, continues for another week or two, and then disappears by the sixth to eighth week of illness. During the second to third week, antibodies specific for the *Mycoplasma* begin their appearance, in the IgM, IgG, IgA, and s-IgA categories. The IgG antibodies are the most durable, persisting in significant titers for up to a year following infection. There is evidence that the s-IgA antibodies are the best correlate of protective immunity; they are detectable for about 4 weeks in nasal secretions.

Early in *M. pneumoniae* infections, the suppression of T cell function is reflected by a state of anergy to intradermal injections of a variety of antigens. This anergic state lasts for several weeks and can be confusing in patient management, for example, when a previously positive tuberculin test result is converted to negative. Later lymphocytes reactive to the mycoplasmal antigens can be detected by in vitro systems. Immunologic memory cells persist for 4 to 10 years, mediating the protective immune state. After this period of time in older subjects, reinfection and repeated disease can occur. In preschool children, this response is immature, and reinfections may occur within 18 months.

Evidence suggests that the pathologic changes seen in the lung tissue are in fact the histologic expression of host immune responsiveness. In a hamster model of infection, it has been found that the peribronchial lymphocytes produce IgM and IgG antibodies. The local presence of these antibodies, together with complement, is lytic to the mycoplasmal cells. The cellular reaction products also are responsible for recruitment of polymorphonuclear leukocytes to areas of infection. In the hamster, administration of antithymocyte globulin before experimental infection completely ablates the changes of "pneumonia." A counterpart to this observation is a report that immunodeficient patients infected with *M. pneumoniae* had prolonged illnesses but failed to show any evidence of pulmonary infiltrates in their chest radiographs. Evidence of this kind has led to the development of hypotheses concerning the need for children to be infected more than once before their immune responsiveness is adequate to produce a full-blown reaction, in turn allowing them to have mycoplasmal pneumonia. If correct, this theory provides a ready explanation for why young children have frequent asymptomatic infections when the age of peak incidence of mycoplasmal pneumonia is not until 10 years.

PATHOGENESIS

The pathogenesis of *M. pneumoniae* disease has been deduced from studies in experimental model systems in correlation with clinical and pathologic information. Infectious droplets of respiratory secretions from patients, when inhaled by susceptible contacts, initiate colonization of the recipients' respiratory mucosae. The organisms apparently penetrate the mucous layer using their properties of motility and ability to secrete a neuraminidase. Sialic

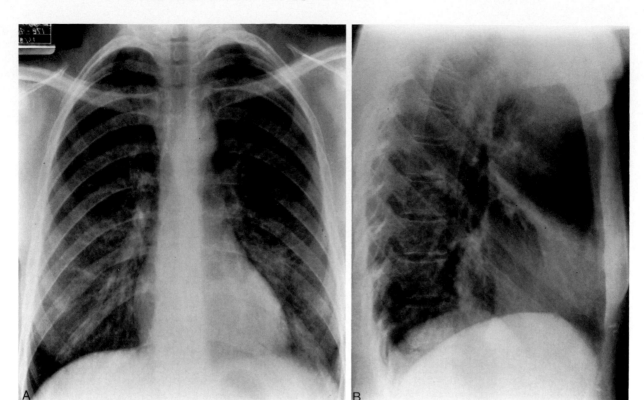

Figure 23–5. *A*, A peribronchial infiltrate is seen in segments of the right middle lobe and left lower lobe; *B*, lateral view.

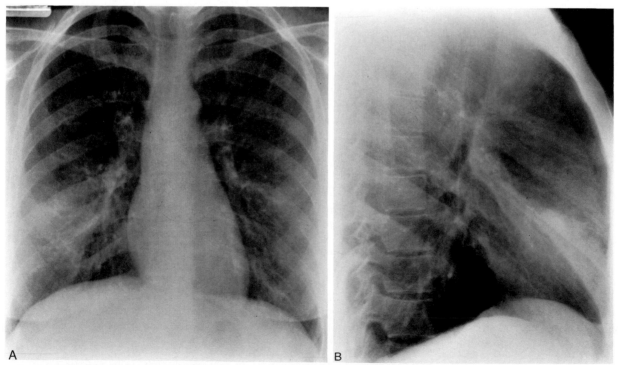

Figure 23–6. *A*, An interstitial infiltrate is present in the lateral segment of the right middle lobe; *B*, lateral view.

acid moieties on the host-cell membrane are the attachment site, and anchoring of the mycoplasma is then mediated by the P-1 attachment protein. For the next 2 to 3 weeks, doubling of the organisms by binary fission occurs approximately every 3 hours, resulting in colonization of the nasopharynx, pharynx, and tracheobronchial tree.

Parasitized respiratory mucosal epithelial cells, both ciliated and nonciliated, are injured by release of peroxide from the organisms and possibly by lipopolysaccharides in the mycoplasmal membranes. The physiologic effect of this injury is disruption and eventual cessation of organized ciliary motility, with consequent disturbance of mucociliary clearance similar to that occurring in pertussis. It has been shown that this pathophysiologic disturbance persists for up to a year following recovery from the infection.

In the absence of antimycoplasmal antibodies, the organisms resist phagocytosis by alveolar macrophages. The host immune response begins with recruitment of B lymphocytes to the peribronchial area and hilar lymph nodes, with subsequent proliferation and secretion of IgM and IgG antibodies, under the direction of T lymphocyte helpers. The presence of antibody enables phagocytosis of organisms by macrophages and recruited polymorphonuclear leukocytes to begin, and, coupled with complement, antibody-mediated lysis of mycoplasmas occurs. As indicated earlier, s-IgA antibodies also are stimulated, and the presence of these antibodies is the closest correlate of protective immunity against future infection. The immune state fades after a few years, and reinfection can take place.

CLINICAL MANIFESTATIONS

The usual clinical picture of *M. pneumoniae* disease is that of an influenza-like syndrome, with the predominant symptoms being fever, malaise, headache, scratchy sore throat, and cough. Unlike influenza viral disease, which becomes fully manifest in 24 to 48 hours, the mycoplasmal disease develops gradually over several days to a week or more. It is usually at this time that patients first seek medical attention. Physical findings may be few: temperature rarely exceeds 38.5BC; pharyngeal erythema without exudate is common; and evidence of tracheobronchitis may be elicited by palpating the trachea with the patient's neck hyperextended, resulting in a complaint of tenderness or the initiation of a coughing paroxysm. In patients with pneumonia, radiographic changes may precede any signs by several days. Findings in the chest include small areas of dullness to percussion over atelectatic areas or fluid accumulations, crackles (usually posteriorly located at the lung bases), and localized wheezing. Evidence of otitis media may be seen in younger children, whereas older children and adults may show signs of bullous myringitis or sinusitis.

A number of nonrespiratory manifestations have been described as complications of *M. pneumoniae* disease. Rashes are the most common, usually macular or papular lesions on the lower extremities. Erythema multiforme and erythema multiforme major (Stevens-Johnson syndrome) with varicella-like eruptions also have been described. Less common are central nervous system syndromes, including cerebellar ataxia, transverse myelitis, Guillain-Barré syndrome, and peripheral neuropathies. Other conditions seen less commonly include skeletal myositis, pericarditis, myocarditis, hemolytic anemia, and arthritis. Thromboembolic phenomena may produce a variety of other findings.

ROENTGENOGRAPHIC FINDINGS

Chest radiographic changes in *M. pneumoniae* pneumonia are nonspecific and can mimic a wide variety of other diseases and conditions. Most frequent are bronchopneumonic infiltrates, generally in one of the lower lobes. The thickening of the bronchial submucosa due to cellular infiltration allows the air column to be seen against the infiltrative radiopacity as "tram lines" when bronchial branches are projected in sagittal section or as "doughnuts" when they are projected in cross section (Fig. 23–5). Another pattern that may be seen alone or in combination with the signs of bronchial thickening is a change of interstitial infiltration (Fig. 23–6). Small areas of subsegmental or segmental atelectasis are common, sometimes resulting in plate-like shadows (Fig. 23–7). Rarely, segmental or lobar consolidation occurs (Fig. 23–8).

Pleural effusions are not infrequent but generally tend to be small and transient (Fig. 23–9). Rarely, they may be massive, suggesting a different diagnosis (Fig. 23–10).

Two other types of changes bear mention. One of these consists of diffuse nodular densities, similar to the appearance of miliary tuberculosis (Figs. 23–11 and 23–12). Enlargement of hilar nodes may be seen in combination with parenchymal infiltrative changes or alone mimicking sarcoidosis (Figs. 23–13, 23–14, 23–15, and 23–16).

Although the protean manifestations of *M. pneumoniae* pneumonia are nonspecific for this disease, they are nevertheless useful in evaluating the sick patient who has limited physical findings, and they can support the diagnosis in combination with clinical and epidemiologic information.

LABORATORY FINDINGS

Laboratory data are useful in excluding diagnoses of infections other than those caused by *M. pneumoniae*, and some can provide a definitive diagnosis. The leukocyte total and differential cell counts usually are normal, an exception being the counts for patients with sickle cell anemia, who may show poly-

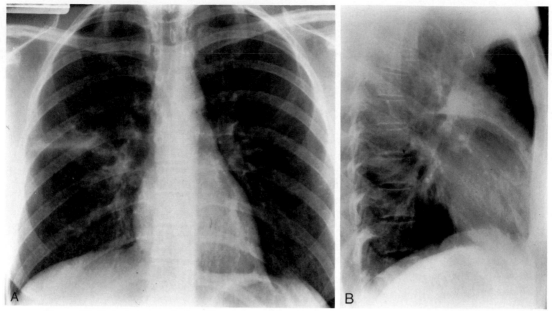

Figure 23–7. *A,* An area of plate-like atelectasis is seen in the right midlung field; *B,* lateral view.

morphonuclear leukocytosis (Shulman et al, 1972). The erythrocyte sedimentation rate is elevated, and C-reactive protein may be present. Various biochemical determinations may be abnormal if complications of the infection occur. For example, in the presence of myositis, sharp elevations of creatine phosphokinase are seen; with hemolytic anemia, elevation of serum bilirubin levels is evident.

Intradermal tests with tuberculin and other antigens are unreliable during *M. pneumoniae* disease. T-helper lymphocyte suppression occurs, leading to a transient state of anergy. If the differential diagnosis includes tuberculosis, it is well to repeat the skin tests after 2 to 3 months of convalescence.

Examination of the sputum may provide some

diagnostic clues. Gram stain shows no bacteria or a low number of mixed species. The cellular content is better determined with a cytologic stain, such as the Papanicolaou method. Large numbers of polymorphonuclear cells and macrophages are seen, together with sheets of desquamated ciliated epithelial cells.

Serologic tests of several kinds may be useful. The rapid or "bedside" cold agglutinin test is easily performed (Garrow, 1958). Four drops of whole blood are placed in a sodium citrate blood collection tube (light blue rubber stopper), which is then chilled in crushed ice for 30 to 60 sec. Holding the tube by the stopper, it should be rotated under a good light source so that a film of blood coats the tube wall. Definite cell clumping corresponds to a standard

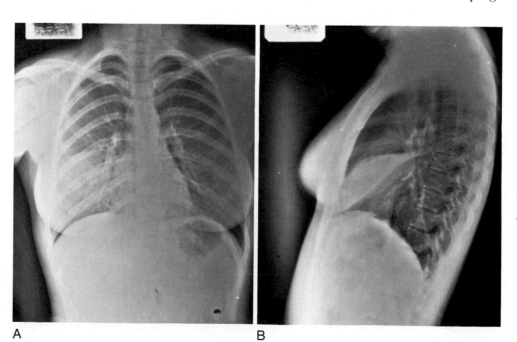

Figure 23–8. *A,* Consolidation of the right middle lobe; *B,* lateral view. (Reproduced with permission from Clyde WA Jr: In Gallagher J et al [eds]: Medical Care of the Adolescent. 3rd ed. New York, Appleton-Century-Crofts, Inc, 1976.)

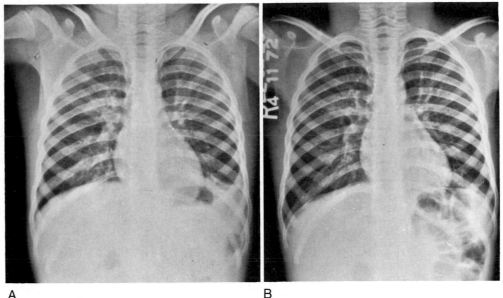

Figure 23–9. *A,* A small left pleural effusion. *B,* Clearing of the effusion 4 days later. (Reproduced with permission from Clyde WA Jr: In Gallagher J et al [eds]: Medical Care of the Adolescent. 3rd ed. New York, Appleton-Century-Crofts, Inc, 1976.)

A   B

titration of 1:64 or greater. False-positive reactions must be excluded by warming the tube, which should make the agglutination pattern disappear. Diseases causing false-positive reactions include measles, adenovirus infection, infectious mononucleosis, and several tropical diseases. Cold agglutinins are seen in about half of *M. pneumoniae* infections, so their absence does not exclude the diagnosis. In mycoplasmal pneumonia, the frequency of cold agglutinins rises to 70 per cent. Because of the rapid rise and fall of this IgM antibody response, negative reactions may convert to positive over the course of a few days. The standard cold agglutinin titration should be performed on paired serums obtained acutely and 1 to 2 weeks later; rises (or falls) in titer greater than or equal to fourfold are considered significant.

A number of specific serologic tests for *M. pneumoniae* have been described, the most widely available

of which is the complement fixation method. This test should be done using paired serums collected 2 to 3 weeks apart; again, titer changes greater than or equal to fourfold are considered significant. Because *M. pneumoniae* infections are so prevalent in the population, it is difficult to interpret a single titer. Levels 1:128 or greater suggest recent infection.

The gold standard for diagnosis of *M. pneumoniae* infection remains recovery of the organism from respiratory secretions, but this procedure is not widely available in diagnostic laboratories. Because available methods require 1 to 3 weeks, culture is of no value in therapeutic decision making. Newer rapid diagnostic methods are under evaluation and appear

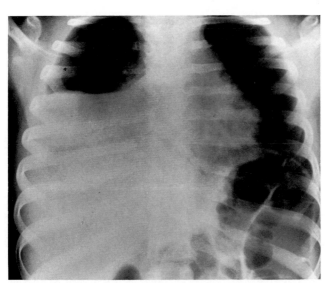

Figure 23–10. A massive right pleural effusion.

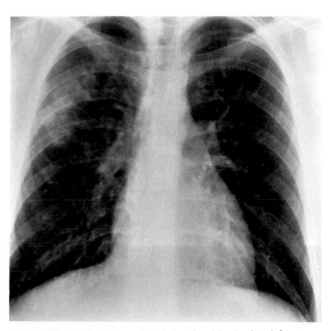

Figure 23–11. A pattern of nodular densities in the right upper lobe.

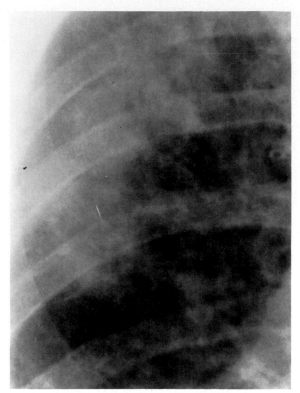

Figure 23–12. Close-up of the nodular densities shown in Figure 23–11.

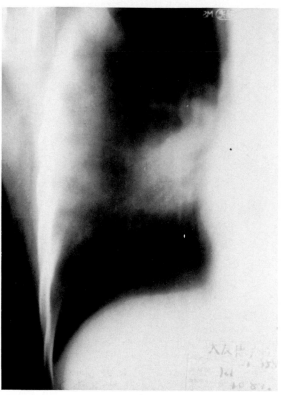

Figure 23–14. Tomogram of right hilum from the patient shown in Figure 23–13. (Reproduced with permission from Niitu Y: *M. pneumoniae* respiratory diseases: clinical features—children. Yale J Biol Med 56:493–503, 1983; photograph courtesy of Y Niitu.)

promising. One is based on detection of mycoplasmal antigen in respiratory secretions using a radio-labeled DNA probe that is specific for *M. pneumoniae* ribosomal RNA. Another uses monoclonal antibodies to "capture" the mycoplasmal antigens from specimens. These methods will need thorough testing under field conditions before their dependability can be established.

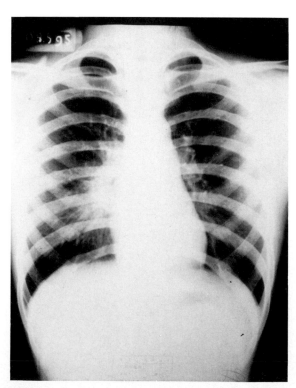

Figure 23–13. Right hilar adenopathy. (Reproduced with permission from Niitu Y: *M. pneumoniae* respiratory diseases: clinical features—children. Yale J Biol Med 56:493–503, 1983; photograph courtesy of Y Niitu.)

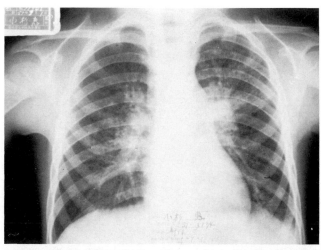

Figure 23–15. Bilateral hilar adenopathy and infiltration. (Reproduced with permission from Niitu Y: *M. pneumoniae* respiratory diseases: clinical features—children. Yale J Biol Med 56:493–503, 1983; photograph courtesy of Y Niitu.)

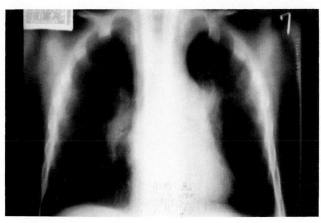

Figure 23–16. Tomogram of the patient in Figure 23–15. (Reproduced with permission from Niitu Y: *M. pneumoniae* respiratory diseases: clinical features—children. Yale J Biol Med 56:493–503, 1983; photograph courtesy of Y Niitu.)

DIAGNOSIS

Mycoplasma pneumoniae should be considered in every case of pneumonia because it is such a common cause of this disease. A combination of epidemiologic, clinical, and roentgenographic data usually are sufficient for empirical therapy. Support of the diagnosis is provided by excluding classic bacterial disease and by using the cold hemagglutinin test, specific serologic tests, and mycoplasma culture (Clyde, 1988).

From the discussion of clinical manifestations and radiographic findings, it is apparent that *M. pneumoniae* can mimic a very wide variety of other infectious as well as noninfectious causes (Table 23–1). However, reports of a new *Chlamydia* species involved in the atypical pneumonia syndrome possibly make this organism the most significant in the differential diagnosis (Grayston et al, 1986; Leigh and Clyde, 1987). This chlamydial agent is spread person-to-person, has the same age distribution as mycoplasmal pneumonia, and is said to be indistinguishable from it clinically.

MANAGEMENT

Like other mycoplasmas, *M. pneumoniae* is sensitive to tetracyclines but resistant to all penicillins and several other antibiotics whose mode of action is to interfere with cell-wall synthesis. Unlike other mycoplasmas, this organism is also very sensitive to the macrolide antibiotics. For children below the age of 8 years, erythromycins are the drugs of choice; above this age, tetracycline is an equally effective alternative. Treatment should be given for 2 weeks, because relapses can occur with shorter courses. With severe infections, hospital admission for oxygen and respiratory support may be required.

PREVENTION

Several candidate vaccines have been field tested as a means of controlling *M. pneumoniae* disease, particularly in the armed forces, in which this disease is a major problem among recruits (Denny et al, 1971). None of these products is licensed for use, because they either have undesirable side effects or suboptimal efficacy. The prophylactic use of tetracycline has been studied in families; this approach fails to reduce the rate of secondary infections in household contacts.

PROGNOSIS

Generally *M. pneumoniae* disease is a benign and self-limiting process in which the treatment is designed mainly to reduce the morbidity of the infection. Secondary bacterial infections are very rare, as is a fatal outcome. Long-term sequelae are unknown, except for reports of residual pleural abnormality and delayed mucociliary clearance lasting up to a year following the infection. Some evidence suggests that mycoplasmal pneumonia in older children and adults may trigger hyperreactive airways disease, but this finding is not well documented.

REFERENCES

Alexander ER, Foy HM, Kenny GE et al: Pneumonia due to *Mycoplasma pneumoniae*. Its incidence in the membership of a cooperative medical group. N Engl J Med 275:131, 1966.

Broughton RA: Infections due to *Mycoplasma pneumoniae* in childhood (a review with 233 literature citations). J Ped Infect Dis 5:71, 1986.

Clyde WA Jr: Mycoplasmal infections. In Wentworth BB (ed): Diagnostic Procedures for Bacterial Infections. 7th ed. Washington, DC, American Public Health Association, 1988.

Clyde WA Jr and Fernald GW: Mycoplasmas: the pathogens' pathogens. Cell Immunol 82:88, 1983.

Denny FW, Clyde WA Jr, and Glezen WP: *Mycoplasma pneumoniae* disease: clinical spectrum, pathophysiology, epidemiology and control. J Infect Dis 123:74, 1971.

Eaton MD, Meiklejohn G, and van Herick W: Studies on the etiology of atypical pneumonia. I. A filterable agent transmissible to cotton rats, hamsters and chick embryos. J Exper Med 79:649, 1944.

Garrow DH: A rapid test for the presence of increased cold agglutinins. Brit Med J 2:206, 1958.

Grayston JT, Kuo C-C, Wang S-P et al: A new *Chlamydia psittaci*

Table 23–1. DIFFERENTIAL DIAGNOSIS OF *MYCOPLASMA PNEUMONIAE* PNEUMONIA

Problem Type	Entities
Infectious	
Viral	Influenza A or B
	Adenovirus types 3, 4, 7 (adults)
	Respiratory syncytial virus (to age 6)
Bacterial	*Chlamydia* sp. "TWAR"
	Streptococcus pneumoniae
	Mycobacterium tuberculosis
	Bordetella pertussis
Fungal	*Histoplasma capsulatum*
	Coccidioides immitis
	Blastomyces dermatitidis
Physiologic	Asthma
Aspirational	Gastric contents, foreign body
Chemical	Drugs

TWAR, the first two chlamydial isolates (*TW*-183, *AR*-39).

strain, TWAR, isolated in adult respiratory tract infections. N Engl J Med 315:161, 1986.

Leigh MW and Clyde WA Jr: Chlamydial and mycoplasmal pneumonias. Semin Respir Infect 2:152, 1987.

Murphy TF, Henderson FW, Clyde WA Jr et al: Pneumonia: an eleven year study in a pediatric practice. Am J Epid 113:12, 1981.

Reimann HA: An acute infection of the respiratory tract with atypical pneumonia. A disease entity probably caused by a filterable virus. JAMA 111:2377, 1938.

Shulman ST, Bartlett J, Clyde WA Jr, and Ayoub EM: The unusual severity of mycoplasmal pneumonia in children with sickle cell disease. N Engl J Med 287:164, 1972.

24

ROBERT H. PARROTT, M.D.

INFLUENZA

THE VIRUS

Influenza illness has been defined epidemiologically for centuries; influenza viruses were the first viral agents proved to be respiratory tract pathogens. Nonetheless, the terms *influenza* and *flu* are among the most overused diagnoses for nondescript infectious diseases in both lay and medical circles. Perhaps this overuse is because the spectrum of clinical response to influenza infection is broad and the most practical clue to the probable diagnosis of influenza is epidemiologic—the knowledge that influenza infection is prevalent in the community.

Influenza viruses are members of the Orthomyxovirus family. They are essentially spherical virions, 80 to 120 nm in diameter but may be elongated when first recovered from an infected host. They contain eight ribonucleic acid segments surrounded by an envelope of lipoprotein.

There are three influenza viruse types distinct in their nucleoprotein and matrix antigens: A, B, and C. The envelope surrounding the ribonucleic acid segments has periodic projections or spikes that house the hemagglutinin (HA) and neuraminidase (NA) antigens, which are the basis for the World Health Organization (WHO) nomenclature for influenza subtypes. In humans, there are three distinct HA proteins, H1, H2, and H3, and two NA proteins, N1 and N2. Primarily among A serotypes but also among the B serotypes, variation in antigenic composition occurs from time to time. The changes may be major, such as a complete shift in either HA or NA or both HA and NA at once. Minor mutations or "antigenic drift" may take place within a single type of HA or NA. Kilbourne (1973) believes that pandemic or epidemic severity "reflects principally the extent of antigenic change from pre-existing virus"; Table 24–1 displays both the WHO nomenclature for influenza A viruses and shows the basis

for Kilbourne's belief. This antigenic shifting largely accounts for the ability of influenza to produce epidemics even in populations of persons who have previously experienced influenza infection or immunization and has serious implications for the preparation and availability of effective vaccines. In 1988 and 1989 the projected prevalent strains in the United States were H3N2 subtypes, which began to appear in 1968, and H1N1 subtypes, which probably were present from 1918 to 1956 and reappeared in 1977.

EPIDEMIOLOGY AND IMMUNITY

Influenza infection often occurs in epidemics that may sweep through a community in a matter of 1 or

Table 24–1. ANTIGENIC VARIATIONS IN HEMAGGLUTININ (HA) AND NEURAMINIDASE (NA) OF THE VIRUS AND PANDEMIC SEVERITY OF INFLUENZA

Year	Virus		Change in	Extent of Change	Result
1918	H1*	N1	?	?	Pandemic (severe)
192?	H1†	N1	HA	+ +	No pandemic
			NA	+	
1947	H1	N1	HA	+ +	Pandemic (mild)
			NA	+	
1957	H2	N2	HA	+ + +	Pandemic (severe)
			NA	+ + +	
1968	H3	N2	HA	+ + +	Pandemic (moderate)
1977	H1	N1	HA	+ + +	Pandemic (moderate among persons born after 1956)
			NA		

*Formerly H–sw₁.
†Formerly H–O.
(Updated from Kilbourne ED: The molecular epidemiology of influenza. J Infect Dis, 127:478, 1973. University of Chicago Press, Publisher.)

2 months. Morbidity in a susceptible population may be high and is particularly severe in infants and persons over 65 years of age. The incidence of infection and illness is highest, however, in children of school age. Type-specific and subtype-specific immunity after natural infection exists, based on anti-HA and anti-NA antibodies, but is not of high order; children may become infected several times within a matter of years by the same or related strains. Detectable strain-specific serum antibodies, however, do occur and persist. There is evidence that antibody developed against earlier strains may rise during a subsequent infection with a related strain of influenza virus. Perhaps this recurrence of antibody is the reason that the incidence of influenza infection and clinical illness is lower in older persons than in school-age children. When an H1N1 influenza strain ("Russian" influenza) unexpectedly began to circulate in 1977, illness was manifest primarily in persons young enough never to have been exposed to earlier H1N1 viruses.

Influenza A virus activity was demonstrated in infants and young children from metropolitan Washington, D.C., during each of 17 successive years. Overall, 14 per cent of 812 croup patients and 5 per cent of 5313 hospitalized patients with respiratory infection showed evidence of influenza A or B virus infection. Infection with influenza A virus was about four times more common than infection with influenza B virus. Influenza A infections were particularly common between 1968 and 1974, after the appearance of the H3N2 virus subtype. During the peak month of a composite of 11 consecutive influenza A virus outbreaks, influenza A virus infection was demonstrated in 70 per cent of croup patients and in 36 per cent of all patients hospitalized for respiratory disease. During the peak month of a composite of six consecutive influenza B virus outbreaks, influenza B virus infection was demonstrated in 27 per cent of croup patients and in 10 per cent of all patients hospitalized for respiratory disease. In Houston between 1975 and 1976, influenza viruses were the most important cause of illness that brought children to an ambulatory care setting, but several influenza-infected children were admitted to hospital with nonspecific febrile illnesses or central nervous system involvement.

LABORATORY DIAGNOSIS

Laboratory demonstration of influenza virus infection may consist of either demonstration of the virus or antigen in throat washings and swabbings or evidence of a significant rise in serum antibody during convalescence from illness. Influenza antigen can be identified rapidly in exfoliated cells on a slide if sensitive antibody is available in a fluorescent antibody test. Enzyme immunoassay (EIA) shows promise for rapid diagnosis. Chick embryo has been the traditional laboratory host for the isolation of influenza viruses. The clinical specimen is preferably inoculated into the amniotic sac of chick embryos 10 to 11 days old. The amniotic fluid is harvested in 2 or 3 days and tested for hemagglutinins with chicken or guinea pig red blood cells. The inoculation of monkey kidney cell cultures, however, and the subsequent development of hemadsorption, which occurs with influenza virus–infected tissue culture, is a simpler and more sensitive method for most influenza strains. Type-specific animal serums are used to identify the virus recovered in egg or tissue culture. Serums obtained from patients early and about 3 weeks after the onset of illness are tested for antibodies to influenza virus by complement fixation, hemagglutination inhibition, EIA, or tissue culture neutralization methods.

PATHOGENESIS, PATHOLOGY

One of the predominant pathogenic characteristics of influenza viruses in susceptible hosts, such as chick embryos, ferrets, or humans, is a peculiar affinity for epithelial cells of the respiratory tract mucosa. Typically, influenza virus infection destroys ciliated epithelium, and there is metaplastic hyperplasia of the tracheal and bronchial epithelium with associated edema. The alveoli may become distended with a hyaline-like material.

During influenza infection, there is the development of type- and subtype-specific serum and secretory antibody, an elevation in interferon levels in secretions and serum, a brief lymphopenia, a depression in delayed hypersensitivity in general but an increase in influenza virus–specific cell-mediated responses, and some depression in the capacity of polymorphonuclear and mononuclear cells to respond to chemotaxis.

CLINICAL FEATURES

Infection in humans may be subclinical or may be accompanied by mild, moderate, or severe clinical manifestations. In most cases of overt illness, the throat and nasal mucous membranes are dry, and there is a dry cough with a tendency toward hoarseness. There is fever of sudden onset accompanied by flushed facies, photophobia with retrobulbar pain, myalgia, hyperesthesia, and sometimes prostration. In uncomplicated cases, these symptoms last for 4 or 5 days. Usually, a child with influenza infection has a more sudden onset of these "toxic" signs than do children with parainfluenza, respiratory syncytial virus, or adenovirus infection.

Subglottic croup is a common manifestation, especially in infants. Complications of influenza infection include severe viral pneumonia, often hemorrhagic, and encephalitis or encephalopathy. Influenza infection, particularly that due to type B, has been found in significant numbers of children with

Reye syndrome. Influenza virus infection has also been associated with sudden infant death syndrome. Bacterial infection due to *Haemophilus influenzae*, beta-hemolytic streptococci, or, especially, *Staphylococcus aureus* may complicate influenza infections, apparently with a higher frequency than in other viral illnesses. Pneumonia is the principal clinical manifestation of bacterial invasion.

TREATMENT AND PREVENTION

Antibiotics should not be used in uncomplicated influenza.

VACCINE

Multivalent inactivated type A and B influenza virus vaccines are available for immunization. To be effective, such vaccines must contain antigens similar to those that will be encountered in nature within a few months to a year following vaccine administration. Because influenza viruses show progressive antigenic variation, suitable vaccine strains are likely to be those recovered in the recent past. Worldwide surveillance is maintained with the hope of identifying major antigenic shifts so that new strains can be included in vaccines.

There is increasing recognition that influenza infections produce more illness in infants and children than was previously believed. Also, children are a major link in the spread of influenza infection throughout the community. Broad use of an effective vaccine in children, particularly those of school age, might well reduce the spread of virus and lessen the total impact of influenza in a community. However, potential control of influenza illness and spread in normal children probably awaits development of live attenuated vaccines, because some reports show that annual revaccination with inactivated vaccine offers no long-term advantage to school-age children.

Studies to determine an optimal dosage of killed vaccine for children in the 1976 immunization program showed that (1) dose of "whole virus" vaccine that regularly produced antibody also produced an undesirable level of local and febrile reactions, and (2) children responded with fewer reactions and with reasonable antibody levels to a strain to which they had no prior exposure after two doses of "split product" vaccine given 4 weeks apart.

These studies thus helped determine dosage of such vaccines in the future. Current schedules typically recommend (1) split or subvirion vaccine for individuals less than 13 years of age, (2) two doses 4 weeks apart of a vaccine against a strain to which an individual has never previously been exposed, (3) half the current adult dosage for infants and children 6 to 35 months of age. The vaccine should be administered in the fall in temperate climates because influenza occurs during the winter months; vaccine is more effective in the months immediately following administration and loses effectiveness toward the end of a year.

The vaccine should be administered intramuscularly in the deltoid muscle in adults and older children and in the anterior lateral aspect of the thigh in infants and small children. Killed influenza vaccine should be used for (1) infants and children 6 months of age or older who would be at high risk if they contracted influenza, (2) medical care providers or household contacts of the infants and children listed in (1), (3) children and adolescents who are receiving long-term aspirin therapy and thus might have an increased risk of acquiring Reye syndrome as a result of influenza virus infection, and (4) other children whose families may wish to reduce their chances of acquiring influenza. Recent specific recommendations have been made for (1) *targeted high-risk children*. According to the American Academy of Pediatrics, this category includes children with the following conditions: chronic pulmonary disease, including those with moderate to severe asthma, bronchopulmonary dysplasia, and cystic fibrosis; those with hemodynamically significant disease; those receiving immunosuppressant therapy; and those with sickle cell disease and other hemoglobinopathies. (2) *Other high-risk children.* Children with diabetes, chronic renal and metabolic diseases, and symptomatic HIV infection and those receiving long-term aspirin therapy belong in this category.

A high-risk child could acquire influenza from persons in the home, but these children and other children in health care facilities could also become infected by physicians, nurses, and other personnel who have extensive contact with them. Thus immunization is recommended for primary care and certain specialty clinicians and staff of long-term care facilities and intensive care units, particularly neonatal intensive care units, and for providers of home care to high-risk persons.

The only specific contraindication for the use of inactivated influenza vaccine is anaphylactic hypersensitivity to eggs. Children with such an allergy who are otherwise at high risk should be considered for the use of amantadine prophylaxis when influenza A is prevalent.

Special consideration is needed for immunosuppressed and other immunocompromised children. Immune response may be limited and is best accomplished during periods of remission or other reason for cessation of immunosuppressive drugs. There is little or no effect on renal function and no effect on allograft rejection in chronic renal disease or renal transplant recipients. There may be temporary brief impairment in air flow in asthma patients, but influenza-immunized children have fewer influenza-related hospitalizations.

Because formulations and content of vaccines are likely to change, the physician is advised to consult the most recent statements from the Public Health Service Advisory Committee on Immunization Prac-

Table 24–2. DOSAGES OF AMANTADINE PER DAY IN A SINGLE OR DIVIDED DOSE

	Adults and Children 10–12 years	Children ≥ 10 Years Under 45 kg	Children 1–9 Years
Prophylaxis	100 mg	4.4 mg/kg	4.4 mg/kg
Not to exceed	100 mg	100	100
Treatment	200 mg	4.4 mg/kg	4.4 mg/kg
Not to exceed	200 mg	150	200

tices or the American Academy of Pediatrics' Committee on Infectious Diseases.

Several research groups are developing potential attenuated influenza vaccines with inhibitor-resistant, cold-adapted, or temperature-sensitive strains. Prototypes of such vaccines have been shown to be attenuated for adults and older children. However, mild residual pathogenicity has been demonstrated in infants who had no prior experience with any influenza virus. Further attenuated prototypes are under study.

AMANTADINE

The synthetic amine amantadine has been shown to be effective in preventing and possibly ameliorating influenza A but not influenza B infection. Prophylactic use of amantadine is being recommended, preferably in conjunction with immunization, for adults and older children at high risk for serious influenza and also for adults whose activities are essential to community function and for selected health personnel. To prevent infection the drug must be used before exposure. Because specific viral diagnosis before individual patient use is impractical, one should consider prophylactic or potential therapeutic use when influenza A infection is known to be prevalent in a particular community. Some relief of symptoms is reported if amantadine is given within 48 hours of onset of the symptoms.

Prophylactic use of amantadine is recommended as an adjunct to late vaccination for high-risk persons to reduce the spread of infection and to maintain care for high-risk persons in the home, for immunodeficient persons as a supplement to the protection afforded by vaccine, and for persons for whom influenza vaccine is contraindicated. Therapeutic use is strongly considered for the aforementioned groups as well as for an infant or child with severe croup or pneumonia, the cause of which has been proved or is strongly suspected to be influenza A infection.

In June 1988, the Immunization Practices Advisory Committee of the U.S. Public Health Service suggested dosages of amantadine per day in a single or divided dose, which are given in Table 24–2. The drug has not been studied or prescribed widely in infants and children, and the ratio of therapeutic dose to toxic dose is potentially narrow. However, pending further controlled studies, careful selective use in high-risk children seems warranted.

RIBAVIRIN

Ribavirin is a synthetic nucleoside whose primary action leads to intracellular virustasis of most susceptible viruses, including influenza A and B in vitro. In 1981 Knight and colleagues used this antiviral agent by aerosol and detected improvement in college-age students with influenza. Although ribavirin aerosol has been approved for general use in the United States and Canada only for the treatment of respiratory syncytial virus in infants, studies are under way to explore its potential use against influenza.

REFERENCES

Immunization Practices Advisory Committee: Prevention and control of influenza. MMWR 37:361, 1988.

Kilbourne ED: The molecular epidemiology of influenza. J Infect Dis 127:478, 1973.

Knight V and Gilbert BE: Ribavirin aerosol treatment of influenza. Infect Dis Clin N Am 1(2):441, 1987.

Murphy BR and Webster RG: Influenza viruses. In Fields BN et al (eds): Virology. New York, Raven Press, 1985.

25

BRONCHIECTASIS

First described by Laennec in 1819 in *Traité de l'auscultation médiate,* bronchiectasis is a now uncommon disorder in developed nations, restricted in large degree to the pediatric population. Vaccines effective against measles and pertussis and advances in antimicrobial therapy (especially antituberculous agents) have led to a decline in the incidence of bronchiectasis, so much so that it has been called an "orphan disease" (Barker and Bardana, 1988). As these infections have become less important as primary causative agents in bronchiectasis, other more obscure factors have been identified that predispose an individual to this disorder. Improvements in computed tomographic techniques have facilitated early diagnosis and provided a noninvasive means of evaluating the extent of the disease. The same advances that led to the decline in the incidence of bronchiectasis have greatly improved the prognosis for most patients, with an ever-increasing number avoiding surgery. Though uncommon, bronchiectasis continues to be associated with a significant morbidity.

INCIDENCE

Accurate estimates of the incidence of bronchiectasis are not available. Typically, diagnostic studies are pursued only in those patients with persistent symptoms and signs, both clinical and radiographic, of the disorder. Many patients who are asymptomatic or only mildly symptomatic but who are at risk for the development of bronchiectasis because of recurrent pneumonia, recent pertussis or measles infection, or protracted and poorly controlled asthma probably escape detection for lack of further investigation. Likewise, less well-known risk factors for bronchiectasis (right middle lobe syndrome; adenoviral, herpes, and mycoplasmal pneumonia) may be overlooked.

Available data suggest that the incidence of bronchiectasis is quite low. Biering (1956) studied 151 patients in Copenhagen following pneumonia or pertussis possibly complicated by pneumonia and found only one child (0.7 per cent) to have bronchiectasis. Ruberman and colleagues (1957) evaluated with bronchoscopy 69 patients with persistent abnormalities on chest radiographs out of 1711 young adults

(18 to 25 years of age) treated for pneumonia at a U.S. army hospital. They found 29 (1.7 per cent) to have bronchiectatic changes. Clark (1963) found an incidence of bronchiectatic changes of 1.06 per 10,000 children living in northeastern Scotland. Most series indicate a male to female ratio of about 1:1.4.

Field (1969), in examining yearly admission rates for bronchiectasis at five hospitals in Great Britain between 1938 and 1961, noted a dramatic decrease in admission rates, from an average of 48 per 10,000 total pediatric admissions in 1952 to 10 per 10,000 total pediatric admissions in 1960. She speculated that improved treatment of lower respiratory tract infections made possible by the increased availability of broad-spectrum antibiotics during that period accounted for the decreased incidence. Other contributing factors include the prevention of measles and pertussis through immunization and the marked decrease in primary pulmonary tuberculosis in the pediatric population brought about by better public health measures and improved treatment regimens for this disease. Though its incidence in developed countries has been reduced as a result of these factors, bronchiectasis remains a common problem in developing countries, and even within certain populations (namely, the poor and medically indigent) in industrial societies.

PATHOLOGY

It was Laennec who, in 1819, provided the first pathologic description of bronchiectasis, based on examination of post-mortem specimens.

> *Sometimes it exists in one or in several branches, or even over almost the whole extent of one lung, without any other change in the appearance of the affected bronchia, than increase of volume: thus, ramifications which in the natural state would scarcely admit a fine probe, acquire a diameter equal to that of a crow-quill, or goosequill, or even a finger. . . . At other times, the dilated bronchia lose their natural shape, and present themselves under the form of a cavity, capable of containing a hempseed, a cherry-stone, an almond, or even a walnut.*

Surgical resection, curative for many patients, has provided specimens for detailed pathologic study.

Early on, the macroscopic abnormality is that of fusiform or cylindric dilation of subsegmental bronchi. Also described are alternating areas of dilation and constriction, called *varicose bronchiectasis* (Reid, 1950). In later stages, saccular dilation occurs. There is often accompanying atelectasis of the involved lobe, with pleural thickening and adhesions (Ogilvie, 1941). In addition, the bronchi are often tortuous and filled with mucopurulent material. The small distal airways may be obliterated as the result of long-standing obstruction, being replaced by a discrete cord of fibrous tissue containing muscle, elastic tissue, capillaries, and occasionally plates of cartilage (Reid, 1950).

Microscopically, there is a continuum of changes, the severity of which depends on the nature and duration of the etiologic event. Associated with early (fusiform or cylindric) disease is focal destruction of elastic tissue, edema, and infiltration of inflammatory cells in the surrounding parenchyma. As the process progresses, there is continued inflammatory infiltration, damage to the muscle layers, and eventually destruction of the supportive cartilage surrounding the airways. It is in the last-mentioned stage that, having lost their supportive structures, the airways take on a saccular appearance.

Ogilvie (1941) and later Whitwell (1952) reviewed that histologic changes associated with bronchiectasis and found a loss of cilia in surrounding areas. The affected area itself is no longer lined by columnar epithelium, containing instead cuboidal cells and, in more advanced (saccular) disease, squamous epithelium, which is often heaped up but may also be ulcerated, fibrosed, or denuded. There is associated hypertrophy of bronchial glands, lymphoid hyperplasia, and hypertrophy of mucous glands, occasionally to the point of bronchial obstruction.

Vascular changes are also associated with bronchiectasis. Liebow and co-workers (1949) were able to demonstrate marked enlargement of bronchial arteries in surgical specimens from patients with bronchiectasis. Further, they found anastomoses between the bronchial and pulmonary arteries, typically located near distal subsegmental bronchi that had undergone saccular bronchiectatic change. Just proximal to the anastomoses, the pulmonary arteries took on a spiral configuration. The investigators hypothesized that the enlargement and anastomoses are the result of engorgement of the bronchial capillary bed (in response to local inflammation) near the pulmonary arterial vessels.

The potential clinical significance of enlarged bronchial arteries underlying areas of weakened, eroded bronchial wall is not difficult to imagine. Further damage could easily lead to erosion into the high-pressure bronchial circulation and pulmonary hemorrhage. Liebow and colleagues, however, propose that the anastomoses may actually be beneficial, in that the high-pressure flow from the bronchial side may help shunt blood (desaturated) within the pulmonary system away from bronchiectatic areas to areas with more normal gas exchange capability, thereby decreasing intrapulmonary shunting.

PATHOGENESIS

Since Laennec's original description of bronchiectasis, much has been learned about this disorder, including the identification of clinical conditions that may predispose one or may themselves lead to bronchiectasis. Though several mechanisms have been proposed to explain the loss of normal bronchial anatomy, the exact process remains obscure. It seems likely that the pathogenesis of bronchiectasis is multifactorial, with the different factors taking on different degrees of importance in each patient.

The various mechanistic theories have been divided into four groups (Wigglesworth, 1955; Davis et al, 1983). The *pressure-of-secretion theory* proposes that thick secretions first obstruct, then mechanically distend the airway in such a way that the dilation persists after clearance of the obstruction. The *atelectasis theory* suggests that bronchial dilation is the result of increasingly negative intrapleural pressure brought about by collapse of lung parenchyma surrounding the bronchus in question. Somewhat similar, the *traction theory* contends that fibrosis and scarring from parenchymal disease exert traction on the bronchial walls. Finally, the *infection theory* holds that it is largely infection and the inflammatory response to infection that result in damage to the supportive structures of the bronchial wall and subsequent bronchiectasis. Of these theories, only the infection theory is supported by animal models of this disease.

In an attempt to investigate the pathogenesis of bronchiectasis, Tannenberg and Pinner (1942) produced bronchial obstruction by both intrabronchial (foreign body) and extrabronchial (ligation) means in rabbits. This bronchial obstruction quickly resulted in atelectasis, but even with long-standing obstruction, bronchiectasis did not occur in the absence of infection. Further, they found that atelectasis resulted in constriction, not dilation, of the bronchi. Cheng (1954) likewise ligated the bronchi of rats, producing distal infection in all. He found that antibiotic treatment prevented the develoment of bronchiectasis. Croxatto and Lanari (1954) first ligated and then later reestablished the lumen of the left main stem bronchus in dogs. They concluded that early dilation was the result of entrapment of secretions and was reversible with relief of the bronchial obstruction. Irreversible dilation (i.e., bronchiectasis) was the result of bronchial wall alterations from the pressure of entrapped secretions, concomitant infection, or both.

These studies suggest that atelectasis and traction play minimal, if any, roles in the pathogenesis of bronchiectasis. Bronchial obstruction with retention of secretions and infection appear to be the major factors in its development in most cases. The exact relationship of these processes to each other and to subsequent bronchiectasis, however, remains to be defined.

ETIOLOGY

INFECTION

Among the various entities that predispose one to the development of bronchiectasis, infection is by far the most common, and, until relatively recently, tuberculosis was the most common infectious agent responsible for postinfectious bronchiectatic changes. The hilar and peribronchial lymphadenopathy associated with it results in bronchial obstruction, which, when coupled with parenchymal damage from that or from subsequent infections with other organisms, can lead to bronchial wall destruction and bronchiectasis. Histoplasmosis may incite a similar chain of events (Rosenzweig and Stead, 1966). With the decline in the incidence of tuberculosis, its role in the pathogenesis of bronchiectasis has likewise decreased.

Pertussis and, more commonly, measles complicated by pneumonia have been associated previously with subsequent development of bronchiectasis, although there are no reliable estimates of its incidence following either infection. Lees (1950), in examining the incidence of bronchiectasis and atelectasis in 150 consecutive cases of pertussis, found that only four patients (2.6 per cent) developed bronchiectatic changes; three of these later had spontaneous resolution. This result occurred despite an incidence of atelectasis of 43 per cent, further calling into question the role of atelectasis in the pathogenesis of bronchiectasis. Fawcitt and Parry (1957) similarly reviewed 956 cases of pertussis and 897 cases of measles and found atelectasis in 48 per cent and 28 per cent, respectively. At a later follow-up, 17 per cent of the pertussis patients and 15 per cent of the measles patients had residual atelectasis. Six of these children were evaluated with bronchography, one with measles, four with pertussis, and one with both. Of these, one was normal (the child with both measles and pertussis), four had bronchiectatic changes, and one had no dilation, but a crowding of bronchi was noted. They concluded that permanent residual change was rare following pertussis and measles.

In any case, it may not be the primary infection that is responsible for such changes but concomitant or subsequent infection with other agents, particularly adenovirus and herpesvirus, that mediates the injury resulting in bronchiectasis (Kaschula et al, 1983; Warner and Marshall, 1976). A number of investigators (Herbert et al, 1977; Becroft, 1971, 1979; Simila et al, 1981; Lang, 1969) have documented bronchiectasis in 20 to 64 per cent of children following pneumonia from adenovirus (types 1,3,4,7, and 21) alone. Other infectious agents that have been linked to the development of bronchiectasis include *Aspergillus fumigatus* (Wang et al, 1979) and *Mycoplasma pneumoniae* (Goudie et al, 1983; Whyte and Williams, 1984; Halal et al, 1977), as well as other microorganisms that may cause chronic necrotizing bronchopneumonia.

CONGENITAL AND GENETIC DISORDERS

By far the most common genetically transmitted disorder that results in bronchiectasis is cystic fibrosis, which is likely the result of chronic bronchial obstruction with inspissated mucus, infection, and inflammation; a structural defect has not been proven. A complete discussion of this disorder can be found in Chapter 47.

Williams and Campbell in 1960 described five patients with onset of lung disease, including bronchiectasis, in infancy. Autopsy findings in one of the children were remarkable for near-total absence of supportive cartilage in segmental and subsegmental bronchi. There have since been 14 additional cases reported, including 11 more by Williams and co-workers (1972). Mitchell and Bury (1975) describe a case in which, in addition to deficiency of cartilage, obliterative bronchiolitis was noted. They suggest that, although infection plays an important role in the outcome of these patients, it is lack of cartilage that is primarily responsible for the bronchiectasis. Wayne and Taussig (1976) described the disorder in two siblings, suggesting a familial occurrence of this syndrome.

Tracheobronchomegaly is characterized by a markedly dilated trachea, which may be equal in size to the vertebral column on a chest radiograph. Bronchoscopy confirms the tracheobronchial dilation and often reveals the airway walls to be floppy and redundant, with occasional outcroppings or diverticula (Katz et al, 1962). In contrast to the deficiency of cartilage found in Williams-Campbell syndrome, this disorder is attributed to a developmental abnormality of tracheobronchial elastic tissue and muscle.

Evidence is accumulating that Marfan syndrome, long associated with spontaneous pneumothorax, may also be associated with bronchiectasis. Wood and colleagues (1984) reviewed the records and radiographs of 100 patients with Marfan syndrome and found two who had bronchiectasis; eight others had frequent respiratory infections. They suggest that connective tissue weakness in Marfan syndrome makes these individuals susceptible to the development of bronchiectasis.

Although most often associated with emphysematous changes, alpha$_1$-antiproteinase deficiency is also associated with bronchiectasis. Varpela and colleagues (1978) screened 60 consecutive patients with bronchiectasis and found six (10 per cent) to have the Pi^{mz} genotype (compared to 2.7 per cent in controls). No other genotypic variants were found. It is interesting to speculate that in patients with active, ongoing inflammatory processes (e.g., cystic fibrosis, chronic pneumonia), a relative deficiency of antiproteinase activity may be present as a result of high local concentrations of endogenous (e.g., neutrophil elastase) and exogenous proteinases. Although the patients thus far described with bronchiectasis associated with decreased alpha$_1$-antiproteinase levels have been adults, it would seem reasonable to screen for this disorder in children with severe bronchiectasis that does not have an obvious cause.

In addition to these disorders, there may also be a very small group of patients whose bronchiectasis is truly congenital. These individuals appear to have had a developmental abnormality that has resulted in cystic deformity of the airway. Over time, recurrent infections result in further deformity and frank bronchiectasis.

CILIARY ABNORMALITIES

With the decline of tuberculosis, pertussis, and measles, abnormalities of ciliary structure and function have emerged as important causes of bronchiectasis. Kartagener syndrome, the most well known, is recognizable clinically as the triad of situs inversus, sinusitis, and bronchiectasis. Also associated with it is abnormal ciliary function, which is responsible for the suppurative aspects of the syndrome.

Three patterns of ciliary ultrastructural abnormality have been described in patients with disorders of ciliary function (Davis et al, 1983), the most common being total or partial absence of dynein arms. Absence of the radial spokes and loss of central tubules have also been reported. These abnormalities are congenital and are thought to be transmitted in an autosomal-recessive manner. Wakefield and Waite (1980) have reported a variety of ciliary abnormalities among Polynesians, a group with a relatively high incidence of bronchiectasis.

Ciliary abnormalities can also be acquired as the result of infection. Corbeel and co-workers (1981) studied the ciliary ultrastructure of five children with recurrent pulmonary infections. They found multiple architectural abnormalities that reverted to normal following recovery from infection. Carson and colleagues (1985) similarly found transient ultrastructural abnormalities in children acutely infected with a variety of respiratory viruses. There is also evidence that high levels of elastase present in the sputum of many patients with bronchiectasis reduce ciliary beat frequency (Smallman et al, 1984). These changes may contribute to the development of bronchiectasis by impairing mucociliary clearance and thus perpetuate the inflammatory process. Disorders of ciliary structure and function are discussed in detail in Chapter 45.

IMMUNODEFICIENCIES

Among the many forms of immunodeficiency, those most commonly associated with bronchiectasis involve deficiency of one or more classes of immunoglobulins. Deficiency of IgG, either in total or of one or more subclasses (most often IgG$_2$), is often associated with recurrent respiratory tract infections and the potential development of bronchiectasis. The availability of immunoglobulin replacement therapy makes screening for such deficiencies important. A normal serum level of total IgG does not preclude a deficiency in one of the subclasses; IgG subclasses should be evaluated separately.

Though relatively common, IgA deficiency is infrequently associated with bronchiectasis (Chipps et al, 1978). However IgA deficiency may be associated with IgG$_2$ subclass deficiency and recurrent pyogenic pulmonary infections (Oxelius et al, 1981). Immunoglobulin replacement must be monitored closely in these patients, as they may become immunized against IgA.

Deficiencies of complement and abnormalities of neutrophil function may also lead to recurrent pulmonary infections.

Other immunologic abnormalities have been described in association with bronchiectasis. Hilton and Doyle (1978) found that 42 of 53 patients (79 per cent) with bronchiectasis had at least one abnormality of immunoglobulins, typically an elevation in serum levels of IgA, IgG, or IgM; eight patients (15 per cent) had elevations of all three classes. Hilton and co-workers (1979) evaluated serums from 14 patients with bronchiectasis and found evidence suggesting the presence of circulating immune complexes, a finding also noted in cystic fibrosis patients (Church et al, 1981). It is unclear whether these abnormalities are mediators of, or responses to, long-standing bronchial infection and pulmonary parenchymal damage.

FOREIGN BODY ASPIRATION

The prolonged presence of a foreign body within the airway can result in chronic obstruction and inflammation, both major factors in the development of bronchiectasis. In a review of 500 patients with bronchiectasis, Kürklü and colleagues (1973) found eight (1.6 per cent) to have a long-retained foreign body as the cause. Aytaç and colleagues (1977) reviewed 462 cases of foreign body aspiration in children and found chronic infection, bronchiectasis, or both in 3.5 per cent.

RIGHT MIDDLE LOBE SYNDROME

Persistent right middle lobe atelectasis, a relatively frequent reason for referral to the pediatric pulmonary subspecialist, can be associated with the development of bronchiectasis. Bertelsen and colleagues (1980) reported a 10-year study of 135 patients (predominantly adults) with isolated right middle lobe atelectasis. Of 46 patients with nonmalignant disease who underwent bronchography, eight (17 per cent) had bronchiectasis. Although direct extrapolation of these results to the pediatric population is not possible, the results would support the prompt evaluation and vigorous treatment of children with persistent middle lobe atelectasis.

ASTHMA

Asthma has been proposed as both a predisposing factor and an indicator of poor prognosis in patients with bronchiectasis. The reasons for these effects are unclear. Field (1949) and Clark (1963) describe asthma in 6.9 and 7.8 per cent, respectively, of children with bronchiectasis. Strang (1956) noted wheezing in 50 of 209 children (24 per cent) with bronchiectasis, although only eight (3.8 per cent) had "clear cut attacks of spasmodic asthma." Varpela and co-workers (1978) evaluated 48 consecutive adult patients with bronchiectasis and found 11 (22 per cent) to have asthma and 50 per cent to have bronchial histamine hyperreactivity.

On follow-up, Strang found that of 26 patients treated surgically whose wheezing was mild (nocturnal, associated with upper respiratory infections or exercise only), 14 had the wheezing resolved after surgery. Those patients who had frank attacks of wheezing before surgery continued to have significant symptoms of reactive airways disease and did poorly from the standpoint of continued cough, sputum production, and intermittent fever. This despite postoperative bronchograms documenting the absence of bronchiectasis. Field (1969), in a long-term follow-up of bronchiectasis, also found that those whose wheezing persisted after surgery did less well than those whose wheezing subsided.

OTHER

Heroin intoxication and overdose have been associated with the development of bronchiectasis. In early reports, bronchiectasis was thought to have been the result of aspiration of vomitus superimposed on heroin-induced pulmonary edema. Banner and colleagues (1976), however, proposed that it is an infectious process (typically viral) that, in conjunction with pulmonary edema, results in bronchiectatic changes.

Developmental abnormalities of the lung, such as intralobar pulmonary sequestration or bronchogenic cyst, may promote the development of bronchiectasis by causing extrinsic obstruction of the airway.

Chronic sinusitis has previously been associated with bronchiectasis. Whether chronic aspiration of purulent sinus drainage leads to bronchiectasis or chronic expectoration of purulent sputum causes recurrent contamination of the sinuses or both is not known. However, with the increased recognition of sinus disease and the availability of appropriate an-

tibiotic therapy, both the incidence of chronic sinusitis and its association with lower respiratory tract disease have diminished.

Severe or recurrent aspiration may lead to the development of bronchiectasis. Anatomic abnormalities, such as a tracheoesophageal fistula, or neurologic deficits, such as cerebral palsy, may be associated with chronic aspiration and the subsequent development of bronchiectasis. Aspiration following general anesthesia, especially for tonsillectomy and adenoidectomy, has in the past been linked to bronchiectasis, although, happily, this outcome is now uncommon.

Pulmonary injury from inhalation of noxious gases may predispose one to bronchiectasis. Anhydrous ammonia and sulfur dioxide have both been implicated in this regard. Concomitant or subsequent infection may be important cofactors for these events.

Racial predilections to bronchiectasis have been suggested, specifically among children of Australian aboriginal, Inuit (Eskimo), and Polynesian origin. Except for Polynesians (in whom ciliary abnormalities have been identified), the higher incidence of bronchiectasis among these groups is related not to inherent biologic factors but to socioeconomic conditions.

PRESENTATION

AGE

The majority of children with bronchiectasis present in the preschool and early school-age years. Field (1949) found that 40 per cent of the 160 patients in her review presented before 7 years of age, with 20 per cent presenting between age 6 and 7 years. Strang (1956) observed that 75 per cent of the 209 children in his series presented before age 6 years. Likewise, Fernald (1978), in reviewing 38 cases of childhood bronchiectasis, noted that 63 per cent were diagnosed before age 6 years. Of the 116 children with bronchiectasis reviewed by Clark (1963), 84 per cent presented before age 6 and 50 per cent before age 3.

SYMPTOMS

The most common symptoms seen in children with established bronchiectasis are listed in Table 25–1. Cough, not surprisingly, is an almost universal finding and can often be dated from an actue respiratory illness. The incidence of sputum production is likely much higher than listed, because many patients present before an age when sputum is normally expectorated. Hemoptysis, when noted, is generally characterized as mild, slight, or streaking. Other symptoms noted with less frequency include weight loss (although most children with bronchiectasis maintain adequate weight gain) and intermittent fever. The duration of symptoms before presentation

Table 25–1. FREQUENCY OF SYMPTOMS AT PRESENTATION IN CHILDHOOD BRONCHIECTASIS

Symptom	%
Cough	97
Sputum	46
Wheezing	21
Chest Pain	20
Hemoptysis	14
Dyspnea	7.2

(Adapted from the combined data of Field CE: Pediatrics 4:2, 1949; Clark NS: Br Med J 1:80, 1963; and Strang C: Ann Int Med 44:630, 1956.)

in some cases has been greater than 10 years, but Field (1949) found a median duration of approximately 3 years.

The same symptoms may be observed on an intermittent basis in children developing bronchiectasis. Frequently present, a history of recurrent pneumonia, especially when restricted to a single lobe or segment, should prompt a careful evaluation for developing bronchiectasis as well as for potential causative factors.

CLINICAL SIGNS

The frequencies of different physical findings noted at presentation in children with bronchiectasis are listed in Table 25–2. Except in diffuse disease, the auscultatory findings are usually localized to the involved areas. In addition to these physical findings, Field (1949) described various deformities of the chest wall, the most common being a linear area of depression circumscribing the lower third of the chest wall (Harrison's sulcus). She also found postural deformities (rounded shoulders, lordosis, protuberant abdomen) to be common.

In our experience, clubbing is much less frequent than the table would indicate, perhaps because of the inclusion of data from older series of patients. The degree of digital clubbing is related more to duration of disease and frequency of intercurrent pulmonary infections than to type or extent of bronchiectasis (Whitwell, 1952; Laurenzi, 1970). When present, clubbing is reversible with medical and, when appropriate, surgical management. Field (1969) found that at long-term follow-up the incidence of clubbing had fallen from 43.7 per cent to 6.5 per cent, although

Table 25–2. FREQUENCY OF CLINICAL SIGNS NOTED AT PRESENTATION IN CHILDHOOD BRONCHIECTASIS

Clinical Signs	%
Crackles	82
Dullness to percussion	47
Clubbing	46
Suppression	35
Bronchial breath sounds	19
Cyanosis	5

(Adapted from the combined data of Field CE: Pediatrics 4:2, 1949; Clark NS: Br Med J 1:80, 1963; and Strang C: Ann Int Med 44:630, 1956.)

she points out that the death of the most severely affected patients may have influenced the change in these figures.

DIAGNOSIS

Although not diagnostic, bronchiectasis can be suspected on the basis of abnormalities on chest radiographs. Nonspecific findings said to be suggestive of bronchiectasis (Fraser and Paré, 1979) include (1) segmental accentuation and loss of definition of lung markings (Fig. 25–1); (2) loss of lung volume, manifested by crowding of lung markings (Fig. 25–2); (3) cysts up to 2 cm in diameter, sometimes with air-fluid levels; (4) a "honeycomb" pattern of cystic changes (in severe cases); and (5) compensatory hyperinflation of other lung segments. Another finding is the "tram-track" sign, parallel linear markings that represent thickened bronchial walls viewed in their longitudinal dimension (see Fig. 25–1). When seen in cross section, they appear as thick-walled circles.

Regardless of how suggestive the clinical picture or findings on plain radiographs are, bronchography remains the definitive study against which all other diagnostic methods are compared (Fig. 25–3). Although good results have been reported using blind passage of an endotracheal tube in awake, sedated children (Wilson et al, 1972), bronchography in the past was often done under general anesthesia with direct endotracheal intubation. The child is rotated through various positions to bring the contrast to the desired area. In experienced hands, this procedure can yield important diagnostic information with little associated morbidity. Levy and co-workers (1983) reviewed their experience with 110 bronchoscopies, including 18 bronchograms. Bronchography was performed for the purpose of confirming bronchiectasis in 11 patients, and findings were positive in seven. Although there were three deaths in these 110 patients, all deaths were attributed to the underlying disease.

With technologic advances and improvements in technique, flexible fiberoptic bronchoscopy has become an extremely valuable diagnostic modality for the pediatric pulmonary subspecialist. When combined with the instillation of contrast material via the bronchoscope, selective bronchography can be carried out without the need for general anesthesia. Lundgren and colleagues (1982) found that this technique allowed direct visualization of the area and provided a means for obtaining bacteriologic and histopathologic samples. In addition, bronchography could be carried out in a more deliberate, selective fashion, making possible sequential evaluation of adjacent bronchi. In our experience, as little as 2 ml of contrast material is sufficient to adequately visualize the airways of a preschool child using bronchoscopically directed bronchography. It is the practice at our center, however, to reserve bronchography for those children who, having failed medical man-

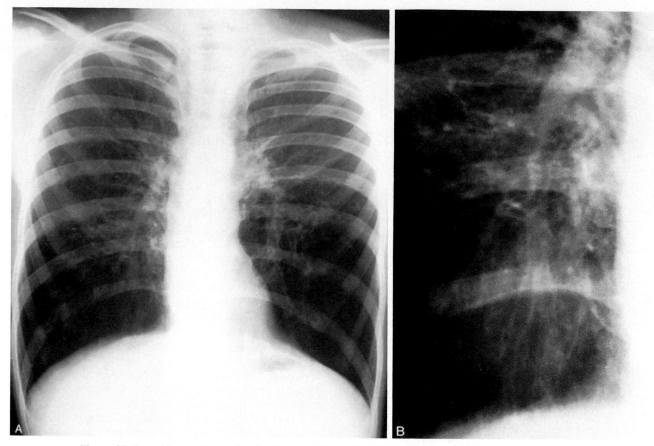

Figure 25–1. *A,* Chest radiograph of a 17-year-old boy with bilateral lower lobe bronchiectasis of unknown origin. Lung markings are accentuated, and there is hyperinflation of adjacent lung segments. *B,* Enlargement of the area in the right lower lobe, demonstrating the "tram-track" sign.

agement, are considered candidates for surgical resection and therefore need accurate definition of both the location and the extent of the disease.

Much interest has been shown in the use of computed tomography (CT) in the evaluation of bronchiectasis. Naidich and co-workers (1982) used CT to evaluate six patients with confirmed bronchiectasis. They described four findings characteristic of that disease: (1) air-fluid levels in distended bronchi, (2) a linear array or cluster of cysts, (3) dilated peripheral bronchi, and (4) thickened bronchial walls (Fig. 25–4). Subsequently, other investigators have found CT to have poor sensitivity, especially for mild disease (Müller et al, 1984; Phillips et al, 1986; Cooke et al, 1987), or to be unable to determine segmental location (Mootoosamy et al, 1985). However, using medium-thickness cuts (4 mm) at medium-slice intervals (5 mm), Joharjy and co-workers (1987) found a specificity of 100 per cent for all types of bronchiectasis and sensitivities of 100 per cent for cystic and 94 per cent for cylindrical disease when compared with bronchograms in 20 patients. Although bronchography remains the gold standard, with appropriate technique, CT may be useful in patients for whom bronchography would be unduly risky.

Smith (1983) evaluated two patients with bronchiectasis and five with cystic fibrosis using magnetic resonance imaging (MRI). Although secretion-filled

bronchiectatic lung and areas of inflammation were easily identifiable, the role of this imaging technique in the primary evaluation of bronchiectasis remains to be determined.

Its exact usefulness is somewhat controversial, but lung scintigraphy appears to be a useful screening measure when combined with plain chest radiography. Sutherland and co-workers (1980) found marked reductions in ventilation and less severe reductions in perfusion in 36 patients with bronchiectasis. In their hands, scintigraphy had a sensitivity of 89 per cent for bronchiectasis, as compared with 71 per cent for chest radiographs. This result agrees quite well with the findings of Vandevivere and colleagues (1980). They evaluated 76 children with chest radiographs, bronchography, and lung scintigraphy. The sensitivity for chest radiographs was 73 per cent and for lung scintigraphy 92 per cent. When combined, the sensitivity rose to 96 per cent. Both these groups concluded that lung scintigraphy is a useful screening test for bronchiectasis when combined with a chest radiograph.

As might be expected, bronchiectatic lesions are most commonly identified in the lower lobes, especially the left lower lobe (Table 25–3). The upper lobes are less commonly involved, probably because mucociliary clearance is facilitated by gravity. Multi-

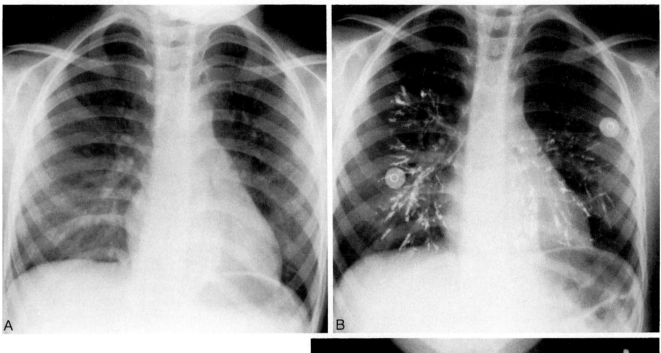

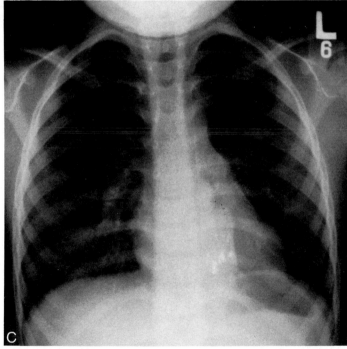

Figure 25–2. *A,* Chest radiograph of a 4-year-old girl with left lower lobe bronchiectasis. There is atelectasis and crowding of lung markings in that area. *B,* Bronchogram of the same patient. There is a slight increase in the diameter of the airways in the left lower lobe and obvious crowding of the airways. *C,* Chest radiograph taken 4 days after the bronchogram, demonstrating marked delay in clearance of contrast from the affected areas. The patient underwent left lower lobectomy without incident and is doing well approximately 1 year after surgery.

lobar involvement is common, with left lower lobe and lingula the most common combination.

Once the presence of bronchiectasis is reasonably well established, it becomes important to attempt to determine its cause and to identify predisposing factors. Viral and bacteriologic studies not only provide epidemiologic data but also may guide therapy. Flexible fiberoptic bronchoscopy can be invaluable in obtaining appropriate microbiologic specimens, evaluating for the presence of a foreign body, obtaining samples of respiratory epithelium for ciliary studies, and providing information regarding endobronchial anatomy. Evaluation for immunodeficiency, cystic

fibrosis, aspiration, mycobacterial or fungal disease, or other predisposing factors is also important and should proceed as guided by the clinical picture (Table 25–4).

TREATMENT

Once the diagnosis of bronchiectasis has been reasonably well established, consideration can begin regarding therapy (Fig. 25–5). We feel comfortable initiating therapy based on compatible findings on history and physical examination and changes on

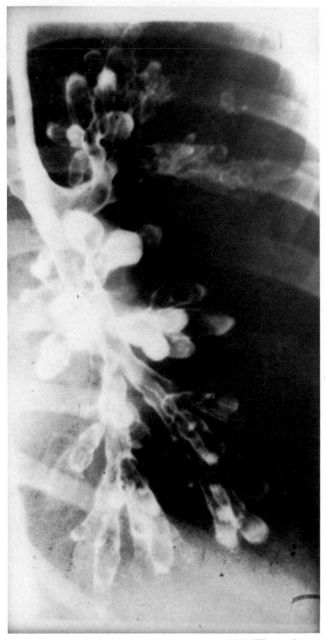

Figure 25–3. Bronchogram from a patient with Williams-Campbell syndrome, demonstrating severe saccular bronchiectasis.

chest radiograph suggestive of bronchiectasis. If a causative or predisposing factor has been identified, appropriate intervention should, of course, be instituted. Otherwise, the therapy of bronchiectasis varies little from patient to patient. The emphasis is on removal of excess secretions, treatment of intercurrent infection, and good nutrition. Surgical management, utilized less frequently than in the past because of improved medical management, may offer significant benefits to those children with localized disease but persistent symptoms.

MEDICAL THERAPY

Although currently out of favor in the treatment of patients with chronic obstructive pulmonary dis-

ease, chest percussion and postural drainage (or chest physiotherapy) are effective in facilitating clearance of secretions in those patients whose bronchiectasis is associated with excessive sputum production (greater than 30 ml per day) (Murray, 1979). Bateman and colleagues (1979) have shown that in patients with excessive sputum production, physiotherapy results in more rapid and complete clearance of a radioactive aerosol than coughing alone. Some studies have shown improvement in pulmonary function following chest physiotherapy (Tecklin and Holsclaw, 1975; Cochrane et al, 1977), but others have shown improvement only in clearance of secretions (Mazzocco et al, 1985). Cascade cough may also be helpful in those children old enough to master this technique.

The role of aerosol therapy is not clear. Bland aerosol therapy has not been shown to be beneficial. Mucolytic agents, such as N-acetylcysteine, may not penetrate the mucous blanket enough to be effective and, more important, may be potent bronchial irritants. There is some evidence, however, that beta-adrenergic agonists improve mucociliary clearance. Wood and co-workers (1975) documented improved tracheal mucociliary transport following administration of terbutaline to 14 adults with cystic fibrosis. Care must be taken, however, if bronchodilators are given, as reduction in bronchomotor tone may result in an impaired cough reflex and airway obstruction from pooled secretions and "floppy" airways. Bronchoscopy and bronchial lavage are not recommended for routine pulmonary toilet but may be appropriate in selected cases with specific indications.

Although antibiotic therapy is clearly indicated for acute infections (increased cough and sputum production, fever, malaise, etc.), its use on a continuous basis is generally discouraged. Long-term antibiotic therapy may be of benefit to those individuals whose bronchiectasis has an underlying cause (e.g., cystic fibrosis, immotile cilia syndrome), those who experience a marked increase in pulmonary symptoms on withdrawal of antibiotics, or those who have frequent bouts of lower respiratory tract infection. Evidence is also emerging that long-term antibiotic therapy may reduce sputum concentration of elastase, a potential mediator of ongoing inflammation and lung injury (Stockley et al, 1984).

Whenever possible, antibiotic therapy should be directed at specific pathogens and guided by sputum cultures and sensitivity studies. Pending the outcome of microbiologic studies, empiric antibiotic therapy should be directed against those organisms commonly found in the sputum of patients with bronchiectasis: *Haemophilus influenzae, Streptococcus pneumoniae,* and *Staphylococcus aureus.* Organisms found less commonly include *Pseudomonas aeruginosa* and *Proteus vulgaris.*

In addition to oral antibiotic therapy, there has been interest in the use of aerosolized antibiotics in patients with bronchiectasis. Stockley and co-workers (1985) found that despite no response to oral amoxicillin and emergence of resistance, there was a de-

Figure 25–4. *A*, Posteroanterior radiograph showing marked changes of cystic bronchiectasis, especially in the right lower lobe. *B*, Section through the right lower lobe. Numerous dilated bronchi are grouped together in the right lower lobe; the appearance resembles a cluster of grapes. *C*, Enlargement of *B* on the left side. Thick-walled bronchi can be seen in the anterior portion of the left lower lobe, extending toward the lung periphery (*middle arrows*). These bronchi have a "tram-track" appearance, indicative of cylindric bronchiectasis. In the posterior portion of the left lower lobe, several dilated bronchi are aligned in a row, resembling a string of cysts (*lower arrows*). This finding is indicative of cystic bronchiectasis. Note the solitary thick-walled bronchus adjacent to its accompanying pulmonary artery (*white arrowhead*). *D*, Enlargement of a section obtained at a slightly higher level than that shown in *B* on the right side. In the superior segment of the right lower lobe and the middle lobe, several dilated bronchi are aligned in a linear fashion, resembling a string of pearls (*arrows*). (Reproduced with permission from Naidich DP et al: Computed tomography of bronchiectasis. J Comp Assist Tomography 6:437, 1982.)

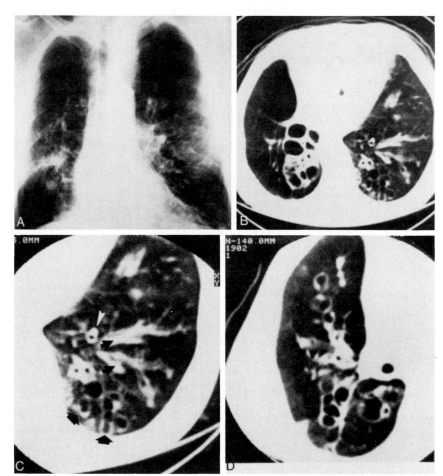

Table 25–3. DISTRIBUTION OF INVOLVEMENT IN CHILDHOOD BRONCHIECTASIS

Location	%
RIGHT LUNG	
Upper lobe	21
Middle lobe	47
Lower lobe	51
LEFT LUNG	
Upper lobe	14
Lingula	55
Lower lobe	72

(Adapted from the combined data of Field CE: Arch Dis Child 44:551, 1969; Clark NS: Br Med J 1:80, 1963; and Glauser et al: Acta Pediatr Scand 165:1, 1966.)

Table 25–4. SUGGESTED BASIC EVALUATION FOR PATIENTS WITH BRONCHIECTASIS GROUPED BY POTENTIAL CAUSES*

Infection
Sputum or bronchoalveolar lavage fluid (BALF) for bacterial/ mycobacterial/fungal cultures
Nasopharyngeal swab/wash and/or BALF for viral culture
Skin tests (PPD, fungal, control)
†Serologic studies

Immunodeficiency
Complete blood count with differential
Quantitative immunoglobulins (including IgE)
IgG subclasses
†Total hemolytic complement
†Tests of white blood cell function (nitroblue tetrazolium dye test, chemotactic assays, etc.)

Cystic Fibrosis
Sweat test

Aspiration
Barium swallow
Extended esophageal pH monitoring

Ciliary Dysfunction
Nasal/tracheal epithelium for light microscopy (ciliary motion) and electron microscopy (ciliary ultrastructure)

*Other studies may also be indicated, depending on history and physical findings.
†If indicated by history and/or physical examination.

crease in sputum production and purulence and an increase in peak expiratory flow rate with the use of aerosolized amoxicillin, with no adverse side effects noted. They speculate that high local antibiotic concentrations may be necessary for a good response.

An important factor in the outcome of medical therapy is regular ongoing medical care. Routine immunizations should be carried out (provided a contraindicating immunodeficiency is not present), and respiratory tract illnesses should be vigorously

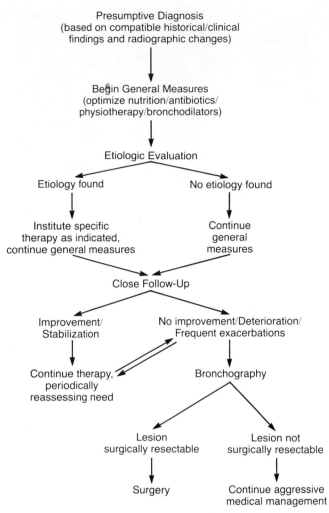

Figure 25–5. Suggested algorithm for evaluation and treatment of bronchiectasis.

treated. Cherniack and co-workers (1967), in a study of 63 adult patients with bronchiectasis, found that the rate of deterioration of pulmonary function was related to the frequency of lower respiratory tract infections.

SURGICAL THERAPY

Paralleling the reduced incidence of bronchiectasis has been a decline in the number of patients coming to operation for treatment of that disease. This decline is a reflection not only of decreased incidence but also of more effective medical management. Still, there are children whose disease is unresponsive to aggressive medical management who are best served by surgical intervention.

Several large series have shown that, in skilled hands and with careful selection, resection for bronchiectasis is well tolerated and offers a reasonably good chance for improvement in symptoms. Sanderson and co-workers (1974) reviewed 393 patients (88 of them less than 15 years of age) and compared outcomes in the surgically and conservatively treated

groups. They found that surgically treated patients overall had better outcomes, although with milder disease the difference between the groups was less striking. Wilson and Decker (1982) reported their experience with 195 children, 84 of whom underwent surgery. They found that at an average follow-up of 10 years, 75 per cent of the surgically treated group were well or much improved (including 67 per cent who were asymptomatic). In contrast, the medically treated group was largely unchanged (69 per cent). The complication rate was low in both series and consisted for the most part of relatively minor problems (also see "*Complications*").

Most investigators agree that aggressive medical therapy should be carried out for at least 2 years before considering surgery. In addition, Wilson and Decker (1982) advocate deferring surgery until between 6 and 12 years of age to allow for full progression of any subtle bronchiectatic changes present. It is our practice, however, to recommend surgical resection sooner, after 6 to 9 months of aggressive medical management. We believe this approach more fully takes advantage of potential compensatory lung growth that may occur in young children following pulmonary resection.

One area of controversy involves the preservation of the apical segment in lower lobe resections, which is usually done to retain as much functioning pulmonary tissue as possible or to help prevent displacement of the remaining parenchyma. However, the apical segment is often the site of residual disease following resection of the basal segments. Wilson and Decker (1982) have concluded that this segment can be preserved with good results provided it is dem-

Table 25–5. SUGGESTED INDICATIONS FOR SURGICAL TREATMENT OF BRONCHIECTASIS

Clear-cut Indications
1. Localized disease, producing severe symptoms:
   (a) profuse sputum
   (b) fetid breath
   (c) severe cough or other symptoms that interfere with a normal life pattern
2. Threatening hemorrhage from a demonstrated focal, segmental, or lobar source
3. Resectable disease of significant severity associated with failure to thrive
4. Resectable disease of a demonstrated site of recurrent, acute lower respiratory infections

Less Clear-cut Indications
1. Evidence of unstable disease associated with significant progression or extension of resectable disease
2. Bronchiectasis not easily or totally resectable but associated with failure to thrive
3. Bronchiectasis not easily or totally resectable associated with life-threatening or truly disabling symptoms:
   (a) profuse sputum
   (b) fetid breath
   (c) hemorrhage
   (d) severe, recurrent, focal infection episodes
4. Localized disease, producing minimal to moderate symptoms

(Adapted and reproduced with permission from Wilson JF and Decker AM: The surgical management of childhood bronchiectasis. Ann Surg 195:354, 1982.)

onstrated to be completely free of disease by bronchography.

Depending on the cause of bronchiectasis, surgical resection is an option even in patients with bilateral disease. Such patients generally undergo resection in two stages, with the more severely affected area being removed first. Occasionally, the second resection can be deferred because of satisfactory improvement achieved with the first procedure. George and colleagues (1978) reviewed their experience with 99 such patients over 40 years. In a follow-up study, 84 per cent of their patients had satisfactory to excellent results. With very careful patient selection and compulsive attention to pulmonary toilet, both preoperatively and postoperatively, pulmonary resection can even be beneficial in patients with bronchiectasis as a consequence of cystic fibrosis (Marmon et al, 1983; Mearns et al, 1972).

The most important factor in determining outcome following pulmonary resection for bronchiectasis is patient selection. Davis and co-workers (1983) have suggested that children with localized disease accompanied by significant persistent symptoms are the best surgical candidates. Wilson and Decker (1982) have provided more detailed indications for surgical treatment (Table 25–5).

COMPLICATIONS

Along with the decline in incidence and the improved treatment of bronchiectasis has come a marked decline in the complications from it. Common in the preantibiotic era but rare now are brain and lung abscess; empyema and pyopneumothorax; bronchopleural fistula; severe atypical pneumonia; hemoptysis; amyloidosis; and, in advanced disease, cor pulmonale (Perry and King, 1940).

Serious complications from surgical therapy are uncommon, but less severe problems are more common. In their series of 272 surgical procedures, Sanderson and colleagues (1974) had an overall complication rate of 30.5 per cent, including one intraoperative death (Table 25–6). In a later, smaller

Table 25–6. COMPLICATIONS FOLLOWING SURGICAL RESECTION FOR BRONCHIECTASIS

Sanderson et al (1974)	
Total Procedures	272 (100%)
Deaths	1 (0.4%)
Air leak/atelectasis	64 (24%)
Bronchitis	7 (2.5%)
Bronchopleural fistula	7 (2.5%)
Empyema (5 with fistula)	11 (4%)
Wilson and Decker (1982)	
Total Procedures	96 (100%)
Deaths	0 (0%)
Air leak/atelectasis	4 (4.2%)
Bronchopleural fistula	1 (1%)
Respiratory insufficiency	1 (1%)
Chylothorax	1 (1%)

(Adapted from Sanderson JM et al: Thorax 29:407, 1974; and Wilson JF and Decker AM: Ann Surg 195:354, 1982.)

series Wilson and Decker (1982) had an overall complication rate of 9.4 per cent.

PROGNOSIS

Although obviously dependent on causative factors, the prognosis for children with bronchiectasis is, in general, quite good. Several of the same medical advances that led to a decline in bronchiectasis have made a major impact on its treatment and subsequent outcome.

Clark (1963) reviewed the outcome in 116 children at 5 to 14 years after diagnosis. In 79 of the children, repeat bronchograms had been performed at intervals from 6 months to 8 years. Of these children, 46 (58 per cent) showed no change, 27 (34 per cent) had deteriorated, and 7 (9 per cent) had improved. Only 15 of the 27 patients who had deteriorated demonstrated involvement of previously normal airways. There were five deaths, two postoperatively. Of the 80 children treated surgically, 55 per cent recovered completely and 16 per cent had only minimal symptoms. In the medically treated group (6 of whom were considered candidates for surgery), 81 per cent were improved, although 12 of these patients had only mild disease initially. Field (1949) found similar results in her initial follow-up series.

In a later review of outcome, Field (1969) concluded that patients generally improve during puberty (even to the point of becoming asymptomatic) and for the most part remain stable thereafter. Individuals may, however, show an increased susceptibility to respiratory tract infections (sinusitis, upper respiratory infection, bronchitis) and not uncommonly will have prolonged coughing spells after acute minor episodes. Exceptions include patients with severe disease initially and those with concomitant asthma, all of whom show persistent symptoms or even steady deterioration.

Landau and colleagues (1974) evaluated pulmonary mechanics in 69 children and young adults with bronchiectasis. Their results suggest that generalized small airways obstruction is common in bronchiectasis that has been present since childhood, independent of the treatment modality used. They found that the maximum expiratory flow volume (MEFV) curve was most useful and sensitive in detecting this expiratory airway obstruction.

Finally, from the standpoint of social functioning (employment, marriage, and family life), there is general agreement that the majority of patients with bronchiectasis can lead relatively normal lives if they are provided with appropriate medical support and care (Field, 1969; Ellis et al, 1981; Landau, 1974).

REFERENCES

Aytaç A, Yurdakul Y, Ikizler C et al: Inhalation of foreign bodies in children. J Thorac Cardiovasc Surg 74:145, 1977.

Banner AS, Muthuswamy P, Shah RS et al: Bronchiectasis follow-ing heroin-induced pulmonary edema: rapid clearing of pulmonary infiltrates. Chest 69:552, 1976.

Barker AF and Bardana EJ: Bronchiectasis: update of an orphan disease. Am Rev Respir Dis 137:969, 1988.

Bateman JRM, Newman SP, Daunt KM et al: Regional lung clearance of excessive bronchial secretions during chest physiotherapy in patients with stable chronic airways obstruction. Lancet 1:294, 1979.

Becroft DMO: Bronchiolitis obliterans, bronchiectasis and other sequelae of adenovirus type 21 infection in young children. J Clin Pathol 24:72, 1971.

Becroft DMO: Pulmonary sequelae of epidemic type 21 adenovirus infection: a 13-year follow-up. Arch Dis Child 54:155, 1979.

Bertelsen S, Struve-Christensen E, Aasted A, and Sparup J: Isolated middle lobe atelectasis: aetiology, pathogenesis, and treatment of the so-called middle lobe syndrome. Thorax 35:449, 1980.

Biering A: Childhood pneumonia, including pertussis, pneumonia, and bronchiectasis: a follow-up study of 151 patients. Acta Paediatr 45:348, 1956.

Carson JL, Collier AM, and Hu SS: Acquired ciliary defects in nasal epithelium of children with acute viral upper respiratory infections. N Engl J Med 312:463, 1985.

Cheng KK: The experimental production of bronchiectasis in rats. J Pathol Bacteriol 57:89, 1954.

Cherniack NS, Dowling HF, Carton RW, and McBryde VE: The role of acute lower respiratory infection in causing pulmonary insufficiency in bronchiectasis. Ann Intern Med 66:489, 1967.

Chipps BE, Talamo RL, and Windelstern JA: IgA deficiency, recurrent pneumonias, and bronchiectasis. Chest 73:519, 1978.

Church JA, Jordan SC, Keens TG, and Wang C-I: Circulating immune complexes in patients with cystic fibrosis. Chest 80:405, 1981.

Clark NS: Bronchiectasis in childhood. Br Med J 1:80, 1963.

Cochrane GM, Webber BA, and Clarke SW: Effects of sputum on pulmonary function. Br Med J 2:1181, 1977.

Cooke JC, Currie DC, Morgan AD et al: Role of computed tomography in diagnosis of bronchiectasis. Thorax 42:272, 1987.

Corbeel L, Cornillie F, Lauweryns J et al: Ultrastructural abnormalities of bronchial cilia in children with recurrent airway infections and bronchiectasis. Arch Dis Child 56:929, 1981.

Croxatto OC and Lanari A: Pathogenesis of bronchiectasis: experimental study and anatomic findings. J Thoracic Surg 27:514, 1954.

Davis PB, Hubbard VS, McCoy K, and Taussig LM: Familial bronchiectasis. J Pediatr 102:177, 1983.

Ellis DA, Thornley PE, Wightman AJ et al: Present outlook in bronchiectasis: clinical and social study and review of factors influencing prognosis. Thorax 36:659, 1981.

Fawcitt J and Parry HE: Lung changes in pertussis and measles in childhood: a review of 1894 cases with a follow-up study of the pulmonary complications. Br J Radiol 30:76, 1957.

Fernald GW: Bronchiectasis in childhood: a 10-year survey of cases treated at North Carolina Memorial Hospital. N Carolina Med J 39:368, 1978.

Field CE: Bronchiectasis in childhood. I. Clinical survey of 160 cases. Pediatrics 4:21, 1949.

Field CE: Bronchiectasis: third report on a follow-up study of medical and surgical cases from childhood. Arch Dis Child 44:551, 1969.

Fraser R and Paré J: Diagnoses of Diseases of the Chest. 2nd ed. Philadelpia, WB Saunders Co, 1979.

Gamsu G, Platzker A, Gregory G et al: Powdered tantalum as a contrast agent for tracheobronchography in the pediatric patient. Radiology 107:151, 1973.

George SA, Leonardi HK, and Overholt RH: Bilateral pulmonary resection for bronchiectasis: a 40-year experience. Ann Thorac Surg 28:48, 1978.

Glauser EM, Cook CD, and Harris GBC: Bronchiectasis: a review of 187 cases in children with follow-up pulmonary function studies in 58. Acta Pediatr Scand 165:1, 1966.

Goudie BM, Kerr MR, and Johnson RN: Mycoplasma pneumonia complicated by bronchiectasis. J Infect 7:151, 1983.

Halal F, Brochu P, Delage G et al: Severe disseminated lung disease and bronchiectasis probably due to *Mycoplasma pneumoniae*. Can Med Assoc J 117:1055, 1977.

Herbert FA, Wilkinson D, Burchak E, and Morgante O: Adenovirus type 3 pneumonia causing lung damage in childhood. Can Med Assoc J 116:274, 1977.

Hilton AM and Doyle L: Immunological abnormalities in bronchiectasis with chronic bronchial suppuration. Br J Dis Chest 72:207, 1978.

Hilton AM, Moore M, Howat JMT, and Kimber I: Characterization of circulating immune complexes in bronchiectasis by gel filtration. Clin Allergy 9:65, 1979.

Joharjy IA, Bashi SA, and Adbullah AK: Value of medium-thickness CT in the diagnosis of bronchiectasis. AJR 149:1133, 1987.

Kaschula ROC, Druker J, and Kipps A: Late morphologic consequences of measles: a lethal and debilitating lung disease among the poor. Rev Infect Dis 5:395, 1983.

Katz I, LeVine M, and Herman P: Tracheobronchiomegaly: the Mounier-Kuhn syndrome. Am J Roentgenol 88:1084, 1962.

Kürklü EU, Williams MA, and le Roux BT: Bronchiectasis consequent upon foreign body retention. Thorax 28:601, 1973.

Laennec RTH: De l'auscultation médiate, un Traité du diagnostic des maladies des poumons et du coeur, fonde, principalement sur ce noveau moyen d'exploration. Paris: Brosson et Chande, 1819.

Landau LI, Phelan PD, and Williams HE: Ventilatory mechanics in patients with bronchiectasis starting in childhood. Thorax 29:304, 1974.

Lang WR, Howden CW, Laws J, and Burton JF: Bronchopneumonia with serious sequelae in children with evidence of adenovirus type 21 infection. Br Med J 1:73, 1969.

Laurenzi GA: A critical reappraisal of bronchiectasis. Med Times 98:89, 1970.

Lees AW: Atelectasis and bronchiectasis in pertussis. Br Med J 2:1138, 1950.

Levy M, Glick B, Springer C et al: Bronchoscopy and bronchography in children. Am J Dis Child 137:14, 1983.

Liebow AA, Hales MR, and Lindskog GE: Enlargement of the bronchial arteries, and their anastomoses with the pulmonary arteries in bronchiectasis. Am J Pathol 25:211, 1949.

Lundgren R, Hietala S, and Adelroth E: Diagnosis of bronchial lesions by fiber-optic bronchoscopy combined with bronchography. Acta Radiol (Diagn) 23:231, 1982.

Marmon L, Schidlow D, Palmer J et al: Pulmonary resection for complications of cystic fibrosis. J Pediatr Surg 18:811, 1983.

Mazzocco MC, Owens GR, Kirilloff LH, and Rogers RM: Chest percussion and postural drainage in patients with bronchiectasis. Chest 88:360, 1985.

Mearns MB, Hodson CJ, Jackson ADM et al: Pulmonary resection in cystic fibrosis: results in 23 cases, 1957–1970. Arch Dis Child 47:499, 1972.

Mitchell RE and Bury RG: Congenital bronchiectasis due to deficiency of bronchial cartilage (Williams-Campbell syndrome). J Pediatr 87:230, 1975.

Mootoosamy IM, Reznek RH, Osman J et al: Assessment of bronchiectasis by computed tomography. Thorax 40:920, 1985.

Müller NL, Bergin CJ, Ostrow DN, and Nichols DM: Role of computed tomography in the recognition of bronchiectasis. AJR 143:971, 1984.

Murray J: The ketchup-bottle method. N Engl J Med 300:1155, 1979.

Naidich DP, McCauley DI, Khouri NF, Stitik FP, and Seigelman SS: Computed tomography of bronchiectasis. J Comput Assist Tomogr 6:437, 1982.

Ogilvie AG: The natural history of bronchiectasis. Arch Intern Med 68:395, 1941.

Oxelius V, Laurell A, Lindquist B et al: IgG subclasses in selective IgA deficiency. N Engl J Med 304:1476, 1981.

Perry KMA and King DS: Bronchiectasis: a study of prognosis based on a follow-up of 400 patients. Am Rev Tuberc 41:531, 1940.

Phillips MS, Williams MP, and Flower CDR: How useful is computed tomography in the diagnosis and assessment of bronchiectasis? Clin Radiol 37:321, 1986.

Reid LM: Reduction in bronchial subdivision in bronchiectasis. Thorax 5:233, 1950.

Rosenzweig DY and Stead WW: The role of tuberculosis and other forms of bronchopulmonary necrosis in the pathogenesis of bronchiectasis. Am Rev Respir Dis 93:769, 1966.

Ruberman W, Shauffer I, and Biondo T: Bronchiectasis and acute pneumonia. Am Rev Tuberc 76:761, 1957.

Sanderson JM, Kennedy MCS, Johnson MF, and Manley DCE: Bronchiectasis: results of surgical and conservative management. Thorax 29:407, 1974.

Simila S, Linna O, Lanning P et al: Chronic lung damage caused by adenovirus type 7: a ten year follow-up study. Chest 80:127, 1981.

Smallman LA, Hill SL, and Stockley RA: Reduction of ciliary beat frequency in vitro by sputum from patients with bronchiectasis: a serum proteinase effect. Thorax 39:663, 1984.

Smith FW: The value of NMR imaging in pediatric practice. Pediatr Radiol 13:141, 1983.

Stockley RA, Hill SL, and Brunett D: Nebulized amoxicillin in chronic purulent bronchiectasis. Clin Ther 7:593, 1985.

Stockley RA, Hill SL, and Morrison HM: Effect of antibiotic treatment on sputum elastase in bronchiectatic outpatients in a stable clinical state. Thorax 39:414, 1984.

Strang C: The fate of children with bronchiectasis. Ann Int Med 44:630, 1956.

Sutherland JM, Palser RF, Pagtakhan RD, and McCarthy DS: Xenon-133 ventilation and perfusion studies in bronchiectasis. J Can Assoc Radiol 31:242, 1980.

Tannenberg J and Pinner M: Atelectasis and bronchiectasis: an experimental study concerning their relationship. J Thorac Surg 11:571, 1942.

Tecklin JS and Holsclaw DS: Evaluation of bronchial drainage in patients with cystic fibrosis. Phys Ther 55:1081, 1975.

Vandevivere J, Spehl M, Dab I et al: Bronchiectasis in childhood: comparison of chest roentgenograms, bronchography and lung scintigraphy. Pediatr Radiol 9:193, 1980.

Varpela E, Koistinen J, Korhola O, and Keskinen H: Deficiency of alpha$_1$-antitrypsin and bronchiectasis. Ann Clin Res 10:79, 1978.

Varpela E, Laitinen LA, Keskinen H, and Korhola O: Asthma, allergy and bronchial hyperreactivity to histamine in patients with bronchiectasis. Clin Allergy 8:273, 1978.

Wakefield SJ and Waite D: Abnormal cilia in Polynesians with bronchiectasis. Am Rev Respir Dis 121:1003, 1980.

Wang JLF, Patterson R, Mintzer R et al: Allergic bronchopulmonary aspergillosis in pediatric practice. J Pediatr 94:376, 1979.

Warner JO and Marshall WC: Crippling lung disease after measles and adenovirus infection. Br J Dis Chest 70:89, 1976.

Wayne KS and Taussig LM: Probable familial congenital bronchiectasis due to cartilage deficiency (Williams-Campbell syndrome). Am Rev Respir Dis 114:15, 1976.

Whitwell F: A study of the pathology and pathogenesis of bronchiectasis. Thorax 7:213, 1952.

Whyte KF and Williams GR: Bronchiectasis after mycoplasma pneumonia. Thorax 39:390, 1984.

Wigglesworth FW: Bronchiectasis: an evaluation of present concepts. McGill Med J 24:189, 1955.

Williams H and Campbell P: Generalized bronchiectasis associated with deficiency of cartilage in the bronchial tree. Arch Dis Child 35:182, 1960.

Williams HE, Landau LI, and Phelan PD: Generalized bronchiectasis due to extensive deficiency of bronchial cartilage. Arch Dis Child 47:423, 1972.

Wilson JF and Decker AM: The surgical management of childhood bronchiectasis. Ann Surg 195:354, 1982.

Wilson JF, Peters GN, and Fleshman JK: A technique for bronchography in children. Am Rev Respir Dis 105:564, 1972.

Wood JR, Bellamy D, Child AH, and Citron KM: Pulmonary disease in patients with Marfan syndrome. Thorax 39:780, 1984.

Wood RE, Wanner A, Hirsch J, and Farrell PM: Tracheal mucociliary transport in patients with cystic fibrosis and its stimulation by terbutaline. Am Rev Respir Dis 111:733, 1975.

26

M. INNES ASHER, M.B., CH.B., and PIERRE H. BEAUDRY, M.D.

LUNG ABSCESS

A lung abscess is a circumscribed, thick-walled cavity in the lung that contains purulent material resulting from suppuration and necrosis of the involved lung parenchyma. The diagnosis is usually inferred from characteristic roentgenographic findings.

Lung abscess used to be a common childhood occurrence, particularly when tonsillectomy was done using crude anesthesic technique and little attention was paid to the possibility of aspiration of infected material. In the absence of antibiotic therapy for the treatment of lung infections, aspiration of infective material as well as pneumonias often progressed to abscess formation. The decrease in incidence has resulted in a decreased overall attention to the management of the condition. Thus, there are no prospective well-controlled studies of its management.

Like all conditions in children, lung abscess must be evaluated in the context of the interaction between the host and the etiologic agent. Various classifications of lung abscess have been proposed. The division into putrid and nonputrid types was introduced in the mistaken belief that it distinguished anaerobic from aerobic infection. The distinctions multiloculated and uniloculated, and aspirational and hematogenous were fruitless attempts to correlate size or origin with outcome. In order to provide useful direction in the identification of the suspected etiologic agent and in the appropriate investigation and management, we choose to retain the classifications primary and secondary. A *primary abscess* is that occurring in an otherwise healthy child. A *secondary abscess* is that occurring in a child who is otherwise compromised, e.g., because of serious infection including extensive bronchopneumonia, such as staphylococcal pneumonia, immunodeficiency or immunosuppression, predisposition to repeated aspiration of material into the lungs, prematurity, or being newborn (Table 26–1). Surprisingly, the development of an abscess subsequent to the aspiration of a foreign body is very rare.

EPIDEMIOLOGY

Lung abscesses due to *Staphylococcus aureus* occurred frequently during the epidemic of Asian influenza in 1956, but an increased incidence during other epidemics of viral respiratory disease has not been reported. The true incidence and prevalence of lung abscess, which is now considered a rare condition, have never been accurately established. In Montreal, Canada, in a predominantly white and urban population who have easy access to modern medical care, Asher and co-workers (1982) identified 31 cases of lung abscess during a 19-year period; 14 of these cases were primary and 17 secondary, in a

Table 26–1. CONDITIONS PREDISPOSING TO THE DEVELOPMENT OF SECONDARY LUNG ABSCESS IN CHILDREN

Condition	Examples
Serious infection	Bronchopneumonia Meningitis Osteomyelitis Septicemia Infected eczema Septic arthritis Abdominal wall abscess Peritonsillar abscess Endocarditis
Immunodeficiency or immunosuppression disorder	Measles Burns Prematurity Blood dyscrasias Leukemia Hepatitis Dysgammaglobulinemia Nephrotic syndrome Chronic granulomatous disease Steroid therapy Malnutrition
Condition leading to repeated aspiration	Seizure disorders Mental deficiency Altered consciousness Dysphagia Periodontitis Riley-Day syndrome
Other (miscellaneous or rare)	Cystic fibrosis Misplaced central nervous catheter Alpha$_1$-antitrypsin deficiency Foreign body in respiratory tract Eroded foreign body in the esophagus

total of 232,570 admissions to their hospital. This represents an occurrence rate of 1.3 per 10,000 hospital admissions or 0.7 per 100,000 admissions per year. In a similar population at the Children's Hospital of Eastern Ontario, three children with lung abscesses were identified in 7 years from a child population base of 450,000, which gives a rate of 0.67 per 100,000 children or an incidence of 0.95 per million per year.

Lung abscesses can occur in a child at any age, although they are very rare in the neonatal period. It appears that primary lung abscesses are less common than secondary abscesses and occur with the same frequency from 1 month to 15 years. Secondary abscesses occur more often in younger children. Both primary and secondary abscesses appear to be more common in males than in females, in a proportion of 1.6:1.

A seasonal variation in prevalence has been observed with primary lung abscess, which occurs predominantly in the winter or spring, as do episodes of bronchopneumonia in children. Whether there is a seasonal variation of secondary abscesses is not known, but because they are so much influenced by underlying conditions in the host, the same seasonal variation as with primary abscesses may not be expected.

Lung abscesses are reported in asthmatic children, but there is no clear evidence that this is out of proportion to the incidence of asthma in the general population.

ETIOLOGY

Organisms implicated in lung abscess cover nearly the entire microbiological spectrum: bacteria, fungi, viruses, and protozoa (Table 26–2). In most cases, however, one or more pathogenic bacteria are cultured. *S. aureus* is by far the organism most commonly reported from culture in both primary (62 per cent) and secondary (35 per cent) abscesses and is usually penicillin resistant. It is of interest that anaerobic organisms have not been reported in primary abscesses but seem to occur exclusively in secondary abscesses. The following organisms have been reported in lung abscess in adults but have yet to be described in children: *Campylobacter fetus, Corynebacterium equi, Legionella micdadei, Legionella pneumophila, Pasteurella multocida, Petriellidium boydii, Streptococcus milleri, Pseudomonas pseudomallei, Actinomyces,* and *Entamoeba histolytica.* In the neonatal period, group B streptococci, *Klebsiella pneumoniae,* and *Escherichia coli* have been reported repeatedly.

Infections with *Mycobacterium tuberculosis, Histoplasma capsulatum,* and *Coccidioides immitis* can progress to cavitation with secondary pulmonary disease but rarely do with initial pulmonary disease. However, although a tuberculous cavity in the lung may at first be mistaken for a lung abscess, its prior contents are caseous, not purulent. This condition is uncommon

Table 26–2. SPECTRUM OF ORGANISMS ASSOCIATED WITH LUNG ABSCESS

Type of Abscess	Organisms
Primary	*Staphylococcus aureus* *Haemophilus influenzae* types B, C, F, and nontypable *Streptococcus viridans, pneumoniae* Alpha-hemolytic streptococci *Neisseria* sp. *Mycoplasma pneumoniae*

Secondary	Aerobes
	  All those listed for primary abscess
	  Haemophilus aphropilus, parainfluenzae
	  Streptococcus group B, *intermedius*
	  Klebsiella pneumoniae
	  Escherichia coli, freundii
	  Pseudomonas pyocyanea, aeruginosa, denitrificans
	  Aerobacter aeruginosa
	  Candida
	  Rhizopus sp.
	  Aspergillus fumigatus
	  Nocardia sp.
	  Eikenella corrodens
	  Serratia marcescens
	Anaerobes
	  Peptostreptococcus constellatus, intermedius, saccharolyticus
	  Veillonella sp., *alkalenscens*
	  Bacteroides melaninogenicus, oralis, fragilis, corrodens, distasonis, vulgatus, ruminicola, asaccharolyticus
	  Fusobacterium necrophorum, nucleatum
	  Bifidobacterium sp.

before adolescence. When it does occur earlier in childhood, it may follow primary pulmonary tuberculosis by a shorter interval than in adolescents or adults.

PATHOLOGY

A lung abscess arises from aspiration of infective material, antecedent primary bacterial infection of the lung, hematogenous seeding of the lung by pyogenic organisms, or spread of infection from a neighboring organ. It begins as a focus of inflammation followed by central necrosis. At first the enclosing wall is poorly defined, but with time and progressive fibrosis it becomes more discrete. The cavity may or may not be filled with suppurative debris, depending on the presence or absence of a communication with the air passages. The cardinal histologic change is suppurative destruction of the lung parenchyma with central cavitation.

The pathophysiology of lung abscess in childhood has not been discussed recently in the literature. The bronchial circulation near the abscess has been found to be significantly altered in sheep with lung abscesses. Whether the same phenomenon occurs in children is not known. The abscess is a space-occupying lesion in the lung parenchyma and therefore compresses surrounding structures and restricts the respiratory system. When the abscess is small, changes in ventilation and perfusion due to compression may well be minimal and symmetrical, and restriction of the respiratory system will not be clinically detectable. With a larger abscess there may be larger alterations in ventilation and perfusion, and hypoxemia may be clinically detectable as tachypnea. A restrictive type of impairment may become obvious with increasing size of the abscess or because of pleural reaction and chest pain. The loss of lung volume caused by the abscess decreases the pulmonary compliance, so retractions of chest soft tissues are seen subsequent to wider fluctuations in negative pleural pressure.

CLINICAL MANIFESTATIONS

Features of both primary and secondary abscess in children are fever, often up to 40°C, which is almost always present; malaise and weight loss, which are common; and vomiting, which is uncommon. The most common symptoms referable to the respiratory system are, first, cough, and then, in decreasing frequency, chest pain, dyspnea, sputum production, and hemoptysis. A putrid odor of the breath is occasionally noted in secondary lung abscess. Children receiving steroids and newborn infants may have no fever or a subnormal temperature. As expected, neonates show less specific signs of illness, such as apnea, grunting, respiratory distress, diarrhea, and even hematemesis. At the time of admission to hospital, children may have been sick for days or several weeks.

The heart rate is usually increased. Signs localizing disease to the chest and within the chest are sometimes absent in lung abscess, particularly in very young children. When present, they may include increased respiratory rate, retractions, decreased movement of the chest, suppressed breath sounds, dullness to percussion, fine crackles, and bronchial breathing. Clubbing of the digits is rarely seen, with only one such case reported in the past 3 decades.

ROENTGENOGRAPHIC MANIFESTATIONS

The abscess usually appears as a thick-walled cavity in the lung and may be solitary or multiple. Primary abscesses are almost always solitary (Fig. 26–1), and secondary abscesses may be solitary or multiple. Solitary abscesses occur more often in the right lung than in the left, with the upper and lower lobes being affected with equal frequency. Abscesses vary in size from 2 to 20 cm or more in diameter. An intrapulmonary abscess without communication with the bronchial tree is roentgenographically opaque. The abscess cavity becomes visible when air entering from a bronchus creates an air-fluid level over the pus. An air-fluid level is often present, and abscess contents

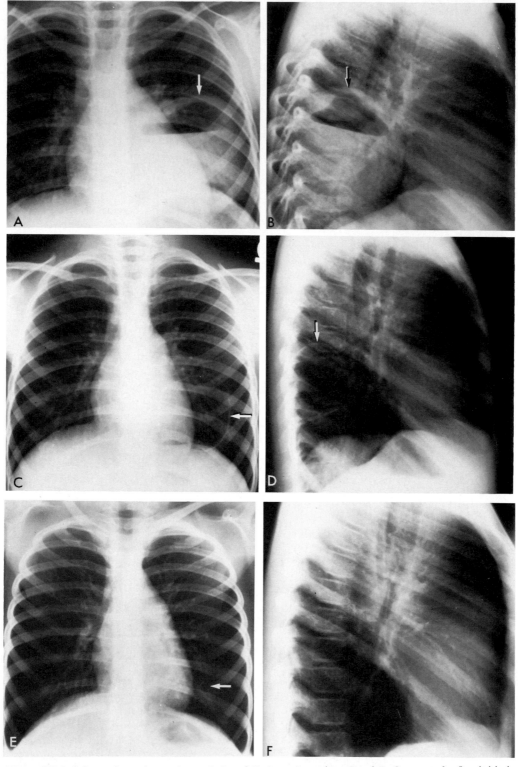

Figure 26–1. Primary lung abscess *(arrows)*. *A* and *B*, At presentation. *C* and *D*, One month after initiation of therapy. *E* and *F*, One year later.

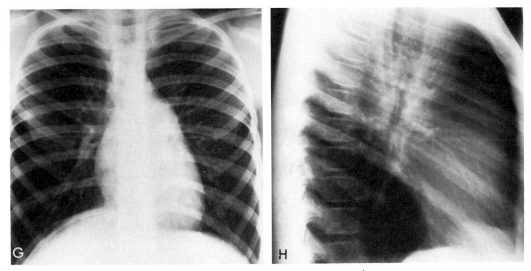

Figure 26–1 *Continued G* and *H*, Two years later.

are usually uniloculated but may be multiloculated (Fig. 26–2). Compressive atelectasis is often seen around the abscess, especially if it is large. When the abscess is near the pleural surface, overlying pleural thickening is seen, and occasionally there is a small amount of pleural fluid. Hilar and mediastinal adenopathy have been reported with secondary lung abscess.

LABORATORY FINDINGS

The white blood cell count is usually mildly increased but has been reported to reach 32,700/mm³, with a predominance of polymorphonuclear leukocytes. In neonates, juvenile forms are observed more commonly. The erythrocyte sedimentation rate may be normal but usually is mildly increased, and values up to 58 mm in 1 hour have been reported.

Blood cultures rarely detect the organism in primary lung abscess but occasionally may be positive in secondary lung abscess.

The determination of the organism responsible for lung abscesses remains most difficult. Direct percutaneous aspiration of material in the abscess is undoubtedly the most reliable mode of identification of the etiologic agent, but this technique is difficult unless the abscess is peripheral and in most situations appears unwarranted. Other indirect means, relying on the microbiologic evaluation of pulmonary secretions, are either as technically hazardous or unreliable (Table 26–3). Added to this situation is the lack of sputum production in most children. One is often forced to rely on a broad knowledge of the most common causative agents and to treat the abscess

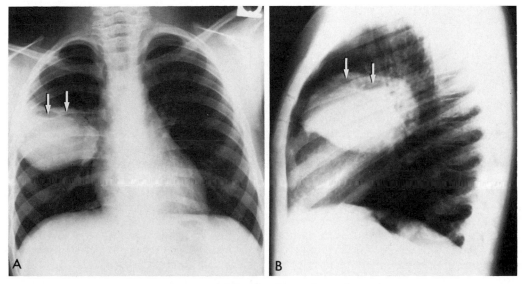

Figure 26–2. Multiloculated lung abscess *(arrows)*.

Table 26–3. RELIABILITY OF IDENTIFICATION OF THE CAUSATIVE ORGANISM IN LUNG ABSCESS

Technique of Obtaining Specimen	Results of Bacteriologic Study	
	FALSE-POSITIVE	FALSE-NEGATIVE
Transtracheal aspiration	Infrequent	Infrequent
Wire brushing through a fiberoptic bronchoscope	Frequent	Frequent
Sputum expectoration	Frequent	Frequent

accordingly. Should one opt to rely on sputum examination, a positive microscopic identification in the absence of bacterial growth must be considered an alert that an anaerobic organism is present.

DIAGNOSIS

The presence on the chest roentgenograph of a thick-walled cavity in the lung, with or without an air-fluid level, is characteristic and is often the first indication of a lung abscess. In a minority of cases, especially when the lesion is peripheral, it may be difficult to distinguish between a lung abscess and an empyema with a bronchopleural fistula. Oblique or decubitus views may sometimes be necessary to help distinguish between the two conditions. Although ultrasonography may also be helpful, computed tomographic (CAT) scan is particularly valuable when conventional roentgenographic features fail to confirm the diagnosis. A CAT scan offers better demonstration of the three-dimensional shape of the lesion and improves the visualization of the pleuropulmonary interface.

Infection of the lungs with *Echinococcus granulosa* occasionally resembles a lung abscess. Congenital cyst or adenomatous malformation of the lung must also be considered, particularly in neonates. If the lesion on the chest roentgenograph fails to show a cavity and has a homogeneous density, the possibilities of simple pneumonia, neoplasm, and loculated empyema must be entertained. Tomography has been used to define a cavity if present, and xerotomography may provide even better definition. Although magnetic resonance imaging appears to be effective in identifying lung abscess in children, its role in the diagnosis of this condition has yet to be defined.

MANAGEMENT

Antibiotics are the mainstay of therapy and should be directed primarily against penicillinase-producing *S. aureus*. In primary lung abscess, streptococci and *Hemophilus influenzae* are sometimes reported, and therefore therapy should aim to treat all of these organisms. In secondary lung abscess, the same approach should be taken, with the possible role of anaerobic organisms in this condition kept in mind. Most anaerobes responsible for aspiration lung abscess are quite sensitive to penicillin and sensitive to a lesser extent to semisynthetic penicillins and cephalosporins. Until recently, there was no clinical evidence that clindamycin was superior to penicillin in treatment of anaerobic infections in the lung. A prospective study in adults suggests that this situation may be changing.

There have been no prospective trials of antibiotic regimens in lung abscess in children. In primary lung abscess, we favor a combination of flucloxacillin and cefuroxime, eliminating one of these drugs if the offending organism and its sensitivities are identified. In secondary lung abscess, the addition of penicillin is necessary unless the infection is clearly aerobic. In unusual cases of secondary lung abscess, in which other organisms are suspected and found, specific antimicrobial therapy directed against the responsible organisms is indicated.

There are no clear guidelines about the length of antibiotic therapy required. It would seem reasonable to use parenteral therapy until an effective program of oral therapy can be established, which should be continued until the child is asymptomatic. Initial response to therapy usually takes several days, and complete resolution of the symptoms 1 to 3 weeks.

There is no evidence that drainage of the abscess is necessary for satisfactory and complete resolution, although this has been advocated by some authors if fever persists for more than 1 week. Children with primary abscess do well with antibiotic therapy alone. Surgical treatment is indicated if there is clinical deterioration despite appropriate antibiotic therapy. One must keep in mind that bronchoscopy, which is sometimes used for drainage, may not be an innocuous procedure. In addition to the risks of general anesthesia in a sick child, there is a small risk of massive aspiration of pus into other parts of the bronchial tree. This complication occurred in an adult after rupture of the abscess during aspiration using a fiberoptic bronchoscope. Bronchoscopy was recommended initially for use in adults with lung abscess in order to rule out malignancy and tuberculosis and facilitate drainage of the abscess. However, the same concern about pulmonary malignancy does not apply to children, and tuberculosis can now be diagnosed by other means. Bronchoscopy is indicated if there is a history of foreign body aspiration. Given the wide range of antibiotics available, the need to drain the abscess has not been substantiated in the recent past. Whether bronchoscopic drainage hastens immediate improvement is not known, and improvement has been satisfactory in primary lung abscess without such intervention.

Other approaches have been used in an attempt to drain the abscess cavity in the unusual event of failure of antibiotic therapy. Percutaneous drainage with an indwelling catheter (pneumonotomy) has been used with some success in the treatment of primary lung abscess refractory to medical therapy. Complications of this procedure are uncommon but include the development of empyema and bronchopleural fistula. Postural drainage and percussion have often been used in the management of lung abscess in the belief that they help to drain the abscess. There is little information about their success in doing so, and less about their benefit.

Lobectomy is rarely used in lung abscess but should be reserved for massive expansion of the abscess associated with compression of the surrounding structures and attendant symptoms.

COMPLICATIONS

Complications of lung abscess today are exceedingly rare, even in secondary lung abscess, in which one case of associated empyema has been reported. Overexpansion of the abscess with mediastinal shift has been reported in one neonate and tension pneumothorax in two others. Spontaneous rupture of the abscess with seeding to other parts of the lung has been reported in one adult.

The institution of aggressive investigations or therapy has led to some complications. Transtracheal aspiration has been complicated by hemoptysis and subcutaneous emphysema in children and by cardiac arrhythmias, bilateral pneumothorax, fatal hemorrhage, inadequate oxygenation, and intratracheal blood clots in adults. Lobectomy has been followed by empyema and pleural effusion. Fiberoptic bronchoscopy has been complicated by massive intrabronchial aspiration of abscess contents in one adult. Percutaneous aspiration of the abscess theoretically can be complicated by pneumothorax, but this event has not been reported.

COURSE AND PROGNOSIS

The outcome of lung abscess has dramatically improved since the introduction of antibiotics. In primary abscess, once adequate antibiotic therapy has been started, the fever resolves in about 1 week in most children but may last as long as 3 weeks. After complete clinical resolution of the illness, which averages 2 weeks, resolution of the cavity as seen on roentgenographs may take a variable amount of time; complete resolution may occur in 1 month but may take months or years, as is illustrated in Figure 26–1. The rate of resolution of the cavity does not depend on its original size. During the resolution of the roentgenographic changes, children are well and do not seem prone to repeated lower respiratory tract disease. Pulmonary function evaluations (measurement of lung volumes and expiratory flow rates), made on the average of 9 years after the primary lung abscess, have failed to show abnormalities

(Asher et al, 1982). This favorable outcome is very similar to that previously reported in survivors of staphylococcal pneumonia complicated by abscess, empyema, pyopneumothorax, or pneumatocele.

The outlook in secondary lung abscess is more variable and depends on the underlying condition. However, the prognosis for a solitary cavity seems more favorable than for multiple abscesses.

The availability of a wide range and a greater specificity of antibiotics has made the management of lung abscess, when it occurs, effective and much simpler. Drainage or excision of the abscess, with the attendant morbidity and mortality, seems no longer justified except in unusually complicated situations. Nevertheless, this condition still remains a challenge to pediatricians. The roentgenographic appearance is often dramatic and promotes considerable alarm in the attending physician, unfortunately leading to overtreatment in some cases.

REFERENCES

Arneborn P, Lindquist BL, and Sjöberg L: Severe pulmonary infection by *Haemophilus aphrophilus* in a non-compromised child. Scand J Infect Dis 17:327, 1985.

Asher MI, Spier S, Beland M et al: Primary lung abscess in childhood. The long-term outcome of conservative management. Am J Dis Child 136:491, 1982.

Balikian JP and Mudarris FF: Hydatid disease of the lungs. A roentgenologic study of 50 cases. Am J Roentgenol Radium Ther Nucl Med 122:692, 1974.

Bartlett JG and Gorbach SL: Penicillin or clindamycin for primary lung abscess? Ann Intern Med 98:546, 1983.

Bigler RD, Atkins RR, and Wing ER: *Yersinia enterocolitica* lung infection. Arch Intern Med 141:1529, 1981.

Blyth DF and Pirie D: Haematogenous amoebic lung abscess. A case report. S Afr Med J 53:147, 1978.

Brook I: Bacteriology and treatment of gram-negative pneumonia in long-term hospitalized children. Chest 79:432, 1981.

Brook I and Finegold SM: Bacteriology and therapy of lung abscess in children. J Pediatr 94:10, 1979.

Bujak JS, Ottesen EA, Dinarello CA, and Brenner VJ: Nocardiosis in a child with chronic granulomatous disease. J Pediatr 83:98, 1973.

Canny GJ, Marcotte JE, and Levison H: Lung abscess in cystic fibrosis. Thorax 41:221, 1986.

Ceruti E, Contreras J, and Neira M: Staphylococcal pneumonia in childhood. Am J Dis Child 122:386, 1971.

Charan NB, Turk GM, and Dhand R: The role of bronchial circulation in lung abscess. Am Rev Respir Dis 131:121, 1985.

Cohen JR, Amorosa JK, and Smith PR: The air-fluid level in cavitary pulmonary tuberculosis. Radiology 127:315, 1978.

Cohen MD, Eigen H, Scott PH et al: Magnetic resonance imaging of inflammatory lung disorders: preliminary studies in children. Pediatr Pulmonol 2:211, 1986.

Diggory P and Ross BA: Lung abscess resulting from gross inflorescence. Thorax 39:480, 1984.

Dowling JN, Kroboth FJ, Karpf M et al: Pneumonia and multiple lung abscesses caused by dual infection with *Legionella micdadei* and *Legionella pneumophila*. Am Rev Respir Dis 127:121, 1983.

Groff DB and Marquis J: Transtracheal drainage of lung abscesses in children. J Pediatr Surg 12:303, 1977.

Groff DB and Rapkin RH: Primary lung abscess in childhood. J Med Soc NJ 71:649, 1974.

Hammer DL, Aranda CP, Galati V, and Adams FV: Massive intrabronchial aspiration of contents of pulmonary abscess after fibreoptic bronchoscopy. Chest 74:306, 1978.

Irwin RS, Garrity FL, Erickson AD et al: Sampling lower respiratory tract secretions in primary lung abscess. A comparison of the accuracy of four methods. Chest 79:559, 1981.

Jackson CL and Judd AR: The role of bronchoscopy in the treatment of pulmonary abscess. J Thorac Surg 10:179, 1940.

Kitagawa S, Kaplan SL, and Seilheimer DK: Lung abscess due to *Haemophilus influenzae* type C. Am J Dis Child 133:650, 1979.

Kosloske AM, Ball WS, Butler C, and Musemeche CA: Drainage of pediatric lung abscess by cough, catheter, or complete resection. J Pediatr Surg 21:596, 1986.

Levine MM, Ashman R, and Heald F: Anaerobic (putrid) lung abscess in adolescence. Am J Dis Child 130:77, 1976.

Liechty E, Kleiman MB, Ballantine TVN, and Grosfeld JL: Primary *Hemophilus influenzae* lung abscess with bronchial obstruction. J Pediatr Surg 17:281, 1982.

Lorenzo RL, Bradford BF, Black J, and Smith CD: Lung abscesses in children: diagnostic and therapeutic needle aspiration. Radiology 157:79, 1985.

McCracken GH Jr: Lung abscess in childhood. Hosp Pract 13:35, 1978.

Maklad NF, Ting YM, and Ravikrishnan KP: Xerotomography of peripheral lung lesions. Chest 69:516, 1976.

Mark PH and Turner JAP: Lung abscess in childhood. Thorax 23:216, 1968.

Moore TC and Battersby JS: Pulmonary abscess in infancy and childhood: Report of 18 cases. Ann Surg 151:496, 1960.

Morton JR, Mihalas LS, Leung P, and Strieder DJ: Corticosteroids and malnutrition. Aspergillus lung abscess in an asthmatic child. Chest 78:667, 1980.

Norman WJ, Moule NJ, and Walrond ER: Lung abscess: a complication of malposition of a central venous catheter. Br J Radiol 47:498, 1974.

Okafor BC: Lung abscess secondary to esophageal foreign body. Ann Otol Rhinol Laryngol 87:568, 1978.

Oleske JM, Starr SE, and Nahmias AJ: Complications of peritonsillar abscess due to *Fusobacterium necrophorum*. Pediatrics 57:570, 1976.

Palmer PE: Pulmonary tuberculosis—usual and unusual radiographic presentations. Semin Roentgenol 14:204, 1979.

Powell KR: Primary pulmonary abscess. Am J Dis Child 136:489, 1982.

Räsänen J, Bools JC, and Downs JB: Endobronchial drainage of undiagnosed lung abscess during chest physical therapy. A case report. Phys Ther 68:371, 1988.

Rohlfing BM, White EA, Webb WR, and Goodman PC: Hilar and mediastinal adenopathy caused by bacterial abscess of the lung. Radiology 128:289, 1978.

Rosenfeld S and Granoff DM: Pulmonary cavitation and Pi SZ alpha$_1$-antitrypsin deficiency. J Pediatr 94:768, 1979.

Saadah HA and Dixon T: *Petriellidium boydii (Allescheria boydii)*. Necrotising pneumonia in a normal host. JAMA 245:605, 1981.

Samies JH, Hathaway BN, Echols RM, et al: Lung abscess due to *Corynebacterium equi*. Report of the first case in a patient with acquired immunodeficiency syndrome. Am J Med 80:685, 1986.

Sandweiss DA: Empyema or abscess? Is ultrasound a diagnostic aid? Chest 75:297, 1979.

Scully RE, Mark EJ, McNeely WF, and McNeely BU: Case records of the Massachusetts General Hospital. Case 36–1987. A 14-year-old girl with diabetic ketoacidosis and pneumonitis with cavitation. N Engl J Med 317:614, 1987.

Siegel JD and McCracken GH: Neonatal lung abscess. A report of six cases. Am J Dis Child 133:947, 1979.

Siegler DIM: Lung abscess associated with *Mycoplasma pneumoniae* infection. Br J Dis Chest 67:123, 1973.

Spencer CD and Beaty HN: Complications of transtracheal aspiration. N Engl J Med 286:304, 1976.

Steyer BJ and Sobonya RE: *Pasteurella multocida* lung abscess. A case report and review of the literature. Arch Intern Med 144:1081, 1984.

Targan SR, Chow AW, and Guze LB: *Campylobacter fetus* associated with pulmonary abscess and empyema. Chest 71:105, 1977.

Waitkins SA, Ratcliffe JG, and Roberts C: *Streptococcus milleri* found in pulmonary empyemas and abscesses. J Clin Pathol 38:716, 1985.

Williford ME and Godwin JD: Computed tomography of lung abscess and empyema. Radiol Clin North Am 21:575, 1983.

Wise MB, Beaudry PH, and Bates DV: Long-term follow-up of staphylococcal pneumonia. Pediatrics 38:398, 1966.

Yellin A, Yellin EO, and Lieberman Y: Percutaneous tube drainage: the treatment of choice for refractory lung abscess. Ann Thorac Surg 39:266, 1985.

27

REYNALDO D. PAGTAKHAN, M.D., and
MARK D. MONTGOMERY, M.D.

PLEURISY AND EMPYEMA

In Chapter 40 we review the anatomic features of the pleura and the physiology of liquid movement across it in health and disease, present a classification of pleural effusions based on pathophysiology and chemistry of their contents, and discuss the management of noninflammatory, hemorrhagic, and chylous effusions. This chapter considers the etiologic spectrum, pathogenesis, functional pathology, diagnosis, management, and prognosis of inflammatory pleural disorders.

ETIOLOGY AND PATHOGENESIS

Inflammation of the pleural membranes (pleurisy, pleuritis) is usually a consequence of diseases elsewhere in the body and, rarely, of disturbances residing primarily in the pleura. The inciting process may be infection, neoplasm, trauma, pulmonary vascular obstruction, systemic granulomatous disease, or a generalized inflammatory disorder affecting serous membranes. Table 27–1 classifies the clinical disor-

Table 27–1. ETIOLOGIC SPECTRUM OF PLEURISY AND EMPYEMA

Origin and Nature of Inflammation	Illustrative Clinical Disorders
Primary in Pleura	
Neoplasm	Primary pleural mesothelioma
Trauma	Following cardiothoracic surgery, lung aspiration and percutaneous pleural biopsies, thoracic irradiation therapy
Contiguous Structures	
Lung infection	Pneumonia (aerobic and anaerobic bacterial, tuberculous, fungal, viral, mycoplasmal, echinococcal), bronchopleural fistula
Chest wall and subdiaphragmatic infection	Chest wall contusion and abscess, intra-abdominal abscess (subphrenic and hepatic), acute hemorrhagic pancreatitis, pancreaticopleural fistula
Mediastinal infection and neoplasm	Acute mediastinitis (secondary to esophageal rupture); mediastinal tumors
Systemic Diseases	
Septicemia	Distant sites of suppuration
Malignancy	Lymphoma, leukemia, neuroblastoma, hepatoma, multiple myeloma
Vascular obstruction	Pulmonary infarction
Connective tissue or collagen disorders	Systemic lupus erythematosus, polyarteritis, Wegener's granulomatosis, rheumatoid arthritis, scleroderma, rheumatic fever
Granulomatous disease	Sarcoidosis

ders that may cause pleurisy and empyema according to the original site and nature of the inciting process. Infection from adjacent pulmonary and subdiaphragmatic foci reaches the pleura by contiguous spread. Bacteria occasionally reach the pleural cavity via a bronchopleural fistula, through a traumatic breach of the chest wall, or by way of the circulation from distant sites of suppuration. Neoplastic involvement of the pleura may be primary or metastatic. Metastases may occur through parenchymal lung involvement or directly into the pleura. Neoplasms may also obstruct lymphatic channels and interfere with pleural drainage, particularly clearance of proteins from the pleural cavity. Trauma following certain diagnostic and therapeutic cardiothoracic procedures irritates the pleura, which may become secondarily infected. Pulmonary embolism (thrombus, fat, or gas) results in focal parenchymal necrosis that spreads to involve the pleural surface, causing pleurisy with or without effusion. Connective tissue disorders such as systemic lupus erythematosus and rheumatoid arthritis may involve the pleura as part of the more widespread inflammatory process.

Irrespective of the inciting process, the initial exudative stage of pleural inflammation is characterized by accumulation of a small amount of thin fibrin along with a few polymorphonuclear cells. Liquid exudation into the pleural cavity is minimal or not detectable (dry or plastic pleurisy). The liquid remains uninfected for some time, even in those cases in which the inciting underlying disorders are infectious in nature. Subsequently, permeability of the pleural capillaries is greatly enhanced, resulting in considerable accumulation of fibrin exudates (pleurisy with effusion). Because exudates have high protein concentration, the pleural liquid oncotic pressure is increased, thereby favoring further transport of liquid into the pleural cavity. These changes ulti-

mately exceed lymphatic drainage, and significant pleural effusion ensues. When the underlying disturbance is a bacterial infection, frank empyema may ensue. The development of an empyema can be divided into three stages. The first stage, in which the pleural fluid glucose and pH are normal, is simply parapneumonic effusion. The second stage is the fibrinopurulent phase, which is characterized by increased accumulation of fibrin and polymorphonuclear leukocytes and by bacterial invasion of the pleural cavity. The pleural fluid pH and glucose decrease and lactate dehydrogenase (LDH) rises during this stage. Also, the effusions tend to loculate. The third stage is reached when the purulent pleural exudate becomes thick. This is called *empyema*. It may be associated with a penetrating putrid odor characteristic of anaerobic infection. The bacterial agent, however, may not be identified if antimicrobial therapy had been given before evacuation of empyema. If the fibrinopurulent effusion is not drained in time, fibroblasts grow from both pleural surfaces and form an inelastic membrane that restricts lung expansion. Thus the nature of the underlying clinical disorder, stage of pleurisy, specific type of infecting agent, and start of antimicrobial therapy determine the degree and final character of the pleural exudate.

Primary neoplasms of the pleura, which include benign and malignant mesothelioma, are rare causes of exudative pleural effusions in children. Metastatic involvement of the pleura may arise directly from pulmonary parenchymal lesions or through contiguous spread of a metastatic lung lesion. The neoplastic masses may obstruct the lymphatic channels, thereby decreasing removal of proteins from the pleural space. Pleural irritation may follow certain diagnostic procedures (e.g., needle aspiration of the lung and percutaneous pleural biopsy) or therapeutic procedures (e.g., radiation therapy for mediastinal malignancy, cardiothoracic operations). Fortunately, the risk of occurrence of secondary purulent pleurisy due to medical intervention is low.

Thoracoabdominal infections constitute the major origin of pleurisy with effusion. Up to 20 per cent of children with viral and mycoplasma pneumonia develop effusions, which are usually transient and of minor importance. On occasion, however, the effusions may be massive and cause respiratory distress, necessitating prompt drainage, or may be recalcitrant and cause prolonged morbidity in infants with concurrent malnutrition. Nonetheless, the effusions usually remain thin.

Pulmonary tuberculosis usually causes dry pleurisy until the caseous materials containing the tuberculous antigen leak into the pleura via the pleural circulation. Considerable effusion then occurs as a result of the specific allergic reaction of the pleural membranes. The onset of effusion is within 6 months of the primary infection and is coincident with the development of cell-mediated immunity. The cellular character of the exudate is lymphocytic. Effusion is usually on the side of the primary parenchymal focus. Bilateral effusions indicate hematogenous dissemination from some remote focus. Frank tuberculous empyema is rare, occurring in only about 2 per cent of cases of tuberculous pleurisy, particularly those complicated by bronchopleural fistula.

Nontuberculous bacterial pneumonias constitute the most frequent origin of inflammatory pleural effusions, also referred to as parapneumonic effusions. Such an effusion may loculate owing to pleural adhesions or may be purulent. Table 27–2 lists in order of descending prevalence the predominant aerobic and anaerobic isolates of empyema. In any given patient, either or both types may be isolated, but the actual occurrence rate is difficult to ascertain. The opportunity to establish a specific etiologic agent may depend on the patient's age, nature of the underlying disease, standard of laboratory culture methods, and start of antimicrobial therapy.

The advent of the antimicrobial era has brought about not only a significant drop in the overall

Table 27–2. BACTERIOLOGY OF NONTUBERCULOUS EMPYEMA

Aerobic bacteria
  Staphylococcus aureus
  Haemophilus influenzae
  Streptococcus pyogenes
  Diplococcus pneumoniae
  Escherichia coli
  Klebsiella sp.
  Pseudomonas aeruginosa
Anaerobic bacteria
  Microaerophilic streptococci
  Fusobacterium nucleatum
  Bacteroides melaninogenicus
  Bacteroides fragilis
  Peptococcus
  Peptostreptococcus
  Catalase-negative, non–spore-forming,
    gram-positive bacilli

incidence of bacterial infection but also a shift in bacteriologic predominance. Thus staphylococci have emerged as the single most common aerobic pathogen of empyema. Infants and children are prone to develop septicemia from staphylococcal pneumonia, perhaps because they have appreciably low serum titers of coagulase-reacting factor. Clinical settings that favor consideration of staphylococcal empyema include the presence of superficial skin lesions, osteomyelitis, lung abscess, bronchopleural fistula, and cystic fibrosis. Another common aerobic isolate is *Haemophilus influenzae,* associated with otitis media and pneumonia in older children. This agent has become the most common cause of empyema in children less than 2 years of age. Paracolon bacteria and pneumococci are common in infants. *Pseudomonas* is encountered with increased frequency in debilitated patients requiring prolonged respirator therapy.

Anaerobic pleuropulmonary infections, which remain uncommon in children, have their distinctive clinical settings. More than 90 per cent of the patients manifest periodontal infections and have altered consciousness and dysphagia. Thus aspiration of a large volume of oropharyngeal secretions occurs in the presence of disturbed clearing mechanisms. It is therefore not surprising that the three predominant pleural anaerobic isolates—namely, microaerophilic streptococci, *Fusobacterium nucleatum,* and *Bacteroides melaninogenicus* (see Table 27–2)—compose the normal flora of the upper respiratory tract and that localization of the primary pulmonary disease (e.g., lung abscess and necrotizing pneumonia) is usually in gravity-dependent lung segments. The clinical course is generally insidious and indolent. Mediastinal and subdiaphragmatic foci of infections are also common sites of origin for anaerobic empyema.

Except for septicemia from contiguous or distant sites of suppuration, systemic origins of pleurisy generally produce nonpurulent effusion. Effusion secondary to pulmonary embolism of venous thrombi, fat, or gas is rare in childhood, although it may be a serious consequence of malignancy. Pleurisy may be associated with connective tissue disorders, such as lupus erythematosus and rheumatoid arthritis, and is part of the more widespread inflammatory process.

In summary, various clinical disorders of protean inflammatory origins can induce pleurisy and empyema. Certain clinical settings are distinctive for specific bacterial isolates.

FUNCTIONAL PATHOLOGY

Pulmonary disability is a function of duration, rapidity of onset, and extent of pleural involvement and is modified by concurrent complications and the status of cardiopulmonary reserve. Early in the phase of pleurisy, chest pain on inspiration diminishes thoracic excursion, induces rapid shallow breathing, and increases the ratio of dead space to tidal volume. As a result of hypoventilation, hypoxemia and hypercapnia ensue. Later, significant effusion displaces the mediastinum, which reduces lung volume and impedes venous return. With concurrent complication, such as pneumatocele in staphylococcal infection, ventilation-perfusion imbalance is further compromised and the work of breathing is aggravated. Reflex bronchospasm may occur. Thus severe pleural disease may produce striking abnormalities in lung volume, air flow, and pulmonary blood flow with ensuing disturbances of gas exchange.

DIAGNOSIS

HISTORY AND PHYSICAL EXAMINATION

Physicians are first alerted to a diagnosis of pleurisy as they listen to a narration of symptoms produced by pleural inflammation per se and those due to the underlying clinical disorder. Symptoms of direct pleural involvement include chest pain, chest tightness, and dyspnea. Older children may complain of sharp pleuritic pain on inspiration or with cough, which is due to stretching of the parietal pleura. The locus of pleurisy determines the site of pain, which may be felt in the chest overlying the site of inflammation, or may be referred to the shoulder if the central diaphragm is involved or to the abdomen if the peripheral diaphragm is involved. Severe chest pain inhibits respiratory movement and causes dyspnea. As effusion increases and separates the pleural membranes, pleuritic pain becomes a dull ache and may disappear. However, a large accumulation of pleural liquid also causes dyspnea. Dyspnea and cough may vary with changes in body position.

Patients may present with manifestations related to the underlying inciting process. High fever, chills, vomiting, anorexia, lethargy, and severe prostration suggest an infectious etiologic agent (e.g., staphylococcal empyema). Abdominal distention may be present owing to partial paralytic ileus. A symptomless period may intervene between the apparent improvement of an underlying pneumonia and the onset of the pleural complication. Relentless pneumonia in the presence of pancreatitis suggests pancreaticopleural fistula. A history of rapid reaccumulation of effusion associated with weight loss should suggest a malignancy. Pleurisy with effusion is one of the hallmarks of systemic lupus erythematosus and may occur in other connective tissue disorders. Thus, systemic manifestations of pleurisy vary with the nature of the underlying disorders and their protean clinical picture. Moreover, steroid therapy may mask the common constitutional symptoms.

Attention to the chest findings on physical examination is important, particularly if only a small amount of pleural exudate is present. Pleural rub due to roughened pleural surfaces may be the only finding early in the disease and may be heard during inspiration or expiration. As pleural effusion increases, the pleural rub is lost. Thus the presence of pleural rub indicates absence of significant pleural effusion. Diminished thoracic wall excursion, dull or flat percussion, decreased tactile and vocal fremitus, diminished whispering pectoriloquy, fullness of the intercostal spaces, and decreased breath sounds are easily demonstrated over the site involved in an older child with moderate effusion. Breath sounds in a neonate can come through loud and clear because of the small chest volume. The trachea and the cardiac apex are displaced toward the contralateral side. Splinting of the involved hemithorax may result in scoliosis concave to the affected side.

History taking and physical examination do not stop after admission of the patient to the hospital. Events in the clinical course during hospitalization may suggest emergency of certain complications of empyema. Expectoration of an increasing quantity of purulent sputum with or without hemoptysis may herald the onset of bronchopleural fistula and ensuing pyopneumothorax. Bronchopleural fistula may be due to rupture of neglected empyema into the lung or rupture of pulmonary suppuration into the pleura. Findings of chest wall abscess and costal chondritis indicate extension of the process (empyema necessitans). Muffling of the heart tones and pericardial rub indicate extension into the pericardium. Another complication is acute mediastinitis, which with its clinical picture of increasing toxicity is as serious as pericarditis. Thus vigilant patient care is essential for early detection of certain complications.

CHEST ROENTGENOGRAM

A chest roentgenogram is most useful in substantiating the physical findings of pleural effusion, irrespective of its nature and underlying cause (see also Chapter 40). Obliteration of the costophrenic sinus (Fig. 27–1, *arrow*) may be the earliest radiologic sign of minimal liquid accumulation, best demonstrated in the decubitus position. Moderate effusion causes layering of liquid density along the lateral chest wall. In the absence of pleural adhesions, the liquid density shifts with change in body position from upright to decubitus. With the affected hemithorax placed inferiorly, even small amounts of free fluid in the pleural cavity shift with the change in body position. The decubitus radiograph allows a semiquantitative assessment of the effusion. A fluid layer between the inside of the chest wall and the lung of less than 10 mm thickness is probably not clinically significant. Therapeutic thoracentesis is indicated for a fluid layer greater than 10 mm. Failure of the liquid to shift indicates loculation, as commonly seen in staphylococcal empyema. Ultrasonography can differentiate pleural thickening from an effusion, preventing fruitless attempts at diagnostic thoracen-

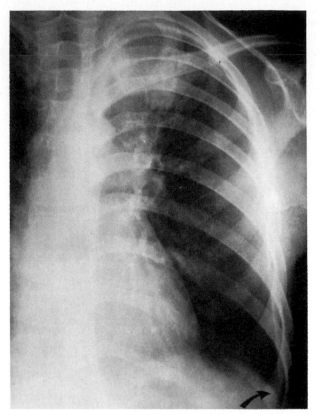

Figure 27–1. Chest radiograph of a child with tuberculous pleural effusion, demonstrating obliteration of the costophrenic sinus *(arrow)* and layering of liquid along the lateral chest wall. Also seen are left upper lobe consolidation and left hilar node enlargement.

tesis, and identify the best site for thoracentesis or insertion of the thoracotomy tube. Massive effusion may occupy one hemithorax, which demonstrates a uniform water density and displacement of the mediastinum toward the contralateral side (Fig. 27–2) and thereby obscures an underlying parenchymal lesion. A lateral decubitus chest radiograph with the affected side placed superiorly produces a medial pleural fluid layer allowing visualization of the underlying lung.

A chest roentgenogram is also important in documenting the presence of pyopneumothorax, which appears in the upright view as an air-liquid level extending to the lateral portion of the hemithorax. This condition can be differentiated from a huge lung abscess by obtaining a decubitus view. The contents of a lung abscess, as opposed to an empyema, are more viscous, resulting in little change in fluid level position with change in posture. Furthermore, an empyema usually creates an obtuse angle where it meets the chest wall, in contrast to the acute angle produced by an abscess. Computed axial tomography (CAT scan) may be extremely helpful in making a differential diagnosis.

Further thoracic imaging techniques are required to demonstrate bronchopleural fistula. One approach is by sinography. Radiopaque contrast material is injected into the affected pleura through a needle or existing chest tube (Fig. 27–3). As the patient coughs, the contrast material opacifies the fistula and spreads throughout the bronchial tree. This is the procedure of choice for peripherally situated small fistulas. Selective bronchography is employed to delineate multiple, centrally located fistulas.

LABORATORY INVESTIGATIONS

Examination of the Pleural Liquid

The pleural liquid may provide the only evidence on which to make a specific etiologic diagnosis or exclude others (see also Chapter 40). Thus thoracentesis is mandatory. It must be performed by experienced personnel after careful planning. The proce-

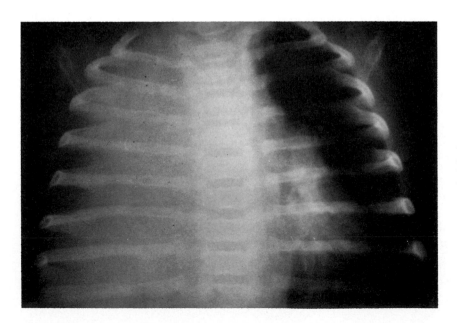

Figure 27–2. Chest radiograph of a child with staphylococcal empyema, demonstrating complete opacification of the right hemithorax with displacement of the heart and mediastinum to the left.

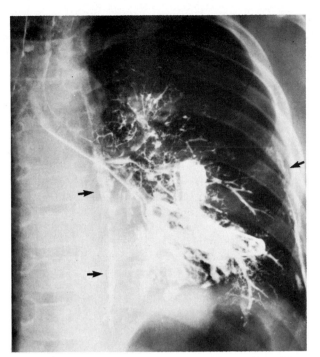

Figure 27–3. Pleurogram of a child with bronchopleural fistula, demonstrating the contrast material in the pleural cavity *(arrows)* and airways. Lipiodol was injected through a chest tube.

dure is explained to patients old enough to comprehend. Local anesthetic is used. Size and length of the needle are determined by chest wall thickness and anticipated character of the fluid. Interposing a three-way stopcock between needle and syringe allows a large quantity of liquid to be removed without danger of air entry. In addition to guidance from the chest roentgenogram, the point of maximum dullness must be ascertained to localize the site of needle entry. The seventh posterolateral intercostal space is sufficient for most cases of nonloculated effusions. Loculated effusions can be located and aspirated using the ultrasonographic technique for guidance. Once inserted, the needle is clamped at skin level to prevent inadvertent shifting. Vigorous cough is dangerous, and if it occurs the needle should be withdrawn quickly. A postthoracentesis chest film is obtained to look for any complication or underlying parenchymal disease.

The gross appearance of the liquid is noted, and a Gram stain is made. The remainder of the specimen is sent for cytologic examination, biochemical studies, pH and P_{CO_2} determinations, and microbiologic cultures. Thin and clear pleural effusions suggest noninfectious inflammatory exudates, which must be differentiated from transudates (see Table 40–2, Chapter 40). Nontraumatic sanguineous exudates may be due to underlying malignancy, pulmonary infarction, pancreaticopleural fistula, connective tissue disorder, or tuberculosis. Thick, purulent effusion is diagnostic of empyema. If it is putrid, anaerobic infection is incriminated. Thin, clear effusions, however, do not rule out an infectious basis. Gram stain is particularly useful if the patient had prior

antimicrobial therapy. Cytologic findings of malignant cells are diagnostic. In addition to biochemical studies for protein and lactic dehydrogenase, which separate exudate from transudate, determination of amylase helps establish a diagnosis of underlying pancreatitis (amylase concentration is elevated). Countercurrent immunoelectrophoresis (CIE) has proved useful for the diagnosis of certain bacterial antigens (e.g., staphylococcal) in the body fluids, including pleural liquid. It may provide a presumptive etiologic diagnosis for certain infectious pleural effusions in the event that Gram stain and culture results are negative. A definitive etiologic diagnosis rests on the result of microbiologic cultures, which are positive in approximately two thirds of children with empyema.

Infectious pleural effusions developing during the course of bacterial pneumonias may be categorized as (1) empyema—that is, purulent with positive Gram stain and/or culture result—or (2) nonempyema. Nonempyemic effusions either remain free or loculate, depending on the stage of pleurisy. Table 27–3 compares empyema, loculated exudates, and nonloculated effusions according to gross appearance, bacteriologic confirmation, biochemical characteristics, and P_{CO_2} and pH determinations. The specimen for pH and P_{CO_2} determinations must be collected anaerobically and placed in ice during its transport to the blood gas laboratory. Arterial pH is determined simultaneously, because it influences pleural liquid pH. It appears that pleural liquid pH can discriminate free-moving, nonloculated effusions (pH>7.30) from loculated exudates and frank empyema (pH<7.30). Thus low pleural liquid pH may have therapeutic and prognostic importance. It is imperative to emphasize, however, that the diagnostic use of pleural liquid pH below and above 7.30 is valid only with effusions due to nontuberculous bacterial pneumonias. Tuberculous and other, noninfectious inflammatory exudates may also have a low pleural liquid pH, and their differentiation must be based on clinical information and results of other laboratory tests.

Pleural Biopsy

Parietal pleural biopsy is indicated in patients with unexplained inflammatory pleural effusion. The procedure may be performed either percutaneously at the bedside, with a specially designed needle, or by open thoracotomy under general anesthesia. A variety of special cutting needles have been used, namely, Cope, Abrams, Ballestero, Vim-Silverman, and Harefield. The Harefield needle allows aspiration of liquid at the time of pleural biopsy. The tissue specimen includes portions of intercostal muscles and adjoining parietal pleura approximately 4 mm in diameter and is sent for histologic and culture studies. The liquid in the pleural space prevents the needle from puncturing the lung. Thus the biopsy is most easily accomplished at the time of initial thoracentesis, when there is the least chance of lacerating the underlying lung.

Table 27–3. PHYSICAL AND CHEMICAL CHARACTERISTICS OF PARAPNEUMONIC PLEURAL EFFUSIONS

Characteristics	Empyema	Loculated Exudates	Nonloculated Effusions
Appearance	Purulent and predominantly turbid	Nonpurulent and predominantly less turbid	Nonpurulent and predominantly less turbid
Gram stain and/or culture	Positive	Negative	Negative
Glucose (mg/dL)	Majority <50 (mean = 36)	Majority <50 (mean = 36)	Majority >100 (mean = 134)
Protein (g/dL)	Invariably >3 (mean = 4.7)	Invariably >3 (mean = 6.0)	Majority <3 (mean = 2.7)
P_{CO_2} (mm Hg)	Majority >60 (mean = 100)	Majority >60 (mean = 71)	Majority <40 (mean = 45)
pH (units)	Invariably <7.30 (mean = 6.93)	Invariably <7.30 (mean = 6.94)	Invariably >7.30 (mean = 7.38)

(Modified from Potts DE, Levin DC, and Sahn SA: Pleural fluid pH in parapneumonic effusions. Chest 70:328, 1976.)

The greatest value of percutaneous parietal biopsy is in clinical disorders that cause widespread involvement of the pleural surface (e.g., tuberculosis, tumors).

Technique. The technique of percutaneous pleural biopsy is as follows: The patient is seated and adequately supported. The appropriate site for needle entry is infiltrated to the parietal pleura with local anesthesia. A small incision is made on the skin to facilitate introduction of the trocar. The Harefield needle, with the notch closed, is carefully advanced into the pleural space. The pleural effusion is aspirated. Thereafter, the needle with the notch open is withdrawn slowly while lateral pressure is applied in the direction of the notch, which is indicated by the small rounded knob on the hub of the needle. A catch is felt as the notch becomes engaged on the parietal pleura. The inner cutting core is advanced, obtaining the specimen, and the needle is then withdrawn. Careful technique is associated with a minimal occurrence of complications such as pneumothorax and hemothorax. Because morbidity from the procedure is low and repetition of the biopsy increases the diagnostic yield, a second biopsy is indicated if an etiologic diagnosis has not been established by means of the first.

OTHER INVESTIGATIONS

Additional appropriate tests are carried out to elucidate a suspected underlying disease state. For example, a positive Mantoux reaction, particularly a recent conversion, strongly suggests tuberculosis; a negative skin reaction does not rule it out. Examination of bronchopulmonary secretions obtained by sputum induction, by gastric fluid aspiration, and during bronchoscopy may be indicated. Certain immunologic tests (e.g., anti-DNA) are indicated to clarify the causative role of some connective tissue or collagen disorders. Blood culture is performed when sepsis is suspected. A negative sweat test result rules out cystic fibrosis.

Roentgenograms of other organs are ordered when underlying malignancy is a consideration. Also, a second physical examination may reveal findings that lead to a specific diagnosis.

MANAGEMENT

Treatment of inflammatory pleural disorders is aimed at specific management of the underlying cause and relief of functional disturbances caused by the inciting clinical disorder, pleural involvement, and concurrent complication. Therapy is medical and surgical. A prompt and specific etiologic diagnosis is optimal for management.

General supportive measures include bed rest for the acutely ill child and chloral hydrate for restlessness and irritability. Fluid management must be sufficient to replace increased losses due to fever and tachypnea. Supplemental oxygen should be administered to the child with hypoxia or increased work of breathing. It is imperative to recognize that irritability may be due to pain, high fever, distressing cough, or hypoxia. Relief of sharp pain occurring with every phase of respiration—characteristic of dry pleurisy—demands immediate attention. Mild cases promptly respond to such simple measures as local heat and oral analgesics. Acetaminophen is also indicated for very high fever to minimize discomfort and avert febrile convulsion, particularly in young infants. Severe pleuritic pain may require the use of oral codeine sulfate, which will also suppress dry cough due to irritation of the airways. Alternative analgesic measures include topical ethyl chloride spray and intravenous calcium gluconate; response in some patients to these drugs indicates that muscle spasm may play a role in the genesis of pain. Lying on the affected side may provide temporary relief by splinting the involved thorax. Excruciating pain, as may occur in pleuritis due to neoplasm, requires an exceptional approach. Repeated subcutaneous morphine injection may be indicated in terminal cases. Moreover, intercostal nerve block using 1 to 2 ml of 1 per cent lidocaine solution has been tried. It is injected via a 23-gauge, 2-inch-long needle into the area near the nerves involved. This technique may provide relief of pleuritic pain for 12 to 24 hours.

The stage of effusion following dry pleurisy usually provides permanent relief from pain. However, accumulation of an excessive amount of pleural liquid necessitates thoracentesis to relieve dyspnea. Repeated thoracentesis and, eventually, continuous chest-tube drainage are indicated if rapid reaccumulation of effusion induces dyspnea and dominates the clinical picture, as commonly occurs in neoplasm. Although most effusions due to a noninfectious inflammatory process require only drainage to relieve dyspnea, additional specific measures may be indicated in the presence of certain underlying systemic diseases. Systemic and intrapleural instillation of chemotherapeutic agents and mediastinal irradiation of the involved nodes or primary tumor sites control pleural effusion in lymphoma. Prednisone ameliorates dyspnea as well as cough, anorexia, and weight loss in sarcoidosis. Steroids increase the rate with which tuberculous effusion resolves and fever returns to normal, but definitive proof of their value on eventual ventilatory function has not been shown. If steroids are to be used to help alleviate dyspnea, concomitant antituberculous chemotherapy is essential. Tuberculous effusions usually clear within 6 months on isoniazid and rifampin therapy. Indeed, asymptomatic noninfectious pleural exudates need only management of the underlying disorder. Improvement in the underlying systemic disease is paralleled by resolution of the accompanying pleural exudation.

Pleural effusions due to infection require specific antimicrobial treatment and certain surgical considerations. Antimicrobial therapy should be initiated on the strength of a positive response to Gram stain or grossly purulent liquid. Initial choice of antimicrobial agents is based on a consideration of the clinical data, the bacterial epidemiology in the community, and known pharmacologic properties of the drugs. Dosage must be adequate, and administration initially should be intravenous. Infection may be polymicrobial, so more than one antimicrobial drug must be given initially. Subsequent changes in antimicrobial coverage are guided by the results of culture and sensitivity tests. A guide to antimicrobial therapy of nontuberculous bacterial pleurisy and empyema is presented in Table 27–4. Duration of drug treatment must be long enough to prevent relapse. Physicians must always be aware of the potential side effects of the drugs on various target organs and must be prepared to use alternative drugs at the appropriate time.

With specific antimicrobial therapy and timely provision of appropriate pleural drainage, patients should recover completely from an episode of bacterial pleurisy and empyema. Rational choice of a surgical procedure requires knowledge of the specific etiologic agent and clinical course of the disease. Table 27–5 lists current surgical considerations in the management of pleurisy and empyema. Thoracentesis is performed to relieve dyspnea during the acute stage and is repeated as required; it may be all that is necessary for free-moving effusions with pH above 7.30 and LDH less than 1000 units/L. Progressive decline in pH or increase in LDH may mandate closed-tube thoracostomy. Localized exudates with pH below 7.30 and massive effusion associated with overwhelming sepsis, such as secondary to H. influenzae or Staphylococcus aureus infection, require immediate closed thoracotomy. Immediate closed-tube thoracostomy is indicated if examination of the pleural fluid reveals frank pus, positive Gram stain, pH less than 7.20 or more than 0.05 units below arterial pH, or if serum LDH is greater than 1000 units/L. The application of negative pressure to the tube enhances obliteration of the empyema space and re-expansion of the lung. Clinical improvement may be expected in 48 hours. Drainage may be stopped when the patient becomes asymptomatic, without waiting for the complete resolution of the roentgenographic abnormalities. In contrast, the thick loculated empyema that is usually secondary to anaerobic pneumonitis or tardily diagnosed staphylococcal infection requires prolonged open thoracotomy drainage. Introduction of streptokinase into the empyema cavity has been shown to lyse adhesions, thus enhancing drainage. The usual method is to dilute 250,000 units of the drug in 100 ml of normal saline. This solution is injected into the cavity via the chest tube, which is clamped for 4 hours before resuming drainage. Patients with this kind of empyema tend to remain febrile for an average of 3

Table 27–4. A GUIDE TO ANTIMICROBIAL THERAPY OF BACTERIAL PLEURISY AND EMPYEMA

Infecting Agent	Drug and Dosage (per kg per day) Route and Duration*
A. Aerobic bacteria	
1. Staphylococci	1.a. Methicillin, 200–400 mg divided in 3–4 doses IV initially; for 3–4 weeks
	b. Cloxacillin, 100–200 mg divided in 3–6 doses IV initially; for 3–4 weeks
2. Haemophilus influenzae	2.a. Ampicillin, 100–200 mg divided in 2–4 doses IV initially; for 1–2 weeks or
	b. Chloramphenicol, 50–100 mg divided in 4 doses IV initially; for 1–2 weeks or
	c. Cefuroxime, 75–225 mg divided in 3 doses IV initially for 1–2 weeks
3. Pneumococcus and streptococci	3. Penicillin G, 50,000–300,000 units divided in 3–4 doses IV or IM; for 7–10 days
4. Escherichia coli and Klebsiella	4. Gentamicin, 5–7 mg divided in 2–3 doses IV; for 14 days or longer
5. Pseudomonas	5.a. Carbenicillin, 100–600 mg divided in 4 doses IV; for 10 days or longer or
	b. Ticarcillin, 400 mg, divided in 4 doses IV for 10 days or longer
	c. Tobramycin, 5–7 mg divided in 2 doses
B. Anaerobic bacteria	
1. Bacteroides fragilis	1. Chloramphenicol, same as A.2.b
2. All except B. fragilis	2.a. Penicillin G, same as A.3
	b. Ampicillin, same as A.2.a

*The lower dose in the dosage range and less frequent intervals of administration are recommended for neonates.
Duration of therapy for anaerobic pneumonitis requires an adjustment if the lung lesions go on to cavitate. Often, 6 to 12 weeks are required before the lung lesions clear or only a small stable residual disease is left.
IV, intravenously; IM, intramuscularly; CNS, central nervous system; kg, kilogram body weight.

Table 27–5. SURGICAL MANAGEMENT OF BACTERIAL PLEURISY AND EMPYEMA

Procedure	Rationale and Comments
Thoracentesis (needle aspiration)	For prompt relief of dyspnea and initial step for diagnostic study of the liquid. May be repeated two or three times and most of effusion removed during tap.
Intercostal tube drainage (closed thoracotomy)	For massive, relatively thin effusion in the presence of overwhelming toxicity (e.g., secondary to lung abscess).
Tube thoracotomy with rib resection (open thoracotomy)	For symptomatic thick, encapsulated empyema not controlled by antibiotics and when early obliteration of empyema cavity is expected (e.g., postlobectomy empyema).
Open flap drainage	For larger symptomatic empyema (e.g., postpneumonectomy empyema). Easy to care for technique for septic and debilitated patients.
Pleural decortication	For removal of restrictive fibrous tissue layer on surface of lungs. Indicated for symptomatic chronic empyema with lung entrapment.
Extrapleural thoracoplasty	To obliterate pleural cavity and lessen space into which lung has to expand. May be a deforming procedure and now very rarely indicated.

weeks after the first drainage, and most fatalities (10.6 per cent) have been ascribed to delay in beginning or failure to obtain optimal surgical drainage.

The procedures of open flap drainage, pleural decortication, and thoracoplasty now almost never need to be done. Perhaps the only remaining indication for these procedures is concurrent bronchopleural fistula, which if recalcitrant may require grafting with pedicled muscle. Concurrent extrapulmonary complications (e.g., pericarditis) are managed appropriately.

PROGNOSIS

The outlook in inflammatory pleural disorders basically depends on the nature of the underlying clinical problem, nature and extent of pleural disease, age of the patient, start of therapy, and occurrence of complications. Malignant pleurisy carries an extremely grave prognosis, whereas viral and *Mycoplasma* pleural diseases generally resolve spontaneously with time. Patients with empyema have a more prolonged and complicated hospital course and may require longer follow-up after returning home than do patients with nonempyemic, free-moving pleural liquid. Empyema carries a far higher mortality in infants under 2 years of age if treatment is delayed. Prompt and adequate therapy during the acute phase should result in complete recovery. Complications such as bronchopleural fistula and tension pneumatocele are rare but may delay onset of full recovery.

Noninfectious pleurisy and effusions resolve with the resolution of the underlying systemic clinical problems. The outcome of bacterial pleurisy and empyema has remarkably improved in recent years. Only 30 years ago, the mortality from empyema approximated 100 per cent; now, virtually no death should occur with prompt therapy. Most recent series report case fatality rates of 6 to 12 per cent, with the highest among infants less than 1 year of age. Fibro-

thorax is extremely rare. In contrast to adults, infants and children have a remarkable ability to resolve pleural thickening with no effect on subsequent lung growth and function.

REFERENCES

Bartlett JG and Finegold SM: Anaerobic infections of the lung and pleural space. Am Rev Respir Dis 110:56, 1974.

Bechamps GJ, Lynn HB, and Wenzl JE: Empyema in children: review of Mayo Clinic experience. Mayo Clin Proc 45:43, 1970.

Berger HW and Mejia E: Tuberculous pleurisy. Chest 63:88, 1973.

Bergh NP, Ekroth R, Larsson S, and Nagy P: Intrapleural streptokinase in the treatment of haemothorax and empyema. Scand J Thorac Cardiovasc Surg 11:265, 1977.

Cho C, Hiatt WD, and Behbehan AM: Pneumonia and massive pleural effusion associated with adenovirus type 7. Am J Dis Child 126:92, 1973.

Dorman JP, Campbell D, Grover F, and Trinkle JK: Open thoracostomy drainage of postpneumonic empyema with bronchopleural fistula. J Thorac Cardiovasc Surg 66:979, 1973.

Eichenwald HF: Antimicrobial therapy in children. Curr Probl Pediatr 4:3, 1974.

Fine NL, Smith LR, and Sheedy PF: Frequency of pleural effusions in mycoplasma and viral pneumonias. N Engl J Med 288:790, 1970.

Freij BJ, Kusmiesz H, Nelson JD, and McCracken GH: Parapneumonic effusions and empyema in hospitalized children: a retrospective review of 227 cases. Pediatr Infect Dis 3:578, 1984.

Griz A and Giammona ST: Pneumonitis with pleural effusion in children due to *Mycoplasma pneumoniae*. Am Rev Respir Dis 109:665, 1974.

Hsu JT, Bennett GM, and Wolff E: Radiologic assessment of bronchopleural fistula with empyema. Diagn Radiol 103:41, 1972.

Kissane JM: Pathology of Infancy and Childhood. 2nd ed. St. Louis, CV Mosby Co, 1975.

Krugman S and Ward R: Infectious Diseases of Children and Adults. 5th ed. St. Louis, CV Mosby Co, 1973.

Lampe RM, Chottipitayasunondh T, and Sunakorn P: Detection of bacterial antigen in pleural fluid by counterimmunoelectrophoresis. J Pediatr 88:557, 1976.

Light RW: Parapneumonic effusions and empyema. Semin Respir Med 9:37, 1987.

Lincoln EM, Davies PA, and Bovornkitti S: Tuberculous pleurisy with effusion in children. Am Rev Tuberc 77:271, 1958.

Potts DE, Levin DC, and Sahn SA: Pleural fluid pH in parapneumonia effusions. Chest 70:328, 1976.

Sahn SA, Lakshminarayan S, and Char DG: "Silent" empyema in a patient receiving corticosteroids. Am Rev Respir Dis 107:873, 1973.

Shackelford PG, Campbell J, and Feigin RD: Countercurrent immunoelectrophoresis in the evaluation of childhood infections. J Pediatr 85:478, 1974.

Stiles QR, Lindesmith GG, Tucker BL et al: Pleural empyema in children. Ann Thorac Surg 10:37, 1970.

Thornton GF: The role of corticosteroids in the management of tuberculous infections. In Johnson JE III (ed): Rational Therapy and Control of Tuberculosis. Gainesville, University of Florida Press, 1970.

Weick JK, Killy JM, Harrison EG et al: Pleural effusion in lymphoma. Cancer 31:848, 1973.

Wise MB, Beaudry PH, and Bates DV: Long term follow-up of staphylococcal pneumonia. Pediatrics 38:398, 1966.

Wolfe WG, Spick A, and Bradford WD: Pleural fluids in infants and children. Am Rev Respir Dis 98:1027, 1968.

NONINFECTIOUS DISORDERS OF THE RESPIRATORY TRACT

28

ROBERT B. MELLINS, M.D.

LUNG INJURY FROM HYDROCARBON ASPIRATION AND SMOKE INHALATION

LUNG INJURY FROM HYDROCARBON ASPIRATION

Hydrocarbon toxicity resulting from the ingestion of petroleum solvents, dry-cleaning fluids, lighter fluids, kerosene, gasoline, and liquid polishes and waxes (mineral seal oil) has continued to be a common occurrence in small children during the past 25 years (Mellins et al, 1956; Eade et al, 1974; Pearn et al, 1984; Klein and Simon, 1986). The decrease in the frequency of kerosene poisoning during this period may reflect the concomitant decrease in the use of kerosene space heaters. (Whether a reversal of this trend will follow the recent increase in use of space heaters remains to be seen.) The availability of an increasing number of cleaning fluids, furniture polishes, and liquid floor waxes within the home and all too frequently within the easy reach of toddlers also accounts for the persistence of hydrocarbon poisoning.

Although central nervous system (CNS) abnormalities (including weakness, confusion, and coma), gastrointestinal irritation, myocardiopathy, and renal toxicity all occur, the most common as well as the most serious complication is pneumonitis. Deaths from hydrocarbon poisoning are almost always from pneumonitis rather than from CNS toxicity.

PATHOLOGY

Pathologic changes in the lungs in fatal cases have included necrosis of bronchial, bronchiolar, and alveolar tissue, atelectasis, interstitial inflammation, hemorrhagic pulmonary edema, vascular thromboses, necrotizing bronchopneumonia, and hyaline membrane formation (Klein and Simon, 1986). Injury to the myocardium has also been reported (James et al, 1971). Studies of experimental hydrocarbon aspiration in rats have had conflicting results. Early studies revealed an acute alveolitis that is most

severe at 3 days, subsides at 10 days, and is followed by a chronic proliferation phase that may take weeks to resolve (Gross et al, 1963). These experimental studies, when taken in conjunction with the observation in humans that the chest roentgenographic abnormalities are present for some time after the physical findings have cleared, suggest that the pulmonary lesions may also persist for some time in humans. More recent studies of kerosene aspiration in rats have demonstrated hyperemia within 1 hour with vascular engorgement of both large and small blood vessels (Scharf et al, 1981). At 24 hours there was a focal bronchopneumonia with microabscess formation. By 2 weeks the process was largely resolved, although some vascular engorgement and rare peribronchial inflammation persisted.

PATHOPHYSIOLOGY

Low surface tension facilitates the spread of hydrocarbons along mucous membranes and, coupled with choking and gagging, probably accounts for the aspiration of hydrocarbon liquids into the lungs. Low viscosity and high volatility may facilitate deep penetration into the lungs.

Experimental evidence suggests that hydrocarbons increase the minimum surface tension, presumably by altering surfactant, thus predisposing to alveolar instability, small-airway closure, and atelectasis (Giammona, 1967). These alterations in the lung would account for the combination of hyperinflation and atelectasis seen on the chest roentgenogram, as well as the hypoxemia. Because they are liquid solvents, hydrocarbons possibly injure cells by disrupting cell membranes. The observation that there is a decrease in the ability to clear bacteria after experimental kerosene poisoning suggests that hydrocarbon aspiration also impairs pulmonary defense mechanisms.

The studies by Scharf and co-workers (1981) provide evidence that challenges the view that the pathogenesis can be attributed simply to an increase in

Supported in part by NIH grant HL 07421.

449

surface tension. They found an *increase* in total lung capacity and lung compliance by 24 hours; these returned to control levels by 2 weeks. When lung compliance was normalized for the increase in total lung capacity, the specific compliance did not change over the 2-week period. There was no evidence of closed lung units under control conditions to explain the subsequent increase in total lung capacity after kerosene inhalation. A change in the elastic fibers of the lung after inhalation is one possible explanation for these findings. Relaxation of contractile elements within the interstitial cells of the alveolar walls and elsewhere is another possibility. Indeed, the vascular engorgement that was so prominent a feature of the reaction to injury may also have resulted from muscle relaxation.

Initially, considerable controversy centered around how much of the toxicity resulted from aspiration as opposed to gastrointestinal absorption with subsequent transport to the lungs and other organs by the blood. The bulk of evidence now suggests that the pulmonary lesions are caused by aspiration and not by gastrointestinal absorption (Richardson and Pratt-Thomas, 1951; Gerarde, 1959; Huxtable et al, 1964; Giammona, 1967; Wolfe et al, 1970; Wolfsdorf and Kundig, 1972; Dice et al, 1982). Experimental evidence suggests that the hydrocarbons are removed by the first capillary bed they encounter (Bratton and Haddow, 1975; Wolfsdorf, 1976), again reinforcing the notion that pulmonary damage occurs from aspiration, not from pulmonary excretion following gastrointestinal absorption. Indeed, the liver and the lungs filter out sufficient amounts of kerosene to protect the brain from damage (Bratton and Haddow, 1975).

Although drowsiness, tremor, and occasionally convulsions have been presumed to result from direct injury of the CNS, it seems more reasonable to attribute CNS involvement to hypoxia from lung damage (Bratton and Haddow, 1975). Fatalities are rarely attributed to CNS involvement per se. The available experimental evidence indicates that small amounts of hydrocarbons, when aspirated, may produce more serious disease than larger amounts retained in the stomach.

CLINICAL FINDINGS

Intercostal retractions, grunting, cough, and fever may appear within 30 min of aspiration or may be delayed for a few hours. Initially, auscultation of the chest may reveal only coarse or decreased sounds. When severe injury occurs, hemoptysis and pulmonary edema develop rapidly, cyanosis becomes more severe, and death may occur within 24 hours of aspiration. Roentgenographic signs of chemical pneumonitis, when present, are evident by 2 hours after ingestion in 88 per cent of cases and within 12 hours in 98 per cent (Daeschner et al, 1957). The findings vary from punctate, mottled densities to pneumonitis or atelectasis or both and tend to be more prominent in dependent portions of the lung (Fig. 28–1A). Air trapping with overdistention of the lungs, pneumatoceles, and pleural effusions may also develop (Fig. 28–1B). The radiographic abnormalities reach their maximum by 72 hours and then usually clear within a few days. Occasionally, the roentgenographic findings are said to persist for several weeks. There is a very poor correlation among clinical symptoms, physical findings, and radiographic abnormalities. In general, the radiographic changes are more prominent than the findings on physical examination and tend to persist for a longer period. Pneumatoceles, when they occur, are likely to do so after a patient has become asymptomatic and are detected incidentally on follow-up chest radiographs. They require several months for spontaneous resolution.

Blood gas studies reveal hypoxemia without hypercapnia, suggesting that ventilation-perfusion abnormalities, rather than alveolar hypoventilation, are the primary physiologic defect. Destruction of the epithelium of the airways together with bronchospasm caused by surface irritation accounts for the ventilation-perfusion abnormalities.

Long-term follow-up studies of the pulmonary function in patients who have had hydrocarbon pneumonitis indicate that there is residual injury to the small airways. An evaluation of 17 asymptomatic children conducted 8 to 14 years after an episode of hydrocarbon pneumonitis showed some abnormality in lung function in 14 of the subjects. The most common abnormalities seen were an elevated ratio of residual volume to total lung capacity, an increased slope of phase III, reduced forced expiratory volume in 1 sec (FEV_1) and flow rates at 50 and 25 per cent of the vital capacity, and a high volume of isoflow. These findings have been interpreted as reflecting small-airway obstruction or loss of elastic recoil (Gurwitz et al, 1978). Other studies indicate that when radiographic changes accompany the ingestion of hydrocarbons, evidence of abnormal lung function could be detected 10 years later in otherwise asymptomatic subjects; these included a significantly higher volume of isoflow (Viso $\dot{V}$) and a significantly lower delta $\dot{V}max_{50}$, interpreted as indicating residual small airways disease. Nevertheless, airway reactivity appeared to be normal (Tal et al, 1984).

MANAGEMENT

Because large volumes of hydrocarbon appear to do less damage when ingested into the gastrointestinal tract than when aspirated into the lungs, it seems reasonable to avoid emetics or gastric lavage. Studies in animals and humans have failed to demonstrate either a therapeutic or prophylactic role for adrenocorticosteroids in this condition (Hardman et al, 1960; Albert and Inkley, 1968; Steele et al, 1972; Marks et al, 1972; Wolfsdorf and Kundig, 1973).

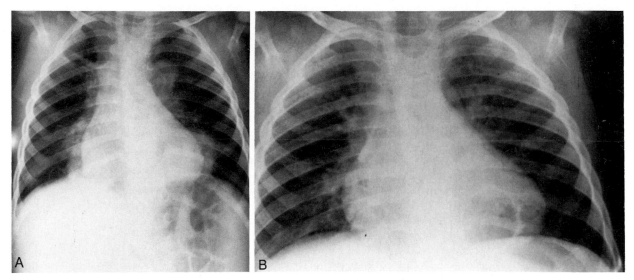

Figure 28–1. Hydrocarbon pneumonia. *A*, Confluent sequential infiltrate is present in the left lower lobe. *B*, Three weeks later, pneumatoceles are apparent; the large pneumatocele in the left lower lobe is at the site of the previous infiltrate. (From Felman AH: Radiology of the Pediatric Chest. New York, McGraw-Hill Book Co, 1987.)

Although superimposition of bacterial infection is always of concern, there is no good evidence to suggest that this occurs often. Because leukocytosis and pyrexia are common findings after hydrocarbon aspiration, it is extremely difficult, perhaps impossible, to tell whether bacterial superinfection has occurred. One thoughtful review concludes that bacterial complications do not occur in the majority of patients (Eade et al, 1974). Until there is further evidence on this subject, we believe that antimicrobial therapy should be reserved for patients who are severely compromised by undernutrition, debilitation, or underlying disease or in whom the pneumonia is especially severe. Nor do we believe that focusing on the possibility of infection should obscure or delay initiation of other forms of therapy when pulmonary disease is severe. Because airway closure and collapse may be a significant part of the disease, the use of some form of continuous distending airway pressure of the lungs would seem to be desirable, especially because such a measure may make it possible to reduce the concentration of inspired oxygen necessary to maintain a reasonable Pa_{O_2}. The use of bronchodilators would also seem to be reasonable for relief of bronchospasm.

Prevention of the accidental ingestion of products containing hydrocarbons should be a high priority. Education of parents to keep potentially toxic materials out of the reach of young children would seem to be self-evident.

HYDROCARBON "SNIFFING"

Deliberate inhalation of volatile hydrocarbons to induce a state of euphoria is common among teenage boys; chronic inhalation is a problem in poor and socially deprived children. The euphoria of mild intoxication may be accompanied by mild nausea and vomiting. More prolonged exposure may lead to violent excitement followed by CNS depression, unconsciousness, and coma. Large doses of halogenated hydrocarbons, especially when combined with exertion, excitement, and hypercapnia, may be associated with severe arrhythmias and death. Medullary depression and respiratory paralysis are generally accepted as the mechanism of death in most gasoline inhalation fatalities. Strong psychological dependence may develop in some sniffers. Lung injury per se from hydrocarbon sniffing has not been described.

RESPIRATORY COMPLICATIONS OF SMOKE INHALATION

A great deal of the morbidity and mortality of victims of fires is now recognized to result from pulmonary injuries due to smoke inhalation. The severity of the lung injury depends on (1) the nature of the material involved in the conflagration and the products of incomplete combustion that are generated and (2) whether the victim has been confined in a closed space. Although we will focus in this section on the serious consequences of smoke inhalation from fires, it is worth pointing out that some of the same compounds that are generated in fires are now considered part of the industrial pollution of the environment. Thus the lung injury that occurs in victims of smoke inhalation may represent an extreme form of a challenge to which we are all exposed in smaller doses.

PATHOGENESIS

In a general way, the pathogenesis of lung injury from smoke inhalation includes thermal and chemical factors. Because the upper air passage is such an effective heat exchanger, it is likely that most of the heat from inhaled smoke is dissipated by the time the inhaled material reaches the carina. On theoretical grounds, it is conceivable that continuous oxidation of incompletely combusted material as it descends into the lung may result in thermal injury of the small and more peripheral lung units.

Depending on the material involved in fires, a wide variety of noxious gases may be generated. These include the oxides of sulfur and nitrogen, acetaldehydes, hydrocyanic acid, and carbon monoxide. Irritant gases such as nitrous oxide or sulfur dioxide may combine with water in the lungs to form corrosive acids. Aldehydes that form from the combustion of furniture and cotton materials induce denaturation of protein, cellular damage, and pulmonary edema. The combustion of wood is also likely to generate considerable quantities of carbon monoxide (CO). Plastics, if heated to sufficiently high temperatures, may be the source of very toxic vapors. Thus, chlorine and hydrochloric acid may be generated from polyvinylchloride; hydrocarbons, aldehydes, ketones, and acids from polyethylene; and isocyanate and hydrogen cyanide from polyurethane (Witten et al, 1988). Although the particulate matter carried in the smoke (soot) probably does not of itself produce injury, toxic gases may be absorbed on the surface of the particles and carried into the lungs; the soot particles may also be responsible for inducing reflex bronchoconstriction.

Carbon Monoxide Poisoning

Carbon monoxide poisoning is an especially serious complication of smoke inhalation and is likely to occur soon after exposure. The mechanism of toxicity results from the reversible combination of CO with hemoglobin to form carboxyhemoglobin (HbCO), leading to severe hypoxia. Under normal conditions, the HbCO concentration in the blood is less than 1 per cent. Because the HbCO concentration is higher in smokers (ranging as high as 5 to 10 per cent) for the same exposure, smokers may end up with more intense CO poisoning. CO not only has a high affinity for hemoglobin but also shifts the oxyhemoglobin dissociation curve to the left, making it necessary for the oxygen tension in the tissues to decrease to very low levels before appreciable amounts of oxygen are released in the hemoglobin (Root, 1965). For this reason, the toxicity of CO poisoning is greater at high altitude and in the presence of anemia. It is important to emphasize that although the oxygen content of the arterial blood is low in CO poisoning, the oxygen tension (Pa_{O_2}) is not reduced. Because the carotid body is believed to respond to the Pa_{O_2}, ventilation may not be stimulated until serious acidosis has resulted. This, together with the fact that HbCO is bright red, makes the clinical diagnosis very difficult. The reduction in hemoglobin available to oxygen in carbon monoxide poisoning is much more serious than an equivalent reduction in anemia because there is a left shift as well as a change in the shape of the oxygen dissociation curve, which therefore requires a considerably lower oxygen tension at the tissue level before oxygen is unloaded. Carbon monoxide also binds to myoglobin in muscle and to cytochrome oxidases in cells and thus may block cellular oxidation, resulting in anoxia of cells.

PATHOLOGY

Various pathologic lesions have been described in patients after smoke inhalation. Part of the variation in pathologic lesions described may be attributed to differences in the toxic products generated in fires. However, many of the changes may not result simply from the direct chemical injury to the respiratory tract. Rather, they may reflect secondary circulatory, metabolic, or infectious complications of surface burns or may be induced by tracheostomy tubes, the administration of oxygen, the use of mechanical ventilator, and the administration of intravenous fluids in volumes in excess of maintenance needs.

The use of animal models to study the pathologic process has been of limited value because steam rather than the toxic products present in smoke has usually been used, and the modifying effects of the upper air passages have been eliminated by the use of tracheal cannulas. The lesions following smoke inhalation are likely to resemble those seen after the inhalation of toxic gases, such as phosgene or chlorine. Inhalation of small amounts of these gases results in alveolar and bronchiolar epithelial damage leading to an obliterative bronchiolitis. Severe exposure also produces damage to the alveolar capillaries, with hemorrhage, edema, and the formation of hyaline membranes.

A group of infants carefully studied after exposure to smoke in a newborn nursery (Cox et al, 1955) was found to have necrosis of bronchial and bronchiolar epithelium with vascular engorgement and edema and with the formation of dense membranes or casts that partially obstructed the large and small airways. Bronchiolitis and bronchopneumonia were present in some, as well as interstitial and alveolar edema. There was carbonaceous material in the alveoli, with alveolar hemorrhage.

Electron microscopic studies of 10 fatal cases of smoke inhalation following a hotel fire revealed interstitial and alveolar edema as well as engorgement of alveolar vessels (Burns et al, 1986). Carbon particles were seen within alveolar macrophages. Type I pneumocytes showed greater injury than the pulmonary endothelial cells.

Patients who died after severe surface burns have had necrotizing bronchitis and bronchiolitis with intra-alveolar hemorrhage and hyaline membrane formation and massive pulmonary edema. In these patients, it is difficult to know how much to attribute to direct pulmonary injury from smoke rather than to the complex metabolic, infectious, and circulatory derangements that complicate surface burns.

PATHOPHYSIOLOGY

Severe damage to the upper air passages leads to stridor, with increases in both inspiratory and expiratory resistance. Bronchiolitis and alveolitis are likely to lead to impaired gas exchange, exaggerating the hypoxemia. Depending on the severity and the distribution of the airway obstruction, there may be atelectasis or air trapping with hyperinflation. The latter is especially likely to occur because of premature closure of small airways. Reduced surfactant activity may predispose to atelectasis.

Although reflex bronchoconstriction is likely to contribute to the increase in airway resistance, it is difficult to assess the magnitude of its contribution because airway resistance is already high as a result of bronchial and bronchiolar edema and inflammation.

Impaired chemotactic and phagocytic function of the alveolar macrophage after smoke inhalation has been demonstrated in adult humans and experimental animals. The clinical relevance of this finding with respect to the pathogenesis as well as the increased susceptibility to infection remains to be established.

A summary of the evidence that pulmonary edema plays a prominent role in the pathophysiology of lung injury from smoke inhalation has been provided recently (Witten et al, 1988). Double-indicator dilution studies have demonstrated increased extravascular lung water without a concomitant increase in pulmonary capillary pressure (wedge pressure) in studies in adult patients. Studies in an experimental model of smoke inhalation injury in sheep have revealed an increase in lung lymph and an increase in the lymph to plasma ratio of protein, suggesting increased permeability of the alveolar-capillary membrane (Traber et al, 1986).

Pulmonary insufficiency from inhalation injury and burns results from several factors: cytoxic damage from multiple products of incomplete combustion, hypoxic cellular damage, pulmonary surfactant inactivation, oxygen radical dependent lung injury, aggregation of cellular elements of blood, and release of vasoactive substances altering microvascular perfusion or permeability (Shirani et al, 1988).

CLINICAL FINDINGS

The initial assessment of a victim of a fire should focus on CNS damage due to hypoxemia. Hypoxemia, whether the result of asphyxia or of CO poisoning, may produce irritability or depression. If there is any change in the state of the sensorium, oxygen should be administered while blood gas studies, including the level of carbon monoxide, are being conducted in the laboratory.

The clinical manifestations of carbon monoxide poisoning vary with the level of HbCO. Mild varieties of intoxication lead to headache, diminution in visual acuity, irritability, and nausea. More severe intoxication (generally in excess of 40 per cent HbCO) produces confusion, hallucination, ataxia, and coma. Carbon monoxide may increase cerebral blood flow, the permeability of cerebral capillaries, and the pressure in the cerebrospinal fluid. There is also reason to believe that CO may have some long-term effects on the CNS.

To what extent the complications in smoke inhalation injuries result from hypoxia or anoxia directly or secondarily to CO poisoning is not clear. CO poisoning unrelated to smoke inhalation has been associated with myocardial injury in adults, as indicated by elevated myocardial enzymes. Patients dying of CO poisoning have had pulmonary hemorrhage and edema. It is not clear, however, whether these complications result from anoxia per se or from left heart failure or pulmonary aspiration. Muscle necrosis with myoglobinuria and acute renal failure has been reported with CO poisoning (Zimmerman and Truxal, 1981). Finally, CO poisoning may produce cutaneous erythema, edema, blister, and bullae that may be mistaken for cutaneous burns.

CO levels may be reduced by half in less than an hour when the patient is breathing pure oxygen. If severe CO poisoning is suspected, it may be necessary to administer oxygen by mask with nonrebreathing valves in order to achieve concentrations close to 100 per cent. Furthermore, if clinical or arterial blood gas studies suggest alveolar hypoventilation, mechanical control of ventilation will also be necessary.

Maximum inspiratory and expiratory flow volume curves and flexible fiberoptic nasopharyngoscopy or bronchoscopy has been found to be helpful in the early assessment of the extent of tracheobronchial injury and the likelihood of subsequently developing airway obstruction (Herdon et al, 1987).

Although there may be some delay in the clinical evidence of respiratory tract injury resulting from smoke inhalation, manifestations of respiratory distress (including tachypnea, cough, hoarseness, and stridor) and auscultatory evidence of respiratory tract damage (including decreased breath sounds, wheezes, rhonchi, and rales) are usually present by 12 to 24 hours and perhaps sooner. Roentgenographic evidence of pulmonary disease is usually not very helpful in the early diagnosis, because positive findings may lag several hours or more behind auscultatory evidence of damage. In older individuals, abnormal retention of ^{133}Xe in the lungs at 90 sec on lung scans has been used as a sensitive test of early lung injury; these patients also have decreased airflow rates and elevated airflow resistance.

There is a growing consensus that clearance of inhaled aerosol containing technetium-labeled diethylenetriaminepentacetate ([99m]TcDTPA) may be used as an index of pulmonary epithelial cell injury. Thus injury to the alveolar capillary membrane by smoke inhalation may be detected early by increased clearance of ^{99m}TcDTPA. The experimental basis for this has already been published (Witten et al, 1988); unfortunately, a preliminary study in patients has not confirmed this (Clark et al, 1988).

Respiratory insufficiency may occur early in the course of smoke inhalation, not only as the result of asphyxia and CO poisoning, but also as the result of airway obstruction. This may occur from edema anywhere along the laryngotracheobronchial tree or at the alveolar level. It may be difficult to localize the level of obstruction; therefore, whenever there is clinical evidence of severe obstruction, the upper airways should be assessed by direct or indirect laryngoscopy before swelling of the head, neck, or oropharynx and trismus make this examination difficult. Fiberoptic bronchoscopy may be very useful to evaluate the extent of mucosal damage, but intense vasoconstriction in hypovolemic patients may mask this (Shirani et al, 1988).

Measurements of Pulmonary Function

Although studies of pulmonary function measurements in the pediatric age group are not available, reports in adults indicate their usefulness in recognizing abnormalities early and in following course and severity of disease. Positive ^{133}Xe scintiphotographic scans and abnormal single-breath nitrogen test results indicating maldistribution of ventilation have been noted within the first 72 hours after smoke inhalation (Petroff et al, 1976). Smoke inhalation results in severe airway obstruction within 9 hours, with reduced forced vital capacity and FEV_1; improvement then gradually occurs. Maximum improvement has taken as long as 5 months, indicating the prolonged nature of the lung injury. For patients with surface burns, the reduction in forced vital capacity and FEV_1 correlates with the extent of surface burns and reflects chest wall restriction and perhaps increased lung water (Whitener et al, 1980).

TREATMENT

As already indicated, the initial treatment should focus on reversing CO poisoning, if present, by administration of humidified oxygen. Subsequently, the administration of oxygen may be important because of the hypoxemia resulting from bronchiolitis and alveolitis with premature closure of small airways. Constant distending airway pressure, whether administered positively at the mouth or negatively around the body, may also be necessary to maintain reasonable levels of Pa_{O_2} without using excessively high concentrations of inspired oxygen.

Intubation of the trachea may be necessary when there are (1) severe burns of the nose, face, or mouth, because of the likelihood that nasopharyngeal edema and obstruction will develop; (2) edema of the vocal cords with laryngeal obstruction; (3) difficulty in handling secretions; and (4) progressive respiratory insufficiency requiring mechanical assistance to ventilation. Although there is considerable disagreement about when to perform tracheostomy, in general it makes more sense to perform the procedure in patients in whom the obstruction is proximal to the larynx, and to use nasotracheal intubation if lower portions of the respiratory tract are involved. Regardless of whether the glottis is bypassed by endotracheal tube or tracheostomy tube, small amounts of constant positive airway pressure or positive end-expiratory pressure may be helpful to minimize edema and improve oxygenation.

In addition to the increase in airway resistance resulting from edema in and around the walls of the airways, it is likely that some reflex bronchoconstriction occurs from irritation of airway receptors. For this reason, it seems reasonable to administer bronchodilators such as isoproterenol or theophylline or some of the relatively selective bronchodilators, such as terbutaline or albuterol.

As in many other conditions, the role of chest physiotherapy is yet to be clearly defined. Nevertheless, the encouragement of deep breathing and cough or gentle endotracheal suction in the presence of endotracheal intubation coupled with postural drainage would seem to be reasonable.

Although the use of corticosteroids is frequently advocated in the hope of suppressing inflammation and edema, most control studies evaluating their use in other conditions, such as pneumonitis resulting from aspiration of gastric contents or hydrocarbons, have failed to demonstrate a significant effect. Thus it is difficult to marshal strong support for the use of corticosteroids based on the experience with other forms of chemical injury to the lung. Furthermore, the long-term use of steroid therapy in victims of fires is likely to be deleterious because it increases the susceptibility to infection. To what extent the cerebral edema that complicates asphyxial injury responds to corticosteroids is also not clear. Until further evidence is available, it may not be unreasonable to give one large dose of corticosteroids early in the course of smoke inhalation and then to focus on other therapeutic modalities, including the use of bronchodilators, constant distending airway pressures, and mechanical support of ventilation. Whether cyclooxygenase inhibitors will have a useful role is still not clear. At the experimental level, ibuprofen but not indomethacin when given immediately after smoke inhalation injury prevented the development of pulmonary edema (Shinozawa et al, 1986).

The available evidence indicates that the use of antimicrobial agents does not prevent the subsequent development of infection and may only predispose to the emergence of resistant organisms. Because fever, white blood cell count, and erythrocyte sedimentation rate all may be elevated as a result of smoke inhalation, and because the chest roentgenogram may show nonspecific opacities that represent either atelectasis or edema, it may be extremely difficult to establish the presence of an infection in the absence of positive blood cultures. Under these circumstances, it would seem preferable, at present, to reserve the use of antimicrobial therapy for those patients in whom there is clinical deterioration in spite of supportive therapy. Because the prevention of infection is clearly an important part of the therapy in victims of fires, aseptic care of the trachea and humidifying equipment is essential.

THE RELATION OF PULMONARY INJURY FROM SMOKE INHALATION TO THE PULMONARY COMPLICATIONS OF SURFACE BURNS

It is our present view that pulmonary damage from smoke inhalation declares itself during the first 24 hours. Individuals with widespread surface burns may develop pulmonary complications after several days, but it is our current notion that these late complications are not the result of direct chemical or thermal injuries to the respiratory tract from smoke inhalation. We think it more than likely that the late pulmonary injury is attributable to complex metabolic, infectious, or circulatory derangements complicating the surface burns (Herndon et al, 1987). Because of the present tendency to administer fluids aggressively to patients who are victims of fires, especially when there are surface burns with loss of serum proteins, it seems likely that some of the increase in pulmonary opacities seen in chest roentgenograms after 2 or 3 days may represent pulmonary edema that is, in part at least, the result of aggressive fluid therapy. There may be an advantage to maintaining colloid cosmotic pressure with salt-poor albumin infusion. Extensive circumferential burns of the thorax and abdomen may lead to unyielding eschar, producing restriction of thoracic and abdominal wall movement with concomitant impairment of ventilatory function. Prospective studies of burned patients with inhalation injury has failed to reveal any beneficial effects of corticosteroids or aerosolized antimicrobial agents.

REFERENCES

Lung Injury from Hydrocarbon Aspiration

Albert WC and Inkley SR: The efficacy of steroid therapy in the treatment of experimental kerosene pneumonitis. Am Rev Respir Dis 98:888, 1968.
Bergeson PS, Hales SW, Lustgarten MD, and Lipson HW: Pneumatoceles following hydrocarbon ingestion. Am J Dis Child 129:49, 1975.
Bratton L and Haddow JE: Ingestion of charcoal lighter fluid. J Pediatr 87:633, 1975.
Daeschner CW, Blattner RJ, and Collins VP: Hydrocarbon pneumonitis. Pediatr Clin North Am 4:243, 1957.
Dice WH, Ward G, Kelley J, and Kilpatrick WR: Pulmonary toxicity following gastrointestinal ingestion of kerosene. Ann Emerg Med 11:138, 1982.

Eade NR, Taussig LM, and Marks MI: Hydrocarbon pneumonitis. Pediatrics 54:351, 1974.
Gerarde HW: Toxicological studies on hydrocarbons. V. Kerosene. Toxicol Appl Pharmacol 1:462, 1959.
Giammona ST: Effects of furniture polish on pulmonary surfactant. Am J Dis Child 113:658, 1967.
Gross P, McNerney JM, and Babyak MA: Kerosene pneumonitis: an experimental study with small doses. Am Rev Respir Dis 88:656, 1963.
Gurwitz D, Kattan M, Levison H, and Culham JAG: Pulmonary function abnormalities in asymptomatic children after hydrocarbon pneumonitis. Pediatrics 62:789, 1978.
Hardman G, Tolson R, and Baghdassarian O: Prednisone in the management of kerosene pneumonia. Indian Pract 13:615, 1960.
Huxtable KA, Bolande RP, and Klaus M: Experimental furniture polish pneumonia in rats. Pediatrics 34:228, 1964.
James JW, Kaplan S, and Benzing G: Cardiac complications following hydrocarbon ingestion. Am J Dis Child 121:431, 1971.
Klein BL and Simon JE: Hydrocarbon poisonings. Pediatr Clin North Am 33:41, 1986.
Marks MI, Chicoine L, Legere G, and Hillman E: Adrenocorticosteroid treatment of hydrocarbon pneumonia in children—a cooperative study. J Pediatr 81:366, 1972.
Mellins RB, Christian JR, and Bundesen HN: The natural history of poisoning in childhood. Pediatrics 17:314, 1956.
Pearn J, Nixon J, Ansford A, and Corcoran A: Accidental poisoning in childhood: five year urban population study with 15 year analysis of fatality. Br Med J 288:44, 1984.
Poklis A and Burkett CD: Gasoline sniffing: a review. Clin Toxicol 11:35, 1977.
Richardson JA and Pratt-Thomas HR: Toxic effects of varying doses of kerosene administered by different routes. Am J Med Sci 221:531, 1951.
Scharf SM, Heimer D, and Goldstein J: Pathologic and physiologic effects of aspiration of hydrocarbons in the rat. Am Rev Respir Dis 124:625, 1981.
Steele RW, Conklin RH, and Mark HM: Corticosteroids and antibiotics for the treatment of fulminant hydrocarbon aspiration. JAMA 219:1434, 1972.
Tal A, Aviram M, Bar Ziv J, and Scharf SM: Residual small airways lesions after kerosene pneumonitis in early childhood. Eur J Pediatr 142:117, 1984.
Wolfe BM, Brodeur AE, and Shields JB: The role of gastrointestinal absorption of kerosene in producing pneumonitis in dogs. J Pediatr 76:867, 1970.
Wolfsdorf J: Kerosene intoxication: an experimental approach to the etiology of the CNS manifestation in primates. J Pediatr 88:1037, 1976.
Wolfsdorf J and Kundig H: Kerosene poisoning in primates. S Afr Med J 46:619, 1972.
Wolfsdorf J and Kundig H: Dexamethasone in the management of kerosene pneumonia. Pediatr Res 7:432, 1973.
Wyse DG: Deliberate inhalation of volatile hydrocarbon: a review. Can Med Assoc J 108:71, 1973.

Respiratory Complications of Smoke Inhalation

Burns TR, Greenberg SD, Cartwright J, and Jackimczyk JA: Smoke inhalation: an ultrastructural study of reaction to injury in the human alveolar wall. Environ Res 41:447, 1986.
Clark WR, Grossman ZD, Ritter-Hrncirik BS, and Warner F: Clearance of aerosolized 99Tc-diethylenetriaminepentacetate before and after smoke inhalation. Chest 94:22, 1988.
Cox ME, Heslop BF, Kempton JJ, and Ratcliff RA: The Dellwood fire. Br Med J 1:942, 1955.
Grunnet ML: Long-term nervous system effects resulting from carbon monoxide exposure. In Physiological and Toxicological Aspects of Combustion Products. International Symposium. Washington, DC, National Academy of Sciences, 1976.
Herndon DN, Langner F, Thompson P, et al: Pulmonary injury in burned patients. Surg Clin North Am 67:31, 1987.
Lloyd EL and MacRae WR: Respiratory tract damage in burns. Br J Anaesth 43:365, 1971.
Mellins RB and Park S: Respiratory complications of smoke inhalation in victims of fires. J Pediatr 87:1, 1975.

Petroff PA, Hander EW, Clayton WH, and Pruitt BA: Pulmonary function studies after smoke inhalation. Am J Surg 132:346, 1976.

Quinby WC Jr: Restrictive effects of thoracic burns in children. J Trauma 12:646, 1972.

Root WS: Carbon monoxide. In Fenn WO and Rahn H (eds): Handbook of Physiology, Section 3: Respiration. Vol II. Washington, DC, American Physiological Society, 1965.

Shinozawa Y, Hales C, Jung W, and Burke J: Ibuprofen prevents synthetic smoke-induced pulmonary edema. Am Rev Respir Dis 134:1145, 1986.

Shirani KZ, Moylan JA, and Pruitt BA Jr: Diagnosis and treatment of inhalation injury in burn patients. In Loke J (ed): Pthophy-

siology and Treatment of Inhalation Injuries. Vol 34. Lung Biology in Health and Disease. Marcel Dekker, New York, 1988.

Traber DL, Herndon DN, Stein MD, et al: The pulmonary lesion of smoke inhalation in an ovine model. Circ Shock, 18:311, 1986.

Whitener DN, Whitener LM, Robertson KJ et al: Pulmonary function measurements in patients with thermal injury and smoke inhalation. Am Rev Respir Dis 122:731, 1980.

Witten ML, Quan SF, Sobonya RE, and Leman RJ: New developments in the pathogenesis of smoke inhalation-induced pulmonary edema. West J Med 148:33, 1988.

Zimmerman SS and Truxal B: Carbon monoxide poisoning. Pediatrics 68:215, 1981.

29

JEROME H. MODELL, M.D.

DROWNING AND NEAR-DROWNING

Drowning is one of the three leading causes of accidental death in the United States (Zugzda, 1969, 1973). Unfortunately, there are no national statistics that reflect the large group of persons who "near-drown" and then either recover uneventfully or suffer permanent neurologic damage. One report noted an 89 per cent survival rate in 121 patients admitted to three hospitals from 1963 to 1980 who had a diagnosis of near-drowning (Modell et al, 1980). If these figures are extrapolated to the national population by using published mortality data, as many as 1,226,000 patients may have been treated for near-drowning during the past 25 years. In addition, many persons are resuscitated at the scene of the accident and are never admitted to a hospital. Therefore, this figure of more than 1 million victims is probably an underestimation.

The highest incidence of drowning occurs in the second decade of life (Press et al, 1968). Most of the victims were healthy and had a normal life expectancy before their accidents. Unlike patients who are treated for a progressive, incapacitating illness, near-drowned victims, after successful therapy, usually have a normal life span of health and productivity.

Approximately 65 per cent of those who died from drowning were unable to swim (Webster, 1967). More than half of those who drown in swimming pools in the United States are children under the age of 10 (Webster, 1967). These statistics emphasize the importance of early swimming instruction, water safety instruction, and proper pool fencing. Approximately one third of drowned victims were adequate swimmers who overexerted themselves by attempting to

swim distances beyond their capabilities; these victims either swam long distances underwater after hyperventilating or disregarded boating and fishing safety rules, e.g., failed to use life preservers and then had to try to swim to shore (Press et al, 1968). Therefore, it is important not only to offer proper swimming instruction early but also to emphasize continually the potential hazards of inadequate safety measures for water sports. Unfortunately, in spite of intensified instructional efforts, loss of life from aquatic accidents continues. It is necessary, therefore, to understand in depth the pathophysiologic changes that occur during near-drowning to ensure an orderly approach to resuscitation.

Ten per cent of drowned victims do not actually aspirate water (Cot, 1931) but die from acute asphyxia while submerged, perhaps because of reflex laryngospasm or breath-holding. No two near-drowned victims aspirate exactly the same quantity of water. The type of water aspirated can be fresh water, seawater, or brackish water. No two near-drowned victims are exactly alike physiologically. The state of health of two victims immediately before the same type of accident may have differed considerably, and various quantities of water may have been aspirated. Some patients may have submerged after maximal inhalation, and others after maximal exhalation. Thus, the length of time before irreversible hypoxia occurs may vary. The circumstances of the accident also influence pathophysiologic effects. Some patients may have been submerged in very cold water, and others in warm water. One patient may succumb in the water from physical exhaustion.

Another may hyperventilate before entering the water and then, swimming underwater, may lose consciousness from cerebral hypoxia. Still another may fall into the water, receive a blow to the head, and suffer a concussion. A victim may have become severely ill or may have died of some disease and then subsequently may have fallen into the water. For example, an elderly patient may suffer a myocardial infarction during swimming, may lose consciousness, and then may aspirate fluid as a terminal event. All these factors must be considered when describing an individual patient (Davis, 1971). Therefore, review of the pathophysiologic studies of drowning and near-drowning should serve as valuable background for understanding the problems that arise in treating the individual patient.

PATHOPHYSIOLOGY

CHANGES IN BLOOD GAS, ACID-BASE, AND PULMONARY STATUS

The single most important consequence of near-drowning is hypoxemia (Modell et al, 1966). The degree and duration of hypoxemia depend on the length of submersion and on whether or not the patient aspirates fluid. Initially, hypoxemia is accompanied by hypercarbia and acidosis (Modell et al, 1966). A mammal responds to total immersion in liquid by holding its breath or closing its vocal cords, or both (Coryllos, 1938; Lougheed et al, 1939). Approximately 10 per cent of drowned humans die without actually aspirating fluid (Cot, 1931). Experiments using anesthetized, intubated dogs demonstrate that when laryngospasm is simulated by occluding the endotracheal tube, the carbon dioxide tension increases only 3 to 6 mm Hg per minute, and the pH decreases approximately 0.05 unit per minute. However, arterial oxygen tension (Pa_{O_2}) drops precipitously from the normal control values that existed immediately before tracheal obstruction to approximately 40 mm Hg after 1 min of obstruction, to 10 mm Hg after 3 min, and to 4 mm Hg after 5 min (Modell et al, 1972). In another study, Kristoffersen and co-workers (1967) reported that a decrease in Pa_{O_2} to 10 to 15 mm Hg was uniformly fatal in dogs. However, Modell and colleagues (1972) have shown that 80 per cent of dogs anesthetized with barbiturates could be resuscitated by ventilating their lungs with air 5 min after the onset of tracheal obstruction, even though their mean Pa_{O_2} was 4 mm Hg. Whether the barbiturate anesthetic protected these animals is speculative. However, some investigators report that barbiturates can protect the brain against hypoxia (Michenfelder and Theye, 1973).

In two studies reported in 1961, Craig demonstrated the importance of hypoxia as a cause of death in persons who hyperventilate before swimming underwater. In studying the breaking point of breath-holding in human volunteers simulating underwater

swimming, he found that point to be 87 sec at rest, at which time the carbon dioxide tension of alveolar air (PA_{CO_2}) was 51 mm Hg and the oxygen tension (PA_{O_2}) was 73 mm Hg. After hyperventilation, breath-holding could be maintained for 146 sec. In this instance, the PA_{CO_2} rose to only 46 mm Hg but the PA_{O_2} dropped to 58 mm Hg. When exercise followed hyperventilation, the breath-holding point dropped to 85 sec and the PA_{CO_2} remained fairly constant at 49 mm Hg. However, the PA_{O_2} dropped further to 43 mm Hg. Craig postulated that if the swimmer hyperventilates before swimming underwater, the Pa_{CO_2} remains low. The swimmer therefore consciously represses the urge to breathe, then suffers cerebral hypoxia, loses consciousness, and begins to breathe while submerged (Craig, 1961a).

In treating 91 human victims of near-drowning, my colleagues and I have seen 10 patients (12 per cent) who probably suffered near-drowning without aspiration (Modell et al, 1976). This diagnosis was based on the patients' histories and on the fact that on admission to the hospital, their Pa_{O_2} levels were over 80 mm Hg while they spontaneously breathed room air. In these cases, mouth-to-mouth resuscitation had been given promptly at the scene of the accident, and spontaneous ventilation had returned rapidly. In some, closed-chest cardiac massage had also been necessary. If victims of near-drowning without aspiration are ventilated artificially before circulation ceases or before irreversible damage to the cardiovascular and central nervous systems occurs, recovery will be dramatic and complete. If spontaneous ventilation begins while the patient is still underwater, however, aspiration will occur and treatment will be more complicated.

When a near-drowning victim aspirates, even though the initial hypercarbia may be reversed rapidly by increasing the patient's minute alveolar ventilation, and even though respiratory acidosis may disappear, the patient frequently is left with persistent arterial hypoxemia and metabolic acidosis (Modell, Davis, Giammona et al, 1968). A Pa_{O_2} as low as 17 mm Hg (Modell et al, 1980) and a pH as low as 6.77 (Modell et al, 1976) have been reported. The metabolic acidosis frequently requires the administration of sodium bicarbonate. In 76 patients who had bicarbonate levels calculated after near-drowning, 55 had levels of 20 mEq/L or less. In 10 patients, the levels were as low as 6 to 10 mEq/L (Modell et al, 1976). The arterial hypoxemia that occurs can be profound and will persist as long as significant intrapulmonary pathologic conditions continue unless aggressive therapy is instituted.

Although hypoxia occurs when either fresh water or seawater is aspirated, the factors contributing to hypoxia may differ between the two fluids. In either case, pulmonary compliance decreases (Colebatch and Halmagyi, 1961, 1962, 1963; Halmagyi and Colebatch, 1961). However, after the aspiration of seawater, the primary problem is fluid-filled but perfused alveoli (Modell et al, 1967). They respond as they would in atelectasis and produce a large intrapulmonary shunt. Because seawater is hypertonic, fluid is drawn from the plasma into the alveoli. For example, in animals that aspirate 22 ml/kg seawater, an average of 33 ml/kg can be drained by gravity from the lungs after 5 min (Modell et al, 1973). On the other hand, when experimental animals aspirate fresh water, significant amounts of fluid cannot be drained from the lungs because the fluid is absorbed into the circulation (Modell and Moya, 1966). When fresh water is aspirated, the surface tension properties of pulmonary surfactant are altered (Giammona and Modell, 1967). As a result, the alveoli become unstable and atelectasis occurs, which, in turn, produces an intrapulmonary shunt and hypoxemia (Modell, Moya, Williams, and Weibley, 1968). Other factors that might contribute to pulmonary edema and to the alteration of ventilation-perfusion ratio ($\dot{V}/\dot{Q}$) in patients who aspirate fresh water are pulmonary hypertension and cerebral hypoxia (Moss et al, 1972).

Various microscopic findings have been reported after fluid aspiration. With electron microscopy, no changes were seen in rats that had aspirated small quantities of fresh water (Halmagyi, 1961). On the other hand, when lungs of rats were perfused through the trachea with large quantities of fresh water, the alveolar septa widened, the capillaries collapsed, the number of red blood cells decreased, the endothelial and septal cell nuclei became engorged, the mitochondria became swollen, and the cell outlines were obliterated (Reidbord and Spitz, 1966). After aspiration of small quantities of seawater, the lung weight increased and intra-alveolar hemorrhages were seen (Halmagyi, 1961). After aspiration of large volumes of seawater, however, the changes were less marked than those observed after the aspiration of large quantities of fresh water (Reidbord and Spitz, 1966). Thus the microscopic changes that occur differ when very small or very large quantities of different types of water are aspirated. This finding may account for some of the differences reported in autopsies of human drowning victims.

Another condition commonly found at autopsy performed soon after drowning is hyperexpansion of the lungs with areas that resemble those occurring in acute emphysema (Davis, 1971). This could result from the rupture of alveoli when the airway pressure fluctuates widely during violent ventilatory efforts against a closed glottis or when a column of water obstructs the airway during submersion. If the patient survives for at least 12 hours after near-drowning only to die later, the lungs frequently show evidence of bronchopneumonia, multiple abscesses, mechanical injury, and deposition of hyaline material in the alveoli (Fuller, 1963a, 1963b; Modell, Davis, Giammona, et al, 1968).

Placing positive end-expiratory pressure (PEEP) on the airway of anesthetized animals after near-drowning with seawater markedly increases the Pa_{O_2} in animals that either breathe spontaneously or are ventilated mechanically (Modell et al, 1974). These studies suggest that the use of PEEP increases functional residual capacity, which minimizes intrapulmonary shunting and ventilation-perfusion abnormalities and promotes better oxygenation.

Similar studies of freshwater aspiration demonstrated an improvement in Pa_{O_2} when mechanical ventilation was combined with PEEP. However, no consistent improvement in Pa_{O_2} was seen when PEEP of 10 cm H_2O was applied in spontaneously breathing animals (Ruiz et al, 1973). Subsequent studies demonstrated that applying continuous positive airway pressure (CPAP) in dogs that breathed spontaneously after the aspiration of fresh water resulted in a variable response. In some, the shunting was completely reversed, whereas in others as much as 40 per cent of the cardiac output was still shunted (Bergquist et al, 1980). The difference in results between the studies performed with fresh water and with seawater may be that in order to overcome surfactant changes after the aspiration of fresh water, the alveoli must be inflated mechanically by higher peak inspiratory pressure before PEEP or CPAP can effectively keep alveoli inflated. On the other hand, because pulmonary surfactant characteristics are normal after seawater aspiration, the spontaneous respiration of the animal might be sufficient to inflate the alveoli, and PEEP or CPAP might help to keep them partially inflated.

It should be emphasized that in two of the three studies described in the previous paragraphs (Modell et al, 1974; Ruiz et al, 1973), PEEP was set at 10 cm H_2O in all animals. Clinically, it is our practice to titrate PEEP or CPAP to produce the minimal degree of pulmonary venous admixture or intrapulmonary shunt without decreasing cardiac output (Kirby et al, 1975). It has been demonstrated in human victims of near-drowning that titration of CPAP does improve $\dot{V}/\dot{Q}$ and arterial oxygenation, not only when ventilation is controlled but also during spontaneous ventilation with intermittent mandatory breaths from a ventilator, as needed, to clear carbon dioxide (Modell and Downs, 1976).

BLOOD VOLUME AND SERUM ELECTROLYTES

In addition to the acute pulmonary effects and the changes in blood gas tensions and acid-base balance that occur, aspiration of hypotonic (fresh water) or hypertonic (seawater) fluid can result in a number of changes in other systems. The extent and direction of these changes depend on the quantity and nature of the fluid aspirated.

In general, the greater the volume of water that is aspirated, the greater are the changes. If 11 ml/kg of fluid or less is aspirated, it is unlikely that persistent changes will occur in any system other than those caused by fluid in the lungs (Modell, 1968). However, if more than 11 ml/kg of hypotonic fluid is aspirated, the blood volume increases in direct proportion to the quantity of the fluid aspirated (Modell, 1968). Conversely, blood volume decreases linearly as the quantity of aspirated seawater increases (Modell et al, 1967). In instances of total immersion, blood volume may increase as much as 160 per cent after freshwater aspiration (Modell and Moya, 1966) and may decrease to approximately 65 per cent of the normal value after seawater aspiration (Modell et al, 1967). Tabeling and Modell (1983) reported that even though blood volume increased acutely when 11 or 22 ml/kg of fresh water was aspirated, by 60 min after aspiration, blood volume was lower than it had been before aspiration. This change likely reflects the redistribution of the hypotonic fluid to body tissues and to the lungs as edema fluid.

Most patients do not aspirate enough fluid to cause life-threatening changes in blood volume. Thus, although it is important to check the effective circulating blood volume by measuring the patient's central venous pressure and pulmonary artery occlusion pressure (PAOP) as appropriate, blood volume changes requiring urgent treatment usually are not seen. Any significant decrease in the effective circulating blood volume usually results from the loss of fluid from the vascular space into the lung. In victims of severe near-drowning, significant amounts of fluid can be lost into the lung as pulmonary edema and requires fluid replacement.

Changes that occur in serum electrolyte concentrations after drowning and near-drowning also depend on both the type and the volume of water aspirated and are inversely proportional to changes in blood volume. Experiments have shown that if dogs aspirate 22 ml/kg of fresh water or less, significant changes in extracellular serum electrolytes do not persist (Modell and Moya, 1966). Another study demonstrated that less than 15 per cent of human drowning victims who died in the water had serum electrolyte concentrations indicating the aspiration of more than 22 ml/kg of water (Modell and Davis, 1969). This might explain why significant changes in serum electrolyte concentrations have not been reported in near-drowned humans.

My colleagues and I studied electrolyte concentrations in 83 patients who near-drowned in fresh water, seawater, or brackish water (Modell et al, 1976). In the freshwater victims, mean concentrations were as follows: serum sodium, 138 mEq/L; serum chloride, 97 mEq/L; and serum potassium, 3.9 mEq/L. Victims of seawater near-drowning had these mean concentrations: serum sodium, 146 mEq/L; serum chloride, 103 mEq/L; and serum potassium, 3.9 mEq/L. The ranges of values for both groups together were as follows: serum sodium, 126 to 160 mEq/L; serum chloride, 86 to 126 mEq/L; and serum potassium, 2.4 to 6.3 mEq/L. Although the seawater victims showed a slight to moderate increase in the concentrations of extracellular serum electrolytes, in no case were these concentrations life threatening. This finding suggests that immediate therapy for electrolyte

changes after near-drowning is seldom necessary and that each patient's electrolyte status should be evaluated before corrective therapy is initiated.

HEMOGLOBIN AND HEMATOCRIT VALUES

In instances of seawater aspiration, one might predict an increase in the hemoglobin and hematocrit values of whole blood because of hemoconcentration and, after freshwater aspiration, a decrease resulting from hemodilution. However, when the hemoglobin and hematocrit values of 83 near-drowned victims were analyzed, the mean value for hemoglobin in victims near-drowned in fresh water was 13.2 g/100 ml. The value was 13.4 g/100 ml for those near-drowned in seawater (Modell et al, 1976). Likewise, there was no difference in the mean hematocrit concentrations between the two groups of patients. Marked changes in hemoglobin and hematocrit values rarely are reported, which further substantiates the hypothesis that near-drowned humans do not aspirate huge quantities of fluid.

When large volumes of fresh water are absorbed, hemolysis of red blood cells can occur and can cause plasma hemoglobin to increase. This hemolysis is not due solely to hypotonicity but is strongly related to the Pa_{O_2}. When 44 ml/kg of distilled water was injected rapidly into the superior vena cava of animals and they were permitted to breathe spontaneously so that Pa_{O_2} remained within reasonable limits, the plasma hemoglobin levels were not significantly elevated. On the other hand, when tracheal obstruction was combined with the infusion of the same quantity of water, plasma hemoglobin concentrations in excess of 1000 mg/100 ml were noted (Modell et al, 1972). This further emphasizes the importance of establishing adequate arterial oxygenation in near-drowned victims.

CARDIOVASCULAR SYSTEM

The cardiovascular system of most near-drowned humans shows remarkable stability. Experimental evidence suggests that changes in cardiovascular function during near-drowning are caused predominantly by changes in Pa_{O_2} and acid-base balance (Noble and Sharpe, 1963; Modell and Moya, 1966; Modell et al, 1967, 1976; Modell, Davis, Giammona et al, 1968; Modell, Moya, Williams, and Weibley, 1968). Variations in blood volume and serum electrolyte concentrations also can contribute to cardiovascular changes. However, less than 15 per cent of drowned victims aspirate enough water to cause such changes (Modell and Davis, 1969).

A wide variety of electrocardiographic changes have been reported in experimental studies of drowning and near-drowning in both fresh water and seawater. The early literature emphasizes that ventricular fibrillation occurs secondary to freshwater drowning (Swann et al, 1947; Swann and Brucer, 1949). It has been shown, however, that death from ventricular fibrillation does not occur in dogs that aspirate 22 ml/kg of fresh water or less (Modell and Moya, 1966). On the other hand, when at least 44 ml/kg was aspirated, ventricular fibrillation occurred in as many as 80 per cent of the animals studied (Modell and Moya, 1966). Only two cases of documented ventricular fibrillation after near-drowning have been reported in humans (Middleton, 1962; Redding, 1965).

Arterial blood pressure after near-drowning has been reported to be normal, high, or low (Rath, 1953; Dumitru and Hamilton, 1963; Fainer, 1963; Modell, 1963; Munroe, 1964). Changes from normal pressure seem to be secondary to the state of oxygenation, acid-base balance, cardiac function, and the level of circulating catecholamines. Measurements of central venous pressure and PAOP usually reflect the effective circulating blood volume. Low values in near-drowned victims usually indicate an acute decrease in blood volume, which occurs when plasma is lost into the lungs.

When sublethal volumes of fresh water are aspirated experimentally, cardiac output has been shown to decrease and then to return toward normal. But when animals are mechanically ventilated, and especially when mechanical ventilation and PEEP are administered simultaneously, a significant decrease in cardiac output recurs (Bergquist et al, 1980). In this case, the magnitude of the decrease in cardiac output when mechanical ventilation and 15 cm H_2O PEEP are applied can be greater than 50 per cent of the normal value. Therefore, even though mechanical ventilation and PEEP restore the Pa_{O_2} to almost normal, oxygen delivery is marginal. In this animal model, attempting to drive the heart with dopamine does not restore a normal cardiac output, but increasing the effective circulating blood volume with a rapid infusion of crystalloid does restore cardiac output to normal levels with only a minimal change in intrapulmonary shunt. Thus, the Pa_{O_2} remains high, the cardiac output is restored to normal, and the oxygen delivery is increased (Tabeling and Modell, 1982).

RENAL FUNCTION

Renal function remains intact in most patients who are resuscitated after near-drowning, although albuminuria, hemoglobinuria, oliguria, or anuria can occur (Rath, 1953; Fuller, 1963b; Kvittingen and Naess, 1963; King and Webster, 1964; Munroe, 1964; Redding and Pearson, 1964; Gambino, 1969). Renal damage also may progress to acute tubular necrosis (Fuller, 1963b). It is not known whether this is secondary to severe lactic acidosis, hypoxemia, or both, or to the biochemical effects of the aspirated water. In any event, such severe changes are rare. Attention must be paid to renal function to permit

early therapy and to help prevent permanent damage.

EFFECT OF TEMPERATURE

The temperature of the water in which a person is submerged is important, because immersion of the face in water colder than 20°C may evoke the *diving reflex:* bradycardia, peripheral vasoconstriction, and preferential perfusion of the heart and brain (Gordon, 1972). Immersion of the whole body in cold water leads to significant hypothermia that protects the patient by prolonging the length of time that hypoxia can be tolerated before the irreversible destruction of tissue occurs. On the other hand, profound hypothermia (< 25 to 28°C) may precipitate ventricular dysrhythmia that by itself can lead to death.

NEUROLOGIC FUNCTION

The question is frequently asked, How long can a person remain submerged and still be resuscitated? There are reports of individuals being resuscitated after submersion in fresh water for 10 min (Ohlsson and Beckman, 1964), 20 min (Ohlsson and Beckman, 1964), 22 min (Kvittingen and Naess, 1963), and 40 min (Siebke et al, 1975) and in seawater for 17 min (King and Webster, 1964). All of these patients were hypothermic, and three of them suffered prolonged neurologic deficits. However, approximately 1 year later, all functioned normally.

The possibility of resuscitating a near-drowned victim who may have a prolonged neurologic deficit is always present. However, the cases just cited indicate the tremendous variation in the human capacity to tolerate submersion and subsequent hypoxemia and should encourage physicians and rescuers to maintain resuscitative efforts as long as possible. In a series of 81 survivors from a total of 91 near-drowned victims, my colleagues and I have seen only two patients who had residual neurologic damage (Modell et al, 1976). In both instances, the patients were still in a state of cardiac arrest when brought to the emergency room.

THERAPY

The prime objective of emergency therapy for near-drowned victims is to restore arterial blood gas and acid-base levels to normal as rapidly as possible. Thus immediate rescue and initial therapy of near-drowned victims are crucial to the outcome. Although, theoretically, the use of appliances would facilitate rescue in the water, such items are rarely available at the scene of the accident. Because the degree of hypoxia increases rapidly with continuing apnea, it is imperative that emergency measures be taken to initiate ventilation. Some rescuers can deliver mouth-to-mouth or mouth-to-nose respiration while the victim is still in the water. Others find this impossible because of limited swimming ability.

Artificial respiration should be given to apneic near-drowned victims as soon as possible. Many external chest compression methods to administer artificial ventilation have been reported during the years. Yet there is little question that the most effective methods available are still mouth-to-mouth and mouth-to-nose ventilation (Safar et al, 1958). To ensure adequate ventilation with these methods, the rescuer must obtain an adequate airway by clearing the patient's mouth of foreign objects and by supporting the airway by elevating the jaw and soft tissues. Placing an appliance, such as a nasopharyngeal, oropharyngeal, or endotracheal airway, is necessary occasionally. However, in most patients an adequate airway can be achieved without such devices. Furthermore, inserting an appliance in a partially responsive patient may precipitate laryngospasm or vomiting, and the latter may lead to the aspiration of stomach contents.

Recently, some have advocated that an abdominal thrust (Heimlich maneuver) should either replace or precede mouth-to-mouth ventilation. Heimlich (1981) suggests that using this procedure eliminates aspirated water from the lungs and airways and washes out bacteria and particulate material. Because humans usually do not aspirate large quantities of water and any fresh water that is aspirated is absorbed rapidly, reports of water gushing out of the patient's mouth with this technique likely describe liquid forced from the stomach. If this liquid is aspirated, it further complicates the pulmonary injury. Werner and colleagues (1982) showed experimentally that the abdominal thrust was not helpful after seawater aspiration. Gordon and Terranova (1981) report a case in which the Heimlich maneuver clearly was effective; the effectiveness of the technique, however, was in removing an aspirated foreign body (a piece of celery) from a near-drowned child's trachea. Use of the Heimlich maneuver in this circumstance was consistent with the recommendations of the American Heart Association (1987). Both Orlowski (1987) and Ornato (1986) point out the possible complications of using the Heimlich maneuver in near-drowned patients: aspiration of stomach contents and delay in ventilation and oxygenation. Therefore, the abdominal thrust should be reserved for patients in whom solid material obstructs the larynx and thus prevents establishing a clear airway and applying effective mouth-to-mouth ventilation.

Victims of drowning and near-drowning frequently swallow large quantities of water before losing consciousness. Thus, another important reason to ensure a free airway is to prevent pressure from overdistending the stomach during resuscitation. If gastric distention does occur, the patient may regurgitate and then may aspirate acidic gastric contents, which may cause aspiration pneumonitis (Wynne and Modell, 1977). During the initial phase of resuscitation, extreme care should be taken to avoid causing aspiration of gastric contents.

If a victim has not aspirated water and if effective ventilation is established before permanent circulatory or neurologic changes occur, the prognosis is excellent. If water has been aspirated, as discussed earlier in this chapter, persistent alterations of pulmonary function occur. In general, time should not be wasted trying to drain water from the lungs of a victim near-drowned in fresh water (Ruben and Ruben, 1962). On the other hand, because seawater is hypertonic, fluid is drawn from the circulation into the lungs of such a victim (Modell et al, 1967, 1974). It has been shown that the survival rate in animals that have aspirated large quantities of seawater can be increased if their lungs are drained by gravity (Modell et al, 1974). Because drowned and near-drowned humans rarely aspirate large quantities of water, it is more important to initiate artificial ventilation than to drain fluid. However, if the victim of a seawater accident can be placed in a head-down position to promote drainage by gravity without delaying or interfering with artificial ventilation, this procedure is, of course, preferable.

If near-drowned victims remain hypoxic after initial resuscitation, supplemental oxygen must be given as soon as possible. When the proper equipment for mechanical ventilation is available, it should replace mouth-to-mouth resuscitation. A method of positive-pressure ventilation that also can supply a high concentration of inspired oxygen should be used. Hand-operated units frequently are preferable to pressure-cycled units in an emergency, because most automatic devices are pressure limited, and in a patient who has a very low pulmonary compliance, the apparatus can be shut off before adequate volumes of inspiratory gases are delivered. This is particularly true if a patient requires simultaneous closed-chest cardiac massage. The pressure generated by chest compression frequently cycles the ventilator before an adequate tidal volume is delivered. In selecting a device to replace mouth-to-mouth ventilation, consider whether the appliance or mechanical ventilator can produce PEEP; most emergency resuscitators cannot be adapted to produce PEEP. However, as was stated earlier, the use of PEEP significantly increases the Pa_{O_2} of victims of near-drowning.

If the patient does not have an effective heartbeat, closed-chest cardiac massage should be instituted immediately. In this situation, the presence or absence of ventricular fibrillation should be confirmed to determine whether electrical defibrillation is indicated.

Even when a patient breathes spontaneously after rescue or begins to breathe after initial resuscitation, the rescuer should not be lulled into a false sense of security. A patient who can converse with the rescuer still may have an extremely low Pa_{O_2}. Supplemental oxygen therapy should be continued until actual measurement of Pa_{O_2} confirms it to be unnecessary. Because the pulmonary lesion may not be readily reversible if the patient has aspirated water, and because the rescuer cannot always determine at the scene of the accident whether water has been aspirated, any near-drowned victim should be taken to a hospital for further evaluation and therapy. During transport to the hospital, supplemental oxygen should be given, regardless of the patient's apparent clinical condition. Ventilatory and circulatory assistance should be provided as indicated.

Initial hospital therapy should emphasize pulmonary care, which may range from simply increasing the fractional concentration of inspired oxygen (FI_{O_2}) in a spontaneously breathing patient to providing continuous ventilatory support by establishing a patent airway with an endotracheal tube that is connected to a mechanical ventilator. Although strict guidelines that establish when endotracheal intubation is necessary are not available, in one series of 20 near-drowned victims, all of whom had normal chest roentgenograms on admission to the hospital, only one required endotracheal intubation, even though some patients had oxygen tensions as low as 50 mm Hg (Modell et al, 1976). In retrospect, perhaps this one patient could have been treated more conservatively as well. Current recommendations are that patients who are awake, alert, and cooperative on arrival at the hospital do not need endotracheal intubation unless their pulmonary lesions do not respond to levels of CPAP that can be delivered with a mask or unless they require mechanical breaths. All comatose patients must have tracheal intubation. Patients with a blunted level of consciousness should be evaluated individually. Even when the chest roentgenogram is normal, arterial blood gases must be monitored with serial analyses, because the findings from the chest roentgenogram frequently lag behind the actual intrapulmonary status (Modell et al, 1976).

Approximately 70 per cent of near-drowned victims have a significant degree of metabolic acidosis accompanying their hypoxia (Modell et al, 1976). Therefore, I recommend empirically that if a patient is unresponsive and if results of arterial blood gas analysis are not immediately available, sodium bicarbonate (1.0 mEq/kg) should be given to the near-drowned victim. Of course, samples of arterial blood must be taken as soon as possible to evaluate Pa_{O_2}, Pa_{CO_2}, pH, and bicarbonate level. These values determine the extent of ventilatory support needed, the appropriate FI_{O_2} required, the amount of additional bicarbonate to be administered, and the pattern of mechanical ventilatory support necessary to produce normal carbon dioxide elimination and acid-base balance and adequate oxygenation.

It has been shown that adding PEEP, both with and without concomitant mechanical ventilation, can increase Pa_{O_2} significantly in both animals and humans after the aspiration of seawater (Modell et al, 1974). Similarly, PEEP combined with mechanical ventilation has been shown to increase Pa_{O_2} significantly in freshwater near-drowned victims (Ruiz et al, 1973; Rutledge and Flor, 1973). CPAP produces similar results when applied to the airway of some spontaneously breathing victims of freshwater aspiration, but in others, mechanical breaths must be added to improve $\dot{V}/\dot{Q}$ matching and Pa_{O_2} (Bergquist et al, 1980). The exact amount of PEEP or CPAP that is supplied to any patient should be determined individually. The amount of pressure is increased incrementally, and the effect on intrapulmonary shunt, Pa_{O_2} and cardiovascular function is then assessed. An optimal level will be reached when the lowest intrapulmonary shunt or intrapulmonary venous admixture is achieved without adverse effects on circulation. If this level of PEEP or CPAP is exceeded, Pa_{O_2} may decrease rather than increase. If access to mixed venous blood by which to calculate shunt is not available, titration of CPAP can be accomplished by monitoring Pa_{O_2} in patients whose cardiovascular status is stable. The use of positive airway pressure frequently permits a physician to maintain adequate arterial oxygenation with a lower FI_{O_2} and thus to minimize the possibility of oxygen toxicity. CPAP is usually preferred over PEEP for spontaneously breathing patients because there is less work of breathing. However, because the mean intrathoracic pressure is greater with CPAP, it may have a greater effect on venous return.

Many clinicians fear that an increase in PEEP or CPAP always decreases cardiac output. Although a decrease can occur with hypovolemia, if effective circulating blood volume is normal, cardiac output actually may increase as Pa_{O_2} improves (Downs et al, 1973).

Bronchospasm after the aspiration of fluid can be treated by administering a bronchodilating agent intravenously, e.g., aminophylline. Pulmonary edema frequently is seen after near-drowning with aspiration. Applying PEEP or CPAP is excellent therapy for pulmonary edema, and once airway pressure has been titrated to an optimal level, it should not be removed abruptly or pulmonary edema will recur.

Many physicians initially advocated the use of steroids and prophylactic broad-spectrum antibiotics to treat the pulmonary lesion of near-drowned victims (Modell, Davis, Giammona et al, 1968; Sladen and Zauder, 1971). Evidence now suggests that steroid therapy does not improve arterial oxygenation in or survival of animals that have aspirated hydrochloric acid (Chapman, Downs, Modell, and Hood, 1974; Chapman, Modell, Ruiz et al, 1974; Downs et al, 1974). Similar studies with a model of freshwater drowning also failed to demonstrate any significant improvement in either arterial oxygenation or survival with the use of steroids (Calderwood et al, 1975). Retrospective analysis of a large series of consecutive near-drowned humans also failed to demonstrate any superiority of therapy using steroids and prophylactic antibiotics (Modell et al, 1976). Routine use of broad-spectrum antibiotics may disrupt bacterial flora normally found in the airway and thereby encourage secondary infection with organisms such as *Pseudomonas*. It is better to treat infection with specific antibiotics when it occurs, rather than to administer antibiotics prophylactically, the one exception being a patient who aspirates fluid known to be grossly contaminated.

Many near-drowned victims vomit during either the accident or the emergency resuscitation and aspirate solid debris or particles of undigested food. Serial physical examinations and chest roentgenograms prove helpful in diagnosing regional or lobar atelectasis caused by the aspiration of particulate matter. If regional atelectasis occurs, bronchoscopic examination is indicated. With use of the fiberoptic bronchoscope, the presence of foreign material in the airway can be confirmed without interrupting mechanical ventilatory support. This minimizes the period of hypoxia that might otherwise occur during bronchoscopic examination.

Although the patient's hematocrit should be determined, unless it is markedly abnormal or unless hemolysis is obvious in the plasma fraction after freshwater aspiration, the problems in treating the patient will be limited almost exclusively to ventilation, oxygenation, and acid-base balance; significant fluid and electrolyte disturbances are unlikely to occur.

All near-drowned victims should be monitored closely. At the minimum, vital signs should be monitored frequently in every patient: pulse, respiration, blood pressure, and temperature. It is imperative that in all near-drowned victims serial determinations also be made of arterial blood gas tensions and pH; arterial catheters facilitate blood sampling for these determinations. Monitoring oxygen saturation with a pulse oximeter gives real-time data on oxygen delivery to the tissue being monitored and thus documents gas exchange, blood flow, and oxygen delivery. Electrocardiographic monitoring and urine output should be observed closely in patients who require any type of prolonged support. If the patient shows any circulatory instability, venous pressure should be monitored. However, central venous pressure is only an approximate guide in the complete assessment of cardiac function and blood volume balance, because this pressure reflects only what may be happening proximal to the right ventricle.

It frequently is necessary to distinguish the effects of hypovolemia from those of cardiac failure when hypotension and a low cardiac output are present. These conditions suggest placing a Swan-Ganz pulmonary arterial catheter so that PAOP can be measured (Swan et al, 1970). The latter value is a better indicator of the function of the left side of the heart and is more useful therefore in determining whether the patient requires additional fluid or supplemental cardiac support. A catheter in the pulmonary artery permits analysis of mixed venous blood so that the arterial-venous oxygen content difference can be monitored. When oxygen consumption is reasonably constant, this value indirectly indicates whether cardiac output is increasing, decreasing, or stabilizing (Colgan and Mahoney, 1969; Gustafson and Nordström, 1970). Pulmonary venous admixture also can be measured, and if a pulmonary catheter with a

thermodilution tip is used, serial determinations of cardiac output can be obtained.

In addition to monitoring the patient with serial determinations of Pa_{O_2}, Pa_{CO_2}, pH, and bicarbonate level, laboratory evaluation should include hemoglobin, hematocrit, and serum electrolyte determinations; urinalysis; culture of tracheal secretions; and chest roentgenograms. These evaluations should be made routinely, and other tests should be added as appropriate.

If serum electrolyte concentrations are abnormal, administering the appropriate physiologic salt solution is indicated. Because most of these patients do not have marked abnormalities of serum electrolyte levels, a "routine" approach to fluid administration is not advised. In general, intravenous fluid therapy should begin with lactated Ringer's solution, which should be replaced by the specific fluid required. If clinical signs and results of monitoring indicate hypovolemia, giving crystalloid, volume expanders, or, in rare cases, blood should be considered. After near-drowning in seawater, administering blood is rarely necessary, because usually there is no loss of red blood cells. On the other hand, volume expanders may have to be given to replace plasma lost into the lungs. After aspiration of large quantities of fresh water, hemolysis of red blood cells can occur. This is most marked during severe hypoxemia. Hemoglobin and hematocrit concentrations of whole blood may not reflect the extent of hemolysis immediately on admission to the hospital. Serial determinations of these values sometimes show a gradual decrease (Modell, Davis, Giammona et al, 1968). Pulmonary edema almost always accompanies near-drowning, so a physician may be faced with the necessity of giving fluid to replace blood volume in such a patient. This requires constant, simultaneous attention to both effective circulating blood volume and pulmonary status. It may be necessary to infuse fluid while applying PEEP or CPAP to maintain an acceptable effective circulating blood volume.

The two most important drugs in treating near-drowned victims are oxygen and bicarbonate solution. If proper attention is paid to balancing the effective circulating blood volume with fluid replacement according to urine output and central venous pressure and PAOP measurements, vasopressor therapy will rarely have to be considered for near-drowned patients. It may occasionally be advisable to use drugs that primarily stimulate the beta receptors in order to increase the cardiac output temporarily until blood volume can be stabilized. Prolonged use of any type of vasopressor is not suggested. At best, it should be considered a "crutch" rather than a specific mode of therapy. In addition, diuretics may be helpful in promoting renal output, particularly in patients with high concentrations of plasma hemoglobin. Potent diuretics also have been recommended to help mobilize intrapulmonary water in order to shorten the course of pulmonary insufficiency (Sladen et al, 1968). Use of diuretics for this purpose is potentially hazardous, however, because hypovolemia may result.

Deliberately induced hypothermia (Ohlsson and Beckmann, 1964) and exchange transfusions (Kvittingen and Naess, 1963) have been advocated on occasion in the treatment of the near-drowned patient. The rationale for inducing hypothermia is that it will decrease cerebral oxygen consumption. However, to be effective, hypothermia should be induced before hypoxia occurs, but this is not possible in near-drowned patients. Therefore, the rationale for using induced hypothermia is questionable.

Some physicians have recommended exchange transfusions for freshwater near-drowned victims because of a potentially high plasma hemoglobin level that might adversely affect the kidneys (Kvittingen and Naess, 1963). Because patients with plasma hemoglobin levels in excess of 500 mg/dL have not been reported (Modell, Davis, Giammona, et al, 1968), exchange transfusion is probably not necessary and may only further delay the institution of proper therapy.

In two separate series, patients were categorized according to neurologic status on admission to the hospital. In these series, irrespective of whether patients suffered a cardiac arrest at the scene, all children who were awake on admission to the hospital and all but one whose level of consciousness was described as "blunted" survived with no apparent residual abnormality. Of the patients who were still comatose on admission, 44 per cent survived with normal function in both studies; the remainder either died or suffered brain damage (Conn et al, 1980; Modell et al, 1980). Conn and colleagues (1980) believed that cerebral salvage can be improved with what they described as H.Y.P.E.R. therapy. I am not sure that all the components of H.Y.P.E.R. therapy are necessary, and because they present potential complications of their own, I am reluctant to endorse them until a prospective study demonstrates their combined efficacy. A follow-up retrospective study on H.Y.P.E.R. therapy does not support the use of this therapy and reports that it may actually increase morbidity and mortality (Bohn et al, 1986). I recommend the following for patients who are still comatose when admitted to the hospital: placement of an intracranial pressure (ICP) monitor; hyperventilation to decrease cerebral blood flow and, thereby, to decrease ICP; maintenance of a normal Pa_{O_2}; and aggressive measures to decrease ICP if it exceeds 20 mm Hg, e.g., fluid restriction, diuresis, and barbiturate-induced coma. If movement or coughing by the patient is reflected in an increased ICP, muscle paralysis with pancuronium bromide should be added. It should be emphasized that this approach is empiric, and there are no controlled studies to document that it improves cerebral salvage from near-drowning. This approach differs from that of Conn and associates in that it (1) does not include induced hypothermia or steroids and (2) reserves the administration of barbiturates and potent diuretics for those

patients with an increased ICP. In the presence of these recommendations, many clinicians have stopped monitoring ICP in near-drowned patients because increased ICP is thought to be a late sign of irreversible brain damage. Nevertheless, this area requires further investigation (Modell, 1986).

In summary, the near-drowned victim must be treated immediately for ventilatory insufficiency, hypoxia, and resulting acidosis. The cause and pathophysiologic changes of pulmonary insufficiency vary according to the type and volume of fluid aspirated. Success or failure of the overall resuscitative effort frequently depends on the adequacy of prompt emergency resuscitation and on effective intensive pulmonary care. Each patient should be evaluated and treated individually, because abnormalities of multiple organ systems can occur, the degree and form of which vary considerably.

REFERENCES

American Heart Association: Textbook of Advanced Cardiac Life Support. Dallas, American Heart Association, 1987.

Bergquist RE, Vogelhut MM, Modell JH et al: Comparison of ventilatory patterns in the treatment of freshwater near-drowning in dogs. Anesthesiology 52:142, 1980.

Bohn DJ, Biggar WD, Smith CR et al: Influence of hypothermia, barbiturate therapy, and intracranial pressure monitoring on morbidity and mortality after near-drowning. Crit Care Med 14:529, 1986.

Calderwood HW, Modell JH, and Ruiz BC: The ineffectiveness of steroid therapy for treatment of fresh-water near-drowning. Anesthesiology 43:642, 1975.

Chapman RL Jr, Downs JB, Modell JH, and Hood CI: The ineffectiveness of steroid therapy in treating aspiration of hydrochloric acid. Arch Surg 108:858, 1974.

Chapman RL Jr, Modell JH, Ruiz BC et al: Effect of continuous positive-pressure ventilation and steroids on aspiration of hydrochloric acid (pH 1.8) in dogs. Anesth Analg 53:556, 1974.

Colebatch HJH and Halmagyi DFJ: Lung mechanics and resuscitation after fluid aspiration. J Appl Physiol 16:684, 1961.

Colebatch HJH and Halmagyi DFJ: Reflex airway reaction to fluid aspiration. J Appl Physiol 17:787, 1962.

Colebatch HJH and Halmagyi DFJ: Reflex pulmonary hypertension of fresh-water aspiration. J Appl Physiol 18:179, 1963.

Colgan FJ and Mahoney PD: The effects of major surgery on cardiac output and shunting. Anesthesiology 31:213, 1969.

Conn AW, Montes JE, Barker GA, and Edmonds JF: Cerebral salvage in near-drowning following neurological classification by triage. Can Anaesth Soc J 27:201, 1980.

Coryllos PN: Mechanical resuscitation in advanced forms of asphyxia. A clinical and experimental study in the different methods of resuscitation. Surg Gynecol Obstet 66:698, 1938.

Cot C: Les Asphyxies Accidentelles (submersion, electrocution, intoxication oxycarbonique). Étude clinique, thérapeutique et préventive. Paris, Éditions Médicales N. Maloine, 1931.

Craig AB Jr: Causes of loss of consciousness during underwater swimming. J Appl Physiol 16:583, 1961a.

Craig AB Jr: Underwater swimming and loss of consciousness. JAMA 176:255, 1961b.

Davis JH: Autopsy findings in victims of drowning. In Modell JH (ed): The Pathophysiology and Treatment of Drowning and Near-drowning. Springfield, Ill, Charles C Thomas, 1971.

Downs JB, Chapman RL Jr, Modell JH, and Hood CI: An evaluation of steroid therapy in aspiration pneumonitis. Anesthesiology 40:129, 1974.

Downs JB, Klein EF Jr, and Modell JH: The effect of incremental PEEP on Pa_{O_2} in patients with respiratory failure. Anesth Analg 52:210, 1973.

Dumitru AP and Hamilton FG: A mechanism of drowning. Anesth Analg 42:170, 1963.

Fainer DC: Near drowning in sea water and fresh water. Ann Intern Med 59:537, 1963.

Fuller RH: The clinical pathology of human near-drowning. Proc R Soc Med 56:33, 1963a.

Fuller RH: The 1962 Wellcome prize essay. Drowning and the post-immersion syndrome. A clinicopathologic study. Milit Med 128:22, 1963b.

Gambino SP: Personal communication. January 13, 1969.

Giammona ST and Modell JH: Drowning by total immersion. Effects on pulmonary surfactant of distilled water, isotonic saline, and sea water. Am J Dis Child 114:612, 1967.

Gordon BA: Drowning and the diving reflex in man. Med J Aust 16:583, 1972.

Gordon BJ and Terranova GJ: Heimlich maneuver in cold-water drowning. Connecticut Med 45:775, 1981.

Gustafson I and Nordström L: Central venous PO_2 and open-heart surgery. Acta Anaesthesiol Scand 37(Suppl):112, 1970.

Halmagyi DFJ: Lung changes and incidence of respiratory arrest in rats after aspiration of sea and fresh water. J Appl Physiol 16:41, 1961.

Halmagyi DFJ and Colebatch HJH: The drowned lung. A physiological approach to its mechanism and management. Aust Ann Med 10:68, 1961.

Heimlich HJ: The Heimlich maneuver: first treatment in human drowning victims. Emerg Med Serv 10:58, July/August 1981.

King RB and Webster IW: A case of recovery from drowning and prolonged anoxia. Med J Aust 1:919, 1964.

Kirby RR, Downs JB, Civetta JM et al: High level positive end expiratory pressure (PEEP) in acute respiratory insufficiency. Chest 67:156, 1975.

Kristoffersen MB, Rattenborg CC, and Holaday DA: Asphyxial death: the roles of acute anoxia, hypercarbia and acidosis. Anesthesiology 28:488, 1967.

Kvittingen TD and Naess A: Recovery from drowning in fresh water. Br Med J 5341:1315, 1963.

Lougheed DW, Janes JM, and Hall GE: Physiological studies in experimental asphyxia and drowning. Can Med Assoc J 40:423, 1939.

Michenfelder JD and Theye RA: Cerebral protection by thiopental during hypoxia. Anesthesiology 39:510, 1973.

Middleton KR: Cardiac arrest induced by drowning: attempted resuscitation by external and internal cardiac massage. Can Med Assoc J 86:374, 1962.

Modell J: Die physiologischen Grundlagen fŕ die Behandlung von Ertrunkenen. Therapiewoche 43:1928, 1968.

Modell JH: Resuscitation after aspiration of chlorinated fresh water. JAMA 185:651, 1963.

Modell JH: Treatment of near-drowning—is there a role for HYPER therapy? Crit Care Med 14:593, 1986.

Modell JH and Davis JH: Electrolyte changes in human drowning victims. Anesthesiology 30:414, 1969.

Modell JH and Downs JB: Patterns of respiratory support aimed at pathophysiology. 1976 ASA Refresher Course Lectures, 1976.

Modell JH and Moya F: Effects of volume of aspirated fluid during chlorinated fresh water drowning. Anesthesiology 27:662, 1966.

Modell JH, Calderwood HW, Ruiz BC et al: Effects of ventilatory patterns on arterial oxygenation after near-drowning in sea water. Anesthesiology 40:376, 1974.

Modell JH, Davis JH, Giammona ST et al: Blood gas and electrolyte changes in human near-drowning victims. JAMA 203:337, 1968.

Modell JH, Gaub M, Moya F et al: Physiologic effects of near drowning with chlorinated fresh water, distilled water and isotonic saline. Anesthesiology 27:33, 1966.

Modell JH, Graves SA, and Ketover A: Clinical course of 91 consecutive near-drowning victims. Chest 70:231, 1976.

Modell JH, Graves SA, and Kuck EJ: Near-drowning: correlation of level of consciousness and survival. Can Anaesth Soc J 27:211, 1980.

Modell JH, Kuck EJ, Ruiz BC, and Heinitsch H: Effect of intravenous vs. aspirated distilled water on serum electrolytes and blood gas tensions. J Appl Physiol 32:579, 1972.

Modell JH, Moya F, Newby EJ et al: The effects of fluid volume in seawater drowning. Ann Intern Med 67:68, 1967.

Modell JH, Moya F, Williams, HD, and Weibley TC: Changes in blood gases and A-aDO_2 during near-drowning. Anesthesiology 29:456, 1968.

Moss G, Staunton C, and Stein AA: Cerebral etiology of the "shock lung syndrome." J Trauma 12:885, 1972.

Munroe WD: Hemoglobinuria from near-drowning. J Pediatr 64:57, 1964.

Noble CS and Sharpe N: Drowning: its mechanism and treatment. Can Med Assoc J 89:402, 1963.

Ohlsson K and Beckman M: Drowning—reflections based on two cases. Acta Chir Scand 128:327, 1964.

Orlowski JP: Vomiting as a complication of the Heimlich maneuver. JAMA 257:512, 1987.

Ornato JP: The resuscitation of near-drowning victims. JAMA 256:75, 1986.

Press E, Walker J, and Crawford I: An interstate drowning study. Am J Public Health 58:2275, 1968.

Rath CE: Drowning hemoglobinuria. Blood 8:1099, 1953.

Redding JS: Treatment of near drowning. Int Anesthesiol Clin 3:355, 1965.

Redding JS and Pearson JW: Management of drowning victims. GP 29:100, 1964.

Reidbord HE and Spitz WU: Ultrastructural alterations in rat lungs. Changes after intratracheal perfusion with freshwater and seawater. Arch Pathol 81:103, 1966.

Ruben A and Ruben H: Artificial respiration. Flow of water from the lung and the stomach. Lancet 1:780, 1962.

Ruiz BC, Calderwood HW, Modell JH, and Brogdon JE: Effect of ventilatory patterns on arterial oxygenation after near-drowning with fresh water: a comparative study in dogs. Anesth Analg 52:570, 1973.

Rutledge RR and Flor RJ: The use of mechanical ventilation with positive end-expiratory pressure in the treatment of near-drowning. Anesthesiology 38:194, 1973.

Safar P, Escarraga LA, and Elam JO: A comparison of the mouth-to-mouth and mouth-to-airway methods of artificial respiration with chest-pressure arm-lift methods. N Engl J Med 258:671, 1958.

Siebke H, Breivik H, Rød T, and Lind B: Survival after 40 minutes' submersion without sequelae. Lancet 1:1275, 1975.

Sladen A and Zauder HL: Methylprednisolone therapy for pulmonary edema following near drowning. JAMA 215:1793, 1971.

Sladen A, Laver MB, and Pontoppidan H: Pulmonary complications and water retention in prolonged mechanical ventilation. N Engl J Med 279:448, 1968.

Swan HJC, Ganz W, Forrester J et al: Catheterization of the heart in man with use of a flow-directed balloon-tipped catheter. N Engl J Med 283:447, 1970.

Swann HG and Brucer M: The cardiorespiratory and biochemical events during rapid anoxic death. VI. Fresh water and sea water drowning. Tex Rep Biol Med 7:604, 1949.

Swann HG, Brucer M, Moore C, and Vezien BL: Fresh water and sea water drowning: a study of the terminal cardiac and biochemical events. Tex Rep Biol Med 5:423, 1947.

Tabeling BB and Modell JH: Drowning and near-drowning: its pathophysiology and treatment. In Tinker J and Rapin M (eds): Care of the Critically Ill Patient. New York, Springer-Verlag, 1982.

Tabeling BB and Modell JH: Fluid administration increases oxygen delivery during continuous positive pressure ventilation after fresh-water near-drowning. Crit Care Med 11:693, 1983.

Webster DP: Pool drownings and their prevention. Public Health Rep 82:587, 1967.

Werner JZ, Safar P, Blichei NG et al: No improvement in pulmonary status by gravity drainage or abdominal thrusts after sea water near drowning in dogs. Anesthesiology 57 (Suppl):A81, 1982.

Wynne JW and Modell JH: Respiratory aspiration of stomach contents. A review. Ann Intern Med 87:466, 1977.

Zugzda MJ: Personal communications. July 25, 1969, and November 2, 1973.

30

ARNOLD C. G. PLATZKER, M.D.

GASTROESOPHAGEAL REFLUX AND RESPIRATORY ILLNESS

Aspiration constitutes one of the most serious challenges to the integrity of the developing airways. Pediatricians have long recognized that infants and children are particularly at risk for aspiration and contamination of the airways as a result of faulty or dysfunctional swallowing. Although aspiration is more common in newborn infants, especially premature neonates, it continues to be a major health hazard for older infants and children into the preschool years. It has not been until the past decade that along with pediatric conditions heightening the risk of aspiration (e.g., congenital anomalies of the palate and upper respiratory tract and swallowing disorders), disorders of the esophageal motility, cardiac sphincter tone, and gastric emptying have become recognized as frequent causes of acute and chronic respiratory disease in infancy and childhood. Interestingly, in the 1967 Pediatric Clinics of North America edition dedicated to topics in pediatric gastroenterology there was no mention of gastroesophageal reflux (GER). Although the association between the disorders of gastrointestinal motility and acute and chronic respiratory disease in infants and children is now well accepted, the mechanism by which GER precipitates respiratory illness in infants and children remains incompletely understood. In fact, at the present time, there is no clear documentation of a relationship between GER-associated respiratory illness and aspiration. GER is a very common occurrence in pediatric patients. In adults, GER occurs in approximately one third of the population, but in only 10 per cent of adults with GER does it ever cause respiratory symptoms. GER is probably an even more common phenomenon in infants and children, although it may be a less frequent cause of significant symptoms or respiratory illness than in adults. However, because of the lack of extensive prospective studies, the incidence of GER and of GER-related respiratory illness in infants and children is unknown. This chapter reviews the current understanding of the pathophysiologic relationship between GER and reactive airways disease and discusses the concepts of diagnostic, therapeutic, and preventive care for GER.

PATHOGENETIC CONSIDERATIONS

Although the pathophysiology of the respiratory symptoms associated with GER has yet to be clarified, three mechanisms have been proposed primarily on studies in animals and adult humans. Mendelson was first to associate respiratory disease as a consequence of GER. He described an "asthma-like" syndrome following gastroesophageal reflux and aspiration of acidic gastric contents during the induction of obstetric anaesthesia. Subsequent investigations in animals have documented the esophageal and airway mucosal injury from GER and aspiration and have confirmed the physiologic response and respiratory consequences of aspiration of various amounts of gastric juice. Aspiration of small amounts of gastric juice (>1.0 ml/kg of pH <2.5) can result acutely in marked respiratory embarrassment and pneumonia. Aspiration of less than 1.0 ml/kg of gastric juice has been shown to result in significant but less violent clinical respiratory illness, acutely, characterized by an obstructive bronchitis or asthma-like syndrome. With chronic aspiration, the pathologic picture may evolve into a chronic interstitial pneumonia. Over time, continued acid soiling of the airways and lungs results in interstitial thickening and fibrosis of the lungs. In pediatric patients, chronic though often more mild respiratory symptoms are commonly associated with GER. This has led to the proposal of a second hypothesis, that of "silent" or microaspiration to explain the respiratory symptoms and pathologic findings associated with GER. In this theory, a small amount of soiling of the upper airway by acidic gastric fluid provokes bronchospasm by stimulating the irritant receptors in the trachea and upper airway. The aspirate is isolated and confined to the upper airway through the normal protective mechanisms of cough and vagally mediated bronchospasm and the offending aspirate is removed from the respiratory tract by mucociliary clearance. Each episode of GER is followed by a swallow, although the exact role of the post-GER swallow has not been determined. It has been demonstrated, however, that after infusion of acid into the esophagus, esophageal pH rises toward neutral pH following a swallow and that successive swallows induce esophageal peristaltic waves that effectively clear the esophagus of acid and restore esophageal pH neutrality. Virtually all acid is cleared from the esophagus within two peristaltic sequences, and the remaining acid is effectively neutralized by swallowed saliva. Unfortunately, aspiration of saliva from the mouth abolishes esophageal acid clearance (Helm et al, 1984). More significant consequences of GER occur when gastric reflux is associated with defects in swallowing, cough, or mucosal clearance mechanisms. With defects in these "protective" mechanisms, aspiration of the contents of the oral cavity is frequent and the respiratory symptoms are likely to result as much from aspiration from "above" as from GER.

In the final mechanism proposed to explain the respiratory illness associated with GER, distal esophageal reflux of acidic gastric juice or distention of the esophagus triggers esophageal stretch, pH or thermal mucosal receptors resulting in reflex bronchoconstriction. Interest in this hypothesis may be due to the difficulty and lack of success in documenting penetration of the airway by gastric contents in most patients with GER. Studies to test this hypothesis that distal esophageal reflux of gastric juice alone is sufficient to induce reflex bronchospasm in animals models of GER have been plagued with conflicting results. Investigations have focused on both animls with intact esophageal mucosa and on those with chronic acid reflux esophagitis. In the former, most studies have been unable to document a consistent temporal relationship between acid infused into the distal esophagus and changes in airway mechanics (Boyle et al, 1985). In one study, 0.1 N hydrochloric acid (HCl) infused into the distal esophagus of kittens appeared to stimulate only a very mild increase in the bronchomotor tone. In this study, the induction of esophagitis provoked no greater increase in bronchomotor tone following infusion of acid into the distal esophagus than observed in kittens without esophagitis, although with esophagitis, lower esophageal sphincter tone was decreased. In infants referred for the diagnosis of GER and associated respiratory illness, our group has performed measurements of esophageal manometry and pH with concurrent measurement of airway mechanics and respiratory resistance. We have not been able to confirm any change in airway mechanics during or following distal esophageal acidification with 0.1 N HCl regardless of the state of injury of the esophageal mucosa. Significant respiratory illness was present in all of the patients selected for study, and clear clinical findings and positive imaging studies supported the diagnosis of GER.

DIAGNOSTIC CONSIDERATIONS

ASPIRATION FROM ABOVE

Establishing the diagnosis of GER presents a very difficult task in many cases. This disorder must be distinguished from all other disorders that are associated with aspiration. The aspiration of nasal or sinus secretions and oropharyngeal contents is considered to be aspiration coming from above, whereas aspiration of gastric contents is referred to as aspiration from "below." Respiratory illness due to aspiration from above may be caused by infectious drainage from the sinuses or oral cavity gaining entrance into the airway when the infant or child is supine. It occurs most commonly during sleep and when airway clearance mechanisms are thought to be depressed. Thus acute or chronic sinobronchitis may be misinterpreted as GER. However, two other categories of conditions lead to aspiration from above: congenital craniofacial or upper airway malformations and neurologic or muscular disorders. These latter two categories of disorders are grouped together as *oral and pharyngeal dysphagia-related aspiration* (Table 30–1). This type of aspiration occurs as a result of weakness or dysfunction of the bulbar musculature leading to swallowing dyskinesia and aspiration during the process of swallowing. In craniofacial anomalies, the defect in swallowing is anatomic, and the congenital deformity of the face or cranium interferes with the swallowing process. A poor palatal seal with the posterior pharyngeal wall during swallow (e.g., cleft palate) and an abnormal communication between the respiratory and digestive tracts (e.g., tracheoesophageal fistula, larygotracheal cleft) are typical examples of this type of swallowing dysfunction leading to a heightened risk of aspiration. Some of these disorders are also associated with a heightened risk of GER. Thus for a physician to select an appropriate and effective therapeutic strategy, diagnostic studies must focus on whether one or both of these disorders are responsible for the patient's respiratory illness.

Table 30–1. ORAL AND PHARYNGEAL DYSPHAGIA-RELATED ASPIRATION

Congenital Malformations
Choanal atresia
Cleft lip and palate
Cysts or tumors
Laryngotracheal cleft
Macroglossia
Pharyngeal diverticulum
Pierre Robin syndrome
Tracheoesophageal fistula

Neurologic or Muscular Abnormalities
Bulbar paralysis
Cerebral palsy
Cricopharyngeal achalasia
de Lange syndrome
Familial dysautonomia
Isolated cranial nerve paralysis
Möbius syndrome
Myasthenia gravis
Myotonic dystrophy
Pharyngeal incoordination
Suprabulbar paralysis
Werdnig-Hoffmann disease

DISORDERS OF GASTROESOPHAGEAL MOTILITY AND SPHINCTER TONE

Although as already discussed, the respiratory disease may not be the result of actual aspiration, GER-related respiratory illness is defined as aspiration from below. It comprises a complex of problems that have abnormalities in gastroesophageal motility as their common basis. Although the overriding physiologic feature of GER is lowered distal esophageal pressure (LES), the mean resting LES is reduced in patients with GER. There are large swings in LES rising as high as 60 cm H_2O. In pediatric patients with GER, only slightly greater than 10 per cent of the episodes of GER occur while there is continuous reduction in the resting LES. More than half of the GER episodes occur during a transient increase in intra-abdominal pressure that exceeds the resting level of LES. These transient episodes are thought to occur during wakefulness, when a patient's activity is sufficient to provoke a rise in intra-abdominal pressure, such as when straining, crying, coughing, or during a Valsalva maneuver with passing stool. Only a third of the episodes of GER occur during a brief period of complete relaxation of LES. These episodes do not occur in association with swallowing or esophageal peristalsis. In normal infants and children, only 1 per cent of GER episodes occur against a background of reduced LES; the vast majority of GER episodes occur during a transient relaxation of LES. Thus these two factors—frequent spontaneous relaxation of LES and frequent, sometimes unexplained, episodes in which intra-abdominal pressure exceeds LES—differentiate abnormal GER from asymptomatic GER in normal infants and children. Finally, when pathologic GER occurs, the refluxate is more frequently acidic in patients (66 per cent compared with 34 per cent in normal individuals).

Surprisingly, the tone of the LES is affected only partially by neural blockade and to a different degree in each species studied. Cervical vagotomy has no effect on LES tone. However, LES relaxation is neurally mediated under normal conditions. It is probable that inappropriate relaxation of the LES tone may be an important factor in the development of GER. Because LES tone decreases normally only in association with esophageal peristalsis, a decline in LES pressure in the absence of peristalsis is considered inappropriate and results in GER. Table 30–2 lists the agents responsible for modulating, positively or negatively, the tone of the LES.

A second mechanism protecting against GER and propagation of esophageal reflux into the airway of pediatric patients is the tone or the competence of the upper esophageal sphincter (UES). The UES, like the cardioesophageal sphincter, is thought to be another critical sphincter mechanism protecting against soiling of the airway from below. Very little is known about UES function or the control of its tone in humans. There have been no studies of UES function in normal infants and children, nor in

Table 30–2. AGENTS AUGMENTING OR LOWERING LES TONE

Agents Augmenting LES Tone	Agents Lessening LES Tone
Gastrin	Methylxanthine compounds
Motilin	Theophylline
Substance P	Caffeine
Prostaglandin F_2	Chocolate
Adrenergic agonists	Beta-adrenergic agonists
Cholinergic agents	Alpha-adrenergic antagonists
Bethanechol	Glucagon
Methacholine	Secretin
Histamine	Cholecystokinin
Gastric alkalinization	Anticholinergic agonists
Metoclopramide	Gastric acidification
Indomethacin	Fatty meal
5-Hydroxytryptamine	Narcotic agents
High-protein meal	Ethanol
	Dopamine
	Valium
	Peppermint
	Prostaglandins E_1, E_2, A_2

pediatric patients with GER. Our knowledge of the anatomy and function of this sphincter is derived largely from studies of animals and adult humans. Anatomically, the UES is formed by the cricopharyngeus and the inferior pharyngeal constrictor muscles, which maintain the tone of the sphincter by "firing" continuously under vagal control. The activity of this sphincter is directly proportional to upper esophageal intraluminal pressure. The tone of the UES increases with acidification of the lower esophagus and with distention of the esophagus. In addition, with either upper esophageal distention or lower esophageal acidification, a secondary esophageal peristalsis is initiated. This secondary peristalsis is a centrally mediated reflex affecting the striated portion of the esophageal musculature, with secondary peristalsis in the smooth muscle portions of the esophagus being initiated locally solely by esophageal distention and requiring no central input.

There are other considerations in this complex relationship between passage of food from the mouth into the small intestines and the protective mechanisms preventing contamination of the parallel respiratory tract during this process of digestion. These factors include swallowing, epiglottis/vocal cord function, and gastric emptying. A more complete discussion of these factors is beyond the scope of this chapter.

SYMPTOMS

The presenting gastrointestinal symptoms of GER are often not clearly defined in the history because they are frequently subtle. Even when patients are old enough to assist in supplying the history, they may not localize the complaints to the gastrointestinal tract. It is uncommon for an infant or child with this disorder to experience overt emesis, and when emesis does occur, this symptom may be overlooked and called a "wet burp." The gastrointestinal symptoms are often misinterpreted as behavioral or associated with problems with other organ systems. For example, irritability in an infant as a result of retrosternal discomfort resulting from reflux esophagitis may be misinterpreted as hunger if the irritability improves with feeding. Rarely, the diagnosis of GER in such an infant may elude the pediatrician until the infant has a complete investigation for associated respiratory complaints or presents with clearly recognizable gastrointestinal findings such as hematemesis or melena.

On the other hand, the respiratory symptoms and findings are usually overt but still may be confusing, and it may be difficult to document their relationship to GER. The respiratory symptoms and respiratory illness associated with GER must be differentiated from respiratory illness due to aspiration from above. This is particularly true in those disorders in which GER and aspiration may coexist. The common theme in these disorders is either muscle weakness or incoordination. That is, a small premature infant may experience GER on a developmental basis but may also have a dyskinetic or dysfunctional swallow (more commonly termed *oropharyngeal dysphagia*, difficulty in initiating a swallow) also secondary to immaturity of the swallowing mechanism (common before 34 weeks' gestation) or resulting from perinatal injury to cranial nerves V, VII, X, and XII. These cranial nerves are involved in both the afferent and efferent limbs of the central nervous system control of swallow. In both premature and full-term infants, nerves X and XII can be injured as a result of abnormal intrauterine head position or more commonly by a difficult delivery during which the neck is hyperextended in an effort to deliver the anterior shoulder. Swallowing may also be compromised in infants and children with anoxic encephalopathy (e.g., cerebral palsy), congenital myopathies, or failure to thrive.

Perhaps the major reason for the apparent difficulty in identifying infants and children with GER is that GER is prevalent in patients suffering from respiratory illnesses. The symptoms of GER-related respiratory illness are similar to or masked by the symptoms of the patient's primary illness. For example, infants with apnea and GER may manifest only increased frequency of apneic episodes, whereas patients with asthma and GER may experience only more severe or unresponsive wheezing. Therefore, the awareness of a linkage between a particular illness and GER is key to the successful identification and treatment of this disorder. Table 30–3 lists the disorders with which GER may be associated.

The most common respiratory symptoms of GER are wheezing and nighttime coughing (Table 30–4). However, the particular presenting symptoms may be age dependent. Infants who in the first 3 months have GER may also experience intermittent or frequent apnea. In some, apnea presents as a life-threatening event (formerly called near-miss sudden infant death syndrome [SIDS]) that may even require

Table 30–3. DISORDERS ASSOCIATED WITH GASTROESOPHAGEAL REFLUX

Asthma
Bronchopulmonary dysplasia
Tracheoesophageal fistula
Anoxic encephalopathy
Neurologic impairment
Myopathies
Cystic fibrosis
Achalasia
Failure to thrive
Hiatus hernia
Infant apnea

full resuscitation to reestablish spontaneous breathing. Although GER does not cause apnea, it may cause increased frequency of episodes of apnea in infants already at risk for apnea. Effective medical or surgical treatment of GER may be accompanied by reduction in the frequency of apneic episodes but not their elimination. Wheezing and nighttime coughing are frequently unresponsive to treatment with bronchodilator medications. In infants and children with very severe respiratory symptoms, recurrent pneumonia and otitis media are common. Some infants and children present with stridor or hoarseness, suggesting that during episodes of reflux, gastric juice has risen to the level of the UES or vocal cords and has caused inflammation and edema of the pharynx and vocal cords. Less commonly, infants present with anemia and hemoptysis or melena, suggesting that GER has resulted in hemorrhagic esophagitis. In its most extreme presentation, GER may first come to the attention of a pediatrician when an infant is brought to the office for evaluation of failure to thrive, which in GER may be due to inadequate caloric intake from chronic esophagitis and dysphagia. In the chronic, long-term respiratory illness of GER, diffuse pulmonary fibrosis may result from chronic soiling and inflammation of the airway and lung parenchyma.

Table 30–4. CLINICAL FINDINGS IN GASTROESOPHAGEAL REFLUX

Common
Frequent emesis
Colic
Nighttime coughing
Wheezing
Recurrent pneumonia
Recurrent otitis media
Esophagitis

Uncommon
Apnea
Near-miss sudden infant death syndrome
Failure to thrive
Stridor
Abnormal head, neck, and thorax positioning

Rare
Hoarseness
Hemoptysis
Anemia
Pulmonary fibrosis

DIAGNOSIS

The goal of the diagnostic evaluation of patients suspected of having respiratory illness resulting from GER is the demonstration of GER and time-related abnormalities in ventilatory function or penetration of the vocal cords by refluxate while ruling out other causes of aspiration. This goal is rarely achieved, primarily because of the difficulty in confirming the association of aspiration with GER. The diagnostic studies now available are frequently found to lack sufficient sensitivity, and few centers are equipped to perform the sophisticated measurements of gastro-esophageal function and concurrent ventilatory function necessary to establish the diagnosis of GER and to verify its relationship to the cause of an infant's respiratory symptoms.

Table 30–5 lists the laboratory diagnostic studies that may be used for establishing or confirming the clinical diagnosis of GER and its associated respiratory illness. An upper gastrointestinal series of roentgenograms using barium sulfate as the contrast medium is the most often used, but not necessarily always the most definitive, of the diagnostic studies. However, it is a widely available radiologic examination. With the use of fluoroscopy, the barium swallow provides sufficient structural detail of the upper gastrointestinal tract to aid in the diagnosis of structural defects. Thus lesions impinging on the esophagus, such as vascular rings or slings, may often be clearly defined on fluoroscopy as a pulsating narrowing or stricture of the esophageal barium column. Abnormal communication between the airway and esophagus may also be defined with positive-contrast roentgenograms. Finally, the upper gastrointestinal series is helpful in the study of swallowing, esophageal motility, cardiac sphincter function, GER, and gastric emptying. The technique for performing this study varies widely. When evaluating an infant with this technique, it is important to feed the barium to the infant by bottle in order to look for the presence of oral or pharyngoesophageal dysphagia. Some radiologists prefer to pass a feeding tube and infuse the barium into the distal esophagus. This practice should be discouraged if a complete study is to be obtained. During the study, if the patient cries vigorously, if excessive pressure is placed on the patient's abdomen, or if the patient is positioned in the head-down position, a positive result may be seen in a patient who normally does not have significant reflux. It is also possible that the extent of the reflux, if present, may be exaggerated.

The limitations of the barium swallow include the static nature of the study (i.e., only one swallow is studied) and the use of only a thickened swallowing medium (not fluid or solids). The barium swallow is also not sufficiently sensitive to detect microaspiration and is appropriate for the study of gastroesophageal function only during the wakeful state. Thus the barium swallow is frequently not the final nor the only diagnostic study used for confirming the diagnosis of GER in infants or children with respiratory illness. Support for this statement is documented in the false-positive diagnostic rate for this study in excess of 30 per cent and the false-negative rate of 14 per cent. Finally, the barium swallow is not suitable for the combined study of ventilation and gastroesophageal function.

The gastric scintiscan may be used to complement or confirm the results of the barium swallow. It is more sensitive than the barium swallow and therefore has an occasional problem of false-positive results, but it is only rarely associated with false-negative results. This study is performed using a ^{99m}Tc sulfur colloid-tagged meal. In this study, the isotope may be mixed with formula or a mixed fluid-solid meal. The isotopic meal is either ingested orally or administered by nasogastric tube into the lower esophagus or stomach. Detectors under the infant or child monitor the progress of the tagged meal through the esophagus into the stomach and its transit time in the stomach. Reappearance of radioactivity in the esophagus and its subsequent appearance in the peripheral lung fields is an indication that reflux and pulmonary aspiration have taken place. This study when carefully performed may allow discrimination between aspiration during deglutition and aspiration after GER. Reflux is confirmed when a vertical column of radioactivity reappears above the diaphragm. With this study, continuous monitoring of the progress of the radioactive meal is critical to the sensitivity of the study. Ideally, accumulation and decay of radioactivity should be monitored by computer as well as the scintillation camera to permit second-to-second replay and quantitation of the events. In this way, a continuous and uninterrupted picture of the passage of the radioactive meal through the upper gastrointestinal tract is possible. Prolonging the study time for at least 4 hours allows accurate measurement of gastric emptying time and recognition of the role of delayed gastric emptying or of gastric outlet obstruction in the patient's clinical problem. This length of study time should allow complete emptying of the stomach. Disadvantages of this technique include the failure to provide high-quality resolution of the esophageal and gastric surface anatomy and the difficulties with interpretation in the presence of congenital anomalies affecting the upper gastrointestinal or upper respiratory tract or both, such as esophageal atresia and tracheoesophageal fistula, laryngotracheal clefts, rings, slings, hiatus hernia, or pyloric stenosis. In some patients with poor distal esophageal motility following surgical correction of congenital esophageal atresia and tracheoesophageal

Table 30–5. DIAGNOSTIC STUDIES TO CONFIRM THE DIAGNOSIS OF GASTROESOPHAGEAL REFLUX

Barium swallow (e.g., upper gastrointestinal series)
Gastric scintiscan
Esophageal pH
Esophageal manometrics
24-hour esophageal pH/motility study

fistula, the very abnormal distal esophageal transit time may be misinterpreted as GER.

Esophagoscopy and bronchoscopy are of little value in the diagnosis of GER and respiratory illness. Esophagoscopy may disclose thickening and inflammatory change in the lower esophageal mucosa. Microscopic examination of the biopsy of the mucosa may reveal intraepithelial eosinophils, supporting a diagnosis of esophagitis. However, this diagnostic technique does not provide confirmation of a linkage of GER and the respiratory illness experienced by the patient. Bronchoscopy and tracheal lavage, on the other hand, may reveal inflammatory change in the airway mucosa and the presence of lipid-laden macrophages in the lavage, but this procedure, although confirming the presence or absence of pulmonary aspiration, contributes little information about the origin of the aspirate. The aspirate may result from dysphagia (aspiration from above), rather than from GER (aspiration from below).

As long ago as 1958, Tuttle described a method for detecting incompetence of the gastrocardiac sphincter mechanism. He determined that the concurrent measurement of distal esophageal pressure and pH would be the most sensitive method for recognizing incompetence of the sphincter mechanism. In the past 10 years, this test has been modified for use in infants and children. Arndorfer and colleagues have also developed a double-lumen sleeve catheter that permits concurrent monitoring of upper and lower esophageal pressure at the LES and UES, as well as esophageal pH. This study permits the detection of reflux, the determination of the height of reflux, and the competence of the UES as well as the LES. This study was initially performed with acid first introduced into the stomach through the catheter, which was then withdrawn into the distal esophagus to monitor the time course of esophageal pH after an initial clearance of residual acid from the esophagus by perfusion of a small amount of saline into the esophagus. The study technique has evolved, and the length of monitoring of esophageal manometry and pH has been increased. In 1985, at an American Thoracic Society Conference on Aspiration Hazards to the Developing Lung, the panel on Swallowing and Upper Gastrointestinal Function proposed that the method be standardized to include the following:

1. Placement of the pH probe in the distal esophagus, using LES pressure determined manometrically as the landmark (Cohen, 1985).

2. Monitoring of pH for at least 6 hours, including one cycle of rapid-eye-movement (REM) sleep and feeding.

3. Standardized position (not in an infant seat) without medication.

4. Simultaneous monitoring of pharyngeal and esophageal function and possibly LES function to determine mechanisms of reflux clearance.

5. Standardized scoring methods; either the Euler or Herbst method could be used. Normal values should be more definitively established.

The panel further recommended that respiratory function should be monitored along with the manometric and pH monitoring to establish a temporal relationship between reflux and respiratory symptoms or alterations in respiratory function.

With the availability of the portable esophageal pH probe with microprocessor recorder, the study of ambulatory esophageal pH monitoring is now standardized and should be performed over a 24-hour period. Although there are few normal values published for this study in infants and children, these values are usually reported as total time or per cent of the study time with pH less than 4.0, number of episodes of pH less than 4.0 in a 24-hour period, and the number of episodes greater than 5 min. Each of these values is also broken down into the supine or sleep time and the upright or awake time. Table 30–6 lists the normal values for infants, children, and adults. Figure 30–1 illustrates the radiologic confirmation of the placement of the esophageal probe for a 24-hour study of esophageal pH. The recording accompanying the roentgenogram illustrates the monitoring of upper and lower esophageal pH in an infant with GER and chronic lung disease. Note that shortly after the beginning of the tracing, there are two episodes of GER during which the pH of the lower esophagus falls below 2 but the upper esophagus remains above 6. Both of these episodes occurred immediately after feeding, and the esophageal pH gradually returned to baseline values during the postprandial period. After these two episodes are GER episodes with reflux of gastric juice to the level of the upper probe, causing a decrease in upper esophageal pH below 4.0. In this infant, reflux occurred for 23 per cent of the time and occurred for almost one third of the time during meals when supine and for 20 per cent of the time when held upright. However, with episodes of GER there was no temporally related change in lung mechanics. This infant had unexplained chronic lung disease and was oxygen dependent. A chest roentgenogram revealed chronic right upper and middle lobe infiltrates. Barium swallow failed to reveal a defect in swallowing. The gastric scintiscan failed to confirm delayed gastric emptying but confirmed the presence of GER. A small amount of radioactivity was detected over the right upper lung fields, suggesting that aspiration followed the episode of GER. In only a few patients will the diagnostic studies be as helpful or definitive. This illustrative case is, however, a fitting example of how each of the diagnostic studies may be used in evaluation of a patient in an attempt to confirm the diagnosis of GER and respiratory illness.

Several other diagnostic studies are appropriate in some instances in which a diagnosis of GER is being considered. In an infant or child receiving assisted ventilation through an uncuffed endotracheal tube or a tracheostomy and experiencing frequent unexplained exacerbations of respiratory disease, GER is often a diagnostic consideration. Study of the tracheal aspirate for reducing substances (if the patient is

Table 30–6. 24-HOUR ESOPHAGEAL MONITORING IN ASYMPTOMATIC INFANTS, CHILDREN, AND ADULTS

	Infants* <15 days	Infants* >5 months	Children† >1 year	Adults‡
% Time pH <4.0	1.20 ± 0.91‖	4.18 ± 2.6		0.7 ± 0.23
Episodes (24 hr)	7.73 ± 6.51	19.98 ± 16.1	20.16 ± 8.64	0.6 ± 1.2§
Episodes >5 min	0.64 ± 0.51	3.24 ± 2.41		2.86 ± 2.68

*Vandeplas and Sacre-Smits (1987).
†Sondheimer and Haase (1988).
‡Fink and McCallum (1984).
§Johnson and DeMeester (1974).
‖Reported as mean ± 1 standard deviation

receiving gastric feedings) or lipid-laden macrophages has been advocated. In an older child with a tracheostomy, cytologic examination of the tracheal aspirate may contain vegetable fibers when aspiration has taken place. Each of these studies, if positive, merely confirms that aspiration is likely to have occurred. They do not rule out the possibility that contamination of the respiratory tract may be the result of a congenital or, rarely, an acquired abnormal connection between the upper respiratory and gastrointestinal tracts. When any of these test results are positive, further investigation with the imaging and respiratory function and upper gastrointestinal manometric and pH studies is indicated.

THERAPY

MEDICAL

Although medical therapy for GER has changed little in the past decade, it is still the initial therapy of choice in infants and children. Infants have been found to respond favorably to positioning. When infants are placed prone with the head of the crib elevated, gravity aids esophageal motility and emptying of the stomach. The head-down supine position and the upright position in an infant seat encourage or increase reflux in an infant at high risk for GER. Thickening of the feedings is also indicated in small infants with GER. Although thickened feedings reduce the overt findings of GER such as emesis, they are not uniformly considered to be effective in reducing episodes of reflux. Those encouraging thickened feedings contend that rice cereal must be added to the formula until the formula is the consistency of raw honey in order for this therapy to be effective. This usually requires 2 to 3 teaspoons of rice cereal per ounce of formula. Augmenting positioning and thickened feedings, the addition of smaller but more frequent feeding and withholding feedings for several hours before bedtime may improve the effec-

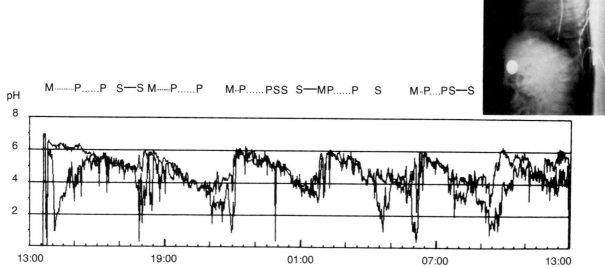

Figure 30–1. Chest roentgenogram, lateral view, showing the double lumen pH probe with the lower sensor resting in the esophagus immediately cephalad to the level of the diaphragm and the upper lumen sensor at the level of the upper esophageal sphincter *(arrow)*. The pH tracing reveals multiple episodes of gastroesophageal reflux resulting in the fall of the esophageal pH. Shortly after 1300 hours only the lower esophageal reflux is recorded, with a fall in pH below 2. At 2330 hours another episode of reflux to the level of the upper esophageal sphincter is recorded beginning with *(M)* through the entire postprandial period *(P....P)* and during sleep in the supine position *(SS)*. At 0900 a fall in both the lower and the upper esophageal pH below 4 is recorded, with the onset of the drop in pH associated with feeding, *(M)* beginning of the feeding through the postprandial period *(P)*, and continuing during supine positioning *(S)* after feeding. No change was recorded in total respiratory resistance with any episode of reflux.

tiveness of medical therapy by reducing postprandial stomach volume and minimizing the volume of the potential refluxate.

Three pharmacologic approaches have been used for the treatment of GER. Medications to improve sphincter tone and increase esophageal motility and gastric emptying are agents with cholinergic activity, such as metoclopramide and bethanechol. Bethanechol has the potential for causing increased bronchomotor tone and is thus not generally a useful drug in infants and children with GER and reactive airway disease as the major respiratory finding. Metoclopramide (0.1 mg/kg four times daily) has been found to be effective in improving delayed gastric emptying and has been reported to be an effective medication for improving gastroesophageal motility and sphincter tone. Although the medication has been reported to cause extrapyramidal side effects manifested as acute dystonic reactions, these rarely are seen with the prescribed dosage. Benadryl is effective in the treatment of these side effects.

A second class of medications for treating infants and children with GER are the H$_2$ receptor antagonists. These agents are used to reduce gastric acidity by decreasing the release of gastric juice. Ranitidine and cimetidine are the most frequently used medications in this class. They are frequently used in conjunction with antacids. The effectiveness of this form of therapy in GER of infancy and childhood is not uniformly endorsed. When GER is complicated by esophagitis or upper gastrointestinal bleeding, the use of antacids and H$_2$ antagonists is clearly indicated.

SURGICAL

Surgery is indicated for the treatment of GER when medical therapy has not led to an improvement in the gastrointestinal and respiratory findings of GER. There are three conditions in which medical management frequently fails and surgical management is considered. These disorders are tracheoesophageal fistula following complete surgical repair, profound (usually perinatal) neurologic injury, and severe bronchopulmonary dysplasia. Unfortunately, many of the infants with GER and severe respiratory illness who fail to respond to medical management are also quite malnourished. These infants are poor surgical candidates and are at risk for postoperative problems with wound healing, respiratory infection, and failure or slippage of the fundoplication and recurrence of GER. In this instance, surgery is best postponed. Patients should be treated with total parenteral nutrition and all feedings should be discontinued. The goals of therapy in the preoperative period are to effect improvement in nutrition, prevent further GER and aspiration, and reduce or eliminate symptoms and findings of airway and parenchymal lung disease. Nasogastric drainage is maintained as an adjunct to keep the stomach empty and reduce the risk of GER and further aspiration.

In preparation for antireflux surgery, treatment of airway disease is very important. This may include antibiotics for treatment of pneumonia, chest percussion, postural drainage, and in infants, pharyngeal suctioning to aid in clearance of pulmonary secretions. Bronchodilator medications are better administered as an aerosol rather than per gastrum. Both methylxanthine and beta-adrenergic bronchodilator medications have the side effect of reducing distal esophageal pressure and encouraging esophageal reflux. With beta-adrenergic agonist aerosol treatments, systemic absorption of the medications is minimized. Continuous monitoring of oxygen and carbon dioxide tension and oxygen saturation is helpful in defining which infants will also benefit from continuous oxygen therapy.

The appropriate surgical procedure for the treatment of GER depends on the constellation of pathologic gastrointestinal findings. With GER alone, a simple fundoplication is indicated. When the patient also has delayed gastric emptying, fundoplication and pyloroplasty should be considered. Fonkalsrud and colleagues (1987) reported that in more than 50 per cent of infants and children who were less than 18 years of age and were referred for fundoplication, GER was complicated by delayed gastric emptying. A final consideration is whether a gastrostomy should be placed. This procedure is indicated when GER is complicated by oral or pharyngeal dysphagia. In these patients, long-term gastrostomy feedings are advisable to avoid the risk of worsening respiratory disease from continued aspiration from above.

In follow-up of infants and children receiving surgical treatment for GER, specific complications and long-term sequellae have been described. Although in adults nearly 50 per cent experience continued symptoms after fundoplication, less than one third of the infants and children undergoing antireflux surgery experience side effects from the surgical procedure. The frequency of long-term problems includes inability to vomit or even burp in 28 per cent, gas bloating in approximately 36 per cent, slow eating in 32 per cent, and choking on some solids in 25 per cent. In a large series of 335 infants and children treated surgically with a partial fundoplication procedure, Ashcraft and associates (1981) reported that 9 per cent required reoperation. Of these, 10 patients experienced a "slipped" wrap or disrupted fundoplication, 6 an incisional hernia or dehiscence, 4 a hiatal hernia, and 3 a bowel obstruction. Other follow-up studies confirm these findings. Finally, in a worldwide survey conducted by Bettex and colleagues (1979), including 3917 operative procedures, a 1.3 per cent fatality rate was reported.

The concensus now is that fundoplication is an appropriate treatment for pediatric patients with GER and respiratory illness unresponsive to an adequate course of appropriate medical therapy. The most favorable outcome and the lowest morbidity are achieved when surgery is postponed until the patient is adequately nourished. Surgery should be delayed in malnourished infants or children until patients have had adequate nutritional rehabilitation with total parenteral nutrition as determined by consistent weight gain and skin-fold thickness. During this period of parenteral nutrition, patients should not be fed by mouth and a program of respiratory care, as already outlined, should be undertaken.

REFERENCES

Arndorfer RC, Steff JJ, Dodds WJ et al: Improved infusion system for intraluminal esophageal manometry. Gastroenterology 73:23, 1977.

Ashcraft KW, Goodwin C, Amoury RA, and Holder TM: Early recognition and aggressive treatment of gastroesophageal reflux following repair of esophageal atresia. J Pediatr Surg 12:317, 1977.

Ashcraft KW, Holder TM, and Amoury RA: Treatment of gastroesophageal reflux in children by Thal fundoplication. J Thorac Cardiovasc Surg 82:706, 1981.

Asoh R and Goyal RK: Monometry and electromyography of the upper esophageal sphincter in the opossum. Gastroenterology 74:514, 1978.

Bailey DJ, Andres JM, Danek GD, and Pinero-Carrero VM: Lack of efficacy of thickened feedings as treatment for gastroesophageal reflux. J Pediatr Gastroenterol Nutr 5:716, 1986.

Berezin S, Newman LJ, Schwarz SM, and Spiro AJ: Gastroesophageal reflux associated with nemaline myopathy of infancy. Pediatrics 81:111, 1988.

Berquist WE and Ament ME: Upper GI function in sleeping infants. Am Rev Respir Dis 131(Suppl):S26, 1985.

Berquist WE, Rachelefsky GS, Rowshan N et al: Quantitative gastroesophageal reflux and pulmonary function in asthmatic children and normal adults receiving placebo, theophylline, and metoclopramide sulfate therapy. J Allergy Clin Immunol 73:253, 1984.

Bettex M, Oesch-Amrein I, and Kuffer F: Mortality after operation for hiatus hernia. In Rickham PP, Hecker WCh, Prevot J et al (eds): Causes of postoperative death in children. Baltimore, Williams & Wilkins Co, 1979.

Blumhagen JD, Rudd TG, and Christie DL: Gastroesophageal reflux in children: radionuclide gastroesophagography. Am J Roentgenol 135:1001, 1980.

Boerema I: Hiatus hernia: repair by right-sided, subhepatic, anterior gastropexy. Surgery 65:884, 1969.

Boonyaprapa D, Alderson PO, Garfinkel DJ et al: Detection of pulmonary aspiration in infants and children with respiratory disease: concise communication. J Nucl Med 21:314, 1980.

Boyle JT, Tuchman DN, Altschuler SM et al: Mechanisms for the association of gastroesophageal reflux and bronchospasm. Am Rev Respir Dis 131(Suppl):16, 1985.

Byrne WJ, Euler AR, Ashcraft E et al: Gastroesophageal reflux in the severely retarded who vomit: criteria for and results of surgical intervention. Surgery 91:95, 1982.

Christie DL: Pulmonary complications of esophageal disease. Pediatr Clin North Am 31:835, 1984.

Christie DL, O'Grady LR, and Mack DV: Incompetent lower esophageal sphincter and gastroesophageal reflux in recurrent acute pulmonary disease of infancy and childhood. J Pediatr 93:23, 1978.

Cohen S: Swallowing and upper gastrointestinal function: specific gastrointestinal considerations. Am Rev Respir Dis 131(Suppl):S61, 1985.

Danus O, Casar C, Larrain A, and Pope CE II: Esophageal reflux—an unrecognized cause of recurrent obstructive bronchitis in children. J Pediatr 89:220, 1976.

Darling DB, McCauley RGK, Leonidas JC, and Schwartz AM: Gastroesophageal reflux in infants and children: correlation of radiologic severity and pulmonary pathology. Radiology 127:735, 1978.

Dodds WJ: Instrumentation and methods for intraluminal esophageal manometry. Arch Int Med 136:515, 1976.

Dodds WJ, Dent J, Hogan WJ et al: Mechanisms of gastroesophageal reflux in patients with reflux esophagitis. N Engl J Med 307:1547, 1982.

Dodds WJ, Hogan WJ, Miller WN et al: Effect of increased intra-abdominal pressure on lower esophageal sphincter pressure. Am J Dig Dis 20:298, 1975.

Eastwood GL, Castell DD, and Higgs RH: Experimental esophagitis in cats impairs lower esophageal sphincter pressure. Gastroenterology 69:146, 1975.

Enzmann ER, Harell GS, and Zboralske FF: Upper esophageal responses to intraluminal distention in man. Gastroenterology 72:1292, 1977.

Euler AR: Use of bethanechol for the treatment of gastroesophageal reflux. J Pediatr 96:321, 1980.

Euler AR and Ament ME: Detection of gastroesophageal reflux in the pediatric age patient by esophageal intraluminal pH probe measurement (Tuttle test). Pediatrics 60:55, 1977.

Euler AR and Byrne WJ: Twenty-four hour esophageal intraluminal pH probe testing: a comparative analysis. Gastroenterology 80:957, 1981.

Exarhos ND, Logan WD, Abbott OA, and Hatcher CR: The importance of pH and volume in tracheobronchial aspiration. Dis Chest 47:167, 1965.

Feigelson J, Girault F, and Pecau Y: Gastro-oesophageal reflux and esophagitis in cystic fibrosis. Acta Paediatr Scand 76:989, 1987.

Fink SM and McCallum RW: The role of prolonged esophageal pH monitoring in the diagnosis of gastroesophageal reflux. JAMA 252:1160, 1984.

Foglia RP, Fonkalsrud EW, Ament ME et al: Gastroesophageal fundoplication for the management of chronic pulmonary disease in children. Am J Surg 140:72, 1980.

Fonkalsrud EW, Berquist W, Vargas J et al: Surgical treatment of gastroesophageal reflux syndrome in infants and children. Am J Surg 154:11, 1987.

Ghaed N and Stein MR: Assessment of a technique for scintographic monitoring of pulmonary aspiration of gastric contents in asthmatics with gastroesophageal reflux. Ann Allergy 42:306, 1979.

Guiffre RM, Rubin S, and Mitchell I: Antireflux surgery in infants with bronchopulmonary dysplasia. Am J Dis Child 141:648, 1987.

Harding R and Titchen DA: Chemosensitive vagal endings in the esophagus of the cat. J Physiol 247:52, 1975.

Harnsberger JK, Corey JJ, Johnson DG, and Herbst JJ: Long-term follow-up of surgery for gastroesophageal reflux in infants and children. J Pediatr 102:505, 1983.

Harrington RA, Hamilton CW, Brogden RN et al: Metoclopramide: an updated review of its pharmacological properties and clinical use. Drugs 25:451, 1983.

Helm JF, Dodds WJ, Pelc LR et al: Effect of esophageal emptying and saliva on clearance of acid from the esophagus. N Engl J Med 310:284, 1984.

Herbst JJ, Minton SD, and Book LS: Gastroesophageal reflux causing respiratory distress and apnea in newborn infants. J Pediatr 95:763, 1978.

Herbst JJ, Book LS, Johnson DG, and Jolly S: The lower esophageal sphincter in gastroesophageal reflux. J Clin Gastroenterol 1:119, 1979.

Higgs RH, Smyth RD, and Castell DO: Gastric alkalinization: effect on lower-esophageal sphincter pressure and serum gastrin. N Engl J Med 291:486, 1974.

Hopper AO, Kwong LK, and Stevenson DK et al: Detection of gastric contents in tracheal fluid of infants by lactose assay. J Pediatr 102:415, 1983.

Hyams JS, Leichtner AM, Zamett LO, and Walters JK: Effect of metoclopramide on prolonged intraesophageal pH testing in infants with gastroesophageal reflux. J Pediatr Gastroenterol Nutr 5:716, 1986.

Johnson DG: Current thinking on the role of surgery in gastroesophageal reflux. Pediatr Clin North Am 32:1165, 1985.

Johnson DG, Jolley SG, Herbst JJ, and Cordell LJ: Surgical selection of infants with gastroesophageal reflux. J Pediatr Surg 16:587, 1981.

Johnson LF: 24 hour pH monitoring in the study of gastroesophageal reflux. J Clin Gastroenterol 62:325, 1974.

Jolley SG, Herbst JJ, Johnson DG et al: Esophageal pH monitoring during sleep identifies children with respiratory symptoms from gastroesophageal reflux. Gastroenterology 80:1501, 1981.

Jona JZ, Sty JR, and Glicklich M: Simplified radioisotope technique for assessing gastroesophageal reflux in children. J Pediatr Surg 16:114, 1981.

Kennedy JH: "Silent" gastroesophageal reflux: an important but little known cause of pulmonary complications. Dis Chest 42:42, 1962.

Logan WJ and Bosma JF: Oral and pharyngeal dysphagia in infancy. Pediatr Clin North Am 14:47, 1967.

Lopes JM, Tabachnik E, Muller NL et al: Total airways resistance and respiratory muscle activity during sleep. J Appl Physiol 54:773, 1983.

McCauley RG, Darling DB, Leonidas JC, and Schwartz AM: Gastroesophageal reflux in infants and children: a useful classification and reliable physiologic technique for its demonstration. Am J Roentgenol 130:47, 1978.

Macfadyen UM, Hendry GMA, and Simpson H: Gastro-oesophageal reflux in near-miss sudden infant death syndrome or suspected recurrent aspiration. Arch Dis Child 58:87, 1983.

Machida HM, Forbes DA, Gall DG, and Scott RB: Metoclopramide in gastroesophageal reflux. J Pediatr 112:483, 1988.

Mansfield LE and Stein MR: Gastroesophageal reflux and asthma: a possible reflex mechanism. Ann Allergy 41:224, 1978.

Mansfield LE, Hameister HH, Spaulding HS et al: The role of the vagus nerve in airway narrowing caused by intra-esophageal hydrochloric acid provocation and esophageal distention. Ann Allergy 47:431, 1981.

Mendelson CL: The aspiration of stomach contents into the lungs during obstetric anesthesia. Am J Obstet Gynecol 52:191, 1946.

Meyers WF and Herbst JJ: Effectiveness of positioning therapy for gastrocsophageal reflux. Pediatrics 69:768, 1982.

Meyers WF, Roberts CC, Johnson DG, and Herbst JJ: Value of tests for evaluation of gastroesophageal reflux in children. J Pediatr Surg 120:515, 1985.

Moran JR, Block SM, Lyerly AD et al: Lipid-laden alveolar macrophage and lactose assay as markers of aspiration in neonates with lung disease. J Pediatr 112:643, 1988.

Moran TJ: Experimental aspiration pneumonia. IV. Inflammatory and reparative changes produced by intratracheal injections of autologous gastric juice and hydrochloric acid. Arch Pathol 60:122, 1955.

Nissen R: Gastropexy and "fundoplication" in surgical treatment of hiatal hernia. Am J Dig Dis 6:954, 1961.

Orenstein SR, Magill HL, and Brooks P: Thickening of infant feedings for therapy of gastroesophageal reflux. J Pediatr 110:181, 1987.

Orenstein SR and Whittington PF: Positioning for prevention of infant gastroesophageal reflux. J Pediatr 103:534, 1983.

Orenstein SR, Whitington PF, and Orenstein DM: The infant seat as treatment for gastroesophageal reflux. N Engl J Med 309:760, 1983.

Parker AF, Christie DL, and Cahill JL: Incidence and significance of gastroesophageal reflux following repair of esophageal atresia and tracheoesophageal fistula and the need for antireflux procedures. J Pediatr Surg 14:5, 1979.

Pieretti R, Shandling B, and Stephens CA: Resistant esophageal stenosis associated with reflux after repair of esophageal atresia. A therapeutic approach. J Pediatr Surg 9:355, 1974.

Reich SB, Earley WC, Ravin TH et al: Evaluation of gastropulmonary aspiration by a radioactive technique: concise communication. J Nucl Med 18:1079, 1977.

Russell COH, Hill LD, Holmes ER III et al: Radionuclide transit: a sensitive screening test of esophageal dysfunction. Gastroenterology 80:887, 1981.

Scott RB, O'Loughlin EV, and Gail DG: Gastroesophageal reflux in patients with cystic fibrosis. J Pediatr 106:223, 1985.

Simonsson BG, Jacobs FM, and Nadel JA: The role of the autonomic nervous system and the cough reflex in the increased responsiveness of airways in patients with obstructive airways disease. J Clin Invest 46:1812, 1967.

Sondheimer JM: Upper esophageal sphincter and pharyngoesophageal motor function in infants with and without distal gastroesophageal reflux. Gastroenterology 85:301, 1983.

Sondheimer JM: Gastroesophageal reflux.: update on pathogenesis and diagnosis. Pediatr Clin North Am 35:103, 1988.

Sondheimer JM and Haase GA: Simultaneous pH recordings from multiple sites in children with and without distal gastroesophageal reflux. J Pediatr Gastroenterol Nutr 7:46, 1988.

Sondheimer JM and Morris BA: Gastroesophageal reflux among severely retarded children. J Pediatr 94:710, 1979.

Spaulding HS, Mansfield LE, Stein MR et al: Further investigation of the association between gastroesophageal reflux and bronchoconstriction. J Allergy Clin Immunol 69:516, 1982.

Spitzer AR, Boyle JT, Tuchman DN, and Fox WW: Awake apnea associated with gastroesophageal reflux: a specific clinical syndrome. J Pediatr 104:200, 1984.

Stanciu C and Bennett JR: Upper esophageal sphincter yield pressure in normal subjects and in patients with esophageal reflux. Thorax 29:459, 1974.

Sutphen JL, Dillard VL, and Pipan ME: Antacid and formula effects on gastric acidity in infants with gastroesophageal reflux. Pediatrics 78:55, 1986.

Thal AP: A unified approach to surgical problems of the esophagastric junction. Ann Surg 168:542, 1968.

Thomas D, Rothberg RM, and Lester LA: Cystic fibrosis and gastroesophageal reflux in infancy. Am J Dis Child 139:66, 1985.

Tuchman DN, Boyle JT, Pack AI et al: Comparison of airway responses following tracheal or esophageal acidification in the cat. Gastroenterology 87:872, 1984.

Tunnell WP, Smith EI, and Carson JA: Gastroesophageal reflux in childhood. The dilemma of surgical success. Ann Surg 197:560, 1983.

Tuttle SG and Grossman MI: Detection of gastroesophageal reflux by simultaneous measurement of intraluminal pressure and pH. Proc Soc Exp Biol Med 98:225, 1958.

Vandeplas Y and Sacre-Smits L: Continuous 24-hour esophageal monitoring in 285 asymptomatic infants 0–15 months old. J Pediatr Gastroenterol Nutr 6:220, 1987.

Werlin SL, Dodds WJ, Hogan WJ, and Andorfer RC: Mechanisms of gastroesophageal reflux in children. J Pediatr 97:244, 1967.

Widdicombe JG: Respiratory reflexes from the trachea and bronchi of the cat. J Physiol 123:55, 1954.

Wilkinson JD, Dudgeon DL, and Sondheimer JM: A comparison of medical and surgical treatment of gastroesophageal reflux. J Pediatr 99:202, 1981.

Winter HS, Madara JL, and Stafford RJ: Intraepithelial eosinophils: a new diagnostic test for reflux esophagitis. Gastroenterology 83:818, 1982.

Wynne JW and Modell JH: Respiratory aspiration of stomach contents. Ann Intern Med 87:466, 1977.

Wynne JW, Ramphal R, and Hood CI: Tracheal mucosal damage after aspiration. A scanning electron microscope study. Am Rev Respir Dis 124:728, 1981.

31

ARNOLD M. SALZBERG, M.D., JAMES W. BROOKS, M.D.,
and THOMAS M. KRUMMEL, M.D.

FOREIGN BODIES IN THE AIR PASSAGES

Foreign bodies aspirated into and retained in the tracheobronchial tree in infancy and childhood may threaten life and produce severe lung damage. Since 1960 at the Medical College of Virginia Hospitals, a total of 131 foreign bodies in the respiratory tract have been reported in 131 children (Tables 31–1 and 31–2). The spectrum of foreign bodies encountered between 1976 and 1981 is typical of the overall experience (Table 31–3).

DIAGNOSIS

Foreign body aspiration is often accompanied by sudden, violent coughing, gagging, wheezing, vomiting, cyanosis, and brief episodes of apnea. If the foreign body is small and not obstructive, these findings may be minimal. After the initial dramatic symptoms, an annoying cough and wheezing persist without respiratory distress, unless the trachea is involved.

Physical examination can be helpful in diagnosis and localization. Observation may demonstrate unilateral thoracic overexpansion from obstructive emphysema or underexpansion from atelectasis. Wheezing can be heard with and without the stethoscope, and decreased breath sounds over the affected side are constant.

Fluoroscopy and chest roentgenogram in various projections are indispensable. A radiopaque foreign body offers no problem in identification (Fig. 31–1). The usual radiologic finding associated with nonopaque foreign bodies is atelectasis or obstructive emphysema, except for those occasions when a lateral chest roentgenogram may demonstrate the object in a well-outlined air tracheogram (Fig. 31–2). Fluoroscopy and lateral decubitus chest roentgenograms may

document the dynamics of air trapping and may localize the obstructive emphysema (Fig. 31–3). After the first 24 hours, the roentgenographic findings may progress from those of partial to complete atelectasis; the situation may be complicated by pneumonitis (Fig. 31–4).

Occasionally, the initial symptoms and physical findings may be minimal or overlooked and the presenting problem is persistent, localized, recurrent pneumonia that does not completely clear with adequate therapy. Bronchoscopy should be done if the possibility of foreign body exists, especially if hemoptysis is concurrent.

Respiratory distress may accompany obstructing foreign bodies of the high esophagus and pharyngoesophageal junction, and this area should be scrutinized endoscopically if roentgenograms are suggestive and dysphagia occurs.

TREATMENT

Foreign bodies in the tracheobronchial tree should be removed promptly by bronchoscopy under general anesthesia. Early extraction reduces local damage and distal parenchymal complications.

The Jackson bronchoscope, designed in the early twentieth century, was the standard bronchoscopic instrument until the availability of the Hopkins rod lens system in the early 1970s. The ventilating bronchoscope surrounding the Storz-Hopkins telescope provides a closed, safe, efficient route for general anesthesia and mechanical ventilation. A separate channel in the bronchoscope sheath permits the

Table 31–1. RESPIRATORY FOREIGN BODIES: DISTRIBUTION BY LOCATION

	1960–1975	1976–1988
Trachea	10 (18%)	7 (9%)
Right main stem bronchus	27 (49%)	44 (58%)
Left main stem bronchus	18 (33%)	25 (33%)
Total	55	76

Table 31–2. RESPIRATORY FOREIGN BODIES: ENDOSCOPIC EXTRACTION BEFORE AND AFTER THE STORZ-HOPKINS BRONCHOSCOPE

	1960–1975*	1976–1988†
Bronchoscopic extraction	50 (91%)	74 (97%)
Thoracotomy	4 (7%)	1 (1%)
Mortality	1 (2%)	0 (0%)
Total	55	75

*Jackson bronchoscope.
†Storz-Hopkins bronchoscope.

476

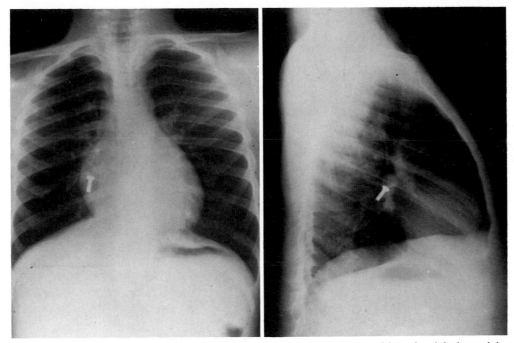

Figure 31–1. Posteroanterior and lateral roentgenograms of a screw aspirated into the right lower lobe of the lung.

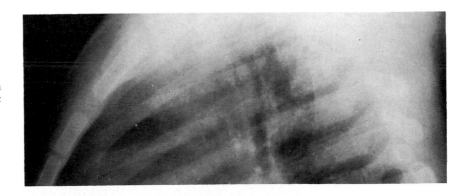

Figure 31–2. Lateral chest roentgenogram showing an aspirated peanut in the thoracic trachea just proximal to the carina.

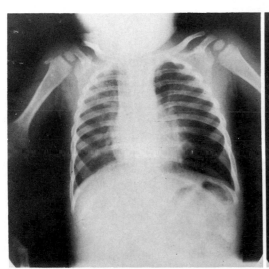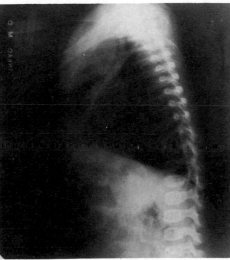

Figure 31–3. Air trapping of the left lower lobe of the lung due to an aspirated peanut.

Table 31–3. FOREIGN BODY IN THE RESPIRATORY TRACT, 1976–1981: DISTRIBUTION BY TYPE

Type	Number of Cases
Nut(s)	18
Plastic	7
Pin or screw	4
Seed	3
Bone	2
Coin	1
Thermometer	1
Total	36

insertion of foreign body forceps without obstruction of vision and permits manipulation under magnification. Even under these superior circumstances, extraction is often difficult and tedious, especially with foreign objects that tend to crumble, such as peanuts.

Following removal of a foreign body from the lower airway, edema of the glottis due to manipulation or of the bronchus due to contact or chemical bronchitis can be annoying. Corticosteroid therapy for 24 to 48 hours and a course of antibiotic therapy should be helpful. Postoperative chest films may demonstrate a pneumothorax, which on rare occasions follows overenthusiastic anesthesia or excessive coughing. Chest-tube drainage becomes necessary under these circumstances.

In less than 5 per cent of our patients, endoscopic extraction was not possible in spite of repeated attempts, and thoracotomy with bronchotomy became necessary. No unusual morbidity followed these procedures (Fig. 31–5). Failure of bronchoscopy on two

occasions would seem to be an indication for open operation, because nonoperative resolution is highly unlikely and delay is associated with pulmonary morbidity.

Small respiratory foreign bodies have been removed using a Fogarty catheter (Fig. 31–6) and by means of inhalation of bronchodilators with postural drainage.

Despite the various technical manipulations possible through the Storz-Hopkins bronchoscopic equipment, large tracheal foreign bodies pose an additional threat. Such large foreign bodies may be lost during extraction through the narrow subglottic area; thus uncontrolled, they may migrate within the airway, rotate on their axis, and produce acute airway obstruction with the ever present threat of cardiopulmonary arrest and cerebral hypoxia.

To obviate this potential morbidity and mortality, simultaneous bronchoscopy with an elective tracheostomy, through which the foreign body may be withdrawn, appears to be a rational option.

RESULTS

At the Medical College of Virginia Hospitals, 131 respiratory foreign bodies in as many children have been seen since 1960; their management with the Jackson and the Storz-Hopkins bronchoscopes is compared retrospectively.

From 1960 to 1975, the Jackson bronchoscope was used in 55 patients. Ten foreign bodies were tracheal (18 per cent), 27 right sided (49 per cent), and 18 left sided (33 per cent). Thoracotomy was necessary

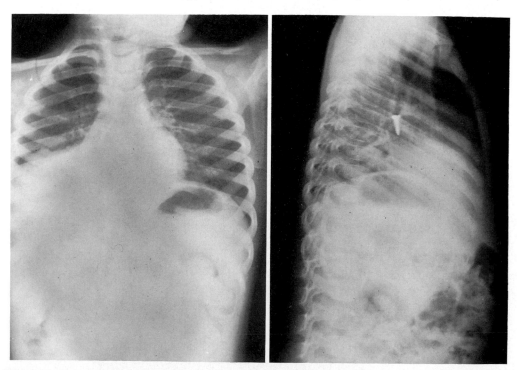

Figure 31–4. Atelectasis and pneumonia of the right lower lobe of the lung due to a screw aspirated into the right lower lobe approximately 96 hours before these roentgenograms were made.

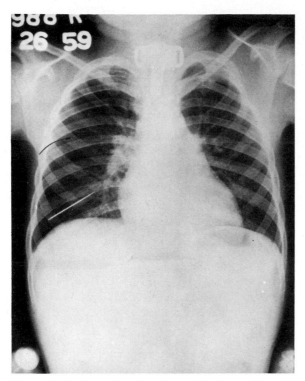
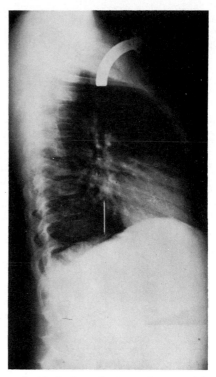

Figure 31–5. An aspirated sewing needle that could not be located with the bronchoscope, thus requiring thoracotomy for successful removal.

in 4 of the 55 cases (7 per cent), with one death occurring from a balloon in the trachea during transport to the hospital. Fifty of 55 foreign bodies were extracted bronchoscopically (91 per cent).

Since 1976, the Storz-Hopkins bronchoscope has been used in 76 patients without mortality. Seven foreign bodies were tracheal (9 per cent), 44 right sided (58 per cent), and 25 left sided (33 per cent). Thoracotomy was necessary in one case in 1981 but has not been required since. One metallic needle foreign body remains electively retained in peripheral pulmonary parenchyma. In this most recent group, bronchoscopic removal of respiratory foreign bodies was accomplished in 74 of 76 patients (97 per cent).

Contemporary bronchoscopic equipment and corresponding advances in anesthetic technique have improved the capability of foreign body removal and diminished the incidence of thoracotomy.

CONCLUSION

It is apparent that foreign bodies in the tracheobronchial tree are particularly life threatening in the pediatric population. Parents should be made aware

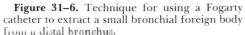
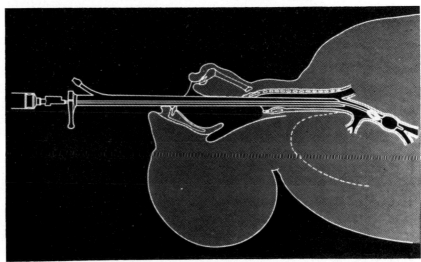

Figure 31–6. Technique for using a Fogarty catheter to extract a small bronchial foreign body from a distal bronchus.

of the hazards and of the necessity to exclude small objects from the environment and peanuts and fruit seeds from the diet of small children.

REFERENCES

Aytac A, Yurdakul Y, Ikizler C et al: Inhalation of foreign bodies in children. Report of 500 cases. J Thorac Cardiovasc Surg 74:145, 1977.

Brown BSJ, Ma H, Dunbar JS et al: Foreign bodies in the tracheobronchial tree in childhood. J Can Assoc Radiol 14:158, 1963.

Camarata SJ and Salyer JM: Management of foreign bodies in air passages and esophagus under general anesthesia. Am Surg 31:725, 1965.

Carter R: Bronchotomy: the safe solution for an infarcted foreign body. Ann Surg 10:93, 1970.

Daniilidis J, Symeonidis B, Triardis K et al: Foreign body in the airways. A review of 90 cases. Arch Otolaryngol 103:570, 1977.

Hight EW, Philippart AI, and Hertzler JH: The treatment of retained foreign bodies in the pediatric airway. J Pediatr Surg 16:694, 1981.

Holinger LD and Callins WP: Endobronchial foreign body removal. Arch Otolaryngol 103:563, 1977.

Hunsicher RC and Gartner WS: Fogarty catheter technique for removal of endobronchial foreign body. Arch Otolaryngol 103:103, 1977.

Jackson C: Grasses as foreign bodies in bronchus and lung. Laryngoscope 62:897, 1972.

Kim IG, Brummitt WM, Humphrey A et al: Foreign body in the airway: A review of 202 cases. Laryngoscope 83:347, 1973.

Law D and Kosloske AM: Management of tracheobronchial foreign bodies in children: a reevaluation of postural drainage and bronchoscopy. Pediatrics 58:362, 1976.

Lejeune FE: Foreign bodies in the tracheobronchial tree and esophagus. Surg Clin North Am 46:1501, 1966.

Majd NS, Mofenson HC, and Greensher J: Lower airway foreign body aspiration in children. Clin Pediatr 16:13, 1977.

Swensson EE, Rah KH, Kim MC et al: Extraction of large tracheal foreign bodies through a tracheostoma under bronchoscopic control. Ann Thorac Surg 39:251, 1985.

32

WILLIAM M. THURLBECK, M.B., F.R.C.P.(C), and
JOHN A. FLEETHAM, M.B., B.S., F.R.C.P.(C)

USUAL INTERSTITIAL PNEUMONIA
(Cryptogenic or Idiopathic Fibrosing Alveolitis)

Various terms have been used to describe interstitial inflammatory disease of the lung associated with interstitial fibrosis: organizing interstitial pneumonia, idiopathic pulmonary fibrosis, chronic interstitial pneumonitis, idiopathic diffuse interstitial fibrosis of the lung, bronchiolar emphysema, muscular cirrhosis of the lung, chronic diffuse sclerosing alveolitis, and Hamman-Rich syndrome. *Cryptogenic or idiopathic fibrosing alveolitis* or just *fibrosing alveolitis* is most commonly used at present, although as Liebow (1975) has pointed out, these are not completely satisfactory terms in that they stress only one possible outcome of lung injury, and he thus preferred "usual" interstitial pneumonia. It is now apparent that a useful purpose can be served by classifying the interstitial pneumonias into several categories. This chapter deals with the "usual" form of interstitial pneumonia, and Chapter 33 deals with described variants.

DEFINITION AND PATHOLOGY

Fibrosing alveolitis is characteristically heterogeneous in both gross and microscopic appearances.

On gross examination, parts of the lung may appear normal, whereas others may have a fine, multicystic appearance, with cysts 0.5 to 10 mm in diameter (honeycomb lung). These cysts, when under the pleura, impart a hobnail appearance resembling that of cirrhosis of the liver. This represents the advanced stage of the condition and is usually more severe in the lower and peripheral zones of the lung. Histologically, varying degrees of fibrosis are present. In about one quarter of cases, fibrosis is focal and most alveoli are normal; in another one quarter there is more fibrous tissue than normal lung, and in the remainder most of the lung biopsy specimen is fibrotic (Crystal et al, 1976). Varying degrees of proliferation of smooth muscle also occur. Interstitial inflammation is always present but varies in severity. Most of the inflammatory cells are lymphocytes, plasma cells, or macrophages, and there may be nodular collections of lymphocytes. Neutrophils and eosinophils are usually found but are not commonly prominent. These are usually found in the cyst-like spaces. Active-appearing granulation tissue may be found in alveolar spaces, but its presence should raise the possibility of cryptogenic organizing pneumonia or bronchiolitis obliterans organizing pneumonia (see Chapter 33). The final result is gross disorganization of the lung, so that the periphery of the lung consists of small cystic spaces lined by bronchiolar cells and type I and type II alveolar epithelial cells. The spaces are separated from each other by dense connective tissue (Figs. 32–1 and 32–2).

The exact mode of development of the lesion is uncertain, but it is postulated that an initial injury to the alveolar wall results in destruction of the alveolar basement membrane and formation of an exudate in the alveolar spaces. Loose fibrous (granulation) tissue results and may form intraluminal buds that partially fill air spaces. These may obliterate lumens of air spaces or become reepithelialized and incorporated into the walls of air spaces (Basset et al, 1986). Another mechanism is infolding or collapse of alveolar walls so that there is permanent apposition of alveolar walls. Type II alveolar epithelial cells proliferate over the top of the apposed walls, combining the folded or collapsed alveolar walls into a single septum (Katzenstein, 1985). Consequently, there is loss of distal air spaces (alveolar ducts and sacs) and dilation of the proximal part of the acinus (respiratory bronchioles), which becomes lined largely by continuous bronchiolar epithelium. This causes the microcystic appearance of the lung, but in reality the majority of the "cysts" connect with airways and are dilated distal airways. The best term for this lesion is *bronchiolectasis*. Because the airway connections are imperfect, bronchiolar secretions accumulate in many of the spaces.

The characteristic histologic feature of usual interstitial pneumonia is heterogeneity of lesions. In the same biopsy specimen, indeed in adjacent microscopic fields, there may be normal lung, equivocal interstitial pneumonia, obvious interstitial pneumonia with little fibrosis, mild fibrosis, and honeycombing.

ETIOLOGY

Honeycomb lung or end-stage lung (Genereux, 1975) may represent the pulmonary outcome of a wide variety of insults. The many conditions that may lead to honeycomb lung are listed in Table 32–1. Honeycomb lung should not be confused with usual interstitial pneumonia because honeycomb lung is nonspecific, whereas usual interstitial pneumonia has specific diagnostic features.

The etiology of idiopathic fibrosing alveolitis is unknown. In about 5 per cent of patients, it occurs as a familial autosomal dominant condition (Swaye et al, 1969; Solliday et al, 1973). The age of onset of this familial disease varies from early infancy to adulthood. A number of different studies have reported an excess of HLA-B12, HLA-B7, and HLA-B8 in patients with usual interstitial pneumonia (Turton et al, 1978). Viral infection may play a role, and the original cases of Hamman-Rich syndrome were noted to occur following a severe viral respiratory infection (see "Acute Interstitial Pneumonia"). There is some indirect evidence that fibrosing alveolitis is an immunologically mediated disease (Crystal et al, 1981). Identical lung lesions may be found in patients with rheumatoid arthritis, scleroderma, dermatomyositis, and systemic lupus erythematosus. Rheumatoid factor and antinuclear factor are often present despite the clinical absence of rheumatoid arthritis and

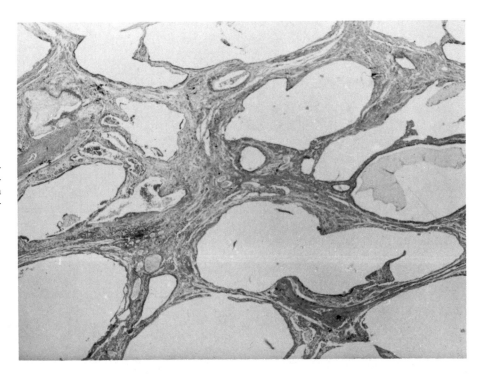

Figure 32–1. The normal lung architecture is grossly disorganized and replaced by cystic spaces 0.5 to 2 mm in diameter and separated from one another by dense fibrous tissue (× 30).

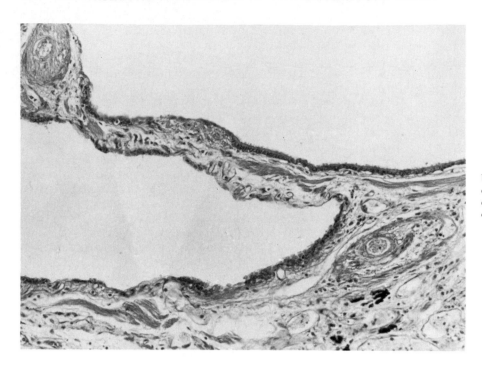

Figure 32–2. The air spaces are lined by bronchiolar epithelium, and there is dense interstitial fibrosis. Note the presence of smooth muscle and the scattering of inflammatory cells (× 150).

systemic lupus erythematosus (Turner-Warwick and Haslam, 1971). In addition, deposition of immunoglobulin in the lungs and circulating immune complexes may be found in these patients (Dreisin et al, 1978).

CLINICAL MANIFESTATIONS

The condition is relatively uncommon in children. It is a similar condition to that in adults but is usually a more acute illness and if untreated more predictably fatal. Ten children with fibrosing alveolitis presenting at birth to 6 years of age have been reported

Table 32–1. CAUSES OF HONEYCOMB LUNG (END-STAGE LUNG)

Environmental Causes
Inorganic dusts
Organic dusts (hypersensitivity pneumonitis)
Noxious gases
Drugs
Radiation

Collagen-Vascular Diseases
Rheumatoid arthritis
Progressive systemic sclerosis
Systemic lupus erythematosus

Sarcoidosis

Inherited Disorders
Neurofibromatosis

Miscellaneous Causes
Celiac disease
Whipple's disease
Renal tubular acidosis
Weber-Christian disease
Histiocytosis X
Hermansky-Pudlak syndrome

and compared with an additional 31 children previously reported with this condition (Hewitt et al, 1977). More recently, 10 children (age range 6 months to 14 years) with fibrosing alveolitis have been reviewed (Chetty et al, 1987). The familial form of the disease occurs in about the same proportion of children to adults as the nonfamilial form. In adults, the condition is more common in men than in women, but the sex incidence is about equal in children. In the familial variant, females are more commonly affected.

The patients typically present with an insidious onset of dyspnea, which first appears on exertion but is progressive and later occurs at rest. Cough is often present and usually unproductive unless there is a coexistent bronchopulmonary infection. Anorexia, poor weight gain, failure to thrive, polyarthralgia, fatigue, and nonspecific pleuritic and substernal chest pain may develop as the disease progresses. Hemoptysis and spontaneous pneumothorax (Gaensler et al, 1972) are recognized complications of the disease and occasionally provide the presenting complaint. Physical examination may be unremarkable, particularly in the early stages of this disease. The most common findings are rapid, shallow breathing and bibasilar end-inspiratory crackles. Digital clubbing and central cyanosis occur as the disease progresses. The appearance of peripheral edema, hepatomegaly, an increased pulmonic second sound, and venous distention indicates the presence of right ventricular failure, which is common in the terminal stages of the disease and is of serious import.

The appearance on chest radiograph varies depending on the stage of disease and the rapidity of onset. Chest radiographs may be entirely normal even when there are clinical symptoms and physiologic abnormalities. The typical radiographic appearance is a diffuse reticulonodular infiltrate, more striking in the lower zones of the lung (Fig. 32–3). As the disease progresses, lung volume diminishes and small cystic lesions surrounded by thickened tissue (honeycomb lung) become evident. Pleural involvement is unusual.

The computed tomographic (CAT) appearance may be specific (Müller et al, 1986). Reticular densities correlate with fibrosis, and cystic spaces may be seen, corresponding to honeycomb lung; these both are characteristically subpleural. A CAT scan is also a good predictor of disease activity and is seen as air space opacification (Müller et al, 1987). Air space opacifications are patchy and also occur dominantly in subpleural regions.

DIAGNOSIS

No laboratory studies yield pathognomonic findings. Many patients with idiopathic fibrosing alveolitis have elevated sedimentation rates or hypergammaglobulinemia, but there is little evidence to suggest that these parameters correlate with the activity of the lung disease. Antinuclear factor and rheumatoid factor are present in 30 to 50 per cent of cases. Polycythemia is often present when hypoxemia has been either prolonged or severe.

Pulmonary function studies help to document the severity of the functional impairment and provide useful indices with which to monitor any response to therapy (Keogh and Crystal, 1980). However, most physiologic parameters correlate poorly with disease activity and are unhelpful in terms of both etiology and pathogenesis. Characteristically, patients with diffuse interstitial fibrosis have restrictive lung disease. All lung volumes are reduced, but the relative proportions are preserved. Tests of expiratory flow may also show reduced values, but when found, they are usually due to diminished lung volumes. When correction is made for the reduced lung volumes, the expiratory flow rate is often supernormal, reflecting the increased elastic recoil of the lung. Lung compliance is typically diminished; the pressure-volume curve is flattened and displaced downward. Diffusing capacity is often markedly reduced and may be abnormal before any other radiologic or physiologic findings.

Blood gas analysis usually shows reduced arterial P_{O_2} and compensated respiratory alkalosis with low arterial P_{CO_2}. The hypoxemia is usually mild at rest but may decrease dramatically on exercise. It is due primarily to ventilation-perfusion inequality, but there is some evidence that impaired diffusion may exacerbate the hypoxemia on exercise. The cause of the hyperventilation in these patients is unclear but may be intrapulmonary reflexes or stimulation of the peripheral chemoreceptors by the hypoxemia. Arterial P_{CO_2} becomes normal as the disease progresses and ultimately is raised in the terminal stages of the illness.

Definitive diagnosis by ruling out the other causes of diffuse interstitial lung disease requires a lung biopsy. Open lung biopsy is the procedure of choice. Conventional wisdom dictates that biopsy of the lingular or right middle lobe is inadvisable because these may be the site of the worst and most chronic lesions. However, a recent study has shown that they are equally as good as other sites (Miller et al, 1987). These authors considered that the site of biopsy should be dictated by the CAT appearance. Interpretation of tissue obtained by a transbronchial bi-

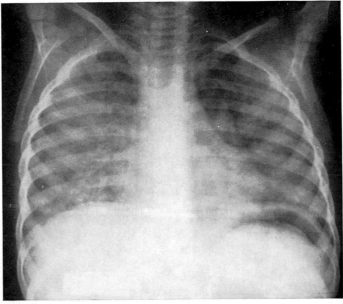

Figure 32–3. There are diffuse reticulonodular densities in the middle and lower zones of the lungs (× 150). (Courtesy of Dr. WW Waring.)

opsy is often difficult, as the amount of tissue is small and the specimen may not be representative of the disease process. Significant rates of false-positive and false-negative results have been documented (Wall et al, 1981).

COURSE AND COMPLICATIONS

Characteristically, the disease is slowly progressive, with increasing disability. Complete and permanent arrest of the condition is unusual. Pulmonary hypertension and right ventricular failure occur late in the disease. Most children die in respiratory failure, the terminal episode usually being precipitated by a superimposed acute infection. In adults, the median survival from the time symptoms are first reported is less than 6 years (Carrington et al, 1978).

TREATMENT

The therapeutic approach is generally symptomatic and supportive, with emphasis on the prevention and prompt treatment of respiratory infections. Low-flow oxygen may improve exercise tolerance in hypoxemic patients, but there is no evidence that this improvement changes their ultimate survival. A therapeutic trial of corticosteroids is indicated in all patients with usual interstitial pneumonia. Children appear more likely to respond than adults (Hewitt et al, 1977). An appropriate course of oral corticosteroids is prednisone, 1 mg/kg/day for an 8-week period. The results of therapy should be objectively monitored by serial pulmonary function studies and chest radiographs or CAT scans. If there is significant improvement, corticosteroid therapy should be cautiously tapered after 6 months to 1 year of treatment. If there is no improvement, corticosteroid therapy should be rapidly tapered. The role of immunosuppressive drugs such as azathioprine, cyclophosphamide, and penicillamine in the therapy of idiopathic fibrosing alveolitis is controversial. In view of the significant side effects of these cytotoxic agents, their widespread use should await the outcome of randomized trials. Total heart-lung transplantation has now been successfully achieved in usual interstitial pneumonia and may soon be indicated in selected patients.

ACUTE INTERSTITIAL PNEUMONIA

Although most cases of usual interstitial pneumonia have a slowly progressive course, some are rapidly progressive. Thus they resemble the original cases described by Hamman and Rich (1944). Katzenstein and colleagues (1986) have pointed out that such cases have generally been included among cases of fibrosing alveolitis in the past; thus, we have included this topic in this chapter rather than the next one.

In a prospective study, Pratt and associates (1979) described 12 cases of what they described as the accelerated version of interstitial pneumonitis. They described 12 patients (nine men, three women) with an average age of 62 years (range 27 to 75 years) who died 1 to 18 months after the onset of the disease (mean 4.7 months). In this series, five had overt collagen-vascular disease and four had evidence of immunologic disorders. More recently, Katzenstein and co-workers (1986) have studied rapidly progressive cases, determined on the basis of the lung biopsy appearance. They reported eight patients with an average age of 28 years and a range of 13 to 50 years. The clinical features were of sudden onset and rapid progression, with death in 23 days to 2 months in five patients and within 3½ to 6 months in another two. One patient survived. Of the five women, two were pregnant. In six, there was a virus-like prodrome. None had associated collagen-vascular disease. Bilateral diffuse infiltrates were seen on the chest radiographs. The biopsy specimens showed a thickened, edematous, fibroblastic stroma with numerous mitoses and extensive type II epithelial cell hyperplasia with nuclear atypicality. Residual hyaline membranes were seen in six of the eight cases. In four cases, squamous metaplasia of bronchiolar epithelium was seen spreading to the surfaces of adjacent air spaces. Organizing thrombi were seen in small arteries in five subjects. As opposed to usual interstitial pneumonia, the lesions were uniform throughout the biopsy sample and all of the apparent same age in appearance. The lesion resembles that of the proliferative phase of the adult respiratory distress syndrome and, indeed, the early phases of bronchopulmonary dysplasia. None of the usual causes of the adult respiratory distress syndrome could be identified, and the authors postulated that the lesion represented a response to a massive, unknown, respiratory insult.

REFERENCES

Basset F, Ferrans VJ, Soler P et al: Intraluminal fibrosis in interstitial lung disorders. Am J Pathol 122:443, 1986.
Carrington CB, Gaensler EA, Coutu RE et al: Natural history and treated course of usual and desquamative interstitial pneumonia. N Engl J Med 298:801, 1978.
Chetty A, Bhuyan UN, Mitra DK et al: Cryptogenic fibrosing alveolitis in children. Ann Allergy 58:336, 1987.
Crystal RG, Fulmer JD, Roberts WC et al: Idiopathic pulmonary fibrosis. Clinical, histologic, radiographic, physiologic, scintigraphic, cytologic and biochemical aspects. Ann Intern Med 85:769, 1976.
Crystal RG, Gadek JE, Ferrans VJ et al: Interstitial lung disease: current concepts of pathogenesis, staging and therapy. Am J Med 70:542, 1981.
Dreisin RB, Schwarz MI, Theofilopoulos AN, and Stanford RE: Circulating immune complexes in the idiopathic interstitial pneumonias. N Engl J Med 298:353, 1978.
Gaensler EA, Carrington CB, and Coutu RE: Chronic interstitial pneumonias. Clinical Notes on Respiratory Diseases 10:3, 1972.
Genereux GP: The end-stage lung: pathogenesis, pathology, and radiology. Radiology 116:279, 1975.
Hamman L and Rich A: Acute diffuse interstitial fibrosis of the lung. Bull Johns Hopkins Hosp 74:177, 1944.

Hewitt CJ, Hull D, and Keeling JW: Fibrosing alveolitis in infancy and childhood. Arch Dis Child 52:22, 1977.

Katzenstein A-L A: Pathogenesis of "fibrosis" in interstitial pneumonia: an electron microscopic study. Hum Pathol 16:1015, 1985.

Katzenstein A-L A, Myers JL, and Mazur MT: Acute interstitial pneumonia. A clinicopathologic, ultrastructural, and cell kinetic study. Am J Surg Pathol 10:256, 1986.

Keogh BA and Crystal RG: Pulmonary function testing in interstitial pulmonary disease. Chest 78:856, 1980.

Liebow AA: Definition and classification of interstitial pneumonias in human pathology. Hum Pathol Prog Respir Res 8:1, 1975.

Miller RR, Nelems W, Müller NL et al: Lingular and right middle lobe biopsy in assessment of diffuse lung disease. Ann Thorac Surg 44:269, 1987.

Müller NL, Miller RR, Webber WR et al: Fibrosing alveolitis: CT pathologic correlation. Radiology 169:585, 1986.

Müller NL, Staples CA, Miller RR et al: Disease activity in idio-pathic pulmonary fibrosis: CT and pathologic correlation. Radiology 165:731, 1987.

Pratt DS, Schwartz MI, May JJ, and Dreisin RB: Rapidly fatal pulmonary fibrosis; the accelerated variant of interstitial pneumonitis. Thorax 34:587, 1979.

Solliday NH, Williams JA, Gaensler EA et al: Familial chronic interstitial pneumonia. Am Rev Respir Dis 108:193, 1973.

Swaye P, Van Ordstrand HS, McCormack LJ et al: Familial Hamman-Rich syndrome. Report of eight cases. Chest 55:7, 1969.

Turner-Warwick M and Haslam P: Antibodies in some chronic fibrosing lung diseases. 1. Nonspecific autoantibodies. Clin Allergy 1:83, 1971.

Turton CWG, Morris LM, Lawler SD, and Turner-Warwick M: HLA in cryptogenic fibrosing alveolitis. Lancet 1:507, 1978.

Wall CP, Gaensler EA, Carrington CB, and Hayes JA: Comparison of transbronchial and open biopsies in chronic infiltrative lung disease. Am Rev Respir Dis 123:280, 1981.

33

JOHN A. FLEETHAM, M.B., B.S., F.R.C.P.(C), and
WILLIAM M. THURLBECK, M.B., F.R.C.P.(C)

DESQUAMATIVE INTERSTITIAL PNEUMONIA AND OTHER VARIANTS OF INTERSTITIAL PNEUMONIA

There are several morphologically distinct variants of interstitial pneumonia, and it is important to recognize these variants. It is particularly important to distinguish cryptogenic organizing pneumonia (bronchiolitis obliterans organizing pneumonia) and desquamative interstitial pneumonia, the most common variants, because their prognostic implications are very different from those of fibrosing alveolitis (see Chapter 32). It is also true that in the past, distinctions have not been made among the various types of interstitial pneumonia, and they have been grouped together as fibrosing alveolitis or Hamman-Rich syndrome. Thus some of the reports in the literature concerning fibrosing alveolitis are hard to interpret because they likely include several separate histologic and, perhaps, clinical entities.

DESQUAMATIVE INTERSTITIAL PNEUMONIA

Like fibrosing alveolitis, desquamative interstitial pneumonia (DIP) is much more common in adults than in children, but at least 34 cases have been reported in children, and the youngest child had symptoms dating from the age of 2½ weeks (Howatt et al, 1973). In adults, idiopathic fibrosing alveolitis is about four times more common than DIP (Gaensler et al, 1972), and the same proportion exists in children (Stillwell et al, 1980). DIP is defined and diagnosed using histologic criteria. The main diagnostic criterion of DIP is the presence of a large number of macrophages that fill up the air spaces (Fig. 33–1E). Occasionally the macrophages may fuse to form giant cells. There usually is retention of lung structure; alveoli can be recognized (Fig. 33–1F), but they are lined by hyperplastic type II cells. A mild interstitial mononuclear infiltrate is usually present, and there is generally a mild degree of interstitial fibrosis. In some instances, fibrosis may be prominent, with distortion of lung parenchyma and formation of cyst-like spaces. Nodular accumulations of lymphocytes occur, often near bronchioles but also near the pleura within parenchyma. Eosinophilic intranuclear inclusions have been described in 5 to 80 per cent of cases (Liebow et al, 1965; Patchefsky et al, 1971). They occur in both the alveolar lining cells and the desquamated cells. They have been described as virus-like, but electron microscopic studies have shown that these inclusions correspond to degenerative changes and consist of myelin figures (McNary and Gaensler, 1971) and that there is clumping of the chromatin at the nuclear membrane. Many observers believe that there is a transition between DIP and fibrosing alveolitis, and cases have been recorded showing the development of fibrosing alveolitis some years after lung biopsy had revealed classic DIP (McCann and Brewer, 1974). Nonetheless, the great differences in prognosis make it important to differentiate the two conditions.

ETIOLOGY

The cause of DIP is unknown, but because of the overlap between this disease and idiopathic fibrosing alveolitis, an immunologic mechanism is often invoked. Onset of disease may be signified by symptoms resembling those of an acute respiratory infection, suggesting a viral etiology. Histologic features identical to those in DIP have been found after exposure to asbestos, nitrofurantoin, and tungsten carbide dust. These features, however, probably represent responses to diffuse alveolar damage and probably do not implicate these agents as specific etiologic causes in most cases of DIP.

CLINICAL FEATURES

The incidence is about equal in males and females and the age of onset is most often in the first year of life. In general, the clinical features are similar to those of fibrosing alveolitis. The onset in most cases is insidious, but in two reported cases the onset appeared to be related to influenza in the family. All members of the family were affected, but the two DIP patients had dyspnea. Dyspnea is the most striking feature, and in young children, tachypnea and tachycardia are prominent findings. An irritating nonproductive cough, poor appetite, easy fatigability, and weight loss are common in older children. Physical findings may be entirely normal despite the presence of functional abnormalities. A mild pyrexia may occur, and then, as the disease progresses, the patient may develop tachypnea, clubbing, central cyanosis, and bibasilar end-inspiratory crackles (Rosenow et al, 1970).

RADIOLOGIC FINDINGS

The roentgenographic features may be normal in about 10 per cent of cases of DIP, despite the presence of symptoms and functional abnormalities (Epler et al, 1978). In about two thirds of cases, an almost unique roentgenographic picture is seen (Gaensler et al, 1972): a faint triangular haziness radiating out from the hila, along the heart borders to both bases, but sparing the costophrenic angles.

The opacities have been described as having a ground-glass appearance. In children, however, the shadows are likely to be more irregularly distributed (see Fig. 33–1A to D), although the ground-glass characteristic is usually present. Thus, in the 16-year-old boy reported in the original series of cases, lesions were first seen in the left upper lobe with no involvement of the diaphragmatic region (Liebow et al, 1965); the process then evolved in a pattern more characteristic of adult disease. The radiologic changes clear more slowly than the symptoms when patients are treated with corticosteroids.

LABORATORY FINDINGS

Routine laboratory studies are usually normal and of no diagnostic or prognostic value. A mild leukocytosis with or without eosinophilia is sometimes found. Antinuclear factor, rheumatoid factor, and dysgammaglobulinemia are found much less frequently than in idiopathic fibrosing alveolitis (Patchefsky et al, 1973).

The pulmonary function abnormalities in DIP are similar to those in idiopathic fibrosing alveolitis (see Chapter 32). These consist of a restrictive pattern, low CO-diffusing capacity, and arterial hypoxemia that becomes more marked on exercise. These changes tend to be less severe than in fibrosing alveolitis.

TREATMENT AND COURSE

The clinical course of DIP in children appears similar to that in adults, and some pediatric patients may recover without specific therapy. The majority of cases in children respond to corticosteroid therapy even when there is severe respiratory distress. One 8-year-old child appeared to be in extremis, yet 3 weeks after commencement of prednisone therapy she was breathing normally without oxygen, and 10 years later she was free of pulmonary symptoms (Bhagwat et al, 1970). Premature discontinuation of steroid therapy can result in relapse, but in these cases reinstitution of steroids in high dosages is usually followed by improvement; this occurred in the patient whose radiologic features are described in this chapter (Liebow et al, 1965). Response to corticosteroids is not uniform, and the disease may be slowly progressive, with increasing disability. Stillwell and associates (1980) reviewed 28 children with DIP treated with corticosteroids and reported that 17 (61 per cent) survived. Tal and associates (1984) reported three consecutive infant siblings with DIP. No cause was determined, and all three infants died before the age of 4 months despite corticosteroid treatment. The presence of alveolitis with minimal alveolar-capillary damage in the lung biopsy specimen is a good prognostic sign. Once the diagnosis of DIP has been established by biopsy, gallium scans or

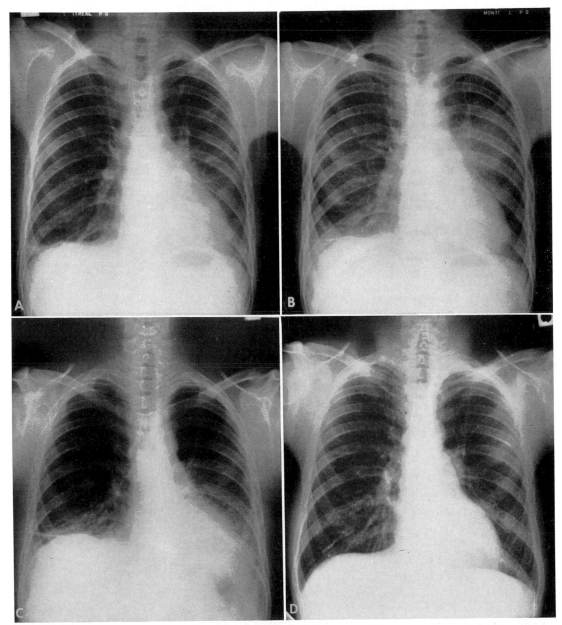

Figure 33–1. Radiographs and histologic sections of an 11-year-old boy with desquamative interstitial pneumonia. The symptoms dated from an onset of influenza and responded to steroids. An initial biopsy was done on presentation, and a second biopsy was done 3 years later. Physiologically, the patient showed mild restrictive lung disease. The patient remained reasonably well until he was killed in an automobile accident 5 years later. (From Bates DV, Macklem PT, and Christie RV: Respiratory Function in Disease. 2nd ed. Philadelphia, WB Saunders Co, 1971. Reproduced courtesy of Dr. David Bates.)

Radiologic examination *(A to D)*. At the time of initial presentation, the chest roentgenogram *(A)* shows loss of volume of both lower lobes, and there is a similar change in the lingular segment. The pulmonary infiltrations become more obvious in the radiograph taken in January of the following year *(B)*. Some improvement is noted by October of the same year *(C)*, and there is almost complete resolution in November, 2 years later *(D)*.

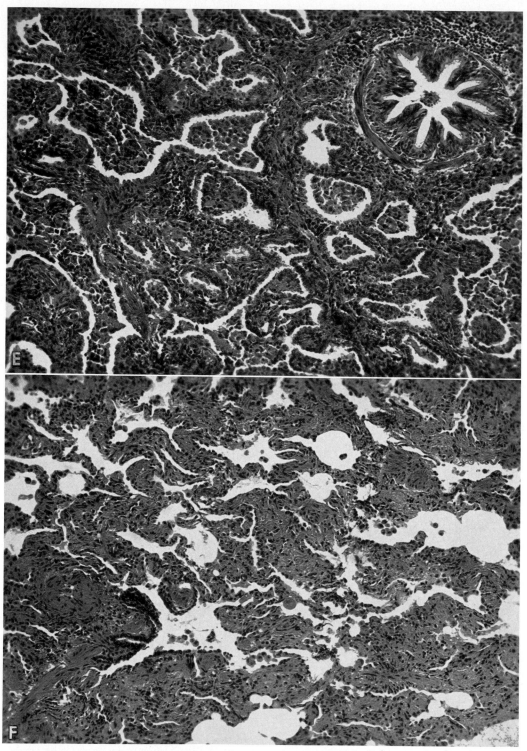

Figure 33–1. *Continued* Histologic specimen from the initial biopsy *(E)* illustrates the relative preservation of the architecture of the lung. The alveolar spaces can still be recognized as such, but they are lined by columnar (type II) epithelial cells. The air spaces contain many of the characteristic desquamated cells, which are macrophages. The specimen from the second biopsy performed 3 years later *(F)* shows extensive resolution of the proliferation of the cells lining the air spaces and absence of cells within the air spaces. There is modest interstitial pulmonary fibrosis, but the lung architecture is essentially intact.

bronchoalveolar lavage can be used to monitor the intensity of the alveolitis and make rational therapeutic decisions (Crystal et al, 1981). The natural history and treated course of idiopathic fibrosing alveolitis and DIP have been well documented in adults (Carrington et al, 1978) and are presumed to be the same in children. In their study of adults with both diseases, Carrington and associates (1978) found that 22 per cent of 40 adult DIP patients improved without treatment and 61 per cent with corticosteroid therapy; in contradistinction, none of 53 patients with idiopathic fibrosing alveolitis improved without treatment, and only 11 per cent improved with corticosteroid therapy. Chloroquine has been reported to be effective in the treatment of two infants with DIP (Leahy et al, 1985; Springer et al, 1987). This drug should be considered in patients who have DIP that fails to respond to corticosteroids.

LYMPHOID INTERSTITIAL PNEUMONIA

Lymphoid interstitial pneumonia (LIP) is less common than DIP, and few cases have been reported in children. It is likewise defined morphologically and is characterized by an exquisitely interstitial infiltrate of lymphocytes and plasma cells. Lymphocytes are present in all cases and are usually the dominant cells, although plasma cells occasionally may be prominent. Touton-type giant cells sometimes occur in poorly formed granulomas. There is a distinct overlap among LIP, Sjögren syndrome, Waldenström macroglobulinemia, and involvement of the lung by lymphoma; Gibbs and Seal (1978) have referred to these disorders as "primary lymphoproliferative conditions of the lung."

CLINICAL FEATURES

Because the number of cases in children is so few, the precise features of pediatric LIP are uncertain, and the following remarks refer to LIP in both adults and children.

Lymphoid interstitial pneumonia is encountered more commonly in females than in males and may occur as early as 15 months of age. O'Brodovich and associates (1980) described two brothers who developed LIP in early childhood. Dysproteinemia is a commonly associated feature. In a review of 13 cases, Strimlan and co-workers (1978) found that 10 patients (77 per cent) had dysgammaglobulinemia, including 8 with hypergammaglobulinemia and 2 with hypogammaglobulinemia. Church and associates (1981) reported three children with LIP and hypogammaglobulinemia. LIP has been associated with various immune disorders, including pernicious anemia, chronic active hepatitis, myasthenia gravis, juvenile rheumatoid arthritis, and Sjögren syndrome. This last association led Liebow and Carrington (1973) to suggest that LIP may be a variant of Sjögren syndrome that occurs principally in the lungs. Lymphoid interstitial pneumonia may "transform" into lymphoma, and a case of LIP with associated Sjögren syndrome that developed into lymphomatoid granulomatosis has been described (Weisbrodt, 1976). Recently, LIP has become well recognized as a complication of acquired immune deficiency syndrome (AIDS) in children (Joshi et al, 1985; Joshi and Oleske, 1986), as well as in adults (Solal-Celigny et al, 1985; Greicho and Chinoy-Acharya, 1985) (see Chapter 74).

The onset of LIP is insidious, with a slowly progressive course. Dyspnea, cough, and weight loss are the usual presenting complaints, but in an occasional patient a definite episode of pneumonia has preceded the onset of other symptoms. Fever, malaise, and pleuritic chest pain are less common. Physical signs are usually minimal but may include cyanosis, tachycardia, digital clubbing, hepatosplenomegaly, and bibasilar end-inspiratory crackles. Pulmonary function data consistently demonstrate a restrictive defect, with a low CO-diffusing capacity (Strimlan et al, 1978).

RADIOLOGIC FINDINGS

Findings on chest roentgenograms are nonspecific but usually show a reticulonodular pattern, which is characteristically linear and is more obvious at the bases, where it has a fern-like or feathery appearance. Alveolar infiltrates reflecting heavy interstitial infiltration may occur as the disease progresses. Pneumothorax, hilar lymphadenopathy, and pleural effusion are uncommon. Honeycomb lung may develop eventually in the advanced stages of LIP.

TREATMENT AND PROGNOSIS

The clinical course of LIP is variable, and consequently its outcome is difficult to predict. Some patients, especially those with associated Sjögren syndrome, have good response to corticosteroid therapy. A therapeutic trial of corticosteroids is therefore justified in all patients with LIP. However, any response should be documented by serial pulmonary function studies. Immunosuppressive drugs, such as cyclophosphamide and chlorambucil, have been tried in this disorder, but such therapy should be considered experimental at present.

GIANT CELL INTERSTITIAL PNEUMONIA

A rare variant of interstitial pneumonia, giant cell interstitial pneumonia (GIP) is characterized by the presence of many large, rather bizarre multinucleated cells in the alveolar spaces (Liebow, 1975). These cells are "cannibalistic," i.e., they engulf other cells. In addition, discrete desquamated macrophages fill the alveolar spaces, and the alveoli are lined by type II cells; there is also an interstitial infiltrate of monocytes, predominantly lymphocytes.

Few cases have been reported in detail (Reddy et al, 1970; Sokolowski et al, 1972). The clinical presentation has been similar to that of fibrosing alveolitis or DIP—progressive dyspnea, cough, chest pain, fatigue, and weight loss, with clubbing and fine basilar crackles being found at physical examination. In children, GIP has been associated with evidence of immunologic dysfunction (Reddy et al, 1970).

The chest roentgenogram usually shows bilaterally patchy nodular infiltrates involving the mid-lung fields or upper zones of the lung, with the apices and costophrenic angles generally being spared. In other cases, flame-shaped opacities have been described; in yet others, the roentgenogram has resembled that seen in DIP.

The majority of patients have benefited from steroid treatment, but the result has not been uniform. It seems likely that this rare condition is a variant of DIP.

BRONCHIOLITIS OBLITERANS AND ORGANIZING PNEUMONIA (CRYPTOGENIC ORGANIZING PNEUMONIA)

The term *bronchiolitis obliterans* implies inflammation of the bronchioles with occlusion of the airways. Bronchiolitis obliterans occurs in a nonspecific pattern and has various causes and associations, including toxic fume exposure, infections, drugs, collagen diseases, allergic reactions, and proximal obstruction (Epler and Colby, 1983). It may be a prominent feature of eosinophilic pneumonia, and there is a distinct overlap among rheumatoid arthritis, eosinophilic pneumonia, and bronchiolitis obliterans (Cooney, 1981). No cause is apparent in the majority of patients, when it is then described as idiopathic. The subject of bronchiolitis and bronchiolitis obliterans is covered in more detail in Chapter 18.

Inhalation of toxic gases such as nitrogen dioxide may initially cause a noncardiogenic pulmonary edema and acute respiratory distress. After a latent period of several weeks during which the patient may be relatively asymptomatic, bronchiolitis obliterans without organizing pneumonia may develop. Corticosteroid therapy may not be helpful in these patients (Charan et al, 1979). Postinfectious bronchiolitis obliterans is usually encountered in children, especially after viral or *Mycoplasma* infections (Hardy et al, 1988). Patients present with cough, tachypnea, fever, diffuse wheezing, and localized crackles. Chest radiographs are usually abnormal, with both interstitial and peribronchial infiltrates.

Histologically, there is a bronchiolitis obliterans with and without organizing pneumonia (Laraya-

Cuasay et al, 1977). Response to corticosteroid treatment is variable. Bronchiolitis obliterans with and without organizing pneumonia occurs in connective tissue disorders such as rheumatoid arthritis and drug reactions, notably to penicillamine. These patients present with cough, dyspnea, crackles, and physiologic evidence of airflow obstruction. Chest radiographs are often normal, and corticosteroid treatment is sometimes helpful (Geddes et al, 1977).

During the past few years, a well-defined entity has emerged, called either *bronchiolitis obliterans and organizing pneumonia* (Epler et al, 1985; Katzenstein et al, 1986) or *cryptogenic organizing pneumonia* (COP) (Davidson et al, 1983). We prefer the latter term because bronchiolitis obliterans may not be present in 70 per cent of cases, and the characteristic granulation tissue is found in alveolar ducts and sacs rather than airways. There has been considerable confusion about these terms in the past. Bronchiolitis obliterans and interstitial pneumonia was one of the original variants of interstitial pneumonia described by Liebow, but in no great detail. He and his associates (Gosink et al, 1973) described various cases of bronchiolitis obliterans, some of which probably included bronchiolitis obliterans and organizing pneumonia. We have included it in this chapter because it is primarily a restrictive lung disease and clinically is included in the differential diagnosis of usual interstitial pneumonia (UIP) and other infiltrative lung diseases.

The presence of abundant loose granulation tissue in alveoli, alveolar ducts, and sacs resembling the Masson bodies described in organizing lobar pneumonia is characteristic of COP (Fig. 33–2A). In one third or more of cases, the loose granulation tissue is seen in respiratory bronchioles or even membranous bronchioles, where it characteristically protrudes as a "tongue" into the lumen (Fig. 33–2B). In the air spaces in patients with COP, the connective tissue is characteristically within the lumen; in UIP, the young connective tissue is seen in the walls of air spaces when it is present. Interstitial inflammation is not a prominent feature, nor is interstitial fibrosis. The lesions all are at the same stage and are scattered and peribronchiolar in position. This is in contrast to UIP, in which the lesions are very varied in appearance and differ in position within the biopsy.

Patients with COP present with a nonproductive cough and progressive dyspnea. Many have a history of preceding flu-like symptoms. As opposed to UIP, in COP the history is short and patients present after an average lapse of 3 months.

Radiologically, the appearance is reasonably diagnostic. There are multiple poorly defined nodular (alveolar filling) opacities, together with a reticulonodular pattern (Guerry-Force et al, 1987; Müller et al, 1987 [these are the same cases]). Data concerning pulmonary function abnormalities are conflicting. On one hand, it has been suggested that there is a less severe restrictive defect, with the DL_{CO} less commonly abnormal, and there is more frequent evidence of

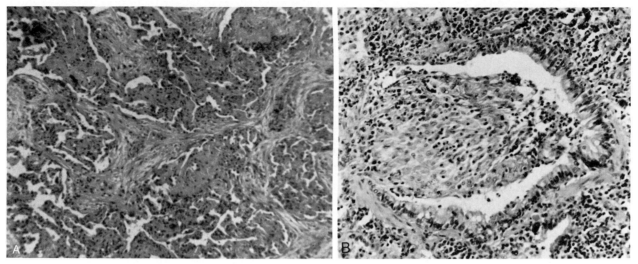

Figure 33–2. *A,* Cryptogenic organizing pneumonia. Note the loose granulation tissue within the lumens of the alveolar ducts. *B,* A "tongue" of loose granulation tissue protrudes into the lumen of a bronchiole (bronchiolitis obliterans).

airflow obstruction in COP than in UIP (Katzenstein et al, 1986). Other investigators, however, find no significant differences in pulmonary function between the conditions (Guerry-Force et al, 1987), although there are trends in the direction of the previous report.

The distinction between these two diagnoses is important because unlike UIP, COP has a favorable prognosis and response to treatment. In a review of 50 patients, Epler and associates (1985) reported complete recovery in 65 per cent of patients undergoing corticosteroid treatment and only two deaths related to progressive disease. In another series, the mortality was 30 per cent, and in these patients the course was short, with an average survival of 3 months (Katzenstein et al, 1986). In the majority of patients, this disorder does not evolve into a chronic disease.

REFERENCES

Bhagwat AG, Wentworth P, and Conen PE: Observations on the relationship of desquamative interstitial pneumonia and pulmonary alveolar proteinosis in childhood: a pathologic and experimental study. Chest 58:326, 1970.

Carrington CB, Gaensler EA, Coutu RE et al: Natural history and treated course of usual and desquamative interstitial pneumonia. N Engl J Med 298:801, 1978.

Charan NB, Myers CG, Lakshminarayan S, and Spencer TM: Pulmonary injuries associated with acute sulfur dioxide inhalation. Am Rev Respir Dis 119:555, 1979.

Church JA, Isaacs H, Saxon A et al: Lymphoid interstitial pneumonitis and hypogammaglobulinemia in children. Am Rev Respir Dis 124:491, 1981.

Cooney TP: Interrelationship of chronic eosinophilic pneumonia, bronchiolitis obliterans, and rheumatoid disease: a hypothesis. J Clin Pathol 34:129, 1981.

Crystal RG, Gadek JE, Ferrans VJ et al: Interstitial lung disease: current concepts of pathogenesis, staging and therapy. Am J Med 70:542, 1981.

Davidson AG, Heard BE, McAllister WC, and Turner-Warwick MEH: Cryptogenic organizing pneumonia. Q J Med 52 (New Series):382, 1983.

Dreisin RB, Schwarz MI, Theofilopoulos AN, and Stanford RE: Circulating immune complexes in the idiopathic interstitial pneumonias. N Engl J Med 298:353, 1978.

Epler GR and Colby TV: The spectrum of bronchiolitis obliterans. Chest 83:161, 1983.

Epler GR, Colby TV, McLoud TC et al: Bronchiolitis obliterans organizing pneumonia. N Engl J Med 312:151, 1985.

Epler GR, McCloud TC, Gaensler EA et al: Normal chest roentgenograms in chronic diffuse infiltrative lung disease. N Engl J Med 298:934, 1978.

Gaensler EA, Carrington CB, and Coutu RE: Chronic interstitial pneumonias. Clinical Notes on Respiratory Diseases 10:3, 1972.

Geddes DM, Corrin B, Brewerton DA et al: Progressive airway obliteration in adults and its association with rheumatoid disease. Q J Med 46:427, 1977.

Gibbs AR and Seal RME: Primary lymphoproliferative conditions of the lung. Thorax 33:140, 1978.

Gosink BB, Friedman PJ, and Liebow AA: Bronchiolitis obliterans. Roentgenologic pathologic correlations. Am J Roentgenol Radium Ther Nucl Med 117:816, 1973.

Greicho MH and Chinoy-Acharya P: Lymphoid interstitial pneumonia associated with the acquired immune deficiency syndrome. Am Rev Respir Dis 131:952, 1985.

Guerry-Force ML, Müller NL, Wright JL et al: A comparison of bronchiolitis obliterans with organizing pneumonia, usual interstitial pneumonia and small airways disease. Am Rev Respir Dis 135:705, 1987.

Halprin GM, Ramirez RJ, and Pratt PC: Lymphoid interstitial pneumonia. Chest 62:418, 1972.

Hardy KA, Schidlow DV, and Zaeri N: Obliterative bronchiolitis in children. Chest 93:360, 1988.

Howatt WF, Heidelberger KP, LeGlovan DP, and Schnitzer B: Desquamative interstitial pneumonia: case report of an infant unresponsive to treatment. Am J Dis Child 126:346, 1973.

Joshi VV and Oleske JM: Pulmonary lesions in children with the acquired immunodeficiency syndrome: a reappraisal on data in additional cases and follow-up study of previously reported cases. Hum Pathol 17:641, 1986.

Joshi VV, Oleske JM, Minnefor AB et al: Pathologic finding in children with the acquired immunodeficiency syndrome. Hum Pathol 16:241, 1985.

Katzenstein ALA, Myers JL, Prophet WD et al: Bronchiolitis obliterans and usual interstitial pneumonia. Am J Surg Pathol 10:373, 1986.

Laraya-Cuasay LR, DeForest A, Huff D et al: Chronic pulmonary complications of early influenza virus infection in children. Am Rev Respir Dis 116:617, 1977.

Leahy F, Pasterkamp H, and Tal A: Desquamative interstitial pneumonia responsive to chloroquine. Clin Pediatr (Phila) 24:230, 1985.

Liebow AA: Definitions and classification of interstitial pneumonias in human pathology: alveolar interstitium of the lung. International Symposium, Paris, 1974. Prog Respir Res 8:1, 1975.

Liebow AA and Carrington CB: Diffuse pulmonary lymphoreticular infiltrations associated with dysproteinemia. Med Clin North Am 57:809, 1973.

Liebow AA, Steer A, and Billingsley JG: Desquamative interstitial pneumonia. Am J Med 39:369, 1965.

McCann BG and Brewer DB: A case of desquamative interstitial pneumonia progressing to "honeycomb lung." J Pathol 112:199, 1974.

McNary WF and Gaensler EA: Intranuclear inclusion bodies in desquamative interstitial pneumonia. Electron microscopic observations. Ann Intern Med 74:404, 1971.

Müller NL, Guerry-Force ML, Staples CA et al: Differential diagnosis of bronchiolitis obliterans with organizing pneumonia. Clinical, functional and radiologic findings. Radiology 162:151, 1987.

O'Brodovich HM, Moser MM, and Lu L: Familial lymphoid interstitial pneumonia: a long-term follow-up. Pediatrics 65:523, 1980.

Patchefsky AS, Banner M, and Freundlich LM: Desquamative interstitial pneumonia: significance of intranuclear viral-like inclusion bodies. Ann Intern Med 74:322, 1971.

Patchefsky AS, Fraimow W, and Hoch WS: Desquamative interstitial pneumonia: pathological findings and follow-up in 13 patients. Arch Intern Med 132:222, 1973.

Reddy PA, Gorelick DF, and Christianson CS: Giant cell interstitial pneumonia. Chest 58:319, 1970.

Rosenow EC, O'Connell EJ, and Harrison EG: Desquamative interstitial pneumonia in children. Am J Dis Child 120:344, 1970.

Sokolowski JW, Cordray DR, Cantow EF et al: Giant cell interstitial pneumonia: report of a case. Am Rev Respir Dis 105:417, 1972.

Solal-Celigny P, Condere LJ, Herman D et al: Lymphoid interstitial pneumonia in acquired immunodeficiency syndrome–related complex. Am Rev Respir Dis 131:956, 1985.

Springer C, Maayan C, Katzir Z et al: Chloroquine treatment in desquamative interstitial pneumonia. Arch Dis Child 62:76, 1987.

Stillwell PC, Norris DG, O'Connell EJ et al: Desquamative interstitial pneumonitis in children. Chest 77:165, 1980.

Strimlan CV, Rosenow EC, Weiland LH, and Brown LR: Lymphocytic interstitial pneumonitis. Ann Intern Med 88:616, 1978.

Tal A, Maor E, Bar-Ziv J, and Gorodischer R: Fatal desquamative interstitial pneumonia in three infant siblings. J Pediatr 104:873, 1984.

Weisbrodt IM: Lymphomatoid granulomatosis of the lung, associated with a long history of benign lymphoepithelial lesions of the salivary glands and lymphoid interstitial pneumonitis. Report of a case. Am J Clin Pathol 66:792, 1976.

34

HARRIS D. RILEY, JR., M.D.

PULMONARY ALVEOLAR PROTEINOSIS

Pulmonary alveolar proteinosis or phospholipidosis is a syndrome of unknown cause characterized by progressive dyspnea and cough. It was first described in 1958 by Rosen and co-workers, who reported 27 instances of the disorder, and was considered a new disease. However, retrospective studies suggest that the condition may have existed as early as 1941. In 1969, Davidson and Macleod reviewed the literature and stated that 139 cases had been reported up to that time, 100 from the United States and 39 from other parts of the world, especially Great Britain and France. Four were children and 7 teen-agers, but 85 of the patients were between the ages of 30 and 50 years. Since that time, sporadic cases, usually in adults, have been described, and by 1976, at least 260 cases had been described in the world literature. Of the patients initially described by Rosen and colleagues, two were children, 2 years 4 months and 15 years of age, respectively. However, the number of cases occurring in infants and children among the total cases described is small. Danigelis and Markar-

ian reported in December 1969 that only 10 cases in the pediatric age group had been described, and Colon and associates in 1971 reported 23 cases occurring in children. Sunderland and co-workers (1972) stated that 34 cases in children 15 years of age or less had been cited in the world literature. Pulmonary alveolar proteinosis has now been described as a cause of chronic neonatal respiratory distress. In several instances, it was observed that symptoms began in the first week of life.

PATHOLOGY

The gross pathologic appearance of the lungs is characteristic, although the extent and distribution of the disease may vary. Multiple firm gray or yellow nodules of various sizes are often located subpleurally throughout the lungs, and the weight of the lungs is increased. The bronchial tree appears normal, and there is usually evidence of alveolar wall damage.

Although hyperplasia of the alveolar epithelium is usually present, inflammation and fibrous thickening of the interalveolar septa are conspicuously absent, and in the absence of infection, fibrous tissue organization to the stage of honeycombing has never been reported. The most striking feature is the microscopic appearance, which is characterized by interalveolar deposition of granular, eosinophilic, periodic acid–Schiff (PAS)-positive proteinaceous material (Fig. 34–1). Special stains have shown the presence of carbohydrates, protein, and increased amounts of phospholipids in the alveolar debris. The material in the alveoli, which has been identified as a lipoprotein with many chemical similarities to pulmonary surfactant but with different physical properties, is thought to be derived from granular pneumocytes.

These pathologic findings are believed by some investigators to result from the transformation of alveolar pneumocytes, which increase in both size and number and project into the alveolar lumen. These cells subsequently slough and degenerate, and the alveolar accumulation leads to an alveolar-capillary block type of diffusion defect and an increase in pulmonary venous shunt. In addition to the interference with gaseous exchange, a major effect of alveolar proteinosis is impairment of pulmonary defense against microorganisms. The disorder may represent an atypical response of the lungs to various types of injury rather than a single disease entity. Other workers have postulated that the alveolar deposits represent a response to an infectious agent or to a toxic substance in the environment, such as quartz crystals. Pulmonary changes similar to those in humans with this disease have been produced in pathogen-free rats exposed to quartz inhalation. The disease has also been considered to be caused by (1) an abnormal generation of a surface-active substance, which is normally present in small amounts in the lung, (2) a plasma infiltrate secondary to inherent defects in the pulmonary alveolar capillaries, or (3) deficient pulmonary cellular clearance, a concept that has received some support from the studies of Ramirez and Harlan (1968). All attempts to isolate a bacterial or parasitic agent have been unsuccessful, and the alveolar accumulation does not impair migration of macrophages. Certain pathologic changes in the lungs are similar to changes produced by infection with *Pneumocystis carinii*. Plenk and co-workers (1960) reported the presence of complement-fixing antibodies to *P. carinii* in four of nine patients, but the organism was not recovered in any instance; patients with pulmonary alveolar proteinosis are susceptible to secondary infection by this parasite.

PATHOGENESIS

Many theories on the pathogenesis of pulmonary alveolar proteinosis have been advanced. Although the data are not conclusive, it is likely that overproduction of the surfactant-like material by the granular pneumocyte (type II cell) may be the primary pathogenetic event. Others have postulated that the underlying cause is defective clearance of the lipoproteinaceous material by alveolar macrophages. Pulmonary macrophages from affected patients have been shown to exhibit decreased adherence, chemotaxis, and candidacidal activity in vitro. A defect in bacterial phagocytosis and killing has subsequently been demonstrated. These defects in the function of alveolar macrophages may be related to the high incidence of serious and unusual infections in this disorder. Current evidence suggests that the dysfunction of the alveolar macrophages is secondary to the overingestion of the material in alveoli. It has been suggested that the disorder may be a syndrome that can result from any of several abnormalities in the reprocessing of pulmonary surfactant. There is evidence that it may be a nonspecific response to various injuries to the alveolar macrophage or type II pneumocyte or both, including exposure to certain dusts and chemicals and occurrence of hematologic diseases or infections.

In 1965, Liebow and co-workers first described desquamative interstitial pneumonia, a disease also of unknown cause, characterized by proliferation of alveolar lining cells with desquamation of alveolar cells into the distal air spaces. These workers believed

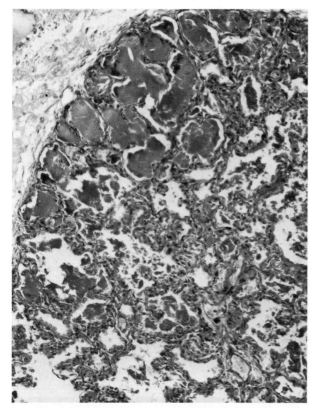

Figure 34–1. Photomicrograph of a typical section of the lung in a 3-month-old infant with pulmonary alveolar proteinosis. Peripheral alveoli are filled with dense, periodic acid–Schiff (PAS)-positive homogeneous material with acicular spaces. (Reproduced with permission from Wilkinson RH, Blanc WA, and Hagstrom JWC: Pulmonary alveolar proteinosis in three infants. Pediatrics 41:510, 1968.)

it to be a separate entity from pulmonary alveolar proteinosis but pointed out that the two diseases had striking similarities. Bhagwat and associates (1970) reported the case of a 9-month-old infant with necropsy findings that resembled both desquamative interstitial pneumonia and pulmonary alveolar proteinosis. They also experimentally produced similar histopathologic changes of both disorders in the same rabbit lung. These investigators have suggested that pulmonary alveolar proteinosis and desquamative interstitial pneumonia may have a common pathogenesis or that they may represent different stages or components of a single disease, previous sensitization to an unknown agent being an important factor in determining which components of the disease process will predominate.

There is no definitive correlation of pulmonary alveolar proteinosis with exposure to various inhalants, occupation, race, nationality, or geographic location. It has been postulated that pulmonary alveolar proteinosis may be another manifestation, perhaps earlier or to a less evocative insult, of the same spectrum of reactions that includes desquamative interstitial pneumonia and diffuse interstitial fibrosis. In one patient, lung biopsy showed typical pulmonary alveolar proteinosis without thickening or inflammatory infiltration of the alveolar septa. The patient died 12 years later of pulmonary insufficiency secondary to lung fibrosis.

Kunstling and colleagues (1976) have detailed the pathologic and pathogenetic findings and relationships of diseases that are characterized by proliferation of granular pneumocytes along the alveolar surface and, in some instances, shedding into the alveolar spaces.

There is increasing evidence that impairment of immunocompetence may be important in the pathogenesis of pulmonary alveolar proteinosis. Familial occurrence of the disease has also been observed.

CLINICAL MANIFESTATIONS

The clinical manifestations of pulmonary alveolar proteinosis are extremely varied. The usual clinical picture is characterized by progressive dyspnea and cough, which in older children may produce yellow sputum; cyanosis, fatigue, and weight loss are also characteristic. In pediatric cases, which often manifest before 1 year of age, vomiting and diarrhea may be the earliest manifestations. The onset may be abrupt or insidious and not infrequently is ushered in by a febrile illness. Hemoptysis occasionally occurs. Physical findings are relatively few and usually consist of only a few scattered crackles and, rarely, clubbing of the fingers and toes. The disease, in some instances, may assume a comparatively chronic course; in such instances, growth failure is common.

The vital capacity is reduced to a variable degree. The maximum breathing capacity is normal or slightly reduced. The oxygen saturation of the he-

moglobin of the arterial blood may be normal or reduced.

An increasing number of patients, especially children, with pulmonary alveolar proteinosis and evidence of impaired immunologic capacity have been encountered. The immunologic abnormalities include low serum IgA levels, lymphopenia, and thymic aplasia. It is not surprising that a variety of opportunistic infections occur in these patients. *Nocardia* infections are common. Other fungal infections, including aspergillosis, histoplasmosis, cryptococcosis and mucormycosis, have been observed frequently. However, tuberculosis, other bacterial infections, cytomegalovirus, and *Pneumocystis* infections have also been described. Prompt diagnosis and proper treatment of such complicating infections are key aspects of management. An association with leukemia and hematologic malignancies has been observed.

The disease may be suspected from changes noted on the chest roentgenogram. There typically is a fine, diffuse, feathery perihilar increase in lung density radiating in a butterfly pattern similar to that seen in pulmonary edema, but without cardiac enlargement (Fig. 34–2). The infiltration occasionally assumes a slightly nodular pattern but is more homogeneous than that usually seen in idiopathic pulmonary hemosiderosis. The roentgenographic changes are due to the presence of the alveolar fluid.

If sputum specimens can be obtained, PAS-positive material may be demonstrated by cytologic examination. Elevation of the serum lactic acid dehydrogenase (LDH) in the absence of hepatic disease is

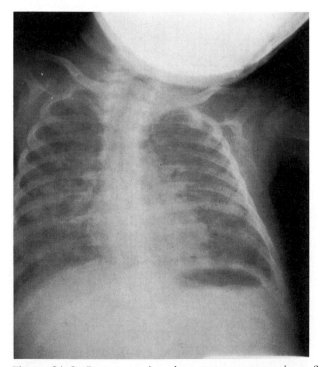

Figure 34–2. Posteroanterior chest roentgenogram in a 3-month-old infant with pulmonary alveolar proteinosis, showing diffuse, feathery infiltration. (Reproduced with permission from Wilkinson RH, Blanc WA, and Hagstrom JWC: Pulmonary alveolar proteinosis in three infants. Pediatrics 41:510, 1968.)

reported to occur commonly; the LDH level returns to normal in patients who recover. Lung biopsy is the more commonly used method of making the diagnosis ante-mortem.

Pulmonary alveolar proteinosis must be differentiated from diseases of the heart with associated pulmonary edema, from the pulmonary disorders characterized by fibrosis, and from sarcoidosis and fungal infections of the lungs. *P. carinii* infection can present a similar clinical picture. Lung biopsy is necessary to clarify the diagnosis in most instances.

PROGNOSIS

The prognosis is generally unfavorable. In adults, the disease may remain stable for considerable periods, and spontaneous improvement may occur; however, death eventually occurs in about one half of the patients from progressive filling of alveoli or from secondary infection. In children, the mortality to date is more than 75 per cent, with the duration of illness ranging from a few days to several months. Secondary bacterial and mycotic infections are particularly common in infants and children and are frequently the cause of death.

TREATMENT

Various methods of treatment have been attempted. Some degree of reversibility in certain patients is suggested by the clearing of pulmonary roentgenographic changes and improvement in gaseous exchange following aerosol therapy with proteolytic enzymes or pulmonary lavage with saline, heparinized saline, or *N*-acetylcysteine, alone or in combination. Of these, whole-lung bronchopulmonary lavage appears to be the most promising. Only one lung is irrigated at a time, and several liters of solution and several separate irrigations may be necessary. Irrigation should yield large quantities of surfactant and alveolar macrophages. When there is progression of symptoms, functional impairment, and roentgenographic evidence of alveolar filling, lavage is indicated. Total-lung lavage has been carried out successfully by Moazam and associates (1985) in a 15-week-old infant using a double-lumen Swan-Ganz catheter as a tracheal divider while the patient was oxygenated through a rigid bronchoscope. In very small patients or those with marked impairment of pulmonary function, lavage may be carried out with the assistance of cardiopulmonary bypass or the extracorporeal membrane oxygenator. Antibiotics appear to be indicated only if there is secondary bacterial infection. In contrast to the results in desquamative interstitial pneumonia, adrenocorticosteroids seem to have no demonstrable benefit.

REFERENCES

Bedrossian CW, Luna MA, Conklin RH, and Miller WC: Alveolar proteinosis as a consequence of immunosuppression. A hypothesis based on clinical and pathologic observations. Hum Pathol 11(Suppl 5):527, 1980.

Bhagwat AG, Wentworth P, and Conen PE: Observations on the relationship of desquamative interstitial pneumonia and pulmonary alveolar proteinosis in childhood: a pathologic and experimental study. Dis Chest 58:326, 1970.

Claypool WD, Rogers RM, and Matuschak GM: Update on the clinical diagnosis, management, and pathogenesis of pulmonary alveolar proteinosis (phospholipidosis). Chest 85:550, 1984.

Coleman M, Dehner LP, Sibley RK et al: Pulmonary alveolar proteinosis: an uncommon cause of chronic neonatal respiratory distress. Am Rev Respir Dis 121:583, 1980.

Colón AR, Lawrence RD, Mills SD, and O'Connell EJ: Childhood pulmonary alveolar proteinosis. Am J Dis Child 121:481, 1971.

Cugell DW: Pulmonary alveolar proteinosis. JAMA 234:80, 1975.

Danigelis JA and Markarian B: Pulmonary alveolar proteinosis including pulmonary electron microscopy. Am J Dis Child 118:871, 1969.

Davidson JM and Macleod WM: Pulmonary alveolar proteinosis. Br J Dis Chest 63:13, 1969.

Golde DW: Alveolar proteinosis and the overfed macrophage (editorial). Chest 76:119, 1979.

Heppleston AG and Young AE: Alveolar lipo-proteinosis: an ultrastructural comparison of the experimental and human forms. J Pathol 107:107, 1972.

Hocking WG and Golde DW: The pulmonary-alveolar macrophage. N Engl J Med 301:580, 1979.

Hudson AR, Halprin GM, Miller JA, and Kilburn KH: Pulmonary interstitial fibrosis following alveolar proteinosis. Chest 65:700, 1974.

Kunstling RR, Goodwin RW Jr, and DesPrez RM: Diffuse interstitial pulmonary fibrosis (cryptogenic fibrosing alveolitis). South Med J 69:479, 1976.

Liebow AA, Steer A, and Billingsley JC: Desquamative interstitial pneumonia. Am J Med 39:369, 1965.

Moazam F, Schmidt JH, Chesrown SE et al: Total lung lavage for pulmonary alveolar proteinosis in an infant without the use of cardiopulmonary bypass. J Pediatr Surg 20:398, 1985.

Plenk HP, Swift SA, Chambers WL, and Peltzer WE: Pulmonary alveolar proteinosis—a new disease? Radiology 74:928, 1960.

Prakash UBS, Barham SS, Carpenter HA et al: Pulmonary alveolar phospholipoproteinosis: experience with 34 cases and a review. Mayo Clin Proc 62:499, 1987.

Ramirez RJ: Pulmonary alveolar proteinosis, treatment by massive bronchopulmonary lavage. Arch Intern Med 119:147, 1967.

Ramirez RJ and Harlan WR Jr: Pulmonary alveolar proteinosis. Nature and origin of the alveolar lipid. Am J Med 45:502, 1968.

Reyes JM and Putong PB: Association of pulmonary alveolar lipoproteinosis with mycobacterial infection. Am J Clin Pathol 74:478, 1980.

Rosen SH, Castleman B, and Liebow AA: Pulmonary alveolar proteinosis. N Engl J Med 258:1123, 1958.

Spitler L, Keuppers F, and Fundenberg HH: Normal macrophage function in pulmonary alveolar proteinosis. Am Rev Respir Dis 102:975, 1970.

Sunderland WA, Campbell RA, and Edwards MJ: Pulmonary alveolar proteinosis and pulmonary cryptococcosis in an adolescent boy. J Pediatr 80:450, 1972.

Webster JR Jr, Battifora H, Furey C et al: Pulmonary alveolar proteinosis in two siblings with decreased immunoglobulin A. Am J Med 69:786, 1980.

Wilkinson RH, Blanc WA, and Hagstrom JWC: Pulmonary alveolar proteinosis in three infants. Pediatrics 41:510, 1968.

35

EDWIN L. KENDIG, JR., M.D.

IDIOPATHIC PULMONARY ALVEOLAR MICROLITHIASIS

Idiopathic pulmonary alveolar microlithiasis is a rare disease; fewer than 200 cases have been reported in the English-language literature. The condition is more commonly diagnosed in adults between 30 and 50 years of age. Although cases in children have been rare, the disease has occurred in premature twins.

The disease has been reported from many areas of the world, with Caucasian and Oriental patients predominating. There has been no history of unusual environmental exposure to toxic substances or airborne agents. No recognized infectious agent has been identified, and no geographic clustering of patients has been demonstrable.

The familial incidence of pulmonary alveolar microlithiasis was first reported by Mikhailov (1954), and in more than one half of the reported cases a familial incidence has been demonstrated, almost always among siblings. There is probably no sexual predominance.

The pathogenesis of the disease is as yet undefined. The only extrapulmonary changes in specimens obtained at autopsy are those consistent with cor pulmonale and anoxemia.

The disease is characterized by the intra-alveolar deposition of calcific granules, usually varying in size from about 0.1 to 0.3 mm in diameter. The deposits initially are most prominent in the lung bases and gradually involve more and more of the alveoli. The deposits are laminated onionskin granules consisting of various calcium and phosphate complexes. Other substances may be present in small amounts. Pleural abnormalities occasionally occur. Computed tomography and ^{99m}Tc diphosphonate scans may be used to verify very diffuse calcification noted on chest roentgenogram.

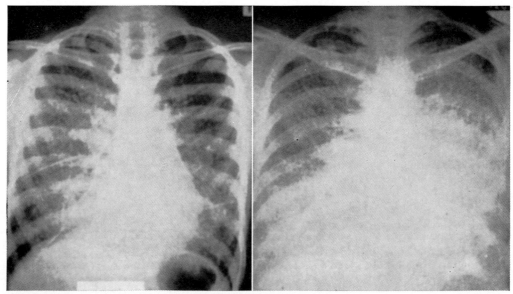

Figure 35–1. *A,* Roentgenogram taken in February 1954, showing minute miliary dissemination ("sandstorm") except at the apex and peripheral parts of both lungs. Hairline densities can be seen from the hilus to the peripheral parts. *B,* Roentgenogram taken in April 1964. Minute miliary dissemination has become confluent at the hilus and striated at the peripheral parts of both lungs. (Reproduced with permission from Oka S, Shiraishi K, Ogata K et al: Pulmonary alveolar microlithiasis. Am Rev Respir Dis 93:612, 1966.)

In adults, reduction in residual pulmonary volume is present, with an inexorably progressive reduction in pulmonary function until death results from pulmonary insufficiency, cor pulmonale, or both, with right-sided heart failure. The disease is usually fatal by midadult life, although an occasional patient may survive somewhat longer.

Children with the disease are commonly asymptomatic, although an occasional patient has had chronic cough; hemoptysis has been reported in one patient (Thind and Bhatia, 1978). As far as can be determined, there has been no report of the expectoration of an identifiable microlith in children, although this does occur on occasion in adults. Although physical findings are usually nonspecific or normal, at least one patient has exhibited evidence of pulmonary involvement at the time of diagnosis (Onadeko et al, 1977). When pulmonary insufficiency is great enough, clubbing of the fingers and cyanosis result.

The diagnosis is usually made by the characteristic "sandstorm" changes on chest roentgenogram (Fig. 35–1). The lesions generally are greatest in the lung bases and gradually involve more of the lungs in adult life, until almost all the alveoli are involved. In adults with long-standing disease, emphysematous blebs may occasionally be present. In the United States, one of the most common diseases from which idiopathic pulmonary alveolar microlithiasis must be differentiated is healed disseminated histoplasmosis. The differentiation can be readily accomplished by means of chest roentgenograms and other appropriate studies (see earlier discussion).

The diagnosis can be confirmed with open biopsy of the lung. Because of the familial incidence, roentgenograms of other members of the family should be obtained.

There is no known specific treatment, and when it occurs in childhood, the disease pursues an inexorably progressive course culminating in death, usually in early adult life. Bronchopulmonary lavage has been recommended, but Palombini (1981) reported failure in the only documented case in which this form of therapy was attempted. Supportive and symptomatic treatment is indicated when necessary. Appropriate counseling and sympathetic support must be included in the overall management.

REFERENCES

Brown ML, Swee RG, Olsen RJ, and Bender CE: Pulmonary uptake of [99mTc] diphosphonate in alveolar microlithiasis. AJR 131:703, 1978.

Caffrey PR and Altman RS: Pulmonary alveolar microlithiasis occurring in premature twins. J Pediatr 66:758, 1965.

Chalmers AG, Wyatt J, and Robinson PJ: Computed tomographic and pathological findings in pulmonary alveolar microlithiasis. Br J Radiol 59:408, 1986.

Clark RB and Johnson FC: Idiopathic pulmonary alveolar microlithiasis. Pediatrics 28:650, 1961.

Fulcihan FJD, Abboud RT, Balikian JP, and Nucho CKN: Pulmonary alveolar microlithiasis; lung function in five cases. Thorax 24:84, 1969.

Hossein E: Pulmonary alveolar microlithiasis. Mich Med 72:691, 1973.

Mikhailov V: Pulmolithiasis endalveolaris et interstitialis difusa. Klin Med (Mosk) 32:31, 1954.

Oka S, Shiraishi K, Ogata K et al: Pulmonary alveolar microlithiasis. Am Rev Respir Dis 93:612, 1966.

Onadeko BO, Beetlestone CA, Cooke AR et al: Pulmonary alveolar microlithiasis. Postgrad Med J 53:165, 1977.

O'Neill RP, Cohn JE, and Pellegrino FD: Pulmonary alveolar microlithiasis—a family study. Ann Intern Med 67:957, 1967.

Palombini BC, da Silva Porto N, Wallau CU, and Camargo JJ: Bronchopulmonary lavage in alveolar microlithiasis. Chest 80:242, 1981.

Prakash USB, Barhan SS, Rosenow EC et al: Pulmonary alveolar microlithiasis: a review including ultrastructural and pulmonary function studies. Mayo Clin Proc 58:290, 1983.

Shigeno C, Fukunaga M, Morita R et al: Bone scinitigraphy in pulmonary alveolar microlithiasis: a comparative study of radioactivity and density distribution. Clin Nucl Med 7:103, 1982.

Sosman MC, Dodd GD, Jones WD, and Pillmore GU: Familial occurrence of pulmonary microlithiasis. Am J Roentgenol 77:947, 1957.

Thind GS and Bhatia JL: Pulmonary alveolar microlithiasis. Br J Dis Chest 72:151, 1978.

Thurairajasingam S, Dharmasena BD, and Kasthuriratna T: Pulmonary alveolar microlithiasis. Australas Radiol 19:175, 1975.

36

DOUGLAS C. HEINER, M.D.

PULMONARY HEMOSIDEROSIS

The term *pulmonary hemosiderosis* indicates an abnormal accumulation of iron as hemosiderin in the lungs. It results from bleeding into the lungs and is much more likely to follow diffuse alveolar hemorrhage than bleeding from large arteries or arterioles. It may be primary in the lungs or secondary to cardiac or systemic disease. In most instances in which the disease is primary, the cause is unknown, but a significant proportion of cases occurring in infants and a small percentage in older children appear to be related to the ingestion of cow's milk and occasionally other foods. Pulmonary hemosiderosis in adults is commonly secondary to cardiac disease involving left ventricular failure or pulmonary venous hypertension such as occurs in mitral stenosis. This elevation of venous pressure may result in recurrent or chronic capillary oozing of blood into the alveoli with resultant hemosiderosis (brown induration) of the lungs. In children, on the other hand, primary pulmonary hemosiderosis is more common than the secondary varieties. The majority of all primary cases occur during childhood.

Although the first description of the pathologic features of brown induration of the lungs was by Virchow in 1864, the clinical picture of idiopathic pulmonary hemosiderosis was not reported until Ceelen's description in 1931. The first ante-mortem diagnosis was recorded by Waldenström in 1940, and knowledge of the disease has since been amplified by many authors. In Europe, the idiopathic form is frequently referred to as Ceelen disease or Ceelen-Gellerstedt disease.

It seems likely that several disease processes may lead to primary as well as to secondary pulmonary hemosiderosis, and as time progresses, the diagnosis of idiopathic pulmonary hemosiderosis should apply to a smaller and smaller proportion of patients. At present, it is convenient to classify and describe pulmonary hemosiderosis as follows:

Primary pulmonary hemosiderosis:
1. Isolated
2. With cardiac or pancreatic involvement
3. With glomerulonephritis (Goodpasture syndrome)
4. With sensitivity to cow's milk

Secondary pulmonary hemosiderosis:
1. With primary cardiac disease
2. With primary collagen-vascular disease or systemic vasculitis
3. With bleeding disorder
4. With granulomatosis

ISOLATED PRIMARY PULMONARY HEMOSIDEROSIS

This diagnosis refers to those instances in which no cause and no significant associated disease are apparent. It may occur at any age but affects chiefly children and young adults. It is commonly referred to as idiopathic pulmonary hemosiderosis.

SYMPTOMS AND PHYSICAL FINDINGS

The most helpful clinical signs are iron deficiency anemia; recurrent or chronic pulmonary symptoms including cough, hemoptysis, dyspnea, wheezing, and, often, cyanosis; and characteristic abnormalities on chest roentgenograms. Hemoptysis in children is an especially helpful clue to the diagnosis, although one must be aware that sometimes it is difficult to determine the origin of blood when children are both coughing and vomiting. In some infants, swallowed blood from the lungs is vomited without coughing, so the possibility of a pulmonary source of bleeding should be kept in mind when diagnosing unexplained hematemesis in children, particularly when there are roentgenographic abnormalities in the lungs.

Any of the features previously noted may be the first manifestation of the disease. For example, subjects in whom the initial single abnormal finding was apparently an asymptomatic iron deficiency anemia have been recorded. Others have had hemoptysis, persistent cough, or another pulmonary symptom before anemia was apparent. Pulmonary symptoms may occur with or without detectable roentgenographic abnormalities, or there may be striking roentgenographic changes before pulmonary symptoms or other features are clearly manifest. The clinical picture is usually characterized by recurrent episodes of pulmonary bleeding during which there is fever, tachycardia, tachypnea, leukocytosis, an elevated

498

sedimentation rate, abdominal pain, and often other findings suggesting a bacterial pneumonia. Pneumonia occasionally appears to be confirmed by positive sputum or throat cultures, and only long-term follow-up combined with an awareness of the possibility of pulmonary hemosiderosis leads to the correct diagnosis. Poor weight gain and easy fatigability are common in subjects with moderate to severe disease.

One of our patients had two serious episodes of pulmonary hemorrhage, each immediately following vigorous physical exercise. It is of interest that exercise-induced pulmonary hemosiderosis is known to occur in racehorses (Cook et al, 1988). Drinking ice water or cold drinks repeatedly led to an exacerbation of symptoms in another of our pediatric patients. Exacerbations sometimes occur in humans during pregnancy (Michaeli et al, 1987). Another factor that should be considered is exposure to inhaled chemicals or administered drugs. Trimellitic anhydride (Zeiss et al, 1987) and D-penicillamine (Sternlieb et al, 1975) are documented examples.

Physical findings vary, depending on the status of the patient at the time of examination. Pallor, dyspnea, bronchial or suppressed breath sounds, crackles, rhonchi, wheezing, and an emphysematous chest may be noted. Liver or spleen enlargement is sometimes found and may be transient.

LABORATORY AND ROENTGENOLOGIC FINDINGS

The anemia is typically microcytic and hypochromic, and the serum iron concentration is low in spite of an excessive accumulation of iron in the lungs. Trace labeling of red blood cells with radioisotopes has shown that large volumes of blood may exude into the lungs, the iron subsequently becoming largely sequestered in macrophages, where it is unavailable for use in the formation of new red blood cells. Animal experiments suggest, however, that there may be slow utilization of hemosiderin iron from the lungs for hematopoiesis, and it is possible that in human pulmonary hemosiderosis the rate of deposition of iron in the lungs in most instances merely exceeds the rate of use. The fact that symptoms, radiologic abnormalities, and anemia sometimes clear completely indicates that in remission there may be significant net removal of iron from the lungs.

There is a variable hematologic response to oral or intramuscular administration of iron. Some patients have a good reticulocyte and hemoglobin response, but others appear to have defective hematopoiesis while the disease process is active. Many have reticulocytosis during periods of active pulmonary bleeding whether or not iron therapy is administered, and this finding, along with mild jaundice and an elevated urobilinogen excretion, may lead to an erroneous diagnosis of hemolytic anemia. This diagnosis seems even more credible in the few subjects who have a positive direct Coombs test result, suggesting that anti–red blood cell antibodies are adherent to the erythrocyte surfaces. Circulating cold agglutinins may also be found and, like a positive Coombs test result, suggest the presence of an unusual immune response.

Increased serum levels of IgG, IgA, IgM, and IgE are commonly found (Heiner and Rose, 1970; Valassi-Adam et al, 1975; Scully et al, 1988; Sher and Heiner, 1988). On the other hand, we have found that about 15 per cent of patients have an isolated deficiency of IgA or IgG4 or both, suggesting that a deficiency of either of these immunoglobulins may increase the likelihood of overt disease.

A partial deficiency of C4 has been described in two subjects with primary pulmonary hemosiderosis (Mamlok et al, 1987). It is of interest that IgG4 deficiency is a common concomitant of C4 deficiency (Wedgwood et al, 1986; Bird and Lachmann, 1988). How either of these deficiencies could predispose to diffuse alveolar bleeding is unknown at this time.

Another correlation that has been noted is the association of celiac disease with primary pulmonary hemosiderosis (Rieu et al, 1983; Wright et al, 1983). Both of these diseases have an increased incidence of IgA and IgG4 deficiency.

Eosinophilia has been present in one eighth to one fifth of the reported cases, but experience suggests that eosinophil counts fluctuate markedly in this disease and that the likelihood of finding eosinophilia is proportional to the number of times it is looked for in a given case. If frequent differential leukocyte or absolute eosinophil counts are obtained, more than this proportion of subjects will be found to have eosinophilia.

Stool guaiac test results frequently are positive, presumably because of swallowed blood from the tracheobronchial tree. Reasonable evidence for this presumption comes from the fact that most patients with pulmonary hemosiderosis produce bloody sputum, some of which is obviously swallowed. In addition, the gastric juice usually contains iron-laden macrophages (siderophages) from the lungs even when there is no obvious hemoptysis.

The finding of siderophages in the stomach in the presence of otherwise unexplained pulmonary disease is good presumptive evidence of pulmonary hemosiderosis (Fig. 36–1). It is the simplest reliable diagnostic laboratory test in infants and young children. The Prussian blue reaction with potassium ferrocyanide and hydrochloric acid is a reliable stain, the hemosiderin granules within macrophages acquiring an easily recognized deep blue color. Siderophages may also be found in the sputum or in washings of the tracheobronchial tree, or within the alveoli of biopsy specimens obtained by needle aspiration or open operation. Most workers accept siderophages in gastric or bronchial secretions as diagnostic if typical clinical features are present and are not accompanied by evidence of extrapulmonary disease.

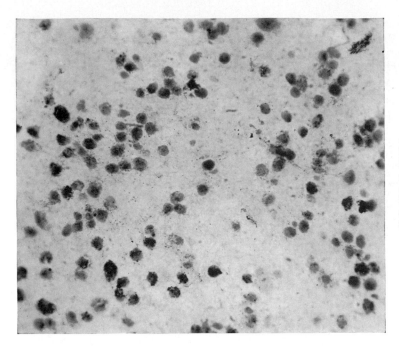

Figure 36–1. Siderophages in gastric washings of a 15-year-old boy with chronic pulmonary disease, recurrent hemoptysis, and iron deficiency anemia. Bronchial washings showed similar iron-laden macrophages. There was no evidence of cardiovascular, renal, collagen, or purpuric disease, but multiple precipitins to cow's milk were present in high titer. Chronic cough and hemoptysis ceased coincidentally with removal of milk from the diet. (Prussian blue stain × 150.)

Searches should be made for elevated levels of serum antibodies to cow's milk, for IgA and/or IgG4 deficiency, and for circulating antiglomerular basement antibody. These values can be obtained by study of peripheral blood and can facilitate a specific diagnosis of pulmonary hemosiderosis with sensitivity to cow's milk, humoral immunodeficiency, or Goodpasture syndrome. Each diagnosis has therapeutic implications.

A diagnosis by biopsy is considered necessary by some workers. The pathologic findings obtained with light microscopy of lung tissue have been summarized in detail by Soergel and Sommers (1962). They include alveolar epithelial hyperplasia and degeneration with excessive shedding of cells, large numbers of siderocytes, various amounts of interstitial fibrosis and mast cell accumulation, elastic fiber degeneration, and sclerotic vascular changes. Most of these features are present in the specimen shown in Figure 36–2. Vasculitis is usually absent but, if found, suggests that the disorder may not be primary but rather may be secondary to a systemic vascular disease.

Immunofluorescent studies reveal fibrinogen or fibrin in the alveolar spaces, but immunoglobulin deposits and complement are usually not demonstrable. Electron microscopy has revealed focal ruptures of the capillary basement membranes, with collagen deposition and hydropic changes in the pneumocytes but normal endothelial cells. These findings are thought to distinguish the histologic features of primary or idiopathic pulmonary hemosiderosis from those of Goodpasture syndrome, in which linear deposition of immunoglobulin and complement along the basement membrane has been shown by immunofluorescence, and vascular damage with wide endothelial gaps and a diffusely fragmented basement membrane with a thin electron-dense margin

has been shown by electron microscopy. However, some subjects with Goodpasture syndrome do not have demonstrable immunoglobulin deposits in the lungs, and some patients with idiopathic pulmonary hemosiderosis have immunofluorescent evidence of linear immunoglobulin deposition in the renal glomeruli without clinical evidence of renal disease. Hence, there may be some overlapping between these two diseases, especially in young adult patients.

Lung biopsy is justified in infants or young children in whom clinical findings are atypical or if the diagnosis is still in doubt after all simpler procedures have been done, including a careful search for siderophages in several specimens of gastric juice, sputum, or bronchial washings. Needle aspiration biopsy may be as risky as or more risky than open biopsy under anesthesia. The author observed one subject in whom the clinical picture suggested primary pulmonary hemosiderosis with active pulmonary lesions and in whom needle biopsy was performed under local anesthesia. The procedure was considered benign when it was done but seemed to be the turning point to deterioration with a rapidly progressive downhill course, massive pulmonary hemorrhage, and a fatal termination several hours later. Postmortem examination confirmed the clinical diagnosis. Other authors have suggested that needle biopsy is not without danger in this disease.

Roentgenographic abnormalities vary from minimal transient infiltrates to massive parenchymal involvement with secondary atelectasis, emphysema, and hilar lymphadenopathy. The findings are somewhat variable from patient to patient and may change in a given subject with each new bleeding or with clinical remission. Diffuse, soft perihilar infiltrates are common. In some subjects, the appearance is similar to that of pulmonary edema. In others it is

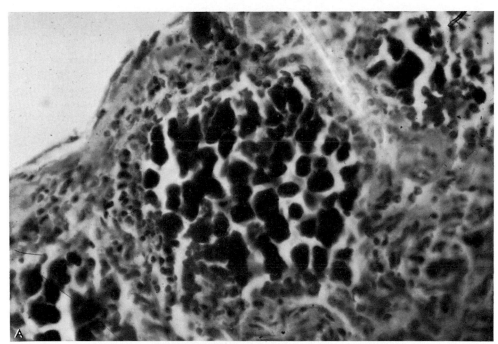

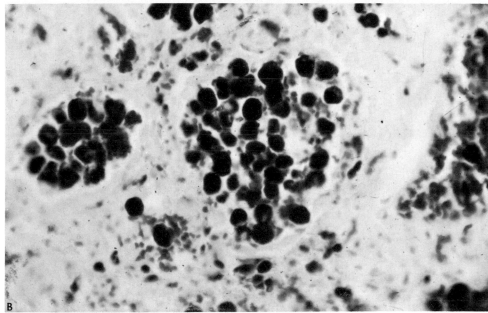

Figure 36–2. Microscopic sections of lung from a 3-year-old boy with pulmonary hemosiderosis who died several hours after a diagnostic needle biopsy of the lung. *A,* Hematoxylin and eosin stain showing iron-containing macrophages filling an alveolus, marked alveolar epithelial proliferation, fibrosis, and fresh intraalveolar bleeding. *B,* Prussian blue stain showing hyperplastic alveolar walls and alveoli containing red blood cells and many deeply stained iron-laden macrophages (× 500).

more like bronchial or lobar pneumonia, and in still others it may resemble the findings in miliary tuberculosis, Gaucher disease, or Wegener granulomatosis. Thus, there frequently is thickening of interlobar septa, with horizontal lines and fine nodulations suggesting interstitial fibrosis. The resulting reticular or reticulonodular pattern may be widespread but is often present chiefly in the lower lobes, and in patients who survive, it is likely to persist for months or years after acute infiltrative lesions have cleared. Illustrative roentgenograms are shown in Figures 36–3 and 36–4.

Pulmonary function tests have demonstrated impaired diffusion, decreased compliance (stiff lungs), and airway obstruction. The findings are most marked during and immediately after active intrapulmonary bleeding. One may find reductions in vital capacity, total lung capacity, 1-sec forced expiratory volume, maximal breathing capacity, and arterial oxygen tension, with variable changes in arterial carbon dioxide tension and decreased arterial oxygen saturation in some subjects.

An interesting and helpful observation was made by Ewan and co-workers (1976), who demonstrated an increase in single-breath carbon monoxide (CO) uptake associated with intrapulmonary hemorrhage. The increase is due to the marked affinity of hemoglobin for CO, which is highly diffusible even into blood-filled alveoli, and reflects an increased total lung content of hemoglobin at the time of CO inha-

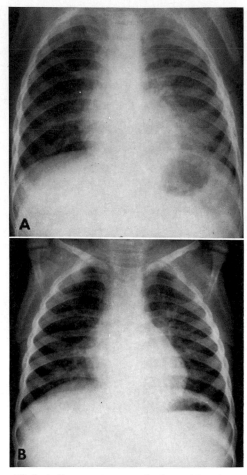

Figure 36–3. *A*, Roentgenogram of a boy with primary pulmonary hemosiderosis of 2 years' duration during an exacerbation at 27 months of age. Note the soft perihilar infiltrates, most evident along the left cardiac border. *B*, The same patient 4 months later when asymptomatic. Note the decrease in soft infiltrates but a prominent bilateral reticulonodular pattern suggesting interstitial fibrosis.

lation. Fresh bleeding is indicated by a concurrent increase in single-breath CO uptake.

Cardiac catheterization has revealed variable findings. Some patients show no abnormalities, and others have pulmonary arterial hypertension and even right ventricular failure as a result of cor pulmonale. Significant abnormalities in pulmonary function and demonstrated pulmonary hypertension indicate a more guarded prognosis than if these physiologic parameters are normal, although most deaths are due to active bleeding rather than to pulmonary or cardiac insufficiency.

COMPLICATIONS

The potential danger of needle biopsy in idiopathic pulmonary hemosiderosis has been mentioned. With the use of radioiodinated serum albumin for pulmonary scanning, severe reactions have been recorded. They were perhaps due to iodine sensitivity associated with the use of oral Lugol solution to block

thyroidal uptake of radioiodine. One subject has been reported to have had an exacerbation of pulmonary symptoms when given aerosolized Isuprel for wheezing; he improved markedly when the inhalation therapy was discontinued. One must be on guard against requesting unnecessary studies and should be alert for untoward reactions to drugs. Sudden unexpected death occasionally occurs, in some subjects during the first apparent episode of pulmonary bleeding. In such cases there may be minimal or no frank hemoptysis, the diagnosis being first suspected at post-mortem examination. The usual cause of death is respiratory failure or shock associated with massive intrapulmonary hemorrhages.

TREATMENT

When possible, treatment should be preceded by vigorous attempts to rule out known factors that might be important in causing or aggravating idiopathic hemosiderosis. These include appropriate studies to detect heart disease, diffuse collagen-vas-

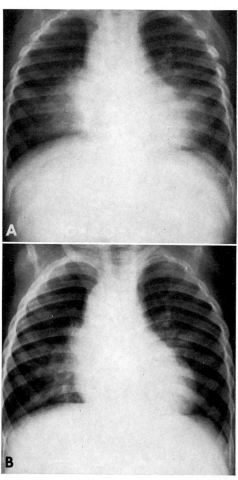

Figure 36–4. *A*, Roentgenogram of a boy with primary pulmonary hemosiderosis at 2 years of age, showing diffuse, soft perihilar infiltrates, somewhat suggestive of pulmonary edema. *B*, The same patient 6 months later, showing less pronounced infiltrates in the right middle lobe and left hilar regions and some horizontal septal lines suggesting fibrosis.

cular disease, and thrombocytopenic purpura. Attempts should be made to uncover sensitivity to drugs, inhaled substances, and foods. Acute crises should be treated with oxygen. Severely dyspneic patients may benefit from its administration by intermittent positive pressure, and persistent bleeding occasionally may be reversed by more prolonged periods of positive end-expiratory pressure (PEEP) breathing. Blood transfusions are indicated to correct severe anemia or shock. The blood should be obtained from a healthy nonallergic donor and carefully cross-matched. It should be given under close supervision, because several acutely ill patients have been thought to do less well during and immediately after transfusions. Adrenocorticotropic hormone (ACTH), 10 to 25 units daily, or methylprednisolone, 1 mg/kg every 6 hours by intravenous infusion, is recommended. Critically ill subjects are probably best kept on intravenous fluid therapy with nothing by mouth for 24 to 48 hours. After this, foods may be introduced, and prednisone or methylprednisolone, 1 to 2 mg/kg/day, may be given orally instead of ACTH or intravenous corticosteroids. After a clinical remission has been well established, the corticosteroid level can be gradually decreased until the drug is discontinued or until pulmonary symptoms recur. If maintenance corticosteroid therapy is necessary, an attempt should be made to establish the minimum dose that will suppress symptoms but will not produce undesirable side effects. The drug should be continued at this dose for 3 months before discontinuation is again attempted. Steroid side effects can be minimized by administering the corticosteroid as a single dose every second day at breakfast. If pulmonary disease recurs, round-the-clock corticosteroid therapy should be reinstituted or the alternate-day dosage increased. Control of the disease should be judged on the basis of symptoms, hematologic studies, and roentgenographic findings. Many subjects with idiopathic pulmonary hemosiderosis are in constant danger of relapse and even death; hence, careful long-term medical supervision is indicated.

Several additional approaches to therapy are worth consideration. The first is a concerted effort to provide a hypoallergenic diet. There is evidence that milk restriction may be of benefit in infants who are regularly ingesting cow's milk at the time of diagnosis and who have skin test or laboratory evidence of excessive immunologic responses to cow's milk (see p. 505). In older children and adults, milk restriction usually has proved to be of little or no obvious benefit. If "idiopathic" pulmonary hemosiderosis is in fact usually an allergic or "immunoallergic" disorder, the situation may be analogous to gastrointestinal food allergies in which milk sensitivity is common in infants but is much less important in older persons. A trial period of 2 or 3 months of a milk-free diet is innocuous and should always be considered, particularly if there was chronic rhinitis, recurrent or persistent otitis media, atopic dermatitis, wheezing, or frequent respiratory symptoms early in life while the child was ingesting relatively large amounts of milk. Subjects in whom the onset of symptoms occurs only later in life, when milk intake has been reduced, are unlikely to respond to a milk-free diet; nevertheless, it is my belief that meticulous efforts to identify allergens, including the judicious use of diets from which likely allergens have been eliminated, may be fruitful. In two referred children whose serum was studied, exacerbations were induced repeatedly by both cow's milk and soy formulas; serum contained precipitating antibodies to both substances. In other children, recurrences of pulmonary infiltrates have followed the ingestion of pork or peanuts. Recording of the food and beverages ingested for the 24 hours before the onset of each exacerbation may give a clue to an allergenic food. Efforts to quantitate reaginic and precipitating antibodies to food proteins and to demonstrate a decrease in total serum IgE on elimination of a dietary item followed by an increased IgE when the food is again ingested may prove helpful in individual cases. My associates and I have recently studied a child with this disease who had no demonstrable precipitins to cow's milk but by radioimmunoassay was shown to have excessively high levels of IgG4 antibodies to several milk proteins; there was dramatic improvement when cow's milk was removed from her diet, and an exacerbation followed the unauthorized ingestion of ice cream. Another child had no increase of any antibodies to cow's milk but was found to have high levels of IgG4 antibodies to peanut antigens. He did not respond to a milk-free diet but has improved considerably since peanuts and peanut butter have been excluded from his diet. No challenges with peanuts have occurred or been recommended in this case.

The second measure to consider is the use of an additional immunosuppressant drug, such as azathioprine, cyclophosphamide, or chlorambucil. Azathioprine (Imuran) has been administered most frequently. The dose ranges from 1.2 to 5 mg/kg/day; 2 or 3 mg/kg/day is the usually recommended initial dose. Under most circumstances, this would be given in combination with prednisone in doses of 5 to 20 mg every 6 hours during active disease. The steroids are then shifted as the clinical course permits to single doses of 10 to 40 mg administered every second morning. Each immunosuppressive drug may be expected to have the effect of lowering the required dose of the other, thereby minimizing undesirable side effects. Each may be increased at times of exacerbation or decreased in the presence of side effects.

An attempt should be made to discontinue all drugs after a year has elapsed in which no symptoms, anemia, or roentgenographic evidences of disease activity have occurred and pulmonary function tests have been normal. There should be little hesitation, however, in reinstituting single- or double-drug immunotherapy if the disease again becomes active.

We have encountered three subjects who had primary pulmonary hemosiderosis and had a marked deficiency or absence of IgA in the serum and secretions. Another case has been reported in the literature. One of our patients with deficiencies of both IgA and IgG4 had two almost fatal episodes of bleeding and each time showed sudden dramatic improvement after blood transfusions, suggesting that replacement of IgA and perhaps of concomitantly missing IgG subclasses was beneficial. We recommend intravenously administered gamma globulin replacement therapy in subjects with symptomatic immunoglobulin deficiencies.

A final measure that may be worthy of trial in subjects who respond poorly to other measures or who have chronic pulmonary symptoms or persistent roentgenographic findings is the use of the iron-chelating drug deferoxamine (desferrioxamine). This agent has been found to be useful in removing excessive accumulations of tissue iron from subjects who have idiopathic hemochromatosis and in whom repeated phlebotomies are not feasible, as well as in those with transfusion hemosiderosis, acute iron toxicity, and other conditions. Although experience to date suggests that hemosiderin sequestered in pulmonary macrophages is quite resistant to deferoxamine chelation, Cavalieri (1963) was encouraged by the use of the drug. Current evidence indicates that urinary iron excretion in subjects with excessive iron accumulation is proportional to the number of grams of deferoxamine administered up to 1.6 g daily, or about 26 mg/kg/day. The drug seems to be most effective when given intramuscularly in divided doses 8 hours apart. Levels of 24-hour urinary iron excretion should be studied for several days before and after institution of chelate therapy. An increase of daily urinary iron excretion by more than 3 or 4 mg per gram of administered deferoxamine or by 8 to 10 mg/24 hours is evidence that excessively accumulated iron is being removed. An increase in serum iron levels should also occur, and if iron deficiency anemia is present, it may improve. Periodic checks of 24-hour urinary iron excretion should be made with any long-term chelate therapy in order to indicate its continued value.

PRIMARY PULMONARY HEMOSIDEROSIS WITH CARDIAC OR PANCREATIC INVOLVEMENT

Some patients with idiopathic pulmonary hemosiderosis have been found at post-mortem examination to have inflammatory infiltrates in the myocardium. These have varied from minimal scattered lesions to extensive myocardial disease. If significant myocardial disease is present when the pulmonary disease is discovered, it may be difficult or impossible to decide whether the pulmonary hemosiderosis is a primary or secondary phenomenon. Distinctive alterations may be demonstrated on lung biopsy and may help in the differential diagnosis. From a clinical point of view, when myocarditis is the primary disorder, the heart should be large and other evidence of congestive failure should be present early in the course of the disease. However, if the heart is normal in size at the time pulmonary hemosiderosis is recognized and then enlarges, one can assume that the lung disease is primary rather than secondary to myocarditis.

The treatment of idiopathic pulmonary hemosiderosis is the same whether or not myocarditis is present, with one exception. If congestive failure is detected, it should be treated appropriately with digitalis, diuretics, and other measures of recognized value.

One subject has been reported to have developed both exocrine pancreatic deficiency and diabetes mellitus, his clinical course suggesting elements of hemochromatosis as well as idiopathic pulmonary hemosiderosis. A second subject with idiopathic pulmonary hemosiderosis developed diabetes, bilateral penetrating corneal ulcerations, and myocarditis. In such cases, it may be extremely difficult to decide whether the pulmonary disease is most appropriately classified as the primary disorder or is simply a major secondary manifestation of a more generalized connective tissue or "immunoallergic" disease. At present, pulmonary hemosiderosis may be classified as primary or idiopathic if it is the major manifestation and if the associated findings do not fit any well-recognized syndrome such as polyarteritis nodosa.

PRIMARY PULMONARY HEMOSIDEROSIS WITH GLOMERULONEPHRITIS (GOODPASTURE SYNDROME)

In 1918, Goodpasture described a patient with pulmonary bleeding and glomerulonephritis. Although it is not certain that his patient had primary pulmonary hemosiderosis, the name *Goodpasture syndrome* has been applied to the triad of primary pulmonary hemosiderosis, proliferative or membranous glomerulonephritis, and antibody to glomerular basement membrane antigen. It is sometimes difficult to differentiate this disease from isolated pulmonary hemosiderosis. Several investigators have pointed out differences in the clinical picture and in pathologic findings in the lungs. Thus it is known that Goodpasture syndrome usually occurs in young adult males and is rare or nonexistent in infants. It is more likely to be fatal than is isolated pulmonary hemosiderosis, although neither disease has a generally good prognosis. Examination of lung tissue in Goodpasture syndrome has been reported to show necrotizing alveolitis with degenerative changes of the alveolar capillary basement membranes, occasional arteritis, and relatively little alveolar epithelial proliferation or hemosiderosis, all of which are somewhat in contrast to the findings in isolated pulmonary disease. The finding by immunofluorescence of immunoglobulin and complement deposits along the alveolar septal walls has been thought to be more characteristic of Goodpasture syndrome, as has ultrastructural evidence of diffuse vascular disease with wide endothelial gaps and fragmented capillary basement membranes having electron-dense margins. Linear immunofluorescence of renal glomeruli has generally been considered characteristic of Goodpasture syndrome, but even this sign is not present in all patients with idiopathic pulmonary hemosiderosis associated with glomerulonephritis. In any event, the clinical disease usually is characterized by initial pulmonary involvement with hemoptysis, iron deficiency anemia, and typical siderophages. Thus in the early stages, before evidence of renal disease appears, the disease may be clinically indistinguishable from isolated pulmonary hemosiderosis. Death may result either from the renal disease or from pulmonary hemorrhage. In a few subjects, renal disease becomes apparent before or concomitantly with the pulmonary disease.

Treatment is similar to that described for isolated pulmonary hemosiderosis, corticosteroids being the most helpful single therapeutic agent. Results of therapy are much better when kidney lesions have not progressed to the point of renal insufficiency. If a remission occurs, careful follow-up is mandatory, and attempts should be made to suppress recurrent pulmonary or renal disease as soon as either appears. Patients whose disease does not remit with immunosuppressive drugs should have plasma exchanges to lower or eliminate circulating antibodies to basement membranes. These should remove 50 to 65 ml of plasma per kilogram of body weight and replace with normal plasma or an equivalent amount of intravenous gamma globulin. This will result in remission in the majority of cases. There have been reports of cessation of pulmonary hemorrhaging in subjects with Goodpasture syndrome following bilateral nephrectomy. This is reserved for those subjects who fail to respond to high-dose corticosteroids and plasma exchange.

PRIMARY PULMONARY HEMOSIDEROSIS WITH SENSITIVITY TO COW'S MILK

In 1962, four patients were described as fulfilling the criteria for primary pulmonary hemosiderosis in that each had recurrent pulmonary disease, hemoptysis, iron deficiency anemia, and iron-laden macrophages in gastric or bronchial washings or at lung biopsy (Heiner et al, 1962). Additional distinctive features included unusually high titers of serum precipitins to multiple constituents of cow's milk, positive intradermal skin tests to various cow's milk proteins, chronic rhinitis, recurrent otitis media, and growth retardation. In each patient, the symptoms improved when cow's milk was removed from the diet and returned when it was reintroduced. Since this report, the author has attended additional subjects with proven pulmonary hemosiderosis and multiple precipitins to cow's milk at high titer who improved after removal of milk from the diet. Serum samples from other patients with an established diagnosis have been sent to me, and about half of these have been found to have multiple precipitins to cow's milk. Each of the patients with precipitins was believed by his physician to have much less hemoptysis or none at all and to show general improvement when cow's milk was removed from his diet. An almost immediate clearing of chronic rhinitis and cough in several subjects who were given a milk-free diet seems to have provided an early clue that a lasting improvement in the pulmonary status would result. Most of the subjects having an important element of sensitivity to cow's milk were small infants, although one was 15 years of age.

A few subjects with this disorder have mild to moderate enlargement of the liver or spleen. Others have hypertrophy of the tonsils and adenoids, sometimes of sufficient degree to cause respiratory obstruction with secondary pulmonary hypertension and cor pulmonale. In addition, there often is an increase in the levels of serum immunoglobulins, IgG, IgM, IgA, and IgE. These findings, in conjunction with high levels of precipitating antibodies to food proteins, suggest a general stimulation of the immunologic apparatus. This is further substantiated by the fact that these findings usually return to normal on institution of a milk-free diet.

It should be emphasized that not all subjects with primary pulmonary hemosiderosis have unusual precipitins to cow's milk, and some without them do not change dramatically when on a milk-free diet. Nevertheless, several subjects with proven diagnoses but without multiple precipitins have been believed by competent pediatricians to clearly improve on a milk-free diet, and the one who was challenged with milk reintroduction had an immediate recurrence of symptoms. This suggests that in at least some subjects with pulmonary hemosiderosis and clinical sensitivity to milk, demonstrable precipitins may not be an essential part of the disease. One must conclude either that antibodies in subprecipitating quantities can be etiologic factors or that antibodies per se may simply indicate a vigorous immune response and may be unrelated to the pathogenesis of the hypersensitive state. The point is unsettled. A few subjects continue to have active pulmonary disease with bleeding and succumb while on a milk-free diet. This suggests either multiple etiologies or diverse exacerbating factors. In some instances, it may be impossible to sort out etiologic and aggravating factors, but every effort should be made to relate these to relapses, and their avoidance to remissions. The characteristic remitting nature of all forms of primary pulmonary hemosiderosis makes this task particularly challenging.

There are several similarities between subjects having pulmonary hemosiderosis with sensitivity to cow's milk and infants with milk-induced gastrointestinal bleeding and iron deficiency anemia. Both groups are likely to have multiple precipitins to cow's milk in high titer, and both are usually recognized to have the disorders between the ages of 6 months and 2 years. Symptoms and abnormal bleeding can be repeatedly induced in each group by the ingestion of cow's milk, and symptom-free intervals without bleeding occur with a milk-free diet. There seems to be a direct relation between the amount of milk ingested and the severity of symptoms and bleeding in both groups. In both cases, rather large amounts of cow's milk are usually ingested and untoward reactions to the milk occur only after hours or days, not immediately as occurs with IgE-mediated allergy. Some patients in each category become less sensitive to cow's milk as they grow older. One observable difference is that most patients with milk-induced gastrointestinal bleeding and iron deficiency anemia usually do not have positive intradermal skin test results to milk proteins, whereas those with milk-related pulmonary hemosiderosis do. However, neither group commonly has reaginic antibodies to milk demonstrable by Prausnitz-Küstner reactions or by the radioallergosorbent test (RAST). The diseases in both groups are associated with high levels of IgG antibodies to cow's milk proteins. IgG4 antibodies are nonprecipitating, and their presence may inhibit precipitin reactions in agar. Hence it is worthwhile to search for high levels (more than two standard deviations above the normal mean) of IgG antibodies by enzyme-linked immunosorbent assay (ELISA) or radioimmunoassay in precipitin-negative patients. Low to moderate levels of IgE antibodies are usually present, perhaps enough to facilitate basophil and mast cell chemical mediator release in the lungs with subsequent leakage of blood into the alveoli.

The treatment of subjects with milk-related pulmonary hemosiderosis is identical with that described previously under "Idiopathic Pulmonary Hemosiderosis." Cow's milk and its products should be removed from the diet until a complete remission has been attained. Subsequent challenge with cow's milk in selected subjects who have not been critically ill may be justified. This must be done cautiously beginning with 1 tablespoon and daily increments as follows:

Day 1:	15 ml	Day 4:	4 oz
Day 2:	1 oz	Day 5:	8 oz
Day 3:	2 oz	Day 6:	16 oz

then 16 to 32 oz daily for 1 mo.

If respiratory tract symptoms or abnormalities in pulmonary function recur when milk is reintroduced and then resolve when it is again eliminated, a milk-free diet should be maintained indefinitely. The same may be said if a significant drop in total serum IgG, IgA, IgM, or IgE follows elimination of cow's milk from the diet and a subsequent rise follows milk reintroduction. An aliquot of serum should be frozen near the time of diagnosis, after 1 to 2 months on a milk-free diet, and following 1 month of challenge or within a week of challenges that induce symptoms. All three serums should be retested in one assay under identical conditions in order to validate milk-related variations in immunoglobulin levels. Some subjects with precipitins or high IgG antibodies have appeared able to tolerate milk after a symptom-free interval on a milk-free diet for several months or years. Nevertheless, recurrent pulmonary infiltrates or abnormalities in pulmonary function have been found in several such subjects, suggesting that a milk-free diet should have been continued.

The possibility that foods other than cow's milk may play a role in occasional instances of pulmonary hemosiderosis should be considered. If a food comes under suspicion as a result of history, skin tests, or immunologic studies, trial elimination of the food is warranted. Carefully supervised challenges may also be warranted in selected cases. A technique that is helpful in identifying other offending dietary constituents is prescribing a protein-free synthetic diet such as Vivonex (Eaton Laboratories) for 2 weeks. If symptoms become quiescent, well-cooked meats, vegetables, and fruits are added one at a time at intervals of 4 days. They are given twice daily in generous proportions. If no exacerbation of symptoms is noted, cereals, eggs, fish, and other foods can also be added in this manner. Pork, soy, and peanut are finally added. One must search for a relation between the ingestion of a specific food and the occurrence of respiratory tract symptoms, new pulmonary infiltrates, an increase in CO uptake, or the recurrence of iron-laden macrophages. If any of these reappear after a food challenge and disappear when the food is again avoided, that food should be completely withheld from the diet.

PULMONARY HEMOSIDEROSIS SECONDARY TO HEART DISEASE

Any form of heart disease that results in a chronic increase in pulmonary venous and capillary pressure may theoretically lead to diapedesis of red cells into the alveoli and secondary pulmonary hemosiderosis. The most common defect causing this sequence of events is mitral stenosis, but the sequence has occurred in chronic left ventricular failure of several varieties. If significant heart disease is present, therefore, one must consider this in the interpretation of iron-laden macrophages in gastric and bronchial washings, in sputum, and even in lung biopsies. In these instances, the burden of proof is on the person who suggests an origin other than cardiac. According to some authors, even the pathologic findings in biopsy sections may look enough like those of idiopathic pulmonary hemosiderosis to be difficult to distinguish. Others, however, report distinctive features in hemosiderosis secondary to heart disease and list concentric hypertrophy of pulmonary arterioles, thickened alveolar capillary basement membranes, and an interstitial diapedesis of red blood cells as findings that are not seen in the primary pulmonary forms of the disease.

If mitral stenosis, cor triatriatum, or infradiaphragmatic drainage of the pulmonary veins is present in association with pulmonary hemosiderosis, a vigorous program of medical therapy followed by surgical repair of the obstructive lesion is mandatory, because reversal of the disease process is otherwise unlikely. Special diagnostic procedures, including echocardiography and cardiac catheterization with measurement of the gradient across the mitral valve or other sites of obstruction and selective angiocardiograms to define precisely the pathologic anatomy, may be necessary to establish an accurate diagnosis.

If chronic myocardial disease or another cause of left ventricular failure is primarily at fault, every effort must be made to determine the cause of the disorder and to provide appropriate medical and surgical therapy.

We have followed one instructive case of pulmonary hemosiderosis due to cardiac disease. A girl with cyanotic congenital heart disease—specifically, a single ventricle with pulmonary hypertension—had frequent respiratory infections in early childhood. When 7 years old, she began to have recurrent episodes of severe hemoptysis. From then on she had marked persistent pulmonary infiltrates, with two near-fatal pulmonary bleeds at age 9. Soon thereafter she was referred to us for evaluation because of the unusual severity of pulmonary disease and hemoptysis. Gastric washings contained many iron-laden macrophages. Tests for precipitins to cow's milk and a milk RAST were negative. Immediate reactions to skin prick and intradermal tests with milk were normal. Because of the poor prognosis and the possibility that the patient might be hypersensitive to an unknown food or environmental allergen, we instituted high-dose prednisone therapy. The patient showed remarkable improvement over several days, and after 10 days, we changed the prednisone therapy to an alternate-day schedule with gradual dose reduction. When the dose fell below 30 mg on the alternate-day schedules, however, cough and increased dyspnea ensued; lowering the dose to below 25 mg repeatedly resulted in hemoptysis. After 4 years of alternate-day prednisone therapy, on which the patient did quite well, we reevaluated her serum antibodies using two new radioimmunoassay techniques; these tests revealed excessively high levels of IgD and IgG4 antibodies to purified beta-lactoglobulin. Armed with this information, we eliminated cow's milk from her diet. The patient immediately noted decreased cough, decreased nasal stuffiness, and increased exercise tolerance. Soon thereafter we were able to lower the steroid dose to half the previous level, and the patient could climb a flight of stairs and walk to school, activities she had not been able to perform since age 7. During the 3 years following elimination of cow's milk from her diet, she has had one episode of hemoptysis, which followed the unauthorized ingestion of ice cream at a party. This experience has taught us that hypersensitivity to a food can aggravate the pulmonary vascular disease that accompanies certain congenital heart defects.

PULMONARY HEMOSIDEROSIS AS A MANIFESTATION OF DIFFUSE COLLAGEN-VASCULAR OR PURPURIC DISEASE

In a number of recorded instances, the lesions of polyarteritis nodosa have been limited to a few organs, including pulmonary involvement with hemosiderosis. In such instances, it may initially be impossible to distinguish this disease from primary pulmonary hemosiderosis except by biopsy. Nevertheless, with or without therapy, the passage of time may result in involvement of other organs, leading to a suspicion of polyarteritis and also providing material that is more accessible for biopsy. Pulmonary hemosiderosis sometimes occurs as part of Wegener granuloma, which is considered by some to be a variant of polyarteritis nodosa involving chiefly the nasal septum, lungs, spleen, liver, and kidney. Other connective tissue diseases, including lupus erythematosus, rheumatic fever, and rheumatoid arthritis, have occasionally occurred in association with pulmonary hemosiderosis, often with a diffuse vasculitis. Treatment of diffuse collagen-vascular disease with pulmonary hemosiderosis is much the same as that outlined for idiopathic pulmonary hemosiderosis. It should also include any measures or precautions indicated for the management of the connective tissue disease itself.

Several subjects have been reported to have pulmonary hemosiderosis in association with anaphylactoid purpura, and others in association with thrombocytopenic purpura. When either occurs, treatment must be directed at the basic disease as well as at the pulmonary complication. Splenectomy is likely to be particularly helpful in thrombocytopenic purpura with pulmonary hemosiderosis if an early and lasting remission does not occur with steroid therapy alone or with intravenously administered gamma globulin.

REFERENCES

Anspach WE: Pulmonary hemosiderosis. Am J Roentgenol 41:592, 1939.

Apt L, Pollycove M, and Ross JF: Idiopathic pulmonary hemosiderosis: a study of the anemia and iron distribution using radio-iron and radiochromium. J Clin Invest 36:1150, 1957.

Azen EA and Clatanoff DV: Prolonged survival in Goodpasture's syndrome. Arch Intern Med 114:453, 1964.

Beckerman RC, Taussig LM, and Pinnas JL: Familial idiopathic pulmonary hemosiderosis. Am J Dis Child 133:609, 1979.

Beirne GJ and Brennan JT: Glomerulonephritis associated with hydrocarbon solvents: mediated by anti-glomerular basement membrane antibody. Arch Environ Health 25:365, 1972.

Bird P and Lachmann PJ: The regulation of IgG subclass production in man: low serum IgG4 in inherited deficiencies of the classical pathway of C3 activaion. Eur J Immunol 18:1217, 1988.

Boat TF, Polmar SH, Whitman V et al: Hyperreactivity to cow milk in young children with pulmonary hemosiderosis and cor pulmonale secondary to nasopharyngeal obstruction. J Pediatr 87:23, 1975.

Bowley NB, Hughes JBM, and Steiner RE: The chest x-ray in pulmonary capillary haemorrhage: correlation with carbon monoxide uptake. Clin Radiol 30:413, 1979.

Breckinridge RL Jr and Ross JS: Idiopathic pulmonary hemosiderosis: a report of familial occurrence. Chest 75:636, 1979.

Byrd RB and Gracey DR: Immunosuppressive treatment of idiopathic pulmonary hemosiderosis. JAMA 226:458, 1973.

Campbell S: Pulmonary haemosiderosis and myocarditis. Arch Dis Child 34:218, 1959.

Case Records of the Massachusetts General Hospital (Case 17-1976). N Engl J Med 294:944, 1976.

Cavalieri S: Desferrioxamine with corticosteroids in a case of idiopathic pulmonary hemosiderosis. Fracastoro 56:389, 1963.

Cavalieri S and Mariotti M: Study of two cases of idiopathic pulmonary hemosiderosis. Minerva Pediatr 15:683, 1963.

Ceelen W: Die Kreislaufstörungen der Lungen. In Henke F and Lubarsch O (eds): Handbuch der speziellen pathologischen Anatomie und Histologie. Vol. 3. Berlin, J Springer, 1931.

Cook CD and Hart MC: Cited by Hill LW: Some advances in pediatric allergy in the last ten years. Pediatr Clin North Am 11:17, 1964.

Cook WR, Williams RM, Kirker-Head CA, and Verbridge DJ: Upper airway obstruction (partial asphyxia) as the possible cause of exercise-induced pulmonary hemorrhage in the horse: an hypothesis. Equine Vet J 8:11, 1988.

DeGowin RL, Sorensen LB, Charleston DB et al: Retention of radio iron in the lungs of a woman with idiopathic pulmonary hemosiderosis. Ann Intern Med 69:1213, 1968.

Dolan CJ Jr, Srodes CH, and Duffy FD: Idiopathic pulmonary hemosiderosis. Electron microscopic, immunofluorescent, and iron kinetic studies. Chest 68:577, 1975.

Donald KJ, Edwards RL, and McEvoy JD: Alveolar capillary basement membrane lesions in Goodpasture's syndrome and idiopathic pulmonary hemosiderosis. Am J Med 59:642, 1975.

Elgenmark O and Kjellberg SR: Hemosiderosis of the lungs—typical roentgenological findings. Acta Radiol 29:32, 1948.

Ewan PW, Jones HA, Rhodes CG, and Hughes JMB: Detection of intrapulmonary hemorrhage with carbon monoxide uptake. Application in Goodpasture's syndrome. N Engl J Med 295:1391, 1976.

Gellerstedt N: Über die essentielle anamisierende Form der braunen Lungeninduration. Acta Pathol Microbiol Scand 16:386, 1939.

Gilman PA and Zinkham WH: Severe idiopathic pulmonary hemosiderosis in the absence of clinical or radiologic evidence of pulmonary disease. J Pediatr 75:118, 1969.

Glockner WM, Dienst C, Kindler J, and Sieberth HG: [Plasma exchange in rapidly progressive glomerulonephritis (author's transl)]. Dtsch Med Wochenschr 106:1616, 1981.

Goodpasture EW: Significance of certain pulmonary lesions in relation to the etiology of influenza. Am J Med Sci 158:863, 1919.

Heiner DC and Rose B: Elevated levels of γE (IgE) in conditions other than classical allergy. J Allergy 45:30, 1970.

Heiner DC, Sears JW, and Kniker WT: Multiple precipitins to cow's milk in chronic respiratory disease. A syndrome including poor growth, gastrointestinal symptoms, evidence of allergy, iron deficiency anemia, and pulmonary hemosiderosis. Am J Dis Child 103:634, 1962.

Holland HH, Hong R, Davis NC, and West CD: Significance of precipitating antibodies to milk proteins in the serum of infants and children. J Pediatr 61:181, 1962.

Holzel A: Primary hemosiderosis followed by exocrine and endocrine pancreatic deficiencies. Proc Roy Soc Med 61:302, 1968.

Hukill PB: Experimental pulmonary hemosiderosis. The liability of pulmonary iron deposits. Lab Invest 12:577, 1963.

Hwang Y-F and Brown EB: Evaluation of deferoxamine in iron overload. Arch Intern Med 114:741, 1964.

Idiopathic pulmonary haemosiderosis (editorial). Lancet 1:979, 1963.

Irwin RS, Cottrell TS, Hsu KC et al: Idiopathic pulmonary hemosiderosis. An electron microscopic and immunofluorescent study. Chest 65:41, 1974.

Johnson JR and McGovern VJ: Goodpasture's syndrome and Wegener's granulomatosis. Australas Ann Med 11:250, 1962.

Kennedy WP: Idiopathic pulmonary hemosiderosis. Am Rev Respir Dis 99:967, 1969.

Kilman JW, Clatworthy HW, Hering J et al: Open pulmonary biopsy compared with needle biopsy in infants and children. J Pediatr Surg 9:347, 1974.

Krieger I and Brough JA: Gamma-A deficiency and hypochromic anemia due to defective iron mobilization. N Engl J Med 276:886, 1967.

Leatherman JW: Immune alveolar hemorrhage. Chest 91:891, 1987.

Lewis EJ, Schur PH, Busch GJ et al: Immunopathologic features of a patient with glomerulonephritis and pulmonary hemorrhage. Am J Med 54:507, 1973.

Lexow P and Sigstad H: Glomerulonephritis with initial lung purpura. Acta Med Scand 168:405, 1960.

Livingstone CS and Boczarow B: Idiopathic pulmonary hemosiderosis in a newborn. Arch Dis Child 42:543, 1967.

Lockwood CM, Boulton-Jones JM, and Wilson CB: Plasmapheresis: the role of this new technique in the recovery of a patient with Goodpasture's syndrome and severe renal failure. Presented at the Sixth International Congress of Nephrology, Florence, Italy, June 8–12, 1975. Bologna, Poligrafici Luigi Parma, 1975.

Loftus LR, Rooney PA, and Webster CM: Idiopathic pulmonary hemosiderosis and glomerulonephritis. Report of a case. Dis Chest 45:93, 1964.

McCanghey WT and Thomas BJ: Pulmonary hemorrhage and glomerulonephritis. The relation of pulmonary hemorrhage to certain types of glomerular lesions. Am J Clin Pathol 38:577, 1962.

MacGregor CS, Johnson RS, and Turk KAD: Fatal nephritis complicating idiopathic pulmonary haemosiderosis in young adults. Thorax 15:198, 1960.

Maddock RK Jr, Stevens LE, Reemtsma K, and Bloomer HA: Goodpasture's syndrome. Cessation of pulmonary hemorrhage after bilateral nephrectomy. Ann Intern Med 67:1258, 1967.

Mamlok V, Mamlok RJ, Kalia A, and Goldman AS: Partial deficiency of the fourth component of complement in patients with idiopathic pulmonary hemosiderosis. Clin Res 35:66A, 1987.

Matsaniotis N, Karpouzas J, Apostolopoulou E, and Messaritakis J: Idiopathic hemosiderosis in children. Arch Dis Child 43:307, 1968.

Michaeli J, Kornberg A, Menashe M et al: Exacerbation of idiopathic pulmonary hemosiderosis in pregnancy. Eur J Obstet Gynecol Reprod Biol 25:153, 1987.

Nomura S and Kanoh T: Association of idiopathic pulmonary haemosiderosis with IgA monoclonal gammopathy. Thorax 42:696, 1987.

O'Donohue WJ Jr: Idiopathic pulmonary hemosiderosis with manifestations of multiple connective tissue immune disorders: treatment with cyclophosphamide. Am Rev Respir Dis 109:473, 1974.

Ognibene AJ: Rheumatoid disease with unusual pulmonary manifestations. Pulmonary hemosiderosis, fibrosis and concretions. Arch Intern Med 116:567, 1965.

Ploem JE, DeWail J, Verloop NAC, and Punt K: Sideruria following a single dose of desferrioxamine. Br J Haematol 12:396, 1966.

Rieu D, Ariole P, Lesbros D et al: Idiopathic pulmonary hemosiderosis and celiac disease in a child. Case report. Presse Med 12:2931, 1983.

Rose GA and Spencer H: Polyarteritis nodosa. Q J Med 26:43, 1957.

Saltzman PW, West M, and Chomet B: Pulmonary hemosiderosis and glomerulonephritis. Ann Intern Med 56:409, 1962.

Scully RE, Mark EJ, McNeely WF, and McNeely BU: Case Records of the Massachusetts General Hospital. 319:227, 1988.

Sher L and Heiner DC: Immunoglobulin isotype levels in primary pulmonary hemosiderosis. J Allergy Clin Immunol 81:289, 1988.

Soergel KH and Sommers SC: Idiopathic pulmonary hemosiderosis and related syndromes. Am J Med 32:499, 1962.

Steiner B: Immunoallergic lung purpura treated with azathioprine, and with splenectomy. Helv Acta Paediatr 24:413, 1969.

Sternlieb I, Bennet B, and Scheinberg IW: D-penicillamine-induced Goodpasture's syndrome in Wilson's disease. Ann Intern Med 82:673, 1975.

Thaell JF, Greipp PR, Stubbs SE, and Siegal GP: Idiopathic pulmonary hemosiderosis: two cases in a family. Mayo Clin Proc 53:113, 1978.

Thomas HM and Irwin RS: Classification of diffuse intrapulmonary hemorrhage. Chest 68:483, 1975.

Valassi-Adam H, Rouska A, Karpouzas J, and Matsaniotis N: Raised IgA in idiopathic pulmonary hemosiderosis. Arch Dis Child 50:320, 1975.

Walsh JR, Mass RE, Smith FW, and Lange V: Desferrioxamine effect on iron excretion in hemochromatosis. Arch Intern Med 113:435, 1964.

Wedgwood RJ, Ochs HD, and Oxelius V-A: IgG subclass levels in the serum of patients with primary immunodeficiency. Monogr Allergy 20:80, 1986.

Wilson CB, Marquardt H, and Dixon FJ: Radioimmunoassay (RIA) for circulating antiglomerular basement membrane (GBM) antibodies. Kidney Int 6:114A, 1974.

Wilson JF, Heiner DC, and Lahey ME: Studies on iron metabolism. IV. Milk-induced gastrointestinal bleeding in infants with hypochromic microcytic anemia. JAMA 189:568, 1964.

Wright PH, Buxton-Thomas M, Keeling PW, and Kreel L: Adult idiopathic pulmonary haemosiderosis: a comparison of lung function changes and the distribution of pulmonary disease in patients with and without coeliac disease. Br J Dis Chest 77:282, 1983.

Zeiss CR, Levitz D, Leach CL et al: A model of immunologic lung injury induced by trimellitic anhydride inhalation: antibody response. J Allergy Clin Immunol 79:59, 1987.

Ziai M: Anemia, shortness of breath and asthma in an infant. Clin Pediatr 14:976, 1975.

37

THOMAS A. HAZINSKI, M.D.

ATELECTASIS

The term *atelectasis*, which means imperfect expansion, is used to refer to nonaerated but otherwise normal lung parenchyma. Atelectasis was first described by Laennec (1819) from necropsy findings and was produced experimentally in 1845 by Traube (1846). This chapter deals with *acquired* atelectasis and refers to postnatal collapse of a segment, lobe, or lobes of the lung.

CAUSES

Some of the causes of atelectasis are shown in Table 37–1. Acquired atelectasis may occur under a variety of circumstances: (1) *bronchial obstruction* due to problems in the bronchial lumen, such as mucus plugs or foreign bodies; problems in the wall of the bronchus, such as mucosal edema, inflammation, tumors, or smooth muscle spasm; or peribronchial factors, such as pressure from nodes or tumors; (2) direct local *pressure on parenchymal tissue* from contiguous masses, enlargement of heart or adjacent vascular structures, or misplaced viscera, such as diaphragmatic hernia or eventration of the diaphragm; (3) *increased intrapleural pressure* from exudate, blood, pus, or air in the pleural space; (4) *abnormal alveolar surface tension* following alteration of the alveolar lining layer; (5) *neuromuscular disease,* such as weakness of the diaphragm in Guillain-Barré syndrome, postoperative respiratory depression, or congenital anomalies, such as amyotonia congenita.

PATHOPHYSIOLOGY

When an airway becomes occluded, air is trapped in lung units ventilated by that airway, and the trapped gases are absorbed into the blood perfusing that part of the lung (Rahn, 1959–1960). The rate at which absorption occurs depends on the solubility of the constituent gases: atmospheric air, nitrogen, and helium are absorbed in 2 to 3 hours; 100 per cent oxygen is absorbed in a few minutes, leading to rapid lung unit collapse within 6 minutes (Benumof, 1979). This observation may explain why atelectasis is so common in the postoperative period when high concentrations of oxygen are used.

The rate and extent of collapse are further modified by collateral ventilation through intra-alveolar pores and through bronchiole-alveolar communications. The presence of interalveolar pores described by Kohn (1893) has been confirmed in several studies. A different and even more significant collateral ventilating mechanism has been described by Lambert, who found short, epithelium-lined communications, approximately 30 μ in diameter, between the distal bronchioles and neighboring alveoli (1957). These tubules are about three times the diameter of most interalveolar pores and can aerate hundreds of alveoli adjacent to a peripheral bronchiole.

Atelectasis may also occur without airway obstruction because of surfactant deficiency or surfactant dysfunction. Surfactant deficiency is seen in its purest form in hyaline membrane disease in premature

Table 37–1. CAUSES OF ATELECTASIS
IN INFANTS AND CHILDREN

Intrabronchial Obstruction
Foreign body
Mucus plugs
Cystic fibrosis
Asthma

Bronchial Wall Damage or Disease
Airway stenosis
Airway inflammation and edema due to aspiration or inhalation
  injury
Airway edema
Bronchial tumors
Granuloma
Papillomas

Extrinsic Bronchial Compression
Tumors
Lymph nodes
Cardiomegaly
Vascular rings
Lobar emphysema

Surfactant Deficiency or Dysfunction
Hyaline membrane disease
Adult respiratory distress syndrome (ARDS)
Pneumonia
Pulmonary edema
Near-drowning

Compression of Normal Lung Tissue
Chylothorax
Hemothorax
Pneumothorax
Tumors

infants, but surfactant dysfunction may also occur in near-drowning and in adult respiratory distress syndrome (ARDS). Surfactant can directly vary alveolar surface tension with changes in lung volume, thereby preventing collapse of small alveoli at low lung volumes and facilitating alveolar collapse at high lung volumes. The property of variable surface tension is attributable to the phospholipid component of surfactant, but other lipids, proteins, and calcium are present in natural surfactant and are required for normal function (Wright and Clements, 1987).

In addition, evidence indicates that the lung contains smooth muscle fibers that are interwoven with elastic fibers in the most distally located portion of the air passages, including the alveolar sacs. This "myoelastic" element may be responsible for maintaining a state of contraction of pulmonary tissue similar to the continuous tone provided by smooth muscle elsewhere. This tendency toward lung collapse is balanced (at functional residual capacity) by the tendency of the chest wall to spring outward. This phenomenon explains why lung collapse accompanies pneumothorax even though the surfactant system is intact.

Nonobstructive atelectasis may also occur during episodes of alveolar hypoventilation, as demonstrated in sedated preoperative patients (Tockics et al, 1987).

FUNCTIONAL CONSEQUENCES

The four most important functional consequences of bronchial obstruction are hypoxemia, secretion stasis, overexpansion of adjacent lung units, and pulmonary edema on reexpansion.

After the collapse of a segment or lobe, ventilation of the alveoli served by that airway decreases, whereas perfusion of the area may be only slightly decreased, resulting in a low $\dot{V}A/\dot{Q}$ area in the involved portion of the lung (Fig. 37–1). If the obstructed area is large enough, hypoxemia may result because of an increase in venous admixture; hypoxemia may persist even when positive pressure ventilation is applied and ventilation to the previously obstructed unit is restored.

Another important change that occurs after virtually complete obstruction of a bronchus is the accumulation of secretions distal to the obstructed area, which creates a favorable site for the growth of microorganisms. As the secretions accumulate, they may distend a collapsed segment to more than its normal size. Later, with the absorption of fluid, the affected portion contracts, and typical plate-like infiltrates are identified radiographically.

The mechanical effect of the collapsed segment may also result in the distention of adjacent unobstructed alveoli. This compensatory overdistention may be so prominent radiographically that small collapsed areas will not be noticed clinically or on roentgenograms. This is especially true for areas or segments adjacent to the heart, in which small triangular paracardiac shadows may be unnoticed. The heart and the mediastinum may shift toward the atelectatic lung to fill the space previously occupied by expanded lung. If overinflation is a prominent feature of the chest radiograph, it is sometimes difficult to determine whether atelectasis or emphysema is the primary abnormality, especially in a young infant, in whom congenital malformations are a possibility.

Acute pulmonary edema following reexpansion of a large area of atelectasis has been reported following treatment of a large pneumothorax or pleural effusion (Mahfood et al, 1988). The edema usually affects only the reexpanded lung and occurs within 1 to 36 hours after the reexpansion procedure. Appropriate respiratory support, including oxygen, diuretics, and in severe cases intubation and positive pressure ventilation, is necessary. The mechanisms responsible for reexpansion pulmonary edema are unknown. A review found a mortality of 20 per cent in adults (Mahfood et al, 1988).

SPECIFIC CAUSES

Extrabronchial obstruction leading to atelectasis can be caused by compression of adjacent bronchi by hilar and mediastinal lymph nodes. Such nodal enlargement may result from infection of the lungs and pleura or, rarely, from descending drainage into the bronchi from an infection in the upper respiratory tract. The most common agents are tuberculosis and atypical strains and respiratory viruses, such as Ep-

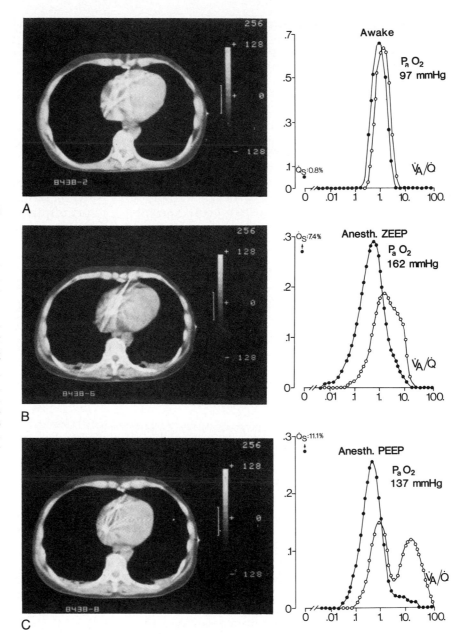

Figure 37–1. Transverse computed tomographic (CT) scans of the chest and $\dot{V}A/\dot{Q}$ distributions (O: ventilation; •: blood flow, l/min) in patient 7 in the awake state *(A)*; during anesthesia with mechanical ventilation *(B)* with zero end-expiratory pressure (ZEEP); and after the addition of a positive end-expiratory pressure (PEEP) of 10 cm H_2O *(C)*. Note the absence of any lung tissue changes and the unimodal $\dot{V}A/\dot{Q}$ distribution, with almost no shunt, in the awake state. Note also the appearance of densities in the dependent lung regions and shunt during anesthesia. The densities but not the shunt were reduced by PEEP. A distinct "high $\dot{V}A/\dot{Q}$" mode also became evident. Pa_{O_2} is presented in *A*, *B*, and *C*. (Reproduced with permission from Tockics L, Hedenstierna G, Strandberg A et al: Lung collapse and gas exchange during general anesthesia: effects of spontaneous breathing, muscle paralysis, and positive end-expiratory pressure. Anesthesiology 66:157, 1987.)

stein-Barr virus and cytomegalovirus. Other causes are immunodeficiency syndromes including AIDS; lymphoreticular malignancies; and metastasis from malignancy in other organs, such as Wilms tumor, neuroblastoma, retinoblastoma, osteogenic sarcoma, and teratoma of the testes (Krushner et al, 1980; Baldeyrou et al, 1984).

Compression of an airway by a markedly enlarged heart may produce atelectasis. In infants and young children with acyanotic congenital heart disease, the distended pulmonary arteries and an enlarged left atrium result in airway obstruction. The most common sites affected are the left upper bronchus, left main bronchus, and middle bronchus (Stanger et al, 1969).

Primary malignant tumors of the lung are extremely rare in children, but they may cause atelec-

tasis. The most common primary tumor is bronchial carcinoid (McDougall et al, 1980), but mucoepidemal carcinomas and undifferentiated mesenchymal tumors may also occur (Dehner, 1989). These lesions cause atelectasis by compressing normal lung tissue or by causing bronchial obstruction.

Congenital anomalies of the diaphragm (eventration or hernia) may permit sufficient pressure on the bronchi by displaced viscera to produce atelectasis of the parenchyma supplied by the compressed bronchus. Symptoms are minimal or absent and may go unnoticed for years. Occasionally bleeding, intestinal obstruction, or intercurrent infection may lead to the diagnosis.

Intrabronchial obstruction may be endogenous or exogenous. An example of the former is granulomatous tissue, polyps, papillomas, or mucous obstruction secondary to cystic fibrosis, asthma, or bronchiectasis (Finer and Etches, 1989). Exogenous obstruction may be caused by aspiration of a foreign body (Wiseman, 1984; Musemeche and Kosloske, 1986; Rothmann, 1980). Foreign bodies aspirated into the lung usually enter a noninfected lung with healthy bronchi. The sequence of events in this circumstance will depend on the patient's age, state of consciousness, and health; the nature of aspirated material; the promptness of correct diagnosis; and the speed and success of appropriate therapy. Metallic aspirants may produce obstruction because of their size and shape, but vegetable matter is particularly irritating and can result in obstruction due to mucosal swelling. Some of these vegetable products, such as peanuts, beans, corn, peas, and watermelon seeds, swell to many times their size and constitute a most serious problem; the diagnosis is often missed initially because the foreign body is not visible on roentgenogram and the history is incomplete. Foreign bodies may also cause chronic atelectasis if small fragments remain after initial bronchoscopic removal (Wiseman, 1984; Wood and Ganderer, 1984).

SIGNS AND SYMPTOMS OF BRONCHIAL OBSTRUCTION

The signs and symptoms of bronchial obstruction will vary with the acuity of the pulmonary collapse. In general, atelectasis that occurs during the course of tuberculosis, lymphoma, neoplasm, asthma, or infections such as bronchiolitis, bronchitis, bronchopneumonia, and sinobronchitis produces no change in the clinical picture unless the obstructed area is large. Large areas of obstruction are rare in the course of these pulmonary infections. Because of the diminished aeration of lung associated with obstruction, the symptoms of tachypnea, dyspnea, cough, and stridor may be present.

Occasionally, a localized constant wheeze, diminished breath sounds, and impaired resonance may suggest atelectasis; in these patients diagnosis is con-

firmed by chest roentgenogram. Careful observation may reveal a difference in respiratory expansion; there may be diminished expansion and contraction of the ribs over the atelectatic area and fullness and widened intercostal spaces over the adjacent, overdistended portion of the lung. Displacement of the heart and the mediastinum and elevation of the diaphragm are detectable only if the atelectasis involves a large area. In young infants, the mobility of the mediastinum may shift the position of the trachea toward the atelectatic lung.

When a previously well child aspirates a foreign body, there may be definite evidence of acute respiratory disturbance. Although coughing, choking, and gagging may occur at the time of aspiration, these signs may not be taken seriously until secondary signs of infection and obstruction become prominent. If a large bronchus is involved, cyanosis or asphyxia may occur. A wheeze is heard, sometimes without the use of a stethoscope. If the obstruction is at the site of the main bronchus, bilateral wheezing will be evident; otherwise the wheeze is localized in the obstructed area. In many instances, and especially if the obstructed area is limited to a segment or a subsegment, the incident of choking may be followed by an asymptomatic period of many days. Then infection in the area of atelectasis results in fever, cough, tachypnea, and malaise. At this point, the clinical picture is that of pneumonitis with atelectasis; the severity of the pneumonitis is related to the virulence of the infecting organism and the nature of the aspirated foreign body.

IDENTIFICATION OF ATELECTASIS

The clinician must remember that atelectasis is a *sign* of disease and does *not* per se suggest a specific diagnosis. Once atelectasis is identified, its differential diagnosis must be considered. The most valuable diagnostic tool is the roentgenogram of the chest (Figs. 37–2 and 37–3). The earliest roentgenographic evidence of atelectasis may be linear infiltrates with

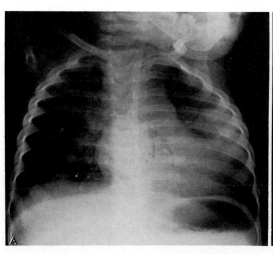
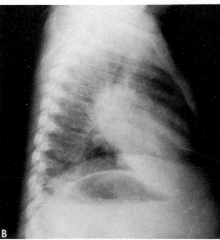

Figure 37–2. A homogeneous density is seen in the left midlung field *(A)*, which on lateral view *(B)* is apparently segmental, involving the entire lingula. This corresponds to the bronchoscopic findings as reported. These roentgenographic findings remained unchanged for many months. Tuberculous cause was clearly established.

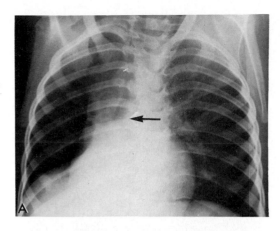

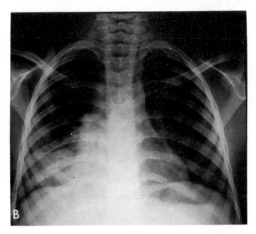

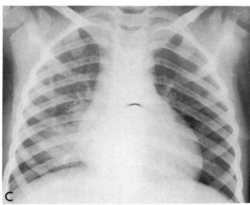

Figure 37–3. *A,* There is a homogeneous dense shadow above the right diaphragm extending from the periphery to the heart border, bounded superiorly by a straight edge at the level of the fifth rib anteriorly, consistent with atelectasis. There is hypoaeration in the right lung above this area. There is also displacement of the heart and mediastinum to the right (even discounting the effect of some torsion to the right). Bronchoscopy determined that the bronchi to the right middle and lower lobes were obstructed. *B,* Four days later, after bronchoscopy and suction of caseous material from the right middle and lower lobes, there is partial expansion of the atelectatic segment. The costophrenic angle is clear. The shadow is less dense in the right base, but there is still displacement of the heart and mediastinum. Note the large dense shadow in the right hilar area. *C,* One month later, after a second bronchoscopy and suction of large amounts of cloudy fluid material, the atelectasis has almost completely cleared and the mediastinal structures have almost returned to normal position.

fissure lines extending beyond their normal areas. Shortly afterward, as a lung segment becomes atelectactic or airless, the fissure lines shift upward or downward and the segment contracts to a much smaller size. This progression of change is best exemplified in atelectasis of the right middle lobe, especially if the atelectasis has been present over a period of time; the lobe may become so small that it is seen radiographically as a dense band suggesting pleural thickening rather than a completely atelectatic lobe.

The position of the diaphragm may be of diagnostic aid; it is usually unaffected in lobar pneumonia and is displaced downward and often flattened on the side of pleural effusion; it sometimes cannot be visualized if fluid overlies it. In these instances, ultrasonography may be useful in determining whether or not the opacity represents fluid or collapsed lung. For proper interpretation and diagnosis of atelectasis, roentgenograms should be obtained in both lateral and posteroanterior views. Films taken during inspiratory and expiratory phases of respiration are also helpful, especially when aspiration of a nonopaque foreign body is a likely cause of atelectasis; however, even in these cases, the chest radiograph may be normal (Musmeche and Kosloske, 1986). Computerized tomography can be most helpful, especially in the interpretation of round, peripheral atelectasis areas that may be mistaken for masses or tumors (Doyle and Lawler, 1984; Hanke and Kretzchmar, 1980).

Atelectasis may occur in any lobe or segment of the lung. When all causes for obstruction of the airway are considered, the right lower and left lower lobes are most frequently collapsed. The age of the patient and the cause of the atelectasis determine the frequency of lobe obstruction. The right middle lobe is most vulnerable when there is enlargement of the hilar lymph nodes; it is also the most commonly affected lobe in asthmatic patients (Fig. 37–4). Some researchers have referred to this predisposition as the *right middle lobe syndrome* (Livingston et al, 1987). Aspirated material in young supine infants more often produces right upper lobe obstruction, probably because of the supine position of the baby and because of the sharp angulation of the right upper lobe bronchus, which tends to trap aspirated material rather than permit expulsion into the main bronchus.

The diagnosis of atelectasis is usually made easily by physical examination and roentgenograms, but the radiographic appearance may mimic hemothorax or chylothorax, especially in the patient recovering from thoracic abdominal surgery. In contrast to the fluid-filled chest, the heart and the mediastinum are displaced toward the affected side and the diaphragm is elevated in massive atelectasis (Fig. 37–5). Dullness and markedly diminished breath sounds are also present. If the unventilated lung is normally perfused, hypoxemia will be present.

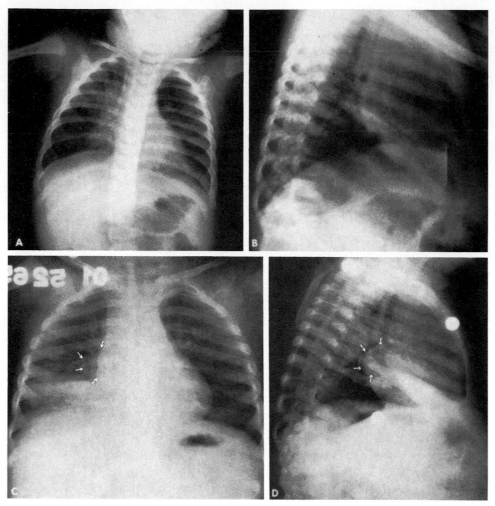

Figure 37–4. *A,* There is an increase in the bronchovascular markings extending from the right root, and some patchy infiltration is seen in the hilar area along the heart border and extending upward into the right upper lobe. *B,* In the lateral view there is a mottled density in the medial aspect of the lung extending from the bronchial bifurcation and overlying the heart shadow, but this density is not definitely segmental in distribution. *C,* There is some displacement of trachea, heart, and mediastinum to the right. A rounded, fairly dense area in the right hilar area suggests nodal enlargement. There is a homogeneous shadow above the diaphragm extending as a wedge-shaped shadow to the periphery. The costophrenic angle is clear. *D,* A shrunken right middle density may be seen, suggesting atelectasis of the entire right middle lobe with questionable hilar density surrounding the apex of the lobe. These films were taken during 2 months of recurrent pneumonia that failed to respond to antibiotics. Bronchoscopy was negative. Atelectasis may be due to disturbed respiration from disease of the central nervous system in this hydrocephalic infant.

TREATMENT

The treatment of atelectasis depends on its cause, duration, and severity. Atelectasis associated with acute infections of the lower respiratory tract is usually short-lived and clears with antimicrobial treatment or spontaneous resolution of the infection. This progression is especially common in acute bronchitis, bronchiolitis, and pneumonia in normal infants. In such instances, atelectasis may not resolve for 6 weeks or so, and specific treatment is usually unnecessary. When atelectasis persists for longer than 6 to 8 weeks, chest physiotherapy, maintenance of moisture in the air, and sometimes bronchodilator therapy are indicated.

In hospitalized patients, lobar atelectasis that occurs following surgery or during mechanical venti-

lation may be treated medically with chest physiotherapy and bronchodilators. Bronchoscopy is sometimes used to reexpand the affected lobe, but little evidence suggests that such intervention is more effective than medical treatment in this group of patients (Marini et al, 1979). When atelectasis occurs in a patient who has had chronic or recurrent pulmonary disease, the bronchi may be damaged, and the secretions in such areas may be retained or expelled more slowly. These children require careful investigation of the underlying cause of recurrent or persistent atelectasis. Although the most likely cause of chronic atelectasis is infection, congenital or acquired immunologic deficiencies should also be considered. Cultures for the etiologic agent should be ordered; postural drainage with chest percussion should be used, and the administration of a broncho-

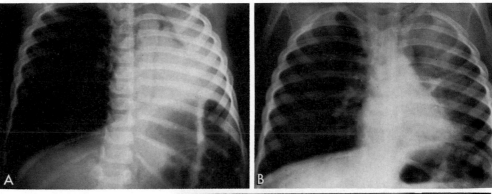

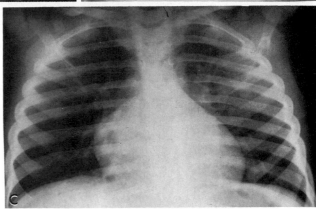

Figure 37–5. *A*, Complete shift of the heart and mediastinal structures into the left hemithorax, where there is a homogeneous density filling the chest. Signs are suggestive of massive atelectasis of the left lung. A peanut was removed from the left main stem bronchus by bronchoscopy, immediately clearing the obstruction *(B)*. Within a few days the patient completely recovered *(C)*.

dilator is often helpful. In those with recurrent episodes of pulmonary obstruction, positive pressure breathing exercises may be of value. Adequate medical treatment must always be given a proper trial before bronchoscopy is done.

In general, the goal of therapy in obstructive atelectasis is to locate the cause of bronchial obstruction, to remove it as soon as possible by appropriate methods, and to maintain normal gas exchange.

When the cause of atelectasis is benign, such as mucus plugging, most patients recover spontaneously with the use of simple mechanical measures, such as coughing and positioning. Active treatment consists of removal of the obstruction and maintenance or improvement of gas exchange by oxygen therapy, bronchodilator inhalation, and use of mucolytic solutions. Ventilation with positive pressure may be required after careful evaluation of the airway obstruction. It is important to remember that atelectasis may clear spontaneously and that good general care of the patient and encouragement of deep inspiration are desirable for a short time before invasive therapeutic measures are used.

Successful medical management of respiratory infections with antibiotics, greater therapeutic use of rigid and flexible bronchoscopes (Wood, 1985; Ward et al, 1987; Shinwell et al, 1989; Black et al, 1984), and skillful and effective thoracic surgery offer an optimistic outlook for most children with acute or subacute atelectasis. When atelectasis persists for many months, the affected portion of the lung parenchyma becomes susceptible to recurrent infection and abscess formation or to development of fibrosis. If medical treatment and bronchoscopy have been ineffective in reaerating the lung, surgical removal of the lobe or segment should be considered both for diagnostic and therapeutic purposes. Many factors will influence the ultimate choice of surgical removal versus medical treatment of the diseased portion of the lung: the age of the patient, the location of the diseased lobe or segments, the extent of damage to the lung, the result of pulmonary function studies, the underlying cause of the atelectasis, the presence of infection, and the general health of the child.

COMPLICATIONS AND PROGNOSIS

Acute and subacute atelectasis are usually benign and respond to therapy. A fatal outcome is likely only when the underlying cause of the atelectasis is life threatening, such as chest trauma, or when the extensive loss of gas exchanging surface area goes unrecognized or is unresponsive to treatment. For example, an unrecognized or untreated foreign body aspiration or an intraoperative mucus plug may be fatal by causing complete collapse of an entire lung. Chronic atelectasis has also been implicated in the pathogenesis of chronic pulmonary fibrosis (Burkhardt, 1989).

REFERENCES

Baldeyrou P, Lemoine G, Zucker JM, and Schweisguth O: Pulmonary metastases in children: the place of surgery. A study of 134 patients. J Pediatr Surg 19:121, 1984.

Benumof JL: Mechanism of decreased blood flow to atelectatic lung. J Appl Physiol 46:1047, 1979.

Black RE, Choi KJ, Syme WC et al: Bronchoscopic removal of aspirated foreign bodies in children. Am J Surg 148:778, 1984.

Burkhardt A: Alveolitis and collapse in the pathogenesis of pulmonary fibrosis. Am Rev Respir Dis 140:513, 1989.

Dehner LP: Tumors and tumor-like lesions of the lung and chest wall in childhood: clinical and pathologic review. In Stocker JT (ed): Pediatric Pulmonary Disease. New York, Hemisphere Publishing Corp, 1989.

Doyle TC and Lawler GA: CT features of rounded atelectasis of the lung. AJR 143:225, 1984.

Finer NN and Etches PC: Fiberoptic bronchoscopy in the neonate. Pediatr Pulmonol 7:116, 1989.

Hanke R and Kretzchmar R: Rounded atelectasis. Semin Roentgenol 15:174, 1980.

Kohn HH: Zur Histologie des indurirenden fibrinosen Pneumonie. Munch Med Wochenschr 40:42, 1893.

Krushner DC, Weinstein HJ, and Kirkpatrick JA: The radiologic diagnosis of leukemia and lymphoma in children. Semin Roentgenol 15:316, 1980.

Laennec RTH: Diseases of the Chest (1819). 4th ed. Translated by John Forbes in 1834. London.

Lambert MW: Accessory bronchiolo-alveolar channels. Anat Rec 127:472, 1957.

Livingston GL, Holinger LD, and Luck SR: Right middle lobe syndrome in children. Int J Pediatr Otorhinolaryngol 13:11, 1987.

McDougall JC, Unni K, Gorenstein A, and O'Connell EJ: Carcinoid and mucoepidermoid carcinoma of bronchus in children. Ann Otol Rhinol Laryngol 89:425, 1980.

Mahfood S, Hix WR, Aaron BL et al: Reexpansion pulmonary edema. Ann Thorac Surg 45:340, 1988.

Marini JJ, Pierson DJ, and Hudson LD: Acute lobar atelectasis: a prospective comparison of fiberoptic bronchoscopy and respiratory therapy. Am Rev Respir Dis 119:971, 1979.

Musemeche CA and Kosloske AM: Normal radiographic findings after foreign body aspiration. When the history counts. Clin Pediatr (Phila) 25:624, 1986.

Rahn H: The role of N₂ gas in various biological processes, with particular reference to the lung. Harvey Lect 55:173, 1959–1960.

Rothmann BF: Foreign bodies in the larynx and tracheobronchial tree in children. A review of 225 cases. Ann Otol 89:434, 1980.

Shinwell ES, Higgins RD, Auten RL, and Shapiro DL: Fiberoptic bronchoscopy in the treatment of intubated neonates. Am J Dis Child 143:1064, 1989.

Stanger P, Lucas RV, and Edwards JE: Anatomic factors causing respiratory distress in acyanotic congenital cardiac disease. Special reference to bronchial obstruction. Pediatrics 43:760, 1969.

Tockics L, Hedenstierna G, Strandberg A et al: Lung collapse and gas exchange during general anesthesia: effects of spontaneous breathing, muscle paralysis, and positive end-expiratory pressure. Anesthesiology 66:157, 1987.

Traube L: Die Uraschen und die Beschaffenheit der jenigen Veranderungen, welche das Lungenparenchym nach Durchschneidung der Nn. Vagi erleidet. Kritischexperimenteller Beitrag zur Lehre von der Pneumonie und Atelektase. Beitr Exp Pathol Physiol 1:65, 1846.

Ward RF, Arnold JE, and Healy GB: Flexible minibronchoscopy in children. Ann Otol Rhinol Laryngol 96:645, 1987.

Wiseman NE: The diagnosis of foreign body aspiration in childhood. J Pediatr Surg 19:531, 1984.

Wood R: Clinical applications of ultrathin flexible bronchoscopes. Pediatr Pulmonol 1:244, 1985.

Wood RE and Gauderer MWL: Flexible fiberoptic bronchoscope in the management of tracheobronchial foreign bodies in children: the value of a combined approach with open tube bronchoscopy. J Pediatr Surg 19:693, 1984.

Wright JR and Clements BJ: Metabolism and turnover of lung surfactant. Am Rev Respir Dis 135:426, 1987.

38

ROBERT B. MELLINS, M.D.

PULMONARY EDEMA

One by-product of the availability of potent diuretics and the modern trend toward intensive care and monitoring of patients with serious illnesses has been a greater appreciation of the significance of fluid movement into the lung as a complication of a variety of conditions. This, coupled with an improved understanding of the pathogenesis of pulmonary edema, summarized in several reviews (Staub, 1974; Guyton et al, 1975; Levine and Mellins, 1975; Staub and Taylor, 1984; Drake and Laine, 1988), has enhanced our ability to treat a variety of illnesses in which pulmonary edema develops.

Supported in part by NIH grants HL 07421, HL 24997, and HL 14218 (SCOR), with additional support from the New York Lung Association.

ANATOMIC CONSIDERATIONS

Certain structural features of the lung are worth pointing out because they have a bearing on gas exchange during pulmonary edema. The capillaries are placed eccentrically within the alveolar septum (Fig. 38–1A). In some areas, the basement membranes of the capillary endothelium and the alveolar epithelium are fused with no additional space between them, even during edema formation. This situation would seem to be ideal for preserving gas exchange, at least until such time as the alveoli themselves are filled with liquid. In other areas, there is an interstitial space between the endothelial and epithelial basement membranes that contains a ground substance and connective tissue elements,

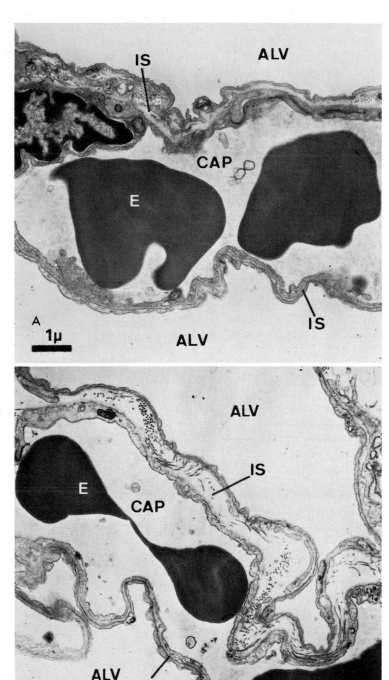

Figure 38–1. *A*, The normal alveolar septum in which the epithelial and endothelial basement membranes are fused in some areas and separated by an interstitial space of connective tissue in others. *B*, The alveolar septum in pulmonary edema. The areas where the basement membranes are fused remain thin; only the areas with a connective tissue interstitial space widen. *ALV*, alveolar lumen; *CAP*, capillary; *E*, erythrocyte; *IS*, interstitial space. (Reproduced with permission from Mellins RB, Levine OR, Skalak R, and Fishman AP: Interstitial pressure of the lung. Circ Res 24:197, 1969.)

including collagen, elastin, microfibrils, and fibroblasts. In addition to supplying support to the capillary network, this widened portion of the alveolar-capillary membrane provides a channel for water and protein en route to the lymphatics and larger interstitial fluid spaces (Fig. 38–1*B*). As long as water can be confined to these channels, gas exchange can be preserved.

Pulmonary capillaries, like muscle capillaries, have a continuous endothelium with relatively tight intercellular junctions. The bronchial microvasculature, much like visceral capillaries, is discontinuous, with intercellular fenestrations or gaps. Whether these gaps account for increased fluid movement across the bronchial but not the pulmonary capillaries—for example, in response to bradykinin, as shown by Pietra and co-workers (1971)—remains to be determined. It may be that the role of the bronchial circulation in the genesis of pulmonary edema has been underestimated.

At the ultrastructural level, the available evidence from tracer studies indicates that the alveolar epithelial membrane contains tighter cellular junctions than does the capillary endothelial membrane. Thus edema in diseases that alter pulmonary vascular permeability is likely to be confined initially to the interstitial and lymphatic spaces; alveolar edema results only when the volume that can be handled by these is overwhelmed. Electron-microscopic studies have revealed pores between endothelial cells of approximately 40 Å that are large enough to restrain macromolecules. Whether pinocytotic vesicles can account for the movement of larger molecules across the endothelial cell (vesicular shuttle) is not clear. Also the extent to which pores can enlarge as the result of pressure or injury is unclear.

Although the alveoli are generally conceived as spheric, increasing evidence indicates that a polyhedral model is closer to reality. Figure 38–2 shows that surfactant removed from the lung does indeed assume a polyhedral shape. From the point of view of fluid movement in the lung, the importance of this shape is that the walls of the alveolar septa are flat, except at the corners where the septa meet. Thus it is only at the corners, where the alveolar air-liquid interface is curved, that the force exerted by surface tension can lower alveolar fluid and interstitial fluid pressures as predicted by the Laplace relationship (Fig. 38–3). The lower interstitial pressures at the corners favor movement of interstitial fluid that has traversed the alveolar capillary wall toward the corners, where it is then picked up by the terminal lymphatics and eventually returned to the systemic venous system.

Pulmonary blood vessels have been defined anatomically and physiologically. Anatomically, the vessels have been classified traditionally by their morphologic characteristics as arteries, arterioles, capillaries, veins, or venules. Physiologically, these divisions are included under two broad classifications based on their behavior relative to the hydrostatic pressures of the interstitium surrounding the vessels, the interstitial fluid pressure. These are the alveolar vessels and the extra-alveolar vessels. The alveolar vessels are in the alveolar walls or septa and behave as if they were exposed to alveolar pressure. These vessels may collapse if airway pressures exceed vascular pressures (zone I conditions of West). Extra-alveolar vessels lie in the larger interstitial spaces and behave as if surrounded by a pressure that is as negative as or more negative than pleural pressure (Bhattacharya and Staub, 1984) and that tends to vary with pleural pressure. In addition, there are vessels lying in the intersections of alveolar septal walls (corner vessels) that are exposed to more negative pressures than the alveolar vessels, at least in part because of the acute radius of curvature found at the alveolar corners, as described previously (see Fig. 38–3). The functional classification is important because it predicts the pressures surrounding the vessels participating in fluid exchange, and it is used in subsequent analyses of fluid movement and edema in this chapter. Unfortunately, there is no clear-cut correlation between the functional and the anatomic classifications. Although fluid movement occurs at the level of the arterioles and venules (Iliff, 1971), it is generally considered that the bulk of fluid movement occurs at the level of the capillaries, with one calculation being 76 per cent from alveolar vessels (Gropper et al, 1988).

In addition, receptors appear to be present in the pulmonary interstitium that are responsible for stimulating breathing, the so-called J receptors.

FACTORS RESPONSIBLE FOR FLUID MOVEMENT

The factors responsible for fluid accumulation are shown in Figure 38–4. These include intravascular and interstitial hydrostatic and colloid osmotic pressures, permeability characteristics of the fluid exchanging membrane, and lymphatic drainage.

The equilibrium of fluid across fluid-exchanging membranes is generally expressed as follows:

$$Q_f = K_f (Pmv - Ppmv) - \sigma(\pi mv - \pi pmv)$$

wherein
Q_f = the net transvascular flow;

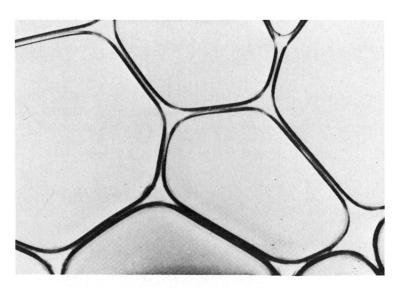

Figure 38–2. Surfactant foam obtained from the lung by bronchial rinsing assumes a polyhedral shape. (Reproduced with permission from Reifenrath R: The significance of alveolar geometry and surface tension in the respiratory mechanics of the lung. Resp Physiol 24:115, 1975.)

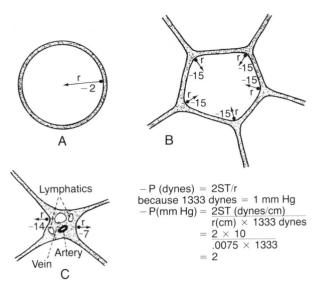

$$-P \text{ (dynes)} = 2ST/r$$
because 1333 dynes = 1 mm Hg
$$-P \text{(mm Hg)} = \frac{2ST \text{ (dynes/cm)}}{r(cm) \times 1333 \text{ dynes}}$$
$$= \frac{2 \times 10}{.0075 \times 1333}$$
$$= 2$$

Figure 38–3. Effect of surface tension on the alveolar fluid and interstitial fluid pressure. *A*, Assuming a spheric model of the alveolus with a radius of 75 microns and a surface tension of 10 dynes/cm, we calculate that the fluid lining the alveolus would be pulled away with a pressure of minus 2 mm Hg. *B*, Assuming a polyhedral model with the radius of curvature at the corners of 10 microns, the negative pressure in the corners would be minus 15 mm Hg. The pressure at the angles (not shown) where the alveolar air-liquid interface is cylindric and where $-P = ST/r$ would be minus 7.5 mm Hg. *C*, Dynamics at alveolar angles adjacent to interstitial spaces surrounding larger blood vessels and lymphatics; pressures of minus 7 to minus 14 mm Hg can be calculated, depending on the radius of curvature at the angles. (Modified from Guyton AC et al: In Lung Liquids. Ciba Symposium 38. New York, American Elsevier Publishing Co, 1976.)

K_f = the filtration coefficient of the fluid-exchanging vessels and includes both the contribution of the permeability of the vessels and the surface area across which fluid exchange occurs;

P_{mv} = microvascular hydrostatic pressure;

P_{pmv} = perimicrovascular (interstitial fluid) hydrostatic pressure;

π_{mv} = colloid osmotic pressure in the microvasculature;

π_{pmv} = colloid osmotic pressure in the perimicro-

vasculature, the interstitial fluid colloid osmotic pressure; and

σ = the reflection coefficient and describes the transvascular protein osmotic pressure difference; it is a measure of the resistance of the membrane to the flow of protein.

The walls of the pulmonary circulation are not a perfect semipermeable membrane. They possess pores that are larger than protein molecules. Fluid filtering through a pore will drag some protein with it. The larger the protein relative to the size of the pore, the less protein will be dragged. When the protein is the same size as or larger than the pore, the reflection coefficient σ is one. As the size of the protein becomes progressively smaller, σ approaches zero (Drake and Laine, 1988).

The term microvasculature is used because, as previously indicated, fluid exchange is not limited to the capillaries alone. In the following discussion, each of the previously cited factors and the pathophysiologic influences on them are described in detail.

VASCULAR FORCES

The pressure in the pulmonary microvasculature, Pmv (generally but not precisely referred to as pulmonary capillary pressure), is estimated to be about 7 mm Hg with peak pressure under exercise conditions in the adult rising to 20 mm Hg. For technical reasons, this pressure is extremely difficult to measure in vivo. The pulmonary wedge pressure is really a measure of left atrial pressure. Pmv is believed to be above left atrial pressure by approximately 40 per cent of the difference between left atrial (LA) pressure and pulmonary arterial (PA) pressure. An increase in either PA or LA pressure will tend to increase the hydrostatic pressure, favoring movement out of the fluid-exchanging vessels. For example, Pmv may be increased by the elevation in LA pressures in left-sided heart failure or by increases in PA pressure as seen in large left-to-right shunts. Because of the large capacity of the pulmonary vascular bed, considerable elevation in blood flow can occur (as in

Figure 38–4. Factors affecting fluid accumulation in the lung.

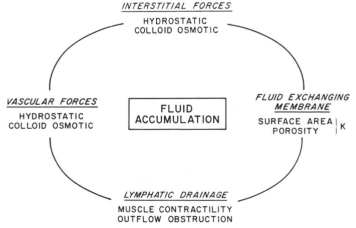

INTERSTITIAL FORCES
HYDROSTATIC
COLLOID OSMOTIC

VASCULAR FORCES
HYDROSTATIC
COLLOID OSMOTIC

FLUID ACCUMULATION

FLUID EXCHANGING MEMBRANE
SURFACE AREA
POROSITY | K

LYMPHATIC DRAINAGE
MUSCLE CONTRACTILITY
OUTFLOW OBSTRUCTION

exercise or shunts) without raising PA pressures appreciably. At the experimental level, ligation of one pulmonary artery, directing all flow through the contralateral lung, results in only a slight elevation of PA pressure at rest. A clinical illustration of the capacity of the pulmonary vascular bed to handle an increase in blood flow was provided by a 5-month-old infant we studied, who had congenital absence of the left lung and total anomalous pulmonary venous connection to the right atrium. Surgical correction of pulmonary venous obstruction reduced PA pressures to normal, despite the continued diversion of the total cardiac output to the right lung (Boxer et al, 1978). Pmv will also vary depending on the resistance to blood flow on the arterial and venous sides of the pulmonary capillary bed.

Because the pulmonary vascular membrane is only very slightly permeable to proteins, the plasma proteins normally are responsible for osmotic pressure (pmv) well in excess of the pulmonary microvascular hydrostatic pressure. The plasma colloid osmotic pressure may be markedly reduced in clinical conditions in which the plasma proteins are low, e.g., malnutrition, nephrosis, and massive burns, and thus may facilitate edema formation.

It should also be emphasized that the rapid infusion of non–colloid-containing fluids not only raises vascular hydrostatic pressure but also lowers the colloid osmotic pressure because of hemodilution. However, the infusion of colloid-containing fluids may raise microvascular hydrostatic pressure because of the absorption of fluid throughout the body, thus limiting its usefulness as a therapeutic agent in edema.

The interplay between maturation and surfactant on alveolar interstitial pressure has been demonstrated by studies in isolated lungs of mature and immature rabbits (Raj, 1987). The pressure and alveolar wash phospholipids were lower in the immature lung but rose toward the higher levels of pressure of the mature lung following surfactant replacement.

INTERSTITIAL FORCES AND MECHANICAL INTERDEPENDENCE

Although it is still a matter of controversy, we believe that the weight of evidence provided by Guyton and associates (1975) and Brace (1981) favors the conclusion that the interstitial hydrostatic pressure throughout the lung is normally negative (relative to alveolar pressure), a conclusion that is confirmed by experimental studies (Bhattacharya and Staub, 1984). The degree of negativity that one calculates using the classic Starling formulation depends on the values one uses for the perimicrovascular or interstitial colloid osmotic pressure. Because the concentration of protein in the lymph from the lung is relatively high compared with that in lymph from an extremity, some have assumed that the

protein concentration in the perimicrovascular space is also high. For most organs it is reasonable to think that lymph fluid collected before a lymph node is traversed is a representative sample of interstitial fluid, and indeed this conclusion may be true in the lung under conditions of high flow. However, with lesser degrees of lymph flow, the perivascular and peribronchial spaces do not seem to be very well mixed (Taylor, 1981). Contributions of the caudal mediastinal lymph node to lung lymph have called into question some estimates of tissue colloid osmotic pressure based on studies of lung lymph. Also, considering the delicate nature of the lymphatic walls and the fact that lymphatics can generate considerable pressures, it seems likely that concentration of the protein occurs in the lung lymphatics and that the protein concentration in the pulmonary interstitial spaces may be considerably lower than in the lung lymph. This concentrating ability of the lymphatics together with its pumping action would seem to be necessary for the maintenance of a negative interstitial fluid pressure and a dry lung. A negative interstitial fluid pressure appears to be maintained by a low effective microvascular pressure, lymphatic removal of interstitial fluid and protein, low microvascular permeability, and low filtration coefficient (Brace, 1981).

Some studies on the manner in which pleural pressures are transmitted to the interstitium of the lung have special relevance to the development of pulmonary edema, especially in diseases that affect the lung nonuniformly. As previously indicated, the pressure surrounding the corner and extra-alveolar vessels is believed to be less than pleural pressure and to become considerably more negative at high lung volumes (Permutt, 1973). In disease, these negative pressures may be amplified manyfold because of "mechanical interdependence" of lung units (Mead et al, 1970; Macklem and Murphy, 1974). When the expansion of some units of the lung lags behind surrounding lung units because of disease, the force (pleural pressure) per unit area distending the lagging unit is increased. Amplification of transpulmonary (distending) pressures by mechanical interdependence is seen in increased respiratory resistance, decreased lung compliance, and expansion of the lung from the airless state. Mechanical interdependence can act on diseased areas of the lung to produce distending pressures that are exceedingly high. When transmitted to the interstitial space around blood vessels, these pressures can enhance edema formation and can cause the rupture of vessels. Indeed, this mechanism may be central in the formation of hyaline membranes. These considerations become especially important because various forms of constant distending pressures are used therapeutically. Although only 5 to 10 cm H_2O may be applied, if the pressure does not distend some areas of the lung as quickly as others, the pressure surrounding lagging units may be considerably greater because of amplification. Two other approaches that have led to much the same conclusions have been provided by Reifenrath (1975), who suggests that it is mechanical interdependence that is primarily responsible for lung stability, and Smith-Ericksen and Bo (1979), who have demonstrated that although a pleural pressure is poorly transmitted to the alveolar interstitial space in the normal lung with open airways, it is well transmitted when there is airway closure.

MICROVASCULAR FILTRATION COEFFICIENT AND VASCULAR PERMEABILITY

Several groups of workers have attempted to characterize the ease with which water crosses the pulmonary fluid-exchanging vessels by calculating K_f, the filtration coefficient. K_f includes both the surface area of the membrane and its porosity. For the most part, the data to date indicate that K_f is in the range of 0.03 to 0.2 ml/min/mm Hg/100 gm (Drake and Laine, 1988). At least two kinds of questions should be addressed. First, is the pulmonary capillary more or less leaky than fluid-exchanging vessels in other tissues? Second, is the lung of the young animal more or less leaky than the lung of the adult?

Some studies have suggested that the K_f of the pulmonary capillaries is about one tenth that of the muscle capillaries (Levine et al, 1967). Other studies provide evidence that the filtration coefficient of the pulmonary vessels is approximately the same as that of the skeletal muscle capillaries (Perl et al, 1975).

Some of the apparent differences in K_f obtained by different workers (Staub, 1974) may be explained by Guyton's observations that normally there is a great deal of resistance to the flow of fluid in the narrow interstitial spaces of the alveolar septal wall, resulting in a very low "effective" pulmonary capillary filtration coefficient. As fluid accumulates and the septum widens, the resistance falls and the "effective" filtration coefficient is higher. Other differences may relate to various estimates of perimicrovascular hydrostatic and colloid osmotic pressure; the fact that there is likely to be inhomogeneity of both of these adds to the complexity.

Early experimental evidence suggested that the microvascular permeability to protein is greater in the young than in the adult dog (Taylor et al, 1967; Boyd et al, 1969) and that the filtration coefficient of the puppy lung is greater than that of the adult dog lung (Levine et al, 1973). However, uncertainties about the difference in magnitude of the interstitial forces, the lymphatic drainage, and the surface area of the alveolar capillary membrane in the immature and mature lung make it difficult to calculate K_f with any precision. Using measurements of extravascular water and permeability surface area products, Brigham and co-workers (1978) have concluded that microvascular permeability to small hydrophilic molecules in newborn lambs is similar to that in adult sheep. Bland (1986) has summarized the data dem-

onstrating no difference in lung microvascular permeability to protein before and after birth in lambs. However, fluid filtration pressures and microvascular surface area per unit mass are greater in newborn lungs than in adult lungs (Bland, 1986).

Our understanding of the factors that alter microvascular membrane permeability is primitive. Contrary to much that is written, there is evidence that hypoxia alone does not alter permeability in either the mature (Goodale et al, 1970) or the immature animal (Hansen et al, 1984). Histamine causes increased leakage of fluid from both the systemic and pulmonary vascular beds (Brigham, 1978), and the increased permeability is reversed by antihistamines and catecholamines (Marciniak et al, 1978). There is also some evidence that antihistamines are able to reverse the increase in vascular permeability produced by bradykinin. The role of potent vasoactive chemical mediators with known permeability effects, such as bradykinin and the prostaglandins, is just beginning to be studied. Current research on mechanisms of permeability is focused on a variety of vasoactive factors, including proteases in plasma and formed elements in blood and in the interstitium. On the basis of reports currently available, it is reasonable to say that all of these are involved. Future studies will no doubt help us to understand what stimulates these factors and what controls them.

Whatever the particular vasoactive agents involved in increasing microvascular permeability, the list of clinical entities in which increased lung water content is secondary to increased permeability is growing. Because the only Starling force holding fluid in the vascular compartment is the osmotic pressure generated by the protein concentration gradient across the capillary membrane, even slight decreases in this gradient (consequent to movement of protein from inside to outside the vessel) have profound effects on net water balance. An increase in microvascular hydrostatic pressure produces a much greater outward flow of water when the protein gradient is reduced because of altered permeability, so the combination of increased permeability and high left atrial pressures represents an especially difficult clinical challenge.

LYMPHATIC CLEARANCE

Whether there is fluid accumulation in the lung depends on the balance between fluid filtration into the lung and lymphatic clearance. Early in the onset of interstitial edema, lymphatic drainage of fluid is an important protective mechanism preventing alveolar flooding. Studies using experimentally induced permeability-type edema by intravenous infusion of Pseudomonas aeruginosa indicate that under acute experimental conditions lymph flow can increase tenfold without overflow of edema fluid into the alveolar space. Furthermore, there is experimental evidence to indicate that under conditions of chronic edema the ability of the lymphatics to clear fluid may increase severalfold, presumably as the result of proliferation.

The concentration of protein in lymph is generally high. Although our focus is on pulmonary edema, a major role of the lymphatics is to return the interstitial protein back to the circulation. Because the lymphatics ultimately drain into the great veins, elevation of systemic venous pressure might be expected to increase fluid accumulation not only by raising pressure in the fluid-exchanging vessels but also by impairing lymphatic drainage. Impairment of clearance by this mechanism may occur under conditions of chronic right-sided heart failure, especially if lymphatic valve incompetence occurs. Although some experimental work provides indirect evidence that the pulmonary lymphatics can actively generate high pressures (Pang and Mellins, 1975), other experimental studies on unanesthetized sheep indicate that lung lymph flow falls even at relatively low outflow pressures (Drake et al, 1985). The latter studies indicate that elevated central venous pressures are likely to lead to excess accumulation of fluid in the lung only when accompanied by increased filtration rate. Other studies suggest that the maximum flow of lymph from edematous lungs is limited by the resistance of the extrapulmonary lung lymph drainage system.

Although earlier work had indicated that increased motion or ventilation of the lung increased the lymphatic fluid drainage, suggesting a passive milking action, it now appears that the contribution of active contractions of the smooth muscle of the lymphatics is also significant. To what extent drugs that affect smooth muscle also affect lymphatic pumping is unknown but could be appreciable.

Active contraction of the lymphatics, together with the presence of lymphatic valves, helps to explain how fluid moves "uphill" from the negative pressures in the pulmonary interstitium to a pressure of zero or above in the great veins.

SURFACE TENSION

Surface tension on the inner surface of the alveolus tends to pull fluid away from the alveolar epithelium with a force of at least -2 mm Hg (see Fig. 38–3A). This figure is based on the assumption that the alveolar surface is spheric and that the surface tension is 10 dynes per cm, which is low presumably because of the presence of the surfactant. However, because the alveoli are polyhedral, there are many angles at which two alveoli come together and corners at which more than two alveoli abut. Although the shape of the alveolar air-liquid interface is spheric in the corners as well as in crypts in the alveolar walls, it is cylindric at the angles, and therefore $-P = ST/r$ would be the appropriate formula to use at the angles. Because the radii of curvature at the angles and corners of the alveoli are much smaller, the

pressures are much more negative (see Fig. 38–3B). Surface tension at the alveolar air-liquid interface would be expected to expand the perivascular space and to lower perimicrovascular pressure, thus promoting the formation of interstitial edema. The effect of the change in radius of curvature of the alveolar air-liquid interface on surface forces is further illustrated in Figure 38–5. Initially, as fluid collects in the corners, the radius of curvature becomes greater and the pressure becomes less negative (Fig. 38–5B). Once the fluid layer becomes spheric throughout the inner surface of the alveoli, additional fluid will decrease the radius, and the pressure will become more negative (Fig. 38–5C). This process explains why the filling of an alveolus with fluid is self-accelerating once there is a critical amount of fluid in it.

From the foregoing reasoning, Guyton and associates (1975) have concluded that for alveoli of normal size, the interstitial fluid pressure around alveoli (and around alveolar vessels) would have to be at most -2 mm Hg to prevent alveolar flooding; for smaller alveoli, the interstitial pressure would have to be still more negative.

Surface tension at the alveolar air-liquid interface opposes the transmission of alveolar pressure to the fluid-exchanging vessels (Mellins et al, 1969). Therefore, the beneficial effects of positive-pressure breathing in the treatment of pulmonary edema probably do not relate to an increase in the pressure surrounding the fluid-exchanging vessels, but rather to (1) an increase in intrathoracic pressures, impeding venous return to the thorax, thus lowering the hydrostatic pressures within the pulmonary vascular bed, and (2) the prevention of airway collapse, thus enhancing blood gas exchange.

PROTECTION AGAINST EDEMA

A variety of clinical observations have indicated that vascular hydrostatic pressures must be raised 15 to 20 mm Hg, or plasma colloid osmotic pressures must be reduced an equivalent amount, before edema develops. Several factors contribute to this protection against edema. The interstitial fluid pressure, which, as we have noted previously, is below alveolar pressure, is not a fixed value but will rise to approximately zero with minimal amounts of fluid filtration into the lung. With increased fluid filtration,

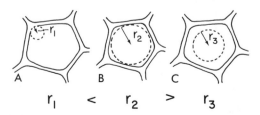

Figure 38–5. Effect of fluid accumulation on the radius of curvature at the alveolar air-liquid interface. See text for description.

it may increase further by 4 or 5 mm Hg and thus oppose fluid movement. At the same time, the filtered fluid will dilute the interstitial plasma protein, thus lowering the interstitial colloid osmotic pressure. Lymphatic drainage of fluid and protein also contributes to this "margin of safety." The ability of the lymphatics to concentrate protein by filtering fluid through their walls, although still an area of controversy, probably also contributes by keeping the interstitial osmotic pressure low. The interstitial space itself, especially around the bronchi and blood vessels (bronchovascular cuffs), can sequester fluid (as much as 500 ml in the adult) and thus can provide an additional safety factor before fluid floods the alveoli (Matthay, 1985). In addition, surfactant, by keeping surface tension low, tends to prevent the lowering of alveolar interstitial pressure.

PATHOPHYSIOLOGIC CONSEQUENCES OF EDEMA

The effect of pulmonary edema on the function of the lung is complex. Increased pulmonary blood volumes without edema result in a mild fall in lung compliance, i.e., increased lung recoil, at normal or high lung volumes (Levine et al, 1965); however, there is a decrease in lung recoil at low lung volumes, which leads to premature airway closure and an increase in the resistance of the peripheral airways (Macklem, 1976). Increase in interstitial edema does not further reduce the compliance at high lung volumes until the extravascular fluid volumes increase at least threefold (Hauge et al, 1975).

Although peribronchiolar cuffs of fluid would be expected to lead to increases in airway closure and airway resistance, morphometric studies provide no support for the notion that interstitial lung edema compresses airways (Michel et al, 1987). They suggest that alveolar or airway lumenal edema may be responsible for the increase in resistance with edema. Studies in adult animals have shown some increase in total airway resistance (Levine et al, 1965). If the small airways contribute a relatively greater proportion of the total airway resistance in infants than in adults, one might expect edema to lead to a greater increase in airway resistance in infants. Indeed, airway obstruction has been a presenting sign of a group of infants with ventricular septal defects and left-to-right shunts (Hordof et al, 1977). In addition, some children with interstitial edema as a result of left atrial obstruction, e.g., cor triatriatum, have also presented with a history of recurrent asthmatic attacks. To minimize the markedly increased work of moving their stiff lungs, a pattern of rapid, shallow breathing is used. It is also believed that stimulation by edema of vagal juxta-alveolar receptors, or J receptors, within the interstitium contributes to the hyperventilation as well as the tachypnea and dyspnea so characteristic of early pulmonary edema. It is not clear whether increased ventilation enhances or impedes fluid accumulation. Increased ventilation is known to promote the removal of excess water by the lymphatics. However, if there are inhomogeneities of disease within the lung, mechanical amplification of pressures could lead to enhanced edema formation, as we have already indicated.

Initially, edema fluid collects around the larger blood vessels and airways. Airway resistance increases, perhaps as suggested previously because of airway lumenal edema. The airways are narrowed and more likely to close at higher than normal lung volumes. Alveolar gas exchange is impaired. At this stage, there is hypocapnia as the result of the J reflex hyperventilation, whether or not there is hypoxemia. As edema worsens and alveolar flooding occurs, there is further hypoxemia as the blood shunts past nonventilating alveoli. Respiratory acidosis may supervene if the patient is depressed by sedation or if exhaustion develops. The extent to which bronchial mucosal edema intensifies the increase in airway resistance when pulmonary edema is accompanied by elevated systemic venous pressure is not known. With alveolar flooding and disruption of the normal alveolar lining, resistance to airflow increases, dynamic and static compliance are reduced, and there is increasing inhomogeneity of airflow. One can account for most of the clinical findings, e.g., rales and diffuse wheezing, on the basis of interstitial, airway, and alveolar edema. Mediator release and airway smooth muscle constriction are probably not of importance in hemodynamic pulmonary edema (Snapper, 1985). In permeability-type edema, e.g., adult respiratory distress syndrome (ARDS), lung compliance may be very reduced, and even with mechanical ventilators, it may be very difficult to ventilate the lung without using very high pressures.

The rightward shift of the oxygen dissociation curve produced by the increased red blood cell 2,3-diphosphoglyceric acid seen with chronic hypoxemia may not occur with acute pulmonary edema, thus limiting the unloading of oxygen at the tissue level. Respiratory alkalosis, more commonly seen in older children and adults with pulmonary edema, may shift the oxygen dissociation curve to the left, which also impairs oxygen unloading.

Pulmonary edema has been shown to impair intrapulmonary antibacterial activity in vivo, and the antibacterial activity of alveolar macrophages harvested from edematous lungs has also been shown to be impaired (La Force et al, 1973).

The dynamics of pleural fluid formation are discussed in Chapter 40. Clinical studies have suggested that left heart failure with pulmonary edema is associated with larger pleural effusions than right heart failure (Weiner-Kronish et al, 1985), the reverse result of some experimental studies in dogs (Mellins et al, 1970). There is general consensus, however, that the greatest amounts of pleural fluid are seen with combined left and right heart failure. Greater amounts of pulmonary edema will also result from elevation of left atrial and hence pulmonary artery pressures when systemic venous pressures are also elevated (Laine et al, 1986).

RESOLUTION OF PULMONARY EDEMA

How quickly pulmonary edema resolves once the basic condition producing the edema is reversed depends on (1) whether the fluid is confined to the interstitium, from which it can be cleared in hours, or is also located in the alveolar space, from which it may take days to clear; and (2) whether the alveolar fluid has high or low concentration of protein. In high-pressure edema, protein concentration is relatively low, and therefore this fluid can be cleared more quickly than when there is high protein concentration.

The relative contribution of the pulmonary and bronchial circulations and lymphatics to clearing of alveolar and interstitial edema is uncertain. The relatively slow clearance of alveolar fluid has been attributed to the tight alveolar epithelial junctions. Because alveolar fluid has cleared even when the protein concentration is extremely high and large osmotic pressure-restraining fluid is in the alveolar compartment, it has been proposed that active metabolic processes might be involved (Matthay, 1985). Active transport of chloride ion across alveolar epithelial cells toward the lumen in the fetus and active transport of sodium in the reverse direction postnatally have been demonstrated. Presumably, water follows these processes passively. The observations that catecholamines enhance fluid clearance and amiloride, an inhibitor of sodium entry, retards fluid movement into the apical surface of the epithelium are consistent with this view (Matthay, 1985). Nevertheless, the active sites, e.g., alveolar or bronchial epithelium, transcellular or paracellular, remain to be elucidated.

Protein clearance from the alveolar spaces is relatively slow, and the mechanisms, including metabolic degradation and macrophage ingestion, remain unclear. Protein clearance from the interstitial space is believed to occur primarily by lymphatic clearance, but direct penetration into the circulation either before or after metabolic degradation has not been excluded as a potential mechanism.

The presence of protein in the alveolar and interstitial spaces may serve as a stimulant for the attraction of inflammatory cells, which can occur during the development of pulmonary edema, whether there has been lung injury and hence increased alveolar-capillary permeability. Circulating monocytes and alveolar macrophages appear and play a major role in the clearance of inflammatory edema of the lung (Henson et al, 1984).

In summary, a wide variety of mechanisms and sites exist for protein and electrolyte clearance and fluid removal, including pulmonary and bronchial circulations, lymphatics, active transport of ions, mac-

romolecular metabolism and degradation, and mononuclear cell activity. The relative contribution of each has yet to be assessed.

ETIOLOGIC CONSIDERATIONS

INCREASED HYDROSTATIC PRESSURE IN THE PULMONARY MICROVASCULATURE

A variety of clinical conditions are associated with increased hydrostatic pressures in the pulmonary vascular bed, either as the result of elevation of vascular pressures distal to the lung or as the result of increased blood flow and pulmonary arterial hypertension. Those conditions resulting from elevation of pressures distal to the lung include left-sided heart failure, congenital hypoplastic left heart syndrome, cor triatriatum, mitral stenosis, congenital obstruction of pulmonary venous drainage, and pulmonary veno-occlusive disease.

Pulmonary edema as a result of left-sided heart failure is seen in severe aortic stenosis, in coarctation of the aorta (usually accompanied by a left ventricular overload in infants), in intrinsic myocardial disease (cardiac glycogen storage diseases, endocardial fibroelastosis, anomalous left coronary artery, viral and rheumatic myocarditis), and in large congenital arteriovenous fistulas. Pulmonary edema is a frequent complication of acute renal disease when systemic hypertension is accompanied by expansion of the extracellular fluid in excess of urine output; chronic renal disease may also predispose an individual to pulmonary edema by producing hypoproteinemia.

A variety of congenital heart lesions, including ventricular septal defects and patent ductus arteriosus, are associated with increased blood flow and pressure in the pulmonary vascular bed, leading to vascular engorgement and edema. When the burden on the left ventricle becomes too great as a result of the large left-to-right shunt, and left-sided heart failure supervenes, pulmonary vascular pressures are increased by both high flow and increased left atrial pressures.

Pulmonary edema is sometimes seen as a complication of surgically performed systemic-to-pulmonary artery shunts for congenital lesions with insufficient pulmonary blood flow, such as Fallot tetralogy. This complication is more likely to occur following a Waterston-type shunt procedure than a Blalock procedure, because the range between an insufficient shunt and one that is too great is very narrow in the former.

Overzealous administration of fluids may also intensify the development of pulmonary edema by raising hydrostatic pressures and diluting plasma proteins. To what extent the inappropriate secretion of antidiuretic hormone complicates and intensifies the development of pulmonary edema in diseases is not known. This secretion has been reported to occur with severe pneumonia (Mor et al, 1975) and asthma (Baker et al, 1976) and could accompany other diseases.

DECREASED PLASMA COLLOID OSMOTIC PRESSURE

For any given level of vascular pressure, pulmonary edema is more likely to develop when the plasma proteins are low. This condition is seen with severe malnutrition, massive burns, protein-losing enteropathies, and nephrosis. It can also be seen in patients with a variety of other conditions when withdrawal of multiple blood samples for diagnostic purposes is coupled with the administration of large amounts of non–colloid-containing fluids.

DECREASED INTERSTITIAL HYDROSTATIC PRESSURE

As previously emphasized, because of mechanical interdependence of adjacent lung units, when inflation of some units lags behind that of others, large negative interstitial pressures can be generated around and within the lagging units. We believe that these negative pressures can be transmitted to the fluid-exchanging vessels (when there is airway closure), enhancing edema formation, especially in obstructive lung diseases such as asthma and bronchiolitis as well as in the respiratory distress syndrome (RDS). Although one might argue that all pressures, including the vascular pressures, would fall a similar amount, at least three factors keep vascular pressures high relative to interstitial pressures:

1. The decrease in intrathoracic pressures will enhance venous return, increasing cardiac output.

2. As pulmonary microvascular pressures decrease below alveolar pressure, alveolar vessels will be compressed and perfusion obstructed; this process, in turn, will increase afterload on the right ventricle. Any decrease in emptying of the right ventricle will lead to an increase in end-diastolic volume, which in turn will lead to an increase in the force of contraction maintaining forward flow by raising intravascular hydrostatic pressures.

3. Exposure of the surfaces of the left ventricle to large negative pleural pressures is analogous to imposing an afterload. Theory would predict that as a consequence, end-diastolic filling pressures will increase, which will be reflected in elevated left atrial and pulmonary microvascular pressures. It should also be recalled that when airway resistance is high, e.g., during croup, large negative alveolar pressures may be generated during inspiration (Newth et al, 1972), and these too would be expected to be transmitted to the fluid-exchanging vessels.

These considerations have special relevance to a variety of clinical conditions in which there is a lag in the expansion of the lung in spite of the development of very negative intrathoracic pressures (Stalcup and Mellins, 1977). One such example is in a child with heart failure complicating hypertrophied tonsils and adenoids (Luke et al, 1966; Bland et al, 1969; Cayler et al, 1969). Although many have assumed that cor pulmonale with right-sided heart failure is the principal complication, we, like others (Levin et al, 1975), have been struck by the clinical and radiographic findings of pulmonary edema in several children with this condition. At the bedside, one cannot but be impressed with the severe intercostal retractions during inspiration. Indeed, this inspiratory pattern comes very close to simulating a Müller maneuver, i.e., a strong inspiration against a closed glottis or obstructed upper airway. The negative pressures surrounding and restraining the left ventricle are analogous to an afterload and would be expected to raise the pressures on the left side of the heart relative to pleural pressures. Thus, we believe, the large negative intrathoracic pressures are at least in part responsible for cardiomegaly, pulmonary vascular engorgement, and edema.

A dramatic example of the change in heart size following removal of the tonsils and adenoids is shown in Figure 38–6. Part A shows the chest roentgenogram of a 3-year-old boy with chronic hypertrophied tonsils and adenoids at the time of presentation with clinical evidence of left-sided and right-sided heart failure. Figure 38–6B shows the improvement following removal of the tonsils and adenoids. The obstruction in this condition has been attributed solely to the size of the tonsils and the adenoids; however, the fact that the obstruction is considerably less during wakefulness than during sleep indicates that oropharyngeal muscle control is also a contributing factor. Indeed, it may be that variations in this control, especially during sleep, rather than simply the size of the tonsils and adenoids, explain why some children have cardiopulmonary difficulty but others with apparently just as much hypertrophy of the tonsils and adenoids do not.

Coordination of the activity of the respiratory muscles (diaphragm and chest wall muscles) and the upper airway muscles is well recognized. Thus flaring of the alae nasi commonly occurs when there is increased chemical drive to breathe. Synchronization of the upper airway muscles, especially of those in the tongue with the other muscles of respiration, is believed to be important in maintaining the patency of the upper airways. When contraction of the upper airway muscles is out of phase, there is collapse of the oropharyngeal air space, and upper airway resistance is greatly increased. Clinical and experimental studies suggest that this process is more likely to occur during sleep. The factors responsible for coordination of all the respiratory muscles are complex and incompletely understood; they are likely to be highly relevant to this and other clinical conditions (Strohl, 1981). Because there is very little one can do at present to facilitate coordination of respiratory muscles, therapy has focused on removing a com-

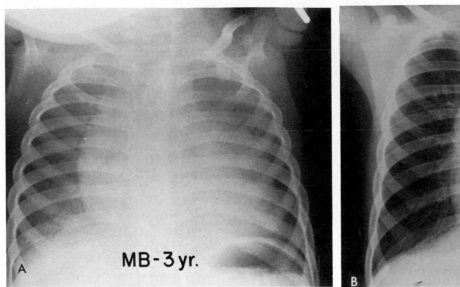
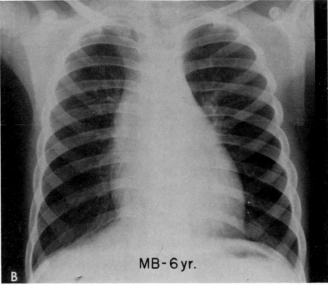

Figure 38–6. Chest roentgenogram before *(A)* and after *(B)* removal of tonsils and adenoids.

pounding problem, namely, hypertrophy of tonsils and adenoids. Failure of upper airway obstruction to disappear following removal of the tonsils and adenoids in some children suggests that oropharyngeal muscle control may be the predominant factor in these patients.

Although there is considerable controversy as to whether conditions with severe inspiratory obstruction, e.g., croup and epiglottitis, do predispose the patient to pulmonary edema, edema may develop only in those in whom there is airway closure so that very negative pressures are transmitted to the interstitium surrounding the fluid-exchanging vessels of the lung.

Sudden marked lowering of the interstitial fluid pressure may be the mechanism responsible for edema in at least nine patients, mostly young adults, who have been reported with the sudden development of pulmonary edema following reexpansion of pneumothorax (Childress et al, 1971; Waqaruddin and Bernstein, 1975). This development has occurred in some after conventional closed underwater drainage but in others after application of very negative pressures by suction. Although the mechanism has not been established, it seems likely that very negative interstitial pressures as the result of the simultaneous occurrence of bronchial occlusion or some factor restraining lung expansion and very negative pleural pressures is the cause (Childress et al, 1971). In most of the reported patients, lung collapse had been present for some time before reexpansion. Whether this factor alone restrains rapid expansion, as, for example, by a decrease in surfactant in the collapsed area, remains unclear.

Experimental studies of reexpansion pulmonary edema in rabbits (Pavlin et al, 1981) provide evidence that increased vascular permeability to protein occurs. Although the mechanism for injury of the vascular membrane is not known, increased stretch or tension of the alveolar septal walls is one likely explanation for the protein and water accumulation during reexpansion of lungs that have been collapsed for several days. Pavlin and co-workers reported that alterations in vascular pressures did not take place, and, interestingly, that once the lung expanded, very negative suction (-100 mm Hg) did not result in pleural pressures lower than -7 to -10 cm H_2O. Studies suggesting that cytotoxic products of O_2 metabolism could play a role in reexpansion pulmonary edema include the demonstration that collapsed lung tissue has decreased mitochondrial superoxide dismutase (SOD) and cytochrome oxidase (Jackson et al, 1988); these changes could enhance O_2 free radical production during the reoxygenation that accompanies reexpansion.

INCREASED VASCULAR PERMEABILITY IN FLUID-EXCHANGING VESSELS

The permeability of a membrane can be increased in at least two ways: the total number of pores may increase or the diameter of the pores may increase. The distinction between pulmonary edema induced by increases in hydrostatic pressure and that induced by increases in permeability, although clinically useful, is sometimes blurred by the observation that as intravascular pressures rise the pores may be stretched, thus altering permeability. It is our impression that relatively large pressures, i.e., pressures in excess of 30 mm Hg, are necessary to produce the stretched-pore phenomenon. It may be, however, that the sensitivity of the methods available to detect small increments in the rate of fluid movement is not sufficient to demonstrate the phenomenon at lower pressures.

A variety of clinical conditions are believed to alter

the permeability of the alveolar capillary membrane, presumably by damage to epithelial or endothelial cells. In addition, there is now increasing evidence that the release of potent chemical mediators may be involved in the genesis of pulmonary edema in these conditions. For example, histamine, prostaglandins, bradykinin, as well as a variety of toxic oxygen radicals, are capable of increasing vascular permeability under some circumstances. These agents may be responsible for pulmonary edema when released by autoimmune mechanisms in hypersensitivity pneumonitis or alveolitis, as well as in Goodpasture syndrome and systemic lupus erythematosus. Whether idiopathic pulmonary hemosiderosis falls into this group remains unknown.

The inhalation of a variety of noxious gases, many of which may be generated during fires, produces denaturation of proteins, cellular damage, and pulmonary edema. These include the oxides of sulfur and nitrogen, hydrocyanic acid, and several aldehydes. The inhalation of herbicides, such as paraquat, has been associated with the development of pulmonary edema, presumably on the basis of a change in permeability. Even before morphologic evidence of alveolar injury is apparent, there is an increase in surface tension, presumably as the result of inactivation or impaired synthesis of pulmonary surfactant (Robertson, 1973).

In victims of fires, the auscultatory evidence of pulmonary edema resulting from inhalation of smoke with damage to the alveolar capillary membrane is always manifest within 24 hours and usually precedes roentgenographic changes (Mellins and Park, 1975). The diffuse haziness on chest roentgenograms that first appears several days following massive burns probably results from the loss of plasma proteins coupled with the administration of large amounts of intravenous fluids, or from other circulatory complications (see Chapter 28).

A variety of circulating toxins, for example, snake venom, produce pulmonary edema by altering the alveolar capillary membrane. Experimental evidence has been presented indicating that gram-negative bacteremia can produce a sustained increase in lung vascular permeability as well as a transient elevation of pulmonary vascular pressures (Brigham et al, 1974). Although the lymphatics have been shown to have the ability to clear large volumes of filtered fluid and protein in this condition, eventually this mechanism can also be overwhelmed. Therefore, fluid therapy should be adjusted to keep vascular pressures low when permeability is increased.

CLINICAL CAUSES OF PULMONARY EDEMA

Although clinical causes of pulmonary edema have been classified as resulting from hemodynamic or permeability alterations, it is appreciated increasingly that in many instances a combination of the two is present. There are a number of clinical conditions in which the mechanisms responsible for pulmonary edema are not clear. In some of these, one suspects that alterations in vascular pressures in conjunction with increases in permeability may be responsible.

Uremia. Uremia may lead to pulmonary edema as the result of overhydration, expansion of the blood volume, and elevation of the pulmonary microvascular pressures, compounded by anemia and reduced colloid osmotic pressures. In addition, vascular permeability may be altered as the result of increased metabolic products of uremia.

Neurogenic Pulmonary Edema. This condition is seen following head trauma, subarachnoid hemorrhage, brain tumors, and meningitis. The mechanism responsible for pulmonary edema following lesions of the brain is not fully understood but appears to result from a combination of hemodynamic and permeability altering factors (Malik, 1985). Neurogenic pulmonary edema may develop acutely over minutes to hours or may be delayed. Following acute head injury or sudden increases in intracerebral pressure, acute sympathetic discharge has been documented (Nathan and Reis, 1975). The discharge has the effect of acutely increasing left ventricular afterload. Cardiac output is maintained in this circumstance at the expense of increased left ventricular, and hence left atrial, filling pressures. This increase in pressure will lead to increased pulmonary microvascular hydrostatic pressure, which in turn will cause fluid to move into the lung interstitium (Theodore and Robin, 1976). Although this analysis favors microvascular hypertension as the primary cause of neurogenic pulmonary edema, studies of sheep in which lymph is collected and its protein content measured suggest that microvascular permeability is also increased (Bowers et al, 1979); high protein content has been noted in humans as well (Carlson et al, 1979). The more delayed forms of neurogenic pulmonary edema are characterized by normal pulmonary wedge and pulmonary arterial pressures and high protein content, suggesting that they result primarily from altered vascular permeability. Thus factors raising pulmonary vascular pressure as well as factors altering vascular permeability are part of the pathogenesis. Ordinarily, neurogenic pulmonary edema may resolve with only supplemental oxygen. If positive ventilatory pressures, especially PEEP, are required, they should be administered cautiously, because they can interfere with cerebral venous return, thus leading to further cerebral edema.

Adult Respiratory Distress Syndrome. A variety of conditions referred to as shock lung or adult respiratory distress syndrome (ARDS) result in edema by mechanisms that are not entirely clear. One can speculate that the release of a variety of vasoactive substances alters pulmonary capillary permeability. Although hypoxia, especially when accompanied by acidosis, is believed to enhance pulmonary edema, one thoughtful review comes to the conclusion that there is no good experimental evidence that hypoxia per se alters pulmonary capillary permeability (Staub, 1974). However, high concentrations of oxygen are known to produce lung damage and edema. Experimental evidence from studies of endotoxemia in animals consisting of an increased lymph to plasma protein ratio and an increase in lymph flow in the absence of an increase of vascular surface has led to the conclusion that there are alterations in alveolar capillary permeability. In spite of 2 decades of research on the pathogenesis of ARDS, the etiology remains poorly understood. However, a number of factors have been considered. Sepsis, whether related to endotoxin or the neutrophil response, is believed to be a major cause of lung injury. Although toxic products released by neutrophils, including toxic oxygen radicals, are believed to play a role, the evidence remains indirect. Several products of arachidonic acid metabolism have also been considered as potential mediators of acute lung injury, including both cyclooxygenase and lipoxygenase pathways. A variety of other factors, including complement, platelets, or clotting factors and kinins, have also been considered, but their precise role remains undefined.

High-Altitude Pulmonary Edema. The pathogenesis of high-altitude edema remains unclear. It affects some highlanders who return home after a brief stay at sea level. It also affects some sea-level dwellers soon after arriving at a high altitude. Fatigue, dyspnea, cough, and sleep disturbances are common and may progress rapidly to severe tachypnea, shock, and death unless rapid descent to a lower altitude or administration of oxygen occurs. Some researchers have assumed that, in addition to a constitutional predisposition of some individuals to pulmonary hypertension with hypoxia (Hultgren et al, 1971), nonuniform increases in precapillary resistance are responsible for the very high pressures seen in at least some pulmonary capillaries (Viswanathan et al, 1969). The absence of a satisfactory animal model has been a handicap to the study of the pathogenesis. Nevertheless, some studies of bronchoalveolar lavage and pulmonary edema fluid have demonstrated a high protein content and an increased percentage of alveolar macrophages (but not neutrophils), suggesting that increased permeability also plays a role in the pathogenesis (Schoene, 1985).

Narcotics. Heroin and other narcotics have also been associated with pulmonary edema. Pulmonary capillary wedge pressure has been elevated in some patients (Paranthaman and Khan, 1976) but has been normal in others. The protein concentration in pulmonary edema fluid from the trachea has been very close to serum levels, suggesting alterations in pulmonary capillary permeability (Katz et al, 1972). Whether hypoxia and acidosis or neurogenic pulmonary edema as the result of cerebral edema plays a role is not known. Clinical and roentgenographic signs of pulmonary edema have occurred following the intravenous administration of paraldehyde (Sinal

and Crowe, 1976); although a direct toxic action on the pulmonary vascular bed has been proposed, the cause remains obscure.

Salicylate-Induced Pulmonary Edema. Pulmonary edema has been seen as a late complication of severe salicylate poisoning. Experimental studies in sheep indicate that salicylate pulmonary edema is due not to increased vascular pressure but rather to increased vascular permeability (Bowers et al, 1977). Insofar as these studies can be applied to the human, the researchers suggest that aspirin can cause pulmonary edema in doses considered therapeutic for some diseases. Although the mechanisms responsible for the altered vascular permeability remain unknown, at least two effects of salicylates could affect vascular integrity: alterations in platelet function and inhibition of prostaglandin synthesis.

Neonatal Respiratory Distress Syndrome. A number of factors contribute to pulmonary edema after preterm birth (Bland, 1987). These include the presence of excess fetal lung liquid at birth; high pulmonary vascular pressures and blood flow, especially if there is a ductus arteriosus; low interstitial pressures, in part the result of high alveolar surface tension; low plasma protein concentration (and hence low plasma osmotic pressure); increased epithelial permeability; lung endothelial injury from inflammation and as a result of therapy; high airway pressures; and high inspired oxygen concentrations. It has also been hypothesized that impaired ion transport by type II lung epithelial cells may also predispose to edema. High airway pressures increase the epithelial protein leak in mechanically ventilated lambs (Jobe et al, 1985) and may also damage the endothelium. In addition to mechanical stress, injury may also result from the release of vasoactive substances and from toxic oxygen radicals. Finally, the immature lung is deficient in elastase and alpha$_1$-antitrypsin inhibitors (Merritt et al, 1983). Thus increased alveolar capillary permeability in the newborn infant may result from excessive levels of proteases released from inflammatory cells, resulting in pulmonary edema. Confirmation of increased pulmonary permeability in hyaline membrane disease has been demonstrated by Jeffries and colleagues (1984), using [99m]technetium DPTA.

In neonatal RDS, pleural pressures can be inferred to be very negative, at least during part of the inspiratory cycle, from the bedside observations of pronounced inspiratory retractions. The lungs, which are stiff, at least in part because of surfactant deficiency, have an increased tendency to collapse. The patient must develop very negative pleural pressures to ventilate these stiff lungs. However, the highly compliant chest wall of the newborn infant may limit the magnitude of negative pressures that can be generated spontaneously. Insofar as negative pleural pressures are generated, interstitial or perimicrovascular pressures will become more negative, enhancing edema. However, in the absence of surfactant, surface forces will become extremely large at low lung volumes. At the alveolar level, there will be a lowering of the interstitial pressure surrounding at least some of the fluid-exchanging vessels. Areas of microatelectasis will be subjected to increased distending pressures from adjacent inflated lung. Because the forces are operating over a smaller area in the collapsed lung, they will be amplified by mechanical interdependence. However, the very negative interstitial pressures generated in the perimicrovascular space will favor edema formation.

There are at least two possible explanations for the development of hyaline membranes in neonatal RDS: (1) if amplified pressures are applied to the surface of units of lung with complete airway closure and if there is diminution or absence of collateral ventilation, as probably occurs in small infants, the absorption of gas will result in sufficiently low alveolar pressures to induce transudation of fluid and hemorrhagic atelectasis (Pang and Mellins, 1975), and (2) release or altered metabolism of vasoactive substances associated with the events of birth may increase vascular permeability. The observation in neonatal RDS of blood pressure instability with hypotension, a hypercoagulable state, defective fibrinolysis, hypoproteinemia, and systemic and pulmonary edema provides indirect evidence that the vasoactive products of uncontrolled protease activity can play an important role in the pathogenesis of RDS, including the abnormal movement of fluid and protein into the lung.

Ongoing inflammation and edema in those infants who do not show normal resolution of hyaline membrane disease but progress to bronchopulmonary dysplasia (BPD) have been attributed to increased numbers of inflammatory cells in the lung, increased and unrestrained protease activity, vasoactive substances, and in all probability, various cytokines (O'Brodovich and Mellins, 1985). Other neonatal conditions in which edema plays a major role include group B-hemolytic streptococcal sepsis and patent ductus arteriosus, especially in the preterm infant.

Overhydration and Obstructive Airways Disease. In the past, it has been customary to advocate increased fluid intake for patients with asthma and bronchiolitis. The rationale that increased fluid intake will loosen secretions and facilitate their expectoration has never been established. The very negative intrathoracic pressures seen in acute asthma would have the effect of increasing the transmural pulmonary artery pressures favoring fluid filtration (Permutt, 1973). We have argued that the very negative intrathoracic pressures, especially in the presence of airway obstruction, would be transmitted to some of the fluid-exchanging vessels and thus would promote pulmonary edema (Stalcup and Mellins, 1977). Although airway inflammation is recognized as an important part of the pathogenesis of asthma, it is not clear to what extent edema of the airways per se plays an appreciable role in the airway obstruction. Nevertheless, we have seen dramatic reversal of CO_2 retention in some patients with asthma and

bronchiolitis following the use of powerful diuretics. Because these diuretics could also change vascular compliance and pressures, the mechanism for the response is not clear. Nevertheless, because these patients had been overhydrated as part of the therapy, we have challenged the generally accepted view that these patients should receive "two times maintenance fluids" and have instead recommended that after deficits have been replaced, only normal maintenance fluids be given.

CLINICAL CONSIDERATIONS

DIAGNOSIS OF PULMONARY EDEMA

In a general way, small increases in lung fluid are too subtle to detect by currently available clinical methods, e.g., auscultation and chest radiology, until the extravascular fluid volume has increased considerably. Nevertheless, in adult humans and dogs, the chest radiograph has been used to diagnose edema when extravascular lung water is increased by 35 per cent. The presence of crackles does not usually occur until edema fluid has moved from the alveoli to the terminal airways and is produced by the sudden opening of peripheral lung units (alveolar ducts or terminal bronchioli).

When the fluid moves up to larger airways, rhonchi and wheezes are to be expected. The contribution of bronchial wall edema and bronchospasm to rhonchi and wheezes is not known.

Under conditions of chronic edema formation, lymphatics and interstitial accumulations of fluid may be visible as Kerley lines (see "Radiographic Findings"). Because pulmonary edema can lead to airway obstruction in children, airway closure is more likely to occur at high lung volumes, producing air trapping. Thus low diaphragms may be a useful sign of interstitial edema, provided there are no other reasons for airway obstruction. Other signs that are useful in following the severity of pulmonary engorgement and edema include the rapidity and shallowness of breathing, the magnitude of inspiratory intercostal retractions, and changes in body weight. Grunting is a common accompaniment of pulmonary edema and represents a useful maneuver to prevent lung collapse (Pang and Mellins, 1975).

Once the magnitude of pulmonary edema is sufficiently severe to lead to persistent airway closure or alveolar flooding, it is very difficult to separate edema, atelectasis, and inflammation on chest roentgenograms.

Although the distinction between cardiogenic or high-pressure edema and permeability or low-pressure edema has been based on the finding of a low pulmonary wedge pressure in the latter, it is now clear that Pmv may be elevated in the presence of a normal left atrial or wedge pressure and that there are limitations to using the wedge pressure to separate hemodynamic or cardiogenic edema from permeability or noncardiogenic edema (Allen et al, 1987).

RADIOGRAPHIC FINDINGS

Although most of the radiographic signs of pulmonary edema are nonspecific, improved radiographic techniques, in conjunction with improved understanding of the pathophysiology of pulmonary edema, have enhanced the usefulness of the chest roentgenogram in the diagnosis of pulmonary edema (Hublitz and Shapiro, 1974; Pistolesi et al, 1985), at least in the adult.

The Kerley A and B lines represent interlobular sheets of abnormally thickened or widened connective tissue that are tangential to the x-ray beam; the A lines are in the depths of the lung near the hilum, and the B lines are at the periphery or surface of the lung (Fig. 38–7). These are more properly referred to as septal lines. Although thickening may occur from a variety of processes, including fibrosis, pigment deposition, and pulmonary hemosiderosis, when they are transient these lines are usually caused by edema. These septal lines of edema are more clearly visible in older children and adults with chronic edema (see Fig. 38–7) than in infants, presumably because they are wider.

Perivascular and peribronchial cuffing are also radiographic signs of interstitial edema fluid. Another radiographic sign of early pulmonary edema is prominent upper lobe vessels, which appear in conjunction with basal interstitial edema. For hydrostatic reasons, perivascular edema is greatest at the bases, and the normal tethering action of the lung is therefore less in this region. With increased resistance to the lower lobe vessels, there is redistribution to the upper lobes. This sign is, of course, of limited value in infants because they are most likely to be in the supine position. The recognition of interstitial pulmonary edema depends on the highest quality radiographic techniques, including short exposure times.

More severe forms of pulmonary edema commonly produce a perihilar haze, presumably because the large perivascular and peribronchial collections of fluid are in this location. A reticular or lattice-like pattern may also be present and is more common at the base in the upright individual.

Although studies in children are limited, a summary of findings that allows separation of cardiogenic or hemodynamic edema, renal or overhydration edema, and injury or ARDS edema has been provided in adults (Pistolesi et al, 1985). Thus there is an inverted base-to-apex redistribution of blood flow in cardiac patients. The progressive recruitment of connective tissue spaces by edema fluid in both cardiac and renal disease gives rise to hilar blurring, peribronchial cuffing, and a hazy pattern of increasing lung density. The lower serum albumin levels in renal patients, and therefore the lower interstitial proteins, produce a more rapid clearance of the

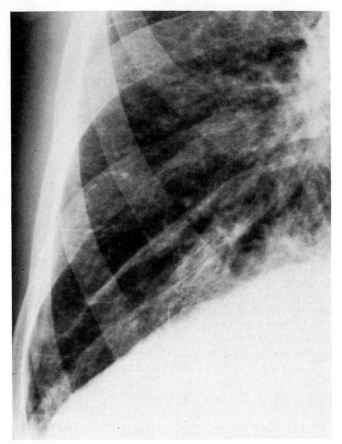

Figure 38–7. Chest roentgenogram of an 18-year-old with congenital mitral stenosis, demonstrating horizontal septal lines of edema (Kerley B lines) at the periphery of the lung.

peripheral fluid, leading to central distribution in renal failure. By contrast in ARDS, protein-rich fluid initially formed in the periphery clears more slowly. Furthermore, the alveolar capillary injury itself predisposes to alveolar flooding. Hence in ARDS there is more likely to be a patchy peripheral distribution of edema and a paucity of such findings as septal lines and peribronchial cuffing.

One major difference between the chest radiograph of the young child as contrasted with the adult during early vascular engorgement and pulmonary edema is the increased lung volume (low diaphragm) in the child. Although we had originally attributed this increased volume to compression of peripheral airways by interstitial edema and vascular engorgement (competition for space), morphometric studies in adult dogs offer little support for this mechanism (Michel et al, 1987). Unfortunately, there are not comparable studies in the very young animal. Other potential mechanisms include transient bronchoconstriction mediated by vagal reflex and increase in airway fluid and formation of bronchial froth (Ishii et al, 1985).

The extent to which thin section computed tomography and magnetic resonance imaging will increase our diagnostic abilities in following patients with pulmonary edema remains to be seen.

Initially, vascular engorgement may lead to an *increase* in the diffusing capacity (DL_{CO}) by increasing the extent to which the lung is perfused and respiratory alkalosis. As interstitial edema collects, there may be an increase in closing volume, a decrease in maximum expiratory flow, an increase in ventilation-perfusion inhomogeneity, and a decrease in arterial P_{O_2}. With alveolar flooding, there is further air trapping, increased vascular resistance (as the result of pressure on alveolar capillaries), decreased lung volumes, decreased lung compliance, decreased DL_{CO}, and progressive hypoxemia (increased right-to-left shunting), rising Pa_{CO_2}, and increased dead-space ventilation.

MEASUREMENT OF LUNG WATER AND PROTEIN

In the experimental animal, weighing the lung before and after drying with correction for blood water remains the most precise way to measure lung water.

The double-indicator dilution technique depends on one tracer that is confined to the vascular space and another tracer that diffuses into the perfused tissue. The difference in the sum of the two time concentration curves has been used to calculate the lung water. Unfortunately, it can only measure that portion of the lung that is perfused and therefore may underestimate the total lung water.

Magnetic resonance imaging and positron-emission tomography are newer techniques being evaluated. They are noninvasive and do not require exposure to ionizing radiation.

When patients with pulmonary edema are intubated, collections of airway fluid may represent a reasonable sample of alveolar fluid. When hemodynamic alterations are primarily responsible for the edema, the ratio of protein in the edema to that in the blood in the adult is <0.6, whereas when lung injury or alterations in permeability are the cause, the ratio is >0.7 (Fein et al, 1979); comparable studies have not been done yet in children.

OTHER TESTS OF LUNG INJURY

Although the measurement of endothelial cell injury has been assessed by the removal and metabolism of a variety of substances, these tests are not sufficiently far along to be very sensitive or specific. Nevertheless, it remains an area of active research in the hope of providing clinically useful early indices of lung injury.

THERAPY

Reversing hypoxemia remains the essential first step. When this cannot be done by simply increasing the O_2 concentration of the inspired mixture, mechanical ventilation may be necessary. Mechanical aid not only reduces the oxygen consumption by reducing the work of breathing but also, when coupled with positive end-expiratory pressure (PEEP), improves oxygenation by preventing collapse of lung units. The positive intrathoracic pressure generated by positive pressures at the mouth may reduce fluid filtration in the lung by impeding venous return and therefore decreasing pulmonary vascular volume and pressure. The experimental evidence reviewed previously suggests that when vascular volume and pressures are maintained, positive-pressure ventilation may actually enhance fluid accumulation in the lung. The improved oxygenation suggests that the fluid must be sequestered in interstitial spaces that do not impair gas exchange.

Reduction of fluid filtration in the lung is the second most important step. Although an increase in colloid osmotic pressure by infusion of colloid would seem to be a logical approach, the concomitant rise in vascular pressure as vascular volume is increased, secondary to the movement of water from the tissues to the vascular compartment, may undermine this effort. Thus lowering vascular pressures by use of diuretics and drugs that reduce vascular resistance or afterload is advantageous.

When pulmonary edema results from heart failure, with elevation of pulmonary microvascular pressures, several therapeutic approaches are helpful. These include (1) measures that improve cardiac contractility and allow the heart to achieve an increased stroke volume at a lower filling pressure, e.g., use of oxygen and digitalis; (2) measures that reduce preload, including the sitting position, rotating tourniquets, and positive-pressure ventilation; (3) measures that reduce both preload and afterload primarily by relieving anxiety, e.g., use of morphine; (4) measures that improve contractility and afterload and also produce bronchodilation, e.g., use of aminophylline; (5) measures that decrease plasma volumes and left atrial pressure and increase plasma colloid osmotic pressures, e.g., administration of diuretics; (6) measures that decrease systemic or pulmonary vascular pressures or both, such as vasodilators; and (7) measures that reduce excessive salt and water intake. These measures are all very helpful in reducing the microvascular pressures in the lung regardless of whether the cause of the edema is hemodynamic or altered vascular permeability. As shown in Figure 38–8, small reductions in microvascular pressures can achieve large reductions in pulmonary edema when increased vascular permeability is the primary cause of the edema.

A variety of cardiovascular drugs have been found to be useful in the treatment of pulmonary edema, especially combinations of drugs that improve cardiac output and drugs that reduce systemic vascular pressures or afterload, thus reducing pressures in the fluid-exchange vessels of the lung. Inotropic agents are very useful in individuals who are hypotensive or

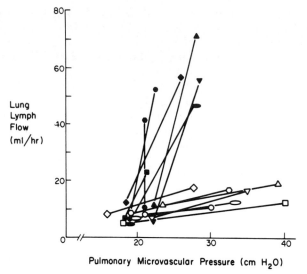

Figure 38–8. Relation of lung lymph flow to pulmonary microvascular pressures during hemodynamic edema *(open symbols)* and during permeability edema produced by infusion of *Pseudomonas (closed symbols)*. For a given reduction in vascular pressures, there is a much greater reduction in lung lymph flow in permeability edema than in hydrostatic edema. (Reproduced with permission from Brigham KL et al: Increased sheep lung vascular permeability caused by Pseudomonas bacteremia. J Clin Invest 54:792, 1974.)

have low cardiac output. By improving cardiac contractility, especially on the left side, they reduce the back pressure into the lung. Of the common cardiovascular drugs now used to treat hemodynamic pulmonary edema, the cardiac glycosides remain the only ones the effect of which is exclusively inotropic. Most of the newer drugs now used to improve cardiac contractility, e.g., dopamine or dobutamine, also have effects on the systemic or pulmonary vasculature (see review by Colucci et al, 1986 for details). When pulmonary edema is primarily the result of myocardial dysfunction, sympathomimetic drugs such as dopamine or dobutamine are especially helpful because of their inotropic action, which results from the stimulation of myocardial beta-adrenergic receptors. When the systemic vascular resistance is also low, e.g., during septic shock, dopamine, the endogenous precursor of norepinephrine, may be especially effective because at least in high doses it increases systemic vascular resistance. However, when systemic vascular resistance is high, for example, during heart failure as a result of cardiomyopathy, the synthetic agent dobutamine may be the drug of choice because it can raise cardiac output without increasing systemic vascular resistance and may, in fact, produce systemic vasodilation.

When pulmonary edema is accompanied by systemic vasoconstriction, nitroprusside is especially useful because it can lower both systemic and pulmonary vascular resistance, thus decreasing afterload and also pulmonary vascular pressures; its potent hypotensive effects, however, require very close cardiovascular monitoring. If the pressure fall is too great, admin-

istration of volume may be required to raise cardiac output. The addition of nitroprusside to dopamine is especially useful because it counteracts the vasoconstrictive effects of dopamine without blocking its powerful inotropic effect. Another group of promising drugs that has both inotropic and vasodilatory effects is the phosphodiesterase inhibitors, e.g., amrinone. These drugs are neither glycosides nor sympathomimetic agents. The drug can be given intravenously or orally and in patients with heart failure can result in marked increases in cardiac output as well as reductions in cardiac filling pressures and systemic vascular resistance (Colucci et al, 1986). Despite its favorable hemodynamic effects, the use of this drug has been limited by a variety of side effects, including dose-dependent but reversible thrombocytopenia. A closely related drug, milrinone, has very similar inotropic and vasodilator effects with apparently fewer side effects. Among the drugs that may be useful on a long-term basis, one could list the angiotensin-converting enzyme inhibitors, e.g., captopril, which lowers systemic vascular resistance.

Except when patients are already hypotensive or volume depleted, diuretics may be very helpful in pulmonary edema. They work by increasing venous capacitance initially, and then by promoting salt and water excretion, thus reducing pressures in the fluid-exchanging vessels of the lung.

When it is possible to anticipate alterations in one or another of the factors responsible for fluid accumulation in the lung, the best overall plan for fluid management would seem to be to replace fluid deficits while correcting acid-base abnormalities and then to administer maintenance needs, carefully calculated to take into consideration decreased or increased losses.

When a decreased plasma colloid osmotic pressure is a complicating factor of pulmonary edema, intravenous administration of albumin may be helpful. However, because albumin will initially promote the absorption of fluid from the entire body, vascular pressures may rise transiently, thus minimizing the gain. For this reason, colloid administration must be done slowly and cautiously, probably in conjunction with the administration of diuretics. It should also be borne in mind that although too large a vascular volume may promote edema formation by elevating vascular hydrostatic pressure, too small a vascular volume may lead to poor perfusion of vital organs. This problem may occur during periods when venous return is impaired by the positive intrathoracic pressures that accompany mechanical ventilation.

In addition to the general therapeutic measures already discussed, treatment of neurogenic pulmonary edema should focus on the reduction in intracranial pressure, when this is possible, and on the pharmacologic reduction in systemic arterial blood pressure.

The treatment of pulmonary edema resulting from altered pulmonary permeability is on less secure ground. Thus some have advocated large doses of corticosteroids and nonsteroid anti-inflammatory drugs in patients with ARDS. When pulmonary edema is a complication of severe shock with disseminated intravascular coagulation, low-molecular-weight dextran and heparin have been used. Whenever increased capillary permeability is responsible for pulmonary edema, the rate and volume of intravenous fluids should be adjusted to keep vascular pressures low. Because there is an increase in vascular permeability to plasma proteins, the potential therapeutic effectiveness of raising intravascular osmotic pressure by administering colloid is markedly reduced. The drug furosemide appears to lower microvascular pressures by two separate mechanisms: (1) it increases venous capacitance, and (2) it lowers vascular volume and hence pressure as a result of diuresis. Thus the initial improvement in oxygenation may occur because of its vasoactive effect before any diuresis occurs. Because toxic oxygen radicals are believed to play a role at least in some cases of lung injury, antioxidants are also being evaluated. Positive or increased end-expiratory pressure may improve arterial oxygenation in permeability-type edema just as it does in hemodynamic edema by reducing intrapulmonary shunt, but this action does not necessarily result in a reduction in edema. Because PEEP may lead to a reduction in cardiac output, barotrauma, and an increase in edema, one suggested approach (Prewitt et al, 1981) is to use the least PEEP that achieves adequate arterial oxygen saturation during ventilation with relatively nontoxic oxygen concentrations. Meanwhile, adequate cardiac output can be maintained without raising the vascular pressures in the fluid-exchanging vessels of the lung by using vasoactive agents like nitroprusside that lower afterload.

A recurrent theme throughout this chapter has been the potential role of vasoactive substances in the genesis or clearance of pulmonary edema by altering vascular pressures and permeability as well as active ion transport across the alveolar capillary membrane. Although the information about them is still very limited, we have chosen to emphasize their importance because we believe that a more fundamental understanding of their role in the genesis of pulmonary edema is likely to lead to more specific forms of therapy.

REFERENCES

Allen SJ, Drake RE, Williams JP et al: Recent advances in pulmonary edema. Crit Care Med 15:963, 1987.
Baker JW, Yerger S, and Segar WE: Elevated plasma antidiuretic hormone levels in status asthmaticus. Mayo Clin Proc 51:31, 1976.
Bhattacharya J and Staub NC: Interstitial fluid pressure gradient measured by micropuncture in the excised dog lung. J Appl Physiol 56:271, 1984.
Bland JW, Edwards FK, and Brinsfield W: Pulmonary hypertension and congestive heart failure with chronic upper airway obstruction. Am J Cardiol 23:830, 1969.
Bland RD: Lung fluid balance before and after birth. In Johnston BM and Gluckman PD (eds): Respiratory Control and Lung Development in the Fetus and Newborn (Reproductive and Perinatal Medicine Ser No 3). Ithaca, NY, Perinatology Press, 1986.
Bland RD: Pathogenesis of pulmonary edema after birth. Adv Pediatr 34:175, 1987.
Bowers RE, Brigham KL, and Owen PJ: Salicylate pulmonary edema: the mechanism in sheep and review of the clinical literature. Am Rev Respir Dis 115:261, 1977.
Bowers RE, McKeen CE, Park BE, and Brigham KL: Increased pulmonary vascular permeability follows intracranial hypertension in sheep. Am Rev Respir Dis 119:637, 1979.
Boxer RA, Hayes CJ, Hordof AJ, and Mellins RB: Agenesis of the left lung and total pulmonary venous connection: hemodynamic studies before and after complete surgical correction. Chest 74:106, 1978.
Boyd RDH, Hill JR, Humphreys RW et al: Permeability of lung capillary to macromolecules in fetal and newborn lambs and sheep. J Physiol (Lond) 201:567, 1969.
Brace RA: Progress toward resolving the controversy of positive vs. negative interstitial fluid pressure. Circ Res 49:281, 1981.
Brigham KL: Lung edema due to increased vascular permeability. In Staub NC (ed): Lung Water and Solute Exchange. (Lung Biology in Health and Disease Ser, vol 7.) New York, Marcel Dekker, Inc, 1978.
Brigham KL, Sundell H, Harris TR et al: Lung water and vascular permeability in sheep. Newborns compared with adults. Circ Res 42:851, 1978.
Brigham KL, Woolverton WC, Blake LH, and Staub N: Increased sheep lung vascular permeability caused by Pseudomonas bacteremia. J Clin Invest 54:792, 1974.
Carlson RW, Schaeffer RC Jr, Michaels SG et al: Pulmonary edema following intracranial hemorrhage. Chest 75:731, 1979.
Cayler GG, Johnson EE, Lewis BE et al: Heart failure due to enlarged tonsils and adenoids. Am J Dis Child 118:708, 1969.
Childress ME, Moy G, and Mottram M: Unilateral pulmonary edema resulting from treatment of spontaneous pneumothorax. Am Rev Respir Dis 104:119, 1971.
Colucci WS, Wright RF, and Braunwald E: New positive inotropic agents in the treatment of congestive heart failure. N Engl J Med 314:290, 349, 1986.
Drake RE and Laine GA: Pulmonary microvascular permeability to fluid and macromolecules. J Appl Physiol 64:487, 1988.
Drake RE, Giesler M, Laine GA et al: Effect of outflow pressure on lung lymph flow in unanesthetized sheep. J Appl Physiol 58:70, 1985.
Fein A, Grossman RE, Jones JG et al: The value of edema fluid protein measurement in patients with pulmonary edema. Am J Med 67:32, 1979.
Fishman AP: Pulmonary edema. The water-exchanging function of the lung. Circulation 46:390, 1972.
Goodale RL, Goetzman B, and Visscher MB: Hypoxia and iodoacetic acid and alveolocapillary barrier permeability to albumin. Am J Physiol 219:1226, 1970.
Gropper MA, Bhattacharya J, and Staub NC: Filtration profile in isolated zone 1 and zone 3 dog lungs at constant high alveolar pressure. J Appl Physiol 65:343, 1988.
Guyton AC, Taylor AE, and Granger HJ: Circulatory Physiology II: Dynamics and Control of the Body Fluids. Philadelphia, WB Saunders Co, 1975.
Guyton AC, Taylor AE, Drake RE, and Parker JC: Dynamics of subatmospheric pressure in the pulmonary interstitial fluid. In Lung Liquids, Ciba Symposium 38. New York, American Elsevier Publishing Co, 1976.
Hansen TN, Hazinski TA, and Bland RD: Effects of asphyxia on lung fluid balance in baby lambs. J Clin Invest 74:370, 1984.
Hauge A, Gunnar B, and Waaler BA: Interrelations between pulmonary liquid volumes and lung compliance. J Appl Physiol 38:608, 1975.
Henson PM, Larsen GL, and Henson JE et al: Resolution of pulmonary inflammation. Fed Proc 43:2799, 1984.
Hordof AJ, Mellins RB, Gersony WM, and Steeg CN: Reversibility of chronic obstructive lung disease in infants following repair of ventricular septal defects. J Pediatr 90:187, 1977.
Hublitz UF and Shapiro JH: The radiology of pulmonary edema. CRC Crit Rev Clin Radiol Nucl Med 5:389, 1974.

Hultgren HN, Grover RF, and Hartley LH: Abnormal circulatory response to high altitude in subjects with a history of high-altitude pulmonary edema. Circulation 44:759, 1971.

Iliff L: Extra-alveolar vessels and edema development in excised dog lungs. Circ Res 28:524, 1971.

Ishii M, Matsumoto N, and Fuyuki T: Effects of hemodynamics edema formation on peripheral vs. central airway dynamics. J Appl Physiol 59:1578, 1985.

Jackson RM, Brannen AL, Vaal CF, and Fulmer JD: Superoxide dismutase and cytochrome oxidase in collapsed lungs: possible role in reexpansion edema. J Appl Physiol 65:235, 1988.

Jeffries AL, Coates G, and O'Brodovich HM: Pulmonary epithelial permeability in hyaline membrane disease. N Engl J Med 311:1075, 1984.

Jobe A, Jacobs H, Ikegami M et al: Lung protein leaks in ventilated lambs: effect of gestational age. J Appl Physiol 58:1246, 1985.

Katz S, Aberman A, Frand UI et al: Heroin pulmonary edema. Am Rev Respir Dis 106:472, 1972.

La Force FM, Mullane JF, Boehme RF et al: The effect of pulmonary edema on antibacterial defenses of the lung. J Lab Clin Med 82:634, 1973.

Laine GA, Allen SJ, and Katz J et al: Effect of systemic venous pressure elevation on lymph flow and lung edema. J Appl Physiol 61:1634, 1986.

Levin DL, Muster AJ, Pachman LM et al: Cor pulmonale secondary to upper airway obstruction. Chest 68:166, 1975.

Levine OR and Mellins RB: Liquid balance in the lung and pulmonary edema. In Scarpelli E and Auld PA (ed): Pulmonary Physiology of the Fetus, Newborn and Child. Philadelphia, Lea & Febiger, 1975.

Levine OR, Mellins RB, and Fishman AP: Quantitative assessment of pulmonary edema. Circ Res 27:414, 1965.

Levine OR, Mellins RB, Senior RM, and Fishman AP: The application of Starling's law of capillary exchange to the lungs. J Clin Invest 46:934, 1967.

Levine OR, Rodriguez-Martinez F, and Mellins RB: Fluid filtration in the lung of the intact puppy. J Appl Physiol 34:683, 1973.

Luke MJ, Mehrizi A, Folger GM Jr, and Rowe RD: Chronic nasopharyngeal obstruction as a cause of cardiomegaly, cor pulmonale and pulmonary edema. Pediatrics 37:762, 1966.

Macklem PT: Influence of left atrial pressure on lung mechanics. Paper presented at the International Congress on Cardiac Lung. Sponsored by European Society of Cardiology and European Society for Clinical Respiratory Physiology. Florence, December 1976.

Macklem PT and Murphy B: The forces applied to the lung in health and disease. Am J Med 57:371, 1974.

Malik AB: Mechanisms of neurogenic pulmonary edema. Circ Res 57:1, 1985.

Marciniak DL, Dobbins DC, Maciejko JJ et al: Antagonism of histamine edema formation by catecholamines. Am J Physiol 234:H180, 1978.

Matthay M: Pathophysiology of pulmonary edema. Clin Chest Med 6:301, 1985.

Mead J, Takishima T, and Leith D: Stress distribution in lungs: a model of pulmonary elasticity. J Appl Physiol 28:596, 1970.

Mellins R and Park S: Respiratory complications of smoke inhalation in victims of fires. J Pediatr 87:1, 1975.

Mellins RB, Levine OR, and Fishman AP: Effect of systemic and pulmonary venous hypertension on pleural and pericardial fluid accumulation. J Appl Physiol 29:564, 1970.

Mellins RB, Levine OR, Skalak R, and Fishman AP: Interstitial pressure of the lung. Circ Res 24:197, 1969.

Merritt TA, Cochrane CG, Holcomb K: Elastase and a_1-proteinase inhibitor activity in tracheal aspirates during respiratory distress syndrome. J Clin Invest 72:656, 1983.

Michel RP, Zocchi L, Rossi A et al: Does interstitial lung edema compress airways and arteries? A morphometric study. J Appl Physiol 62:108, 1987.

Mor J, Ben Galim E, and Abrahamov A: Inappropriate antidiuretic hormone secretion in an infant with severe pneumonia. Am J Dis Child 129:133, 1975.

Nathan MA and Reis DJ: Fulminating arterial hypertension with pulmonary edema from release of adrenomedullary catecholamines after lesions of the anterior hypothalamus in the rat. Circ Res 37:226, 1975.

Newth CJL, Levison H, and Bryan AC: The respiratory status of children with croup. J Pediatr 81:1068, 1972.

O'Brodovich HM and Mellins RB: State of the art bronchopulmonary dysplasia: unresolved neonatal acute lung injury. Am Rev Respir Dis 132:694, 1985.

Pang LM and Mellins RB: Neonatal cardiorespiratory physiology. Anesthesiology 43:171, 1975.

Paranthaman S and Khan F: Acute cardiomyopathy with recurrent pulmonary edema and hypotension following heroin overdosage. Chest 69:117, 1976.

Pavlin J, Nessly ML, and Cheney FW: Increased pulmonary vascular permeability as a cause of re-expansion edema in rabbits. Am Rev Respir Dis 124:422, 1981.

Perl W, Chowdhury P, and Chinard FP: Reflection coefficients of dog lung endothelium to small hydrophilic solutes. Am J Physiol 228:797, 1975.

Permutt S: Physiologic changes in the acute asthmatic attack. In Austen KF and Lichtenstein LM (eds): Asthma: Physiology, Immunopharmacology and Treatment. New York, Academic Press, 1973.

Pietra GG, Szidon JP, Leventhal MM, and Fishman AP: Histamine and interstitial pulmonary edema in the dog. Circ Res 29:323, 1971.

Pistolesi M, Miniati M, Milne ENC et al: The chest roentgenogram and pulmonary edema. Clin Chest Med 6:315, 1985.

Prewitt RM, McCarthy J, and Wood LDH: Treatment of acute low pressure pulmonary edema in dogs. J Clin Invest 67:409, 1981.

Raj JU: Alveolar liquid pressure measured by micropuncture in isolated lungs of mature and immature fetal rabbits. J Clin Invest 79:1579, 1987.

Reifenrath R: The significance of alveolar geometry and surface tension in the respiratory mechanics of the lung. Resp Physiol 24:115, 1975.

Robertson B: Paraquat poisoning as an experimental model of the idiopathic respiratory distress syndrome. Bull Physiopathol Respir (Nancy) 9:1433, 1973.

Robin ED, Cross CE, and Zelis R: Pulmonary edema. N Engl J Med 288:239, 1973.

Schoene RB: Pulmonary edema at high altitude. Clin Chest Med 6:491, 1985.

Sinal SH and Crowe JE: Cyanosis, cough and hypotension following intravenous administration of paraldehyde. Pediatrics 57:158, 1976.

Smith-Ericksen N and Bo G: Airway closure and fluid filtration in the lung. Br J Anaesth 51:475, 1979.

Snapper JR: Lung mechanics in pulmonary edema. Clin Chest Med 6:393, 1985.

Stalcup SA and Mellins RB: Mechanical forces producing pulmonary edema in acute asthma. N Engl J Med 297:592, 1977.

Staub NC: Pulmonary edema. Physiol Rev 54:678, 1974.

Staub NC and Taylor AE: Edema. New York, Raven Press, 1984.

Strohl KP: Upper airway muscles of respiration. Am Rev Respir Dis 124:211, 1981.

Taylor AE: Capillary fluid filtration. Starling forces and lymph flow. Circ Res 49:557, 1981.

Taylor PM, Boonyaprakob U, Waterman V et al: Clearance of plasma proteins from pulmonary vascular beds of adult dogs and pups. Am J Physiol 213:441, 1967.

Theodore J and Robin ED: Speculations on neurogenic pulmonary edema (NPE). Am Rev Respir Dis 113:405, 1976.

Van der Zee H, Malik AB, Lee BC, and Hakim TS: Lung fluid and protein exchange during intracranial hypertension and role of sympathetic mechanisms. J Appl Physiol 48:273, 1980.

Viswanathan R, Jain SK, and Subramanian S: Pulmonary edema of high altitude. III. Pathogenesis. Am Rev Respir Dis 100:342, 1969.

Waqaruddin M and Bernstein A: Re-expansion pulmonary oedema. Thorax 30:54, 1975.

Weiner-Kronish JP, Matthay MA, Cullen PW et al: Relationship of pleural effusions to pulmonary hemodynamics in patients with congestive heart failure. Am Rev Respir Dis 132:1253, 1985.

A. AVITAL, M.D., and
V. CHERNICK, M.D.

39

EMPHYSEMA AND ALPHA₁-ANTITRYPSIN DEFICIENCY

The antiprotease capacity of human serum was first recognized in 1897 (Camus and Gley, 1897). A few years later the proteolytic activity of inflammatory exudates was described (Opie, 1905) and allocated to blood leukocytes. It was suggested even at that time that human serum has a protective activity against enzymatic damage. This protective inhibitory activity was later ascribed to the a_1-globulin peak in serum (Jacobsson, 1955). Laurel and Eriksson (1963) noted that in three out of five adult patients, severe alpha₁-antitrypsin deficiency was associated with chronic obstructive pulmonary disease. The familial nature of this deficiency was described 2 years later in a report of the onset of the pulmonary symptoms in the third or fourth decade (Eriksson, 1965). The first report of the deficiency in association with emphysema in a child was in 1971 (Talamo et al, 1971). Severe alpha₁-antitrypsin deficiency has also been described in infants with onset of liver disease in the early months of life that progresses to cirrhosis (Sharp et al, 1969). Some children have been described with a combination of cirrhosis and chronic obstructive lung disease (Glasgow et al, 1973; Kaiser et al, 1975).

Alpha₁-antitrypsin is now known to inhibit a number of other proteolytic enzymes with serine at their active sites and is therefore also known as alpha₁-protease inhibitor (A_1Pi) or SERPINS (serine protease inhibitors). The name *alpha₁-antitrypsin* (A_1AT) has been maintained for historical reasons and because of its common usage in the literature.

BIOLOGIC ASPECTS

Alpha₁-antitrypsin is the major a_1-globulin in human serum and is a glycoprotein with a molecular weight of 52,000 daltons. It is composed of a single 394 amino acid polypeptide chain with three carbohydrate side chains (including galactose, mannose, N-acetylglucosamine, fucose, and sialic acid) amounting to about 12 per cent of the total molecular weight (Carrell et al, 1982) (Fig. 39–1). It is a globular molecule with important salt bridges between amino acids 290–342 and 264–387. A number of variants,

caused primarily by single amino acid substitutions, have been identified. These variants (more than 35) are classified according to the Pi (protease inhibitor) system, which is based on differences in charge and electrophoretic mobility of the molecule. Letters early in the alphabet indicate rapid movement toward the anode, and letters near the end of the alphabet indicate slower mobility. When an appropriate letter has been used, a number or name (of a city) is added.

The most common form of alpha₁-antitrypsin has been assigned the letter "M" (intermediate mobility) and consists of at least four common subtypes (Table 39–1). Other important variants are "S" and "Z," in which a substitution of glutamine for valine occurs at position 264 (Owen and Carrell, 1976) and lysine for glutamine at position 342 (Yoshida et al, 1976), respectively (see Fig. 39–1). A_1AT is synthesized in the liver and to a minor extent in mononuclear phagocytes and is secreted into the serum, in which its half-life is 4 to 6 days. One direct proof of the origin of A_1AT is the observation that after liver transplantation in deficient patients, A_1AT levels returned to normal and had the Pi M phenotype of the donor (Sharp, 1971). The normal concentration in serum is 150 to 350 mg/dL (30 to 70 mM/L). About 40 per cent of the protein is found in plasma, and most of the remaining 60 per cent is in the extravascular compartment. It appears in pulmonary alveolar macrophages; on the surface of polymorphonuclear leukocytes; along human airways; in platelets, granules, and megakaryocytes; and in many bodily fluids, including nasal secretion, saliva, tears, colostrum, lymph, perilymph, cerebrospinal fluid, amniotic fluid, synovial fluid, semen, and cervical mucus. The transport of A_1AT across the placenta appears to be minimal. The concentration in newborn serum is approximately 70 per cent of normal adult mean values, and the Pi type of the cord serum is that of the fetus rather than the mother (Talamo, 1975). A_1AT is an acute phase reactant, and its concentration may double or triple as a result of various nonspecific inflammatory processes; pregnancy; neoplasia; smoking; stress of surgery; and administration of estrogens, steroids, or typhoid vaccine. This increase probably reflects an increase in synthesis rather than a decrease in excretion (Resendes, 1987).

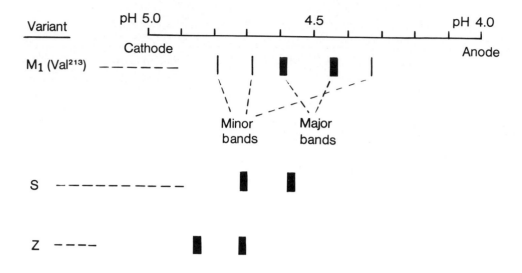

Figure 39–1. Schematic structure of the most common $M_1(Val^{213})$ normal variant of alpha₁-antitrypsin, showing the amino acid substitution of the S and Z variants.

In deficiency states, patients show a smaller rise in serum concentration with stress.

A_1AT is the major protease inhibitor in human plasma, with 95 per cent of the total trypsin inhibitory capacity (Catz and Cox, 1979). The enzymes inhibited by A_1AT include all the serine-containing proteases, such as polymorphonuclear leukocyte elastase, collagenase, macrophage cathepsin, plasmin tissue kallikrein, thrombin, factor IX, pancreatic elastase, renin, chymotrypsin, and trypsin. A_1AT has been called the "suicide" protein because once it forms a complex with the protease, it is cleared by the reticuloendothelial system and excreted by the liver through catabolism. The inhibitory site for neutrophil elastase is centered at residue 358, and the reaction with the protease is essentially irreversible. The Z protein has a shorter life span, but its decreased release from liver cells accounts for the low plasma level in Pi Z individuals. Removal of sialic acid from the M protein resulted in an extremely rapid removal of A_1AT from the circulation (Jeppsson et al, 1978).

GENETICS

Laurell and Eriksson (1963) found that the sister of one of the three original patients with A_1AT deficiency and widespread pulmonary lesions also had the same lung lesion and suggested that the defect may be inherited. A year later Eriksson (1964) published family studies and reinforced the theory of autosomal recessive inheritance. Subsequent studies showed that A_1AT variants are inherited as codominant alleles with the haplotype from both parents being equally expressed, determining both the serum concentration of the protein and its electrophoretic mobility (Fagerhol and Laurell, 1967; Fagerhol and Gedde-Dahl, 1969; Fagerhol and Cox, 1981).

The A_1AT gene is composed of seven exons and six introns located over 12 kb of DNA segments (q 31 to 32.3) on chromosome 14 (Schroeder et al, 1985). All the structural information for the A_1AT protein is coded for by the last four exons. The normal gene codes for a 418 amino acid precursor protein; a terminal 24 amino acid peptide is cleaved before the secretion of the mature 394 amino acid protein. The A_1AT gene is expressed in two major sites: the hepatocyte and the mononuclear phagocyte. The hepatocyte is the main manufacturer of A_1AT and contains approximately two-hundredfold more A_1AT mRNA transcripts per cell than the mononu-

Table 39–1. A_1AT COMMON VARIANTS, SERUM LEVELS, AND RISK FOR ORGAN INVOLVEMENT

Name	Variant Change AA	Site	Serum Level (mg/dL)	Allelic Frequency	Risk for Involvement in Lung	Liver
NORMAL LEVELS						
M_1 (Val²¹³)			150–350	0.44–0.49	—	—
M_1 (Ala²¹³)	Ala	213	150–350	0.20–0.23	—	—
M_2	His	101	150–350	0.14–0.19	—	—
M_3	Asp	376	150–350	0.10–0.11	—	—
DEFICIENT						
S	Val	264	100–200	0.02–0.04	—	—
Z	Lys	342	15–50	0.01–0.02	yes	yes
NULL						
Pi(-)			0	rare	yes	—
DYSFUNCTIONAL						
pittsburgh	Arg	358	normal	rare	—	—
					(bleeding diathesis)	

clear phagocyte. The hepatocyte mRNA is shorter (1.4 kb) than the two forms found in monocytes (1.6 and 1.9 kb) (Perlino et al, 1987).

The mRNA is translated on ribosomes bound to the rough endoplasmic reticulum. The A_1AT polypeptide proceeds through the membrane of the endoplasmic reticulum to the Golgi apparatus, where the carbohydrate side chains are added and the protein starts folding into its three-dimensional globular configuration. The carbohydrate side chains are attached to amino acids 46, 83, and 247 (see Fig. 39–1), and those chains can be biantennary (with two "antennae" of N-acetylglucosamine-galactose-sialic acid coming off the terminal mannose) or triantennary. In general, at positions 46 and 247 the side chains are biantennary, whereas at position 83, 65 per cent are biantennary and 35 per cent are triantennary (Mega et al, 1980). These different side chains and the length of the polypeptide chain are the causes of the two major and the three minor bands of A_1AT that appear on polyacrylamide isoelectric focusing (Fig. 39–2).

Alpha₁-antitrypsin has a globular structure 6.7 nm by 3.2 nm, with the three carbohydrates on the external surface of the molecule. The internal structure has 30 per cent alpha helixes and 40 per cent beta-pleated sheets. There are two main salt bridges within the molecule, between Lys^{290}-Glu^{342} and Glu^{264}-Lys^{387}, bridges that play a role in the pathogenesis of some deficiency states.

The active site of A_1AT against the proteases is centered at residues Met^{358}-Ser^{359} as an external loop protruding from the molecule (Loebermann et al, 1984). This site is highly attractive to the active site (pocket) of neutrophil elastase, neutralizing it tightly in a suicide interaction with a very low dissociation rate.

Approximately 34 mg of A_1AT is produced per day per kg body weight. During inflammatory states or treatment with anabolic steroid, the A_1AT gene is up-regulated, resulting in increased production. No stimuli are known to repress the gene. The two parental A_1AT genes are co-dominantly expressed, and each A_1AT molecule from each parent functions autonomously (Fagerhol, 1969). The A_1AT variants can be classified according to serum level and function state into four groups.

Normal. A_1AT level is within normal range (150 to 350 μg/dL), and its function is normal. Most of these variants migrate to the M region on standard electric focusing gels, are centered at approximately pH 4.5, and are called *common normal M family variants* (see Table 39–1) (Frants and Eriksson, 1976). They include M (Val²¹³), which is the most common allele in the white population in the United States; M_1 (Ala²¹³) with just a change in amino acid, which can be recognized only by restriction fragment length polymorphism analysis; and M_2 and M_3, which are less frequent and have a single base change. All M types, whether inherited in a homozygous or heterozygous form with each other, give normal serum levels and antielastase activity. There are at least 47 other rare normal varieties, most of which have been discussed in single case reports (Brantly et al, 1988).

Deficient Variants. In this group, the serum levels of A_1AT are lower than normal, and the main types are S and Z variants. The S type is more common than the Z type; its allelic frequency in the United States is 0.02 to 0.03 and even higher (0.13) in Spain and Portugal (Goedde et al, 1973; Martin et al, 1976). From the clinical point of view, this variant is not important, because even the homogenous form secretes 40 to 60 per cent of normal A_1AT levels (100 to 200 mg/dL), the S protein has normal antielastase activity, and the lung is generally not involved. Heterozygous MS subjects have 80 per cent of normal A_1AT blood levels. The sequence of the exons in the gene for the S variant is identical to that of the normal M_1 (val²¹³) variant except for a change in exon III (GAA becomes GTA), which causes a substitution of valine for glutamine at position 264 of the A_1AT molecule.

The Z variant was described originally by Laurell and Eriksson (1963) and is associated with both lung and liver involvement. The sequence of the exons in the Z gene is identical to that of the M_1 (ala²¹³) gene except for a change in DNA from GAG to AAG, which causes a change from glutamine to lysine at position 342 (Nukiwa et al, 1986). This change in DNA causes a change in migration of the Z variant toward the cathode on isoelectric focusing (see Fig. 39–2).

The allelic frequency of the Z variant is 0.01 to 0.02 among white persons in the United States (Dykes et al, 1984), higher (0.026) in Scandinavia (Sveger, 1976), and very rare among blacks and in Asian populations (Fagerhol and Tenfjord, 1968). In homozygous variants, the serum levels are 10 to 15 per

Figure 39–2. Polyacrylamide gel electrophoresis of serum, showing the major and minor bands of the common normal variant M_1(Val²¹³) and the major bands of the pathologic S and Z types.

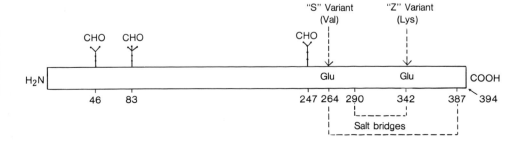

cent (15 to 50 mg/dL) of normal A_1AT levels (Fagerhol and Laurell, 1970). Heterozygous MZ subjects have approximately 55 per cent of normal serum levels, whereas the levels for heterozygous SZ subjects are approximately 37 per cent of normal. A functional impairment in the A_1AT Z molecule prevents it from irreversibly inhibiting neutrophil elastase. The change in amino acids at position 342 blocks the formation of the internal salt bridge from position 290 to 342 (Loebermann et al, 1984), and the folding of the protein in the rough endoplasmic reticulum is slower than normal, causing aggregation of adjacent Z molecules. These aggregated A_1AT molecules form globules easily seen in hepatocytes of homozygous patients (Sharp et al, 1969) and result in the lowered secretion of A_1AT into the serum.

There are at least nine other rare deficiency variants (Brantly et al, 1988), such as M malton (Cox, 1976), with plasma levels similar to homozygous Pi ZZ. This variant tends to predispose a person to emphysema. The heterozygous type M malton Z has also been described with emphysema (Allen et al, 1986).

Null Variants. This rare group has no measurable A_1AT in serum and is always associated with emphysema before the age of 30. Patients who have these variants rarely live to age 40 (Talamo et al, 1973; Bernheim et al, 1976; Bamforth and Kalsheker, 1988). The genetic explanation for the null variant is different for each type. For example, in Null (bellingham) a change in one base (*AAG*) on exon II forms a stop codon (*TAG*), explaining the absence of A_1AT mRNA (Satoh et al, 1988). In Null (granite falls), a deletion in a single base on exon II (TAC) causes the G base from the next codon to form the sequence TAG, and again no A_1AT can be produced.

Dysfunctional Variants. One variant with dysfunctional A_1AT has been described (pittsburgh) with normal blood level of A_1AT, reduced antielastase capacity, and bleeding diathesis. This A_1AT molecule has a mutation at position 358 (active site) with Arg^{358} instead of Met^{358}. This variation causes a migration closer to the cathode than the normal M variant on isoelectric focusing gel and a functional impairment with a reduced inhibition of neutrophil elastase but a very potent antithrombin activity even in the heterozygous form.

LABORATORY DIAGNOSIS

Diagnostic procedures in the laboratory include functional tests, serum electrophoresis, and gene identification. Most hospital laboratories can perform functional tests of A_1AT and simple electrophoresis. For more complex electrophoresis procedures and precise gene identification serum, samples may have to be sent to highly specialized laboratories. These tests can be described in more detail.

Functional Tests. Functional spectrophotometric assays based on the ability of serum to inhibit trypsin activity on synthetic substrates were the first to be developed. Another technique is radioimmunodiffusion, in which a serum sample is placed in the central well of an agar gel plate containing A_1AT antibody. The diameter of precipitation is a function of the concentration of the antigen.

Electrophoresis of A_1AT. The initial diagnostic test, which is also the simplest, is a serum paper or gel protein electrophoresis that shows the presence or absence of the α_1-globulin peak (Fig. 39–3). Because A_1AT is the major α_1-globulin in human serum, the absence of a peak in the α_1 region is suggestive of the deficiency. Before 1976, the A_1AT deficiency variants were identified primarily by acid starch gel electrophoresis, with a migration at pH 5 of A_1AT more toward the anode than the other serum proteins. The deficient type Z variant migrated more slowly than normal, and the variants were first named according to their relative mobility (F = fast, M = medium, S = slow, Z = most cathodal). Subsequently, variants were named alphabetically according to their mobility in starch.

Thin layer polyacrylamide gel isoelectric focusing of serum at pH 4.5 (see Fig. 39–2) is efficient and sensitive enough to detect the subtypes of the alleles. Typically the normal M_1 (val^{213}) variant will show two major bands (both 394 amino acids but one with three biantennary carbohydrate side chains, the other with two biantennary and one triantennary side chains) and three minor bands, two of the minor bands with deleted 5 N terminal amino acids and one with a different carbohydrate side chain.

Crossed immunoelectrophoresis is a two-stage process. First, acid starch gel electrophoresis and banding separation of A_1AT are done. The bands are then transferred to an agarose gel containing its corresponding antibody, and a second electrophoresis at right angles is performed that produces precipitation peaks according to the A_1AT variants.

A_1AT Gene Analysis. Sequencing of the exons of the A_1AT gene gives a direct and definitive approach for the identification of A_1AT variants. The A_1AT gene is cloned, split into pieces, and sequenced (Nukiwa et al, 1986).

Restriction fragment-length polymorphism uses restriction endonuclear DNA-cutting enzymes at specific sequences, separating the resulting fragments by size and identifying them using a labeled A_1AT gene probe.

Oligonucleotide hybridization analysis, using short labeled sequences of DNA complementary to a specific region of exon of the A_1AT gene, allows the identification of single base difference in mutations within the A_1AT gene, for example, the Z mutation in exon V coding for residue 342 (Kidd et al, 1983). The problem is that it can identify only limited segments of DNA. This method can be used to detect homozygous as well as heterozygous A_1AT deficiency prenatally and postnatally.

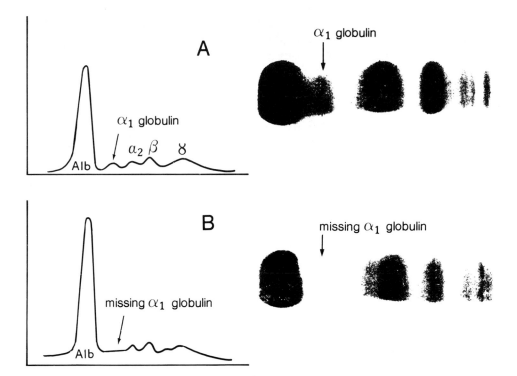

Figure 39–3. Agarose serum protein electrophoresis of human serum. Note that the serum from the normal subject *(A)* shows an a_1-globulin peak that is notably absent in the serum from the patient suffering from alpha₁-antitrypsin deficiency *(B)*. *Alb,* albumin.

PATHOGENESIS

Several lines of evidence support the neutrophil elastase inhibitor imbalance theory as the cause of lung destruction that characterizes the emphysema of A_1AT deficiency. Epidemiologic studies associate decreased serum levels of A_1AT (less than 80 mg/dL) with increased risk for development of emphysema (Gadek and Crystal, 1983a). Emphysema will develop in all patients with the null-type variant (with no detectable serum A_1AT) and in 85 per cent of the patients with homozygous type Z (15 to 50 mg/dL), who not only have low levels of A_1AT but also are disadvantaged by the fact that the Z protein is a less potent inhibitor of neutrophil elastase (Larsson, 1978). Heterozygous SZ, MZ, and MS subjects (with 37, 57, and 80 per cent of normal serum levels, respectively) and homozygous SS subjects (60 per cent of normal serum levels) (Laurell and Jeppsson, 1975) may develop emphysema, but they are probably not at a much higher risk than the general population (Gadek, Fells, Zimmerman et al, 1981).

A_1AT levels on the epithelial surface of the respiratory tract are approximately 10 per cent of the serum levels and are therefore very low in A_1AT-deficient patients (Wewers, Casolaro, Sellers et al, 1987; Wewers, Casolaro, and Crystal, 1987). The antineutrophil elastase capacity of the lower respiratory tract fluid is also markedly depressed in such patients.

Emphysema has been induced in rats a few hours after intratracheal injections of papain, an enzyme with elastolytic properties (Gross et al, 1964). Emphysema has also been induced in hamsters after inhalation of papain; the induction of emphysema could be prevented by intratracheal injection of human A_1AT but not by increasing serum trypsin inhibitory capacity (Martorana and Share, 1976).

The lower respiratory tract is continuously exposed to aging granulocytes that die and release their enzymatic content, including elastase and collagenase, into pulmonary tissue. The elastase degrades elastin in alveolar septa; in fact, purified granulocyte elastase has been shown to localize in alveolar septa after tracheal installation. Thus it seems logical to conclude that lung destruction depends on the equilibrium between sufficient amounts of functional A_1AT and the amount of elastase along the alveolar lining. Any infection or toxic injury to the lung that might increase the number of granulocytes or alveolar macrophages could enhance the release of elastase and hasten the progression of elastin destruction in deficient individuals.

Smoking is another high-risk factor for the development of emphysema in the A_1AT-deficient patient. An increased number of polymorphonuclear leukocytes and macrophages are found in the lungs of smokers compared with the lungs of nonsmokers. Alveolar macrophages from smokers, in contrast to those from nonsmokers, will release elastase into a serum-free culture medium (Rodriguez et al, 1977). The antielastase activity of A_1AT obtained from the bronchoalveolar lavage from smokers is reduced twofold from that of nonsmokers (Gadek et al, 1979). Cigarette smoke causes oxidation of methionine at the active site (Met^{358}) of A_1AT, resulting in a two thousandfold reduction in its ability to inhibit neutrophil elastase (Johnson and Travis, 1979; Johnson and Travis, 1978; Travis et al, 1980; Carp and Janoff, 1978). Similar changes in antielastase activity can be induced by cellular oxidants (Carp and Janoff, 1979), ozone (Johnson, 1980), or chemical means (Abrams et al, 1981). A_1AT can be inactivated by a variety of enzymes that cause cleavage at or near the active site, including enzymes from bacteria (Morihara et al, 1979), macrophages, and serum proteases.

Cigarette smoke thus increases the burden of oxidants from neutrophils and their elastase while reducing the production of A_1AT and its antielastase potency. Therefore, it accelerates the development of emphysema and significantly shortens the life span of patients with deficient or absent A_1AT (Houstek et al, 1973).

CLINICAL ASPECTS

The vast majority of individuals with familial emphysema and A_1AT deficiencies are variants Z and null. A few have been described with types SZ, SS, PZ, and M malton Z. There is a threshold level of serum A_1AT (approximately 35 per cent of normal) below which emphysema generally occurs (Gadek and Crystal, 1983a). Epidemiologic studies have demonstrated that individuals with A_1AT deficiency and serum levels below 50 mg/dL have an 80 per cent or greater chance of developing emphysema (Larsson, 1978; Kueppers and Black, 1974).

In most individuals with familial emphysema and A_1AT deficiency there is a subtle increase in dyspnea usually beginning near the end of the third decade of life. The first case report in childhood of pulmonary emphysema associated with A_1AT deficiency homozygous Z type was published in 1971. This case involved a 13-year-old girl with evidence of emphysema in lung biopsy specimens since the age of 7 years (Figs. 39–4 and 39–5) (Talamo et al, 1971). Two other cases showed earlier pulmonary presentation (2 and 6 years), had low levels of A_1AT in the Pi ZZ range, but did not have Pi typing. Pi null subjects have been documented with emphysema in their early twenties (Talamo et al, 1973; Bernheim et al, 1976). Dyspnea is generally progressive, especially during exercise, and is not associated with cough or sputum production. Digital clubbing occurs in severely affected patients. Chest radiographs demonstrate increasing hyperaeration of the lungs, beginning at the lung bases. Pulmonary function studies show a progression to irreversible chronic obstructive lung disease. Carbon monoxide diffusion is reduced, residual volume can be significantly increased, but vital capacity and blood gases usually are affected only in the later stages of the disease. Radio-labeled pulmonary scanning in the early stages demonstrates diminished perfusion at the lung bases in the upright position. As the disease progresses, recurrent infections with bronchitis and bronchiectasis may become superimposed on the diffuse emphysematous process. Clearly the progression of the disease can be hastened by smoking or recurrent pulmonary infections.

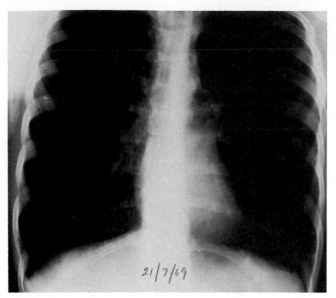

Figure 39–4. An anteroposterior chest roentgenogram of a 13-year-old female with Pi Z alpha₁-antitrypsin deficiency and biopsy evidence of panacinar emphysema. A striking degree of radiolucency is present.

Several Pi ZZ individuals reported to be totally asymptomatic in their fifth decade when studied in the pulmonary function laboratory showed a variety of physiologic abnormalities, including impairment in expiratory flow rates, hypoxemia, decreased carbon monoxide diffusing capacity, and increased alveolar-arterial oxygen tension differences.

Studies of the distribution of A_1AT deficiency in persons with asthma have been conflicting. A high proportion of MS and S variants have been reported in asthmatic patients (Fagerhol and Hauge, 1969; Arnaud et al, 1976), but others have found a normal distribution of A_1AT variants in patients with asthma (Szczeklik et al, 1974; Katz et al, 1976). If there is any association between A_1AT deficiency and asthma, it may be connected with the S allele. Heterozygous MZ individuals may be at a higher risk to develop chronic obstruction pulmonary disease (COPD) in the presence of the other risk factors, such as grain-dust exposure (Horne et al, 1986).

The pathologic change in the lung in patients with severe A_1AT deficiency is quite characteristic, showing diffuse panacinar emphysema. This process appears to begin at the lung bases and then to advance progressively toward the apices. In a few cases, bronchiectatic segments have been found superimposed on the underlying emphysema.

LIVER INVOLVEMENT

The association of A_1AT deficiency and liver disease was reported in 1969 (Sharp et al, 1969). The involvement begins in infancy with hepatocellular damage and obstructive jaundice (Eriksson, 1985); it occurs in approximately 12 per cent of homozygous

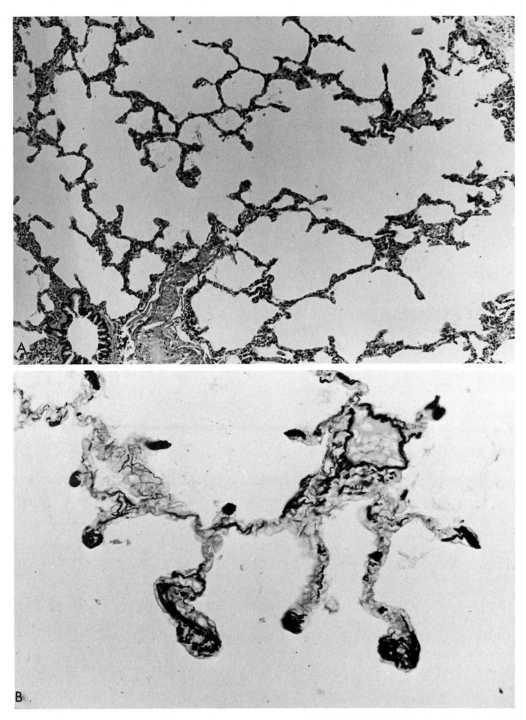

Figure 39–5. A biopsy specimen of a lingula of a 13-year-old girl with Pi ZZ alpha₁-antitrypsin deficiency and respiratory failure. *A,* Section showing ruptured alveolar walls (hematoxylin and eosin stain, x115). *B,* Section showing recoiled elastin at points of rupture (aldehyde-fuchsin stain, x460). (Reproduced with permission from Talamo RC et al: Symptomatic pulmonary emphysema in childhood associated with hereditary alpha₁-antitrypsin and elastase inhibitor deficiency. J Pediatr 79:20, 1971.)

Z variants (Sveger, 1976). The majority improve, but 10 to 15 per cent develop cirrhosis (Sveger, 1976). Higher rates of severe liver complications have also been reported (Psacharopoulos et al, 1983). For the purpose of genetic counseling, the risk for two MZ-variant parents to have a ZZ-variant child with severe liver disease is small, on the order of 1 to 2 per cent.

It appears that certain families have a higher incidence of liver disease. The liver disease appears frequently as "neonatal hepatitis syndrome," with delayed jaundice, failure to thrive, hepatosplenomegaly, and severe portal hypertension. Liver function tests show conjugated hyperbilirubinemia. Thirteen to 30 per cent of infants with neonatal hepatitis syndrome were found to have the Z variant of A_1AT deficiency (Cottrall et al, 1974; Moroz et al, 1976). Breast-feeding may offer some protection against severe liver disease (Udall et al, 1985). Within the hepatocyte, globular inclusion bodies contain aggregated A_1AT. Globular inclusion bodies are also found in hepatocytes of heterozygous patients but in a smaller number. This difference may be the reason for an increased prevalence of cryptogenic cirrhosis in MZ-phenotype patients (Hodges et al, 1981; Carlson and Eriksson, 1985). The prevalence of hepatoma is also significantly greater among homozygous or heterozygous Z variants than among control subjects (Carlson and Eriksson, 1985; Eriksson et al, 1986).

OTHER DISORDERS

Reports on A_1AT deficiency and other disorders are controversial, with some studies showing an increased frequency of heterozygous Z variants in patients with rheumatoid arthritis (Cox and Huber, 1976; Buisseret et al, 1977) and other studies showing no difference (Michalski et al, 1986).

Immune complex formation with Z protein leaking from dying liver cells and complement may deposit on basement membranes. Renal disease, pancreatitis, panniculitis, peptic ulcer, and cutaneous vasculitis have been reported in association with A_1AT deficiency (Kennedy et al, 1986; Smith et al, 1987; Brandrup and Ostergaard, 1978).

THERAPY

All the A_1AT-deficient patients, especially the homozygous variants, should avoid exposure to noxious agents that are known to accelerate the progression of lung disease, such as passive or active cigarette smoke, industrial dust and smoke, grain-dust exposure, and any form of atmospheric pollution. They should seek early treatment for respiratory tract infections. There is no evidence for the use of prophylactic antibiotics in these patients.

Pulmonary physical therapy and breathing exercises are of benefit when recurrent infections and bronchiectasis are features of the disease.

Bronchodilators should be used only when their benefit can be demonstrated, such as in the presence of superimposed infection or coexistent asthma. There is no evidence that corticosteroids are beneficial in A_1AT deficiency.

In the last 10 years, several therapeutic strategies have been used for augmentation therapy, in an attempt to maintain serum A_1AT levels above 80 mg/dL. Because the major source of A_1AT is the hepatocyte, numerous trials to increase the endogenous production and release of A_1AT have been directed toward stimulation of the liver with pharmacologic agents. Typhoid vaccine administration transiently increased A_1AT levels in MZ heterozygous individuals but not in homozygous variants (Kueppers, 1968). Because A_1AT levels increase in pregnancy, attempts to mimic the hormonal changes with estrogen-progesterone medications were made but were also unsuccessful (Laurell et al, 1967). Danazol, a synthetic testosterone without major androgenic properties, has been tried (600 mg for 30 days) in seven patients with severe emphysema and A_1AT deficiency (six ZZ variants, one M duarte Z) and one asymptomatic SZ variant (Eriksson, 1983). Five of the patients had an increase in serum levels but never more than 50 mg/dL. Another extensive trial of danazol in 43 homozygous Z variants showed an average and insufficient increase of 53 per cent over the pretreatment levels (Wewers et al, 1986). Trial therapy with tamoxifen citrate (an intracytoplasmic estrogen receptor binder) in three A_1AT SZ variants induced a 50 to 70 per cent increase of A_1AT levels over base line expectations but was not effective in homozygous Z variants (Eriksson, 1983; Wewers, Brantly, Casolaro et al, 1987).

Because the liver is the major site of A_1AT production, liver transplantation is theoretically the best endogenous way to increase and maintain serum A_1AT levels. It was tried successfully (producing normal donor type and sufficient levels of A_1AT) in a few homozygous Z variants (Gordon et al, 1986; Van Thiel et al, 1982). However, this procedure is invasive, has its own risks, and is dependent on appropriate donors.

Since 1981, several trials of replacement therapy have been reported (Gadek, Klein, Holland et al, 1981; Gadek and Crystal, 1983b; Wewers, Casolaro, and Crystal, 1987; Wewers, Casolaro, Sellers et al, 1987). Five homozygous Z variants were first treated with 4 g of a human A_1AT enriched plasma at weekly intervals for 4 weeks (Gadek, Klein, Holland et al, 1981). Serum levels were maintained over 70 mg/dL, and bronchoalveolar lavage showed effective antielastase activity. Since then trials have been reported with more purified preparations (Prolastin) on more patients and for longer periods. Weekly intravenous infusion of 60 mg/kg A_1AT produced average serum levels of 163 mg/dL (twice the threshold level known to protect the lung against protease destruction) and resulted in a fourfold increase in A_1AT levels in the lung and a twofold increase in neutrophil antielastase activity (Wewers, Casolaro, Sellers et al, 1987). However, the two major drawbacks of A_1AT replacement therapy are the frequent (weekly) need for treatment and the costs of the treatment ($21,840 US/year for a 70-kg adult). Higher doses of A_1AT (240 mg) administered once every 4 weeks (Hubbard et al, 1988) maintained serum A_1AT above threshold 21 out of 28 days between infusions. In three of the 21 patients treated, bronchoalveolar lavage was performed and showed A_1AT levels and antielastase capacity above threshold values. After 6 months of treatment, no change in lung function could be observed in the 21 treated patients (Wewers, Casolaro, Sellers et al, 1987). To demonstrate that such therapy can delay or halt the progressive deterioration in lung function would require a large study population treated early and followed for several years.

In one study, A$_1$AT (20 mg/kg) was administered to three dogs as an aerosol using an ultrasonic nebulizer (Smith and Spragg, 1988). Bronchial lavage fluid obtained 6 hours after inhalation contained large amounts of A$_1$AT. This approach may provide an alternative to protective therapy against proteolytic destruction of the lung in A$_1$AT-deficient patients, but appropriate clinical trials need to be done.

REFERENCES

Abrams WR, Cohen AB, Damiano VV et al: A model of decreased functional α$_1$-proteinase inhibitor. J Clin Invest 68:1132, 1981.

Allen MB, Ward AM, and Perks WH: Alpha$_1$-antitrypsin deficiency due to M malton Z phenotype: case report and family study. Thorax 41:568, 1986.

Arnaud P, Chapuis-Cellier C, Souillet G et al: High frequency of deficient Pi phenotypes of α$_1$-antitrypsin in non-atopic infantile asthma. Trans Assoc Am Physiol 89:205, 1976.

Bamforth FJ and Kalsheker NA: Alpha$_1$-antitrypsin deficiency due to Pi null: clinical presentation and evidence for molecular heterogeneity. J Med Genet 25:83, 1988.

Bernheim JL, Arnaud P, Cellier C et al: Apparent total α$_1$-antitrypsin deficiency. Isr J Med Sci 12:678, 1976.

Brandrup F and Ostergaard PA: Alpha$_1$-antitrypsin deficiency associated with persistent cutaneous vasculitis: occurrence in a child with liver disease. Arch Dermatol 114:921, 1978.

Brantly M, Nukiwa T, and Crystal RG: Molecular basis of alpha$_1$-antitrypsin deficiency. Am J Med 84(suppl 6A):13, 1988.

Buisseret PD, Pembrey ME, and Lessof MH: Alpha$_1$-antitrypsin phenotypes in rheumatoid arthritis and ankylosing spondylitis. Lancet 2:1358, 1977.

Camus L and Gley E: Action du serum sanguin sur quelques ferments digestifs. C R Soc Biol (Paris) 49:825, 1897.

Carlson J and Eriksson S: Chronic "cryptogenic" liver disease and malignant hepatoma in intermediate alpha$_1$-antitrypsin deficiency identified by a Pi Z-specific monoclonal antibody. Scand J Gastroenterol 20:835, 1985.

Carp H and Janoff A: Possible mechanisms of emphysema in smokers. In vitro suppression of serum elastase-inhibitory capacity by fresh cigarette smoke and its prevention by antioxidants. Am Rev Respir Dis 118:617, 1978.

Carp H and Janoff A: In vitro suppresion of serum elastase-inhibitory capacity by reactive oxygen species generated by phagocytosing polymorphonuclear leukocytes. J Clin Invest 63:793, 1979.

Carrell RW, Jeppsson JO, Laurell CB et al: Structure and variation of human α$_1$-antitrypsin. Nature 298:329, 1982.

Catz E and Cox DW: α$_1$-antitrypsin deficiency: the spectrum of pathology and pathophysiology. Perspect Pediatr Pathol 5:1, 1979.

Cottrall K, Cook PJL, and Mowat AP: Neonatal hepatitis syndrome and alpha$_1$-antitrypsin deficiency: an epidemiological study in southeast England. Postgrad Med J 50:376, 1974.

Cox DW: A new deficiency allele of alpha$_1$-antitrypsin: Pi M malton. In Peeters H (ed): Protides of the Biological Fluids. Oxford, Pergamon Press, 1976.

Cox DW and Huber O: Rheumatoid arthritis and alpha$_1$-antitrypsin. Lancet 1:1216, 1976.

Dykes DD, Miller SA, and Polesky HF: Distribution of α$_1$-antitrypsin variants in a US white population. Hum Hered 34:308, 1984.

Eriksson S: Pulmonary emphysema and alpha$_1$-antitrypsin deficiency. Acta Med Scand 175:197, 1964.

Eriksson S: Studies in α$_1$-antitrypsin deficiency. Acta Med Scand 177(suppl 432):1, 1965.

Eriksson S: The effect of tamoxifen in intermediate alpha$_1$-antitrypsin deficiency associated with the phenotype Pi SZ. Ann Clin Res 15:95, 1983.

Eriksson S: Liver disease in alpha$_1$-antitrypsin deficiency. Scand J Gastroenterol 20:907, 1985.

Eriksson S, Carlson J, and Velez R: Risk of cirrhosis and primary liver cancer in alpha$_1$-antitrypsin deficiency. N Engl J Med 314:736, 1986.

Fagerhol MK: Quantitative studies on the inherited variants of serum α$_1$-antitrypsin. Scand J Clin Lab Invest 23:97, 1969.

Fagerhol MK and Cox DW: The Pi polymorphism: genetic, biochemical and clinical aspects of human alpha$_1$-antitrypsin. Adv Hum Genet 1:1, 1981.

Fagerhol MK and Gedde-Dahl T Jr: Genetics of the Pi serum types. Family studies of the inherited variants of serum alpha$_1$-antitrypsin. Human Hered 19:354, 1969.

Fagerhol MK and Hauge HE: Serum Pi types in patients with pulmonary diseases. Acta Allerg (Kobenhavn) 24:107, 1969.

Fagerhol MK and Laurell CB: the polymorphism of "prealbumins" and α$_1$-antitrypsin in human sera. Clin Chim Acta 16:199, 1967.

Fagerhol MK and Laurell CB: The Pi system-inherited variants of serum α$_1$-antitrypsin. In Steinberg A and Bearn A (eds): Progress in Medical Genetics. Vol III. New York, Grune & Stratton, 1970.

Fagerhol MK and Tenfjord OW: Serum Pi types in some European, American, Asian and African populations. Acta Path Microbiol Scand 72:601, 1968.

Frants RR and Eriksson AW: α$_1$-antitrypsin: common subtypes of pi M. Hum Hered 26:435, 1976.

Gadek JE and Crystal RG: α$_1$-antitrypsin deficiency. In Stanbury JB, Wyngaarden JB, Fredrickson DS et al (eds): The Metabolic Basis of Inherited Diseases. 5th ed. New York, McGraw-Hill Book Co, Inc, 1983a.

Gadek JE and Crystal RD: Experience with replacement therapy in the destructive lung disease associated with severe alpha$_1$-antitrypsin deficiency. Am Rev Respir Dis 127:45, 1983b.

Gadek JE, Fells GA, and Crystal RG: Cigarette smoking induces functional antiprotease deficiency in the lower respiratory tract of humans. Science 206:1315, 1979.

Gadek JE, Fells GA, Zimmerman RL et al: Anti-elastases of the human alveolar structures: Implications for the protease-antiprotease theory of emphysema. J Clin Invest 68:889, 1981.

Gadek JE, Fulmer JD, Gelfand JA et al: Danazol-induced augmentation of serum α$_1$-antitrypsin levels in individuals with marked deficiency of this anti-protease. J Clin Invest 66:82, 1980.

Gadek JE, Klein HG, Holland PV et al: Replacement therapy for alpha$_1$-antitrypsin deficiency. J Clin Invest 68:1158, 1981.

Glasgow JFT, Lynch MJ, Hercz A et al: α$_1$-antitrypsin deficiency in association with both cirrhosis and chronic obstructive lung disease in two sibs. Am J Med 54:181, 1973.

Goedde HW, Hirth L, Benkmann HG et al: Population genetic studies of serum protein polymorphisms in four Spanish populations: part 2. Hum Hered 23:135, 1973.

Gordon RD, Shaw BWJ, Iwatsuki S et al: Indications for liver transplantation in the cyclosporine era. Surg Clin North Am 66:541, 1986.

Gross P, Pfitzer EH, Tolker E et al: Experimental emphysema: its production with papain in normal and silicotic rats. Arch Environ Health 11:50, 1964.

Hodges JR, Millward-Sadler GH, Barbatis C et al: Heterozygous MZ alpha$_1$-antitrypsin deficiency in adults with chronic hepatitis and cryptogenic cirrhosis. N Engl J Med 10:557, 1981.

Horne SL, Tennent RK, Cockcroft DW et al: Pulmonary function in Pi M and MZ grain workers. Chest 89:795, 1986.

Houstek J, Copova M, Zapletal A et al: Alpha$_1$-antitrypsin deficiency in a child with chronic lung disease. Chest 64:773, 1973.

Hubbard RC, Sellers S, Czerski D et al: Biochemical efficacy and safety of monthly augmentation therapy in α$_1$-antitrypsin deficiency. JAMA 260:1259, 1988.

Ihrig J, Schwartz HJ, Rynbrandt DJ et al: Serum trypsin inhibitory capacity and Pi phenotypes: prevalence of α$_1$-antitrypsin deficiency in an allergy population. Am J Clin Pathol 64:297, 1975.

Jacobsson K: Studies on the trypsin and plasmin inhibitors in human blood serum. Scand J Clin Lab Invest 7(suppl 14):55, 1955.

Jeppsson JO, Laurell CB, Nosslin B et al: Catabolic rate of α_1-antitrypsin of Pi types S and M malton and of asialylated M protein in man. Clin Sci Mol Med 55:103, 1978.

Johnson D and Travis J: Structural evidence for methionine at the reactive site of human alpha$_1$-proteinase inhibitor. J Biol Chem 253:7142, 1978.

Johnson D and Travis J: The oxidative inactivation of human α_1-antiprotease inhibitor: further evidence of methionine at the reactive center. J Biol Chem 254:4022, 1979.

Johnson DA: Ozone inactivation of human α_1-proteinase inhibitor. Am Rev Respir Dis 121:1031, 1980.

Kaiser D, Rennert OM, Joller-Jemelka H et al: Alpha$_1$-antitrypsin Mangel: Kombination von Lungenemphysem und Lebercirrhose in frühen Kindesalter. Klin Wochenschr 53:117, 1975.

Katz RM, Lieberman J, and Siegel SC: Alpha$_1$-antitrypsin levels and prevalence of Pi variant pheonotypes in asthmatic children. J Allergy Clin Immunol 57:41, 1976.

Kennedy JD, Talbot IC, and Tanner MS: Severe pancreatitis and fatty liver progressing to cirrhosis associated with Coxsackie B4 infection in a three year old with alpha$_1$-antitrypsin deficiency. Acta Paediatr Scand 75:336, 1986.

Kidd VJ, Wallace RB, Itakura K et al: α_1-antitrypsin deficiency detection by direct analysis of the mutation in the gene. Nature 304:230, 1983.

Kueppers F: Genetically determined differences in the response of alpha$_1$-antitrypsin levels in human serum to typhoid vaccine. Hum Genet 6:207, 1968.

Kueppers F and Black LF: α_1-antitrypsin and its deficiency. Am Rev Respir Dis 110:176, 1974.

Larsson C: Natural history and life expectancy in severe alpha$_1$-antitrypsin deficiency. Acta Med Scand 204:345, 1978.

Laurell CB and Eriksson S: The electrophoretic α_1-globulin pattern of serum in α_1-antitrypsin deficiency. Scand J Clin Lab Invest 15:132, 1963.

Laurell CB and Jeppsson JO: Protease inhibitors in plasma. Chapter 5. In Putnam FW (ed): The Plasma Protein: Structure, Function and Genetic Control. New York, Academic Press, 1975.

Laurell CB, Kullander S, and Thorell J: Effect of administration of a combined estrogen-progestin contraceptive on the level of individual plasma proteins. Scand J Clin Lab Invest 21:337, 1967.

Loebermann H, Tokuoka R, Deisenhofer J et al: Human α_1-proteinase inhibitor: crystal structure analysis of two crystal modifications, molecular model and preliminary analysis of the implications for function. J Mol Biol 177:531, 1984.

Martin JP, Sesboue R, Charlionet R et al: Genetic variants of serum α_1-antitrypsin (Pi types) in Portuguese. Hum Hered 26:310, 1976.

Martorana PA and Share NN: Effect of human alpha$_1$-antitrypsin on papain-induced emphysema in the hamster. Am Rev Respir Dis 113:607, 1976.

Mega T, Lujan E, and Yoshida A: Studies on the oligosaccharide chains of human α_1-protease inhibitor: II. Structure of oligosaccharides. J Biol Chem 255:4057, 1980.

Michalski JP, McCombs CC, Scopelitis E et al: Alpha$_1$-antitrypsin phenotypes including M subtypes, in pulmonary disease associated with rheumatoid arthritis and systemic sclerosis. Arthritis Rheum 29:586, 1986.

Morihara K, Tsuzuki H, and Oda K: Protease and elastase of pseudomonas aeruginosa: inactivation of human plasma α_1-proteinase inhibitor. Infect Immun 24:188, 1979.

Moroz SP, Cutz E, Cox DW et al: Liver disease associated with alpha$_1$-antitrypsin deficiency in childhood. J Pediatr 88:19, 1976.

Nukiwa T, Satoh K, Brantly ML et al: Identification of a second mutation in the protein-coding sequence of the Z type alpha$_1$-antitrypsin gene. J Biol Chem 34:15989, 1986.

Opie EL: Enzymes and antienzymes of inflammatory exudates. J Exp Med 7:316, 1905.

Owen MC and Carrell RW: Alpha$_1$-antitrypsin: molecular abnormality of S variant. Br Med J 1:130, 1976.

Perlino E, Cortese R, and Ciliberto G: The human α_1-antitrypsin gene is transcribed from two different promoters in macrophages and hepatocytes. EMBO J 6:2767, 1987.

Psacharopoulos HT, Mowat AP, Cook PJL et al: Outcome of liver disease associated with alpha$_1$-antitrypsin deficiency (Pi Z). Arch Dis Child 58:882, 1983.

Resendes M: Association of α_1-antitrypsin deficiency with lung and liver diseases. West J Med 147:48, 1987.

Rodriguez RJ, White RR, Senior RM et al: Elastase release from human alveolar macrophages: comparison between smokers and non-smokers. Science 198:313, 1977.

Satoh K, Nukiwa T, Brantly M et al: Emphysema associated with complete absence of α_1-antitrypsin in serum and the homozygous inheritance of stop codon in α_1-antitrypsin coding exon. Am J Hum Genet 42:77, 1988.

Schroeder WT, Miller MF, Woo SLC et al: Chromosomal localization of the human variant alpha$_1$-trypsin gene (Pi) to 14q 31–32. Am J Hum Genet 37:868, 1985.

Sharp HL: Alpha$_1$-antitrypsin deficiency. Hosp Pract 6:83, 1971.

Sharp HL, Bridges RA, Krivit W, and Freier EF: Cirrhosis associated with α_1-antitrypsin deficiency: a previously unrecognized inherited disorder. J Lab Clin Med 73:934, 1969.

Smith KC, Pittelkow MR, and Su WPD: Panniculitis associated with severe α_1-antitrypsin deficiency. Arch Dermatol 123:1655, 1987.

Smith RM and Spragg RG: Production and administration to dogs of aerosols of alpha$_1$-proteinase inhibitor. Am J Med 84(suppl 6A):48, 1988.

Sveger T: Liver disease in alpha$_1$-antitrypsin deficiency detected by screening of 200,000 infants. N Engl J Med 294:1316, 1976.

Szczeklik A, Turowska B, Czerniawska-Mysik G et al: Serum α_1-antitrypsin in bronchial asthma. Am Rev Respir Dis 109:487, 1974.

Talamo RC: Basic and clinical aspects of the alpha$_1$-antitrypsin. Pediatrics 56:91, 1975.

Talamo RC, Langley CE, Reed CE et al: α_1-antitrypsin deficiency: a variant with no detectable α_1-antitrypsin. Science 181:70, 1973.

Talamo RC, Levison H, Lynch MJ et al: Symptomatic pulmonary emphysema in childhood associated with hereditary α_1-antitrypsin and elastase inhibitor deficiency. J Pediatr 79:20, 1971.

Travis J, Beatty K, Wong PS et al: Oxidation of alpha $_1$-proteinase inhibitor as a major contributing factor in the development of pulmonary emphysema. Bull Eur Physiopathol Respir 16(suppl):341, 1980.

Udall JN Jr, Dixon M, Newman AP et al: Liver disease in alpha$_1$-antitrypsin deficiency: a retrospective analysis of the influence of early breast- versus bottle-feeding. JAMA 253:2679, 1985.

Van Thiel DH, Schade RR, Starzl TE et al: Liver transplantation in adults. Hepatology 2:637, 1982.

Webb DR, Hyde RW, Schwartz RH et al: Serum α_1-antitrypsin variants. Am Rev Respir Dis 108:918, 1973.

Wewers MD, Brantly MC, Casolaro MA et al: Evaluation of tamoxifen as a therapy to augment alpha$_1$-antitrypsin concentration in Z homozygous alpha$_1$-antitrypsin deficient individuals. Am Rev Respir Dis:135:401, 1987.

Wewers MD, Casolaro MA, and Crystal RG: Comparison of alpha$_1$-antitrypsin levels and antineutrophil elastase capacity of blood and lung in a patient with the alpha$_1$-antitrypsin phenotype null-null before and during alpha$_1$-antitrypsin augmentation therapy. Am Rev Respir Dis 135:539, 1987.

Wewers MD, Casolaro MA, Sellers SE et al: Replacement therapy for alpha$_1$-antitrypsin deficiency associated with emphysema. N Engl J Med 316:1055, 1987.

Wewers MD, Gadek JE, Keogh BA et al: Evaluation of danazol therapy for patients with Pi ZZ alpha$_1$-antitrypsin deficiency. Am Rev Respir Dis 134:476, 1986.

Yoshida A, Lieberman J, Gaidulis L et al: Molecular abnormality of human alpha$_1$-antitrypsin variant (Pi ZZ) associated with plasma activity deficiency. Proc Natl Acad Sci USA 73:1324, 1976.

REYNALDO D. PAGTAKHAN, M.D., and
VICTOR CHERNICK, M.D.

40

LIQUID AND AIR IN THE PLEURAL SPACE

Disorders of the pleura constitute an important cause of morbidity and mortality in infants and children. Their prompt recognition and appropriate management can avert the occurrence of a more serious cardiorespiratory catastrophe. In this chapter we discuss the anatomic features of the pleural "space," the physiology of liquid transport in the potential space, and the various noninflammatory disorders of liquid accumulation and their management. (Inflammatory disorders of the pleura are discussed in Chapter 27.) Finally, the process of gas accumulation in the pleural space due to leakage of air from the alveoli and the treatment of this problem are considered.

LIQUID IN THE PLEURAL SPACE

ANATOMIC FEATURES

The pleural membranes cover the outer surface of the lungs (visceral pleura) and the inner surface of the thoracic wall (parietal pleura). They are in intimate contact, with only a thin film of liquid between the two surfaces. The membranes are lined with a single layer of ciliated, flat mesothelial cells, 6 to 7 μ thick, along with a connective tissue layer of collagen and elastic fiber, 30 to 40 μ thick. Between the connective tissue layer and the limiting membrane of the lung lies a region, 20 to 50 μ thick, of blood vessels and lymphatics. Branches of the pulmonary artery supply the visceral pleura, and branches of the intercostal arteries supply the parietal pleura. Lymphatic vessels are located in the subepithelial layer of the parietal pleura. The parietal pleura drains into the internal mammary system ventrally, the intercostal lymph node dorsally, and the mediastinal lymph nodes inferiorly. The entire visceral pleura drains into the mediastinal nodes. The thoracic and right lymphatic ducts then drain into the systemic venous circulation.

PHYSIOLOGY OF LIQUID IN THE PLEURAL SPACE

The pleural membranes are permeable to liquid. Normally, complete emptying of the pleural liquid does not occur, and a small but measurable amount (approximately 1.0 ml) of liquid remains. A rational understanding of excess pleural liquid accumulation in various disease states requires a knowledge of normal liquid transport into and out of the pleural cavity. Close to 90 per cent of the original amount of pleural liquid filtered out of the arterial end of the capillaries is reabsorbed at the venous end. The remainder (10 per cent) of the filtrate is returned via the lymphatics. The imbalance between filtration and reabsorption forces determines the direction of liquid movement. Starling described a classic approach to convective (bulk) liquid movement between vascular and extravascular compartments, which can be expressed as

$$\dot{Q}_V = K_f [(P_c - P_{is}) - (\pi_{pl} - \pi_{is})]$$

where $\dot{Q}_v$ = rate of net liquid movement per unit surface area of capillary; K_f = capillary filtration coefficient; P_c = capillary hydrostatic pressure; P_{is} = hydrostatic pressure in interstitial space (equivalent to intrapleural pressure); π_{pl} = plasma oncotic pressure; and π_{is} = interstitial space oncotic pressure (equivalent to oncotic pressure of pleural liquid).

Liquid movement across the pleural capillaries obeys the foregoing law of transcapillary liquid exchange. The filtration coefficient (K_f) is an index of capillary wall permeability that depends on the structural integrity of the intercellular junctions of the endothelial lining. The oncotic pressure (π) is a function of the molal concentration of protein, mainly albumin. Normal plasma with a protein concentration of 7.0 g/100 ml has an oncotic pressure of 32 to 35 cm H_2O, whereas pleural liquid with a protein concentration of 1.77 g/100 ml has an estimated oncotic pressure of about 5.8 cm H_2O). The mean hydrostatic pressures (P_c) in the parietal and visceral pleural capillaries are 30 and 11 cm H_2O, respectively. The intrapleural pressure (equivalent to P_{is}) at resting lung volume is about 5 cm H_2O subatmospheric, so there is a net pressure of 9 cm H_2O (filtration pressure) at the parietal pleural capillary level tending to drive liquid into the pleural space. In contrast, a net driving pressure of -10 cm H_2O (absorption pressure) is acting on the visceral pleural

545

capillaries, driving liquid from the pleural space into the capillaries (Table 40–1). Net liquid absorption from the pleural space occurs because absorption pressure is slightly greater than filtration pressure. Increased negative pressure develops in the liquid between the contact points of visceral and parietal pleura because of increased stretching and deformation at these sites. Ultimately, the negative pleural liquid pressure equilibrates with the absorption pressure. Thus the pleural space is kept only nearly liquid free, a state that represents an equilibrium between filtration and absorption.

The pleural liquid is sterile and contains an average of nearly 2.0 g/100 ml proteins. Particulate matter from the pleural liquid is returned to the systemic circulation via the lymphatics or directly into the pleural capillaries. Large molecular-weight particles, such as proteins and erythrocytes, are cleared solely via the lymphatic channels in the parietal pleura through preformed stomas formed by direct continuity of the endothelial cells of lymphatic vessels with pleural mesothelial cells. Clearance of proteins occurs independently of net liquid movement. A major propelling force in the transport of pleural content into the circulation is respiratory movement. Hypoventilation is known to decrease absorption of particulate matter from the pleural space. Smaller ions, such as sodium, and low-molecular-weight dyes, such as methylene blue, are rapidly absorbed directly into the visceral pleural circulation. Pleural absorption of both liquid and small particles is hastened by the augmentation of intercostal and diaphragmatic activity, e.g., deep breathing exercises, which result in increased vascular and lymphatic uptake owing to dehiscences formed between mesothelial cells of the visceral pleural.

Normally, the pleural liquid is alkaline. The pH of the liquid is determined by several factors, namely (1) pH, P_{CO_2}, and bicarbonate of arterial blood, (2) P_{CO_2} of the local pleural tissue, (3) metabolism of cells in the pleural liquid, and (4) transfer of H^+, CO_2, and bicarbonate between the pleural cavity and the surrounding blood and tissue.

ACCUMULATION OF EXCESS PLEURAL LIQUID

Etiology and Pathogenesis

The normal state of a nearly liquid-free pleural cavity represents an equilibrium between pleural liq-uid formation (filtration) and removal (absorption). Fundamentally, excess liquid accumulates in the pleural cavity (effusion) whenever filtration exceeds removal mechanisms as a result of either (1) increased filtration associated with normal or impaired absorption or (2) normal filtration associated with inadequate removal. Thus disequilibrium may be due to disturbances in Starling forces that govern filtration and absorption or to alterations in lymphatic drainage, or both.

Various clinical disorders can alter vascular filtration and absorption in the pleural capillaries as well as lymphatic flow (Table 40–2). The capillary filtration coefficient (K_f) may be increased because of damage to the basement membrane as a result of inflammation (e.g., pleural infection, rheumatoid arthritis, systemic lupus erythematosus, pulmonary infarction) or because of direct toxic damage to the endothelium. Local blood flow may increase, resulting in an increase in capillary hydrostatic pressure (P_c). Moreover, protein is lost from the capillaries and accumulates in the pleural cavity, thereby increasing pleural fluid oncotic pressure (π_{is}). The net consequence of these changes is increased liquid and protein transudation into the pleural cavity that exceeds the normal capacity of lymphatic drainage. Hydrostatic pressure (P_c) may also be increased because of systemic venous hypertension (e.g., pericarditis, right-sided heart failure from overinfusion of blood or fluid, superior vena cava syndrome) or because of pulmonary venous hypertension (e.g., congestive heart failure). The resulting increased pleural liquid accumulation (hydrothorax) is due not only to increased driving pressure in the systemic capillaries but also to a higher filtration coefficient. The creation of a markedly subatmospheric pleural pressure (e.g., following thoracentesis), even in the presence of a normal hydrostatic pressure in the pleural capillaries, may also result in increased fluid filtration from the pleural capillaries. This mechanism explains recurrences of effusion following repeated thoracenteses and the increasing effusion that occurs in tuberculosis, with visceral pleural thickening and fibrosis and permanently atelectatic lungs.

Oncotic pressure (π) determines how effectively fluid is reabsorbed. Net absorption by the visceral pleura is reduced to zero by an increase in pleural liquid protein concentration higher than 4 g/100 ml (e.g., infection) in the presence of normal plasma

Table 40–1. STARLING RELATIONSHIP IN PARIETAL AND VISCERAL PLEURA

	Parietal Pleura	Visceral Pleura
Force Moving Liquid into Pleural Space (cm H_2O)		
Capillary hydrostatic pressure	30	11
Interstitial hydrostatic pressure (pleural pressure)	5	5
Oncotic pressure of pleural liquid	6	6
Total (cm H_2O)	41	22
Force Moving Liquid into Pleural Capillaries (cm H_2O)		
Plasma oncotic pressure	32	32
Net Force (cm H_2)	9 (out)	10 (in)

Table 40–2. PATHOPHYSIOLOGY OF PLEURAL LIQUID ACCUMULATION

Primary Mechanism	Clinical Disorders	Pleural Effusion
ALTERED STARLING FORCES		
Increased capillary permeability (K_f)	Pleuropulmonary infection; circulating toxins; systemic lupus erythematosus; rheumatoid arthritis; sarcoidosis; tumor; pulmonary infarction; viral hepatitis	Exudate
Increased capillary hydrostatic pressure (P_c)	Overhydration; congestive heart failure; venous hypertension; pericarditis	Transudate
Decreased hydrostatic pressure of the interstitial space (P_{is})	Trapped lung with chronic pleural space; postthoracentesis	Transudate
Decreased plasma oncotic pressure (π_{pl})	Hypoalbuminemia; nephrosis; hepatic cirrhosis	Transudate
Increased oncotic pressure of interstitial space (π_{is})	Pulmonary infarction	Exudate
INAPPROPRIATE LYMPHATIC FLOW		
Inadequate outflow	Hypoalbuminemia; nephrosis	Transudate
Excessive inflow	Hepatic cirrhosis with ascites; peritoneal dialysis	Transudate
Impaired flow (mediastinal lymphadenopathy and fibrosis; thickening of parietal pleura; obstruction of thoracic duct; developmental hypoplasia or defect)	Mediastinal radiation, superior vena caval syndrome, pericarditis; tuberculosis; lymphoma, mediastinal hygroma; hereditary lymphedema, congenital chylothorax	Exudate or transudate or chyle
Disruption of diaphragmatic lymphatics	Pancreatitis; subphrenic abscess	Exudate
VASCULAR LEAK	Trauma; spontaneous rupture; vascular erosion by neoplasm; hemorrhagic disease	Blood

protein concentration. When plasma oncotic pressure is significantly reduced (e.g., in hypoalbuminemia or nephrosis), parietal pleural filtration is increased and visceral pleural absorption is reduced even with normal concentration of pleural protein. If lymphatic channels are unable to provide adequate drainage, pleural effusion ensues. Lymphatic drainage, however, may be impeded as a result of (1) systemic venous hypertension, (2) mediastinal lymphadenopathy (e.g., lymphoma or fibrosis), (3) thickening of parietal pleura (e.g., tuberculosis), (4) obstruction of thoracic duct (e.g., chylothorax), and (5) developmental hypoplasia of lymphatic channels (e.g., hereditary lymphedema). On occasion, the lymphatic system is overloaded by absorption of peritoneal fluid (e.g., liver cirrhosis with ascites, peritoneal dialysis) via the diaphragmatic lymphatics. The result is escape of excess lymphatic fluid under increased pressure into the pleural cavity, where pressure is normally subatmospheric.

From the foregoing discussion, it is evident that a single clinical disorder may cause a pleural effusion through one or several mechanisms. Moreover, it is possible that clinical disorders may coexist. These facts may explain the varying character of pleural effusion seen clinically.

Classically, pleural effusions have been classified as transudate and exudate. This classification can be of great value, because certain disease states produce transudates almost exclusively (e.g., congestive heart failure) and others produce exudates (e.g., pleural infections). A transudate occurs when the mechanical forces of hydrostatic and oncotic pressures are so altered as to favor liquid filtration in excess of absorption. The pleural surfaces are not directly involved by the underlying disorder. In contrast, exudates result either from inflammatory diseases that affect the pleural surfaces, causing increased capillary permeability, or from disorders that impede lymphatic drainage. The pleural liquid protein concentration distinguishes the type of effusion; in transudative effusion the concentration is < 3 g/100 ml, and in exudative effusion the concentration is > 3 g/100 ml. Another approach classifies exudates as having any one of the following features: a pleural liquid to serum protein ratio greater than 0.5; a pleural liquid lactic dehydrogenase (LDH) level greater than 200 I.U.; or a pleural liquid to serum LDH ratio greater than 0.6 (Table 40–3).

Pleural effusion may also be classified as chylothorax (Table 40–4), chyliform, or hemothorax. *Chylothorax* refers to an accumulation of chyle in the pleural cavity and results from obstruction of either the thoracic duct or left subclavian vein (e.g., neoplastic, parasitic, and inflammatory conditions), from congenital lymph fistula of undetermined cause, or from traumatic rupture of lymphatic channels (e.g., following extracardiac vascular operations or diaphragmatic hernia repair); chylothorax is the most common type of pleural effusion in the newborn period. When the type of pleural liquid only assumes the appearance of chyle (milky white and opalescent) but does not demonstrate fat globules (pseudochyle), the effusion is called *chyliform;* the milky appearance represents the fatty degeneration of pus and endothelial cells. It may be seen in long-standing cases of

Table 40–3. CHEMICAL SEPARATION OF TRANSUDATES AND EXUDATES

Type of Effusion	Pleural Liquid Concentration		Pleural/Serum Concentration Ratio	
	PROTEIN	LDH	PROTEIN	LDH
Transudate	<3 gm/100 ml	<200 I.U.	<0.5	<0.6
Exudate	≥3 gm/100 ml	≥200 I.U.	≥0.5	≥0.6

LDH, lactic dehydrogenase.

purulent effusion. Frank blood in the pleural cavity is referred to as *hemothorax;* it may be caused by trauma to the chest wall, vascular erosion by neoplasm (e.g., pleural mesothelioma), spontaneous rupture of a subpleural bleb or the great vessels (patent ductus arteriosus, coarctation of aorta), or strangulated diaphragmatic hernia.

Functional Pathology

The degree of dysfunction is determined by the severity and rapidity of development of pleural effusion as well as by the nature of the underlying disorder and the status of cardiopulmonary function. Moderate to large pleural effusions increase elastic resistance to distention, thereby reducing lung volume on the ipsilateral side. Thus the vital capacity is reduced. Airflow remains normal, because the nonelastic resistance is usually unaffected. The corresponding hemidiaphragm is depressed, and contralateral lung function and vascular flow may be compromised by mediastinal displacement. Thus alveolar gas exchange may be seriously impaired and cardiac function may be disturbed. Malnutrition secondary to loss of chyle (rich in proteins, lipids, and fat-soluble vitamins) and shock due to blood loss are additional hazards.

Diagnosis

History and Physical Examination. Pleural effusion is usually secondary to an underlying disorder. The basic disease determines most of the systemic symptoms. Until accumulation of pleural liquid increases enough to cause cardiorespiratory difficulties (e.g., dyspnea, orthopnea), a pleural effusion may be asymptomatic. Thus attention to the chest findings on physical examination is important, particularly if only a small amount of liquid is present. Pleural rub may be the only finding during the early phase.

Table 40–4. CERTAIN PHYSICAL AND CHEMICAL CHARACTERISTICS OF CHYLE

Sterile
Ingested lipophilic dyes stain the effusion
Cells predominantly lymphocytes
Sudan stain: fat globules
Total fat content exceeds that of plasma
   (e.g., up to 660 mg/100 ml)
Protein content = ½ or same as that of plasma
   (usually ≥ 3.0 gm/100 ml)
Electrolytes = same as plasma
Blood urea nitrogen = same as plasma
Glucose = same as plasma

Diminished thoracic wall excursion, dull or flat percussion, decreased tactile and vocal fremitus, diminished whispering pectoriloquy, fullness of the intercostal spaces, and decreased breath sounds are easily demonstrated over the site in the older child with moderate effusion. (Breath sounds in the neonate can come through loud and clear because of his small chest volume.) The trachea and the cardiac apex are displaced toward the contralateral side. Careful physical examination, even in the neonate, will enable the physician to suspect a pleural effusion.

Chest Roentgenogram. In general, a minimum of approximately 400 ml of pleural liquid is required for roentgenographic visualization in upright views of the chest. A small quantity of pleural liquid is seen best at end-expiration as a straight radiodense line. It should be differentiated from the undulating outline of soft tissues unaffected by the respiratory phase. Lateral decubitus films taken with the patient lying on the affected side can detect as little as 50 ml of liquid or even less if the radiographs are properly exposed. It is demonstrable as a layering of liquid density in the dependent portion of the thoracic cavity. Decubitus films may also demonstrate an infrapulmonary pleural effusion (Figs. 40–1 and 40–2). When effusion is moderate, chest radiographs demonstrate uniform water density and widened interspaces on the affected side with displacement of the mediastinum to the contralateral hemithorax. A roentgenogram taken after thoracentesis may demonstrate the underlying parenchymal involvement that was obscured by the effusion.

Examination of the Pleural Liquid. Evacuation of liquid by thoracentesis confirms the clinical and radiologic diagnosis of effusion. The specimen may provide the only evidence on which to make the diagnosis of certain specific disease states or to exclude others.

The gross appearance of the liquid may be a clue to the cause of the effusion. Thus a pale yellow liquid suggests a transudate. Aspiration of chylous liquid suggests injury to the lymphatic channels (e.g., after surgery or in neoplasm or tuberculosis) or spontaneous anatomic leakage of chyle (e.g., congenital chylothorax). The characteristic milky appearance in congenital chylothorax is seen only after oral feedings have been started. A bloody fluid implies vascular erosion from a malignant tumor or damage to intercostal or chest wall vessels from blunt thoracic trauma. Brisk and massive bleeding is apt to be seen when the systemic circulation is involved, because systemic pressure is sixfold higher than the pulmonary pressure. A purulent specimen indicates bacterial infection of the pleura (see Chapter 27).

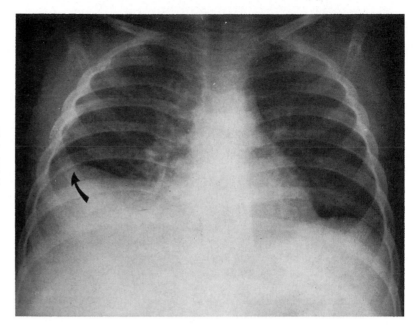

Figure 40–1. Upright chest radiograph of a child with nephrotic syndrome, demonstrating right infrapulmonary pleural effusion. The right hemidiaphragm shows peak elevation laterally *(arrow)* and relative lucency of the costophrenic sinus, signs that indicate an infrapulmonary location of the liquid.

Total counts of red and white blood cells are of negligible value and need not be done routinely, unless chest trauma is suspected, in which case eosinophilia may be present. Differential cell counting can identify tumor cells and is done if a neoplasm is suspected. Aliquots are sent for cytologic studies for malignant cells, for biochemical determinations (pH, fat content, protein and LDH concentrations along with their serum determinations), and for immunologic (CIE) and microbiologic studies (cultures and Gram stain) to rule out infection.

Summary. Physical and chemical characteristics of pleural liquid differentiate inflammatory pleural effusion from transudate, chyle, or frank blood caused by a variety of clinical disorders. In the group of conditions associated with noninflammatory pleural

effusion, the pleural membranes remain basically healthy. The underlying primary mechanisms are fundamentally a result of physical imbalance between increased liquid formation and inappropriate lymphatic flow. Pleural transudation occurs as a consequence of any of the following alterations in Starling forces: (1) increased pulmonary capillary hydrostatic pressure, (2) decreased plasma oncotic pressure, and (3) markedly subatmospheric pleural pressure. These changes favor increased liquid filtration at the parietal pleural surface. Liquid accumulates in the pleural cavity because lymphatic drainage is inadequate to cope with the increased liquid load. A transudate may also occur as a result of excessive lymphatic inflow and pressure at the level of the diaphragmatic lymphatic channels. Impaired lymphatic flow may

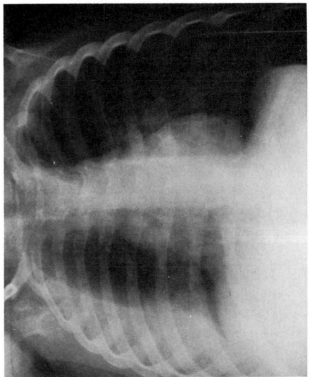

Figure 40–2. Decubitus chest radiograph with right side dependent of the same patient as in Figure 40–1, confirming the presence of free-flowing right pleural effusion.

produce either a transudate or an exudate, depending on the dominant underlying or concurrent pathologic process. Thoracic duct obstruction can produce pure chylous effusion. Chylothorax in later childhood may also be traumatic. In contrast, overt trauma and underlying pathologic states are usually not recognizable in neonatal chylothorax. A bloody pleural liquid is almost invariably a result of noninflammatory vascular leak (trauma); rarely in childhood is it caused by vascular erosion secondary to neoplasm.

Management

Treatment of transudative, hemorrhagic, and chylous pleural effusions is directed at supportive therapy of the functional disturbances and at specific management of the underlying disorder. Evacuation of a transudate following the initial diagnostic thoracentesis is indicated only for relief of dyspnea and other cardiorespiratory disturbances caused by mediastinal displacement. Intercostal tube drainage is provided when repeated thoracenteses are necessary, because repeated needle drainage is upsetting to a child. Diuretics administered to some patients may slow reaccumulation of transudate and thereby may decrease or eliminate the need for frequent thoracentesis. Specific treatment of the underlying disorder emphasizes the need for thorough history taking and meticulous physical examination to arrive promptly at an accurate clinical diagnosis. Cardiovascular and renal causes (e.g., congestive heart failure, nephrosis) as well as lymphatic disorders causing inappropriate lymphatic flow are managed accordingly. Pleural transudation due to fluid overload (e.g., from intravenous infusion or peritoneal dialysis) may require only a diuresis or may resolve spontaneously.

The treatment of hemothorax associated with shock requires immediate expansion of vascular volume and direct surgical repair of bleeders. Smaller bleeds should be evacuated, because healing is often associated with pleural adhesions. Fibrinolytic enzymes instilled into the pleural cavity may help if clots have formed. Chest pain is relieved by analgesics.

Chylothorax poses unique problems in management. Immediate and repeated thoracentesis is required for life-threatening cardiorespiratory embarrassment. In the absence of a life-threatening situation, initial treatment for neonatal and most cases of surgical traumatic chylothorax includes (1) single thoracentesis with complete drainage of chyle, (2) use of medium-chain triglyceride (MCT) as the major source of dietary fat, and (3) replacement of nutrient losses. Some cases of traumatic chylothorax would immediately require direct surgical intervention. The use of an MCT diet and avoidance of fatty meals containing long-chain fatty acids significantly reduces lymph flow (up to tenfold) because MCT is absorbed directly into the portal venous blood and contributes little to chylomicron formation. Cessation

of chylous effusion occurs largely toward the end of the second week of treatment. In an occasional patient in whom chyle reaccumulates rapidly, a subsequent trial of fasting and parenteral hyperalimentation (via a vein other than the left subclavian) is indicated. The nonsurgical treatment program is continued for a duration of 4 to 5 weeks to allow sufficient time for closure of lymphatic channel fistulae. Concurrently, intravenous solutions containing proteins and electrolytes are infused to replace protein loss and prevent hypovolemia. Vitamin supplements are added to avoid deficiency states. With the foregoing therapeutic program, most patients respond favorably with progressive weight gain and cessation of chylothorax; only a few cases are recalcitrant and require thoracotomy.

AIR IN THE PLEURAL SPACE

In this section we consider the physiology of gas in the pleural space, and the process, clinical spectrum, diagnosis, and treatment of gas accumulation in the pleural cavity and adjacent tissues because of leakage of air from the alveoli.

BASIC CONSIDERATIONS

The pleural membranes are permeable to gas. In view of the nature of dissociation curves for oxygen and carbon dioxide, the partial pressures of gases in the venous blood at sea level are: $p_{O_2} = 40$, $P_{CO_2} = 46$, $P_{N_2} = 573$, and $P_{H_2O} = 47$. They add up to 706 mm Hg, that is, 54 mm Hg (73 cm H_2O) less than atmospheric pressure (at sea level). Because the total gas pressure in the venous blood is about 73 cm H_2O subatmospheric and the intrapleural pressure at resting lung volume is approximately 5 cm H_2O subatmospheric, there exists a pressure gradient of about 68 cm H_2O favoring continuing absorption of gas from the pleural space into the circulation. Thus any gas volume within the pleural space diffuses out of it until all of the gas disappears (provided there is no continuing air leak to the pleural space from the atmosphere), and normally the pleural space is kept totally gas-free.

When there is a pneumothorax, this process of absorption can be hastened considerably (approximately sevenfold) if the gas is loculated (there is no continuous air leak) by breathing 100 per cent oxygen. Oxygen breathing will wash out nitrogen from the body without significantly increasing venous P_{O_2}. Because under ordinary circumstances arterial blood is nearly completely saturated with oxygen during air breathing, oxygen breathing changes arterial oxygen content by increasing only the amount of oxygen dissolved in plasma. The increase in dissolved oxygen that occurs with a change from air to oxygen breathing is approximately 1.5 volumes per cent. Because arteriovenous oxygen content difference remains on average 5 volumes per cent, and the steep part of the oxyhemoglobin dissociation curve is in effect, breathing 100 per cent oxygen will raise venous P_{O_2} only from 40 to, say, 50 mm Hg. This rise in venous P_{O_2} is accomplished while P_{N_2} goes to nearly zero, and therefore the total venous gas pressure is approximately 143 mm Hg or some 617 mm Hg (800 cm H_2O) less than atmospheric pressure. Thus 100 per cent oxygen breathing will hasten the absorption of loculated gas.

CLINICAL CONSIDERATIONS

Etiology and Pathogenesis

Intrapleural accumulation of air (pneumothorax) ensues whenever the pleural space develops a free communication with the atmosphere, either from a chest wall defect through the parietal pleura or from alveolar rupture, or both. A chest wall defect can result from surgical procedures or from a penetrating injury from a missile or projectile. Thoracic trauma, including compressive blunt injury from vehicular accidents, falls, and external cardiac massage, can rupture the lung. Infants and children are prone to internal injury from blunt trauma because of the greater compressibility of the chest wall. Thus laceration or transection of major airways has been reported to accompany chest trauma even without fractured rib fragments or obvious external injury.

Fundamentally, three factors determine the extent of alveolar distention, namely (1) degree of transpulmonary pressure exerted, (2) duration of pressure applied, and (3) ratio of inexpansible to expansible portion of the lung. Alterations of these factors with concomitant lung rupture can occur during the patient's own respiratory efforts. More commonly, lung rupture occurs during resuscitation and artificial ventilation and in the presence of incomplete airways obstruction and parenchymal consolidation seen in a variety of lower respiratory tract diseases. Positive intra-alveolar inflation pressure increases air volume but decreases blood volume in the adjacent vessels. Given this disporportionate change in blood volume and air volume, the tissue that tethers the perivascular sheath to the alveolar wall tends to attenuate. Because the mechanical forces in the alveolar wall and the tethering elements are angular to each other, rupture of the base of the alveoli occurs when the critical shear or traction force is exceeded, allowing gas to escape into the perivascular space. The escaping air dissects along perivascular planes centrifugally to the hilum, where it ruptures into the mediastinum (pneumomediastinum) and then ruptures through the visceral pleura into the pleural space. Alternatively, when under tension in the interstitial space, air may rupture directly through the visceral pleura into the pleural space. When the air leak is confined to the interstitium of the lung, the condition is known as pulmonary interstitial emphysema (Fig. 40–3).

Chest roentgenograms demonstrating pneumothorax and pneumomediastinum are illustrated in Figures 40–4 and 40–5, respectively. When under sufficient pressure, air may dissect out of the thorax along subcutaneous tissue planes (subcutaneous emphysema) or into the peritoneal cavity (pneumoperitoneum) (see Fig. 40–5). Air may become loculated in lobar fissures to produce pulmonary pseudocysts. Less commonly, air that ruptures into the mediastinum may dissect into the pericardial space (pneumopericardium). Table 40–5 lists the clinical entities that result from air leak due to lung rupture. In the neonatal period, lung rupture can result from prolongation of the high transpulmonary pressure required during the first few breaths to open an airless lung, which opens sequentially. Prolonged application of high transpulmonary pressure across the normally aerated portions of the lung occurs because some of the airways may be occluded by aspirated blood, mucus, meconium, or squamous epithelium. The incidence of spontaneous pneumothorax in the newborn period is about 1 per cent. The newborn is particularly susceptible to uneven alveolar distention because the pores of Kohn, which normally allow interalveolar air distribution, are underdeveloped.

Hyaline membrane disease (HMD) with multiple areas of atelectasis can also lead to rupture of alveoli. Spontaneous air leak occurs in about 5 to 8 per cent of patients with HMD. There is conflicting evidence as to whether a continuous distending pressure during spontaneous ventilation increases the incidence of lung rupture in HMD. Continuous negative pressure is not associated with an increase in the incidence of air leak in HMD above the incidence of spontaneous air leak, but nasal continuous positive airway pressure (CPAP) has been associated with an increased incidence in some studies. The introduction of positive end-expiratory pressure (PEEP) during artificial ventilation has significantly increased the incidence of air leak in HMD.

The pathogenesis of pneumothorax in the older child can be disease specific. In cavitary or progressive tuberculosis, subpleural caseous infiltrates undergo liquefaction, resulting in pleural necrosis and rupture. Although an inflammatory response is elicited that attempts to seal off the rupture, bronchopleural fistula often persists. Pneumothoraces sometimes seen in miliary pulmonary tuberculosis are unexplained. Pulmonary metastases of a sarcoma have been postulated to grow very rapidly, outgrow their blood supply, and become necrotic, thereby rupturing the bronchus and pleural space and creating a bronchopleural fistula. Alternatively, tumor emboli cause lung infarction and necrosis and eventually air leak. Primary or metastatic pulmonary tumor may also cause lung rupture by ball-valve obstruction of an airway. In cystic fibrosis, pneumothorax results from rupture of subpleural blebs and large bullae—a result of chronic air trapping in patients with long-standing, more advanced obstructive lung disease. Rupture of blebs and bullae usually

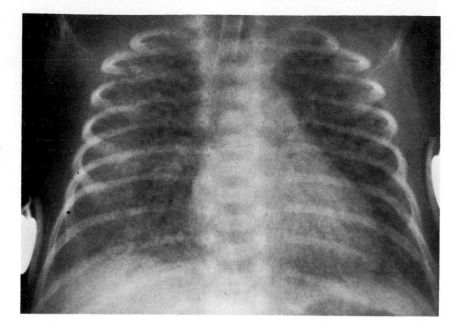

Figure 40–3. Chest radiograph of a neonate with hyaline membrane disease, demonstrating interstitial emphysema of the right lung.

occurs during exacerbation of pulmonary infection. In asthma, it is postulated that the visceral pleura is thinner and thus has increased susceptibility to rupture at transpulmonary pressures that would not allow rupture under normal circumstances. Moreover, mucoid impaction may be associated with expiratory obstruction, leading to overdistention and rupture of alveoli.

Functional Pathology

Irrespective of the age of the patient and the underlying cause of pneumothorax, massive or continued air leak elevates the intrapleural pressure to above atmospheric—so-called tension pneumothorax. The ipsilateral lung collapses because its elastic recoil can no longer be counteracted by the outward pull of a previously subatmospheric pleural

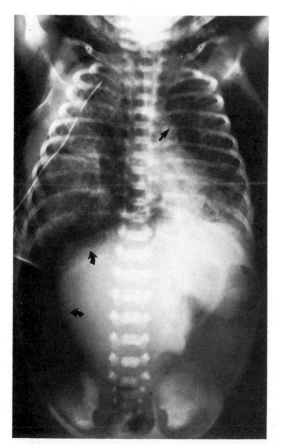

Figure 40–5. Chest radiograph of a neonate with hyaline membrane disease, demonstrating pneumomediastinum *(small arrow)*, massive subcutaneous emphysema, and pneumoperitoneum that is pushing the liver down *(two large arrows)*.

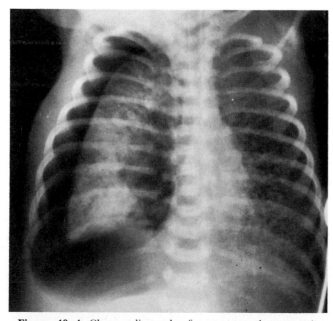

Figure 40–4. Chest radiograph of a neonate, demonstrating right pneumothorax.

Table 40–5. CLINICAL SPECTRUM OF AIR LEAK PHENOMENA SECONDARY TO RUPTURE OF ALVEOLI

Interstitial emphysema
Pneumomediastinum
Pneumothorax
Subcutaneous emphysema
Pneumoperitoneum
Pneumopericardium
Pulmonary pseudocyst
Pulmonary venous gas embolism

pressure. The contralateral lung is overexpanded during inspiration and develops a greater retractive force, thereby pulling the mediastinum toward it during expiration, impeding venous return to the heart. Because ventilation is impaired, greater inspiratory efforts develop in an attempt to generate sufficient negative pleural pressure to ventilate the normal lung, thereby aggravating the tension pneumothorax, shifting the mediastinum further, and severely impeding systemic venous return to the heart. Hypoxemia and hypercapnia result. Compensatory tachycardia occurs and further decreases diastolic filling and ventricular output, with cardiac standstill imminent unless pulmonary tamponade is decompressed. Lung collapse per se does not contribute in a major way to poor gas exchange because there is a redistribution of pulmonary blood flow to the normal lung with lower vascular resistance.

In addition to the intrapleural pressure developed and the inherent elastic recoil of the lung, the degree of lung collapse also varies with the cause of pneumothorax and the presence of visceroparietal adhesions. Chronic lung disease that decreases lung elastic recoil as well as concomitant pleural adhesions will restrain total collapse.

Diagnosis

Symptoms of pneumothorax vary according to the extent of lung collapse, degree of intrapleural pressure, rapidity of onset, and age and respiratory reserve of the patient. A patient may present suddenly in cardiorespiratory collapse without any clinical warning or antecedent roentgenographic change, or may be asymptomatic with the diagnosis initially made on the basis of a chest roentgenogram. Early recognition of lung rupture requires keen awareness of its possibility, particularly when dealing with diseases and clinical situations known to be associated with this complication (Table 40–6). Pneumothorax may also be a spontaneous event, unrelated to any known cause, particularly in the newborn infant.

In an otherwise normal neonate, symptoms of spontaneous pneumothorax are often subtle, and physical findings are misleading, because no abnormal physical findings may be immediately discernible. Certain clinical features, however, have been seen on close observation: the infant is unusually irritable; tachypnea with a respiratory rate above 60 per minute is invariably seen; and chest bulging is usually noticeable, especially if unilateral pneumothorax is present. A shift of the cardiac impulse away from the site of the pneumothorax is a useful sign but often cannot be confidently detected. As well, it is difficult to appreciate diminished air entry on the ipsilateral side because of the small size of the newborn chest. Grunting, retraction, and cyanosis are noted late in the progression of the complication.

In a newborn with underlying lung disease requiring some form of mechanical respiratory assistance, certain observations are useful to note. Rapid increase in inspiratory pressure reading on the respirator accompanied by sudden deterioration should immediately suggest a diagnosis of tension pneumothorax, which necessitates prompt needle decompression. Changes in vital signs include decreases in heart rate, blood pressure, and respiratory rate and narrowing of pulse pressure. An ominous clinical presentation is cardiorespiratory arrest. Even when deterioration is gradual, auscultation is often unreliable, because breath sounds from the remaining expansible areas of the lungs are clearly transmitted across the small newborn chest during mechanical ventilation. It is obvious that serial chest roentgenograms taken every 12 to 24 hours are essential during the early phase of ventilatory treatment of the newborn even in the absence of clinical signs of pneumothorax, because these signs can occur without forewarning. Moreover, in the presence of interstitial emphysema, pneumomediastinum, or hyperlucency of any lung zone, particularly when the infant is receiving continuous distending pressure, the clinician must be alert to the increased threat of impending serious air leak and pneumothorax.

Although certain limitations of physical examination of the chest have been alluded to, periodic physical reappraisal remains important and must be done whenever clinical worsening or deterioration in arterial gas tensions, or both, are observed. Additional nonroentgenographic tools for monitoring infants for the presence of pneumothorax in high-risk

Table 40–6. CONDITIONS ASSOCIATED WITH ALVEOLAR RUPTURE

First breath

Diagnostic and therapeutic maneuvers
  Thoracentesis
  Aspiration lung biopsy
  Percutaneous pleural biopsy
  Cardiothoracic surgery
  Resuscitation
  Ventilator therapy, especially with PEEP

Lower respiratory tract diseases

  Hyaline membrane disease
  Aspiration syndrome
  Asthma
  Cystic fibrosis
  Tuberculosis (cavitary; miliary)
  Pneumonia and bronchiolitis
  Malignancy (primary or metastatic)

Blunt thoracic trauma

PEEP, positive end-expiratory pressure.

situations, e.g., in hyaline membrane disease or meconium aspiration, and during mechanical ventilation, should be utilized; they include continuous electrocardiographic (ECG) display on the oscilloscope or intermittent ECG recording. A sudden decrease (40 per cent or more) or variability in the QRS voltage seen in the left precordial and standard leads I, II, and III should alert one to the occurrence of a pneumothorax. Care must be taken to avoid misdiagnosis from electronic artifacts, such as a change in standardization. Chest transillumination utilizing a powerful fiberoptic light probe has been effectively applied to diagnosis of pneumothorax at the bedside and has a distinct advantage on that basis. Wider application of these techniques can indicate the necessity for an early radiologic examination.

Roentgenographic confirmation is essential when the physical findings are minimal and cardiorespiratory function is only modestly altered. An anteroposterior chest film supplemented by a horizontal-beam cross-table lateral view with the patient supine or in the decubitus position can detect even relatively small amounts of intrapleural or mediastinal air. Pneumothorax has to be differentiated from lung cyst and lobar emphysema, in both of which the lower border of the radiolucency is crescentic; in addition, attenuated lung markings are seen in lobar emphysema. A skin fold is seen as a radiodense line extending beyond the skeletal chest wall boundary into the surrounding soft tissues, and lung markings may appear lateral to this line. A congenital diaphragmatic hernia can readily be identified in the following way: a nasogastric tube with a radiopaque tip is used for decompression and is then left in place while a radiograph is taken; if the tip is seen on the radiograph to be in the thoracic cavity, a diaphragmatic hernia is present.

In an older child, certain disease conditions—bronchiolitis, asthma, cystic fibrosis, pertussis syndrome, hydatid cyst, progressive primary pulmonary tuberculosis, metastatic sarcoma, staphylococcal pneumonia, and blunt thoracic injury—alert the clinician to the risk of pneumothorax. The diagnosis is suspected when a patient suddenly develops severe cardiorespiratory collapse or, less seriously, sudden pain in the chest or referred to the shoulder associated with dyspnea, cyanosis, and rapid shallow breathing. Contributory factors to the foregoing clinical setting include frequent paroxysms of cough, severity of the underlying lung disease, and the use of respirator therapy. The presence of pneumothorax is not as difficult to detect in older children as it is in the newborn infant, because it is easier to ascertain abnormal physical findings in the older child. Nonetheless, it must be realized that in children with diffuse, obstructive lung disorders the physical signs of the underlying disease may be similar to those of the pneumothorax and may be quite unchanged by the addition of this complication, except for the shift of the trachea and the apex beat. Even the latter may be difficult to locate in light of the overinflation. The scratch sign—loud and harsh sound heard over the midsternum when the affected side is stroked with a dull instrument or finger—may be elicited.

Radiologic confirmation during full expiration is helpful. Bullae, massive lung cyst, or partial obstruction with secondary overinflation may be mistaken for a chronic pneumothorax. Careful attention to details of the patient's history and assessment of the lung edge on chest film usually clarify the diagnosis. Another consideration is traumatic diaphragmatic hernia, which usually occurs on the left because of the shielding effect of the liver on the right and possible inherent weakness of the left leaf of the diaphragm. Attention should be directed to the convex shadow cast by the upper border of the stomach and to the linear opacities representing the bowel wall. Definitive diagnosis is made with a chest roentgenogram taken following a barium swallow. Errors in diagnosis may lead to trauma to the stomach, spleen, or other abdominal organs located in the chest cavity or to the development of a tension pneumothorax during attempts to insert a needle into an intrapulmonary air space.

Arterial gas tensions and pH may be normal initially, with P_{CO_2} even below normal at times. In the presence of unrelieved tension, however, acidosis, hypoxemia, and hypercapnia are invariably present.

Management

The functional consequences of a tension pneumothorax or of even a small pneumothorax in patients with respiratory insufficiency pose an immediate threat to life unless the intrapleural air is immediately evacuated. Effective management requires early clinical recognition and prompt radiologic investigation. Frequent utilization of electrocardiographic monitoring and chest transillumination hastens confirmation of the diagnosis and increases the chances of successful treatment.

A rational approach to therapeutic management of air leak complications should take into account clinical severity, presence and nature of the underlying lung disease, gestational and postnatal age, precipitating event, and history of recurrence. Attention must be directed equally to the treatment of the underlying disease process. With a small, nonprogressive, asymptomatic or mildly symptomatic pneumothorax in the term newborn infant that is not associated with any underlying disease, expectant care is frequently satisfactory, because the gas will eventually be absorbed. Conservative measures include frequent small feedings, mild sedation to minimize crying, and oxygen-enriched air. Spontaneous resolution is achieved in an average period of 48 hours (range 1 to 3 days). Absorption of the loculated pneumothorax is hastened sevenfold by oxygen inhalation, which increases the pressure gradient of gases between the pleura and the venous blood. Administration of high concentrations of oxygen to premature infants should always be closely monitored because of the dangers of retrolental fibroplasia. In the absence of a definitive roentgenographic picture that excludes the usual differential diagnoses, it is best to defer needle aspiration unless clinical worsening indicates a contrary approach. Needle perforation of a tension pulmonary cyst, congenital lobar emphysema, or a traumatic tear of the lung can add or lead to tension pneumothorax, resulting in a more precarious clinical situation.

In the presence of underlying disease, such as meconium aspiration or HMD, direct mechanical evacuation of intrapleural air should be performed unless the size of the pneumothorax is very small, the underlying disorder is mild, and the clinical status is stable. However, close clinical and blood gas monitoring are integral parts of management. Appropriate measures must be taken as soon as clinical or biochemical deterioration is detected.

Mechanical evacuation of air from the pleural cavity is achieved by direct needle aspiration via a catheter attached to a one-way flutter valve (Heimlich valve) requiring no underwater seal or suction or via an underwater seal tube drainage with suction applied. The choice depends on the clinical circumstances. Direct needle aspiration using the second or third intercostal space along the midclavicular line is warranted for prompt decompression of a severe tension pneumothorax.

For a neonate with minimal underlying disease and small to medium-sized pneumothorax, an Argyle thoracic semirigid catheter size French 12 is used. The catheter is mounted on a trocar to facilitate its introduction, and it has terminal and side holes for better air evacuation and a radiopaque sentinel line for radiographic visualization. With strict asepsis and under local anesthesia, the catheter is inserted through a small skin incision over the anterior second or third intercostal space just lateral to the midclavicular line and is introduced deeply enough to ensure that the side holes are within the pleural cavity (surgical emphysema may develop if the side holes lie immediately underneath the skin). The catheter is then secured to the skin, using a purse-string suture technique. After the initial evacuation of intrapleural air with a syringe, a Heimlich valve is fitted directly onto the external end of the catheter, requiring no adaptor. The valve allows air to escape but prevents its reflux and functions equally well in the presence of fluid that may drain. Fluid can cause sticking of the one-way rubber valve, which therefore should be cleaned at least once every 12 hours or whenever any significant fluid drainage occurs. The connection between the catheter and the valve is sealed off with adhesive tape, and the area around the tube insertion is similarly sealed. The entire setup is then attached to the anterior chest wall, with care taken to ensure that the distal end is unimpeded.

An underwater seal system, however, has to be used when there is a large or continued air leak that exceeds the outflow capacity of the Heimlich valve; when the patient is receiving intermittent positive pressure ventilation, particularly with concomitant application of a continuous distending pressure at end-expiration; and when associated fluid drainage interferes with the free exit of air. Care is taken to ensure that the drainage tube is no deeper than 2 cm under water; if it is deeper, air will not drain until a higher pressure builds up in the pleural space. Suction is applied at a pressure of -5 to -15 cm H_2O.

Shortly after the procedure, a chest film should be taken to assess expansion of the lungs. The drainage tube is left in place for an average period of 3 days. The time to extubate is crucial, and once the decision has been made, extubation must be a sequential process. First, suction is discontinued after continued air leak has ceased. Cessation of air leak is recognized by cessation of air bubbling in the drainage tube under the water seal during the respiratory cycle. Patency of the tube is assured by observing the swing of the water meniscus, which normally oscillates during respiration. After cessation of air leak is established and complete lung expansion is confirmed by roentgenography, the tube is withdrawn. The tube should *not* remain in place clamped for an extended period before its withdrawal.

Pneumomediastinum seldom causes severe cardiorespiratory difficulty. However, if the gas does not decompress by extension to the pleural or subcutaneous spaces, high pressures may result. In rare circumstances, direct decompression of the mediastinum may be achieved by placement of a needle behind the sternum from below (xiphoid approach) or by a small incision at the sternal notch.

Pulmonary interstitial emphysema may be treated by increasing inspired O_2 concentration and by reducing ventilator pressures. Occasionally, selective bronchial intubation of the normal side may be used to decompress the affected lung. Very high-frequency, low-pressure ventilation has been used with some success in patients with bilateral disease. Occasionally, interstitial emphysema of the lung persists as loculated gas spaces and necessitates surgical removal, particularly in small premature infants requiring ventilator therapy for HMD.

Pneumopericardium may be managed conservatively by lowering ventilatory flow rates and end-expiratory pressure. If the cardiac size is markedly reduced or there is rapid onset of hypotension associated with muffled heart tones, bradycardia, and cyanosis, immediate pericardiocentesis is indicated to relieve cardiac tamponade.

Pneumoperitoneum from alveolar rupture must be differentiated from that due to a perforated viscus, which requires immediate surgical intervention. When the pneumoperitoneum is associated with extensive pulmonary air leak in an infant who is otherwise in relatively good condition, conservative medical therapy utilizing high inspired oxygen and adjustment of ventilator pressures may suffice. Paracentesis is done when increased abdominal pressure adds to dyspnea.

The therapeutic approach to management for the neonate just outlined applies to any pediatric patient. Drainage by a one-way flutter valve usually suffices for the older child with mild or moderately symptomatic spontaneous pneumothorax. Special considerations, however, are taken in the management of older children in whom the predisposing or underlying clinical conditions may be asthma, tuberculosis, metastatic sarcoma, or cystic fibrosis. Immediate closed thoracotomy with insertion of a water-seal intercostal tube is the treatment of choice for pneumothorax complicating acute asthma or progressive pulmonary tuberculosis, because any further reduction in pulmonary function should be avoided. In tuberculosis, too much suction is avoided, because it can sometimes keep the fistula patent. In the older child with a large fistula, subsequent decortication may be necessary.

Management of the complication in patients with cystic fibrosis involves several considerations. In the first attack of a small asymptomatic unilateral pneumothorax, expectant care in the hospital and treatment of acute pulmonary infection are usually followed by resolution. In the case of bilateral pneumothorax, one may elect to decompress initially only the side associated with greater lung collapse in anticipation of spontaneous resolution on the other, less severely involved side. If spontaneous resolution in either situation does not occur or if the initial episode is a large pneumothorax, mechanical drainage is done. Whenever feasible, use of a portable device (e.g., Heimlich valve) is recommended, because it permits early mobilization, which is particularly important in this group of children. Otherwise, the underwater seal system under suction is used. The underwater seal system is indicated whenever the pneumothorax reduces lung volume by 50 per cent or more or is increasing in size and causing dyspnea in a patient with poor respiratory reserve. After most of the intrapleural air has been evacuated, pleurodesis is recommended for those patients with persistent or recurrent pneumothorax, because major pulmonary surgery is a great risk for them. The sclerosing agent favored by most is quinacrine hydrochloride, which is instilled into the pleura at a dose of 100 mg in 15 ml of saline, with the patient positioned for an hour with the affected side down; this procedure is repeated daily until four doses have been given. If this approach fails, open thoracotomy with segmental resection and pleurectomy are undertaken, except in patients with far-advanced respiratory insufficiency and cor pulmonale. A similar surgical procedure is indicated in any child with chronic pneumothorax (longer than 3 months), irrespective of cause.

Prognosis

Prognosis is a function of the severity (i.e., with or without tension) and type (i.e., spontaneous, traumatic, or associated with parenchymal disease) of pneumothorax, the nature of the underlying lung disorder, and the promptness of diagnosis and evacuation of the intrapleural air. Preparedness is the key factor to an excellent outcome. Thus in hospital areas where high-risk patients are cared for, that is, in intensive care units for newborns, infants, and older children, and in emergency departments, an equipment tray containing a 50-ml syringe, a three-way stopcock, an 18-gauge needle, a kidney basin, and a bottle of sterile saline should always be at hand. Medical and nursing personnel should have an ongoing program of preparedness and should be able to intervene promptly and appropriately when the need arises.

REFERENCES

Liquid in the Pleural Space
Badrinas F, Rodriguez-Roisin R, Rives A, and Picada C: Multiple myeloma with pleural involvement. Am Rev Respir Dis 110:82, 1974.
Black LF: The pleural space and the pleural fluid. Mayo Clin Proc 47:493, 1972.
Chernick V and Reed MH: Pneumothorax and chylothorax in the neonatal period. J Pediatr 76:624, 1970.
Dines D, Pierre RV, and Franzen S: The value of cells in the pleural fluid in the differential diagnosis. Mayo Clin Proc 50:571, 1975.
Dippel WF, Doty DB, and Ehrenhaft JL: Tension hemothorax due to patent ductus arteriosus. N Engl J Med 288:353, 1973.
Hyde R, Hall C, and Hall WJ: New pulmonary diagnostic procedures. Am J Dis Child 126:292, 1973.
Kosloske AM, Martin LW, and Schubert WK: Management of chylothorax in children by thoracentesis and medium-chain triglyceride feedings. J Pediatr Surg 9:365, 1974.
Light RW and Luchsinger PC: Metabolic activity of pleural liquid. J Appl Physiol 34:97, 1973.
Light RW, Macgregor MI, Luchsinger PC, and Ball WC: Pleural effusions: diagnostic separation of transudates and exudates. Ann Intern Med 77:507, 1972.
Mellins RB, Levine DR, and Fishman AP: Effect of systemic and pulmonary venous hypertension on pleural and pericardial fluid accumulation. J Appl Physiol 29:564, 1970.
Moskowitz H, Platt RT, Schachar R, and Mellins H: Roentgen visualization of minute pleural effusion. Radiology 109:33, 1973.
Murchison WG, Harper WK, and Putnam JS: Traumatic diaphragmatic hernia: late presentation as bloody pleural effusion. Chest 66:734, 1974.
Nelson DG and Loudon RG: Sarcoidosis with pleural involvement. Am Rev Respir Dis 108:647, 1973.
Staub NC: Pathogenesis of pulmonary edema. Am Rev Respir Dis 109:358, 1974.
Wang N: The preformed stomas connecting the pleural cavity and the lymphatics in the parietal pleura. Am Rev Respir Dis 111:12, 1975.

Air in the Pleural Space
Aranda JV, Stern L, and Dunbar JS: Pneumothorax with pneumoperitoneum in a newborn infant. Am J Dis Child 123:163, 1972.
Berg TJ, Pagtakhan RD, Reed MH et al: Bronchopulmonary dysplasia and lung rupture in hyaline membrane disease: influence of continuous distending pressure. Pediatrics 55:51, 1975.
Dines DE, Cortese D, Brennan MD et al: Malignant pulmonary neoplasms predisposing to spontaneous pneumothorax. Mayo Clin Proc 48:541, 1973.
Glauser FL and Bartlett RH: Pneumoperitoneum in association with pneumothorax. Chest 66:536, 1974.
Heimlich HJ: Valve drainage of the pleural cavity. Dis Chest 53:282, 1968.

Kattwinkel J, Taussig LM, McIntosh CL et al: Intrapleural instillation of quinacrine for recurrent pneumothorax. JAMA 226:557, 1973.

Katz S and Horres AD: Medullary respiratory neuron response to pulmonary emboli and pneumothorax. J Appl Physiol 33:390, 1972.

Kirkpatrick BV, Felman AH, and Eitzman DV: Complications of ventilator therapy in respiratory distress syndrome. Am J Dis Child 128:496, 1974.

Kuhns LR, Bednarck FJ, Wyman ML et al: Diagnosis of pneumothorax or pneumomediastinum in the neonate by transillumination. Pediatrics 56:355, 1975.

Kuritzky P and Goldfarb AL: Unusual electrocardiographic changes in spontaneous pneumothorax. Chest 70:535, 1976.

Lackey DA, Ukrainski CT, and Taber P: The management of tension pneumothorax in the neonate using the Heimlich flutter valve. J Pediatr 84:438, 1974.

Macklin CC: Transport of air along sheaths of pulmonic blood vessels from alveoli to mediastinum. Arch Intern Med 64:913, 1939.

Malan AF and Heese H de V: Spontaneous pneumothorax in the newborn. Acta Pediatr Scand 55:224, 1966.

Merenstein GB, Dougherty K, and Lewis A: Early detection of pneumothorax by oscilloscope monitor in the newborn infant. J Pediatr 80:98, 1972.

Ogata ES, Gregory GA, Kitterman JA et al: Pneumothorax in the respiratory distress syndrome: incidence and effect on vital signs, blood gases, and pH. Pediatrics 58:177, 1976.

Pomerance JJ, Weller MH, Richardson CJ et al: Pneumopericardium complicating respiratory distress syndrome: role of conservative management. J Pediatr 84:883, 1974.

Summers RS: The electrocardiogram as a diagnostic aid in pneumothorax. Chest 63:127, 1973.

Wilson JL: Factors involved in the production of alveolar rupture with mechanical aids to respiration. Pediatrics 13:146, 1954.

Liquid and Air in the Pleural Space

Agostoni E: Mechanics of the pleural space. Physiol Rev 52:57, 1972.

Grosfeld JL and Ballantine TVN: Surgical respiratory distress in infancy and childhood. Curr Probl Pediatr 6:1, 1976.

Murray JF: The Normal Lung: The Basis for Diagnosis and Treatment of Pulmonary Disease. Philadelphia, WB Saunders Co, 1976.

41

C. WARREN BIERMAN, M.D., and
DAVID S. PEARLMAN, M.D.

ASTHMA

Asthma is a disorder of the tracheobronchial tree characterized by mild to severe obstruction of airflow. In a given patient, the obstruction may improve spontaneously or may subside only after intensive therapy. Symptoms varying from recurrent paroxysms of dyspnea to coughing are generally episodic and paroxysmal and may last for hours to days or persist for months to years. A predominant feature of asthma is heightened airway irritability, manifested by hyperreactivity of the trachea and bronchi to irritants (Boushey et al, 1980; Townley et al, 1975). So characteristic is this feature that asthma has been termed "reactive airways disorder."

The clinical hallmark of asthma is wheezing, a squeaking expiratory sound made through the partially obstructed larger airways. Cough also is characteristic of asthma and may be the predominant symptom (Cloutier and Loughlin, 1981). However, asthma may occur without discernible wheezing (McFadden, 1975a; Corrao et al, 1979; Koenig, 1981). In the absence of recurrent episodes of overt wheezing, the diagnosis may be missed, especially in children. All too frequently, children are considered to have "recurrent pneumonia," "recurrent" or "chronic" bronchitis, or simply "recurrent colds with chest congestion" (Taussig et al, 1981). Because of frequent misconceptions about the etiology of asthma and its course and prognosis, asthma is a greatly undertreated disorder in children, and its physical, psychological, and socioeconomic morbidity is unnecessarily high (Speight et al, 1983; Pearlman, 1984).

EPIDEMIOLOGY

Although a great deal has been written about the prevalence of asthma in children, the published papers are confusing because their authors have not agreed on a single definition of asthma or on a uniform method of obtaining epidemiologic information. Prevalence estimates for asthma derived from patient/parent questionnaires, for example, are much lower than those based on physician assessment (Williams and McNicol, 1969). As a result, the prevalence is greatly underestimated, and the morbidity and prognosis in children are considered to be more favorable than they really are (Smith, 1978; Slavin and Smith, 1988).

Although general surveys estimate the prevalence of asthma in the general population to be less than 5 per cent (Wilder, 1973; Speizer, 1976; Gregg, 1977;

Some of the material appears in a slightly different form in Allergic Diseases from Infancy to Adulthood. 2nd ed. Philadelphia, WB Saunders Co, 1988.

Smith, 1978), other surveys suggest an incidence in children ranging from 7 per cent (Rhyne et al, 1971) to 19 per cent (Williams and McNicol, 1969). The wide variation results from a difference in the techniques used to obtain data, e.g., physician evaluation versus patient/parent questionnaires. Other factors relate to geographic differences, with particularly low rates reported in children from Scandinavian countries (Gregg, 1977; Smith, 1978); to racial differences, with low incidence in Eskimo and American Indian populations and variable reports of lower incidence among blacks (Gregg, 1977; Smith, 1978); and to environmental differences (Smith, 1961, 1975). Differences in prevalence of asthma reported in various parts of the United States (Wilder, 1973) may reflect differences in diagnostic criteria. Conflicting data relating to socioeconomic status may reflect the problems of crowding and poverty in lower socioeconomic groups or the availability of better medical care in higher socioeconomic groups.

Asthma frequently begins in childhood, although estimates of the incidence of asthma in various age groups vary widely. Most children develop asthma before age 8, perhaps half before age 3 (Wilder, 1973; Gregg, 1977; Slavin and Smith, 1988). Before puberty, asthma occurs one-and-one-half to three times as frequently in boys as in girls. In adolescence, this difference between the sexes tends to equalize (Gregg, 1977; Smith, 1978; Slavin and Smith, 1988), whereas adult-onset asthma appears to occur more frequently in women.

The familial association among asthma, allergic rhinitis, and atopic dermatitis suggests that these disorders may have a common genetic basis. Attempts to define the heritability of asthma, however, have led only to speculation about a genetic basis. The highly frequent association between these three disorders and laboratory or clinical evidence of "allergy" at first complicated the analysis of an already complex issue. Schwartz (1952) was among the first to point out that the likelihood for the development of asthma depends more on a family history of asthma per se than on a family history of other "allergic" disorders. The familial or genetic "tendency" appears to come from both sides of the family: the likelihood of asthma is greater if one parent has asthma than if neither does and greater still if both parents are asthmatic (VanArsdel and Motulsky, 1959). Although this familial association has generally been interpreted in genetic terms, there is at least some suggestion that there may be alternative explanations, reflecting, for example, familial transmission of infectious agents that precipitate disease (Smith, 1978).

Studies of twins have shown that if one twin has asthma, the likelihood of the other having asthma is much greater, with identical twins having a greater tendency for asthma concordance than fraternal twins (Lubs, 1971). Even with identical twins, however, concordance rates are less than 50 per cent. Consequently, it is generally accepted that there is a heritable "propensity" to develop asthma, but that environmental factors also are critical determinants for the development of the disease.

Family studies of the relationship between asthma and IgE-mediated diseases have revealed further the separability of various phenomena associated with so-called allergic disorders. For example, in family constellations in which asthma occurs, there is a higher incidence of asthma and of allergic rhinitis than in the population at large (Cooke and VanderVeer, 1916; Rooney and Williams, 1971; Smith, 1978). However, various patterns pertinent to these associations are revealed: some family members have allergic rhinitis without asthma, others have asthma and allergic rhinitis, others may have asthma without allergic rhinitis, and still others share no clinical stigmata of allergy at all (Sibbald et al, 1980). Thus in spite of frequent associations between asthma and allergic factors and among various allergic (atopic) disorders, allergy and disorders commonly associated with allergy can "sequester" within families separately from one another. In general, the greater the number of these family factors present within a family, the younger the child will be when allergic diseases, including asthma, occur (Cooke and VanderVeer, 1916). Thus allergic factors may be associated with asthma, but "allergy" is not a prerequisite for the development of asthma.

Although the separability of asthma and "allergy" is recognized, the strong association between these two factors in the pediatric age group also is striking. In many estimates, two thirds to three fourths of all children with asthma are "allergic" (Rackemann and Edwards, 1952; Williams et al, 1958; Ford, 1969; Davis, 1976). A number of environmental factors may precipitate asthma and initiate airway hyperreactivity. The onset of asthmatic symptoms in both childhood and adult life is commonly associated with viral respiratory tract infection, respiratory syncytial virus in particular being a major culprit in childhood (Rooney and Williams, 1971; McIntosh et al, 1973). Other viral organisms that are more likely to be associated with asthma include parainfluenza virus, rhinovirus, coronavirus, adenovirus, and influenza virus (McIntosh et al, 1973; Mitchell et al, 1976). There also are high associations between bronchiolitis in infancy and the subsequent development of asthma (Rooney and Williams, 1971; McIntosh, 1976) and between bronchiolitis and the development of airway hyperreactivity with or without overt asthma (Gurwitz et al, 1981). Studies of Welliver and colleagues (1980) raise the possibility that the development of IgE antibody to respiratory virus plays a strategic role in inducing an allergic response to virus. Although viral organisms may play an etiologic role in instigating asthma in some children, clearly not all respiratory syncytial or other respiratory virus infections lead to asthma, nor does it appear that respiratory viral infection is a prerequisite for the development of asthma. Exposure to allergic factors, industrial irritants, and even psychological factors have been claimed to instigate asthma. It would appear that various kinds of environmental factors may be associated with the onset of asthma and that once asthma develops, these same and other factors may play a role in precipitating or aggravating symptoms.

Despite the relatively high prevalence of asthma, mortality rates for asthma in childhood fortunately are extremely low. The mortality rate for asthmatics is less than 0.1 per cent per year, a relatively low yet significant rate. In addition, asthma deaths appear to be increasing in many Western countries (Asthma Deaths, 1986). Considering the relatively lower mortality rates in children with asthma than in adults and the presumed prevalence of asthma in childhood, the overall mortality rate in childhood probably is less than 1 in 20,000 asthmatic children per year (authors' estimate). Nevertheless, children do die of asthma, and there is an unquestionable risk of death in severely asthmatic children. Analyses of causes of death in children with asthma indicate that the major causes are the failure of the physician, parent, or patient to appreciate the severity of asthma, which results in inadequate or delayed treatment, and the use of inappropriate medications, such as sedatives that depress respiration (Richards and Patrick, 1965; Fischer and Ghory, 1975). Morbidity in asthma, however, is extraordinarily high. In an analysis covering the years 1959 to 1961, Schiffer and Hunt (1963) found that more than 7.5 million school days were lost because of asthma each year. Children spent more than 11 million days in bed because of their asthma; and annually there were more than 24 million days in which activity had to be restricted because of asthma. According to 1971 statistics on asthmatic children and adults, each asthmatic spent almost 6 days in bed each year because of asthma and lost at least 1 school or work day; activity was restricted on an average of 15 days a year for each asthmatic. Children with moderately severe to severe asthma tend to perform poorly in school, undoubtedly because of lost time at school, restriction of activity, and loss of sleep. The effects of these symptoms on adjustment and function in adult life are not known, but asthma plays a significant and inadequately appreciated role in adult life as well.

PATHOLOGY

Examination of post-mortem lung specimens of patients who died of asthma shows marked hyperinflation with smooth muscle hyperplasia of bronchial and bronchiolar walls, thick tenacious mucus plugs often completely occluding the airways, markedly thickened basement membrane, and variable degrees of mucosal edema and denudation of bronchial and bronchiolar epithelium (Fig. 41–1). Eosinophilia of the submucosa and secretions is prominent whether or not allergic (IgE-mediated) mechanisms are present. Plasma cells that contain IgG, IgM, and IgA may be seen, and in some patients plasma cells that contain IgE also are seen. Occasionally, the inflammatory response is indicative of infection, a finding more common in adults, especially those with concurrent chronic bronchitis. Mucus plugs contain layers of shed epithelial cells, which may form creola bodies (sloughed epithelial clumps) and eosinophils, and may contain polymorphonuclear neutrophils, lymphocytes, and plasma cells. Charcot-Leyden crystals from eosinophils and mucous casts of the airways with epithelial cell clumps (Curschmann spirals) also are observed. Toxic products from eosinophils, in particular, may play an important role in the destructive changes observed (Frigas and Gleich, 1986). The mucosal edema with separated columnar cells and stratified nonciliated epithelium, which replace ciliated epithelium, results in abnormal mucociliary clearance. Mast cells often are absent, possibly reflecting degranulation and discharge of the chemical mediators. Submucous gland hypertrophy and increased goblet cell size are not constant features of asthma, being more characteristic of chronic bronchitis. The long-recognized inflammatory nature of the bronchial response with desquamation of the bronchial epithelium has only recently been emphasized in the contexts of both pathophysiology and important clinical therapeutic implications (see subsequent discussion). The development of bronchial hyperresponsiveness, considered to be an important pathogenetic feature in patients with current symptomatic asthma, has been attributed to "late" cellular inflammatory responses initiated by allergic and other nonimmune mechanisms (Cockroft, 1985; Larsen, 1985; Hargreave et al, 1986).

The thickened basement membrane is a striking feature of asthma and has been reported even in "mild" asthmatics, sometimes associated with deposition of various immunoglobulins. Part of the apparent thickening is due actually to submembrane deposition of collagen and various other materials. Basement membrane thickening is thought to occur early in the disease, but its pathogenetic significance remains to be determined. All of these findings have been observed in symptom-free asthmatic individuals who died accidental deaths (Fig. 41–2). On the one hand, although an occasional patient may show localized bronchiectasis and small focal areas of alveolar destruction, these are not characteristic of asthma, and there is little evidence that asthma leads to destructive emphysema. On the other hand, "distensive emphysema," a clinically significant diminution in pulmonary elasticity, may be a concomitant of long-standing alveolar hyperinflation. Bronchiectasis is rare in asthma but may occur in association with allergic bronchopulmonary aspergillosis when it involves the proximal branches and in a small number of patients with similar disorders. Incomplete reversibility of airflow limitation seen in some asthmatics suggests that some of the pathologic changes noted may, in fact, have long-term clinical implications.

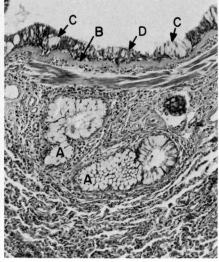

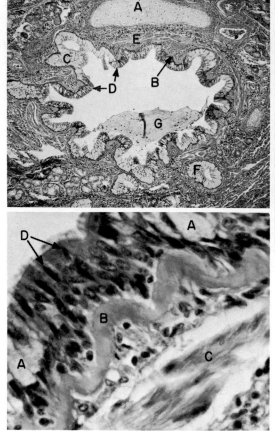

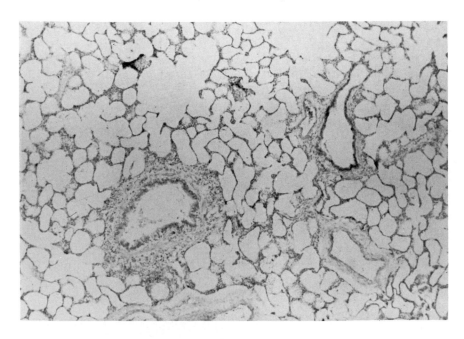

Figure 41–1. Sections of asthmatic lung. *Top left,* Cross section of bronchus (×66) showing *A,* cartilage; *B,* basement membrane, which is thickened; *C,* epithelium containing many goblet cells; *D,* area of many ciliated epithelial cells; *E,* connective tissue; *F,* mucous gland; *G,* mucus plug. *Top right,* Bronchial epithelium (×136) showing *A,* mucous glands; *B,* hyaline basement membrane; *C,* goblet cells; *D,* ciliated cells. *Bottom left,* Bronchial epithelium (×700) showing *A,* goblet cell; *B,* basement membrane; *C,* connective tissue; *D,* ciliated respiratory epithelial cells.

PATHOPHYSIOLOGY

Airflow limitation in asthma results from a combination of obstructive processes. This combination, principally mucosal edema, bronchospasm, and mucous plugging, can be seen or can be inferred from the pathologic findings in asthma. The relative roles these processes play in producing obstruction may differ, however, according to the age of the child, the size and anatomy of various portions of the airway, the type of agent precipitating obstruction, and the duration and severity of asthma.

Airway obstruction results in increased resistance to airflow through the trachea and bronchi and in decreased flow rates due to narrowing and premature closure of the smaller airways. These changes lead to

Figure 41–2. Pulmonary changes in a toddler who died of aminophylline suppository intoxication. Note the infiltration of cells around the bronchus with sloughing of epithelial cells into the bronchial lumen. The alveoli all appear normal.

a decreased ability to expel air and result in hyper-inflation. Although pulmonary overdistention benefits respiration by helping to maintain airway patency, the work of breathing increases because of the altered pulmonary mechanics. To a certain extent, increasing lung volumes can compensate for pulmonary obstruction, but compensation is limited as tidal volume approaches the volume of pulmonary dead space, with resultant alveolar hypoventilation (McFadden, 1976, 1980b; Permutt, 1977).

Changes in resistance to airflow are not uniform throughout the tracheobronchial tree, and because of regional differences in this resistance, the distribution of inspired air is uneven, more air flowing to the less resistant portions. The pulmonary circulation also is affected by hyperinflation, which induces increased intrapleural and intra-alveolar pressures and uneven circulation to the alveoli. The increased intra-alveolar pressure, decreased ventilation, and decreased perfusion (the last through hypoxic vasoconstriction) lead to variable and uneven ventilation-perfusion relationships within different lung units. The ultimate result is early reduction in blood oxygenation, even though carbon dioxide is eliminated effectively because of its ready diffusibility across alveolar capillary membranes. Thus early in asthma, hypoxemia is common in the absence of CO_2 retention, even in asymptomatic asthmatic children. The hyperventilation resulting from the hypoxemic drive causes a fall in Pa_{CO_2}. However, as the obstruction becomes more severe and the number of alveoli being adequately ventilated and perfused decreases, a point is reached at which CO_2 retention occurs (i.e., respiratory failure).

Alterations in pH homeostasis result from respiratory and metabolic factors. Early in the course of acute asthma, respiratory alkalosis may occur because of hyperventilation. Coincidentally, metabolic acidosis occurs because of the increased work of breathing, increased oxygen consumption, and increased cardiac output. Metabolic acidosis is a problem, especially in young children, who have little glycogen reserve and inadequate caloric intake because of anorexia or vomiting and fever. When respiratory failure is superimposed, respiratory acidosis may result in a precipitous fall in pH. In an attempt to perfuse the lung adequately, pulmonary arterial pressure may increase to match increasing intra-alveolar pressure, possibly resulting in pulmonary hypertension and right heart strain.

Hyperinflation is matched by increased residual volume and decreased vital capacity. Pulmonary hyperventilation may be severe and prolonged and may cause permanent anatomic changes ("barrel chest," pectus excavatum or carinatum, and "asthmatic pseudo-rickets"), particularly in young children with soft and developing rib cages (Gilliam et al, 1970).

The site and degree of obstruction may differ in a given patient from one asthma attack to another. In most patients with asthma, both larger and smaller airways are obstructed. Some patients may have small airway obstruction primarily or even exclusively (McFadden, 1975b). Even in a patient whose asthma involves the entire tracheobronchial tree, there may be a difference in how the large and small airways respond to inciting agents. Thus in acute, relatively short-lived asthmatic episodes, the large airways may be involved predominantly. Obstruction of smaller airways occurs more slowly (Cade et al, 1971). Also, relief of obstruction, either with treatment or with time, occurs more promptly in larger than in smaller airways (Cade et al, 1971). Indeed, chronic partially irreversible small airway obstruction may occur in asymptomatic asthmatic children (Weng and Levison, 1969).

In short attacks of acute asthma, bronchospasm, mucosal edema, or both probably predominate. Mucous secretions become far more important as a cause of obstruction as the inflammation becomes more intense and prolonged, for example, during a respiratory viral infection, when damage to and sloughing of epithelial cells impair mucociliary function and increase reflex bronchoconstriction.

The severity, location, and sites of obstruction are related also to age. In the early months of postnatal life, peripheral bronchioles enlarge, and alveoli multiply rapidly. Respiratory surface area doubles by age 18 months and trebles by age 3 years, so only a small reserve for gas exchange is present in the very young child. Conducting airways increase in size from infancy to adulthood. In young children, the small airways account for about 50 per cent of the airways resistance. In children above the age of 5 years and in adolescents and adults, 80 per cent of resistance lies in airways larger than 2 mm in diameter. Thus any change in small airways resistance induced by asthma seriously affects the young child, whereas considerable increase in small airways resistance may occur without symptoms in the older child (Simons and Chernick, 1988). The amount of smooth muscle in the wall of the peripheral airways is scanty in the infant and increases throughout early childhood. Moreover, there are more mucous glands per square centimeter of mucosa in the major bronchi in normal infants than in normal children, and the adult distribution of mucous glands is not reached until later childhood. Accordingly, mechanical obstruction from edema, mucus, and cellular infiltrates, which is slow to reverse, is a much more important component of airways obstruction in the infant than bronchospasm, which is more easily reversed. This difference is reflected in the higher numbers of young children requiring hospitalization for control of asthma.

ETIOLOGY

The influence of factors such as wind, temperature, weather changes, exposure to animals, and emotional changes has been recognized for centuries (Maimonides, cited in Muntner, 1963). The spasmodic nature of asthmatic attacks and the inability to account for episodic symptoms at autopsy fortified an impression that asthma was related to physical and psychological "nervous" factors that induced "bronchial spasms." In 1915, Eppinger and Hess postulated that asthma was a disease of neurologic origin and was due to an autonomic imbalance, specifically, an overactivity or dominance of the parasympathetic over the sympathetic components of the nervous system.

With the discovery of antibodies and the recognition that they could both protect against and cause disease, a relationship between asthma in humans and anaphylaxis in guinea pigs was suspected (Meltzer, 1910). When a skin-sensitizing substance with antibody-like activity was discovered, it was related to certain clinical diseases, including asthma and hay fever. This common relationship among presence of skin-sensitizing antibody, asthma, and hay fever and the strong familial occurrence of these disorders led to their inclusion under a single descriptive term—atopy, meaning "strangeness." Atopic disorders were considered to be familial and presumably genetic in origin, more or less confined to humans, and often associated with the peculiar skin-sensitizing antibody (atopic reagin). Once an association between these disorders and atopic reagin was appreciated, it was a natural step to assume that the production of atopic reagin was the basis for the development of these disorders, a concept still held by some physicians today.

Rackemann in 1917 divided asthma into two categories: "extrinsic" asthma, which was thought to be precipitated by allergens external to the body, and "intrinsic" asthma, which was thought to be related to bacterial allergens, present within the body. This concept has since been modified, so intrinsic asthma today is ordinarily considered to be nonallergic, that is, asthma that is not IgE-mediated.

In the vast majority of asthmatic children, specific IgE antibody can be demonstrated to a variety of allergens. Often there is a relationship between the presence of specific antibody and the development of symptoms on exposure to the corresponding antigens. However, IgE antibody is not always associated with asthma (Aas, 1970). Rarely are allergic factors exclusive precipitants of asthma in children or adults. Szentivanyi (1968) pointed out that a common denominator in asthma is the hyperreactivity of the tracheobronchial tree to various chemical mediators of inflammation. These mediators in turn may be activated or liberated by numerous mechanisms. He postulated that the constitutional basis for asthma may be a defect of autonomic regulation in counterbalancing the bronchial obstructive effect of these mediators, specifically arising through a deficit in beta-adrenergic receptor function. Various other theories, including alterations of mucosal permeability through interruption of tight junctions between epithelial cells (Hogg, 1981) or cholinergic hyperreactivity through increased irritant receptor sensitivity (Nadel, 1977) or abnormality of mechanisms associated with calcium flux (Cerrina et al, 1981), have also

been proposed. These theories are not mutually exclusive, and indeed, each may be applicable to the general syndrome of "asthma." Whatever the explanation for the etiology of asthma, it is apparent that the clinical and pathologic features of asthma, the mediators involved, and the responses to pharmacotherapeutic agents are similar, whether or not "allergy" is implicated as an important factor in the disorder. Although the clinical syndrome of asthma and evidence of hyperreactivity are frequently associated with the ability to produce IgE antibody, there is strong evidence for separate inheritances of asthma and the propensity for IgE antibody formation (Sibbald et al, 1980). Children who develop asthma early in life with viral respiratory tract infection frequently develop allergic asthma when they grow older. Conversely, children with allergic asthma who continue to have asthma in adulthood often appear to lose evidence of IgE-mediated disease. Thus the common denominator in patients with asthma appears to be airway hyperreactivity to various chemical mediators of inflammation or neurohormonal regulators of airflow in the tracheobronchial tree. There appears to be far better correlation of the severity of asthma and the medication required for its control with the degree of airway hyperreactivity to histamine, methacholine, or both than with allergic factors, even in an allergic asthmatic (Makino, 1966; Cockroft, Killian, Mellon, and Hargreave, 1977; Hargreave et al, 1981). Airway hyperreactivity is not a universal finding in asthma, however, and its role in the etiology of asthma is unclear. Nevertheless, airway hyperresponsiveness does have important pathogenetic and clinical implications (Pearlman, 1984).

Increased airway reactivity can be induced by infectious agents (principally viral) (Little et al, 1978); allergens (Cockroft, Ruffin, Dolovich, and Hargreave, 1977); industrial exposures based on mechanisms that are not necessarily allergic (Lam et al, 1979); and atmospheric pollutants (Holtzman et al, 1979). Once hyperreactivity occurs, it becomes nonspecific in the sense that there is then oversensitivity to various mediators as well as to various precipitating agents. The degree of airway hyperreactivity varies among asthmatics and is known to increase and decrease from time to time in a given asthmatic, in part because of the degree of exposure to agents that initially induced heightened airway reactivity (Cockroft, Killian, Mellon, and Hargreave, 1977; Lam et al, 1979).

Asthma occurs in families, suggesting that it may be transmitted genetically, although the genetic transmission is not clear. For example, the development of asthma is greater in identical than in nonidentical twins, but concordance is less than 50 per cent (Lubs, 1971). This fact suggests that environmental factors may be equal in importance to inherited factors and that airway hyperreactivity and clinical asthma develop when "predisposed" individuals are infected by viruses such as respiratory syncytial virus (Rooney and Williams, 1971; McIntosh et al,

1973). There may be numerous inciting factors that have not yet been identified. Once airway hyperreactivity occurs, it is often retained, even in individuals who are asymptomatic for prolonged periods (Townley et al, 1975). Whatever the basis for the development of airway hyperreactivity, recognition of the abnormality has made it easier to understand why various apparently unrelated precipitating factors may play such an important role in asthma.

ASTHMA-RELATED CHEMICAL MEDIATORS

Numerous pharmacologic agents are activated or liberated in inflammation. Many are probably important in asthma (Fig. 41–3). These substances may act directly on target cells and induce bronchospasm, mucosal edema, or mucous secretion, or they may act indirectly through activation of other mediators or through recruitment of mediator cells. Mediator cells may increase or decrease inflammation by either accentuating or inactivating inflammatory mediator substances. The inflammatory process that results in asthma is a complex process involving numerous pharmacologically active substances with diverse interrelationships.

Three different cells are known to possess both high-affinity receptors for the Fc portion of IgE and the metachromatic granules that contain histamine (Wasserman, 1988). Although basophils have long been differentiated from mast cells, it was only later that two subtypes of mast cells were recognized (Metcalfe, 1983). One, the "typical" or connective tissue type, is prominent in loose connective tissue on serosal surfaces and in skin. The other, the "atypical" or mucosal mast cell, is richly represented in gastrointestinal mucosa and perhaps in other mucosal and epithelial locations as well.

Basophils arise in the bone marrow from precursors in the polymorphonuclear leukocyte series and are most closely related to eosinophilic polymorphonuclear leukocytes. Basophils, similar to mast cells, possess on their surfaces 50,000 to 100,000 receptors for the Fc portion of IgE. They have larger but fewer nonheparin-containing metachromatic granules (Metcalfe et al, 1984). The cells generally are found only in the marrow or peripheral blood (0.1 to 2 per cent) but can be identified in tissue in various inflammatory situations, most particularly in contact dermatitis (Dvorak and Dvorak, 1975).

These cells are the principal sources of preformed histamine and mediators derived from arachidonic acid, such as slow-reacting substance of anaphylaxis (SRS-A). As Figure 41–4 indicates, these cells also liberate or activate various other substances that induce eosinophil or neutrophil chemotaxis, act on platelets, or activate kinins. Intensive studies have focused on the release or activation of mediators from these cells by an allergen-induced IgE antibody-dependent reaction. The reader is referred elsewhere for detailed analyses of these mechanisms (Wasserman, 1988).

The interaction between IgE antibody located on the surface of mast cells or basophils and the antigen serves to activate antibody and the cellular receptors to which the antibody is attached. This activation leads to the activation of a chymotrypsin-like esterase and of methyl transferases in the cell membranes, which in turn leads to methylation of membrane phospholipids. Calcium influx follows, permitting secretion of histamine and activation of arachidonic acid metabolites (including SRS-A). This secretory process is energy dependent and does not destroy the cell. The number of recognized pharmacologi-

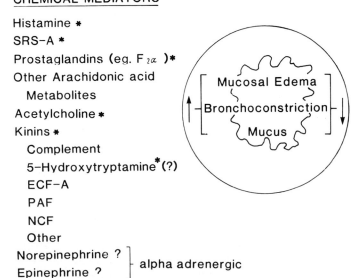

Figure 41–3. The pharmacologic basis of asthma. Asterisk (*) indicates hypersensitivity (10- to 7000-fold) shown in asthmatics.

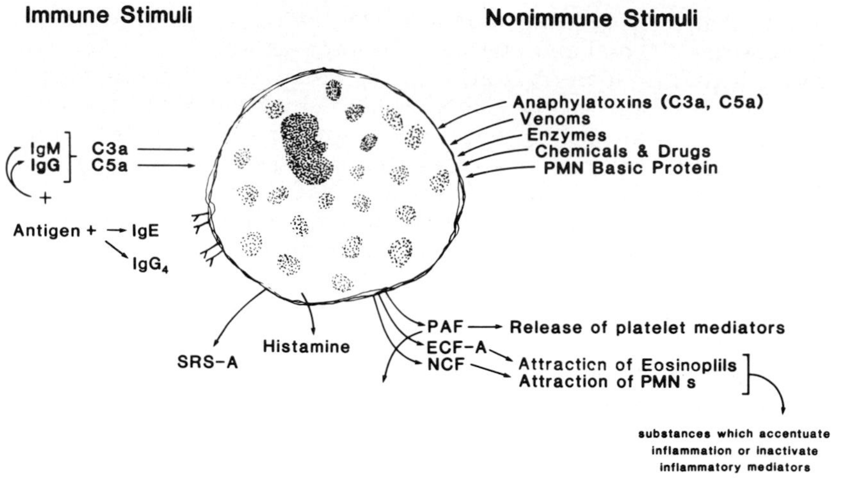

Immune Stimuli   **Nonimmune Stimuli**

Figure 41–4. Mast cell mediators released by various stimuli.

cally active agents, liberated or activated, grows yearly as new identification techniques are developed. Cyclic nucleotides modify the process: increased intracellular concentration of adenosine 3′, 5′-cyclic monophosphate (cAMP) inhibits mediator activation and secretion, whereas increased concentration of guanosine 3′, 5′-cyclic monophosphate (cGMP) tends to increase mediator release and activation. Pharmacologic agents appear to alter this reaction by altering intracellular concentrations of cyclic nucleotides.

Inflammation may be modified also by such substances as histamine and arachidonic acid metabolites, including certain prostaglandins, which may act to inhibit mediator activation and release. Chemotactic factors derived from arachidonic acid eosinophil chemotactic factor of anaphylaxis (ECF-A) and neutrophil chemotactic factor (NCF) recruit cells that play a further role in inflammation. Eosinophils contain histaminase, which degrades histamine, and arylsulfatase, which inactivates SRS-A. Eosinophils also may elaborate substances such as the eosinophilic basic protein, which destroys ground substance and serves to intensify the inflammatory process. The attraction of neutrophils that release lysosomal enzymes may cause direct tissue damage or activate kinins and arachidonic acid metabolites, which promote inflammation indirectly. Platelet aggregation, caused by platelet-activating factor (PAF) derived from mast cells, results in the release of 5-hydroxytryptamine (serotonin) (5-HT), thromboxanes, and other active agents that also may play an important role in inflammation. Thus the mast cell stimulated by IgE antibody-antigen reaction can release pharmacologic mediators that stimulate target cells, activate or liberate other mediators, or recruit cells that may intensify or modify the inflammatory process.

Mediators can be activated or can be released from mast cells also by nonimmune mechanisms (see Fig. 41–4). The resulting inflammatory response is indistinguishable from that induced by "allergic" (immune) factors. The intensity and duration of the stimulus and the interplay between the pharmacologic mediators are important determinants of the

process. The type of stimulus can determine the resulting tissue changes. For example, some patients who have bronchospasm to hyperventilation or exercise may react by cholinergic and other pathways rather than through activation or liberation of mediators from mast cells or basophils, although various mechanisms also may be involved (Deal et al, 1978, 1979; Weiler-Ravell and Godfrey, 1981).

VASOACTIVE-SPASMOGENIC MEDIATORS

Histamine

Histamine is an imidazole derivative with a molecular weight of 111. It is found preformed predominantly in mast cells and basophils in association with a proteoglycan backbone of mast cell granules. Histamine is released and circulates in blood at concentrations of 100 to 300 picograms/ml (Dyer et al, 1982), which are maximal in the early morning (Barnes et al, 1980). Histamine exerts its activities through interaction with two types of receptive substances, H_1 and H_2 receptors (Black et al, 1972). It induces bronchoconstriction directly through activation of H_1 receptors but also can do so indirectly through stimulation of cholinergic pathways. It may also have a weak bronchodilating effect through H_2 receptor activation. Histamine causes vasodilation and increases venular permeability, predominantly H_1 actions. It also stimulates mucous release, alters chemotaxis of eosinophils (increases chemotaxis through H_2 activation), and stimulates prostaglandin synthesis. Histamine inhibits further histamine release through a feedback mechanism that can be blocked by H_2-receptor antagonists. Increases in blood levels of histamine occur in physical urticaria, asthma, anaphylaxis, and systemic mastocytosis (Brown et al, 1982). A third histamine receptor has been described with receptors primarily in the brain and lung (Arrang et al, 1987). Its function is not currently known.

Arachidonic Acid Metabolites

The conversion of membrane phospholipids to arachidonic acid leads eventually to the generation of a variety of pharmacologically active agents with numerous properties of potential importance in asthma (Fig. 41–5) (MacGlashan et al, 1982). Slow-reacting substance of anaphylaxis actually appears to be composed of leukotriene derivatives of arachidonic acid (i.e., leukotriene C, D, and E), which are potent bronchoconstrictors generated from mast cells or basophils and other cells as well. In fact, SRS-A is not generated as rapidly as histamine is released, and bronchoconstriction from this substance occurs later and is more prolonged than histamine-induced bronchoconstriction. The bronchoconstrictive effects of SRS-A are disproportionately greater in the more distal airways than in the proximal, larger airways; SRS-A also can increase vascular permeability and stimulate the synthesis of prostaglandins. They are potent producers of wheal and flare responses (Soter et al, 1983). LTD_4 is most potent and LTE_4 least (Lewis and Austen, 1981).

Prostaglandins

Prostaglandins also are products of the arachidonic acid pathway (McCarthy, 1979; Robinson, 1981). Numerous specific prostaglandins can be generated, depending somewhat on the cells from which they originate (Weksler, 1981). Prostaglandins PGG_2, PGH_2, PGF_2-alpha, and PGD_2 as well as thromboxane A_2 all induce bronchoconstriction, whereas PGE_2 is capable of inducing bronchodilation. Vasodilation is produced by PGE_1 and PGI_2 (prostacyclin). Chemotaxis is stimulated by PGE_2. PGD_2 and PGI_2 induce

platelet aggregation, presumably with subsequent mediator release from platelets. PGI_1 also has been reported to produce an itching sensation and vasodilation when injected in the skin. Prostaglandins also can increase or decrease cyclic AMP formation and stimulate cyclic GMP formation, thereby modulating the activation and release of other mediators. Their effects are competitive, as are their direct actions on target cells, so prostaglandins have been considered to have normal homeostatic functions in the regulation of tracheobronchial patency. Other metabolites of arachidonic acid (HETE, HHT) stimulate cellular movement and are chemotactic (see Fig. 41–5). Aspirin and other nonsteroidal anti-inflammatory agents affect the production of arachidonic metabolites at various points in the metabolic pathway. Aberrations in this pathway induced by such agents are thought by some to be the underlying mechanism in asthma induced by aspirin and other nonsteroidal anti-inflammatory drugs (Szczeklik et al, 1975, 1976; Abrishami, 1977). Human mast cells generate prostaglandin D_2 as products of cyclo-oxygenase action (Lewis et al, 1982).

Platelet-Activating Factor

Platelet-activating factor, a phosphorylcholine derivative (acetylglyceryl ether phosphorylcholine), is a low-molecular-weight compound or series of compounds that is also generated with activation of mast cells and basophils (Demopoulos et al, 1979). It aggregates platelets and, in so doing, may stimulate discharge or generation of mediators from platelets, such as 5-HT, which is a potent pulmonary vasoconstrictor with potential bronchoconstrictive activity in

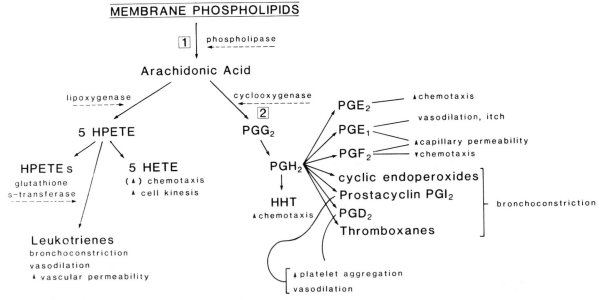

Figure 41–5. The products of arachidonic metabolism. *HETE*, hydroxyeicosatetraneoic acid; *HPETE*, hydroperoxyeicosatetraenoic acid; *HHT*, heptadecatrienoic acid; *PG*, prostaglandin. *Boxed 1* indicates site of inhibition by glucocorticoids; *Boxed 2* indicates site of inhibition by acetylsalicylic acid and other nonsteroidal anti-inflammatory agents. (Data from various sources; see Weksler, 1981; Goetzl, 1980; and Michaelides, 1980, in list of references at end of chapter.)

asthmatics. Also PAF induces immediate skin blanching, pain, pruritus, erythema, and edema when injected into the skin in amounts as small as 50 picograms that can be associated with local lymphocyte infiltration (Humphrey et al, 1982). It directly induces constriction of smooth muscle in the lungs and intestines and induces vasoconstriction (Humphrey et al, 1982). It may alter pulmonary blood flow and may cause abnormal cardiac rhythms (Halonen et al, 1980). In addition, PAF can induce pulmonary hypertension, increase pulmonary resistance, and decrease dynamic compliance (Wasserman, 1988).

Adenosine

Activation of mast cells consumes adenosine triphosphate (ATP) and thereby generates *adenosine*. This purine nucleoside is released parallel with histamine from activated mast cells (Marquardt et al, 1984). On its release, adenosine is metabolized via adenosine deaminase to inosine and hypoxanthine or may be taken up into cells and phosphorylated to AMP. Circulating levels of adenosine approximate 0.3 μm (Mills et al, 1976) and may rise tenfold on induction of asthma or hypoxia (Mentzer et al, 1975). Adenosine is a potent vasodilator and causes bronchoconstriction in asthmatics but not in healthy subjects (Holgate et al, 1984). Adenosine is unique in its ability to enhance mast cell mediator release through its action on a mast cell receptor specific for this nucleoside (Marquardt and Wasserman, 1985). Adenosine action on the mast cell receptor and its ability to induce bronchospasm can be inhibited by therapeutic concentrations of theophylline, a known adenosine receptor blocker.

Enzymatic Mediators

Kallikreins are enzymes that cleave peptide precursors of kinins and in so doing form active kinins. *Basophil kallikrein of anaphylaxis (BK-A)*, identified in basophils, is a protein with a molecular weight of approximately 400,000 daltons. It generates kinin from kininogen in a process involving the Hageman factor. Kallikreins are present in and can be elaborated by various other cells, including polymorphonuclear neutrophils (PMNs), so the attraction of various cells by chemotactic mediators liberated from mast cells and basophils has the potential to generate other potent mediators of inflammation, such as the kinins (Schwartz et al, 1982).

Kinins

Kinins are pharmacologically very active agents with many histamine-like activities, particularly their ability to produce vasodilation and increase capillary permeability (Wilhelm, 1971). Kinins also induce contraction of some smooth muscle, but their role in inducing bronchoconstriction in asthma is unclear. Three major kinins have been identified: bradykinin,

a nonapeptide; lysyl-bradykinin; and methionyl-lysyl-bradykinin. Kinins can be generated by various tissues and enzymes, including clotting factors. Hageman factor (coagulation factor XII) activation leads to the generation of prekallikrein activators, which in turn produce kallikrein (Kaplan and Austen, 1975; Irani et al, 1986).

Lymphokines

Numerous factors that may play an important role in lymphocyte-mediated inflammation are elaborated by lymphocytes (Wasserman, 1988). These include mitogenic factors; interferon, which can enhance antigen-induced mediator release (Ida et al, 1977); chemotactic factors; and substances that can induce vasodilation and perhaps increase capillary permeability. It is possible that they play a role in the delayed response (6 to 8 hours after exposure) to antigen.

Complement

Activation of complement generates various active agents, including chemotactic factors and substances (anaphylatoxins) capable of inducing mediator release from mast cells (Fearon and Austen, 1976). Complement can be activated by immune and nonimmune mechanisms (Fig. 41–6).

Acetylcholine

Acetylcholine is the principal parasympathetic nervous system mediator, and it plays an important role in homeostatic mechanisms regulating bronchial tone. It is a bronchoconstrictor, and in individuals with asthma, sensitivity to acetylcholine and its derivatives characteristically is greatly increased, up to a thousandfold in some patients (Townley et al, 1965). Its role as a mediator in asthma has been controversial for many years, particularly because atropine is not usually effective in controlling asthma. Cholinergic activity not only induces bronchoconstriction but also may cause increased mucus secretion and can intensify mediator release through stimulation of cyclic GMP (Tauber et al, 1973). Cholinergic mechanisms may play a role in antigen-induced bronchoconstriction, in which histamine may act indirectly to stimulate acetylcholine (Yu et al, 1972); exercise-induced asthma; asthma aggravated by psychogenic factors (McFadden et al, 1969); and asthma intensified by viral bronchial infections (Empey et al, 1976).

Sympathomimetic Agents

Sympathomimetic agents are considered the physiologic antagonists of the mediators of inflammation. Bronchomotor tone is maintained largely through the competing activities of acetylcholine and sympathomimetic agents (particularly epinephrine). Bronchodilation by epinephrine is mediated through activation of beta-adrenergic receptors. The tracheo-

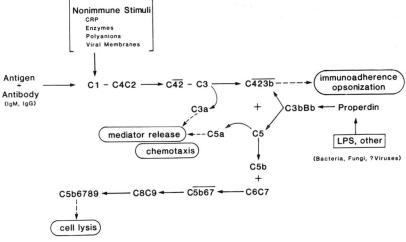

Figure 41–6. Complement pathways.

bronchial trees of many asthmatics contain alpha receptors, through which sympathomimetic agents also can induce bronchoconstriction. Szentivanyi (1968) pointed out that asthmatics behave as if they have reduced beta-adrenergic receptor responsiveness and hypothesized that the major defect in asthma and perhaps other atopic disorders is an autonomic imbalance with a deficit in beta-adrenergic function, leaving the bronchial tree unable to counterbalance the bronchoconstricting effects of neurohormones such as acetylcholine and various inflammatory mediators.

Although the long-term use of beta-adrenergic drugs may induce subsensitivity of beta-adrenergic receptor function (Morris et al, 1977), beta-adrenergic hyporesponsiveness occurs even if such stimulants are not used (Brooks et al, 1979). Many asthmatics also appear to have enhanced alpha-adrenergic receptor function (Henderson et al, 1979). In these patients, activation of adrenergic receptors may induce bronchoconstriction and enhance mediator release through increase in cyclic GMP production (Kaliner et al, 1976). Thus both epinephrine and norepinephrine may have a "paradoxical" effect on the tracheobronchial tree, in that both may induce bronchoconstriction and bronchial obstruction rather than bronchodilation.

CELLULAR INTERACTION

Neutrophil Chemotactic Mediators

Neutrophil chemotactic mediator molecules generated during mast cell activation are capable of altering neutrophil migration. Some, including PGD_2, leukotriene B_4, several monohydroxy fatty acids, and platelet-activating factor, are not specific for neutrophils but rather are broadly chemotactic or chemokinetic, acting on various migratory cell types.

A high-molecular-weight (660 Kd), neutral isolec-

tric-point protein (HMW-NCF) has been identified in the blood of patients with antigen or exercise-induced bronchospasm (Atkins et al, 1976) or experimentally induced physical urticaria (Wasserman et al, 1977). In patients developing a second, late bronchospastic response to antigen, a second peak of HMW-NCF has been noted (Nagy et al, 1982). This factor is specific for neutrophils, and after its appearance in serum, a transient inhibition of neutrophil chemotactic responsiveness termed *deactivation* occurs (Center et al, 1979). Other specific neutrophil-directed chemotactic activities, termed *inflammatory factors of anaphylaxis*, have been partially isolated from the granules of rodent mast cells (Oertel and Kaliner, 1981).

Eosinophil-Associated Mediators

The association of eosinophils with allergic diseases has long been noted. Evidence indicates that this association, in addition to providing diagnostic information, also has pathogenetic implications (Wasserman, 1988).

Several peptides and proteins are responsible for eosinophil-induced inflammation. These include the major basic protein (MBP) (Gleich et al, 1976), eosinophil cationic peptide (Olsson and Venge, 1974), eosinophil-derived neurotoxin (Durach et al, 1981), and an eosinophil membrane–associated enzyme (Weller et al, 1983). These toxins damage tracheal epithelium, trigger mast cell and basophil secretion, damage central nervous system neurons, and induce LTC_4 production (Weller et al, 1983) and PAF production (Lee et al, 1984).

Purinergic Mechanisms

An additional nonadrenergic noncholinergic (NANC) inhibitory mechanism in the tracheobronchial tree has been identified (Richardson, 1977). Relaxation of bronchial smooth muscle occurs following stimulation of tracheobronchial nerve fibers in the presence of atropine. This response is not blocked by adrenergic blocking agents. Little is known about this inhibitory system, but ATP is believed to be the inhibitory transmitter released from the involved neurons, hence the term purinergic. A defect in this system could lead to bronchial hyperreactivity in much the same way as that postulated for beta-adrenergic receptor hyporesponsiveness in asthma.

Immune Reactants Implicated in Asthma

IgE Antibody. Skin-sensitizing antibody (atopic reagin) associated with asthma belongs to a special class of immunoglobulins designated IgE. IgE occurs in most individuals. In the majority of the population, antigenic exposure ordinarily results in little specific IgE antibody synthesis. However, some individuals may respond with a vigorous IgE antibody synthesis. In such individuals, it is not unusual to find that specific IgE antibody levels rise in response to various inhalant and food substances that are ordinarily considered innocuous. IgE antibody responses appear to be controlled genetically both in terms of absolute serum concentration and in the quantity induced by exposure to specific antigens (Buckley, 1988). Whereas in some children there is little question that IgE antibody–mediated mechanisms are important in the precipitation of asthma, the facility with which an individual manufactures IgE antibody on the one hand and the ease with which he develops asthma on the other are frequently associated but separable phenomena. IgE antibody is of particular importance in allergic asthma because of its ability to bind to receptors of mast cells and basophils and, on interaction with antigen, to induce liberation and activation of potent mediators of inflammation. Extraordinarily small quantities of IgE are required for mediator release, so IgE antibody interaction is an especially potent activator of inflammatory mediators.

IgE antibody has a molecular weight of approximately 190,000 daltons and is heat labile in the sense that heating at 56° C for several hours inactivates its receptor-binding activity (Ishizaka and Ishizaka, 1975). It is ordinarily present in serum in extremely low concentrations (approximately 50 ng/ml or less), although in some individuals this concentration may be more than a hundredfold greater. IgE antibody can be synthesized in a large part of the lymphoid system, but its predominant sites of manufacture are on the mucosal surfaces of the upper and lower respiratory tract and the gastrointestinal tract, in which tissues and their secretions it also tends to be concentrated. Its serum half-life is only about 2.5 days, but its tissue half-life is around 3 weeks. Because it is synthesized at mucosal surfaces and specifically at the points of entry of inhaled and ingested allergens, IgE antibody rarely may be available to participate locally in allergic reactions to inhaled or ingested allergens without being present in sufficient

concentrations to be detected elsewhere (Huggins and Brostoff, 1975). However, in most individuals in whom IgE antibody appears to be of clinical significance, sufficient antibody is formed to be detectable in serum and in skin. Classically, the presence of this kind of antibody is sought by allergy skin testing, in which a small amount of antigen is introduced superficially into the skin by prick, puncture, or injection. If IgE antibody is present, the procedure results in a wheal and erythema reaction induced by liberated histamine within 15 to 20 minutes. Unfortunately, excessively high concentrations of antigenic material can induce a wheal and erythema-like reaction in the absence of antibody, and all too often it is assumed the specific antibody is present when in fact the reaction is a result of nonimmune-mediated irritation.

Serologic tests are available for assaying IgE antibody (Buckley, 1988). The best known and most widely available of these tests, the radioallergosorbent test (RAST), is less sensitive than skin tests. Other variants include an enzyme modification of the test, which obviates the use of radioactive materials. The concentration of immunoglobulin E can be assessed by a radioactive method, radioimmunosorbent test (RIST), or paper radioimmunosorbent test (PRIST). Children with asthma tend to have higher levels of IgE than nonasthmatic or nonallergic children. There is an extremely wide scatter of IgE levels in asthmatic individuals, however, and IgE levels neither confirm nor deny the diagnosis of asthma. Although high IgE levels are more commonly associated with specific IgE antibody to various inhaled allergens, IgE antibody often is present and is of clinical significance even when immunoglobulin levels are low or within the normal range. However, even in children with historical and laboratory evidence of allergic asthma, IgE antibody to some allergens plays no apparent role in a child's asthma in spite of positive skin reactions and RAST results (Aas, 1970). In addition, some children with IgE antibody to various antigens may have allergic rhinitis due to IgE antibody–dependent mechanisms but at the same time have asthma that does not relate to specific IgE antibody.

Other Immune Reactants. In some individuals, a heat-stable skin-sensitizing antibody has been identified and implicated as a factor in asthma (Heiner, 1988). This antibody has a shorter half-life in skin than IgE antibody and has been called *short-term sensitizing* or *STS* antibody. Some have claimed that intradermal skin testing is more efficient in picking up reactions with this kind of antibody than a more superficial puncture or prick test and that the RAST, which utilizes specific anti-IgE serum to identify antibody, is incapable of identifying this kind of antibody. There is reason to believe that IgG_4 may represent STS antibody (Stanworth and Smith, 1973). The importance of this kind of antibody in asthma and allergy is unclear.

Various other kinds of immune reactants can activate or liberate inflammatory mediators and by inference may be involved in asthma. For example, activation of complement by mechanisms dependent on IgG and IgM antibodies results in the release of histamine and other mediators of inflammation, as illustrated in Figure 41–4. Involvement of such antibody-dependent mechanisms in asthma is conjectural. However, considering (1) the hyperreactivity of asthmatic airways to various chemical mediators of inflammation and (2) the fact that the interaction between antigen and IgG and IgM antibodies, as well as other kinds of immune reactants, most certainly occurs in the respiratory tract (e.g., to infectious agents), it is highly likely that immune mechanisms involving antibodies other than IgE play some role in asthma. In unusual forms of asthma, such as allergic bronchopulmonary aspergillosis, there are high concentrations of aspergillus organisms within the bronchi, immune complexes (IgG and IgM antibody), cell-mediated mechanisms, and IgE-dependent immune mechanisms. All these factors have been implicated in the production of allergic inflammation and the bronchial obstruction associated with asthma (Schatz et al, 1979). Figure 41–6 also indicates that, as with mediator release from mast cells, complement activation and complement-derived mediator release can be induced by both immune and nonimmune mechanisms. It seems likely that inflammation induced by cell-mediated immune mechanisms also plays a role in at least some forms of asthma.

PRECIPITATING AND AGGRAVATING FACTORS IN ASTHMA

Allergens. In some individuals with asthma, it is possible to induce an asthmatic reaction to substances in which IgE and possibly other skin-sensitizing antibodies can be demonstrated. In others, allergens may play only an ancillary or a negligible role. Allergic reactions may induce bronchoconstriction directly, may increase tracheobronchial sensitivity in general, or may be obvious or subtle precipitating factors. In addition, the role played by an allergen may appear to be inconsistent and therefore historically confusing or unclear as an asthma precipitant, related not only to intensity of exposure but to the degree of airway hyperreactivity, which may change from time to time (Fig. 41–7). Although "immediate" responses to allergens via IgE antibody–induced mediator release are striking, it may be that "late" reactions (which occur 4 to 12 hours after antigen contact and which appear to be mediated also by IgE antibody–related mechanisms) are more important in the disease. Allergens that can induce asthma include foods (mainly in early life), animal allergens, mold spores, pollens, insects (mainly by inhalation but also by sting), infectious agents (especially fungi but perhaps viruses, as discussed subsequently), and, occasionally, drugs.

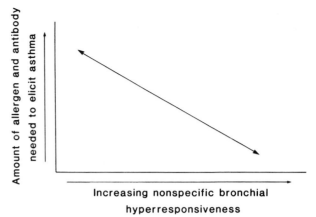

Figure 41–7. Relationship between bronchial hyperreactivity and the amount of allergen exposure required to induce bronchial obstruction. As the degree of nonspecific bronchial responsiveness increases, the amount of antigen-antibody reacting required to induce obstruction diminishes. Thus a casual encounter with an allergen in a highly sensitive individual with marked nonspecific bronchial hyperresponsiveness may induce asthma, but intense antigen exposure may be required to do so in the asthmatic with relatively little IgE antibody or relatively little nonspecific bronchial hyperresponsiveness. (Modified from Cockroft DW et al: Determination of allergen-induced asthma: dose of allergen, circulating IgE antibody concentration, and bronchial responsiveness to inhaled histamine. Am Rev Respir Dis 120:1053, 1979.)

Irritants. Numerous upper and lower respiratory irritants have been implicated as precipitants of asthma. These include paint odors, hairsprays, perfumes, chemicals, air pollutants, cigarette smoke (also cigar and pipe smoke), cold air, cold water, cough, and positive ions. Some allergens may act as irritants. As indicated previously, some irritants such as ozone and industrial chemicals also may initiate bronchial hyperresponsiveness by inducing inflammation. Active and passive exposure to cigarette and cigar smoke, in addition to acting as precipitants and aggravators of asthma, also can be associated with an accelerated irreversible loss of pulmonary function (Barter and Campbell, 1976; Murray and Ferguson, 1983).

Weather Changes. Atmospheric changes commonly are associated with an increase in asthmatic activity. The mechanism of this effect has not been defined.

Infections. By far, the most common infectious agents responsible for precipitating or aggravating asthma are viral respiratory pathogens. In some instances, however, fungal infections (e.g., bronchopulmonary aspergillosis), bacterial infections (e.g., pertussis), and parasitic infestations (e.g., toxocariasis and ascariasis) can be important triggers. The importance of viral infections as precipitants and possible initiators of asthma and bronchial hyperreactivity cannot be overemphasized. Various mechanisms have been implicated to explain the role of viruses in asthma and other allergic diseases, including IgE-mediated mechanisms (Welliver, 1986).

Exercise. Strenuous exercise ordinarily associated with breathlessness, such as running, bicycle riding, and cross-country skiing (downhill skiing generally is not associated with this problem), may induce bronchial obstruction in the vast majority (at least 70 to 80 per cent) of individuals with asthma. In some instances, exercise is a major asthmatic precipitant, whereas in others it is a minor or an insignificant one altogether. Exercise can be a subtle though significant problem associated with only cough or excessive breathlessness. Exercise can induce late asthmatic responses, but it is unclear whether these responses are associated with bronchial hyperreactivity.

Emotional Factors. The influence of the psyche on asthma is unquestioned, and in some instances suggestion has been shown to alter airway resistance significantly. Emotional upsets clearly aggravate asthma in some individuals. However, there is no evidence indicating that psychological factors are the basis for asthma. The elegant studies of Kinsman and associates (1977) strongly indicate that coping styles of patients, their families, and their physicians can intensify or lead to more rapid amelioration of asthma. Conversely, denial of asthma by patients, parents, or physicians may delay therapy to the point that reversibility of obstruction is more difficult. Psychological factors have been implicated in deaths from asthma in children (Strunk et al, 1985). The influence of psychosocial factors on compliance and the effect of hostility or fear on the ability or propensity to comply are yet other important facets of treatment failure or success.

Just as psychological factors may influence the course of asthma in a given patient, it is important to recognize that asthma itself can strongly influence the emotional state of the patient, of the family, and of other individuals associated with the patient. Indeed, asthma probably is more frequently "somato-psychic" than it is "psychosomatic".

Gastroesophageal Reflux. Reflux of gastric contents into the tracheobronchial tree can aggravate asthma in children as well as in adults and is one of the causes of nocturnal asthma. There also is suggestive information that gastroesophageal reflux (GER) may increase airway reactivity.

Allergic Rhinitis, Sinusitis, and Upper Respiratory Tract Inflammation. Acute or chronic sinusitis can be associated with aggravation of asthma and can be a cause of recalcitrant asthma (Slavin, 1986). Evidence from experimental animal studies also suggests that sinusitis may be capable of increasing bronchial responsiveness. It is probable that allergic rhinitis also can aggravate asthma through irritant or "reflex" mechanisms. Irritation of the upper respiratory tract by any of a variety of mechanisms appears capable of triggering asthmatic symptoms.

Nonallergic Hypersensitivity to Drugs and Chemicals. Though allergic sensitivity to aspirin has been reported on occasion with manifestations that include asthma, aspirin and nonsteroidal anti-inflammatory drugs (NSAIDs), such as indomethacin and ibuprofen, are more likely to exacerbate asthma on a nonallergic basis. Aspirin ingestion may diminish pulmonary functions in up to one third of children and adolescents with severe asthma (Rachelefsky et al, 1975). In many instances, this effect may be subtle. Consequently, as a general rule, it is wise to restrict aspirin and aspirin-containing products for all individuals who have asthma. Patients who react to aspirin are likely to react to other NSAIDs that should be avoided, but most are able to tolerate acetaminophen. The importance of sensitivity to tartrazine (FD & C Yellow No. 5), a common dye found in many foods and drugs, in aspirin-sensitive or other asthmatics is unclear, but early reports that it can induce asthma have not been confirmed. Metabisulfite can be an important precipitant or aggravator of asthma, both by allergic and nonallergic mechanisms (Bush et al, 1986). A small proportion of severe asthmatics appear to be extremely sensitive, but it is probable that all asthmatics are sensitive to some degree to sulfur dioxide that is released from metabisulfite.

Endocrine Factors. Aggravation of asthma occurs in some patients in relation to the menstrual cycle, beginning shortly before menstruation. Whether this reflects changes in water and salt balance, irritability of bronchial smooth muscle, or other factors is unknown. The use of birth control pills occasionally also aggravates asthma. Hyperthyroidism has been reported to worsen or precipitate asthma severely in an occasional patient. Treatment of hyperthyroidism usually ameliorates the asthma.

Sleep or Nocturnal Asthma. Sleep or nocturnal asthma is a risk factor for asthma severity and even death in some asthmatics. Although nocturnal asthma may result from late phase reactions to earlier allergen exposure, GER, or sinusitis in some patients, these conditions are not present in most patients with severe nocturnal asthma. Nocturnal asthma does not appear to be related to recumbency or to sleep per se. One possible explanation is an exaggeration of a normal circadian variation in bronchomotor tone (Barnes, 1986). Abnormalities in central nervous system control of respiratory drive, in particular with defective hypoxic drive, also may be present in some patients and can pose serious risks to those with asthma (Martin, 1984; Lancet Commentary, 1983).

Interaction of Various Precipitating Factors. Not infrequently, concurrent exposure to various precipitating or aggravating factors may induce additive effects in asthma. For example, some individuals experience exercise-induced asthma only when exercising in cold air or during a pollen allergy season. Others recognize increased symptoms from specific allergen exposure after respiratory infections. As indicated previously, this may be due to increased bronchial responsiveness caused by inflammation (allergic or infectious).

Patterns of Asthma. In some children, one precipitating factor may be clearly responsible for the asthma. Viral respiratory tract infections may be the predominant or apparently exclusive precipitant of asthma, particularly in early life, or the child may have overt symptoms only in relation to exposure to certain animals or with strenuous exercise. However, the occurrence of a single precipitant in childhood asthma is the exception rather than the rule. Moreover, patterns of reactivity may change. Thus young children with "wheezy bronchitis" or "asthmatic bronchitis" with a predisposition for making IgE antibody eventually develop allergen-induced asthmatic symptoms to potential allergens in their environment. Exercise may be only a minor factor when a child is young but may become a major one as the child grows older and engages in more strenuous physical activities.

The importance of various precipitating or aggravating factors may differ with age in children, and this changing pattern of factors may continue into adulthood (Table 41–1). Thus exercise-induced asthma may not be viewed as a problem in many adults with asthma who have learned in childhood that exercise induces symptoms and consequently have developed a life style that avoids exercise. Allergic factors that precipitated asthma in childhood may no longer cause symptoms in adolescence or adulthood even though the patient continues to have asthma. Patterns also may change with treatment. For example, asthma in a patient who has major allergic reactions to animal danders may assume a "nonallergic" pattern when danders are excluded from the environment.

NATURAL HISTORY AND PROGNOSIS

Knowledge of the natural history of asthma is incomplete because it has been obtained largely from patient/parent questionnaires rather than from long-term prospective studies. Published studies are also difficult to compare because each author has employed his or her own criteria for classifying severity or loss of asthma. This has led to a widespread notion that children usually "outgrow" their asthma in adolescence. Children with asthma appear to have less severe symptoms in general as they enter adolescence, but one half continue to have asthma (Rackemann and Edwards, 1952; Buffum and Settipane, 1966; Kuzemko, 1980).

A substantial number of childhood asthmatics who appear to lose symptomatology have recurrences of asthma in adulthood, when it may become more severe once again (Rackemann and Edwards, 1952; Martin et al, 1980). Two studies illustrate this point. In 1945, Flensborg, reporting on 300 childhood asthmatics at the end of 15 to 20 years of follow-up, found that approximately 40 per cent of the patients had had no asthma for 1 to 2 years. Ryssing contacted the majority of these same patients in 1959 and found also that approximately 40 per cent of the patients had been free from asthma for at least 1 to 2 years. However, this was not the same 40 per cent of the group! In many instances, patients who were asthma-free in 1945 had remained asthma-free to 1959, but in other instances, patients reported by Flensborg to have been asthma-free for 1 to 2 years, and therefore to have "lost" their asthma, had asthma again in 1959. Other investigators also have observed recurrences of symptomatic asthma years after apparent loss of symptoms and have pointed out the importance of long-term follow-up for childhood asthma (Blair, 1977; Martin et al, 1980).

Careful studies of children with asthma based both on history and on assessment of pulmonary function indicate that many children who lose overt symptoms have persistent airway obstruction (Levison et al, 1974). Weng and Levison (1969) reported that the majority of children with asthmatic symptoms in their clinic who were asthma-free for months had significant airway obstruction and lower than normal arterial oxygen saturation. Similar findings have been reported by others (Jones and Jones, 1966; Blackhall, 1970). Nonspecific airway hyperreactivity, associated with and perhaps fundamental to asthma, is present in formerly asthmatic patients who are free from clinical asthma (Townley et al, 1975; Martin et al, 1980), suggesting the possibility of recurrence of asthma later in life. Indeed, up to one half of adults with asthma date the onset of their disease to childhood. The recurrence of overt asthma after years of freedom from symptoms is not unusual. Thus asthma is often a lifelong disease with periodic exacerbations and remissions. All too often it is the pediatrician who is "outgrown" rather than the asthma (Fig. 41–8) (Levison et al, 1974).

Table 41–1. PRECIPITANTS OF ASTHMA AT VARIOUS AGES

Precipitant	Infancy	Early Childhood	Later Childhood	Early to Middle Adulthood
Respiratory infection (mainly viral)	+ + + +	+ + +	+(+)	+ + +
Allergens				
Foods	+	+	(+)	(+)
Household inhalants	+	+ + +	+ + +	+ + +
Outdoor (seasonal) inhalants		+ +	+ + +	+ + +
Irritants	+	+ +	+ +	+ +
Exercise	(+)	+ +	+ + +	+ +
Aspirin and other nonsteroid anti-inflammatory drugs	?	?	(+)	+
Emotional factors	(+)	(+)	(+)	(+)

(Reproduced with permission from Bierman CW and Pearlman DS [eds]: Allergic Diseases from Infancy to Adulthood. 2nd ed. Philadelphia, WB Saunders Co, 1988.)

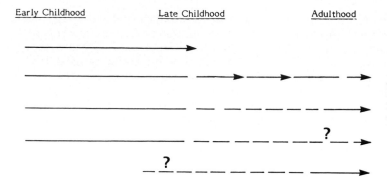

Figure 41–8. Natural history of childhood asthma. *Solid arrow* indicates active asthma. *Dotted arrow* indicates airway hyperreactivity but no overt asthma (there may be subclinical asthma with evidence of chronic intermittent airway obstruction).

The likelihood for children with asthma to improve and to lose symptoms altogether appears to be much greater if the asthma is mild and if the child is free from symptoms between attacks (Dawson et al, 1969; Blair, 1977; Martin et al, 1980). Whether the age of onset of childhood asthma has prognostic implications is not clear. Some investigators report that asthma that develops before 3 years of age has a worse prognosis than asthma that develops later (Williams and McNicol, 1969; McNicol and Williams, 1973a), whereas others do not find such a relationship (Blair, 1977). It is claimed that children with nonallergic asthma ("wheezy bronchitis") are more likely to outgrow asthma before adulthood than children who have asthma in which allergic factors play an important role (McNicol and Williams, 1973a). An association with other manifestations of atopic disease also appears to relate to more severe and more persistent asthma (McNicol and Williams, 1973b; Blair, 1977). Asthma has a tendency to remit by or at puberty, with somewhat earlier ages of remission in girls than boys (Flensborg, 1945).

In children and adolescents, asthma frequently is a completely "reversible" obstructive airways disease, and indeed no abnormalities in pulmonary functions can be detected in many asthmatic patients when they become symptom free. However, there is a significant subpopulation of asthmatic children and adults who, even in the absence of symptoms for prolonged periods of time, have persistent abnormalities in pulmonary functions, with chronic hyperinflation, decreased pulmonary flow rates, or both, with or without mild hypoxemia. The potential reversibility of abnormal pulmonary functions—even in severely asthmatic children—toward or to normal by intensive therapy was demonstrated by Tooley and colleagues (1965). However, it is clear that in many children and adults with severe asthma, normal pulmonary functions cannot be maintained without continuous intensive therapy, including corticosteroids. Reversibility of pulmonary function abnormalities with therapy is transient in that withdrawal of constant therapy usually leads to the return of pulmonary functions to initial abnormal baselines (Cade and Pain, 1973).

As noted previously, even severe asthma generally does not progress to emphysema. However, asthma appears to progress to chronic nonreversible obstructive disease in some individuals with the disorder. Chronic mucus plugging, tracheobronchial ciliary dysfunction, smooth muscle hyperplasia, and persistent hyperinflation possibly may lead to pulmonary abnormalities in adult life. Recent findings of residual pulmonary function abnormalities following respiratory viral infections early in life (Kattan et al, 1977) and the fact that viral respiratory tract infections occur more commonly in asthmatic children than in their nonasthmatic siblings (Minor et al, 1974) further confuse the issue. Similar arguments may be made with regard to irreversible pulmonary changes in asthmatic adults. In addition, passive or active smoking in asthmatic children as well as adults has been shown to be related to more rapid decline in small airways function in comparison with nonasthmatics (Barter and Campbell, 1976). Thus it is not clear that asthma per se leads to irreversible pulmonary changes. Evidence suggests, however, that asthma significantly predisposes patients to irreversible damage from various noxious environmental agents (Pearlman, 1984).

Because the natural course of continued bronchial obstruction is not known, a therapeutic dilemma arises about the extent to which asthma should be treated. Should the patient be treated until pulmonary function is totally normal or until he or she can function reasonably and normally even though pulmonary functions are abnormal? Whether intensive therapy early in the course of asthma or persistent therapy to achieve constant pulmonary normality can prevent any irreversible changes later, in childhood or adulthood, needs to be determined.

Although deaths have been attributed to overuse of isoproterenol and similar inhaled bronchodilators, as well as inappropriate administration of sedatives and misuse of aminophylline and theophylline, by far the greatest contributor to death from the disease is undertreatment. The underdiagnosis of the severity of asthma by physicians, hospital personnel, and attendants undoubtedly contributes to the fact that an emergency room constitutes a risk factor for death in asthmatics! The lability of asthma, regardless of severity, also is a risk factor, as are respiratory infections, nocturnal asthma, history of respiratory failure, and marked diurnal variation in airflow limitation

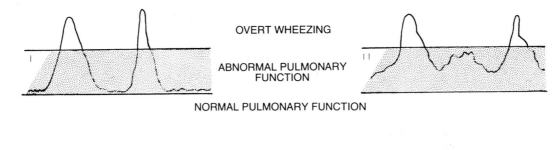

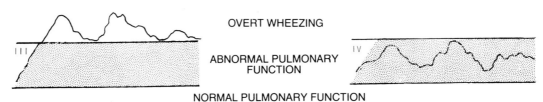

Figure 41–9. Iceberg concept of asthma. The "ocean floor" represents pulmonary normality, and the surface of the ocean represents the point at which asthmatic symptoms (e.g., wheezing) are obvious. (Reproduced with permission from Bierman CW and Pearlman DS [eds]: Allergic Diseases from Infancy to Adulthood. 2nd ed. Philadelphia, WB Saunders Co, 1988.)

with low pulmonary functions in the morning ("morning dippers"). It is important to recognize that some patients cannot perceive severe airflow obstruction, especially when it occurs gradually. Such patients must be taught to recognize warning signs of airflow obstruction. A simple device for measuring airflow, such as a portable peak flow meter, will help the patient to recognize the development of severe asthma. Finally, psychological factors have been implicated in deaths from asthma, particularly in sudden deaths in asthmatic adolescents (Strunk et al, 1985; Benatar, 1986; Asthma Deaths, 1986).

PRESENTATION OF ASTHMA

The asthmatic classically presents with wheezing, a high-pitched sound heard mostly on expiration. The sound is due to air rushing through the larger airways, which are narrowed. Associated symptoms often include cough, which is sometimes extreme to the point that it induces gagging and vomiting; shortness of breath; a feeling of "tight chest"; complaints of chest congestion; poor exercise tolerance; "recurrent chest colds"; "recurrent" or "chronic" bronchitis; or, occasionally, "recurrent pneumonia." Patients may present with many of these symptoms even though wheezing cannot be detected either overtly or on cursory examination (although, in most instances, careful examination including a forced-expiratory maneuver will elicit wheezing). It is well known that "all is not asthma that wheezes," and that causes of airway obstruction with wheezing in childhood are numerous (see "Differential Diagnosis"). Nevertheless, the vast majority of children with recurrent wheezing do in fact have asthma. So common is recurrent wheezing as a presentation of asthma that its cause can be considered "probable asthma" until proven otherwise.

In recent years, particularly with the extensive use of pulmonary function measurements, it has become apparent also that "not all asthma wheezes." Because airflow through small airways is laminar (and therefore does not produce a wheezing sound) rather than turbulent (which does produce a wheezing sound), significant peripheral airway obstruction may exist in the absence of wheezing. In most patients with asthma, asthmatic obstruction tends to be generalized, so that wheezing is detectable. However, significant airway obstruction may persist for prolonged periods after other obvious signs of asthma have cleared. Asthma also may manifest in some individuals with subtle symptoms and signs, without surfacing overtly as obvious paroxysms of airway obstruction. It is important to appreciate the chronicity of airway obstruction after acute asthmatic paroxysms (McFadden, 1975b) and to recognize that asthmatics may have different patterns. Wheezing can be regarded as the tip of the asthmatic "iceberg," with much that is not obvious occurring below the clinical surface.

It is useful in considering asthmatic patterns to view asthma as an iceberg, with various shapes of the iceberg possible. Auscultation (looking below the surface) may elicit wheezes before they are otherwise clinically apparent. Before wheezing can be detected, however, there may be significant airway obstruction detectable only by measurement of pulmonary function. Using this concept, several kinds of asthmatic patterns emerge. For illustrative purposes four kinds of patterns are considered; they are illustrated in Figure 41–9. In some instances *(Example 1)*, asthmatic paroxysms develop and subside rapidly, as in the brief encounter with an allergen or exercise-induced asthma in some patients. Airway obstruction may occur within minutes, with overt asthmatic symptoms correspondingly appearing over a period of minutes or perhaps hours and airway obstruction resolving more or less completely in a similar time. There may be relatively few of these episodes, perhaps a half dozen per year or less, with no symptoms or functional impairment between episodes. Symptoms, on the other hand, may last for a few days to a week at a time. These patterns are typical of the milder forms of asthma, which in turn probably represent a third to a half of all cases of childhood asthma. *Example 2* illustrates a pattern of asthma superficially resembling that in Example 1 in that there may be only five or six attacks of asthma each year. However, in Example 2 there is evidence of persistent airway obstruction, with some functional impairment and subtler asthmatic symptoms between overt episodes. *Example 3* is typical of many children with severe asthma, in whom overt symptoms occur more or less constantly, although varying in degree (at least, in the absence of adequate therapy). This pattern is typical of probably less than 5 per cent of children with asthma. An alternative pattern is illustrated in *Example 4*, in which the "asthmatic iceberg" never "surfaces" with wheezing or other obvious asthmatic symptoms, but nonetheless continuous though variable airway obstruction, functional impairment, and more subtle signs of airflow limitation persist. These two patterns (Examples 2 and 4) are probably more typical of children who are considered to have moderate to moderately severe asthma and account for a sizeable portion of asthma in children, perhaps as much as 50 per cent.

Various other patterns or combinations of patterns may occur. For example, the shape of the asthmatic iceberg in Example 1 could be much broader, with airway obstruction beginning with an upper respiratory tract infection, taking at least a couple of days before the asthma becomes apparent, and also requiring many days to resolve completely. Or the pattern may be similar to this without overt asthmatic symptoms, with significant subclinical airway obstruction occurring in association with a respiratory tract infection and lasting days to weeks. The pattern also may change in a given individual with time, reflecting growth, the development of newly acquired allergic sensitivities, or a change in exposure to recognized factors. The same child may have short-lived airway obstruction after exercise, whereas a viral infection of the respiratory tract may induce symptoms of airway obstruction for many days. Patterns can be altered also by therapy.

It is important to recognize such patterns because the type and duration of pharmacotherapy appropriate for one pattern may be inappropriate for another. Thus for Example 1, treatment lasting hours to days may be appropriate, whereas in the other patterns, round-the-clock bronchodilator therapy may need to be supplemented by a course of steroidal anti-inflammatory agents. Moreover, recognition of prodromal signs or symptoms of overt asthma is of therapeutic importance, for there is reason to believe that early treatment of asthma is more successful than late treatment. In addition, there is suggestive

evidence that greater normalization of pulmonary functions is associated with less frequent and less severe episodes of asthma (Haynes et al, 1976).

It is important not only for physicians but also for parents and older children to recognize these patterns. Treatment should be instituted with the onset of signs of asthma or evidence of increasing pulmonary obstruction (measurable in the physician's office or, in some instances, at home with simple peak flow devices) and should be continued until clinical and laboratory measurements indicate that pulmonary obstruction has cleared or has reached an acceptable level.

It is important to remember that asthma is a chronic disorder that may become clinically obvious only periodically, one in which the severity of airway obstruction is frequently underestimated by physician and patient alike.

DIAGNOSIS

CLINICAL DIAGNOSIS

History

Although patients with asthma may present in a variety of ways, most have certain common historical features, and asthma often can be diagnosed on the basis of history alone. Asthma is characterized by episodes of respiratory obstruction, with expiratory obstruction predominating over inspiratory obstruction. This obstruction usually is manifested by wheezing, a musical high-pitched sound produced by airflow turbulence in the large airways. However, asthma can occur without wheezing if the obstruction involves small airways predominantly—a form termed *occult asthma* (Petty, 1977). Wheezing, although predominantly expiratory, also occurs with inspiration when asthma worsens and may disappear altogether as obstruction becomes more severe and airflow is limited. Inspiratory wheezing per se is not characteristic of asthma and suggests higher obstruction in the laryngeal area, such as that induced by croup or a foreign body.

Wheezing usually is accompanied by coughing. Occasionally, coughing may be the only symptom. Asthmatic attacks are episodic at first, with symptom-free intervals between, but as the disease becomes more chronic, such intervals may diminish progressively.

Usually, symptoms are more severe at night or in the early morning and improve through the day. A history of symptomatic improvement after an injection of epinephrine, inhaled or oral adrenergic drugs, or oral theophylline suggests the diagnosis of asthma. A typical "attack" usually lasts 3 to 7 days and may clear spontaneously (although lung function may not return to normal for several weeks).

Symptoms vary with age. The infant or young child may have a history of recurrent bronchitis, bronchiolitis, or pneumonia, persistent coughing with colds, recurrent "croup," or just a chronic chest "rattle." Older children often develop a "tight" chest with colds, recurrent "chest congestion," or persistent coughing or wheezing. Respiratory symptoms may be precipitated or exacerbated also by exposure to irritants, animals, molds or dusty areas, pollens, tobacco smoke, or cold air, or by exercise. Often the precipitating factor is not recognized.

Physical Examination

The physical examination should focus on overall growth and development; on the condition of the entire respiratory tract including the upper airway, ears, and paranasal sinuses as well as the chest; and on other associated signs of allergic disease.

Growth. Weight and height should be recorded and plotted on a growth grid. Asthma can affect growth, as can its therapy. Growth retardation may be caused by injudicious use of steroids but can also result from the chronic hypoxemia of uncontrolled asthma. When growth is retarded, the patient may have a growth spurt when the asthma is brought under control. Blood pressure should be recorded, because steroids, adrenergic agents, and possibly theophylline may elevate blood pressure. Cardiac rate and rhythm should be scrutinized for similar reasons.

Respiratory Mechanics and Chest Examination. The physician should observe respiratory rate and color of lips and nail beds and should look for evidence of finger clubbing (not a concomitant of asthma), dyspnea or prolongation of expiration, retractions, or use of accessory muscles to lift the shoulders in breathing. A round-shouldered posture with an increase in anteroposterior diameter results from hyperinflation. In children who develop asthma in early childhood there may be a "pseudorachitic" chest deformity from long-standing airway obstruction. In the small child, the lungs are best examined first, when the child is cooperative and has not been frightened by an otoscope or tongue blade.

Examination of the lungs frequently reveals rhonchi or unequal breath sounds, which may clear at least partly on changing position or coughing. Compression of the chest during expiration may induce latent wheezes. Although wheezing can be elicited frequently with a forced expiratory maneuver, occasionally there is only prolongation of expiration without wheezing. Often it is difficult to persuade the older child or adolescent to exhale forcefully to induce latent wheezes, because the patient has discovered intuitively that such a maneuver may induce coughing that can increase bronchospasm. It is important to note air exchange: some patients with severe asthma do not wheeze because too little air is exchanged to generate a wheezing sound. Wheezing from the lower respiratory tract should be differentiated from similar sounds that can emanate from the laryngeal area in (normal) older children with sufficient forced expiration. When hyperinflation is marked, the heart and liver both may be displaced downward as the diaphragm is depressed, shifting the point of cardiac maximal impact, decreasing precardiac dullness, and making the liver palpable. Examination of the heart is important because both the disease and its therapy may alter rate and rhythm. Wheezing and pulmonary rhonchi, however, may make this examination difficult.

Associated Signs of Allergy. The recognition of signs of upper respiratory allergy, which often coexists with asthma, may aid in achieving better control of asthma by identifying aggravating factors (e.g., sinusitis) or coexistent physical disability (e.g., serous otitis with conductive deafness). Because nasal polyps occur rarely in the child with uncomplicated asthma, their presence suggests cystic fibrosis in the young child or paranasal sinusitis with aspirin sensitivity in the adolescent. ("Allergy" is an unusual cause of nasal polyposis.) Eardrums should be examined with a pneumatic otoscope for serous otitis. The conjunctivae should be examined for edema, inflammation, and tearing. A slit-lamp examination for cataracts also is indicated in the child who is receiving chronic treatment with corticosteroids. The texture of the skin and subcutaneous tissue should be noted, as it relates to nutrition and fluid balance, and flexor creases and other areas of skin should be examined for active or healed atopic dermatitis.

DIFFERENTIAL DIAGNOSIS

Table 41–2 lists the common conditions to be differentiated from asthma at various stages of childhood. Almost all can coexist with asthma. A comprehensive list of conditions associated with wheezing is found elsewhere (Siegel et al, 1978).

Laryngotracheobronchomalacia. A congenital disorder of cartilage, laryngotracheobronchomalacia, can coexist with asthma. Symptoms increase with respiratory infections. The condition usually subsides spontaneously by 2 years of age.

Cystic Fibrosis. Cystic fibrosis should be suspected in any infant who has recurrent bronchial infection with poor growth. A diagnosis of cystic fibrosis does not rule out asthma, because the two may exist in the same patient. Control of asthma and other allergic respiratory disease may lead to overall improvement of the patient with cystic fibrosis.

Chronic Diseases due to Respiratory Viral Infections. Both adenovirus and respiratory syncytial virus infections may cause chronic pulmonary disease in infants. The ultimate prognosis for such children is not known at present, although several prospective studies are now in progress.

Foreign Body. The presence of a foreign body must be distinguished from asthma at any age. *The sudden onset of persistent, unremitting wheezing is due to a foreign body until proven otherwise.* Some foreign bodies may not induce symptoms immediately because of their composition and the regions in which they lodge. For instance, an aspirated peanut may

Table 41–2. DIFFERENTIAL DIAGNOSIS OF ASTHMA

Condition	Relative Frequency of Occurrence			
	INFANCY	CHILDHOOD	ADOLESCENCE	ADULTHOOD
Laryngomalacia-tracheomalacia-bronchomalacia	+ +	±	–	–
Cystic fibrosis	+ + +*	+*	±	±†
Chronic viral infection	+ + +	+ +		
Foreign body	+ +	+ + +	±	±
Croup	+ +	+	–	–
Epiglottitis	+ + +	+	–	–
Pertussis	+ + +	+	–	–
Congenital anomalies	+ + +	+	–	–
Hyperventilation syndrome	–	+	+ +	+ +
Bronchiectasis	+	+	+	+
Mitral valve prolapse	–	–	+	+
Laryngeal (physical or psychological)	–	–	±	±
Tumors (extra- or intralumenal)	–	–	–	+
COPD (includes emphysema, chronic bronchitis)	–	–	–	+ +*
Cardiac	–	–	–	+
Pulmonary embolism	–	–	–	±
Collagen-vascular	–	–	±	±
Aspiration syndromes	+	±	±	+

*Often coexists with an element of "asthma." Information obtained from various sources.
†Many patients with cystic fibrosis are now living into adulthood. The minus sign denotes never or extremely rare.
COPD, Chronic obstructive pulmonary disease.
(Reproduced with permission from Bierman CW and Pearlman DS [eds]: Allergic Diseases from Infancy to Adulthood. 2nd ed. Philadelphia, WB Saunders Co, 1988.)

cause progressive symptoms not only because it induces progressive inflammation per se but also because it may induce allergic sensitization leading to a progressive allergic reaction to peanut antigens. Inflammation caused by a foreign body may progress to localized bronchiectasis. If a foreign body is suspected, chest radiographs should be taken during inspiration and expiration, followed by fluoroscopy or bronchoscopy, or both if necessary.

Croup and Acute Epiglottitis. Croup is a common condition caused by respiratory virus; acute epiglottitis is a fulminating infection due to *Hemophilus influenzae*. Often children with asthma have a history of recurrent croup. In both croup and epiglottitis, however, "wheezing" is mainly inspiratory.

Hyperventilation Syndrome. This condition is more likely to occur in adolescence than in childhood; it may be mistaken for asthma or may coexist with it. Typically, the patient is anxious and complains of marked dyspnea and difficulty getting enough air to breathe in spite of excellent air exchange on auscultation and an absence of wheezing. Often there are associated complaints of headache and tingling of the fingers and toes. Pulmonary function tests are helpful in differentiating hyperventilation syndrome from asthma if the patient's cooperation can be obtained. (The patient sometimes will refuse to perform the maneuvers because of fear of "smothering.") Immediate therapy consists of giving reassurance and having the patient rebreathe into a paper bag to elevate Pa_{CO_2}. Long-term therapy involves evaluation of the cause of anxiety and psychotherapy if appropriate. "Laryngeal wheezing" is another condition with a possible psychosomatic etiology that must be differentiated from asthma.

Mitral Valve Prolapse. Mitral valve prolapse oc-

curs in slender asthenic adolescents and is more common in females than in males. Patients with this condition have symptoms of chest pain during or following strenuous exercise; it is this symptom that could be taken for asthma induced by exercise. On physical examination, the diagnosis may be suspected if systolic "clicks" are heard in the mitral area and may be confirmed by echocardiography (Devereaux et al, 1976). An exercise test would rule out exercise-induced asthma but should be performed only with continuous cardiac monitoring.

LABORATORY DIAGNOSIS

Table 41–3 lists laboratory tests useful in diagnosing asthma.

CBC. Often the complete blood count is normal. Eosinophilia, if present, does not indicate an allergic etiology, because eosinophil counts may vary with adrenal function and severity of asthma. Nor does a leukocytosis greater than 15,000 cells/mm³ necessarily indicate infection; both the "stress" of acute asthma and the injection of epinephrine can induce leukocytosis.

Cytologic Examination of Sputum and Nasal Mucus. Examinations of sputum and nasal mucus are simple, noninvasive tests. Asthma in older children and adults is characterized by abundant, thick, tenacious sputum. In young children, sputum rarely is observed because it is ordinarily swallowed. When obtained, it usually is white or "clear"; it may contain small yellow plugs (often containing eosinophils), even when infection is not present. On microscopic examination, eosinophils usually are present, along with other findings listed in Table 41–3. There is

Table 41–3. LABORATORY FINDINGS IN ASTHMA

Test	Possible Findings in Asthma	Comments
Complete blood count	Leukocytosis (occasional)	Induced by infection, epinephrine administration, "stress" (?)
	Eosinophilia (frequent)	Varies with medication, time of day, adrenal function; not necessarily related to "allergy"; often higher in "intrinsic" than "extrinsic" asthma
Sputum examination	White or clear with small yellow plugs	
	Eosinophils	Present in both "intrinsic" and "extrinsic" asthma
	Charcot-Leyden crystals	Derived from eosinophils
	Creola bodies	Clusters of epithelial cells
	Curschmann's spirals	Threads of glycoprotein
Nasal smear	Eosinophils	Predominance suggests concomitant nasal allergy in children
	Lymphocytes, PMNs, macrophages	Predominant cells in upper respiratory infections
	PMNs with ingested bacteria	Suggests rhinitis or sinusitis
Quantitative serum immunoglobulin levels		
IgG, IgA, IgM	Often normal; may be abnormal	Various patterns seen
IgE	Sometimes elevated in "allergic" asthma; often normal	
	Presence of Aspergillus precipitin	Suggestive but not diagnostic of bronchopulmonary aspergillosis
Sweat test	Normal in asthma	Performed to rule out cystic fibrosis (CF), especially in infants with growth retardation and/or recurrent pneumonia; positive result does not rule out asthma, which can coexist with CF
Chest x-ray	Hyperinflation, atelectasis, infiltrates, pneumomediastinum, pneumothorax	Should be done once in every asthmatic child; should always be considered on hospitalization for asthma
Lung function tests	Decreases in FEV_1, FVC, $FEF_{50-75\%}$, PEFR, and FEV_1/FVC	Useful for following course of disease and response to treatment
Response to β_2 bronchodilators	15% improvement in FEV_1 and/or PEFR	Safest diagnostic test for asthma (see text for dosage)
Exercise tolerance tests	Decrease in lung function after 6 min of exercise	Useful to diagnose asthma in children; results often abnormal when resting lung function is normal
Bronchial challenge tests		
Methacholine inhalation (Mecholyl) test, histamine inhalation test	20% fall in FEV_1 in asthmatic	Should be performed only by specialist, occasionally used to diagnose asthma
Antigen inhalation test	20% fall in FEV_1 immediately after challenge; possible delayed response 6–8 hours later	Potentially dangerous—can induce anaphylaxis; should be performed only by specialist; rarely necessary
Allergy skin tests	Positive reactions if patient is allergic to factors tested	Performed to identify potential allergic factors in asthma; only the likely factors (indicated by history) should be tested for
RAST	Same significance as allergy skin tests	More expensive than allergy skin tests

PMN, polymorphonuclear neutrophils; RAST, radioallergosorbent test.
(Reproduced with permission from Bierman CW and Pearlman DS [eds]: Allergic Diseases from Infancy to Adulthood. 2nd ed. Philadelphia, WB Saunders Co, 1988.)

eosinophilia in the sputum in both nonallergic and allergic asthma.

By contrast, nasal secretions are obtained readily in children. Predominance of eosinophils suggests accompanying nasal allergy in children, although adolescents and adults can have nasal eosinophilia in the absence of allergy (Mullarkey et al, 1980). A predominance of PMNs and lymphocytes occurs with viral respiratory infections; PMNs and ingested bacteria are seen frequently in patients with sinusitis.

Serum Tests. Determining quantitative levels of immunoglobulin G, M, and A is useful only to rule out immunodeficiency symptoms in children with recurrent or chronic infection. In children with asthma, IgG levels usually are normal, IgA levels occasionally are low, and IgM levels may be elevated. Systemic steroids, however, can depress IgG and perhaps IgA levels. IgE determinations are rarely needed. A normal IgE level does not rule out allergy,

and an elevated level does not diagnose it. However, the serum IgE level may be useful if it is elevated in the young child with recurrent bronchitis in whom there is a question of the role of "allergy" in inducing or exacerbating the symptoms. In the child with shifting pulmonary infiltrates, a marked elevation of serum IgE level should occasion tests for precipitating antibody to *Aspergillus* and agents causing hypersensitivity pneumonitis.

Sweat Test. A sweat test should be carried out on infants and children with chronic respiratory symptoms to rule out cystic fibrosis. However, cystic fibrosis also may have a significant reactive airways component, which should be treated.

Radiographs. All children with asthma should have a chest radiograph at some time to rule out parenchymal disease, congenital anomaly, and foreign body. A chest radiograph should be obtained or at least considered for every child admitted to a hospital with asthma. Radiographic findings in asthma may range from normal to hyperinflation with peribronchial interstitial infiltrates and atelectasis. In a 3-year study of children hospitalized for asthma, the following abnormalities were seen: 76 per cent had hyperinflation with increased bronchial markings (Fig. 41–10A); 20 per cent had infiltrates, atelectasis, pneumonia, or a combination of the three (Fig. 41–10B); and 5.4 per cent had pneumomediastinum (Fig. 41–10C), often with infiltrates (Eggleston et al, 1974). Pneumothorax occurs rarely (Fig. 41–10D).

Paranasal sinus radiographs also should be considered for children with persistent nocturnal coughing and headaches.

Lung Function Tests. Pulmonary function tests are objective, noninvasive, and extremely helpful in diagnosis and follow-up of patients with asthma. A simple mechanical spirometer from which a forced expiratory volume in 1 sec (FEV_1) and a forced vital capacity (FVC) can be calculated or a Wright Pediatric Peak Flow Meter for younger children is useful in office practice. Children as young as 2 years can be taught to perform pulmonary function maneuvers with a birthday party favor (Fig. 41–11). Results can be compared with normal standards (Table 41–4).

Bronchial Challenge Tests. Airway hyperreactivity to substances such as methacholine or histamine forms the basis of a diagnostic test for asthma (Chai

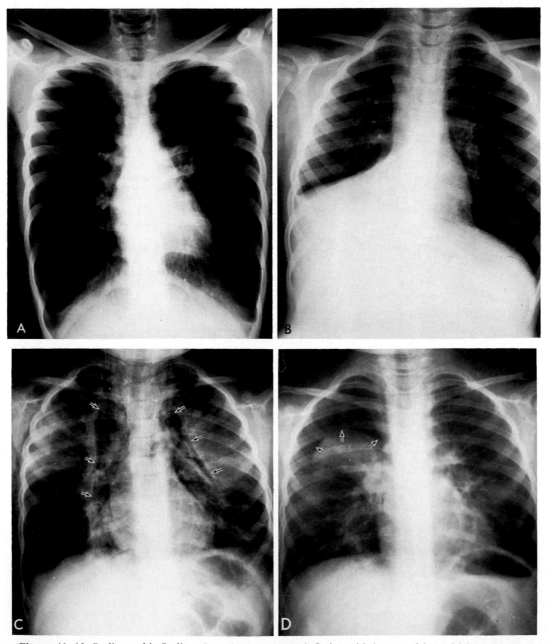

Figure 41–10. Radiographic findings in asthma. *A,* Hyperinflation with increased bronchial markings. *B,* Atelectasis involving a complete lobe. *C,* Massive pneumomediastinum complicating asthma. *D,* Pneumothorax secondary to paroxysmal coughing in asthma.

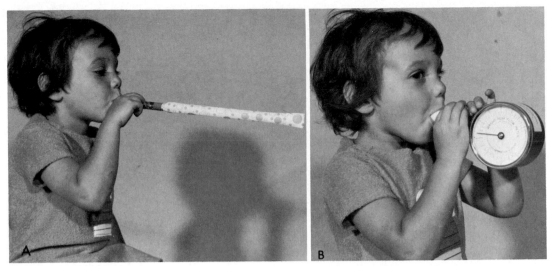

Figure 41–11. Use of party favor to teach lung function maneuver to small children.

Table 41–4. AVERAGE (50%) PULMONARY FUNCTION VALUES IN CHILDREN

Height		FVC (liters)		FEV₁	$FEF_{25-75\%}$		PEFR	
cm	in	Boys	Girls	(liters)	L/min	L/sec	L/min	L/sec
100	39.4	1.00	1.00	.70	55	.91	100	1.67
102	40.2	1.03	1.00	.75	60	1.00	110	1.83
104	40.9	1.08	1.07	.82	64	1.06	120	2.00
106	41.7	1.14	1.10	.89	70	1.17	130	2.17
108	42.5	1.19	1.19	.97	75	1.25	140	2.33
110	43.3	1.27	1.24	1.01	80	1.33	150	2.50
112	44.1	1.32	1.30	1.10	86	1.43	160	2.67
114	44.9	1.40	1.36	1.17	90	1.50	174	2.90
116	45.7	1.47	1.41	1.23	96	1.60	185	3.08
118	46.5	1.52	1.49	1.30	100	1.67	195	3.25
120	47.2	1.60	1.55	1.39	105	1.75	204	3.40
122	48.0	1.69	1.62	1.45	110	1.83	215	3.58
124	48.8	1.75	1.70	1.53	118	1.97	226	3.77
126	49.6	1.82	1.77	1.59	121	2.01	236	3.93
128	50.4	1.90	1.84	1.67	127	2.12	247	4.11
130	51.2	1.99	1.90	1.72	132	2.20	256	4.27
132	52.0	2.07	2.00	1.80	139	2.32	267	4.45
134	52.8	2.15	2.06	1.89	142	2.37	278	4.63
136	53.5	2.24	2.15	1.98	149	2.48	289	4.82
138	54.3	2.35	2.24	2.06	153	2.55	299	4.98
140	55.1	2.40	2.32	2.11	159	2.65	310	5.17
142	55.9	2.50	2.40	2.20	163	2.72	320	5.33
144	56.7	2.60	2.50	2.30	170	2.83	330	5.50
146	57.5	2.70	2.59	2.39	173	2.88	340	5.67
148	58.3	2.79	2.68	2.48	180	3.00	351	5.85
150	59.1	2.88	2.78	2.57	183	3.05	362	6.03
152	59.8	2.97	2.88	2.66	190	3.17	373	6.22
154	60.6	3.09	2.98	2.75	195	3.25	384	6.40
156	61.4	3.20	3.09	2.88	200	3.33	394	6.57
158	62.2	3.30	3.18	2.98	205	3.42	404	6.73
160	63.0	3.40	3.27	3.06	210	3.50	415	6.92
162	63.8	3.52	3.40	3.18	215	3.58	425	7.08
164	64.6	3.64	3.50	3.29	220	3.67	436	7.28
166	65.4	3.78	3.60	3.40	225	3.75	446	7.43
168	66.1	3.90	3.72	3.50	230	3.83	457	7.62
170	66.9	4.00	3.83	3.65	236	3.93	467	7.78
172	67.7	4.20	3.83	3.80	241	4.01	477	7.95
174	68.5	4.20	3.83	3.80	246	4.10	488	8.13
176	69.3	4.20	3.83	3.80	251	4.18	498	8.30

(Data from Polgar G and Promadhat V: Pulmonary Function Testing in Children: Techniques and Standards. Philadelphia, WB Saunders Co, 1971.)

et al, 1975; Spector and Kinsman, 1979). Methacholine and histamine responsiveness are similar when tested in the same individual and may be more sensitive than an exercise test in diagnosing nonspecific bronchial hyperresponsiveness (Hargreave et al, 1981).

Inhalation of an antigen to which the patient has a positive skin reaction has been employed to test the relevance of skin test results to the child's asthma and the effect of drugs (Chai, 1979) and other therapy (Aas, 1970) on the bronchial response. Often this inhalation test induces a biphasic reaction, an initial fall in lung function followed in 6 to 8 hours by more severe bronchospasm. The consequence of this late asthmatic reaction can be an increase in bronchial hyperactivity that may persist for days or weeks and is thought to be due to the infiltration of inflammatory cells, especially eosinophils (Wasserman, 1988). Because bronchial challenge with antigen is a potentially dangerous procedure, and because the information can often be obtained by other means, such as correlating the child's history with the amount of specific antibody measured by RAST or with results of specific skin tests, bronchial challenge tests using antigen are rarely indicated in children. Bronchial challenge tests should be performed only by specialists who have had training in their use.

However, bronchial provocation tests using histamine, methacholine, or hypertonic saline to diagnose bronchial hyperreactivity (BHR) are not associated with late reactions. Table 41–5 provides guidelines for bronchial provocation using methacholine or histamine. The end point is a 20 per cent fall in FEV_1 (PD_{20}) sustained for 3 minutes (Shapiro et al, 1982).

Exercise Tolerance Test. In children 6 years of age through adulthood, a treadmill exercise test provides useful information about the individual's ability to exercise and to participate in sports and normal recreational activities. It also measures functionally how well drugs have controlled the asthma. In addition, the exercise test can be useful in diagnosing asthma in children with histories suggestive of exercise-induced bronchospasm.

One can minimize the influence of factors such as environmental temperatures and humidity by performing the test in an environmentally controlled laboratory, in which ambient temperature and humidity can be maintained within a constant range. Cardiac monitoring during exercise testing is important to safety, even in children. A monitor in which both pulse and cardiac rhythm can be observed in the form of continuous electrocardiogram (ECG) is preferred, so that a tracing can be made in the event of aberrant rhythm or other cardiac abnormality. Readily available should be drugs for treating asthma and resuscitation equipment and supplies, including syringes, intravenous sets, oxygen, a defibrillator, and a hand-controlled respirator with face mask or its equivalent (Cropp, 1979).

Pulmonary function should be measured 5 min before and immediately before exercise. During ex-

Table 41–5. METHACHOLINE OR HISTAMINE BRONCHIAL CHALLENGE

Equipment
1. Compressed-air tank with regulator pressure gauge.
2. Rosenthal-French Dosimeter.
3. DiVilbiss Nebulizer No. 646.
4. Methacholine or histamine phosphate in solution with buffered saline at the following concentrations:
   a. 0.075 mg/ml
   b. 0.15 mg/ml
   c. 0.31 mg/ml
   d. 0.62 mg/ml
   e. 1.25 mg/ml
   f. 2.5 mg/ml
   g. 5.0 mg/ml
   h. 10.0 mg/ml*
   i. 25.0 mg/ml*
5. Pulmonary function testing equipment.
6. Have aerosolized bronchodilator (metaproterenol, isoetharine, or albuterol) on hand to reverse severe drop if necessary.

Technique
1. Obtain two baseline readings of pulmonary function 5 min apart.
2. Have the patient inhale buffered saline after pressing the reset button.
3. The patient should inhale for as long as the "valve open" light is on.
4. The reset button must be pressed again before another breath can trigger the control unit.
5. The dose should be inhaled five times, and each inhalation should be held for 5 sec.
6. After each solution has been inhaled, spirograms should be obtained at 1.5 and 3 min.
7. Have the patient inhale the weakest dose of metacholine or histamine (0.075 mg/ml) and follow the same procedure.
8. Have the patient inhale the next stronger dose (0.15 mg/ml) and follow the same procedure; repeat with next stronger dose.
9. Bronchial challenge is stopped when a dose triggers a sustained 20% decrease in pulmonary function; the dose that has triggered it is noted.

*Histamine in this concentration may induce side effects, such as headache and flushing.

ercise, peak flow measurements taken at 2 min and 4 min provide information about the degree of bronchodilation induced by exercise. Other pulmonary function parameters are difficult to obtain without interrupting treadmill exercise. Following exercise, serial pulmonary function measurements should be obtained for at least 20 min to determine the severity of exercise-induced asthma. Calculations of $\dot{V}_{50}$ or $FEF_{25-75\%}$ should include an isovolume correction to compensate for changing lung volumes. A decrease of more than 10 per cent in peak expiratory flow rate, of more than 12 per cent in FEV_1, or of more than 15 per cent in $FEF_{25-75\%}$ is diagnostic of exercise-induced asthma. Table 41–6 contains guidelines for performance of an exercise tolerance test.

Allergy Testing. Allergy testing—skin testing or RAST—is indicated in patients in whom specific allergic factors are believed to be important and probably in all children with severe asthma to rule out allergic factors that might contribute significantly to the asthma (e.g., danders from domestic animals in the home). Testing is done with allergens selected on the basis of history of known or potential allergen exposures.

INDICATIONS FOR TESTING. After a detailed dietary

Table 41–6. PROCEDURE FOR EXERCISE TOLERANCE (TREADMILL) TEST

1. Measure pulmonary function (PEFR and spirogram) 5 min before start of test.
   Note: Do not perform exercise test if subject's baseline functions are decreased by 20 per cent or more from those on previous visit or if subject is coughing or wheezing.
2. Prepare areas of subject's skin for application of electrodes at third intercostal space on each side and in midsternal areas; apply electrodes.
3. Connect cable to electrodes. Check ECG tracing. Reposition electrodes if necessary.
4. Loosely attach cable to subject's forearm, holding it in place with rubber tourniquet. DO NOT wrap cable around treadmill handle.
5. Repeat pulmonary function readings immediately before beginning test.
6. Start the treadmill at a walking pace. Gradually increase elevation to 10 per cent and increase the speed until subject's heart rate is stabilized at the target pulse rate.
   Note: Adults (older than 20 years) should run at a speed that keeps the heart rate at no more than 80 per cent of maximum as indicated on the table below.
7. Subject should run for 6 min. PEFR should be determined at 2 min and 4 min from start of running.
8. After subject has run for 6 min, obtain spirogram and PEFR immediately and at 3, 5, 10, 15, and 20 min. If subject experiences wheezing or significant difficulty breathing, administer aerosolized bronchodilator, e.g., two inhalations of albuterol.
9. Calculate maximum drop in lung function, using lowest postexercise values and highest pre-exercise values.
10. To calculate $FEF_{25-75\%}$ or $\dot{V}_{50}$, use isovolume correction calculation derived from the lowest postexercise values.

PREDICTED HEART RATES ACCORDING TO AGE

Age (years)	Maximum Heart Rate (beats/min)	Percentage of Predicted Maximum				
		95	90	85	80	75
5	206 ± 10	196	185	175	165	155
10	202 ± 10	192	182	172	162	152
15	198 ± 10	188	178	168	158	149
20	194 ± 10	184	175	165	155	146
25	191 ± 10	181	172	162	153	143
30	187 ± 10	178	168	159	150	140

and environmental history is taken, skin testing is a logical procedure for identifying allergens that may be causing or exacerbating asthmatic symptoms. Skin tests should be limited to most likely allergens as suggested by the history.

FACTORS AFFECTING SKIN REACTION. Skin test results may vary with age, drug therapy, and inherent skin factors. For example, a positive skin reaction in an infant may appear as a small wheal with a minimal flare, compared with a large wheal with "pseudopods" and a dramatic surrounding flare in an older child or adult. This difference may result from the presence of only small amounts of skin-fixed specific IgE and low skin histamine content in the infant. Drugs affecting skin test results include antihistamines (particularly hydroxyzine, which may inhibit skin reactions for up to 72 hours, or longer-acting antihistamines, such as astemizole, which can suppress skin reactions for weeks). Other asthma drugs, such as oral adrenergic agents, cromolyn sodium, and theophylline, may decrease the size of but will not block skin reactions. Topical and systemic corticosteroids do not affect skin reactions. Positive (histamine) and negative (saline) control tests should be included to detect inherent skin factors that may affect the reaction to allergen, such as dermatographism and possible interference from drugs.

RAST. The RAST makes use of the affinity of IgE antibody for antigen that has been bound to a cellulose disc. A radio-tagged or enzyme-linked anti-IgE detects the quantity of specific IgE bound to the disc. The RAST is no more specific than the antigen employed (hence, no more specific than a skin test) and should be reserved for special situations in which

skin tests are impractical, as in the patient with generalized dermatitis, the very young child, and the rare patient who is too ill for direct testing or must continue to receive medications with antihistaminic activity (e.g., tricyclic antidepressants).

THERAPEUTIC CONSIDERATIONS

PHILOSOPHY OF MANAGEMENT

A comprehensive approach to treatment of asthma in children requires an understanding of the disease, the manner in which it manifests in children, and the ways it may affect physical and psychological growth and development. *The ultimate goal is to prevent disability and to minimize physical and psychological morbidity.* This goal includes facilitation of the child's social adjustments in the family, school, and community and of normal participation in recreational activities and sports. Asthma control is achieved in steps and should begin with early diagnosis and appropriate management of acute episodes. Irritant and allergic factors should be identified and eliminated from the child's environment. *Education of the parents and child concerning the long-term nature of asthma and the management of exacerbations is an essential part of asthma therapy.* Unnecessary and illogical restrictions of the child's and family's life styles should be avoided. Associated conditions that exacerbate asthma and predispose to school absenteeism or interfere with school performance must be recognized and treated. The ultimate goal should be "functional" normality, in which the patient can participate fully in activities with family and peers with minimal restrictions and the fewest adverse effects from treatment.

Achieving these goals requires time, knowledge, and experience. The demands on the physician will vary depending on the severity of the disease, the age of the patient, and the resources of the family. The family physician or pediatrician *who is willing to devote the time* can care adequately for the child with mild or moderate asthma. Nevertheless, many such patients, as well as patients with severe asthma and chronic obstructive pulmonary changes, will benefit from referral to a specialist, who has the knowledge, experience, and time to initiate appropriate therapy, provide long-term follow-up, and act as an adviser to the primary care physician. Such a referral should emphasize prompt and effective treatment of acute attacks and should minimize the need for hospitalization (or reduce the length of hospital stay when hospitalization is necessary). A team approach that includes regular communication among the parents or patient or both, the referring physician, and the specialist is essential for consistent and comprehensive long-term care.

Compliance by patient and family is the keystone of any therapy. Compliance is influenced by many factors: the physician's attitude, the family's and patient's understanding of the disease, and peer pressures. It is in compliance that psychological factors are of overwhelming importance. The child's attitude toward asthma and willingness to comply with recommendations reflect the parents' attitude toward the disease. The physician's guidance can prevent overprotection or neglect by helping the family of the younger child to cope with such aspects of asthma as the inconvenience of a round-the-clock medication schedule and environmental control. As children grow, physicians and families should give them the responsibility for taking medication, although *physicians should help by providing the most convenient medication schedule possible*—ideally one that avoids the need to take medication in school. When medication is needed at school, the patient should be permitted to take it privately without embarrassment. The physician should aid the patient and family in making decisions about such activities as sports, overnight visits, and camping trips, taking care to avoid overprotection while ensuring appropriate control of asthma. The physician also can help to change the attitudes of teachers, principals, and coaches (and in some cases, school nurses) by educating them about the needs of the individual child and by showing them how the school program can be adjusted to the child's physical capacity, so that the child is not penalized or singled out for ridicule.

When a child or the parents fail to comply, the physician should try to find out the reasons for noncompliance and to work out a reasonable solution acceptable to the patient and the family.

PHARMACOLOGY OF ASTHMA DRUGS

Current treatment of asthma involves drugs of four major classes: adrenergic agents, methylxanthines, cromolyn sodium, and adrenocorticosteroids. This section deals with the clinical pharmacology of each of these classes. In the next section, ways in which these agents may be prescribed to control asthma are discussed.

Adrenergic Drugs

The activity of adrenergic drugs in asthma was first appreciated with the introduction of epinephrine (adrenaline) into clinical practice early in the twentieth century. Because it was inactive orally, a search for an oral adrenergic agent led to the introduction in 1924 of ephedrine, a drug still widely used in orally active asthma preparations. The division by Ahlquist (1948) of adrenoceptors into alpha and beta types and the subsequent classification of beta receptors by Lands and colleagues (1967) into β_1 and β_2 subtypes led to the synthesis of long-acting agents with specific activity in asthma.

Approximately 20 years ago, *isoproterenol* became the preferred drug for aerosolized use because of its greater potency and specificity for beta receptors. Isoproterenol, however, has the disadvantage of being short acting because it is actively transported into cells by the uptake-2 process for catecholamine, where it is inactivated by catechol-O-methyl transferase (COMT). Because isoproterenol activates β_1 as well as β_2 receptors, it has marked cardiovascular effects even at therapeutic doses. The first pulmonary-selective drug, *isoetharine* (1969), was distinctly more active on bronchial muscle than on heart muscle. Its main disadvantage is its short duration of action, which is due to its basic catechol structure. *Metaproterenol*, the first noncatechol analogue, was synthesized in Germany. It is 10 to 40 times less active than isoproterenol, but its bronchodilating effect, when administered by inhalation, is accompanied by only minor systemic effects because it is relatively slowly absorbed from the lung. Its bronchodilating action persists for about 4 hours. Metaproterenol is available as tablets and syrup for oral administration and as a metered-dose inhaler and solution for aerosol administration. *Albuterol* (salbutamol), the first highly selective β_2-stimulant bronchodilator with a duration of action of 4 to 6 hours, was developed in England and came into general clinical use in 1969 (1981 in the United States). It is available as tablets and solution for oral administration as well as a solution and metered-dose inhaler for aerosol administration. *Terbutaline*, available in tablets, a metered-dose inhaler, and a solution for parenteral use in the United States, is similar to albuterol in duration and specificity. Other β_2-specific agents include bitolterol mesylate, fenoterol (available in Canada), and pirbuterol acetate, available in metered-dose inhalers.

Pharmacology

ABSORPTION. Modified adrenergic agents (saligenin or resorcinol derivatives) are absorbed when administered orally, whereas catecholamines must be administered parenterally or by aerosol because they are inactivated by COMT in the lung and by sulfokinase in the gastrointestinal tract.

DISTRIBUTION. Once absorbed, adrenergic drugs are distributed rapidly to the vascular compartment and transported selectively by the uptake-2 process into the intracellular compartment of cells containing beta-adrenergic receptors, such as bronchial smooth muscle and mast cells.

METABOLISM. The catecholamine beta-adrenergic agonists form a substrate for COMT, which, along with monoamine oxidase, methylates and deaminates the drugs for excretion in urine. The catecholamines are rapidly metabolized intracellularly at the membrane level; resorcinol derivatives, such as metaproterenol and terbutaline, and saligenin derivatives, such as albuterol, have longer half-lives because they are not metabolized by COMT but are inactivated by hepatic metabolism to glucuronides and intestinal sulfokinases or are excreted unchanged. Accordingly, the resorcinol and saligenin derivatives have longer and more specific beta-adrenergic activity on smooth muscle and mast cells.

EXCRETION. Metabolic products of catecholamines as well as modified adrenergic agents are excreted primarily by the kidneys as glucuronides, sulfates, and various forms of mandelic acid.

Mode of Action. The adrenergic agents with β_1 and β_2 receptor activity initiate their response on the receptor site of the bronchial smooth muscle cell or mast cell. The activated receptor mediates a transfer reaction through a membrane subcoupler unit and a catalytic subunit to induce adenylate cyclase generation. Adenylate cyclase acts as a catalyst for the intracellular conversion of adenosine triphosphate (ATP) to adenosine 3',5'-cyclic monophosphate (cAMP). The increased levels of cellular cAMP mediate the cellular response, i.e., bronchodilation, inhibition of mediator release, or glycolysis.

Side Effects. The action of these relatively specific β_2 agents in vivo depends on the route of delivery. Systemic administration may produce side effects, such as muscular tremor and some cardiovascular effects, in addition to bronchodilation, whereas administration by aerosol in the usual dose induces bronchodilation with minimal tremor and cardiovascular effects.

The inhalation of isoproterenol causes marked tachycardia, of metaproterenol only mild tachycardia, and of albuterol and terbutaline minimal change in pulse rate (unless dosage exceeds 600 to 800 μg). Oral administration of metaproterenol, albuterol, or terbutaline produces a dose-related increase in pulse rate.

Skeletal muscle tremor invariably accompanies systemic administration of β_2 agents. A dose of 4 mg albuterol or 5 mg terbutaline doubles baseline tremor when administered for the first time. Tremor tends to decrease with chronic use.

Methylxanthines

Pharmacologists in both the United States and Germany in 1922 discovered that naturally occurring methylxanthines were bronchodilators, and that dimethylxanthines (theophylline and theobromine) were more active than trimethylxanthine (caffeine). As early as 1931, an oral bronchodilator containing theophylline and theobromine was marketed for pediatric use. Intravenous aminophylline was found to be effective in treating severe asthma in 1938 and has been employed widely since. However, it was not until the late 1960s that the knowledge of the clinical pharmacology of these agents, along with the widespread availability of therapeutic monitoring, made this class safe and effective in treating asthma in children.

Pharmacology

ABSORPTION. Theophylline is relatively insoluble in water, but its solubility can be increased if it is combined with ethylenediamine (aminophylline) or a similar substance. Because of this low solubility, theophylline was thought to be poorly absorbed from the stomach and small intestines. However, pharmacokinetic studies have demonstrated that it is well absorbed, even when taken with food.

DISTRIBUTION. A two-compartment pharmacologic model appears to account for the distribution of theophylline between the gastrointestinal tract and plasma.

METABOLISM. Theophylline is metabolized primarily in the liver, probably utilizing enzyme systems that degrade troleandomycin but not bilirubin and probably not phenobarbital. Serum half-life of theophylline varies widely with such factors as age, diet, illness, and cigarette smoking but averages approximately 4 hours in children. *Certain drugs, e.g., erythromycin, troleandomycin (TAO), Lincocin, and cimetidine, also can interfere with metabolism, significantly increasing the serum half-life of theophylline.* Metabolism of this drug is greatly decreased in infants younger than 4 months. In addition, wide inter- and intrasubject variation makes therapeutic monitoring an essential part of theophylline therapy.

EXCRETION. Theophylline is metabolized virtually completely by the liver, but at least one metabolite retains some biologic activity. The metabolites are excreted entirely by the kidneys.

Mode of Action. Methylxanthines were once believed to competitively inhibit a phosphodiesterase that converts adenosine 3',5'-monophosphate to the biologically inert 5'-AMP. This action has been disproved, and current theory postulates that theophylline may inhibit adenosine-induced bronchoconstriction (Holgate et al, 1984).

The effectiveness and toxicity of theophylline appear to relate to serum concentration. In general a serum concentration of 5 to 10 μg/ml is required for effectiveness. Significant and sufficient therapeutic effects can be achieved at lower blood levels than 10 μg/ml in many children. If the concentration is above 20 μg/ml, the likelihood of significant drug toxicity is greatly increased. Adverse effects on the central nervous system may occur (effect on memory) at levels substantially less than 20 μg/ml. The average dosages required to achieve a serum concentration of theophylline in the range of 10 to 20 μg/ml are as follows: for children 1 to 8 years old, 25 mg/kg; for children 8 to 16 years, 20 mg/kg; for children 16 and older, 12 mg/kg. One should remember, however, that *there are marked variations in theophylline metabolism and therefore in individual patient requirements.*

Preparations. A plethora of theophylline preparations are available. These range from solutions, suspensions, and anhydrous or microcrystalline preparations to timed-release beads and compressed tablets. The reader is advised to become thoroughly familiar with a few preparations and to use them appropriately. The following factors may influence the choice of specific preparations: (1) anhydrous theophylline equivalence, (2) route of administration, (3) rate of dissolution of oral timed-release preparations, (4) the patient's individual theophylline metabolic rate, and (5) patient compliance in following the dosage schedule. Most available preparations are intended for oral administration. Theophylline ethylenediamine (aminophylline) is available for intravenous use. For rectal administration, both aminophylline suppositories and rectal solutions are available. The *rectal suppositories* are erratically absorbed, are potentially hazardous because of easy overdosage, and therefore *are not recommended.* Rectal solutions by contrast are readily and rapidly absorbed and may be useful in patients who cannot retain oral preparations because of vomiting due to viral infection or other causes. However, they should not be administered to a patient who is vomiting until a serum level test confirms that theophylline intoxication is not causing the vomiting.

Oral preparations are available as liquids (for small children who cannot take other formulations) and "immediate-release" and "sustained-release" tablet forms. Liquid preparations and "immediate-release" tablets and capsules are particularly useful for intermittent therapy. Sustained-release preparations, available as timed-release granules and compressed tablets, have dissolution times ranging from 8 to 12 hours. Dosage requirements vary widely in patients, depending on such factors as age and individual theophylline half-life; it is therefore preferable to select the preparation that best controls the asthma with an 8-hour or 12-hour dosage schedule.

Patients with rapid theophylline metabolism (i.e., in whom the drug has a short half-life) will require the frequent administration of nonsustained-release drugs or the use of sustained-release preparations. Those with a slow metabolism (i.e., in whom the drug has a long half-life) may require only two or three doses per day of regular theophylline.

The final factor to consider before prescribing the specific drug is whether the patient is likely to comply with a particular schedule. The dosage times must be reasonable, the liquid must be palatable, and the patient must be old enough to swallow the granules or sustained-release tablets without chewing or crushing them. Theophylline combined with other drugs (ephedrine, barbiturate, antihistamine, guaiacolate) is still available and may be useful in patients with mild asthma, but it is far wiser to prescribe a single-entity theophylline preparation and add other agents as symptoms necessitate. Theophylline formulations that release over a 24-hour span are useful in adolescents and adults (Bierman et al, 1988).

Side Effects. The methylxanthines are coronary artery dilators and can stimulate the myocardium directly. They also induce pulmonary vascular dilation, cause cerebral vascular constriction, and increase vascular resistance. They can enhance the cardiotoxic effects of epinephrine and other adrenergic drugs. Theophylline is an active diuretic and may aggravate water and saline depletion in small children who are vomiting. Theophylline also has central nervous system effects and can interfere with school performance and short-term memory (Furukawa et al, 1988). Theophylline overdose results in gastric irritation, gastrointestinal hemorrhage in rare instances, and central nervous system symptoms, such as agitation, convulsions, coma, respiratory failure, and vasomotor collapse (Mitenko and Ogilvie, 1973). Because nausea and vomiting are centrally induced side effects of theophylline, they can be induced with *any* route of administration of the drug.

Cromolyn Sodium

Cromolyn sodium was synthesized in 1965 as an analogue of khellin, a substance extracted from a Near Eastern plant used in ancient times to treat colic. It is a member of the chromone group of chemicals and is not related to corticosteroids, theophylline, or adrenergic drugs. Its primary action is in prophylaxis of asthma by reduction of the bronchial reactivity induced by irritants, antigens, and exercise. Cromolyn is as effective as theophylline in asthma prophylaxis in children and adolescents with mild to moderate asthma (Furukawa et al, 1984) and is safer than theophylline because it is not absorbed from the gastrointestinal tract and has no central nervous system side effects.

Pharmacology. Cromolyn sodium is a unique chemical because its bibasic structure inhibits gastrointestinal absorption and facilitates excretion.

ABSORPTION AND DISTRIBUTION. A maximum of 8 per cent of an inhaled dose of cromolyn sodium reaches the tracheobronchial tree (Bernstein, 1981). The remainder lodges in the hypopharynx and is swallowed. Because cromolyn is a highly polarized molecule and is insoluble in lipids, it does not cross the mucosa of the gastrointestinal tract readily. Less than 1 per cent of an orally ingested dose is absorbed (Cox et al, 1970). Cromolyn is also absorbed poorly from the lung. A mean peak concentration of 9.52 μg/ml is reached in the first 15 min after inhalation of 20 mg of cromolyn (Bernstein, 1981).

METABOLISM. No biotransformation occurs either in animals or in man. Cromolyn is excreted intact with no intermediate metabolites.

EXCRETION. Approximately 85 per cent of an inhaled dose of cromolyn is excreted in the bile and urine within 1 hour after inhalation, and 95 per cent is excreted within 6 hours.

Mode of Action. Cromolyn appears to be a unique immunopharmacologic agent because it diminishes IgE antibody–induced release of inflammatory mediators from sensitized mast cells. It is not an antihistamine and does not appear to act directly on smooth muscle or through adenylate cyclase, although some studies suggest that it may inhibit phosphodiesterase degradation of cAMP. Cromolyn also appears to decrease bronchial reactivity to irritants such as sulfur dioxide.

Side Effects. The major side effect of cromolyn sodium is transient airway irritation and coughing on inhalation of the powder, which may be very annoying to patients who have hyperreactive airways. However, the aerosol formulations (solution and metered-dose inhalers) are free of this side effect (Shapiro and Koenig, 1985). Maculopapular rashes, urticaria, and various allergic reactions to cromolyn have been reported in a few patients. Toxic reactions to cromolyn are uncommon with clinically attainable dosage levels. Even when the drug was administered intravenously in doses far exceeding the amount normally absorbed in the human through inhalation, no adverse effects occurred (Weinberger and Hendeles, 1988). Cromolyn has no known teratogenic or carcinogenic side effects.

Corticosteroids

The remarkable anti-inflammatory action of the adrenal corticosteroids was discovered by Hench in 1948, who reported dramatic short-term effectiveness in treating rheumatoid arthritis. Thereafter corticosteroids were employed widely in various diseases. Both acute asthma and chronic asthma were found to respond well to cortisone. Steroids were recognized as the only antiasthmatic drugs that could reverse severe asthma unresponsive to bronchodilators. It was almost a decade later that their major side effects became apparent, including severe retardation of linear growth in children. Since then, the major thrust in steroid clinical pharmacology has been to find a method to provide the benefits of effective steroid therapy with minimal adverse effects. In asthma this has been accomplished in two ways: first, by the administration of steroids with short half-life in the morning every second day in sufficient dosage to control asthma, and second, by the use of inhaled forms, which have potent topical but minimal systemic effects. Both methods are effective in increasing the therapeutic index of corticosteroids.

Pharmacology. Exogenous corticosteroids affect carbohydrate metabolism and suppress function of the hypothalamic-pituitary-adrenal gland axis. In addition to their anti-inflammatory actions, these drugs may suppress growth, induce involution of thymus and lymph nodes, cause eosinopenia and lymphocy-

topenia, mobilize free fatty acids, and produce redistribution of lipids within the body.

The anti-inflammatory actions appear to be related to the direct effect on capillary walls and to the indirect effect of reducing the number of inflammatory cells at the site of inflammation. In addition, steroids reduce numbers of circulating eosinophils, monocytes, and lymphocytes and stabilize neutrophil lysozymes.

Corticosteroids also appear to prevent release of cell membrane–derived arachidonic acid, which forms a substrate for both lipoxygenase and cyclooxygenase systems. Thus they may inhibit formation of both prostaglandin and leukotriene derivatives (SRS-A mediators).

ABSORPTION. Corticosteroids are absorbed with oral, topical, intramuscular, intravenous, or inhalational administration. Many steroids are conjugated to improve water solubility and thereby enhance their absorbability, especially from the gastrointestinal tract. Both phosphate and hemisuccinate conjugates enhance or increase the rate of absorption. Aerosolized topical steroids are relatively poorly absorbed but have potent local anti-inflammatory effects in the lungs.

DISTRIBUTION. It appears that approximately 70 per cent of orally administered steroid is absorbed and converted to an active steroid compound in the first 4 to 6 hours after administration. Binding to transcortin and transport are influenced directly by the level of transcortin in the circulation. Steroid bound by transcortin is in equilibrium with the free or unbound steroid, the pharmacologically active form of the drug. An increase in free or non–protein-bound steroid correlates with increased pharmacologic effect.

METABOLISM. A small amount of steroid enters the cells and binds to an intracellular transport mechanism, making its way finally to the nucleus. There it appears to alter messenger RNA transcription to enhance the synthesis of specific proteins and enzymes. The rate of metabolism or degradation varies significantly among asthmatics. Previous steroid therapy may increase the metabolic degradation rates, and liver disease may slow it. Concomitant administration of other drugs, such as barbiturates, may induce microsomal hepatic enzymes and increase the metabolic degradation of corticosteroids.

EXCRETION. Steroids are excreted after glucuronide conjugation in part by biliary excretion but primarily by the kidneys.

Mode of Action. Corticosteroids may have both mineral corticoid and glucocorticoid activities. The anti-inflammatory effect and the effectiveness of steroids in asthma are associated primarily with the glucocorticoid effects.

Corticosteroids appear to act in asthma in a variety of ways. They may restore responsiveness to and act synergistically with catecholamines to increase mast cell and smooth muscle intracellular cAMP, hence decreasing the release of mediators and promoting bronchodilation. Corticosteroids decrease edema, possibly through stabilization of lysozymes. They also appear to suppress allergic mediator formation by inhibiting release of arachidonic acid precursors of potent bronchoconstrictor substances, such as prostaglandin $F_{2\alpha}$ and SRS-A (leukotrienes C, D, and E).

Side Effects. The therapeutic benefits of corticosteroids are marred by their potential adverse effects, which include excessive weight gain, hypertension, and cataracts. The mechanisms of these adverse effects are complex and have been reviewed elsewhere (Morris and Selner, 1980). More commonly, steroids encourage hyperglycemia by diminishing insulin responsiveness of peripheral tissues, decrease growth by diminishing tissue responsiveness to growth hormone, increase protein metabolism (causing osteoporosis), prevent peripheral uptake of amino acids, and interfere with the normal hypothalamic-pituitary-adrenal gland (HPA) feedback mechanism.

The following principles aid in reducing adverse effects from long-term steroid therapy: (1) use steroids with short half-lives (prednisone, prednisolone, methylprednisolone), which are less likely to suppress the HPA axis; (2) use the lowest possible dose; (3) administer steroids in the morning in a single dose (nocturnal administration of exogenous glucocorticoid will suppress the HPA axis significantly); (4) change to every-other-day administration, using two-and-one-half times the minimal daily dose as the initial dose and then reducing it gradually; (5) use inhaled steroids such as beclomethasone dipropionate, flunisolide, or triamcinolone acetonide, in place of oral steroids.

Other Drugs

Expectorants, antibiotics, sedatives, tranquilizers, and antihistamines are sometimes prescribed for asthma. All expectorants depend on adequate hydration for effective action. Iodides, the traditional expectorants of the past, are unacceptable for use in children because of their many adverse effects (American Academy of Pediatrics, 1976). Expectorants, such as glyceryl guaiacolate, add little, at best, to hydration. Antibiotics are indicated only when there is substantial evidence of bacterial or mycoplasmal infection. Troleandomycin, sometimes prescribed in severe chronic asthma, should be used with utmost caution in children because of its many adverse effects, including inhibition of theophylline metabolism. *Sedatives and tranquilizers are contraindicated in asthma therapy.* Anxiety, which is related to airways obstruction, dyspnea, and hypoxemia, is most effectively relieved by adequate asthma therapy. *Antihistamines* may be useful for therapy of allergic rhinitis in asthmatic patients. There is evidence that some of the newer agents with antihistaminic action, such as ketotifen fumarate, azelastine hydrochloride, terfenadine, and astemizole, may be useful for asthma (Simons, 1985).

OFFICE MANAGEMENT OF ASTHMA

The effective management of asthma in the office should focus on (1) identification and elimination of exacerbating or aggravating factors, (2) pharmacologic therapy, (3) provision for maximum physical exercise, (4) immunotherapy (hyposensitization) when appropriate for major allergens that cannot be eliminated or avoided, and (5) education of the patient and family about the disease.

Environmental Control. Allergic and irritant factors that exacerbate asthma should be identified and removed from the child's environment. Major allergic or irritant factors in the home or school, suggested by a detailed history and confirmed by skin tests, should be eliminated or avoided to the extent possible within the framework of normal physical and psychological growth and development. Although the removal of important allergic and irritant factors from the home is essential, the physician must be flexible and reasonable. Often effective environmental control may involve a compromise between what is medically desirable and what is emotionally or economically acceptable to the family and child.

Maximum Physical Exercise. Participation in normal family, school, and community functions requires reasonably normal exercise tolerance. Regular exercise should be encouraged. The child with asthma does particularly well in such sports as swimming, downhill skiing, gymnastics, and soccer (playing some positions). Acceptance as a normal team member strengthens the ego and builds self-respect. Pretreatment with appropriate medication and a warm-up consisting of a short period of mild exercise before active exercise are especially helpful.

Hyposensitization. Allergy injection therapy (immunotherapy) is indicated for major environmental allergens, such as pollen antigens, that cannot be avoided. Many children and adolescents have allergic rhinitis, for which hyposensitization has proved efficacious. Injection therapy also can ameliorate the allergic component of asthma in children (Warner et al, 1978).

Management of the Acute Attack

Acute asthma in children can occur as a mild illness that responds promptly to bronchodilators, or it can develop into a medical emergency over a matter of a few hours, especially in the young child who is unable to retain oral medication and fluids. In such a child, wheezing that decreases with time in the face of persistently increasing respiratory distress may reflect progressive obstruction of airways and decreased air exchange and is an ominous sign. If the child's asthma fails to respond to home treatment, he or she should be seen on an emergency basis in the physician's office or a hospital emergency room.

For acute asthma, the drugs of choice are epinephrine by injection or aerosolized adrenergic agents (Table 41–7). Epinephrine may be repeated two or

Table 41-7. ADRENERGIC DRUGS FOR TREATMENT OF ACUTE ATTACK

Drug	Administration*	Dosage		Frequency	Notes
		CHILD	ADULT		
Terbutaline	Subcutaneous	0.01 mg/kg	0.25 ml	20 min (×2)	
Epinephrine aqueous 1:1000 sol (1 mg/ml)	Subcutaneous	0.01 mg/kg	0.3 ml	20 min (×3)	
Suspension epinephrine 1:200 (Sus-Phrine) (5 mg/ml)	Subcutaneous	0.005 ml/kg	0.2 ml	Single dose	To follow treatment, if appropriate (see text).
Isoetharine 1:100 (10 mg/ml)	Nebulized aerosol	0.25 to 0.60 ml in 2.0 ml saline	0.25 to 1.0 ml in 2.0 ml saline	30 min (×3)	
Metaproterenol 1:20 (50 mg/ml)	Nebulized aerosol	0.1 to 0.2 ml in 2.5 ml saline	0.2 to 0.3 ml in 2.5 ml saline	30 min (×3)	‡
Albuterol 1:200 (5 mg/ml)	Nebulized aerosol	0.02 ml/kg up to 0.5 ml (100 μg/kg)	0.5 to 1.0 ml in 2.0 ml saline	30 min (× 3)	‡
Terbutaline 1:1000 (1 mg/ml)	Nebulized aerosol	1 ml in 1 ml saline†	2.0 ml in 1.0 ml saline	30 min (×3)	‡

*In moderately severe or severe attack, it is best to administer drug via or concomitant with oxygen.
†Authors' recommendation.
‡Safety and effectiveness of the inhaled solution in patients younger than 12 years have not been established.
(Reproduced with permission from Bierman CW and Pearlman DS [eds]: Allergic Diseases from Infancy to Adulthood. 2nd ed. Philadelphia, WB Saunders Co, 1988.)

three times at 20-min intervals if necessary, or aerosolized agents may be administered by an oxygen-driven or ultrasonic nebulizer for 5 to 10 min at 30-min intervals.

Increasingly, aerosolized bronchodilators have become the treatment of choice. Becker and co-workers (1983) compared inhaled albuterol (0.02 ml/kg of a 0.5-per cent solution, maximum dosage 1 ml) with injected epinephrine in 40 children with acute asthma. Although the two drugs provided similar clinical improvement, epinephrine was associated with severe adverse effects but albuterol was not. Except for metaproterenol, pediatric dose-response curves have not been carried out with adrenergic drugs (Shapiro et al, 1987).

Patients responding incompletely to adrenergic agents may benefit from short bursts (5 to 7 days) of prednisone or methylprednisolone. These short bursts will provide more rapid returns to normal pulmonary functions without significant adverse effects (Shapiro et al, 1983). *Intermittent positive-pressure breathing (IPPB) should not be used,* because it might induce or worsen pneumomediastinum or pneumothorax (Alveolar rupture, 1978). If the child can cooperate, pulmonary function testing (either spirometry or peak flow measurements) before and after therapy provides an objective measurement of response to treatment. The most common physician error is underestimating the degree of obstruction and overestimating the response to medication with a stethoscope. In general, pressurized adrenergic hand nebulizers containing albuterol, terbutaline, or metaproterenol are helpful in acute asthma. However, they should be used with particular caution in children because of the potential for abuse. Adrenergic aerosols can be administered through compressed-air devices in the home on the same basis. When an adequate trial of appropriate therapy fails

to relieve the asthma significantly, the patient should be admitted to the hospital (see "Hospital Management of Asthma").

Management of Mild Asthma. Mild asthma, in which the patient has only intermittent episodes of asthma but is completely symptom free between episodes, can often be managed by aerosolized adrenergic solutions. In the small child, an adrenergic bronchodilator (see Table 41-7) can be administered by an electric compressor-driven nebulizer. In the older child and adult, metered-dose inhalers can be used alone or with a spacer device, minimizing the need to coordinate inspiration with activation of the pressurized canister. Often even an adolescent who has difficulty with coordination of inspiration will benefit from the use of a spacer.

Oral administration of adrenergic agents, theophylline, or both represents an alternative form of therapy for acute attacks, although oral adrenergic agents and theophylline are associated with increased systemic adverse effects compared with inhaled adrenergic drugs.

Aminophylline suppositories should be avoided because of erratic and slow absorption and potential overdosage. Rectal theophylline preparations, in the marketed solution form, however, are well absorbed and can be used for short periods in place of oral theophylline. Cromolyn sodium may be effective if used before anticipated exposure to known allergens (e.g., cat dander) or before exercise, but it should be discontinued during acute attacks.

Management of Moderate Asthma. Asthma that interferes with activity, sleep, or exercise and is characterized by persistently abnormal lung functions requires a regular maintenance medication for control. Either aerosolized cromolyn or sustained-release theophylline can be employed as a first-line, maintenance drug (Table 41-8). Both appear to be equiv-

Table 41–8. PHARMACOTHERAPY OF MODERATE ASTHMA

Drug	Formulation	Dosage	Frequency	Comments
Theophylline	Timed-release spansule/tablet	16–24 mg/kg/day	8–12 h	Follow theophylline levels.
Cromolyn sodium	Turboinhaler	20 mg	Begin qid; reduce to tid or bid	Used for prophylaxis of asthma.
	Aerosol solution	20 mg		
	MDI*	2 mg (2 inhalations)		
Adrenergic agents				
Albuterol	MDI	2 inhalations	q 4–6 h	‡
	Nebulizer solution	0.2 ml/kg up to 1 ml	q 4–6 h	‡
	Oral solution/tablets	0.1 mg/kg maximum of 4 mg	q 6–8 h	Few data on children under 6.†
Metaproterenol	MDI	2 inhalations	q 4–6 h	‡
	Nebulizer solution	0.1–0.2 ml in 2 ml saline	q 4–6 h	‡
	Oral solution tablets	1.3–2.6 mg/kg/day; maximum of 20 mg tid	q 6–8 h	Few data on children under 6.
Terbutaline	MDI	2 inhalations	q 4–6 h	‡
	Tablets	2.5–5 mg	q 4–6 h	Few data on children under 12.
	Ampules	0.25 mg IM or SC	Repeat in 20 mins X 1	
Bitolteral mesylate	MDI	2 inhalations	q 4–6 h	‡
Pirbuterol acetate	MDI	2 inhalations	q 4–6 h	
Isoetharine	1 per cent	0.30–0.75 ml	q 4–6 h	
	MDI	2 inhalations	q 4–6 h	
Ipratropium bromide	MDI	2 inhalations	qid	‡ Marketed for those with chronic bronchitis but effective in some with asthma.
Steroids	See Table 41–9.			Short bursts used occasionally when not adequately responsive to nonsteroidal bronchodilators.

*MDI, metered-dose inhaler.
†Drug used round-the-clock or prn as appropriate (see text).
‡Safety and effectiveness in patients below 12 years of age have not been established, according to manufacturer.
(Reproduced with permission from Bierman CW and Pearlman DS [eds]: Allergic Disease from Infancy to Adulthood. 2nd ed. Philadelphia, WB Saunders Co, 1988.)

alent in asthma control in children with moderate asthma (Furukawa et al, 1984). Cromolyn does not have the side effects of theophylline, including adverse effects on school performance (Rachelefsky et al, 1986), and does not require the regular monitoring of serum concentrations that is obligatory for theophylline. Cromolyn, however, is not a bronchodilator and is not effective in acute asthma. Cromolyn may be administered as a metered-dose aerosol, as a powder by a turboinhaler, or as a solution by motor-driven nebulizer. The initial dosage of four times daily may be reduced to thrice or even twice daily once the medication's effect has been achieved (usually in a 4-week period).

When theophylline is prescribed as a primary drug, a timed-release formulation is administered every 8 to 12 hours in a dose that provides a peak concentration of less than 20 μg/ml (we prefer to keep peak levels less than 15μg/ml). A back-up adrenergic agent is appropriate for exacerbation of acute asthma, or one can be added to the long-term therapeutic regimen. Exacerbations of acute asthma are treated as previously described, adding short bursts of short-acting steroids as necessary. Increasingly, aerosolized steroids are prescribed as first-line drugs in Europe, Canada, and Australia. A multicenter study comparing them with conventional therapy is under way in the United States.

Management of Severe Asthma. In severe asthma, the patient continues to have incapacitating dyspnea, cough, and obstructed airways in spite of treatment as described for moderate asthma. Long-term corticosteroid therapy is essential to the treatment of such patients as an adjunct to other therapy. After controlling the asthma with a burst of short-acting steroids (prednisone, prednisolone, methylprednisolone), the patient may be placed on every-other-day steroids, beginning with 2.5 times the minimal daily steroid dosage that controlled the asthma, or on inhaled steroids (beclomethasone dipropionate, triamcinolone acetonide, or flunisolide) (Table 41–9). Inhaled steroids are usually initiated with a dosage of three inhalations four times daily. The dosage of oral or inhaled steroids is slowly reduced to the smallest one that will control the asthma. Often the frequency of inhaled steroids can be reduced to thrice daily, and occasionally to twice daily. Oral candidiasis, the major complication of aerosolized steroid therapy, can be minimized by rinsing the mouth with water after each treatment.

When a patient has received oral steroids for a prolonged period, prednisone should be tapered

Table 41–9. PHARMACOTHERAPY OF SEVERE
ASTHMA

Theophylline, adrenergic drugs, cromolyn: as outlined in Table
41–8 for moderately severe asthma.

Steroids including prednisone, prednisolone, methylprednisolone:
Begin at 30 to 40 mg/day (once daily in AM or split into 2 to 3
doses/day). Taper to lowest daily (early AM) dose that controls
asthma and maintains adequate lung functions. Short bursts (3
to 10 days) used occasionally may suffice without long-term
therapy. Long-term therapy involves shifting to every second
day (qod), using 2.5 times the lowest daily dosage that
controlled asthma. (Give before 8 AM.) Dosage reductions should
be attempted at 2-week intervals. Reassess dosage
requirements periodically.

*Aerosolized steroids including beclomethasone dipropionate,
triamcinolone acetonide, flunisolide:* Begin with 2 to 3
inhalations, four times daily (qid), and reduce to lowest dosage
that controls asthma. Dosage reductions should be attempted at
2-week intervals. Reassess dosage requirements periodically.
Larger doses may be required in patients with resistant
diseases.

(Reproduced with permission from Bierman CW and Pearlman
DS [eds]: Allergic Diseases from Infancy to Adulthood. 2nd ed.
Philadelphia, WB Saunders Co, 1988.)

slowly when attempting to replace the oral steroids
with aerosolized steroids, because the HPA axis may
take up to a year to recover normal responsiveness.
If the patient is on alternate-day or aerosolized steroid therapy, short courses of daily steroid therapy
should be considered for acute exacerbations of
asthma, major surgery, and acute, severe illness in
general.

When systemic steroids cannot be changed to
every-other-day dosage or to aerosolized steroids,
TAO has been found to have a unique steroid-
sparing effect. This effect is exclusively associated
with methylprednisolonc therapy (Spector et al,
1974). Methylprednisolone and TAO have been
found useful in treating steroid-dependent children
between 7 and 13 years of age (Eitches et al, 1985).
In 11 steroid-dependent children, TAO therapy resulted in improved clinical and pulmonary function
within 7 days of initial treatment. Side effects of
treatment were increased cushingoid features, abdominal pain, and increased liver enzyme concentrations. After a methylprednisolone reduction to the
lowest effective dosage, TAO was begun at 14 mg/
kg/day with a weekly reduction over 4 weeks to 3.5
mg/kg/day and a concomitant reduction of methylprednisolone. Patients on daily steroids were shifted
to every-other-day dosages, if possible, and those on
oral steroids were shifted to aerosolized steroids. *TAO
affects the metabolism of theophylline, so that the theophylline
dosage should be reduced 30 to 50 per cent to avoid toxicity.*
Weekly liver tests, spirometry, and theophylline
serum levels should be performed on patients who
are taking TAO.

Further studies in adults recommend a starting
dosage of 250 mg once daily, which should be shifted,
if possible, to every other day with the methylprednisolone every other day. Those patients whose
asthma cannot be controlled on every-other-day steroids should be considered TAO failures, and TAO
should be discontinued (Wald et al, 1986).

The mechanism of action of TAO is not clear; it
does not act as an antibiotic. Although it appears to
have a steroid-sparing action, responsive patients
become cushingoid at lower steroid dosages. Also
TAO has a direct adverse effect on the liver and
induces abnormal liver chemistry findings in some
patients. However, neither its steroid-sparing nor
hepatic action explains its effectiveness.

Methotrexate has been effective in a pilot program
of adult patients whose asthma was resistant to steroids. This technique should be considered experimental at present (Mullarkey et al, 1988).

Comment on Drug Therapy

Recommendations given here are intended as
guidelines only. Drug therapy must be individualized
to the child's age, severity of disease, and ability to
tolerate the drug. It must be readjusted regularly for
growth and changes in disease severity, with use of
lowest dosage and least toxic drugs compatible with
"functional normality."

HOSPITAL MANAGEMENT OF ASTHMA

Status asthmaticus, or acute severe asthma that is
resistant to appropriate outpatient therapy, is a life-
threatening medical emergency that requires
prompt, systematic, and aggressive management in
the hospital. The initiation of early, appropriate
therapy shortens hospitalization and reduces complications. The younger child is at particular risk for
status asthmaticus (Fig. 41–12).

Therapy

General Treatment. The child with status asthmaticus should be managed in an intensive care unit or
a similar facility in which the patient's overall condition and vital signs, symptoms, and progress can be
monitored closely by a physician, nurse, respiratory
therapist, and consultant anesthesiologist team. Although the management of each child with status
asthmaticus must be individualized, certain general
principles apply to all patients with this disease
(see "Management Protocol for Acute Bronchial
Asthma"). Some hospitals may not be equipped to
carry out all of the following recommendations, but
most of these general principles can be instituted in
any facility caring for such children.

While an appropriate history is being obtained and
physical examination is being performed, humidified
oxygen should be administered and an intravenous
infusion should be initiated. Pulmonary function tests
(FVC/FEV$_1$ or PEFR) may be performed if the child
is old enough and can cooperate. Arterial or arterialized blood gases, serum electrolytes, and serum
theophylline should be measured as soon as possible.

In the history, details about the acute illness—its

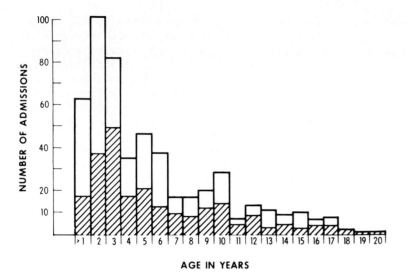

Figure 41–12. Number of admissions for asthma to a children's hospital according to age at admission. Hatched areas represent girls, nonhatched represent boys. Note predominance of male admissions in childhood.

duration, progression, manifestations, and initiating factors—as well as information on the duration of asthma and the details of previous acute episodes should be noted. The patient's fluid balance (intake, vomiting, and urination), medication (including the names, dosages, and exact time of all medications administered within 24 hours), and any corticosteroid drugs administered within 12 months should be documented.

On physical examination, the general appearance and level of activity, respiratory effort, presence or absence of wheezing, tachycardia, tachypnea, skin turgor, and color of mucous membranes are important clinical parameters that provide information about pulmonary obstruction, hypoxemia, and fluid balance. Fever, acute otitis media, pharyngitis, or signs of pneumonia indicate a need for bacterial cultures and possibly for treatment with antibiotics.

A chest radiograph provides information on pulmonary problems, such as pneumonia, atelectasis, pneumomediastinum, pneumothorax, and the presence of a foreign body, that might complicate management.

Oxygenation. Humidified oxygen delivered by nasal cannula, face mask, or mechanical ventilator at a final concentration (FI_{O_2}) to maintain Pa_{O_2} of 80 to 100 mm Hg (at sea level, with proportionally lower values at higher altitudes) is an important adjunct in managing status asthmaticus. *All patients who require hospitalization because of refractory asthma have hypoxemia.* Certain drugs (e.g., epinephrine) that are employed frequently in treatment may increase the myocardial oxygen need when the arterial oxygen is low. In addition, the potential toxicity of such medications is increased under conditions of hypoxemia and acidosis. Leukotriene mediators, which appear to be so important in severe asthma, also may reduce coronary artery blood flow and induce myocardial depression (Lewis and Austen, 1981). The appropriate use of oxygen supports the myocardium and helps prevent arrhythmias.

Hydration. Administration of intravenous fluids is essential for treatment of status asthmaticus. A child so affected often is dehydrated on admission to the hospital because of vomiting, inadequate fluid intake, and greater insensible water loss from the increased work of breathing. Fluid therapy should be designed to replace deficits as well as to provide normal maintenance requirements (Table 41–10). Excessive fluid administration should be avoided, however, because pulmonary edema and hypervolemia with water intoxication may result (Segar and Chesney, 1981).

Overhydration may increase microvascular hydrostatic pressure and reduce plasma colloid osmotic pressure. These changes can lead to formation of pulmonary edema in the child who has asthma with substantial negative pleural pressure (Stalcup and Mellins, 1977).

Correction of Acidosis. If the patient is in severe

Table 41–10. GUIDELINES FOR INTRAVENOUS FLUID THERAPY IN STATUS ASTHMATICUS

Hydration (initial)
5 per cent glucose in normal saline, 12 ml/kg or 360 ml/m² for first hour

Depletion Repair
Normal saline, 10–15 ml/kg or 300–500 ml/m² in 24 hours
Water (5 per cent glucose in water), 10–15 ml/kg or 300–500 ml/m² in 24 hours

Maintenance
Fluids: 5 per cent glucose in water, 50 ml/kg or 1500 ml/m² in 24 hours, depending on age
Electrolytes: Potassium, 2 mEq/100 ml of maintenance IV fluid
Sodium, 3 mEq/100 ml of maintenance IV fluids

Buffers
If pH is below 7.30 and base deficit is greater than 5 mEq/L, correct to normal range with IV sodium bicarbonate according to the following calculation:
bicarbonate (mEq) = negative base excess (mEq) × 0.3 × body weight (kg)
Administer half the calculated dose initially and the other half after repeating blood gas determinations.

(Reproduced with permission with Bierman CW and Pearlman DS [eds]: Allergic Diseases from Infancy to Adulthood. 2nd ed. Philadelphia, WB Saunders, 1988.)

distress, the serum pH should be determined as soon as possible and should be corrected using the formula shown in Table 41–10. Give one half of the calculated dose initially and the other half after repeating blood gas determinations.

Aminophylline (Theophylline Ethylenediamine) Therapy. Aminophylline or theophylline is an effective bronchodilator for children with status asthmaticus (Pierson et al, 1971) and has become the most frequently administered intravenous drug for severe asthma. If the patient has not been receiving theophylline and has a zero theophylline level, a loading dose is usually administered followed by a maintenance dosage.

If the patient has an adequate serum theophylline level, obviously an initial loading dose should not be administered, and only a maintenance dosage should be given. Intravenous aminophylline treatment, consisting of a fourth of the calculated dose administered intravenously every 6 hours, may be preferred when consistent infusion is not practical (Maselli et al, 1970).

During intravenous aminophylline therapy, serum theophylline concentrations should be monitored for safety and effectiveness. Levels should be maintained above 10 μg/ml and below 20 μg/ml. Such levels should be obtained after the loading dose has equilibrated (approximately 1 hour after administration) and again after 6, 12, and 24 hours of intravenous therapy. Additional determinations of levels should be obtained if the patient has persistent heartburn, nausea, vomiting, seizures, nervousness, anxiety, insomnia, headache, diarrhea, irritability, or cardiac arrhythmia, to rule out theophylline intoxication (Weinberger et al, 1976). Also theophylline can drive the respiratory center and increase the pulse rate.

Use of Adrenergic Agonists. For acute asthma, these agents are the mainstay in treatment, often used also as "add ons" for those on maintenance theophylline. Whereas subcutaneously injected epinephrine is commonly employed in treating acute asthma, its short duration of action and side effects (stimulation of β_1 as well as β_2 receptors) make it less desirable than drugs that can be administered by aerosol (Becker et al, 1983). Inhalation of this class of drugs is preferred generally, in fact, to injection. However, a patient with severe obstruction (PEFR<25 per cent of predicted) is likely to have a more rapid recovery after subcutaneous medication because of greater dilation of both larger and more peripheral small airways (Tashkin et al, 1980; Pliss and Gallagher, 1981). Multiple injections of epinephrine, although not cumulative in their action, have a sustaining therapeutic effect (Ownby and Anderson, 1986). Ben-Zvi and colleagues (1983) found that a single injection of epinephrine resulted in two to three times more failures than multiple injections. However, a single injection of Sus-Phrine (1:200 epinephrine suspension) had the same beneficial results at 1 hour as did multiple injections but with fewer side effects, and it has been recommended for

initial therapy. Although the child may respond poorly to beta-adrenergic agents on hospital admission, he or she will become progressively more responsive as other therapy is administered.

Aerosolized metaproterenol solution (Shapiro et al, 1987), terbutaline, or albuterol (salbutamol) in 3 ml saline (Beck et al, 1985) should be given every half hour for the first 2 hours and at longer intervals as the patient improves. These drugs are administered by low-pressure ultrasonic or wall-mounted nebulizer for 5 to 10 min every half hour ($\times$4), then as indicated by the patient's condition. The pulse should be monitored, and treatment should be stopped when the pulse is $\geq$190 beats/min. Continuous administration of aerosolized beta-adrenergic drugs (e.g., terbutaline, 1 to 2 mg/hr) has been employed successfully in the treatment of acute asthma in children and adults.

Positive pressure ventilation (IPPB) is contraindicated in children because of the danger of inducing greater bronchoconstriction, pneumomediastinum, and pneumothorax. Hypokalemia is a potential complication of beta-adrenergic therapy even with inhalation (Haalboon et al, 1985); hence, serum electrolyte levels should be monitored.

Corticosteroid Therapy. Patients requiring hospitalization, those already on steroids or previously on long-term oral steroids, and those on aerosolized steroids in the previous 6 weeks, should receive corticosteroids immediately. Short-term intravenous administration of steroids in high doses rarely, if ever, causes adverse effects. Recommendations of steroid dosages are found in the management protocol (see Table 41–10).

Corticosteroids accelerate the recovery from status asthmaticus, with a maximal effect occurring 2 to 3 days after the beginning of treatment. Pierson and co-workers (1971) documented better arterial oxygen tensions in children who were treated with glucocorticosteroids compared with children who received a placebo. In a study of children with acute asthma, steroid therapy improved small airways obstruction 24 hours after it was instituted but had minimal effectiveness on large airways obstruction, as compared with placebo-treated children (Shapiro et al, 1983). This finding may explain why several published studies have failed to show any beneficial effects of steroid therapy on lung function, because these studies employed measurements of airflow only in large airways (Luksza, 1982).

Another important effect of steroids appears to be the increase in effectiveness of beta-adrenergic drugs, an effect that may occur earlier than previously appreciated (Arnaud et al, 1979). Even in hospitalized infants with "bronchiolitis," there is evidence that steroids enhance the effectiveness of beta-adrenergic drugs (Tal et al, 1983). The beneficial effect of steroids in the treatment of acute severe asthma also has been well documented in adults (Littenberg and Gluck, 1986).

Antibiotic Therapy. Antibiotics are indicated only

in children in whom bacterial diseases are suspected (Shapiro et al, 1974). Viral respiratory infections induce acute severe asthma far more frequently than do bacterial infections, and current antibiotics are not effective in treating viral infections. There are no special indications for the use of antibiotics in asthma or other allergic disorders.

Asthma is frequently accompanied by patchy atelectasis that is often misinterpreted on a radiograph as bronchopneumonia (Eggleston et al, 1974). Leukocytosis of 15,000/mm³ or more may occur in severe asthma in the absence of a demonstrable infection, particularly after administration of epinephrine.

Use of Sedatives. Patients with severe asthma have good reason to experience extreme anxiety, and their anxiety is the result of respiratory distress and hypoxemia rather than the cause of them. *Sedatives are contraindicated in patients with status asthmaticus.*

Anticholinergic Drug Therapy. Anticholinergic agents, atropine sulfate, atropine methylnitrate, and ipratropium bromide, have been used in treatment of acute and chronic asthma with some success, although results have been variable. Relatively few data exist on the use of these agents in acute severe asthma in children, but data in adults suggest that they probably add little to the therapy of acute severe asthma and may disproportionately increase undesirable effects (Karpel et al, 1986). However, Beck and colleagues (1985) did find a small but significant beneficial effect from combining ipratropium bromide with albuterol in children.

Follow-up Therapy

In the Hospital. Arterial blood gas determinations should be repeated regularly until asthma is adequately controlled, the patient's P_{O_2} is stable in room air, and blood gas homeostasis has been established. As a further guide to therapy, airway function should be monitored regularly in children old enough to cooperate. A spirogram from which the FVC and FEV_1 can be measured is the preferred method, but a peak expiratory flow rate (PEFR) is equally useful if spirometry is not available. After 24 hours, theophylline, corticosteroids, and antibiotics, if indicated, may be administered orally if the patient is improving (Table 41–11). Nebulized adrenergic agents should be used every 4 hours.

Outpatient Therapy. Although status asthmaticus often can be controlled sufficiently that a child can be discharged from the hospital at 36 to 48 hours, full recovery from asthma may take several weeks.

Table 41–11. ORAL THERAPY FOR SEVERE ASTHMA

Drug	Dosage
Theophylline	5 mg/kg q 6 hr with dosage adjusted on basis of serum theophylline level
Prednisone/ methylprednisone	30–40 mg/day for 2 days, then decreased by 4–5 mg/day until discontinued

As a patient improves, do not diminish therapy too rapidly. Patients should be discharged while receiving round-the-clock bronchodilators and a tapering dose of prednisone administered as a single dose at 8 AM daily. Tapering may take up to 7 to 10 days at a reduction of 5 mg/day. Follow-up is important. Complete recovery from severe asthma may take far longer than is generally appreciated (McFadden, 1975a).

MANAGEMENT PROTOCOL FOR ACUTE BRONCHIAL ASTHMA

I. Patients with Acute Severe Asthma
  A. Adrenergic Therapy
    1. *Epinephrine 1-1000,* 0.01 ml/kg (maximum of 0.3 ml), subcutaneously, every 15 to 20 min, for up to three doses. Maximum dose of 0.6 ml the first hour, and q 4 hr. Last dose should be Sus-Phrine (epinephrine suspension 1:200) (Shake Well), 0.005 ml/kg, subcutaneously, then q 6 to 12 hr, *or*
    2. Sus-Phrine (Shake Well), 0.005 ml/kg, subcutaneously, q 6 to 12 hr (20 per cent is released immediately). Maximum single dose 0.2 ml, *or*
    3. *Terbutaline,* 0.01 mg/kg (maximum of 0.25 mg), subcutaneously, repeat in 20 min (maximum of 0.5 mg/4 hr), *or*
    4. *Aerosolized adrenergic agents,* see Table 41–7, may be used if PEFR or FEV_1 is greater than 40 per cent of predicted.
  B. Oxygen, humidified, to maintain Pa_{O_2} between 80 and 100 mm Hg.
  C. Response to treatment: if unresponsive in 1 hour, consider admitting to hospital and proceed as follows.
  D. Corticosteroids, if patient not immediately responsive, start steroids.
II. Patients with Early Status Asthmaticus
  A. Draw blood sample for stat studies, serum theophylline level, arterial blood gas values, pHa, serum electrolyte levels, complete blood count, and differential.
  B. Aminophylline
    1. Obtain stat theophylline level on all patients. For patients with 0 level, use loading dose of 7.0 mg/kg over 15 min. If level is under 10 μg/ml, give a sufficient dose to reach a therapeutic level. The maintenance infusion should be initiated at a rate of 0.85 mg/kg/hr for those 1 to 6 years old, 0.65 mg/kg/hr for those 7 to 16 years old, and 0.45 mg/kg/hr for those older than 16 years for a level between 10 and 15 μg/ml. Repeat levels at 1, 6, 12, and 24 hours of intravenous therapy.
    2. In the patient who has not received theophylline-containing medication, a loading dose is usually given followed by mainte-

nance therapy. The loading dose in a patient not taking oral theophylline ranges from 5 to 7 mg/kg diluted in 25 to 50 ml of saline and given over 20 min. *An initial loading dose should not be administered to a patient who is receiving an oral theophylline preparation if the initial serum theophylline concentration is unknown.*

C. Intravenous fluids: these are administered as 5 per cent glucose in normal saline for hydration with fluids as appropriate for maintenance and depletion repair.
 1. Initial hydration—12 ml/kg or 360 ml/m² for the first hour (5 per cent glucose in normal saline).
 2. Maintenance—50 ml/kg/24 hr depending on age or 1500 ml/m²/24 hr (5 per cent glucose in water).
 3. Depletion repair—normal saline, 10 to 15 ml/kg/24 hr or 300 to 500 ml/m² and water (5 per cent glucose in water), 10 to 15 ml/kg/24 hr or 300 to 500 ml/m²/24 hr.
 4. Maintenance of normal pH and electrolyte concentrations—the following is recommended for maintenance of normal potassium and sodium concentrations:
  a. Potassium—2 mEq/100 ml of maintenance intravenous fluids (after urination established).
  b. Sodium—3 mEq/100 ml of maintenance intravenous fluids.
  c. Buffers—if pH is below 7.30 and base deficit is greater than 5 mEq/L, correct to normal range with intravenous sodium bicarbonate as follows:
   (1) mEq bicarbonate = negative base excess × 0.3 × kg (body weight)
   (2) Administer half the calculated dose initially and the other half after repeating blood gas determinations.

D. Corticosteroids
 1. Hydrocortisone hemisuccinate, 7 mg/kg stat and 7 mg/kg/24 hr.
 2. Solu-Medrol (paraben-free methylprednisolone sodium succinate) or equivalent, 2 mg/kg stat, I.V., slowly over 10 min and 4 mg/kg/24 hr.
 3. Dexamethasone phosphate, 0.3 mg/kg stat and 0.3 mg/kg/24 hr.
 4. Betamethasone, 0.3 mg/kg stat and 0.3 mg/kg/24 hr by constant infusion or divided into four 6-hour doses.

E. Diagnostic Studies
 1. Posteroanterior and lateral x-ray of chest
 2. Urinalysis
 3. Nose, throat, and sputum cultures

III. Patients with Advanced Status Asthmaticus
 A. Admit to Intensive Care Unit.
 B. Corticosteroids, as noted.
 C. Vital Signs
  1. Record and evaluate blood pressure, pulse, respiratory rates, and pulsus paradoxus.
  2. Observe for sternocleidomastoid contraction and supraclavicular indrawing every 15 min.
  3. Repeat blood gas analysis, pHa every 30 to 60 min, and Na, K, and Cl every hour as appropriate.
 D. Antibiotics, as indicated for obvious bacterial infection.
 E. Medical Staff Coordination
  1. The same physician should evaluate the patient *at least* hourly for several hours.
  2. Document review of vital observations and that medications and fluids are given on schedule.
  3. Associated staff physicians should be kept current on patient's condition.
  4. Alert controlled ventilation team (pediatrician, allergist, critical care physician, and pediatric pulmonologist or anesthesiologist) in the event of impending respiratory failure, if the Pa_{CO_2} is increasing by 5 mm Hg/hr.

IV. Patients with Acute Respiratory Failure
 A. Follow protocol noted in II and III.
 B. If the patient is stuporous or unconscious or if the patient's condition is rapidly deteriorating (e.g., an increase in Pa_{CO_2} of 5 mm Hg or more per hour), proceed as follows:
  1. Assemble controlled ventilation team.
  2. Examine bag and mask and ensure readiness to resuscitate patient.
  3. Have endotracheal tubes, tracheostomy set, cutdown set, and good suction equipment at the bedside.
 C. Intravenous isoproterenol, via a calibrated constant infusion pump, beginning with 0.1 μ/kg/min, increasing the dosage 0.1 μ/kg/min every 15 to 20 min until clinical improvement or tachycardia (200/min) develops, as observed by electrocardiography (ECG) monitoring (Downs et al, 1973). *This step is not for children who are past their early teens.*
 D. *Mechanical ventilation* may be necessary if the patient is unresponsive to isoproterenol, unable to receive it, or comatose.
  1. Endotracheal intubation, neuromuscular paralysis, sedation, and mechanical ventilation with a volume ventilator, with constant monitoring of ECG and frequent blood gas determinations are necessary.
  2. Once asthma is controlled with the aforementioned medications, the patient can be provided assisted ventilation and usually extubated in 24 to 48 hr (Simons et al, 1977).
 E. Additional Options: the following options are available if controlled ventilation is unsuccessful, prolonged, or complicated:

1. The use of halothane anesthesia (O'Rourke and Crane, 1982).
2. Bronchopulmonary lavage (Rogers et al, 1972).
3. Extracorporeal membrane oxygenation (Zapol et al, 1977).
4. Ether anesthesia (Robertson et al, 1985) should be seriously considered (Mansmann, 1983, 1987).
5. Because of its lesser myocardial depression and arrhythmogenic potential than halothane, the administration of isoflurane should be entertained (Bierman et al, 1986).

V. Follow-up Therapy
  A. Monitor pulmonary function and blood gas values.
  B. Change patient's therapy to oral theophylline and corticosteroids (prednisone, 1 to 2 mg/kg is initiated as a single morning dose for at least 5 days or tapered gradually over 7 to 10 days).
  C. Continue aerosolized adrenergic agents.
  D. Taper steroid therapy as rapidly as patient's condition permits.
  E. Discharge patient as soon as stable and on oral medication.
  F. Follow up within 1 week of hospital discharge.

COMPLICATIONS

Complications of asthma comprise those related to the lungs and those remote from the lungs. Pulmonary complications include (1) acute respiratory failure, (2) atelectasis, and (3) pneumomediastinum and pneumothorax. Extrapulmonary complications include (1) vasopressin excess, (2) flaccid paralysis of an arm or leg, (3) sudden alteration in theophylline metabolism, and (4) cardiac arrhythmias. Pulmonary and extrapulmonary factors may combine to cause acute respiratory failure, resulting in cardiorespiratory arrest with brain damage or death.

PULMONARY COMPLICATIONS

Respiratory Failure

Respiratory failure occurs in a small but significant number of children admitted to the hospital with status asthmaticus. Most commonly, respiratory failure develops insidiously in the hospitalized asthmatic child, frequently because the physician has failed to recognize the severity of the asthma. Clinical criteria for the diagnosis of respiratory failure in children include decrease or absence of pulmonary breath sounds, severe retractions and use of accessory muscles, cyanosis in 40 per cent oxygen, decreased response to pain, and poor skeletal muscle tone. Pulsus

paradoxicus also may be a warning sign. *Arterial blood gas tensions and pH must be monitored frequently in the distressed child.* Impending respiratory failure cannot be diagnosed from clinical signs alone.

The presence of an elevated Pa_{CO_2} confirms the diagnosis of respiratory failure, but a rapid rise in Pa_{CO_2} (e.g., from 35 to 40 mm Hg in 1 hour) in an exhausted child who is receiving optimal therapy should be considered respiratory failure and additional treatment should be provided.

Respiratory failure can be managed in some children with intravenous isoproterenol, but ultimately its management is with endotracheal intubation, mechanical ventilation, and continuation of intravenous and aerosolized bronchodilator therapy.

Intravenous Isoproterenol. Therapy with intravenous isoproterenol must be carried out in a properly equipped intensive care unit with continuous cardiac monitoring, a regularly calibrated constant-infusion pump, and an intra-arterial catheter for monitoring blood gas tension. Use of this agent should be restricted to children younger than 14 years of age because of the increased frequency of cardiac arrhythmias in older adolescents and adults. If the physician elects to treat an older child with intravenous isoproterenol, the *anesthesiologist should first be consulted so that all facilities for mechanical ventilation are immediately available.* This precaution is especially important for the child who has received excessive quantities of beta-adrenergic agents before admission, in whom isoproterenol may precipitate worsening of respiratory failure. After an initial dose of 0.1 µg/kg/min delivered by a constant-infusion pump, the isoproterenol dose is increased at the rate of 0.1 µg/kg/min every 15 to 20 min until there is clinical involvement or until tachycardia of 200 beats/min or an arrhythmia develops. Hazards include cardiac arrhythmias, myocarditis, and subendocardial necrosis. An essential part of therapy is a staff thoroughly familiar with this treatment, because 10 to 30 per cent of patients still require mechanical ventilation (Parry et al, 1976).

Mechanical Ventilation. Endotracheal intubation, neuromuscular blockade, and sedation are required for mechanical ventilation. A volume-controlled ventilator with constant monitoring of EKG and an intra-arterial line for frequent blood gas determinations must be employed to produce adequate alveolar ventilation. Once stabilized, the patient can be shifted to intermittent mandatory ventilation. Generally, patients can be weaned from mechanical ventilation in 24 to 48 hours. The possibility of pneumomediastinum, pneumothorax, cardiac arrhythmias, and unintentional extubation makes this a complicated procedure that should be performed only in adequately equipped and staffed tertiary care centers.

Atelectasis

Approximately one fourth of all hospitalized asthmatic children have pulmonary complications, such as pneumonia and atelectasis. In a study of 465 children hospitalized for asthma, 20 per cent had pulmonary infiltrates involving multiple lobes. Perihilar interstitial infiltrates varied in severity from increased bronchovascular markings to shaggy diffuse peribronchial pneumonia. Atelectasis of all or part of a lobe was the next most common complication, occurring in 10 per cent of admissions and involving the right middle lobe most frequently. The right middle lobe is particularly susceptible to atelectasis because of anatomic factors—the right main stem bronchus tends to twist with hyperinflation, resulting in its partial occlusion. Why right middle lobe atelectasis develops in girls more often than in boys has not yet been elucidated (Eggleston et al, 1974).

Treatment of atelectasis should be conservative. In most cases it will resolve with control of asthma and appropriate physical therapy, postural drainage, and chest clapping. With persistent atelectasis, the presence of a foreign body, anatomic defect, or obstruction by peribronchial lymph nodes must be considered. *Rarely* is bronchoscopy or bronchography indicated. Care must be taken with the use of positive pressure, which may facilitate the development of pneumothorax or pneumomediastinum.

Pneumomediastinum and Pneumothorax

During acute asthma, 5 per cent of patients develop pneumomediastinum (Eggleston et al, 1974). Shearing forces superimposed on hyperinflation cause air to rupture alveolar bases and to dissect along blood vessel sheaths (Bierman, 1967). This complication results in a worsening clinical course and is associated with reduced venous return, decreased cardiac output, and a fall in blood pressure. Air dissects along great vessel sheaths to the mediastinum and pericardium, along the aorta to the intestinal wall, or along fascial planes into the neck. While this air remains under high pressure, there are symptoms of worsening asthma and an absence of cardiac dullness on percussion. Relief is often associated with escape of this air into the relatively low-pressure subcutaneous tissue of the neck and axilla (Fig. 41–13). Subcutaneous emphysema is a late sign of extrapleural air.

Pneumothorax occurs rarely in childhood asthma. It may be self-limited if small or may severely compromise breathing and may be a cause of sudden death. A tension pneumothorax that results from a pulmonary rupture into the pleural space needs decompression with a chest tube and underwater suction. However, a pneumothorax secondary to dissection of air into the pleural space from the pneumomediastinum is less serious and may be treated conservatively. Often it will clear with treatment of the asthma.

EXTRAPULMONARY COMPLICATIONS

Vasopressin Excess (Inappropriate Antidiuretic Hormone Secretion)

The release of antidiuretic hormone (ADH) is regulated through such mechanisms as (1) pain, fear,

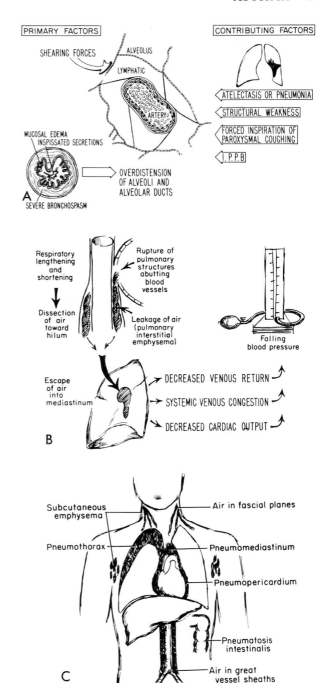

Figure 41–13. Mechanism of pneumomediastinum in acute asthma.

and drugs acting on higher central nervous system centers, (2) a drop in arterial pressure, (3) an increase ≥280 mOsm/L in plasma concentration of nondiffusible solute perfusing the hypothalamus, and (4) a stretch receptor in the left atrium. With decreased filling of the left atrium, vagal stimulation of the hypothalamus causes secretion of vasopressin. During status asthmaticus ADH levels are elevated irrespective of the serum sodium concentration, and the ADH level falls as the patient improves (Segar and Chesney, 1981).

The diagnosis of vasopressin excess rests on the

Table 41–12. CAUSES OF DEATH FROM ASTHMA

Failure of physician or patient to appreciate severity
    Lack of objective measurements
    Lack of intensified therapy
Inappropriate therapy given
    Too late because of delay by patient or physician
    Too little (e.g., low steroid dose or recent discontinuation)
    Too much (e.g., beta agonists, theophylline, sedative abuse)
Progressive Unresponsive Asthma
Prolonged Attack
Pulmonary Complications
    Infection (often undiagnosed)
    Pneumothorax
    Barotrauma
    Aspirations of gastric contents
    Malfunction of ventilator
Cardiac Complications
    Arrhythmias
    Hypotension
    Myocardial toxicity
    Sudden cardiac arrest
Underlying Cardiopulmonary Disease
Hemodynamic
    Hypovolemia, shock
    Pulmonary edema

following criteria: hyponatremia with hypo-osmolality of the plasma, continuing renal excretion of sodium, absence of any evidence of dehydration, urinary osmolality that is greater than plasma osmolality, and normal renal and adrenal function.

Therapy for this condition comprises treatment of the underlying severe asthma; water restriction with daily monitoring of body weight, plasma electrolyte concentration and osmolarity, urine volume, and urine osmolality; and in rare instances (with central nervous system involvement), administration of hypertonic saline (20 ml/100 kcal of 1.5 per cent NaCl) plus furosemide.

Irreversible Pulmonary Changes

An increasing number of patients with severe asthma in childhood are recognized as having chronic nonreversible obstructive disease in adult life (see "Natural History and Prognosis"). The pathogenetic mechanism that leads to irreversibility is unknown.

Sudden Alteration in Theophylline Metabolism. Theophylline clearance may be decreased by a number of factors. Aminophylline should be used cautiously in febrile patients, and dosage should be regulated by serial monitoring of serum theophylline concentrations in order to avoid theophylline toxicity. The theophylline requirement may increase because of third compartment filling secondary to edema and inappropriate ADH secretion. This condition could lead to sudden theophylline toxicity when the patient's pulmonary function improves.

Flaccid Paralysis. In 1974, Hopkins reported ten children with flaccid paralysis after acute asthma severe enough to require hospitalization. The paralysis developed during the recovery phase from asthma. In all patients, paralysis was permanent and involved one arm or one leg. To date, 19 children

with this syndrome from Australia, England, Sweden, and the United States have been reported in the medical literature (Shapiro et al, 1979); we have knowledge of at least four other unreported cases in North America.

Patients had similar characteristics as follows: (1) all were between 1 and 11 years of age; (2) all had asthma that was severe enough to require hospitalization; (3) all developed paralysis 4 to 11 days after onset of asthma (average = 5 days); (4) all had only one affected limb; more frequently it was the arm rather than the leg; (5) all had flaccid paralysis that affected only the motor nerves with no sensory involvement; and (6) all had progressive paralysis that was permanent (Commentary, 1980). All reported patients had been immunized for poliomyelitis, and no polio virus was obtained on culture. Although this paralysis is presumed to be a disease of viral etiology, no pathogenetic virus has yet been identified in these patients. There also is no explanation why these phenomena occurred only in children who had severe asthma.

Transient phrenic nerve paralysis also has been reported in status asthmaticus, possibly as a complication of assisted ventilation (Rohatigi et al, 1980).

Cardiorespiratory Arrest with Brain Damage. Permanent hypoxic brain damage due to cardiorespiratory arrest can be a complication of severe asthma and is particularly unfortunate because it is preventable with appropriate therapy. In virtually all cases, it has been the result of the parent's or the physician's failure to recognize the severity of asthma and to institute appropriate therapy (Bierman et al, 1975).

Death. Table 41–12 lists the causes of death associated with asthma in children. Virtually all are potentially preventable and can be avoided with appropriate education and treatment (Strunk and Mrazek, 1986).

REFERENCES

Aas K: Bronchial provocation tests in asthma. Arch Dis Child 45:221, 1970.
Abrishami MA: Aspirin intolerance: a review. Ann Allergy 39:28, 1977.
Ahlquist RP: A study of the adrenotropic receptors. Am J Physiol 153:586, 1948.
Alveolar rupture (editorial): Lancet 2:137, 1978.
American Academy of Pediatrics Committee on Drugs: Adverse reactions to iodide therapy of asthma and other pulmonary diseases. Pediatrics 57:272, 1976.
Arnaud A, Vervoet D, and Dogue P: Treatment of acute asthma: effect of intravenous corticosteroids and beta-2 agonists. Lung 156:43, 1979.
Arrang JM, Garbag M, Lancelot JC et al: Highly potent and selective ligands for histamine H-3 receptors. Nature 327:117, 1987.
Asthma deaths. NER Allergy Proc 7:421, 1986.
Atkins PC, Norman P, Werner H et al: Release of neutrophil chemotactic activity during immediate hypersensitivity reactions in humans. Ann Int Med 86:415, 1976.
Barnes P et al: Nocturnal asthma and changes in circulating epinephrine, histamine, and cortisol. N Engl J Med 303:263, 1980.

Barnes PJ: Nocturnal asthma: underlying mechanisms and implications for therapy. Immunol Allergy Pract 3:9, 1986.

Barter CE and Campbell AH: Relationship of constitutional factors and cigarette smoking to decrease in 1-second forced expiratory volume. Am Rev Respir Dis 113:305, 1976.

Beck R, Robertson C, Galdes-Sebaldt M, and Levinson H: Combined salbutamol and ipratropium bromide by inhalation in the treatment of severe asthma. J Pediatr 107:605, 1985.

Becker AB, Nelson NA, and Simons FER: Inhaled salbutamol (albuterol) vs. injected epinephrine in the treatment of acute asthma in children. J Pediatr 102:465, 1983.

Benatar SR: Fatal asthma. N Engl J Med 314:423, 1986.

Ben-Zvi Z, Lam C, Spohm WA et al: An evaluation of repeated injections of epinephrine for the initial treatment of acute asthma. Am Rev Respir Dis 127:101, 1983.

Bernstein IL: Cromolyn sodium in the treatment of asthma: changing concepts. J Allergy Clin Immunol 68:247, 1981.

Bierman CW: Pneumomediastinum and pneumothorax complicating asthma in children. Am J Dis Child 114:42, 1967.

Bierman CW, Pierson WE, Shapiro GG, and Furukawa CT: Is a continuous "therapeutic" theophylline blood level necessary for optimal theophylline therapy? Am J Med 85:17, 1988.

Bierman CW, Pierson WE, Shapiro GG, and Simons FER: Brain damage from asthma in children. J Allergy Clin Immunol 55:126, 1975.

Bierman MI, Brown M, Muren O et al: Prolonged isoflurane anesthesia in status asthmaticus. Crit Care Med 14:832, 1986.

Black JW et al: Definition and antagonism of histamine H_2 receptors. Nature 236:385, 1972.

Blackhall M: Ventilating function in subjects with childhood asthma who have become symptom free. Arch Dis Child 45:363, 1970.

Blair H: Natural history of childhood asthma. Arch Dis Child 52:613, 1977.

Boushey HA, Holtzman MJ, Sheller JR et al: Bronchial hyperreactivity. Am Rev Respir Dis 121:389, 1980.

Brooks SM, McGowan K, Bernstein IL et al: Relationship between numbers of beta adrenergic receptors in lymphocytes and disease severity in asthma. J Allergy Clin Immunol 63:401, 1979.

Brown MJ et al: A novel double isotope technique for the enzymatic assay of plasma histamine: application to estimation of mast cell activation assessed by antigen challenge in asthmatics. J Allergy Clin Immunol 69:20, 1982.

Buckley RH: IgE antibody in health and disease. In Bierman CW and Pearlman DS (eds): Allergic Diseases from Infancy to Adulthood. 2nd ed. Philadelphia, WB Saunders Co, 1988.

Buffum WP and Settipane GA: Prognosis of asthma in childhood. Am J Dis Child 112:214, 1966.

Bush RK, Taylor SL, and Busse W: A critical evaluation of clinical trials in reactions to sulfites. J Allergy Clin Immunol 78:191, 1986.

Cade JF and Pain MCF: Pulmonary function during clinical remission of asthma. How reversible is asthma? Aust N Z J Med 3:545, 1973.

Cade JF, Woolcock AJ et al: Lung mechanics during provocation of asthma. Clin Sci 40:381, 1971.

Center DM, Soter NA, Wasserman SI, and Austen KF: Inhibition of neutrophil chemotaxis in association with experimental angioedema in patients with cold urticaria: a model of chemotactic deactivation in vivo. Clin Exp Immunol 35:112, 1979.

Cerrina J, Denkar A, Alexander G et al: Inhibition of exercise-induced asthma by a calcium antagonist. Am Rev Respir Dis 123:156, 1981.

Chai H: Antigen and methacholine challenge in children with asthma. J Allergy Clin Immunol 64:575, 1979.

Chai H, Fan RS, and Froehlich IA: Standardization of bronchial inhalation challenge procedures. J Allergy Clin Immunol 56:323, 1975.

Cloutier MM and Loughlin GM: Chronic cough in children: a manifestation of airway hyperreactivity. Pediatrics 67:6, 1981.

Coca AF and Cooke RA: On the classification of the phenomena of hypersensitiveness. J Immunol 8:163, 1973.

Cockroft DW: The bronchial late response in the pathogenesis of asthma and its modulation by therapy. Ann Allergy 55:857, 1985.

Cockroft DW, Killian DN, Mellon JJA, and Hargreave FE: Bronchial reactivity to inhaled histamine: a clinical survey. Clin Allergy 7:235, 1977.

Cockroft DW, Ruffin RE, Dolovich J, and Hargreave FE: Allergen-induced decrease in non-allergic bronchial reactivity. Clin Allergy 7:503, 1977.

Commentary: post-asthmatic pseudopolio in children. Lancet 1:860, 1980.

Cooke RA and VanderVeer A Jr: Human sensitization. J Immunol 1:201, 1916.

Corrao WM, Braman SS, and Irwin RS: Chronic cough as the presenting manifestation of bronchial asthma. N Engl J Med 300:633, 1979.

Cox JSG, Beach JE, and Blair AM: Disodium cromoglycate. Adv Drug Res 5:115, 1970.

Cropp GJA: The exercise bronchoprovocation test: standardization of procedures and evaluation of response. J Allergy Clin Immunol 64:627, 1979.

Davis JB: Asthma and wheezy bronchitis in children: skin test reactivity in cases, their parents and siblings: a controlled population study of sex differences. Clin Allergy 6:329, 1976.

Dawson B, Illsley R, Horobin G, and Mitchell R: A survey of childhood asthma in Aberdeen. Lancet 1:827, 1969.

Deal EC Jr, McFadden ER Jr, Ingram RH Jr, and Jaeger JJ: Effects of atropine on potentiation of exercise-induced bronchospasm by cold air. J Appl Physiol 45:238, 1978.

Deal EC Jr, McFadden ER Jr, Ingram RH Jr, and Jaeger JJ: Hyperpnea and heat flux: initial reaction sequence in exercise-induced asthma. J Appl Physiol 46:476, 1979.

Demopoulos CA, Pinkard RN, and Hanahan DJ: Platelet-activating factor. Evidence for 1-O-alkyl-2-acetyl-snglyceryl-3-phosphorylcholine as the active component. J Biol Chem 254:935, 1979.

Devereaux RB, Perloff JK, Reichele N, and Josephson MF: Mitral valve prolapse. Circulation 54:3, 1976.

Downs JJ, Wood DW, Harwood I et al: Intravenous isoproterenol infusion in children with severe hypercapnia due to status asthmaticus. Crit Care Med 1:63, 1973.

Durach DT, Ackerman SJ, Loegering DA et al: Purification of human eosinophil-derived neurotoxin. Proc Natl Acad Sci (USA) 78:5165, 1981.

Dvorak HF and Dvorak AM: Basophilic leukocytes: structure, function, and role in disease. Clin Haematol 4:651, 1975.

Dyer J et al: Measurement of plasma histamine: description of an improved method and normal values. J Allergy Clin Immunol 70:82, 1982.

Eggleston PA, Ward BH, Pierson WE, and Bierman CW: Radiographic abnormalities in acute asthma in children. Pediatrics 54:442, 1974.

Eitches RW, Rachelefsky GS, Katz RM et al: Methylprednisolone and troleandomycin in treatment of steroid-dependent asthmatic children. Am J Dis Child 139:264, 1985.

Empey DW, Laitinen LA, Jacobs L et al: Mechanisms of bronchial hyperreactivity in normal subjects after upper respiratory tract infection. Am Rev Respir Dis 113:131, 1976.

Eppinger H and Hess L: Vagotonia: a clinical study in vegetative neurology. Nervous and Mental Disease Monographs, No 20, 1915 (English translation).

Fearon DT and Austen KF: The human complement system: biochemistry, biology and pathobiology. Essays Med Biochem 2:1, 1976.

Fischer TJ and Ghory JE: Asthma as a lethal disease: the Cincinnati experience. J Asthma Res 13:27, 1975.

Flensborg EW: The prognosis of bronchial asthma arisen in infancy after the nonspecific treatment hitherto applied. Acta Paediatr 33:4, 1945.

Ford RM: Aetiology of asthma: a review of 11,551 cases (1958 to 1968). Med J Aust 56:628, 1969.

Frigas E and Gleich GJ: The eosinophil and the pathophysiology of asthma. J Allergy Clin Immunol 77:527, 1986.

Frigas E, Loegering DA et al: Elevated levels of the eosinophil granule major basic pattern in the sputum of patients with bronchial asthma. Mayo Clin Proc 56:345, 1981.

Furukawa CT, DuHamel TR, Weimer L et al: Cognitive and behavioral findings in children taking theophylline. J Allergy Clin Immunol 81:83, 1988.

Furukawa CT, Shapiro GG, Bierman CW et al: A double blind study comparing the effectiveness of cromolyn sodium and sustained-release theophylline in childhood asthma. Pediatrics 74:453, 1984.

Gilliam GL, McNicol KN, and William HE: Chest deformity, residual airways obstruction and hyperinflation, and growth in children with asthma. II. Significance of chronic chest deformity. Arch Dis Child 45:789, 1970.

Gleich GJ, Loegering DA, Mann KG et al: Comparative properties of the Charcot-Leyden crystal protein and the major basic protein from human eosinophils. J Clin Invest 57:633, 1976.

Goetzl EJ: Mediators of immediate hypersensitivity derived from arachidonic acid. N Engl J Med 303:822, 1980.

Gregg I: Epidemiology. In Clark TJH and Godfrey S (eds): Asthma. Philadelphia, WB Saunders Co, 1977.

Gurwitz D, Corey M, and Levison H: Pulmonary function and bronchial reactivity in children after croup. Am Rev Respir Dis 122:95, 1980.

Gurwitz D, Mirdorff C, and Levison H: Increased incidence of bronchial reactivity in children with a history of bronchiolitis. J Pediatr 98:551, 1981.

Haalboon JRE, Deenstra M, and Struyvenberg A: Hypokalaemia induced by inhalation of fenoterol. Lancet 1:1125, 1985.

Halonen M, Palmer JD, Lohman IC et al: Respiratory and circulatory alterations induced by acetylglyceryl ether phosphoryl-choline, a mediator of IgE anaphylaxis in the rabbit. Am Rev Respir Dis 122:915, 1980.

Hargreave FE, Dolovich J, O'Byrne PA et al: The origin of airway hyperresponsiveness. J Allergy Clin Immunol 5:825, 1986.

Hargreave FE, Ryan G, Thomson NC et al: Bronchial responsiveness to histamine or methacholine in asthma: measurement and clinical significance. J Allergy Clin Immunol 68:347, 1981.

Haynes RL, Ingram RH Jr, and McFadden ER Jr: An assessment of the pulmonary response to exercise in asthma and an analysis of the factors influencing it. Am Rev Respir Dis 114:739, 1976.

Heiner DC: Non-IgE antibody in disease. In Bierman CW and Pearlman DS (eds): Allergic Diseases from Infancy to Adulthood. 2nd ed. Philadelphia, WB Saunders Co, 1988.

Henderson WR, Shelhamer JH, Reingold DB et al: Alpha-adrenergic hyperresponsiveness in asthma. N Engl J Med 300:642, 1979.

Hogg JC: Bronchial mucosal permeability and its relationship to airways hyperreactivity. J Allergy Clin Immunol 67:421, 1981.

Holgate ST et al: Pharmacological modulation of airway caliber and mediator release in human models of bronchial asthma. In Austen KF, Lichenstein LM and Kay AB (eds): Asthma: Physiology, Immunopharmacology and Treatment. London, Academic Press, 1984.

Holtzman MJ, Cunningham JH, Sheller JR et al: Effect of ozone on bronchial reactivity in atopic and nonatopic subjects. Am Rev Respir Dis 120:1059, 1979.

Hopkins TJ: A new syndrome: poliomyelitis-like illness associated with acute asthma in childhood. Aust Paediatr J 10:273, 1974.

Huggins KG and Brostoff J: Local production of specific IgE antibodies in allergic rhinitis patients with negative skin tests. Lancet 2:148, 1975.

Humphrey DM, Handham DJ, Pinkard RN: Induction of leukocytic infiltrates in rabbit skin by acetylglyceryl ether phosphorylcholine. Lab Invest 47:227, 1982.

Ida S, Hooks JJ, Siraganian RP et al: Enhancement of IgE-mediated histamine release from human basophils: role of interferon. J Exp Med 145:892, 1977.

Ihle JN et al: Biologic properties of homogeneous interleukin 3. I. Demonstration of WEHI-3 growth factor activity, mast cell growth factor activity, P cell-stimulating factor activity, colony-stimulating factor activity, and histamine-producing cell-stimulating factor activity. J Immunol 131:282, 1983.

Irani AA, Schechter NM, Craig SS et al: Two types of human mast cells that have distinct neutral protease composition. Proc Natl Acad Sci (USA) 83:4464, 1986.

Ishizaka T: Analysis of triggering events in mast cells for immunoglobulin E-mediated histamine release. J Allergy Clin Immunol 67:90, 1981.

Ishizaka T and Ishizaka K: Biology of immunoglobulin E. Molecular basis of reaginic activity. Progr Allergy 19:60, 1975.

Jones RHT and Jones RS: Ventilatory capacity in young adults with a history of asthma in childhood. Br Med J 2:976, 1966.

Kaliner M, Orange RP, and Austen KF: Immunological release of histamine and slow reacting substance of anaphylaxis from human lung. J Exper Med 136:556, 1976.

Kaplan AP and Austen KF: Activation and control mechanisms of Hageman factor-dependent pathways of coagulation, fibrinolysis, and kinin generation and their contribution to the inflammatory response. J Allergy Clin Immunol 56:491, 1975.

Karpel JP, Appel D, Breidbart D, and Fusco MJ: A comparison of atropine sulfate and metaproterenol sulfate in the emergency treatment of asthma. Am Rev Respir Dis 133:727, 1986.

Kattan M, Keens TG, Lapierre JG et al: Pulmonary function abnormalities in symptom-free children after bronchiolitis. Pediatrics 59:683, 1977.

Kinsman RA, Dahlem NW, Spector S, and Standenmeyer H: Observations on subjective symptomatology, coping behavior, and medical decision in asthma. Psychosomat Med 39:102, 1977.

Koenig P: Hidden asthma in childhood. Am J Dis Child 135:1053, 1981.

Kraemer MJ, Furukawa CT, Shapiro GG et al: Altered theophylline clearance during an influenza B outbreak. Pediatrics 69:476, 1982.

Kuzemko JA: Natural history of childhood asthma. J Pediatr 97:886, 1980.

Lam S, Wong R, and Yeung M: Nonspecific bronchial reactivity in outpatient asthma. J Allergy Clin Immunol 63:28, 1979.

Lancet commentary: Asthma at night. Lancet 1:220, 1983.

Lands AM, Arnold A, McAuliff JP et al: Differentiation of receptor systems activated by sympathomimetic amines. Nature 214:597, 1967.

Larsen GL: Late phase reactions: observations on pathogenesis and prevention. J Allergy Clin Immunol 76:665, 1985.

Lee TC, Lenihan DJ, Malone B et al: Increased biosynthesis of platelet-activating factor in activated human eosinophils. J Biol Chem 259:5526, 1984.

Levison HS, Coolins-Williams C, Bryan AC et al: Asthma current concepts. Ped Clin North Am 21:951, 1974.

Lewis RA and Austen KE: Medication of local homeostasis and inflammation by leukotrienes and other mast cell–dependent compounds. Nature 293:103, 1981.

Lewis RA et al: Prostaglandin D_2 generation after activation of rat and human mast cells with anti-IgE. J Immunol 129:1627, 1982.

Littenberg B and Gluck EH: A controlled trial of methylprednisolone in the emergency treatment of acute asthma. N Engl J Med 314:150, 1986.

Little JN, Hall WJ, Douglas RG Jr et al: Airway hyperreactivity and peripheral airway dysfunction in influenza A injection. Am Rev Respir Dis 118:295, 1978.

Lubs ML: Allergy in 7,000 twin pairs. Acta Allergol 26:249, 1971.

Luksza ARP: Acute severe asthma treated without steroids. Brit J Dis Chest 76:15, 1982.

McCarthy JA: Prostaglandins, an overview. Adv Pediatrics 25:121, 1979.

McFadden ER Jr: Exertional dyspnea and cough as preludes to acute attacks of bronchial asthma. N Engl J Med 292:555, 1975a.

McFadden ER Jr: The chronicity of acute attacks of asthma—mechanical and therapeutic implications. J Allergy Clin Immunol 56:18, 1975b.

McFadden ER Jr: Respiratory mechanics in asthma. In Weiss EB and Segal MS (eds): Bronchial Asthma: Mechanisms and Therapeutics. Boston, Little, Brown & Co, 1976.

McFadden ER Jr: Asthma: airways reactivity and pathogenesis. Semin Respir Med 1:287, 1980a.

McFadden ER Jr: Asthma: pathophysiology. Semin Respir Med 1:297, 1980b.

McFadden ER Jr, Lyons HA, Bleecker ER, and Luparello T: The mechanism of action of suggestion in the induction of acute asthmatic attacks. Psychosomat Med 31:134, 1969.

MacGlashan DW Jr, Schleimer RP, Peters SP et al: Generation of leukotrienes by purified human lung mast cells. J Clin Invest 70:747, 1982.

McIntosh K: Bronchiolitis and asthma: possible common pathogenetic pathways. J Allergy Clin Immunol 57:595, 1976.

McIntosh K, Ellis EF, Hoffner LS et al: The association of viral and bacterial respiratory infections with exacerbations of wheezing in young asthmatic children. J Pediatr 82:578, 1973.

McNicol KN and Williams HB: Spectrum of asthma in children. I: clinical and physiological components. Br Med J 4:7, 1973a.

McNicol KN and Williams HB: Spectrum of asthma in children. II: allergic components. Br Med J 4:12, 1973b.

Makino S: Clinical significance of bronchial sensitivity to acetylcholine and histamine in bronchial asthma. J Allergy 38:127, 1966.

Mansmann HC Jr: A 25-year perspective of status asthmaticus. Clin Rev Allerg 1:147, 1983.

Mansmann HC Jr: A 29-year perspective of status asthmaticus in children. In An International Symposium on Status Asthmaticus and Asthma Deaths. NER Allergy Proc 1987.

Marquardt DL, Gruber HE, Wasserman SI: Adenosine release from stimulated mast cells. Proc Natl Acad Sci (USA) 81:6192, 1984.

Marquardt DL and Wasserman SI: Adenosine binding to rat mast cells—pharmacologic and functional characterization. Agents Actions 16:453, 1985.

Martin AJ, McLenna LA, Landau LI, and Phelan RD: The natural history of childhood asthma to adult life. Br Med J 1:1397, 1980.

Martin RJ: Cardiorespiratory Disorders During Sleep. Mount Kisco, NY, Futura Publishing Co, Inc, 1984.

Maselli R, Casal GL, and Ellis EF: Pharmacologic effects of intravenously administered aminophylline in asthmatic children. J Pediatr 76:777, 1970.

Meltzer SJ: Bronchial asthma as a phenomenon of anaphylaxis. JAMA 55:1021, 1910.

Mentzer RM, Rubio R, and Berne RM: Release of adenosine by hypoxic canine lung tissue and its possible role in pulmonary circulation. Am J Physiol 229:1625, 1975.

Metcalfe DD: Effector cell heterogeneity in immediate hypersensitivity reactions. Clin Rev Allergy 1:311, 1983.

Metcalfe DD, Bland CE, and Wasserman SI: Biochemical and functional characterization of proteoglycans isolated from basophils of patients with chronic myelogenous leukemia. J Immunol 132:1943, 1984.

Michaelides DN: Immediate hypersensitivity: the immunochemistry and therapeutics of reversible airway obstruction: a review. Immunol Allergy Pract 2:133, 1980.

Mills GC et al: Purine metabolism in adenosine deaminase deficiency. Proc Natl Acad Sci (USA) 73:2867, 1976.

Minor TE, Baker JW, Dick EC et al: Greater frequency of viral infections in asthmatic children as compared with their nonasthmatic siblings. J Pediatr 85:472, 1974.

Mitchell I, Inglis H, and Simpson H: Viral infection in wheezing bronchitis and asthma in children. Arch Dis Child 51:707, 1976.

Mitenko P and Ogilvie RI: Rational intravenous doses of aminophylline. N Engl J Med 289:600, 1973.

Morris HG and Selner JC: Endocrine aspects of allergy. In Bierman CW and Pearlman DS (eds): Allergic Diseases of Infancy, Childhood, and Adolescence. Philadelphia, WB Saunders Co, 1980.

Morris HG, Rusnak SA, and Barzens K: Leukocyte cyclic adenosine hemophosphate in asthmatic children: effects of adrenergic therapy. Clin Pharmacol Ther 22:352, 1977.

Mullarkey MF, Blumenstein BA, Andrade WP et al: Methotrexate in the treatment of corticosteroid-dependent asthma: a double-blind crossover study. N Engl J Med 318:603, 1988.

Mullarkey MF, Hill JS, and Webb DR: Allergic and nonallergic rhinitis: their characterization with attention to the meaning of nasal eosinophilia. J Allergy Clin Immunol 65:122, 1980.

Muntner S (ed): Medical Writings. Vol 1. Philadelphia, JB Lippincott Co, 1963.

Murray AB and Ferguson AC: Dust-free bedrooms in the treatment of asthmatic children with house dust or house dust mite allergy: a controlled trial. Pediatrics 71:418, 1983.

Nadel JA: Autonomic control of airway smooth muscle and airway secretions. Am Rev Respir Dis 115:117, 1977.

Nagy L, Lee TH, and Kay AB: Neutrophil chemotactic activity in antigen-induced late asthmatic reaction. N Engl J Med 306:497, 1982.

Oertel H and Kaliner M: The biologic activity of mast cell granules. III. Purification of inflammatory factors of anaphylaxis (IF-A) responsible for causing late-phase reactions. J Immunol 127:1398, 1981.

Olsson I and Venge P: Cationic proteins of human granulocytes. Blood 44:235, 1974.

O'Rourke PP and Crane RK: Halothanein status asthmaticus. Crit Care Med 10:341, 1982.

Ownby DR and Anderson J: Response to epinephrine in children receiving oral B-agonists. Am J Dis Child 140:122, 1986.

Parry WH, Martorano F, and Cotton EK: Management of life-threatening asthma with intravenous isoproterenol infusions. Am J Dis Child 130:39, 1976.

Paterson NAM et al: Release of chemical mediators from partially purified human lung cells. J Immunol 117:1356, 1976.

Pearlman DS: Bronchial asthma. A perspective from childhood to adulthood. Am J Dis Child 138:459, 1984.

Pearlman DS and Scoggin C: Asthma. In Abrams R and Wexler P (eds): Medical Problems in Pregnancy, Concepts and Management. Boston, Little, Brown & Co, 1983.

Permutt S: Physiologic changes in the acute asthmatic attack. In Lichtenstein LM et al (eds): Asthma: Physiology, Immunopharmacology and Treatment. New York, Academic Press, 1977.

Petty TL: Pulmonary rehabilitation. Resp Care 22:68, 1977.

Phipatanakul CS and Slavin RG: Bronchial asthma produced by paranasal sinusitis. Arch Otolaryngol 100:109, 1974.

Pierson WE, Bierman CW, Stamm SJ et al: Double-blind trial of aminophylline in status asthmaticus. Pediatrics 46:642, 1971.

Pinckard RN, McManus LM, Demopoulos CA et al: Molecular pathobiology of acetyl glyceryl ether phosphorylcholine: evidence for the structural and functional identity with platelet-activating factor. J Retic Soc 28(Suppl):45, 1980.

Pliss LB and Gallagher EJ: Aerosol vs. injected epinephrine in acute asthma. Ann Emerg Med 10:353, 1981.

Polgar G and Promadhat V: Pulmonary Function Testing in Children: Techniques and Standards. Philadelphia, WB Saunders Co, 1971.

Post-asthmatic pseudopolio in children (commentary). Lancet 1:860, 1980.

Rachelefsky GS, Coulson A, Siegel SC, and Stiehm EK: Aspirin intolerance in chronic childhood asthma: detected by oral challenge. Pediatrics 56:443, 1975.

Rachelefsky GS, Wo J, Adelson MA, et al: Behavior abnormalities and poor school performance due to oral theophylline use. Pediatrics 78:1133, 1986.

Rackemann FM: A clinical study of one hundred and fifty cases of bronchial asthma. Arch Intern Med 22:517, 1917.

Rackemann FM and Edwards MC: Asthma in children. A follow-up study of 688 patients after an interval of twenty years. N Engl J Med 246:815, 1952.

Razin E, Stevens RL, Akiyama F et al: Culture from mouse bone marrow of a subclass of mast cells possessing a distinct chondroitin sulfate proteoglycan with glycosaminoglycans rich in N-acetylgalactosamine-4,6 disulfate. J Biol Chem 257:7229, 1982.

Rhyne MB, Nathanson CA, Mellits ED, and Rodman AD: Determination of the Prevalence and Special Needs of Children with Bronchial Asthma or Atopic Dermatitis (final report for US Dept. HEW). Baltimore, The Johns Hopkins University Press, 1971.

Richards W and Patrick JR: Death from asthma in children. Am J Dis Child 110:4, 1965.

Richardson JB: The neural control of human tracheobronchial smooth muscle. In Lichtenstein LM et al (eds): Asthma: Physiology, Immunopharmacology and Treatment. New York, Academic Press, 1977.

Robertson CE, Sinclair CJ, Steedman D et al: Use of ether in life-threatening acute severe asthma. Lancet 1:182, 1985.

Robinson DR: Prostaglandins and inflammation. NESA Proc 2:79, 1981.

Rogers RM, Braunstein MS, and Shuman JF: Role of bronchopulmonary lavage in the treatment of respiratory failure: a review. Chest 62S:95S, 1972.

Rohatigi N, Fields A, and Sly RM: Status asthmaticus complicated by phrenic nerve paralysis. Ann Allergy 45:177, 1980.

Rooney JC and Williams H: The relationship between proved viral bronchiolitis and subsequent wheezing. J Pediatr 79:744, 1971.

Rossing TH, Fanta CH, Goldstein DH et al: Emergency treatment of asthma: Comparison of the acute effects of parenteral and inhaled sympathomimetics and infused aminophylline. Am Rev Respir Dis 122:365, 1980.

Ryssing E: Continued follow-up investigations concerning the fate of 298 asthmatic children. Acta Paediatr 48:255, 1959.

Schatz M, Patterson R, and Fink J: Immunologic lung disease. N Engl J Med 300:1310, 1979.

Schiffer CG and Hunt EP: Illness among Children. Children's Bureau Publication No 405. Washington, DC, US Dept. HEW, 1963.

Schwartz LB, Schratz JJ, Vik D et al: Metabolism of human C3 by human mast cell tryptase. J Allergy Clin Immunol 69:94S, 1982.

Schwartz M: Heredity in Bronchial Asthma. Copenhagen, Einar Minksgaard, 1952.

Segar WE and Chesney RW: Disorders of electrolyte metabolism. Pediatr Ann 10:P288, 1981.

Shapiro GG and Koenig P: Cromolyn sodium: a review. Pharmacotherapy 5:156, 1985.

Shapiro GG, Bierman CW, Furukawa CT, and Pierson WE: Double-blind dose-response study of metaproterenol inhalant solution in children with acute asthma. J Allergy Clin Immunol 79:378, 1987.

Shapiro GG, Chapman JI, Pierson WE, and Bierman CW: Poliomyelitis-like illness after acute asthma. J Pediatr 94:767, 1979.

Shapiro GG, Eggleston PA, Pierson WE et al: Double-blind study of the effectiveness of a broad spectrum antibiotic in status asthmaticus. Pediatrics 53:867, 1974.

Shapiro GG, Furukawa CT, Pierson WE, and Bierman CW: Methacholine bronchial challenge in children. J Allergy Clin Immunol 69:365, 1982.

Shapiro GG, Furukawa CT, Pierson WE et al: Double-blind evaluation of methylprednisolone versus placebo for acute asthma episodes. Pediatrics 71:510, 1983.

Sibbald B, Horn MEC, Brain EA, and Gregg I: Genetic factors in childhood asthma. Thorax 35:671, 1980.

Siegel SC, Katz RM, and Rachelefsky GS: Asthma in infancy and childhood. In Middleton E and Reed CE (eds): Allergy: Principles and Practice. St. Louis, CV Mosby Co, 1978.

Simons FER: Antihistamines (H_1 receptor antagonists) in asthma. In The Child with Asthma. Report of the Sixth Canadian Ross Conference in Pediatrics. Montreal, Quebec, 1985.

Simons FER and Chernick V: Principles of diagnosis and treatment of lower respiratory tract disease. In Bierman CW and Pearlman DS (eds): Allergic Diseases from Infancy to Adulthood. 2nd ed. Philadelphia, WB Saunders Co, 1988.

Simons FER, Pierson WE, and Bierman CW: Respiratory failure in childhood status asthmaticus. Am J Dis Child 131:1097, 1977.

Slavin RG: Recalcitrant asthma: have you looked for sinusitis? J Respir Dis 7:61, 1986.

Slavin RB and Smith LJ: Epidemiologic considerations in atopic disease. In Bierman CW and Pearlman DS (eds): Allergic Diseases from Infancy to Adulthood. 2nd ed. Philadelphia, WB Saunders Co, 1988.

Smith JM: Prevalence and natural history of asthma in school children. Br Med J 1:711, 1961.

Smith JM: Studies of the prevalence of asthma in childhood. Allergol Immunopathol 3:127, 1975.

Smith JM: Epidemiology and natural history of asthma, allergic rhinitis, and atopic dermatitis (eczema). In Middleton E and Reed CE (eds): Allergy: Principles and Practice. St. Louis, CV Mosby Co, 1978.

Soter NA et al: Local effects of synthetic leukotrienes (LTC_4, LTD_4, LTE_4, and LTB_4) in human skin. J Invest Dermatol 80:115, 1983.

Spector SL and Kinsman RA: More implications of reactivity characteristics to methacholine and histamine in asthmatic patients. J Allergy Clin Immunol 64:587, 1979.

Spector SL, Katz FH, and Farr RS: Troleandomycin: effectiveness in steroid-dependent asthma and bronchitis. J Allergy Clin Immunol 54:367, 1974.

Speight ANP, Lee DA, and Hey EN: Underdiagnosis and undertreatment of asthma in childhood. Br Med J 286:1253, 1983.

Speizer FE: Epidemiology, prevalence and mortality in asthma. In Weiss EB and Segal MS (eds): Bronchial Asthma: Mechanisms and Therapeutics. Boston, Little, Brown & Co, 1976.

Stalcup SA and Mellins RB: Mechanical forces producing pulmonary edema in acute asthma. N Engl J Med 297:592, 1977.

Stanworth DR and Smith AK: Inhibition of reaginmediated PCA reactions in baboons by the human IgG_4 subclass. Clin Allergy 3:37, 1973.

Strunk RC and Mrazek DA: Deaths from asthma in childhood. Can they be predicted? N Engl Reg Allergy Proc 7:454, 1986.

Strunk RD, Mrazek DA, Fuhrmann GS, and LaBreoque JF: Physiologic and psychological characteristics associated with deaths due to asthma in childhood. JAMA 254:1193, 1985.

Szczeklik A, Gryglewski RJ, Czerniawska-Mysik G et al: Relationship of inhibition of prostaglandin biosynthesis by analgesico of asthma attacks in aspirin-sensitive patients. Br Med J 1:67, 1975.

Szczeklik A, Gryglewski RJ, Czerniawski-Mysik G et al: Aspirin-induced asthma. J Allergy Clin Immunol 58:10, 1976.

Szentivanyi A: The beta adrenergic theory of the atopic abnormality in bronchial asthma. J Allergy 42:203, 1968.

Tal A, Bavilsk C, Yohai D et al: Dexamethasone and salbutamol in the treatment of acute wheezing in infants. Pediatrics 71:13, 1983.

Tashkin DP, Trevor E, Chopra SK, and Taplin GV: Sites of airway dilatation terbutaline. Comparison of physiologic tests with radionuclide lung images. Am J Med 68:14, 1980.

Tauber AL, Kaliner M, Steehschulte DJ, and Austen KF: Immunologic release of histamine and slow reacting substance of anaphylaxis from human lung V: Effects of prostaglandins on release of histamine. J Immunol 111:27, 1973.

Taussig LM, Smith SM, and Blumenfeld R: Chronic bronchitis in childhood—what is it? Pediatrics 67:1, 1981.

Tooley WH, Demuth C, and Nadel JA: The reversibility of obstructive changes in severe childhood asthma. J Pediatr 66:517, 1965.

Townley RE, Ryo UY, Kolotkin SM, and Kang B: Bronchial sensitivity to methacholine in current and former asthmatic and allergic rhinitis and control patients. J Allergy Clin Immunol 56:429, 1975.

Townley RG, Dennis M, and Itkin IH: Comparative action of acetyl beta-methylcholine, histamine, and pollen antigens in subjects with hay fever and patients with bronchial asthma. J Allergy 36:121, 1965.

VanArsdel PP Jr and Motulsky AG: Frequency and heritability of asthma and allergic rhinitis in college students. Acta Genet Stat Med 9:101, 1959.

Wald JA, Friedman BF, and Farr RS: An improved protocol for the use of troleandomycin (TAO) in the treatment of steroid dependent asthma. J Allergy Clin Immunol 78:36, 1986.

Warner JO, Price JF, Soothill JF, and Hey EN: Controlled trial of hyposensitization to Dermatophagoides pteronyssinus in children with asthma. Lancet 2:912, 1978.

Wasserman SI: The mast cell and the inflammatory response. In Pepys J and Edwards AM (eds): The Mast Cell: Its Role in Health and Disease. San Francisco, Fearon Pitman Publishers, Inc, 1979.

Wasserman SI: Chemical mediators of inflammation. In Bierman CW and Pearlman DS (eds): Allergic Diseases from Infancy to Adulthood. 2nd ed. Philadelphia, WB Saunders Co, 1988.

Wasserman SI, Austen KF, and Soter NA: The function and physiochemical characterization of three eosinophilotactic activities released into the circulation by cold challenge of patients with cold urticaria. Clin Exp Immunol 47:570, 1982.

Wasserman SI, Soter NA, Center DM et al: Cold urticaria: Recognition and characterization of a neutrophil chemotactic factor which appears in serum during experimental cold challenge. J Clin Invest 60:189, 1977.

Weiler-Ravell D and Godfrey S: Do exercise- and antigen-induced asthma utilize the same pathways? Antigen provocation in patients refractory to exercise-induced asthma. J Allergy Clin Immunol 67:391, 1981.

Weinberger M and Hendeles L: Pharmacologic management. In Bierman CW and Pearlman DS (eds): Allergic Diseases from Infancy to Adulthood. 2nd ed. Philadelphia, WB Saunders Co, 1988.

Weinberger MW, Matthay RA, Ginihansky EJ et al: Intravenous aminophylline dosage: use of serum theophylline measurement for guidance. JAMA 235:2110, 1976.

Weksler BB: Arachidonic acid cascade: the cyclooxygenase pathway. NESA Proc 2:56, 1981.

Weller PA, Lee CW, Foster DW et al: Generation and metabolism of 5-lipoxygenase pathway leukotrienes by human eosinophils: predominant production of leukotriene C_4. Proc Natl Acad Sci (USA) 80:7626, 1983.

Welliver RC: Allergy and the syndrome of chronic Epstein-Barr virus infection (editorial). J Allergy Clin Immunol 78:278, 1986.

Welliver RC, Kaul A, and Ogra RL: The appearance of cell-bound IgE in respiratory-tract epithelium after respiratory-syncytial-virus infection. N Engl J Med 303:1198, 1980.

Weng TR and Levison H: Pulmonary function in children with asthma at acute attack and symptom-free status. Am Rev Respir Dis 99:719, 1969.

Wilder CS: Prevalence of Selected Chronic Respiratory Conditions: United States, 1970 (Ser 10, No 84), National Center for Health Statistics. Rockville, Md, US Dept. HEW, 1973.

Wilhelm DL: Kinins in human disease. Ann Rev Med 22:63, 1971.

Williams DA, Lewis-Faning E, Rees L et al: Assessment of the relative importance of the allergic, infective and psychological factors in asthma. Acta Allergol 12:376, 1958.

Williams HB and McNicol KN: Prevalence, natural history and relationship of wheezy bronchitis and asthma in children: an epidemiological study. Br Med J 2:321, 1969.

Yu DYE, Galant SP, and Gold W: Inhibition of antigen induced bronchoconstriction by atropine in asthmatic patients. J Appl Physiol 32:823, 1972.

Zapol WM, Snider MT, and Schneider RC: Extracorporeal membrane oxygenation for acute respiratory failure. Anesthesiology 46:272, 1977.

42

C. WARREN BIERMAN, M.D., WILLIAM E. PIERSON, M.D., and F. STANFORD MASSIE, M.D.

NONASTHMATIC ALLERGIC PULMONARY DISEASE

An increasing number of substances associated with home, hobbies, vocations, and medications are capable of inducing non–IgE-mediated allergic pneumonitides, which may be subdivided into three major categories on the basis of pathophysiologic features, mechanism of tissue injury, and etiologic agent. *Hypersensitivity pneumonitis*, or extrinsic allergic alveolitis, the most common and best-characterized of these diseases, occurs primarily in nonatopic individuals. *Allergic bronchopulmonary disease*, by contrast, occurs exclusively in allergic patients who usually have chronic asthma; it has characteristics of both IgE-mediated allergy and hypersensitivity pneumonitis. *Pulmonary hypersensitivity reactions* to chemicals or drugs may resemble asthma, hypersensitivity pneumonitis, or allergic bronchopulmonary disease and may occur with equal frequency in "nonallergic" and "allergic" individuals.

In all of these diseases, symptoms of severe non-wheezing dyspnea, coughing, fever, and malaise may occur hours to days after exposure to the allergen. Because symptoms are delayed, neither physician nor patient may relate them to the causative agent. Yet early diagnosis is important, because early recognition and prompt therapy may prevent the development of such irreversible lung damage as pulmonary fibrosis or saccular bronchiectasis.

The number of substances and agents capable of causing such lung disease has been steadily increasing since the first of these disease states was recognized 20 years ago. Undoubtedly, many additional causes of "idiopathic" chronic lung disease have yet to be identified. In patients with such symptoms, a detailed history of home, school, occupation, and hobbies may identify the cause. Early recognition and prompt therapy may avoid years of disability and ultimate death from respiratory failure.

HYPERSENSITIVITY PNEUMONITIS (EXTRINSIC ALLERGIC ALVEOLITIS)

*Hypersensitivity pneumonitis** is a term that was introduced by Fink and co-workers in 1968 to characterize a group of pulmonary diseases resulting from the inhalation of organic dust particles of less than 10 μ in diameter, which include mold spores, bacterial products, avian droppings, and other proteins of animal origin. It is the term most frequently employed in the United States. *Extrinsic allergic alveolitis** was introduced by Pepys in 1969 in England. Although this term is not anatomically appropriate, because these diseases are associated with bronchiolar as well as alveolar involvement and occasionally with sarcoid-like granulomas (Gandevia, 1973), it has become generally accepted in the European literature.

These diseases may result from a number of unrelated organic dusts and occur only after intense or

---

*For purposes of this chapter, *extrinsic allergic alveolitis* and *hypersensitivity pneumonitis* are used interchangeably.

prolonged exposure, but they share common anatomic, histologic, and immunologic features (Salvaggio, 1980):

1. They involve peripheral airways exclusively.

2. Histologic examination shows that mononuclear cells infiltrate interstitial and alveolar areas, granulomas form, and pulmonary alveolar macrophages are "activated."

3. Immunologic changes include high titers of precipitating antibodies against the dust antigens; serum complement is not activated; and IgE antibody levels and peripheral eosinophil counts remain normal, although concentrations of other classes of immunoglobulins may be elevated.

Classification of the currently recognized diseases that occur with inhalation of organic dusts is given in Table 42–1.

CLINICAL FEATURES

Extrinsic allergic alveolitis, or hypersensitivity pneumonitis, can occur as an acute intermittent systemic and respiratory illness or as an insidious and progressive respiratory disease. The intensity and frequency of exposure to the etiologic antigens may determine whether the disease is acute or chronic (Fink, 1976).

The Acute Form

Chills, fever, malaise, cough and dyspnea, basilar rales, leukocytosis, pulmonary infiltrates, and restrictive-type pulmonary function test defects usually begin 4 to 6 hours after exposure to the causative organic dust. Symptoms and signs are frequently mistaken for infectious pneumonitis. Temperature may be as high as 40°C (104°F). Rapid respirations and moist crepitant rales may be heard predominantly at the lung bases, and there usually is no wheezing and minimal hyperinflation. These abnormalities ordinarily resolve within 12 to 18 hours but occasionally may persist for several days, unless terminated by corticosteroid therapy.

The Insidious Form

With prolonged and continuous exposure to the offending dust, cough and dyspnea may be progressive without acute episodes. Dyspnea on exertion, anorexia, weight loss, and fatigue may occur without fever, and positive findings may be limited to fine basilar rales and, rarely, clubbing of the fingers. The course in a child is shown in Figure 42–1 (Cunningham et al, 1976).

RADIOGRAPHIC STUDIES

In the acute form of the disease, the chest roentgenogram shows a diffuse, interstitial infiltrate of the alveolar walls and adjacent lobular septa, fine reticular densities with multiple small nodules, and patchy infiltration at the lung bases (Fig. 42–2) (Marinkovich, 1975; Fink, 1981). Chronic disease is manifested radiographically as a diffuse interstitial fibrosis with coarsening of the bronchovascular markings that is particularly prominent in the upper lobes. Hyperinflation is rare. Because none of these findings is specific for hypersensitivity pneumonitis, the chest

Table 42–1. CLASSIFICATION OF HYPERSENSITIVITY PNEUMONITIS

Type of Exposure	Disease	Source	Antigen
Environment	Humidifier lung Ventilation system disease	Home or work humidifers and air-conditioning systems	Thermophilic actinomycetes, ameba, various fungi
Hobbies and pets	Pigeon breeder's disease Bird fancier's lung	Pigeon, parakeet, or parrot droppings	Avian protein antigen
Occupation	Bagassosis	Moldy sugarcane	*Thermoactinomyces vulgaris*
	Cheese worker's disease	Cheese mold spores	*Penicillium casei*
	Enzyme worker's lung	Bacterial products (inhalation)	*Bacillus subtilis* enzyme
	Farmer's lung	Moldy hay, oats, corn	*Micropolyspora faeni* and *Thermoactinomyces vulgaris*
	Mushroom worker's disease	Compost	
	Malt worker's lung	Germinating barley	*Aspergillus clavatus, A. fumigatus*
	Maple bark disease	Moldy maple bark	*Cryptostroma corticale*
	Mill worker's disease	Mill dust, wheat flour	*Sitophilus granarius* (weevil)
	Poultry worker's disease	Poultry sheds	Chicken dander
	Sequoiosis	Moldy redwood sawdust	*Graphium pullularia*
	Wood worker's lung	Moldy wood chips	*Alternaria* species
	Suberosis	Moldy cork dust	*Penicillium frequentans*
Chemicals	Isocyanate hypersensitivity pneumonitis	Isocyanates	Toluene diisocyanate
	Porcelain refinisher's lung	Paint catalyst	Diphenyl methane diisocyanate
	Epoxy resin worker's lung	Epoxy resin	Phthalic anhydride
	Plastic worker's lung	Trimellitic anhydride	Trimellitic anhydride
Animals	Laboratory worker's lung	Rodent urine	Rodent proteins
	Furrier's lung	Hair dust	Dander proteins
Medications	Pancreatic extract lung	Pancreatic enzymes (inhalation)	Pig pancreatic protein
	Pituitary snuff taker's lung	Pituitary powder (inhalation)	Ox or pig protein

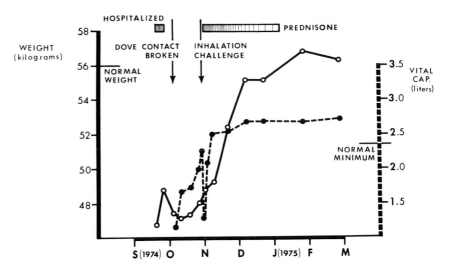

Figure 42–1. Clinical course of a child with hypersensitivity pneumonitis due to exposure to dove antigens. (Reproduced with permission from Cunningham AS, Fink JN, and Schlueter DP: Childhood hypersensitivity pneumonitis due to dove antigens. Pediatrics 58:441, 1976.)

roentgenogram must be correlated with the clinical features.

LABORATORY FINDINGS

Blood Studies and Cultures

During the acute phase, there may be leukocytosis as great as 25,000 cells/mm³, with a predominance of segmented forms of polymorphonuclear leukocytes and up to 10 per cent eosinophils. These findings return to normal when the acute symptoms subside. In the chronic form, the blood count is usually normal. Serum immunoglobulin levels may be elevated. IgE is usually normal, except in atopic individ-

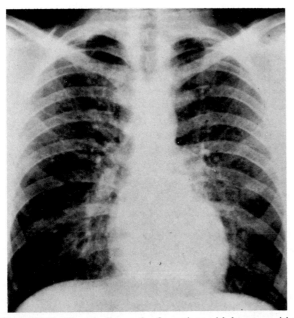

Figure 42–2. Chest radiograph of a patient with hypersensitivity pneumonitis. Note fine reticulonodular infiltrates of both lungs. (Reproduced with permission from Warren CPW and Tse KS: Extrinsic allergic alveolitis owing to hypersensitivity to chickens. Am Rev Respir Dis 109:672, 1974.)

uals with bird fancier's lung or allergic bronchopulmonary aspergillosis (A.B.A.). Nonspecific serologic findings, such as the presence of rheumatoid factor and positive mononucleosis spot test results, may be seen in those with the acute illness. The erythrocyte sedimentation rate occasionally is elevated. Smears and cultures of the throat, sputum, and blood are negative for pathogenic organisms. Leukocytosis and other nonspecific abnormal findings are usually absent in the chronic intermittent exposure form of the disease (Fink, 1984; Levy and Fink, 1985).

Pulmonary Function

Restrictive impairment to ventilation is the primary abnormality of hypersensitivity pneumonitis. Forced vital capacity (FVC) is reduced in acute episodes and may return to normal during remissions. It is irreversibly reduced in the chronic phase of the disease because of pulmonary fibrosis. Pulmonary compliance is decreased owing to increased stiffness of the lung, and carbon monoxide diffusion is diminished, indicating an alveolar-capillary blockade with reduced gas transfer. Functional residual capacity and total lung capacity are low. Arterial blood gases reveal diminished Pa_{O_2} and decreased oxygen saturation, which fall further with exercise.

Arterial P_{CO_2} is usually diminished, and the pH is slightly elevated, with a mild to moderate respiratory alkalosis during acute episodes. Renal compensation allows the pH to return to normal (Schlueter et al, 1969; Slavin, 1976; Fink, 1976). Airway resistance measured by plethysmography, forced expiratory volume at 1 sec (FEV₁), and midmaximal flow rates are usually normal unless the patient is atopic and has superimposed asthma.

In insidious hypersensitivity pneumonitis, some patients also have increased residual volumes, decreased flow rates, and loss of pulmonary elasticity as found in emphysema (Fink, 1976).

Immune Responses

Antigens that induce hypersensitivity pneumonitis appear to be of appropriate size (10 μ) for reaching the bronchial tree, where they are processed by pulmonary macrophages. The antigens are nondigestible by lysosomal enzymes, are particulate in nature, are capable of directly activating complement, and have an adjuvant effect on pulmonary immune responses (Fink, 1984). In the serum of patients with hypersensitivity pneumonitis, precipitating IgG antibodies characteristically are found to organic dust–containing fungal antigens, thermophilic actinomycetes, or avian proteins (Fig. 42–3). These antibodies may be detected in up to 50 per cent of asymptomatic, similarly exposed individuals, and therefore their presence per se is not indicative of disease. Epidemiologic studies have suggested that they simply reflect predominant antigen exposure. Early studies postulated that they were responsible for a type III or local Arthus hypersensitivity reaction in the lung. Although type III reactions appear to occur in these diseases, recent experimental and human studies have implicated monocytes and lymphocytes (and presumably type IV reactions) in the pathogenesis of the pulmonary reaction. Precipitating antibodies may play a protective role in antigen-clearing mechanisms. Antibody titers generally are higher in symptomatic individuals. Cross-reactions have been noted between various organic dust antigens and are believed to indicate a wide degree of exposure to the antigens capable of inducing hypersensitivity pneumonitis in patients with the disease. Patients with farmer's lung disease have been found to have broad immune responses with elevated specific antibodies to a panel of respiratory viruses and *Mycoplasma* compared with normal individuals, perhaps indicating wide antigenic exposure or unknown peculiarities in host responsiveness.

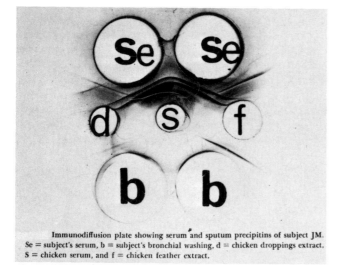

Immunodiffusion plate showing serum and sputum precipitins of subject JM.
Se = subject's serum, b = subject's bronchial washing, d = chicken droppings extract,
S = chicken serum, and f = chicken feather extract.

Figure 42–3. Serum and bronchial precipitins to chicken proteins in a patient with hypersensitivity pneumonitis. (Reproduced with permission from Warren CPW and Tse KS: Extrinsic allergic alveolitis owing to hypersensitivity to chickens. Am Rev Respir Dis 109:672, 1974.)

Serum complement has been reported to be decreased in asymptomatic, but not in symptomatic, pigeon breeders on inhalation challenge with pigeon antigens; however, in other studies, alveolar fluid levels of complement from patients with hypersensitivity lung disease did not differ from levels from patients with idiopathic pulmonary fibrosis or normal controls. Furthermore, extracts of *Micropolyspora faeni*, important in farmer's lung disease, have been found to consume complement in vitro in the absence of detectable antibodies. The immunopathogenic role of complement activation directly by causative antigens (alternative pathway?) or through antigen-antibody interaction (classic pathway) requires further elucidation (Marx and Flaherty 1976; Olenchock and Burrell, 1976).

Cellular Immune Studies

Peripheral blood lymphocytes and bronchoalveolar lavage (BAL) T cells from patients with hypersensitivity pneumonitis undergo blast transformation and release lymphokines when cultured in vitro with appropriate fungal or avian antigens. In contrast, lymphocytes from asymptomatic individuals do not react in this manner even though there may be serum-precipitating antibodies present to the antigens. In pigeon breeder's disease, BAL T cells are increased with normal T and B cell ratios and helper and suppressor cell ratios. Abnormalities in T cell immunoregulation with decreased suppressor cell function exist and may be important in the pathogenesis of hypersensitivity pneumonitis. In animal models of hypersensitivity pneumonitis, lymphocytes appear to be of prime importance. Animal transfer experiments with infusion of sensitized lymphocytes were followed by pulmonary lesions on antigen challenge by inhalation. In most studies, serum transfer was less likely to induce typical lesions after inhalation challenge (Fink, 1981; Levy, 1985).

Genetic control of the pulmonary response is suggested by studies in animals and humans. Human leukocyte antigen (HLA) linkage has not been confirmed, however. Pulmonary damage appears to develop after an immune response that combines both antigen-specific humoral antibodies and cellular hypersensitivity, with mononuclear cells releasing lymphokines. Complement activation in the lung and irritant effects of the thermophilic agents also may be important. Cellular hypersensitivity to organic dusts may lead to hypersensitivity pneumonitis, after being triggered by a nonspecific inflammatory process, such as a respiratory infection (Reynolds, 1977).

Skin Tests. Prick or intracutaneous skin tests are useful with pigeon-derived antigens (pigeon serum and dropping extracts) in pigeon breeder's disease, as are the other bird proteins in chicken sensitivity lung disease (Pepys, 1974; Fink, 1976). Skin testing may also be helpful in pituitary snuff taker's lung and in pancreatic extract lung. It cannot be used satisfactorily in hypersensitivity pneumonitis from

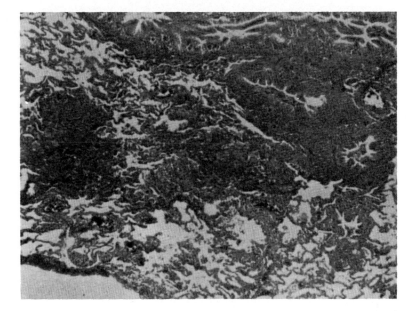

Figure 42–4. Appearance of a typical section of lung obtained by biopsy from a patient with "pigeon fancier's disease." Note the diffuse involvement as well as the large nodular cellular aggregates. At higher magnification, these were seen to contain chronic inflammatory cells, including plasma cells, lymphocytes, rare multinucleated giant cells, and large sheets of finely vacuolated histiocytes. Most of the alveolar septa were thickened by similar cells. (Reproduced with permission from Van Arsdel PP Jr and Thune R: Infiltrative lung disease and hypersensitivity to organic dusts. Yale J Biol Med 40:501, 1967.)

thermophilic actinomycetes because extracts of these agents are irritating and may give nonspecific, false-positive reactions.

Rarely, an immediate wheal-and-flare reaction occurs 15 min after skin testing. An erythematous, occasionally ecchymotic reaction usually occurs 4 to 8 hours later. Biopsy examination of the skin test site shows a mild infiltration of polymorphonuclear leukocytes and plasma cells surrounding the vessels, consistent with an Arthus type of response (Pepys, 1969; Fink, 1976).

Inhalation Challenge Studies

On inhalation challenge with extracts of causative agents, patients with hypersensitivity pneumonitis develop chills, fever, malaise, leukocytosis, restrictive pulmonary changes, and a fall in Pa_{O_2} 4 to 8 hours after exposure (Pepys, 1974; Fink, 1976). Because these reactions may be severe, inhalation challenge must be done in the hospital and with great caution, and a severe reaction should be terminated with corticosteroids. Challenge material must be pure, because extracts contaminated with endotoxin can produce a nonspecific response (Slavin, 1976). In some patients, careful reexposure to areas suspected of containing offending antigens, such as a pigeon coop, barn, or place of employment, may be necessary.

Lung Biopsy

As with serologic, radiologic, and pulmonary function test results, the histologic findings in patients with hypersensitivity pneumonitis vary, depending on whether the disease is acute or chronic (Fink, 1976). Lung biopsy specimens from patients with acute hypersensitivity pneumonitis reveal interstitial pneumonia, with involvement of the alveolar walls

and bronchioles, and positive results of fluorescent staining for immunoglobulin and complement (Wenzel et al, 1971). Infiltrations with lymphocytes, plasma cells, and occasional clusters of histiocytes containing foamy cytoplasm may be seen, in association with intra-alveolar proteinaceous fluids and increased numbers of alveolar macrophages. Focal sarcoid-type noncaseating granulomas with Langhans-type giant cells, bronchiolitis, and minimal vasculitis may also be present (Seal et al, 1968; Fink and Sosman, 1974; Hensley et al, 1974).

In chronic hypersensitivity pneumonitis, fibrosis and destruction of lung parenchyma predominate over lymphocyte and plasma infiltration of alveolar walls (Fig. 42–4). Severe fibrosis is associated with cystic changes and obliteration of bronchioles by collagen deposition and granulation tissue (Fink, 1976).

None of these findings is specific for hypersensitivity pneumonitis, and the features of biopsy material must be correlated with other clinical and laboratory findings.

EXPERIMENTAL STUDIES

Experimental hypersensitivity pneumonitis has been induced in many animals, including rats, guinea pigs, rabbits, horses, and monkeys, to a number of antigens, including extracts of pigeon guano, bagasse, thermophilic actinomycetes, and *Aspergillus* spores.

All features of human disease have been reproduced in rabbits (Moore and Fink, 1975). Rabbits exposed by aerosol to large quantities of pigeon antigens developed a humoral, but not cellular, immunologic response, and their lungs remained normal histologically. A single intravenous injection of killed BCG vaccine in oil facilitated the induction of pulmonary cell-mediated hypersensitivity to the inhaled antigen as well as the development of pulmonary lesions. Further, in animals with histologically normal lungs, a decrease in complement levels occurred after aerosolized pigeon antigen challenge, but this did not occur in the BCG-treated animals. Transfer of sensitivity by lymphoid cells in rabbits also resulted in alveolar, interstitial, and peribronchial lesions (Richerson, 1983; Fink 1983).

DIAGNOSIS

The diagnosis of hypersensitivity pneumonitis depends on a high index of suspicion and a thorough history, with particular attention to the patient's home environment, hobbies, and work. A physician may be misled by the fever, leukocytosis, and pulmonary infiltrates that occur in the acute form and may attribute clinical improvement to antibiotics rather than to hospitalization and change in environment. The recurrence of symptoms on return to the previous environment should be the key to the diagnosis.

Patients with insidious-onset disease do not relate their symptoms to an exposure to antigen. In patients who smoke and have chronic bronchitis, the diagnosis may easily be missed. These patients are at risk of progressing to chronic pulmonary fibrosis. In these patients, the insidious onset and progressive nature of dyspnea without other systemic symptoms should encourage the physician to examine the patient's environment, culturing for air-borne fungi when appropriate and performing serologic tests for precipitins to these fungi. Inhalation challenge or open-lung biopsy with specific immunologic studies may be necessary to confirm the diagnosis.

THERAPY

Careful avoidance of reexposure to causative agents and corticosteroid therapy will achieve remission of the acute form. Steroid therapy should begin with a single early morning dose of 40 mg of prednisone, with a gradual daily dose reduction. Chest x-ray films and lung function tests should be carefully monitored. If long-term steroid therapy is necessary, an alternate-day regimen should be tried. Avoiding reexposure may be difficult, because occupation or life style may need to be changed. Lack of compliance may be followed by recurrence or progression of pulmonary disease.

SPECIFIC SYNDROMES

Hypersensitivity Pneumonitis Related to Home Environment

Interstitial Lung Disease Due to Contamination of Forced-Air Systems. In the home and office environments, humidifiers and air-conditioning systems present specific hazards of hypersensitivity pneumonitis. In 1970, Banaszak and associates recognized hypersensitivity pneumonitis in four patients as a result of contamination of a home air conditioner with thermophilic fungi. Since then, many patients have been reported to have had either chronic or acute hypersensitivity pneumonitis secondary to either home or office heating or air-conditioning systems. The etiologic antigens identified to date are *Thermoactinomyces candidus, T. vulgaris, T. sacchari*, and *Mucor faeni*.

In an epidemiologic survey of 272 subjects, Banaszak and co-workers (1974) performed culture studies of the homes for thermophilic fungi, performed pulmonary function tests, took chest roentgenograms, and performed serum studies for precipitating antibodies to a group of fungi. Thermophilic fungi were recovered in culture from 74 per cent of the homes. Significantly higher concentrations were found in homes with symptomatic subjects. Substantially more precipitating antibodies were identified among the symptomatic group, although there was not good correlation between presence of precipitating antibodies, degree of pulmonary involvement, and chest roentgenogram abnormalities. Of eight subjects whose disease resulted from chronic exposure to actinomycetes-contaminated home humidifiers, three had persistent lung disease in spite of recognition and therapy (Fink, 1976). In children with persistent respiratory problems, the chronic use of humidifiers or vaporizers should be suspected as the cause of disease (Hodges et al, 1974; Seabury et al, 1976).

Disease Due to Hobbies

Pigeon Breeder's Disease. Pigeon breeder's disease is the most common and best-studied pediatric hypersensitivity pneumonitis (Fink, 1983). It has been reported after long-standing exposure to avian antigens from pigeons, parrots, doves, parakeets (budgerigars), and chickens. Hypersensitivity pneumonitis has been reported after exposure to mice, rats, gerbils, and guinea pigs. There usually is an insidious onset with a prolonged course. Weight loss is a common sign. Clinical features include cough, dyspnea, basilar rales, absence of wheezing, abnormal chest x-ray films with infiltrates, and restrictive lung disease with reduced FVC and diffusing capacity. A history of exposure to avian antigens is reported, with a variable duration from 6 weeks to 7 years. Skin testing with pigeon serum or extracts of feathers and droppings may reveal both an immediate and a late onset of skin reaction. Precipitating antibodies to avian proteins are present in the serum. Careful inhalation challenge with bird-derived extracts in a hospitalized patient is followed by an acute syndrome with cough, dyspnea, and rales 4 to 8 hours after exposure, with abnormal pulmonary function studies. Lung biopsy specimen reveals a chronic interstitial mononuclear infiltration. Therapy consists of elimination of birds and a course of corticosteroids. These produce clearing of the abnormal signs and normal chest x-ray film findings, if exposure has not been sufficient to produce pulmonary fibrosis.

The course of illness in one such patient is demonstrated in Figure 42–1, and chest roentgenograms obtained before and after therapy are noted in Figure 42–5.

OCCUPATIONAL HYPERSENSITIVITY PNEUMONITIS

As outlined in Table 42–1, hypersensitivity pneumonitis may be seen in workers exposed to organic dust containing thermophilic actinomycetes or other fungi from sugar cane (bagassosis), cheese, laundry detergent enzymes *(Bacillus subtilis)*, moldy hay (farmer's lung disease), mushroom compost, or wood dust; in chemical workers exposed to isocyanates and phthalic and trimellitic anhydrides; in animal workers exposed to laboratory rodents; in furriers; and in individuals exposed to medications containing pig or cow proteins. Clinical features of hypersensitivity pneumonitis have been reported in parents caring for children with cystic fibrosis (pancreatic enzymes) and in patients with diabetes insipidus (pituitary snuff). Synthetic vasopressin (Pitressin) has significantly reduced the incidence of this latter problem.

A high index of suspicion and a careful environmental history are essential to the diagnosis of any individual with chronic cough and interstitial pneumonitis. Failure to recognize a relationship between environmental exposure to causative agents and preventable chronic lung disease may lead to insidious

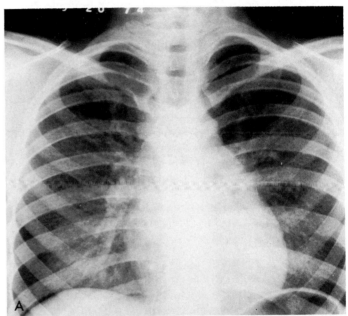
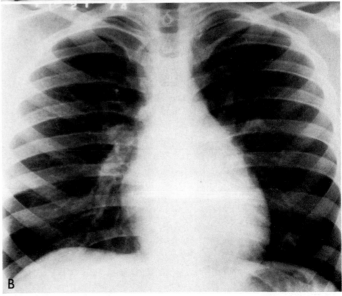

Figure 42–5. Chest radiographs of a child with hypersensitivity pneumonitis due to exposure to doves in the home taken during the acute *(A)* and convalescent *(B)* periods. (Reproduced with permission from Cunningham AS, Fink JN, and Schlueter DP: Childhood hypersensitivity pneumonitis due to dove antigens. Pediatrics 58:436, 1976.)

pulmonary deterioration, with fibrosis as the end result.

ALLERGIC BRONCHOPULMONARY ASPERGILLOSIS

DEFINITION

ABA is an immune bronchial disease occurring in asthma sufferers. Pulmonary infiltrates and eosinophilia in blood and sputum are characteristic. It was first described in adults in England in 1952 and in children in 1970. It may be distinguished from other forms of lung disease due to *Aspergillus fumigatus* such as invasive or septicemic aspergillosis, aspergilloma, IgE-mediated asthma from *A. fumigatus* sensitivity, and hypersensitivity pneumonitis due to *A. clavus*, growing in barley, in malt worker's lung.

Aspergillus is found year-round in air; soil; decaying vegetation, such as cut grass, potting soil, and mulches; basements; bedding; house dust; and swiming pool water. Individuals with episodic bronchial obstructive disease, such as patients with asthma and, occasionally, patients with cystic fibrosis, are susceptible to colonization of the bronchial tree with *A. fumigatus*. Presumably because of thick, tenacious mucus and possibly other host factors, ABA may develop. There have been occasional reports of at least two family members having the disease. HLA studies have revealed no genetic predisposition.

Clinical symptoms include anorexia, malaise, fever, attacks of wheezing, and productive cough with solid sputum plugs. Rales over areas of pulmonary infiltrates and wheezing may be heard on auscultation of the chest. Laboratory studies reveal a profound eosinophilia frequently greater than $1000/mm^3$ and elevated IgE level as high as 80,000 ng/ml. Most reported patients have been adults, but the diagnosis should be suspected in wheezing children ever under 2 years of age who exhibit recurrent infiltrates, eosinophilia, and *A. fumigatus* in the sputum (Imbeau et al, 1978; Rickett et al, 1984; Slavin, 1985).

DIFFERENTIAL DIAGNOSIS

The differential diagnosis of ABA is listed in Table 42–2. Steroid-dependent asthmatic patients should be investigated carefully for the presence of ABA. Other causes for the pulmonary infiltrate with eosinophilia syndrome should be considered. ABA appears to be increased in patients with cystic fibrosis, with increased IgE, with atopy, and with positive skin test reactions to *A. fumigatus*. Positive sputum cultures for *A. fumigatus* may be noted in this disease, with a frequency of 20 to 50 per cent. Ten per cent of 100 cystic fibrosis patients ages 2 to 34 years had features indicating ABA (Laufer et al, 1984). Differentiating features of ABA and hypersensitivity pneumonitis are listed in Table 42–3.

Table 42–2. DIFFERENTIAL DIAGNOSIS OF ALLERGIC BRONCHOPULMONARY ASPERGILLOSIS

Poorly controlled asthma with mucoid impaction/atelectasis
Pneumonitis, viral or bacterial
Tuberculosis with eosinophilia
Sarcoidosis
Pulmonary infiltrates with eosinophilia syndrome
Parasitism
Churg-Strauss vasculitis
Pulmonary neoplasm
Hypersensitivity pneumonitis
Cystic fibrosis
Immotile cilia syndrome

RADIOGRAPHIC FEATURES

Radiographic features are variable, depending on the severity of asthma and the degree of tissue damage resulting from the disease. The initial chest roentgenogram of a child with ABA and a follow-up film taken 7 years later are shown in Figure 42–6.

Acute changes may vary from small areas of consolidation with patchy areas of atelectasis to large areas of consolidation with atelectasis of an entire lobe. Frequently there are homogeneous shadows 2 to 3 cm in length, caused by bronchi filled with secretions, and "tram lines" or parallel hairline shadows extending from the hilum, indicating dilated bronchi. The atelectasis resulting from mucous plugs may result in a mediastinal shift to the affected side. *Chronic changes* consist of ring shadows 1 to 2 cm in diameter due to dilated bronchi; circular shadows 2 to 3 cm in diameter representing cavities; and tubular shadows, parallel lines wider than a bronchus separated by a translucent zone, due to saccular bronchiectasis, which is characteristically proximal and frequently involves the upper lobes (McCarthy et al, 1971).

All of the abnormal radiographic findings seen in allergic bronchopulmonary aspergillosis are more severe in the upper lobes than in the lower lobes. Progressive loss of volume, fibrosis, and bronchiectasis develop in some patients (Imbeau et al, 1978).

Lung scans using ^{87m}Sr are characteristic, with localization of the radionuclide in radiographic abnormalities. Such a "positive" scan in a patient with chronic pulmonary disease should suggest occult allergic bronchopulmonary aspergillosis (Adiseshan and Oliver, 1973).

LABORATORY FINDINGS

Blood Studies and Cultures

General findings in ABA include eosinophilia in peripheral blood and sputum and marked elevation of serum IgE (Patterson et al, 1973). Expectorated sputum frequently contains brownish plugs from which fungal mycelia and *A. fumigatus* grow readily on culture.

Table 42–3. DIFFERENTIAL DIAGNOSIS OF HYPERSENSITIVITY PNEUMONITIS (HP) AND ALLERGIC BRONCHOPULMONARY ASPERGILLOSIS (ABA)

Diagnostic Feature	HP	ABA
Nature of patient	Nonatopic (nonallergic)	Atopic (allergic)
Symptoms and physical findings	Cough, dyspnea, fever, no wheezing, weight loss, rales at lung bases	Asthma, fever, ± hemoptysis, chest pain
Skin tests	± (positive immediate and late reactions in some cases of pigeon breeder's lung)	+ (immediate and late responses)
Blood count	Normal or lymphopenia	Eosinophilia
Immunoglobulins	Elevated IgG and IgA, IgG precipitating antibodies	Elevated IgE, IgG precipitating antibodies
Sputum	Normal	Eosinophilia, mycelia
Chest x-ray film	Pulmonary interstitial infiltrates	Pulmonary lobar infiltrates
Complications	Pulmonary fibrosis	Atelectasis, proximal bronchiectasis, fibrosis (late)
Pulmonary function tests	Restrictive	Obstruction (restrictive late)
Inhalation challenge tests	Late restriction (± immediate/late obstruction) (positive immediate and late reactions in some cases of pigeon breeder's lung)	Immediate and late obstruction
Immune mechanism	Immune complexes and delayed hypersensitivity	Immediate hypersensitivity and immune complexes, (± delayed hypersensitivity)
Treatment	Avoidance, corticosteroids	Bronchodilators, corticosteroids

(Modified with permission from Slavin RG: Allergic bronchopulmonary aspergillosis. In Middleton E Jr, Reed CE, and Ellis EF [eds]: Allergy: Principles and Practice. St. Louis, CV Mosby Co, 1983.)

Pulmonary Function Studies

Like chest roentgenograms, pulmonary function values vary with the activity and severity of the disease. They range from mild obstructive airway changes to severe airway obstruction that is not reversed by isoproterenol, hyperinflation, increased total lung capacity, and decreased diffusing capacity (Safirstein et al, 1973).

During acute "flares" of ABA, there are significant reductions in total lung capacity, vital capacity, FEV_1, and DL_{CO} all of which return to normal with steroid therapy (Nichols et al, 1979).

Immunologic Findings

Serologic Studies. Precipitin tests performed by immunodiffusion or radioimmunoelectrophoresis reveal the presence of IgG precipitating antibodies in the majority of patients (Safirstein et al, 1973), and up to three arcs have been found in more than 90 per cent. By contrast, in aspergillosis with tissue invasion, a broader humoral response occurs, with up to eight precipitin arcs (Bardana et al, 1975; Citron, 1975).

Marked elevations of serum IgE (10,000 to 30,000 IU/ml) are characteristic of ABA during acute pulmonary infiltrations (Patterson et al, 1973). Some but not all of the IgE is specific for *Aspergillus* antigens (Patterson and Roberts, 1974). Exacerbations of ABA are associated with sharp increases in total serum IgE, which subsequently decrease with prednisone therapy. The increase in IgE levels frequently precedes pulmonary infiltrates and clinical symptoms. Acute asthma in these same patients, by contrast, is not associated with increased IgE (Wang et al, 1979). Histamine release studies have suggested that both IgE and IgG, anti-*Aspergillus* antibodies, may be cytophilic for human basophils (Bardana et al, 1975; Citron, 1975).

Inhalation Challenge Studies

Inhalation challenge with *A. fumigatus* has been shown experimentally to result in a dual reaction—an immediate reaction and a delayed reaction—in contrast to only a delayed reaction in hypersensitivity pneumonitis (McCarthy and Pepys, 1971).

The immediate reaction occurs within minutes and consists of "tickling" in the throat, eyes, or ears; dry, repetitive coughing; and tightness of the chest with wheezing. Lung function testing shows asthma or increased asthma with a decrease of 500 ml or more in the FEV_1. The late reaction occurs after about 3 to 8 hours and consists of a productive cough, wheezing, dyspnea, malaise, headache, anorexia and flu-like sensation, and an inability to sleep. Signs of airway obstruction reappear or become clinically worse in association with a decline of 500 ml or more in FEV_1 after initial recovery. Pyrexia and leukocytosis are maximal 24 hours after the test.

The early reaction may be prevented by pretreatment with cromolyn or reversed by isoproterenol; the late reaction is less frequently prevented by cromolyn, is infrequently reversed by isoproterenol, and may require corticosteroid treatment. Inhalation challenge should be performed only when the patient will be in the hospital for 24 hours after challenge, and concentrations of inhaled antigens are determined by quantitative skin testing.

PATHOLOGIC FEATURES

Bronchiectasis involving segmental bronchi with sparing of distal branches, particularly in the upper lobes, is characteristic (Fig. 42–7). Inspissated mucus contains Curschmann spirals, Charcot-Leyden crystals, eosinophils, fibrin, and mononuclear cells. Fungal hyphae may be seen, *A. fumigatus* may be cultured,

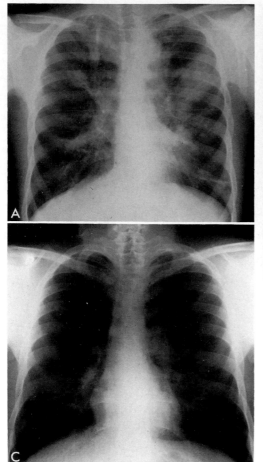

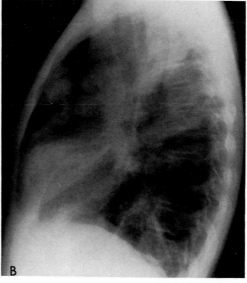

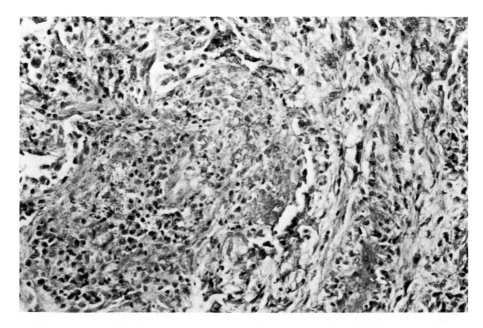

Figure 42–6. *A* and *B*, Roentgenograms of a 13-year-old boy with allergic bronchopulmonary aspergillosis. Note atelectasis in the left base and the left lingula. There is consolidation of the right upper lobe and both midlungs with dilated bronchi in apical segments of both upper lobes. Note bullous lesion of right suprahilar area. *C*, In same patient at age 19 years, lungs are clear except for enlarged inferior right hilar density and lobe linear streaking (probable fibrosis) in the left lower lobe.

Figure 42–7. Appearance of a typical section of lung taken by biopsy from a child with allergic bronchopulmonary aspergillosis. The bronchial wall on the right is severely involved, with total destruction of the epithelial lining and only remnants of smooth muscle. The alveolar lumens are filled with inflammatory exudate and cellular debris. Other areas of this biopsy specimen contained some multinucleated giant cells, eosinophils, and mononuclear cells. (Courtesy of Dr. Joel E Hass.)

but there is no invasion of bronchial walls. A granulomatous bronchiolitis sometimes is seen. Microabscesses containing *A. fumigatus*, eosinophilic pneumonia, lipid pneumonia, lymphocytic interstitial pneumonia, desquamative interstitial pneumonia, fibrosis, bronchiolitis obliterans, or bronchocentric granulomatosis may be reported from pathology specimens of patients with ABA. Bronchoprovocation tests with *A. fumigatus* and bronchography have attendant risks and are not generally necessary for diagnosis. Lung biopsy is best reserved for questionable cases, when other diseases must be ruled out.

DIAGNOSIS

Diagnostic aids for ABA are outlined in Table 42–4. All asthmatic patients with pulmonary infiltrates should have skin testing with *A. fumigatus* antigen. A dual reaction with an immediate (10 to 15 min) and a late (4 to 8 hours) reaction occurs in a third of patients with ABA. The immediate response is IgE mediated; the late response also may be largely IgE mediated, because biopsy specimens of the late reaction fail to show vasculitis, as in a true Arthus reaction, despite the presence of IgG, IgM, IgA, and C3. Similarly, immediate and late immune reactions are believed to be pathogenetic for the bronchial disease that occurs. When levels of IgE-Af or IgG-Af antibodies or both are compared between ABA patients and asthmatic patients who are *A. fumigatus* skin test positive but have no evidence of ABA, ABA patients are found to have at least twice the levels of antibody as asthmatic individuals without ABA. This *A. fumigatus* antibody "index" is helpful in diagnosis and follow-up of ABA patients. Antibodies are measured by radioimmunoassy (RIA) and enzyme-linked immunosorbent assay (ELISA) techniques. Total IgE concentration is elevated at least twofold over baseline measurements in all patients with acute infiltrates and is a useful aid in following disease activity (Greenberger, 1984).

Table 42–4. CRITERIA FOR DIAGNOSIS OF ALLERGIC BRONCHOPULMONARY ASPERGILLOSIS

Primary
Obstructive airway disease
Eosinophilia > 1000/mm³
Immediate skin test positive reaction to *Aspergillus fumigatus*
Serum precipitating antibodies against *A. fumigatus*
Elevated serum IgE level
History of transient or fixed pulmonary infiltrates
Central bronchiectasis in upper lobes
Elevated serum IgE/IgG antibodies to *A. fumigatus*

Secondary
Positive sputum culture for *A. fumigatus*
History of golden brown sputum plugs
Late skin test reactivity to *A. fumigatus* (4 to 8 hours)
Decline in total IgE level after prednisone therapy

TREATMENT

Once the diagnosis of an acute or exacerbated stage is determined, corticosteroid therapy is begun (Table 42–5). After initiation of prednisone therapy, pulmonary infiltrates should disappear. A decline in total serum IgE level of up to 35 per cent may be noted within 6 weeks. A decrease in peripheral eosinophilia and asthma symptoms accompanies improvement. Prednisone decreases the inflammatory response and aids in removal of the fungus by relieving airway obstruction. Antifungal agents, cromolyn sodium, and topical inhalant steroids have been used but are not effective. Corticosteroid-dependent asthma and ABA in fibrotic stages are less responsive to prednisone because of the damage to the bronchial tree already present. In order to prevent these stages, follow-up with frequent total serum IgE levels and chest x-rays as outlined in Table 42–5 is essential. A declined and stabilized serum IgE level and a clearing of pulmonary infiltrates for at least 6 months are noted in the remission stage. Prednisone can then be tapered and discontinued. A sharp rise in serum IgE level and a new pulmonary infiltrate herald an exacerbation. Prednisone should be instituted and given as in the acute stage. Bronchodilator therapy should be continued through all stages. Heavy mold spore exposure and allergen immunotherapy with *Aspergillus* should be avoided. The prognosis of patients with ABA is good if the condition is detected early and treated with prednisone; however, a long-term study of patients with untreated ABA revealed progressive declines in lung functions. Clinicians should maintain a high index of suspicion for ABA in asthmatic patients (Massie, 1988).

OTHER IMMUNOLOGIC LUNG DISEASE

As in hypersensitivity pneumonitis, occupational factors are associated with an ever increasing number of pulmonary diseases that may involve immunologic mechanisms (Salvaggio, 1982). However, hypersensitivity pneumonitis has been studied in depth, and its pathophysiology is now understood. Many of the pulmonary syndromes considered here are not so well characterized or the mechanism of lung damage is not clear but appears to involve the immune system (symposium, 1982).

In general, only a small portion of the persons exposed actually develop symptoms. However, the problem is growing. It is estimated that 15 per cent of all adult males who develop asthma in Japan do so because of exposure to industrial vapors, dusts, gases, or fumes (Kobayashi, 1974). Exposure of workers in the enzyme detergent industry to *B. subtilis* enzymes resulted in respiratory symptoms in 2 per cent of employees (Commentary, 1976). Exposure to gum acacia used in color printing resulted in respi-

Table 42–5. TREATMENT AND FOLLOW-UP OF ALLERGIC BRONCHOPULMONARY ASPERGILLOSIS

Prednisone, 0.5 mg/kg, at 8 AM every day for 2 weeks (40 to 60 mg/day in adults); check for improvement in pulmonary infiltrates.
Prednisone, 0.5 mg/kg, at 8 AM every other day for 3 months after clearing of infiltrates.
Taper every-other-day dose (5 mg/month) over 3 months with continued improvement.
Obtain total serum IgE levels monthly for 2 years, then every 2 months.
Obtain chest x-ray films every 4 months for 2 years, every 6 months for 2 years, and yearly thereafter.
Reinstitute daily prednisone with twofold rise in serum IgE level and new pulmonary infiltrates.

ratory symptoms among 20 to 50 per cent of the workers studied (Fowler, 1952).

Numerous industrial materials and drugs are known to produce pulmonary disease. The types of reactions are obstructive, with asthma-like syndromes (e.g., aspirin, industrial chemicals); restrictive, with diffuse pulmonary disease suggesting pneumonitis (e.g., nitrofurantoin); and combined obstructive and restrictive (e.g., metal fumes). Mediastinal and hilar changes have been reported from phenytoin and corticosteroids, and respiratory muscle paralysis has been reported from a number of antibiotics. An asthma-like syndrome, a late-onset asthma with chills and fever, and a restrictive lung disease or hypersensitivity pneumonitis have been reported with trimellitic anhydride, isocyanate, and sodium diazobenzene sulfate exposure (Schatz and Patterson, 1983; Zeiss et al, 1977). Table 42–6 lists these syndromes (Schotz and Patterson, 1983).

PATHOGENESIS AND PATHOGENETIC MECHANISMS

Occupational lung disease may be induced by irritant, pharmacologic, or IgE-mediated allergic factors. Atopy is often a predisposing factor in the development of these pulmonary symptoms. For example, in printers who developed acacia lung disease, those who were atopic developed asthma with one-half the exposure necessary to produce it in those who were not. In general, it appears that many occupational agents lead to the development of hy-peractive airways (Chan-Yeung, 1977) and that this hyperactive state may persist after exposure to the occupational agent is discontinued.

Exposure to an irritant such as acid sulfates, sulfur dioxide, ammonia, or hydrochloric acid can induce coughing, bronchitis, and asthma, presumably through a vagal reflex mechanism.

Nonallergic factors such as air pollutants, exercise, and cigarette smoking can significantly increase respiratory disability in susceptible patients. Such air pollutants as sulfur dioxide and acid sulfates can increase exercise-induced bronchoconstriction in both asthmatic and atopic nonasthmatic persons. Patients exposed to ozone during exercise exhibit a higher pulmonary reactivity than when exposed at rest. Cigarette smoke adversely affects mucociliary clearance and increases the time required for pulmonary clearance of iron oxide. It also decreases clearance of PMNs from the lungs (MacNee, 1989). The heightened bronchial lability appears to be mediated by irritant receptors in the large airways.

Many industrial materials, such as toluene diisocyanate (TDI), may act as irritants in the majority of subjects, who react to concentrations of 0.5 ppm, but can induce asthma in other workers at concentrations of 0.001 ppm (Butcher et al, 1978), suggesting that it may act as an allergen as well as an irritant.

Some substances may act as pharmacologic agents in inducing certain forms of occupational asthma. Inhalation of cotton dust, for example, not only can induce asthma in exposed workers who have byssinosis but also can induce similar symptoms in healthy volunteers. Extracts of cotton, flax, and hemp can

Table 42–6. COMMON CAUSES OF CHEMICAL- AND DRUG-INDUCED IMMUNOLOGIC LUNG DISEASES

| | | **Chemicals** | |
NAME	SOURCE	SUBSTANCE	TYPE REACTION
Cedar worker's disease	Western red cedar sawdust	Plicatic acid	Obstructive, restrictive, or both
Coffee worker's disease	Coffee bean dust	Chlorogenic acid	Restrictive
Meat wrapper's asthma	Plastic wrap	Organic copolymers of polyvinyl chloride	Obstructive
Metal fume fever	Plastic wrap	Zinc salts	Restrictive and obstructive
Polymer fume fever	Industrial exposure	Polytetrafluoroethylene	Obstructive
TDI diseases	Polyurethane plastics	Toluene diisocyanate	Obstructive
Trimellitic anhydride disease	Plastics, epoxy resins, paint manufacturing	TMA—human protein conjugate	Obstructive, restrictive, or both
Silicosis, asbestosis	Mining, manufacturing, etc.	Alveolar macrophage damage by silica or asbestos	Restrictive
		Drugs	
Aspirin asthma	Oral medication	Acetylsalicylic acid	Obstructive
Blood transfusion lung	Multiple transfusions	Donor HLA antigens	Restrictive
Pulmonary drug reaction	Ingested medication	Nitrofurantoin	Restrictive

also release histamine from nonsensitized human lung, suggesting a direct mast cell effect (Bouhuys and Lindell, 1961). Other agents with pharmacologic actions include organic phosphate insecticides, which have an anticholinesterase action, and agents such as TDI, which has a beta-adrenergic blocking action. Both of these types of agents could induce asthma by a non–IgE-mediated pharmacologic pathway.

Castor bean allergy, green coffee bean allergy, and asthma related to platinum salts are examples of clear-cut IgE-mediated asthma. Allergy can be demonstrated by immediate wheal-and-flare prick test reactions, radioallergosorbent test (RAST) reactions, Prausnitz-Küstner assays, and in vitro histamine release procedures (Davis et al, 1977; Karr et al, 1978; Pepys et al, 1979).

CLINICAL FEATURES

As noted in Table 42–6, the clinical manifestations of chemical and pulmonary drug reactions vary from acute bronchospasm, as in meat-wrapper's asthma and polymer fume fever, to restrictive pulmonary disease with interstitial pneumonitis, as in nitrofurantoin pulmonary hypersensitivity, or both, as in the disease seen in sawmill workers who inhale western red cedar sawdust. Because these reactions may take such diverse forms and because the number of chemical agents capable of inducing such reactions is growing steadily, physicians must increasingly be aware of the environmental chemicals to which their patients are exposed.

LABORATORY FEATURES

In vitro tests are available for a few drugs. Cellular and humoral immune responses to cromolyn sodium have been demonstrated in a few patients with allergic reactions to the drug (Sheffer et al, 1975). Immunopathologic mechanisms have not been delineated, however, in the majority of drug-induced pulmonary reactions (Rosenow, 1976).

Inhalation bronchial challenge is used in diagnosing immediate and late pulmonary reactions to a number of occupational antigens, such as chemical vapors, drugs, and enzymes (Butcher et al, 1976).

A detailed review of these individual diseases is beyond the scope of this chapter. Table 42–6 lists common causes of chemical- and drug-induced lung disease. Interested readers are referred to various reviews of these disorders (Butcher and Salvaggio, 1986; Chan-Yeung, 1986; Barkman and Salvaggio, 1988).

REFERENCES

Adiseshan N and Oliver WA: Strontium lung scans in the diagnosis of pulmonary aspergillosis. Am Rev Respir Dis 108:441, 1973.

Banaszak EF, Barboriak J, Fink J et al: Epidemiologic studies relating thermophilic fungi and hypersensitivity lung syndromes. Am Rev Respir Dis 110:585, 1974.
Banaszak EF, Thiede WH, and Fink JN: Hypersensitivity pneumonitis due to contamination of an air-conditioner. N Engl J Med 283:271, 1970.
Bardana EJ Jr: Measurement of humoral antibodies to aspergilli. Ann NY Acad Sci 221:64, 1974.
Bardana EJ Jr, Gerber JD, Graig S, and Cianciulli FD: The general and specific immune response to pulmonary aspergillosis. Am Rev Respir Dis 112:799, 1975.
Barkman HW Jr, and Salvaggio JE: Occupational asthma. In Bierman CW and Pearlman DS: Allergic Diseases from Infancy to Adulthood. 2nd ed. Philadelphia, WB Saunders Co, 1988.
Bouhuys A and Lindell SE: Release of histamine by cotton dust extracts from human lung tissue in vitro. Experientia 17:211, 1961.
Butcher BT and Salvaggio JE: Occupational asthma. J Allergy Clin Immunol 78:547, 1986.
Butcher BT, Salvaggio JE, Weill H, and Ziskind MM: Toluene diisocyanate (TDI) pulmonary disease: immunologic and inhalation challenge studies. J Allergy Clin Immunol 58:89, 1976.
Butcher BT, Karr RM, O'Neil CE et al: Toluene diisocyanate (TDI) pulmonary disease: studies of mediators and inhalation challenge testing in sensitized workers. J Allergy Clin Immunol 61:138, 1978.
Chan-Yeung M: Fate of occupational asthma. Am Rev Respir Dis 116:1023, 1977.
Chan-Yeung M and Lam S: State of art: occupational asthma. Am Rev Respir Dis 133:686, 1986.
Citron KM: Respiratory fungus allergy and infection. Proc R Soc Med 68:587, 1975.
Commentary: Biologic effects of proteolytic enzyme detergents. Thorax 31:621, 1976.
Cunningham AS, Fink JN, and Schlueter DP: Childhood hypersensitivity pneumonitis due to dove antigens. Pediatrics 58:436, 1976.
Davis RJ, Butcher BT, O'Neil CE, and Salvaggio JE: The in vitro effect of toluene diisocyanate on lymphocyte cyclic adenosine monophosphate production by isoproterenol, prostaglandin and histamine. J Allergy Clin Immunol 60:223, 1977.
Fink J: Hypersensitivity pneumonitis. In Kirkpatrick CE and Reynolds HY (eds): Lung Biology and Health Disease. Vol. 1. New York, Marcel Dekker Inc, 1976.
Fink JN: Immunologic lung diseases. Hosp Pract 16:53, 1981.
Fink JN: Pigeon breeder's disease. Clin Rev Allergy 1:497, 1983.
Fink JN: Hypersensitivity pneumonitis. J Allergy Clin Immunol 74:1, 1984.
Fink JN and Sosman AJ: Allergic lung disease not mediated by IgE. Med Clin North Am 58:157, 1974.
Fink JN, Sosman AJ, Barboriak JJ et al: Pigeon breeder's disease. A clinical study of a hypersensitivity pneumonitis. Ann Intern Med 68:1205, 1968.
Fink JN, Banaszak EF, Barboriak JJ, et al: Interstitial lung disease due to contamination of forced air systems. Ann Intern Med 84:406, 1976.
Fowler PBS: Printer's asthma. Lancet 2:755, 1952.
Gandevia B: Hypersensitivity disorders of the lungs and bronchi. Ann Clin Lab Sci 3:386, 1973.
Greenberger PA: Allergic bronchopulmonary aspergillosis. J Allergy Clin Immunol. 74:645, 1984.
Hensely GT, Fink JN and Barboriak JJ: Hypersensitivity pneumonitis in the monkey. Arch Pathol 97:33, 1974.
Hodges GR, Fink JN, and Schlueter DP: Hypersensitivity pneumonitis caused by a contaminated cool mist vaporizer. Ann Intern Med 80:501, 1974.
Imbeau SA, Nichols D, Flaherty D et al: Allergic bronchopulmonary aspergillosis. J Allergy Clin Immunol 62:243, 1978.
Karr RM, Lehrer SB, Butcher BT, and Salvaggio JE: Coffee worker's asthma. J Allergy Clin Immunol 62:143, 1978.
Kobayashi S: Occupational asthma due to inhalation of pharmacologic dusts in Japan. In Yamamura Y et al (eds): Allergology. Amsterdan, Excerpta Medica Foundation, 1974.
Lauter P, Fink JN, Bruns WT, et al: Allergic bronchopulmonary aspergillosis and cystic fibrosis. J Allergy Clin Immunol 73:44, 1984.

Levy MB and Fink JN: Hypersensitivity pneumonitis. Ann Allergy 54:167, 1985.

MacNee W, Wiggs B, Belzberg AS, and Hogg JC: The effect of cigarette smoking on neutrophil kinetics in human lungs. N Engl J Med 321:924, 1989.

Marinkovich VA: Hypersensitivity alveolitis. JAMA 321:944, 1975.

Marx JJ and Flaherty DK: Activation of the complement sequence of extracts of bacteria and fungi associated with hypersensitivity pneumonitis. J Allergy Clin Immunol 57:328, 1976.

Massie FS: Hypersensitivity pneumonitis and allergic bronchopulmonary aspergillosis. In Bierman CW and Pearlman DS (eds): Allergic Diseases from Infancy to Adulthood. WB Saunders Co, Philadelphia, 1988.

McCarthy DS and Pepys J: Allergic bronchopulmonary aspergillosis. Clin Allergy 1:414, 1971.

McCarthy DS, Simon G, and Hargreaves FE: Radiological appearance in allergic bronchopulmonary aspergillosis. Clin Radiol 21:366, 1970.

Moore VL and Fink JN: Immunologic studies in hypersensitivity pneumonitis—quantitative precipitins and complement fixing antibodies in symptomatic and asymptomatic pigeon breeders. J Lab Clin Med 85:540, 1975.

Nichols D, Dopico GA, Braun S et al: Acute and chronic pulmonary function changes in allergic bronchopulmonary aspergillosis. Am J Med 67:631, 1979.

Olechock SA and Burrell B: The role of precipitins and complement activation in the etiology of allergic lung disease. J Allergy Clin Immunol 58:76, 1976.

Patterson R and Roberts M: IgE and IgG antibodies against *Aspergillus fumigatus* in sera of patient with bronchopulmonary allergic aspergillosis. Int Arch Allergy 46:150, 1974.

Patterson R, Fink JN, Pruzansky JJ et al: Serum immunoglobulin levels in pulmonary allergic aspergillosis and certain other lung diseases with special reference to immunoglobulin E. Am J Med 54:16, 1973.

Patterson R, Roberts M, Roberts RC et al: Antibodies of different immunoglobulin classes against antigens causing farmer's lung. Am Rev Respir Dis 114:315, 1976.

Pepys J: Hypersensitivity disease of the lungs due to fungi and other organic dusts. Monogr Allergy No 4, Basel, Switzerland, S Karger, 1969.

Pepys J: Immunologic approaches in pulmonary disease caused by inhaled materials. Ann NY Acad Sci 221:27, 1974.

Pepys J, Pariser W, Cronwell O, and Hughes EG: Passive transfer in man and monkey of type 1 allergy due to heat labile and heat stable antibody to complex salts of platinum. Clin Allergy 9:99, 1979.

Reynolds HY, Fulmer JD, and Kazierowski JA: Analysis of cellular and protein content of bronchoalveolar lavage fluid from patients with idiopathic pulmonary fibrosis and chronic hypersensitivity pneumonitis. J Clin Invest 59:165, 1977.

Richerson HB: Hypersensitivity pneumonitis—pathology and pathogenesis. Clin Rev Allergy 1:469, 1983.

Ricketti AJ, Greenberger PA, Mintzer RA, and Patterson R: Allergic bronchopulmonary aspergillosis. Chest 86:773, 1984.

Rosenow EC III: Drug-induced hypersensitivity disease of the lung. In Kirkpatrick CE and Reynolds HY (eds): Lung Biology and Health Disease. Vol. 1: Immunologic and Infectious Reactions in the Lung. New York, Marcel Dekker, Inc, 1976.

Safirstein BH, D'Souza MF, Simon G et al: Five-year follow-up of allergic bronchopulmonary aspergillosis. Am Rev Respir Dis 108:450, 1973.

Salvaggio JE: Diagnosis and management of hypersensitivity pneumonitis. Hosp Pract 15:93, 1980.

Salvaggio JE: Overview of occupational immunologic lung disease. J Allergy Clin Immunol 70:5, 1982.

Schlueter DP, Fink JN, and Sosman AJ: Pulmonary functions in pigeon breeders' disease. Ann Intern Med 70:457, 1969.

Schatz M and Patterson R: Hypersensitivity pneumonitis—general considerations. Clin Rev Allergy 1:451, 1983.

Slavin RG: Allergic bronchopulmonary aspergillosis. Clin Rev Allergy 3:167, 1985.

Seabury J, Becker B, and Salvaggio J: Home humidifier thermophilic actinomycete isolates. J Allergy Clin Immunol 57:174, 1976.

Seal RME, Hapke EJ, Thomas GO et al: The pathology of acute and chronic stages of farmer's lung. Thorax 23:469, 1968.

Sheffer AL, Rocklin RE, and Goetzl EJ: Immunologic components of hypersensitivity reactions to cromolyn sodium. N Engl J Med 293:1220, 1975.

Slavin RG: Immunologically mediated lung diseases, extrinsic allergic alveolitis and allergic bronchopulmonary aspergillosis. Postgrad Med 59:137, 1976.

Slavin RG: Allergic bronchopulmonary aspergillosis. Clin Rev Allergy 3:167, 1985.

Symposium Proceedings on Occupational Lung Disease. J Allergy Clin Immunol 70:1, 1982.

Wang JLF, Patterson R, Roberts M, and Ghory AC: The management of allergic bronchopulmonary aspergillosis. Am Rev Respir Dis 120:87, 1979.

Wenzel FJ, Emanuel DA, and Gary RL: Immunofluorescent studies in patients with farmer's lung. J Allergy Clin Immunol 48:224, 1971.

Zeiss CR, Patterson R, Pruzansky JJ, et al: Trimellitic anhydride—induced airway syndromes: Clinical and immunologic studies. J Allergy Clin Immunol 60:96, 1977.

43

JAMES W. BROOKS, M.D.

TUMORS OF THE CHEST

Neoplasms of the chest in children may be categorized as follows:

1. Pulmonary
   a. Benign
   b. Malignant
   c. Metastatic
2. Mediastinal
   a. Primary
   b. Thymus tumors
   c. Teratoid
   d. Neurogenic
   e. Lymph node

f. Vascular-lymphatic
g. Fatty
h. Thyroid and parathyroid
3. Cardiac and pericardial
4. Diaphragmatic
5. Chest wall

DIAGNOSIS OF PULMONARY OR MEDIASTINAL TUMOR

Children who have symptoms of pulmonary involvement that do not disappear promptly when treated in the usual manner by expectorants and antibiotics must be suspected of having a space-occupying lesion. Posteroanterior and lateral chest roentgenograms are mandatory whenever respiratory symptoms persist.

Indeed, it might seem logical for all children to have a routine chest roentgenogram within the first 6 months of life. Certainly a physical examination in an adult patient is no longer considered complete without a chest roentgenogram. Why should children be excluded from this advanced form of diagnosis? Without such refinement, how can we expect to help those with potentially curable lesions? Only by such techniques can obstructive emphysema (Fig. 43–1), atelectasis (Fig. 43–2), and actual solid masses be seen at a stage of development when active resectional surgery may offer some hope of cure (Figs. 43–3 to 43–7).

In addition to having a probing history and complete physical examination, children with respiratory symptoms should have other studies.

It is impossible to obtain *sputum* voluntarily from an infant, but swabs from the posterior portion of the pharynx may be studied. In older children, however, sputum can be collected. A small catheter placed through the nose and adjusted into the trachea, thereby producing cough, will allow one to collect sputum through the catheter (Fig. 43–8). Any sputum thus collected should be studied by smear and culture for routine bacteria, acid-fast bacilli, and fungi; bacteria should be tested for *antibiotic* sensitivity. Cytologic analysis for tumor cells should be carried out.

The tuberculin (PPD or tine) *skin test* should be applied. Coccidioidin, blastomycin, and histoplasmin skin tests may be applied, although they are not as accurate as complement-fixation studies.

Protein electrophoresis may show hypogammaglobulinemia to be a primary or secondary etiologic factor in recurrent pulmonary infectious processes. *Complement-fixation blood studies* for fungal infections are generally more reliable than skin tests. Pulmonary complications of hematologic disorders, such as leukemia, Hodgkin's disease, and lymphosarcoma, may be properly identified by examination of the peripheral *blood smear*.

Examination of the bone marrow may give diagnostic evidence of blood dyscrasia, such as leukemia or myeloma, or even metastatic malignancy.

Cystic fibrosis as a cause of chronic recurrent pulmonary inflammatory disease may be suggested or ruled out by *sweat chloride determination* (see Chapter 47).

Roentgenologic examination of the chest with fluoroscopy and cinefluoroscopy, special views such as apical lordotic and right and left oblique, and planigrams may be necessary for final definition. *Cinefluoroscopy* allows repeated examination of the thoracic organs in motion (function) without subjecting an infant to excessive radiation exposure. During this examination and at the time of *fluoroscopy*, studies with barium in the esophagus will aid in determining any displacement of the posterior mediastinum. Body section

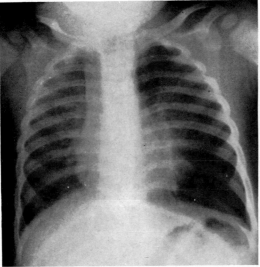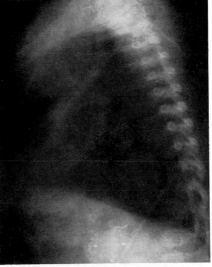

Figure 43–1. Obstructive emphysema of the left lower lobe bronchus caused by partial occlusion of the lumen. The left diaphragm is flattened, mediastinal and cardiac shadows are displaced toward the right, the left upper lobe is compressed, and there is increased radiolucency of the left lower lobe.

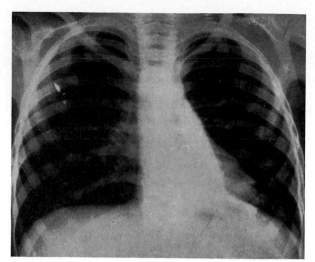

Figure 43–2. Total atelectasis of the left lower lobe secondary to an inflammatory stricture of the left lower lobe bronchus. A retrocardiac position tends to confuse diagnosis in some cases.

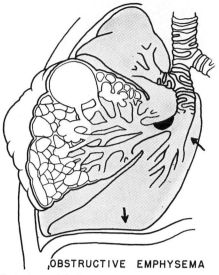

OBSTRUCTIVE EMPHYSEMA

Figure 43–4. A partial obstruction leads to the retention of air in the pulmonary parenchyma distal to the obstructed bronchus. Retention of air will cause an ipsilateral compression of the adjacent, normally aerated lung tissue, widening of intercostal spaces, descent of the diaphragm, a shift of the mediastinum away from the lung with the partially obstructing lesion, and a wheeze accompanied by decreased breath sounds over the affected lung.

radiography *(planigraphy)* can aid in the exact definition of mediastinal and lung masses; however, because young children are often unable to cooperate by ceasing all movement during filming, this procedure is less applicable than in adults. The bony thorax and aerated lung present obstacles to ultrasonic transmission, limiting the usefulness of *ultrasonography* in this situation. Real-time or B-mode scanning, however, can serve to clarify otherwise confusing radiographic findings. The most practical applications are in locating and assisting in the needle aspiration of pleural fluid collections (Fig. 43–9). Mediastinal, pulmonary, and diaphragmatic densities are best detailed with *computerized axial tomography (CAT) of the thorax,* which has added a new dimension to the accurate study of all these areas (Figs. 43–10 to 43–12). Its specific value will be better judged as

more information is obtained from its now widespread use.

Magnetic resonance imaging (MRI) is beginning to have an impact on thoracic diagnostic work-up. It can discriminate masses in the mediastinum from vascular structures better than CAT and is more sensitive in detecting intraspinal extension. Computed tomography demonstrates calcifications and bronchial abnormalities that are not seen on MRI. Magnetic resonance imaging is an important new diagnostic tool because it involves no ionizing radia-

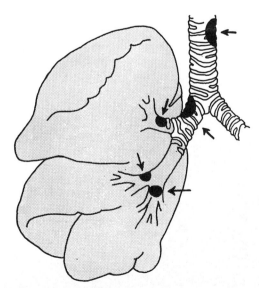

Figure 43–3. A diagram illustrating locations of lesions within the lumens of the major bronchi. The location of such lesions dictates the area of pulmonary involvement, unilaterality or bilaterality, and the extent of signs and symptoms.

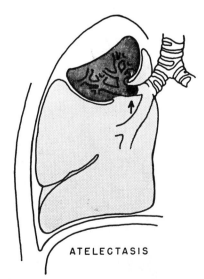

ATELECTASIS

Figure 43–5. Persistence of the lesion with ultimate total obstruction gives rise to atelectasis, an absence of breath sounds over the affected lung tissue, an overexpansion of the surrounding lung tissue, and a shift of the diaphragm to a more normal position, with a return of the mediastinum to midline. Bronchial secretions may actually decrease in amount.

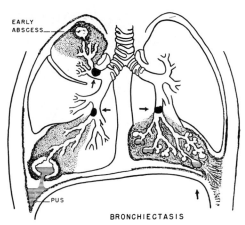

Figure 43–6. The persistence of an obstructing lesion leads to permanent destructive changes in the pulmonary parenchyma distal to the lesion, such as abscess formation, chronic pneumonitis with fibrosis, pleurisy, empyema, and bronchiectasis with parenchymal contracture secondary to fibrosis.

tion, has no complicating side effects, and is noninvasive and painless.

Diagnostic pneumoperitoneum (introduction of air into the peritoneal cavity, thereby outlining the diaphragm) may aid in the diagnosis of abnormalities adjacent to the diaphragm; congenital diaphragmatic hernias may also be visualized (Fig. 43–13).

Angiocardiograms outlining the cardiac chambers and pulmonary arteries will point up any displacement due to masses in the lung, mediastinum, or pericardium. Certain lesions may be studied better by *venous angiography* outlining the major veins of the mediastinum. The use of aortograms will assist in ruling out such vascular causes of symptoms such as vascular ring, congenital aneurysm, congenital vascular malformations of the pulmonary tree, and sequestration. *Thoracic aortograms* are used to define bronchial arteries in patients with massive hemoptysis. Once the bleeding vessel has been identified,

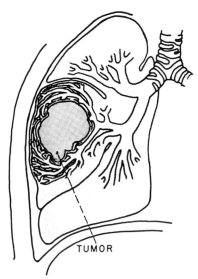

Figure 43–7. If the tumor is within the pulmonary parenchyma, pressure on the adjacent lung and bronchi will give a surrounding zone of pneumonitis that may actually show incomplete, temporary improvement with antibiotic therapy.

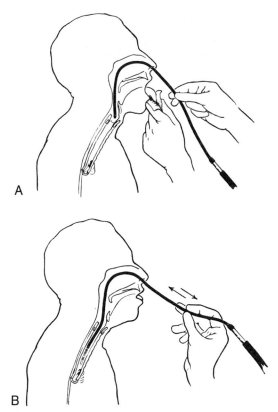

Figure 43–8. A diagram illustrating the placement of a rubber catheter through the nose into the posterior pharynx *(A)*, followed by its insertion into the trachea *(B)* through the opened epiglottis at a time of deep inspiration or cough to obtain bronchial secretions.

embolization with Gelfoam often successfully stops the hemoptysis.

Bronchograms are extremely useful in the study of the trachea, major bronchi, and lobar and segmental bronchi. Intraluminal lesions, obstructive lesions, and lesions causing displacement of bronchial segments may be identified (Fig. 43–14). Air bronchograms may show sufficient detail to dispense with contrast liquid materials (Fig. 43–15).

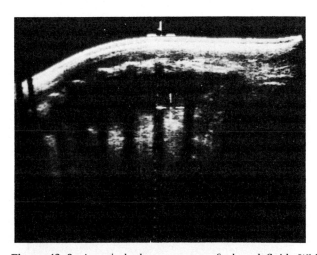

Figure 43–9. A typical ultrasonogram of pleural fluid. With such accurate localization, needle aspiration is easily carried out.

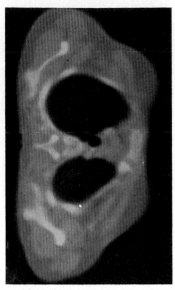

Figure 43–10. A CAT scan showing multiple bilateral pulmonary metastases.

Bronchoscopy is the best available procedure for the study of tracheobronchial and pulmonary disease. This procedure enables visual study of the vocal cords, larynx, trachea, and major bronchi and their important segmental orifices. Congenital anatomic abnormalities may be visualized; *biopsy* of lesions within the lumen can be performed for a definitive diagnosis; prognosis in extensive lesions is evaluated by study of the carina and trachea. *Aspiration of secretions* is an important therapeutic contribution. Study of secretions and washings must include cytologic studies for malignant cells, routine bacterial smear, culture and sensitivity studies, acid-fast smear and cultures, and fungal smear and cultures. (See discussion of bronchoscopy in Chapter 4.)

Biopsy of palpable lymph nodes may aid in the diagnosis of abnormal processes in the lung. Most important are the scalene lymph nodes, which drain the pulmonary parenchyma. Regardless of palpability, these nodes should be sampled in those cases of

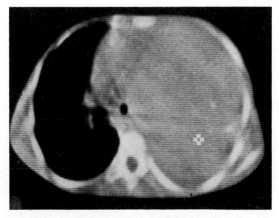

Figure 43–11. A CAT scan of a child with small-cell carcinoma.

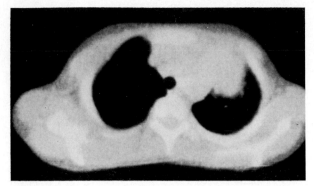

Figure 43–12. A CAT scan of the mediastinum and lung in a child with Hodgkin's disease.

pulmonary disease in which the diagnosis is uncertain and thoracotomy is contemplated. Scalene lymph node biopsy and mediastinoscopy with biopsy of available mediastinal nodes as distal as the carina are of great help in the diagnosis of sarcoidosis, in lymphatic malignancies such as Hodgkin's disease and lymphosarcoma, and in primary neoplasms of the lung and mediastinum. Biopsy specimens of mediastinal lymph nodes in the pediatric age group may best be obtained not by the cervical suprasternal notch approach, but rather by an anterior mediastinotomy with removal of either the second or third right or left costal cartilage.

Lymph nodes obtained at the time of biopsy should be subjected to histologic study, and a portion should be sent to the bacteriology laboratory for routine bacterial smear and culture, studies for sensitivity of the organism to antibiotics, acid-fast smear and culture, and fungal smear and culture (Fig. 43–16).

The use of a thoracoscope to obtain biopsy specimens of lesions on the mediastinal, pleural, or diaphragmatic surfaces can satisfactorily avoid thoracotomy in selected cases.

When all other methods have failed to produce a definitive diagnosis, *thoracotomy* should be considered. A limited incision may first be made, and *biopsy of the lung* may be performed. If the situation appears to be an inoperable problem, biopsy may afford useful information (Fig. 43–17). Thoracotomy should not be unnecessarily delayed when definitive diagnosis has not been made.

PULMONARY TUMORS

In the pediatric age group, all forms of primary pulmonary tumors are unusual.

BENIGN PULMONARY TUMORS

Hamartoma

The term *hamartoma* was coined in 1904 by Albrecht, who defined it as a tumor-like malformation formed by an abnormal mixing of the normal com-

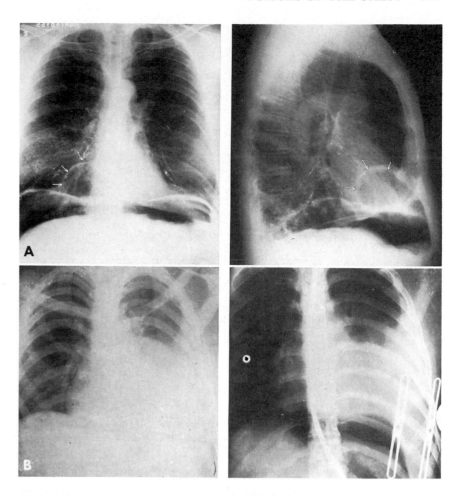

Figure 43–13. *A*, Diagnostic pneumoperitoneum showing congenital diaphragmatic Morgagni hernia. *B*, An outline of a normal diaphragm with intrapleural or pneumonic density above.

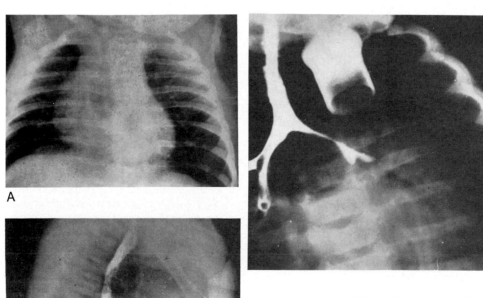

Figure 43–14. *A* and *B*, Anterior and lateral chest roentgenograms in an infant with a congenital bronchogenic cyst at the carina and clinical respiratory distress. *C*, A contrast tracheobronchogram delineates a narrowing of the left main bronchus and a displacement of the right main bronchus.

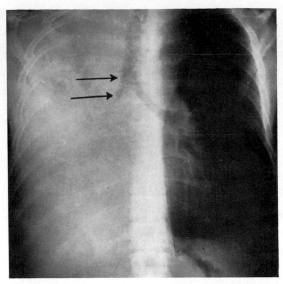

Figure 43–15. An air bronchogram showing a complete block of the right main bronchus in a patient with total right lung atelectasis.

ponents of the organ. Hamartomas of the lung consist largely of cartilage and also include variable quantities of epithelium, fat, and muscle (Fig. 43–18). They are usually located in the periphery of the lung, but involvement of intermediate and primary bronchi has been reported. Developmental derangement is apparently responsible for their occurrence.

The incidence of hamartoma in all patients is 0.25 per cent (Lindskog and Liebow, 1962), but only six have been reported in children; four of these were discovered at autopsy, and two were successfully removed.

Although rare cases of endobronchial hamartoma have been reported in adults, none has been seen in children.

Unlike harmartomas in adults, which are usually asymptomatic and small, the rare tumor found in infancy has been large and symptomatic and has contributed to the death of the infant (prematurity combined with respiratory inadequacy). At least four of the six reported hamartomas showed obvious progressive intrauterine development and had attained considerable size at the time of birth.

Recognition and prompt removal of such large intrapulmonic tumors are necessary for survival. Difficult resuscitation or early demise may, however, make a timely operation impossible.

Although solid masses seen on chest roentgenograms in infants may lead one to suspect hamartoma, the diagnosis cannot be substantiated without thoracotomy. Surgical removal is the treatment of choice.

Holder and Christy (1964) have collected from the literature 32 cases of cystic adenomatoid malformation of the lung in newborn infants. These authors suggest that the entity be designated *adenomatoid hamartoma*; although this is a form of congenital cystic disease of the lung resulting from abnormal growth of normal lung components, it is not a true hamartoma.

Mesodermal Tumors

Polypoid Intrabronchial Mesodermal Tumors. As far as can be determined, chondromas, granular cell myoblastomas, and mesenchymomas have not been reported in the pediatric age group.

Benign Parenchymal Tumors. Plasma cell granuloma of the lung has been reported infrequently in pediatric patients, with the greatest number between 8 and 12 years of age. Many patients are asymptomatic; others show signs of pulmonary infection. Roentgenographic appearance is frequently interpreted as tumor. Calcification is common. Regional lymph nodes may be enlarged. Because the lesion is benign, surgical removal should conserve pulmonary tissue.

Study of the literature has revealed no case of sclerosing hemangioma in children.

Bronchial Adenoma. Bronchial adenoma is a neoplasm arising from either the cells of the mucous glands of the bronchi or the cells lining the excretory ducts of these glands.

Two histologic types are defined. The *carcinoid type* (90 per cent) has histologic resemblance to carcinoid tumor of the small bowel; it is composed of somewhat oval cells filled almost entirely by nucleus. The cells, which have barely detectable lumina, are arranged in a quasi-acinar fashion and are piled up in several layers. The tumor is very vascular and is surrounded by a thin capsule of fibrous tissue that is not invaded by the tumor cells. Metaplastic epithelium of the bronchial mucosa covers the intrabronchial component. The tumor is frequently shaped like a dumbbell, with the smaller component intrabronchial and the larger one intrapulmonic. Though considered benign, bronchial adenomas have a definite malignant potential; lymph node metastasis is more frequent (15 per cent) than distant blood-borne metastasis. The *cylindromatous type* (10 per cent) is made up of cuboidal or flattened epithelial cells, arranged in two layers, which form core-like structures of the cylinders. Histologically, it closely resembles mixed tumor of the salivary glands and basal cell carcinoma of the skin. There is a 40 per cent chance of malignancy.

Approximately 21 cases of bronchial adenoma, all apparently of the carcinoid type, have been reported in the pediatric age group. There were no metastases, and the carcinoid syndrome was not described.

The most prominent symptoms and signs are recurrent and refractory pneumonitis, elevated temperature, cough, and chest pain due to bronchial obstruction with associated distal infection. Hemoptysis and wheeze are not as common in children as in adults. The right main bronchus is most commonly involved, and the diagnosis can usually be made by biopsy performed at bronchoscopy. The tumor occurs five times more commonly in males. Although the youngest recorded patient was a 10-month-old infant, all the other pediatric tumors were seen in children at least 8 years of age (Fig. 43–19).

No case of peripheral bronchial adenoma has come to our attention.

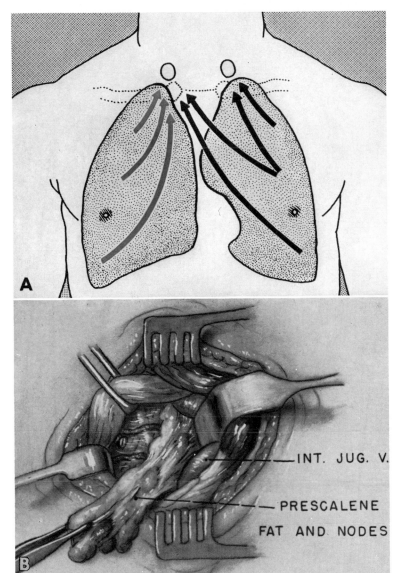

Figure 43–16. *A,* Disease within the right lung usually drains into the right scalene lymph node group. Disease within the left lung may drain to either scalene node group in a pattern similar to that indicated on the illustration. Generally, left lung disease requires bilateral scalene node biopsy, whereas right lung disease requires only right scalene node biopsy. Regardless of the side of lung disease, all palpable nodes in the scalene node area should be examined by biopsy. *B,* The scalene group of nodes is contained in the fat pad bounded medially by the internal jugular vein, inferiorly by the subclavian vein, and superiorly by the posterior belly of the omo-hyoid muscle. The base of the triangle is formed by the anterior scalene muscle. Retraction of the internal jugular vein is essential in order to get all nodes in this group.

Thoracotomy and resection of a segment, lobe, or total lung, according to the degree of involvement, is indicated. Treatment by bronchoscopy is not effective, because complete removal of the tumor cannot be thus carried out. Rarely, a bronchial adenoma can be removed by bronchial resection.

Tracheal Tumors

Papilloma of the Trachea and Bronchi. These lesions, the cause of which is not known, may be single but are more frequently multiple. The tendency for papillomas to disappear spontaneously at puberty has suggested a hormonal relationship.

Symptoms depend on the location and size of the tumor. The lesions may be attached by a pedicle and may oscillate in and out of orifices during inspiration and expiration (flutter valve). Single, slow-growing, high lesions within the trachea may be asymptomatic for years. Dyspnea and stridor are the most common

symptoms, occurring in 63 per cent of the cases. Cough, at first dry and later productive, is another common symptom.

Wheeze, audible at the open mouth, is the earliest sign of papilloma of the trachea. This eventually develops into stridor and is associated with slowly increasing dyspnea. Such secondary changes as obstructive emphysema, atelectasis, pneumonia, lung abscess, and bronchiectasis may occur in the distal parts of the tracheobronchial tree; empyema may also occur. Unless diverted, the usual course is one of increasing dyspnea that terminates in asphyxia.

These tumors should be removed because of their tendency to obstruct. Distal pulmonary infection or death from asphyxia may result. Ogilvie (1953) has reported two instances of malignancy arising from tracheobronchial papillomas.

Excision is the treatment of choice. Owing to the frequent multiplicity of the papillomas, treatment may be difficult and tedious, requiring numerous

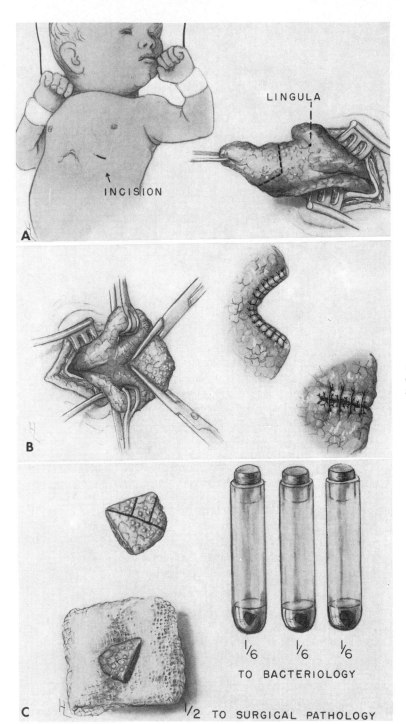

Figure 43–17. An adequate lung biopsy with specimens for bacteriology and pathology laboratories is essential. In general, a small open thoracotomy has many advantages over the blind needle biopsy technique.

endoscopic procedures. Electrocoagulation can be used, and x-ray therapy has been most beneficial when there are multiple papillomas. The prognosis is good, but these lesions have a tendency to recur, and constant vigilance with follow-up by periodic bronchoscopy is indicated.

Fibroma of the Trachea. Nine cases of fibroma of the trachea have been recorded in infants (Gilbert et al, 1953).

Angioma of the Trachea. Six children with benign

angioma have been reported by Gilbert and colleagues (1953). Congenital hemangioma of the trachea may cause death by the compromise of a vital structure, bleeding complications, intractable cardiac failure from atrioventricular shunting of blood within the tumor, or malignant change. In infants and children, these tumors are usually below the vocal cords, sessile, flat, and associated with dyspnea. Ninety per cent of the recorded patients have been 6 months of age at the time of the onset of symptoms,

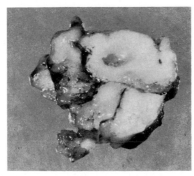

Figure 43–18. A hamartoma removed from the right upper lobe of an adult. Note the predominance of cartilage.

and females predominate over males two to one. Fifty per cent of the infants have hemangiomas elsewhere.

The onset is insidious, with symptoms of respiratory obstruction such as stridor, retraction, dyspnea, wheezing, and sometimes cyanosis and cough. The symptoms tend to be intermittent and labile. Fever and leukocytosis are usually absent, but superimposed infection may produce fever and an elevated

white blood cell count. The best diagnostic tools are roentgenogram and endoscopy. Biopsy is not advisable at the time of endoscopy, because bleeding may cause asphyxia or an exsanguinating hemorrhage. Tracheostomy with x-ray therapy is probably the best form of treatment.

Leiomyoma of the Lung

Grossly, these tumors cannot be differentiated from other benign tumors of the lung. Leiomyomas of the lung are usually asymptomatic unless there is partial or complete bronchial obstruction. In a review of the world literature, Guida and co-workers (1965) found only one case in a child. This 6-year-old had a tumor in the right lower lobe; it was successfully treated by lobectomy.

Lipoma

Review of the literature reveals no cases of lipoma of the bronchus or lung in the pediatric age group.

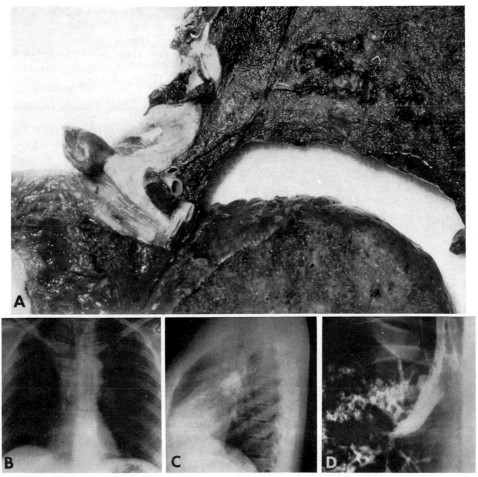

Figure 43–19. A bronchial adenoma (carcinoid type) *(A)* and total obstruction of the right upper lobe bronchus with resultant distal atelectasis *(B and C)*. Recurrent pneumonitis, cough, and hemoptysis had occurred. Diagnostic biopsy at the time of bronchoscopy. *D,* Obstruction of the right upper lobe bronchus is demonstrated with bronchograms. Treated by performing a right upper lobectomy.

Neurogenic Tumors

Of the 32 patients with proven primary intrapulmonic neurogenic tumors recorded in the world literature, three were children. One had a neurofibroma, and the other two had neurilemomas.

MALIGNANT PULMONARY TUMORS

Bronchogenic Carcinoma. Primary tumors of the lung are rare in the pediatric age group. Forty-seven cases of bronchogenic carcinoma are reported in children under 16 years of age (Hartman and Shochat, 1983).

The youngest patient was a 5-month-old girl with cystic lung disease and malignancy in the left lung, reported by Schwyter in 1928.

Every cell type except alveolar cell carcinoma, giant cell carcinoma, and carcinosarcoma has been seen in the pediatric age group.

The most common bronchial tumors in childhood are carcinoids, with 18 cases in the English literature (Lack et al, 1983).

Despite the rarity of primary pulmonary neoplasms in children, this diagnosis should be considered in young patients with solitary pulmonary masses or persistent, atypical pulmonary symptoms (Hartman and Shochat, 1983).

Fibrosarcoma of the Bronchus. Review of the literature reveals only five cases of primary fibrosarcoma of the bronchus in the pediatric age group. Three were in girls and two in boys.

Fever, probably due to bronchial obstruction and distal infection, is the most common symptom; hemoptysis is relatively uncommon. Diagnosis in these cases should be established by bronchoscopy. Resection is the treatment of choice, because recurrence is common when any other mode of therapy is used. As a rule, metastasis occurs by way of the blood stream, but lymph node involvement is possible.

Leiomyosarcoma. Ten cases of primary leiomyosarcoma (Jimenez et al, 1986) and four cases of nonspecific primary sarcoma of the lung have been reported in children. Cough, dyspnea, and signs of obstructive pneumonitis are usually present. Surgery is indicated (Fig. 43–20).

Multiple Myeloma. Multiple myeloma is usually limited to the medullary space. Extramedullary plasma cell tumors are relatively uncommon (myeloma or solitary plasmacytoma of the lung parenchyma). In a review of the literature, Sekulich and co-workers (1965) found only 19 cases since 1911; one of these was a plasmacytoma in a 3-year-old girl. Cytologic examination of sputum may be diagnostic.

Chorioepithelioma. A case of chorioepithelioma of the lung in a 7-month-old white girl has been reported by Kay and Reed (1953). The presenting symptoms were fever, dyspnea, and anorexia; massive hemoptysis then occurred. Roentgenogram showed almost complete opacity of the right side of the chest. Pneumonectomy was performed, but the child died several hours postoperatively. This rare lesion has other scattered case reports in the English literature.

SYSTEMIC NEOPLASMS AFFECTING THE LUNG

Myeloid and lymphatic leukemia may have a pulmonary component, but isolated pulmonary disease has not been recorded. Similarly, Hodgkin's disease and lymphosarcoma may involve the lung during the course of the disease, but neither occurs as an isolated pulmonary lesion.

METASTATIC PULMONARY TUMORS

Primary sarcomas occur much more frequently in children than do primary carcinomas. The literature does not contain a report of a primary carcinoma in an infant with metastases to the lung; however, there are a number of references to primary sarcomas with pulmonary involvement by metastases. Primary sarcoma of the kidney (Wilms), primary malignant skeletal tumors (chondrosarcoma and osteogenic sarcoma), Ewing tumor, reticulum cell sarcoma, and soft tissue sarcomas (fibrosarcoma, rhabdomyosarcoma, liposarcoma, malignant neurilemoma, and synovioma) may metastasize to the lung. In general, the indications for resection of metastatic pulmonary disease should be based on (1) unilateral pulmonary involvement and (2) evidence of local control of the primary malignancy for a period of 1 year before pulmonary resection.

However, recent developments in the chemotherapeutic management of pulmonary sarcomas in children have produced data that strongly support an aggressive approach to this malignancy, whether primary or metastatic. Vigorous attack using chemotherapy, irradiation, and surgical resection of unilateral or bilateral pulmonary metastases is now advocated regardless of the interval between the diagnosis of the primary sarcoma and the recognition of the pulmonary metastasis. Conventional chest radiography, planigraphy, and in particular CAT scan of the lungs serve to map bilateral pulmonary lesions in preoperative evaluation and postoperative follow-up. Repeated thoracotomies for removal of recurrent lesions are acceptable.

MEDIASTINAL TUMORS

The mediastinum, the portion of the body that lies between the lungs, is bounded anteriorly by the sternum and posteriorly by the vertebrae. It extends superiorly from the suprasternal notch and terminates inferiorly at the diaphragm. Cysts or tumors that arise within the mediastinum may originate from

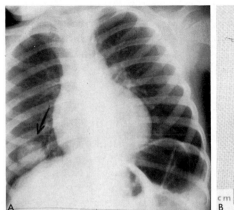
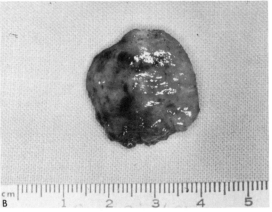

Figure 43–20. *A,* A 3-year-old white male with an increasing mass in the right lower lobe of the lung. *B,* The shelled-out leiomyosarcoma after a lower lobectomy. No recurrence after 1 year.

any of the structures contained therein or may be the result of developmental abnormalities. The mediastinum is lined on both sides by parietal pleura and contains all structures of the thoracic cavity except the lungs. At times the lungs may herniate into the mediastinum. For ease of definition of sites of disease, the mediastinum may be thought of as divided into four compartments (Fig. 43–21): (1) the

superior mediastinum—the portion of the mediastinum above a hypothetical line drawn from the junction of the manubrium and gladiolus of the sternum (angle) to the intervertebral disc between the fourth and fifth thoracic vertebrae; (2) the anterior mediastinum—the portion of the mediastinum that lies anterior to the anterior plane of the trachea; (3) the middle mediastinum—the portion containing the heart and pericardium, the ascending aorta, the lower segment of the superior vena cava bifurcation of the pulmonary artery, the trachea, the two main bronchi, and the bronchial lymph nodes; (4) the posterior mediastinum—the portion that lies posterior to the anterior plane of the trachea.

SIGNS AND SYMPTOMS OF MEDIASTINAL TUMOR

A great number of lesions (even very large ones) in the mediastinum remain asymptomatic for a considerable period and are discovered only through the use of routine chest roentgenograms. The patient becomes aware of lesions within the mediastinum only when pressure is exerted on sensitive structures of the mediastinum or when the structures are displaced; therefore, the severity of symptoms depends on the size and location of the tumor, the rapidity of its growth, and the presence or absence of actual invasion of organs. Symptoms resulting from mediastinal lesions may become manifest according to the degree of functional disturbance of the various organs in the mediastinum.

Respiratory Symptoms. In a mediastinal lesion in a child, respiratory symptoms are the most important. They are the result of direct pressure on some portion of the respiratory tract. This pressure causes narrowing of the trachea or bronchi or compression of the lung parenchyma (Fig. 43–22). Dry cough may be present; stridor or wheeze may occur at the same time or may precede it. The compression may be sufficient to produce enough occlusion to cause distal obstructive emphysema or atelectasis, pneumonitis,

Figure 43–21. *A,* The mediastinal compartment as seen from the left hemithorax. *B,* Mediastinal compartments as seen from the right hemithorax.

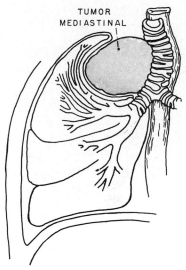

Figure 43-22. A diagram illustrating a large mediastinal tumor or cyst with pressure on the tracheobronchial tree as well as on the pulmonary parenchyma. Such a condition might possibly give rise to pulmonary symptoms.

or chronic recurrent lower respiratory tract infections with associated fever and leukocytosis. The dry cough may be replaced by a productive one with mucoid sputum; if infection occurs, the secretion will become purulent. The unilateral nature of the wheezing and respiratory complaints serves to rule out asthma, bronchiolitis, and chronic recurrent infections secondary to cystic fibrosis or hypogammaglobulinemia but will not eliminate the possibility of endobronchial or endotracheal lesions; nor can the possibility of a foreign body in the tracheobronchial tree be discarded. Bronchoscopy is necessary in order to make this differentiation.

If the lesion in the mediastinum exerts pressure on the recurrent laryngeal nerve, hoarseness and a brassy cough result. Dyspnea, which may be progressive, is a common symptom of mediastinal tumors. Acute episodes of dyspnea with associated pneumonitis may occur when there is tracheal or bronchial obstruction, leading to distal infection. Hemoptysis occurs in less than 10 per cent of mediastinal tumors in children.

Gastrointestinal Symptoms. Symptoms referable to the gastrointestinal tract result primarily from pressure on the esophagus. Regurgitation of food and dysphagia with a slight sensation of sticking in the lower esophagus are common. Displacement of the esophagus usually does not cause dysphagia; however, if there is fixation of the mass secondary to infection, hemorrhage, or malignant degeneration, thereby causing interference with the peristaltic activity of the esophagus, dysphagia will occur. Vomiting is rare when the tumor is benign but may occur when it is malignant; it is then the result of the systemic effects of the malignancy.

Neurologic Symptoms. Older children often describe a feeling of vague intrathoracic discomfort, fullness, or ache caused by pressure on the sensitive

intercostal nerves. Such pain may be mild or severe and is common in tumors of neurogenic origin. The appearance of herpes zoster indicates involvement of an intercostal nerve, but this is not common in the pediatric age group. When lesions impinge on the pleura, the pain may be pleuritic. Erosion of vertebrae causes a boring pain located in the interscapular area. A malignant lesion that invades the brachial plexus causes severe pain in the upper extremities; the presence of Horner syndrome indicates involvement of the cervical sympathetics. Inflammation, intracystic hemorrhage, or malignant degeneration causing pressure on the phrenic nerve may result in hiccups. Certain dumbbell tumors of the spinal cord and mediastinum may exhibit symptoms referable to spinal cord pressure.

Vascular Symptoms. Benign lesions of the mediastinum rarely cause obstruction of the great vessels in the mediastinum; however, obstruction is a common finding in malignant mediastinal tumors and carries a poor prognosis. Superior vena caval involvement gives rise to a dilatation of veins in the upper extremity, head, and neck. As the obstruction progresses, cyanosis of the head and neck area occurs in association with bounding headaches and tinnitus. Either innominate vein may be involved, causing unilateral venous distention and edema of the upper extremity, head, and neck (ipsilateral). Pressure on the inferior vena cava is less common, but when it is present there may be associated edema of the lower extremities.

Miscellaneous Symptoms. Fever is uncommon in mediastinal lesions unless there is secondary infection in the tracheobronchial tree; it may also be present with Hodgkin's disease, lymphosarcoma, and breakdown of malignant disease. Weight loss, malaise, anemia, and anorexia are uncommon unless there is malignancy.

Physical Findings. Often there are no unusual physical findings; wheeze, rhonchi, or rales may be present. There may be dullness to percussion over the area of mediastinal enlargement, extending laterally from each sternal border or posteriorly between the scapulae and above the diaphragm. Occasionally there is tenderness over the chest wall, when a mediastinal tumor exerts pressure on the parietal pleura in that area.

DIAGNOSTIC PROCEDURES

The diagnostic procedures used for suspected lung lesions also apply for mediastinal tumors. However, the widespread use of and rapid improvements in CAT scan and MRI have greatly aided the understanding of lesions and adjacent mediastinal structures. Solid mass lesions can more easily be differentiated from fluid-containing lesions as well as from the combination in a single lesion.

Certain situations unique to mediastinal tumors will be mentioned.

A tumor or lesion of the mediastinum should never be aspirated preoperatively when operation is clearly indicated. If a neoplasm is present, needle aspiration may cause spread of the tumor cells. This procedure should be reserved for inoperable tumors and for emergencies in which tremendous cystic enlargement may jeopardize the child's life or may interfere with anesthesia induction.

The trial use of x-ray therapy for undiagnosed mediastinal lesions is not warranted. Deep x-ray therapy may be administered in dosage sufficient to produce shrinkage of hyperplasia of the thymus, the mediastinal nodes in Hodgkin's disease, and lymphosarcoma. The danger of radiation-induced thyroid carcinoma, however, makes the use of deep x-ray therapy for the shrinkage of hyperplasia of the thymus inadvisable. Peripheral lymph node biopsy is preferable in suspected cases of Hodgkin's disease or lymphosarcoma. If such lymph nodes are not diagnostic, thoracotomy is then indicated.

Hydatid disease is not common in the United States, and only when it is present in the lung adjacent to the mediastinum can mediastinal tumor be simulated. The precipitin and skin test results are positive in hydatid disease with an active hydatid cyst. Hooklets may often be found in the sputum of patients so affected.

Mediastinal abscess is rarely confused with a neoplasm of the mediastinum. With abscess there is usually a history of trauma, foreign body in the esophagus, or use of surgical or gastroscopic instruments in the area. High fever, tachycardia, dyspnea, extreme weakness, and prostration usually develop rapidly; thus, the signs and symptoms of acute infection are paramount. The development of a fluid level in the mediastinum is diagnostic of mediastinal abscess if the preceding physical findings are also present. Intensive antibiotic therapy and prompt surgical drainage are indicated. There may be masses in the neck secondary to extension from lesions within the mediastinum.

PRIMARY MEDIASTINAL CYSTS

Lesions occurring within the mediastinum may be predominantly cystic or predominantly solid. Cystic lesions are usually benign, and solid lesions have higher malignant potential.

Primary mediastinal cysts probably represent abnormalities in embryologic development at the site of the foregut just when separation of esophageal and lung beds occurs (Fig. 43–23).

Structures that arise from the foregut are the pharynx, thyroid, parathyroid, thymus, respiratory tract, esophagus, stomach, upper part of the duodenum, liver, and pancreas; thus, abnormal development at this stage may give rise to bronchogenic cysts, esophageal duplication cysts, and gastroenteric cysts.

Bronchogenic Cysts. Maier (1948) has classified

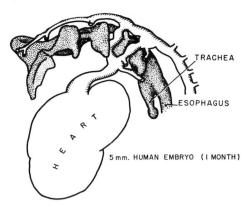

Figure 43–23. The foregut, lying between the tracheal and esophageal buds, is the probable site of embryologic maldevelopment, which gives rise to the growth of foregut cysts.

bronchogenic cysts according to location (Fig. 43–24) as tracheal, hilar (Fig. 43–25), carinal (Fig. 43–26), esophageal, and miscellaneous (Fig. 43–27).

Bronchogenic cysts are usually located in the mid-mediastinum but have been described in all mediastinal subdivisions. Under microscopic examination, bronchogenic cysts may contain any or all of the tissues normally present in the trachea and bronchi (fibrous connective tissue, mucous glands, cartilage, smooth muscle, and a lining formed by ciliated pseudostratified columnar epithelium or stratified squamous epithelium). The fluid inside the cyst is either clear water-like liquid or viscous gelatinous material. The amylase content of the fluid is very high.

Bronchogenic cysts are usually asymptomatic. There may, however, be frequent upper respiratory tract infections, vague feelings of substernal discomfort, and respiratory difficulty (cough, noisy breathing, dyspnea, and possibly cyanosis). Bronchogenic cysts may communicate with the tracheobronchial tree and show varying air-fluid levels accompanied by the expectoration of purulent material. If communication with the tracheobronchial tree is present, it may be visualized using bronchoscopy and bronchography. Hemoptysis may occur when there is infection and communication of the cyst with the tracheobronchial tree.

On x-ray examination, the bronchogenic cyst is usually a single, smooth-bordered, spherical mass (Fig. 43–28). It has a uniform density similar to that of the cardiac shadow. Calcification is unusual. Fluoroscopic examination of the cyst may demonstrate that it moves with respiration (it is attached to the tracheobronchial tree); its shape may alter during the cycles of respiration. Evidence of bone erosion with bronchogenic cysts is not recorded.

When the bronchogenic cyst is located at the carina, it may cause severe respiratory distress owing to compression of either one or both major bronchi (see Figs. 43–14 and 43–29). Early diagnosis and prompt removal are necessary.

The recorded incidence of bronchogenic cyst varies greatly. For example, Gross (1964) found one bronchogenic cyst out of a total of 33 cysts and tumors of

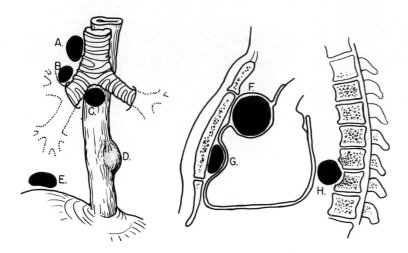

Figure 43–24. A diagram of the location of bronchogenic cysts, as suggested by Maier (1948); *B* and *C* are the sites most commonly recorded.

the mediastinum, whereas Heimburger and Battersby (1965) found seven cases (20 per cent) in their series of 36 cysts and tumors. When the latter researchers combined the results of five series from the literature, they found an incidence of 10 per cent.

A review of the literature by Dobbs and co-workers (1957) revealed 10 cases of intrapericardial bronchogenic cysts.

Bronchogenic cyst should be treated by surgical removal. Its exact diagnosis can rarely be confirmed before thoracotomy. Removal is indicated because the lesion represents an undiagnosed thoracic mass; because inflammation and intracystic hemorrhage may cause symptoms of severe respiratory distress, complicating removal; and finally, because continued growth will embarrass surrounding vital structures.

Esophageal Cysts (Duplication). Esophageal cysts are located in the posterior mediastinum; they are usually on the right side and are intimately associated in the wall of the esophagus (Fig. 43–30). They occur more frequently in males than in females.

There are two types of esophageal cysts; the more characteristic type resembles adult esophagus with the cyst lined by noncornified stratified squamous epithelium having a well-defined muscularis mucosae and striated muscle in the wall. Intimate association in the muscular wall of the esophagus is not accompanied by communication with the lumen of the esophagus.

The second type is lined by ciliated mucosa, thus resembling the fetal esophagus. Esophageal cysts may be associated with mild dysphagia and regurgitation but most frequently are asymptomatic. Barium esophagogram shows smooth indentation of the esophagus. On esophagoscopy there is indentation of the normal mucosa by a pliable, movable, soft extramucosal mass. Removal by thoracotomy is indicated for the same reasons as noted in discussion of the therapy of bronchogenic cysts.

Gastroenteric Cysts. The third type of cyst arising from the foregut is the gastroenteric. This lies against the vertebrae, posterior or lateral to and usually free of the esophagus, and usually in the posterior mediastinum with the main attachment posterior. It may

be recalled that the fetal esophagus is lined by columnar epithelium, much of which is ciliated, and this is only gradually converted to the stratified epithelium of the definitive organ. The change is generally complete or almost complete at birth (Arey, 1974). Thus, if a cyst arises from the embryonic esophagus, it has a ciliated lining.

The enteric nature of a posterior mediastinal cyst is presumably certain if microscopic examination reveals a frank gastric or intestinal type of epithelium, but in general a better index of the nature and origin of such a cyst is the presence of well-developed muscularis mucosae, tela submucosa, and two or even three main muscle coats. Gastric glands are most common, but esophageal, duodenal, or small-intestinal glands may be found. At operation, the cyst sometimes seems grossly "stomach-like" or "bowel-like." The significant fact is that cysts encountered in the posterior mediastinum show a highly developed mesodermal wall and even the presence of Meissner and Auerbach plexuses, whereas the lining epithelium varies in type from case to case, from columnar ciliated to typical small-intestinal.

Two types of gastroenteric cysts have been described: (1) acid-secreting cysts, which are functionally active, and (2) cysts in which the mucosa has no functional activity.

Males are predominantly affected with this abnormality. Unlike other foregut cysts, posterior gastroenteric cysts are usually symptomatic. The symptoms are usually due to pressure on thoracic structures or rupture into bronchi with massive hemoptysis and death. Calcification also is frequent. Ossification has been reported by Steele and Schmitz (1945) in a cyst from a 15-year-old girl.

If the lining is gastric, dyspnea is the usual presenting symptom and occurs early. Actual peptic perforation of the lung with hemorrhage has been recorded.

Hemoptysis in young infants is difficult to distinguish from hematemesis; it may follow ulceration of a gastroenteric cyst (with gastric lining) of the mediastinum, with subsequent erosion into the lung. Gastric epithelium associated with intestinal or res-

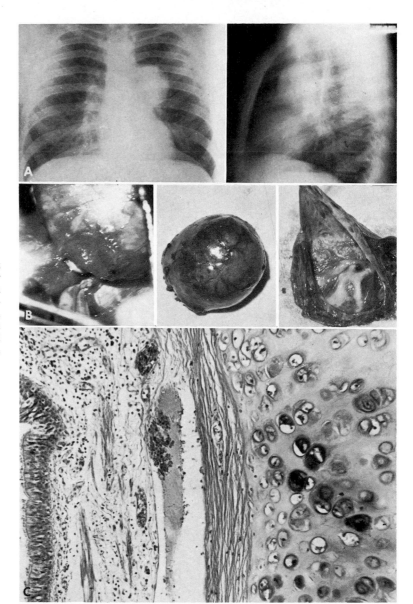

Figure 43–25. *A*, Typical left hilar bronchogenic cyst with a rounded, smooth border, and a density similar to cardiac density. *B*, At the time of thoracotomy, a solid stalk was found attached to the left main bronchus. The cyst was unilocular and contained thick, yellowish mucoid material. The wall was thin with typical trabeculations. *C*, Microscopic study revealed cartilage, smooth muscle, and pseudostratified, ciliated, columnar epithelium.

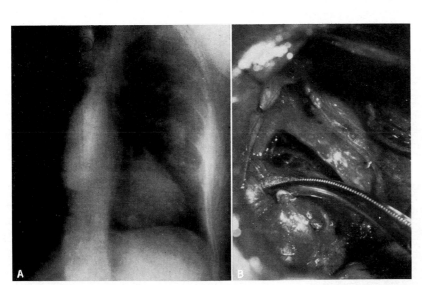

Figure 43–26. *A*, An overexposed posteroanterior chest radiograph shows a carinal bronchogenic cyst. *B*, At the operation, the location is clearly seen at the carina. A solid fibrous stalk is attached at the carina and is separated just beneath the instrument dissector.

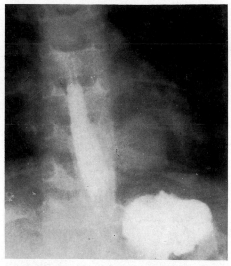

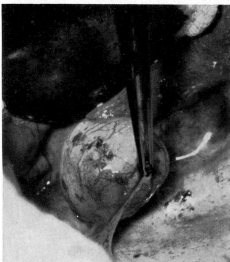

Figure 43–27. A bronchogenic cyst in a child. The cyst is located retropleurally, overlying the distal thoracic aorta, and not attached to the respiratory tract or esophagus.

piratory epithelium is apparently less secretory. Many functional cysts may lose their functional activity when the secretory areas of the mucosa are destroyed. Renin, pepsin, chlorides, and free hydro-

chloric acid have been demonstrated in the contents of some of the cysts.

Posterior gastroenteric foregut cysts of the mediastinum are frequently associated with two other types of congenital anomalies, mesenteric abnormalities and vertebral abnormalities. Both types may occur in the same case. In the embryo, the notochord and the entoderm are at one time in intimate contact; thus, this combined developmental anomaly may result from abnormal embryonic development.

Penetration of the diaphragm by a cyst arising primarily from the thorax may occur; conversely, penetration of the diaphragm by the free end of an intramesenteric intestinal duplication is also possible.

A survey of the literature on mediastinal cysts combined with vertebral anomalies reveals that hemivertebra, spina bifida anterior, or infantile scoliosis has been reported in 61 per cent of 18 cases. Most of these vertebral lesions involve the upper thoracic and lower cervical vertebrae, and the cyst tends to be caudad to the vertebral lesion. Planigrams may be necessary for diagnosis.

The presence of spina bifida anterior, congenital scoliosis, Klippel-Feil syndrome, or similar but less well-defined lesions in the cervical or dorsal vertebra suggests enteric cysts in the mediastinum or in the abdomen.

In a survey by Abell (1956), four such gastroenteric cysts (3 per cent) were present in a series of 133 tumors of the mediastinum; they composed 10 per cent of the mediastinal cysts in this series. All produced symptoms, were present in patients from 7 months to 5 years old, were located in the posterior mediastinum, were associated with abnormalities of the cervical or dorsal spine, and were resected successfully.

Pericardial Coelomic Cysts. These mesothelial cysts are developmental in origin, and formal genesis is related to the pericardial coelom. The primitive pericardial cavity forms by the fusion of coelomic spaces on each side of the embryo. During the process, dorsal and ventral parietal recesses are formed. Dorsal recesses communicate with the pleu-

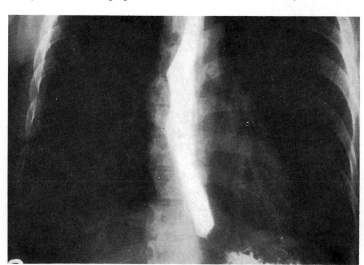

Figure 43–28. An esophagogram of a hilar bronchogenic cyst with an esophageal indentation.

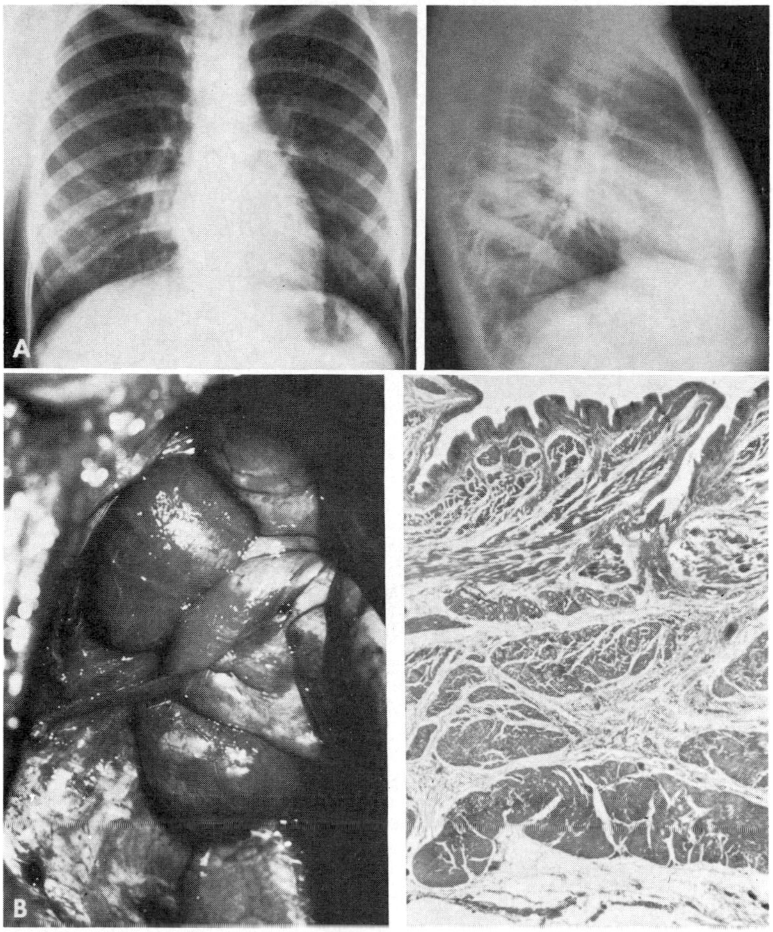

Figure 43–29. *A,* A bronchogenic cyst in a child whose mother had tuberculosis. The child was treated with antituberculous drugs for 1 year without change. *B,* A dumbbell-shaped bronchogenic cyst was found in the region of the inferior pulmonary vein during an operation. The microscopic section shows a wall with ciliated epithelium, no cartilage, and a smooth muscle wall of two layers.

roperitoneal coelom, and the ventral recesses end blindly at the septum transversum. Persistence of segments of the ventral parietal recess accounts for most pericardial coelomic cysts.

The cysts are usually located anteriorly in the cardiophrenic angles, more frequently on the right, and occasionally on or in the diaphragm (Fig. 43–31). They are usually asymptomatic and are discovered on routine chest roentgenogram. Rarely do they reach sufficient size to cause displacement of the heart or to produce pressure on the pulmonary tissue. Infection is unusual.

Pericardial cysts are usually unilocular. The walls are thin, and the intersurfaces are smooth and glistening, lined by a single layer of flat mesothelial cells. The mesothelium is supported by fibrous tissue with attached adipose tissue.

These cysts are usually not diagnosed in the pediatric age group. There are no recorded cases of asymptomatic pericardial coelomic cysts in children.

Intrathoracic Meningoceles. Intrathoracic meningoceles are not true mediastinal tumors or cysts; they are diverticuli of the spinal meninges that protrude through the neuroforamen adjacent to an intercostal nerve and manifest beneath the pleura in the posterior medial thoracic gutter. The wall represents an extension of the leptomeninges, and the content is cerebrospinal fluid. Enlargement of the intervertebral foramen is common; vertebral or rib anomalies

adjacent to the meningocele are also frequent. The most commonly associated anomalies are kyphosis, scoliosis, and bone erosion or destruction. The wall of these cysts is formed by two distinct components, the dura mater and the arachnoidea spinalis, with small nerve trunks and ganglia occasionally incorporated in it.

Of the 46 reported cases of intrathoracic meningocele, 4 were in the pediatric age group.

A threefold syndrome of generalized neurofibromatosis (von Recklinghausen disease), kyphoscoliosis, and intrathoracic meningocele may occur, but thoracic meningocele as an isolated defect is much less frequent. This lesion is usually asymptomatic; it occurs on the right side approximately three times more often than on the left. Rarely, the lesion may be bilateral. In patients with neurofibromatosis, posterior sulcus tumors are usually meningoceles and rarely neurofibromas.

On x-ray examination, the lesion is a regular, well-demarcated intrathoracic density located in the posterior sulcus; associated congenital anomalies of the spine and thorax may be noted. On fluoroscopic examination, pulsations may be noted in the sac. Diagnosis may be confirmed by myelograms.

When diagnosis is established, no therapy is indicated unless the lesion is symptomatic.

Operative complications such as empyema, men-

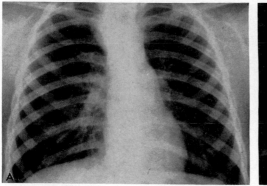
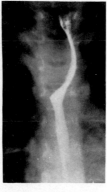
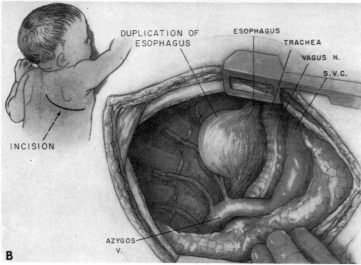

Figure 43–30. *A,* A posteroanterior chest roentgenogram taken of a child with an upper respiratory tract infection. A mass is seen in the posterior superior mediastinum presenting into the right hemithorax. At the time of an esophagogram, the esophagus is seen displaced toward the left by a smooth mass. *B, C,* and *D,* Drawings of findings at the operation. Note the plane of separation from the mucosa of the esophagus and the lack of communication with the esophageal lumen. *E,* An opened operative specimen, the cavity of which was filled with mucoid fluid. The lining of the duplication was typical squamous cell.

ingitis, and spinal fluid fistula have been greatly reduced since the advent of antibiotic therapy.

TUMORS OF THE THYMUS

Normally the thymus is located in the anterior superior mediastinum, but abnormalities of the thymus have been reported in all areas of the mediastinum. Abnormalities of the thymus in children are (1) hyperplasia, (2) neoplasms, (3) benign thymomas, (4) cysts, (5) teratoma, and (6) tuberculosis.

Hyperplasia of the Thymus. Thymic masses are the most common of the mediastinal masses in children; of these, hyperplasia of the thymus is most frequent.

The function of the thymus is still not clear, but recent studies suggest that it may in some way be involved in the determination of immunologic individuality. The thymus varies greatly in size. Steroids, infection, androgens, and irradiation may make the thymus smaller; those stimuli that cause it to increase in size are not understood. As in other ductless glands, local variations in size are probably related to chance.

In a review of normal chest roentgenograms, Ellis, Kirklin, Hodgson, and colleagues (1955) found that a recognizable thymic shadow was almost always present during the first month of life; there was great variation in the size and shape. The mediastinal shadow in these young infants seemed to be proportionally wider than in older children and adults because of the proportionally larger heart and thymic shadow. Between 1 and 12 months, the thymic shadow was still present if it had been seen earlier. Between 1 and 3 years, very little of the thymic shadow remained. Two per cent of children more than 4 years of age still have a recognizable thymus on x-ray examination. It does not contain calcium, and there are transmitted pulsations on fluoroscopy. Cervical extension of the thymus gland is common. If the thymus is located in the superior thoracic inlet, its enlargement may cause tracheal compression (Fig. 43–32).

The distinction between obstruction and an enlarged gland is established by high-quality x-ray films, with the lateral view taken during full inspiration with the child's head in a neutral position. Both esophageal and angiographic studies can be used to rule out vascular ring. In cases of vascular ring obstruction, most patients find that their distress is relieved by hyperextension of the head.

Treatment of an enlarged thymus causing respiratory obstruction may be carried out in one of three ways. First, the thymus responds rapidly to small doses (70 to 150 R) of irradiation; however, the

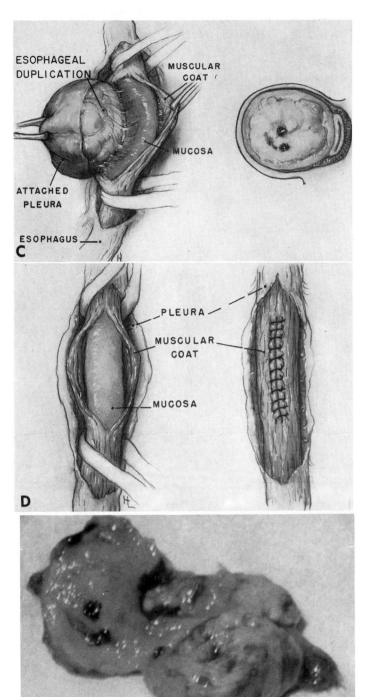

Figure 43–30. *Continued.*

danger of carcinogenic effect has caused this method of treatment to be abandoned. Second, corticosteroids cause a rapid decrease in the size of the thymus, usually within 5 to 7 days. After cessation of corticosteroid therapy, the gland may reach a size greater than that before treatment was instituted. Such a response may also be used in distinguishing between a physiologic enlargement of the thymus and a neoplasm (Fig. 43–33). Third, surgery may be indicated both for the treatment of respiratory obstruction and for diagnosis.

Neoplasm of the Thymus. Malignant thymic tumors in children are quite rare. Lymphosarcoma is by far the most frequent; primary Hodgkin's disease of the thymus and carcinoma have been described. In none has there been an associated myasthenia gravis.

Benign Thymoma. Rarely, benign thymic tumors have been reported in children (Fig. 43–34).

Thymic Cysts. Multiple small cysts of the thymus are frequently observed in necropsy material, but large thymic cysts are rare (Fig. 43–35). Fridjon

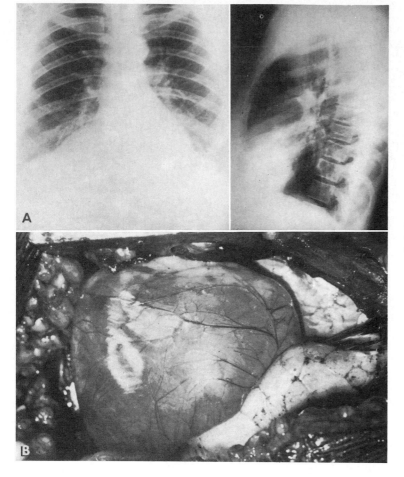

Figure 43–31. *A,* The typical location of a pericardial cyst in posteroanterior and lateral chest films at the right cardiophrenic angle. *B,* A large cyst seen at the time of a thoracotomy.

(1943) described a large cyst in the thymus of a 1-day-old infant. Thymic cysts have been resected from the neck (Fig. 43–36).

Teratoma of the Thymus. Teratoma of the thymus in a 2-day-old white girl was described by Sealy and co-workers (1965); she suffered progressive respiratory distress and underwent operation at 7 weeks of age.

Tuberculosis of the Thymus Gland. A single case

of tuberculosis involving only the thymus gland has been described in a stillborn infant.

TERATOID MEDIASTINAL TUMORS

Teratoid tumors of the mediastinum may be classified as (1) benign cystic teratomas, (2) benign teratoids (solid), or (3) teratoids (carcinoma).

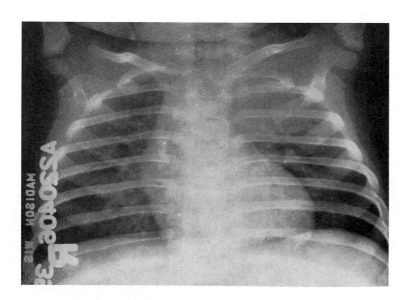

Figure 43–32. Mild respiratory distress in an infant with an enlarged thymus. Gradual improvement occurred with age and no specific therapy.

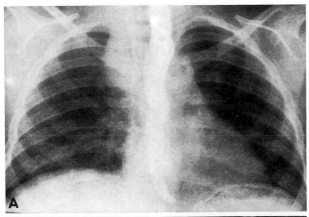

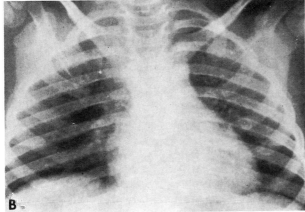

Figure 43–33. *A,* An enlarged thymus in an infant. *B,* A reduction in size can be seen after 7 days of steroid therapy.

Benign Cystic Teratoma. Teratoma of the anterior mediastinum probably results from faulty embryogenesis of the thymus or from local dislocation of tissue during embryogenesis.

Benign cystic teratoma (mediastinal dermoid cyst) contains such elements of ectodermal tissue as hair, sweat glands, sebaceous cysts, and teeth. Other elements, including mesodermal and entodermal tissue, may also be found when benign cystic teratoid lesions are subjected to comprehensive examination; thus, such tumors are more properly classified as teratoid than dermoid cysts.

Cystic teratomas are more common than solid ones. These lesions are predominantly located in the anterior mediastinum and may project into either hemithorax, more commonly the right. In children, females are affected more often than males. Malignant degeneration is less common than in the solid form of teratoid tumor.

It seems reasonable to assume that most, perhaps all, mediastinal teratomas are present at birth; however, Edge and Glennie (1960) reported two adult patients from whom large teratoid tumors were removed 2 years and 4 years after routine chest roentgenograms were normal.

These cystic masses usually cause symptoms because of pressure on or erosion into the adjacent respiratory system. Symptoms usually include vague chest discomfort associated with cough, dyspnea, and pneumonitis. Infection may cause a sudden exacerbation of symptoms, and rupture into the lung may occur with expectoration of hair; rupture into the pleura or pericardium may also occur.

The lesion is usually in the anterior mediastinum. On x-ray film, the lesion is well outlined, with sharp borders; definite diagnosis is not possible unless teeth can be demonstrated in the mass. Calcification, which is not unusual, appears as scattered masses rather than as diffuse, small densities. Cystic swelling in the suprasternal notch may occur.

Benign cystic teratomas should be removed. In cases in which infection, perforation, intracystic hemorrhage, or malignant degeneration has occurred, complete removal may be difficult or impossible, owing to adherence to surrounding vital structures.

Benign Solid Teratoid Tumors and Malignant Teratoid Tumors. Teratoma is the most common tumor occurring in the anterior mediastinum of infants and children (Fig. 43–37). The solid tumors in the teratoid group are much more complex and have a greater propensity for malignant change (Fig. 43–38). The incidence of malignancy is about 20 per cent.

Benign solid teratoid tumors have well-differentiated structures that are rarely observed in malignant tumors. The connective tissue stroma of malignant teratoma is usually poorly arranged, but that of benign teratoma is dense and of the adult type. In the benign type, nerve tissue, skin, and teeth may be found. Skin and its appendages are usually present and remarkably well formed. Hair follicles preserve their normal slightly oblique position relative to the free surface and are always accompanied by well-developed sebaceous glands. Sweat glands, often of the apocrine type, are frequently located near the sebaceous glands. Smooth muscle closely resembling arrectores pilorum is occasionally encountered.

Mesodermal derivatives, such as connective tissue, bone, cartilage, and muscle arranged in organoid pattern, are frequently found. When present, hematopoietic tissue is found only in association with cancellous bone. Smooth muscle is most often observed as longitudinal or circular bundles in organoid alimentary structures. Occasionally, it is also seen in bronchial walls.

Entodermal derivatives, representing such structures as intestine, and respiratory and pancreatic tissue are also present.

In a review of mediastinal tumors, Ellis and DuShane (1956) found 27.6 per cent teratomatous tumors in infants. Of this group of 16 teratomatous tumors, 8 were benign teratomas, 5 were teratoid cysts, and 3 were teratoid carcinoma.

The symptoms, signs, and roentgenographic findings in these cases are identical with those in teratoid cysts unless malignant spread has occurred.

The final diagnosis of malignancy can be determined only after removal and histologic study of the tumor. Malignant degeneration usually involves only one of the cellular components.

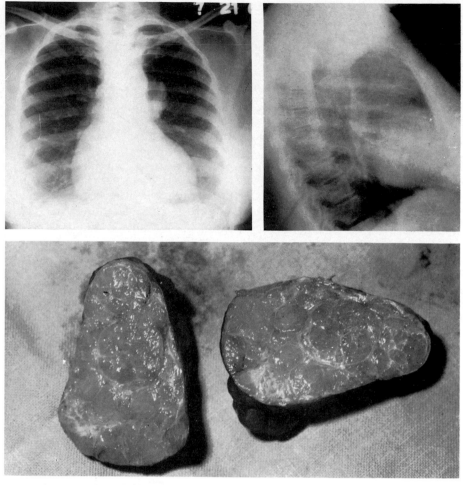

Figure 43–34. A benign thymoma located in the anterior superior mediastinum.

Heuer and Andrus (1940) reviewed 217 cases of teratoid tumors and found that only 5.5 per cent were discovered before the patients reached 12 years of age. Both benign and malignant teratoid tumors may occur within the pericardial sac.

NEUROGENIC MEDIASTINAL TUMORS

Neurogenic tumors, by far the most common tumors with posterior mediastinal origin, may be classified as follows:

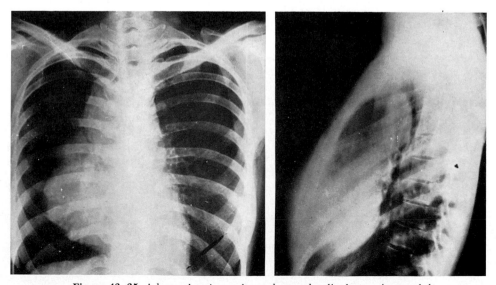

Figure 43–35. A large thymic cyst located near the diaphragm in an adult.

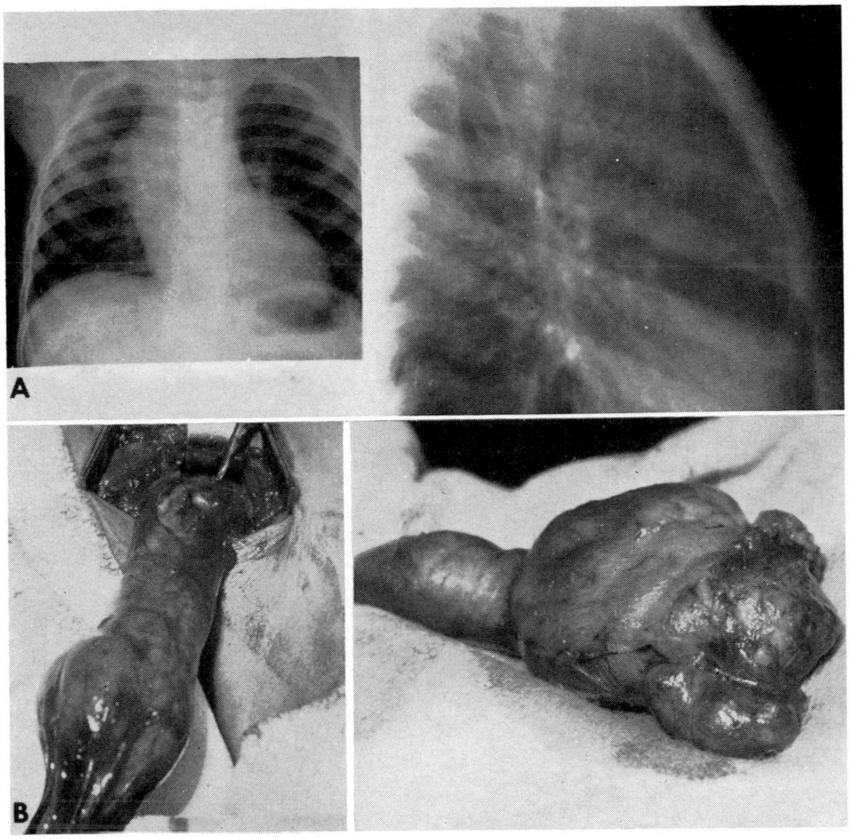

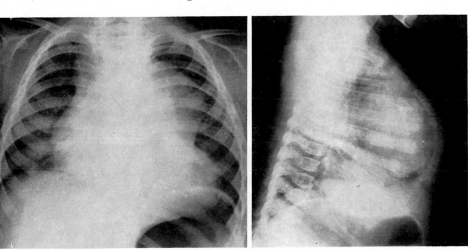

Figure 43–36. *A*, A large thymic cyst in a 4-year-old boy that was evident as a mass in the right side of the neck clinically as well as on a chest roentgenogram. Removal required a thoracotomy and a supraclavicular incision. *B*, A thymic cyst as seen after a thoracotomy and at the time of removal through a neck incision.

1. Neurofibroma and neurilemoma
    a. Malignant schwannoma
2. Tumors of sympathetic origin
    a. Neuroblastoma
    b. Ganglioneuroma
    c. Ganglioneuroblastoma
    d. Pheochromocytoma
3. Chemodectoma

Benign neurofibromas, neurilemomas, and malignant schwannomas are extremely unusual in the pediatric age group and when present are most often asymptomatic (Fig. 43–39).

A neuroblastoma is a malignant tumor arising from the adrenal medulla and occasionally from ganglia of the sympathetic nervous system; it consists of uniform cell layers with or without pseudorosettes. The cells have a dark nucleus and scant cytoplasm and are separated by an eosinophilic fibrillar stroma. Cellular differentiation is sometimes very poor. Although a primary neuroblastoma may cause the first clinical signs or symptoms, metastases in the bone, skin, or lymph nodes may be the first indication of its presence.

The ganglioneuroma is a benign tumor made up of mature ganglion cells, few or many, in a stroma of nerve fibers.

Ganglioneuroblastoma is a tumor composed of various proportions of neuroblastoma and ganglioneuroma.

Ganglioneuroma and ganglioneuroblastoma are

Figure 43–37. A large, solid, benign teratoma in an infant. Note the anterior mediastinal position and the forward displacement of the sternum.

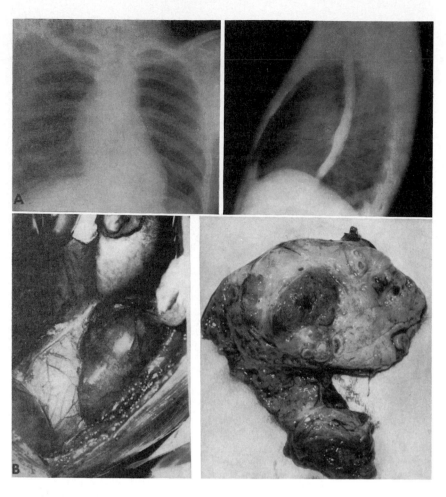

Figure 43–38. *A,* Posteroanterior and lateral radiographs of an anterior malignant teratoma in an older child. *B,* Note the anterior mediastinal position, with the teratoma wedged between the heart and the sternum.

more likely to occur after the age of 2 years. The more malignant forms, such as neuroblastoma, frequently occur before the age of 2 years. Ganglioneuroma is more common in children than in adults; respiratory symptoms are rare (Fig. 43–40).

Tumors of nerve origin usually occur in the upper two thirds of the hemithorax and tend to extend locally. They may grow into the lower part of the neck and across the midline through the posterior mediastinum to the opposite hemithorax, descend through the diaphragm into the upper part of the abdomen or into the intercostal spaces posteriorly, and involve one or several of the vertebral foramina. Ganglioneuroblastoma rarely metastasizes to lymph nodes.

A large number of neurogenic tumors, more often the benign type, may be asymptomatic. Symptoms such as radicular pain, paraplegia, motor disturbances, and Horner syndrome may occur.

Upper respiratory tract infections, dyspnea, elevated temperature, weight loss, and asthenia may occur. Neurogenic tumors of the neuroblastoma group usually occur in younger children, and respiratory symptoms, thoracic pain, and fever are more common (Fig. 43–41).

On x-ray examination, neurogenic tumors are round, oval, or spindle shaped and are characteristically located posteriorly in the paravertebral gutter.

On thoracic roentgenograms, a ganglioneuroma appears as an elongated lesion and may extend over a distance of several vertebrae. Typically, a neurofibroma tends to be more rounded in outline. Calcifications within the tumor may be seen, more commonly in the malignant forms. Even though not demonstrated on x-ray examination, calcification may be found at the time of histologic examination. Bone lesions, such as intercostal space widening, costal deformation, vertebral involvement, and metastatic bone disease, are not unusual with neurogenic tumors.

The therapy for neurogenic tumors of the thoracic cavity is surgery. Every case of ganglioneuroma reported in a study by Schweisguth and co-workers (1959) was amenable to resection. In malignant neurogenic tumor, all possible tumor growth should be excised and postoperative irradiation therapy should be instituted. X-ray therapy must be given judiciously, because growth disturbances, pulmonary fibrosis, and other sequelae may develop. In the hourglass type of tumor, laminectomy must precede thoracotomy.

Mediastinal chemodectomas are usually located anteriorly; they are likely to be associated with similar tumors in the carotid body and elsewhere. There is a tendency for these tumors to be multiple.

Mediastinal pheochromocytomas are extremely

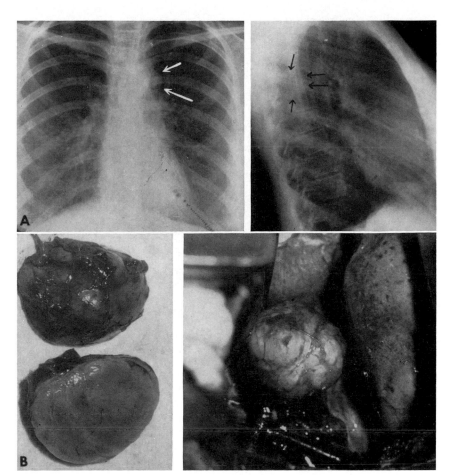

Figure 43–39. *A*, Neurofibroma seen posteriorly located in posteroanterior and lateral films. *B*, Note the solid nature of the lesion, its round smooth outline, and its attachment to the intercostal nerve.

rare and have not been recorded in the pediatric age group.

In Heimburger and Battersby's (1965) series of mediastinal tumors in childhood, 25 per cent of 36 tumors were of the neurogenic type. Ellis and Du-Shane (1956) reported 32 per cent neurogenic tumors in a review of primary mediastinal cysts and neoplasms in infants.

MEDIASTINAL LYMPH NODE ABNORMALITIES

Abnormalities of the lymph nodes in the mediastinum may be classified as follows:
1. Leukemia
2. Hodgkin's disease
3. Lymphosarcoma

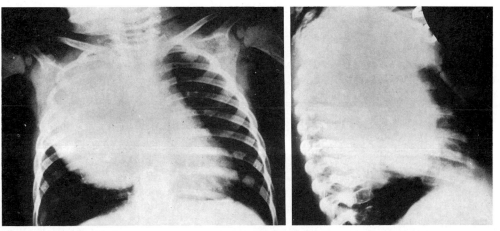

Figure 43–40. A large ganglioneuroma in an infant. The benign lesion was removed, with a good follow-up result.

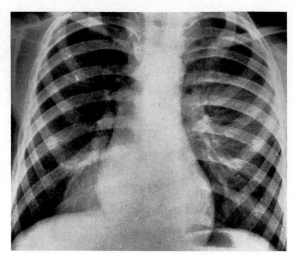

Figure 43–41. A neuroblastoma in a 6-year-old boy.

4. Sarcoidosis
5. Inflammatory disorders
   a. Tuberculosis
   b. Fungus
   c. Nonspecific

Any lymph node enlargement in a child should be viewed with suspicion. Lymphatic tumors are one of the more frequently observed malignant growths in childhood. The diagnosis is made by biopsy. Tumors of the Hodgkin's lymphosarcoma and reticulum cell sarcoma group are found primarily in children more than 3 years of age, with a peak incidence from 8 to 14 years. More than 95 per cent of children with primary lymphatic malignancy have lymph node enlargement as the presenting sign. Tonsillar hypertrophy and adenoidal hyperplasia, pulmonary hilar enlargement, splenomegaly, bone pain, unexplained fever, anemia, infiltrative skin lesions, and, rarely, central nervous system symptoms may also be present. The diagnosis should be sought through the study of peripheral blood smears, lymph node biopsy, or bone marrow examination.

Surgery has limited value in lymphosarcoma, because the disease is usually widespread. However, when the lesions are apparently isolated in the neck, axilla, mediastinum, or gastrointestinal tract, surgery may be of great benefit. With few exceptions, all the tumors in this group are radiosensitive; however, they are not curable by x-ray therapy.

In most cases of mediastinal malignancy, bilateral hilar enlargement as well as bilateral mediastinal enlargement is present. The lymph node enlargement may rarely be unilateral and relatively localized. In such cases, routine study of the blood smear, scalene lymph node biopsy, and bone marrow studies may not provide the diagnosis, and open thoracotomy may be necessary. In such cases, complete lymph node removal should be carried out if technically feasible.

Inflammatory Disorders. Lymph node enlargement in the hilus of the lung or mediastinum may be secondary to tuberculous, fungal, or bacterial lung disease. Diagnosis is usually confirmed by means of sputum culture, examination of washings from the tracheobronchial tree taken at the time of bronchoscopy, scalene node biopsy, and skin tests correlated with the general clinical picture. The same is true in sarcoidosis. In sarcoidosis there may be involvement of the eye, skin, peripheral lymph nodes, mediastinal or hilar lymph nodes, and the lung parenchyma. It is possible to establish the diagnosis with this clinical picture and scalene node biopsy in approximately 80 to 85 per cent of the cases of sarcoidosis.

Although nonspecific symptomatic or asymptomatic enlargement of the mediastinal lymph nodes may occur, a cause can usually be found. For example, histoplasmosis may produce the clinical picture outlined.

Veneziale and co-workers (1964) have described angiofloccular hyperplasia of the mediastinal lymph nodes. Although this rare, benign, localized lymph node enlargement may occur in extrathoracic locations, it most often occurs as an isolated asymptomatic mediastinal or pulmonary hilar tumor. Grossly, the tumors are moderately firm and usually well encapsulated. Calcification may occur but is unusual. On microscopic examination, the two main features of these lymphoid masses are a diffuse follicular replacement of the lymph node architecture and much follicular and interfollicular vascular proliferation. Sixty per cent of patients with this entity are asymptomatic. When symptoms occur, they may include cough, fatigue, chest pain, and fever. Surgical excision is the treatment of choice and is usually successful.

VASCULAR LYMPHATIC ABNORMALITIES OF THE MEDIASTINUM

Vascular-lymphatic abnormalities of the mediastinum may be classified as (1) cavernous hemangioma, (2) hemangiopericytoma, (3) angiosarcoma, or (4) cystic hygroma.

Vascular tumors of the mediastinum in children are rare, and preoperative diagnosis is unusual. Vascular tumors may occur at any level in the mediastinum but are more frequent in the upper portion of the thorax and in the anterior mediastinum. They are uniformly rounded in appearance and are moderately dense. Calcification within the tumor is unusual. They are usually asymptomatic.

Cystic hygromas are relatively rare but occur more often in infants and children than in adults. These tumors consist of masses of dilated lymphatic channels containing clear, watery fluid; they are lined with flat endothelium and are usually multilocular. They may appear to be isolated in the mediastinum (Fig. 43–42) but more often have an associated continuation into the neck. They may be rather large and unilateral, with lateral masses in the superior mediastinum. In 1948, Gross and Hurwitt reported

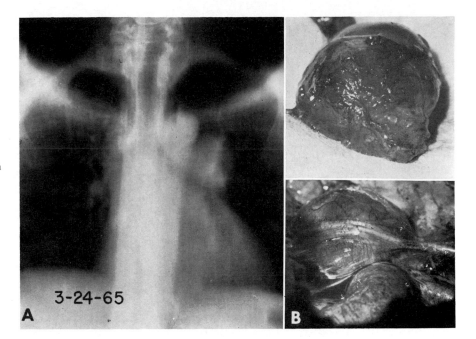

Figure 43–42. A large lymphatic cyst in the anterior mediastinum.

21 cases of cervical mediastinal hygromas and only 8 cases of isolated mediastinal hygromas.

Diagnosis of a cervicomediastinal hygroma is made by physical examination of the cervical swelling and x-ray examination of the chest. Periodic fluctuation in size frequently occurs in cervical hygromas. This is even more characteristic of the combined cervico-mediastinal lesions; in these, the cervical component may increase in size during inspiratory movements. X-ray films and fluoroscopic examination may show descent of the mass into the mediastinum on inspiration with prominence in the neck during expiration.

Cystic hygroma confined to the mediastinum is usually discovered at autopsy or as an unanticipated finding on x-ray examination. The soft and yielding nature of the cysts allows them to attain considerable size without producing symptoms. On x-ray film there is a somewhat lobulated, smoothly outlined mass; however, it is usually not possible to distinguish hygromas from other benign tumors or cysts of the mediastinum by this method.

When respiratory infections occur, hygromas often become infected. Such infections are usually controlled by chemotherapy or by incision and drainage. A mediastinal or blood stream infection may result, however, or infection may be followed by local fibrosis and the disappearance of the mass. Spontaneous or posttraumatic hemorrhage into a cyst may result in extension of the cyst; this may cause sudden tracheal compression, a surgical emergency. Malignant change in hygroma has not been reported.

Surgical excision is the treatment of choice. Mediastinal hygromas can usually be excised with little difficulty because tissue planes around the cysts are well developed.

Chylothorax may result when there is cervical hygroma with involvement of the thoracic duct.

MEDIASTINAL LIPOMA AND LIPOSARCOMA

Intrathoracic lipoma is rare in children. Lipomas of the mediastinum have been divided into three groups according to their location and form: (1) tumors confined within the thoracic cage, (2) intra-thoracic lipomas that extend upward into the neck, and (3) intrathoracic lipomas with an extrathoracic extension forming a dumbbell configuration.

Of the lipomas reported in the world literature, 76 per cent were intrathoracic, 10 per cent cervicomediastinal, and 14 per cent of the dumbbell type. Only 15 occurred in the pediatric age group, and these were intrathoracic. Four cases of liposarcoma of the mediastinum in children have been reported. Although these tumors usually do not metastasize, their invasiveness and tendency to recur place them in the malignant group.

In general, lipomas of the subcutaneous tissue are benign, whereas those of the retroperitoneal area and deep somatic soft tissue are usually malignant. The tumors of the mediastinum seem to have an incidence and behavior similar to those of lipomas in the peritoneal region.

Radical surgical excision is the procedure of choice. Repeated surgical attacks may serve as a method of extended control, and x-ray therapy may be added for palliative purposes.

THYROID AND PARATHYROID DISORDERS

Substernal thyroid is a common anterior superior mediastinal tumor in the adult age group but apparently does not occur before puberty. Ectopic thyroid in the mediastinum does occur in children, and in such cases blood supply is derived from a mediastinal vessel.

Parathyroid adenoma with a typical syndrome of hyperparathyroidism does not occur before puberty.

PRIMARY CARDIAC AND PERICARDIAL TUMORS

Primary tumors of the heart in infants may cause cardiac enlargement or enlargement of the cardiac silhouette, giving rise to symptoms in the lungs or esophagus. Most frequently, the signs and symptoms of congestive heart failure are much more prominent than those of tumors of the respiratory system or esophagus.

Rhabdomyoma appears to be the only cardiac tumor showing a definite predilection for the younger age groups. This is particularly true of children with tuberous sclerosis, in whom rhabdomyoma of the heart is prone to occur. Such tumors are not considered true neoplasms and probably represent an area of developmental arrest in the fetal myocardium. It is not unusual for rhabdomyoma to regress spontaneously without having caused any appreciable impairment of cardiac function.

Myxoma is by far the most common primary tumor of the heart, accounting for slightly more than 50 per cent of all primary cardiac tumors. It may be encountered at almost any age. The signs and symptoms vary widely but ultimately lead to cardiac failure that does not respond to the usual medical management. Most myxomas are located in the atria, more frequently on the left than on the right. They tend to proliferate and project into the chambers of the heart, preventing normal cardiac filling by obstruction to the mitral or tricuspid valve. The origin appears to be in the atrial septa.

Primary sarcoma of the heart is less common than myxoma but may occur at any age. It does not, as a rule, proliferate into the lumina of the heart; it infiltrates the wall of the myocardium and frequently extends into the pericardial cavity.

Other primary tumors of the heart are angioma, fibroma, lipoma, and hamartoma. All are rare and usually produce prominent circulatory symptoms.

Primary neoplasms of the pericardium are rare. On histologic examination, the predominant tumors are mesotheliomas (endotheliomas) and sarcomas, but leiomyomas, hemangiomas, and lipomas occasionally occur.

A single instance of a large cavernous hemangioma of the pericardium has been described in an 8-year-old girl; it was successfully removed.

TUMORS OF THE DIAPHRAGM

Tumors involving the diaphragm may cause chest pain and discomfort or pulmonary compression; thus, they may simulate mediastinal or primary pulmonary neoplasms. Primary tumors of the diaphragm are extremely rare in the pediatric age group.

Benign tumors of the diaphragm that have been reported, though not necessarily in children, are lipoma, fibroma, chondroma, angiofibroma, lymphangioma, neurofibroma, rhabdomyofibroma, fibromyoma, and primary diaphragmatic cyst.

Malignant tumors of the diaphragm that have been reported are fibrosarcoma, rhabdomyosarcoma, myosarcoma, leiomyosarcoma, and fibromyosarcoma. None of these tumors appears to have been reported in children.

PRIMARY TUMORS OF THE CHEST WALL

Figures 43–43 and 43–44 illustrate findings seen in two forms of chest wall tumors.

Lipoma of the chest wall is common in adults but rare in the pediatric age group. As noted previously, these may be dumbbell in shape, presenting on the chest wall with a large intrathoracic component. Chest roentgenogram will aid in its definition.

Extensive cavernous hemangiomas of the thoracic wall are seen in infancy or childhood. They may be isolated or associated with similar lesions in other tissues, including the lung. In these cases, the diagnosis of Osler-Weber-Rendu syndrome is suggested. Intrathoracic extension of these lesions may occur.

In von Recklinghausen disease, multiple cutaneous and subcutaneous nodules are present. Patients with this disease should be carefully studied for the possible coexistence of mediastinal neurofibromas or intrathoracic meningocele.

Chondroma and chondrosarcoma are the principal bony tumors of the chest wall; 80 per cent of these occur in the ribs or sternum, usually in the anterior extremity of a rib near the costochondral junction. They may also occur in the sternum, scapula, clavicle, or vertebral bodies. There may be few, if any, symptoms. Radiographic examination reveals a discrete expansion of the bone with an intact, thinned-out cortex.

Chondrosarcoma of the rib occurs more frequently in males; it is usually seen in the posterior half and paravertebral portion of the rib, but it sometimes involves the transverse process and the vertebral body either primarily or secondarily. The direction of growth occasionally appears to be entirely internal, thus simulating the radiologic appearance of a primary pleural or mediastinal tumor. However, there usually is an externally visible and palpable tumefaction. This usually occurs during the middle decades of life.

Solitary plasmacytoma, a lesion histologically similar to multiple myeloma but localized to a single bone, may involve any part of the thoracic cage; it may involve the vertebrae, rarely attacks the ribs, and may involve the lung itself. In solitary plasma-

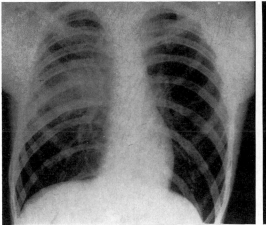

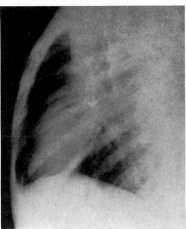

Figure 43–43. Reticulum cell sarcoma in the chest wall of an 8-year-old white boy. He survived for more than 18 months.

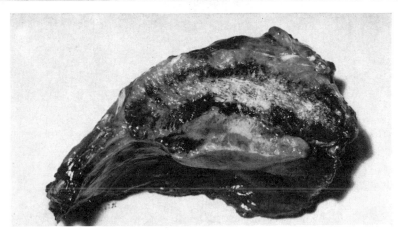

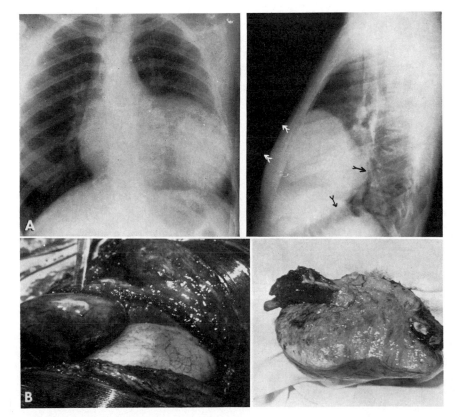

Figure 43–44. A desmoid tumor of the chest wall in a child 18 months after patent ductus surgery. The desmoid was in the line of the posterior lateral incision.

cytoma, the bone is thinned and may be greatly expanded.

Ewing tumor is sometimes primary in a rib and is unusual before the second decade of life.

REFERENCES

General

Arey LB: Developmental Anatomy. Revised 7th ed. Philadelphia, WB Saunders Co, 1974.

Ariel IM and Pack GT: Cancer and Allied Diseases of Infancy and Childhood. Boston, Little, Brown & Co, 1960.

Azizkhan RG, Dudgeon DL, Buck JR et al: Life threatening airway obstruction as a complication to the management of mediastinal masses in children. J Pediatr Surg 20:816, 1985.

Benson CD, Mustard WT, Ravitch MM et al: Pediatric Surgery. Vol. I. Chicago, Year Book Medical Publishers, 1962.

Culham JAG: Special procedures in pediatric chest radiology. Pediatr Clin North Am 26:661, 1979.

Fellows KE, Stigol L, Shuster S et al: Selective bronchial arteriography in patients with cystic fibrosis and massive hemoptysis. Radiology 114:551, 1975.

Felson B: Fundamentals of Chest Roentgenology. Philadelphia, WB Saunders Co, 1960.

Gilbert JG, Mazzarella LA, and Feit EJ: Primary tracheal tumors in the infant and adult. Arch Otolaryngol 58:1, 1953.

Glenn WWL: Thoracic and Cardiovascular Surgery. 4th ed. New York, Appleton-Century-Crofts, 1983.

Greenfield LJ: Complications in Surgery and Trauma. Philadelphia, JB Lippincott Co, 1984.

Gryminski T, Krakowka P, and Lypacewica G: The diagnosis of pleural effusion by ultrasonic and radiologic techniques. Chest 70:33, 1976.

Haller JO, Schneider M, Kassner EG et al: Sonographic evaluation of the chest in infants and children. Am J Roentgenol 134:1019, 1980.

Hinshaw HC and Murray JF: Diseases of the Chest. 4th ed. Philadelphia, WB Saunders Co, 1980.

Ivancev K, Halldorsdottir A, Laurin S et al: Computed tomography in the diagnosis and treatment of mediastinal abnormalities in children. Acta Radiol 29:115, 1988.

Jones PG and Campbell PE: Tumours of Infancy and Childhood. London, Blackwell Scientific Publications; Philadelphia, JB Lippincott Co, 1976.

Keith A: Human Embryology and Morphology. 6th ed. Baltimore, Williams & Wilkins Co, 1948.

Kirks DR and Korobkin M: Computed tomography of the chest in infants and children. Techniques and mediastinal evaluation. Radiol Clin North Am 19:409, 1981.

Kreel L: Computed tomography of the thorax. Radiol Clin North Am 16:575, 1978.

Laurin S, Williams JL, and Fitzsimmons JR: Magnetic resonance imaging of the pediatric thorax: initial experience. Eur J Radiol 6:36, 1986.

Lindskog GE and Liebow AA: Thoracic and Cardiovascular Surgery. 3rd ed. New York, Appleton-Century-Crofts, 1962.

Muhm JR: Role of computed tomography in evaluation of intrathoracic lesions. J Thorac Cardiovasc Surg 79:469, 1980.

Ochsner A Jr, Lucas GL, and McFarland GB Jr: Tumors of the thoracic skeleton, review of 134 cases. J Thorac Cardiovasc Surg 52:311, 1966.

Odom JA, De Muth WE, and Blakemore WS: Chest wall chondrosarcoma in youth. J Thorac Cardiovasc Surg 50:550, 1965.

Parish JM, Rosenow EC, and Muhm JR: Mediastinal masses: clues to interpretation of radiologic studies. Postgrad Med 76:173, 1984.

Ravin CE: Thoracocentesis of loculated pleural effusions using grey scale ultrasonic guidance. Chest 71:666, 1977.

Rubin EH: The Lung as a Mirror of Systemic Disease. Springfield, Ill, Charles C Thomas, 1956.

Rubin EH and Rubin M: Thoracic Diseases, Emphasizing Cardiopulmonary Relationships. Philadelphia, WB Saunders Co, 1961.

Ryckman FC and Rodgers BM: Thoracoscopy for intrathoracic neoplasia in children. J Pediatr Surg 17:521, 1982.

Sabiston DC and Spencer FC: Gibbon's Surgery of the Chest. 4th ed. Philadelphia, WB Saunders Co, 1982.

Schaffer AJ and Avery ME: Diseases of the Newborn. 4th ed. Philadelphia, WB Saunders Co, 1977.

Shin MS and Gray PW Jr: Pitfalls in ultrasonic detection of pleural fluid. J Clin Ultrasound 6:421, 1978.

Ultrasound in Pediatrics. New York, Churchill-Livingstone, 1981.

Benign Pulmonary Tumors

Albrecht EE: Verh Dtsch Ges Pathol 7:153, 1904.

Archer FL, Harrison RW, and Moulder PV: Granular cell myoblastoma of the trachea and carina treated by resection and reconstruction. J Thorac Surg 45:539, 1963.

Baker DC Jr and Pemington CL: Congenital hemangioma of the larynx. Laryngoscope 66:696, 1956.

Blackman J, Cantril ST, Lund TK, and Sparkman D: Tracheobronchial papillomatosis, treated by roentgen irradiation. Radiology 73:598, 1959.

Borkowsky W, Martin D, and Lawrence HS: Juvenile laryngeal papillomatosis with pulmonary spread. Regression following transfer factor therapy. Am J Dis Child 138:667, 1984.

Campbell JS, Wiglesworth FW, Latarroca R, and Wilde H: Congenital subglottic hemangiomas of the larynx and trachea in infants. Pediatrics 22:727, 1958.

Cavin E, Masters JH, and Moody J: Hamartoma of the lung. J Thorac Surg 35:816, 1958.

Doermann P, Lunseth J, and Segnitz RH: Obstructing subglottic hemangioma of the larynx in infancy. Review of the literature and report of a deceptive case. N Engl J Med 258:68, 1958.

Ferguson CF and Flake CG: Subglottic hemangioma as a cause of respiratory obstruction in infants. Trans Am Bronchoesoph [A] 41:27, 1961.

Fishman L: Papilloma of the trachea. J Thorac Cardiovasc Surg 44:264, 1962.

Guida PN, Fultcher T, and Moore SW: Leiomyoma of the lung. J Thorac Surg 49:1058, 1965.

Holder TM and Christy MG: Cystic adenomatoid malformation of the lung. J Thorac Surg 47:590, 1964.

Jones CJ: Unusual hamartoma of the lung in the newborn infant. Arch Pathol 48:150, 1949.

Kauffman SL and Stout AP: Histiocytic tumors (fibrous xanthoma and histiocytoma) in children. Cancer 14:469, 1961.

Kumis FD and Conn JH: Endobronchial hamartoma. J Thorac Surg 50:138, 1965.

Littler ER: Asphyxia due to hemangioma in the trachea. J Thorac Cardiovasc Surg 45:552, 1963.

Ogilvie OE: Multiple papillomas of the trachea with malignant degeneration. Arch Otolaryngol 58:10, 1953.

Oleszczuk-Raszke K and Cremin HJ: Computed tomography in pulmonary papillomatosis. Br J Radiol 61:160, 1988.

Pearl M and Woolley MW: Pulmonary xanthomatous postinflammatory pseudotumors in children. J Pediatr Surg 8:255, 1973.

Smoller S and Maynard A DeL: Adenoma of the bronchus in a nine year old child. Am J Dis Child 82:587, 1951.

Stein AS and Volk BM: Papillomatosis of the trachea and lung. Arch Pathol 124:127, 1959.

Taylor TL and Miller DR: Leiomyoma of the bronchus. J Thorac Cardiovasc Surg 57:284, 1969.

Thomas MR: Cystic hamartoma of the lung in a newborn infant. J Pathol Bacteriol 61:599, 1949.

Verska JJ and Connolly JE: Bronchial adenomas in children. J Thorac Cardiovasc Surg 55:411, 1968.

Ward DE Jr, Bradshaw HH, and Prince TC: Bronchial adenoma in children. J Thorac Surg 27:295, 1954.

Primary and Metastatic Malignant Pulmonary Tumors

Archer RL, Grogg SE, and Sanders SP: Mucoepidermoid bronchial adenoma in a 6 year old girl: a case report and review of the literature. J Thorac Cardiovasc Surg 94:452, 1987.

Baldeyrou P, Lemoine G, Zucker JM, and Schweisguth O: Pulmonary metastases in children: the place of surgery. A study of 134 patients. J Pediatr Surg 19:121, 1984.

Bartley JD and Arean VM: Intrapulmonic neurogenic tumors. J Thorac Surg 50:114, 1965.

Beardsley JM: Primary carcinoma of the lung in a child. Can Med Assoc J 29:257, 1933.

Beattie EJ Jr: Surgical treatment of pulmonary metastases. Cancer 54:2729, 1984.

Beattie EJ, Martini N, and Rosen G: The management of pulmonary metastases in children with osteogenic sarcoma with surgical resection combined with chemotherapy. Cancer 35:618, 1975.

Berman L: Extragenital chorionepithelioma with report of a case. Am J Cancer 38:23, 1940.

Brandt B III, Heintz SE, Rose EF, and Ehrenhaft JL: Bronchial carcinoid tumors. Ann Thorac Surg 39:63, 1984.

Cayley CK, Mersheimer W, and Caez HJ: Primary bronchogenic carcinoma of the lung in children. J Dis Child 82:49, 1951.

Cliffton EE and Pool JL: Treatment of lung metastasis in children with combined therapy. J Thorac Cardiovasc Surg 54:403, 1967.

de Parades CG, Pierce WS, Groff DB, and Waldhausen JA: Bronchogenic tumors in children. Arch Surg 100:574, 1970.

Dowell AR: Primary pulmonary leiomyosarcoma. Ann Thorac Surg 17:384, 1974.

Dyson BC and Trentalance AE: Resection of primary pulmonary sarcoma. J Thorac Surg 47:577, 1964.

Feldman PA: Sarcoma of the lungs, a report of three cases. Br J Tuberc Chest Dis 51:331, 1957.

Giritsky AS, Etcubanas E, and Mark JBD: Pulmonary resection in children with metastatic osteogenic sarcoma. J Thorac Cardiovasc Surg 75:354, 1978.

Harris WH and Schattenberg HH: Anlagen and rest tumors of the lung. Am J Pathol 18:955, 1942.

Hartman GE and Shochat SJ: Primary pulmonary neoplasms of childhood: a review. Ann Thorac Surg 36:108, 1983.

Herring N, Templeton JY III, Haup GJ, and Theodos PA: Primary sarcoma of the lung. Dis Chest 42:315, 1962.

Hollinger PH, Johnston KC, Gosswiller N, and Hirsch EC: Primary fibrosarcoma of the bronchus. Dis Chest 37:137, 1960.

Jimenez JF: Pulmonary blastoma in childhood. J Surg Oncol 34:87, 1987.

Jimenez JF, Uthman EO, Townsend JW et al: Primary bronchopulmonary leiomyosarcoma in childhood. Arch Pathol Lab Med 110:348, 1986.

Kay S and Reed WG: Chorioepithelioma of the lung in a female infant seven months old. Am J Pathol 29:555, 1953.

Killingsworth WP, McReynolds GS, and Harrison AW: Pulmonary leiomyosarcomas in a child. J Pediatr 42:466, 1963.

Kirks DR and Korobkin M: Computed tomography of the chest wall, pleura, and pulmonary parenchyma in infants and children. Radiol Clin North Am 19:421, 1981.

Kyriakos M and Webber B: Cancer of the lung in young men. J Thorac Cardiovasc Surg 67:634, 1974.

Lack EE, Harris GB, Eraklis AJ, and Vawterg F: Primary bronchial tumors in childhood. A clinicopathologic study of six cases. Cancer 51:492, 1983.

Lembke J, Havers W, Doetsch N et al: Long-term results following surgical removal of pulmonary metastases in children with malignomas. Thorac Cardiovasc Surg 34:137, 1986.

McNamara JJ, Paulson DL, Kinglsey WB et al: Primary leiomyosarcoma of the lung. J Thorac Cardiovasc Surg 57:635, 1969.

Marks P: Multiple thoracostomy from metastatic pulmonary neoplasm. Thorax 29:248, 1974.

Martini N, Huvos AG, Miké V et al: Multiple pulmonary resections in the treatment of osteogenic sarcoma. Ann Thorac Surg 12:271, 1971.

Merrit JW and Parker KR: Intrathoracic leiomyosarcoma. Can Med Assoc J 77:1031, 1957.

Muhm JR, Brown LR, and Crowe JK: Detection of pulmonary nodules by computed tomography. Am J Roentgenol 128:267, 1977.

Noehren TH and McKee FW: Sarcoma of the lung. Dis Chest 25:633, 1954.

Ochsner S and Ochsner A: Primary sarcoma of the lung. Ochsner Clin Rep 3:105, 1957.

Randell WS and Blades B: Primary bronchogenic leiomyosarcoma. Arch Pathol 42:543, 1946.

Remy J, Arnaud A, Fardou H et al: Treatment of hemoptysis by embolization of the bronchial arteries. Radiology 122:33, 1977.

Rosen G, Tan C, Exelby P et al: Vincristine, high-dose methotrexate with citrovorum factor rescue, cyclophosphamide, and Adriamycin cyclic therapy following surgery in childhood osteogenic sarcoma. Proc Am Assoc Cancer Res 15:172, 1974.

Schaller RT Jr, Haas J, Schaller J et al: Improved survival in children with osteosarcoma following resection of pulmonary metastasis. J Pediatr Surg 17:546, 1982.

Sekulich M, Pandola G, and Simon T: A solitary pulmonary mass in multiple myeloma: report of a case. Dis Chest 48:100, 1965.

Shaw RR, Paulson DL, Kee JL, and Lovett VF: Primary pulmonary leiomyosarcomas. J Thorac Cardiovasc Surg 41:430, 1961.

Sherman RS and Malone BH: A study of muscle tumors primary in the lung. Radiology 54:507, 1950.

Simpson JA, Smith F, Matz LR et al: Bronchial adenoma: a review of 26 cases. Aust NZ J Surg 44:110, 1974.

Stout AP and Himidi GM: Solitary (localized) mesothelioma of the pleura. Ann Surg 133:50, 1951.

Verska JJ and Connolly JE: Bronchial adenomas in children. J Thorac Cardiovasc Surg 55:411, 1968.

Watson WL and Anlyan AJ: Primary leiomyosarcoma of the lung. Cancer 7:250, 1954.

Mediastinal Tumors

Abell MR: Mediastinal cysts. Arch Pathol 61:360, 1956.

Ackerman LR and Taylor FH: Neurogenic tumors within the thorax. Cancer 4:669, 1951.

Adkins RB Jr, Maples MD, and Hainsworth JD: Primary malignant mediastinal tumors. Ann Thorac Surg 38:648, 1984.

Adler RH, Taheri SA, and Waintraub DG: Mediastinal teratoma in infancy. J Thorac Surg 39:394, 1960.

Archer O, Pierce JC, and Good RA: Role of the thymus in the development of the immune response. Fed Proc 20:26, 1961.

Arciniegas E, Hakimi M, Farooki ZQ, and Green EW: Intrapericardial teratoma in infancy. J Thorac Cardiovasc Surg 79:306, 1980.

Arger PH, Mulhern CB, Littman PS et al: Management of solid tumors in children: contribution of computed tomography. AJR 137:251, 1981.

Arnason BG, Jankovic BD, and Wadsman BH: A survey of the thymus and its relation to lymphocytes and immune reactions. Blood 20:617, 1962.

Bale PM: A congenital intraspinal gastroenterogenous cyst in diastematomyelia. J Neurol Neurosurg Psychiatr 36:1011, 1973.

Bednav B: Malignant intrapericardial tumor of heart (translation). Cas Lek Cesk 48:1355, 1950.

Barnard ED and James LS: The cardiac silhouette in newborn infants: a cinematographic study of the normal range. Pediatrics 27:13, 1961.

Bernatz PE, Harrison EG, and Clagett OT: Thymoma: a clinicopathologic study. J Thorac Cardiovasc Surg 42:424, 1961.

Bill AH Jr, Bracher G, Creighton SA et al: Common malignant tumors of infancy and childhood. Pediatr Clin North Am 6:1197, 1959.

Blades B: Mediastinal tumors: report of cases treated at Army thoracic surgery centers in the U.S. Ann Surg 123:749, 1946.

Bower RJ and Kiesewetter WB: Mediastinal masses in infants and children. Arch Surg 112:1003, 1977.

Bowie PR, Teixeira DHP, and Carpenter B: Malignant thymoma in a nine year old boy presenting with pleuropericardial effusion. J Thorac Cardiovasc Surg 79:777, 1979.

Bremmer JL: Diverticuli and duplications of the intestinal tract. Arch Pathol 38:132, 1944.

Brewer LA III and Dolley FS: Tumors of the mediastinum: a discussion of diagnostic procedure and surgical treatment based on experience with 44 operated cases. Am Rev Tuberc 60:419, 1949.

Bunin NJ, Hvizdala E, Link M et al: Mediastinal nonlymphoblastic lymphomas in children: a clinicopathologic study. J Clin Oncol 4:154, 1986.

Burnett WE, Rosemond GP, and Bucher RM: The diagnosis of mediastinal tumors. Surg Clin North Am 32:1673, 1952.

Caffey J and Silbey R: Regrowth and overgrowth of the thymus after atrophy induced by oral administration of adrenocortico-steroids to human infants. Pediatrics 26:762, 1960.

Callahan WJ and Simon AL: Posterior mediastinal hemangioma associated with vertebral body hemangioma. J Thorac Cardiovasc Surg 51:283, 1966.

Castleberry RP, Kelly DR, Wilson ER et al: Childhood liposarcoma. Report of a case and review of the literature. Cancer 54:579, 1984.

Cicciarelli EH, Soule EH, and McGoon DC: Lipoma and liposarcoma of the mediastinum, a report of fourteen tumors including one lipoma of the thymus. J Thorac Surg 47:411, 1964.

Claireaux AE: An intrapericardial teratoma in a newborn infant. J Pathol Bacteriol 63:743, 1951.

Clark DE: Association of irradiation with cancer of the thyroid in children in adolescence. JAMA 157:107, 1955.

Cohen AJ, Sbaschnig RJ, Hochholzer L et al: Mediastinal hemangiomas. Ann Thorac Surg 43:656, 1987.

Cohn SR, Geller KA, Birns JW et al: Foregut cysts in infants and children: diagnosis and management. Ann Otol Rhinol Laryngol 91:622, 1982.

Conklin WS: Tumors and cysts of the mediastinum. Dis Chest 17:715, 1950.

Conti EA, Patton GD, Conti JE, and Hempelmann LH: The present health of children given x-ray treatment to the anterior mediastinum in infancy. Radiology 74:386, 1960.

Cruickshank DB: Primary intrathoracic neurogenic tumors. J Fac Radiol Lond 8:369, 1957.

Dieter RA Jr, Riker WL, and Hollinger P: Pedunculated esophageal hamartoma in a child. J Thorac Cardiovasc Surg 59:851, 1970.

Dobbs CH, Berg R Jr, and Pierce EC II: Intrapericardial bronchogenic cysts. J Thorac Surg 34:718, 1957.

Duprez A, Corlier R, and Schmidt P: Tuberculoma of the thymus. J Thorac Cardiovasc Surg 44:115, 1962.

Edge JR and Glennie JS: Teratoid tumors of the mediastinum found despite previous normal chest radiography. J Thorac Cardiovasc Surg 40:172, 1960.

Ellis FH Jr and DuShane JW: Primary mediastinal cysts and neoplasms in infants and children. Am Rev Tuberc Pulm Dis 74:940, 1956.

Ellis FH Jr, Kirklin JW, and Woolner LB: Hemangioma of the mediastinum: review of literature and report of case. J Thorac Surg 30:181, 1955.

Ellis FH Jr, Kirklin JW, Hodgson JR et al: Surgical implications of the mediastinal shadow in thoracic roentgenograms of infants and children. Surg Gynecol Obstet 100:532, 1955.

Emerson GL: Supradiaphragmatic thoracic duct cysts. N Engl J Med 242:575, 1950.

Fallon M, Gordon ARG, and Lendrum AC: Mediastinal cysts of fore-gut origin associated with vertebral abnormalities. Br J Surg 41:520, 1954.

Ferguson JO, Clagett OT, and McDonald JR: Hemangiopericytoma (glomus tumor) of the mediastinum: review of the literature and report of case. Surgery 36:320, 1954.

Filler RM, Simpson JS, and Ein SH: Mediastinal masses in infants and children. Pediatr Clin North Am 26:677, 1979.

Filler RM, Traggis DG, Jaffe N, and Vawter GF: Favourable outlook for children with mediastinal neuroblastoma. J Pediatr Surg 7:136, 1972.

Flege JB Jr, Valencia AG, and Zimmerman G: Obstruction of a child's trachea by polypoid hemangioendothelioma. J Thorac Cardiovasc Surg 56:144, 1968.

Forsee JH and Blake HA: Pericardial celomic cyst. Surgery 31:753, 1952.

Fridjon MH: Cysts of the thymus in a newborn baby. Br Med J 2:553, 1943.

Friedman NB: Tumors of the thymus. J Thorac Cardiovasc Surg 53:163, 1967.

Gaebler JW, Kleman MB, Cohen M et al: Differentiation of lymphoma from histoplasmosis in children with mediastinal masses. J Pediatr 104:706, 1984.

Garland HL: Cancer of the thyroid and previous radiation. Surg Gynecol Obstet 112:564, 1961.

Gebauer PW: Case of intrapericardial teratoma. J Thorac Surg 12:458, 1953.

Gerami S, Richardson R, Harrington B, and Pate JW: Obstructive emphysema due to mediastinal bronchogenic cysts in infancy. J Thorac Cardiovasc Surg 58:432, 1969.

Godwin JT, Watson WL, Pool JL et al: Primary intrathoracic neurogenic tumors. J Thorac Surg 20:169, 1950.

Gondos B and Reingold IM: Mediastinal ganglioneuroblastoma. J Thorac Surg 47:430, 1964.

Griffiths SP, Levine OR, Baker DH, and Blumenthal S: Evaluation of an enlarged cardiothymic image in infancy: Thymolytic effect of steroid administration. Am J Cardiol 8:311, 1961.

Grosfeld JL, Ballatine TVN, Lowe D, and Baehner RL: Benign and malignant teratomas in children: analysis of 85 patients. Surgery 80:297, 1976.

Grosfeld JL, Weber TR, and Vane DW: One-stage resection for massive cervicomediastinal hygroma. Surgery 92:693, 1982.

Gross RE: Thoracic surgery for infants. J Thorac Surg 48:152, 1964.

Gross RE and Hurwitt ES: Cervical mediastinal cystic hygromas. Surg Gynecol Obstet 87:599, 1948.

Gross RE, Holcomb GW, and Farber S: Duplications of the alimentary tract. Pediatrics 9:449, 1952.

Haller JA, Mazur DO, and Morgan WW: Diagnosis and management of mediastinal masses in children. J Thorac Cardiovasc Surg 58:385, 1969.

Handorf CR: Intrathoracic lipoma in children. South Med J 75:1403, 1982.

Hardy LM: Bronchogenic cysts of the mediastinum. Pediatrics 4:108, 1949.

Hedblom CA: Intrathoracic dermoid cysts and teratomata, with report of six personal cases and 185 cases collected from the literature. J Thorac Surg 3:22, 1933.

Heimburger IL and Battersby JS: Primary mediastinal tumors of childhood. J Thorac Cardiovasc Surg 50:92, 1965.

Herlitzka HA and Gayle JW: Tumor and cysts of the mediastinum. Arch Surg 76:697, 1958.

Heuer GJ: The thoracic lipomas. Ann Surg 98:801, 1933.

Heuer J and Andrus W: The surgery of mediastinal tumors. Am J Surg 50:146, 1940.

Hollingsworth RK: Intrathoracic tumors of the sympathetic nervous system. Surg Gynecol Obstet 82:682, 1946.

Hopkins SM and Freitas EL: Bilateral osteochondroma of the ribs in an infant, an unusual cause of cyanosis. J Thorac Surg 49:247, 1965.

Hurwitz A, Conrad R, Selvage IL, and Oberton EA: Hypertrophic lobar emphysema secondary to a paratracheal cyst in an infant. J Thorac Cardiovasc Surg 57:412, 1966.

Issa PY, Brihi ER, Janin Y, and Slim MS: Superior vena cava syndrome in childhood: report of ten cases and a review of the literature. Pediatrics 71:337, 1983.

Jellen J and Fisher WB: Intrapericardial tertoma. Am J Dis Child 51:1397, 1936.

Jones JC: Esophageal duplications or mediastinal cysts of enteric origin. West J Surg 55:610, 1947.

Karl SR and Dunn J: Posterior mediastinal teratomas. J Pediatr Surg 20:508, 1985.

Kauffman SL and Stout AP: Lipoblastic tumors of children. Cancer 12:912, 1959.

Kenny JB and Carty HM: Infants presenting with respiratory distress due to anterior mediastinal teratomas: a report of three cases and a review of the literature. Br J Radiol 61:241, 1988.

Kent EM, Blades B, Valle AR, and Graham EA: Intrathoracic neurogenic tumors. J Thorac Surg 13:116, 1944.

Kessel AWL: Intrathoracic meningocele, spinal deformity and multiple neurofibromatosis. J Bone Joint Surg 33B:87, 1951.

King RM, Telander RL, Smithson WA et al: Primary mediastinal tumors in children. J Pediatr Surg 17:512, 1982.

Kirwan WO, Walbaum PR, and McCormack RJM: Cystic intrathoracic derivatives of the pregut and their complications. Thorax 28:424, 1973.

Koop CP, Kiesewetter WB, and Horn RC: Neuroblastoma in childhood: an evaluation of surgical management. Pediatrics 16:652, 1955.

Kuipers F and Wieberdink J: An intrathoracic cyst of enterogenic origin in a young infant. J Pediatr 42:603, 1953.

Lack EE, Weinstein HJ, and Welch KJ: Mediastinal germ cell

tumors in childhood: a clinical and pathological study of 21 cases. J Thorac Cardiovasc Surg 89:826, 1985.

Ladd WE and Scott HW Jr: Esophageal duplications or mediastinal cysts of enteric origins. Surgery 6:815, 1944.

Laipply TC: Cysts and cystic tumors of the mediastinum. Arch Pathol 39:153, 1945.

Lambert AV: Etiology of thin-walled thoracic cysts. J Thorac Surg 10:1, 1940.

Leagus CJ, Gregorski RF, Crittenden JJ et al: Giant intrapericardial bronchogenic cyst. J Thorac Cardiovasc Surg 52:581, 1966.

LeGolvan DP and Abell MR: Thymomas. Cancer 39:2142, 1977.

Lillie WE, McDonald JR, and Clagett OT: Pericardial celomic cysts and pericardial diverticula: Concept of etiology and report of cases. J Thorac Surg 20:494, 1950.

Longino LA and Meeker E Jr: Primary cardiac tumors in infancy. J Pediatr 43:724, 1953.

McLetchie NGB, Purves JK, and Saunders RL: Genesis of gastric and certain intestinal diverticula. Surg Gynecol Obstet 99:135, 1954.

Maier HC: Bronchogenic cysts of the mediastinum. Ann Surg 127:476, 1948.

Maier HC and Sommers SC: Mediastinal lymph node hyperplasia, hypergammaglobulinemia, and anemia. J Thorac Cardiovasc Surg 79:860, 1980.

Maksim G, Henthorne JC, and Allebach HK: Neurofibromatosis with malignant thoracic tumor and metastasis in a child. Am J Dis Child 57:381, 1939.

Marsten JL, Cooper AG, and Ankeney JL: Acute cardiac tamponade due to perforation of a benign mediastinal teratoma into the pericardial sac. J Thorac Cardiovasc Surg 51:700, 1966.

Mayo P: Intrathoracic neuroblastoma in a newborn infant. J Thorac Surg 45:720, 1963.

Mixter CG and Clifford SH: Congenital mediastinal cysts of gastrogenic and bronchogenic origin. Ann Surg 90:714, 1929.

Murphy SB: Current concepts in cancer: childhood non-Hodgkin's lymphoma. N Engl J Med 299:1446, 1978.

Myers RT and Bradshaw HH: Benign intramural tumors and cysts of the esophagus. J Thorac Surg 21:470, 1951.

Nanson EM: Thoracic meningocele associated with neurofibromatosis. J Thorac Surg 33:650, 1957.

Neal AE and Menten ML: Tumors of the thymus in children. Am J Dis Child 76:102, 1948.

Nicholls MF: Intrathoracic cyst of intestinal structure. Br J Surg 28:137, 1940.

Olken HG: Congenital gastroenteric cysts of the mediastinum, review and report of a case. Am J Pathol 20:997, 1944.

Page US and Bigelow JC: A mediastinal gastric duplication leading to pneumonectomy. J Thorac Cardiovasc Surg 54:291, 1967.

Patcher MR: Mediastinal non-chromaffin paraganglioma. J Thorac Surg 45:152, 1963.

Perry TM and Smith WA: Rhabdomyosarcoma of the diaphragm, a case report. Am J Cancer 35:416, 1939.

Pickardt OC: Pleuro-diaphragmatic cyst. Ann Surg 99:814, 1934.

Pirawoon AM and Abbassioun K: Mediastinal enterogenous cyst with spinal cord compression. J Pediatr Surg 9:543, 1974.

Pohl R: Meningokele im Brustraum unter dem Bilde eines intrathorakalen Rundschattens. Röntgenpraxis 5:747, 1933.

Raeburn C: Columnar ciliated epithelium in the adult oesophagus. J Pathol Bacteriol 63:157, 1951.

Ranström S: Congenital cysts of the esophagus. Acta Otolaryngol 33:486, 1945.

Rath J and Touloukian RJ: Infarction of a mediastinal neuroblastoma with hemorrhagic pleural effusion. Ann Thorac Surg 10:552, 1970.

Reiquam CW, Beatty EC, and Allen RP: Neuroblastoma in infancy and childhood. Am J Dis Child 91:588, 1956.

Richards GE Jr and Reaves RW: Mediastinal tumors and cysts in children. J Dis Child 95:284, 1958.

Sabiston DC and Scott HW: Primary neoplasms and cysts of the mediastinum. Ann Surg 135:777, 1952.

Saini VK and Wahi PL: Hour glass transmural type of intrathoracic lipoma. J Thorac Surg 47:600, 1964.

Sakulsky SB, Harrison EG, Dines DE, and Payne WS: Mediastinal granuloma. J Thorac Cardiovasc Surg 54:279, 1967.

Salyer WR and Eggleston JC: Thymoma. A clinical and pathological study of 65 cases. Cancer 37:229, 1976.

Schowengerdt CG, Suyemoto R, and Main FB: Granulomatous and fibrous mediastinitis. J Thorac Cardiovasc Surg 57:365, 1969.

Schwartz H II and Williams CS: Thoracic gastric cysts, report of two cases with review of the literature. J Thorac Surg 12:117, 1942.

Schweisguth O, Mathey J, Renault P, and Binet JP: Intrathoracic neurogenic tumors in infants and children: a study of forty cases. Ann Surg 150:29, 1959.

Scott OB and Morton DR: Primary cystic tumor of the diaphragm. Arch Pathol 41:645, 1946.

Sealy WC, Weaver WL, and Young WG Jr: Severe airway obstruction in infancy due to the thymus gland. Ann Thorac Surg 1:389, 1965.

Seybold WD, McDonald JR, Clagget OT, and Harrington SW: Mediastinal tumors of blood vascular origin. J Thorac Surg 18:503, 1949.

Seydel GN, Valle ER, and White ML Jr: Thoracic gastric cysts. Ann Surg 123:377, 1946.

Shackelford GD and MacAlister WH: The aberrant positioned thymus. Am J Roentgenol 120:291, 1974.

Shurin SB, Haaga JR, Wood RE, and Ittleman FP: Computed tomography for the evaluation of thoracic masses in children. JAMA 246:65, 1981.

Skinner GE and Hobbs ME: Intrathoracic cystic lymphangioma, report of two cases in infants. J Thorac Surg 6:98, 1936.

Siegel MJ, Nadel SN, Glazer HS, and Sagel SS: Mediastinal lesions in children: comparison of CT and MR. Radiology 160:241, 1986.

Singleton AO: Congenital lymphatic disease—lymphangiomata. Ann Surg 105:952, 1937.

Sochberg LA and Robinson AL: Primary tumor of the pericardium involving the myocardium, surgical removal. Circulation 1:805, 1950.

Soloman RD: Malignant teratoma of the heart: report of a case with necropsy. Arch Pathol 52:561, 1951.

Soto MV: Un caso de lipoma de la cara toracica del diafragma. J Int Coll Surg 6:146, 1943.

Starer F: Successful removal of an anterior mediastinal teratoma from an infant. Arch Dis Child 27:371, 1952.

Steel JD and Schmitz J: Mediastinal cyst of gastric origin. J Thorac Surg 14:403, 1945.

Stich MH, Rubinstein J, Freidman AB, and Morrison M: Mediastinal lymphosarcoma in an infant. J Pediatr 42:235, 1953.

Stout AP: Ganglioneuroma of the sympathetic nervous system. Surg Gynecol Obstet 84:101, 1947.

Stowens D: Neuroblastomas and related tumors. Arch Pathol 63:451, 1957.

Svien HJ, Seybold WD, and Thelen EP: Intraspinal and intrathoracic tumor with paraplegia in a child; report of case. Proc Staff Meet Mayo Clin 25:715, 1950.

Swift WA and Neuhof H: Cervicomediastinal lymph angioma with chylothorax. J Thorac Surg 15:173, 1946.

Tarney TJ, Chang CH, Nugent RG, and Warden HE: Esophageal duplication (foregut cyst) with spinal malformation. J Thorac Cardiovasc Surg 59:293, 1970.

Touroff ASW and Sealey HP: Chronic chylothorax associated with hygroma of the mediastinum. J Thorac Surg 26:318, 1953.

Thompson DP and Moore TC: Acute thoracic distress in childhood due to spontaneous rupture of a large mediastinal teratoma. J Pediatr Surg 4:416, 1969.

Veneziale CM, Sheridan LA, Payne WS, and Harrison EG Jr: Angiofollicular lymph node hyperplasia of the mediastinum. J Thorac Surg 47:111, 1964.

Weichert RF III, Lindsey ES, Pearce CW, and Waring WW: Bronchogenic cyst with unilateral obstructive emphysema. J Thorac Cardiovasc Surg 59:287, 1970.

Weimann RB, Hallman GL, Bahar D, and Greenberg SD: Intrathoracic meningocele. J Thorac Surg 46:40, 1963.

Weinstein EC, Payne WS, and Soule EH: Surgical treatment of desmoid tumor of the chest wall. J Thorac Surg 46:242, 1963.

Welch CS, Ettinger A, and Hecht PL: Recklinghausen's neurofibromatosis associated with intrathoracic meningocele: report of case. N Engl J Med 238:622, 1948.

White JJ, Kaback MM, and Haller JA: Diagnosis and excision of an intrapericardial teratoma in an infant. J Thorac Cardiovasc Surg 55:704, 1968.

Williams KR and Burgord TH: Surgical treatment of granulomatous paratracheal lymphadenopathy. J Thorac Surg 48:13, 1964.

Willis RA: An intrapericardial teratoma in an infant. J Pathol Bacteriol 58:284, 1946.

Wilson JR and Bartley TD: Liposarcoma of the mediastinum. J Thorac Surg 48:486, 1964.

Wilson JR, Wheat MW Jr, and Arean VM: Pericardial teratoma. J Thorac Surg 45:670, 1963.

Wyllie WG: Myasthenia gravis. Proc R Soc Med 39:591, 1946.

Ya Deau RE, Clagett OT, and Divertie MB: Intrathoracic meningocele. J Thorac Surg 49:202, 1965.

Yater WM: Cyst of the pericardium. Am Heart J 6:710, 1931.

Cardiac Tumors

Arciniegas E, Hakimi M, Farooki ZQ et al: Primary cardiac tumors in children. J Thorac Cardiovasc Surg 79:582, 1980.

Graham HV, Von Hartitzsch B, and Medina JR: Infected atrial myxoma. Am J Cardiol 38:58, 1976.

Kilman JW, Craenen J, and Hoiser DM: Replacement of entire atrial wall in an infant with a cardiac rhabdomyoma. J Pediatr Surg 8:317, 1973.

Powers JC, Falkoff M, Heille RA et al: Familial cardiac myxoma. J Thorac Cardiovasc Surg 79:782, 1980.

Rogers EW, Weyman AE, Nobler J, and Bruins SC: Left atrial myxoma infected with *Histoplasma capsulatum*. Am J Med 64:683, 1978.

Simcha A, Wells BG, Tynan MJ, and Waterston DJ: Primary cardiac tumors in childhood. Arch Dis Child 46:508, 1971.

Van De Hauwaert LG: Cardiac tumours in infancy and childhood. Br Heart J 33:125, 1971.

Diaphragm and Chest Wall Tumors

Anderson LS and Forrest JV: Tumors of the diaphragm. Am J Roentgenol 119:259, 1973.

Bolanowski PJP and Groff DB: Thoracic wall desmoid tumor in a child. Ann Thorac Surg 15:632, 1973.

Grundy GW and Miller RW: Malignant mesothelioma in childhood. Report of 13 cases. Cancer 30:1216, 1972.

44

EMMANUEL CANET, M.D., and
MICHEL A. BUREAU, M.D., F.R.C.P.(C), F.C.C.P.

CHEST WALL DISEASES AND DYSFUNCTION IN CHILDREN

GENERAL CONSIDERATIONS

Since Lavoisier's stipulation in 1791 that respiration is essentially a phenomenon of oxygen (O_2) consumption and carbon dioxide (CO_2) production, the chest wall has been recognized to be the vital pump responsible for the movement of gases from the atmosphere into the lungs and from the lungs to the air. Today much is known about the adaptability of the vital pump to satisfy the changing metabolic needs under various physiologic and pathologic conditions (e.g., rest, exercise, hyperthermia). Also, the vital pump participates in numerous functions such as singing, talking, wind instrument playing, coughing, sneezing, and hiccupping.

Among human subjects from premature infants to the elderly, the characteristics of the respiratory pump vary considerably in bony structure and chest wall musculature, because of anatomic differences in the configuration of the chest and differences in pathologic processes involving the neuromuscular apparatus. The most important disease conditions causing dysfunction of the chest wall are reviewed in this chapter.

The Strategy of Breathing. The inspiratory and expiratory muscles that, respectively, expand and reduce the volume of the chest cage take advantage of two possibilities in the strategy of breathing. They may fix the rib cage and predominantly move the diaphragm like a piston; this type of inspiration and expiration is called *diaphragmatic breathing*, the dominant pattern of quiet breathing chosen spontaneously by most people in the supine position either awake or asleep. An alternative is *dominant thoracic breathing*, which consists of relative fixation of the position of the diaphragm by isometric contraction (with the aid of the abdominal muscles) and elevation of the ribs by the action of the inspiratory muscles of the rib cage; this type of breathing is chosen preferentially in the sitting or erect posture. Under voluntary control anyone can perform both of these maneuvers of breathing, but in certain clinical situations (e.g., quadriplegia, diaphragmatic palsy) only one type of breathing can be achieved. A mixture of the two types is the usual breathing pattern in normal humans (Fig. 44–1).

Neural Control of the Chest Wall. Considering the diversity in the basic metabolic demand to breathe and the various chest wall conditions, the respiratory system requires a remarkable feedback system, one that will inform the respiratory centers about the magnitude of the task to be accomplished as well as the capacity of the pump to perform the mechanical work of inspiration and expiration. The information

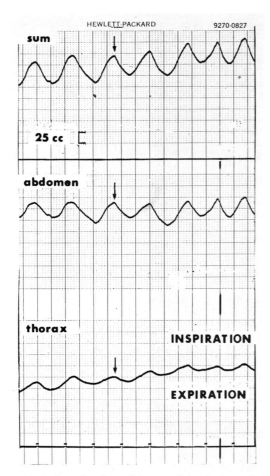

Figure 44–1. Coordination of thoracoabdominal ventilation in a 4-day-old term newborn. In supine position, breathing is due mainly to abdominal expansion with a minor contribution from thoracic expansion. These motions of thorax and abdomen are well coordinated.

fed to the center before a breath occurs must include data on the mechanical properties of the chest wall, the respiratory muscles, and the lungs. Only then can the respiratory centers smoothly coordinate the actions of the chest wall components, and only then will a normal breath occur. Despite numerous adverse clinical conditions, the gas convection (tidal volume) into and out of the lung is maintained, thereby satisfying metabolic needs. But patients must overcome adverse conditions affecting chest wall function in their strategies of breathing—conditions ranging from the pliable chest wall of the preterm infant to the scoliotic chest and from the feeble chest in neuromuscular disease to the fixed chest wall of arthritis or obesity.

The Mechanoreceptors of the Respiratory Apparatus. Even before a breath is taken, the respiratory centers must receive information about the magnitude of the task associated with the inspiration of the tidal air. In this endeavor, each successive breath is preprogrammed, so that the required respiratory muscles can be mobilized sequentially, taking into account the capacity of the muscles to perform the work demanded. The respiratory centers are in-

formed about the chest wall status by reflexes in the diaphragm, the chest wall muscles, and the intercostal and costosternal joints. The most important sensory input to the chest wall comes from the muscle spindles, which may initiate both the local spinal arc reflex and the centrally mediated reflexes. These propriosensitive receptors detect the force applied to the chest wall and the workload that is required to breathe. Additional sensory information is obtained by the costosternal and costovertebral joints, which sense any alteration in the position of the rib cage and the tension applied across the joint space, thereby informing the center about the level of the chest wall inflation. In other words, these reflexes inform the center about the level of the functional residual capacity (FRC).

Information pertaining to the airway status (irritant receptors) and the lung condition itself (J receptors in the lung, stretch receptors in the alveolar wall) is also provided for all assessments of the breathing load. Integration of this information allows the respiratory center specific control of inspiration, specific control of expiration, and specific fine control of the end of inspiration and expiration.

Control of the Chest Wall During Inspiration. Control of inspiration implies that the respiratory centers select the muscle to be recruited and determine the intensity of the muscle contraction as well as the duration of the inspiratory effort (T_i). As shown in Figure 44–1, the end product of these choices is that for each breath there is a defined tidal volume (V_t) and a total duration of the cycle (T_{tot}) (the sum of the duration of the inspiration [T_i] and the duration of the expiration [T_e]). The ratio of V_t / T_i is the mean inspiratory flow, reflecting in large part the intensity of the drive of breathing. The intensity of the effort is reflected more by the pressure (P_{di}) generated across the diaphragm to breathe than by V_t. This P_{di} is normally a small proportion of the maximum pressure ($P_{di\ max}$) that one can produce with a forceful inspiration.

Recruitment of the Accessory Muscles and the Diaphragm. In normal resting conditions, the diaphragm is the principal muscle used for inspiration. The accessory inspiratory muscles fixate the chest wall in a stable condition, opposing the inward forces produced when the diaphragm contracts for inspiration. A failure to fixate the wall would result, as it does in the case of chest wall weakness (e.g., Werdnig-Hoffman disease), in an inward motion of the chest wall or a "sucking in of the chest wall rather than fresh air" (Bryan and Wohl, 1979). With proper chest wall–diaphragm coordination, the rib cage muscles keep their tonic action, while the diaphragmatic contraction displaces the diaphragm caudally and inspires air into the lung. That inspiration lasts until the reflexes of the chest wall and the lungs tell the respiratory center to terminate inspiration.

When the workload of inspiration is increased, two phenomena occur to meet the increased demand. First, additional accessory inspiratory muscles are recruited, thereby producing an upward motion of the ribs (a bucket handle motion) that results in a more pronounced chest expansion. This added contribution of the inspiratory muscles produces an increased rate of volume inspiration, in other words a higher V_t / T_i. This rate increase, however, does not necessarily result in a higher V_t because, as a counterpart, the T_i may have been shortened. Progressive increase in workload, because of disease or an artificial workload, almost invariably results in an increase in the V_t / T_i (Fig. 44–2).

Chest Wall Muscles in the Switch from Inspiration to Expiration. The switch from inspiration to expiration is not accomplished by an abrupt "switching off" of the inspiratory muscle activity. Inspiration terminates with a kind of inspiratory hold, accomplished by a progressive phasing out of the inspiratory muscles, which thereby extend their tonic activity into early expiration and results in a relatively smooth braking of the early phase of passive expiration.

Control of Expiration and Control of FRC. Although lung deflation is driven by the elastic recoil of the lungs and chest wall, expiration is not really passive, and the control of expiration is intertwined with the control of FRC. Unless a patient is paralyzed and artificially ventilated, expiration actually is fairly active and finely controlled by the respiratory centers. First, the rate of lung deflation is established, controlled by the rate of decline of the inspiratory muscle activity during expiration. Second, the glottis constricts or dilates to modulate the rate of the expiratory flow. The narrowing of the glottis is commonly used even in normal breathing; it reduces flow rate and creates a natural airway distending pressure in the

Table 44–1. GUIDELINES FOR ASSESSMENT OF CHEST WALL FUNCTION

Clinical Evaluation
  & Chest wall configuration, e.g., scoliosis, overdistention
  & Pattern of spontaneous breathing:
    Rate and amplitude of breathing
    Thoracic and/or abdominal breathing
    Coordination or paradoxical thoracic and abdominal expansion
  & Specific maneuvers:
    Maximal variation in thoracic circumference
    Maximal excursion of diaphragm (inspection and percussion)
    Cough maneuver—feeble or strong?
Laboratory Evaluation
  & Electromyographic studies of various respiratory muscles
  & Roentgenograms (in supine position):
    Cinefluoroscopic studies of diaphragmatic and rib cage movements
    Plain roentgenograms in full expiration and inspiration
  & Real-time ultrasonography
  & Pulmonary function tests:
    Pressures: PI_{max}, PE_{max}, P_{di}
    Volumes: vital capacity, inspiratory and expiratory reserve volume, RV, TLC
    Coordination of breathing studied by magnetometers on thorax and abdomen

lung—a kind of "auto-PEEP." Third, the T_e is determined by the respiratory centers.

The FRC, which is the lung volume at which expiration ends, is finely regulated by (1) prolongation of the inspiratory muscle tonic action during expiration, so as to elevate the lung volume; (2) glottic closure, causing a back pressure into the lung volume; and (3) control of T_e—that is, as the expiratory time shortens, the expiration is terminated before full emptying of the lung can occur, thus increasing FRC.

ASSESSMENT OF CHEST WALL FUNCTION

Clinical Evaluation. Bedside evaluation of the chest wall by inspection and percussion can provide a clinician with essential information about chest wall function in a particular patient. Rate and amplitude of breathing, pattern of spontaneous breathing, maximal excursion of the diaphragm (by percussion during inspiration), maximal expansion of the circumference of the rib cage, the pattern of the chest wall motion during quiet and maximal breathing, the strength of cough maneuvers, and the symmetry and configuration of the chest all should be evaluated (Table 44–1).

Laboratory Evaluation. More precise qualitative and quantitative assessments of chest wall function can be obtained and are particularly useful in the long-term follow-up of patients with chest wall disorders. The physiology of each group of respiratory muscles can be studied with electromyography using superficial or needle electrodes. One can evaluate muscle activity during resting breathing or maximal stimulation in order to detect the level of muscle fatigue. With these methods, the electrophysiologic

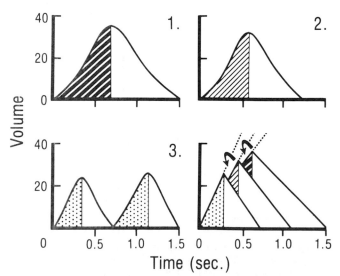

Figure 44–2. Schematic representation of the timing of the respiratory cycle and the progressive change in the strategy of breathing in patients with lung disease. In each panel, the shaded area represents the duration of inspiration (T_i) and the clear area the duration of expiration (T_e). *Panel 1,* Quiet breathing. *Panel 2,* Mild hyperventilation. *Panel 3,* Moderate to severe distress. The *lower right panel* illustrates graphically the progressive increase toward rapid shallow breathing. V_T decreases and the time of the total respiratory cycle decreases as V_T/T_i (*dotted lines*) increases.

condition of each group of inspiratory and expiratory muscles can be determined. Real-time ultrasonography is the initial means for evaluation of diaphragmatic movement in infants and children.

Simple cineradiologic studies of the rib cage and diaphragm motion during breathing maneuvers or plain roentgenograms taken on inspiration and expiration can give semiquantitative information about chest wall motion and its two components, the diaphragm and the rib cage. These studies should be done with the patient in a supine position, in order to minimize the misleading passive diaphragmatic motion due to the gravitational traction of the intra-abdominal organs, which may mimic downward motion of the diaphragm if the patient is upright.

With pulmonary function tests, the strength of inspiratory and expiratory muscles can be assessed by simple devices measuring the maximal mouth pressures generated by inspiratory or expiratory maneuvers against an occluded mouthpiece. The strength of the inspiratory and expiratory muscles is indicated by the maximal inspiratory and expiratory pressures taken, respectively, at residual volume (PI_{max}) and at total lung capacity (PE_{max}). The strength of the diaphragm itself can be evaluated by measuring the pressure generated across the diaphragm (transdiaphragmatic pressure, P_{di}); measurements of P_{di} require the simultaneous measurement of pressures on each side of the diaphragm, pressure in the stomach, and pressure in the lower third of the esophagus (thereby measuring the combined strength of all muscles participating in these efforts).

Finally, measurements of lung volume and flow rates can be used as indirect but practical means of assessing chest wall function. Chest wall dysfunction generally leads to changes in lung volume and flow rates. Specifically, measurement of vital capacity can serve as a bedside quantitative evaluation of the restrictive defect resulting from chest wall weakness. In subjects with the polyradiculitis of the Guillain-Barré syndrome or with myasthenia gravis, such measurements of vital capacity with portable spirometers (electronic, volumetric, Wright spirometers) may be used to monitor progressive deterioration of ventilation and to guide clinicians in efforts to maintain adequate ventilation.

FAILURE OF THE CHEST WALL TO ACHIEVE ADEQUATE VENTILATORY OUTPUT

Fatigue of the Chest Wall

The respiratory muscles may become fatigued in either an acute or chronic condition. Fatigue of the respiratory pump results from an imbalance between the energy supply to the inspiratory muscles and the demand of work to be accomplished. Loss of energy supply to the muscles because of hypotension, or very low O_2 tension, also reduces the energy available for chest wall muscle activity and favors the development of respiratory muscle fatigue. The fatigued muscle shows characteristic electromyographic discharges, which appear when the respiratory muscle fails to meet the demand of breathing. The muscle cannot perform the work needed, and unless another muscle takes over, the vital pump fails and respiratory failure occurs. In an attempt to avoid fatigue, a patient may opt to diminish the effort and to use less force per breath, thereby reducing the V_t. The patient will compensate for the decreased V_t by taking more breaths per minute (see Fig. 44–2). In this pattern transdiaphragmatic pressure as a proportion of the maximal transdiaphragmatic pressure achievable ($P_{di}/P_{di\ max}$) is reduced, and as the respiratory rate increases, T_i is also reduced, thereby departing from the fatigue critical threshold.

Tension-Time as Determinant of Threshold of Fatigue. Any condition in which the *duration* of the muscle contraction (diaphragm and/or accessory muscles) is prolonged predisposes to fatigue. Any condition in which the required levels of *pressure* to be generated by the respiratory muscles are increased causes the respiratory apparatus to fatigue. Children with croup or epiglottitis present the ideal setting for fatigue because of the combination of long T_i and large P_{di} needed to produce adequate ventilation. With any given breathing condition, two important components, pressure and time, determine the tension–time index, which allows one to position the breathing pattern in relation to the critical level of function of the muscles or the threshold of muscle fatigue (Fig. 44–3).

In normal circumstances, the T_i over the T_{tot} would be approximately 35 per cent of the cycle. Because T_i represents the time during which the inspiratory muscle actively contracts, the longer the T_i the higher is the cost in energy. The shorter the inspiration duration, the lower is the energy expenditure. Thus one can predict that as fatigue is approached, T_i must be shortened to depart from the critical fatigue zone.

The magnitude of the inspiratory effort is measured by transdiaphragmatic pressure (P_{di}) as a proportion of the maximum transdiaphragmatic pressure one can produce ($P_{di\ max}$). This effort may be related to the fatigue threshold of the respiratory pump. For instance, as measured by the P_{di}, each normal breath lies in the range of 10 per cent of the maximum breathing effort that can be produced by the inspiratory muscles. As long as P_{di} is below 40 per cent of the maximum that can be produced, an individual can breathe indefinitely without muscle fatigue. When P_{di} exceeds 40 per cent of its maximum fatigue will occur with a variable delay.

Signs and Symptoms of Respiratory Muscle Exhaustion. With adequate knowledge and careful bedside observation of the patient at risk for respiratory muscle exhaustion, one can quite easily recognize the progression of fatigue and can intervene before a catastrophic but predictable respiratory arrest occurs.

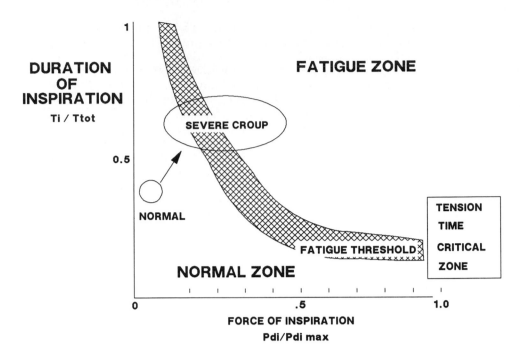

Figure 44–3. Schematic representation of the relationship between the duration of inspiration and the force of inspiration in positioning the breathing in regard to the threshold of fatigue. The shaded zone reflects the variability among individuals in the threshold of fatigue. Normal subjects having a low T_i/T_{tot} and a low inspiratory effort can sustain breathing indefinitely. With disease, the fatigued zone could be reached because of the increase in inspiratory force or inspiratory duration. Patients with croup experience an increase in both inspiratory force and inspiratory duration, which favors the occurrence of fatigue.

These signs and symptoms are based on the progressive loss of the nonrespiratory function of breathing as well as an inappropriate respiratory rate and pattern of breathing, and a few warning signs (Table 44–2).

First, with respiratory distress, a progressive loss of the nonventilatory function of breathing occurs. One must take note of any progressive loss in the capacity to pause breathing voluntarily, eat, drink, talk, or cough. All these usual functions require a critical ventilatory reserve. Coughing (other than a superficial cough), for example, requires a deep breath, an inspiratory hold, and a prolonged forceful expiration. This requires both energy and ventilatory reserves. A loss of coughing capacity or other nonbreathing functions of the respiratory apparatus therefore indicates that a patient has lost ventilatory reserve (or force reserve) and is at great risk for exhaustion or respiratory arrest.

The simple respiratory rate is a remarkable sign. In acute diseases, one should follow the change in respiratory rate. As the load to breathe increases, the subject adopts an increased respiratory rate, thereby avoiding the critical threshold of fatigue. However, a very rapid breathing rate cannot be sustained indefinitely; it may lead to respiratory muscle exhaustion. Adults, for example, cannot sustain rates above 50 breaths/min without risk of fatigue. In our experience, rates of 70 to 75 breaths/min or greater in children 4 to 14 years of age lead to exhaustion and cannot be sustained without risk of failure. For younger children, a rate of 90 can be tolerated in children with bronchiolitis, whereas a rate of 100 to 120 can be sustained by neonates with lung disease.

The regularity of breathing as well as the pattern of the thorax and abdominal movements are critical features to observe in a patient at risk for fatigue. For instance, breathing that becomes increasingly more rapid and shallow and is interrupted by a deep breath with a pause is a sign of fatigue. Although pauses are normal in healthy subjects with a low breathing rate, they are inappropriate in respiratory distress and could be a sign of exhaustion, being brief resting pauses for the exhausted inspiratory muscles. One equivalent of a resting pause to relieve fatigue is the *respiratory alternans*, in which deep thoracic breathing alternates with deep abdominal breathing and is associated with paradoxical tho-

Table 44–2. CLINICAL SIGNS AND SYMPTOMS OF RESPIRATORY MUSCLE FATIGUE

Loss of respiratory reserve needed to perform nonventilatory functions
    Inability to eat/drink/cry
    Reluctance to pause breathing voluntarily
Major use of accessory muscles
    Sternocleidomastoid muscles, pectoral
Increase of respiratory rate to critical level
    Adolescents:] 55 breaths/min
    Children, 4–10 years:] 70–75 breaths/min
    Infants, 1–3 years:] 90 breaths/min
    Neonates:] 120 breaths/min
Signs reflecting options taken to relieve fatigue
    Reduced T_i and decreased P_{di}: very shallow breathing
    Deep breaths with a brief pause to rest the muscles
    Respiratory alternans
Appearance of warning signs indicating pending respiratory arrest
    Cyanotic spell
    Cyanosis with brief cough or brief pause
    Inappropriate pause
    Sustained paradoxical thoracic/abdominal movement
    Drooling in absence of airway obstruction (cannot pause to swallow)
    Central nervous system signs (confusion)

racic/abdominal excursion. This means that to rest the fatigued diaphragm, an individual takes a thoracic breath while the diaphragm rests, and the abdomen paradoxically draws in as the chest expands. The reverse movement of large abdominal breaths with thoracic drawing inward indicates a rest being given to the accessory muscles. All these are signs of advanced fatigue.

In the extreme, major warning signs occur and should suggest measures to help the respiratory apparatus before an arrest occurs. These are extremely shallow breathing, pauses with cyanosis, and complete incapacity to cough.

Acute and Chronic Respiratory Muscle Fatigue. Acute fatigue is characterized by progressive exhaustion of the respiratory muscles, leading within minutes or hours to respiratory insufficiency. For pediatricians, the best examples of conditions leading to acute fatigue are patients with croup or epiglottitis. For these patients, the time to work (T_i) is too long and the time to rest (T_e) between each breath is too short in regard to the high inspiratory force they require. When severe, such high $P_{di}/P_{di\,max}$ and high T_i/T_{tot} lead to acute fatigue (Fig. 44–3). In these circumstances, complete respiratory arrest is preceded by respiratory pauses and cyanotic spells. The only therapy for such respiratory failure is to relieve the load of breathing against the narrowed airway by intubation. Surprisingly, immediately after the intubation, the exhausted respiratory muscles will recuperate and, within 5 to 10 minutes, will be capable of sustained spontaneous breathing.

Chronic respiratory muscle fatigue is not as easily identified as the acute form. In certain clinical conditions in which the mechanical load of breathing is high, such as in patients with long-standing severe scoliosis or patients with weakness of the respiratory muscles (e.g., Duchenne muscular dystrophy), researchers have found that therapy involving intermittent rest of the respiratory muscles improved patients' respiratory condition. The clear benefit of providing overnight mechanical support to rest the respiratory muscles led to the recognition that these muscles must be in a state of chronic fatigue. In such conditions, periodic mechanical support in the form of nasal continuous positive airway pressure (CPAP), nasopharyngeal ventilation, or chest wall cuirass is less invasive than intubation or tracheostomy.

Methods to Improve Respiratory Muscle Performance. Adequate nutrition is essential for the respiratory muscles. Patients with a chronic condition (e.g., cystic fibrosis or severe asthma) are commonly malnourished, a state that can lead to muscle atrophy and loss of respiratory muscle capacity to perform the work of breathing. An adequate O_2 supply is also needed for the muscles to perform their work. Thus nutritional support and O_2 supplementation may improve respiratory muscle function. To help the chronically fatigued respiratory muscles, periodic ventilatory support is useful for the sequential resting of the respiratory apparatus (as discussed earlier).

Finally, drugs such as caffeine and theophylline are advocated to increase the performance of respiratory muscles.

CAUSES OF CHEST WALL DYSFUNCTION

Chest wall movement should be envisioned as the result of a chain of effectors that successively transmit the drive to breathe from the respiratory center to the upper motor neurons of the central nervous system, the lower motoneuron, and finally the respiratory muscle fibers. The central drive to breathe is transformed into a mechanical force resulting from contractions of respiratory muscles, which move the chest wall and generate inspiratory and expiratory pressure responsible for air movement into and out of the lungs. Thus, motion of the chest wall may be impaired by physiologic disturbances occurring at the various levels of effectors, namely the upper and lower motor neurons, the muscular fibers, and the mechanical architecture of the bony structure of the thorax. Table 44–3 shows the systemic conditions that cause disturbances at these different levels. They are briefly described here, but more detailed discussions of the major diseases appear later in this chapter.

Table 44–3. CAUSES OF CHEST WALL DYSFUNCTION ACCORDING TO SITE OF DEFECT

Site of Defect	Causes
Central drive of breathing	Congenital or acquired
Upper motor neuron	Hemiplegia
	Cerebral palsy
Lower motor neuron	Quadriplegia
	Poliomyelitis
	Guillain-Barré syndrome
	Tetanus
	Progressive spinal atrophy (Werdnig-Hoffman paralysis)
	Traumatic nerve lesions
	Phrenic nerve paralysis
Neuromuscular junction	Myasthenia gravis
	Botulism
	Antibiotic intoxication
Respiratory muscles	Duchenne muscular dystrophy
	Myotonic dystrophy
	Muscle dysfunction due to connective tissue disease
	Friedreich ataxia
	Congenital myopathies
	Metabolic myopathies
	Steroid myopathy
	Diaphragmatic malformation (eventration, hernia)
Chest wall bony structures	Scoliosis
	Rib cage abnormality
	Overinflated chest in obstructive disease
	Fixation of thoracic wall in connective tissue disease
	Thoracic burns
	Obesity
	Eventration
Diaphragmatic disorders	Malformation (hernia, eventration)

Neurologic diseases, at the level of the central nervous system (upper motor neurons) or at the level of peripheral innervation of the chest wall (lower motor neurons), may lead to secondary dysfunction of the muscular components of the chest wall. The best examples of these entities are hemiplegia, quadriplegia, poliomyelitis, progressive spinal atrophy (Werdnig-Hoffman paralysis), and polyradiculitis (Guillain-Barré syndrome).

Muscular disease from various types of muscular dystrophy and myasthenia gravis results in failure of the respiratory muscles to produce an adequate contraction. Also, various conditions (e.g., severe prematurity) and systemic diseases (e.g., connective tissue disease, severe malnutrition) may lead to a loss in respiratory muscle mass and thereby may diminish the power of the neuromuscular apparatus of the chest wall; this weakness results in poor movement of the chest wall and consequently contributes to ventilatory failure.

Malformation of the chest wall architecture, either congenital or acquired, impairs the transformation of the muscle contraction into adequate pressure required by the vital pump to ventilate properly. The chest wall functions as a system of levers, and various anatomic distortions of the chest wall cause a loss of efficiency of the respiratory apparatus, which when extreme results in ventilatory failure. Conditions such as scoliosis, bronchiolitis, and advanced cystic fibrosis diminish ventilatory efficiency because malpositioning of the respiratory muscles makes it difficult to generate adequate inspiratory pressure in a distorted or overdistended chest. Finally, obesity causes an additional mechanical load on both the thoracic and abdominal components of the chest wall and limits its performance capacity.

Increased Resistance of the Chest Wall to Breathing. Most diseases leading to chest wall dysfunction increase the resistance of the chest wall to breathing either at rest or during exercise. A study of scoliotic subjects showed that the compliance of the respiratory system, particularly of the chest wall, was reduced in proportion to the degree of the chest deformity. Similarly, in obese subjects, the accumulation of fat over the thoracic and abdominal walls leads to a loss of the elastic properties of the respiratory system. Even in individuals with impairment of only the innervation (e.g., polyomyelitis) or muscular dysfunction (Duchenne muscular dystrophy, Steinert's disease), the elastic properties of the respiratory system are decreased and the performance of the respiratory system is diminished.

Functional Similarities Among the Various Causes of Chest Wall Dysfunction. Despite their major differences in pathogenesis, the various entities that cause chest wall dysfunction share some clinical and physiologic features. Chest wall dysfunction leads to restrictive pulmonary disease with reduced pulmonary volume, reduced absolute values of flow rates, reduced strength of inspiratory (PI_{max}) and expiratory (PE_{max}) muscles, and decreased ventilatory

performance in response to exercise or to CO_2 (Fig. 44–4). All these diseases reduce the capacity of the chest wall to perform as the vital pump, and affected patients are prone to respiratory insufficiency during critical periods of their lives, such as the time of first breath, periods of pulmonary infection, following general anesthesia, and during the last trimester of pregnancy. The sequence of events leading to respiratory failure in these diseases is illustrated in Figure 44–5.

SKELETAL ANOMALIES

SCOLIOSIS

Scoliosis is not a disease but the result of an underlying pathologic process leading to lateral curvature of the spine. In rare instances, the lateral curvature may be associated with anterior angulation of the spine, and the chest distortion then is called kyphoscoliosis.

The curvature of the spine causes a rotation of the vertebral bodies and distortion of all attached structures. The rotation of the ribs accounts for the characteristic posterior prominence of the rib cage on the convex side of the curve, with anterior flattening and widening of the interspaces. The concave side manifests the opposite deformity. As a consequence of such chest distortions, scoliotic patients suffer from anatomic deformity of the chest and functional pulmonary disability. The effects of scoliosis on pulmonary disability and the reduced life expectancy (see below) have resulted in the development of screening programs in school-age children. The goal of such programs is to detect scoliosis early enough in the course of the disease so that proper therapy can be implemented, thereby avoiding curve progression, subsequent chest wall deformity, and cardiopulmonary dysfunction.

Classification. Etiology determines the basis of the

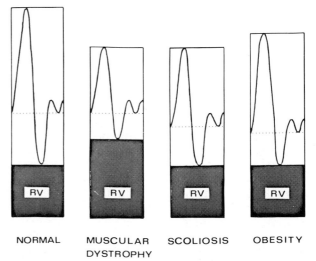

Figure 44–4. Changes in lung volume in diseases characterized by chest wall dysfunction.

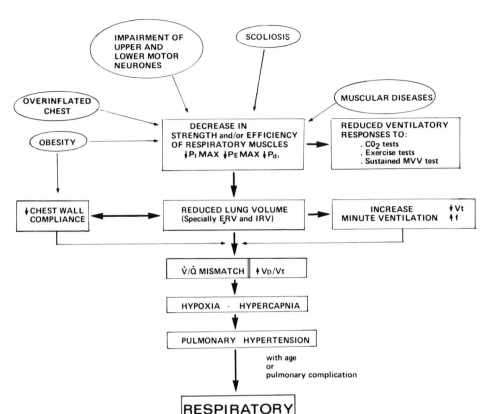

Figure 44–5. Schematic presentation of the pathogenesis of respiratory failure in diseases with chest wall dysfunction.

most commonly used classification of scoliosis (Table 44–4). Idiopathic scoliosis, which accounts for approximately 80 to 85 per cent of all lateral spine curvatures, is categorized into three types—infantile, juvenile, and adolescent—according to the age at which the deformity is first noted. It is defined as a

Table 44–4. CLASSIFICATION OF SCOLIOSIS

Idiopathic (85% of all scoliosis)
  Infantile (¢ 3 years old)
  Juvenile (3–9 years old)
  Adolescent (10 years old to skeletal maturity)
Congenital (5% of all scoliosis)
  Failure of formation (hemivertebra)
  Failure of segmentation
  Mixed
Neuromuscular (5% of all scoliosis)
  Neuropathic
    Lower motor neuron (e.g., poliomyelitis)
    Upper motor neuron (e.g., cerebral palsy)
    Other (e.g., syringomyelia)
  Myopathic
    Progressive (e.g., muscular dystrophy)
    Static (e.g., amyotonia)
    Others (e.g., Friedreich ataxia)
Associated neurofibromatosis (von Recklinghausen disease)
Mesenchymal
  Congenital (e.g., Marfan syndrome)
  Acquired (e.g., rheumatoid disease)
  Others (e.g., juvenile apophysitis)
Trauma
  Vertebral (e.g., fracture, radiation, surgery)
  Extravertebral (e.g., burns, thoracoplasty)
Secondary to irritative phenomenon (e.g., spinal cord tumor)

structural spinal curvature for which no specific cause can be established. Nevertheless, numerous factors are known to cause scoliosis, and a primary etiology for spinal deformity, such as congenital scoliosis or neuromuscular diseases, should be systematically sought. A classification system using radiographic measurement of the severity of the curve (Cobb angle), as well as determination of the curve pattern, based on the level of the apex of the spinal curvature (cervical, high thoracic, thoracic, thoracolumbar, lumbar), and the number of structural curves (single or double) permits comparisons, prognostication, and the development of treatment guidelines.

Prevalence. In the general population, the prevalence of a structural lateral curvature of the spine of 10 degrees or more is approximately 2 to 3 per cent, although it becomes 0.5 and 0.2 per cent for curve magnitudes of greater than 20 degrees and 30 degrees, respectively. Although various female-to-male ratios have been reported, all authors agree that juvenile and adolescent idiopathic scoliosis occur more frequently in girls than boys and that the reverse is true for infantile idiopathic scoliosis. They claim, furthermore, that this female-to-male ratio is augmented with increased curve magnitude.

Natural History. The study of the long-term evolution of previously untreated scoliotic patients forms the basis for our understanding of the natural history of scoliosis. Although the natural evolution of scoliosis is associated with such problems as curve progression, cardiopulmonary impairment, back pain, cosmetic deformity, and neurologic compromise, the natural history of scoliosis varies greatly depending on such factors as specific etiology, age of onset (congenital, infantile, juvenile, or adolescent) (Fig. 44–6), genetic background, and curve pattern.

A summary of the natural history of idiopathic scoliosis in adolescents, derived from studies of large cohorts of untreated adolescents who had severe idiopathic scoliosis and were followed from 1913–1918 to 1963, demonstrates a death rate 2.2 times greater than in a normal group. These deaths, due to cardiopulmonary insufficiency, generally occurred in the fourth or fifth decade of life. Most of the survivors showed significant physical disability characterized by dyspnea, backache, and exercise limitation (Nachemson, 1968; Nilsonne, 1968; Bjure and Nachemson, 1973).

Juvenile scoliosis represents a gradual transition from the characteristics of infantile curvatures to those of adolescents.

Children who have infantile scoliosis and who are untreated and followed to maturity are generally found to have severe and crippling deformities, with a spinal curvature usually exceeding 70 degrees; spontaneous regression of the scoliosis can, however, occur in various proportions (10 to 60 per cent) of patients.

Congenital scoliosis is usually progressive as well and, if untreated, results in severe spinal deformity. The ultimate severity of the curve depends on both the type of anomaly and the site at which it occurs. The most progressive of all anomalies is a concave, unilateral unsegmented bar with a convex hemivertebra.

In both infantile and congenital scoliosis, death may occur before adulthood as a result of cardiopulmonary insufficiency. The vast majority of individuals with scoliosis never develop cardiorespiratory failure, however. In fact, cardiorespiratory failure is rarely reported in childhood. Pulmonary function impairment has been correlated to the degree of spinal curvature, and a Cobb angle greater than 90 degrees is usually a prerequisite for risk of cardiopulmonary failure by way of alveolar hypoventilation, pulmonary arterial hypertension, and cor pulmonale.

The need to prevent curve progression is clearly shown by the long-term follow-up studies of untreated patients who have well-demonstrated deleterious effects of severe spinal deformity. Because prevention of cardiorespiratory failure, cosmetic deformity, and back pain depends on early detection and proper management of scoliosis, school screening programs of 10- to 14-year-olds are advocated. The goal is to detect scoliosis before the adolescent growth spurt. Pilot projects have already established that such school screening decreases the number of curves of severe magnitude and the number of affected patients requiring surgery. The late complications of scoliosis should be reduced thereby as well.

Each individual with scoliosis has his or her own natural history, and prognosticating the risk of spinal curve progression is difficult. Nevertheless, a preliminary identification of the risk factors of progression is possible. (1) For infantile idiopathic scoliosis, a distinction can be drawn between resolving and progressing curves, based on the radiologic assessment of the relationship between the apical vertebra of thoracic curves and its ribs. (2) For other forms of idiopathic scoliosis, a range of factors related to curve progression should be taken into account, including chronological age, pattern and magnitude of the curve, maturity of the patient, and sex. For example, a mild curve ($\leq$ 19 degrees) in a mature boy means that the incidence of progression will be very low, but a large curve (> 20 degrees) in an immature girl means that the risk of progression will be high (20 per cent for a 20-degree curve and 70 per cent for a 30-degree curve).

Signs and Symptoms. In the vast majority, scoliosis is painless and asymptomatic. It is important to complete a careful clinical history and physical examination when scoliosis is detected. The goal is to determine the underlying cause and to evaluate the health, physical fitness, physiologic maturity, and cardiorespiratory symptoms (such as dyspnea, cyanosis, exercise limitation) of the patient. As a general rule, respiratory disability is encountered in patients with spinal angulation of 90 degrees or more. Auscultation of the convex side of the lung usually reveals a normal vesicular sound, while on the concave side the alveolar sounds are decreased. Crackles are occasionally heard at the lower axillary line on the concave side. These are caused by poor aeration of the dependent section of the lung on the concave side. A careful examination of a patient's specific pattern of breathing, maximal thoracic expansion, and diaphragmatic movement should be done. Chest roentgenograms taken on inspiration and expiration are also valuable tools for quantifying the magnitude of the chest wall movement (Fig. 44–7). Specific

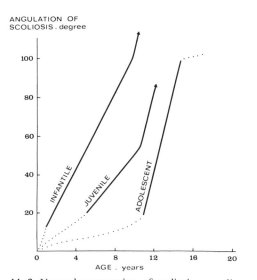

Figure 44–6. Natural progression of scoliosis according to age at the onset of spinal angulation.

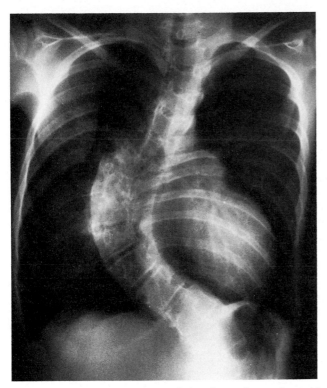

Figure 44–7. Roentgenogram of the chest of a patient with moderate scoliosis (78 degrees). The lung on the convex side (right lung) is larger than that on the concave side (left lung). In comparison to the concave side, the convex hemithorax has a larger minute ventilation and a larger motion of the diaphragm.

roentgenograms of the spine (upright anteroposterior) are required as well for a precise evaluation of the spine (pattern, angle, magnitude, and flexibility of the curvature; integrity of the vertebral bodies) and for a determination of the skeletal maturity.

Pulmonary Function in Scoliosis. The impairment of pulmonary function in scoliosis has been studied by numerous investigators, all of whom generally agree that (1) spinal curvatures of more than 90 degrees greatly predispose the scoliotic individual to cardiorespiratory failure, (2) detectable pulmonary function abnormalities occur when the degree of scoliosis is 50 to 60 degrees, (3) scoliotic lung functions are of the restrictive type, and (4) the duration of the scoliosis correlates with the patient's degree of disability.

Lung Volume. The degree of restrictive lung disease produced by scoliosis is related to the severity of the scoliosis. Among patients with moderate to severe scoliosis, a negative linear correlation has been established between magnitude of the curve and forced vital capacity (FVC) (Fig. 44–8). In some persons with mild scoliosis (e.g., Cobb angle less than 35 degrees), a reduction of lung volume has also been reported, although no correlation between the magnitude of the curve and lung volume has been clearly established. Total lung capacity (TLC) decreases in proportion to the fall in FVC, although the residual volume remains more or less within the predicted normal values, unless the scoliosis has pro-

gressed to a severe degree, in which case residual volume (RV) declines a little. The FRC is slightly diminished as well, and both the RV/TLC and FRC/TLC ratios are increased, not because of an obstructive airway disease but because of the relative decrease in TLC with almost normal RV. In addition, although the absolute values for anatomic and alveolar dead space are believed to remain normal, the ratio of V_d to V_t is increased and plays a major role in the development of alveolar hypoventilation.

The traditional wisdom has been that three factors—reduction of chest wall compliance, impaired lung growth, and/or impaired respiratory muscle strength—account for the effects of scoliosis on lung function. Patients with mild to moderate idiopathic scoliosis have been reported to have a correlation between the decrease in maximum inspiratory pressure and the fall in FVC, even though maximum expiratory pressure was normal (Cooper et al., 1984). This finding suggests that in scoliotic patients with chest deformity, inspiratory muscles work at a mechanical disadvantage, thereby accounting for the reduction in lung volume.

Respiratory Flow Rate and Airway Resistance. In scoliotic patients, expiratory flow rates—as measured by peak flow, maximal midexpiratory flow ($FEF_{25-75\%}$), and FEV in 1 sec (FEV_1)—fall in proportion to the restricted lung volume. The FEV_1/FVC ratios are normal, however, suggesting that the decrease in absolute flow rate is due to the small lung volume rather than to airway obstruction. In particular, the reduced peak flow, which is effort dependent, can be attributed to the disadvantageous working conditions of the respiratory muscles while the airway resistance may be normal or slightly increased. Furthermore, it has been proposed that the chest distortion causes airway distortion, thereby contributing to the slight increase in airway resistance.

Mechanics. Decreased chest wall compliance, cou-

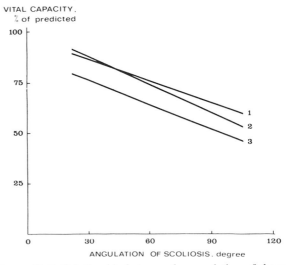

Figure 44–8. Relationship between the angulation of the spine and vital capacity in children and young adults with scoliosis. These regression lines are derived from studies of Westgate (1969), Weber (1975), and Mankin (1964).

pled with reduction of the resting point of the chest wall, plays an important role in the impairment of lung volumes (Bergofsky, 1986). Lung compliance is also reduced, but the reduction is not as great as that of the chest wall. Reduction of lung compliance may be attributed to compression of the lung, reorientation of surface tension forces, and/or alteration of elastic properties of the lung. Moreover, the decrease in compliance in the respiratory system may account for the increased work of breathing as well as the increased O_2 cost of ventilation reported in scoliotic patients.

Chest Wall Movement. Little information is available about breathing strategies and the susceptibility to respiratory muscle fatigue of scoliotic patients. The thoracoabdominal respiratory coordination of these patients is still another area that needs to be explored. Only a few radiologic studies have been carried out, and they show that movements of the diaphragm are not only well preserved in scoliotic subjects, but greater on the side of the convex spinal curve. In addition, measurements of the thoracic wall expansion are reported to vary considerably, from almost no expansion of the chest circumference to normal thoracic movement.

Regional Ventilation and Perfusion. Investigators who have used radioactive gas inhalations (^{133}Xe) to study alveolar ventilation in young subjects with scoliosis have found almost normal values. In effect, the lung on the convex side (the larger lung) receives a greater volume of alveolar ventilation than the lung on the (smaller) concave side. Numerous investigators, however, have also documented air "maldistribution" in severe scoliotic patients and have concluded that alveolar gas maldistribution is correlated with both the angulation of the spine and the age of the patient. Their finding that the closing volume, which is an indirect measurement of air distribution, was abnormal only in older patients is in agreement with the finding of pulmonary air mismatching in adult scoliotic individuals.

Blood Gases. Scoliotic persons commonly exhibit mild hypoxemia with normocapnia, a characteristic presumably related to the ventilation-perfusion ratio ($\dot{V}/\dot{Q}$) mismatch. In severe scoliosis, hypoxemia could also be attributed to diffusion limitation and/or alveolar hypoventilation and, as a consequence, be linked to CO_2 retention. The elevated V_d/V_t ratio contributes to alveolar hypoventilation.

Response to Exercise and to CO_2 Inhalation. Resting ventilation is increased in scoliotic patients, who thereby maintain a normal Pa_{CO_2} level despite an increased V_d/V_t ratio and an abnormal $\dot{V}/\dot{Q}$. But when ventilation of scoliotic patients is challenged by an exercise tolerance test or CO_2 inhalation, the magnitude of the ventilatory response is lower than in normal subjects. Exercise challenge in individuals with mild scoliosis may be the first evidence of respiratory impairment. Reduced respiratory system compliance, increased work of breathing, and a pos-

sibly defective respiratory drive presumably account for their lower ventilatory performances. In scoliotic patients, the effect of exercise on the pulmonary circulation is related to the degree of scoliosis. The mean pulmonary arterial pressure (PAP) increases linearly with O_2 consumption, and the maximal O_2 consumption achieved during exercise testing shows a direct relationship with the vital capacity and the degree of scoliosis. However, in contrast to normal persons, in whom exercise tolerance is usually limited by the circulation, the exercise ability of scoliotic patients is limited by ventilatory factors.

The strategy of breathing adopted by scoliotic patients during hypercapnia or exercise testing combines a reduced V_t and an increased frequency, a pattern similar to that reported in elastic loading experiments performed with healthy subjects. In these conditions of mechanical disadvantage, such a strategy of breathing is adopted to minimize any increase in the work of breathing.

Cardiorespiratory Failure in Scoliosis. In scoliotic patients, cardiorespiratory failure and premature death have been recognized since the time of Hippocrates. The former is rarely reported in scoliotic children, however.

Cardiorespiratory failure generally occurs in scoliotic patients whose curve magnitudes are greater than 90 degrees; it is more likely in those with an upper thoracic curve pattern, an associated thoracic lordosis, a structural abnormality of the vertebral body, or a demonstrable weakness of the respiratory muscles. Severe scoliosis leads to respiratory failure through alveolar hypoventilation, to circulatory failure through pulmonary arterial hypertension, and as a consequence to cor pulmonale. The suggestion has been advanced that alveolar hypoventilation initially occurs at night, especially during rapid-eye-movement (REM) sleep, and that it plays a major role in the development of pulmonary hypertension. Patients with moderate to severe scoliosis should therefore be evaluated for respiratory impairment during sleep, and if needed, overnight noninvasive ventilatory support should be proposed. The area of respiratory impairment during sleep in children with mild to moderate scoliosis has not been studied.

Pathologic Studies. The exact effect of the chest deformity on the growth of the lungs of scoliotic children remains unclear. Nevertheless, post-mortem quantitative studies of lung morphology in such children have led to the proposal that it is the scoliosis that occurs before completion of pulmonary growth that is likely to alter pulmonary development. In effect, because the number of alveoli normally increase until about 8 years of age and maximal alveolar size is not reached until adulthood, the occurrence of scoliosis in children is likely to alter the final gas exchange surface.

Pathologic studies of the lungs of scoliotic children and adults show that they are macroscopically abnormal in appearance because they have been molded by the chest deformity. A microscopic analysis of lung tissue, however, shows little abnormality. In scoliosis of early onset (congenital or infantile), alveolar multiplication is affected, whereas in idiopathic scoliosis (juvenile or adolescent), the alveoli may not enlarge normally.

The number of pulmonary vessels in scoliotic children is also reduced, and in proportion to the status of the lung's development. In addition, there have been reports of smooth muscle hypertrophy in media of pulmonary arteries and arterioles in long-standing scoliotic subjects. This finding, accounting for chronic pulmonary hypertension, probably results from chronic hypoxia or from the abnormal growth of the arteries because of the small lung.

Management. The management of scoliosis depends on the age of the child and the degree of scoliosis, as well as the underlying condition that led to the scoliosis.

CONGENITAL AND INFANTILE SCOLIOSIS. Because it is difficult to stop the progression of the spinal curve in these children and because the consequences of a severely deformed and rigid chest can be catastrophic on a rapidly growing lung, both congenital and infantile scoliosis should be considered to be serious conditions. Most cases of congenital scoliosis are progressive and do not respond to orthoses. For most of the patients, the treatment of choice is therefore based on a spinal fusion performed before severe deformity occurs. For infantile scoliosis that is progressive, active treatment is mandatory and generally based on serial body casting under anesthesia. Failure to control the curve by orthosis warrants surgery involving spinal instrumentation or spinal fusion. More than at any other age, spinal fusions done in infancy to arrest the progression of the curve will result in a short trunk. The consequences are severely restricted lung volume, reduction of the gas exchange surface of the lungs, and failure to thrive. For patients with nonprogressive spinal curves, a close follow-up should be instituted until skeletal maturity is attained.

JUVENILE SCOLIOSIS. For children with nonprogressive spinal curves of less than 20 degrees, a careful follow-up rather than intervention is the rule. A particularly careful follow-up is required at the time of the adolescent growth spurt. Children with a progressive spinal curve should be treated with a brace; those whose curve progression has not stopped or who have spinal curves greater than 40 degrees will require surgical treatment. Whenever possible, fusion should be delayed until the onset of the adolescent growth spurt.

ADOLESCENT SCOLIOSIS. The management of adolescent scoliosis should start with early detection, based on school screening programs before the time of the adolescent growth spurt. In skeletally immature patients with curves of less than 25 degrees, the risk of progression is low and a close follow-up plan may be sufficient. In patients with progressive curves greater than 25 degrees, nonoperative treatment is required. Various nonsurgical means are currently used to stop the spinal curve progression, including bracing, casting, and electrostimulation. Such orthotic management is based on a full-time (24 hours) treatment regimen, the weaning period to begin when spine growth stops. Bracing is cumbersome and limits chest wall expansion. An alternative means of therapy avoiding the adverse effects of bracing by using electrical surface stimulation has been proposed. Many theories about how electrical stimulation works have been proposed, but the mechanism remains unknown. Results comparing the effectiveness of the two techniques in halting curve progression are still controversial. It is nevertheless quite clear that uncontrolled curve progression despite nonoperative treatment or curves of greater than 50 degrees require surgical treatment (spinal fusion). Furthermore, for patients with a severe curve and associated pulmonary disability, preoperative halo gravity traction is usually proposed as a mean of improving respiratory function before surgery.

Postoperative Pulmonary Function in Scoliosis. Pulmonary complications are the principal cause of morbidity and mortality in the period immediately after surgery for scoliosis. Preoperative assessments of pulmonary functions should therefore be done as a guide to prevent postoperative complications. The most frequent respiratory problems reported in the immediate postoperative course of surgery for scoliosis include atelectasis, infiltrates, hemo/pneumothorax, pneumonia, pulmonary edema, upper airway obstruction, pulmonary fat emboli, and, as a consequence, respiratory failure. These complications require specific treatments, such as nasotracheal intubation, mechanical ventilation, chest-tube insertion with drainage, and/or antibiotic therapy. Immediate pulmonary complications result from multiple factors such as the surgical procedure itself, the degree of preoperative pulmonary disability, and the transient limitation of the chest wall expansion as a result of pain and the effect of anesthetics and analgesics. After surgery, a transient reduction of between 10 and 30 per cent of lung volumes and flow rates usually occurs and, at least in part, contributes to postoperative respiratory failure in any patient with severe preoperative pulmonary function impairment. The underlying pathologic conditions associated with scoliosis (e.g., muscle weakness) also play a part in the immediate postoperative course. In scoliosis associated with neuromuscular disease, the loss of respiratory muscle strength, the inability to clear secretions, and the impairment of laryngeal and pharyngeal secretions can increase the risk of immediate postoperative pulmonary complications.

Surgical intervention corrects the spinal curvature, but its effect on lung volume and arterial oxygenation will only become apparent late after surgery. Improvement may not be measurable for 2 years or more after surgery.

ASPHYXIATING THORACIC DYSTROPHY (THORACIC-PELVIC-PHALANGEAL DYSTROPHY)

First described by Jeune in 1954, asphyxiating thoracic dystrophy (ATD) is an autosomal recessive disorder characterized by a narrow, constricted rib cage and generalized chondrodystrophy with short limb dwarfism. Pelvic and phalangeal abnormalities, polydactyly, renal and hepatic disorders, as well as the Swachman syndrome have also been reported in conjunction with ATD.

ATD is usually diagnosed immediately after birth when the thoracic circumference is found to be much smaller than that of the head. Characteristic chest x-ray findings show a narrow and bell-shaped chest cage, with short horizontal ribs and flaring of the costochondral junctions. The clavicles are high. The hypoplastic ribs result in a fixed chest with a very small volume and poorly inflated lungs. Most patients with ATD die soon after birth as a result of respiratory failure, although less severe variants have been reported with clinical courses that vary from respiratory failure in infancy to few or no respiratory symptoms at all. In those patients who survive the neonatal period, respiratory failure may occur during infancy and childhood because of chest constriction, impairment of lung growth, recurrent pneumonia, or atelectasis. Improvement in the bone abnormalities may occur with age, however, thereby justifying life-support procedures in early life, such as long-term mechanical ventilation. In addition, thoracoplasty to enlarge the chest has been attempted with various degrees of success.

Similar severe respiratory distress leading to death in infancy or early childhood has been reported as well in other non-ATD patients with severe rib cage deformities such as thanatophoric dwarfism, achondroplasia, and chondroectodermal dysplasia.

THE CHEST WALL IN OBSTRUCTIVE PULMONARY DISEASE

In obstructive pulmonary disease, overinflation of the chest wall places the diaphragm and the other muscles of breathing in a position disadvantageous to breathing. The diaphragm is flattened, and the inspiratory force generated by contraction of these muscle fibers is lower than that generated by the diaphragm when its position is up with a normal dome. Because the ribs are in a more horizontal position, the inspiratory force generated by the intercostal muscles is also lower than that found with the ribs in their normal oblique position. The result is that the PI_{max} and PE_{max} generated in patients with obstructive pulmonary disease are lower than in normal persons. This is found in children with asthma and cystic fibrosis having moderate pulmonary disease (Table 44–5). In patients with obstructive pulmonary disease, the dysfunction of the chest wall may also be due to reduction in the mass of the respiratory muscles, which along with malnutrition and weight loss is a common finding in adults and children with the advanced form of chronic obstructive pulmonary disease.

MUSCLE DISEASES AFFECTING THE CHEST WALL

Two types of muscular dystrophies commonly lead to respiratory insufficiency before adulthood: Duchenne muscular dystrophy (DMD) and myotonic dystrophy. Other adult forms of muscular dystrophy such as fascioscapulohumeral, limb-girdle, and Becker muscular dystrophy, although they may begin in childhood, generally seem to cause no significant impairment of lung function in their early phases, leading instead to severe pulmonary disability later on in life.

DUCHENNE MUSCULAR DYSTROPHY

DMD is the most common and severe of the muscular dystrophy that afflicts humans. Inherited as an X-linked recessive trait, it has an incidence of approximately 1:3500 male births. Almost one third of the cases result from new mutations. The gene responsible for Duchenne and Becker muscular dystrophy has been localized on the short arm of the X chromosome (Xp21), and a product of the normal gene—a new protein called *dystrophin*—is lacking in DMD, although its role in terms of both function and structure has not yet been clearly defined. The disorder, which almost invariably affects boys, presents with proximal muscle weakness at 2 to 4 years of age. The progress of the disorder is fairly rapid, with the patient becoming confined to a wheelchair around 10 to 12 years of age and invariably dying prematurely before the age of 30, death due to

Table 44–5. STRENGTH OF CHEST WALL APPARATUS IN DISEASE, AS MEASURED BY MAXIMAL INSPIRATORY AND EXPIRATORY PRESSURES*

Disease	Age (years)	PI_{max}† (cm H_2O)	PE_{max}† (cm H_2O)
Asthma‡	6–19	67.9 (111.7)	84.1 (121.0)
Cystic fibrosis‡	7–20	65.2 (107.0)	98.6 (107.3)
Duchenne muscular dystrophy§	7–22	35	36
Myotonic dystrophy§	10–37	36.7 (95.3)	37.6 (95.0)

*Mouth pressures taken at residual volume and total lung capacity, respectively.
†Numbers in brackets are values measured in matched controls.
‡Data from Bureau et al, 1981.
§Data from Bégin et al, 1980.

respiratory failure in 80 per cent of cases. The impairment of pulmonary function in DMD, closely correlated with the progression of the disease, is accelerated by both the loss of ambulation and the progression of scoliosis. In the early phases of the disease, when gait is still preserved, respiratory function values are essentially normal, although a loss in the strength of the respiratory muscles is clearly apparent. In this early stage, resting ventilation, inspiratory and expiratory reserve volumes, and flow rates are normal. At that point, the functioning of the respiratory muscles is adequate for the needs of the affected children, with their low profiles of activity. Even at this stage, however, challenge tests measuring maximal ventilatory performance reveal weaknesses in the respiratory apparatus. The PI_{max} and PE_{max}, for instance, are lower than normal (see Table 44–5), and tests for maximal breathing—carried out by a maneuver of sustained maximal breathing capacity or by ventilatory response to 5 per cent CO_2—establish that children with the disease cannot produce an adequate breathing response. Thus it seems that even early in the course of DMD, the strength of the respiratory muscles is abnormally low, even though the impairment in the maximal ventilation response is not a limiting factor in the patient's daily activity.

The pulmonary disability of patients with DMD is characterized by a restrictive syndrome due to muscle weakness, muscle contractures, and spinal deformity. Serial measurements of lung volumes and maximal static pressure are essential to evaluate the progression of the respiratory system disability. A vital capacity of lower than the 30 to 35 per cent predicted and a PI_{max} of less than 25 cm H_2O can then be recognized as signs of severe inspiratory muscle weakness and impending respiratory failure. Serial measurements of vital capacity reported in absolute value have been found useful. In contrast to normal children, in whom vital capacity increases with linear growth, every patient with DMD experiences a maximum plateau in absolute vital capacity between the ages of 10 and 12 years and a progressive decrease thereafter. This maximum plateau of absolute vital capacity has an important prognostic value; an early plateau at a low absolute vital capacity indicates the possibility of early mortality. Vital capacity expressed as a percentage of its predicted value decreases regularly with age (Fig. 44–9). By the time the patient's gait is lost, there usually is a change in lung volume characterized by a loss in the inspiratory and expiratory reserve volumes; vital capacity decreases and residual volume increases, but FRC remains normal until the late stages of the disease (see Figs. 44–4 and 44–9). Total lung volume, which is almost normal at onset, decreases progressively throughout the course of the disease. Lung volumes are higher in the upright than in the supine position, because in the upright position the gravitational effect of abdominal organs on the diaphragm causes a passive downward displacement of the diaphragm. The ex-

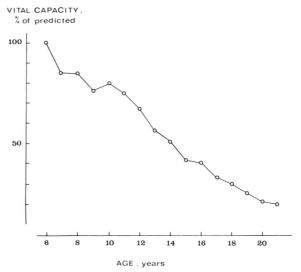

Figure 44–9. Relationship between the fall in vital capacity (in percentage of predicted) and the age of patients with Duchenne muscular dystrophy. (Reproduced with permission from Rideau Y et al: Respiratory function in the muscular dystrophies. Muscle Nerve 4:155, 1981.)

piratory flow rates (peak flow, FEV_1, $FEF_{25-75\%}$) also decrease progressively with progression of the disease. Correction of these low values of flow rate per unit of lung volume (FEV_1/FVC) and readjustment to absolute flow rates on the flow-volume curve demonstrate that the decrease in flow is due to muscle weakness and changes in lung volume, rather than to obstructive pulmonary disease.

Pulmonary mechanics seem to be well preserved in the early phases of DMD. Airway resistance and conductance are normal, and compliance is normal until the advanced stage of the disease. Diffusion capacity is normal or slightly decreased because of the decrease in lung volume. Arterial P_{O_2} and P_{CO_2} are normal or P_{O_2} is low normal. The pattern of breathing in these subjects with weakened chest wall muscles is similar to that expected when the chest of a normal subject is strapped; that is, respiratory frequency is higher than normal and V_t decreases, as a strategy to decrease the work of breathing. The drive to breathe during hypoxia and hypercapnia tests is also preserved, but dystrophic children fail to hyperventilate as much as normal children. In addition, relatively late in the course of the muscle disease, hypoventilation that is uncorrelated with the daytime respiratory function tests occurs during REM sleep. In patients with DMD, the combination of a weak diaphragm with the normal reduction in intercostal and accessory muscle tone in REM sleep probably accounts for these episodes of sleep hypoventilation. Respiratory impairment during sleep should therefore be detected early so that nocturnal hypoxemia can be identified and treated, thereby preventing pulmonary hypertension and cardiorespiratory failure. Ultimately, DMD patients suffer respiratory decompensation, with CO_2 retention and recurrent episodes of pneumonia and/or atelectasis, complicated finally by cor pulmonale. In our experience, subjects with DMD do not exhibit daytime chronic CO_2 retention until the preterminal stage of the disease. In these circumstances, respiratory insufficiency generally becomes fatal during an acute respiratory infection.

Management. In about 75 to 80 per cent of patients with DMD, death is related to respiratory insufficiency. The management of DMD should therefore be directed at slowing down and even stabilizing the progression of respiratory insufficiency and, therefore, preventing secondary skeletal or respiratory disorders. Palliative therapy based on general physiotherapy, surgery, and rehabilitation should aim at prolonging the ambulation. Scoliosis occurs in 50 to 80 per cent of children with DMD. It creates back pain, causes difficulty in positioning the patient, and also contributes to a loss of vital capacity. Management of DMD should therefore also focus on preventing spinal curve progression. Surgical correction is the treatment of choice, because spinal bracing is rarely effective in these patients and may further reduce vital capacity. Surgery should be offered to DMD patients with a Cobb angle of 30 degrees or more, provided their vital capacity is above 35 per cent of the predicted values so as to avoid respiratory failure after surgery.

Respiratory infection is a serious complication in patients with DMD, because expiratory muscle weakness impairs the power to breathe and to clear airway secretions. Afflicted children should avoid contact with individuals with respiratory infection, and preventive immunization is usually recommended. If pneumonia occurs, patients with DMD should be hospitalized for aggressive physical therapy, appropriate antibiotic treatment, and ventilatory support if needed. Deep-breathing exercise, assisted coughing, and forced expiratory maneuvers are recommended. The effectiveness of intermittent positive-pressure breathing and the training of weak respiratory muscles may not be so beneficial, however. Obesity should be curtailed in patients with DMD, and all obese patients should undergo a controlled weight-reduction program. Obesity in these patients increases the work of breathing and further compromises the chest wall disability.

Long-term ventilatory support in patients with DMD is still a subject of controversy and raises ethical difficulties that are not addressed in this chapter. In some patients with DMD, overnight studies show nocturnal hypoventilation that could be treated by noninvasive intermittent positive-pressure ventilation via a nasal mask, for example, and on a nocturnal basis. In combination with prevention of major orthopedic deformity, such therapy will not only improve the quality of life for DMD patients but will prolong life as well. It is the "resting" of the chronically fatigued respiratory muscles as well as the prevention of nocturnal hypoventilation that presumably accounts for this improvement. Whether or not nocturnal ventilatory support before the final stage of the disease actually improves daytime respiratory performance, delaying the decrease of vital capacity to its critical prefatal level, remains controversial. Such therapeutic measures are insufficient as the disease progresses: patients with DMD eventually succumb as a result of respiratory and cardiac failure due to hypoventilation or aspiration pneumonia or secondary to DMD cardiomyopathy. Although spontaneous ventilation using tracheostomy could be useful in the late stages of the disease, it prolongs life beyond the point of incapacitating bulbar weakness. The question then really focuses on the ethical considerations of therapy, what it comprises and what is undue life support in DMD. In our institution, as in many others, we do not recommend a tracheostomy and continuous respiratory support in the late stage of the disease.

MYOTONIC DYSTROPHY

Myotonic dystrophy (MyD) is an autosomal dominant, inherited, progressive disease that occurs with a frequency of between 1:7500 and 1:18,500 people. The most likely site for the MyD gene is on the short arm of chromosome 19. Marked variation in the clinical severity and age of onset has been reported. Myotonia and muscle weakness are the prominent clinical features, but many other organ systems can be affected. Involvement of the respiratory system is the major factor contributing to morbidity and mortality.

Congenital Myotonic Dystrophy. The prominent clinical features of congenital myotonic dystrophy (CMyD) are hypotonia without myotonia, feeding difficulties, and neonatal respiratory distress. The diagnosis is clinical and can be confirmed by examining the mother, CMyD being almost invariably transmitted by the mother. Hydramnios, prematurity, and pulmonary hypoplasia presumably due to the absence of fetal breathing movement account for the intrauterine onset of the disease. The frequently reported respiratory failure at birth is attributed to hyaline membrane disease, perinatal asphyxia, pulmonary hypoplasia, diaphragmatic weakness, or prematurity. Diagnosis of CMyD is delayed until the patient is recognized to be "respirator dependent for unknown reasons," especially if the mother is mildy or subclinically affected. On chest x-ray study of hypotonic infants with respiratory difficulties, hints that might suggest diagnosis of CMyD include thin ribs, possibly due to decreased activity of intercostal muscles during intrauterine life, and right diaphragmatic elevation. Hydrops fetalis with pleural effusions has also been reported. In survivors, features of the classic disease gradually appear during childhood.

It is unclear whether the neonatal-onset form of CMyD differs from the classic disease that begins in childhood. To date, although children with myotonic dystrophy have shown clinical signs of weakness of the chest wall, there have been no studies of pulmonary function in this age group nor quantitative measurements of the strength of the chest wall.

Patients with a later onset of the disease have been more extensively studied. As a predicted consequence of respiratory muscle weakness, a restrictive syndrome is commonly reported in patients with MyD. In mildly affected persons, as well as in those affected with neuromuscular disease and respiratory muscle weakness, studies show a small reduction in vital capacity and TLC and a decrease in the compliance of the respiratory system, attributed at least in part to chest wall stiffness. Even in these mildly affected individuals, the strength of the respiratory muscles is decreased, as evaluated by static maximal inspiratory and expiratory pressures and, in dynamic conditions, by maximal voluntary ventilation (MVV), suggesting that myotonia of the respiratory muscles increases the resistance of the chest wall to breathing and interferes with maximal breathing capacity. Patients with advanced MyD have severe reductions in lung volume and right-sided cardiac insufficiency.

Pathology data confirm the involvement of both the accessory muscles of respiration and the diaphragm in myotonic dystrophy. Electromyogram data are in agreement with this as well, suggesting that reciprocal inhibition among respiratory neurons is enhanced in myotonic dystrophy and that myotonia occurs in the diaphragm when loads oppose its relaxation.

The breathing pattern of affected patients is similar to that described in any patient with a restrictive syndrome due to respiratory muscle weakness; at rest there is an increased frequency of breathing with a smaller tidal volume. Chronic hypercapnia and reduced response to CO_2 rebreathing have also been reported in patients with MyD. The loss in chemical drive may add to the muscle weakness in the genesis of hypercapnia. A recent study (Bégin et al, 1980), however, argues that muscle weakness and fatigability, as well as an alteration in pulmonary mechanics, play the major role in the genesis of respiratory failure, rather than a defect of the central respiratory drive.

Respiratory failure beyond the neonatal period is rare before late adulthood. However, weakness of the respiratory muscles and the muscles of deglutition make these patients prone to postanesthetic failure, repeated aspiration pneumonia, and pulmonary infections.

NEUROMUSCULAR JUNCTION DISEASES

MYASTHENIA GRAVIS

Myasthenia gravis and the myasthenic syndrome, disorders of neuromuscular transmission associated with muscle weakness and fatigability, are attributed to various recognized pathologic mechanisms. Several distinct forms—neonatal, congenital, and juvenile myasthenia gravis—involving different pathogenic mechanisms are found in children.

Neonatal Myasthenia Gravis. This transient disorder affects 10 to 15 per cent of infants born to myasthenic mothers. It results, at least in part, from passively transmitted maternal acetylcholine receptor (AchR) autoantibodies, even if the mother has shown no clinical symptoms. In 80 per cent of affected babies, symptoms of weakness are noted on the first day, usually within hours of birth, and are resolved within 2 to 8 weeks with no recurrence.

The diagnosis relies on a transient improvement of the clinical symptoms after the administration of anticholinesterase medication: for example, edrophonium chloride (0.5 mg IV) or neostigmine methylsulfate (0.1 to 0.2 mg IM). Because paradoxical response—worsening of muscle weakness—is occasionally noted after the injection, mechanical ventilation support should be available when the test is carried out. Electrophysiologic studies and a determination of circulating AchR antibodies are also helpful diagnostic tools.

Major clinical features include feeding and respiratory difficulties, hypotonia, a weak cry, facial weakness, and palpebral ptosis. Antenatal onset of the disease with hydramnios, joint retractions, hypoplasia of the lung, and respiratory distress has also been reported. Respiratory difficulties are related to feeding problems causing aspiration pneumonia; upper airway obstruction due to inability to handle pharyngeal secretions; and/or respiratory muscle weakness and fatigability accounting for feeble cry, tachypnea and superficial shallow breathing, paradoxical inward movement of the abdomen, cyanosis, and apnea. With proper observation of the clinical signs in the neonatal intensive care unit and repeated blood gas analyses, respiratory failure should be detected early. Mechanical ventilation should then be initiated before catastrophic respiratory arrest occurs.

Management relies on anticholinesterase medication (pyridostigmine bromide, starting dose of 1 mg/kg PO [syrup], repeated four to six times a day, adjusted according to severity of the symptoms), as well as adequate feeding and respiratory support until the weakness spontaneously remits. If the response to anticholinesterase is negative, exchange transfusion or plasmapheresis should be proposed. Death due to respiratory failure may occur in the absence of adequate treatment, but the prognosis of the neonatal form of the disease is generally good.

Congenital Myasthenia Gravis. Congenital myasthenia gravis (CMG) is an umbrella term that refers to genetic disorders resulting from various specific defects in neuromuscular transmission. As such, CMG is usually characterized by an autosomal recessive inheritance, absence of myasthenia gravis in the mother, occurrence among siblings, and a wide spectrum in the age of onset. One specific form of CMG related to a defect in acetylcholine synthesis or mobilization is characterized by early onset, fluctuation of symptoms, episodic abrupt crises of muscle weakness, hypoventilation, and apnea responsible for sudden death. Diagnosis relies on family history, clinical symptoms, electrophysiologic studies, a negative determination of circulating AchR antibodies, and a positive response to the anticholinesterase medication test. Negative anticholinesterase tests are possible in some specific forms of congenital myasthenia. As in neonatal myasthenia gravis, antenatal onset of congenital forms has been reported. Management of CMG is based on anticholinesterase medication (if effective) and feeding and respiratory support. Plasmapheresis, exchange transfusion, and thymectomy are not indicated in these forms of the disease that are not immunologically mediated.

Juvenile Myasthenia Gravis. Similar to the adult form, juvenile myasthenia gravis (JMG) is an acquired autoimmune disorder of neuromuscular transmission associated with circulating AchR autoantibodies in 80 to 90 per cent of cases. The juvenile form accounts for 10 per cent of all myasthenia gravis and may present at any age during childhood, even at 6 months of age. Its clinical course, which resembles that of the adult disease, consists essentially of generalized progressive weakness in all muscles and abnormal fatigability on exertion. The disease causes a progressive decrease in the strength of the respiratory muscles, involving accessory respiratory muscles and the diaphragm. Consequently, vital capacity and TLC decrease and RV increases in proportion to the loss of expiratory reserve volume. In patients with a chronic myasthenic disorder, decrease in pulmonary compliance finally occurs. Some fulminant forms with onset of acute respiratory failure have been reported, and anticholinesterase drugs have had a dramatic life-saving effect.

Diagnosis of JMG relies on clinical symptoms, electrophysiologic studies, a positive determination of circulating AchR autoantibodies, and a transient improvement with anticholinesterase medication (edrophonium chloride, 1 to 2 mg IV, followed by 4 mg aliquots until a response is seen, or until a total dose of 10 mg is injected). Management is first based on anticholinesterase medication (pyridostigmine bromide, starting dose of 30 mg PO, repeated four to six times a day and adjusted according to the severity of the symptoms). Thymectomy and immunosuppressant drugs should be proposed for patients who present with juvenile-onset myasthenia with severe generalized weakness that does not respond adequately to anticholinesterase medication. During acute exacerbation of the disease or in the course of respiratory complications, respiratory support may be required for various lengths of time (a few days to several weeks), eventually in association with plasmapheresis. Corticosteroids and/or plasmapheresis may also be used to improve respiratory function before surgery for thymectomy.

BOTULISM

Botulism is a rare cause of neuromuscular transmission blockade in the pediatric population. The toxins (type A, B, or E) produced by *Clostridium botulinum* are responsible for the impaired release of acetylcholine at both the acetylcholine and the neuromuscular junction synapses. A specific entity, infant botulism, has been described in infants of 1 to 6 months of age. The food-borne and wound botulisms of children are similar to the adult forms. Death is usually related to pulmonary complications.

In infant botulism, *Clostridium botulinum* colonizes the infant's intestine and produces the endogeneous toxin that is responsible for the clinical syndrome. Constipation is usually the first symptom; thereafter, neuromuscular dysfunction results in progressive descending muscle weakness, with early bulbar involvement and hypotonia. Acute or progressive respiratory failure is reported in 50 to 90 per cent of affected infants. Respiratory failure results from (1) respiratory muscle weakness and paralysis, causing hypoventilation; (2) bulbar palsy and upper airway muscle weakness, leading to aspiration pneumonia and/or upper airway obstruction; and (3) an inability to clear pulmonary secretions, resulting in pneumonia and atelectasis. Endotracheal intubation should be performed whenever significant depression of the gag reflex is noted, and ventilatory support should be offered if needed. The duration of ventilatory support is variable, but affected infants usually recover fully if treated properly. In infant botulism, antitoxins have no benefit, and as for other forms of the disease, it is recommended that aminoglycoside antibiotics be avoided.

In food-borne botulism, disease is related to the ingestion of the botulism toxin, and symptoms usually occur 16 to 60 hours after toxin ingestion. The first symptoms are related to autonomic involvement; progressive generalized muscle weakness then develops and can result in respiratory failure. Careful monitoring of the clinical symptoms, vital capacity, maximum static inspiratory pressure, and arterial blood gases is useful for assessing the need for ventilatory support. The duration of the disease varies considerably, but the return of head control can still be used in the timing of attempted weanings. As long as appropriate respiratory support is provided, full recovery is the rule, and normal pulmonary function testing at 1 year has been reported for adults. Although specific and prompt antitoxin therapy can be valuable in neutralizing the toxin before all of it is bound to the axon terminals, hypersensitivity reactions are frequent.

FRIEDREICH ATAXIA

Children with Friedreich ataxia suffer from a neuromyotrophy leading to cardiorespiratory death in the second or third decade. These patients have a classic restrictive syndrome, with decrease in vital capacity and TLC and increase in RV because of loss of normal inspiratory and expiratory reserve volumes. In this disease there is a weakness of the respiratory muscles with a decline in PI_{max} and PE_{max}, which along with the progressive scoliosis is responsible for the decrease in lung volume. Unfortunately, there is no specific therapy for this disease, and physicians must aim to minimize the development of scoliosis and to treat recurrent pulmonary complications with physiotherapy and antibiotics.

WERDNIG-HOFFMAN PARALYSIS (AMYOTONIA CONGENITA)

Werdnig-Hoffman paralysis is a heritable form of spinal atrophy also known as severe spinal muscular dystrophy. In this disease, the skeletal and respiratory muscles become progressively paralyzed and atrophic because of degeneration of the lower motor neurons and atrophy of the spinal horns of the medulla. The disease occasionally begins in utero, causing lung hypoplasia, presumably due to a reduction in fetal breathing movements. It is occasionally recognized in the neonatal period, but in two thirds of patients the onset of clinical manifestations occurs in the first 6 months of life. An unusual form of spinal muscle atrophy has also been reported, presenting with respiratory failure secondary to a muscle weakness that first appears in the diaphragm. Although the prognosis varies from person to person, 50 per cent of affected infants die before 1 year of age as a result of respiratory insufficiency. The other 50 per cent progress toward respiratory failure, which usually occurs in adulthood. Because of respiratory muscle atrophy, these infants have a very feeble cry, weak cough, and recurrent pulmonary infections. Physical examination of infants with Werdnig-Hoffman paralysis shows typical paradoxical drawing inward of the chest wall with each diaphragmatic contraction (Fig. 44–10). Roentgenograms of the chest show a reduced intrathoracic volume, a bell-shaped thorax, and a paradoxical position of the diaphragm and thorax. Unfortunately, there is no therapy for this fatal disease. In our institution, we do not implement lifetime assisted ventilatory therapy in such infants.

GUILLAIN-BARRÉ SYNDROME

Guillain-Barré syndrome, an acute inflammatory demyelinating disease of the peripheral nervous system, is believed to be immunologically mediated. It is the most commonly encountered acute neuropathy in the United States (0.6 to 1.9:100,000), with 30 per cent of the cases occurring in persons younger than 20 years. About 80 per cent of the patients have a history of recent illness (cytomegalovirus, Epstein-Barr virus), surgery, or preceding innoculation. Symptoms of progressive weakness develop over several days. The evolution, complete in 2 weeks in 50 per cent of children and 4 weeks in 90 per cent of affected children, is followed by a plateau period of variable duration. Finally, a course of progressive

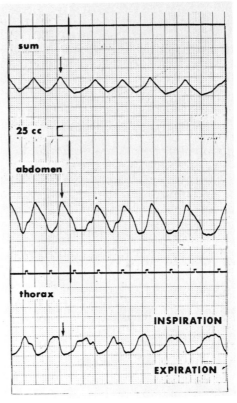

Figure 44–10. Typical paradoxical chest wall and abdominal motion during quiet breathing in an awake child of 3 months with Werdnig-Hoffman spinal atrophy. The abdominal and thoracic motions occur in opposite directions; expansion of the abdomen by diaphragmatic contraction results in severe indrawing of the chest wall (see Figure 44–1 for comparison).

recovery occurs 2 to 4 weeks after the halt of progression. Complete recovery occurs in 80 to 90 per cent of cases.

The polyradiculitis may involve various levels of lower motor neurons. A careful neurologic examination should therefore include a search for bulbar and cranial nerve involvement, which can be complicated by pharyngeal dysfunction. Dysphagia and severe bulbar dysfunction may also lead to aspiration pneumonia and obstructive apnea. Because both the accessory muscles of breathing and the diaphragm are usually affected, frequent and careful monitoring of the ventilatory function—best achieved by repeated measurements of vital capacity—is also recommended. It is also advisable to assess respiratory muscle weakness, because such weakness can lead to impairment of cough and sighing mechanisms, eventually causing pulmonary atelectasis. Reports have indicated that loss of inspiratory and expiratory volumes, resulting in a reduced vital capacity, precedes the loss of respiratory muscle strength, as measured by serial maximal static pressure determinations. This finding has been attributed to the very compliant chest walls of these children.

The most important aspect of managing the acute phase of Guillain-Barré syndrome involves management of patients with acute respiratory failure. Repeated measurements of vital capacity and arterial Pa_{CO_2} are essential aids if appropriate decisions about the use of mechanically assisted ventilation (required in 15 to 20 per cent of affected children) are to be made. Decreases in vital capacity to as low as twice the predicted tidal volume or difficulties in swallowing or handling of pharyngeal secretions are indications for intubation. Mechanical ventilation should be instituted before the level at risk for catastrophic resuscitation is reached. The duration of mechanical ventilation varies widely. When ventilation is required for only a brief period, however, it is best to use nasotracheal intubation rather than a tracheostomy. With the onset of recovery of muscle strength, slow weaning from mechanical ventilation can be started. Recovery of adequate respiratory function is the rule. Reports indicate that early use of plasmapheresis can be beneficial in very severely affected patients.

POLIOMYELITIS

Chest wall dysfunction in poliomyelitis is very similar to that in the other neurologic disease involving the lower motor neurons. Postinfection degeneration of lower motor neurons leads to respiratory muscle atrophy and loss of the chest wall's capacity to move properly. Depending on the distribution and severity of the viral inflammation of the spinal horns or neural nucleus, various permanent sequelae and different forms of restrictive pulmonary disease may occur.

OTHER PARALYTIC DISEASES

Quadriplegia and hemiplegia are known in adults to cause dysfunction of the chest wall and to decrease ventilatory performance. The consequence of the lesion of the motor neurons on breathing in neonates and children has not been evaluated, but there is no reason to believe that impairment of ventilation in children would differ from that in adults. In adults, hemiplegia and quadriplegia reduce the strength of the accessory muscles, and consequently chest expansion is compromised. This results in a decrease of inspiratory and expiratory reserve volumes and leads to decreases in vital capacity and TLC and an elevation in RV. Sustained maximal breathing capacity is reduced in proportion to the thoracic wall impairment. Expiratory flow rates are decreased in absolute values but are normal after correction of flow rates for lung volume (FEV_1/FVC). The coordination of thoracic and diaphragmatic movements is altered because of a loss in intercostal muscle function and paradoxical inward breathing movement of the thorax. Subjects with a complete spinal cord lesion are left with exclusively diaphragmatic breathing. They can perform a maximal breathing capacity that is lower than expected for normal individuals, but recent studies have shown that the performance of breathing can be improved by active training.

DIAPHRAGMATIC PARALYSIS

Unilateral diaphragmatic paralysis usually causes respiratory failure in neonates, whereas it is generally well tolerated in older children and in adults. In neonates, diaphragmatic paralysis generally results from a stretching of the root C3–C5 during birth (breech or face presentation), or injury of the phrenic nerve during thoracic or neck surgery. Tumors of the mediastinum, peripheral neuropathy, and agenesis of the phrenic nerves are less likely causes. Prominent clinical features are unexplained tachypnea, hypoxia, respiratory distress, or failure to wean from ventilatory support after surgery.

On chest x-ray, diaphragmatic paralysis should be suspected in the right hemidiaphragm if it is more than two rib spaces higher than the left hemidiaphragm; paralysis of the left hemidiaphragm results in an elevation of only one or more rib spaces above the right hemidiaphragm. Fluoroscopy or ultrasonography shows little or no diaphragmatic movement (if bilateral) and a paradoxical inspiratory upward motion of the paralyzed hemidiaphragm in a spontaneously breathing subject (if unilateral). Furthermore, repeated evaluations by fluoroscopy, ultrasonography, or electromyography in association with percutaneous stimulation of the phrenic nerve, in addition to their value for diagnosis, aid in the search for indices of improvement in the function of diaphragmatic activity.

Treatment essentially consists of ventilatory support until diaphragmatic activity recovers. In patients with permanent diaphragmatic paralysis and ventilatory failure, unilateral plication of the diaphragm may prevent the paradoxical diaphragmatic movement and improve minute ventilation. In the case of bilateral paralysis, bilateral plication should be avoided. Successful reinnervation after surgical transection of the phrenic nerve has also been reported; to be successful, such reinnervation should be attempted promptly after the diagnosis has been made.

MISCELLANEOUS DISORDERS CAUSING CHEST WALL DYSFUNCTION

OBESITY

Extreme obesity in children and adults leads to premature death of cardiopulmonary origin. The medical literature on this problem in adult subjects is abundant, but only a few reports deal with the cardiopulmonary effects of obesity in children. At first one is tempted to conclude that the effect of obesity on the respiratory system of children is not as dramatic as that reported in adults. In fact, there are fewer than 10 case reports of pickwickian syndrome in the pediatric age group. However, the pulmonary abnormalities described in obese adults result from long-standing obesity from childhood, and pediatricians should regard the lung disorders of obese adults as the long-term sequelae of obesity in their child patients.

In adults, obesity causes abnormalities of lung volume, pulmonary mechanics, work and cost of breathing, pattern of breathing, and ventilatory response to CO_2 inhalation. Most obese subjects are regarded as having simple obesity because their Pa_{CO_2} is normal. Hypercapnic obese subjects do have specific associated features and are referred to as being obese with hypoventilation syndrome (OHS) (Luce, 1980). This later syndrome was originally described by Charles Dickens in *The Pickwick Papers* in 1837 and was reviewed by Burwell in 1956. It is characterized by severe obesity, somnolence, cyanosis, periodic respiration with apneic pauses during sleep, polycythemia, right ventricular hypertrophy, right-sided heart failure, hypoxia, hypercapnia, decrease in FRC and MVV, and a decline in the ventilatory response to CO_2. All these findings usually return to normal after major weight loss.

Only about 10 per cent of adults with simple obesity develop the obesity hypoventilation syndrome. In children, pickwickian syndrome is rare, and most obese children behave like adults with simple obesity.

At rest, obese subjects have increases in O_2 consumption per minute. They adopt a pattern of breathing characterized by an increase in respiratory frequency and a decrease in the tidal volume. This pattern may be chosen because of reduced chest compliance, but it has the consequence of increasing the relative physiologic dead space (V_d/V_t). Thus obese individuals must ventilate more than normal persons for a unit of O_2 consumption, and their ventilatory equivalent $\dot{V}_E/\dot{V}_{O_2}$ is higher than in normal persons. In response to challenges of breathing, obese individuals develop a strategy characterized by a pattern of tachypnea with reduced V_t.

The lung volume is slightly modified by fat tissue load on the chest wall (Figs. 44–4 and 44–11). Inspiratory and expiratory reserve volumes are decreased, as are TLC and vital capacity, whereas RV remains normal or low normal. FRC is lower than normal. Pulmonary mechanics are altered mainly because of the decrease in chest wall compliance with a normal (or low normal) lung compliance. Airway resistance is normal. Studies of air distribution with radioactive ^{133}Xe have shown a $\dot{V}/\dot{Q}$ mismatch in obese subjects; the mismatch is worst in the supine position. Blood gas analysis generally shows low arterial O_2 tension mainly because of $\dot{V}/\dot{Q}$ abnormality. Cardiac function is essentially normal in persons with simple obesity, but studies have also revealed increases in blood volume, left ventricular work, and pulmonary artery pressure.

The only study of obese children reported normal values of lung volume, blood gases, airway resistance, and dynamic compliance (Chaussain et al, 1977). Perhaps a few decades are necessary for the full expression of obesity's effects on the pulmonary volume disturbance. However, an abnormal CO_2 re-

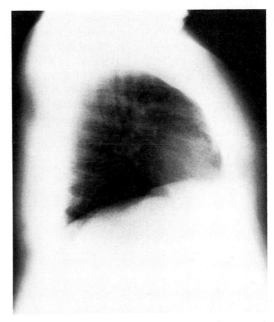

Figure 44–11. A roentgenogram of the chest of a severely obese 15-year-old. The thorax is restricted in a surrounding mass of fatty tissue.

sponse curve is present early in the course of obesity. The CO_2 response in both obese children and obese adults is decreased whether the response is measured in terms of minute ventilation or of alveolar ventilation per unit of increase in P_{CO_2}. The blunted ventilatory output of CO_2 is likely due to the mechanical limitation of the respiratory system of the obese individual rather than a loss in chemosensitivity to CO_2. Indeed, Lourenco (1969) showed that if the CO_2 response is measured by the change in diaphragmatic electromyographic activity instead of by minute ventilation, eucapnic obese subjects do have a higher than normal electromyographic response to CO_2 although they also have a blunted ventilatory response to CO_2. This suggests that the drive is normal or supranormal and that the overactive diaphragm has to work harder than normal to meet the demand of breathing, resulting in a supranormal electromyographic response but a lower than normal ventilatory response to CO_2. With OHS patients, who are CO_2 retainers, the diaphragmatic electromyographic response to CO_2 is lower than normal and is not sufficient to satisfy the demand of breathing and to overcome the mechanical load of fat around the chest wall. Both electromyographic and ventilatory response to CO_2 are blunted, and in the resting condition, CO_2 retention is found. It is still possible that the central sensitivity in OHS patients is reset to a higher CO_2 tolerance; CO_2 sensitivity may be triggered by a respiratory stimulant (e.g., progesterone) or by a major weight loss, either of which results in a decrease in arterial CO_2 tension.

CONNECTIVE TISSUE DISORDERS

Patients with advanced connective tissue diseases usually do not complain of symptoms attributed to chest wall disability. The pulmonary involvement in these diseases mainly consists of pleuroparenchymal lung disease and vasculitis, as has been extensively reviewed by Hunninghake and Fauci (1979). Nevertheless, chest wall involvement by autoimmune processes is recognized in systemic lupus erythematosus (SLE), dermatomyositis, and ankylosing spondylitis and is suspected in rheumatoid arthritis.

Symptoms of chest wall disability may not appear because the patient usually has limited activity and does not challenge the performance of the chest wall. Diaphragmatic weakness and paralysis have been reported in SLE. Dermatomyositis is known to involve all muscles and may therefore cause weakness of the respiratory muscles. In some patients with dermatomyositis, mechanical breathing support is required. In ankylosing spondylitis, the motion of the costovertebral articulations is limited, and affected patients have a typical abdominal breathing pattern. Patients with scleroderma were first believed to have limited thoracic expansion because of thickness of the thoracic wall; however, Sackner and colleagues (1964) showed that chest wall compliance is normal in this disease. In rheumatoid disease, however, the incidence of abnormalities is as high as 40 per cent in the adult population, mostly because of reduction of lung volume and pneumonitis. Bégin and colleagues (1988) reported a series of young adults who had rheumatoid arthritis but normal lungs and who had chest wall dysfunction. The dysfunction was characterized by stiffness of the chest wall, presumed to result from the involvement of the costosternal and costovertebral joint. The limited chest wall expansion resulted in a preferential shift toward a more abdominal breathing pattern. On theoretical grounds, acute myositis of respiratory muscles may also weaken chest wall function. This was reported in an 18-year-old male whose major complaint was dyspnea caused by diaphragmatic and chest wall muscle weakness as the first sign of juvenile rheumatoid arthritis (Brady and Poulson, 1984).

Most of the reports of chest wall involvement in connective tissue diseases are derived from adults, but there is no reason to believe that it does not occur in children, who often have more acute forms of connective tissue disorders than adults.

THE CHEST WALL IN PREMATURE AND FULL-TERM INFANTS

Physicians have learned from bedside observations that the bony structures of the chest wall in premature and full-term infants are much more elastic and deformable than those of adults. In newborns, the lack of rigidity of the chest wall leads to deformation and drawing inward of the ribs and even of the sternum with the simple deep inspiration that occurs in cry, hiccup, or sigh.

The diaphragm and chest wall of a neonate have not reached full maturity at birth. This immaturity causes specific problems that become apparent not in resting healthy conditions but in conditions in which full-term and preterm neonates face an increased load of breathing secondary to pulmonary disease.

Neonatal Diaphragm. The diaphragm of a neonate differs from that of an adult in terms of its position in the chest and its attachment to the chest wall; the muscle fibers of a neonate's diaphragm also differ from those of an adult. In the relaxed condition, the diaphragm of a neonate is positioned higher in the thorax than in an adult, resulting in a smaller radius of diaphragmatic curvature. This anatomic arrangement favors more efficient breathing by the neonate, provided the infant breathes quietly with small diaphragmatic excursion. With large breaths, however, problems occur. In infants, the insertion of the diaphragm to the chest wall is more perpendicular to the wall, an arrangement that favors inward displacement of the lower part of the chest wall with any forceful contraction of the diaphragm. The third difference between the adult and infant diaphragm relates to the proportion of the fatigue-resistant and fatigue-sensitive fibers found in the diaphragm. In brief, the diaphragm of an adult has a larger proportion of type I muscle fibers than in an infant. These are fast-oxidative but fatigue-resistant type I fibers. Of the rest of the adult fibers, 30 per cent are type IIA which are fast-oxidative, fatigue-sensitive fibers. In contrast, the neonatal diaphragm has only 20 per cent of the type I fibers and therefore is less resistant to fatigue.

The Chest Wall. The rib cage of a neonate is a pliable chest wall. One can calculate that contraction of the diaphragm sufficient to produce a pressure of 6 to 8 cm H_2O will suck the chest wall inward during a contraction. That is to say, if there is no muscle action taken to fix the chest wall with each inspiration, a newborn's normal breath will cause automatic inward movement of the chest wall with a proportional reduction of the inspired tidal air. This inward movement, which occurs in patients with Werdnig-Hoffman disease because they cannot fixate the rib cage with their feeble chest wall muscles while the diaphragm contracts, represents energy wastage with each breath. Excessive diaphragm contraction then has to be used to produce the same V_t.

Astute Strategies of the Neonate. To cope with the inherent difficulty of the pliable chest wall, the fatigable diaphragm, and the neonatal insertion of the diaphragm on the rib cage, a neonate in relaxed conditions uses a rapid respiratory rate with limited excursion of the diaphragm. In disease conditions, rather than increasing the depth of each breath, the neonate instead further increases respiratory rate, thereby protecting the diaphragm by a diminished duration of the inspiratory contraction. Another means of protection is to enlarge the resting gas reservoir of the lungs by increasing the level of FRC. This is also accomplished by a rapid rate of breathing, leading to early onset of each inspiration before complete expiration has occurred. Another way of increasing FRC is the use of the glottis during expiration to create a back pressure in the chest or, in other words, an automatic distending pressure or "auto-PEEP."

As a result, the high compliance of the chest wall predisposes infants to a reduction in FRC and enhances the possibility of paradoxical thoracic breathing movement and possibly of respiratory muscle fatigue. The level of FRC is the result of the elastic recoil of the lungs, which exerts an inward force on the thorax that is overcome by the outward force resulting from the rigidity of the thorax. In a premature infant, whose thorax has a weak and deformable bony structure, the recoil of the lungs reduces the intrathoracic resting volume and thereby diminishes FRC.

Lack of rigidity of the thorax explains the drawing inward of the rib cage and sternum found in physiologic conditions (cry, sigh). In disease conditions, which exaggerate the phenomenon, severe drawing inward decreases the efficiency of respiration and reduces the tidal volume, resulting in a paradoxical motion of the lower thoracic wall and the abdominal wall. The upper thorax is overinflated, and the indrawing movements should not be confused with the paradoxical breathing encountered in respiratory muscle fatigue, which is characterized by complete inward motion of upper and lower thorax during diaphragmatic contraction.

Newborns, particularly premature infants, are prone to respiratory muscle fatigue, and nurses and house staff physicians in neonatal intensive care units are aware that minor physical activity (e.g., physiotherapy or crying during blood sampling) often results in apneic spells due to exhaustion of the respiratory system in such patients. Numerous factors may contribute to this fatigability, such as the sleep state, muscle mass, nutrition, lack of rigidity of bony structure of chest wall, and perinatal conditions that stiffen the neonatal lungs.

Therefore, in various clinical conditions, physicians dealing with respiratory disorders must remember that the chest wall of an infant is easily exhausted and that respiratory muscle fatigue may be the cause of respiratory failure.

REFERENCES

General Considerations
Bryan AC: Diaphragmatic fatigue in newborns. Am Rev Respir Dis 119:137, 1979.
Bryan AC and Wohl MEB: Respiratory mechanics in children. In Macklem PT and Mead J (eds): The Handbook of Physiology. Vol. III. Mechanics of Breathing, Part 1. Bethesda, Md, American Physiological Society, 1986.
Bureau MA, Lupien L, and Bégin R: Neural drive and ventilatory strategy of breathing in normal children and in patients with cystic fibrosis and asthma. Pediatrics 68:187, 1981.
Davis GM and Bureau MA: Pulmonary and chest wall mechanics in the control of respiration in the newborn. Clin Perinatal 14:551, 1987.

Davis J: The diaphragm and neuromuscular disease. Am Rev Respir Dis 119:115, 1979.
Davis J, Goldman M, Loh L, and Casson M: Diaphragm function and alveolar hypoventilation. Q J Med 45:87, 1976.
England SJ, Guslits BG, and Bryan AC: Diaphragmatic function in newborn infants. In Sieck GS (ed): Neurology and Neurobiology, vol 26. Respiratory Muscles and Their Neuromotor Control. New York, Alan R. Liss, 1987.
Gerhardt T and Bancalari E: Chest-wall compliance in full-term and premature infants. Acta Paediatr Scand 69:359, 1980.
Grassino A: Respiratory muscle fatigue. Med North Am 22:4208, 1988.
Gravelyn TF: Respiratory rate as an indicator of acute respiratory dysfunction. JAMA 244:1123, 1980.
Macklem PT: Respiratory muscles: the vital pump. Chest 78:753, 1980.
Rochester DF and Arora NS: Respiratory muscle fatigue. Med Clin North Am 67:573, 1983.
Roussos C, Fixley M, Gross D, and Macklem PT: Fatigue of inspiratory muscles and their synergic behavior. J Appl Physiol 46:897, 1979.
Thach BT, Abroms IF, Frantz ID III et al: Intercostal muscle reflexes and sleep breathing patterns in human infants. J Appl Physiol 48:139, 1980.

Scoliosis
Anderson PR, Puno MR, Lovell SL, and Swayze CR: Postoperative respiratory complications in non-idiopathic scoliosis. Acta Anaesthesiol Scand 29:186, 1985.
Bake B, Bjure J, Kasalicky J, and Nachemson A: Regional pulmonary ventilation and perfusion distribution in patients with untreated idiopathic scoliosis. Thorax 27:703, 1972.
Bergofsky EH, Turino GM, and Fishman AP: Cardiorespiratory failure in kyphoscoliosis. Medicine (Baltimore) 38:263, 1959.
Bergofsky EH: Thoracic deformities. In Roussos C and Macklem PT (eds): The Thorax—Lung Biology in Health and Disease. New York, Marcel Dekker, Inc, 1986.
Bjure J and Nachemson A: Non-treated scoliosis. Clin Orthop Rel Res 93:44, 1973.
Bjure J, Grimby G, Kasalicky J et al: Respiratory impairment and airway closure in patient with untreated idiopathic scoliosis. Thorax 25:451, 1970.
Boffa P, Stovin P, and Shneerson J: Lung developmental abnormalities in severe scoliosis. Thorax 39:681, 1984.
Branthwaite MA: Cardiorespiratory consequences of unfused idiopathic scoliosis. Br J Dis Chest 80:360, 1986.
Bunnell WP: The natural history of idiopathic scoliosis. Clin Orthop Rel Res 229:20, 1988.
Ceballos T, Ferrer-Torrelles Castillo F, and Fernandez-Paredes F: Prognosis in infantile idiopathic scoliosis. J Bone Joint Surg 62:863, 1980.
Cobb JR: Outline for the study of scoliosis. Instruct Lect Acad Orthop Surg 51:261, 1961.
Cooper DM, Velasquez Rojas J, Mellins RB et al: Respiratory mechanics in adolescents with idiopathic scoliosis. Am Rev Respir Dis 130:16, 1984.
Davies G and Reid L: Effect of scoliosis on growth of alveoli and pulmonary arteries and on right ventricle. Arch Dis Child 46:623, 1971.
Dollery CT, Gillam PMS, Hugh-Jones P, and Zorab PA: Regional lung function in kyphoscoliosis. Thorax 20:175, 1965.
Golstein LA and Waugh TR: Classification and terminology of scoliosis. Clin Orthop Rel Res 93:10, 1973.
Kafer ER: Idiopathic scoliosis: mechanical properties of the respiratory system and the ventilation response to carbon dioxide. J Clin Invest 55:1153, 1975.
Kafer ER: Idiopathic scoliosis: gas exchange and the age dependence of arterial blood gases. J Clin Invest 58:825, 1976.
Kennedy JD, Robertson CF, Olinsky A et al: Pulmonary restrictive effect of bracing in mild idiopathic scoliosis. Thorax 42:959, 1987.
Kumano K and Tsuyama N: Pulmonary function before and after surgical correction of scoliosis. J Bone Joint Surg [A]64:242, 1982.

Lonstein JE: Natural history and school screening for scoliosis. Orthop Clin North Am 19:227, 1988.

Lonstein JE and Carlson JM: The prediction of curve progression in untreated idiopathic scoliosis during growth. J Bone Joint Surg [A]66:1061, 1984.

Lonstein JE and Winter RB: Adolescent idiopathic scoliosis—nonoperative treatment. Orthop Clin North Am 19:239, 1988.

Makley JT, Herndon CH, Inkley S et al: Pulmonary function in paralytic and nonparalytic scoliosis before and after treatment. J Bone Joint Surg 50:1379, 1968.

Mankin HJ, Graham JJ, and Schack J: Cardiopulmonary function in mild and moderate scoliosis. J Bone Joint Surg 46:53, 1964.

McCarthy RE: Prevention of the complications of scoliosis by early detection. Clin Orthop Rel Res 222:73, 1987.

Muirhead A and Conner AN: The assessment of lung function in children with scoliosis. J Bone Joint Surg [B]67:699, 1985.

Nachemson A: A long-term follow up study of non-treated scoliosis. Acta Orthop Scand 39:466, 1968.

Nilsonne U and Lundgren KD: Long-term prognosis in idiopathic scoliosis. Acta Orthop Scand 39:456, 1968.

Nisbet HIA, Lamarre A, Levison H et al: Thoracic elastance and its components in anesthetized scoliotic children. J Bone Joint Surg 55:1721, 1973.

Olgiati R, Levine D, Smith JP et al: Diffusing capacity in idiopathic scoliosis and its interpretation regarding alveolar development. Am Rev Respir Dis 126:229, 1982.

Prime FJ and Zorab PA: Respiratory function. In Zorab PA (ed): Scoliosis. Springfield Ill, Charles C Thomas, 1969.

Respiratory function in scoliosis (editorial). Lancet 1:84, 1985.

Rom WN and Miller A: Unexpected longevity in patients with severe kyphoscoliosis. Thorax 33:106, 1978.

Sawicka EH and Branthwaite MA: Respiration during sleep in kyphoscoliosis. Thorax 42:801, 1987.

Scadding FH and Zorab PA: The lungs. In Zorab PA (ed): Scoliosis. Springfield Ill, Charles C Thomas, 1969.

School screening for scoliosis (editorial). Lancet 2:345, 1981.

Scott JC and Morgan TH: The natural history and prognosis of infantile idiopathic scoliosis. J Bone Joint Surg 37:400, 1955.

Shannon DC, Riseborough EJ, and Kazemi H: Ventilation perfusion relationships following correction of kyphoscoliosis. JAMA 217:579, 1971.

Shannon DC, Riseborough EJ, Valenca LM, and Kazemi H: The distribution of abnormal lung function in kyphoscoliosis. J Bone Joint Surg 52:131, 1970.

Shneerson JM: The cardiorespiratory response to exercise in thoracic scoliosis. Thorax 33:457, 1978.

Shneerson JM: Pulmonary artery pressure in thoracic scoliosis during and after exercise while breathing air and pure oxygen. Thorax 33:747, 1978.

Shneerson JM and Edgard MA: Cardiac and respiratory function before and after spinal fusion in adolescent idiopathic scoliosis. Thorax 34:658, 1979.

Simon G: The chest radiograph. In Zorab PA (ed): Scoliosis. Springfield, Ill, Charles C Thomas, 1969.

Sleep and scoliosis (editorial). Lancet 1:336, 1988.

Smyth RJ, Chapman KR, Wright TA et al: Ventilatory patterns during hypoxia, hypercapnia, and exercise in adolescents with mild scoliosis. Pediatrics 77:692, 1986.

Szeinberg A, Canny GJ, Rashed N et al: Forced vital capacity and maximal respiratory pressures in patients with mild and moderate scoliosis. Pediatr Pulmonol 4:8, 1988.

Weber B, Smith JP, Briscoe WA et al: Pulmonary function in asymptomatic adolescents with idiopathic scoliosis. Am Rev Respir Dis 111:389, 1975.

Westgate HD: Pulmonary functions in scoliosis. Am Rev Respir Dis 96:147, 1967.

Westgate HD and Moe JH: Pulmonary function in kyphoscoliosis before and after correction by Harrington instrument method. J Bone Joint Surg 51:935, 1969.

Winter RB, Lovell WW, and Moe JH: Excessive thoracic lordosis and loss of pulmonary function in patients with idiopathic scoliosis. J Bone Joint Surg [A]57:972, 1975.

Asphyxiating Thoracic Dystrophy

Finegold MJ, Katzezw H, Granon Genieser N, and Becker MH: Lung structure in thoracic dystrophy. Am J Dis Child 122:153, 1966.

Hull D and Barnes ND: Children with small chests. Arch Dis Child 47:12, 1972.

Jeune M, Carron R, Berau D, and Loaec Y: Polychondrodystrophie avec bloquage thoracique d'évolution fatate. Pediatrie 9:390, 1954.

Oberklaid F, Danks DM, Mayne V, and Campbell P: Asphyxiating thoracic dysplasia. Arch Dis Child 52:758, 1977.

Stokes DC, Phillips JA, Leonard CO et al: Respiratory complications of achondroplasia. J Pediatr 102:534, 1983.

Tahernia CA and Stamps P: "Jeune syndrome" (asphyxiating thoracic dystrophy). Clin Pediatr 16:903, 1977.

Todd DW, Tinguely SJ, and Norberg WJ: A thoracic expansion technique for Jeune's asphyxiating thoracic dystrophy. J Pediatr Surg 21:161, 1986.

Wiebicke W and Pasterkamp H: Long-term continuous positive airway pressure in a child with asphyxiating thoracic dystrophy. Pediatr Pulmonol 4:54, 1988.

Duchenne Muscular Dystrophy

Bach JR, O'Brien J, Krotenberg R, and Alba AS: Management of end stage respiratory failure in Duchenne muscular dystrophy. Muscle Nerve 10:177, 1987.

Bégin R, Bureau MA, Lupien L, and Lemieux B: Control of breathing in Duchenne muscular dystrophy. Am J Med 69:227, 1981.

Bradford DS: Neuromuscular spinal deformity. In Bradford DS, Lonstein JE, Moe JT, O Gilvie JW, and Winter RB (eds): Moe's Textbook of Scoliosis and Other Spinal Deformities. Philadelphia, WB Saunders Co, 1987.

Chelly J and Kaplan JC: La myopathie de Duchenne du gène DMD à la dystrophine. Médecine-Sciences 4:141, 1988.

Delaubier A, Guillou C, Mordelet M, and Rideau Y: Assistance ventilatoire précoce par voie nasale dans la dystrophie musculaire de Duchenne. Agressologie 28:737, 1987.

Ellis ER, Bye PTP, Bruderer JW, and Sullivan CE: Treatment of respiratory failure during sleep in patients with neuromuscular disease. Am Rev Respir Dis 135:148, 1987.

Hapke EJ, Meek JC, and Jacobs J: Pulmonary function in progressive muscular dystrophy. Chest 61:41, 1972.

Heckmatt JZ: Respiratory care in muscular dystrophy. Br Med J 295:1014, 1987.

Inkley SR, Oldenburg FC, and Vignos PJ: Pulmonary function in Duchenne muscular dystrophy related to stage of the disease. Am J Med 56:297, 1974.

Jenkins JG, Bohn D, Edmonds JF et al: Evaluation of pulmonary function in muscular dystrophy patients requiring spinal surgery. Crit Care Med 10:645, 1982.

Kerby GR, Mayer LS, and Pingleton SK: Nocturnal positive pressure ventilation via nasal mask. Am Rev Respir Dis 135:738, 1987.

Miller F, Moseley CF, Koreska J, and Levison H: Pulmonary function and scoliosis in Duchenne dystrophy. J Pediatr Orthop 8:133, 1988.

Monaco AP, Neve R, Lolletti-Feener C et al: Isolation of candidates cDNAS for portions of the DMD gene. Nature 323:646, 1986.

Moseley CF: Natural history and management of scoliosis in Duchenne muscular dystrophy. In Serratrice G, Desnuelle C, Pelissier JF et al (eds): Neuromuscular Diseases. New York, Raven Press, 1984.

Noble-Jamieson CM, Heckmatt JZ, Dubowitz V, and Silverman M: Effects of posture and spinal bracing on respiratory function in neuromuscular disease. Arch Dis Child 61:178, 1986.

Rideau Y, Jawkowski LW, and Grellet J: Respiratory function in the muscular dystrophies. Muscle Nerve 4:155, 1981.

Rideau Y: Acharnement contre une maladie incurable: la dystrophie musculaire de Duchenne. Agressologie 28:733, 1987.

Robertson M: Muscular dystrophy. Mapping the disease phenotype. Nature 327:372, 1987.

Segall D: Noninvasive nasal mask-assisted ventilation in respiratory failure of Duchenne muscular dystrophy. Chest 93:1298, 1988.

Smith PEM, Calverley PMA, Edwards RHT et al: Practical problems in the respiratory care of patients with muscular dystrophy. N Engl J Med 316:1197, 1987.

Smith PEM, Calverley PMA, and Edwards RHT: Hypoxemia during sleep in Duchenne Muscular Dystrophy. Am Rev Respir Dis 137:884, 1988.

Myotonic Dystrophy

Bégin R, Bureau MA, and Lupien L: Control and modulation of respiration in Steinert's myotonic dystrophy. Am Rev Respir Dis 121:281, 1980.

Bégin R, Bureau MA, Lupien L et al: Pathogenesis of respiratory insufficiency in Steinert's muscular dystrophy: the mechanical factor. Am Rev Respir Dis 125:312, 1982.

Bossen EH, Shelburne JD, Durham NC et al: Respiratory muscle involvement in infantile myotonic dystrophy. Arch Pathol 97:250, 1974.

Caughey JE and Pachomov N: The diaphragm in dystrophia myotonia. J Neurosurg Psychiat 22:311, 1959.

Chudley AE and Barmada MA: Diaphragmatic elevation in neonatal myotonic dystrophy. Am J Dis Child 133:1182, 1979.

Farkas-Bargeton E, Barbet JP, Dancea S et al: Immaturity of muscle fibers in the congenital form of myotonic dystrophy: its consequences and its origin. J Neurol Sci 83:145, 1988.

Harper PS: Myotonic disorders. In Engel AG and Banker BQ (eds): Myology—Basic and Clinical. New York, McGraw-Hill Book Co, Inc, 1986.

Jaffe R, Mock M, Abramowicz J, and Ben-Aderet N: Myotonic dystrophy and pregnancy: a review. Obstet Gynecol Surv 41:272, 1986.

Jammes Y, Pouget J, Grimaud C, and Serratrice G: Pulmonary function and electromyographic study of respiratory muscles in myotonic dystrophy. Muscle Nerve 8:586, 1985.

Kilburn KH, Eagan JT, Sieker HO, and Heyman A: Cardiopulmonary insufficiency in myotonia and progressive muscular dystrophy. N Engl J Med 261:1089, 1959.

Osborne JP: Thin ribs on chest x-ray: a useful sign in the differential diagnosis of the floppy newborn. Dev Med Child Neurol 25:343, 1983.

Riley DJ, Santiago TV, Daniele RP et al: Blunted respiratory drive in congenital myopathy. Am J Med 63:459, 1977.

Serisier DE, Mastaglia FL, and Gibson GJ: Respiratory muscle function and ventilatory control (I) in patients with motor neurone disease and (II) in patients with myotonic dystrophy. Q J Med 202:205, 1982.

Simpson K: Neonatal respiratory failure due to myotonic dystrophy. Arch Dis Child 50:569, 1975.

Watters GV and Williams PW: Early onset myotonic dystrophy: clinical and laboratory findings in five families and review of the literature. Arch Neurol 17:137, 1967.

Wesstrom G, Bensch J, and Schollin J: Congenital myotonic dystrophy. Incidence, clinical aspects and early prognosis. Acta Paediatr Scand 75:849, 1986.

Myasthenia Gravis

Bastedo DLA: Acute fulminating myasthenia gravis in children. Can Med Assoc 63:388, 1950.

De Troyer A and Borenstein S: Acute changes in respiratory mechanics after pyridostigmine injection in patients with myasthenia gravis. Am Rev Respir Dis 121:629, 1980.

Engel AG: Myasthenia gravis and myasthenic syndromes. Ann Neurol 16:519, 1984.

Fenichel GM: Clinical syndrome of myasthenia in infancy and childhood. Arch Neurol 35:97, 1978.

Gibson GJ, Pride NB, Davis J, and Loh LC: Pulmonary mechanics in patients with respiratory muscle weakness. Am Rev Respir Dis 115:389, 1977.

Gieron MA and Korthals JK: Familial infantile myasthenia gravis. Report of three cases with follow-up until adult life. Arch Neurol 42:143, 1985.

Gordon N: Congenital myasthenia. Dev Med Child Neurol 28:803, 1986.

Hageman G, Smit LME, Hoogland RA et al: Muscle weakness and congenital contractures in a case of congenital myasthenia. J Pediatr Orthop 6:227, 1986.

Heckmatt J, Placzek M, Thompson A et al: An unusual case of neonatal myasthenia. J Child Neurol 2:63, 1987.

Leventhal SR, Orkin FK, and Hirsh RA: Prediction of the need for postoperative mechanical ventilation in myasthenia gravis. Anesthesiology 53:26, 1980.

Morel E, Eymard B, Vernet-der Garabedian B et al: Neonatal myasthenia gravis: a new clinical and immunologic appraisal of 30 cases. Neurology 38:138, 1988.

Pasternak JF, Hageman J, Adams MA et al: Exchange transfusion in neonatal myasthenia. J Pediatr 99:644, 1981.

Roach ES, Buono G, McLean WT Jr, and Weaver RG Jr: Early-onset myasthenia gravis. J Pediatr 108:193, 1986.

Robertson WC, Chun RWM, and Kornguth SE: Familial infantile myasthenia. Arch Neurol 37:117, 1980.

Rodriguez M, Gomez MR, Howard FM Jr, and Taylor WF: Myasthenia gravis in children: long-term follow-up. Ann Neurol 13:504, 1983.

Seybold ME and Lindstrom JM: Myasthenia gravis in infancy. Neurology (NY) 31:476, 1981.

Snead OC III, Benton JW, Dwyer D et al: Juvenile myasthenia gravis. Neurology 30:732, 1980.

Snead OC III, Kohaut ED, Oh SJ, and Bradley RJ: Plasmapheresis for myasthenic crisis in a young child. J Pediatr 110:740, 1987.

Botulism

Long SS, Gajewski JL, Brown LW, and Gilligan PH: Clinical, laboratory, and environmental features of infant botulism in southeastern Pennsylvania. Pediatrics 75:935, 1985.

Pickett J, Berg B, Chaplin E, and Brunstetter-Shafer M-A: Syndrome of botulism in infancy: clinical and electrophysiologic study. N Engl J Med 295:770, 1976.

Schmidt-Nowara WW, Samet JM, and Rosario PA: Early and late pulmonary complications of botulism. Arch Intern Med 143:451, 1983.

Thompson JA, Glasgow LA, Warpinski JR, and Olson C: Infant botulism: clinical spectrum and epidemiology. Pediatrics 66:936, 1980.

Friedreich Ataxia

Bégin R, Lupien L, Bureau MA, and Lemieux B: Regulation of respiration in Friedreich's ataxia. Can J Neurol Sci 6:159, 1979.

Bureau MA, Ngassam P, Lemieux B, and Trias A: Pulmonary function in Friedreich's ataxia. Can J Neurol Sci 3:343, 1976.

Côté M, Bureau MA, Léger C et al.: Evolution of cardiopulmonary involvement in Friedreich's ataxia. Can J Neurol Sci 6:151, 1979.

Thoren C: Spirometric studies in Friedreich's ataxia. Acta Paediatr Scand 15(Suppl):95, 1964.

Werdnig-Hoffman Paralysis

Bove KE and Iannaccone ST: Atypical infantile spinomuscular atrophy presenting as acute diaphragmatic paralysis. Pediatr Pathol 8:95, 1988.

Dubowitz V: Disorders of the lower motor neurone. In Dubowitz V (ed): Muscle Disorders in Childhood. Philadelphia, WB Saunders Co, 1978.

Pern JH, Gardner-Medwin D, and Wilson J: A clinical study of chronic childhood spinal atrophy: a review of 140 cases. Neurol Sci 38:23, 1978.

Guillain-Barré Syndrome

Dowling PC, Blumberg B, and Cook SD: Guillain-Barré syndrome. In Matthews WB (ed): Handbook of Clinical Neurology. Vol. 7. Neuropathies. Amsterdam, Elsevier Science Publishers BV, 1987.

Eberle E, Brink J, Azen S, and White D: Early predictors of incomplete recovery in children with Guillain-Barré polyneuritis. Pediatrics 86:356, 1975.

Lands L and Zinman R: Maximal static pressures and lung volumes in a child with Guillain-Barré syndrome ventilated by a cuirass respirator. Chest 89:757, 1986.

Loeffel NB, Rossi LN, Mumenthaler M et al: The Landry-Guillain-Barré syndrome. J Neurol Sci 33:71, 1977.

Massam M and Jones RS: Ventilatory failure in the Guillain-Barré syndrome. Thorax 35:557, 1980.

Ropper AH: Management of Guillain-Barré syndrome. In Ropper AH, Kennedy SK, and Zervas NT (eds): Neurological and Neurosurgical Intensive Care. Baltimore, University Park Press, 1983.

Soffer D, Feldman S, and Alter M: Clinical features of the Guillain-Barré syndrome. J Neurol Sci 37:135, 1978.

Diaphragmatic Paralysis

Aldrich TK, Herman JH, and Rochester DF: Bilateral diaphragmatic paralysis in the newborn infant. J Pediatr 97:988, 1980.

Ambler R, Gruenewald S, and John E: Ultrasound monitoring of diaphragm activity in bilateral diaphragmatic paralysis. Arch Dis Child 60:170, 1985.

Brouillette RT, Hahn YS, Noah ZL et al: Successful reinnervation of the diaphragm after phrenic nerve transection. J Pediatr Surg 21:63, 1986.

De Troyer A and Heilporn A: Respiratory mechanics in quadriplegia. The respiratory function of the intercostal muscles. Am Rev Respir Dis 122:591, 1980.

Paralytic Diseases

De Troyer A, De Beyl DZ, and Thirion M: Function of the respiratory muscles in acute hemiplegia. Am Rev Respir Dis 123:631, 1981.

Fugl-Meyer AR and Grimby G: Rib-cage and abdominal volume ventilation partitioning in tetraplegic patients. Scand J Rehabil Med 3:161, 1971a.

Fugl-Meyer AR and Grimby G: Ventilatory function in tetraplegic patients. Scand J Rehabil Med 3:151, 1971.

Greene W, L'Heureux P, and Hunt CE: Paralysis of the diaphragm. Am J Dis Child 129:1402, 1975.

Gross D, Ladd HW, Riley EJ et al: The effect of training on strength and endurance of the diaphragm in quadriplegia. Am J Med 68:27, 1980.

Huldtgren AC, Fugl-Meyer AR, Jonasson E, and Bake B: Ventilatory dysfunction and respiratory rehabilitation in post-traumatic quadriplegia. Eur J Respir Dis 61:347, 1980.

James WS, Minh VD, Minteer MA, and Moser KM: Cervical accessory muscle function in a patient with a high cervical cord lesion. Chest 71:59, 1977.

Laing IA, Teele RL, and Stark AR: Diaphragmatic movement in newborn infants. J Pediatr 112:638, 1988.

McCarthy GS: The effect of thoracic extradural analgesia on the pulmonary gas distribution, functional residual capacity and airway closure. Br J Anaesth 48:243, 1976.

Mortola JP and Sant'Ambrogio G: Motion of the rib cage and the abdomen in tetraplegic patients. Clin Sci Molec Med 54:25, 1978.

Obesity

Burwell CS, Robin ED, Whaley RD, and Brikelman AG: Extreme obesity associated with alveolar hypoventilation—a pickwickian syndrome. Am J Med 21:811, 1956.

Cayler GG, Mays J, and Riley HD: Cardiorespiratory syndrome of obesity (pickwickian syndrome) in children. Pediatrics 27:237, 1961.

Chaussain M, Gamain B, Latorre AM et al: Respiratory function at rest in obese children. Bull Eur Physiopathol Respir 13:599, 1977.

Fadell EJ, Richman AD, Ward WW, and Hendon JR: Fatty infiltration of respiratory muscles in the pickwickian syndrome. N Engl J Med 266:861, 1962.

Farebrother MJB: Respiratory function and cardiorespiratory response to exercise in obesity. Br J Dis Chest 73:211, 1979.

Finkelstein JW and Avery ME: The pickwickian syndrome. Am J Dis Child 106:51, 1963.

Kronenberg RS, Drage CW, and Stevenson JE: Acute respiratory failure and obesity with normal ventilatory response to carbon dioxide and absent hypoxic ventilatory drive. Am J Med 62:772, 1977.

Lourenço RV: Diaphragm activity in obesity. J Clin Invest 48:1609, 1969.

Luce JM: Respiratory complications of obesity. Chest 78:626, 1980.

Melzer E and Souhrada JF: Decrease of respiratory muscle strength and static lung volume in obese asthmatics. Am Rev Respir Dis 121:17, 1980.

Riley DJ, Santiago TV, and Edelman NH: Complication of obesity-hypoventilation syndrome in childhood. Am J Dis Child 130:671, 1976.

Rochester DF and Enson Y: Current concepts in the pathogenesis of obesity-hypoventilation syndrome. Am J Med 57:402, 1974.

Sampson M, Razio E, and Grassino A: Breathing strategy in the obese. Am Rev Respir Dis 121(part 2):399, 1980.

Connective Tissue Disorders

Brady JF and Poulson JM: Diaphragmatic weakness and myositis associated with systemic juvenile rheumatoid arthritis. Can Med Assoc J 130:47, 1984.

Bégin R, Massé S, Cantin A et al: Airway disease in a subset of non-smoking rheumatoid patients: characterization of the disease and evidence for an autoimmune pathogenesis. Am J Med 72:743, 1982.

Bégin R, Radoux V, Cantin A, and Ménard HA: Stiffness of the rib cage in a subset of rheumatoid patients. Lung 166:141, 1988.

Gibson GJ, Edmonds JP, and Hughes GRV: Diaphragm function and lung involvement in systemic lupus erythematosus. Am J Med 63:926, 1977.

Hepper NGG, Ferguson RH, and Howard FM: Three types of pulmonary involvement in polymyositis. Med Clin North Am 48:1031, 1964.

Hunninghake GW and Fauci AS: Pulmonary involvement in the collagen vascular diseases. Am Rev Respir Dis 119:471, 1979.

Sackner MA, Akgun N, Kimbel P, and Lewis DH: The pathophysiology of scleroderma involving the heart and respiratory system. Ann Intern Med 60:611, 1964.

Thompson PJ, Dhillon DP, Ledingham J, and Turner-Warwick M: Shrinking lungs, diaphragmatic dysfunction and systemic lupus erythematosus. Am Rev Respir Dis 132:925, 1985.

Tsanaclis A and Grassino AE: Diaphragm and intercostal muscle behaviour in ankylosing spondylitis during CO_2 rebreathing. Am Rev Respir Dis 119(part 2):336, 1979.

OTHER DISEASES WITH A PROMINENT RESPIRATORY COMPONENT

45

JENNIFER M. STURGESS, Ph.D., and
J. A. PETER TURNER, M.D., F.R.C.P.(C)

THE IMMOTILE CILIA SYNDROME

The immotile cilia syndrome is a recently described human disorder characterized by specific and genetically determined abnormalities of cilia (Afzelius, 1976; Pedersen and Mygind, 1976; Eliasson et al, 1977; Turner et al, 1981). Determination of a ciliary abnormality in this disease has now clarified its variable expression and pleiotropism. Situs inversus is common in affected individuals, so immotile cilia syndrome encompasses the triad of chronic sinusitis, bronchiectasis, and situs inversus totalis that is described as Kartagener syndrome (Kartagener, 1933). The biochemical basis of this disorder is not known, and identification of specific defects depends on electron microscopic examination of cilia in concert with evaluation of ciliary function. Dysfunction of cilia leads to impairment of the mucociliary clearance mechanism that is responsible for the normal transport of mucus and the elimination of inhaled particles from the nasal cavity and lung (Fig. 45–1) (Sturgess, 1979). The characteristic clinical signs are chronic or recurrent upper and lower respiratory disease, including rhinitis, sinusitis, serous otitis, bronchitis, and bronchiectasis.

CILIA

Cilia, complex organelles that are responsible for motility, are ubiquitous in nature. The motility of cilia at epithelial surfaces is coordinated with that of other cilia and supported by cellular functions and secretions to convey fluids and foreign materials. Ciliated cells line the nasal cavity, the paranasal sinuses, the middle ear, and the conducting airways of the lungs. Ciliated epithelia function also in the ependyma of the brain and in the fallopian tubes. The flagella, or tails, of spermatozoa have a core structure identical to that of cilia and thus have the same fundamental characteristics. Cilia represent extensions of specialized epithelial cells, are approximately 6 μ long, and are supported by a series of axial filaments or microtubules composed of the

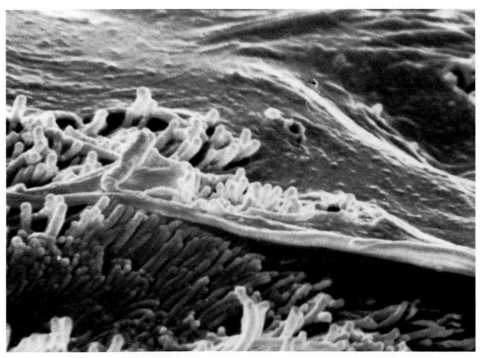

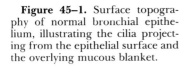

Figure 45–1. Surface topography of normal bronchial epithelium, illustrating the cilia projecting from the epithelial surface and the overlying mucous blanket.

protein tubulin. Cilia move rapidly, at approximately 12 beats/sec in the human trachea. The beat frequency and coordinated wave-like motion of cilia are essential to their effective movement and, hence, to the clearance of mucus and inhaled particulate matter.

In normal cilia, the supporting structures consist of nine microtubular doublets arranged in an outer ring and two single microtubules in the center of the axoneme (Fig. 45–2). The characteristic 9 + 2 pattern is common to all healthy cilia and is maintained by intertubular linkages and accessory proteins (Satir, 1974; Sleigh, 1977). The protein nexin links the outer microtubular doublets in a circumferential pattern. Radial spokes connect the outer microtubular doublets with a central sheath of protein that surrounds the central tubules. Dynein arms, which have ATPase activity, are outer and inner hook-like accessory structures on the microtubular doublets. Ciliary beating results from the sliding of adjacent microtubular doublets. As the nexin links maintain the axonemal structure, the radial spoke linkages convert the sliding of the outer microtubules into a bending movement of the cilia.

PATHOBIOLOGY OF CILIA IN THE IMMOTILE CILIA SYNDROME

The evaluation of bronchial mucosa from patients with immotile cilia syndrome by conventional light microscopy reveals no specific change and shows no features of bronchitis, i.e., hyperplasia of mucus-secreting cells and chronic inflammation. The ciliated cells are numerous, and the cilia are normal in their distribution (Figs. 45–3 and 45–4). With light microscopy, no specific abnormality can be ascribed to the nasal or bronchial mucosa; only with electron microscopy are ciliary defects recognized.

A number of distinct ciliary anomalies have been reported as causes of respiratory disease, including deficiencies in the dynein arms and the radial spoke linkages, and transposition of microtubules (Fig. 45–5). Within one family, the specific ciliary defect appears always identical for the affected subjects, emphasizing the genetic nature of this disorder. How-

ever, the incidence of situs inversus is random within affected families and shows no consistent pattern.

Dynein Arm Defects

The dynein defect is characterized by the lack of dynein arms on the outer microtubular doublets (Afzelius, 1976; Afzelius, 1979). This defect may be exclusive to the outer arms or to the inner arms or may involve both inner and outer arms (Sturgess et al, 1982). A remnant of the outer dynein arm is often attached to the microtubular doublet and is presumed to represent a subunit of this protein complex. From studies with genetic mutants of lower organisms, it is clear that the outer and inner dynein arms have separate genetic determinants. In the absence of dynein, the cilia may be immotile or have abnormal motility (Pedersen and Mygind, 1980; Rossman et al, 1980).

Radial Spoke Defect

A defect in the radial spoke linkages is also recognized as a cause of ciliary immotility (Sturgess et al, 1979). Although the nature of the specific protein responsible for a radial spoke linkage defect is unknown, the lack of the protein results in disorganization of the spoke and disorientation of the central core of the cilia. This type of defect is identified readily on electron microscopy by the eccentric position of the central core. This structural abnormality may be accompanied by the displacement of one of the outer microtubular doublets toward the center of the cilia. With this type of defect, the cilia lack normal motility. The radial spoke includes at least 14 different polypeptides, so defective radial spoke linkages may encompass a number of distinct protein anomalies.

Microtubular Transposition Defect

A defect involving the transposition of one microtubular doublet results from the deficiency of the central tubules in which the central core is replaced by one of the outer microtubular doublets (Sturgess et al, 1980). In this condition, the cilia appear to retain some motility.

Other Defects

Because cilia are composed of more than 200 different polypeptides and protein entities, it is possible that other, as yet undescribed, defects exist. Some of these may be detectable on ultrastructural examination, and others may represent enzymatic abnormalities that elude electron microscopic examination (Herzon and Murphy, 1980). A classification of the currently defined defects is summarized in Table 45–1 (Sturgess and Turner, 1984).

The ultrastructural and functional defects of cilia that are signified early in childhood by respiratory tract disease are manifested also in cilia of the middle ear (Fischer et al, 1978; Jahrsdoerfer et al, 1979), the oviduct (Bleau et al, 1978), and the sperm tails

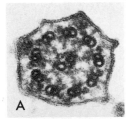
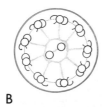

Figure 45–2. *A*, Ultrastructure of a normal bronchial cilium in cross section (× 180,000). *B*, A diagrammatic representation illustrating the major structural components. The nine outer doublet tubules and two central singlet tubules are interconnected by nexin and radial spoke linkages. Outer and inner dynein arms are attached to the complete outer doublet tubules.

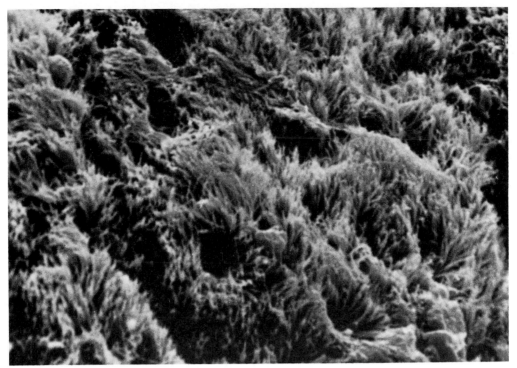

Figure 45–3. Surface topography of the lobar bronchus from a patient with immotile cilia syndrome, illustrating densely packed cilia lining the respiratory tract.

(Eliasson et al, 1977; Afzelius and Eliasson, 1979). Observations of sperm immotility and ultrastructural abnormalities are useful in characterizing the immotile cilia syndrome in postpubescent males. Furthermore, the changes in spermatozoa preclude the possibility that the ciliary anomalies are secondary to infection. The observations of ciliary defects in different organs indicate that this is a multisystem disorder of genetic origin (Sturgess and Turner, 1984).

CLINICAL FEATURES OF THE IMMOTILE CILIA SYNDROME IN CHILDHOOD

Although ciliary abnormalities are presumably present before birth, affected neonates have normal birth weight. Growth and development usually progress within normal percentiles for age. Symptoms may appear in the form of respiratory distress in the neonatal period (Whitelaw et al, 1981). However, in

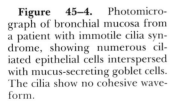

Figure 45–4. Photomicrograph of bronchial mucosa from a patient with immotile cilia syndrome, showing numerous ciliated epithelial cells interspersed with mucus-secreting goblet cells. The cilia show no cohesive waveform.

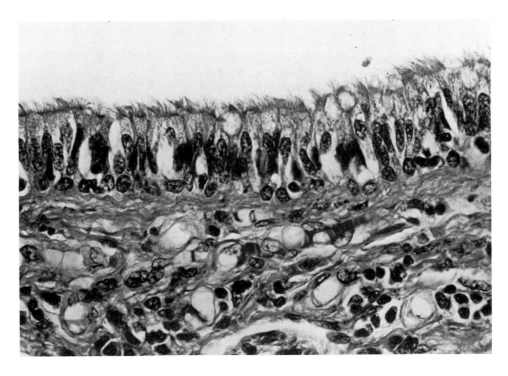

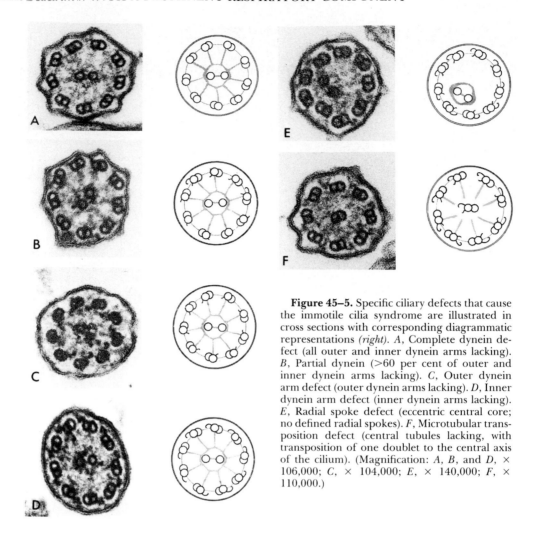

Figure 45–5. Specific ciliary defects that cause the immotile cilia syndrome are illustrated in cross sections with corresponding diagrammatic representations *(right)*. *A,* Complete dynein defect (all outer and inner dynein arms lacking). *B,* Partial dynein (>60 per cent of outer and inner dynein arms lacking). *C,* Outer dynein arm defect (outer dynein arms lacking). *D,* Inner dynein arm defect (inner dynein arms lacking). *E,* Radial spoke defect (eccentric central core; no defined radial spokes). *F,* Microtubular transposition defect (central tubules lacking, with transposition of one doublet to the central axis of the cilium). (Magnification: *A, B,* and *D,* × 106,000; *C,* × 104,000; *E,* × 140,000; *F,* × 110,000.)

the majority of cases, manifestations of respiratory disease may be recognized only in later infancy or early childhood. The severity of symptoms varies considerably (Fig. 45–6) (Rooklin et al, 1980; Turner et al, 1981).

UPPER RESPIRATORY TRACT

Involvement of the nose, paranasal sinuses, and ears occurs in most affected children (Hartline and

Table 45–1. CLASSIFICATION OF DEFECTS IN IMMOTILE CILIA SYNDROME

Dynein defects
Outer arm defect
Inner arm defect
Outer and inner arm defect (complete)
Outer and inner arm defect (partial)
Radial spoke defect
Microtubular transposition
Normal ultrastructural organization with functional impairment

Zelkowitz, 1971; Turner et al, 1981). Nasal congestion or nasal discharge is constant, with little or no seasonal variation. Nasal polyps are not uncommon, being observed in about one third of patients, and may be recognized as early as 2 years of age. Anosmia is an occasional feature that is appreciated only in older children. The radiologic features of sinusitis are seen as early as 6 months of age. Radiography of the sinuses almost always shows complete opacification of the antra with involvement of the ethmoid air cells. There may be involvement to a lesser degree in the frontal sinuses of older subjects. Sinus radiographs demonstrate mucosal thickening with or without fluid levels. The changes are most obvious in the maxillary sinuses.

Ear involvement is variable in severity but present in almost all children suffering from the immotile cilia syndrome (Sethi, 1975). Tympanostomy with insertion of ventilation tubes through the tympanic membrane is a commonly reported procedure in the

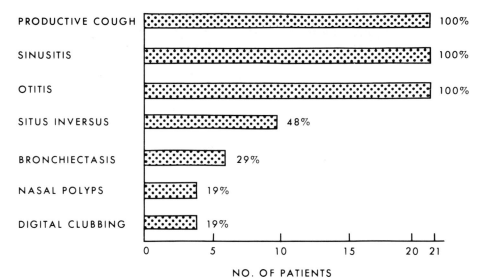

Figure 45–6. Incidence of clinical features of immotile cilia syndrome in 21 children. (Reproduced with permission from Turner JAP et al: Clinical expression of immotile cilia syndrome. Pediatrics 67(6):805–810, June 1981. Copyright American Academy of Pediatrics 1981.)

clinical histories of affected children. Otitis media with aural discharge and even permanent perforation of the tympanic membrane is present in some children. Sclerosis of the mastoid/middle ear region is often present on radiologic examination. Degrees of hearing impairment are detected in the majority of cases in which audiometry has been performed, although subjective complaints of hearing difficulty are documented infrequently.

LOWER RESPIRATORY TRACT

The major symptom of lower airway involvement is recurrent cough, which tends to be more diurnal than nocturnal and is typically productive. Bacteriologic isolates from bronchoscopic aspirate yield various organisms with no consistent pattern of colonization or infection (Turner et al, 1981). The usual bacterial flora are similar to those in adult chronic bronchitis. Wheezing is an uncommon symptom despite the fact that obstructive features are found on pulmonary function assessment.

Clinical findings on examination of the chest are usually nonspecific and relate mainly to the presence of excessive secretions. If bronchiectasis is present, the usual localized findings of fine crepitations may be elicited on auscultation. Bronchiectasis is noted in less than a third of children and, when present, is segmental rather than generalized. The occurrence of bronchiectasis in adults is higher, indicative of progressive pulmonary damage. Digital clubbing may be noted coincident with bronchiectasis.

Chest radiograph abnormalities are observed in all patients (Nadel et al, 1985). The changes are variable, but the characteristic features include bronchial wall thickening and hyperinflation; segmental atelectasis or consolidation is present in some patients, and bronchiectasis may be noted on chest radiographs in older children (Nadel et al, 1985) (Table 45–2).

Bronchography, when indicated, confirms ectasia which may be tubular or saccular. There is a predilection for anatomic middle lobe abnormalities. There is nothing unique in the radiographic appearance to discriminate the immotile cilia syndrome from that due to other causes. The changes have similarities to cystic fibrosis, although they are less severe and less progressive.

SITUS INVERSUS TOTALIS

The manifestation of situs inversus, observed in only 50 per cent of patients with immotile cilia syndrome, is a facultative phenomenon that is an interesting but unexplained aspect of this disease. The incidence appears to be random and shows no familial pattern, in that siblings may or may not exhibit situs inversus despite the similarity of pathologic or clinical findings. The immotile cilia syndrome therefore encompasses the disorder previously diagnosed as Kartagener syndrome, i.e., the clinical triad of situs inversus, chronic sinusitis, and bronchiectasis (Kartagener, 1933).

REPRODUCTIVE TRACT

Because sperm tails have the same fundamental ultrastructure as respiratory cilia, affected males have absence or decrease of sperm motility that may be accompanied by oligospermia (Afzelius and Eliasson,

Table 45–2. CHEST RADIOGRAPH ABNORMALITIES IN IMMOTILE CILIA SYNDROME

Diagnosis	Incidence (%)
Situs inversus	50
Bronchial wall thickening	90
Hyperinflation	97
Segmental loss of volume or consolidation	63
Segmental bronchiectasis	43
Radiologic middle lobe abnormalities	66

1979; Jewett et al, 1980). There is thus a predilection for male infertility in this disorder. Cilia in the fallopian tubes have also been found to be defective in Kartagener syndrome (Bleau et al, 1978). Although fertility may be impaired in females with immotile cilia syndrome, this is not the rule, and the incidence of ectopic pregnancy does not appear to be higher among such patients.

CYTOPLASMIC MICROTUBULAR FUNCTION

Ciliary microtubules are similar in structure to cytoplasmic microtubules, which function as determinants of cell shape and motility, in the ordered movement of intracellular organelles such as in secretion, and in the formation of the mitotic spindle apparatus during cell division. There has been speculation, therefore, that cell functions such as phagocytosis and chemotaxis might be impaired in immotile cilia syndrome (Afzelius et al, 1980). However, there appears to be no significant abnormality of cytoplasmic microtubular function as judged by controlled studies of neutrophil chemotaxis (Corkey et al, 1982).

RESPIRATORY FUNCTION AND CLEARANCE

Pulmonary function studies in subjects with immotile cilia syndrome show variable degrees of airway obstruction (Fig. 45–7). The ratio of residual volume to total lung capacity is increased in almost all patients who have been studied, reflecting the air trapping noted on the chest radiograph. Forced expiratory volume and maximum midexpiratory flow rate are below normal ranges and do not change with the inhalation of bronchodilators. Despite these findings, wheezing is not a common symptom. Arterialized blood gas determinations reveal mild to moderate hypoxemia in room air. The physiologic abnormalities are a result of a mismatch of ventilation and perfusion (Turner et al, 1981). Measurements of the rates of particle transport in the trachea and nasal cavity show mucociliary clearance to be abnormally slow or absent. Such studies are highly specialized and require patient cooperation, so they are applicable only in older children and adults.

The predominant abnormality of pulmonary pathophysiology, therefore, is in mucociliary clearance. It is signified on conventional pulmonary function testing by a ventilation-perfusion imbalance secondary to fixed airway obstruction and air trapping. Despite the high morbidity, the long-term prognosis for children with immotile cilia syndrome appears to be relatively good. Cystic fibrosis shows many similarities in regard to airway disease, but progressive decline of pulmonary function is typical of that disorder. In contrast, pulmonary function was shown in a longitudinal survey of children with immotile cilia syndrome to remain relatively stable (Corkey et al, 1981). The cough mechanism would appear to compensate for the lack of mucociliary clearance in many subjects.

GENETICS AND INHERITANCE

A genetic predisposition to this disorder has been recognized. Immotile cilia syndrome is thought to be a hereditary disorder with autosomal recessive inheritance, on the basis of the lack of clinical signs of respiratory disease among the parents, the increased incidence of consanguineous parentage, the occurrence of several affected siblings, and the lack of affected relatives among families (Rott, 1979; Sturgess et al, 1986). The consistent familial patterns of structural abnormalities suggest that the immotile cilia syndrome is genetically heterogeneous.

Genetic analysis of the immotile cilia syndrome is consistent with autosomal recessive inheritance (Sturgess et al, 1986). There is no evidence of a new autosomal dominant mutation in this disorder. Parents typically have no history of respiratory disease. However, there is little genetic or clinical information on the obligate heterozygotes.

The prevalence of the immotile cilia syndrome has been estimated to be about 1:16,000, based on the population of patients with severe respiratory disease. The incidence of less severe clinical symptoms may not be fully recognized to date. On the basis of autosomal recessive inheritance, approximately 1 in 60 persons in the population would be heterozygous if the syndrome is genetically homogeneous. However, because the ultrastructural variants may reflect different mutations, the combined incidence of heterozygotes for the different mutations is likely to be much higher.

For purposes of genetic counseling, a recurrence risk of 25 per cent is appropriate, based on current evidence. No clinical differences are attributed to the different defects among patients. The immotile cilia syndrome is distributed among different ethnic groups and there appears to be no racial predilection.

DIAGNOSIS OF THE IMMOTILE CILIA SYNDROME

The differential diagnosis in children who have symptoms of persistent or recurrent rhinitis or nasal stuffiness, frequent attacks of serous otitis or otitis media, and recurrent lower respiratory problems such as bronchitis should include immotile cilia syn-

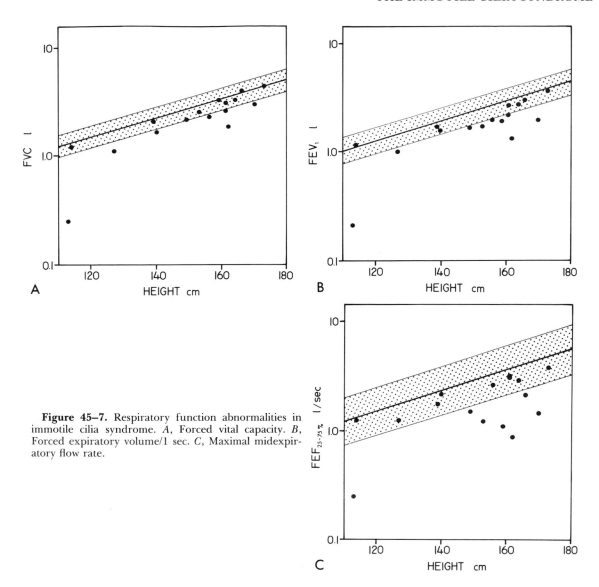

Figure 45–7. Respiratory function abnormalities in immotile cilia syndrome. *A,* Forced vital capacity. *B,* Forced expiratory volume/1 sec. *C,* Maximal midexpiratory flow rate.

drome, particularly if other siblings are similarly affected. Radiologic evaluations of the sinuses show opacification of the antra, and chest radiographs reveal various degrees of involvement ranging from mildly increased bronchovascular patterning to segmental or subsegmental bronchiectasis. Situs inversus is present in only half the affected subjects.

Diagnosis of the ciliary defects rests with the ultrastructural examination of cilia in the transmission electron microscope at magnifications in the order of 100,000 to 150,000×. Bronchial biopsy provides the best source of ciliated cells for definitive diagnosis. However, sampling of nasal cilia by modified cytologic brushing techniques is a noninvasive approach for screening of cilia (Boat et al, 1979; Rutland and Cole, 1980). Nonspecific changes occur sporadically in cilia of the airway epithelium in response to infection. Therefore, for a definitive diagnosis, investigation must include an adequate number of cilia, and the ciliated cells should be derived from at least two different sites in the respiratory tract. The diagnosis may be confirmed by mucociliary clearance studies in the trachea or nasal cavity in vivo or by direct examination of ciliary motility in vitro to identify the nature of the ciliary abnormality.

TREATMENT

No therapeutic modalities are specifically applicable to immotile cilia syndrome. Acute lower respiratory infections should be managed by prompt antibiotic therapy. A prophylactic regimen of antibiotic therapy does not appear to be significantly helpful in most cases. Chest physiotherapy may be important if bronchiectasis is present; otherwise it does not offer much potential, because secretions are usually eliminated by coughing. In this respect, suppression of cough, which is the sole clearance mechanism in the lungs, should be avoided. Surgical resection of affected lung lobes may be considered if saccular bronchiectasis is sufficiently localized. Although there is evidence that beta agonists may enhance beat frequency in normal cilia, their ability to promote clearance by abnormal cilia is doubtful. Development of more specific therapeutic measures will ultimately depend on identification of the biochemical defect(s) in this disease.

REFERENCES

Afzelius BA: A human syndrome caused by immotile cilia. Science 193:317, 1976.

Afzelius BA: The immotile cilia syndrome and other ciliary diseases. Int Rev Exp Pathol 19:1, 1979.

Afzelius BA and Eliasson R: Flagellar mutants in man: on the heterogeneity of the immotile cilia syndrome. J Ultrastruct Res 69:43, 1979.

Afzelius BA, Ewetz L, Palmblad J et al: Structure and function of neutrophil leukocytes from patients with immotile cilia syndrome. Acta Med Scand 208:145, 1980.

Bleau G, Richer CL, and Bousquet D: Absence of dynein arms in cilia of endocervical cells in a fertile woman. Fertil Steril 30:362, 1978.

Boat TF, Wood R, Tanduer B et al: A screening test for the immotile cilia syndrome. Pediatr Res 13:531, 1979.

Camner P, Mossberg B, and Afzelius BA: Evidence for congenitally nonfunctioning cilia in the tracheobronchial tract in two subjects. Am Rev Respir Dis 112:807, 1975.

Corkey CWB, Levison H, and Turner JAP: The immotile cilia syndrome—a longitudinal survey. Am Rev Respir Dis 124:544, 1981.

Corkey CWB, Minta JO, Turner JAP, and Biggar WD: Neutrophil function in the immotile cilia syndrome. J Lab Clin Med 99:838, 1982.

Eliasson R, Mossberg B, Camner P, and Afzelius BA: The immotile cilia syndrome. A congenital ciliary abnormality as an etiologic factor in chronic airways infections and male sterility. N Engl J Med 297:1, 1977.

Fischer TJ, McAdam JA, Entis GN et al: Middle ear ciliary defect in Kartagener's syndrome. Pediatrics 62:443, 1978.

Hartline JV and Zelkowitz PS: Kartagener's syndrome in childhood. Am J Dis Child 121:349, 1971.

Herzon FS and Murphy S: Normal ciliary ultrastructure in children with Kartagener's syndrome. Ann Otol Rhinol Laryngol 89:81, 1980.

Jahrsdoerfer R, Feldman PS, Rubel EW et al: Otitis media and the immotile cilia syndrome. Laryngoscope 89:769, 1979.

Jewett MAS, Greenspan MB, Shier RM, and Howatson AF: Necrospermia or immotile cilia syndrome as a cause of male infertility. J Urol 124:292, 1980.

Kartagener M: Zur pathogenese der bronkiectasien: bronkiectasien bei situs viscerum inversus. Beitr Klin Tuberk 82:489, 1933.

Mossberg B, Afzelius BA, Eliasson R, and Camner P: On the pathogenesis of obstructive lung disease. Scand J Respir Dis 59:55, 1978.

Nadel HR, Stringer DA, Levison H et al: The immotile cilia syndrome: radiological manifestations. Radiology 154:651, 1985.

Pedersen M and Mygind N: Absence of axonemal arms in nasal mucosal cilia in Kartagener's syndrome. Nature 62:494, 1976.

Pedersen H and Mygind N: Ciliary motility in the 'immotile cilia syndrome.' Br J Dis Chest 74:239, 1980.

Rooklin AR, McGready SJ, Mikaelian DO et al: The immotile cilia syndrome: a cause of recurrent pulmonary disease in children. Pediatrics 66:526, 1980.

Rossman CM, Forrest JB, Lee RMKW, and Newhouse MT: The dyskinetic cilia syndrome. Ciliary motility in immotile cilia syndrome. Chest 78:580, 1980.

Rott HD: Kartagener's syndrome and the syndrome of immotile cilia. Hum Genet 46:249, 1979.

Rutland J and Cole PJ: Non-invasive sampling of nasal cilia for measurement of beat frequency and study of ultrastructure. Lancet 2:564, 1980.

Satir P: The present status of the sliding microtubule model of ciliary motion. In Sleigh MA (ed): Cilia and Flagella. New York, Academic Press, 1974.

Schneeberger EE, McCormack J, Issenberg HJ et al: Heterogeneity of ciliary morphology in the immotile syndrome in man. J Ultrastruct Res 73:34, 1980.

Sethi BR: Kartagener's syndrome and its otological manifestations. J Laryngol Otol 89:183, 1975.

Sleigh M: The nature and action of respiratory tract cilia. In Brain JD, Proctor DF, and Reid LM (eds): Respiratory Defense Mechanisms. New York, Marcel Dekker, Inc, 1977.

Sturgess JM: Mucous secretions in the respiratory tract. Pediatr Clin North Am 26:481, 1979.

Sturgess JM, Chao J, Wong J et al: Cilia with defective radial spokes: a cause of human respiratory disease. N Engl J Med 300:53, 1979.

Sturgess JM, Chao J, and Turner JAP: Transposition of ciliary microtubules: another cause of impaired ciliary motility. N Engl J Med 303:318, 1980.

Sturgess JM, Chao J, and Turner JAP: Genetic heterogeneity among dynein deficient cilia. Am Rev Respir Dis 126:302, 1982.

Sturgess JM, Thompson MW, Czegledy-Nagy, E, and Turner JAP: Genetic aspects of immotile cilia syndrome. Am J Med Genet 25:149, 1986.

Sturgess JM and Turner JAP: Ultrastructural pathology of cilia in the immotile cilia syndrome. Perspect Pediatr Pathol 8:133, 1984.

Turner JAP, Corkey CWB, Lee JYC et al: Clinical expressions of immotile cilia syndrome. Pediatrics 67:805, 1981.

Veerman AJP, Van der Baan A, Weltevreden EF et al: Cilia: immotile, dyskinetic, dysfunctional. Lancet 2:266, 1980.

Whitelaw A, Evans A, and Corrin B: Immotile cilia syndrome: a new cause of neonatal respiratory distress. Arch Dis Child 56:432, 1981.

46

JACQUELINE A. NOONAN, M.D.

COR PULMONALE

Pulmonary heart disease, also called cor pulmonale, may complicate pulmonary disorders in children. Cor pulmonale is defined as right ventricular hypertrophy secondary to disease of the lung parenchyma or of the pulmonary vasculature or resulting from abnormalities of pulmonary function. The basic component of cor pulmonale is pulmonary artery hypertension, which is responsible for the development of right ventricular hypertrophy. In most children, pulmonary hypertension results from pulmonary vasoconstriction as a response to hypoxia. Anatomic changes in the pulmonary vessels may be absent or may be limited to medial hypertrophy of the small pulmonary arteries, and if the underlying cause of the hypoxia can be corrected, the pulmonary hypertension is reversible. In some forms of diffuse progressive lung disease, interstitial fibrosis with destruction of the alveolar wall and capillaries may occur, leading to restriction of the pulmonary vascular bed. In such cases, pulmonary artery hypertension may not be completely reversible. When pulmonary hypertension results from pulmonary vascular disease due to multiple pulmonary emboli or from so-called primary pulmonary hypertension, there is little chance for reversibility. In Table 46–1, a simple classification of the causation of cor pulmonale is presented.

PARENCHYMAL LUNG DISEASE

OBSTRUCTIVE AIRWAY DISEASE

Asthma, chronic bronchitis, and fibrocystic disease are common causes of obstructive airway disease in children. Wheezing, prolonged expiration, and overexpanded lungs usually allow ready clinical recognition of obstructive airway disease. Pulmonary function studies show a decrease in vital capacity with increases in residual volume and in functional residual capacity. The obstruction of the small airways may occur because of inflammation of the mucosa, constriction of the bronchiolar smooth muscle, edema of the bronchial tissue, or plugging of the lumen by mucus. In any event, the degree of narrowing is variable among the many small airways, and the distribution of inspired gases is not uniform. This

results in an abnormal ratio between pulmonary blood flow and ventilation and leads to hypoxemia with a decreased arterial P_{O_2}. Because the uninvolved, relatively normal portion of the lungs may hyperventilate in response to hypoxia, the P_{CO_2} may remain quite normal until, with increasing severity of airway obstruction, there is overall alveolar hypoventilation.

Ventricular function is usually normal in patients with mild to moderate lung disease. As the lung disease progresses and reaches the end stage, cor pulmonale occurs as a recognized complication, particularly in fibrocystic disease. The clinical recognition of early cor pulmonale may be very difficult. Tachycardia, tachypnea, hepatomegaly, and cyanosis may be attributed to the pulmonary disease per se. The hyperinflated lungs may mask early cardiac enlargement and also may alter electrical conductance, limiting the value of both the chest roentgenogram and the electrocardiogram. Echocardiography provides a means to detect pulmonary hypertension noninvasively. It is possible to analyze the motion of the pulmonary valve and to measure the thickness of the right ventricular anterior wall, the size of the right pulmonary artery, and the right ventricular systolic time interval ratios, all of which have shown a reasonably good correlation with measured pulmonary artery resistance. These studies, however, require accurate images, which are often difficult to obtain in patients with overexpanded lungs. Morin and co-workers (1980) showed that the degree of airway obstruction could be followed by noting the

Table 46–1. CLASSIFICATION OF COR PULMONALE IN CHILDREN

Hypoxia
  Parenchymal lung disease
    Obstructive airway, e.g., with fibrocystic disease
    Restrictive lung disease, e.g., diffuse interstitial fibrosis
    Other lung disease, e.g., bronchopulmonary dysplasia
  Extrinsic factors
    Upper airway obstruction
    Neuromuscular disorders
    Thoracic cage deformity
    Respiratory center dysfunction
    High altitude
Pulmonary Vascular Disease
  Thromboembolism
  Primary pulmonary hypertension
  Pulmonary veno-occlusive disease

effect of respiration on the echocardiogram with the disappearance of pulsus paradoxus correlating with clinical improvement. Marchandise and colleagues (1987) have reported the noninvasive predication of pulmonary hypertension by Doppler echocardiography to have a higher rate of success than that usually reported with M-mode examination of the pulmonary valve.

Patients with little evidence of pulmonary hypertension at rest may develop significant pulmonary artery hypertension with exercise. Chipps and co-workers (1979) have reported radionuclide scanning to be a potentially valuable noninvasive tool in evaluating both right and left ventricular function with chronic obstructive airway disease during rest and exercise. A decreased right ventricular ejection fraction was found in 13 of 18 patients with cystic fibrosis. Four patients also had evidence of left ventricular dysfunction at rest, and in three others, left ventricular dysfunction was noted during exercise. Abnormal left ventricular function has been demonstrated infrequently in patients with cystic fibrosis. Unlike Chipps and colleagues (1979), Matthay and associates (1980) found normal left ventricular function by radionuclide studies in 22 young adults with cystic fibrosis, and only 9 of these patients had abnormal right ventricular function. Using two-dimensional Doppler echocardiography, Panidis and co-workers (1985) failed to detect evidence of left ventricular dysfunction in 17 consecutive hospitalized patients with cystic fibrosis. Left ventricular dysfunction has, however, been reported and has been attributed to hypoxia, acidosis, or myocardial fibrosis or has occurred as a consequence of abnormal left ventricular septal motion secondary to compression from a markedly dilated right ventricle. Most studies suggest that left ventricular function is preserved in moderately severe lung disease and may remain normal, even in the end stage of obstructive lung disease.

Physical examination is also important in diagnosing cor pulmonale in children with obstructive airway disease. The development of a systolic murmur along the lower left sternal border, indicating tricuspid insufficiency, is strong evidence of pulmonary hypertension. A right-sided gallop is often present when right heart failure occurs. Fluid retention and hepatomegaly are expected when heart failure occurs as a complication of cor pulmonale. The marked overexpansion of the lungs makes auscultation of the heart sounds less reliable in obstructive airway disease than in other pulmonary disorders.

Bronchiectasis may be a complication of obstructive airway disease, such as chronic bronchitis or fibrocystic disease, but so far in my experience cor pulmonale has not been a problem in children with severe localized bronchiectasis. Only mild pulmonary hypertension has been noted at cardiac catheterization, and there is surprisingly little decrease in the arterial P_{O_2}. Liebow and co-workers (1949) have demonstrated communications between the bronchial and pulmonary arteries in bronchiectasis. Moss (1982) pointed out that bronchoarteriography in patients with cystic fibrosis may demonstrate large and tortuous bronchial arteries. Because pulmonary blood flow to the destroyed lung segment is generally markedly reduced, the pulmonary flow and ventilation are fairly well matched and little hypoxemia results. A significant left-to-right shunt, however, may be noted at the pulmonary artery level from the bronchopulmonary anastomoses. Should there be extensive diffuse lung disease in addition to localized bronchiectasis, pulmonary artery hypertension would be expected. In such patients, the presence of a left-to-right shunt would impose an increased burden on the left ventricle, and both right-sided and left-sided heart failure might result.

Because cor pulmonale occurs late in the course of obstructive lung disease, it is not surprising that overt heart failure is an ominous sign. Stern and colleagues (1980) found a mean survival of 8 months for 61 patients with cystic fibrosis when this complication occurred. A similar poor prognosis has been noted by Moss and associates (1975). In the many clinical studies carried out in patients with cystic fibrosis, it is apparent that both right and left ventricular systolic function as assessed by quantitative two-dimensional echocardiography is preserved in patients with moderately severe lung disease, pointing out that the clinical status of a patient is mainly determined by the respiratory rather than cardiac status. This means that the main goal of patient management must be directed at vigorous treatment of the underlying pulmonary disease. As lung disease progresses, alveolar hypoxia occurs. This consequently causes pulmonary artery hypertension and systemic hypoxemia. Hypoxia can often be reversed by the continuous or nocturnal use of oxygen. Spier and colleagues (1984) showed that nocturnal oxygen administration alleviated the hypoxia occurring during sleep without causing significant clinical hypercapnia. A number of vasodilating drugs, such as tolazoline, hydralazine, and nifedipine, have been shown to reduce pulmonary artery pressure and pulmonary vascular resistance in some patients but have not proved effective for long-term management of cor pulmonale. Michael and associates (1984) reported that nifedipine improved exercise tolerance in two patients with cystic fibrosis and cor pulmonale. Both patients, however, died of respiratory failure 2 and 4 months after starting nifedipine therapy. Diuretics are helpful in the management of fluid retention, and digitalis may be helpful in patients with evidence of ventricular dysfunction. When cor pulmonale occurs and the respiratory condition cannot be reversed, the prognosis is very poor. Heart-lung transplantation has been carried out in a few patients with cystic fibrosis, with some limited success.

RESTRICTIVE LUNG DISEASE

In restrictive lung disease, there is impairment of diffusion because of thickening of the alveolar or capillary membrane by transudate, exudate, fibrosis, or granulomatous tissue, which causes an increased diffusion gradient for oxygen from the alveoli to capillary blood. The distribution of gas is uneven and results in a low P_{O_2}. The resulting hypoxemia stimulates hyperventilation, and because the relatively normal lung segments are then overventilated, the P_{CO_2} is usually significantly decreased. The low P_{O_2} causes pulmonary vasoconstriction, which may result in pulmonary artery hypertension. Unfortunately, diffuse pulmonary fibrosis (Hamman-Rich syndrome), chronic pneumonia of various types, sarcoidosis, hemosiderosis, and Wilson-Mikity disease, to name a few of the conditions resulting in restrictive lung disease, may, with increasing severity of the lung process, cause an actual reduction in the total pulmonary capillary bed. Pulmonary artery hypertension in patients with any of these conditions may result from two factors—namely, pulmonary vasoconstriction from hypoxia and actual destruction of part of the pulmonary vascular bed from fibrosis.

Patients with restrictive lung disease have effort dyspnea, fatigue, vague chest pain, and often an irritating, nonproductive cough. On physical examination, respirations are generally shallow and rapid. The lungs may be clear, although some patients have fine, dry rales. Clubbing is often present. Cyanosis is noted on exertion or with crying but in severe cases may be present even at rest. The presence of cyanosis and the absence of striking lung findings on physical examination may lead to a mistaken diagnosis of cyanotic heart disease. The chest roentgenogram usually shows a diffuse infiltrative process but varies, depending on the underlying disease process. If significant pulmonary artery hypertension is present, there is usually definite right ventricular hypertrophy, indicated by the electrocardiogram.

As mentioned elsewhere in this text, it is very important to diagnose the underlying pathologic condition in the lung, because some forms of restrictive lung disease are reversible by proper therapy. If routine laboratory studies and cultures are not productive in establishing a clear-cut, definitive diagnosis, a lung biopsy should be considered early in the course of the disease. Hamman-Rich syndrome, eosinophilic granuloma, desquamative interstitial pneumonitis, and collagen disease all are entities that may respond to steroid therapy, whereas chronic granulomatous disease, such as tuberculosis, histoplasmosis, or other fungal infections, require specific therapy. Establishing a definite diagnosis and instituting proper therapy offer the best chance of reversing the cor pulmonale. Figure 46–1 shows the roentgenogram of a patient with desquamative interstitial pneumonia before and after successful treatment with steroid therapy. Digitalis and diuretics should be used in the presence of suspected or overt congestive heart failure, as well liberal use of oxygen to correct hypoxia.

OTHER LUNG DISEASE

It is not always possible to classify the pulmonary disease as purely obstructive or restrictive, because some conditions result in a combination of these two physiologic derangements. One such entity is pulmonary lymphangiectasis, which is discussed elsewhere in this text. Perhaps the most common cause of chronic lung disease encountered today in infants is that of bronchopulmonary dysplasia (BPD). This form of chronic lung disease follows oxygen and ventilator therapy in the newborn period and is believed to represent a nonspecific reaction of the lungs to a slowly resolving acute injury. Because it occurs in young infants whose pulmonary blood vessels have not yet lost their thick, medial muscle layer, these vessels are especially reactive to hypoxia. Resulting pulmonary vasoconstriction may cause severe pulmonary artery hypertension and may lead to the very rapid development of cor pulmonale. Although oxygen may have contributed to BPD at its origin, supplemental oxygen is needed for these infants if the P_{O_2} is less than 60 mm Hg. This interesting condition, which is characterized by progressive lung changes during the perinatal period, often shows dramatic improvement during early childhood. Recovery from BPD may be complete, or there may be residual changes persisting to adult life.

Almost all infants who are undergoing cardiac catheterization and who have significant BPD have demonstrated pulmonary hypertension that, fortunately, is usually at least partially responsive to oxygen therapy. A study by Brownlee and colleagues (1988) evaluated the acute hemodynamic effects of nifedipine and compared them to those of 95 per cent oxygen in six children with BPD. They noted in those patients with pulmonary artery hypertension that nifedipine achieved a lower pulmonary artery vascular resistance with a greater cardiac output when compared with 95 per cent oxygen. Like other observers, they noted that despite substantial improvement in pulmonary artery pressure, neither nifedipine nor oxygen was able to normalize pulmonary artery pressure or resistance in any of their patients with significant pulmonary artery hypertension. This suggests that in addition to pulmonary vasoconstriction, there is probably also some anatomic loss of vessel cross-sectional area resulting from vascular remodeling or destruction of the lung.

In a recent study by Goodman and co-workers (1988), 17 children who had oxygen-dependent BPD and who showed Doppler echocardiographic evidence of pulmonary hypertension were evaluated by cardiac catheterization. Fifteen of these 17 patients had a mean pulmonary artery pressure greater than 24 mm Hg, while two had normal pulmonary artery pressure despite noninvasive evidence of right ventricular hypertrophy and pulmonary hypertension. Ten of their patients had pulmonary artery hypertension that did not normalize with the use of sup-

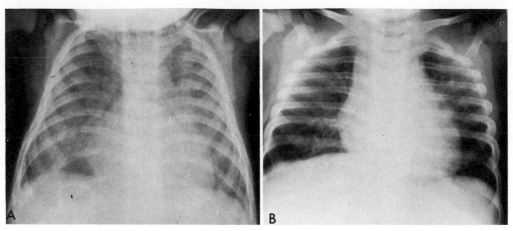

Figure 46–1. Chest roentgenograms of an infant with desquamative interstitial pneumonitis. *A*, Before treatment. *B*, After treatment with steroids.

plemental oxygen. Five of these patients had large collateral pulmonary vessels demonstrated by aortography. Hydralazine was administered to these 10 patients. Two of four patients without collaterals normalized pulmonary artery pressure, but the five patients with large systemic pulmonary collateral vessels showed an unfavorable hemodynamic response to hydralazine. One patient developed pulmonary edema, three patients developed an increase in pulmonary artery pressure or resistance, and no patients showed a favorable response. These authors found an unfavorable prognosis for those infants whose pulmonary artery did not become normal with supplemental oxygen. Fifty percent of such patients died. Thus far, the role of pulmonary collateral circulation in patients with BPD is unknown but should have further study.

Because the natural history of BPD is that of gradual improvement, vigorous treatment to prevent hypoxia by the use of supplemental oxygen and further evaluation of the possible beneficial effects of nifedipine therapy are warranted. Diuretics, especially furosemide, have been beneficial in the management of infants with BPD. Digoxin can also be used if there is evidence of ventricular dysfunction. Figure 46–2 is a roentgenogram of an infant shortly before death at age 6 months due to cor pulmonale resulting from BPD.

EXTRINSIC FACTORS RESULTING IN HYPOVENTILATION

UPPER AIRWAY OBSTRUCTION

Upper airway obstruction causing cor pulmonale is a very important condition to recognize, because it may be reversed by relief of the obstruction. The clinical picture includes noisy respirations with stridor, particularly in the supine position. In addition, somnolence, congestive cardiac failure, and roentgenographic evidence of pulmonary edema are common findings. Although hypertrophied tonsils and adenoids have been the most common cause of upper airway obstruction, micrognathia, glossoptosis, macroglossia, Crouzon disease, Hurler disease, laryngeal web, laryngotracheomalacia, and Pierre Robin syndrome also have been reported as causes. It is significant that many patients reported in the literature have had evidence of mental retardation. Obstructive sleep apnea may occur as a result of upper airway obstruction that is apparent only with sleep (Brouillette et al, 1982).

With upper airway obstruction, generalized hypoventilation of both lungs results. Therefore, there is not only a decreased P_{O_2} but also an elevated P_{CO_2} and, eventually, respiratory acidosis with a lowered pH. In all our patients with this syndrome, severe pulmonary hypertension was demonstrated at cardiac catheterization and was reflected by right ventricular and right atrial hypertrophy on the electrocardiogram. In addition, marked cardiac enlargement and pulmonary congestion were seen on x-ray examination. Severe pulmonary hypertension present during hypoxia and hypercapnia can be promptly reversed

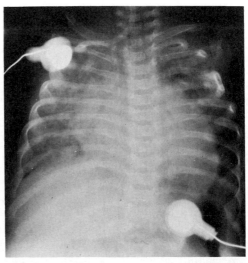

Figure 46–2. Radiograph of a 6-month-old infant with bronchopulmonary dysplasia shortly before death from cor pulmonale.

with relief of the upper airway obstruction. It was interesting to note that in our patients with upper airway obstruction, an elevated wedge or left atrial pressure was found at cardiac catheterization, and in several patients studied there was also an elevation of the end-diastolic pressure in the left ventricle. Hypoxia alone has little effect on left ventricular function. However, the combination of hypoxia plus acidosis has been shown experimentally to be quite detrimental to left ventricular function. It is possible that the pulmonary edema noted on the roentgenogram and the elevated pulmonary wedge pressure reflect left ventricular failure. The exact pathogenesis of the pulmonary edema noted in this syndrome has not yet been clearly defined.

It is essential that this syndrome be considered in any patient presenting with unexplained heart failure, particularly when somnolence is a clinical feature. Many patients reported in the literature were moribund at the time of admission, and four patients have been reported to have died before a correct diagnosis was made. Relief of the upper airway obstruction by removal of the tonsils and adenoids, tracheotomy, or endotracheal intubation should be done promptly. It is very important to be cautious in the use of supplemental oxygen in patients who have an elevated P_{CO_2} and who are hypoxic, because severe respiratory acidosis will quickly result if the hypoxic respiratory drive is inhibited by oxygen therapy. Use of sedation should be avoided until the upper airway obstruction has been relieved. Digitalis and diuretic therapy are recommended in addition to prompt relief of the upper airway obstruction.

NEUROMUSCULAR DISEASES

Inadequate respiration may result in weakness of the respiratory muscles. Werdnig-Hoffmann syndrome, Guillain-Barré syndrome, myasthenia gravis, and poliomyelitis are but a few of the conditions that may result in alveolar hypoventilation, which may in turn lead to hypoxemia and hypercapnia and eventually may cause pulmonary hypertension and cor pulmonale. It is important to obtain serial blood gas determinations in patients with neuromuscular diseases and to use assisted ventilation as soon as it is indicated. Acute respiratory failure and death are probably more common in neuromuscular disease than the development of cor pulmonale.

DEFORMITIES OF THE THORACIC CHEST

Smallness, immobility, or deformity of the chest, from any cause, that renders the chest a poor "bellows" may lead to cor pulmonale. Kyphoscoliosis is the most common thoracic deformity causing cor pulmonale, but because this condition is slowly progressive, symptoms are delayed until adult life and it is seldom a problem in childhood. Pectus excavatum is a very common thoracic deformity, but it rarely results in severe pulmonary dysfunction. There are, however, a number of severe congenital defects that may result in pulmonary insufficiency from so-called asphyxiating thoracic dystrophy. Vigorous physiotherapy and chest exercises should be employed to improve pulmonary function and to prevent or at least postpone the development of cor pulmonale. An associated respiratory infection often results in respiratory failure. If serial blood gases indicate deterioration, treatment with artificial ventilation should be promptly instituted to prevent the development of cor pulmonale or severe respiratory insufficiency.

Diaphragmatic paralysis, usually well tolerated in an older child or adult, may be very poorly tolerated in a newborn. One infant with a paralyzed right diaphragm developed cor pulmonale and marked wasting. Surgical plication of the right diaphragm brought significant clinical improvement. The electrocardiogram returned to normal, as did the pulmonary artery pressure and blood gases. Although Erb palsy associated with diaphragmatic paralysis is usually transient, in its severe form it may lead to cor pulmonale, which can be reversed by proper treatment.

RESPIRATORY CENTER DYSFUNCTION

The name *pickwickian syndrome* has been applied to the development of hyperventilation and cor pulmonale in obese persons. Although obesity itself does interfere with chest expansion because of the marked increase in work required to enlarge the thoracic cavity in the presence of excess weight, only a moderate reduction of vital capacity is expected. It is estimated that about 10 per cent of markedly obese adults actually hypoventilate and are at risk for developing pickwickian syndrome. There is good evidence to implicate a depression of the respiratory center as an important factor in the development of this disorder. Decreased sensitivity of the central nervous system to carbon dioxide inhalation, which does return to normal after weight reduction, has been demonstrated. This is a relatively uncommon syndrome in childhood, but several well-documented cases have been reported. It is interesting that mental retardation has been present in several of the obese children reported to have pickwickian syndrome. Weight reduction is an essential part of treatment for such patients.

Primary alveolar hypoventilation due to central nervous system disease is a rare cause of cor pulmonale. Both brain stem disease and hypothalamic lesions have been associated with hypoventilation. Unfortunately, primary apnea or hypoventilation due to respiratory center dysfunction (Ondine's curse) is rather poorly understood and very difficult to treat.

Respiratory stimulants, in general, are not effective in this syndrome. Mechanical ventilation is often necessary to reverse cor pulmonale. Ondine's curse fortunately is a rare disease, but one that should be kept in mind when an infant develops unexplained cyanosis and deep somnolence. If careful observation of the respiratory pattern and blood gas determinations demonstrate the presence of hypoventilation, mechanical ventilation should be instituted at once to reverse the symptoms. If the central nervous system problem is temporary, such as with drug intoxication, recovery should be expected. In the case of Ondine's curse, the prognosis is more guarded.

During the past few years, sleep apnea has attracted much attention and study (Guilleminault et al, 1976). It is apparent that apnea during sleep may be due to either a central cause or to upper airway obstruction and that in some patients both causes are operative. Sleep apnea may occur in patients with normal lungs, with obesity, with upper airway obstruction, and with chronic obstructive pulmonary disease.

Nocturnal desaturation resulting from an abnormal breathing pattern may result in intermittent pulmonary hypertension during sleep, and unless it is recognized and treated, overt cor pulmonale may result. More studies on the effect of sleep on the pulmonary dynamics of patients with pulmonary problems are needed before we fully understand the risk and implications of nocturnal desaturation (Boysen et al, 1979).

HIGH ALTITUDE

It is well documented that being at altitudes above 10,000 feet results in hypoxia and leads to pulmonary hypertension, which can be reversed on descent to sea level. Children living at high altitudes frequently have abnormal right shift in the mean QRS axis on the electrocardiogram and a raised pulmonary artery pressure at rest, which may in some cases increase markedly with exercise. Most children are asymptomatic despite increased pulmonary artery pressure. Occasionally, however, severe symptoms may occur similar to those noted in primary pulmonary hypertension. One infant had repeated episodes of syncope followed by seizures while living above 10,000 feet. Until she was seen by a pediatric cardiologist, pulmonary hypertension was not considered. At cardiac catheterization, reactive pulmonary artery hypertension and low cardiac output were found. Fortunately, the child became asymptomatic following the family's move to Kentucky, which is closer to sea level. There is an increased incidence of primary pulmonary hypertension among patients living at high altitude, and it is well known that patients with congenital heart disease, particularly those with left-to-right shunts, have a higher pulmonary vascular resistance and smaller left-to-right shunt when at high altitude than when at sea level.

PULMONARY VASCULAR DISEASE

THROMBOEMBOLISM

Pulmonary emboli are uncommon in children but may complicate sickle cell anemia, rheumatic fever, bacterial endocarditis, and schistosomiasis. Chronic cor pulmonale as a complication of multiple pulmonary emboli is even rarer but has been well documented as a complication of ventriculovenous shunt for the treatment of hydrocephalus. Although the cause and pathogenesis of this interesting complication are unknown, several factors have been proposed, including infection, periarteritis of the pulmonary vessels as an autoimmune reaction of the pulmonary vessels to cerebrospinal fluid, and the presence of brain thromboplastin in the circulation predisposing to repeated thromboembolization. Thrombosis of the superior vena cava and right atrium as a complication of the foreign body in the cardiovascular system might well serve as a source for repeated thromboemboli.

Early recognition of the complication of thromboembolism before severe pulmonary hypertension has developed is necessary to reverse the process. The most important part of therapy would be to remove the shunt from the cardiovascular system and substitute a peritoneal or other similar shunt in its place.

Acute cor pulmonale has been reported in children as a result of the development of primary thrombosis of the pulmonary artery, particularly in patients with the nephrotic syndrome. Multiple pulmonary emboli may also occur as a complication of sepsis or severe dehydration. The use of foreign bodies for deep intravenous hyperalimentation increases the risk of thromboembolism in children, particularly if infection occurs.

PRIMARY PULMONARY HYPERTENSION

Primary pulmonary hypertension is a rare but important cause of cor pulmonale in children. In one series of 110 patients with primary pulmonary hypertension, more than one third were under 15 years of age (Wagenvoort and Wagenvoort, 1970). The symptoms develop insidiously and may begin in early infancy. Fatigue, dyspnea on exertion, syncope, and convulsions are common complaints, and congestive cardiac failure is a frequent complication. Because loss of consciousness described as fainting or convulsion may be a predominant presenting symptom, it is not uncommon for a patient to be misdiagnosed as having a convulsive disorder. On physical examination, cyanosis may or may not be present. There typically is evidence of right ventricular hypertrophy with right ventricular lift and a markedly increased pulmonary second sound, often without a significant murmur. Ejection click, systolic ejection murmur, and parasternal diastolic blow as well as a murmur of tricuspid insufficiency all have been described, however. On chest roentgenogram, a prominent pulmonary artery, moderate cardiac enlargement, and decrease in the pulmonary vascularity in the peripheral lung fields are classic findings. An electrocardiogram usually shows evidence of severe right ventricular hypertrophy. Cardiac catheterization and angiocardiography will usually rule out congenital heart disease as the cause of the pulmonary hypertension. A normal wedge pressure helps to rule out left-sided obstructive lesions such as congenital mitral stenosis, cor triatriatum, and stenosis of the pulmonary veins, all of which may mimic primary pulmonary hypertension. Blood gas determinations may show some reduction in the P_{O_2}. The P_{CO_2} is usually quite low, because these patients tend to hyperventilate. Pulmonary artery pressure is markedly elevated and frequently at or near systemic level. The end-diastolic pressure in the right ventricle and the right atrial pressure are elevated if congestive heart failure is present. Cardiac output is generally quite low and fixed, and angiograms show dilated pulmonary vessels with a "pruned" appearance and a slow passage of dye through the lungs.

The cause of this serious disease is unknown. There is, however, a fairly high familial incidence, suggesting that there is some genetic predisposition to its development. Wagenvoort and Wagenvoort (1970) suggest that increased vasomotor tone is the initial factor in primary pulmonary hypertension. Microscopic examinations of the lungs reveal medial hypertrophy of the small pulmonary arteries, with intimal and plexiform lesions becoming more frequent with increasing age. Wagenvoort (1972) believes that the vascular lesions in primary pulmonary hypertension show the same range of vascular alterations as in patients with severe pulmonary hypertension resulting from other causes. He suggests that patients with primary pulmonary hypertension have extreme hyperactivity of the pulmonary vasculature, but what initiates the initial vasoconstriction is unknown.

At present, there is no specific treatment. Digitalis and diuretics are helpful in treating the complications of congestive failure. Intermittent oxygen therapy may improve symptoms. Anticoagulants are worthwhile if one cannot exclude the possibility of multiple pulmonary emboli. The beneficial effect of reducing afterload on the decompensated left ventricle by the use of systemic vasodilators has led many to reason that use of vasodilators in primary pulmonary hypertension might have a similar beneficial effect on the pulmonary bed and right ventricle. Unfortunately, if there already are severe fixed pulmonary vascular changes in the pulmonary arteries, vasodilator therapy is unlikely to be beneficial. The hemodynamic effects of vasodilators in these patients occur mainly in the systemic vascular bed, causing a decline in systemic resistance and a consequent reduction in cardiac output with severe transient hypotension and possible sudden death. Nonetheless, occasional patients appear to benefit both hemodynamically and clinically from vasodilators. Because the prognosis is so poor, a therapeutic trial with various drugs may be justified. Because of the potential for adverse effects, it is important that the pulmonary and systemic arterial pressures be carefully monitored while such drugs are administered. Although no single vasodilator has been shown to be more effective than others, nitrates and nifedipine appear to hold the most promise. Because there is no specific treatment for primary pulmonary hypertension and because the prognosis is so poor, heart and lung transplantation has been performed in a number of patients with primary pulmonary hypertension, and the survivors have been clinically improved. The prospects for this experimental procedure in terms of long-term survival are still uncertain.

When symptoms appear and a definite diagnosis is made, the prognosis is very poor, especially in children; in this age group, death usually occurs within 1 year. Death is frequently sudden and may be precipitated by a diagnostic procedure such as cardiac catheterization or even bone marrow aspiration.

INTRAPULMONARY VENO-OCCLUSIVE DISEASE

A rare disorder that may be confused with primary pulmonary hypertension is intrapulmonary veno-occlusive disease (Wagenvoort, 1976). This condition is associated with pathologic changes and obstruction of the small pulmonary veins and venules. The clinical features are similar to those of other forms of primary pulmonary hypertension and include dyspnea on effort, easy fatigability, chest pain, and syncopal episodes. An occasional patient may present with orthopnea and paroxysmal nocturnal dyspnea, which are rare in patients with primary pulmonary hypertension. Mild arterial unsaturation is frequent.

On physical examination, these patients resemble other patients with severe pulmonary hypertension and demonstrate a loud pulmonary second sound and occasionally the murmur of tricuspid insufficiency or pulmonary insufficiency. In some patients, fine rales may be heard in the lungs, but in patients with primary pulmonary hypertension the lungs are clear. The chest roentgenogram is most useful in distinguishing clinically between primary pulmonary artery hypertension and pulmonary veno-occlusive disease (Fig. 46–3). In both, there is evidence of right ventricular enlargement and a dilated main pulmonary artery. In intrapulmonary veno-occlusive disease, there is a fine and diffuse increase in the interstitial and vascular markings associated with Kerley B lines and visualization of the interlobar fissures. There may occasionally be pleural thickening or an effusion. The radiographic findings are suggestive of pulmonary venous hypertension secondary to a left-sided obstructive lesion of the heart. The roentgenogram may resemble that of a patient

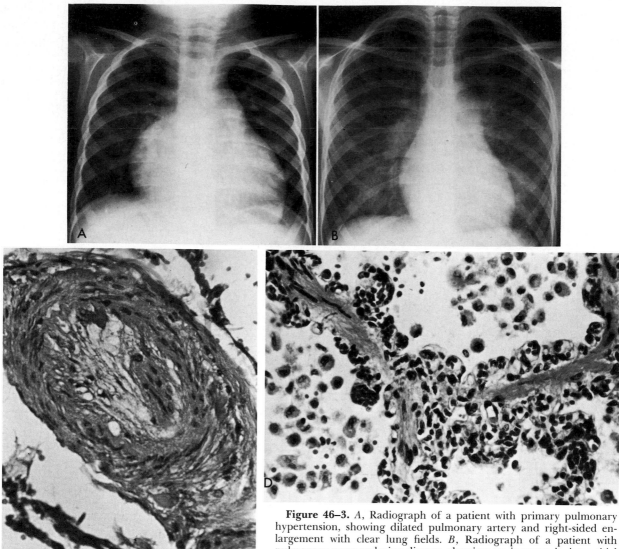

Figure 46–3. *A,* Radiograph of a patient with primary pulmonary hypertension, showing dilated pulmonary artery and right-sided enlargement with clear lung fields. *B,* Radiograph of a patient with pulmonary veno-occlusive disease, showing an increase in interstitial and vascular markings, with Kerley B lines at both bases. *C,* Medial hypertrophy and severe internal proliferation of the pulmonary artery characteristic of primary pulmonary hypertension. *D,* Capillary congestion, interstitial fibrosis, and an increase in inflammatory and heart failure cells characteristic of pulmonary veno-occlusive disease.

with severe mitral stenosis, but there is no evidence of enlargement of the left atrium.

The electrocardiogram is similar to that seen in primary pulmonary hypertension, showing right ventricular hypertrophy. An echocardiogram may be very helpful in ruling out obstructive left-sided heart disease as the possible cause of pulmonary venous congestion. It shows enlargement of the right ventricle, but the left atrium and the left ventricle are normal in size and there is a normal mitral valve.

Cardiac catheterization reveals severe pulmonary artery hypertension with a normal wedge, and the findings are not distinct from those in a patient with primary pulmonary hypertension, except that there is usually some pulmonary venous unsaturation.

On histologic examination, the small pulmonary veins show intimal fibrosis as expected, with pulmonary venous congestion. There are varying degrees

of obstruction of the small veins by thrombi and multiple foci of interstitial fibrosis. Capillary congestion and hemosiderosis and often an increase in inflammatory cells are also seen. Changes in the pulmonary arteries are always less extensive and more recent than those of the veins. The cause of this interesting entity is unknown, although an infectious origin has been proposed in some cases. Most patients, however, have no constitutional symptoms, and in the great majority, the etiologic factor remains obscure. In the patient reported by Rosenthal and co-workers (1973), a genetic factor could be implicated. The prognosis is poor, and all treatment has been ineffective. Of the reported cases, survival after diagnosis was usually less than 2 years, but our patient, shown in Figure 46–3, was dead within 2 months of the onset of clinical symptoms, as was a patient reported by Stoler and associates (1982).

SUMMARY

The cause of cor pulmonale in children is varied and in some cases may be reversed by prompt recognition and therapy. In general, treatment of the underlying lung disease accompanied by relief of hypoxia is the most important part of management. Digitalis is helpful and should be used. Care must be taken to avoid toxicity by strict attention to the potassium level. Diuretics are of great value in relieving the fluid retention of right-sided heart failure. Lasix may be of particular value in reducing the pulmonary congestion that often accompanies pulmonary disease. Oxygen to relieve hypoxia is important but should be administered with care if there is significant CO_2 retention. Mechanical respiratory assistance to correct respiratory insufficiency may be necessary to reverse cor pulmonale in some patients. Cor pulmonale should be considered a serious complication of respiratory disease, and care should be taken to prevent this problem whenever possible.

REFERENCES

Allen HD, Taussig LM, Gaines JA et al: Echocardiographic profiles of the long term cardiac changes in cystic fibrosis. Chest 75:428, 1979.

Abman SH, Wolfe RR, Accurso FJ et al: Pulmonary vascular response to oxygen in infants with severe bronchopulmonary dysplasia. Pediatrics 75:80, 1985.

Bergofsky EH: Cor pulmonale in the syndrome of alveolar hypoventilation. Prog Cardiovasc Dis 9:414, 1967.

Bland JW, Edwards FK, and Brinsfield D: Pulmonary hypertension and congestive heart failure in children with chronic upper airway obstruction. New concepts of etiologic factors. Am J Cardiol 23:830, 1969.

Bove KE and Scott RC: The anatomy of chronic cor pulmonale secondary to intrinsic lung disease. Prog Cardiovasc Dis 9:227, 1966.

Boysen PG, Block AJ, Wynne JW et al: Nocturnal pulmonary hypertension in patients with chronic obstructive pulmonary disease. Chest 76:536, 1979.

Bristow JD, Morris JF, and Kloster FE: Hemodynamics of cor pulmonale. Prog Cardiovasc Dis 9:239, 1966.

Brouillette RT, Fernback SK, and Hunt CE: Obstructive sleep apnea in infants and children. J Pediatr 100:31, 1982.

Brownlee JR, Beekman RH, and Rosenthal A: Acute hemodynamic effects of nifedipine in infants with bronchopulmonary dysplasia and pulmonary hypertension. Pediatr Res 24:186, 1988.

Buchta RM, Park S, and Giammona ST: Desquamative interstitial pneumonia in a seven-week old infant. Am J Dis Child 120:341, 1970.

Cayler GG, Mays J, and Riley HD: Cardiorespiratory syndrome of obesity (pickwickian syndrome) in children. Pediatrics 27:237, 1961.

Chipps BE, Alderson PO, Roland JA et al: Noninvasive evaluation of ventricular function in cystic fibrosis. J Pediatr 95:379, 1979.

Cox MA, Schiebler GL, Taylor WJ et al: Reversible pulmonary hypertension in a child with respiratory obstruction and cor pulmonale. J Pediatr 67:192, 1965.

Cronje RE, Human GP, and Simson IW: Hypoxaemic pulmonary hypertension in children. S Afr Med J 40:2, 1966.

Emery JL and Hilton HB: Lung and heart complications of treatment of hydrocephalus by ventriculoauriculostomy. Surgery 50:309, 1961.

Engelhardt B, Elliott S, and Hazinski TA: Short- and long-term effects of furosemide on lung function in infants with bronchopulmonary dysplasia. J Pediatr 109:1034, 1986.

Enson Y, Giuntini C, Lebois ML et al: The influence of hydrogen ion concentration and hypoxia on the pulmonary circulation. J Clin Invest 43:1146, 1964.

Favara BE and Paul RN: Thromboembolism and cor pulmonale complicating ventriculovenous shunts. JAMA 199:668, 1967.

Finkelstein JW and Avery ME: The pickwickian syndrome. Studies on ventilation and carbohydrate metabolism: case report of a child who recovered. Am J Dis Child 106:251, 1963.

Fishman LS, Samson JH, and Sperling DR: Primary alveolar hypoventilation syndrome (Ondine's curse). Am J Dis Child 110:155, 1965.

Gerald B and Dungan WT: Cor pulmonale and pulmonary edema in children secondary to chronic upper airway obstruction. Radiology 90:679, 1968.

Gervitz M, Eshaghpour E, Holsclaw DS et al: Echocardiography in cystic fibrosis. Am J Dis Child 131:275, 1977.

Gilroy J, Cahalan JL, Berman R, and Newman M: Cardiac and pulmonary complications in Duchenne's progressive muscular dystrophy. Circulation 27:484, 1963.

Goldring RM, Fishman AP, Turino GM et al: Pulmonary hypertension and cor pulmonale in cystic fibrosis of the pancreas. J Pediatr 65:501, 1964.

Goodman G, Perkin RM, Anas NG et al: Pulmonary hypertension in infants with bronchopulmonary dysplasia. J Pediatr 112:67, 1988.

Guilleminault C, Tilkian A, and Dement WC: The sleep apnea syndromes. Ann Rev Med 27:465, 1976.

Heath D: Pulmonary hypertension in pulmonary parenchymal disease. Cardiovasc Clin 4:80, 1972.

Hilton HB and Rendle-Short J: Diffuse progressive interstitial fibrosis of the lungs in childhood (Hamman-Rich syndrome). Arch Dis Child 36:102, 1961.

Hodgman JE, Mikity VG, Tatter D, and Cleland RS: Chronic respiratory distress in the premature infant. Wilson-Mikity syndrome. Pediatrics 44:179, 1969.

Hood WB, Spencer H, Lass RW, and Daly R: Primary pulmonary hypertension: familial occurrence. Br Heart J 30:336, 1968.

Hunt CE and Brouillette RT: Abnormalities of breathing control and airway maintenance in infants and children as a cause of cor pulmonale. Pediatr Cardiol 3:249, 1982.

Husson GS and Wyatt TC: Primary pulmonary vascular obstruction in children. Pediatrics 36:75, 1965.

Jersetz RM, Huszar RJ, and Basu S: Pierre Robin syndrome. Cause of respiratory obstruction, cor pulmonale, and pulmonary edema. Am J Dis Child 117:710, 1969.

Jeune M, Carron R, Berard C, and Loaec Y: Polychondradystrophie avec blocage thoracique d'evolution fatale. Pediatrie 9:390, 1954.

Jordan JD and Snyder CH: Rheumatoid disease of the lung and cor pulmonale: observations in a child. Am J Dis Child 108:174, 1964.

Kelminson LL, Cotton EK, and Vogel JHK: The reversibility of pulmonary hypertension in patients with cystic fibrosis: observations on the effects of tolazoline hydrochloride. Pediatrics 39:24, 1967.

Khoury GH and Howes CR: Primary pulmonary hypertension in children living at high altitude. J Pediatr 62:177, 1963.

Klinke WP and Gilbert JAL: Diazoxide in primary pulmonary hypertension. N Engl J Med 302:91, 1979.

Levin SE, Zamet R, and Schamman S: Thrombosis of the pulmonary arteries and the nephrotic syndrome. Br Med J 1:153, 1967.

Levy AM, Tabakin BS, Hanson JS, and Markewicz RM: Hypertrophied adenoids causing pulmonary hypertension and heart failure. N Engl J Med 277:506, 1967.

Liebow AA, Hales MR, and Lindskog GE: Enlargement of the bronchial arteries, and their anastomoses with the pulmonary arteries in bronchiectasis. Am J Pathol 25:211, 1949.

Luke MJ, Mehrizi A, Folger GM, and Rowe RD: Chronic nasopharyngeal obstruction as a cause of cardiomegaly, cor pulmonale, and pulmonary edema. Pediatrics 37:762, 1966.

Marchandise B, De Bruyne B, Delaunois L et al: Non-invasive prediction of pulmonary hypertension in chronic obstructive pulmonary disease by Doppler echocardiography. Chest 91:361, 1987.

Matthy RA, Berger HJ, Dolan TF et al: Right and left ventricular performance in ambulatory young adults with cystic fibrosis. Br Heart J 43:474, 1980.

Melmon KL and Braunwald E: Familial pulmonary hypertension. N Engl J Med 269:770, 1963.

Menashe VD, Farrehi C, and Miller M: Hypoventilation and cor pulmonale due to chronic upper airway obstruction. J Pediatr 67:198, 1965.

Michael JR, Kennedy TP, Fitzpatrick S et al: Nifedipine inhibits hypoxic pulmonary vasoconstriction during rest and exercise in patients with cystic fibrosis and cor pulmonale. Am Rev Respir Dis 130:516, 1984.

Morin DP, Cottrill CM, Johnson GL et al: Effect of respiration on the echocardiogram in children with cystic fibrosis. Pediatrics 65:44, 1980.

Moss AJ: The cardiovascular system in cystic fibrosis. Pediatrics 70:728, 1982.

Moss AJ, Dooley RR, and Mickey MR: Cystic fibrosis complicated by heart failure. West J Med 122:471, 1975.

Newth CJL, Gow RM, and Rowe RD: The assessment of pulmonary arterial pressures in bronchopulmonary dysplasia by cardiac catheterization and M-mode echocardiography. Pediatr Pulmonol 1:58, 1985.

Noonan JA: Pulmonary heart disease. Pediatr Clin North Am 18:1255, 1971.

Noonan JA: Pulmonary thromboembolism in children. In Mobbin-Uddin K (ed): Pulmonary Thromboembolism. Springfield, Ill, Charles C Thomas, 1975.

Noonan JA and Ehmke DA: Complications of ventriculovenous shunts for control of hydrocephalus. Report of three cases with thromboemboli to the lungs. N Engl J Med 269:70, 1963.

Noonan JA, Walters LR, and Reeves JT: Congenital pulmonary lymphangiectasis. Am J Dis Child 120:314, 1970.

Northway WH, Rosan RC, and Porter DY: Pulmonary disease following respiratory therapy of hyaline-membrane disease. N Engl J Med 276:357, 1967.

Panidis IP, Ren JF, Holsclaw DS et al: Cardiac function in patients with cystic fibrosis by two-dimensional and Doppler echocardiography. J Am Coll Cardiol 6:701, 1985.

Perkin RM and Anas NG: Pulmonary hypertension in pediatric patients. J Pediatr 105:511, 1984.

Pirnar T and Neuhauser EBD: Asphyxiating thoracic dystrophy of the newborn. Am J Roentgenol 98:358, 1966.

Rao BNS, Moller JH, and Edwards JE: Primary pulmonary hypertension in a child: response to pharmacologic agents. Circulation 40:583, 1969.

Rich S, Brundage BH, and Levy PS: The effect of vasodilator therapy on the clinical outcome of patients with primary pulmonary hypertension. Circulation 71:1191, 1985.

Rodman T, Resnick ME, Berkowitz RD et al: Alveolar hypoventilation due to involvement of the respiratory center by obscure disease of the central nervous system. Am J Med 32:208, 1962.

Rosenow EC, O'Connell EJ, and Harrison EG: Desquamative interstitial pneumonia in children. Am J Dis Child 120:344, 1970.

Rosenthal A, Vawter G, and Wagenvoort CA: Intrapulmonary veno-occlusive disease. Am J Cardiol 31:78, 1973.

Rosenthal A, Tucker CR, Williams RG et al: Echocardiographic assessment of cor pulmonale in cystic fibrosis. Pediatr Clin North Am 23:327, 1976.

Rubin IJ and Peter RH: Oral hydralazine therapy for primary pulmonary hypertension. N Engl J Med 302:69, 1979.

Spier S, Rivlin J, Hughes D et al: The effect of oxygen on sleep, blood gases, and ventilation in cystic fibrosis. Am Rev Respir Dis 129:712, 1984.

Stern RC, Borkat G, Hirschfield SS et al: Heart failure in cystic fibrosis. Am J Dis Child 134:267, 1980.

Stoler MH, Anderson VM, and Stuard ID: A case of pulmonary veno-occlusive disease in infancy. Arch Pathol Lab Med 106:645, 1982.

Talner NS, Liu HY, Oberman HA, and Schmidt RW: Thromboembolism complicating Holter valve shunt. A clinicopathologic study of four patients treated with this procedure for hydrocephalus. Am J Dis Child 101:602, 1961.

Thilenius OG, Nadas AS, and Jockin H: Primary pulmonary vascular obstruction in children. Pediatrics 36:75, 1965.

Vogel JHK, Pryor R, and Blount SG: The cardiovascular system in children from high altitude. J Pediatr 64:315, 1964.

Vogel JHK, McNamara DG, Rosenberg HS et al: Influence of altitude on the pulmonary circulation in experimental animals and patients with ventricular septal defects. Clin Res 13:113, 1965.

Wagenvoort CA: Vasoconstrictive primary pulmonary hypertension and pulmonary veno-occlusive disease. Cardiovasc Clin 4:98, 1972.

Wagenvoort CA: Pulmonary veno-occlusive disease; entity or syndrome? Chest 69:82, 1976.

Wagenvoort CA and Wagenvoort N: Primary pulmonary hypertension: a pathologic study of the lung vessels in 156 clinically diagnosed cases. Circulation 42:1163, 1970.

Watkins WD, Peterson MB, Crone RK et al: Prostocyclin and prostaglandin E for severe idiopathic pulmonary artery hypertension (letter). Lancet 10:1083, 1980.

47

IAN MACLUSKY, M.D., and
HENRY LEVISON, M.D.

CYSTIC FIBROSIS

Cystic fibrosis (CF) is the most common, lethal inherited disease of Caucasians. It occurs primarily in people of central and western European origin, with an estimated incidence of around 1:2000 to 1:2600 live births (Wood et al, 1976). Although preceding pathologic descriptions exist, it was not until 1938 that Andersen identified CF as a distinct clinical entity. When first described, CF was thought to be a relatively rare and invariably fatal disease of infancy. Subsequently, as a result of both improved diagnosis with recognition of milder degrees of involvement and improved treatment, there has been a marked increase in life expectancy (Fig. 47–1). Most clinics now report a median life expectancy for patients with CF in excess of 20 years (Corey, 1980). A cure remains elusive, however.

CF is a disease of exocrine gland function involving multiple organs and leading to a diverse range of pathologic and clinical problems (Fig. 47–2). Although most patients have multiple organ involvement, pulmonary disease is the principal cause of both morbidity and ultimate mortality in more than 90 per cent of patients surviving the neonatal period. CF therefore remains one of the major clinical problems confronting pediatricians who treat respiratory disorders.

GENETICS

Despite the marked clinical heterogeneity of CF, family studies have consistently supported an autosomal recessive mode of inheritance. Although primarily a disease of Caucasians, CF has been described in virtually every race, with an approximate incidence of 1:17,000 in blacks (Kulczycki and Schauf, 1974) and 1:90,000 in Orientals (Wright, 1968). In Caucasians, the carrier incidence is around 5 per cent, which is too high to be explained by spontaneous

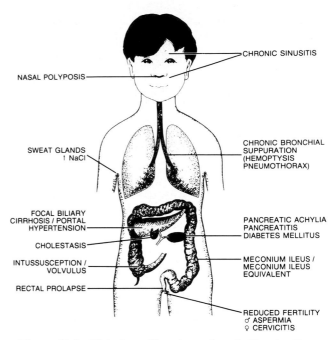

Figure 47–2. Clinical manifestations of cystic fibrosis. (Reproduced with permission from MacLusky IB, McLaughlin FJ, and Levison H: Cystic fibrosis. Curr Probl Pediatr 15(6):11, 1985.)

SURVIVAL OF PATIENTS WITH CF

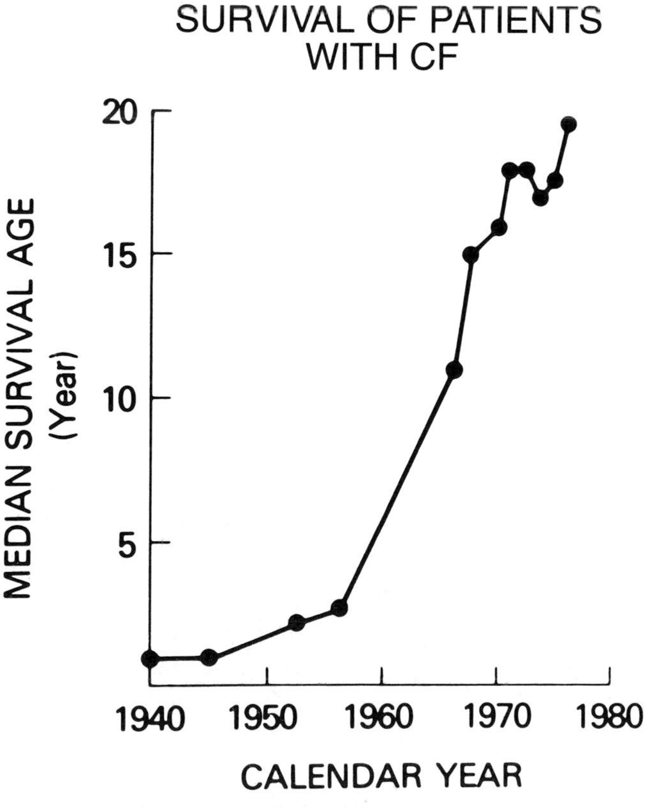

Figure 47–1. Survival of patients with cystic fibrosis in North America. (Reproduced with permission from MacLusky IB, McLaughlin FJ, and Levison H: Cystic fibrosis. Curr Probl Pediatr 15(6):5, 1985. Data after 1960 was obtained from the annual reports of the CF patient registry, Washington, DC, and before 1960 from Warwick WJ and Pogue RE: The prognosis for children with cystic fibrosis based on reasoned approaches to therapy: past, present and future. J Asthma Res 5:277, 1968. Reproduced with permission from Marcel Dekker, Inc.)

mutation. Because CF is a fatal disease, there is presumably a heterozygote advantage. Increased resistance to tuberculosis, syphilis, and increased fertility in male heterozygotes all have been proposed but remain unproven.

The chromosomes of patients with CF show no ultrastructural abnormalities. Advances in molecular biology have, however, allowed for chromosomal localization of the CF gene. Restriction endonucleases are enzymes that cleave DNA molecules at specific sites, dependent on the local base sequence. This results in multiple, pleomorphic DNA fragments, the pattern and structure of which vary depending on the restriction endonuclease used. By using cloning techniques, it is possible to produce sufficient DNA for analysis of these fragments. The fragments can be separated by various techniques, based on molecular size, and characterized by hybridization with various radioisotope-labeled DNA fragments of known sequence (probes). These fragments may be used to study the inheritance of specific factors in large-scale family studies (see Steel, 1984, for a more extensive review of this technique). If one of these fragments lies close to the CF locus, then crossover between the two loci is unlikely to occur during meiosis and the offspring will therefore tend to inherit either both the fragment and the CF gene or neither. By analyzing the incidence of co-inheritance of both CF and a selection of random probes in large-scale studies of affected families, it is possible to estimate statistically the geographic proximity of the CF gene to any of these probes. In 1985, these techniques were used to demonstrate linkage between CF and the genetic determinant for serum paraoxonase, although the chromosomal location of paraoxonase was not known. Tsui and colleagues (1985) subsequently determined that the DNA marker

DOCR1-917, present on the long arm of chromosome 7, showed close linkage to both the CF gene and to paraoxonase. As a result of a large-scale, multinational research effort, many other gene probes have been identified, further localizing the CF gene to a specific region on the long arm of chromosome 7 (Lathrop et al, 1988) (Fig. 47–3).

Once probes sufficiently close to the CF gene were identified by using chromosome "jumping" and chromosome "walking" techniques (mapping overlapping fragments of cloned DNA), it became possible to identify the exact locus of the CF gene. The CF gene has now been characterized as being composed of a segment, approximately 250,000 base pairs in length, located in the region 7q31 (Rommens et al, 1989). A specific trinucleotide deletion (resulting in the loss of phenylalanine from the product protein) has been identified in 70 per cent of patients. The current evidence is that there are at least five distinct possible mutations within the CF gene, resulting in differing degrees of disease expression, which may explain the marked variability in clinical presentation characteristic of the disease (Kerem et al, 1989).

PATHOGENESIS

Whatever the initial clinical presentation, every patient with CF demonstrates the following three distinct abnormalities, albeit to various degrees:

1. An abnormal concentration of inorganic ions in the secretions from serous glands, the most characteristic being elevated concentrations of sodium and chloride in sweat.

2. An increase in the viscosity of secretions from mucus-secreting glands, associated with obstruction and secondary loss of glandular function.

3. An undue susceptibility to chronic endobronchial colonization by specific groups of bacteria.

Although various discrete functional and biochemical abnormalities have been described (Table 47–1), no single abnormality that fully explains all of these observations has yet been identified. Within the constraints of this chapter, it is not possible to do justice to the vast amount of relevant research performed during the past 30 years. We shall briefly review the major findings. Interested readers are referred to more exhaustive reviews (Boat and Dearborn, 1984; Geddes, 1984).

ION TRANSPORT

Sweat from patients with CF characteristically contains elevated levels of both sodium and chloride. Sweat glands isolated from patients with CF continue to show this abnormality in vitro (Yankaskas et al, 1985), suggesting that it arises as an inherent defect rather than as a secondary effect of the underlying disease process or circulating humoral factors. In addition, studies from gastrointestinal, reproductive tract, and pancreatic secretions from pancreatic-suf-

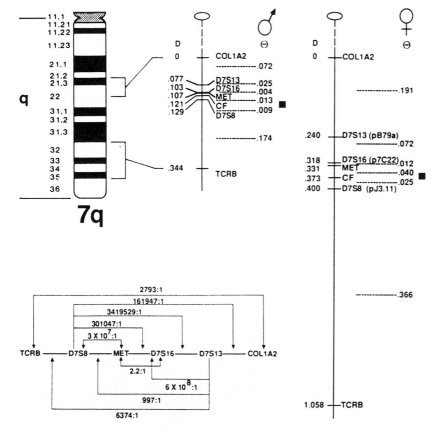

Figure 47–3. A map of chromosome 7q, showing the locations of six linked marker loci and the cystic fibrosis gene under the best supported gene order, as well as the odds against alternative orders. (Reproduced with permission from Lathrop GM: Am J Hum Genet 42:38, 1988.)

Table 47–1. BIOCHEMICAL ABNORMALITIES IN CYSTIC FIBROSIS

Ionic
Block in anionic transport
Abnormal cellular calcium transport

Circulating CF-Specific Factors
Causing abnormal ciliary motility
Blocking sodium chloride reabsorption across the sweat duct

Rheologic
Abnormal mucus glycoproteins

Systemic
Abnormal autonomic responsiveness

ficient patients (Kopelman et al, 1985) have consistently demonstrated reduced water content as a primary abnormality.

Water flow across an epithelium occurs in response to an osmotic gradient created by the active transport of inorganic ions, primarily sodium and chloride. The current model of ion transport across respiratory epithelium is similar to that of other epithelia (Welsh, 1986). The energy for active transport originates from the sodium-potassium ATPase (blocked by ouabain) located on the basolateral membrane of the cell. It extrudes sodium from the cell, setting up the large sodium electrochemical gradient that drives active ion transport. In respiratory epithelial cells that are reabsorbing sodium and fluid from the mucosal surface, the sodium enters the cell through apical sodium channels (blockable by amiloride) and is then extruded out the basolateral membrane (serosal side) by sodium-potassium ATPase (Fig. 47–4). In respiratory epithelial cells that are secreting ions and fluid, the sodium that is extruded out of the cell across the basolateral membrane then reenters the cell along with two chloride and one potassium ion via a cotransporter protein located in the basolateral membrane. The chloride ion accumulates inside the cell above its electrochemical gradient and thus moves out across the apical membrane of the cell. The balance between the active transport of these two ions in any cell will determine whether it is a net fluid-absorbing or fluid-secreting cell.

Abnormalities in ionic transport across CF epithelia

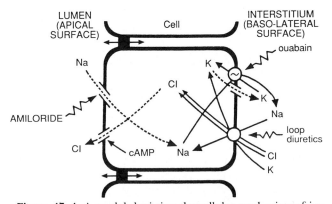

Figure 47–4. A model depicting the cellular mechanism of ion transport by canine tracheal epithelium. See text for discussion. (Adapted from Welsh MJ: Clin Chest Med 7:273, 1986.)

have been consistently observed (Knowles et al, 1986):

1. An elevated potential difference exists between the nasal or tracheal epithelium and the blood. This abnormality is also observed in vitro using primary cultures of affected CF tissues.

2. There is an approximate doubling in the rate of sodium flux from the mucosal to serosal surface of respiratory epithelium.

3. The apical membrane is relatively impermeable to chloride. This likely results from the well-documented failure of the apical chloride channel to open normally in response to agents that stimulate cyclic AMP-dependent protein kinase, beta agonists, and cyclic AMP (Dubinsky, 1987).

4. That the primary defect in cystic fibrosis is due to an intrinsic abnormality in cell membrane function is further supported by the predicted structure of the protein product of the CF gene, called the cystic fibrosis transmembrane conductance regulator (CFTR) (Riordan et al, 1989). This predicted protein has two domains, one of which is capable of spanning the cellular membrane, the other of which is capable of ATP binding. The predicted structure of the CFTR is therefore very similar to previously identified cationic channel proteins. It is reasonable to postulate that the CFTR is involved in regulation of ionic transport across the cell membrane and that structural defects in the CFTR could lead to the abnormalities in anionic transport characteristic of cystic fibrosis.

These observations may explain not only the electrolyte abnormality in CF but also the susceptibility to endobronchial colonization. Ciliary epithelium is covered by a surface fluid comprised of two phases: a "sol" phase surrounding the cilia and a glycoprotein-rich "gel" phase forming a discontinuous blanket overlying the tips of the cilia. An increase in the amount of sodium movement from mucosal to serosal surface combined with a decrease in chloride transport from serosa to mucosa would lead to a relative dehydration of the fluid layer lying above the apices of the cells. A defect in control of depth of the sol phase could thus result in disturbance in mucociliary clearance, making patients susceptible to chronic endobronchial colonization by inhaled organisms. This theory does not explain why patients with CF are preferentially colonized by *Pseudomonas aeruginosa*, however, nor why they have a poorer prognosis than patients with primary ciliary dyskinesia, which is characterized by ineffective ciliary function.

Abnormalities in calcium homeostasis have been observed in CF (Feigal and Shapiro, 1986), although its role in the pathogenesis of the disease is unclear. Elevated levels of calcium have been demonstrated in submaxillary saliva and tears, and increased levels of intracellular calcium are noted in cultured fibroblast from patients with CF. Decreased activity of calcium-ATPase activity has also been described in CF erythrocyte membranes and tissue fibroblasts. Finally, a recent study (Katz et al, 1988) has demonstrated microscopic nephrocalcinosis and hypercalciuria in patients with CF, present even in the neonatal period.

MUCOUS GLYCOPROTEINS

Abnormalities of mucus-secreting glands are one of the primary histologic features of CF, present even in utero. An inherent abnormality in mucous glycoprotein structure therefore has long been searched for.

Mucous glycoproteins form a complex, heterogeneous group of predominately high-molecular-weight, high-carbohydrate molecules, containing numerous sugar side chains. A number of these sugar side chains are highly sulfated, the number varying between the different classes of glycoprotein. It is the ability of mucous glycoproteins to form cross-linking between the sulfhydryl groups of adjacent molecules that is believed to allow for gel formation and hence the viscoelastic properties of mucus secretions.

A number of abnormalities in the glycoprotein structure of secretions from affected CF tissues have been reported. First, increased sulfation of the carbohydrate side chains of glycoproteins has been observed in secretions obtained directly from patients and from in vitro tissue preparations (Cheng et al, 1988). It therefore appears to be an inherent abnormality in CF. Increased sulfation might lead to increased cross-linking between sulfhydryl groups and hence result in increased gel viscosity. Second, elevated levels of both fucose and galactose in the carbohydrate side chains of patients with CF have been described, possibly resulting in a denser, more hyperviscous gel (Wesley et al, 1983). This has not been a universal finding, however, and may simply reflect differences in experimental techniques.

Mucus is an extremely complex, heterogeneous biochemical matrix, with its composition varying between tissues and individuals. We are only beginning to understand the complex factors leading to its formation and the various interactions leading to its specific physicochemical properties. Gel viscosity may be more dependent on the extent of intra- and intermolecular interactions of hydrophilic, covalently bound lipid fractions of the glycoprotein molecules than on the carbohydrate side chains (Slomiany et al, 1988). Gel viscosity is not only dependent on glycoprotein structure and concentration but may also be affected by the concentrations of hydrogen ion, calcium ion, and albumin present in the secretions. The clinical relevance of these observations and the interaction with the documented abnormalities in ion transport therefore remain to be clarified.

INFECTION

Although clearly arising as a consequence of the underlying defect, chronic bronchopulmonary infection is the major cause of the progressive pulmonary damage in CF. The exact mode of acquisition, the clinical significance of the various organisms seen, and the mechanisms of pulmonary damage are still under investigation.

At birth, the lungs of patients with CF are histologically normal. Endobronchial colonization, however, commonly occurs within the first 1 to 2 years of life, the pattern of colonization changing with age and severity of the pulmonary disease (Corey et al, 1984). In the initial stages, colonization is limited to the mucociliary layer of the peripheral airways. Inflammatory changes in the underlying mucosa result, initially with minimal parenchymal involvement. Colonization, once present, tends to be persistent despite aggressive management. With persisting colonization and resulting peribronchial inflammation, there is progressive airway damage, resulting in bronchiolectasis, bronchiectasis, and increasing parenchymal involvement, with microabscess formation and focal hemorrhagic pneumonia. Patients with CF are frequently colonized by multiple organisms (Bauerfeind et al, 1987), most of which may colonize the upper airway of patients who do not have CF or are commonly present in the environment (Fig. 47–5).

STAPHYLOCOCCUS AUREUS

Historically, S. aureus was the principal pathogen found in patients with CF. In recent years, although S. aureus is frequently the initial colonizing agent, patients subsequently become colonized with P. aeruginosa. It is not known whether this shift in bacterial spectrum is due to the widespread use of antistaphylococcal antibiotics or simply is a result of improved nutrition and life expectancy in patients with CF. S. aureus produces a number of well-defined virulence factors (Cohen, 1986). Although colonization is still common, fulminant disease or systemic spread is rare in patients with CF. The mechanism of colonization with S. aureus, as well as its clinical significance and role in the progressive pulmonary disease, remains a matter of debate.

PSEUDOMONAS AERUGINOSA

P. aeruginosa has superseded S. aureus as the principal pathogen in CF; most clinics now report colonization rates in excess of 70 per cent (Bauerfeind et al, 1987; Corey et al, 1984). P. aeruginosa is a ubiquitous organism in the environment, but with the exception of patients with CF, it is usually nonpathogenic to immunocompetent hosts. In CF, colonization by P. aeruginosa is, however, clearly the main cause of the progressive pulmonary disease in the vast majority of patients (Pier, 1985). Steady deterioration commonly follows initial colonization. P. aeruginosa colonization usually occurs within the first decade of life (mean age of colonization in our clinic

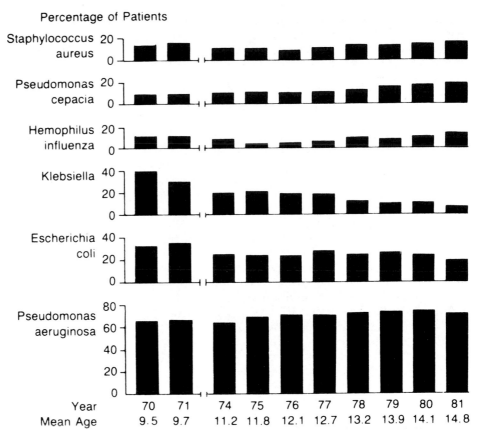

Percentage of Patients

Figure 47–5. Percentage of patients colonized by various organisms who attended the cystic fibrosis clinic, Hospital For Sick Children, Toronto, between 1970 and 1981. (Reproduced with permission from Corey M, Allison L, Prober C et al: J Infect Dis 149:283, 1984. © The University of Chicago Press.)

is 7.5 ± 6.3 SD years). The mode of acquisition in patients with CF is unknown; neither interpatient transmission nor an environmental reservoir has been convincingly demonstrated. Once *P. aeruginosa* colonization has occurred, it is rarely if ever eradicated. For colonization to persist, bacterial adherence has to occur first; persistence depends on malfunction of either local and/or systemic immunity. To date, there is no convincing evidence of a primary systemic immunodeficiency in CF. Most patients demonstrate, if anything, an overactive systemic immune response (see subsequent discussion); despite massive endobronchial colonization at times, systemic spread is rare. Most current evidence thus points to a defect in local immunity as the primary disturbance. *Pseudomonas* is presumably selected as the predominant organism both by specific adhesion properties of the organism and a preferential biochemical environment within the airways of patients with CF.

Mechanisms of Adherence

Although *P. aeruginosa* does not adhere to normal, intact airway epithelium, it does show preferential binding both to damaged epithelium and to airway mucins (Pitt, 1986). Initial colonization is usually by nonmucoid-producing *P. aeruginosa*. Sixty to 90 per cent of patients with CF, however, subsequently become colonized by mucoid strains of *P. aeruginosa* that secrete a mucoexopolysaccharide, commonly referred to as alginate. Nonmucoid strains of *P. aeru-*

ginosa show preferential adherence to both damaged epithelium and surface mucoproteins by means of surface projections called fimbriae. Subsequent mucoid production further mediates adherence, while allowing formation of microcolonies of alginate-embedded organisms that may protect against host defenses. Mucoid-producing strains of *P. aeruginosa* are rare in individuals unafflicted with CF. Mucoid production is an unstable characteristic, many strains reverting to nonmucoid on in vitro culture. It appears that various factors within CF airways preferentially select for mucoid production (Pitt, 1986). First, nonmucoid strains can be stimulated in vitro to produce alginate in the presence of elevated concentrations of calcium, such as occurs within the airway mucus of patients with CF. Second, formation of exopolysaccharide coat may protect *P. aeruginosa* both against opsonophagocytosis and against antibody penetration. Last, mucopolysaccharide may protect against penetration by highly ionized antibiotics, such as the aminoglycosides.

Mechanisms of Damage

P. aeruginosa produces a wide variety of virulence factors, including various proteases, exotoxin A, phospholipase, and pyocyanin (Vasil, 1986). All of these may contribute to cause the airway inflammation and progressive epithelial destruction associated with *P. aeruginosa* colonization. There is, however, increasing evidence to suggest that a significant proportion of the pulmonary damage may be immune mediated (Hoiby, 1987). Patients colonized by *P. aeruginosa* clearly mount an aggressive immune response. Elevated levels of IgG, IgA, and to some degree IgM are characteristically found in chronically colonized patients (Moss, 1987), rising steadily in parallel with advancing pulmonary disease. Indices of inflammation, such as acute phase proteins, erythrocyte sedimentation rate (ESR), and total white blood cell count, also show a progressive rise. In advanced disease, high levels of specific antibodies against *P. aeruginosa* virulence factors are found in both serum and sputum. Despite this aggressive immune response and the fact that most *P. aeruginosa* isolates from patients with CF remain serum sensitive, colonization persists and bacteria within airways reach levels of 10^7 to 10^8 colony-forming units per milliliter. The degree of immune activity may simply reflect the severity of pulmonary colonization. As a consequence of the continued antigen and antibody production, patients with CF are clearly at risk of immune complex formation, however, and hence of immune complex-mediated inflammation (type III hypersensitivity of Coombs and Gell) (Schiotz, 1981). Immune complexes have been demonstrated in serum, in sputum, and in various tissues including lung in as many as 50 per cent of patients with CF (Hoiby, 1986). Although immune complex levels do not have an obvious correlation with the severity of lung disease, the presence of circulating immune complexes and decreased activity of the alternate complement pathway are associated with a more severe prognosis (Wisnieski et al, 1985). Immune complex formation may cause local damage, both by activation of the complement system, supported by the presence of C3 split products in sputum and activated C4 in serum of patients with CF, and by stimulation of polymorphonuclear leukocytes (PMNs) (Hoiby et al, 1987). Sputum from patients with CF contains large numbers of PMNs, and sputum DNA and proteases are primarily of PMN origin (Goldstein and Doring, 1986). Immune complex activation of PMNs results in local tissue damage as a result of release of both superoxide radicals and various granulocyte proteases (Brigham and Meyrick, 1984).

There is evidence of a feed-forward control in PMN activation, because PMN activation leads to release of elastase, which cleaves both free immunoglobulins and immune complexes. These fragments may then act as blocking antibodies, preventing phagocytosis and hence serving to perpetuate *P. aeruginosa* colonization (Tosi et al, 1988).

The Boston group has identified a series of patients with apparent inherent hypogammaglobulinemia (22 per cent under age 10) (Mathews et al, 1980). The cause of the low immunoglobulins is not clear, although it has been suggested that these patients may have reduced epithelial permeability and hence are less exposed to inhaled antigens. Whatever the cause of their deficient immunoglobulins, these patients clearly have a better prognosis than patients with normal or elevated immunoglobulins (Wheeler et al, 1984). Moreover, a preliminary study suggests that anti-inflammatory therapy with long-term systemic corticosteroids had a beneficial clinical effect (Auerbach et al, 1985).

Although immune complex-mediated damage is primarily confined to the lungs, there have been several reports of patients with serum sickness-type illness, arthralgias, nephropathy (Rush et al, 1986), and cutaneous vasculitis (Fradin et al, 1987) apparently due to peripheral deposition of circulating immune complexes.

PSEUDOMONAS CEPACIA

P. cepacia is an aerobic, gram-negative bacillus that is distantly related to *P. aeruginosa*. It is an opportunistic pathogen in hospitalized patients and other compromised hosts. It is an incredibly versatile organism, capable of utilizing a wide variety of nutrients for growth (Goldmann and Klinger, 1986). Outbreaks of nosocomial infection have been described secondary to colonization of both antiseptics and surgical scrub solutions. *P. cepacia* is usually of very low virulence and is virtually nonpathogenic in healthy, immunocompetent individuals. Patients with CF are at significant risk of colonization, however. In 1984, we reported a steady rise in prevalence of *P. cepacia* colonization within our clinic population (Isles et al, 1984), rising from 10 per cent in 1971 to 18 per cent in 1981 and now currently in excess of 30 per cent. Although several other clinics have reported similar experience, there remains a marked variation in incidence between different clinics, some clinics failing to document any episodes of colonization. The high incidence within some clinics suggests that initial colonization frequently occurs around the time of hospitalization. This, plus the observation that siblings of patients colonized by *P. cepacia* are themselves at increased risk of colonization (Tablan et al, 1985), suggest a degree of interpatient transmission. Whether this is by direct transmission or via some intermediary vector such as pulmonary function equipment has not been proved. The Cleveland Clinic has used a program of rigorous isolation of patients colonized with *P. cepacia* to reduce the yearly incidence from 8.2 per cent down to 1.7 per cent within a period of 1 year (Thomassen et al, 1986).

Colonization with *P. cepacia* has been of concern for several reasons. First, the organism is inherently resistant to a wide variety of antibiotics, making treatment of acute exacerbations difficult in colonized patients. Second, a small group of patients, principally adolescent females, have been noted to develop a progressive fulminant bronchopneumonia in association with *P. cepacia*. This is characterized by elevated white blood cell count, ESR, and swinging fevers, with progressive deterioration in pulmonary status. In our initial report, five of eight girls with this clinical picture died (Isles et al, 1984). Several of these patients were, however, colonized with *P. cepacia* for periods before the onset of fulminant disease. Moreover, although *P. cepacia* colonization remains a common finding, since our initial report the incidence of fulminant disease appears to have become less common. We suspect that the fulminant disease may occur as a result of a combination of both *P. cepacia* colonization and some other inciting agent, possibly viral in origin.

P. cepacia colonization is associated with more advanced pulmonary disease. In our clinic, the mean FEV_1 was 62 per cent of predicted values in patients colonized by *P. cepacia*, compared with 73 per cent for patients colonized with *P. aeruginosa* and 85 per cent for patients colonized with neither. It is not clear, however, whether colonization with *P. cepacia* is associated with a more significant rate of decline, or simply that a greater degree of pulmonary damage is required for *P. cepacia* colonization to occur. Although *P. cepacia* colonization may occur in patients with mild disease, colonization usually occurs in older patients with more advanced disease (mean age of acquisition for *P. cepacia* being 13.7 years, compared with 7.5 years for *P. aeruginosa*). The increasing prevalence for colonization may therefore reflect the increased survival of the patient population rather than an increase in interpatient transmission.

OTHER ORGANISMS

A wide variety of other organisms are isolated from patients with CF (Bauerfeind et al, 1987). Examples include *Pseudomonas maltophilia*, *Pseudomonas fluorescens*, several *Actinobacillus* species, *Escherichia coli*, *Klebsiella* species, *Proteus* species, and *Serratia* species. Various anaerobic organisms have also been cultured from thoracotomy specimens in concentrations similar to those of *P. aeruginosa*. *Hemophilus influenzae* is also commonly isolated and is frequently the first organism to colonize the lower respiratory tract. The incidence of infections with the various organisms varies between clinics, and colonization is commonly transient, in most patients eventually being supplanted by *P. aeruginosa* colonization. The exact clinical role of these organisms, particularly in regard to the progressive pulmonary disease, at this point remains speculative.

The role of viral infections in CF is still unclear. Twenty to 30 per cent of episodes of acute exacerbation are associated with viral seroconversion (Stroobant, 1986), principally against respiratory syncytial virus and influenza A (Wang et al, 1984). The incidence of viral seroconversion also correlates directly with both severity and rate of deterioration of pulmonary disease. Viral infection is known to cause epithelial damage, interfering with mucociliary clearance and hence potentiating secondary bacterial infection in normal individuals (Stroobant, 1986). Viral infection may also interact with preceding bacterial colonization, initiating a cytotoxic antigen-antibody complex reaction and impairing local pulmonary and antibacterial defense mechanisms. Viral superinfection may therefore explain the rapid deterioration and fulminant pulmonary disease in some patients (see also "*Pseudomonas cepacia*").

Elevated titers of *Legionella pneumophila* in the serum of patients with CF has also been reported (Efthimiou, 1984). A subsequent study (Wang et al, 1987) suggests that this may be an artifact due to cross-reaction with *P. aeruginosa* antibodies, however.

PULMONARY MANIFESTATIONS

PATHOLOGY

At birth, apart from a mild degree of pleural cell metaplasia, the lungs of patients with CF are morphologically normal. Pathologic changes do develop early in postnatal life, however, being initially localized to the small airways. The initial lesion is dilation and hypertrophy of the mucus-secreting glands (Sturgess, 1982). Subsequent to bacterial colonization there is increasing squamous metaplasia of the bronchial epithelium, mucus plugging of peripheral airways, and ciliary dysgenesis with disorganization and fusion of the cilia into compound cilia. Mucopurulent plugging of bronchi and bronchioles is prominent, with acute and chronic lymphocytic infiltration of the submucosa (Fig. 47–6) (Oppenheimer and Esterly, 1975). Parenchymal involvement is less common, although localized sequential bronchopneumonia is occasionally encountered, primarily in younger patients (Bedrossian et al, 1976). Progressive bronchiectasis develops with increasing age, involving primarily the upper lobes (Tomashefski et al, 1986) and resulting in subsequent airway collapse, air trapping, and focal areas of hemorrhagic pneumonia (Fig. 47–7).

The progressive bronchiectasis and resulting hypoxemia lead to marked pulmonary vascular

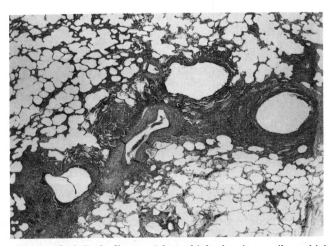

Figure 47–6. Early disease. A bronchiole showing peribronchial inflammation with cellular infiltrates. The pulmonary parenchyma shows minimal involvement.

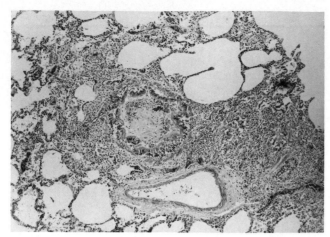

Figure 47–7. More severe disease, with increasing peribronchial inflammation and plugging of the airway by mucopurulent exudate. There is increasing parenchymal involvement, with progression to focal areas of pneumonia.

changes. There is dilation and tapering of the bronchial arteries around areas of bronchiectasis, with new vessel formation creating a rich vascular plexus around the bronchial walls (Mack et al, 1965). A major site for bronchopulmonary shunting is thus created, and rupture of these vessels may lead to massive hemorrhage. As the lung disease progresses, the resultant hypoxemia causes pulmonary artery vasoconstriction, which with time becomes irreversible with changes in the muscularization of the pulmonary vascular tree (Ryland and Reid, 1975). Histologically, there is increasing medial hypertrophy of normally muscular arteries with extension of the muscle distally in the smaller and normally nonmuscular arteries. This can be demonstrated on arteriography as an irregular tapering of the peripheral arteries with dilation and tortuosity of the proximal arteries (Mack et al, 1965).

In advanced disease, there may be extensive pulmonary destruction (Fig. 47–8), but true emphysema afflicts less than 10 per cent of total lung (Sobonya and Taussig, 1986). Bronchiectatic cysts are promi-

nent, particularly within the upper lobes. Rupture of apical cysts into the pleural space is a frequent cause of pneumothoraces.

CLINICAL PRESENTATION

Many children present in infancy with a history of recurrent persistent bronchiolitis (Lloyd-Still et al, 1974), recurrent respiratory tract infections, or overt pneumonia. After diagnosis and institution of appropriate therapy, these patients usually show a significant improvement in clinical status that is commonly maintained until puberty. During this period, however, they develop bacterial colonization with evidence of progressive lung disease as demonstrated by sequential pulmonary function testing and early radiologic changes. The increasing bronchiectasis and resulting bronchorrhea lead to increasing cough, most noticeable on rising in the morning. With progression of the disease, cough becomes an increasing debilitating symptom with increasing frequency, severity, and volume of mucopurulent secretions. Exercise tolerance becomes increasingly limited, paralleling the progressive respiratory impairment. Finger clubbing becomes increasingly obvious and is to a degree proportional to the severity of the pulmonary disease (Fig. 47–9) (Pitts-Tucker et al, 1986). On auscultation there is evidence of decreased breath sounds with diffuse inspiratory crackles due to mucopurulent secretions within the airways. With increasing pulmonary disease, patients frequently experience acute exacerbations of their lung disease (see subsequent discussion). Although hospitalization and intravenous antibiotic therapy usually produce significant symptomatic improvement, the patient's pulmonary status deteriorates steadily, resulting in increasing respiratory embarrassment, reduced or absent exercise tolerance, and progressive cor pulmonale. Death eventually occurs from a combination of respiratory and cardiac failure. There is, however,

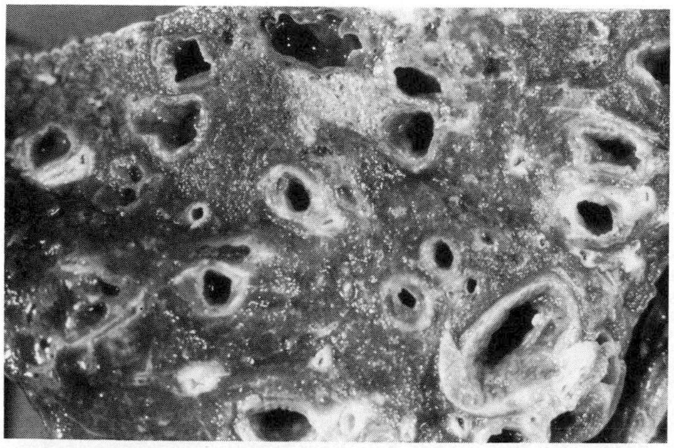

Figure 47–8. Advanced disease, gross pathology. There is diffuse, severe bronchiectatic destruction of both large and small airways, with focal areas of hemorrhagic pneumonia and fibrosis. Increasing alveolar dilation has resulted in the growth of a greater number of cysts and subpleural blebs.

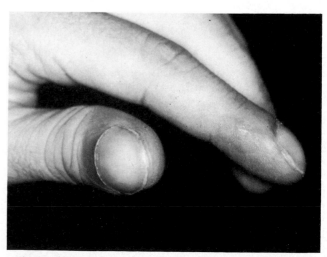

Figure 47–9. Clubbing, showing a loss of nail bed angle and a swelling of the terminal phalanx.

a marked heterogeneity in the rate of progression of pulmonary disease. Some patients may reach end-stage pulmonary failure within the first decade of life (Lloyd-Still et al, 1974), but others may only present in adulthood with "bronchitis," transient hemoptysis, or symptoms of upper respiratory disease and may not progress to significant respiratory impairment until their third or fourth decade of life (Di Sant'Agnese and Davis, 1979).

DIAGNOSIS

Diagnosis first requires clinical suspicion. The majority of children with CF present with a history of recurrent, progressive lower respiratory tract symptoms; bulky, greasy, offensive stools; and malnutrition. Approximately 15 per cent of patients have a history of meconium ileus at birth, whereas only 20 per cent have a positive family history of CF. CF is an extremely pleomorphic disease, and the age of presentation may vary from infancy to adulthood. Any child or adult presenting with one of the clinical stigmata of CF (Table 47–2) requires investigation.

BIOCHEMICAL DIAGNOSIS

Sweat Chloride Concentration

Since the 1950s, demonstration of elevated sweat chloride levels remains the principal method of con-

Table 47–2. CLINICAL FEATURES OF CYSTIC FIBROSIS AT DIAGNOSIS

Age and Clinical Feature	Approximate Incidence (%)
0–2 years	
Meconium ileus	10–15
Obstructive jaundice	
Hypoproteinemia/anemia	
Bleeding diathesis	
Heat prostration/hyponatremia	
Failure to thrive	
Steatorrhea	85
Rectal prolapse	20
Bronchitis/bronchiolitis	
Staphylococcal pneumonia	
2–12 years	
Malabsorption	85
Recurrent pneumonia/bronchitis	60
Nasal polyps	6–36
Intussusception	1–5
13 years +	
Chronic pulmonary disease	70
Clubbing	
Abnormal glucose tolerance	20–30
Diabetes mellitus	7
Chronic intestinal obstruction	10–20
Recurrent pancreatitis	
Focal biliary cirrhosis	15–25
Portal hypertension	2–5
Gallstones	4–14
Aspermia	98

Table 47–3. CAUSES OF ELEVATED SWEAT CHLORIDE IN CHILDHOOD

Cystic fibrosis
Untreated adrenal insufficiency
Glycogen storage disease, type I
Fucosidosis
Hypothyroidism
Nephrogenic diabetes insipidus
Ectodermal dysplasia
Malnutrition
Mucopolysaccharidosis
Panhypopituitarism

firming the diagnosis of CF. The quantitative pilocarpine iontophoresis sweat test (Gibson and Cooke, 1959) is currently the only uniformly accepted method for the diagnosis of CF (Heeley and Watson, 1983). Errors in the collection or analysis of sweat sample may affect the results (Littlewood, 1987), and the test should thus ideally be performed in the laboratory of a regional pediatric center by an experienced technician. A minimum of 50 mg of sweat is required, although greater than 100 mg is preferable for accurate analysis. A positive test should be confirmed, and negative tests should be repeated if clinically indicated (LeGrys and Wood, 1988). Although the test can be performed at any age, it may be difficult to induce adequate sweating in infants younger than 2 months.

In the presence of suggestive clinical features, a sweat chloride level greater than 60 mEq/L is consistent with the diagnosis of CF. Sweat sodium values are slightly higher than chloride values, and a large discrepancy in value should alert the physician to a possible error in assay. Normal sweat chloride levels are less than 30 mEq/L, whereas the majority of patients with CF have levels in excess of 80 mEq/L. The sweat chloride level is higher in adults than children and is usually considered diagnostic if greater than 50 mEq/L in childhood, 60 mEq/L in adults (Stern et al, 1978). Elevated sweat chloride levels have, however, been reported in association with a number of other entities (Littlewood, 1986) (Table 47–3). Most of these conditions are rare and usually are clinically distinct from CF. A study from this institution has shown that malnutrition is a relatively common cause of a mildly elevated sweat chloride (Beck et al, 1986). Improvement in nutritional status usually results in a return to normal values, however.

Borderline Cases

Approximately 1 to 2 per cent of patients have borderline sweat chloride levels (between 50 and 60 mEq/L) (Huff et al, 1979). These patients typically tend to have both pancreatic sufficiency and a milder degree of pulmonary involvement. Some of these patients may have other evidence of CF, such as nasal polyposis, chronic sinusitis, and liver or biliary disease. Sputum colonization by mucoid *Pseudomonas* is highly suggestive of CF, and azoospermia is present in 98 per cent of males. Measurement of nasal epithelial potential difference, when available, may help in diagnosis (Denning et al, 1980). A small group of patients may defy definitive diagnosis. These patients will require continued follow-up, because CF will ultimately lead to progressive pulmonary disease.

Screening Tests

Various neonatal screening tests have been proposed for use in large populations in order to diagnose CF before the onset of overt symptoms. Fecal trypsin or albumin content (Boehringer Mannheim [BM] test), as well as cutaneous chloride (Orion) or electrolyte conductivity (Medtherm) electrodes, all will differentiate patients with CF from normal persons (Denning et al, 1980). The rate of false-positive and false-negative results using these tests is too high for them to be used for routine screening on a clinical basis (Kuzemko, 1986).

Pancreatic obstruction in utero results in "leaking" of pancreatic enzymes into the fetal circulation. Consequently, serum levels of immunoreactive trypsinogen are elevated in virtually every child with CF, including those without steatorrhea. This assay can be performed on dried blood spot samples and is currently employed for wide-scale screening in various parts of the world (Heeley et al, 1982; Wilcken et al, 1983).

Neonatal screening programs are justifiable only if early diagnosis and treatment before the onset of clinical disease significantly improve the long-term outcome. Despite current available therapy, all patients will ultimately develop progressive pulmonary disease. A delay in diagnosis is common. Without neonatal screening, 58 per cent of patients are diagnosed by 1 year of age and 87 per cent by 5 years of age. The mean delay between onset of symptoms and ultimate diagnosis is around 15 to 25 months (Wilcken et al, 1983; Rosenstein et al, 1982). A number of patients therefore suffer significant delay in diagnosis, some with potentially treatable protein-calorie malnutrition and associated progressive lung disease. Indirect evidence suggests that early diagnosis may significantly improve the long-term outcome of these patients (Dankert-Roelse et al, 1987). In addition, early diagnosis would enable genetic counseling for parents before further pregnancies. Whether these advantages outweigh the costs and potential psychosocial problems associated with the small but significant numbers of false-positive and false-negative diagnoses inherent in any screening program remains a matter of debate.

PRENATAL DIAGNOSIS

Genetic

Before identification of the CF gene, it was possible to use DNA probes known to be in close geographic proximity as markers for the gene in families with one or more already affected offspring (see "Genetics"). There are now a sufficient number of probes situated close to the CF locus so that both parents and the affected child will be informative for at least one or more of these probes in over 85 per cent of families (Fig. 47–10). These probes can be used as markers for the CF gene in both parents, and fetal material for DNA analysis can be obtained by chorionic villus sampling at around 12 weeks of gestation. If the fetus shows the same pattern of inheritance for these probes as the affected sibling, there is a 98 per cent probability that the fetus will be affected (Dean et al, 1987). At the time of writing, the exact gene mutation has been identified in 70 per cent of patients with CF. With identification of the major mutations causing CF, carrier detection will become possible in individuals with no prior family history. Prenatal detection will therefore be available for families in which both parents are identified as carriers.

Microvillar Enzymes

A number of enzymes that arise from the epithelial cell microvilli of the fetus and are routinely present in amniotic fluid have been identified. Levels of these enzymes are universally depressed in the presence of a CF-affected fetus, apparently as a result of abnormal intestinal enzyme passage associated with impaired pancreatic maturation (Muller et al, 1987). Decreased levels are also found in other causes of fetal intestinal obstruction, such as imperforate anus and jejunal atresia, as well as trisomies 18 and 21. Moreover, enzyme levels vary markedly during gestation, the best discrimination between normal and

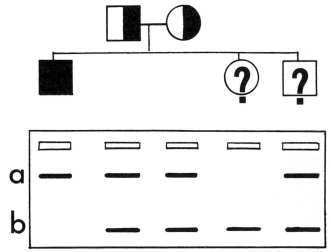

Figure 47–10. An example of genotype assignment by restriction fragment length polymorphism (RFLP) analysis using a linked DNA probe. In this informative family, both parents are heterozygous for the probe, electrophoresis revealing both large (a) and small (b) fragments. The affected son is homozygous for the large fragment (no b), hence demonstrating that the cystic fibrosis gene segregates with the larger DNA fragment (a). Thus the daughter is homozygous normal (no a), and the second son is a carrier for the cystic fibrosis gene (both a and b).

CF-affected fetuses occurring between 17 and 19 weeks of gestation (Boue et al, 1986). Even at this time, the false-positive and false-negative rate is around 2.5 to 5 per cent (Mulivor et al, 1987). This technique should therefore be reserved for use in high-risk pregnancies (1:4 chance) in which either one or both parents are noninformative by genetic analysis (Spence et al, 1987).

ASSESSMENT

CLINICAL

Various clinical scoring systems have been developed to provide both a numerical assessment of patients' status and a way of documenting progress in response to treatment.

The Shwachman-Kulczycki score is the most frequently used (Schwachman and Kulczycki, 1958). In this scoring system, 25 points are given for each of the following categories: activity level, nutritional status, physical examination, and chest radiograph changes. Points are deducted for deterioration in status; 100 is normal, and the lower the number, the worse the clinical condition. Several studies have shown good correlation both between different observers and with formal pulmonary function testing using this scoring system (Lewiston and Moss, 1987).

PULMONARY FUNCTION TESTING

In the initial stages, CF is a disease of the peripheral airways and results in airway obstruction, increased gas trapping, atelectasis, and increasing ventilation-perfusion mismatching. With the progression of the pulmonary infection and resulting chronic inflammation, there is increasing lung destruction and associated fibrosis. Patients with more advanced disease appear increasingly restricted, although gas trapping remains a primary feature.

The majority of patients over the age of 6 years can perform formal pulmonary function testing, and this has proved to be a valid method of monitoring the progression of the disease (Corey et al, 1976). There is no single "best test" that fully documents the disease process, however.

Static Lung Volumes

Early in the disease process, peripheral gas trapping results in an elevated ratio of residual volume to total lung capacity (RV/TLC), as well as an increase in overall lung volume (Levison and Godfrey, 1976). In more advanced disease, the TLC may decline, although the RV/TLC ratio remains elevated (Fig. 47–11). In mild disease, the thoracic gas volume as measured by body plethysmography correlates well with TLC, measured by helium dilution. Progressive gas trapping results in increasing lung volumes not

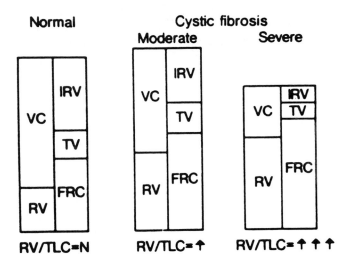

Figure 47–11. Change in lung volumes in cystic fibrosis. Early in the disease, RV increases significantly with a simultaneous small increase in TLC. With advanced disease, a restrictive process may supervene with a fall in TLC, though RV remains increased, leading to a greatly increased RV/TLC ratio. *FRC*, functional residual capacity; *IRV*, inspiratory reserve volume; *RV*, residual volume; *TLC*, total lung capacity; *TV*, tidal volume; *VC*, vital capacity.

in direct continuity with the airways. Helium dilution therefore increasingly underestimates the TLC as the disease progresses (Featherby et al, 1970).

Spirometry

Both the FEV_1 and FEV_1/TLC ratios are useful methods for long-term assessment of pulmonary status, because they both show consistent decreases in the presence of advancing disease. The FEV_1 is a relatively insensitive test for assessing early lung disease and may be normal in patients with clinically significant pulmonary involvement. The $FEF_{25-75\%}$ is a more sensitive indicator of small airways disease than either the FEV_1 or measurements of total airways resistance, although the marked intersubject and intrasubject variability makes a single observation of poor diagnostic value (Laudau and Phelan, 1973). In sequential pulmonary function, the $FEF_{25-75\%}$ will demonstrate deterioration in pulmonary status before changes in FEV_1 or FVC become apparent.

Maximum expiratory flow volume (MEFV) curves are useful in detecting early abnormalities. Convexity of the curve in relation to the volume axis is one of the most sensitive indicators of early obstruction of the peripheral airways (Fig. 47–12) (Mellins, 1969). A modification of the MEFV curve, using inhaled gases of different densities, may be the most sensitive test for demonstrating early abnormalities in small-airway function. The resistance to flow in the large airways is turbulent and hence dependent on gas density. In peripheral airways, the flow is laminar and independent of gas density. In normal individuals, the smaller airways add little to the total airways resistance. Breathing a low-density mixture, such as 20 per cent oxygen and 80 per cent helium (Heli-

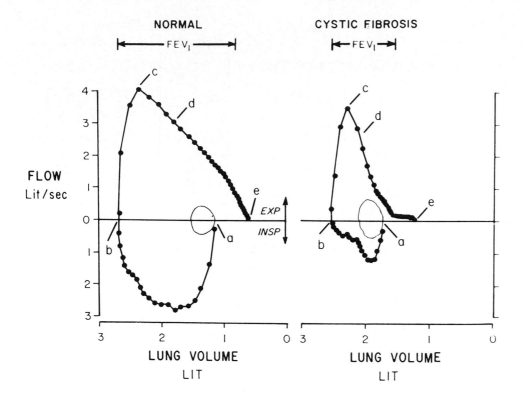

Figure 47–12. Maximal expiratory flow volume curves from a normal 12-year-old boy and a 15-year-old girl with cystic fibrosis. Inspiration (from *a* to *b*) was followed by forced expiration *(b* to *e)*. Peak flow *(c)* is not significantly reduced. There is a fall in the forced vital capacity (FVC) *(b* to *e)*, associated with a marked reduction in the forced expiratory volume in 1 sec (FEV₁). (From Mellins RB: Pediatrics 44:315, 1969. Reproduced by permission of Pediatrics.)

Ox), has marked effect on maximum expiratory flow rates. In diseases such as CF, in which small-airways disease contributes a substantial portion to the overall airways resistance, there is a reduction in the difference between helium-oxygen and air curves (Hutcheon et al, 1974) (Fig. 47–13). Standard spirometry and plethysmographic assessment of lung volume are adequate for routine evaluation of pulmonary disease in the clinical setting (Fig. 47–14).

BLOOD GASES

Extensive regional ventilation-perfusion abnormalities are the characteristic sequelae of the progressive,

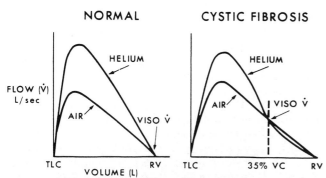

Figure 47–13. Schematic representation of maximal expiratory flow volume curves from a healthy child and a child with cystic fibrosis. The children first inhaled normal air, then a helium-oxygen mixture. The volume of iso flow *(V iso V̇)* is the volume of identical flow, occurring almost at residual volume *(RV)* in the healthy child and at 35 per cent vital capacity *(VC)* in the patient with cystic fibrosis. *TLC*, total lung capacity.

patchy bronchiolitis and mucous plugging in CF. Airways of the lung perfused but not ventilated create an effective right-to-left shunt, whereas ventilated but underperfused airways lead to an increase in functional dead space. Progressive hypoxemia is therefore one of the earliest signs of increasing pulmonary disease and may occur before any other detectable abnormality in lung function (Lamarre et al, 1972). The severity of the hypoxemia closely parallels the deteriorating pulmonary status. A further decline in arterial oxygenation may occur during sleep, possibly secondary to the decrease in functional residual capacity that occurs during rapid-eye-movement (REM) sleep, as well as airway collapse and increased intrapulmonary shunting (Muller et al, 1980). Even with advanced pulmonary disease, patients are usually able to maintain normal levels of P_{CO_2} by increasing minute ventilation to the less affected lung segments. However, patients with progressive pulmonary disease ultimately exhaust their respiratory reserve, subsequently leading to a progressive rise in P_{CO_2}. Hypercapnia usually signifies advanced disease and carries a poor prognosis (Fig. 47–15). Subsequent survival is usually less than 1 year (Wagener et al, 1980).

CHEST RADIOGRAPH

The chest radiograph is normal at birth, although a few individuals may develop rapidly progressive pulmonary disease in the neonatal period. In the initial stages of the disease, the chest radiograph shows hyperinflation and peribronchial thickening,

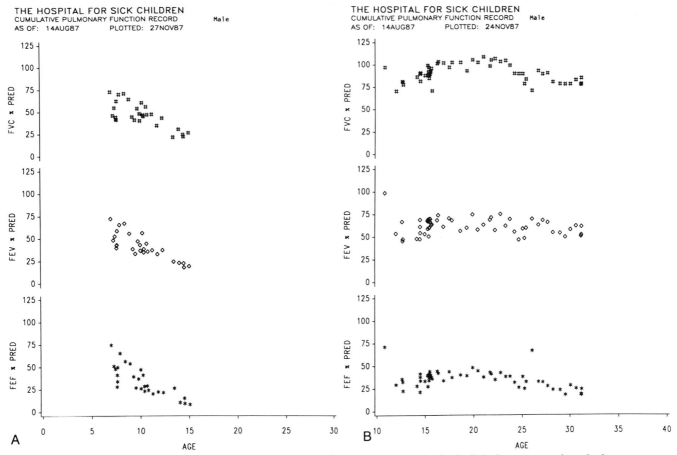

THE HOSPITAL FOR SICK CHILDREN
CUMULATIVE PULMONARY FUNCTION RECORD   Male
AS OF: 14AUG87   PLOTTED: 27NOV87

THE HOSPITAL FOR SICK CHILDREN
CUMULATIVE PULMONARY FUNCTION RECORD   Male
AS OF: 14AUG87   PLOTTED: 24NOV87

Figure 47–14. Examples of sequential pulmonary function, documenting both clinical progress and marked variability in clinical disease in patients with cystic fibrosis. *A,* Patient C.R. presented initially with a mild case of the disease but showed progressive deterioration despite aggressive therapy and repeated hospitalizations and died of progressive respiratory failure at 16 years of age. *B,* Patient J.B. presented with significant pulmonary disease at diagnosis, yet responded well to aggressive management. He has shown minimal progression of the disease over the years and continues to function well, working full time, with only an occasional hospitalization.

seen as pale linear shadows and cuffing of end-on bronchi (Figs. 47–16 and 47–17) (Amodio et al, 1987). Progressive air trapping with frank bronchiectasis may become apparent in the upper lobes. With progression of the disease, pulmonary infiltrates appear, usually forming nodular shadows around 2 to 5 mm in diameter, occasionally associated with segmental or lobar atelectasis (Fig. 47–18). Marked pulmonary hyperexpansion becomes increasingly obvious, with flattening of the diaphragm, thoracic kyphosis, and bowing of the sternum. In advanced disease, cystic lesions are commonly apparent, primarily in the apical segments, and may occasionally lead to spontaneous pneumothoraces (Fig. 47–19) (Friedman, 1987). Obvious abscess formation and areas of cavitation may also develop. With the onset of cor pulmonale, pulmonary hypertension may be manifested by pulmonary artery dilatation and right ventricular hypertrophy, although it is usually masked by the overlying pulmonary hyperinflation.

Several radiologic scoring systems have been developed; the method of Brasfield and colleagues

(1979) can be incorporated in the Schwachman-Kulczycki score (see above).

SPUTUM BACTERIOLOGY

In the majority of pulmonary infections in individuals not affected with CF, sputum culture provides no reliable information on lower respiratory tract colonization. Numerous studies have, however, shown that cultures from expectorated sputum of patients with CF reflect the aerobic flora colonizing the lower respiratory tract as identified from postmortem, thoracotomy, and bronchoscopy specimens (Gilljam et al, 1986). Colonization by some anaerobic organisms may, however, be masked by contamination with oropharyngeal organisms (Barlett and Finegold, 1978). Quantitative sputum cultures should therefore be routinely performed at each clinic visit, both to document change in clinical status and to guide antibiotic therapy during episodes of acute deterioration.

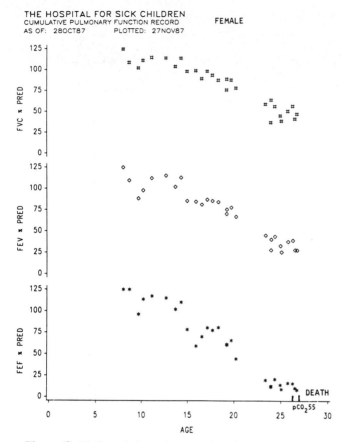

THE HOSPITAL FOR SICK CHILDREN
CUMULATIVE PULMONARY FUNCTION RECORD
AS OF: 28OCT87   PLOTTED: 27NOV87   FEMALE

Figure 47–15. Cumulative pulmonary function record of Patient L.K., a 27-year-old woman with CF who had shown steady deterioration in pulmonary status despite aggressive management. She continued to function well until the last year of her life. Progressive respiratory limitation, however, led eventually to carbon dioxide retention and evidence of cor pulmonale. She continued to show progressive decline, and death occurred 8 months later from intractable cardiorespiratory failure.

TREATMENT

Because of the multiple organ involvement, marked variability in clinical presentation, and lethal nature of the disease, treatment generally concentrates in major regional medical centers where appropriate subspecialty care is available. Although regionalized care may be associated with increased interpatient transmission of viruses, *P. aeruginosa*, and *P. cepacia* (Pedersen et al, 1986), the marked improvement in life expectancy reported by regional centers supports this approach. Patients are examined routinely at least every 3 months (although some clinics suggest up to monthly assessments) for clinical evaluation of nutritional status and pulmonary disease, and quantitative sputum cultures are performed at each visit. Chest radiographs and pulmonary function testing when the patient is old enough should be performed at least every 6 months. Appropriate therapy can therefore be initiated early in the event of any deterioration.

INFECTION

Chronic endobronchial colonization is clearly the primary cause of the progressive pulmonary disease in CF. Antibiotic therapy has long been a mainstay of treatment for CF and appears to be one of the principal reasons for the increased longevity during the past 30 years. Without a clear-cut understanding of the underlying basis for the disease or the exact pathogenic mechanisms of the various organisms, treatment has largely been empirical. It is only relatively recently that there has been a more scientific evaluation of the various therapeutic approaches used. As a consequence, although in general there is a broad unanimity in approach, marked variations remain between different medical centers in both specific approaches to and clinical indications for the various therapies available (Table 47–4).

Prevention

Patients with CF are characteristically colonized by various organisms commonly present in the environment. The exact mode of acquisition of these various organisms is still unknown. *S. aureus* is a common colonizer of the upper respiratory tracts in individuals not suffering from CF. The earlier acquisition of *P. aeruginosa* in patients attending CF centers and the similar phage types found in siblings with the disease may reflect a common environmental reservoir or interpatient transmission. Convincing evidence of interpatient transmission has not been found, however. Without knowing the exact mode of acquisition, it is therefore difficult to design a rational isolation program to prevent *P. aeruginosa* colonization.

There is indirect evidence to suggest interpatient transmission of *P. cepacia* (see "Infection"), but whether acquisition of *P. cepacia* significantly affects the course of the disease is still under investigation. The Cystic Fibrosis Foundation is running a multicenter surveillance program to try and answer some of these questions. Until this information is available, it is difficult to know whether the benefits of a patient isolation program as documented by the Cleveland group outweigh the logistic difficulties and potential psychosocial problems associated with such a program.

Patients colonized with *P. aeruginosa* show a brisk immune response yet fail to clear the organisms. An initial attempt to vaccinate patients with *P. aeruginosa* lipopolysaccharide resulted in more severe disease in the vaccinated patients (Langford and Hiller, 1984). Ongoing research is directed at developing an effective vaccine that would promote phagocytic clearance of *P. aeruginosa* by pulmonary macrophages, although it is unclear how effective this may be in CF.

Long-Term Therapy

Although the rate of deterioration varies markedly between patients, chronic endobronchial colonization

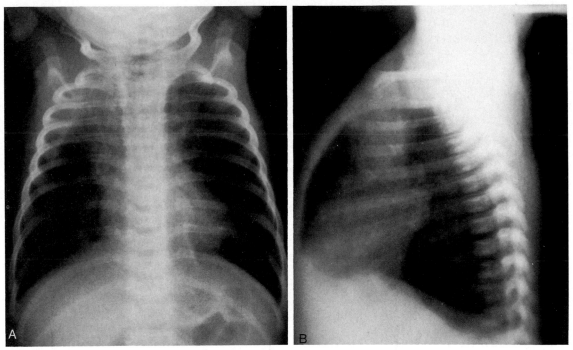

Figure 47–16. Patient C.B., presenting at 3 months of age with clinical bronchiolitis. Chest radiographs show marked hyperinflation, with flattening of the diaphragm and bowing of the sternum, as well as right upper lobe atelectasis.

inevitably leads to progressive pulmonary disease. There is still no consensus about the optimum method of delaying this progression, although various approaches have been suggested (Thomassen et al, 1987).

Antistaphyloccocal. Historically, *S. aureus* was the major pathogen in CF. Coincident with the advent

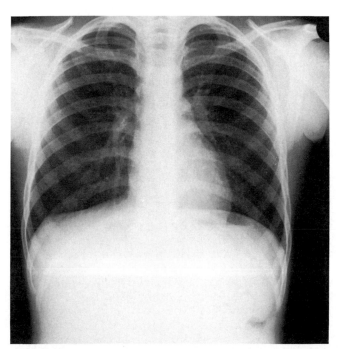

Figure 47–17. Patient C.B., aged 10 years, showing marked improvement, although with mild residual hyperinflation and minimal peribronchial thickening.

of effective antistaphylococcal antibiotics there has been a marked improvement in the life expectancy of patients with CF. Long-term oral antistaphylococcal antibiotics have therefore been used by many clinics as a routine part of therapy, although the approach varies markedly between different clinics. Some routinely employ "prophylactic" antistaphylococcal antibiotics before overt colonization, whereas others confine treatment only to patients with significant lung disease and evidence of colonization. The Danish group treats all patients aggressively at first isolation of *S. aureus*, using 14-day courses of dicloxacillin and fusidic acid, with prolonged therapy or clindamycin in cases of eradication failure (Szaf and Hoiby, 1982). Using this approach, fewer than 1 per cent of patients develop extended colonization. The pattern of virulence of *S. aureus* has, however, changed during the past 30 years, as reflected in the changing spectrum of neonatal disease. Moreover, the widespread use of antistaphylococcal antibiotics has been suggested as one of the factors associated with subsequent colonization by resistant organisms such as *Pseudomonas*. It is hoped that an ongoing multicenter trial may provide a more scientific basis for long-term antistaphylococcal therapy. In the absence of this information, our current policy is to treat only those patients who are colonized with *S. aureus* and who have evidence of significant pulmonary disease.

Antipseudomonal. Until recently, no effective oral antipseudomonal agents were available, necessitating various other therapeutic approaches.

INHALED ANTIBIOTICS. Although inhaled antibiotics have been used for many years, they were not initially subjected to systematic study. Aminoglycosides, carboxypenicillins, and cephalosporins all can be administered by nebulizer. Hodson and colleagues (1981) documented improved pulmonary function and reduced hospitalization in a 6-month placebo control trial of twice-daily aerosolized gentamicin (80 mg) and carbenicillin (1 g) in a group of young adults. A number of subsequent studies have generally confirmed these initial findings. There has been marked variability in protocols, however. Therapeutic regimens have included inhaled amikacin (500 mg b.i.d.), tobramycin (20 mg b.i.d. to 80 mg t.i.d.), ceftazidime (1 g b.i.d.), and colistin (1 million units b.i.d.), and the duration of studies ranges from 3 weeks to 2.5 years (MacLusky et al, 1986). Only 5 to 10 per cent of any nebulized medication is actually inhaled, and lung deposition rates are even less. The amount and pattern of deposition within the airways may vary markedly depending on droplet size, the flow characteristics of the air compressor, and the pattern of breathing and extent of pulmonary disease of the patient (Clarke, 1986). Because of the wide variety of dosages and techniques used in the different studies, it is difficult to determine the most effective therapeutic regimen.

Moreover, there has been no clear unanimity on either clinical indications or duration of therapy. Reported uses have ranged from short-term courses (3 weeks to 3 months) in patients colonized with *P.*

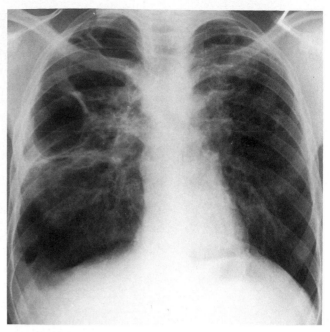

Figure 47–19. Patient C.B., aged 23 years, showing marked hyperinflation and development of massive apical bullae, particularly in the right upper lobe. Chronic parenchymal involvement has resulted in secondary pleural involvement, with pleural thickening, particularly over the upper lobes.

aeruginosa to continuous therapy in all patients irrespective of sputum bacteriology (MacLusky et al, 1986).

It is also clear that not all patients respond to this treatment (in a study at this institution, only 9 of 15 patients colonized with *P. aeruginosa* appeared to show continued response to tobramycin, 80 mg t.i.d. inhaled, during a 2.5-year period). Inhaled antibiotics are an expensive therapy (from $3000 to $6000 per year, depending on drug and dosage used). We therefore need to identify exactly which patients are most likely to respond, as well as exact indications for and optimum duration of therapy.

The potential for interactions between the antibiotics and other inhaled medication has not been fully investigated. Salbutamol (albuterol) does not appear to affect tobramycin activity, and the two can be coadministered. Mucolytics do block antibiotic activity and should not be used concurrently (Alfredsson et al, 1987); the interaction with other inhaled medications such as sodium cromoglycate is not known.

Finally, the short- and long-term risks of inhaled antibiotics have not been fully clarified. Bronchospasm has occasionally been reported following inhaled antibiotics. Of greater significance are the risks of development of allergy not only in the patient but also in family members, particularly when using penicillin derivatives or cephalosporins. Although neither significant nephrotoxicity nor ototoxicity has been reported in any of the trials of inhaled aminoglycosides, there remains the potential for cumulative toxicity, particularly if higher doses or more enhanced delivery systems such as ultrasonic nebulizers

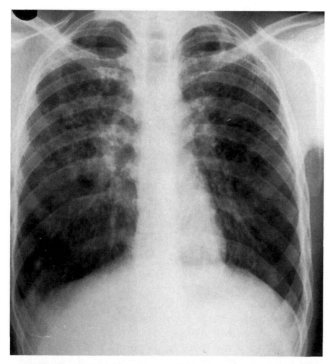

Figure 47–18. Patient C.B., aged 17 years, showing progressive pulmonary disease. There is increasing hyperinflation, bronchial wall thickening, and evidence of early saccular bronchiectasis. There is also increasing parenchymal disease, with nodular infiltrates and loss of the right costophrenic angle due to segmental atelectasis. The ensuing hypoxemia has resulted in pulmonary hypertension, demonstrated by dilation of the proximal pulmonary arteries.

Table 47–4. DRUGS USED IN THE TREATMENT OF CYSTIC FIBROSIS

Drugs	Route	Dose	Schedule
Antibiotics			
Penicillins			
Amoxicillin	PO	50–100 mg/kg/day	q 6 hours
Cloxacillin	PO/IV	50–200 mg/kg/day	q 6 hours
Ticarcillin	IV	200–300 mg/kg/day	q 4–6 hours
Piperacillin	IV	200 mg/kg/day (max 24 g/day)	q 6 hours
Cephalosporins			
Cephalexin	PO	50–100 mg/kg/day	q 6 hours
Ceftazidime	IV	200 mg/kg/day (max 12 g/day)	q 6 hours
Aminoglycosides			
Gentamicin*	IV	10 mg/kg/day	q 8 hours
Tobramycin*	IV	10 mg/kg/day	q 8 hours
Others			
Cotrimoxazole			
Trimethoprim	PO	8 mg/kg/day	q 6–12 hours
Sulfamethoxazole		40 mg/kg/day	
Trimethoprim	IV	5–10 mg/kg/day	q 6–12 hours
Sulfamethoxazole		25–50 mg/kg/day (max adult dose 640 mg trimethoprim/day)	
Chloramphenicol	PO/IV	50–100 mg/kg/day	q 6 hours
Ciprofloxacin	PO	1500 mg/day (adults)	q 12 hours
Bronchodilators			
Salbutamol: (2-mg or 4-mg tabs)	PO	0.1–0.15 mg/kg/dose	q 6 hours
Metered aerosol: (100-μg/puff)	Inhalation	1–2 puffs	q 4–6 hours
0.5% solution	Inhalation	0.01–0.03 ml/kg/dose	q 4–6 hours
Terbutaline:			
Metered aerosol (250-μg/puff)	Inhalation	1–2 puffs	q 4–6 hours
1% solution	Inhalation	0.03 ml/kg/dose (max 1 ml)	q 4–6 hours
Metaproterenol:			
Metered aerosol (750-μg/puff)	Inhalation	1–2 puffs	q 4–6 hours
5% solution	Inhalation	0.01–0.02 ml/kg/dose (max 1 ml)	q 4–6 hours
Fenoterol:			
Metered aerosol (200-μg/puff)	Inhalation	1–2 puffs	q 4–6 hours
0.1% solution	Inhalation	0.01–0.03 ml/kg/day (max 1 ml)	q 4–6 hours
Ipratropium bromide:			
Metered aerosol (20-μg/puff)	Inhalation	2 puffs	q 6–8 hours
Theophylline* (anhydrous):	PO or IV	18–24 mg/kg/day	
Short-acting PO preps			q 6 hours
Long-acting PO preps			q 8–12 hours
Mucolytics			
N-acetylcysteine (20% solution)		1–2 ml	q 8 hours
Cromolyn Sodium			
1% solution	Inhalation	2 ml	q 6 hours
Sclerosing Agents			
Quinacrine	Intrapleural	100 mg in 50 ml normal saline	1/day × 3 days

*Increased drug clearance in patients with CF requires close monitoring of drug levels.

are employed. The reported incidence of resistant organisms is between 0 and 30 per cent (MacLusky et al, 1986) following the use of inhaled antibiotics.

Our practice is to prescribe a 6-month course of inhaled tobramycin (80 mg t.i.d.) to those patients who are colonized with *P. aeruginosa* and who continue to show significant decline or relapse despite aggressive intravenous therapy. Clearly, more research is required to identify exactly which patients are most likely to respond, the optimum antibiotic regimen, and the most effective delivery system before inhaled antibiotics are used indiscriminately.

ORAL ANTIBIOTICS. With the development of the quinolone derivatives, of which ciprofloxacin is currently the most potent antipseudomonal agent, oral antibiotics against *P. aeruginosa* are now available. The exact clinical role has yet to be elucidated (Stutman, 1987). In vitro, ciprofloxacin is one of the most active agents available against *Pseudomonas*, its minimal inhibitory concentration (MIC) for many strains being 100 to 1000 times lower than carbenicillin. Resistance is common following even short courses, however, although the clinical relevance of this is not clear, particularly because many organisms become susceptible again after discontinuation of therapy (Raeburn et al, 1987). There are concerns about the use of these drugs in the pediatric age group, because the parent compound, nalidixic acid, is toxic to growing cartilage. We use ciprofloxacin in 2- to 3-week courses for postpubertal patients either with resistant organisms or as an alternative to hospitalization. This approach will probably change with further information on the clinical effectiveness of these drugs.

REGULAR INTRAVENOUS THERAPY. The Danish group has embarked on a program of regular antimicrobial therapy (Pedersen et al, 1987). All patients colonized with *P. aeruginosa* are evaluated monthly and admitted every 3 months for 14-day courses of antipseudomonal agents. During a decade, the 5-year survival of patients who became colonized with *P. aeruginosa* rose from 54 to 82 per cent with this aggressive approach. There was no control group in their study, however. Moreover, this approach appears to be associated with an increasing incidence of resistant *P. aeruginosa.*

Repeated hospitalization is both expensive and disruptive for families. A number of clinics have therefore set up home intravenous antibiotic programs, both for regular home therapy and also for treatment during episodes of acute deterioration (Kuzemko, 1988). Patients and families can be taught either the technique of intravenous insertion or how to use long-term indwelling central venous lines. With appropriate education, patients seem to tolerate these programs well, with little apparent risk.

The effectiveness of antibiotic therapy alone, as distinct from in-hospital physiotherapy and nutritional management, is still in question (see subsequent discussion). The clinical role of home intravenous antibiotic therapy therefore still needs to be clarified.

STEROIDS. An initial report suggests that long-term systemic corticosteroids may prevent progressive pulmonary deterioration (Auerbach et al, 1985). A multicenter trial is currently assessing the clinical usefulness of this therapy. Because of the significant side effects of long-term corticosteroid therapy, routine clinical use should probably await the results of this trial. Inhaled corticosteroids appear to have no therapeutic effect, except in patients with associated airway hyperreactivity.

Acute Therapy

Patients with CF commonly exhibit episodes of acute deterioration in pulmonary status. The standard therapy is to admit the patient for a 10- to 14-day course of intravenous antibiotics, pulmonary physiotherapy, and nutritional support. Although this approach results in clinical improvement and a return to baseline status in the majority of patients, there still remain several areas of controversy (Nelson, 1985). Michel (1988) reviewed 67 studies on antibiotic therapy of patients with CF, published between 1980 and 1987, and concluded that "no consensus has been reached on indications for antibiotic therapy, the antibiotic to be used, or the dosage schedules." Forty-nine of these studies investigated antipseudomonal therapy.

Indications for Therapy. There are no uniform criteria for exactly what constitutes an acute exacerbation. Typical symptoms are increased cough, sputum production, malaise, anorexia, weight loss, and decreased exercise tolerance. Total white blood cell count and ESR may be elevated, whereas fever is usually low grade or absent. Acute exacerbations are thus frequently characterized by the patient's changing symptoms. Deterioration in pulmonary function

or change in chest radiograph may be the only objective criteria.

Antibiotics to Be Used. The 67 studies reviewed by Michel contained 24 different antibiotic regimens. Although a combination of antibiotics was commonly used in the hope of retarding the development of bacterial resistance, there was little objective evidence to show that two-drug therapy was any more effective than a single drug. In addition, many patients show an improvement in their clinical status despite persistence of organisms that are resistant when assessed in vitro. Michel did not observe any obvious difference in clinical effectiveness between the different regimens, and it must be emphasized that only four of these studies were placebo controlled. Two of these latter four studies (Beaudry et al, 1980; Gold et al, 1987) demonstrated a significant beneficial response in the control group, suggesting that the ancillary therapy associated with hospitalization, such as improved compliance with physiotherapy, bed rest, and improved nutrition, may be of equal importance or at least complementary to antibiotic therapy.

Dosage Schedules. Patients with CF show altered pharmacokinetics and increased clearance for most of the commonly employed antibiotics (Prandota, 1987). In addition, most antibiotics show poor penetration into endobronchial secretions (Levy, 1986). Higher dosages of the most commonly used antibiotics are therefore recommended for patients with CF (see Table 47–4). It must be emphasized that many patients show a beneficial clinical response in spite of the persistence of resistant organisms, and in most studies there was no clear association between clinical response and reduction in endobronchial colonization as characterized by sputum bacteriology.

The usual therapy for an acute exacerbation is to admit patients to the hospital and treat with antibiotics, based on the suspected organisms and subsequent sputum cultures (Govan et al, 1987). Patients colonized with *P. aeruginosa* usually respond to ceftazidime as a single agent or to a combination of an aminoglycoside with a carboxycillin or ureidopenicillin. Piperacillin is commonly associated with febrile or serum sickness-type reactions and should probably only be used in case of resistant organisms or therapeutic failure. There is no consensus on optimum duration of therapy (Boxerbaum, 1982). The majority of patients respond after 1 week of intravenous antibiotic therapy, although some patients may require therapy for 3 or more weeks.

AIRWAY OBSTRUCTION

Airway Hyperreactivity

Diffuse obstruction of the airways with patchy atelectasis and progressive air trapping is characteristic of CF. The primary cause is plugging of airways by mucopurulent secretions. However, 25 to 50 per cent of patients with CF may have evidence of increased airway hyperreactivity when assessed by methacholine, histamine, or cold air challenge (Darga et al, 1986; Mellis and Levinson, 1978; Michell et al, 1978).

The mechanism of airway hyperreactivity appears to differ in patients with CF compared with asthmatic patients. Larger doses of methacholine are required to produce a response, whereas recovery—either spontaneous or following salbutamol therapy—is slower and less complete than in patients with asthma. Patients with CF also show a variable response to exercise challenge, with many patients experiencing dramatic increases in peak expiratory flow rates and only minimal bronchoconstriction following exercise (Skorecki et al, 1976).

The value of bronchodilator therapy in CF therefore remains controversial. Some patients do experience significant bronchodilation in response to inhaled sympathomimetic agents, although other patients may show no benefit and a small number may even experience significant deterioration in lung function (Eber et al, 1988). Therefore, bronchodilator therapy should be used only if either a beneficial clinical or laboratory effect can be demonstrated. Sympathomimetic agents may, however, improve mucociliary function, and our policy has therefore been to prescribe inhaled sympathomimetic agents to the majority of patients immediately before physiotherapy, both to improve mucociliary clearance and to prevent physiotherapy-induced bronchospasm.

Pulmonary Physiotherapy

Pulmonary physiotherapy using standard techniques of percussion and postural drainage has long been a routine part of therapy in most clinics. The techniques have been well described (Gaskell and Weber, 1980). In essence, they use vibration to free up entrapped mucus and, by placing a patient in various positions over a physiotherapy board, use gravity to assist mucociliary clearance from the various dependent lobes. Several mechanical percussors that allow patients to self-administer physiotherapy and hence allow a degree of independence are available. The usual recommended regimen takes 20 to 30 min per session and is performed two to three times daily. Physiotherapy is therefore one of the most time-consuming parts of CF therapy and thus frequently is a major area of noncompliance, particularly among adolescent patients. Approximately 20 per cent of the patients attending our clinic admit to performing no regular physiotherapy.

Although physiotherapy is a traditional part of therapy for CF, there is relatively little scientific evidence supporting its therapeutic role (Sutton et al, 1982). Numerous studies have documented short-term benefits in terms of both sputum production and pulmonary function, as well as deterioration of pulmonary function following its cessation (Desmond et al, 1983). Most studies have been performed on patients who are sputum producers, and it is not clear whether there is any therapeutic value in patients who do not yet produce significant volumes of sputum. Moreover, there is little data documenting either its long-term effectiveness or whether there is any prophylactic value in starting physiotherapy before the onset of significant pulmonary disease.

In an attempt to improve compliance, various techniques have been suggested as possible substitutes for conventional physiotherapy.

The Forced Expiratory Technique (FET). This technique essentially consists of one or two forced expiratory efforts or "huffs" made through an open glottis and performed from midlung volume to low lung volume, followed by a period of relaxed diaphragmatic breathing. During forced expiration, there are compressive forces on the airways downstream (toward the mouth) of the equal pressure point (where intra-airway pressure equals pleural pressure). These compressive forces (choke points) have a vibratory effect on the airways, moving upstream (toward the alveoli) as the lung volume decreases. These compressive forces are therefore believed to aid mucociliary clearance from progressively more distal airways during forced expirations made from mid to low lung volumes (Pryor et al, 1979). Although the technique is effective in some patients (Verboon et al, 1986), we have recently shown it to be less effective than conventional physiotherapy (Reisman, 1988).

Positive Expiratory Pressure (PEP). Several European medical centers have recommended using a PEP mask as an alternative to conventional physiotherapy. The technique uses 10 breaths through a PEP mask against an expiratory pressure of 10 to 15 cm H_2O, followed by a period of forced expiratory coughing (Hofmeyr et al, 1986). It is performed over a period of 20 min, twice daily. This technique is believed to work by causing a pressure gradient to build up behind mucus plugs, forcing secretions toward the large airways. This technique may be used in combination with the FET (Oberwaldner et al, 1986). Reported benefits include increased sputum production and improved oxygenation. Patient compliance may be improved because of the reduced time and equipment required, but it is not clear whether this technique has any therapeutic advantage over conventional physiotherapy.

Exercise. Canny and Levinson (1987) have studied the role of exercise in CF. A regular exercise program improves prognosis and well-being in patients with chronic obstructive pulmonary disease, although the same studies have yet to be performed in patients with CF.

Patients with CF have been noted to have marked increases in expiratory flow rates during exercise, which are believed to be the result of supramaximal flow transients during exercise aiding in clearance of mucus from large, bronchiectatic airways. Preliminary studies have suggested that regular exercise is not only beneficial from a general point of view but may be an effective alternative to conventional physiotherapy in some selected patients (Blomquist et al, 1986). Patients with CF should receive salt supplementation if performing regular exercise at high ambient temperatures because of the risks of developing hyponatremic dehydration.

With increasing pulmonary disease, patients with CF develop a progressive decrease in exercise tolerance because of reduced ventilatory capacity. Patients with CF may, in addition, show significant arterial desaturation during exercise as a result of alveolar hypoventilation, as well as increased intrapulmonary shunting and shortened capillary transit time. Fifty per cent of patients with an FEV_1 of less than 60 per cent predicted may show a significant (greater or equal to 5 per cent) decrease in oxygen saturation during exercise (Canny and Levinson, 1987). Exercise programs should therefore be encouraged but need to be individually tailored, particularly for patients with more advanced pulmonary disease.

Mucolytics

Various mucolytics have been used, both orally and by aerosol, in an attempt to liquefy the hyperviscid airway mucus. The most frequently employed is aerosolized *N*-acetylcysteine. In vitro, this agent breaks the sulfhydryl bonds of the mucous glycoproteins, thereby reducing gel viscosity. It has an offensive smell, may induce bronchospasm, blocks endobronchial antibiotic activity, may cause hemorrhagic tracheitis with prolonged use, and at high doses impairs ciliary function. Moreover, there is little proven efficacy (Ratjen et al, 1985). Thus if used at all, aerosolized *N*-acetylcysteine should be confined to a select group of patients who continue to have marked sputum retention despite aggressive physiotherapy.

Bronchial Lavage

Therapeutic lung lavage was originally proposed by Kylstra (1971) as a means of clearing inspissated mucopurulent secretions from the airways of patients with CF. Although a few centers have continued to use this therapy on a regular basis, there is no unanimity either on the optimum technique or its exact clinical role, if any (Sherman, 1986). Suggested lavage solutions have included saline alone, 4 or 5 per cent *N*-acetylcysteine, and 3.7 per cent sodium bicarbonate. Lavage volumes have ranged from a few milliliters instilled via a fiberoptic bronchoscope into selected pulmonary segments to as much as 18 L instilled via a double-lumen endotracheal tube. Reported benefits are an improvement in patients' well-being, pulmonary function, and arterial blood gas tensions. The long-term effectiveness of repeated lavages has not been documented, however. One retrospective study (Schidlow et al, 1980) compared bronchial lavage versus conventional therapy with intravenous antibiotics and physiotherapy for episodes of acute exacerbations and could identify no

discernible benefits. This study was not randomized, however, and one of the criteria for bronchial lavage was a failure of antibiotic therapy. Bronchial lavage is not more effective than aggressive physiotherapy as first-line therapy in the treatment of lobar atelectasis (Stern et al, 1978).

Bronchial lavage is not an innocuous procedure. General anesthesia is usually required. In the largest reported series, 632 bronchial lavages were performed on 173 patients (Kulczycki, 1981) without mortality or significant long-term morbidity. Significant hypoxemia was common during the procedure, however, as were cardiac arrhythmias and even brief cardiac arrest. Other researchers have reported a 50 per cent incidence of febrile reactions during the procedure (Sherman, 1986). Thus in the absence of demonstrated long-term therapeutic effectiveness, we have reserved bronchoscopy and limited lavage for select patients who have persistent lobar atelectasis and who have failed to respond to conventional physiotherapy.

RESPIRATORY TRACT COMPLICATIONS

UPPER RESPIRATORY TRACT

Nasal Polyps

Nasal polyps are common in patients with CF; the incidence is between 6 and 36 per cent (Stern et al, 1982; David, 1986). The pathogenesis of nasal polyps in CF is unknown but does not appear to be associated with atopy. Polyps from patients with CF do show distinct histologic changes. The peak incidence of nasal polyps is in late childhood and early adolescence, but polyps are noted in children as young as 2 years. Treatment is difficult. Topical or systemic corticosteroids, antihistamines, and local decongestants all have been employed, although with little proven effectiveness (Crockett et al, 1987). Spontaneous regression may occur in many patients. Complete nasal obstruction commonly occurs and necessitates surgical excision. Regrettably, they reoccur within 12 months in up to 60 per cent of patients. In view of the high recurrence rate following excision, some surgeons have recommended a more aggressive approach such as intranasal ethmoidectomy or Caldwell-Luc procedures (David, 1986; Crockett et al, 1987). These more invasive approaches are associated with significant reduction in recurrence rate.

Facial Sinusitis

Radiologic opacification and maldevelopment of the facial sinuses occur in virtually all children with CF (David, 1986). As in other forms of bronchiectatic lung disease, these sinuses are commonly colonized by a spectrum of organisms similar to that in the lower respiratory tract. *P. aeruginosa, S. aureus, H. influenzae,* and anaerobes are the most common organisms isolated in CF. Chronic pansinusitis with facial pain, fevers, and "sinus headaches," however, is relatively rare and is usually encountered in combination with nasal polyposis. Antibiotic therapy is frequently ineffective because of poor penetration into the facial sinuses and the high incidence of antibiotic resistance in the colonizing organisms. Surgical drainage may therefore be required for the small group of patients with significant symptoms.

The incidence of otitis media and middle ear disease is not increased. Hearing loss due to long-term aminoglycoside use remains a risk but appears to be a rare occurrence.

LOWER RESPIRATORY TRACT

As a result of the increasing longevity of patients with CF, the long-term sequelae of chronic bronchopulmonary disease are becoming increasingly common.

Bronchiectasis

Progressive bronchiectasis is characteristic of CF in the vast majority of patients, being too diffuse to warrant surgical management. A small group of patients may present with a localized area of severe bronchiectasis, with the rest of the lung being relatively uninvolved. These patients may present with symptoms such as severe productive cough, malaise, and fevers disproportionate to the general severity of their lung disease. If there is no response to aggressive medical therapy and the symptoms are severe enough, surgical resection of the affected lobe may be warranted (Mearns et al, 1972). There are no clear guidelines about exactly when surgery should be undertaken. Bronchiectasis is usually more extensive than apparent on routine chest radiographs. Exact delineation of the extent and severity of pulmonary disease therefore needs to be performed before surgery is considered. Pulmonary function testing with arterial blood gases will ensure that a patient's respiratory reserve is sufficient to tolerate the extent of the proposed resection. Ventilation-perfusion scans demonstrate the extent of the disease, and computed tomography or bronchography may be used to assess involvement of the adjacent lobes (Maron et al, 1983). If adequate evaluation and aggressive pre- and postoperative therapy are employed, operative morbidity and mortality should be minimal. Although local resection usually results in improved symptoms, it is not clear whether it significantly affects the long-term prognosis.

Atelectasis

Patchy atelectasis is a common finding in CF, although complete lobar collapse occurs in fewer than

5 per cent of patients. The right middle lobe is most commonly involved. The presence of lobar collapse in younger children appears to be associated with more severe disease and is a poor prognostic sign. Treatment is primarily medical, with broad-spectrum antibiotics and aggressive physiotherapy (Stern et al, 1978). Bronchoscopy and lavage should be confined to patients unresponsive to aggressive medical management, although repeat collapse is common.

Pneumothorax

With the progression of the pulmonary disease, air trapping increases and microabscess formation promotes the formation of large apical bullae of up to several centimeters in diameter. Rupture of one of these bullae into the pleural space may lead to pneumothorax (Fig. 47–20). The frequency of spontaneous pneumothoraces increases with age (Penketh et al, 1982), being approximately 19 per cent in patients over 13 years of age. It is thus one of the most common respiratory complications in adulthood.

Small pneumothoraces (10 to 15 per cent in size), if not associated with significant respiratory distress, can usually be managed conservatively. Larger pneumothoraces usually cause significant respiratory embarrassment and hence require treatment with closed

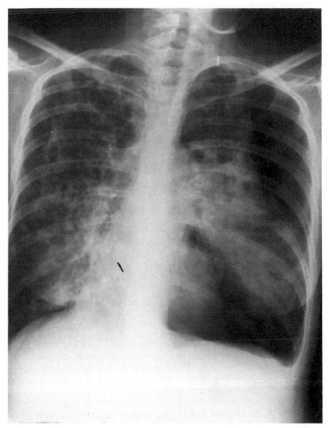

Figure 47–20. Patient L.K. with CF, aged 25 years, showing massive apical bullae and a large left pneumothorax. Although a recurrence was prevented by pleural sclerosis, death occurred 2 years later from progressive cardiorespiratory failure.

thoracotomy and underwater seal drainage. Although spontaneous closure of the air leak usually occurs within 1 to 2 days, up to 50 per cent of patients have a recurrence (McLaughlin et al, 1982). Morbidity and risk of death increase if drainage is needed for periods longer than a week. Our policy has therefore been to perform definitive therapy at the first episode of pneumothorax. Chemical pleurodesis can be performed when leakage ceases. Agents such as talc, tetracycline, or silver nitrate are associated with both a high recurrence rate and marked discomfort, resulting in decreased cough and hence sputum clearance. Intrapleural instillation of quinacrine is better tolerated and has a reduced risk of subsequent recurrences (McLaughlin et al, 1982). Once leakage of air stops, we instill 100 mg of quinacrine in 50 ml of saline via the chest tube and clamp the tube for 1 hour. During this period, the patient is placed in various positions to enhance the distribution of the quinacrine throughout the pleural cavity. After 1 hour, the chest tube is placed back on straight drainage. This is performed on each of 3 sequential days, and then the chest drain is removed. Chemical pleurodesis cannot be performed if air leakage persists. If leakage persists for greater than a week, we then consider open thoracotomy with either pleural abrasion, stripping, or oversewing of the apical bullae.

Some authorities consider previous pleural sclerosis to be an absolute contraindication to lung transplantation because it results in increased operative risks. This condition has presented a difficult therapeutic dilemma in some patients. Therapy has to be individualized, balancing the risks of recurrent pneumothoraces and prolonged chest drainage against the patient's potential for future lung transplantation.

Hemoptysis

Chronic endobronchial bacterial colonization results in progressive bronchiectasis. Within the ectatic airways, the ciliated epithelial lining is replaced by stratified squamous epithelium with discrete areas of granulation tissue. These airways may be traumatized by the paroxysmal coughing, and thus transient hemoptysis is common. With advancing disease, intermittent episodes of blood-stained streaking of sputum occur in up to 60 per cent of patients over 18 years of age (di Sant'Agnese and Davis, 1979). Treatment is aimed primarily at the underlying pulmonary disease, with administration of appropriate systemic antibiotics and correction of any underlying bleeding diathesis. Physiotherapy is usually discontinued until bleeding has stopped.

With the development of severe bronchiectasis, the supplying bronchial blood vessels become dilated and tortuous and develop extensive bronchopulmonary anastomoses. Rupture of one of these vessels into the airways may result in massive hemoptysis (greater than 300 ml in 24 hours) in approximately 5 to 7 per cent of adults (Porter et al, 1983). The incidence of rebleeding is high (around 45 per cent) and may be associated with immediate mortality due to blood loss and asphyxiation. Aggressive therapy is therefore warranted. Bronchoscopy may identify the site of bleeding, and endobronchial balloon tamponade can be successful in arresting the bleeding, although there is a high incidence of rebleeding. Pulmonary resection is curative. Massive hemoptysis is associated with advanced disease, and only limited numbers of patients have sufficient pulmonary reserve to tolerate the resection. Resection is therefore limited to patients who have hemorrhage greater than 600 ml/hr, in whom the site of bleeding can be accurately identified, and who have a FEV_1 of greater than 40 per cent predicted and a Shwachman-Kulczycki score of greater than 55 (Porter et al, 1983).

Selective bronchial angiography with embolization of the affected vessels using Gelfoam pellets can be used in patients with more advanced pulmonary disease. The reported success rate is around 88 per cent, with a recurrence rate of around 23 per cent. Significant complications are unusual (Fellows et al, 1979). Transverse myelitis due to seeding of the pellets via collateral vessels to the spinal cord is the major concern, but it appears to be rare.

Hypertrophic Pulmonary Osteoarthropathy

CF is associated with various musculoskeletal problems (Rush et al, 1986), the severity usually increasing in proportion with advancing pulmonary disease. Hypertrophic pulmonary osteoarthropathy (HPO) is probably the most common sequela, consisting of a triad of arthritis, clubbing, and periosteitis. The long, tubular bones are most commonly involved. Radiographs of the involved area demonstrate subperiosteal new bone formation (Fig. 47–21), although scintography is a more sensitive method for the detection of early HPO. HPO is clearly associated with the severity of pulmonary disease and usually responds to aggressive pulmonary therapy. Treatment of the joint pain itself is symptomatic, using standard anti-inflammatory agents (Phillips and David, 1986).

A non–HPO-related arthritis has also been described in CF. This arthritis was generally asymmetric, usually involving large joints while sparing metacarpophalangeal joints, with an approximate incidence of 2 per cent under the age of 16 (Rush et al, 1986). In the majority of patients, this arthritis is episodic, not related to juvenile rheumatoid arthritis, and does not appear to correlate with the severity of the pulmonary disease. Approximately 40 per cent of patients may develop associated cutaneous rashes, including erythema nodosum, vasculitic nodules, rheumatoid nodules, purpura, and nonpainful cutaneous nodules. This arthritis may therefore reflect peripheral immune complex deposition due to chronic pulmonary infection. Although the condition is generally benign and episodic, a subgroup of these patients develop persistent synovitis and even pro-

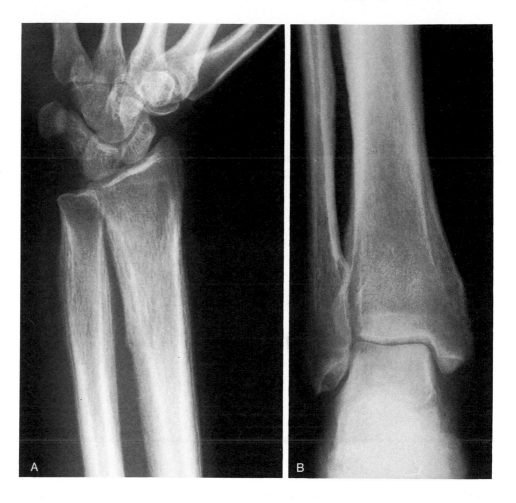

Figure 47–21. Wrist *(A)* and ankle *(B)* radiographs of patient L.K., showing severe hypertrophic pulmonary osteoarthropathy. There is marked periosteal elevation, with laying down of subperiosteal new bone. Subperiosteal laminations indicate ongoing proliferation and active disease.

gressive, symmetric, erosive disease. Treatment is, again, symptomatic with nonsteroidal anti-inflammatory agents.

Occasional, isolated cases of rheumatoid arthritis have also been reported in association with CF.

Allergic Bronchopulmonary Aspergillosis

Allergic bronchopulmonary aspergillosis (ABPA) was originally described in 1967. Several subsequent studies have documented an increased incidence in patients with CF. Although more than 50 per cent of patients with CF may show positive skin tests, precipitating antibiotics, and sputum cultures for both *Aspergillus fumigatus* and *Candida*, the incidence of clinical symptoms due to ABPA appears to be less than 10 per cent (Nelson et al, 1979; Laufer et al, 1984). There is no one specific diagnostic test for ABPA, the diagnosis resting on a combination of objective criteria (Rosenberg et al, 1977). It is occasionally difficult to make the diagnosis of superimposed ABPA in patients with CF because of the significant overlap in radiologic and serologic findings. An elevated serum IgE level, elevated levels of *A. fumigatus*–specific IgG and IgE, along with eosinophilia, positive sputum cultures for *Aspergillus*, and increasing clinical bronchospasm associated with evidence of tubular bronchiectasis on chest radiograph are usually required in combination for a firm diagnosis (Laufer et al, 1984).

Treatment is long-term steroids, initially 0.5 to 1 mg/kg of prednisone daily for 2 weeks, reduced if there is response to the same dose given on alternate days for a minimum of 3 months (Ricketti et al, 1984). Response to therapy can be monitored by changing clinical status and reduced levels of total IgE, specific IgE, and IgG antibodies. Although this treatment is usually effective, repeated courses or even maintenance low-dose prednisone may be required to prevent recurrences.

Despite the frequency of fungal colonization, invasive fungal disease is an extremely rare occurrence.

Gastroesophageal Reflux

Gastroesophageal reflux has been increasingly reported in patients with CF, although the exact incidence is unknown (Scott et al, 1985). Gastroesophageal reflux is known to occur with increased frequency in association with pulmonary disease, presumably as a result of decreased muscle tone or recurrent increases in intra-abdominal pressure associated with coughing. In a series from this institution, which cares for 534 patients, 25 of 75 patients had demonstrable reflux on barium swallow. Pulmonary function was significantly worse in the patients with reflux, although cause and effect could not be demonstrated. Clinical diagnosis may be difficult, because apart from retrosternal discomfort, symptoms of gastroesophageal reflux may be masked by the overlying pulmonary disease. Diagnosis is by barium swallow, esophageal pH probing, or esophagoscopy. The majority of patients respond to medical therapy, which consists of propping up the head of the bed and administering antacids and/or H_2 receptor blockers (Fiegelsen et al, 1987). Occasional patients may not respond or may develop complications such as esophageal stricture and hence require surgical intervention.

CARDIOVASCULAR SEQUELAE

Progressive pulmonary inflammation and associated hypoxemia result in extensive pulmonary vascular remodeling (see also "Pathology"). Consequently, there is increasing pulmonary hypertension leading to progressive right ventricular hypertrophy (cor pulmonale) (Moss, 1982). Overt right-sided cardiac failure eventually occurs, with survival then being less than 1 year. Cardiac failure is a sequela of the chronic, progressive pulmonary vascular disease, and the prognosis does not appear substantially improved by conventional cardiac therapies such as digitalization or diuretic therapy (Stern et al, 1980). Mean survival following onset of overt right ventricular failure is 8 months.

DIAGNOSIS

The diagnosis of cor pulmonale and even overt right ventricular failure may be difficult because of the symptoms of the overlying pulmonary disease. Cardiac catheterization is the gold standard but is rarely performed in patients with CF because of the attendant risks. Pulmonary hyperinflation may limit the value of either chest radiography or standard electrocardiography in assessing right ventricular status. Echocardiography is a valuable technique for measuring both right ventricular wall thickness and right ventricular function (Rosenthal et al, 1976). Pulmonary hyperinflation may limit the echocardiographic "window," however, and satisfactory studies are not feasible in 25 to 50 per cent of patients with CF. Radionuclide angiography does allow early detection of clinical right (and left) ventricular dysfunction, both at rest and during exercise. It has proved reasonably reproducible in patients with CF, is not affected by the presence of concomitant lung disease, and appears useful in serial assessment of cardiac function (Piepsz et al, 1987).

TREATMENT

Improvement in pulmonary status is the most effective therapy for cor pulmonale, but this is not possible in the majority of patients. Most patients will improve with therapy for any acute pulmonary exacerbation, as well as fluid restriction, diuretics, and oxygen. The value of digitalization remains in question.

Pulmonary vasodilator agents may reduce pulmonary vascular resistance in some patients but at the same time may cause increased hypoxemia as a result of increased flow through atelectatic areas, and clinical effectiveness remains in question (Moss, 1982). Aminophylline has no significant therapeutic effect on cardiac function in patients with CF (Canny et al, 1984).

Although the progressive cor pulmonale is clearly linked to the increasing hypoxemia, the value of long-term, domiciliary oxygen remains in question. In chronic obstructive pulmonary disease (COPD), oxygen therapy has been shown to reduce pulmonary vascular resistance and increase cardiac stroke volume. Two independent studies have demonstrated that domiciliary oxygen therapy both reduces mortality and improves overall quality of life in adult patients with COPD (Nocturnal Oxygen Therapy Trial Group, 1980; Report of the Medical Research Council, 1981). However, a double-blind multicenter trial of nocturnal oxygen in patients with CF was unable to demonstrate any effect on the long-term prognosis for patients with cor pulmonale (Zinman et al, 1987). Oxygen therapy in this trial was for only 8 hours at night (Spier et al, 1984), because further desaturation commonly occurs at night. Whether there is a therapeutic place for continuous oxygen in patients with arterial oxygen of less than 60 mm Hg remains a subject for debate.

RESPIRATORY FAILURE

With progression of the pulmonary disease, patients with CF develop increasing hypoxemia. By increasing their minute ventilation, they are able to maintain arterial P_{CO_2} within normal limits until late in the disease process. They are ultimately unable to further increase their minute ventilation, at which point progressive carbon dioxide retention occurs. In the majority of patients, carbon dioxide retention usually arises as an end result of chronic, irreversible pulmonary disease. Assisted ventilation is therefore rarely justified for these patients, because only rarely does sufficient improvement occur to allow extubation, and survival after extubation is usually only for a matter of weeks (Davis and di Sant'Agnese, 1978). This is in contradistinction to elective ventilation, as for surgical procedures. If there has been adequate preoperative assessment and aggressive pre- and postoperative pulmonary management, postoperative morbidity and mortality should be minimal even in the presence of significant lung disease.

NONPULMONARY MANIFESTATIONS OF CYSTIC FIBROSIS

Although pulmonary disease is the major cause of morbidity and ultimate mortality in the majority of patients, CF is a multisystem disease with multiple organ involvement (Fig. 47–22). The degree of other organ involvement has a significant effect on patients' well-being as well as on the course of the pulmonary disease (Park and Grand, 1981).

PANCREATIC

Obstruction of the pancreatic duct commences in utero, resulting in periductal inflammation, fibrosis, and loss of exocrine pancreatic function (Imrie et al, 1979). Pancreatic juice from patients with CF is characteristically low in volume, enzyme, and bicarbonate concentrations, even in the 10 to 15 per cent of patients without overt steatorrhea. Maldigestion of both fat and protein occurs when pancreatic lipase secretion falls below 2 per cent of normal, resulting in clinical steatorrhea (Durie et al, 1984).

Clinical Presentation

Patients with CF commonly present with evidence of protein-calorie malnutrition. The classic presentation is of a sickly infant with a protuberant abdomen, muscle wasting, and progressive failure to thrive despite an apparently voracious appetite. Their stool is commonly described as being frequent, bulky, greasy, and very offensive. Biochemical or clinical evidence of fat-soluble vitamin deficiency may also be present. Approximately 5 per cent of patients present with a particularly severe form of malnutrition, with hypoproteinemia, edema, and anemia. Infants placed on soy-based formula as a result of misdiagnosis of the steatorrhea as secondary to milk allergy and breast-fed babies seem at particular risk (Lee et al, 1974). Significant pulmonary disease also is commonly present in these patients, and the long-term prognosis is usually poor. The severity of malnutrition varies markedly between patients, however. Ten to 15 per cent of patients have sufficient pancreatic function to prevent steatorrhea and hence have normal growth patterns. Growth is also frequently normal in patients with milder disease; they appear to be able to compensate for fecal losses by increased dietary intake.

Diagnosis

Direct Assessment: Pancreatic Stimulation. Pancreatic secretions can be collected by duodenal intubation using a triple-lumen orogastric tube. Maximal

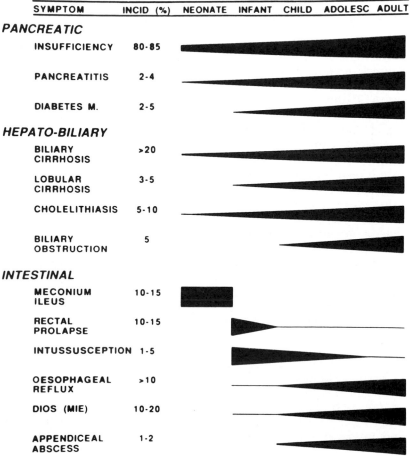

Figure 47–22. Gastrointestinal manifestations of cystic fibrosis. (From Durie PR: In: Willa JP [ed]: Disorders of Gastrointestinal Motility in Childhood. New York, John Wiley & Sons, Ltd, 1988. Reproduced by permission of John Wiley and Sons Limited.)

pancreatic stimulation with pancreozymin and secretin allows quantitative analysis of pancreatic function (Durie et al, 1984). This approach obviously is moderately invasive and is mainly used in patients with questionable pancreatic function. Sequential studies have shown that a number of patients with pancreatic sufficiency, particularly those with low initial levels of pancreatic function, have subsequently become pancreatic insufficient (Durie et al, 1988).

Indirect Assessment

FECAL FAT ASSESSMENT. In patients with steatorrhea, large numbers of fat globules may be readily demonstrated by Sudan red staining of the stool. However, this is neither a definitive nor quantitative test, and formal assessment of fecal fat content needs to be made using a 3- to 5-day stool collection, expressing total fecal fat output as a percentage of oral intake over that period. Fecal fat content is usually less than 2 per cent of intake in normal individuals, but greater than 20 to 30 per cent in patients with pancreatic insufficiency.

PANCREATIC SUBSTRATE ASSAYS. Duodenal intubation and pancreatic stimulation testing are both technically rigorous and moderately invasive. Fecal fat collection is usually easy to perform in bottle-fed infants. It is difficult in breast-fed babies, toddlers, and adolescents because of problems in both fat intake assessment and poor patient compliance with stool collection. Attempts have therefore been made to develop alternative methods to assess pancreatic function by orally administering a substrate that is metabolized into two or more products by pancreatic enzymes. If the initial substrate is not absorbed but one or more of the digestive products are, measurement of the digestion products in blood or urine enables documentation of pancreatic function. The two most common substrates used are N-benzoyl-L-tyrosyl-P-aminobenzoic acid (NBT-PABA), and the pancreolauryl (fluorescein dilaurate) test (Scharpe and Illano, 1987). Both tests discriminate between pancreatic sufficiency and insufficiency, with the pancreolauryl test perhaps having the advantage because of minimal interference with other drugs or serum compounds. There is a degree of overlap between values from pancreatic-sufficient and pancreatic-insufficient patients for both tests, and false results may be obtained in the presence of biliary or intestinal disease. Moreover, neither of the tests provides quantification of residual function in pancreatic-sufficient patients.

SCREENING TESTS. The presence in the stool of either undigested products such as albumin (the BM test) or the absence of pancreatic enzymes such as chymotrypsin has been used as a screening test for the diagnosis of CF. However, none of these assays shows abnormal results in the presence of pancreatic sufficiency (Remtulla et al, 1986), and they also have significant rates of both false-positive and -negative results.

Serum levels of both immunoreactive trypsinogen and lipase are significantly elevated at birth in all patients with CF. Trypsinogen assay appears to provide the best discrimination between patients with CF and normal individuals. In patients with pancreatic insufficiency, there is an exponential decline in serum levels for both enzymes, reaching subnormal levels between 1 and 6 years of age. In pancreatic-sufficient patients, serum levels remain persistently elevated (Durie et al, 1986). Analysis of serum levels of either trypsinogen or lipase may therefore provide a method of discriminating between pancreatic sufficiency and insufficiency in patients over 5 years of age, although again providing no quantification of residual function in pancreatic-sufficient patients.

Complications

Pancreatitis. Patients with residual pancreatic function may suffer from recurrent pancreatitis (Shwachman et al, 1957). Diagnosis may be difficult, because recurrent abdominal pain is common in CF secondary to various other causes (Park and Grand, 1981). Treatment requires parenteral fluids, nasogastric tube suction, and adequate analgesia. Pancreatitis may be recurrent but usually ceases once pancreatic function has been lost.

Diabetes Mellitus. As many as 40 per cent of patients may show evidence of decreased glucose tolerance, with elevated levels of glycosylated hemoglobin (Stutchfield et al, 1987), whereas frank diabetes mellitus is estimated to occur in 7 per cent of adults with CF (Finkelstein et al, 1988). Pancreatic islet cell destruction is believed to occur secondary to progressive pancreatic fibrosis (Soejima and Landing, 1986), the incidence increasing with advancing age. Although requiring insulin therapy, the hyperglycemia is usually easily controlled, and ketosis is rarely encountered. Diabetes has been reported to be associated with more severe pulmonary disease (Finkelstein et al, 1988), although results from our clinic differ. Whether the diabetes is the cause or a consequence of the nutritional and metabolic sequelae of advanced pulmonary disease is not clear. Steroid therapy may also induce diabetes in patients with borderline glucose tolerance. In view of the nutritional problems in CF, dietary management is not recommended, low-dose insulin therapy usually being sufficient to control hyperglycemia. However, with increasing life expectancy in patients with CF, reports of diabetic microangiopathy are now beginning to appear (Dolan, 1986).

GASTROINTESTINAL

Meconium Ileus

Ten to 15 per cent of patients with CF present with meconium ileus in the neonatal period (Park and Grand, 1981). It is believed to be caused by a combination of abnormal pancreatic function and intestinal gland secretions (Hopfer, 1982). The resulting hyperviscid, relatively desiccated meconium contains high levels of calcium and undegraded serum proteins, leading to in utero obstruction of the distal ileum. Meconium ileus is rare except in patients with CF but has occasionally been described in association with pancreatic duct stenosis, partial pancreatic aplasia, and as an isolated event without any other gastrointestinal pathology (Rickham and Boeckman, 1965). Pancreatic insufficiency is not a prerequisite, as meconium ileus has been described in infants with little or no pancreatic involvement.

Diagnosis. The usual clinical picture is of an infant presenting within the first 48 hours of life with evidence of intestinal obstruction. In uncomplicated meconium ileus, flat plate radiographs of the abdomen may show gastric distention with evidence of irregularly distended loops of small bowel containing a characteristic soap bubble appearance as a result of trapping of air in the meconium (Abramson et al, 1987). Air-fluid levels are not always present, the hyperviscid meconium not layering out on the erect film. Fifty per cent of cases are complicated by small or large (or both) bowel atresia, volvulus, or perforation (Fig. 47–23) (Gross et al, 1985). In utero perforation may lead to sterile peritonitis with peritoneal calcifications, meconium pseudocyst, or generalized adhesive meconium peritonitis. Septic peritonitis occurs if perforation is still present at birth. These complications may be diagnosed in utero by ultrasonography.

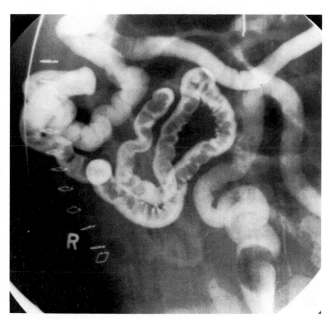

Figure 47–24. A postoperative enema reveals the microcolon with persisting inspissated meconium in the distal small bowel, outlined by the water-soluble contrast.

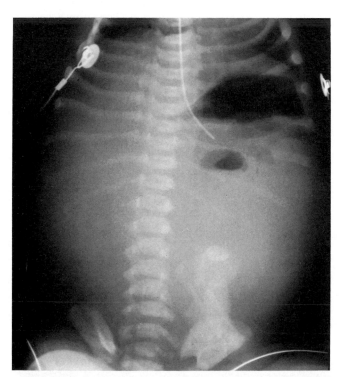

Figure 47–23. Abdominal radiograph of A.B., a patient with CF (24 hours old), presenting with a history of vomiting and failure to pass meconium. The classic features of meconium ileus are masked by evidence of intestinal obstruction with abdominal distention, air fluid levels, and a failure to pass air beyond the proximal small bowel. A laparotomy revealed meconium ileus and a localized volvulus.

Treatment. Before the development of effective surgical therapy, meconium ileus was almost invariably fatal. Even up until the mid-1960s, long-term survival was generally less than 20 per cent. However, subsequent to the development of an effective medical approach for uncomplicated meconium ileus, there has been a marked improvement in life expectancy (Caniano and Beaver, 1987). Gastrografin contains both a hypertonic, radiopaque dye that draws fluid into the bowel lumen and a wetting agent (Tween) that helps breaks up the viscid meconium. Gastrografin enemas are usually successful in alleviating the obstruction, although repeated enemas may be required in some patients (Fig. 47–24). There are risks to this procedure because of the marked fluid and electrolyte shifts and risks of bowel perforation associated with the use of hypertonic enemas (Ein et al, 1987). We therefore now prefer to use a mixture of 25 per cent sodium diatrizoate (Hypaque) with 5 per cent N-acetylcysteine, which, although still hypertonic, is about one third that of Gastrografin. Mortality is now rare in uncomplicated meconium ileus and, because of improved medical and surgical treatment of neonates, is less than 15 per cent in complicated cases (Caniano and Beaver, 1987). The long-term prognosis for survivors beyond the neonatal period appears to be no different from that of patients with uncomplicated pancreatic insufficiency (McPartlin et al, 1972).

Distal Intestinal Obstruction Syndrome (Meconium Ileus Equivalent)

Recurrent distal intestinal obstruction is a common problem in older patients, with an estimated incidence of between 10 and 20 per cent (Rubinstein,

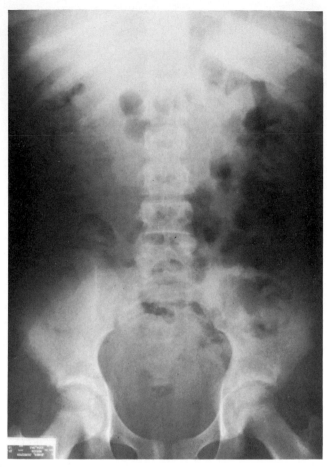

Figure 47–25. Patient J.J., a 15-year-old girl with known cystic fibrosis, presenting with a 3-month history of recurrent, colicky abdominal pain and a firm, tender mass in the right inguinal fossa. A flat-plate radiograph of the abdomen shows massive fecal loading of both the ileum and the ascending colon, indicating a distal intestinal obstruction.

1986). The etiology is unclear. It appears to arise as a combination of abnormal intestinal contents due to pancreatic insufficiency, abnormal intestinal secretions with increased intestinal mucus adherence, and disordered intestinal motility leading to secondary fecal stasis (Durie, 1988). It has occurred in pancreatic-sufficient patients (Davidson et al, 1987).

Diagnosis. Diagnosis is primarily made on clinical grounds. The usual clinical presentation is intermittent crampy lower abdominal pain associated with a palpable mass in the right lower quadrant, although complete intestinal obstruction may occasionally occur. Fecal loading of both colon and terminal ileum is evident on plain radiograph despite a history of apparent regular defecation (Fig. 47–25) (Abramson et al, 1987). Both volvulus and intussusception may complicate distal intestinal obstruction syndrome. Cholecystitis, cholelithiasis, and pancreatitis all appear to occur with increased frequency in CF (Park and Grand, 1981) and need to be included in the differential diagnosis of recurrent abdominal pain. Moreover, acute appendicitis may be masked by the concurrent use of broad-spectrum antibiotics, result-

ing in appendiceal abscess with persisting right lower quadrant pain, mass, and intermittent low-grade fever.

Treatment. Treatment is primarily medical. Mucolytic agents such as *N*-acetylcysteine may be given by enema to disimpact the inspissated material, and maintenance of oral doses may help to prevent recurrence. Stool softeners such as mineral oil or Colace may help alleviate the problem but should not be used concurrently because Colace may potentiate mineral oil absorption. A more effective therapy, particularly in more severe or indolent cases, is the use of a balanced intestinal lavage solution (GoLYTELY) (Cleghorn et al, 1986) that contains polyethylene glycol as a nonabsorbable agent, hence causing minimal transmucosal flux of either fluid or electrolytes. Five to 6 L are administered either orally or via nasogastric tube at a rate of 1 L/hr, until rectal discharge is clear of fecal material. Striking clinical and radiologic improvement usually results (Fig. 47–26), as well as increased time before recurrence of symptoms. However, recurrences do occur. Limited studies on Cisapride, a gastrointestinal prokinetic agent known to increase gastric emptying and small-bowel transit time, suggest that this drug may have a long-term prophylactic value, but further confirmation is required (Durie, 1988).

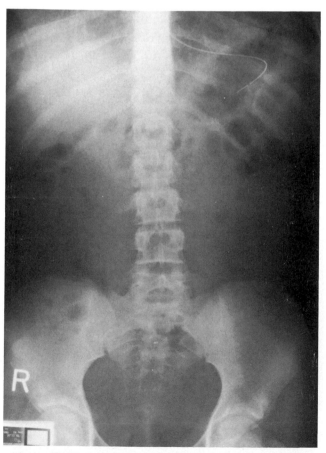

Figure 47–26. Patient J.J., following the administration of 6 L of GoLYTELY through a nasogastric tube. There is marked clearing, although some residual fecal material is still present in the cecum and the ascending colon.

Rectal Prolapse

Rectal prolapse may occur in as many as 20 per cent of patients, most commonly between the ages of 6 months and 2 years, and is frequently recurrent (Stern et al, 1982). The cause is believed to be a combination of poor muscle tone secondary to malnutrition, abnormal intestinal motility, frequent bulky stools due to steatorrhea, and recurrent increases in intra-abdominal pressure due to coughing. Rectal prolapse usually resolves spontaneously on starting pancreatic enzyme supplementation. A surgical approach is rarely required.

NUTRITION

Assessment

There has long been a recognized association between nutritional status and the severity of pulmonary disease in CF. Malnutrition leads to defects in systemic immunity, particularly cell mediated, and hence increases the susceptibility to pulmonary infections even in normal individuals (Martin, 1987). At the same time, pulmonary disease results in decreased intake due to associated anorexia yet increased requirements due to hypoxia and increased work of breathing, resulting in increased risks of malnutrition (Neijens et al, 1984).

Eighty-five per cent of patients with CF have pancreatic lipase production less than 2 per cent of normal maximal values, resulting in maldigestion both of fat and protein, although carbohydrate digestion is minimally affected (Hoffman et al, 1987). Because this dietary fat constitutes 40 per cent of the normal calorie intake in the Western diet, significant calorie deficits result and cannot usually be compensated for by increased carbohydrate intake. The azotorrhea (stool nitrogen being two to two and one-half times normal in most patients with CF), combined with increased protein catabolism due to calorie deprivation, leads to significant protein deficits as well.

Even in patients with pancreatic insufficiency there is marked variability in the severity of steatorrhea. The pancreatic lesion in CF results in production of pancreatic secretions low in volume, enzyme, and bicarbonate concentrations. Patients with CF therefore tend to have low intestinal pH as a result of both relative and absolute gastric acid excess (Youngberg et al, 1987), which results in decreased activity of any residual lipase present. Patients with CF also commonly have lower total circulating bile salt pools, apparently as a result of a combination of increased fecal binding, defective ileal reabsorption (Weber and Roy, 1984), and abnormal gallbladder function (Weizman et al, 1986). The relative severity of these associated defects may explain the variability of steatorrhea in pancreatic-insufficient patients and why some patients may be able, by increasing total calorie intake, to maintain normal growth until the onset of significant pulmonary disease. At that point, with the increased work of breathing and relative anorexia associated with the pulmonary disease, malnutrition may then supervene.

Assessment

Clinical. Patients with CF should have their weight and height assessed at least every 3 months and plotted as per cent predicted against standard growth charts. Weight tends to decline early in malnutrition, growth arrest usually occurring later and signifying severe deficits. Upper limb (triceps and subscapular) skin fold thickness is a good indicator of subcutaneous fat status and can be compared with published normals (Frisancho, 1981).

Biochemical. Malnutrition in CF leads to a wide variety of biochemical abnormalities (Kelleher, 1987). In infancy, hypoalbuminemia usually indicates severe malnutrition. In adulthood, hypoalbuminemia may arise in association with the panhypergammaglobulinemia and secondary fluid retention due to cardiac failure. Albumin levels of less than 38 g/L are usually indicative of significant protein-calorie deficits, however.

The exact role of essential fatty acid deficiency in the pathogenesis of CF remains controversial (Anderson, 1984). Although several reports have documented low levels of linoleic acid in patients with CF (Gibson et al, 1986), correction made no marked effect on either clinical status or pulmonary function (Mischler et al, 1986). Supplementation is warranted in the presence of biochemical deficiency (Kelleher, 1987).

Indirect calorimetry has proved to be helpful in assessing catabolic status in malnourished patients and hence serves to guide nutritional repletion. Although this information is not usually available, these studies have demonstrated resting energy requirements in excess of 150 per cent of normal in patients with significant pulmonary disease or malnutrition (Vaisman et al, 1987). A 3- to 5-day fecal collection with a dietary diary enables calculation of average daily calorie intake. Nutritional repletion needs to be based not only on nutritional status, but ongoing requirements.

Treatment

It is now clear that CF does not have to be synonymous with malnutrition (Littlewood and MacDonald, 1987; Roy et al, 1984). In our clinic, by using a program of aggressive nutritional management, normal growth can be achieved in the vast majority of patients (Fig. 47–27), at least until the onset of advanced pulmonary disease (Gurwitz et al, 1979).

Pancreatic Enzyme Supplementation. Coincident with the introduction of effective pancreatic enzyme supplements in the 1950s there was a marked improvement in life expectancy. Original extracts were

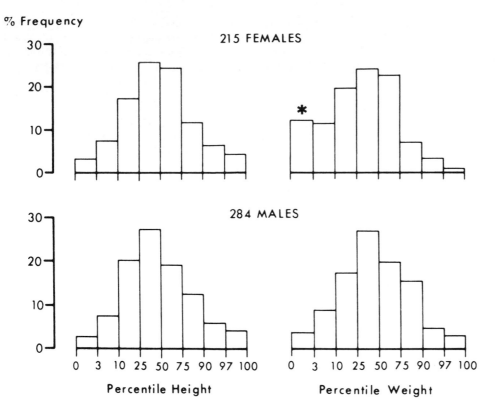

% Frequency

215 FEMALES

284 MALES

Percentile Height

Percentile Weight

Figure 47–27. Percentage frequency distributions of percentile height and percentile weight of patients older than 2 years who attended the Toronto cystic fibrosis clinic in 1978. The asterisk (*) marks a subgroup of females with chronic nutritional deficiencies and significantly worse prognoses. (Reproduced with permission from Gurwitz D, Corey M, Francis PWJ et al: Pediatr Clin North Am 26:606, 1979.)

in powdered form. Because as much as 90 per cent of ingested enzymes may be destroyed by gastric acid, fairly high dosages were required in some patients. Because of the high purine content of pancreatic extracts, patients using these extracts were at risk for hyperuricemia and nephrolithiasis (Bohles and Michalk, 1982). Some patients also have persisting marked steatorrhea despite pancreatic enzyme supplementation. Consequently, various antacid regimens were tried using either bicarbonate or H₂ blockers, with some degree of success (Durie, Bell, Linton et al, 1980). With the development of pH-sensitive polymers, it became possible to encapsulate pancreatic enzymes in acid-resistant microspheres that dissolve only on reaching the alkaline milieu of the small intestine (Braggion et al, 1987). Significantly smaller quantities of enzymes are therefore required to prevent steatorrhea. The dosage of pancreatic enzyme supplementation required by individual patients is variable. In infants, we usually start with the equivalent of 4000 to 8000 units of lipase per 4 oz of formula or per breast, increasing to 24,000 units per meal in children and around 40,000 units per meal in adolescents and adults. The enzyme dosage is varied as necessary to achieve normal growth and prevent clinical steatorrhea. In some patients, this cannot be achieved using pH-sensitive microspheres (Braggion et al, 1987), presumably because residual acidity within the proximal small bowel prevents enzyme release. These patients may therefore require a combination of noncoated enzymes and/or antacids to achieve satisfactory digestion.

Caloric Supplementation. A number of factors

conspire to make patients with CF prone to malnutrition. First, although patients with CF are classically described as having a voracious appetite, 40 per cent of patients actually have calorie intakes below the recommended daily average for age (Littlewood and MacDonald, 1987). Second, pancreatic enzyme supplementation rarely results in complete abolition of steatorrhea, which commonly remains around 10 per cent of intake. Consequently, a number of clinics have in the past recommended a low-fat diet for patients with CF to minimize the persisting steatorrhea. Fat contains two and one-half times more calories per gram than either carbohydrate or protein, and a low-fat diet is relatively unpalatable. It is therefore difficult for patients on this program to ingest sufficient calories to maintain normal growth (Pencharz, 1983). Our clinic therefore emphasizes a high-calorie, high-protein diet, which of course contains significant quantities of fat. The vast majority of patients can achieve normal growth on this diet, at least until adolescence. With the onset of progressive pulmonary disease, resulting in anorexia and increased metabolic demands, patients may become increasingly at risk of malnutrition. This is particularly a problem in adolescent girls, perhaps because of social pressures toward a more asthenic appearance (Gurwitz et al, 1979). Because of the association between nutritional status and progression of pulmonary disease, various stratagems have been proposed to increase calorie intake in patients with increasing malnutrition (Goodchild, 1986).

ORAL SUPPLEMENTS. Various milk-based high-calorie formulas are available for use as dietary supplements. They are relatively unpalatable, require additional enzyme therapy, and will obviously only be effective if used as supplements rather than replacements for a normal daily intake. A fair degree of patient compliance is clearly required. Predigested formulas or medium-chain triglyceride preparations are even less palatable than the milk-based supplement, yet may still require pancreatic enzyme supplementation (Durie, Newth, Forstner, and Gall, 1980).

NASOGASTRIC FEEDING. Some clinics have successfully employed nocturnal feedings of predigested formula delivered via fine Silastic nasogastric feeding tubes. Both parents and older patients can be taught the technique of insertion, and the feeding can be carried out on a long-term at-home basis (Shepherd et al, 1986). We have found dislodgment to be a common problem due to nocturnal coughing, with the risks of aspiration of formula into the lungs, and have therefore been less successful than other clinics in the use of this technique.

INTRAVENOUS FEEDING. Although significant weight gain can be achieved by aggressive intravenous feeding in virtually any patient (Mansell et al, 1984), the clinical role of this therapy is yet to be clarified. Central venous feeding is usually required in order to achieve adequate calorie intake. Although weight gain can usually be rapidly achieved, a significant proportion of this weight gain is due to water retention. A rapid return to baseline may therefore occur after short-term therapy, but with no definite long-term benefits. Both long-term parenteral feeding and intravenous antibiotic therapy have been achieved using indwelling central lines. The risks of infection and thrombosis are significant, however, and the indwelling lines must be meticulously cared for by both patients and their parents.

GASTROSTOMY/JEJUNOSTOMY FEEDING. Selected patients with intractable weight loss despite aggressive nutritional management may respond to nocturnal feedings using an elemental formula delivered by indwelling gastrostomy or jejunostomy tubes (Boland et al, 1986). Although requiring a minimal operative procedure, gastrostomy insertion being performed using an "incisionless" technique under local anesthetic (Mago et al, 1986), neither gastrostomy nor jejunostomy feedings are totally without problems. Gastrostomy feedings may exacerbate gastroesophageal reflux, and both techniques may exacerbate diabetes mellitus and fluid loading in patients with borderline cardiopulmonary status (Levy et al, 1986). Numerous reports have documented improved nutritional status using these techniques. However, no significant improvements in pulmonary function have been documented, although improved nutritional status appears to be associated with a reduced incidence of acute pulmonary exacerbations and an arrest in rates of pulmonary deterioration in some patients (Shepherd et al, 1986). Thus before any program of aggressive nutritional intervention is begun, rigorous patient selection is required to balance the potential benefits against the defined risks of the various available approaches. Moreover, it is clear that in a number of children, malnutrition arises secondary to psychosocial dysfunction rather than organic disease. Therefore, intervention needs to be individualized.

Vitamins. Clinical vitamin deficiency is a relatively rare occurrence, although bleeding diathesis (due to vitamin K deficiency) and neurologic disease (due to vitamin E deficiency) have occasionally been reported. Low serum levels of vitamins A, E, and D all are commonly encountered (Kelleher, 1987).

Vitamin A is stored exclusively in the liver, and serum levels are therefore not good indicators of overall vitamin status. The incidence of clinically significant vitamin A deficiency in CF is not known.

Vitamin D levels have been reported as being both low and normal in patients with CF, possibly reflecting variations in endogenous production associated with exposure to sunlight (Thompson, 1987).

Vitamin E deficiency may lead to increased red cell fragility and decreased red cell survival and may also cause significant neurologic deficits. It has been described even in patients receiving vitamin supplementation (Congden et al, 1981).

Low levels of water-soluble vitamin B_6 have been reported in patients with CF but may occur as a sequela of hepatic disease rather than as a consequence of decreased intake.

Patients with steatorrhea therefore require supplementation with twice the normal daily intake of fat-soluble vitamins, including a water-soluble vitamin E preparation (Littlewood and MacDonald, 1987; Kelleher, 1987).

Minerals

ELECTROLYTES. Hyponatremia and hypokalemia with hypochloremia and metabolic alkalosis may occur as a result of excessive losses in sweat. Infants are primarily afflicted, particularly during the summer months (Beckerman and Taussig, 1979). Symptoms in these patients include anorexia, lethargy, and vomiting associated with decreased oral intake. Treatment is by volume and sodium chloride repletion. Therefore, during the summer months we prophylactically give all infants under the age of 18 months a maintenance oral electrolyte solution containing 1.6 mmol of sodium, 1.6 mmol of potassium, and 2 mmol of chloride per milliliter. Breast-fed babies receive 1.5 ml/kg/day; formula-fed babies, 1 ml/100 ml of formula.

TRACE ELEMENTS. Trace element status appears normal in the vast majority of patients with CF (Kelleher, 1987).

Despite the chronic lung disease and progressive hypoxemia, polycythemia is rarely encountered (Vichinsky et al, 1984). Iron deficiency appears to a relatively common finding, reduced ferritin levels occurring in as many as 30 per cent of patients (Ehrhardt et al, 1987), although the exact cause remains unclear. Iron supplementation may improve hemoglobin levels in some patients, but it may also cause hemolysis in the presence of vitamin E deficiency.

HEPATOBILIARY

Approximately 2 to 5 per cent of patients with CF have clinical evidence of hepatobiliary involvement, the incidence and presentation varying with age.

Liver

Patients may present in the neonatal period with evidence of obstructive jaundice due to plugging of the bile ducts by inspissated bile, which may take as long as 2 to 6 months to resolve. Fatty infiltration of the liver (steatosis) may occur in 30 to 60 per cent of older children but is rarely associated with any clinical disease (Park and Grand, 1981). Steatosis is believed to arise secondary to nutritional disturbance and usually improves with pancreatic enzyme therapy. Steatosis has, however, been described in nutritionally normal patients (Hultcrantz et al, 1986). Focal biliary cirrhosis is pathognomonic for CF, occurring in approximately 10 per cent of older patients, with clinical or biochemical evidence of liver involvement usually occurring late in the disease (Roy et al, 1982). Approximately 2 per cent of patients progress to multilobar cirrhosis presenting with signs of progressive portal hypertension such as hypersplenism and evidence of esophageal varices. Gastrointestinal hemorrhage may be the first presenting sign (Tanner, 1986). Progressive liver failure with abnormal transaminase levels, hypoalbuminemia, hypoprothrombinemia, ascites, and jaundice may eventually occur in a small number of patients.

Gallbladder

Approximately 30 per cent of patients with CF have evidence of abnormal gallbladder function, both histologically and radiologically (either on ultrasonography or by cholangiography). Gallstones may be demonstrated in 5 to 10 per cent of patients. Clinically significant biliary disease seems to occur in only 3.6 per cent of patients. Symptomatic disease includes cholelithiasis, cholecystitis, and occasionally frank cholangitis. Cholecystectomy is usually recommended if symptomatic cholelithiasis is identified, even in the absence of classic biliary colic, because of the risks of progression of the disease (Stern et al, 1986).

Bile Duct

Gaskin and colleagues (1988) found that out of 153 patients with CF, 11 patients had clinical, 14 patients had biochemical, and 36 patients had both clinical and biochemical evidence of hepatic disease. All of the 45 patients with clinical disease had evidence of biliary tract obstruction on hepatobiliary scintigraphy. Percutaneous transhepatic cholangiography was performed on 29 patients. Of these patients, 19 had large gallbladders, 17 also showing evidence of stricture of the distal bile duct. Fourteen patients had sufficient symptoms (recurrent/persistent right upper quadrant or epigastric pain) to warrant surgical correction of the stricture. The authors conclude that stricture of the common bile duct may be a cause of both persistent abdominal pain and progressive liver disease in a significant number of patients with CF. These findings have to be confirmed by other clinics, however.

FERTILITY

Puberty is commonly delayed in patients with CF (Landon and Rosenfeld, 1984; Moshang and Hulsclaw, 1980), presumably secondary to both nutritional factors and the effect of chronic disease.

Males. Approximately 98 per cent of patients with CF are infertile as a result of in utero obstruction of the vas deferens (Taussig et al, 1972). Hormonal functions and hence secondary sexual characteristics are normal, however. Patients may need to be made aware of this feature on reaching puberty, and seminal analysis is arranged as appropriate.

Females. The fertility rate is approximately 20 to 30 per cent of normal in females with CF (Matson and Capen, 1982). The potential for pregnancy exists, and contraceptive advice should be offered to all sexually active females. The optimal form of contraception is still under debate, but the oral contraceptive pill does not appear to adversely affect pulmonary status (Fitzpatrick et al, 1984).

Increasing numbers of patients have successfully carried pregnancy until term, without significant pulmonary deterioration. In advanced disease, however, the hemodynamic stresses of pregnancy and labor may overload an already compromised cardiorespiratory system. Individual counseling therefore needs to be provided for women who have CF and are considering pregnancy. Their current pulmonary status and their preceding rate of decline should be considered (Palmer et al, 1983).

FUTURE CONSIDERATIONS

PREVENTION

Genetic

Isolation of the major mutations of the CF gene will open the way for wide-scale screening of both unrelated carriers and newborn infants (before the onset of clinical disease). However, because of the high incidence of the carrier state in the white population, this screening program will require large resources for both genetic analysis and counseling services for individuals who are identified as heterozygous. Moreover, because the current median life expectancy for patients with CF is in excess of 20 years, many parents may not elect for therapeutic abortion in the presence of an affected fetus. CF is therefore probably going to remain a medical dilemma for many years to come.

Pulmonary Infections

The mechanics of initial bacterial colonization are still not understood. Attempts at vaccination against *P. aeruginosa* have been singularly ineffective. It is hoped that understanding of the mechanisms behind initial bacterial adherence may allow its prevention, hence minimizing or even preventing future pulmonary disease. Whether this will in fact be possible remains speculative.

TREATMENT

Pulmonary Infections

Despite the marked improvements in life expectancy since CF was first described, there appear to be limits to what may be achieved using the currently available therapies. Median life expectancy in our clinic is now around 24 years for women, 28 to 30 years for men. This appears to have reached a plateau, with little significant change during the last decade. The principal cause of death is progressive pulmonary disease secondary to chronic *P. aeruginosa* and *P. cepacia* colonization. Both of these organisms have a great facility for developing antibiotic resistance. Thus although an increasing number of effective antipseudomonal antibiotics may allow increased flexibility in treating acute excerbation, we still remain unable to eradicate the organisms.

Heart-Lung Transplantation

At the time of this writing, more than 250 heart-lung and double-lung transplantations have been performed worldwide (Reitz, 1988), with around 10 per cent of those performed on patients with CF. The overall mortality is reported to be between 30 and 40 per cent, with the longest survival now approaching 2 years after transplantation. The absence of the classic electrochemical abnormalities in the transplanted lungs of these long-term survivors (Alton et al, 1987) suggests that transplantation may indeed be a "cure" for at least the pulmonary disease of CF. Although cor pulmonale is usually present in these patients, it appears reversible with correction of the chronic pulmonary disease. The relative advantages of heart-lung versus double-lung transplants have yet to be elucidated. Single-lung transplantation is contraindicated, because progressive overexpansion of the remaining diseased lung occurs, causing compression of the transplanted normal lung. Even with improved surgical technique and postoperative care, the high risks of complications in

malnourished patients, in patients with previous pleural surgery, and in patients who have progressed to the point of requiring ventilation, together with the difficulty in finding suitable donor organs, mean that transplantation will probably remain a therapeutic option for only a small group of highly selected patients.

SUMMARY

Cystic fibrosis is no longer a purely pediatric disease. With current management, almost 80 per cent of patients should reach adulthood. Increasing numbers of patients are embarking on careers, getting married, and having children. These patients are "survivors," their own health depending on increasingly aggressive therapy. A cure for their illness remains elusive, and a significant number of their fellow patients have died of the disease during childhood. Isolation of the CF gene may improve diagnosis. There are, however, a number of diseases, such as sickle cell disease, for which both the genetic basis and the underlying biochemical defect have been discovered, yet their therapeutic management remains largely unchanged.

Until we better understand the exact pathologic mechanisms behind CF, we will continue to be challenged to minimize and prevent the long-term sequelae and to aid both patients and their families in coping with the medical and psychosocial problems associated with what remains an ultimately fatal disease.

REFERENCES

Introduction

Andersen DH: Cystic fibrosis of the pancreas and its relation to celiac disease, a clinical and pathological study. Am J Dis Child 56:344, 1938.

Corey ML: Longitudinal studies in cystic fibrosis. In Sturgess SM (ed): Perspectives in Cystic Fibrosis. Toronto, Cystic Fibrosis Foundation, 1980.

Wood RE, Boat TF, and Doershuk CF: Cystic fibrosis. Am Rev Respir Dis 113:841, 1976.

Genetics

Kerem BS, Rommeus JM, Buchanan JA et al: Identification of the cystic fibrosis gene: genetic analysis. Science 245:1073, 1989.

Kulczycki L and Schauf V: CF in blacks in Washington, D.C.: Incidence and characteristics. Am J Child 127:64, 1974.

Lathrop GM, Farrall M, O'Connell P et al: Refined linkage map of chromosome 7 in the region of the cystic fibrosis gene. Am J Hum Genet 42:38, 1988.

Rommeus JM, Iannuzzi MC, Kerem BS et al: Identification of the cystic fibrosis gene: chromosome walking and jumping. Science 245:1059, 1989.

Steel CM: DNA in medicine: the tools. Lancet 2:908, 1984.

Tsui LC, Buchwald M, Barker D et al: Cystic fibrosis locus defined by a genetically linked polymorphic DNA marker. Science 230:1054, 1985.

Wright SW and Morton NE: Genetics studies on CF in Hawaii. Am J Hum Genet 20:157, 1986.

Pathogenesis

Boat TF and Dearborn DG: Etiology and pathogenesis in cystic fibrosis. In Taussig LM (ed): Cystic Fibrosis. New York, Thieme-Stratton, Inc, 1984.

Cheng PW, Boucher RC, Yankaskas JM et al: Glycoconjugates secreted by cultured human nasal epithelial cells. In Mastella G and Quinton PM (eds): Cellular and Molecular Basis of Cystic Fibrosis. San Francisco Press, Inc, 1988.

Dubinsky WP: Resolution and reconstitution of the factors controlling chloride permeability in the trachea. Prog Clin Biol Res 254:167, 1987.

Geddes P: Progress in research on cystic fibrosis. Thorax 39:721, 1984.

Feigal RJ and Shapiro BL: Cystic fibrosis—a lethal exocrinopathy with altered mitochondrial calcium metabolism. Ann NY Acad Sci 488:82, 1986.

Katz SM, Krueger LJ, and Falkner B: Microscopic nephrocalcinosis in cystic fibrosis. N Engl J Med 319:263, 1988.

Kopelman H, Durie P, Gaskin K et al: Pancreatic fluid secretion and protein hyperconcentration in cystic fibrosis. N Engl J Med 312:329, 1985.

Knowles MR, Stutts MJ, Yankaskas JR et al: Abnormal respiratory epithelial ion transport in cystic fibrosis. Clin Chest Med 7:285, 1986.

Mastella G and Quinton PM (eds): Cellular and Molecular Traits of Cystic Fibrosis. San Francisco Press, Inc, 1988.

Riordan JR, Rommeus JM, Kerem BS et al: Identification of the cystic fibrosis gene: cloning and characterization of complementary DNA. Science 245:1066, 1989.

Slomiany BL, Nadziejko C, Mizuta K et al: Role of associated and covalently bound lipids in the physicochemical properties of mucus glycoprotein. In Mastella G and Quinton PM (eds): Cellular and Molecular Basis of Cystic Fibrosis. San Francisco Press, Inc, 1988.

Welsh MJ: Mechanisms of airway epithelial ion transport. Clin Chest Med 7:273, 1986.

Wesley A, Forstner J, Quereshi R et al: Human intestinal mucus in cystic fibrosis. Pediatr Res 17:65, 1983.

Yankaskas JR, Knowles MR, Gatzy JT et al: Persistence of abnormal chloride ion permeability in cystic fibrosis nasal epithelial cells in heterologous culture. Lancet 1:954, 1985.

Infection

Auerbach HS, Williams M, Kirkpatrick JA et al: Alternate-day prednisone reduces morbidity and improves pulmonary function in cystic fibrosis. Lancet 2:686, 1985.

Bauerfeind RM, Bertele RM, Harms K et al: Qualitative and quantitative microbiological analysis of sputa of 102 patients with cystic fibrosis. Infection 15:270, 1987.

Brigham KL and Meyrick B: Interactions of granulocytes within the lungs. Circ Res 54:623, 1984.

Cohen ML: *Staphylococcus aureus*: biology, mechanisms of virulence, epidemiology. J Pediatr 108:796, 1986.

Corey M, Allison L, Prober C et al: Sputum bacteriology in patients with cystic fibrosis in a Toronto hospital during 1970–1981. J Infect Dis 149:283, 1984.

Efthimiou J, Hodson M, Taylor P et al: Importance of viruses and *Legionella pneumophila* in respiratory exacerbations of young adults with cystic fibrosis. Thorax 39:150, 1984.

Fradin MS, Kalb RE, and Grossman ME: Recurrent cutaneous vasculitis in cystic fibrosis. Pediatr Dermatol 4:108, 1987.

Goldmann DA and Klinger JD: *Pseudomonas cepacia*: biology, mechanisms of virulence, epidemiology. J Pediatr 108:806, 1986.

Goldstein W and Doring G: Lysosomal enzymes from polymorphonuclear leukocytes and proteinase inhibitors in patients with cystic fibrosis. Am Rev Respir Dis 134:49, 1986.

Hoiby N, Doring G, and Schiotz PO: The role of immune complexes in the pathogenesis of bacterial infections. Ann Rev Microbiol 40:29, 1986.

Hoiby N, Doring G, and Schiotz PO: Pathogenic mechanisms of chronic *Pseudomonas aeruginosa* infections in cystic fibrosis patients. Antibiot Chemother 39:60, 1987.

Isles A, MacLusky I, Corey M et al: *Pseudomonas cepacia* infection in cystic fibrosis: an emerging problem. J Pediatr 104:206, 1984.

Mathews WJ Jr, Williams M, Oliphint B et al: Hypogammaglobulinemia in patients with cystic fibrosis. N Engl J Med 302:245, 1980.

Moss RB: Hypergammaglobulinemia in cystic fibrosis. Chest 91:522, 1987.

Pier GB: Pulmonary disease associated with *Pseudomonas aeruginosa* in cystic fibrosis: current status of the host-bacterium interaction. J Infect Dis 151:575, 1985.

Pitt TL: Biology of *Pseudomonas aeruginosa* in relation to pulmonary infection in cystic fibrosis. J R Soc Med 79(suppl 12):13, 1986.

Rush PJ, Shore A, Coblentz C et al: The musculoskeletal manifestations of cystic fibrosis. Semin Arthritis Rheum 15:213, 1986.

Schiotz PO: Local humoral immunity and immune reactions in the lungs of patients with cystic fibrosis. Acta Pathol Microbiol Immunol Scand (C) (Suppl 276):1, 1981.

Stroobant J: Viral infection in cystic fibrosis. J R Soc Med 79(suppl 12):19, 1986.

Tablan OC, Chorba TL, Schidlow DV et al: *Pseudomonas cepacia* colonization in patients with cystic fibrosis: risk factors and clinical outcome. J Pediatr 107:382, 1985.

Thomassen MJ, Demko CA, Doershuk CF et al: *Pseudomonas cepacia*: decrease in colonization in patients with cystic fibrosis. Am Rev Respir Dis 134:669, 1986.

Tosi M, Zakem H, and Berger M: Elastase impairs neutrophil *Pseudomonas* interaction: implications for chronic lung infection in CF Pediatr Res 23:385A, 1988.

Vasil ML: *Pseudomonas aeruginosa*: biology, mechanisms of virulence, epidemiology. J Pediatr 108:800, 1986.

Wang EL, Prober CG, Manson B et al: Association of respiratory viral infections with pulmonary deterioration in patients with cystic fibrosis. N Engl J Med 311:1653, 1984.

Wang EL, Manson B, Corey M et al: False positivity of *Legionella* serology in patients with cystic fibrosis. Pediatr Infect Dis 6:256, 1987.

Wheeler WB, Williams M, Mathews WJ et al: Progression of cystic fibrosis lung disease as a function of serum immunoglobulin G levels: a five-year longitudinal study. J Pediatr 104:695, 1984.

Wisnieski JJ, Todd EW, Fuller RK et al: Immune complexes and complement abnormalities in patients with cystic fibrosis. Am Rev Respir Dis 132:770, 1985.

Pulmonary Manifestations

Bedrossian CWM, Greenberg SD, Singer DB et al: The lung in cystic fibrosis: a quantitative study including prevalence of pathological findings among different age groups. Hum Pathol 7:196, 1976.

Chow CW, Landau L, and Taussig LM: Bronchial mucus glands in newborn with cystic fibrosis. Eur J Pediatr 139:240, 1982.

Di Sant'Agnese P and Davis PB: Cystic fibrosis in adults. Am J Med 66:121, 1979.

Lloyd-Still JD, Khan KT, and Shwachman H: Severe respiratory disease in infants with cystic fibrosis. Pediatrics 53:678, 1974.

Mack JF, Moss AT, Harper WW et al: The bronchial arteries in cystic fibrosis. Br J Radiol 38:422, 1965.

Oppenheimer ER and Esterly JR: Pathology of cystic fibrosis: review of the literature and comparison with 146 autopsied cases. Perspect Pediatr Pathol 2:241, 1975.

Pitts-Tucker TJ, Miller MG, and Littlewood JM: Finger clubbing in cystic fibrosis. Arch Dis Child 61:576, 1986.

Ryland D and Reid L: The pulmonary circulation in cystic fibrosis. Thorax 30:285, 1975.

Sobonya RE and Taussig LM: Quantitative aspects of lung pathology in cystic fibrosis. Am Rev Respir Dis 134:290, 1986.

Sturgess JM: Morphological characteristics of the bronchial mucosa in cystic fibrosis. In Quinton PM, Martinez JR, and Hopfer U (eds): Fluid and Electrolyte Abnormalities in Exocrine Glands in Cystic Fibrosis. San Francisco Press, Inc, 1982.

Tomashefski JF Jr, Bruce M, Goldberg HI et al: Regional distribution of macroscopic lung disease in cystic fibrosis. Am Rev Respir Dis 133:535, 1986.

Diagnosis

Beck R, Durie PR, Hill JG, and Levison H: Malnutrition: a cause of elevated sweat chloride concentration. Acta Paediatr Scand 75:639, 1986.

Boue A, Muller F, Nezelof C et al: Prenatal diagnosis in 200 pregnancies with a 1-in-4 risk of cystic fibrosis. Hum Genet 74:288, 1986.

Dankert-Roelse JE, Meerman GJT, Martijn A et al: Screening for cystic fibrosis. Acta Paediatr Scand 76:209, 1987.

Dean M, O'Connell P, Leppert M et al: Three additional DNA polymorphisms in the *met* gene and D7S8 locus: use in prenatal diagnosis of cystic fibrosis. J Pediatr 111:490, 1987.

Denning CR, Huag NN, Cuasay LR et al: Cooperative study comparing three methods of performing sweat tests to diagnose cystic fibrosis. Pediatrics 66:752, 1980.

Gibson LF and Cooke RE: A test for concentration of electrolytes in sweat in cystic fibrosis of the pancreas utilizing pilocarpine iontophoresis. Pediatrics 23:545, 1959.

Heeley AF and Watson D: Cystic fibrosis—its biochemical detection. Clin Chem 29:2011, 1983.

Heeley AF, Heeley ME, King DN et al: Screening for cystic fibrosis by dried blood spot trypsin assay. Arch Dis Child 57:18, 1982.

Huff DS, Huang NN, and Arey JB: Atypical cystic fibrosis of the pancreas with normal levels of sweat chloride and minimal pancreatic lesions. J Pediatr 94:237, 1979.

Kuzemko JA: Screening, early neonatal diagnosis and prenatal diagnosis. J R Soc Med 79(suppl 12):2, 1986.

LeGrys VA and Wood RE: Incidence and implications of false-negative sweat test reports in patients with cystic fibrosis. Pediatr Pulmonol 4:169, 1988.

Littlewood JR: The sweat test. Arch Dis Child 61:1041, 1986.

Mulivor RA, Cook D, Muller F et al: Analysis of fetal intestinal enzymes in amniotic fluid for the prenatal diagnosis of cystic fibrosis. Am J Hum Genet 40:131, 1987.

Muller F, Boue J, Nezelof C et al: Intestinal Dysfunction in CF Affected Fetuses. Results of 240 Prenatal Diagnoses Based on Microvillar Enzyme Activities. New York, Alan R Liss, Inc, 1987.

Rosenstein BJ, Langbaum TS, and Metz SJ: Cystic fibrosis: diagnostic considerations. Johns Hopkins Med J 150:113, 1982.

Spence JE, Buffone GJ, Rosenbloom CL et al: Prenatal diagnosis of cystic fibrosis using linked DNA markers and microvillar intestinal enzyme analysis. Hum Genet 76:5, 1987.

Stern RC, Boat TF, Abramowsky LR et al: Intermediate-range sweat chloride concentration and *Pseudomonas* bronchitis: a cystic fibrosis variant with preservation of exocrine pancreatic function. JAMA 239:2676, 1978.

Walton FWF, Hay JG, Munro C et al: Measurement of nasal potential difference in adult cystic fibrosis, Young's syndrome, and bronchiectasis. Thorax 42:815, 1987.

Wilcken B, Towns SJ, and Mellis CM: Diagnostic delay in cystic fibrosis: lessons from newborn screening. Arch Dis Child 58:863, 1983.

Assessment

Amodio JB, Berdon WE, Abramson S et al: Cystic fibrosis in childhood: pulmonary, paranasal sinus, and skeletal manifestations. Semin Roentgenol 22:125, 1987.

Barlett JG and Finegold SM: Bacteriology of expectorated sputum with quantitative culture and wash technique compared to transtracheal aspirates. Am Rev Respir Dis 117:1019, 1978.

Brasfield D, Hicks G, Soong SJ et al: The chest roentgenogram in cystic fibrosis: a new scoring system. Pediatrics 63:24, 1979.

Corey M, Levison H, and Crozier D: Five to seven year course of pulmonary function in cystic fibrosis. Am Rev Respir Dis 114:1085, 1976.

Featherby EA, Weng TR, Crozier DN et al: Dynamic and static lung volumes, blood gas tensions and diffusing capacity in patients with cystic fibrosis. Am Rev Respir Dis 102:737, 1970.

Friedman DJ: Chest radiographic findings in the adult with cystic fibrosis. Semin Roentgenol 22:114, 1987.

Gilljam H, Malmborg A, and Strandvik B: Conformity of bacterial growth in sputum and contamination free endobronchial samples in patients with cystic fibrosis. Thorax 41:641, 1986.

Hutcheon M, Griffin M, Levison H et al: Volume of isoflow: a new test in detection of mild abnormalities of lung mechanisms. Am Rev Respir Dis. 110:465, 1974.

Lamarre A, Reilly BJ, Bryan AC et al: Early detection of pulmonary function abnormalities in cystic fibrosis. Pediatrics 50:291, 1972.

Landau LI and Phelan PD: The spectrum of cystic fibrosis: a study of pulmonary mechanics in 46 patients. Am Rev Respir Dis 108:593, 1973.

Levison H and Godfrey S: Pulmonary aspects of cystic fibrosis. In Mangos JA and Talamo RC (eds): Cystic Fibrosis—Projections into the Future. New York, Stratton Intercontinental Book Corp, 1976.

Lewiston N and Moss R: Interobserver variance in clinical scoring for cystic fibrosis. Chest 91:878, 1987.

Mellins RB: The site of airway obstruction in cystic fibrosis. Pediatrics 44:315, 1969.

Muller N, Frances P, Gurwitz D et al: Mechanisms of hemoglobin desaturation during rapid-eye-movement sleep in normal subjects and in patients with cystic fibrosis. Am Rev Respir Dis 121:463, 1980.

Shwachman H and Kulczycki LL: Long-term study of 105 patients with cystic fibrosis. Am J Dis Child 96:6, 1958.

Wagener JS, Taussig LM, Burrows B et al: Comparison of lung function survival patterns between cystic fibrosis and emphysema or chronic bronchitis patients. In Sturgess JM (ed): Perspectives in Cystic Fibrosis. Proceedings of the Eighth International Congress on Cystic Fibrosis, Toronto, 1980.

Treatment (Infection)

Alfredsson H, Malmborg A, and Strandvik B: *N*-acetylcysteine and 2-mercaptoethane sulphonate inhibit anti-*Pseudomonas* activity of antibiotics in vitro. Eur J Respir Dis 70:213, 1987.

Beaudry PH, Marks MI, McDougall D et al: Is anti-*Pseudomonas* therapy warranted in acute respiratory exacerbations in children with cystic fibrosis. J Pediatr 97:144, 1980.

Boxerbaum B: The art and science of the use of antibiotics in cystic fibrosis. Pediatr Infect Dis 1:381, 1982.

Clarke SW: Aerosols as a way of treating patients. Eur J Respir Dis 69(suppl 146):525, 1986.

Gold R, Carpenter S, Heuter H et al: Randomized trial of ceftazidime versus placebo in the management of acute respiratory exacerbations in patients with cystic fibrosis. J Pediatr 111:907, 1987.

Govan RW, Doherty C, and Glass S: National parameters for antibiotic therapy in patients with cystic fibrosis. Infection 15:86, 1987.

Hodson ME: Antibiotic treatment: aerosol therapy. Chest 94:156S, 1988.

Hodson ME, Penketh ARL, and Batten JC: Aerosol carbenicillin and gentamicin treatment of *Pseudomonas aeruginosa* infection in patients with cystic fibrosis. Lancet 2:1137, 1981.

Kuzemko JA: Home treatment of pulmonary infections in cystic fibrosis. Chest 94:162S, 1988.

Langford DT and Hiller J: Prospective, controlled study of a polyvalent *Pseudomonas* vaccine in cystic fibrosis—three year results. Arch Dis Child 59:1131, 1984.

Levy J: Antibiotic activity in sputum. J Pediatr 108:841, 1986.

MacLusky I, Levison H, Gold R, et al: Inhaled antibiotics in cystic fibrosis: is there a therapeutic effect? J Pediatr 108:861, 1986.

Michel BC: Antibacterial therapy in cystic fibrosis: a review of the literature published between 1980 and February 1987. Chest 94:129S, 1988.

Nelson JD: Management of acute pulmonary exacerbations in cystic fibrosis: a critical appraisal. J Pediatr 106:1030, 1985.

Pedersen SS, Jensen T, Pressler T et al: Does centralized treatment of cystic fibrosis increase the risk of *Pseudomonas aeruginosa* infection? Acta Paediatr Scand 75:840, 1986.

Pedersen SS, Jensen T, Hoiby N et al: Management of *Pseudomonas aeruginosa* lung infection in Danish cystic fibrosis patients. Acta Paediatr Scand 76:955, 1987.

Prandota J: Drug disposition in cystic fibrosis: progress in understanding pathophysiology and pharmacokinetics. Pediatr Infect Dis 6:1111, 1987.

Raeburn JA, Govan JRW, McCrae WM et al: Ciprofloxacin therapy in cystic fibrosis. J Antimicrob Chemother 20:295, 1987.

Stutman HR: Summary of a workshop on ciprofloxacin use in patients with cystic fibrosis. Pediatr Infect Dis 6:932, 1987.

Szaf M and Hoiby N: Antibiotic treatment of *Staphylococcus aureus* infection in cystic fibrosis. Acta Paediatr Scand 71:821, 1982.

Thomassen MJ, Demko CA, and Doershuk CF: Cystic fibrosis: a review of pulmonary infections and interventions. Pediatr Pulmonol 3:334, 1987.

Treatment (Airway Obstruction)

Blomquist M, Freyschuss U, Wiman LG et al: Physical activity and self treatment in cystic fibrosis. Arch Dis Child 61:362, 1986.

Canny GJ and Levison H: Exercise response and rehabilitation in cystic fibrosis. Sports Med 4:143, 1987.

Darga LL, Eason LA, Maximilian D et al: Cold air provocation of airway hyperreactivity in patients with cystic fibrosis. Pediatr Pulmonol 2:82, 1986.

Desmond KT, Schwerk WF, Thomas E et al: Immediate and long term effects of chest physiotherapy in patients with cystic fibrosis. J Pediatr 103:538, 1983.

Eber E, Oberwaldner B, and Zach MS: Airway obstruction and airway wall instability in cystic fibrosis. Pediatr Pulmonol 4:205, 1988.

Gaskell DV and Webber BA (eds): The Brompton Hospital Guide to Chest Physiotherapy. Oxford and London, Blackwell Scientific Publications, 1980.

Hofmeyr JL, Webber BA, and Hodson ME: Evaluation of positive expiratory pressure as an adjunct to chest physiotherapy in the treatment of cystic fibrosis. Thorax 41:951, 1986.

Kulczycki LL: Experience with 632 bronchoscopic bronchial washings (BBW) done on 173 cystic fibrosis (CF) patients during a 16 year period (1965–1980). In Warwick WJ (ed): 1,000 Years of Cystic Fibrosis. Minneapolis, University of Minnesota, 1981.

Kylstra JA, Rausch DC, Hall KD et al: Volume-controlled lung lavage in the treatment of asthma, bronchiectasis, and mucovisicidosis. Am Rev Respir Dis 103:651, 1971.

Mellis CM and Levison H: Bronchial reactivity in cystic fibrosis. Pediatrics 61:446, 1978.

Michell I, Corey M, Woenne R et al: Bronchial hyperreactivity in cystic fibrosis and asthma. J Pediatr 93:744, 1978.

Oberwaldner PT, Evans JC, and Zach MS: Forced expirations against a variable resistance: a new chest physiotherapy method in cystic fibrosis. Pediatr Pulmonol 2:358, 1986.

Pryor JA, Webber BA, Hodson ME, and Batten JC: Evaluation of the forced expiration technique as an adjunct to postural drainage in treatment of cystic fibrosis. Br Med J 2:417, 1979.

Ratjen F, Wonne R, Posselt HG et al: A double-blind placebo controlled trial with oral ambroxol and N-acetylcysteine for mucolytic treatment in cystic fibrosis. Eur J Pediatr 144:374, 1985.

Reisman JJ, Rivington-Law B, Corey M et al: The role of conventional physiotherapy in cystic fibrosis. J Pediatr 113:632, 1988.

Schidlow DV, Simon D, Palmer J et al: Tracheobronchial lavage in cystic fibrosis. In Sturgess JM (ed): Perspectives in Cystic Fibrosis. Proceedings of the VIII International Cystic Fibrosis Congress, Toronto, 1980.

Sherman JM: Bronchial lavage in patients with cystic fibrosis. Pediatr Pulmonol 2:244, 1986.

Skorecki K, Levison H, and Crozier DN: Bronchial lability in cystic fibrosis. Acta Paediatr Scand 65:39, 1976.

Stern RC, Boat TF, Orenstein DM et al: Treatment and prognosis of lobar and segmental atelectasis in cystic fibrosis. Am Rev Respir Dis 118:821, 1978.

Sutton PP, Pavia D, and Bateman JRM: Chest physiotherapy: a review. Eur J Respir Dis 63:188, 1982.

Verboon JML, Bakker W, and Sterk PJ: The value of the forced expiration technique with and without postural drainage in adults with cystic fibrosis. Eur J Respir Dis 69:169, 1986.

Respiratory Tract Complications and Cardiovascular Sequelae

Canny GJ, De Souza ME, Gilday DL, and Newth CJ: Radionuclide assessment of cardiac performance in cystic fibrosis: reproducibility and effect of theophylline on cardiac function. Am Rev Respir Dis 130:122, 1984.

Crockett DM, McGill TJ, Healy GB et al: Nasal and paranasal sinus surgery in children with cystic fibrosis. Ann Otol Rhinol Laryngol 96:367, 1987.

David TJ: Nasal polyposis, opaque paranasal sinuses and usually normal hearing: the otorhinolaryngological features of cystic fibrosis. J R Soc Med 79(suppl 12):23, 1986.

Davis PB and di Sant'Agnese PA: Assisted ventilation for patients with cystic fibrosis. JAMA 239:1851, 1978.

Di Sant'Agnese PA and Davis PB: Cystic fibrosis in adults: seventy five cases, and a review of 232 cases in the literature. Am J Med 66:121, 1979.

Feigelson J et al: Gastro-oesophageal reflux and esophagitis in cystic fibrosis. Acta Paediatr Scand 76:989, 1987.

Fellows KE, Khau KT, Shuster S et al: Bronchial artery embolization in cystic fibrosis: technique and long-term results. J Pediatr 95:959, 1979.

Laufer P, Fink J, Burns T et al: Allergic bronchopulmonary aspergillosis in cystic fibrosis. J Allergy Clin Immunol 73:44, 1984.

McLaughlin FJ, Matthews WJ, Strieder DJ et al: Pneumothorax in cystic fibrosis: management and outcome. J Pediatr 100:863, 1982.

Maron L, Schidlow D, Palmer J et al: Pulmonary resection for complications of cystic fibrosis. J Pediatr Surg 18:863, 1983.

Mearns M, Hodson CJ, Jackson A et al: Pulmonary resection in cystic fibrosis—results in 23 cases, 1957–1970. Arch Dis Child 47:499, 1972.

Moss AJ: The cardiovascular system in cystic fibrosis. Pediatrics 70:728, 1982.

Nelson LA, Collerame ML, and Schwartz RH: Aspergillosis and atopy in cystic fibrosis. Am Rev Respir Dis 120:863, 1979.

Nocturnal Oxygen Therapy Trial Group: Continuous or nocturnal oxygen therapy in hypoxemia chronic obstructive lung disease. Ann Intern Med 93:391, 1980.

Penketh ARL, Knight RK, Hodson ME et al: Management of pneumothorax in adults with cystic fibrosis. Thorax 37:850, 1982.

Phillips BM and David TJ: Pathogenesis and management of arthropathy in cystic fibrosis. J R Soc Med 79(suppl 12):44, 1986.

Piepsz A, Ham HR, Millet E, and Dab I: Determination of right ventricular ejection fraction in children with cystic fibrosis. Pediatr Pulmonol 3:24, 1987.

Porter DK, Van Every MJ, and Anthracite RF: Massive hemoptysis in cystic fibrosis. Arch Intern Med 143:287, 1983.

Report of the Medical Research Council Working Party: Long-term domiciliary oxygen therapy in chronic hypoxic cor pulmonale complicating chronic bronchitis and emphysema. Lancet 1:681, 1981.

Ricketti AJ, Greenberger PA, Mintzer RA, and Paterson R: Allergic bronchopulmonary aspergillosis. Chest 86:773, 1984.

Rosenberg M, Patterson R, Mintzer R et al: Clinical and immunologic criteria for the diagnosis of allergic bronchopulmonary aspergillosis. Ann Intern Med 86:405, 1977.

Rosenthal A, Tucker CR, Williams RG et al: Echocardiographic assessment of cor pulmonale in cystic fibrosis. Pediatr Clin North Am 23:327, 1976.

Rush PJ, Shore A, Coblentz C et al: The musculoskeletal manifestations of cystic fibrosis. Semin Arthritis Rheum 15:213, 1986.

Scott RB, O'Loughlin EV, and Gall DG: Gastroesophageal reflux in patients with cystic fibrosis. J Pediatr 106:223, 1985.

Spier S, Rivlin J, Hughes D, and Levison H: The effect of oxygen on sleep, blood gases, and ventilation in cystic fibrosis. Am Rev Respir Dis 129:712, 1984.

Stern RC, Boat TF, Orenstein DM et al: Treatment and prognosis of lobar and segmental atelectasis in cystic fibrosis. Am Rev Respir Dis 118:821, 1978.

Stern RC, Boat TF, Wood RE et al: Treatment and prognosis of nasal polyps in cystic fibrosis. Am J Dis Child 136:1067, 1982.

Stern RC, Borkat G, Hirschfeld SS et al: Heart failure in cystic fibrosis. Treatment and prognosis of cor pulmonale with failure of the right side of the heart. Am J Dis Child 134:267, 1980.

Zinman R, Corey M, Coates AL et al: Nocturnal oxygen therapy in the treatment of hypoxemic cystic fibrosis patients. Pediatr Pulmonol S1:73, 1987.

Pancreatic/Gastrointestinal

Abramson SJ, Baker DH, Amodio JB, and Berdon WE: Gastrointestinal manifestations of cystic fibrosis. Semin Roentgenol 22:97, 1987.

Caniano DA and Beaver BL: Meconium ileus: a fifteen-year experience with forty-two neonates. Surgery 102:699, 1987.

Cleghorn GJ, Stringer DA, Forstner GG et al: The treatment of distal intestinal obstruction syndrome in cystic fibrosis with a balanced intestinal lavage solution. Lancet 1:8, 1986.

Davidson AC, Harrison K, Steinfort CL, and Geddes DM: Distal intestinal obstruction syndrome in cystic fibrosis treated by oral intestinal lavage, and a case of recurrent obstruction despite normal pancreatic function. Thorax 42:538, 1987.

Dolan TF: Microangiopathy in a young adult with cystic fibrosis and diabetes mellitus (letter). N Engl J Med 314:991, 1986.

Durie PR: Gastrointestinal motility disorders in cystic fibrosis. In Willa JP (ed): Disorders of Gastrointestinal Motility in Childhood. New York, John Wiley & Sons, 1988.

Durie PR, Gaskin KJ, Corey M et al: Pancreatic function testing in cystic fibrosis. J Pediatr Gastroenterol Nutr 3:S89, 1984.

Durie PR, Forstner GG, Gaskin KJ et al: Age-related alterations of immunoreactive pancreatic cationic trypsinogen in sera from cystic fibrosis patients with and without pancreatic insufficiency. Pediatr Res 20:209, 1986.

Durie PR, Kopelman HR, Corey ML et al: Pathophysiology of the exocrine pancreas in cystic fibrosis. In Mastella G and Quinton PM (eds): Cellular and Molecular Basis of Cystic Fibrosis. San Francisco, San Francisco Press, Inc, 1988.

Ein SH, Shandling B, Reilly B, and Stephens CA: Bowel perforation with non-operative treatment of meconium ileus. J Pediatr Surg 222:146, 1987.

Finkelstein SM, Wielinski CL, Elliott GR et al: Diabetes mellitus associated with cystic fibrosis. J Pediatr 112:373, 1988.

Gross K, Desanto A, Grosfeld JL et al: Intra-abdominal complications of cystic fibrosis. J Pediatr Surg 20:431, 1985.

Hopfer U: Pathophysiological considerations relevant to intestinal obstruction in cystic fibrosis. In Quinton PM, Martinez JR, and Hopfer U (eds): Fluid and Electrolyte Abnormalities in Exocrine Glands in CF. San Francisco Press, 1982.

Imrie JR, Fagan DG, and Sturgess M: Quantitative evaluation of the development of the exocrine pancreas in cystic fibrosis and control infants. Am J Pathol 95:697, 1979.

Lee PA, Roloff DW, and Mowatt WF: Hypoproteinemia and anemia in infants with cystic fibrosis. JAMA 228:585, 1974.

McPartlin JF, Dickson JAS, and Swain VA: Meconium ileus: immediate and long-term survival. Arch Dis Child 47:207, 1972.

Park RW and Grand RJ: Gastrointestinal manifestations of cystic fibrosis: a review. Gastroenterology 81:1143, 1981.

Remtulla MA, Durie PR, and Goldberg DM: Stool chymotrypsin activity measured by a spectrophotometric procedure to identify pancreatic disease in infants. Clin Biochem 19:341, 1986.

Rickham PP and Boeckman CR: Neonatal meconium obstruction in the absence of mucoviscidosis. Am J Surg 109:173, 1965.

Rubinstein S, Moss R, and Lewiston N: Constipation and meconium ileus equivalent in patients with cystic fibrosis. Pediatrics 78:473, 1986.

Scharpé S and Illano L: The indirect tests of exocrine pancreatic function evaluated. Clin Chem 33:5, 1987.

Shwachman H, Lebenthal E, and Khaw KT: Recurrent acute pancreatitis in patients with cystic fibrosis with normal pancreatic enzymes. Pediatrics 55:86, 1975.

Soejima K and Landing BH: Pancreatic islets in older patients with cystic fibrosis with and without diabetes mellitus. Pediatr Pathol 6:45, 1986.

Stern RC, Izant FJ, Boat TF et al: Treatment and prognosis of rectal prolapse in cystic fibrosis. Gastroenterology 82:709, 1982.

Stutchfield PR, O'Halloran S, Teale JD et al: Glycosylated haemoglobin and glucose intolerance in cystic fibrosis. Arch Dis Child 62:805, 1987.

Nutrition

Anderson CM: Hypothesis revisited: cystic fibrosis: a disturbance of water and electrolyte movement in exocrine secretory tissue associated with altered prostaglandin (PGE_2) metabolism? J Pediatr Gastroenterol Nutr 3:15, 1984.

Beckerman RC and Taussig LM: Hypoelectrolytemia and metabolic alkalosis in infants with cystic fibrosis. Pediatrics 63:580, 1979.

Bohles H and Michalk D: Is there a risk for kidney stone formation in cystic fibrosis? Helv Paediat Acta 37:267, 1982.

Boland MP, Stoski DS, MacDonald NE, and Soucy P: Chronic jejunostomy feeding with a nonelemental formula in undernourished patients with cystic fibrosis. Lancet 1:232, 1986.

Braggion C, Borgo G, Faggionato P, and Mastella G: Influence of antacid and formulation on effectiveness of pancreatic enzyme supplementation in cystic fibrosis. Arch Dis Child 62:349, 1987.

Congden PJ, Bruce G, Rothburn MM et al: Vitamin status in treated patients with cystic fibrosis. Arch Dis Child 56:708, 1981.

Durie PR, Bell L, Linton W et al: Effect of cimetidine and sodium bicarbonate on pancreatic replacement therapy in cystic fibrosis. Gut 21:778, 1980.

Durie PR, Newth CJ, Forstner GG, and Gall DG: Malabsorption of medium-chain triglycerides in infants with cystic fibrosis: correction with pancreatic enzyme supplements. J Pediatr 96:862, 1980.

Ehrhardt P, Miller MG, and Littlewood JM: Iron deficiency in cystic fibrosis. Arch Dis Child 62:185, 1987.

Frisancho AR: New norms of upper limb fat and muscle areas for assessment of nutritional status. Am J Clin Nutr 34:2540, 1981.

Gibson RA, Teubner JK, Haines K et al: Relationships between pulmonary function and plasma fatty acid levels in cystic fibrosis patients. J Pediatr Gastroenterol Nutr 5:408, 1986.

Goodchild MC: Practical management of nutrition and gastrointestinal tract in cystic fibrosis. J R Soc Med 79:32, 1986.

Gurwitz D, Corey M, Francis PWJ et al: Perspectives in cystic fibrosis. Pediatr Clin North Am 26:606, 1979.

Hoffman RD, Isenberg JN, and Powell GK: Carbohydrate malabsorption is minimal in school-age cystic fibrosis children. Dig Dis Sci 32:1071, 1987.

Hultcrantz R, Mengarelli S, and Strandvik B: Morphological findings in the liver of children with cystic fibrosis: a light and electron microscopical study.

Kelleher J: Laboratory measurement of nutrition in cystic fibrosis. J R Soc Med 80(suppl 15):25, 1987.

Levy L, Durie P, Pencharz P, and Corey M: Prognostic factors associated with patient survival during nutritional rehabilitation in malnourished children and adolescents with cystic fibrosis. J Pediatr Gastroenterol Nutr 5:97, 1986.

Littlewood JM and MacDonald A: Rationale of modern dietary recommendations in cystic fibrosis. J R Soc Med 80(suppl 15):16, 1987.

Mago H, Chen CL, Wesson DE, and Filler RM: Incisionless gastrostomy for nutritional support. J Pediatr Gastroenterol Nutr 5:66, 1986.

Mansell AL, Andersen JC, Muttort CR et al: Short-term pulmonary effects of total parenteral nutrition in children with cystic fibrosis. J Pediatr 104:700, 1984.

Martin TR: The relationship between malnutrition and lung infections. Clin Chest Med 8:359, 1987.

Mischler EH, Parrell SW, Farrell PM et al: Correction of linoleic acid deficiency in cystic fibrosis. Pediatr Res 20:36, 1986.

Neijens HJ, Duiverman EJ, Kerrebijn KF, and Sinaasappel M: Influence of respiratory exacerbations on lung function variables and nutritional status in CF patients. Acta Paediatr Scand (Suppl 317), 38, 1984.

Nielsen OH and Larsen BF: The incidence of anemia, hypoproteinemia, and edema in infants as presenting symptoms of cystic fibrosis. A retrospective survey of the frequency of this symptom complex in 130 patients with cystic fibrosis. J Pediatr Gastroenterol Nutr 1:355, 1982.

Pencharz PB: Energy intakes and low-fat diets in children with cystic fibrosis (editorial): J Pediatr Gastroenterol Nutr 2:400, 1983.

Roy CC, Darling P, and Weber AM: A rational approach to meeting macro- and micronutrient needs in cystic fibrosis. J Pediatr Gastroenterol Nutr 3(suppl 1):S154, 1984.

Shepherd RW, Holt TL, Thomas BJ et al: Nutritional rehabilitation in cystic fibrosis: controlled studies of effects on nutritional growth retardation, body protein turnover, and course of pulmonary disease. J Pediatr 109:788, 1986.

Thompson GN: Determinants of serum vitamin D levels in preadolescent cystic fibrosis children. Acta Paediatr Scand 76:962, 1987.

Vaisman N, Pencharz PB, Corey M et al: Energy expenditure of patients with cystic fibrosis. J Pediatr 111:496, 1987.

Vichinsky EP, Pennathur-Das R, Nickerson B et al: Inadequate erythroid response to hypoxia in cystic fibrosis. J Pediatr 105:15, 1984.

Weber AM and Roy CC: Intraduodenal events in cystic fibrosis. J Pediatr Gastroenterol Nutr 3(suppl 1):S113, 1984.

Weizman Z, Durie PR, Kopelman HR et al: Bile acid secretion in cystic fibrosis: evidence for a defect unrelated to fat malabsorption. Gut 27:1043, 1986.

Youngberg CA et al: Comparison of gastrointestinal pH in cystic fibrosis and healthy subjects. Dig Dis Sci 32:472, 1987.

Hepatobiliary

Abramson SJ, Baker DH, and Berdon WE: Gastrointestinal manifestations of cystic fibrosis. Semin Roentgenol 22:97, 1987.

Gaskin KJ, Waters DLM, Howman-Giles R et al: Liver disease and common-bile-duct stenosis in cystic fibrosis. N Engl J Med 318:340, 1988.

Hultcrantz R, Mengarelli S, and Strandvik B: Morphological findings in the liver of children with cystic fibrosis: a light and electron microscopical study. Hepatology 6:881, 1986.

Park RW and Grand RJ: Gastrointestinal manifestations of cystic fibrosis: a review. Gastroenterology 81:1143, 1981.

Roy CC, Weber AM, Morin CL et al: Hepatobiliary disease in cystic fibrosis: a survey of current issues and concepts. J Pediatr Gastroenterol Nutr 1:469, 1982.

Stern RC, Rothstein FC, and Doershuk CF: Treatment and prognosis of symptomatic gallbladder disease in patients with cystic fibrosis. J Pediatr Gastroenterol Nutr 5:35, 1986.

Tanner MS: Current clinical management of hepatic problems in cystic fibrosis. J R Soc Med 79(suppl 12):38, 1986.

Valman H, France N, and Wallis P: Prolonged neonatal jaundice in cystic fibrosis. Arch Dis Child 46:809, 1971.

Fertility

Fitzpatrick SB, Stokes DC, Rosenstein BJ et al: Use of oral contraceptives in women with cystic fibrosis. Chest 86:863, 1984.

Landon CL and Rosenfeld RG: Short stature and pubertal delay in male adolescents with cystic fibrosis. Am J Dis Child 138:388, 1984.

Matson JA and Capen CV: Pregnancy in the cystic fibrosis patient. J Reprod Med 26:373, 1982.

Moshang T and Holsclaw SS: Menarchal determinants in cystic fibrosis. Am J Dis Child 134:1139, 1980.

Palmer J, Dillon-Baker C, Tecklin JS et al: Pregnancy in patients with cystic fibrosis. Ann Intern Med 99:596, 1983.

Taussig LM, Lobeck CC, Di Sant'Agnese PA et al: Fertility in males with cystic fibrosis. N Engl J Med 287:587, 1972.

Future Considerations

Alton E et al: Absence of electrochemical defect of cystic fibrosis in transplanted lung. Lancet 1(8540):1026, 1987.

Reitz BA: Heart-lung transplantation. Chest 93:451, 1988.

48

LAURA S. INSELMAN, M.D., and
EDWIN L. KENDIG, JR., M.D.

TUBERCULOSIS

From the beginning of history, tuberculosis has created a major health problem throughout the civilized world. This disease has been a serious and constant threat, and, although great strides toward its eradication have been made in many countries, it is still largely uncontrolled in other areas.

Significant progress toward the control of tuberculosis has been made in the United States, but the disease has not been eradicated. In 1986, for example, 22,768 cases of tuberculosis were reported to the Centers for Disease Control (CDC, 1987). This figure represents an increase of 567 cases (3 per cent) over the 1985 total and is a distinct departure from the previously downward trend. Although the number decreased somewhat, by 251 (1.1 per cent) in 1987 and by 332 (1.5 per cent) in 1988, more than 9000 new cases of tuberculosis occurred between 1985 and 1987 (Rieder, 1989). In addition, the proportion of extrapulmonary tuberculosis increased, from 16.1 per cent in 1983 to 18 per cent in 1987 (CDC, 1989a). Although the number of cases of tuberculosis in children younger than 15 years of age decreased slightly, from 1261 in 1985 to 1177 in 1987, the number of new cases in children 5 to 14 years of age increased by approximately 7 per cent during the 3 years (CDC, 1989a; Rieder, 1989). In addition, the increase in new cases in adults is of concern because it represents a source of infection for children.

That tuberculosis can ever be controlled solely by antimicrobial agents seems extremely doubtful. Certainly this control cannot be accomplished with the drugs now available. The present approach must still be aimed at early diagnosis, isolation of infected individuals, and judicious use of available antituberculous drugs and bacille Calmette-Guérin (BCG) vaccine.

To achieve almost complete eradication of tuberculosis nationally, the Advisory Committee for the Elimination of Tuberculosis (ACET) was established in 1987 by the Department of Health and Human Services. The primary goal of the ACET is to virtually eradicate tuberculosis with the aim of decreasing the 1987 case rate from 9.3 cases per 100,000 population to 3.5 cases per 100,000 population by the year 2000 and 0.1 case per 100,000 population by the year 2010 (CDC, 1989b). Attainment of this goal is anticipated

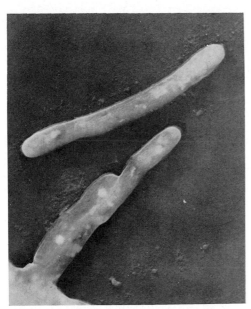

Figure 48–1. Virulent tubercle bacilli (H 37 Rv × 38,000). (From NTA Bulletin, June 1961. Courtesy of the American Lung Association, 1740 Broadway, New York, NY 10019.)

by improved utilization of present means of treatment, control, and prevention of tuberculosis; development of new measures for diagnosis, therapy, and prevention, including drugs that are less toxic, less costly, and more effective, and new diagnostic tests to replace or supplement tuberculin skin testing; and rapid application of these new methods for clinical and epidemiologic use.

ETIOLOGY

In 1882, Koch demonstrated that *Mycobacterium tuberculosis* is the etiologic agent of tuberculosis in humans. This bacterium is a member of the family Mycobacteriaceae, the chief characteristic of which is acid-fastness, i.e., a property that may be defined as resistance to acid decoloration displayed by organisms that have been stained with aniline dyes. The lipid content of the cell wall of the mycobacterium, particularly mycolic acid, is important in this characteristic of acid-fastness. Lipids also appear to be factors in the formation of tubercles.

When examined under the oil-immersion lens of a microscope, acid-fast stained tubercle bacilli appear as slender, bright, refractile red rods, about 4.0 μ in length and 0.5 μ in width. They are slightly curved, may be of various sizes and shapes, and may appear to be beaded or segmented (Fig. 48–1).

Dried tubercle bacilli kept in the dark can survive and remain virulent for many months, but they can be killed by exposure to direct sunlight or ultraviolet rays. In a fluid suspension, they are destroyed by 1 min of boiling or by 15 to 20 min heated at 60° C (140° F). Tubercle bacilli lack chemical constituents that have a demonstrable toxic effect for tissues not sensitized to tuberculin.

EPIDEMIOLOGY

As a result of the large decrease in mortality from the disease and the closing of most sanitariums, many people now believe that tuberculosis is no longer a serious problem in the United States. This is hardly an accurate estimate of the present status of this disease. As noted previously, there are still more than 22,000 new cases of active tuberculosis reported each year, of which 5.3 per cent are in children (Rieder, 1989).

An adult, adolescent, or older child who has active pulmonary tuberculosis has a contagious disease. Spread of the infection is usually accomplished by droplets that contain viable tubercle bacilli, and household contacts, particularly children, are extremely susceptible to this danger. In developing countries, ingestion of milk containing *M. bovis* may also cause disease. In general, children with nonprogressive primary pulmonary tuberculosis should not be considered contagious.

A study at the Medical College of Virginia indicates that contact of an infant with a mother who has supposedly inactive tuberculous disease and whose sputum is negative for tubercle bacilli may not be as safe as previously expected (Kendig, 1960). Of 73 infants in this category, 38 became infected with tuberculosis, and three died with tuberculous meningitis (Table 48–1). For every case, no other tuberculous adult contact could be demonstrated. Although contact of the child with other adults in the household may not be as intimate as that with the mother, the risk does not appear inconsequential. However, the risk of tuberculous infection in the child is much lower when the tuberculous adult is receiving adequate antimicrobial therapy.

Among the more common sources of tuberculous disease in the child are older members of the family, such as grandparents, aunts, and uncles. Baby sitters, housekeepers, household servants, boarders, and frequent visitors in the home may often be the tuberculous contact. For example, careful search of family contacts, household servants, and frequent visitors to the home of a 1-year-old child with a positive reaction to a routine tuberculin skin test was not productive. However, 6 months later, the gardener, with whom the little boy often played, announced that he had been recently diagnosed with tuberculosis. The possibilities of contact with tuberculosis are numerous, and none should be overlooked.

Epidemic spread may occur in population groups largely unexposed to tuberculosis, as has been stressed by Mande and co-workers (1958), who reported 25 such epidemics in schools in France. In 1965, Lincoln reviewed reports of 84 epidemics of

Table 48–1. INFANTS BORN OF TUBERCULOUS MOTHERS WITH SUPPOSEDLY INACTIVE DISEASE

Infected	38
Noninfected	35
Total	73

tuberculosis in school children from 12 countries. The source case is usually a student or one of the school personnel, often a teacher or bus driver.

PREDISPOSING FACTORS

Most individuals infected with *M. tuberculosis* do not develop clinical disease. Some individuals have a greater resistance than others, and the resistance of a given individual may vary from time to time. Important, too, are the relative virulence of the invading organisms and the number of bacilli in the inoculum.

Chronic illness, malnutrition, and chronic fatigue can increase susceptibility to tuberculous disease. Physical trauma can result in rupture of a tuberculous focus with resultant disease in an infected individual who previously received antituberculous chemotherapy or prophylaxis. A quiescent tuberculous lesion can be activated by nontuberculous infections, such as measles, varicella, pertussis, and acquired immunodeficiency; conditions of stress created by surgery; smallpox vaccination; severe viral pulmonary infection; and adrenocorticosteroid therapy. Indeed, any acute infection or alteration in immunity, metabolism, or physiology, e.g., adolescence and pregnancy, can lower resistance. The Medical College of Virginia studies indicate, however, that measles does not exert a deleterious effect on either primary tuberculosis or such serious forms of the disease as tuberculous meningitis if the patient is receiving isoniazid therapy at the time of measles infection. Many studies have also shown that there is no deleterious effect from adrenocorticosteroid therapy if the patient is also receiving isoniazid.

HEREDITY

The higher incidence of tuberculosis in some families is usually the result of more intimate contact with the disease. However, animal studies by Lurie and co-workers (1955) indicate the importance of hereditary factors in the acquisition of tuberculosis.

AGE, RACE, AND SEX

The mortality rate from tuberculosis is elevated during infancy and again at adolescence; it is not as high during the intervening years of childhood. It is also raised in the non-Caucasian population as compared with Caucasians in the United States, but differences in racial immunity are not easily determined. It seems likely that the higher mortality rate in the nonwhite population may be largely the result of social and environmental stress and a greater opportunity for infection.

During the latter part of childhood and during adolescence, girls have a higher incidence of and mortality from tuberculosis than do boys. Except for a higher incidence of disease in older adult males, a difference between the sexes at other age levels does not occur.

DELAYED HYPERSENSITIVITY AND IMMUNITY

After tuberculous infection occurs, an incubation period of 2 to 10 weeks ensues. At the close of this period, the development of cutaneous delayed hypersensitivity is manifested by a positive reaction to the tuberculin skin test. Alteration in the host response to tubercle bacilli also occurs, with an exudation in the tuberculous lesion and a tendency for the infection to become localized. At some less definite time, immunity also develops. This immunity is relative, and the infecting organisms may be so large in number or of such virulence that this partial resistance will be overcome. However, the immunity may be sufficient to protect against the infection. The interaction between delayed hypersensitivity and immunity is complex and involves the activity of T and B lymphocytes, macrophages, and such mediators as lymphokines and prostaglandins.

PATHOGENESIS AND PATHOLOGY

Because the usual mode of tuberculous infection is by inhalation, the primary lesion occurs in the lung parenchyma in more than 95 per cent of cases. It may, of course, occur elsewhere. In a previously uninfected person, the primary lesion is characterized by an accumulation of polymorphonuclear leukocytes initially and epithelioid cell proliferation with formation of the typical tubercle subsequently. Giant cells appear, and the entire area is surrounded by lymphocytes.

Concurrently with the onset of infection, tubercle bacilli are carried by macrophages from the primary focus to the regional lymph nodes. When the primary focus is in the lung parenchyma, the hilar lymph nodes are usually involved, but an apical focus may drain into the paratracheal lymph nodes.

Hypersensitivity of body tissue to tuberculin does not take place immediately but makes its appearance only after a period varying from 2 to 10 weeks. During this time, the primary focus may grow larger, but it is not encapsulated. When hypersensitivity does develop, the perifocal reaction is much more prominent, and the regional lymph nodes enlarge. The primary focus may become caseous but, with the development of acquired resistance, is usually walled off. The caseous material is gradually inspissated and later calcifies. The lesion may completely disappear.

The primary focus is usually single, but the occurrence of two or more lesions is not rare (Fig. 48–2). However, after hypersensitivity develops, the typical

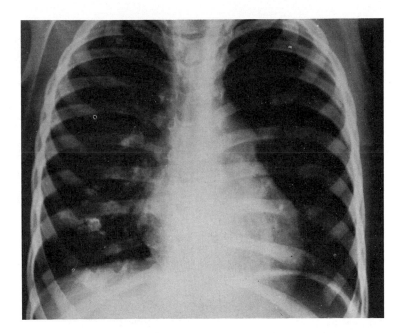

Figure 48–2. Multiple calcified primary foci.

primary complex (parenchymal focus and regional gland involvement) does not occur.

Although the usual tendency in primary pulmonary tuberculosis is toward healing, there may be progression of the primary parenchymal focus. The lesion then continues to enlarge, pneumonitis develops in the surrounding tissue, and overlying pleura may be thickened. Under these conditions, the caseous center may liquefy and empty into one or more bronchi, thereby resulting in a residual cavity and new areas of tuberculous pneumonia, i.e., cavitating primary tuberculosis.

It is during the stage of caseation that acute hematogenous dissemination is most likely to occur. This dissemination may result in widespread miliary lesions in viscera or in isolated foci in lung, bone, eye, brain, kidney, liver, and spleen. Although isolated foci may occur under these conditions, they are more apt to result from the few tubercle bacilli that may reach the blood stream before hypersensitivity develops. This bacillemia may occur directly or through the regional lymph nodes and thoracic duct.

As a rule, progression of the metastatic lesions occurs as a result of seeding from the blood stream. This seeding may be direct, as in miliary or renal tuberculosis, or by contiguity, as in late progression from a previous hematogenous seeding. For example, Rich and McCordock (1933) have demonstrated that tuberculous meningitis is more likely to result from a tuberculoma contiguous to the meninges.

The involved regional lymph nodes also have a tendency to heal but to a lesser extent than does the primary parenchymal focus. Tubercle bacilli may persist for years in the lymph nodes, even though demonstrable areas of calcification in the lymph nodes indicate that at least partial healing has occurred.

As a result of their location, tuberculous hilar lymph nodes, which are hyperemic and edematous, may cause considerable pathologic change, primarily of an obstructive nature. The nodes may encroach on the bronchi, causing occlusion of the airway lumen with resultant atelectasis of the lung distal to the obstruction. Or, more often, a caseous node or mass of nodes may attach to a wall of a bronchus by inflammatory reaction. Infection may progress through the wall and create a fistulous tract. Disease may thus be transmitted through the bronchus to the lung parenchyma. Similarly, too, extrusion of caseous contents from an affected node into a bronchus may produce complete obstruction, with atelectasis of the distal lung parenchyma. A lesion thus created is often a combination of atelectasis and pneumonia, however, and not atelectasis alone. In addition, tuberculous lymph nodes may occasionally invade or compress adjacent structures.

When obstruction of a bronchus is incomplete, a check-valve type of mechanism may result, with air trapping and hyperaeration. Obstruction of part of the wall of a bronchus may lead to a fibrous stricture, with diminished ventilation to that portion of lung distal to the obstruction.

Most complications of primary tuberculosis occur during the first year following the onset of infection. After this time, complications are relatively infrequent until adolescence when pulmonary "adult," or "reinfection," tuberculosis develops and can result in severe disease. Reinfection, or reactivation, pulmonary tuberculosis is twice as frequent in girls as in boys. In Hsu's (1974, 1984) report of 1882 children with tuberculous infection who were given isoniazid chemoprophylaxis, pulmonary tuberculosis developed in only eight cases, and there were no deaths. These results are in marked contrast with two previous studies that were done (Brailey, 1944; Lincoln, 1950) before the availability of isoniazid. Lincoln noted reactivation of pulmonary tuberculosis in 8 per cent of her cases, with a 23.9-per cent mortality rate. Brailey observed a mortality rate of 8.4 per cent in white children and 16 per cent in black children.

It can rarely be determined whether the chronic pulmonary tuberculosis that appears years after primary tuberculosis has healed is the result of activation of a healed primary lesion (endogenous) or the development of an exogenous infection. The presence of increased resistance toward a new infection that follows the primary infection would seem to favor the endogenous cause theory.

DIAGNOSIS

THE TUBERCULIN SKIN TEST

A positive reaction to the tuberculin skin test indicates the presence of tuberculous infection, and the test is, therefore, of great aid in the diagnosis of the disease. Further evaluation, including physical examination and radiographic and laboratory studies, must be performed to determine the presence of disease. The degree of activity, if any, or the severity of the disease process cannot be determined by the size or type of reaction (e.g., induration, vesiculation) of the skin test.

The tuberculin solution utilized in skin testing is available in two forms, purified protein derivative (PPD) and old tuberculin (OT) solution. The PPD is recommended because of its increased specificity and lower cost. It is the protein of the tubercle bacillus obtained from filtrates of heat-killed cultures of tubercle bacilli that have been grown on a synthetic medium and then have been precipitated either by trichloroacetic acid or, in the United States, by neutral ammonium sulfate. The World Health Organization has designated one large batch of PPD (No. 49608, manufactured by Dr. Florence Seibert in 1939) as the international standard tuberculin (PPD-S). PPD is available commercially. When diluted in a buffered diluent, tuberculoprotein is adsorbed in varying amounts by glass and plastics, and a small amount of polysorbate (i.e., Tween 80 at 5 ppm) is added to reduce this adsorption.* To minimize reduction in potency by adsorption, tuberculin should never be transferred from one container to another, and skin tests should be administered immediately after the syringe has been filled.

Unlike PPD, the older OT solution varies somewhat in potency in different batches and is therefore not standardized for administration and interpretation. When refrigerated, OT solution is stable for skin testing for 2 to 4 weeks. OT is no longer available for Mantoux testing but is present in multiple-punc-

*Polysorbate-containing tuberculins are now marketed as Aplisol, 5 international tuberculin units (5 TU) in 10-dose vials (Parke-Davis), and as Tubersol, 5 TU in 10-dose and 50-dose vials and 1 TU and 250 TU in 10-dose vials (Connaught Laboratories). Polysorbate-containing PPD is stable for up to 12 months when refrigerated between 34° F and 46° F in the original container (Connaught Laboratories).

ture tests. Bioequivalency for PPD and OT is as follows: 5 tuberculin units = 0.0001 mg PPD = 0.05 mg OT.

Mantoux (Intracutaneous) Test (Figs. 48–3 and 48–4). A measured amount of tuberculin solution of known concentration is injected intracutaneously. A syringe graduated so that fractional parts of a milliliter may be measured and a short-bevel 26- or 27-gauge needle should be used. Tuberculin is thermostable and can remain on syringes and glassware after ordinary cleansing methods. A syringe for tuberculin testing, therefore, should not be utilized for other skin tests. A separate needle is used for each patient. If the needle and the syringe are not disposable, they should be sterilized by autoclaving or boiling for 30 min.

The testing material (0.1 ml) is injected into the skin on the volar surface of the forearm. If a definite wheal is not present following the injection, a false-negative reaction may result, particularly if the material is injected subcutaneously or if leakage occurs at the site.

The test reaction is interpreted 48 to 72 hours later, and the area of induration is measured at its greatest transverse diameter. Induration less than 5 mm in diameter constitutes a negative reaction. An area of induration measuring at least 10 mm in diameter is considered a positive reaction (Figs. 48–5 and 48–6). If the area of induration measures between 5 and 9 mm in diameter, the reaction is considered doubtful and the patient should be retested. Such a reaction can be considered positive if the child has had intimate contact with active tuberculosis or if the child has signs and symptoms suggestive of tuberculosis.

A doubtful skin test reaction should be repeated with the same dose of tuberculin. If the same degree of reaction occurs, simultaneous testing with 5 TU PPD and the antigens of the nontuberculous mycobacteria (NTM) should be performed to evaluate for

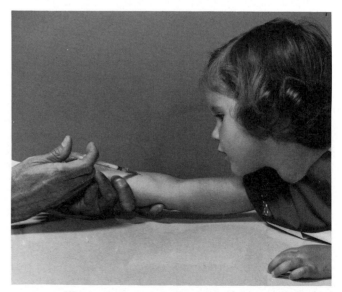

Figure 48–3. Application of the Mantoux test.

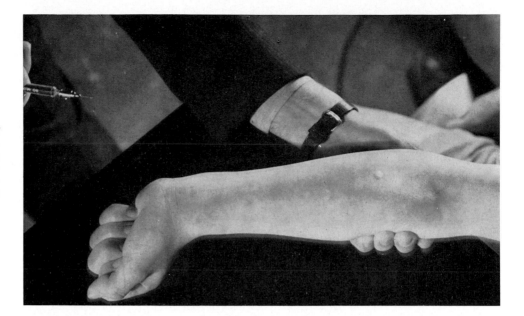

Figure 48–4. Demonstration of the wheal produced by an intracutaneous injection of tuberculin solution (Mantoux test). (Courtesy of the American Lung Association, 1740 Broadway, New York, NY 10019.)

the presence of a heterologous reaction. The NTM antigens are currently not standardized for bioequivalence and are available only for epidemiologic and research purposes from the Centers for Disease Control (Mycobacteriology Branch, Bacteriology Division, U.S. Public Health Service, Atlanta, Georgia). The PPD Battey (PPD-B), prepared from a NTM Group III strain, exhibits high cross-reactivity (low specificity) and is, therefore, recommended as the companion for PPD tuberculin in comparative skin testing. Such tests often result in induration to a tuberculin antigen of 5 to 9 mm in diameter and to a NTM antigen of 15 to 20 mm in diameter. This result suggests that cross-reactivity between tuberculopro-

tein and NTM antigens is present and that the doubtful tuberculin skin test response may be a result of infection by NTM.

The Mantoux test may produce a severe local reaction, including erythema, vesiculation, or ulceration at the site of the injection in individuals with a high degree of sensitivity to tuberculin. Lymphangitis, regional lymphadenopathy, phlyctenular conjunctivitis, and a constitutional reaction with fever may also ensue, although these are unusual occurrences. In an individual known to be sensitive to tuberculin who requires skin testing, 1 TU PPD (first strength) may be utilized, although this dose and its skin test interpretation are not standardized. How-

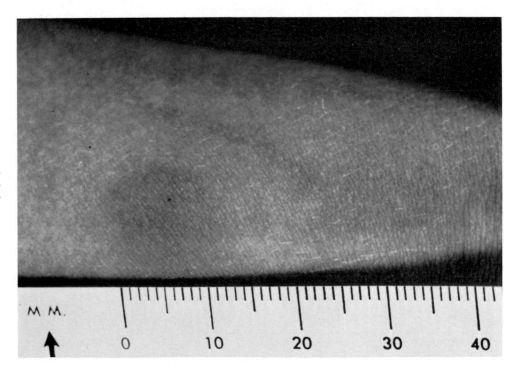

Figure 48–5. A positive reaction to the Mantoux test, measuring 10 mm in diameter of induration.

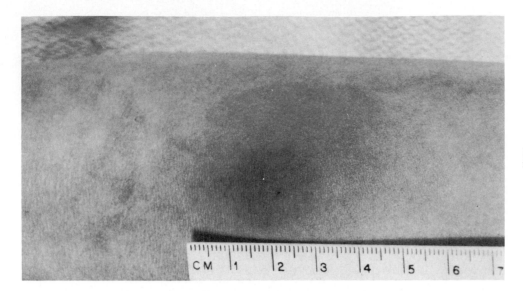

Figure 48–6. Reaction to the Mantoux test measuring 56 mm in diameter of induration.

ever, administration of the higher, intermediate strength PPD may result in augmentation of the sensitivity, with resultant phylctenular conjunctivitis or erythema nodosum.

Skin testing with 5 TU PPD presumably detects almost all individuals infected with tuberculosis. Nonspecific reactions may occur when the amount of tuberculin is increased.

Other tuberculin skin tests, such as Mono-Vacc, Heaf, tine, Aplitest, and Sclavotest, are screening tests that can be utilized for analyzing large segments of the population for tuberculous infection. They use either a solution or a dried preparation of PPD or OT (Table 48–2). However, these multiple-puncture skin tests do not have the advantage of quantitative tuberculin testing afforded by the Mantoux test, and they are more likely to result in false-positive and false-negative reactions than is the Mantoux test. They are, therefore, not recommended for use in high-risk populations. Except for the presence of vesiculation, any induration obtained with a screening test must be verified with a Mantoux test using 5 TU PPD.

Mono-Vacc Test. For screening purposes, the Mono-Vacc test is one of the most practical tests now in use. The test utilizes a device consisting of a nine-point plastic scarifier mounted on the outer side of a ring that fits on the thumb (Fig. 48–7). A plastic tube containing OT solution is sealed around the points. The tube is removed just before application, and the tuberculin solution is squeezed onto the points. The

material is then applied by pressing the points into the skin of the forearm (see Fig. 48–7). An area of induration measuring 5 mm in diameter constitutes a positive reaction, whereas induration of 2 mm is a doubtful response. If vesiculation occurs, the reaction is positive (Fig. 48–8).

Heaf Test. Devised in England and now used rarely in the United States, the Heaf test utilizes a Heaf gun, which makes six simultaneous skin punctures 1 mm deep through a layer of concentrated PPD (100,000 TU/ml) (Fig. 48–9). The reaction is read 3 to 7 days later, and the presence of four or more papules constitutes a positive reaction (Fig. 48–10). The Heaf gun, with disposable needle cartridges (Fig. 48–11), is available as Imotest-tuberculin from Servier Laboratories, in Great Britain.*

Tine Test. The tine test employs a sterilized disposable unit consisting of four tines that have been predipped in an OT concentrate, four times the standard strength of OT, or in PPD (Fig. 48–12). The apparatus is pressed firmly against the skin, held there for approximately 5 sec, and then released. In a strongly positive reaction, a rosette consisting of four confluent areas of induration may result (Fig. 48–13). Fusion of at least two papules is necessary for the reaction to be considered positive.

Studies by Lunn and associates have raised a question as to the accuracy of the tine test (Lunn and Johnson, 1978; Lunn, 1980). Experience both at the Medical College of Virginia and by Rudd (1982) suggests that careful application of the test is mandatory.

Aplitest. As a modification of the tuberculin tine test, the Aplitest uses PPD instead of OT on the tines. The result is interpreted in the same way as that for the tine test.

Sclavotest. This test also utilizes a modification of the tine test with PPD on the prongs, and its interpretation is similar to that of the tine test.

Table 48–2. TYPES OF MULTIPLE-PUNCTURE TUBERCULIN SKIN TESTS

Test	Preparation and Equipment
Mono-Vacc Test	OT, solution, prongs
Heaf Test	PPD, solution, Heaf gun
Tine Test	PPD, solution; OT, dried; prongs
Aplitest	PPD, dried, prongs
Sclavotest	PPD, dried, prongs

OT, old tuberculin; PPD, purified protein derivative.

*Servier Laboratories, Ltd, Fulmer House, Windmill Road, Fulmer, Nr., Slough. Bucks, SL3 6HH, England.

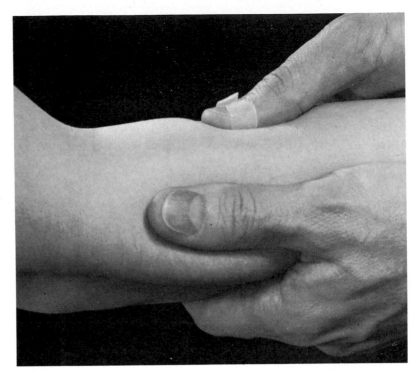

Figure 48–7. Application of the Mono-Vacc test. (Courtesy of Lincoln Laboratories, Inc, Decatur, Ill 62526.)

False-Positive Reactions

False-positive tuberculin skin test reactions may occur. As noted previously, 5 to 9 mm of induration following a 5 TU PPD may reflect infection with NTM and may be a false-positive reaction. This is particularly likely to occur in certain areas of the United States, such as Virginia, where infection with NTM is prevalent.

Other causes of false-positive tuberculin reactions include sensitivity to the preservative used with PPD or OT, resulting in transient erythema that subsides by 24 to 48 hours after application of the test; incorrect administration of the test; incorrect inter-pretation of the test result; and differing potency of tuberculin on the prongs. Previous vaccination with BCG vaccine may also result in a false-positive Mantoux tuberculin skin test reaction. However, experience at the Medical College of Virginia suggests that BCG vaccination performed with the vaccine manufactured by Organon Teknika rarely results in a

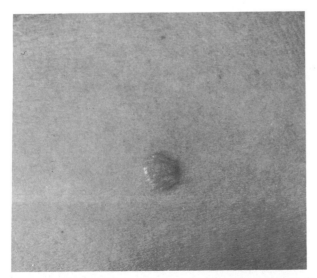

Figure 48–8. A positive reaction to the Mono-Vacc test (× 4). (Courtesy of Lincoln Laboratories, Inc, Decatur, Ill 62526.)

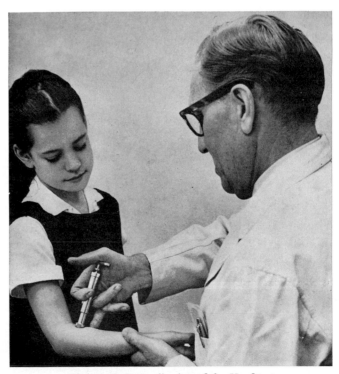

Figure 48–9. Application of the Heaf test.

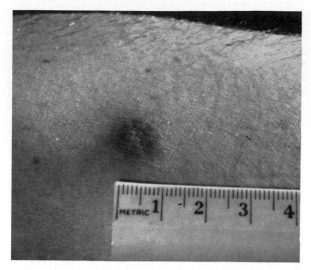

Figure 48–10. Strongly positive (4+) reaction to the Heaf test.

tuberculin skin test reaction measuring more than 10 mm in diameter of induration (Fig. 48–14).*

False-Negative Reactions

False-negative tuberculin skin test reactions may occur during the 2- to 10-week time interval between the initial infection and the development of cutaneous delayed hypersensitivity. A child who is known to have been exposed to a tuberculous adult should not be considered free of infection until a negative tuberculin reaction has been documented at least 10 weeks after contact with the tuberculous adult has ceased.

False-negative tuberculin skin test reactions may also occur with severe systemic tuberculosis, such as

*Organon Teknika, Chicago, Ill.

meningitis or miliary disease; anergy; immunodeficiency; immunosuppression; malnutrition; certain illnesses, such as measles, rubella, mumps, varicella, influenza, infectious mononucleosis, human immunodeficiency viral infection, *Mycoplasma pneumoniae* infection, and sarcoidosis; following the recent administration of live viral vaccine; and adrenocorticosteroid therapy. The tuberculin skin test reaction may be depressed for a month or more following measles or measles vaccination and 1 to 3 weeks following severe rubella infection.

False-negative reactions related to the tuberculin itself may occur. In addition to improper dilutions, bacterial contamination, and exposure to heat or light, adsorption of tuberculoprotein to container walls may be present. It has been demonstrated that 25 per cent of tuberculin in solution is lost 20 min after the syringe has been filled and that 80 per cent is lost by 24 hours. The addition of Tween 80, a surface-active agent, minimizes this adsorption. Incorrect administration and interpretation of the test and differing potency or loss of potency of tuberculin on the prongs can also result in false-negative reactions.

Reading of the tuberculin reaction by parents may be a major cause of inaccurate interpretation. It is strongly advised that all tuberculin skin test reactions be read by a physician or someone with expertise in that area.

Timing of Tests

A routine tuberculin skin test should be administered in children between 12 and 15 months of age, before entry into school, and during adolescence (AAP, 1988). Testing before attendance at summer camp and boarding school may also be useful. An annual skin test is recommended in subpopulations

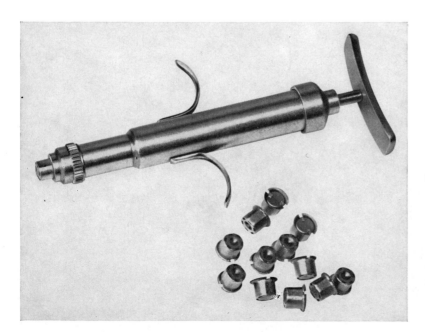

Figure 48–11. The Heaf gun with disposable cartridges.

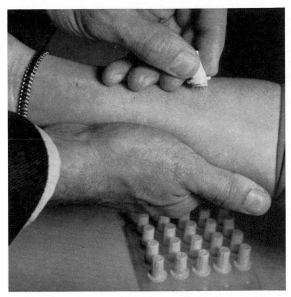

Figure 48–12. Application of the tine test. (Courtesy of Lederle Laboratories, A Division of American Cyanamid Co, Princeton, NJ 08540.)

with high case rates of tuberculosis. A test is, of course, always indicated when there has been known contact with a tuberculous adult. In the latter instance, if the tuberculin skin test reaction is initially negative, the test should be repeated 10 weeks after removal of the tuberculous contact. If the child remains in contact with a tuberculous adult, the tuberculin skin test should be repeated at 3-month intervals.

HISTORY AND PHYSICAL EXAMINATION

In general, tuberculosis in children occurs with minimal or no clinical manifestations, unlike the disease in adults. The classic signs and symptoms of fever, anorexia, malaise, weight loss, failure to thrive,

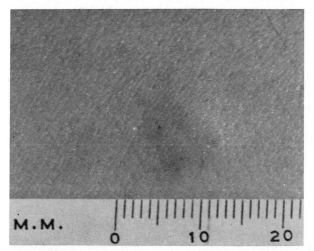

Figure 48–13. A positive reaction to the tine test, with four confluent areas of induration. (Courtesy of Lederle Laboratories, A Division of American Cyanamid Co, Princeton, NJ 08540.)

and cough are frequently absent, particularly in the very young child. Children younger than 10 years of age usually do not have a sufficiently strong cough for sputum production. The only initial indication of tuberculosis in a child may be a positive tuberculin skin test reaction. Therefore, tuberculin skin testing should always be performed in a child with a history of contact with an adult with tuberculosis and in certain conditions (e.g., human immunodeficiency viral infection, corticosteroid therapy) that may predispose the child to the acquisition and development of tuberculosis.

Reviews of 200 children with tuberculous infection at the Medical College of Virginia and of 64 children in an inner city community in New York (Inselman et al, 1981) indicate manifestations of infection ranging from a positive tuberculin skin test reaction without other demonstrable evidence of disease to widespread pulmonary and extrapulmonary tuberculosis. Many children did not exhibit a single symptom or sign that could be associated with any disease process. All cases were diagnosed because a tuberculin skin test was performed routinely or because of known contact with tuberculosis.

Even in progressive tuberculous disease, signs and symptoms may not be as helpful as might be expected. A 3-year-old girl referred to the Medical College of Virginia Hospital with a diagnosis of pulmonary tuberculosis had no history of contact with tuberculosis. Her only symptoms were questionable failure to gain weight during the preceding year and a tendency to cough with exercise. Although the results of her physical examination were unremarkable, a chest roentgenogram indicated atelectasis of the right upper lobe, a thin-walled cavity in the right lower lobe, and miliary tuberculosis (Fig. 48–15).

Although the tuberculin skin test is by far the most useful diagnostic tool, other findings on physical examination may indicate the presence of tuberculosis. These include persistent fever; wheezing; cough; stridor; rales; rhonchi; hepatosplenomegaly; bone tenderness; decreased mobility of an extremity or joint; choroidal tubercles; phlyctenular conjunctivitis; erythema nodosum; lupus vulgaris; cutaneous tuberculids, which represent a hypersensitivity reaction; and cutaneous lesions of acute miliary tuberculosis. The tuberculids and cutaneous miliary lesions have been described in the newborn and are discrete erythematous papules with necrotic or crusted centers (McCray, 1981).

ROENTGENOGRAPHIC EXAMINATION

Once infection with tuberculosis has been established with a positive tuberculin skin test reaction, further procedures must be performed in order to determine the location and degree of severity of the infection. Because more than 95 per cent of primary tuberculous infections occur in the lung parenchyma, a chest roentgenogram, including both anteroposte-

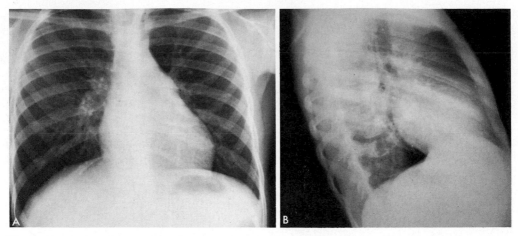

Figure 48–14. A patient vaccinated with BCG (bacillus Calmette-Guérin) in whom tuberculous infection developed later. Roentgenograms show multiple hilar calcifications. Tuberculin reaction (PPD 5TU) measured 12 mm in diameter of induration 3 months after BCG vaccination. At the time of subsequent testing, 3 years later, tuberculin reaction was 52 mm. Roentgenograms taken at that time (A and B) indicate the presence of healed primary tuberculosis. There had been no clinical evidence of the disease.

rior and lateral views, is always indicated (Fig. 48–16).

The primary complex is more likely to be seen on a roentgenogram in infants and small children than in older patients. The complex consists of the primary parenchymal focus, the infected regional lymph nodes, and the connecting lymphatics and occurs following the conversion of a Mantoux tuberculin test from a negative to a positive reaction. The primary parenchymal focus is usually small in comparison with the involved lymph nodes and is frequently not demonstrable on a roentgenogram.

Care should be exercised in positioning the patient for a roentgenogram, as relatively minor rotations of the body can result in distortion of the hilar and mediastinal areas. Hair braids and radiopaque objects, such as necklaces and identification tags, should be removed from the field of view prior to obtaining the roentgenogram.

Films should be obtained during maximal inspiration if possible. Mediastinal widening, an increase in the transverse cardiac diameter, and prominence of pulmonary vasculature will occur during expiration (Fig. 48–17). The diaphragm should be at least as

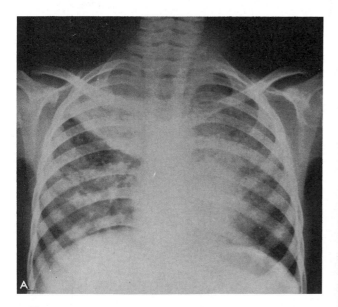

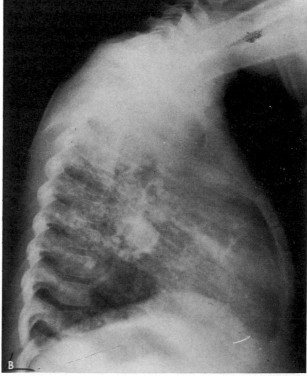

Figure 48–15. Negative findings during a physical examination in a child with atelectasis of the right upper lobe, cavity in the right lower lobe, and miliary tuberculosis. (Reproduced with permission from Kendig EL Jr: Early diagnosis of tuberculosis in childhood. Am J Dis Child 92:558. Copyright 1956, American Medical Association.)

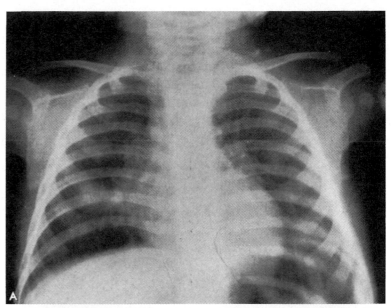

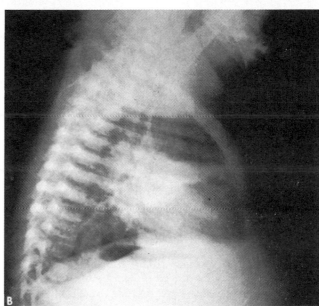

Figure 48–16. Roentgenograms showing the value of a lateral view. Extensive infiltration and hilar adenopathy in the lateral view (primary pulmonary tuberculosis). (See also Fig. 48–21.)

low as the eighth rib posteriorly, even in the smallest infant.

Oblique views of the chest aid in identification of abnormalities in the mediastinum. Apical lordotic films detect lesions in the lung apices. Anteroposterior and lateral films and ultrasonograms may indicate the presence of a pleural effusion. Lateral decubitus views help to determine if an effusion is freely moving or loculated.

RECOVERY OF TUBERCLE BACILLI

While the diagnosis of active tuberculosis is mainly bacteriologic in adults, it is usually epidemiologic and, therefore, indirect in children (Starke, 1988). The diagnosis is established with certainty by the finding of tubercle bacilli in culture, in acid-fast stains, or in both from such specimens as respiratory secretions; sputum; pleural, bronchoalveolar lavage, cerebrospinal, and peritoneal fluids; gastric washings; abscesses; and biopsy material, including lymph nodes, pleura, bone, bone marrow, and liver.

In infants and children, organisms reaching the oropharynx from lung lesions are promptly swallowed. Therefore, examination and culture of gastric contents provide a useful way to detect the presence of tuberculosis. Since the number of tubercle bacilli and the frequency of positive cultures in specimens recovered by gastric lavage are usually small, it is recommended that this procedure be performed on 3 successive days. At the Medical College of Virginia, single gastric cultures of a child with a positive tuberculin skin test reaction and little or no roentgenographic evidence of disease are productive of tubercle bacilli in only about 6 per cent of cases. This number increases when daily culture specimens are obtained and is more than 50 per cent when extensive pulmonary disease is evident roentgenographically.

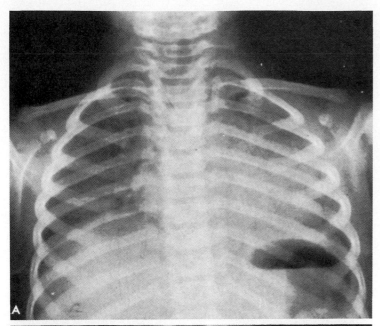

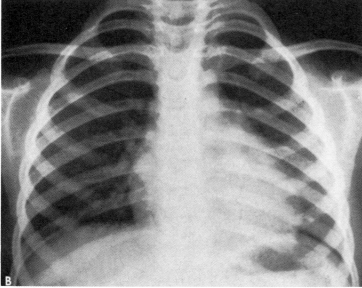

Figure 48–17. Films showing the value of proper technique. The first film (A) was taken during the expiratory phase and the second (B), in the same patient a few minutes later, during the inspiratory phase.

Although the low frequency of positive results of gastric culture in certain situations lessens the value of the procedure as a diagnostic aid, gastric cultures may still be helpful in the diagnosis.

Gastric lavage should be performed early in the morning following an overnight fast. The contents of the stomach are aspirated and placed in a sterile container. The stomach is then irrigated with 20 to 60 ml of sterile water, depending on the size of the child. The gastric washings are aspirated and added to the material in the container. Only sterile water is used because NTM may be present in tap water in certain areas of the United States. Instead of gastric lavage, adolescents may prefer aerosol inhalation to stimulate cough and sputum production, as is now used in adult patients.

The Ziehl-Neelsen, Kinyoun, and fluorescence techniques are different types of acid-fast stains, which can be utilized to identify the tubercle bacillus.

Available culture media include Löwenstein-Jensen, Middlebrook, and BACTEC. The BACTEC system yields culture and susceptibility results within 7 to 10 days. In addition, the presence of caseation necrosis and granulomas in histologic examination of aspirates or biopsy material helps in the diagnosis. Other laboratory studies that may also be helpful in the diagnosis of tuberculosis include the use of DNA probes for *M. tuberculosis*, ELISA testing for antibody in serum or bronchial washings to tubercle bacillus antigens, and radioactively labeled gallium lung scans. The last two techniques may be particularly helpful when culture findings are negative.

BRONCHOSCOPY

Bronchoscopy is indicated in many patients whose roentgenograms show an area of increased density suggestive of segmental obstruction and atelectasis. Bronchoscopy may assist in removing an intrinsic airway obstruction and obtaining secretions for stains and cultures. All personnel performing the procedure should be experienced in the management of children, and satisfactory hospital arrangements should be provided.

PULMONARY FUNCTION TESTS

Although the majority of children with treated pulmonary tuberculosis do not have residual impairment of lung function, pulmonary function tests may be of help in assessing possible risks and benefits of surgery. Severe chronic pulmonary tuberculosis may result in restrictive lung disease and a diminished diffusing capacity. Acute miliary tuberculosis is frequently accompanied by hypoxemia and widening of the alveolar-arterial oxygen gradient.

PRESENTATION OF TUBERCULOSIS

After tuberculous infection has occurred, an incubation period of 2 to 10 weeks ensues, when tubercle bacilli are conveyed from the portal of entry (lung, gastrointestinal tract, skin) by way of the lymphatics to the regional lymph nodes. The lymph nodes become hyperemic and edematous and may later contain areas of caseation. In more than 95 per cent of cases, the portal of entry is the lung and the primary focus is in the lung parenchyma.

At the close of this incubation period, cutaneous delayed hypersensitivity appears, as manifested by a positive tuberculin skin test reaction. At this time, the patient has primary pulmonary tuberculosis. There are few, if any, symptoms, and the diagnosis is usually made by means of a tuberculin skin test performed routinely or because of known contact with tuberculosis.

Approximately three fourths of children with tuberculous infection have normal chest roentgenograms and no physical or laboratory evidence of tuberculous disease (Inselman, 1981). The positive reaction to the tuberculin skin test is the only clue to the presence of tuberculous infection. An additional 18 per cent have roentgenographic evidence of disease (Inselman, 1981), usually with no demonstrable primary parenchymal focus but with an area of increased density in the region of the hilus, which is caused by edematous lymph nodes. Roentgenographic evidence of a primary parenchymal focus with enlarged regional lymph nodes occurs much less often.

Occasionally, the primary lesion is not in the lung parenchyma, and physical and laboratory examination may reveal evidence of tuberculous disease elsewhere. However, manifestations of pulmonary tuberculosis are often present on chest roentgenograms when extrapulmonary disease occurs in children (Inselman, 1981).

Primary tuberculosis tends to heal, but the process may become progressive instead. Destruction at the initial site or erosion of a bronchus with intrabronchial dissemination and metastatic pulmonary lesions can occur. If massive hematogenous seeding develops, widespread formation of tubercles will ensue. With these processes, the patient usually demonstrates symptomatic evidence of worsening of the disease.

Toward the end of the incubation period, a transient bacillemia usually occurs. This may result in formation of tuberculous foci throughout the body, which then remain quiescent for many years. The heaviest distribution of hematogenous seeding is likely to be in the lung, but any organ may be involved. Most of the complications that result later from organisms in these foci are not immediately blood borne. For example, tuberculous meningitis is likely to result from the breakdown of a contiguous tuberculoma, which was previously seeded hematogenously.

MANAGEMENT OF TUBERCULOSIS

The management of tuberculosis includes early diagnosis, isolation of contagious individuals, utilization of antituberculous drugs, and judicious use of BCG vaccination.

An optimum therapeutic result can be achieved only when the diagnosis is established early. Since little reliance can be placed on the basis of symptoms, a tuberculin skin test is necessary to establish the early diagnosis of tuberculosis in childhood. An intracutaneous Mantoux tuberculin test utilizing 5 TU PPD or a multiple-puncture tuberculin screening test should be performed on all children between 12 and 15 months of age, before school entry, and during adolescence. An annual skin test is recommended in subpopulations with high rates of tuberculosis (AAP, 1988). The tuberculin skin test, if properly performed, measured, and recorded, is the major diagnostic tool for the recognition and control of tuberculosis. As indicated earlier, the tuberculin test is, of course, always indicated when there has been known contact with a tuberculous adult. If the tuberculin skin test reaction is initially negative, the test should be repeated 10 weeks following removal of the tuberculous contact. If the child remains in contact with a tuberculous adult, the tuberculin skin test should be repeated at 3-month intervals.

PREVENTIVE THERAPY

When the diagnosis of tuberculosis is established, proper therapy can be promptly instituted for the patient and for the prevention of infection in those in contact with the patient. Results from the United

States Public Health Service Isoniazid Prophylaxis Study indicate that among household contacts of those with active tuberculosis, the prophylactic use of isoniazid is effective in reducing the incidence of tuberculous disease in household contacts by 66 per cent (Ferebee, 1969).

When a child has a positive tuberculin skin test reaction, location and removal of the tuberculous contact from the child must be accomplished as soon as possible. This search entails tuberculin skin tests and chest roentgenograms of all adult contacts, including parents, grandparents, baby-sitters, housekeepers, household servants, and others as applicable. Other children in the home should also have tuberculin skin testing and, if their skin tests are significant, additional studies in order to evaluate the presence of tuberculous infection or disease. Children with tuberculosis who do not produce sputum or do not have endobronchial disease or an open, draining wound are not contagious.

The child should be protected from intercurrent infection because an acute illness or alteration in physiology, immunity, or metabolism may lower resistance. The tuberculin-positive child who has measles, while not receiving antituberculous drug therapy, should be given isoniazid for 8 weeks. The tuberculin-positive child, even though previously treated, who has not had measles should receive the measles vaccine and isoniazid for 8 weeks following administration of the vaccine. Other conditions requiring isoniazid prophylaxis in a child with a positive tuberculin skin test reaction include adrenocorticosteroid therapy, surgical procedures requiring anesthesia, human immunodeficiency viral infection, pertussis, and diabetes mellitus.

In addition, a child exposed to active tuberculosis in the home should receive isoniazid prophylaxis for at least 3 months even if the initial tuberculin skin test reaction is negative. Isoniazid is prescribed because the child may be infected but the tuberculin skin test reaction may not yet have converted. If a repeat tuberculin skin test reaction 3 months later is negative, isoniazid may be discontinued if exposure to active tuberculosis is no longer present. However, if the initial or repeat skin test reaction has 5 mm or more of induration, the child should be considered as having tuberculous infection or disease and should be evaluated and treated accordingly.

Chest roentgenograms at appropriate intervals, as determined by therapy and the child's clinical status, are also necessary.

Analysis of 117 infants born to mothers who had tuberculosis within 2 years of delivery, at the time of delivery, or shortly after birth indicates that removal of the infant from contact with the mother is not always sufficient to prevent later infection in the infant (Kendig, 1960). Even though 73 of these infants were isolated from their respective tuberculous mothers until the mothers' sputum test results were negative, more than one half of these infants became infected with tuberculosis when returned to the home environment. These children had not been given isoniazid prophylaxis or BCG vaccine. It is advised that infants born to mothers with active tuberculosis begin isoniazid prophylaxis immediately in order to prevent infection even if their initial evaluation does not indicate the presence of tuberculous infection or disease. (See "Tuberculosis in the Newborn.")

GENERAL THERAPY

An adequate diet and the usual vitamin supplements for a growing child are necessary, but the advisability of bed rest varies with the type of disease. Children with asymptomatic primary tuberculosis require no limitation of activity, and even those who are acutely ill should be allowed some activity as soon as possible because complete bed rest may result in calcium and nitrogen deficiencies.

GENERAL PRINCIPLES OF ANTIMICROBIAL THERAPY

Antimicrobial therapy for tuberculosis utilizes multiple drugs, including at least one bacteriocidal agent, to destroy tubercle bacilli in both intracellular and extracellular areas. The use of multiple drugs also attempts to prevent the development of drug-resistant strains of tubercle bacilli and the complications of untreated disease.

In the longer therapeutic regimens used previously, both pulmonary and localized extrapulmonary disease were treated with two drugs, while extensive pulmonary disease (e.g., endobronchial, miliary) and systemic disease (e.g., meningitis) were treated with three drugs initially. At least one bacteriocidal drug, usually isoniazid, was always employed.

The newer, short-course regimen utilizes two bacteriocidal drugs, isoniazid and rifampin, with supplementation by pyrazinamide, ethambutol, and streptomycin. Treatment is prescribed for 6 to 9 months. The short-course regimen is as therapeutically effective as the longer regimen for pulmonary tuberculosis, at least in adults; improves patient drug compliance; increases the rate of sputum conversion (in adults); and is more cost effective. The shorter regimen should not be utilized if any of the following occurs: drug intolerance or toxicity to isoniazid or rifampin; drug-resistant tubercle bacilli; inability to eradicate tubercle bacilli in cultures after several months of therapy; absence of clinical improvement within a few months of therapy; and systemic disease, such as human immunodeficiency viral infection, immunosuppression, malignancy, and diabetes mellitus.

The dosages of the antituberculous drugs for both the short-course and longer regimens are listed in Table 48–3. Initial therapy in children should be based on the drug-sensitivity pattern of the source

Table 48–3. DOSAGES OF ANTITUBERCULOUS DRUGS USED IN TREATMENT OF CHILDREN WITH TUBERCULOSIS

Drug	Short-Course Regimen		Longer Regimen*
	*Daily**	*Intermittent*†	
Isoniazid	10–20 mg/kg) (max. 300 mg)	20–40 mg/kg (max. 900 mg)	10–20 mg/kg (max. 300 mg)
Rifampin	10–20 mg/kg (max. 600 mg)	10–20 mg/kg (max. 600 mg)	15–20 mg/kg (max. 600 mg)
Pyrazinamide	15–30 mg/kg (max. 2 g)	50–70 mg/kg	15–30 mg/kg (max. 2 g)
Ethambutol	15–25 mg/kg (max. 1500 mg)	50 mg/kg	15–25 mg/kg (max. 1500 mg)
Streptomycin	20–40 mg/kg (max. 1 g)	25–30 mg/kg	20–40 mg/kg (max. 1 g)
Para-aminosalicylic acid	—	—	200 mg/kg (max. 12 g)
Prednisone	1–2 mg/kg (max. 60 mg)	—	1–2 mg/kg (max. 60 mg)

*Dosages are per 24 hours.

†Dosages are per dose administered twice weekly. When isoniazid and rifampin are used together, the daily dosages of the 2 drugs should not exceed 10 mg/kg for isoniazid and 15 mg/kg for rifampin.

case strain and later availability of the drug-sensitivity pattern of the child's strain. If the sensitivity pattern of the source case strain is unavailable, children with life-threatening forms of tuberculosis should be treated with at least three antimicrobial agents.

There are two suggested short-course regimens (Fig. 48–18). One 9-month regimen consists of daily isoniazid and rifampin for at least 2 months, followed by isoniazid and rifampin either daily or twice weekly for the ensuing 7 months. The 6-month course includes daily isoniazid, rifampin, and pyrazinamide for at least 2 months, followed by isoniazid and rifampin for the ensuing 4 months. Intermittent therapy (twice weekly) is advised only when patient compliance can be assured. The drugs are prescribed for at least 6 months after *M. tuberculosis* no longer grows in culture. The efficacy of therapy is decreased by substitution of ethambutol or streptomycin for pyrazinamide and is not enhanced by continuation of pyrazinamide after the initial 2 months (Bass, 1986). There are currently no pharmacokinetic data for pyrazinamide in children, and until such data become available, use of the 9-month course is favored.

INH + RIF } daily for 2 mo → INH + RIF } daily or twice weekly for 7 mo

(+ EMB if isoniazid-resistance is suspected)

OR

INH + RIF + PZA } daily for 2 mo → INH + RIF } daily or twice weekly for 4 mo

(+ EMB if isoniazid-resistance is suspected)

Figure 48–18. Alternative regimens for short-course chemotherapy of pulmonary and extrapulmonary tuberculosis in children. See text for details. *INH,* isoniazid; *RIF,* rifampin; *PAZ,* pyrazinamide; *EMB,* ethambutol. Pharmacokinetic data for pyrazinamide in children are not available at present; until data are available, use of the 9-month course is favored. Daily medication is advised unless supervised.

If isoniazid resistance is suspected, ethambutol is added initially. However, if resistance to isoniazid is proved, two new drugs, which demonstrate *in vitro* inhibition of the tubercle bacilli, are added or substituted for at least 12 months, with the duration of treatment often individualized. At least one of these new drugs should be bacteriocidal.

ANTIMICROBIAL AGENTS

Isoniazid (INH), rifampin (RIF), pyrazinamide (PZA), ethambutol (EMB), and streptomycin (SM) are the antimicrobial agents of greatest efficacy in the treatment of tuberculosis in childhood. Other drugs, such as para-aminosalicylic acid (PAS), viomycin, cycloserine, ethionamide, kanamycin, and capreomycin have limited value and are employed in the treatment of tuberculosis in children only when multiply drug-resistant tubercle bacilli are present.

Isoniazid

Isoniazid is the most effective antituberculous agent known. It is also the only drug that has been shown to prevent complications of tuberculous disease. Accordingly, it should be included in every therapeutic regimen unless contraindicated because of the presence of drug intolerance, drug toxicity, or drug-resistant tubercle bacilli.

The drug is a hydrazide of isonicotinic acid, has both bacteriocidal and bacteriostatic actions to both intracellular and extracellular bacilli, penetrates the cell membrane, and moves freely into cerebrospinal fluid and caseous tissue. It probably prevents mycolic acid biosynthesis and enzyme activity in tubercle bacilli.

After oral administration, a plasma level 20 to 80 times the usual inhibiting concentration of the drug, which is 0.05 to 0.20 μg/ml, may be attained within a few hours, and effectively high concentrations persist for 6 to 8 hours. The drug may be present in the breast milk of mothers receiving isoniazid therapy and may also cross the placenta. Isoniazid is excreted primarily by the kidneys.

The principal side effects of the drug are neurotoxic, manifested as convulsions or peripheral neuritis, and probably result from competitive inhibition of pyridoxine metabolism. Although pyridoxine deficiencies may be present in young children (Pellock, 1985), adults are more likely to manifest clinical evidence of a deficiency. It is currently recommended that the drug be prescribed for adolescents taking isoniazid in dosages of pyridoxine 25 to 50 mg daily (10 mg for each 100 mg of INH). Other neurotoxic manifestations, which are infrequent, include optic neuritis, ataxia, encephalopathy, and memory loss.

Rarely, isoniazid may be hepatotoxic, but this is more likely to occur when therapy includes rifampin. Although studies appear to show that young children treated with isoniazid have little tendency toward hepatotoxicity, determination of serum bilirubin and liver aspartate aminotransaminase levels are recommended at initiation of treatment, after 8 to 12 weeks of isoniazid therapy, and when therapy is terminated. If elevation of the serum bilirubin or liver transaminase level occurs, these values are followed more closely until they return to normal. The elevated transaminase level is usually transient and decreases to a normal value despite continuation of the drug. Isoniazid is withdrawn from use if the transaminase level rises to above three times its normal value, clinical manifestations of hepatitis occur, or both. Other side effects include gastrointestinal irritation, dermatitis, drug-induced fever, arthralgia, vasculitis, agranulocytosis, anemia, thrombocytopenia, and hypersensitivity.

When phenytoin (Dilantin) is administered with isoniazid, interaction of the drugs may produce central nervous system symptoms, excessive sedation, and incoordination. Careful observation of a patient who is receiving phenytoin is indicated, and occasional reduction of the doses of both phenytoin and isoniazid may be necessary. Isoniazid also potentiates the actions of alcohol, barbiturates, and carbamazepine and decreases the action of ketoconazole. Aluminum-containing antacids decrease its absorption from the gastrointestinal tract, and its interaction with Antabuse can cause psychoses. Overdose can result in hyperglycemia, convulsions, metabolic acidosis, mydriasis, tachycardia, photophobia, urinary retention, hyperpyrexia, and coma.

The dose of isoniazid depends on the type and severity of disease, the presence of susceptible or resistant organisms, and whether the short-course or longer treatment regimen is utilized. Isoniazid is used alone for prophylaxis in the case of a positive tuberculin skin test reaction with no evidence of active primary tuberculosis, i.e., tuberculin skin test conversion. It is the only antituberculous drug that may be used alone. The other drugs, if employed alone, can result in rapid development of resistance of bacilli to them.

Although primary isoniazid-resistant tuberculosis has been reported in children, particularly in those from Southeast Asia and the Caribbean, the significance of this finding has not yet been determined. Certainly, the recommendations that initial therapy in children be based on the drug-susceptibility pattern of the source case strain (Steiner, 1974) should be heeded. Even when in vitro isoniazid resistance occurs, particularly with extrapulmonary tuberculosis, isoniazid at high doses is often included in the therapeutic regimen because high doses may overcome such resistance and because in vitro and in vivo sensitivities may differ.

Isoniazid is available for oral administration in tablets of 50 mg, 100 mg, and 300 mg and in a flavored syrup containing 10 mg/ml. Although children may not absorb the drug well when it is given with food (Notterman, 1986), most clinicians prefer the use of tablets, which can be crushed and administered in jam, preserves, or applesauce. A preparation for parenteral administration (intramuscular or intrathecal) is also available for use in severely ill patients who cannot take the oral preparations. It is administered as one dose per day. A chemical test for the presence of isoniazid in the urine may be of help in determining patient compliance (Eidus and Hamilton, 1964).

Rifampin

Rifampin is a derivative of *Streptomyces mediterranei*. The drug is bacteriocidal to intracellular and extracellular tubercle bacilli and acts by inhibition of DNA-dependent RNA polymerase. It is absorbed in all tissues but enters cerebrospinal fluid only across inflamed meninges. One hour following ingestion, a peak serum level of 8.9 to 11.5 μg/ml can be attained. Rifampin is metabolized by the liver and excreted by the kidneys and gallbladder.

Side effects include hepatotoxicity, which is more likely to occur when therapy includes isoniazid. When both isoniazid and rifampin are used concurrently, the dosages of the two drugs should not exceed 10 mg/kg/day for isoniazid and 15 mg/kg/day for rifampin (CDC, 1980c). Pre-treatment evaluation should include hematocrit, white blood cell and platelet counts, blood urea nitrogen, and serum aspartate aminotransferase and bilirubin concentrations.

Additional side effects of rifampin include gastrointestinal disturbances, dermatoses, thrombocytopenia, reversible leukopenia, anemia, cell-mediated immunosuppression, ataxia, headache, confusion, drowsiness, a reddish-orange color to body secretions (urine, saliva, tears, sweat, sputum, and stool), and a discoloration of contact lenses. Restart of rifampin therapy after a drug-free interval or intermittent rifampin therapy with high doses (more than 10 mg/kg/dose) can cause hepatorenal syndrome, autoimmune anemia, or thrombocytopenia.

The action of rifampin is potentiated with probenecid. Rifampin increases the metabolism by the liver of coumarin, quinidine, digoxin, cyclosporin, methadone, oral hypoglycemic agents, theophylline, chloramphenicol, ketoconazole, corticosteroids, and oral contraceptives, resulting in diminished serum levels and actions of these drugs. Salicylic acid delays its absorption, and its serum level is decreased by ketoconazole. Overdose can cause vomiting, headache, hepatitis, pruritus, periorbital and facial edema, angioedema, drowsiness, and a red-orange color of the skin and secretions although not of the cornea.

The dosage of rifampin is 10 to 20 mg/kg/day, maximum 600 mg/day, or 10 to 20 mg/dose, maximum 600 mg/dose, if intermittent therapy is used. It is available as 150 mg and 300 mg capsules. A rifampin liquid suspension may also be prepared. This suspension is stable for 6 weeks but must be refrigerated. Rifampin is administered as a single oral dose.

Pyrazinamide

Pyrazinamide is used in the treatment of tuberculosis as a supplemental antimicrobial agent in the short-course regimen. It is a synthetic derivative of nicotinamide; penetrates well into tissues and fluid collections, including cerebrospinal fluid; and is excreted by the kidneys. It is well absorbed from the gastrointestinal tract, achieving peak serum levels of 45 µg/ml within 2 hours after ingestion. Pyrazinamide's minimal inhibitory concentration for *M. tuberculosis* is 20 µg/ml at pH 5.5. It is bacteriocidal to intracellular tubercle bacilli only in an acid milieu. There are currently no pharmacokinetic data for pyrazinamide in children.

Adverse effects include hepatotoxicity, which is unusual even when the drug is administered with isoniazid and rifampin; dysuria; arthralgia; gastrointestinal irritation; dermatitis; and drug-induced fever. Hyperuricemia and gout can also occur as a result of inhibition of renal tubular secretion of urate.

Pyrazinamide is available as 500 mg tablets and is administered orally in 3 to 4 divided doses per day. It has no known drug interactions.

Ethambutol

Ethambutol is a bacteriostatic synthetic alcohol that acts by delaying the multiplication of intracellular and extracellular organisms through interference with RNA synthesis. Resistance to the drug develops slowly and, when given in combination with other antimicrobial agents, ethambutol delays the onset of microbial resistance. It is also better tolerated than PAS, with less tendency to produce toxic effects. Ethambutol does not penetrate well into cerebrospinal fluid, even in the presence of inflamed meninges.

Four hours after ingestion, a peak serum level of 5 µg/ml is attained. The drug is stored in red blood cells, from which it is released into the plasma. Ethambutol is excreted by the kidneys primarily and to a lesser extent by the gastrointestinal tract.

Toxicity includes retrobulbar neuritis, with resultant loss of visual acuity, red-green color perception, and peripheral vision; central scotoma; optic neuritis; and diplopia. These effects are infrequent at recommended lower dosages and usually resolve when ethambutol is discontinued. However, retrobulbar neuritis may be irreversible. Monthly or bimonthly screening for visual acuity, color vision, and visual fields is indicated. The drug should be discontinued if there is a two-line loss of visual acuity as measured on the Snellen eye chart, contraction of the visual fields, or loss of color vision. Gastrointestinal disturbances, dermatitis, headache, confusion, and decreased urate excretion resulting in hyperuricemia may also occur. Ethambutol has no known drug interactions.

The drug is supplied in 100 mg and 400 mg tablets and is administered in a single daily oral dose. Dosages of 25 mg/kg/day are utilized during the initial 6 to 8 weeks of therapy and are followed by 15 mg/kg/day. Although the drug is not recommended by the manufacturer for treatment of children younger than age 13 years, it is often given to children in this age group who can be tested for visual acuity and color vision.

Streptomycin

Streptomycin, an aminoglycoside, was isolated from *Streptomyces griseus* in 1944 and was the first effective antimicrobial agent for tuberculosis. The drug is both bacteriocidal and bacteriostatic to extracellular organisms in a medium with alkaline or neutral pH and interferes with protein synthesis in tubercle bacilli. Intracellular penetration by streptomycin is relatively low. The drug inhibits growth of the tubercle bacillus in a concentration of 1.6 µg/ml and rapidly appears in the blood stream following parenteral administration, reaching a peak value of 25 to 50 µg/ml within 2 hours. Streptomycin diffuses into the pleural fluid but does not pass the cerebrospinal fluid barrier to any appreciable extent unless meningeal inflammation is present. The drug is excreted in the urine, with an 80 per cent recovery within 24 hours after administration.

The principal toxic effect of streptomycin is involvement of the eighth cranial nerve. Although loss of vestibular function may be permanent, children usually adjust to this defect without symptoms. Involvement of the auditory branch constitutes a potential danger, but this effect is much less common now than it was in the days of prolonged strepto-mycin therapy. Drug-induced fever, dermatitis, agranulocytosis, anemia, thrombocytopenia, and nephrotoxicity with reduced urinary output and al-buminuria can also occur. Streptomycin acts syner-gistically with cephalosporins, ethacrynic acid, and neuromuscular blocking agents, and its action is potentiated by probenecid.

Streptomycin is administered once or twice daily by intramuscular injection in a dosage of 20 to 40 mg/kg/day, with a maximum daily dosage of 1 g. It is not absorbed from the gastrointestinal tract. Strep-tomycin is supplied in crystalline form, usually as a sulfate, in vials containing 1 g and 5 g.

Para-Aminosalicylic Acid

Para-aminosalicylic acid has bacteriostatic activity against the tubercle bacillus and suppresses the growth and multiplication of extracellular organisms. It is a second-line antituberculous drug. When used in conjunction with isoniazid or streptomycin, PAS acts to delay the emergence of microbial resistance to these drugs. The chief value of PAS lies in the fact that it apparently competes with isoniazid for acetylation in the liver and for inhibition of folate synthesis, thereby increasing the amount of free isoniazid in the blood.

Para-aminosalicylic acid is readily absorbed from the gastrointestinal tract. Two hours following a dose of 4 g, a peak serum level of 75 μg/ml is attained. The drug diffuses to some extent into serous surfaces and reaches the cerebrospinal fluid in small amounts. Para-aminosalicylic acid is excreted by the kidney.

Gastrointestinal disturbances, such as nausea, ab-dominal distress, and anorexia, constitute the prin-cipal adverse manifestations of PAS, but hypokale-mia, a goitrogenic effect, jaundice, leukopenia, hypersensitivity, dermatitis, and drug-induced fever may also occur. The action of PAS is potentiated by probenecid and reduced by salicylates.

Children usually have a much better tolerance for PAS than do adults. The drug is prescribed in a dosage of 200 mg/kg/day. Tolerance is increased in some patients when a smaller dose is employed ini-tially. Para-aminosalicylic acid is better tolerated after meals and is prescribed in three divided doses per day. When sodium, potassium, or calcium salts of PAS are used, the dosage should be correspondingly higher, 250 to 300 mg/kg/day, with a maximum daily dose of 12 g. Para-aminosalicylic acid is supplied as 0.5 g tablets, as a powder, or as a solution of the sodium salt. The solution is rarely used because of instability after 24 hours, and it must be kept in the dark and refrigerated.

Adrenocorticosteroids

Adrenocorticosteroids act to suppress the inflam-matory response of the body with impairment of granulation tissue formation, macrophage activity,

and fibroblastic repair. From the nature of this mech-anism, it appears likely that adrenocorticosteroids would promote progression of tuberculosis. How-ever, this deleterious effect can be overcome by concurrent administration of antituberculous che-motherapy. Adrenocorticosteroids are frequently employed as an adjunct to antituberculous drug therapy in specific situations—endobronchial disease to promote regression of enlarged lymph nodes, miliary disease with cyanosis to reduce alveolocapil-lary block, symptomatic effusions of the pleura or pericardium to enhance fluid resorption, and men-ingitis to decrease intracranial pressure.

Side effects of corticosteroids include suppression of the pituitary-adrenal axis, peptic ulcer, osteopo-rosis, electrolyte imbalance, cataracts, hypertension, obesity, growth suppression, and myopathy. These drugs potentiate the effects of neuromuscular block-ing agents and inhibit the actions of calcium salts. The actions of corticosteroids are inhibited by phe-nytoin, barbiturates, and rifampin.

Prednisone is often used as the oral preparation. For seriously ill patients, intravenous or intramus-cular preparations are administered daily in divided doses.

Other Drugs

Cycloserine, ethionamide, capreomycin, and kan-amycin are other second-line drugs used to treat tuberculosis in the United States. These drugs are utilized for treatment of isoniazid- and rifampin-resistant tuberculosis, but their use in children is limited. Ethionamide and cycloserine are bacterio-static to intracellular and extracellular organisms and are administered orally in doses of 15 to 20 mg/kg/day, maximum 1 g/day. Capreomycin and kanamycin are bacteriocidal to extracellular tubercle bacilli and are administered intramuscularly in doses of 15 to 30 mg/kg/day, maximum 1 g/day. Side effects include hepatotoxicity, gastrointestinal irritation, and hyper-sensitivity for ethionamide; dermatitis, seizures, and psychosis for cycloserine; and auditory and vestibular ototoxicity and nephrotoxicity for capreomycin and kanamycin. These drugs are not given in short-course chemotherapy.

CLASSIFICATION OF TUBERCULOSIS

The classification of tuberculosis as determined by the Committee on Diagnostic Standards of the Amer-ican Thoracic Society (Weg, 1981) is as follows:

0. No tuberculosis exposure, not infected—no his-tory of exposure, negative tuberculin skin test.
I. Tuberculosis exposure, no evidence of infec-tion—history of exposure, negative tuberculin skin test.

II. Tuberculous infection, without disease—positive tuberculin skin test, negative bacteriologic studies (if done), no roentgenographic findings compatible with tuberculosis, no symptoms due to tuberculosis.
III. Tuberculosis: current disease.
    A. Location of disease (predominant site; other sites if significant).
    B. Bacteriologic status.
    C. Chemotherapy status.
    D. Roentgenographic findings.
    E. Tuberculin skin test.
IV. Tuberculosis: no current disease.
    A. Chemotherapy status.
V. Tuberculosis suspect.
    A. Chemotherapy status.

POSITIVE TUBERCULIN REACTION (II. TUBERCULOUS INFECTION, WITHOUT DISEASE)

Delayed cutaneous hypersensitivity develops during the 2- to 10-week period following tuberculous infection, with a resultant positive tuberculin skin test reaction. The primary focus and complex form during this time. The patient, who is asymptomatic, now has tuberculous infection, which may be without (II) or with (III) disease.

If a positive tuberculin skin test reaction occurs without evidence of pulmonary or extrapulmonary tuberculous disease, it is assumed that the primary focus, with associated regional lymph node involvement, is in the lung parenchyma but is too small to be visible on a roentgenogram. The individual is considered to be infected with tuberculosis but does not have clinical disease.

Treatment. There is no antimicrobial agent currently available that will eradicate tubercle bacilli. The aim of antimicrobial therapy is the arrest of the existing tuberculous infection and prevention of complications of the disease. No drug other than

isoniazid can prevent the more serious forms of the disease. Therefore, isoniazid is used to treat tuberculous infection.

All children and adolescents with a positive tuberculin skin test reaction and no evidence of disease who have not previously received prophylaxis should receive isoniazid, 10 to 15 mg/kg/day (maximum dose 300 mg) daily for at least 9 months, if the short-course regimen is utilized, or 12 months, if the longer course is prescribed (Table 48–4). Periodic roentgenograms and the usual precautions are advised (see "Isoniazid"). For pregnant adolescents with a positive tuberculin skin test reaction, it may be preferable to delay isoniazid prophylaxis until after delivery.

Several alternatives are available for prophylaxis for exposure to isoniazid-resistant tubercle bacilli, although none has been evaluated. Either isoniazid or rifampin (10 to 20 mg/kg/day, maximum 600 mg/day) may be given alone or concurrently for 1 year.

PRIMARY PULMONARY TUBERCULOSIS (III. TUBERCULOSIS: CURRENT DISEASE, LYMPHATIC)

The primary complex is composed of the primary focus, the involved regional lymph nodes, and the lymphatics between them. Primary tuberculous disease includes involvement of the primary complex and the progression of any of its components.

Before development of hypersensitivity to tuberculin occurs, the primary focus may become larger but it is not encapsulated. When hypersensitivity develops, the perifocal reaction is much more prominent, and the regional lymph nodes enlarge. Although the primary focus may become caseous, it is usually walled off. The caseous material is gradually inspissated and later calcified, or it may completely disappear. Alternatively, the lesion may become progressively enlarged. The radiographic or clinical presence, or both, of all or part of the primary

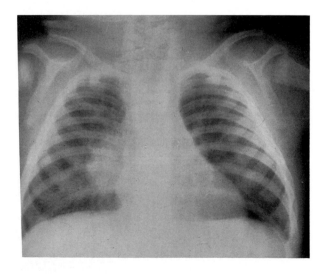

Figure 48–19. Primary pulmonary tuberculosis, with enlarged mediastinal lymph nodes, right. (Reproduced with permission from Kendig EL Jr et al: Isoniazid in treatment of tuberculosis in childhood. Am J Dis Child 88:148. Copyright 1954, American Medical Association.)

Table 48–4. CHEMOTHERAPY OF TUBERCULOSIS

Type or Stage of Disease	Short-Course Regimen		Longer Regimen	
	Drug(s)	Duration of Therapy (months)	Drug(s)	Duration of Therapy (months)
Positive tuberculin skin test reaction	INH	9	INH	12
Primary pulmonary tuberculosis	INH	6–9	INH	12
	RIF	6–9	and	
	PZA	2	RIF	12
			or	
			EMB	12
Progressive primary pulmonary tuberculosis	INH	6–9	INH	12
	RIF	6–9	and	
	PZA	2	RIF	12
			or	
			EMB	12
Tuberculous pneumonia	INH	6–9	INH	12
	RIF	6–9	and	
	PZA	2	RIF	12
			or	
			EMB	12
Endobronchial tuberculosis	INH	6–9	INH	12
	RIF	6–9	RIF	12
	PZA	2	Prednisone	1.5–3
	Prednisone	1.5–3		
Tuberculous pleural effusion	INH	6–9	INH	12–18
	RIF	6–9	and	
	PZA	2	RIF	12–18
	Prednisone	*	or	
			EMB	12–18
			Prednisone	*
Chronic pulmonary tuberculosis	INH	6–9	INH	12–18
	RIF	6–9	and	
	PZA	2	RIF	12–18
			or	
			EMB	12–18
Miliary tuberculosis	INH	9	INH	12–18
	RIF	9	RIF	12–18
	PZA	2	and	
	SM	1–3	PZA	2
	Prednisone	1.5–3	or	
			SM	1–3
			or	
			EMB	3–6
			Prednisone	1.5–3
Tuberculous meningitis	INH	12	INH	12–18
	RIF	12	RIF	12–18
	and		and	
	PZA	2	PZA	2
	and/or		and/or	
	SM	1–3	SM	1–3
	Prednisone	1.5–3	Prednisone	1.5–3
Tuberculosis of superficial lymph nodes	INH	6–9	INH	12–18
	RIF	6–9	and	
	PZA	2	RIF	12–18
			or	
			EMB	12–18
Skeletal, renal, intra-abdominal tuberculosis	INH	9	INH	18–24
	RIF	9	and	
	PZA	2	RIF	18–24
			or	
			EMB	18–24
Neonatal tuberculosis	—	—	INH	12
			RIF	12

*Until fluid is resorbed.
See Table 48–3 for dosages of drugs and chapter text for details.
INH, isoniazid; RIF, rifampin; PZA, pyrazinamide; EMB, ethambutol; SM, streptomycin.

In the most frequently occurring form of primary tuberculosis, the patient's chest roentgenogram shows enlarged mediastinal lymph nodes with no demonstrable primary parenchymal focus (Fig. 48–19). In such instances, when the disease process heals, calcific deposits will often be observed at one or more sites in the lung parenchyma and in the hilus (Ghon complex) (Fig. 48–20). This parenchymal calcification is indicative of a healed primary focus that had never been visible on a roentgenogram. Less common is the primary complex with both a demonstrable primary parenchymal focus and enlarged hilar lymph nodes. Figure 48–21 shows a primary complex with demonstrable involvement of the interfocal zone in the lateral view. Finally, in a small group of patients who have positive tuberculin skin test reactions with no roentgenographic evidence of lung disease, extrapulmonary tuberculous lesions are demonstrable on physical examination or radiographs, or from laboratory study results.

If the primary complex appears on the roentgenogram at all, it appears at the time of onset of the disease. It may progress for 1 to 2 months, diminish in size only after 3 to 4 months, and may remain visible for 6 to 12 months, or even longer. Resolution of the primary complex is apparently not hastened by antimicrobial therapy.

Almost all patients with a primary parenchymal focus have regional lymphadenopathy. As a result of the lymphatic drainage in the mediastinum, a primary focus in the left lung parenchyma may be associated with enlarged lymph nodes in both left and right mediastinum, whereas a focus in the right lung is not associated with lymphadenopathy on the left.

Calcification occurs more frequently in regional lymph nodes than in parenchymal foci probably because of early migration of tubercle bacilli from the parenchymal focus to the regional lymph nodes. The first sign of calcification may appear within 6 months after the diagnosis of primary tuberculosis in an infant and somewhat later in an older child.

The prognosis of unhealed primary tuberculosis depends primarily on the patient's age, the duration of infection, and, to some degree, the extent of the primary lesion. Whenever calcification is seen on the roentgenogram, it may be assumed that the infection is at least 6 months old. The presence of calcification is of good prognostic import, but the amount of calcification and the persistence of roentgenographic evidence of the primary infection are also significant (Fig. 48–22).

Treatment. Primary pulmonary tuberculosis in children should be treated with isoniazid, 10 to 20 mg/kg/day (maximum daily dose 300 mg), and rifampin, 10 to 20 mg/kg/day (maximum daily dose 600 mg), as a daily or an intermittent short-course regimen or as a 1-year, longer regimen (see Tables 48–3 and 48–4). Pyrazinamide, 15 to 30 mg/kg/day (maximum daily dose 2 g), should be added to the short-course regimen if an intermittent short-course

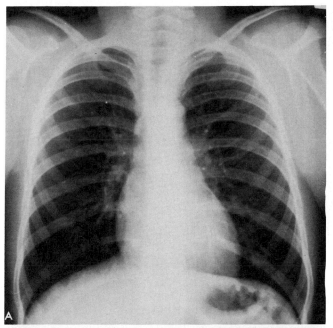
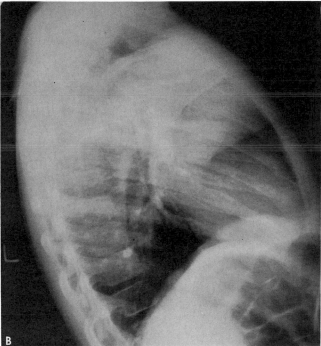

Figure 48–20. Calcific densities indicating the presence and location of the healed primary complex (Ghon complex). The primary parenchymal focus was not visible on the roentgenogram taken during the acute phase of the disease.

complex, whether stable or progressive, represents primary tuberculosis.

Patients with uncomplicated primary tuberculosis may be divided into three groups: (1) those with roentgenographic evidence of mediastinal lymph node enlargement but without a primary parenchymal focus; (2) those with a demonstrable primary parenchymal complex, i.e., both nodes and focus; and (3) those with evidence of primary extrapulmonary tuberculosis.

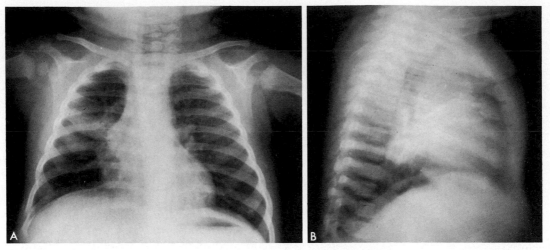

Figure 48–21. A primary complex with demonstrable involvement of the interfocal zone (visible on lateral view, *B*).

regimen is utilized; 6 months of therapy is prescribed; extensive disease is present; or host immunity is naturally impaired, as in the infant.

PROGRESSIVE PRIMARY PULMONARY TUBERCULOSIS (III. TUBERCULOSIS: CURRENT DISEASE, PULMONARY)

Local progression of the pulmonary component of the primary complex occasionally occurs. The area of caseation enlarges and liquefies, and the contents are disseminated into bronchi, thereby setting up new pulmonary foci of disease. This is a severe form of tuberculosis that occurs much more often in young children. Signs and symptoms include persistent fever, anorexia, apathy, loss of weight, cough, tachypnea, and mild respiratory distress. Physical examination of the chest may reveal moist rales over the diseased area. A constant wheeze over the area of obstruction may also be present.

Prompt antituberculous drug therapy for primary pulmonary tuberculosis is almost always successful in preventing this form of tuberculous disease. If the diagnosis of tuberculosis is not made until the disease has reached this stage, the prognosis is less favorable.

Treatment. Pulmonary progression of primary tuberculosis requires an intense therapeutic approach. Antimicrobial therapy consists of isoniazid, 10 to 20 mg/kg/day (maximum daily dose 300 mg); rifampin, 10 to 20 mg/kg/day (maximum daily dose 600 mg); and pyrazinamide, 15 to 30 mg/kg/day (maximum daily dose 2 g), either as a daily or intermittent short-course regimen (see Tables 48–3 and 48–4). If the longer regimen is utilized, isoniazid and rifampin are prescribed for 1 year.

TUBERCULOUS PNEUMONIA (HEMATOGENOUS)

Tuberculous pneumonia of hematogenous origin may also occur. This form makes its appearance near the close of the incubation period and is usually accompanied by few, if any, symptoms. The lesion itself is indistinguishable on a roentgenogram from a primary parenchymal focus (Fig. 48–23). Treatment is the same as that for primary pulmonary tuberculosis (see Tables 48–3 and 48–4).

OBSTRUCTIVE LESIONS OF THE BRONCHUS (ENDOBRONCHIAL TUBERCULOSIS)

The regional lymph nodes draining the primary parenchymal focus are tuberculous. They become hyperemic and edematous, may contain areas of caseation, and may impinge upon the wall of a bronchus to occlude the lumen and cause atelectasis of lung distal to the obstruction. The resulting extrabronchial, or extraluminal, tuberculosis occurs rarely, and, when it does, frequently involves the right middle lobe bronchus.

In contrast, endobronchial tuberculosis occurs more often and results from adherence of infected nodes to an adjacent bronchus, with progression of the infection through the airway wall to the mucosa. Further progression of the disease process, with ulceration of mucosa and formation of granulation tissue, may completely obstruct the bronchial lumen. Occasionally, a tuberculous lymph node penetrates the wall of the bronchus, creates a sinus tract through which caseous material is extruded into the airway, and causes tuberculous bronchitis. Atelectasis results from complete occlusion of the airway (Fig. 48–24) and is more likely to be present in the right lung, particularly the right middle lobe and, to a lesser extent, the right upper lobe. Pneumonia may also be present (Fig. 48–25). In addition, partial airway obstruction with hyperaeration can occur (Fig. 48–26). Rarely, extrusion of large amounts of caseous material into the bronchus will take place, causing complete airway obstruction and asphyxia.

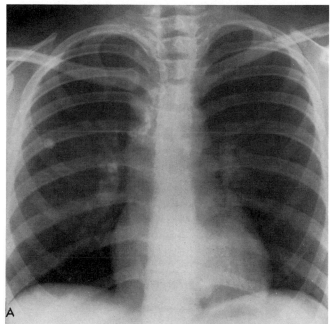

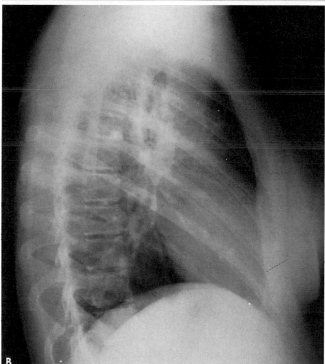

Figure 48–22. A calcified primary complex with no evidence of active tuberculous disease.

With antituberculous chemotherapy, the edematous lymph nodes recede, the lumen of the bronchus again becomes patent, and the atelectic lung re-expands. Bronchoscopy may help remove the caseous material, provide specimens for culture, and more quickly re-expand the atelectic lung.

Treatment. Treatment is essentially the same as that employed for progressive primary pulmonary tuberculosis (see Tables 48–3 and 48–4). In addition, prednisone, 1 mg/kg/day (maximum daily dose 60 mg), prescribed for 6 to 12 weeks early in the course

of the disease appears to promote regression in size of tuberculous lymph nodes. Since sufficient time has not elapsed for fibrosis to occur early in the course of the disease, the anti-inflammatory action of prednisone may allow greater penetration into the lymph node by antituberculous drugs.

Case Report. J.S., a 6-month-old black girl, was enrolled in a study of the therapy of primary tuberculosis at the Medical College of Virginia. The patient was asymptomatic, with a positive tuberculin skin test reaction and right-sided hilar adenopathy on a roentgenogram. Isoniazid, 15 mg/kg/day, was prescribed, and she was seen monthly for follow-up examinations. At the time of her visit after 5 months (at 11 months of age), she had a history of anorexia. Physical examination revealed diminished breath sounds and hyper-resonance over the right side of the chest. A diagnosis of hyperaeration of the right lung was corroborated by a chest roentgenogram. The patient was hospitalized, and bronchoscopy revealed the lumen of the right main bronchus to be almost completely occluded by caseous material. A portion of this material was removed, and daily doses of PAS, 200 mg/kg, and prednisone, 1 mg/kg, were added to the therapeutic regimen. Clinical improvement occurred within 10 days, and the hyperaeration was no longer apparent on the chest roentgenogram after 3 weeks (see Fig. 48–26). Prednisone was continued for 12 weeks, with gradual reduction in dosage before the drug was discontinued. Bronchoscopy before discharge from the hospital showed no evidence of disease. (PAS was used because rifampin, ethambutol, and pyrazinamide were not available in the United States at the time.)

ACUTE MILIARY TUBERCULOSIS

Acute miliary tuberculosis is a generalized hematogenous disease, with formation of multiple tubercles and manifestations that are frequently pulmonary. It is a complication of primary tuberculosis and usually occurs within the first 6 months after the onset of disease. It is more common in infants and young children but may be seen at any age.

The tubercles are millet-sized and relatively uniform and result from the lodging of tubercle bacilli in small capillaries. Necrosis tends to develop in spite of an epithelioid response. The size of the lesions may be determined in part by host resistance. Almost all organs may be involved, although the lungs are almost always affected.

The onset is usually acute with high fever that is most often remittent. The patient appears ill, but symptoms and signs of respiratory disease may be absent. Occasionally, however, respiratory distress is present initially. Hepatosplenomegaly and superficial lymphadenopathy occur in half of the cases. The presence of choroidal tubercles, if seen early, may be of great diagnostic importance.

Approximately 1 to 2 weeks after the onset of

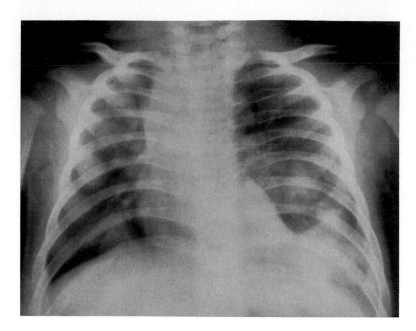

Figure 48–23. Roentgenogram of an infant whose diagnosis was made at 23 days of age, showing several lesions that may be either primary foci or pneumonia of hematogenous origin (indistinguishable on roentgenogram). (Reproduced with permission from Kendig EL Jr: Tuberculosis in the very young. Am Rev Tuberc 70:161, 1954.)

disease, the mottled lesions, which resemble snowflakes, make their appearance on the roentgenogram (Fig. 48–27). Shortly thereafter, fine crepitant rales may be present over the lung fields.

The mortality rate is 100 per cent in untreated cases. Death occurs within 4 to 12 weeks and is usually a result of tuberculous meningitis. In successfully treated cases, fever resolves after 14 to 21 days of therapy. Roentgenographic lesions usually improve within 5 to 10 weeks, but the roentgenogram does not clear until months later.

Treatment. At least three drugs are given initially in treatment of miliary tuberculosis. If the short-course regimen is prescribed, therapy consists of isoniazid, 10 to 20 mg/kg/day (maximum daily dose 300 mg); rifampin, 10 to 20 mg/kg/day (maximum daily dose 600 mg); and pyrazinamide, 15 to 30 mg/kg/day (maximum daily dose 2 g) (see Tables 48–3 and 48–4).

Streptomycin, 20 to 40 mg/kg/day (maximum daily dose 1 g), may be added for 1 to 3 months. If the longer regimen is prescribed, streptomycin for 2 to 3 months; pyrazinamide for at least 2 months; or ethambutol, 15 to 25 mg/kg/day (maximum daily dose 1500 mg), for 3 to 6 months is added to a 12- to 18-month course of isoniazid and rifampin. If acute respiratory distress is present with any of these regimens, prednisone, 1 mg/kg/day (maximum daily dose 60 mg), is frequently included until cyanosis, dyspnea, or both subside.

PLEURAL EFFUSION

A tuberculous pleural effusion is a relatively common early complication of primary pulmonary tu-

berculosis. It is more frequent in the older child but is not rare even in young infants. In a review of 303 children diagnosed with tuberculosis when less than 2 years of age, 3.3 per cent had roentgenographic evidence of pleural effusions, with a 2 male:1 female distribution (Hardy, 1945). The effusion is usually unilateral, and, when bilateral, is frequently secondary to miliary disease.

Most tuberculous pleural effusions occur by extension of the infection from a subpleural focus (Rich, 1951). Hypersensitivity to tuberculin may also be an etiologic factor (Fig. 48–28).

The onset is usually acute, with high fever and chest pain that increases upon deep inspiration. Unilaterally diminished breath sounds, dyspnea, and tachycardia may be present when the effusion is massive, and, rarely, bulging of the intercostal spaces may occur. Fever usually persists for 2 to 3 weeks. Although much of the fluid is usually absorbed by the end of this period, some fluid may persist for a considerably longer period of time.

A patient with a serous pleural effusion and a positive tuberculin skin test reaction must be assumed to have a tuberculous pleural effusion until proved otherwise. A diagnostic thoracentesis should always be performed promptly. Generally, no more than 30 ml of fluid is withdrawn in order to minimize protein and fluid shifts unless the effusion is so massive that respiratory embarrassment occurs. The fluid is usually an exudate, with a protein level above 4 g/dL; has a decreased glucose concentration, which is usually less than 30 mg/dL; and often has an elevated lactic dehydrogenase level. The cellular count varies from 200 to 10,000 cells/mm^3 and is predominantly lymphocytes except in the early stages when poly-

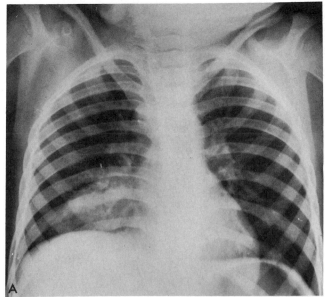

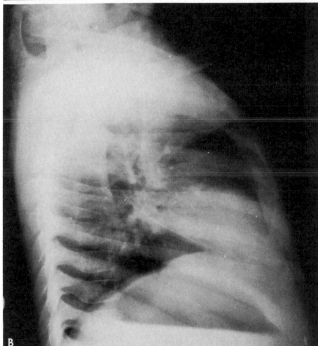

Figure 48–24. Atelectasis of the right middle lobe. Convex borders also suggest either an early atelectasis or an associated pneumonic process.

morphonuclear leukocytes may be present. Acid-fast stain and culture of the fluid for mycobacteria are performed. Cultures grow *M. tuberculosis* in only approximately half the cases because of the small numbers of organisms usually present in the effusion. Pleural biopsy may also help in identifying tubercles on histologic examination and in providing a source for culture and stain.

Although the prognosis depends on the extent and severity of the underlying disease, tuberculous pleural effusions usually resorb completely with minimal sequelae. Complications include spontaneous pneumothorax; caseous pleuritis; empyema, which is

unusual; scoliosis, which results from pleural adhesions; and contraction of a hemithorax.

Treatment. Treatment with short-course chemotherapy is the same as that for primary pulmonary tuberculosis (see Tables 48–3 and 48–4). If the longer regimen is used, isoniazid and either rifampin or ethambutol are prescribed for 12 to 18 months. With either the short-course or the longer regimen, prednisone, 1 mg/kg/day (maximum daily dose 60 mg), can be added to promote fluid resorption.

Antimicrobial therapy is utilized to reduce the progression and complications of tuberculosis and to reduce the incidence of later development of pulmonary tuberculosis. The drugs do not have a direct effect on the effusion.

CHRONIC PULMONARY TUBERCULOSIS (III. TUBERCULOSIS: CURRENT DISEASE, PULMONARY)

Chronic pulmonary tuberculosis usually develops late in the course of infection with tubercle bacilli. It

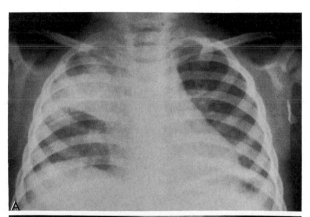

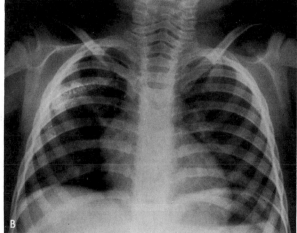

Figure 48–25. Roentgenograms illustrating tuberculous pneumonia associated with atelectasis. *B* shows heavy calcium deposits in the lung parenchyma after clearing of atelectasis and pneumonia. (Reproduced with permission from Kendig EL Jr et al: Isoniazid in treatment of tuberculosis in childhood. Am J Dis Child 88:148. Copyright 1954, American Medical Association.)

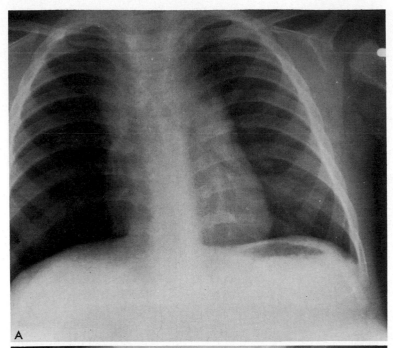

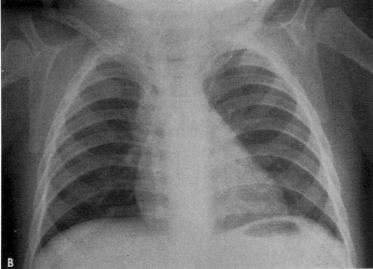

Figure 48–26. *A,* Hyperaeration of the right lung. *B,* Nineteen days after the addition of prednisone to the therapeutic regimen (INH and PAS), the roentgenogram showed complete clearing of the process.

frequently occurs in adolescence rather than in childhood and is more likely to occur during puberty, particularly during the menarchal year. It is characterized by a more acute progression in adolescents when compared with adults with this form of the disease. Although chronic pulmonary tuberculosis can occur exogenously as a result of superinfection, the presence of increased resistance to a second infection with *M. tuberculosis* favors the theory that the majority of cases of chronic pulmonary tuberculosis in children are endogenous, with reactivation of a quiescent infection.

The lesion of chronic pulmonary tuberculosis usually appears in the apical or subapical portion of the lung (Fig. 48–29). Since chronic pulmonary tuberculosis occurs when the tissues have already been sensitized to tuberculin, there is a tendency toward localization of the bacilli and not toward spread through lymphatics. After multiplication of bacilli has occurred, the lesion ulcerates, and liquefied material disseminates through bronchi. If untreated, the disease progresses and destroys large areas of lung. Concomitantly, although rare, tuberculous enteritis and laryngitis may also develop.

Healing occurs by fibrosis and, although not nearly so often at this age, by calcification. Cavities close and obliterate, and, with antituberculous drug therapy, the bronchocavitary junction may re-epithelialize, resulting in "open healing" (Fig. 48–30).

Although symptoms are not a reliable aid to early diagnosis, lassitude, cough, weight loss, anemia, and amenorrhea are indications for a tuberculin skin test. If the tuberculin skin test reaction is positive, a chest roentgenogram should be obtained.

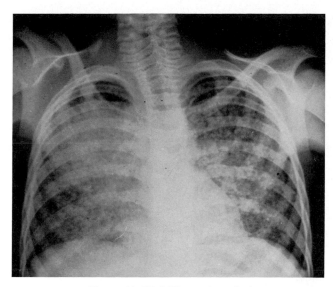

Figure 48–27. Miliary tuberculosis.

Treatment. The lesions of chronic pulmonary tuberculosis in children are extremely unstable, particularly in adolescents, and clinical deterioration can be rapid. Therefore, antituberculous drug therapy should be instituted promptly, and the patient should be carefully monitored. Treatment for chronic pulmonary tuberculosis is not as clear-cut as for other manifestations of tuberculosis. In addition, compliance of adolescents is notoriously poor. Short-course therapy is recommended only when the drugs are prescribed on a daily basis (see Tables 48–3 and 48–4). However, most health-care personnel experienced in the care of adolescents prefer the longer course. Surgical resection of the involved lung may be nec-

essary in cases of advanced disease with extensive caseation necrosis.

OTHER TUBERCULOUS INVOLVEMENT OF THE RESPIRATORY TRACT

Primary tuberculous infection of the tonsils occurred much more frequently in the past than now as a result of ingestion of tubercle bacilli, i.e., *M. bovis,* in milk. However, milk pasteurization and routine tuberculin skin testing of cows have made tonsillar tuberculosis a rarity in developed countries, although this disease may still be seen in other areas of the world.

Tuberculosis of the upper respiratory tract may develop as a result of exposure to tubercle bacilli in respiratory secretions. Tuberculosis of the larynx, middle ear, and mastoid and salivary glands can ensue. A tuberculous retropharyngeal abscess can occur with tuberculosis of the cervical vertebrae, or, rarely, arise from retropharyngeal caseous lymph nodes. A tracheoesophageal fistula can also occur, as exemplified by the following case report.

Case Report. D.J., a 16-month-old girl, was admitted to the Medical College of Virginia Hospital with the diagnoses of primary pulmonary and early miliary tuberculosis. She appeared to improve with isoniazid and PAS during the first 3 months of therapy. However, vomiting and fever subsequently developed, and pneumonic involvement of the right middle lobe was demonstrated on a roentgenogram (Fig. 48–31). Roentgenograms, utilizing a contrast medium swallow, demonstrated a fistula (Fig. 48–32).

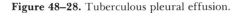

Figure 48–28. Tuberculous pleural effusion.

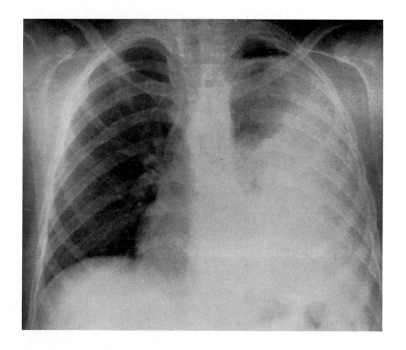

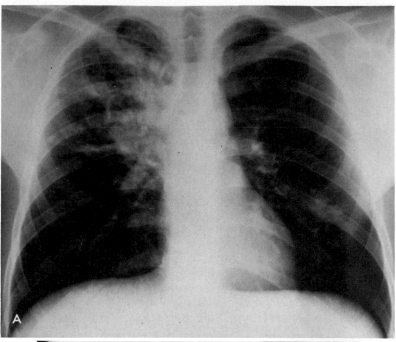

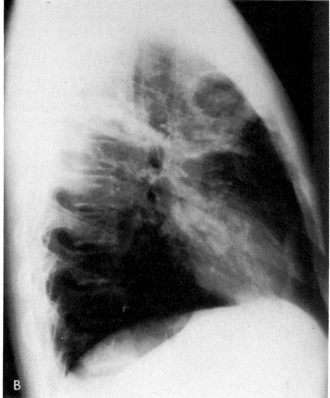

Figure 48–29. Chronic pulmonary tuberculosis with cavitation in a 16-year-old male.

Recovery was uneventful with isoniazid and PAS therapy. (PAS was used because rifampin, ethambutol, and pyrazinamide were not available in the United States at the time.)

EXTRAPULMONARY TUBERCULOSIS

Although pulmonary tuberculosis occurs more frequently in the United States than does extrapulmonary disease, the incidence of extrapulmonary tuberculosis has increased, primarily as a result of infection in the foreign-born population and in those with acquired immune deficiency syndrome (AIDS). Children under 4 years of age are more likely to develop extrapulmonary tuberculosis, particularly meningeal and lymphatic disease. Extrapulmonary tuberculosis is usually secondary to the lung disease as a result of lymphohematogenous dissemination, but it may also be the primary lesion.

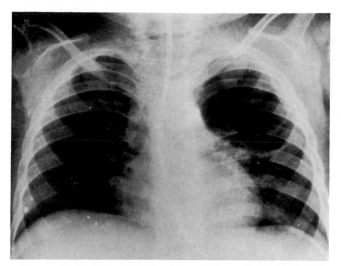

Figure 48–30. "Open healing" in a 16-month-old black male infant with tuberculous meningitis. Diagnosis corroborated at necropsy. (Reproduced with permission from Kendig EL Jr et al: Observations on the effect of cortisone in the treatment of tuberculous meningitis. Am Rev Tuberc 73:99, 1956.)

TUBERCULOSIS OF THE SUPERFICIAL LYMPH NODES (SCROFULA) (III. TUBERCULOSIS: CURRENT DISEASE, LYMPH NODE)

Tuberculosis of the superficial lymph nodes does not occur as frequently as it did prior to routine tuberculin skin testing of cows and pasteurization of milk. When it does occur, it results from the bacillemia that develops at the end of the 2- to 10-week incubation period with deposition of tubercle bacilli in foci in the lymph nodes. Here, the bacilli remain quiescent unless activated by a trigger mechanism.

Usually several lymph nodes are involved. Lymphoid hyperplasia and tubercles develop initially, with subsequent granuloma formation. Caseation and necrosis produce a confluent mass, which, when untreated, causes a sinus tract to form. Calcification is often present in a healed tuberculous lymph node.

Because a trigger mechanism is usually required for activation of disease, the process often occurs in the superficial cervical lymph nodes. Quiescent tubercle bacilli in these nodes are usually activated by acute tonsillitis or adenoiditis. The infection, if bacterial, is controlled by appropriate antibiotics, but the lymphadenopathy persists, and the lymph nodes, which are not painful or tender, continue to enlarge. The affected lymph nodes subsequently adhere to each other and to the overlying skin, which becomes discolored. The caseous material ruptures into the surrounding tissues and eventually drains externally through a sinus tract (Fig. 48–33).

Tuberculosis of the superficial lymph nodes may also result from direct lymphatic drainage from a primary extrapulmonary tuberculous focus. However, this mode of involvement is infrequent.

The differential diagnosis of chronic suppurative lymphadenitis includes acute pyogenic infections, coccidioidomycosis, blastomycosis, histoplasmosis, actinomycosis, brucellosis, infectious mononucleosis, leukemia, lymphoma, Hodgkin's disease, cat-scratch fever, and nontuberculous mycobacterial infection. Infection with nontuberculous mycobacteria may produce a clinical picture identical to that of tuberculous infection. If the tuberculin skin test reaction measures 5 to 9 mm in diameter of induration, it is

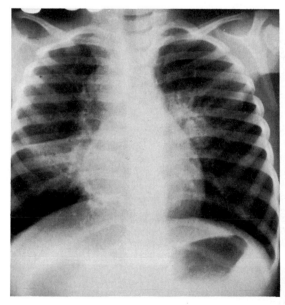

Figure 48–31. Aspiration pneumonia resulting from tracheoesophageal fistula, presumably of tuberculous origin.

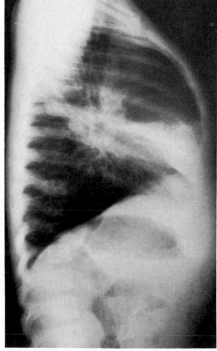

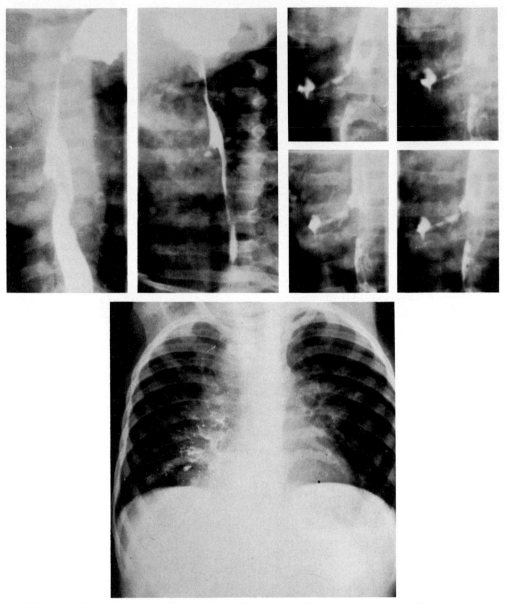

Figure 48–32. A contrast medium swallow demonstrates the tracheoesophageal fistula.

probable that infection with one of the nontuberculous mycobacteria exists.

Treatment. Lymphadenitis should initially be treated with one of the broad-spectrum antibiotics or with penicillin. However, if tuberculosis is suspected by the history or clinical findings; if the tuberculin skin test reaction is positive; and if the lymph nodes measure 2 cm or more in diameter for several weeks, are increasing in size, or showing early signs of suppuration despite antibiotic therapy, prompt excision and antituberculous chemotherapy are indicated. Treatment with the short-course regimen is the same as that for primary pulmonary tuberculosis (see Tables 48–3 and 48–4). If the longer regimen is used, isoniazid and rifampin are prescribed for 12 to 18 months. If the mass of nodes is very large or if complete liquefaction of the node has already oc-

curred and excision cannot be performed, the completely liquefied node should be aspirated. Chemotherapy alone is usually not effective at this stage of the disease. Tonsillectomy is advised only when there are indications for it.

TUBERCULOUS MENINGITIS (III. TUBERCULOSIS: CURRENT DISEASE, MENINGES)

Tuberculous meningitis is the most serious form of tuberculosis. Before the advent of streptomycin it was, presumably, 100 per cent fatal. At present, with the use of isoniazid and two or more additional

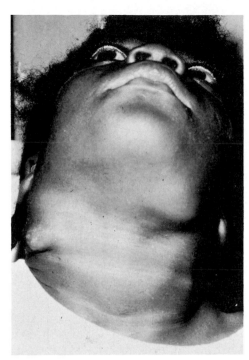

Figure 48–33. Multiple areas of suppurative lymphadenitis. (Reproduced with permission from Kendig EL Jr and Wiley TM: The treatment of tuberculosis in the superficial cervical lymph nodes in children. J Pediatr 47:607, 1955.)

antituberculous chemotherapeutic agents, the disease can almost always be cured if early diagnosis is established. Early treatment usually results in complete recovery, whereas neurologic sequelae and a fatal outcome are more likely if diagnosis and therapy are delayed.

Tuberculous meningitis is caused by the direct extension of a local contiguous lesion (Rich and McCordock, 1933) and is an early complication of tuberculosis. The two principal causes of neurologic sequelae are tuberculous arteritis and obstruction to the flow of cerebrospinal fluid by a thick, gelatinous exudate at the base of the brain.

The clinical course is divided into three stages: (1) nonspecific, generalized symptoms; (2) transitional stage, with early meningeal symptoms and increased intracranial pressure; and (3) severe central nervous system disease and coma.

Tuberculous meningitis is characterized by an insidious onset, although a convulsion may be the first sign. Symptoms are nonspecific, with apathy; lassitude; anorexia; irritability; low-grade fever; and, occasionally, vomiting and constipation early in the course of the disease.

In the second stage, drowsiness increases, and convulsions, opisthotonos, nuchal rigidity, bulging of the fontanel, and ocular paralysis may occur. The patient's condition steadily worsens.

In the final stage, coma, high fever, and an irregular pattern of breathing occur. Hyperglycemia and glycosuria may also be present. Death usually occurs within 3 weeks following the onset of untreated tuberculous meningitis.

The diagnosis is established by a tuberculin skin test, a cerebrospinal fluid examination, and a chest roentgenogram. The tuberculin skin test reaction is negative in up to 40 per cent of cases. Most patients with tuberculous meningitis have some evidence of primary tuberculosis on the chest roentgenogram. The cerebrospinal fluid has a ground-glass appearance with a cellular content of 10 to 1000 cells/mm³. The cells are predominantly polymorphonuclear leukocytes in the early stages of the disease, but lymphocytes are prominent later. The protein level is elevated above 40 mg/dl and results in a turbid sediment upon standing for 24 hours. The glucose concentration is usually decreased. Chloride levels are normal in the early stages and diminish later. On physical examination, the presence of choroidal tubercles, if seen early, may be of great importance in the diagnosis of widespread tuberculous disease.

Absolute diagnosis can be made only by the isolation of tubercle bacilli on smear, culture from the cerebrospinal fluid, or both. In addition, DNA probes can help identify the presence of *M. tuberculosis* in cerebrospinal fluid. However, *therapy should be instituted when the diagnosis is initially suspected* and should not be delayed while awaiting definitive laboratory results.

Treatment. Multiple drugs are used in treatment of tuberculous meningitis. Isoniazid and rifampin are always utilized, with the addition of pyrazinamide, streptomycin, or both (see Tables 48–3 and 48–4). Therapy is administered for 12 months for the short-course regimen and 12 to 18 months, or more, for the longer regimen. Some investigators believe that the duration of treatment should be at least 1 year (Starke, 1988). Isoniazid and rifampin are continued throughout the duration of therapy. Pyrazinamide and streptomycin can be discontinued after 2 to 3 months if a satisfactory clinical and biochemical response occurs. Corticosteroids for 6 to 12 weeks will help to decrease intracranial pressure and prevent the development of hydrocephaly and basilar arachnoiditis. The use of corticosteroids after obstruction to flow in cerebrospinal fluid has occurred often results in dissolution, as exemplified in the following case report.

Case Report. Shortly before the effectiveness of adrenocorticosteroid therapy in prevention and dissolution of cerebrospinal fluid obstruction had become recognized, a 2-year-old black girl had such a block. Cerebrospinal fluid protein was 5600 mg/dl when therapy with cortisone was instituted. After 2 weeeks, the cerebrospinal fluid protein was 650 mg/dl, but, as the drug was decreased in dosage and finally discontinued, the cerebrospinal fluid protein level gradually rose to 5800 mg/dl. When it subsequently became apparent that the obstruction could be controlled by cortisone, the steroid was again added to her regimen of isoniazid, PAS, and streptomycin, and the obstruction rapidly dissolved (Fig. 48–34). (PAS was used because rifampin, ethambutol, and pyrazinamide were not available in the United States at the time.)

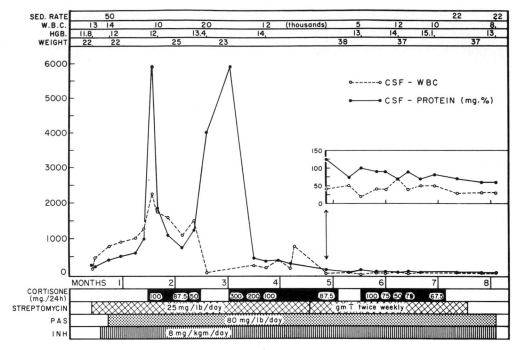

Figure 48–34. Diagram depicting precipitous fall of cerebrospinal fluid protein level when cortisone therapy was instituted. (Reproduced with permission from Kendig EL Jr et al: Observations on the effect of cortisone in the treatment of tuberculous meningitis. Am Rev Tuberc 73:99, 1956.)

The rapidity of the response to antituberculous drug therapy varies considerably. In general, the earlier the diagnosis is made, the more rapid is the response. An affected child may be stuporous, semi-comatose, or even comatose for months and finally attain a complete or almost complete recovery.

SKELETAL TUBERCULOSIS (III. TUBERCULOSIS: CURRENT DISEASE, SKELETAL)

Tuberculosis of the bones and joints usually results from the bacillemia near the close of the incubation period. Clinical disease may develop soon afterwards, or the organism may remain quiescent and reactivate months or years later. The bones most frequently involved are the head of the femur (hip), vertebrae, and phalanges. The pathologic process usually begins in the metaphyseal portions of the epiphyses.

Treatment. Treatment with short-course chemotherapy is the same as that for primary pulmonary tuberculosis, with administration of the drugs for 9 months (see Tables 48–3 and 48–4). If the longer regimen is utilized, isoniazid and either rifampin or ethambutol are prescribed for 18 to 24 months. All superficial and accessible abscesses should be drained. Immobilization is not necessary in the nonweight-bearing structures. If, however, weight-bearing structures, such as the vertebrae and hips, are involved; if joints are unstable; or if neurologic changes are present with spinal disease, then the ability of these bones to bear weight should be prevented by immo-

bilization. Plaster casts and spinal fusion are seldom necessary. Compression of the spinal cord, paravertebral abscess, and progression of the disease even with chemotherapy are indications for surgery.

RENAL TUBERCULOSIS (III. TUBERCULOSIS: CURRENT DISEASE, RENAL)

Tuberculosis of the kidney is of blood-borne origin, and infection occurs either at the time of early bacillemia or as part of generalized miliary tuberculosis. Symptoms and signs usually appear years later.

When the patient does not have associated miliary tuberculosis and has only a positive tuberculin skin test reaction, the most frequent finding is amicrobic pyuria. Albuminuria, hematuria, dysuria, and local renal tenderness may also be present. Culture of urine for *M. tuberculosis* will corroborate the diagnosis, and intravenous pyelograms and renal scans are indicated to determine the area and degree of involvement.

Treatment. Treatment with antituberculous agents, employing either the short-course or longer regimen, is the same as that for skeletal tuberculosis (see Tables 48–3 and 48–4). Since ureteral stricture may appear during therapy, an intravenous pyelogram and ureteral calibration should be performed every 4 to 6 months during treatment and annually during the following 10 years.

INTRA-ABDOMINAL TUBERCULOSIS (III. TUBERCULOSIS: CURRENT DISEASE, ABDOMINAL)

Intra-abdominal tuberculosis is rare in the United States. Tuberculous enteritis may be primary as a result of ingestion of *M. bovis* in milk from tuberculous animals or may be secondary to the spread of *M. tuberculosis* from a pulmonary lesion. Mesenteric and retroperitoneal lymph nodes are usually involved, and, when enlarged, result in abdominal pain and tenderness. Other symptoms include tenesmus, chronic diarrhea, hematochezia, abdominal distention, fever, anemia, and malaise.

Tuberculous peritonitis usually results from rupture of a caseous lesion in a mesenteric lymph node, and, occasionally, from penetration of an intestinal lesion through the outer wall of the intestine. Its onset is insidious, with initially mild abdominal pain, debilitation, and low-grade fever, and later development of vomiting and abdominal distention.

The dosages and duration of chemotherapy, with either the short-course or longer regimen, are the same as those for skeletal tuberculosis (see Tables 48–3 and 48–4). With primary tuberculous enteritis, excision of enlarged or calcified abdominal lymph nodes may be necessary for relief of pain.

OTHER EXTRAPULMONARY SITES OF TUBERCULOSIS

Less frequently occurring forms of extrapulmonary tuberculosis include tuberculosis of the skin, eye, heart, pericardium, endocrine and exocrine glands, genital tract, and tuberculous fistula-in-ano. For consideration of these entities, the reader is referred to publications that deal with tuberculosis in its entirety (Schlossberg, 1988; Lincoln, 1963; Gerbeaux, 1970).

TUBERCULOSIS IN THE NEWBORN

Approximately 300 cases of congenital tuberculosis have been reported in the literature. Although this number represents a small proportion of all childhood tuberculosis, the incidence of congenital tuberculosis may be expected to rise during the next few years as increasing numbers of childbearing women infected with human immunodeficiency virus acquire tuberculosis as an opportunistic infection.

Congenital tuberculosis results from hematogenous dissemination of tubercle bacilli across the placenta or from aspiration or inhalation of infected amniotic fluid prior to or during birth. The diagnosis is made by isolation of *M. tuberculosis* from the infant and either demonstration of a primary tuberculous complex in the liver or exclusion of extrauterine exposure. As with most neonatal diseases, its presenting manifestations in the newborn are nonspecific and include feeding difficulties, poor weight gain, lethargy, irritability, fever, respiratory distress, and hepatosplenomegaly. In addition to acid-fast stain and culture for tubercle bacilli in respiratory secretions, gastric aspirates, urine, bone marrow, and liver biopsy, examination of cerebrospinal fluid should be performed, even if the newborn is asymptomatic, to evaluate the presence of central nervous system disease.

When the mother is known to have active pulmonary tuberculosis, the newborn infant is often separated from her immediately after delivery until maternal infectivity is no longer present and until the infant has been evaluated for the presence of tuberculous infection or disease and either started on chemotherapy or vaccinated with BCG. If isoniazid is instituted, the baby is immediately returned to the mother. Evaluation of 117 infants in Richmond, Virginia, born to mothers who had tuberculosis at the time of delivery, shortly before, or soon after revealed that removal of the infant from contact with the mother without additional measures for the infant was not always enough to prevent later infection in the infant (Fig. 48–35). Even though 75 of the children were isolated from their mothers until the mothers' sputum test results were negative, 38 children became infected with tuberculosis when returned to the home environment (Table 48–5).

An infant born to a mother with tuberculosis should have a roentgenogram of the chest and a Mantoux tuberculin skin test. If the tuberculin skin test reaction is negative and the roentgenogram is normal, isoniazid, 10 mg/kg/day, should be used prophylactically since the infant may have already acquired tuberculous infection. The drug is administered for at least 3 months, at which time another Mantoux tuberculin skin test is performed to determine the presence of skin test conversion. If the reaction becomes positive, the infant is evaluated and treated for active tuberculosis. If the test is negative, isoniazid may be discontinued. However, if there is a question of maternal compliance, isoniazid should be continued in the infant for 12 months. Alternatively, if difficulties in regular, periodic follow-up visits are anticipated initially, BCG vaccine may be administered. In this case, the infant remains separated from the mother until the Mantoux tuberculin skin test reaction becomes positive as a result of the BCG vaccine, which usually takes 6 to 8 weeks.

If the infant has already acquired tuberculous infection, daily doses of isoniazid, 10 mg/kg, and rifampin, 15 mg/kg, should be administered for at least 1 year. Short-course chemotherapy has not been evaluated for treatment of tuberculosis in the newborn.

Although neurotoxicity has not been noted among infants treated with isoniazid, neither the pharmacology of this drug nor its efficacy in chemoprophylaxis for the newborn has been systematically studied. Nevertheless, isoniazid remains the most widely used

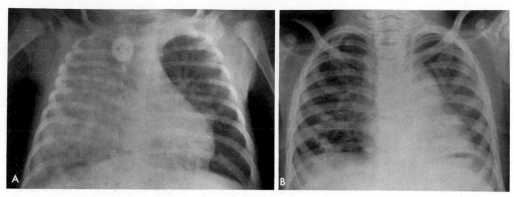

Figure 48–35. Roentgenograms of an infant whose diagnosis was made at 19 days of age, with widespread pulmonary tuberculosis. The patient recovered from the disease. (Reproduced with permission from Kendig EL Jr and Angell FL: Streptomycin and promizole in treatment of widespread pulmonary tuberculosis in a 19-day-old infant, case report. Am Rev Tuberc 61:747–750, 1950.)

antituberculous drug for prophylaxis and treatment of tuberculosis in the newborn.

TUBERCULOSIS DURING PREGNANCY

The occurrence of active tuberculosis during pregnancy represents a risk to the mother, the unborn child, and others living in the home. Tuberculosis is not an indication for a therapeutic abortion, and both mother and fetus have a good prognosis with adequate treatment. Following delivery, the infant is evaluated and treated, as described under "Tuberculosis in the Newborn."

Isoniazid and rifampin are the drugs most frequently prescribed for treatment of active pulmonary tuberculosis during pregnancy, and ethambutol is included if isoniazid resistance is suspected. Either the short-course or longer regimen of treatment may be utilized. Therapy for untreated, inactive pulmonary tuberculosis or isoniazid prophylaxis for a recent conversion of the tuberculin skin test is usually administered post partum. However, since the risk of developing tuberculosis is highest following the first year of infection, isoniazid prophylaxis during pregnancy may be necessary in some individuals and is often prescribed after completion of the first trimester. Pregnant women with previously treated, inactive pulmonary tuberculosis or with tuberculin skin test conversions that are not recent do not need chemotherapy.

Isoniazid, rifampin, ethambutol, and streptomycin cross the placenta. However, only streptomycin has been documented to be teratogenic, with resultant fetal ototoxicity. Presumably the other aminoglycosides, kanamycin and capreomycin, also cause ototoxicity. In addition to these three antimicrobials, pyrazinamide, ethionamide, and cycloserine should be avoided during pregnancy because sufficient data regarding the teratogenicity of these drugs are unavailable.

Antituberculous drugs are present in breast milk in low concentrations. Considerations regarding breast-feeding for a noninfectious mother taking antituberculous drugs should be individualized and include the benefits of breast-feeding and potential risks of drug toxicity to the newborn. The drug levels in breast milk are inadequate for treatment or prophylaxis of tuberculosis in the infant.

PREVENTION OF TUBERCULOSIS

Three methods have been demonstrated to be reasonably effective in preventing tuberculous infection in children: isolation of adults with active tuberculosis, administration of isoniazid to household con-

Table 48–5. EFFECTS OF BCG VACCINATION OF INFANTS OF TUBERCULOUS MOTHERS

Vaccination Status	Maternal Tuberculosis Diagnosed Before Delivery (Number of Infants)	Maternal Tuberculosis Diagnosed After Delivery (Number of Infants)	Total
BCG vaccine			
Infected infants	0	0	0
Noninfected infants	30	0	30
No BCG vaccine			
Infected infants	38 (3 deaths)	8 (1 death)	46
Noninfected infants	37*	4	41
Total Infants	105	12	117

*Three patients died, two with pneumonia (no contact with mother) and one at 2 months of age of undetermined cause.
(From Kendig EL Jr: The place of BCG vaccine in the management of infants born of tuberculous mothers. N Engl J Med 281:520, 1969. Reprinted, by permission, from The New England Journal of Medicine.)

tacts of tuberculous patients, and use of BCG vaccine. Studies by the United States Public Health Service (Ferrebee, 1969) have shown that the use of isoniazid in all household contacts of individuals with tuberculosis reduces the incidence of tuberculous disease in the contacts during the year of prophylactic therapy, and this effect lasts for at least 10 years after discontinuation of such therapy.

BACILLUS CALMETTE-GUÉRIN VACCINE

The BCG vaccine increases resistance to exogenous tuberculous infection. It is used in the United States for children with negative Mantoux tuberculin skin test reactions and negative chest roentgenogram findings, who have repeated exposure to active tuberculosis and unlikely compliance with isoniazid prophylaxis. The vaccine utilizes *M. bovis* as its antigen. It is not standardized throughout the world, thus resulting in variations in immunogenicity, efficacy, and potency. Protection afforded by BCG vaccine against meningeal, cavitary, miliary, and bone and joint tuberculosis is estimated to be at least 75 per cent (Putrali, 1983; Padungchan, 1986; Tidjani, 1986).

Experience at the Medical College of Virginia with the vaccine manufactured by Organon Teknika* has shown that the resultant positive tuberculin skin test reaction has induration that usually measures 5 to 9 mm in diameter and rarely more than 12 to 14 mm in diameter. If the induration measures 15 mm or more in diameter, active tuberculosis is likely to be present, and the patient should be evaluated and treated appropriately (see Fig. 48–14).

To be eligible for BCG vaccination, the patient must have a negative Mantoux tuberculin skin test reaction using 5 TU PPD and a normal chest roentgenogram within the previous 2 weeks. Eight to 12 weeks after vaccination, the tuberculin skin test and chest x-ray should be repeated. At this time, the tuberculin skin test reaction should be positive. If it is not, the vaccination should be repeated.

Two techniques of BCG vaccination are available: multiple-puncture disk and intradermal injection. Although the intradermal injection technique is more widely employed, the multiple-puncture disk method is preferable because of the infrequency of local complications.

Vaccination by the multiple-puncture disk method, as described by Rosenthal (1961), is performed over the deltoid region. The area is cleansed with acetone and allowed to dry thoroughly. Constriction of the arm should not occur. Three drops of BCG vaccine are placed on the skin of the deltoid area using a syringe and 22-gauge needle. The disk is picked up

---

*The Tice Strain for percutaneous administration is manufactured and distributed by Organon Teknika, Chicago, Ill. The Glaxo strain for intradermal use is available from Quad Pharmaceuticals, Inc, 6340 LaPas Trail, Indianapolis, Ind 46268.

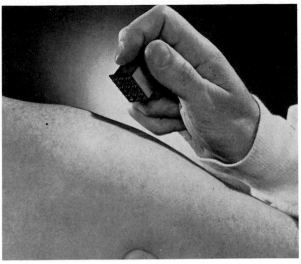

Figure 48–36. A multiple-puncture disk and magnet-type of holder held in position before depressing for BCG vaccination. (Courtesy of SR Rosenthal.)

with a sterile magnetic holder (Fig. 48–36), with the wide margin of the disk extending beyond the magnet and away from the operator. The operator holds the disk at a 30-degree angle and distributes the vaccine over an area approximately 2.5 cm² by tapping with the wide margin of the disk. The points of the disk are dipped into the vaccine as the disk is rotated slightly so that all points become moistened with vaccine. The disk is placed in the center of the vaccine site with the long axis of the holder at a right angle to the arm. The magnet is moved to the center of the disk in order to avoid bending of the disk. The patient's arm is then grasped with the operator's other hand, and the skin over the vaccination area is held taut. With the butt of the magnet in the curve of the operator's index finger, downward pressure is applied so that the points of the disk are penetrated well into the skin (Fig. 48–37). Sufficient pressure is applied so that penetration of the points is readily

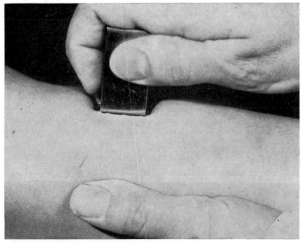

Figure 48–37. A multiple-puncture disk being pressed into the outer aspect of the arm. The disk is pressed downward through a drop of BCG vaccine. (Courtesy of SR Rosenthal.)

felt by the hand. With pressure still exerted, the disk is rocked back and forth and side to side twice. The patient's arm is then released. By maintaining a slight downward pressure on the magnet, the operator slides the magnet off the disk and away from the patient. If the procedure is successful, the disk will be flat on the arm with the points still in the skin. If the points are on top of the skin, the procedure must be repeated. Finally, the disk is again picked up with the magnet with the wide margin of the disk extending beyond the magnet. Through utilization of the wide margin, the vaccine is gently tapped so that each perforation of the skin is covered with vaccine. If too much pressure is applied, the vaccine will be pressed out of the perforations. The vaccine is allowed to dry on the arm without a dressing. The vaccinated area should not be washed for 24 hours (Fig. 48–38).

To ensure a successful result, both children and adults from tuberculous households should receive the two-site method of BCG vaccination. This is a modification of the multiple-puncture disk technique using a larger area of the deltoid region with one vaccination site in the upper portion and a second in the lower one.

The intradermal technique utilizes 0.05 ml of vaccine for neonates and 0.10 ml of vaccine for older children. The resultant scar is a round, raised bleb.

The BCG vaccine is relatively safe, and serious adverse effects are unusual. The most frequent side effects associated with the vaccine include ulceration at the vaccination site and regional lymphadenitis. Such reactions are rare when the multiple puncture technique is utilized and occur in approximately 0.3 per cent of injections of the vaccine at the Medical College of Virginia. Osteomyelitis is associated with some strains with an incidence of one case per one million doses (Snider, 1988). Disseminated BCG in-

fection, which usually accompanies impaired cell-mediated immunity, and lupoid reactions may also develop. The vaccine is contraindicated in pregnancy, immunodeficiency, skin infections, and burns.

REFERENCES

Abernathy RS, Dutt AK, Stead WW, and Moers DJ: Short-course chemotherapy for tuberculosis in children. Pediatrics 72:801, 1983.

American Academy of Pediatrics: Report of the Committee on Infectious Diseases. 21st ed. Elk Grove Village, Ill, 1988.

American Academy of Pediatrics, Section on Diseases of the Chest: The tuberculin test. Pediatrics 54:650, 1974.

American Thoracic Society, Scientific Assembly on Tuberculosis, and Centers for Disease Control, Bureau of State Services, Tuberculosis Control Division: Guidelines for short-course tuberculosis chemotherapy. Morbid Mortal Weekly Report 29:97, 1980.

Anane T, Cernay J, Bensenouci A et al: Résultats comparés des regimens courts et des regimens longs dans la chemeothérapie de la tuberculose de l'enfant en Algérie. Presentation at the African Regional Meeting International Union Against Tuberculosis, Tunis, Tunisia, 1984.

Anderson SR and Smith MHD: The Heaf multiple puncture tuberculin test. Am J Dis Child 99:764, 1960.

Aronson JD: BCG vaccination among American Indians. Am Rev Tuberc 57:96, 1948.

Bailey WC, Albert RK, Davidson PT et al: Treatment of tuberculosis and other mycobacterial diseases. Am Rev Respir Dis 127:790, 1983.

Barclay W, Elbert RH, and Koch-Weser D: Mode of action of isoniazid. Am Rev Tuberc 67:490, 1953; 70:784, 1954.

Bass JB Jr, Farer LS, Hopewell PC, and Jacobs RF: Treatment of tuberculosis and tuberculous infection in adults and children. Am Rev Respir Dis 134:355, 1986.

Beaudry PH, Brickman HF, Wise MB, and MacDougall D: Liver enzyme disturbances during isoniazid chemoprophylaxis in children. Am Rev Respir Dis 110:581, 1974.

Belsey MA: Tuberculosis and varicella infection in children. Am J Dis Child 113:448, 1967.

Bentley FJ, Grzybowski S, and Benjamin B: Tuberculosis in Childhood and Adolescence: with Special Reference to the Pulmonary Form of the Disease. London, The National Association for the Prevention of Tuberculosis, 1954.

Bernstein RE: Isoniazid hepatotoxicity and acetylation during tuberculosis chemoprophylaxis. Am Rev Respir Dis 121:429, 1980.

Blanchard PD, Yao JDC, McAlpine DE, and Hurt RD: Isoniazid overdose in the Cambodian population of Olmsted County, Minnesota. JAMA 256:3131, 1986.

Bobrowitz ID: Ethambutol in pregnancy. Chest 66:20, 1974.

Bolan G, Laurie RE, and Broome CV: Red man syndrome: inadvertent administration of an excessive dose of rifampin to children in a day-care center. Pediatrics 77:633, 1986.

Brailey ME: Prognosis in white and colored tuberculous children according to initial chest x-ray findings. Am J Pub Health 33:343, 1944.

Brasfield DM, Goodloe TV, and Tiller RE: Isoniazid hepatotoxicity in childhood. Pediatrics 58:291, 1976.

Centers for Disease Control: 1987 statistics in the United States. HHS Publication No. (CDC) 89–8322, August 1989a.

Centers for Disease Control: A strategic plan for the elimination of tuberculosis in the United States. MMWR 38:1, 1981.

Centers for Disease Control, Bureau of State Services, Tuberculosis Control Division: Adverse drug reactions among children treated for tuberculosis. Morbid Mortal Weekly Report 29:591, 1980a.

Centers for Disease Control, Bureau of State Services, Tuberculosis Control Division, and Bureau of Laboratories, Bacteriology Division, Mycobacteriology Branch: Primary resistance to anti-

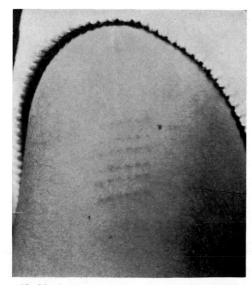

Figure 48–38. Appearance of multiple-puncture BCG vaccination 13 days after vaccination (actual size). (Courtesy of SR Rosenthal.)

tuberculous drugs—United States. Morbid Mortal Weekly Report 29:345, 1980b.

Centers for Disease Control, Bureau of State Services, Tuberculosis Control Division: Follow-up on guidelines for short-course tuberculosis therapy. Morbid Mortal Weekly Report 29:183, 1980c.

Centers for Disease Control: Summary of notifiable diseases, United States, 1986. Morbid Mortal Weekly Report 35:51, 1987.

Centers for Disease Control: Use of BCG vaccines in the control of tuberculosis: a joint statement by the ACIP and the Advisory Committee for Elimination of Tuberculosis. MMWR 37:663, 1988.

Comstock GW, Daniel TM, Snider DE Jr et al: The tuberculin skin test. Am Rev Respir Dis 124:356, 1981.

Comstock GW, Edwards LB, and Livesay VT: Tuberculosis morbidity in the United States Navy: its distribution and decline. Am Rev Respir Dis 110:572, 1974.

Dannenburg AM Jr: Pathogenesis of pulmonary tuberculosis. Am Rev Respir Dis 125:25, 1982.

Debré R and Papp K: About the tuberculin skin test during the course of measles and rubella. C R Soc Biol 95:29, 1926.

de March AP: Tuberculosis and pregnancy. Chest 68:800, 1975.

Dieu JC, Adenis-Lamarre F, Bitar M et al: La rifampicine dans le traitement des formes ganglio-pulmonaires de la tuberculose initiale du nourisson et de l'enfant. Rev Tuberc Pneumol (Paris) 34:320, 1970.

Doster B, Murray FJ, Newman R, and Woolpert SF: Ethambutol in the initial treatment of pulmonary tuberculosis. Am Rev Respir Dis 107:177, 1973.

Dutt AK and Snead WW: Short-course treatment regimens for patients with tuberculosis. Arch Intern Med 140:827, 1980.

Dutt AK, Jones L, and Snead WW: Short-course chemotherapy for tuberculosis with largely twice weekly isoniazid-rifampin. Chest 75:441, 1979.

Edwards LB, Edwards PQ, and Palmer CE: Sources of tuberculin sensitivity in human populations. Acta Tuberc Scand Suppl 47, 1959.

Edwards LB, Palmer CE, Affronti LF et al: Epidemiologic studies of tuberculin sensitivity. II. Response to experimental infection with mycobacteria isolated from human sources. Am J Hyg 71:218, 1960.

Edwards PQ: Tuberculin testing of children. Pediatrics 54:628, 1974.

Edwards PQ and Edwards LB: Story of the tuberculin test from an epidemiologic viewpoint. Am Rev Respir Dis 91(part 2):1, 1960.

Eickhoff TC: The current status of BCG immunization against tuberculosis. Am Rev Med 28:411, 1977.

Eidus L and Hamilton EJ: A new method for the determination of N-acetyl isoniazid in urine of ambulatory patients. Am Rev Respir Dis 89:587, 1964.

Elmendorf DG Jr, Cauthorn WW, Muschenheim C, and McDermott W: The absorption, distribution, excretion and short term toxicity of isoniazid (Nydrazid) in man. Am Rev Tuberc 65:429, 1952.

Engelhard D, Stutman HR, and Marks MI: Interaction of ketoconazole with rifampin and isoniazid. N Engl J Med 311:1681, 1984.

Ferebee SH: Controlled chemoprophylaxis trials in tuberculosis. A general review. Adv Tuberc Res 17:28, 1969.

Ferebee SH and Mount RW: Prophylactic effect of isoniazid on primary tuberculosis in children, a preliminary report: United States Public Health Service Tuberculosis Prophylaxis Trial. Am Rev Tuberc 76:942, 1957.

Filler J and Porter M: Physiologic studies of the sequelae of tuberculous pleural effusion in children treated with antimicrobial drugs and prednisone. Am Rev Respir Dis 88:181, 1963.

Fox AS and Lepow ML: Tuberculin skin testing in Vietnamese refugees with a history of BCG vaccination. Am J Dis Child 137:1093, 1983.

Fox W: Wither short-course chemotherapy? Br J Dis Chest 75:331, 1981.

Gerbeaux J: Primary Tuberculosis in Childhood. Springfield, Ill, Charles C Thomas, 1970.

Ghon A and Kudlich H: Die Eintrittspforten der Infektion vom Standpunkte der pathologischen Anatomie. In Engel S and Pirquet C (eds): Handbuch der Kindertuberckulose. Vol 1. Stuttgart, Georg Thieme Verlag, 1930.

Glassroth J, Robins AG, and Snider DE Jr: Tuberculosis in the 1980's. N Engl J Med 302:1441, 1980.

Goldstein RA, Ang UH, Foellmer JW, and Janicki BW: Rifampin and cell-mediated immune responses in tuberculosis. Am Rev Respir Dis 113:197, 1976.

Grosset J: Sterilizing value of rifampicin and pyrazinamide in experimental short-course chemotherapy. Tubercle 59:287, 1978.

Grosset J: Bacteriologic basis for short-course chemotherapy for tuberculosis. Clin Chest Med 1:231, 1980.

Grossman M, Hopewell PC, Jacobs RF et al: Consensus: management of tuberculin-positive children without evidence of disease. Ped Infect Dis 7:243, 1988.

Grzybowski S, Dorken E, and Bates C: Disparities of tuberculins. Am Rev Respir Dis 100:86, 1969.

Hageman J, Shulman S, Schreiber M et al: Congenital tuberculosis: critical reappraisal of clinical findings and diagnostic procedures. Pediatrics 66:980, 1980.

Hanson ML and Comstock GW: Efficacy of hydrocortisone ointment in the treatment of local reactions to tuberculin skin tests. Am Rev Respir Dis 97:472, 1968.

Hardy JB and Kendig EL Jr: Tuberculous pleurisy with effusion in infancy. J Pediatr 26:138, 1945.

Helms S and Helms P: Tuberculin sensitivity during measles. Acta Tub Scand 35:166, 1958.

Holden M, Dubin RR, and Diamond PH: Frequency of negative intermediate strength tuberculin sensitivity in patients with acute tuberculosis. N Engl J Med 285:1506, 1971.

Houck VN: Tuberculin: past, present, and future. JAMA 222:1421, 1972.

Hsu KHK: Isoniazid in the prevention and treatment of tuberculosis. JAMA 229:528, 1974.

Hsu KHK: Thirty years of isoniozid. Its impact on tuberculosis in children and adolescents. JAMA 251:1283, 1984.

Ibanez S and Ross BG: Quimioterapia abreviada de 6 meses en tuberculosis pulmonar infantil. Rev Chil Pediatr 51:249, 1980.

Illingworth RS and Lorber J: Results of streptomycin treatment in tuberculous meningitis. Lancet 2:511, 1951.

Inselman LS: Tuberculosis in children: lessons in diagnosis. J Respir Dis 5:88, 1984.

Inselman LS: Tuberculosis. In Gellis SS and Kagan BM (eds): Current Pediatric Therapy. 12th ed. Philadelphia, WB Saunders Co, 1986.

Inselman LS, DelaVega CE, and Evans HE: Drug-resistant tuberculosis of the hip in a child. NYS J Med 84:84, 1984.

Inselman LS, El-Maraghy NB, and Evans HE: Apparent resurgence of tuberculosis in urban children. Pediatrics 68:647, 1981.

Israel-Biet D, Venet A, Sandron D et al: Pulmonary complications of intravesical bacille Calmette-Guérin immunotherapy. Am Rev Respir Dis 135:763, 1987.

Jenkins DW and Byrd RB: The tuberculin tine and Mono-Vacc tests in the patient with active tuberculosis. Am Rev Respir Dis 112:140, 1975.

Johnson JR and Davey WN: Cortisone, corticotropin and antimicrobial therapy in tuberculosis in animals and man. Am Rev Tuberc 70:623, 1954.

Johnson WJ: Biological acetylation of isoniazid. Nature 174:744, 1954.

Johnston JA: Nutritional Studies in Adolescent Girls and Their Relation to Tuberculosis. Springfield, Ill, Charles C Thomas, 1953.

Kendig EL Jr: The effect of antihistaminic drugs on the tuberculin patch test. J Pediatr 35:750, 1949.

Kendig EL Jr: The routine tuberculin test—a neglected pediatric procedure. J Pediatr 40:813, 1952.

Kendig EL Jr: Tuberculosis in the very young. Am Rev Tuberc 70:161, 1954.

Kendig EL Jr: Incidence of tuberculous infection in infancy. Am Rev Tuberc 74:149, 1956a.

Kendig EL Jr: Early diagnosis of tuberculosis in childhood. Am J Dis Child 92:558, 1956b.

Kendig EL Jr: BCG vaccination in Virginia. J Pediatr 51:54, 1957.

Kendig EL Jr: Prognosis of infants born of tuberculous mothers. Pediatrics 26:97, 1960.

Kendig EL Jr: Unclassified mycobacteria in children: correlation of skin tests and gastric cultures. Am J Dis Child 101:749, 1961.

Kendig EL Jr: Unclassifed mycobacteria as a causative agent in the positive tuberculin reaction. Pediatrics 30:221, 1962.

Kendig EL Jr: Unclassified mycobacteria: incidence of infection and cause of a false positive tuberculin reaction. N Engl J Med 268:1001, 1963.

Kendig EL Jr: The place of BCG vaccine in the management of infants born of tuberculous mothers. N Engl J Med 281:250, 1969.

Kendig EL Jr: Tuberculosis among children in the United States: 1978. Pediatrics 62:269, 1978.

Kendig EL Jr: Tuberculin testing in the pediatric office and clinic. Pediatrics 64:965, 1979.

Kendig EL Jr: Evolution of short-course antimicrobial treatment of tuberculosis in children, 1951–1984. Pediatrics 75:684, 1985.

Kendig EL Jr: The study of tuberculosis in childhood: the evolution of pediatric pulmonology in North America. Am J Dis Child 141:1075, 1987.

Kendig EL Jr and Burch CD: Short-term antimicrobial therapy of tuberculous meningitis. Am Rev Respir Dis 82:672, 1960.

Kendig EL Jr and Hudgens RO: The effect of rubeola on tuberculosis under antimicrobial therapy. I. Primary tuberculosis treated with isoniazid. II. Tuberculous meningitis treated with isoniazid, streptomycin, and para-aminosalicylic acid. Pediatrics 24:616, 1959.

Kendig EL Jr and Johnson WB: Short-term antimicrobial therapy of tuberculous meningitis. N Engl J Med 258:928, 1958.

Kendig EL Jr and Rogers WL: Tuberculosis in the neonatal period. Am Rev Tuberc 77:418, 1958.

Kendig EL Jr and Wiley TM: The treatment of tuberculosis of the superficial cervical lymph nodes in children. J Pediatr 47:607, 1955.

Kendig EL Jr, Choy SH, and Johnson WH: Observations on the effect of cortisone in the treatment of tuberculous meningitis. Am Rev Tuberc 73:99, 1956.

Kendig EL Jr, Trevathan GE, and Ownby RJ: Isoniazid in treatment of tuberculosis in childhood. J Dis Child 88:148, 1954.

Koplan JP and Farer LS: Choice of preventive treatment for isoniazid-resistant tuberculous infection. JAMA 244:2736, 1980.

Lanier VS, Russel WF Jr, Heaton A, and Robinson A: Concentrations of active isoniazid in serum and cerebrospinal fluid of patients with tuberculosis treated with isoniazid. Pediatrics 21:910, 1958.

Levy H, Wadee AA, Feldman C, and Rabson AR: Enzyme-linked immunosorbent assay for the detection of antibodies against Mycobacterium tuberculosis in bronchial washings and serum. Chest 93:762, 1988.

Light IJ, Saidleman M, and Sutherland JM: Management of newborns after nursery exposure to tuberculosis. Am Rev Respir Dis 109:415, 1974.

Lincoln EM: Course and prognosis of tuberculosis in children. Am J Med 9:623, 1950.

Lincoln EM: Epidemics of tuberculosis. Adv Tuberc Res 14:157, 1965.

Lincoln EM and Sewell EM: Tuberculosis in Children. New York, McGraw-Hill Book Co, Inc, 1963.

Lincoln EM, Davies PA, and Bovornkitti S: Tuberculous pleurisy with effusion in children: a study of 202 children, with particular reference to prognosis. Am Rev Tuberc 77:271, 1958.

Litt IF, Cohen MI, and McNamara H: Isoniazid hepatitis in adolescents. J Pediatr 89:133, 1976.

Long ER: The Chemistry and Chemotherapy of Tuberculosis. 3rd ed. Baltimore, Williams & Wilkins Co, 1958.

Long MW, Snider DE Jr, and Farer LS: U.S. Public Health Service cooperative trial of three rifampin-isoniazid regimens in treatment of pulmonary tuberculosis. Am Rev Respir Dis 119:879, 1979.

Lorber J: Streptokinase as an adjunct in the treatment of tuberculous meningitis. Lancet 1:1334, 1951.

Lorber J: Isoniazid and streptomycin in tuberculous meningitis. Lancet 1:1140, 1954.

Lorber J: Tuberculous meningitis in children treated with streptomycin and PAS. Lancet 1:1104, 1954.

Lorber J: Current results in treatment of tuberculous meningitis and miliary tuberculosis. Br Med J 1:1009, 1956.

Lorriman G and Bentley FJ: The incidence of segmental lesions in primary tuberculosis: with special reference to the effect of chemotherapy. Am Rev Tuberc 79:765, 1959.

Lunn JA: Reason for variable response to tine test. Br Med J 280:223, 1980.

Lunn JA and Johnson AJ: Comparison of the tine and Mantoux tubercular tests. Br Med J 1:1451, 1978.

Lurie MB, Zappasodi P, and Tickner C: On the nature of genetic resistance to tuberculosis in the light of the host-parasite relationship in natively resistant and susceptible rabbits. Am Rev Tuberc 72:297, 1955.

McCray M and Esterly NB: Cutaneous eruptions in congenital tuberculosis. Arch Dermatol 117:460, 1981.

Mande R, Herrault A, Loubry P, and Bouchet C: Les epidémies scolaires de tuberculose. Sem Hop Paris 34:1837, 1958.

Morales SM and Lincoln EM: The effect of isoniazid therapy on pyridoxine metabolism in children. Am Rev Tuberc 75:594, 1957.

Myers JP, Perlstein PH, Light IJ et al: Tuberculosis in pregnancy with fatal congenital infection. Pediatrics 67:89, 1981.

Nemir RL and O'Hare D: Congenital tuberculosis. Review and diagnostic guidelines. Am J Dis Child 139:284, 1985.

Nemir RL, Cardona J, Lacoius A, and David M: Prednisone therapy as an adjunct in the treatment of lymph node-bronchial tuberculosis in childhood. Am Rev Respir Dis 88:189, 1963.

Notterman DA, Nardi M, and Saslow JG: Effect of dose formulation on isoniazid absorption in two young children. Pediatrics 77:850, 1986.

Oseasohn R: Current use of BCG. Am Rev Respir Dis 109:500, 1974.

Padungchan S, Konjanart S, Kasiratta S et al: The effectiveness of BCG vaccination of the newborn against childhood tuberculosis in Bangkok. Bull WHO 64:247, 1986.

Palmer CE and Edwards LB: Geographic variations in the prevalence of sensitivity to tuberculin (PPD-S) and to the Battey antigen (PPD-B) throughout the United States. Bull Int Union Tuberc 32:373, 1962.

Pellock JM, Howell J, Baker H, and Kendig EL Jr: Pyridoxine deficiency in children treated with isoniazid. Chest 87:658, 1985.

Pitchenik AE, Russell BW, Cleary T et al: The prevalence of tuberculosis and drug resistance among Haitians. N Engl J Med 307:163, 1982.

Powell-Jackson PR, Jamieson AP, Gray BJ et al: Effect of rifampicin administration on theophylline pharmacokinetics in humans. Am Rev Respir Dis 131:939, 1985.

Putrali J, Sitrisna B, Rahayoe N et al: A case-control study to evaluate the effectiveness of BCG vaccination in children in Jakarta, Indonesia. Proceedings of the Eastern Regional Tuberculosis Conference of IUAT, Jakarta, Indonesia, 1983.

Rapp RS, Campbell RW, Howell JC, and Kendig EL Jr: Isoniazid hepatotoxicity in children. Am Rev Respir Dis 118:794, 1978.

Rich AR: The Pathogenesis of Tuberculosis. 2nd ed. Springfield, Ill, Charles C Thomas, 1951.

Rich AR and McCordock HA: The pathogenesis of tuberculous meningitis. Bull Johns Hopkins Hosp 52:5, 1933.

Rieder HL, Cauthen GM, Kelly GD et al: Tuberculosis in the United States. JAMA 262:385, 1989.

Robinson A, Myer M, and Middlebrook G: Tuberculin hypersensitivity in tuberculous infants treated with isoniazid. N Engl J Med 252:983, 1955.

Rosenthal SR: BCG Vaccination Against Tuberculosis. Boston, Little, Brown & Co, Inc, 1957.

Rosenthal SR: The disk-tine tuberculin test (dried tuberculin-disposable unit). JAMA 177:452, 1961.

Rosenthal SR, Loewinsohn E, Graham ML et al: BCG vaccination against tuberculosis in Chicago. Pediatrics 28:622, 1941.

Rosenthal SR, Nikurs L, Yordy E et al: Tuberculin tine and Mantoux tests. Pediatrics 30:385, 1965.

Rudd RM, Gellert AR, and Venning M: Comparison of Mantoux, tine and "Imotest" tuberculin tests. Lancet 2:515, 1982.

Sbarbaro JA: Skin test antigens: an evaluation whose time has come. Am Rev Respir Dis 118:1, 1978.

Schaefer G, Zervoudakis IA, Fuchs FF, and Davis S: Pregnancy and pulmonary tuberculosis. Obstet Gynecol 46:706, 1975.

Scharer I and Smith JP: Serum transaminase elevations and other hepatic abnormalities in patients receiving isoniazid. Ann Int Med 71:1113, 1969.

Schlossberg D (ed): Tuberculosis. 2nd ed. New York, Springer-Verlag, 1988.

Sifontes JE: Rifampin in tuberculous meningitis. J Pediatr 87:1015, 1975.

Sinclair DJM and Johnson RN: Assessment of tine tuberculin test. Med Pract 1:1325, 1979.

Sippel JE, Mikhail IA, Girgis NI, and Youssef HH: Rifampin concentrations in cerebrospinal fluid of patients with tuberculous meningitis. Am Rev Respir Dis 109:579, 1974.

Smith MHD: What about short course and intermittent chemotherapy for tuberculosis in children? Pediatr Infect Dis J 1:298, 1982.

Snead WW and Dutt AK: Chemotherapy for tuberculosis today. Am Rev Respir Dis 125:94, 1982.

Snider DE Jr: Pregnancy and tuberculosis. Chest 86:10S, 1984.

Snider DE Jr: TB in children: time for short-course chemotherapy. J Respir Dis 8:70, 1987.

Snider DE Jr, Cohn DL, Davidson PT et al: Standard therapy for tuberculosis 1985. Chest 87:117S, 1985.

Snider DE Jr, Rieder HL, Combs D et al: Tuberculosis in children. Ped Infect Dis J 7:271, 1988.

Starke JR: Modern approach to the diagnosis and management of tuberculosis in children. Pediatr Clin North Am 35:464, 1988.

Starr S and Berkovich S: Effects of measles, gamma globulin modified measles and vaccine measles on the tuberculin test. N Engl J Med 270:386, 1964a.

Starr S and Berkovich S: The depression of tuberculin reactivity during chicken pox. Pediatrics 33:769, 1964b.

Steigman AJ and Kendig EL Jr: Frequency of tuberculin testing. Pediatrics 56:160, 1975.

Steiner P, Rao M, Goldberg R, and Steiner M: Primary drug resistance in children. Drug susceptibility of strains of *M. tuberculosis* isolated from children during the years 1969 to 1972 at the Kings County Hospital Medical Center of Brooklyn. Am Rev Respir Dis 110:98, 1974.

Sweet AY: Personal communication. In Infants of tuberculous mothers: further thoughts. Pediatrics 42:393, 1968.

Tardieu M, Truffot-Pernot C, Carriere JP et al: Tuberculous meningitis due to BCG in two previously healthy children. Lancet 1:440, 1988.

Tidjani O, Amedome A, and Ten Dam HG: The protective effect of BCG vaccination of the newborn against childhood tuberculosis in an African community. Tubercle 67:269, 1986.

Trial of BCG vaccines in South India for tuberculosis prevention. Ind J Med Res 70:349, 1979.

Tuberculosis Vaccines Clinical Trials Committee of the Medical Research Council: BCG and vole bacillus vaccine in the prevention of tuberculosis in adolescents. Br Med J 2:379, 1959.

Vanderhoof JA and Ament ME: Fatal hepatic necrosis due to isoniazid chemoprophylaxis in a fifteen year old girl. J Pediatr 89:867, 1976.

Wallgren A: Pulmonary tuberculosis: relation of childhood infection to the disease in adults. Lancet 1:417, 1938.

Wallgren A: Pulmonary tuberculosis in children. In Miller JA and Wallgren A: Pulmnary Tuberculosis in Adults and Children. New York, Thomas Nelson and Sons, 1939.

Wallgren A: The time table of tuberculosis. Tubercle 29:245, 1948.

Wasz-Höckert O: Variola vaccination as an activator of tuberculous infection. Ann Med Exp Biol Fenn 32:26, 1954.

Weg JG, Farer LS, Kaplan AI et al: Diagnostic standards and classification of tuberculosis and other mycobacterial diseases (14th ed). Am Rev Respir Dis 123:343, 1981.

Weinberger SE and Weiss ST: Pulmonary diseases. In Burrow GN and Ferris TF (eds): Medical Complications During Pregnancy. 3rd ed. Philadelphia, WB Saunders Co, 1988.

Wijsmuller G and Termini J: The tuberculin test: effects of storage and method of delivery on reaction size. Am Rev Respir Dis 107:267, 1973.

Wolinsky E: Non-tuberculous mycobacteria and associated diseases. Am Rev Respir Dis 119:446, 1979.

Zack MB and Fulkerson LL: Clinical reliability of stabilized and nonstabilized tuberculin-PPD. Am Rev Respir Dis 102:91, 1970.

49

EDWARD N. PATTISHALL, M.D., and
EDWIN L. KENDIG, JR., M.D.

SARCOIDOSIS

Sarcoidosis is a multisystem granulomatous disease of unknown cause. It appears to be relatively uncommon among children. In a review of the world literature to February of 1953, McGovern and Merritt (1956) were able to document only 104 cases in children under 16 years of age. Most of these were case reports of only a few children. In the United States, only 12 comprehensive series that include four or more children have been published, for a total of 254 cases. Other published series contain fewer children or describe a particular manifestation of the disease. The largest series includes 69 cases diagnosed at the Medical College of Virginia and 60 cases diagnosed at the University of North Carolina at Chapel Hill (Pattishall, Strope, and Denny, 1986). Many other cases of recognized sarcoidosis in children are undoubtedly still unreported, but the disease must be considered relatively uncommon in children.

The criteria for the diagnosis of sarcoidosis were outlined by James and co-workers (1976) and presented at the Seventh International Conference on Sarcoidosis:

> *Sarcoidosis is a multisystem granulomatous disorder of unknown etiology most commonly affecting young adults and presenting most frequently with bilateral hilar lymphadenopathy, pulmonary infiltration, skin or eye lesions. The diagnosis is established most securely*

when clinicoradiographic findings are supported by histological evidence of widespread noncaseating epithelioid cell granulomas in more than one organ or a positive Kveim-Siltzbach skin test. Immunological features are depression of delayed-type hypersensitivity suggesting impaired cell-mediated immunity and raised or abnormal immunoglobulins. There may also be hypercalciuria with or without hypercalcemia. The course and prognosis may correlate with the mode of onset: an acute onset with erythema nodosum heralds a self-limiting course and spontaneous resolution, while an insidious onset may be followed by relentless progressive fibrosis. Corticosteroids relieve symptoms and suppress inflammation and granuloma formation.

HISTORICAL BACKGROUND

Sarcoidosis was first described in England by Hutchinson in 1875, when he described a girl with "relapsing iritis of inherited gout." Besnier described a case of lupus pernio in 1889, and Tenneson described the histology of lupus pernio in 1892. The first unequivocal case of sarcoidosis was described by Boeck in 1899. He was impressed by the close resemblance of the disease to sarcoma, hence the name *benign sarcoid* (Kerdel and Maschella, 1984). Contributions clarifying certain clinical and pathologic features were also made by Heerfordt (1909), Schaumann (1917), Garland and Thompson (1933), and Longcope and Pierson (1937).

The use of mass radiography, introduced in many countries in an effort to detect tuberculosis (about the time of World War II), led to a significant advance in the knowledge of sarcoidosis. This method, first used in the Armed Forces and later in the general population, led to the finding of a high incidence of presumptive asymptomatic sarcoidosis.

EPIDEMIOLOGY

Incidence and Prevalence

The incidence and prevalence of sarcoidosis in children are unknown. Some researchers have suggested that the incidence in children is as high as in adults and that the prevalence in adults is high because of the chronicity of the disease (Fanburg, 1983; Clark, 1987). In adults, studies of incidence and prevalence have been highly variable and suffer from different methods of case ascertainment, different case definitions, and an unknown population at risk. The incidence and prevalence are influenced by age, race, and geographic location.

Age. Sarcoidosis is encountered more frequently in adults between 20 and 50 years of age, but the disease may occur at any age. Although the youngest patient reported was a 2-month-old infant, most of the cases reported in children have occurred in preadolescents and adolescents. About 68 per cent of patients from both the Medical College of Virginia and the University of North Carolina series were between the ages of 9 and 16. There may be a bimodal distribution of age at diagnosis, with a peak in adolescence and another in early adulthood.

Race. There is a great variation in the racial incidence dependent on the geographic location. In Europe, and particularly in the Scandinavian countries, sarcoidosis is relatively common and occurs largely in the white population. In Japan, there is a relatively high prevalence of sarcoidosis in Orientals. In the United States, sarcoidosis occurs much more commonly in blacks. In three radiographic surveys of the United States Armed Forces, blacks with sarcoidosis outnumbered whites, with the disease in a ratio varying from 7:1 to 26:1. Cummings and co-workers (1956) reported the hospitalization rate for black and white World War II veterans with sarcoidosis to be 40.1 and 3.3:100,000 respectively.

James (1976) has pointed out that in South Africa the Bantus are affected 10 times more frequently than are whites. He concludes that sarcoidosis is most frequently recognized in sophisticated communities with adequate diagnostic facilities and that the racial incidence is the same throughout the world: Blacks predominate in a ratio of 10:1.

Of the 129 children from the Medical College of Virginia and the University of North Carolina, 94 (73 per cent) were black.

Geography. Sarcoidosis has been observed almost everywhere in the world. Sweden has the highest reported incidence of the disease, ranging from 40:100,000 up to 140:100,000. Japan also has a relatively high incidence.

In the United States, reports by Michael and co-workers (1950), Gentry and colleagues (1955) and Cummings and associates (1956) of the birthplace and residence of persons in the Armed Forces indicate that the areas with the highest prevalence are in the South Atlantic and Gulf states, with endemic areas in New England and the Midwest. Nansemond County, Virginia, appears to have the highest incidence of sarcoidosis, with a projected incidence of presumptive disease of 500 per 100,000 population.* The coastal plain of the southeastern section of the United States appears to be a specific area with high incidence. Of the 12 previous large series in children, 10 were from the southeastern or south central United States.

Sex. The sexes appear to be affected with equal frequency. In the Medical College of Virginia and University of North Carolina series, 61 (47 per cent) were females.

Heredity. There have been occasional reports of familial aggregations of cases. These suggest that genetic factors may significantly predispose to the development of sarcoidosis (Brennan et al, 1984). No consistent human lymphocyte antigen (HLA) has been identified in patients tested (Bresnitz and Strom, 1983).

---

*Apperson WE: Unpublished data, Commonwealth of Virginia, Health Dept., Richmond, Va.

ETIOLOGY, PATHOGENESIS, AND IMMUNOLOGY

The cause of sarcoidosis is unknown. A combination of environmental and host factors probably cause the characteristic response. If an exogenous agent is the cause of sarcoidosis, its portal of entry is unknown. The occurrence of mediastinal adenopathy suggests air-borne transmission. Siltzbach (1967) has suggested an environmental origin, because the numerous microbial and chemical sensitivities known to precipitate an attack of erythema nodosum all are of exogenous origin. Investigations have included soil types, proximity to pine forests, exposure to beryllium, and other environmental factors (Bresnitz and Strom, 1983). The only consistent finding has been an association with rural residence. Investigations searching for the active agent in the Kveim-Siltzbach reagent have been fruitless (Teirstein, 1986).

The racial and familial data suggest that host factors may be important as well. An immune dysfunction has been hypothesized and is supported by increased immunoglobulins in patients with sarcoidosis (hyperactive B cells), relative insensitivity to tuberculin as well as other delayed hypersensitivity antigens, and an immune response characterized by an intense alveolitis. Studies by Crystal and colleagues (1983), Hunninghake and Crystal (1981), and Rosen and associates (1978) suggest an intense alveolitis characterized by a mononuclear infiltrate consisting of macrophages and lymphocytes. Activated T cells and macrophages cooperate to increase the number of inflammatory cells that promote a diffuse alveolitis and granuloma formation and ultimately fibrosis. The cause of the initial activation is unknown. It is possible that one or more antigens cause activation in a susceptible host.

An example of the combination of host factors and environmental exposure is the prevalence of sarcoidosis found in mass chest radiographic surveys in London and Ireland. The prevalence per 100,000 of those living in London was 27 for those born in Britain, rising to 97 in Irish men and 213 in Irish women. These figures compare with a rate of 40 for people born and living in Ireland. It has been suggested that this distribution may be due to an exposure of the Irish to some factor to which the indigenous population in London has become relatively immune (James and Williams, 1985).

CLINICAL MANIFESTATIONS

Lesions can occur in almost any tissue or organ. Because symptoms are due primarily to local tissue infiltration and injury by pressure and displacement by sarcoid lesions, the clinical manifestations depend largely on the organ or system involved.

As noted earlier, sarcoidosis most commonly involves the lungs, lymph nodes, eyes, skin, liver, spleen, and, to a lesser extent, phalangeal bones (Table 49–1). In addition, because of the characteristic multisystem involvement, more than one system is usually affected. In the University of North Carolina series, 75 per cent of children had five or more different areas of involvement.

Most of the reported cases are children with symptoms. Only 10 per cent of the children from the Medical College of Virginia and the University of North Carolina were asymptomatic. The symptoms are often nonspecific and most commonly include weight loss, cough, fatigue/lethargy, lymphadenitis, visual disturbances, or skin rashes and less commonly include fever, bone and joint pain, headache, dyspnea, parotid gland enlargement, chest pain, abdominal pain, or nausea.

The physical findings are also due to local infiltration of lesions and most commonly cause peripheral lymphadenopathy, eye changes, skin rashes, liver or spleen enlargement, and less commonly auscultatory findings on chest examination, musculoskeletal abnormalities, parotid gland enlargement, cardiovascular changes, or neurologic changes.

Lungs

Symptoms referable to the chest are usually mild and often consist of a dry, hacking cough. Affected children are likely to have mild to moderate dyspnea. On physical examination, findings may include crackles, rhonchi, wheezing, and decreased breath sounds; however, in most, the physical examination of the chest is normal.

By international convention, the radiographic findings are classified as follows: stage 0—normal chest radiograph; stage 1—bilateral hilar lymphadenopathy, without detectable lung changes (Fig. 49–1); stage 2—bilateral hilar lymphadenopathy with pulmonary infiltrations, which may be fine or coarse miliary nodulation or may have a cotton-wool appearance (Fig. 49–2); and stage 3—fibrosis with formation of bullae and without hilar lymphadenopathy (Fig. 49–3).

The most common roentgenographic finding in children is bilateral hilar lymph node enlargement, with or without lung changes (see Figs. 49–1 and 49–

Table 49–1 COMPARISON OF ORGANS AFFECTED IN THE WORLD GROUP AND MEDICAL COLLEGE OF VIRGINIA SERIES

	McGovern & Merritt (113)	Medical College of Virginia (69)	University of North Carolina (60)
Lungs (parenchyma—hilar lymph nodes)	62	67	56
Peripheral lymphadenopathy	54	38	35
Skin	57	16	24
Eyes	55	16	32
Bones	33	4	2
Spleen	25	11	16
Liver	16	13	20

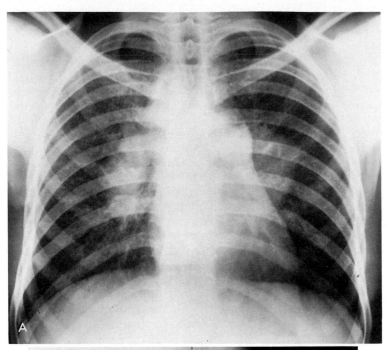

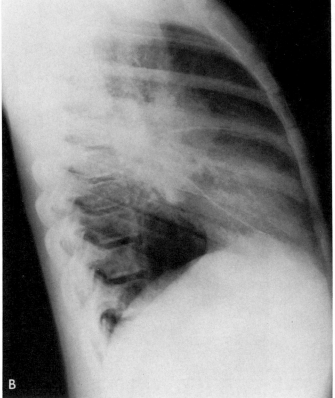

Figure 49–1. Stage 1: bilateral hilar lymph node enlargement.

2). In a worldwide review of sarcoidosis, James and co-workers (1976) noted involvement of the lungs and hilar lymph nodes in 92 per cent of adult cases. In the 128 children from the Medical College of Virginia and the University of North Carolina, 90 per cent of cases had adenopathy (45 per cent with and 45 per cent without parenchymal involvement), whereas 6 per cent had parenchymal involvement

alone and 4 per cent had a normal chest radiograph. The adenopathy was most commonly hilar but occasionally was paratracheal. Atelectasis was noted in three of the cases at the Medical College of Virginia and University of North Carolina and pericardial effusion in another. Pleural effusions have also been reported in children.

Pulmonary function tests most commonly reveal

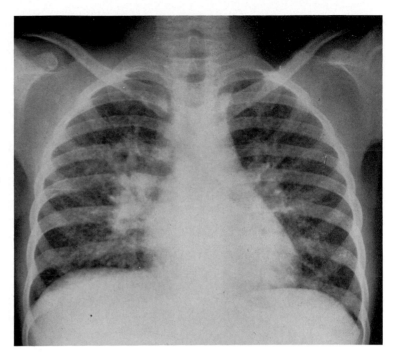

Figure 49–2. Stage 2: bilateral hilar lymph node enlargement and pulmonary infiltration.

changes consistent with restrictive lung disease. There have been few studies of lung function in children. In 50 per cent of the cases tested in the University of North Carolina series, there were restrictive changes. Obstructive changes were also present in a few individuals.

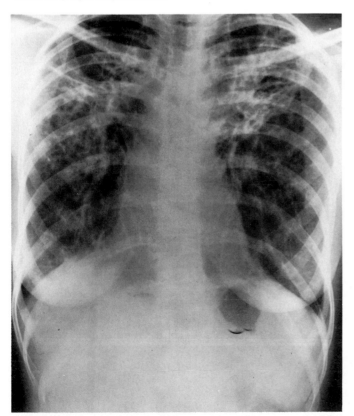

Figure 49–3. Stage 3: sarcoidosis, showing fibrosis with bullae and without hilar lymphadenopathy.

Lymphatics

Similar to the preponderance of adenopathy on chest radiographs, peripheral lymphadenopathy is the most common physical finding in children with sarcoidosis. The nodes are discrete, painless, and freely movable. The typical histologic picture includes epithelioid cell tubercles, showing little or no necrosis (Fig. 49–4).

Peripheral lymphadenopathy occurred in 58 per cent of 127 children from the Medical College of Virginia and the University of North Carolina. Most of the time, a peripheral lymph node yields the typical histologic changes.

Eyes

The ocular involvement of sarcoidosis is usually classified into anterior segment disease, posterior segment disease, and orbital or other disease. Anterior segment disease is the most common, consisting of chronic granulomatous uveitis, acute iritis, and conjunctival granulomas. Secondary complications from inflammation include iris synechiae, iris nodules, corneal band keratopathy, glaucoma, and cataracts (Hoover et al, 1986; Liggett, 1986). Posterior segment disease is less common and consists of periphlebitis, vitreous cells or opacities, macular edema, chorioretinal granulomas, peripheral retinal neovascularization, optic nerve edema, and optic nerve granulomas. Orbital involvement occurs rarely and can cause proptosis. Other ocular syndromes associated with sarcoidosis include Heerfordt syndrome, Lofgren syndrome, and Mikulicz syndrome.

Involvement of the eye with resultant partial or total blindness is one of the most feared lesions. McGovern and Merritt (1956) found in their review

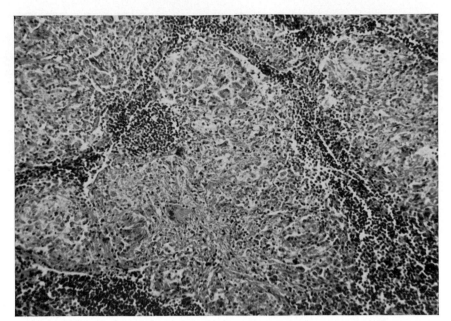

Figure 49–4. The architecture of the node is distorted by numerous solid masses of epithelioid cells with occasional giant cells. The masses are surrounded by lymphocytes. No necrosis or caseation is apparent. Lymphoid follicles are almost absent. (Reproduced with permission from Kendig EL Jr et al: Sarcoidosis: report of three cases in siblings under fifteen years of age. N Engl J Med 26:962, 1959.)

of the world literature that eye lesions in children usually did not appear to be severe; however, they noted one case of partial blindness in their own series. Since that time, it has become clear that the eyes are often involved, and abnormalities of the eyes were the second most common physical findings in the 60 children from the University of North Carolina series. Dresner and colleagues (1986) found that only 44 per cent of patients were referred to an ophthalmologist, even though more than half of those examined manifested signs and symptoms of ocular sarcoidosis. Slit-lamp examination is an integral part of the physical examination.

Skin

Skin lesions in sarcoidosis are common and are varied. Elgart (1986) categorized lesions into specific skin lesions that on biopsy reveal noncaseating granulomas, and nonspecific skin lesions that are secondary processes. The common specific lesions include papules, plaques and nodules (including lupus pernio and psoriasiform lesions), subcutaneous nodules, changes in old scars, and lacrimal and salivary gland enlargement. Uncommon specific lesions include erythroderma, ulcerations, verrucous lesions, pustules, ichthyosis, and nail involvement. Nonspecific lesions include erythema nodosum, erythema multiforme, calcifications, and prurigo. Sarcoid skin lesions may vary in color from waxy and depigmented to reddish blue or violaceous. Their diameter ranges from a few millimeters to more than a centimeter.

Veien and colleagues (1987) described skin changes in 188 adults with sarcoidosis and found that lupus pernio, scar infiltrates, and plaque lesions were the most common and were typically chronic. Although James reported the incidence of skin lesions in adults to be only 9 per cent, such lesions may be more

common in children. In children, skin changes were found in 23 and 42 per cent of the Medical College of Virginia and University of North Carolina series, respectively. Erythema nodosum often accompanies acute sarcoidosis in adults but is rare in children. To our knowledge, lupus pernio has not been reported in children.

The Kidneys and Calcium Metabolism

Kogut and Neumann (1961) found fewer than 10 reported cases of renal involvement in children. However, in more recent series, the involvement appears to be more commonly recognized. Renal involvement can be caused by one or more of the following processes: (1) sarcoid granulomas infiltrating the renal parenchyma, (2) glomerulitis with basement membrane changes, and (3) hypercalcemia with or without nephrolithiasis and nephrocalcinosis. Abnormal urinary findings may include proteinuria, pyuria, hematuria, granular casts, and calciuria. Results of urinalyses were abnormal in 38 per cent of children in the University of North Carolina series. In addition, a high proportion of children had a decreased creatinine clearance, increased serum creatinine, or increased blood urea nitrogen.

Five children in the University of North Carolina series developed nephrolithiasis. Hypercalcemia was present in 31 per cent of children in that series, and hypercalciuria was present in 67 per cent, although only a small number of children were tested. The hypercalcemia and hypercalciuria, once thought to be caused by hyperparathyroidism or abnormal vitamin D responsiveness, appear to be caused by overactivity of calcitriol, which may be due to an extrarenal source of vitamin D (Barbour et al, 1981). The overactivity of calcitriol causes increased intestinal calcium absorption, leading to hypercalcemia and hypercalciuria. Laboratory evaluation of calcium metabolism is important in the evaluation and management of sarcoidosis in children.

Uveoparotid Fever

The syndrome of uveoparotid fever, consisting of ocular disturbances, parotid gland swelling, and often facial nerve palsy, was first described by Heerfordt in 1909. Uveitis is always present at some time in the course of this syndrome. A low-grade fever, gastrointestinal symptoms, and general malaise usually precede the eye involvement. In the world literature reported by McGovern and Merritt (1956), 25 per cent of cases had this syndrome. Since that time it has been reported rarely, and there were no cases in the Medical College of Virginia or the University of North Carolina series.

Bones and Joints

Lytic bone lesions have been described and consist of "punched-out" areas usually located in the metacarpals, metatarsals, and distal phalanges. Bone involvement is usually found in patients with chronic skin lesions. The incidence of osseous lesions in adults has been reported to be 2 to 29 per cent. Among children, 29 per cent of cases in the world literature reported by McGovern and Merritt (1956) had lytic lesions, whereas only about 6 per cent of the Medical College of Virginia and the University of North Carolina series had lytic bone lesions. It appears that bone lesions are not as common as previously suspected.

Joint involvement can cause acute polyarthritis, a chronic arthropathy, and changes associated with bone lesions. Although a transient arthralgia may not be uncommon (eight cases in the Medical College of Virginia series), granulomas are rarely found in joint tissue. In the University of North Carolina series, 14 per cent of children had physical abnormalities of the musculoskeletal system. Because arthropathy and uveitis are relatively common manifestations in young children with sarcoidosis (see below), differentiation from juvenile rheumatoid arthritis may be difficult (Lindsley and Godfrey, 1985; Mallory et al, 1987).

Liver

Although hepatic involvement is found in 60 to 80 per cent of patients by biopsy or autopsy, clinical manifestations are not as apparent (Klatskin, 1976; Neville et al, 1975). Liver enlargement is the usual finding and was present in 37 per cent of cases in the University of North Carolina series and 19 per cent of the Medical College of Virginia series. In the University of North Carolina series, 25 to 50 per cent of children had elevated results on liver function tests (alanine aminotransferase and aspartate aminotransferase). Needle biopsy examination of the liver may be an effective diagnostic aid when physical or laboratory abnormalities are present.

Spleen

Although splenic involvement may be demonstrated by needle biopsy examination, enlargement is almost the only clinical finding. The spleen was palpably enlarged in 27 per cent of the University of North Carolina series and 16 per cent of the Medical College of Virginia series.

Heart

As with other organs, lesions of the myocardium have been described. Although there have been only a few reports of heart involvement, it is probably much underdiagnosed. Silverman and colleagues (1978) found 25 per cent of cases with cardiac involvement at necropsy in adults. Cardiac involvement was found in six of the cases reviewed by McGovern and Merritt but only one patient in the Medical College of Virginia series. Cardiac changes may be secondary to extensive pulmonary involvement or the result of conduction aberrations caused by sarcoid lesions.

Nervous System

Neurosarcoidosis may produce symptoms from involvement of cranial nerves, peripheral nerves, and the central nervous system. Although facial nerve involvement is the most common clinical finding, Oksanen (1986) reported finding central nervous system lesions in 66 per cent, cranial nerve lesions in 24 per cent, and peripheral nerve lesions in 10 per cent of patients with neurosarcoidosis. Optic nerve involvement, pituitary-hypothalamic lesions, meningitis, hydrocephalus, seizures, and psychiatric manifestations have also been reported. Four of the 129 children in the Medical College of Virginia and the University of North Carolina series had neurologic symptoms.

Endocrine Glands

Sarcoidosis may affect the pituitary gland. Diabetes insipidus has been reported in adults, and three of the children in the review by McGovern and Merritt had evidence of diabetes insipidus. None of the Medical College of Virginia or the University of North Carolina series had the disorder.

SUMMARY

The clinical picture of sarcoidosis is widely variable. The most common picture in children from the United States is a black adolescent from the southeast presenting with vague symptoms of weight loss, cough, and fatigue with hilar lymphadenopathy on chest radiograph, peripheral lymphadenopathy, and a large proportion with eye findings, skin involvement, and possibly a calcium metabolism derangement.

SARCOIDOSIS IN VERY YOUNG CHILDREN

Although the onset of sarcoidosis in children is usually between 8 and 15 years of age, the disease has also been reported in 28 children less than 4 years of age, and the clinical manifestations appear to be different in these young children. Although older children usually have involvement in the lungs, lymph nodes, and eyes, Hetherington (1982) reported that children younger than 4 years old usually have involvement of the skin, joints, and eyes without much lung involvement.

LABORATORY MANIFESTATIONS

Among the most common laboratory changes, aside from the radiographic changes that were previously discussed, are hyperglobulinemia, elevated erythrocyte sedimentation rate (ESR), eosinophilia, leukopenia, hypercalcemia, hypercalciuria, and elevated alkaline phosphatase level.

Serum Proteins. Hyperproteinemia is due to an absolute increase in serum globulin, and the ratio of albumin to globulin is frequently reversed. Forty-five per cent of the University of North Carolina children had an elevated total protein, whereas 26 per cent had a decreased serum albumin. In that series, 88 per cent of children tested had elevated gamma globulins. Serum IgG, IgM, and IgA levels all are elevated during the acute phase of the disease.

Hypercalcemia and Hypercalciuria. Hypercalcemia occurs in about 11 per cent of adult patients (James et al, 1976). Serum calcium concentration above 11 mg/100 ml was noted in 7 of the 36 Medical College of Virginia patients and in 17 of the 56 University of North Carolina patients tested. In the University of North Carolina series, 8 of 12 patients tested had hypercalciuria.

Liver Function Tests. Although the serum alkaline phosphatase level can be elevated in sarcoidosis, it is unclear how often this occurs because retrospective interpretation of results is hampered by the use of different measurement units and standards.

The serum glutamic-oxaloacetic transaminase and serum glutamic-pyruvic transaminase may also be elevated in patients with sarcoidosis and are thought to reflect liver involvement. In the University of North Carolina series, 35 to 45 per cent of children tested had elevated transaminase levels.

Eosinophilia. Next to hyperglobulinemia, the most consistent laboratory finding among the Medical College of Virginia patients was eosinophilia. This occurred in about 45 per cent of children tested in the Medical College of Virginia and the University of North Carolina series.

Erythrocyte Sedimentation Rate. Evaluation of the ESR is naturally expected during the acute phase of the disease. Of those children tested in the University of North Carolina series, 74 per cent had an elevated ESR. This is a nonspecific finding that may reflect disease activity.

Leukopenia. Leukopenia was noted in 12 of the 43 Medical College of Virginia patients and in 22 of the 56 children tested in the University of North Carolina series.

Urinary Findings. Abnormal urinary findings are present when there is renal involvement. The abnormalities may include hematuria, pyuria, proteinuria, granular casts, and hypercalciuria.

CORROBORATIVE DIAGNOSTIC PROCEDURES

The diagnosis usually depends on tissue confirmation in a patient with a compatible clinical course. The diagnosis of sarcoidosis cannot be made by any specific laboratory test, and it must be recognized that none of the tests are specific and only supply corroborative evidence of the disease.

Biopsy

Biopsy of a lymph node or other tissue with demonstration of an epithelioid cell tubercle, with little or no necrosis, is essential for diagnosis. Most investigations report cases corroborated by biopsy and include specimens from peripheral lymph nodes, skin, lungs, mediastinal lymph nodes, liver, conjunctiva, minor salivary glands, muscle, bone, and nasal mucosa. Although a mediastinal lymph node has been the "gold standard" tissue for biopsy, in the Medical College of Virginia and the University of North Carolina series a peripheral lymph node was the most common tissue subjected to biopsy and was positive in most children. If no enlarged peripheral lymph node is present, the scalene fat pad is most likely to reveal a lesion compatible with sarcoidosis. Minor salivary glands, conjunctiva, and nasal mucosa are easily accessible for biopsy, and results are especially rewarding when visible lesions are present. A transbronchial biopsy via flexible fiberoptic bronchoscopy is a reasonable method of obtaining lung tissue. Needle aspiration of the liver also appears to be productive in obtaining histologic confirmation of granuloma.

The Kveim Test

The Kveim test represents an attempt to elicit a specific skin reaction by the intracutaneous injection of emulsified sarcoid tissue into patients with suspected sarcoidosis. Methods for preparing Kveim suspension have changed since Williams and Nickerson (1935), Kveim (1941), and Danbolt (1951) first published their work, and the current method of preparation was described by Chase in 1961 and recently reviewed by Teirstein (1986). The intracutaneous test is performed in the manner of a Mantoux test, with the use of 0.15 to 0.2 ml per injection. Biopsy is performed on any nodule that appears at the injection site, no matter how small, after 28 to 42 days. Some studies have shown that about 60 per cent of patients with sarcoidosis have a positive test, and fewer than 1 per cent have false-positive reactions (Hurley and Bartholomeusz, 1971). Other studies have shown a higher false-positive rate. Although Siltzbach (1968) reports a positive Kveim reaction in 16 of 18 children, scarcity of effective Kveim test material limits the usefulness of the test at this time.

Angiotensin-Converting Enzyme

It has been established that serum angiotensin-converting enzyme (ACE) is elevated in patients with active sarcoidosis. The source of the increased level is unknown, although increased production has been documented in granulomas of skin lesions (Takemura et al, 1987) and in alveolar macrophages (Stanislas-Leguern et al, 1986). Although assay of serum ACE does not replace histologic documentation of noncaseating granuloma with exclusion of mycobacterial and fungal causes, the test is a useful adjunct in confirming the diagnosis of sarcoidosis in children. In children, 57 per cent of those tested in the University of North Carolina series had elevated ACE (Pattishall, Strope, and Denny, 1986). Rodriguez and colleagues (1981), at the Medical College of Virginia, found that 80 per cent of children with sarcoidosis had elevated ACE.

Serum levels of ACE must be interpreted with caution because different assay methods with different normal values are used and most laboratories do not have standardized values for children, who are reported to have higher values than adults. When the ACE level is elevated, serial determinations appear to be a useful index to evaluate activity of the disease or to assess the effectiveness of corticosteroid therapy.

Pulmonary Function Tests

Pulmonary sarcoidosis is a restrictive lung disease. In the Medical College of Virginia and University of North Carolina series, most children tested had the characteristic functional changes of restrictive lung disease (Kendig and Brummer, 1976; Pattishall, Strope, Spinola, and Denny, 1986). Some children also have obstructive changes.

Other Tests

A renewed interest in sarcoidosis has resulted from studies using cells obtained by bronchoalveolar lavage. Studies show an increase of three to five times the normal number of lymphocytes and macrophages in the lung, with disproportionate represention by T-lymphocytes (especially helper T cells), which cause the ratio of helper to suppressor cells to be as high as 10:1. The changes are not specific for sarcoidosis but have been used to evaluate disease activity over time in adults. There are no data on the use of this technique in children.

Gallium scanning has also been used as an indicator of disease activity in the lungs. It has not been used in children and appears to have limited clinical utility in adults.

Tests to rule out other diseases include the tuberculin test and complement fixation studies for both histoplasmosis and coccidioidomycosis and should be performed on each patient with suspected sarcoidosis. Although a positive result of either test does not necessarily controvert the diagnosis, it may be an indication that the disease is merely an infection that simulates sarcoidosis.

PROGNOSIS

Sones and Israel (1960), in a review of more than 200 adult patients in Philadelphia, found that sarcoidosis is neither as benign as indicated in some reports nor as malignant as in others. They found survival rates of 88.8 per cent after 5 years of observation and 84.8 per cent after 10 years. Zych and colleagues (1987) found in 960 patients that 20 per cent had an acute course, whereas in 80 per cent the disease was symptomless, often of chronic nature. Spontaneous remission occurred in 62 per cent.

Determination of the prognosis of the disease in children is not easy. Hetherington (1982) reported that long-term sequelae occur in 10 to 20 per cent. Of 28 children followed at the Medical College of Virginia for an average of 9 years, 5 sustained severe damage from the disease; 2 of these are blind, and 3 others developed severe restrictive pulmonary disease (Kendig and Brummer, 1976). One with severe restrictive lung disease has died since the original study on prognosis was reported. In the University of North Carolina series, most had considerable improvement in the clinical manifestations, chest radiographs, and pulmonary function tests; however, 40 per cent were still symptomatic and 35 per cent had physical abnormalities after an average follow-up of about 5 years. Two of those children eventually died of the disease. Therefore, it appears that most children improve; however, significant numbers have severe complications.

Although the presence of skin lesions in children with sarcoidosis has suggested a guarded prognosis in some studies, the outcome of any given case does not seem predictable.

EVALUATION

Sarcoidosis is a multisystem disease and can be manifested in many organs. Because there is no specific test for the disease, arrival at the diagnosis can be frustrating; however, in most instances the diagnosis is not problematic and depends on identifying typical pathologic features in combination with a compatible clinical presentation.

Most commonly, sarcoidosis is suspected after abnormalities are noted on chest radiograph. A complete history and physical examination may lead to specific organ systems that should be investigated. The biopsy is the most important diagnostic procedure. A peripheral lymph node is usually the most accessible tissue for biopsy, but abnormalities of skin, conjunctiva, minor salivary glands, or other tissues suggest histologic evaluation of that abnormality. An ophthalmologic evaluation, including slit-lamp examination, is mandatory. A thorough laboratory evaluation including chest radiograph, serum ACE level, renal function tests, pulmonary function tests, serum and 24-hour urinary calcium, ESR, eosinophil count, liver function tests, and serum proteins may help in defining the disease. To rule out other diagnoses, a tuberculin skin test and complement fixation for coccidioidomycosis and histiocytosis should be performed.

TREATMENT

Once a diagnosis is made, a child should be monitored with periodic clinic visits to evaluate organ system involvement through history and physical examination. Serial chest radiographs, pulmonary function tests, ACE levels, ESR, serum and urinary calcium, and other tests that produced abnormal results at the initial evaluation should be performed to follow the activity of the disease. Periodic ophthalmologic evaluations should also be performed.

Because the cause of sarcoidosis is unknown, there is no known specific therapy. Adrenocorticosteroids are the agents most commonly used to suppress the acute manifestations of the disease. These are usually reserved for acute episodes with progressive lung changes, persistent abnormalities of calcium metabolism, eye changes not controlled by local therapy, disfiguring cutaneous and lymph node lesions, joint involvement, or severe constitutional symptoms.

Zych and colleagues (1987) found spontaneous remission or improvement in 62 per cent of patients, compared with 84 per cent remission or improvement after treatment with adrenocorticosteroids. There are numerous reports of benefits after treatment with adrenocorticosteroids, although most studies suffer from the lack of a controlled design.

Fresh lesions appear more responsive than older ones. Suppressive action is often temporary, but it is beneficial when the unremitting course of the disease will produce loss of organ function. For example, adrenocorticosteroids can reduce the level of serum calcium and may thus help prevent nephrocalcinosis, renal insufficiency, and possibly band keratitis. Whether adrenocorticosteroids should be used in the

treatment of patients whose disease consists only of asymptomatic miliary nodules or bronchopneumonic patches in the lung fields is debatable.

The initial dose of prednisone or prednisolone is 1 mg/kg/day, and of triamcinolone, 0.75 mg/kg/day in three or four divided doses. A gradual reduction in the dose of adrenocorticosteroid is initiated as soon as clinical manifestations of the disease disappear. A maintenance dose of prednisone (15 mg every other day) is continued until a patient has received at least a 6-month total course of treatment. Siltzbach (1968) and Zych and colleagues (1987) reported the frequent occurrence of temporary relapse after the discontinuation of adrenocorticosteroid therapy but noted that improvement usually follows even if the treatment is not resumed.

In the management of ocular sarcoidosis, adrenocorticosteroids in the form of either ointment or drops (0.5 to 1 per cent) are used in conjunction with their systemic form. During the course of such local therapy, the pupils are kept in a state of continuous dilation by use of an atropine ointment (1 per cent).

Adrenocorticosteroid ointment may also be used in the treatment of cutaneous lesions, but better results are obtained when used in conjunction with systemic therapy.

Other drugs occasionally used in the treatment of sarcoidosis in adults (oxyphenbutazone, chloroquine, potassium para-aminobenzoate, and azathioprine) have had little use in children. Cholchicine has been used to treat sarcoid arthritis in children (Rubinstein and Baum, 1986), but the experience is limited and published reports are conflicting.

REFERENCES

Abernathy RS: Childhood sarcoidosis in Arkansas. South Med J 78:435, 1985.
Anderson J, Dent CE, Harper C, and Philpot GR: Effect of cortisone on calcium metabolism in sarcoidosis with hypercalcaemia; possible antagonistic action of cortisone and vitamin D. Lancet 2:720, 1954.
Barbour GL, Coburn JW, Slatopolsky E et al: Hypercalcemia in an anephric patient with sarcoidosis: evidence for extrarenal generation of 1,25-dihydroxyvitamin D. N Engl J Med 305:440, 1981.
Barker DHW: Benign lymphogranulomatosis with apparent involvement of the anterior pituitary. Br J Dermatol 58:70, 1946.
Bauer HJ and Gentz C: The results of mass x-ray examination in Stockholm City during the years 1949–1951. Acta Tuberc Scand 29:22, 1953.
Beier FR and Lahey ME: Sarcoidosis among children in Utah and Idaho. J Pediatr 65:350, 1964.
Berger KW and Relman AS: Renal impairment due to sarcoid infiltration of the kidney; report of a case proved by renal biopsies before and after treatment with cortisone. N Engl J Med 252:44, 1955.
Besnier E: Lupus pernio de la face, synovitis fongueses (scrofulotuberculeuses) symétriques des extrémités supérieures. Ann Dermatol Syphiligr 10:333, 1889.
Boeck C: Multiple benign sarkoid of skin. J Cutan Genitourin Dis 17:543, 1899.
Boman A: Diabetes insipidus vid lymphogranulomatosis benigna. Nord Med 47:675, 1952.
Brennan NJ, Crean P, Long JP, and Fitzgerald MX: High preva-

lence of familial sarcoidosis in an Irish population. Thorax 39:14, 1984.

Bresnitz EA and Strom BL: Epidemiology of sarcoidosis. Epidemiol Rev 5:124, 1983.

Chapman JS: Notes on the secondary factors involved in the etiology of sarcoidosis. Am Rev Tuberc 71:459, 1955.

Chase MW: The preparation and standardization of Kveim testing antigens. Am Rev Respir Dis 84:86, 1961.

Clark SK: Sarcoidosis in children. Pediatr Dermatol 4:291, 1987.

Cummings MM and Dunner E: Pulmonary sarcoidosis. Med Clin North Am 43:163, 1959.

Cummings MM and Hudgins PC: Chemical constituents of pine pollen and their possible relationship to sarcoidosis. Am J Med Sci 236:311, 1958.

Cummings MM, Dunner E, Schmidt RH Jr, and Barnwell JB: Concepts of epidemiology of sarcoidosis. Postgrad Med 19:437, 1956.

Crystal RG, Bitterman PB, Rennard SI et al: Interstitial lung diseases of unknown cause: disorders characterized by chronic inflammation of the lower respiratory tract. N Engl J Med 310:235, 1983.

Danbolt N: On the skin test with sarcoid-tissue-suspension (Kveim's reaction). Acta Derm Venereol 31:184, 1951.

Dressler M: Ueber einem Fall von Splenomegalie, durch Sternalpunktion als Boecksche Krankheit verifiziert. Klin Wochenschr 2:1467, 1938.

Dresner MS, Brecher R, and Henkind P: Ophthalmology consultation in the diagnosis and treatment of sarcoidosis. Arch Intern Med 146:301, 1986.

Dunner E, Cummings MM, Williams JH et al: A new look at sarcoidosis, a review of clinical records of 160 patients with a diagnosis of sarcoidosis. South Med J 50:1141, 1957.

Elgart ML: Cutaneous sarcoidosis: definitions and types of lesions. Clin Dermatol 4:35, 1986.

Fanburg BL: Arcoidosis and other granulomatous diseases of the lung. New York, Marcel Dekker, Inc, 1983.

Garland HG and Thompson JG: Uveoparotid tuberculosis (febris uveoparotid of Heerfordt). Q J Med 2:157, 1933.

Gentry JT, Nitowsky HM, and Michael M Jr: Studies on the epidemiology of sarcoidosis in the United States; the relationship to soil areas and to urban-rural residence. J Clin Invest 34:1839, 1955.

Gilg I: Klinische undersogelser over Boeck's sarcoid (Sarcoidose): behandling og forlob. Ugeskr Laeger 118:46, 1956.

Gleckler WJ: Hypercalcemia and renal insufficiency due to sarcoidosis: treatment with cortisone. Ann Intern Med 44:174, 1956.

Heerfordt CF: Ueber eine "Febris uveoparotidea subschronica," an der Glandula Parotis und der Uvea des Auges lokalisiert und haufig mit Paresen cerebrospinaler Herven kompliaiert. Arch Ophthalmol 70:254, 1909.

Henneman PH, Carroll EL, and Dempsey EF: The mechanism responsible for hypercalciuria in sarcoid. J Clin Invest 33:941, 1954.

Henneman PH, Dempsey EF, Carroll EL, and Albright F: The cause of hypercalciuria in sarcoid and its treatment with cortisone and sodium phytate. J Clin Invest 35:1229, 1956.

Hetherington S: Sarcoidosis in young children. Am J Dis Child 136:13, 1982.

Holt JF and Owens WI: The osseous lesions of sarcoidosis. Radiology 53:11, 1949.

Hoover DL, Khan JA, and Giangiacomo J: Pediatric ocular sarcoidosis. Surv Ophthalmol 30:215, 1986.

Huchinson J: Cases of Mortimer's malady (lupus vulgaris multiplex nonulcerans et nonserpigeneous). Arch Surg (London) 9:307, 1898.

Hunninghake GW and Crystal RG: Pulmonary sarcoidosis: a disorder mediated by excess helper T-lymphocyte activity at sites of disease activity. N Engl J Med 305:429, 1981.

Hurley TH and Bartholomeusz CL: An international Siltzbach-Kveim test study using an Australian (C.S.L.) test material (1966–1969). In Levinsky L and Macholda F (eds): Proceedings of the fifth international congress on sarcoidosis. Prague, Univ. of Karlova, 1971.

Israel HL and Sones M: Sarcoidosis: clinical observations on 160 cases. Arch Intern Med 102:766, 1958.

James DG and Williams WJ: Sarcoidosis and Other Granulomatous Disorders. Philadelphia, WB Saunders Co, 1985.

James DG: Ocular sarcoidosis. Am J Med 26:331, 1959.

James DG: quoted in Siltzbach LE: The Kveim test in sarcoidosis (editorial). Am J Med 30:495, 1961.

James DG: Epidemiology of sarcoidosis. Arch Monaldi 31:25, 1976.

James DG: Sarcoidosis. Part I: making the diagnosis: "All that glitters is not sarcoid." Med Times 108(5):4s, 1980.

James DG and Kendig EL: Childhood sarcoidosis. Sarcoidosis 5:57, 1988.

James DG and Siltzbach LE: Sarcoidosis of the skin. In Madden S: Current Dermatologic Management. St. Louis, CV Mosby Co, 1975.

James DG, Carstares LF, and Neville E: Bone sarcoidosis. (Seventh International Conference on Sarcoidosis and Other Granulomatous Disorders.) Ann NY Acad Sci 278:475, 1976.

James DG, Neville E, and Siltzbach LE: A world wide review of sarcoidosis. (Seventh International Conference on Sarcoidosis and Other Granulomatous Disorders.) Ann NY Acad Sci 278:321, 1976.

James DG, Turiaf J, Hosada Y et al: Description of sarcoidosis: report of the Sub-Committee on Classification and Definition. (Seventh International Conference on Sarcoidosis and Other Granulomatous Disorders.) Ann NY Acad Sci 278:742, 1976.

Jasper PL and Denny FW: Sarcoidosis in children. J Pediatr 73:499, 1968.

Johnson JB and Jason RS: Sarcoidosis of the heart: report of a case and review of literature. Am Heart J 27:246, 1944.

Jones WW and Davies BH (eds): Eighth International Conference on Sarcoidosis and Other Granulomatous Disease. Cardiff, Wales, Alpha Omega Publishing, Ltd, 1980.

Kendig EL Jr: Sarcoidosis in children. Am Rev Respir Dis 84:49, 1961.

Kendig EL Jr: Sarcoidosis among children. J Pediatr 61:269, 1962.

Kendig EL Jr: The clinical picture of sarcoidosis in children. Pediatrics 54:289, 1974.

Kendig EL Jr: Sarcoidosis. Am J Dis Child 136:11, 1982.

Kendig EL Jr and Brummer DM: The prognosis of sarcoidosis in children. Chest 70:351, 1976.

Kendig EL Jr and Niitu Y: Sarcoidosis in Japanese and American children. Chest 77:514, 1980.

Kendig EL Jr and Wiley EJ Jr: Sarcoidosis in children. Postgrad Med J 37:590, 1961.

Kendig EL Jr, Peacock RL, and Ryburn S: Sarcoidosis: report of three cases in siblings under fifteen years of age. N Engl J Med 260:962, 1959.

Kerdel F and Moschella S: Sarcoidosis. J Am Acad Dermatol 11:1, 1984.

Klatskin G: Hepatic granuloma: problems in interpretation. Ann NY Acad Sci 278:427, 1976.

Klatskin G and Gordon M: Renal complications of sarcoidosis and their relationship to hypercalcemia; with a report of two cases simulating hyperparathyroidism. Am J Med 15:484, 1953.

Kogut MD and Neumann LL: Renal involvement in Boeck's sarcoidosis. Pediatrics 28:410, 1961.

Kraus EJ: Sarcoidosis (Boeck-Besnier-Schaumann disease) as a cause of pituitary syndrome. J Lab Clin Med 28:140, 1942.

Krauss L: Genital sarcoidosis: case report and review of the literature. J Urol 80:367, 1958.

Kveim A: Preliminary report on new and specific cutaneous reaction in Boeck's sarcoid. Nord Med 9:169, 1941.

Lieberman J: Serum angiotension-converting enzyme in sarcoidosis. Am J Med 59:365, 1975.

Liggett PE: Ocular sarcoidosis. Clin Dermatol 4:129, 1986.

Lindau A and Lowegren A: Benign lymphogranulomatosis (Schaumann's disease) and the eye. Acta Med Scand 105:242, 1940.

Lindsley CB and Godfrey WA: Childhood sarcoidosis manifesting as juvenile rheumatoid arthritis. Pediatrics 76:765, 1985.

Longcope WT and Freiman DG: A study of sarcoidosis; based on a combined investigation of 160 cases, including 30 autopsies, from the Johns Hopkins Hospital and Massachusetts General Hospital. Medicine 31:1, 1952.

Longcope WT and Pierson JW: Boeck's sarcoid (sarcoidosis). Bull Johns Hopkins Hosp 60:223, 1937.

McGovern JP and Merritt DM: Sarcoidosis in childhood. Adv Pediatr 8:97, 1956.

McSwiney RR and Mills IH: Hypercalcaemia due to sarcoidosis: treatment with cortisone. Lancet 2:862, 1956.

Macholda F (ed): Proceedings of the fifth international congress on sarcoidosis. Prague, University of Karlova, 1971.

Mackensen G: Veranderungen am Augenhintergrund bei Besnier-Boeck-Schaumannscher Erkrankung. Klin Monatsbl Augenheilkd 121:51, 1952.

Maddrey WC, Johns CJ, Boitnott JK et al: Sarcoidosis and chronic hepatic disease: a clinical and pathologic study of 20 patients. Medicine 49:375, 1970.

Mallory SB, Paller AS, Ginsburg BC et al: Sarcoidosis in children: differentiation from juvenile rheumatoid arthritis. Pediatr Dermatol 4:313, 1987.

Mandi L: Thoracic sarcoidosis in childhood. Acta Tuberc Scand 45:256, 1964.

Mankiewicz E: The relationship of sarcoidosis to anonymous mycobacteria. Acta Med Scand 425(Suppl):68, 1964.

Merten DF, Kirks DR, and Grossman H: Pulmonary sarcoidosis in childhood. AJR 135:673, 1980.

Michael J Jr, Cole R, Beeson PB, and Olson B: Sarcoidosis: preliminary report on a study of 350 cases with special reference to epidemiology. Am Rev Tuberc 62:403, 1950.

Mikhail JR, Mitchell DN, Dyson JL et al: Sarcoidosis with genital involvement. Am Rev Respir Dis 106:465, 1973.

Mikhail JR, Shepherd M, and Mitchell DN: Mediastinal lymph node biopsy in sarcoidosis. Endoscopy 11:5, 1979.

Nagle R: Hypercalcemia and nephrocalcinosis in sarcoidosis. J Mt Sinai Hosp 28:268, 1961.

Neville E, Pyasena KHG, and James DG: Granuloma of the liver. Postgrad Med J 51:361, 1975.

Niitu Y, Horikawa M, Suetake T et al: Comparison of clinical and laboratory findings of intrathoracic sarcoidosis of children and adults. (Seventh International Conference on Sarcoidosis and Other Granulomatous Disorders.) Ann NY Acad Sci 278:532, 1976.

Niitu Y, Watanabe M, Suetake T et al: Sixteen cases of intrathoracic sarcoidosis found among school children in Sendai in mass x-ray surveys of the chest. Research Report of Research Institute for Tuberculosis, Leprosy and Cancer, 12:99, 1965.

North AF: Sarcoid arthritis in children. Am J Med 48:449, 1970.

Oksanen V: Neurosarcoidosis: clinical presentations and course of 50 patients. Acta Neurol Scand 73:283, 1986.

Osterberg G: Iritis Boeck (sarkoid of Boeck in iris). Br J Ophthalmol 23:145, 1939.

Pattishall EN, Strope GL, and Denny FW: Pulmonary function in children with sarcoidosis. Am Rev Respir Dis 133:94, 1986.

Pattishall EN, Strope GL, Spinola SM, and Denny FW: Childhood sarcoidosis. J Pediatr 108:169, 1986.

Pautrier LM: Le syndrome de Heerfordt des ophthalmologistes n'est qu'une forme particulière de la maladie de Besnier-Boeck-Schaumann. Ann Dermatol Syphiligr 9:161, 1938.

Pennell WH: Boeck's sarcoid with involvement of the central nervous system. J Nerv Ment Dis 115:451, 1952.

Phillips RW and Fitzpatrick DP: Steroid therapy of hypercalcemia and renal insufficiency in sarcoidosis. N Engl J Med 254:1216, 1956.

Reed WG: Sarcoidosis: a review and report of eight cases in children. J Tenn Med Assoc 62:27, 1969.

Refvem O: Pathogenesis of Boeck's disease (sarcoidosis). Acta Med Scand 149(Suppl 294):1, 1954.

Reisner D: Boeck's sarcoid and systemic sarcoidosis. Am Rev Tuberc 49:437, 1944.

Ricker W and Clark M: Sarcoidosis: a clinicopathologic review of 300 cases, including 22 autopsies. Am J Clin Pathol 19:725, 1949.

Riley EA: Boeck's sarcoid. Am Rev Tuberc 62:231, 1950.

Rodriguez GE, Shin BC, Abernathy RS, and Kendig EL Jr: Serum angiotensin-converting enzyme activity in normal children and in those with sarcoidosis. J Pediatr 99:68, 1981.

Roos B: Cerebral manifestations of lymphogranulomatosis benigna (Schaumann) and uveoparotid fever (Heerfordt). Acta Med Scand 104:123, 1940.

Rosen Y, Athanassiades TJ, Moon S, and Lyons HA: Nongranulomatous interstitial pneumonitis in sarcoidosis: relationship to the development of epithelioid granulomas. Chest 74:122, 1978.

Rubinstein I and Baum GL: Colchicine therapy in sarcoid arthropathy. Pediatrics 78:717, 1986.

Salveson HA: Sarcoid of Boeck, a disease of importance to internal medicine; report of four cases. Acta Med Scand 86:127, 1935.

Scadding JG: Discussion on sarcoidosis. Proc R Soc Med 49:799, 1956.

Scadding JG: Mycobacterium tuberculosis in the aetiology of sarcoidosis. Br Med J 2:16, 1960.

Schabel SI, Stanley JH, and Shelley BE Jr: Pediatric sarcoidosis. JSC Med Assoc 76:419, 1980.

Schaumann J: Etude sur le lupus pernio et ses rapports avec les sarcoides et la tuberculose. Ann Dermatol Syphilig 6(fifth series):357, 1916–1917.

Schmitt E, Appleman H, and Threatt B: Sarcoidosis in children. Radiology 106:621, 1973.

Scholz DA and Keating FR Jr: Renal insufficiency, renal calculi and nephrocalcinosis in sarcoidosis. Am J Med 21:75, 1956.

Sharma OP, Johnson CS, and Balchum OJ: Familial sarcoidosis. Report of four siblings with acute sarcoidosis. Am Rev Respir Dis 104:255, 1971.

Sharma OP, Neville E, Walker AN, and James DG: Familial sarcoidosis: a possible genetic influence. Ann NY Acad Sci 278:386, 1976.

Siltzbach LE: The Kveim test in sarcoidosis (editorial). Am J Med 30:495, 1961.

Siltzbach LE: Sarcoidosis: clinical features and management. Med Clin North Am 51:483, 1967.

Siltzbach LE: Sarcoidosis and mycobacteria. Am Rev Respir Dis 97:1, 1968.

Siltzbach LE (ed): Seventh International Conference on Sarcoidosis and Other Granulomatous Disorders. Ann NY Acad Sci 271:1, 1976.

Siltzbach LE and Greenberg GM: Childhood sarcoidosis. A study of eighteen cases. N Engl J Med 279:1239, 1968.

Silverman KJ, Hutchins GM, and Bulkey BH: Cardiac sarcoid: a clinicopathologic study of 84 unselected patients with systemic sarcoidosis. Circulation 58:1204, 1978.

Sones M and Israel HL: Course and prognosis of sarcoidosis. Am J Med 29:84, 1960.

Stanislas-Leguern G, Mordelet-Dambrine M, Dusser D, and Huesca M: In vitro synthesis of angiotensin-converting enzyme by alveolar macrophages is increased in disseminated sarcoidosis. Lung 164:269, 1986.

Stone DJ and Schwartz A: A long-term study of sarcoid and its modification by steroid therapy. Am J Med 41:528, 1966.

Studdy PR: Biochemical findings in sarcoidosis. J Clin Pathol 33:528, 1980.

Studdy PR and Bird R: Serum angiotensin-converting enzyme (SACE) in sarcoidosis and other granulomatous disorders. Lancet 2:1331, 1978.

Takemura S, Fujioka A, Yasui Y et al: Localization of angiotensin converting enzyme (ACE) in granulomas of sarcoidosis cutaneous lesions. J Dermatol 14:122, 1987.

Teirstein AS: The Kveim-Siltzbach test. Clin Dermatol 4:154, 1986.

Veien NK, Stahl D, and Brodthagen H: Cutaneous sarcoidosis in Caucasians. J Am Acad Dermatol 16:534, 1987.

Walgren S: Pulmonary sarcoidosis detected by photofluorographic surveys in Sweden, 1950–1957. Nord Med 60:1194, 1958.

Walsh FB: Ocular importance of sarcoid; its relation to uveoparotid fever. Arch Ophthalmol 21:421, 1939.

Wegelius C and Wijkstroem S: Mass radiography in Sweden. Nord Med 60:1191, 1958.

Williams RH and Nickerson DA: Skin reactions in sarcoid. Proc Soc Exp Biol Med 33:403, 1935.

Zych D, Krychniak W, Pawlicka L, and Zielinski J: Sarcoidosis of the lung. Natural history and effects of treatment. Sarcoidosis 4:64, 1987.

50

WALTER T. HUGHES, M.D.

HISTOPLASMOSIS

Histoplasmosis is one of the major endemic deep mycotic infections. In the United States, at least 40 million people have been infected with *Histoplasma capsulatum*. Only a small percentage of these individuals develop discernible illness, and the vast majority remain asymptomatic. The infection was first discovered by Dr. Samuel T. Darling. In 1908, he reported the disseminated form of the disease, which he found at autopsy of a patient in Panama. Because he saw the yeast forms in the cytoplasm of histiocytes and because he mistakenly thought the organism was encapsulated and a protozoan, he proposed the name *Histoplasma capsulatum*. The fungal nature of the organism was not recognized until 1934, when De Monbreun isolated the organism from a fatal case. Also in 1934, Dodd and Tompkins reported the first case of histoplasmosis in an infant. For some 40 years after Darling's discovery of histoplasmosis, the disease was believed to be uncommon and usually fatal. However, Christie and Peterson in 1945 and 1946 showed that residual pulmonary calcifications were caused by asymptomatic pulmonary infections from *H. capsulatum*. It was soon realized that there were endemic areas of histoplasmosis where the majority of adult inhabitants had become infected, as evidenced by detectable serum antibody or delayed skin test reaction to *H. capsulatum*. In more recent years, histoplasmosis has become recognized as a potentially life-threatening infection in organ transplant recipients and in immunocompromised patients with cancer, congenital immunodeficiency disorders, and the acquired immune deficiency syndrome (AIDS).

ETIOLOGY

H. capsulatum is a dimorphic fungus that assumes a budding yeast form in infected tissues but grows as a septate hypha in the soil and in the laboratory at room temperature (25°C). Cultures can be converted from mycelial form to yeast form by subculture onto media and incubation at 37°C. The mycelial form of the fungus is septate, with characteristic macroconidia and microconidia. The macroconidia are round spores 8 to 14 μm in diameter, with spike-like projections from the surface that give the appearance of a Teutonic war club (Fig. 50–1A). The yeast form is 1 to 3 μm in diameter, buds from an oval form, and is often found in the cytoplasm of histiocytes (Fig. 50–1B).

EPIDEMIOLOGY

H. capsulatum resides in the soil. It is likely to be found in endemic areas contaminated with bird and bat dung. The organism is transmitted from the soil directly to humans and lower animals. Infection occurs by inhalation of spores. Person-to-person and animal-to-human infections do not occur. Many may become infected by inhalation of spores from the mold (mycelial) form of *H. capsulatum* grown in laboratory cultures.

Outbreaks of histoplasmosis have occurred among spelunkers, dirt-moving equipment operators, poultry breeders, and campers. Digging and turning over the soil provide the opportunity for residual fungal spores to become air-borne. Shady sites underneath trees with bird roosts, in caves, silos, chicken coops, and underneath buildings provide the soil with high acidity and organic content for growth of *H. capsulatum*. Not all such sites, even in endemic areas, are colonized with the fungus. Focal sites serve to harbor the organism so that in heavily endemic areas the incidence of infection in the population may vary from one geographic area to another.

Although histoplasmosis is associated with populations of birds and bats, these animals are usually not infected. Rather, the excretions of these species serve to enrich the soil for growth of *H. capsulatum*.

The endemicity of histoplasmosis in the United States was mapped in an extensive study by Edwards and colleagues (1969). Between 1958 and 1965, military recruits age 17 to 21 years were skin tested with histoplasmin. The results are depicted in Figure 50–2. The states of the Ohio and Mississippi river valleys along with Maryland and Virginia have the highest prevalence of histoplasmin reactors. It must be realized that this landmark study of 275,558 men was carried out more than 20 years ago. More recent data are needed to learn if changes have occurred. Certainly, cases of histoplasmosis have been encountered in recent years in immunocompromised patients who have always resided in nonendemic states

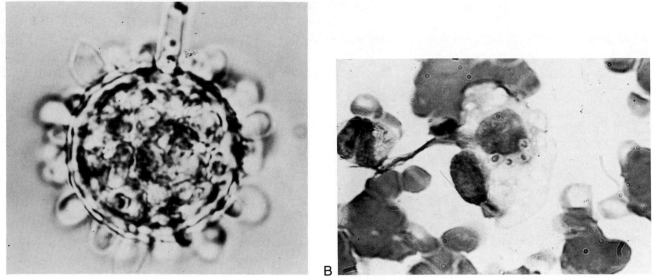

Figure 50–1. *A*, Tuberculate conidia of *Histoplasma capsulatum*. *B*, Yeast forms in the cytoplasm of histiocytes (Giemsa stains) of the marrow.

such as Minnesota, New York, and California. Patients with AIDS are especially susceptible to disseminated histoplasmosis, even when residing outside the endemic area.

The incidence of histoplasmin reactors in endemic areas is related to age of the population. A study of 1068 individuals in Kentucky determined the histoplasmin skin test reactor rates by age. As shown in Figure 50–3, the incidence of positive reactors increases with age.

Histoplasmosis occurs in other countries of temperate and tropical zones.

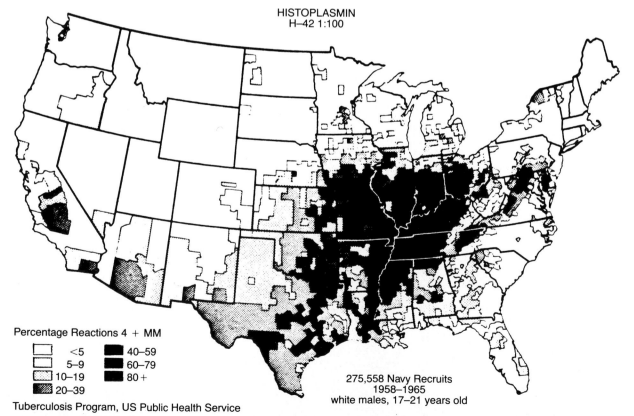

HISTOPLASMIN
H–42 1:100

Percentage Reactions 4 + MM

<5	40–59
5–9	60–79
10–19	80 +
20–39	

Tuberculosis Program, US Public Health Service

275,558 Navy Recruits
1958–1965
white males, 17–21 years old

Figure 50–2. Percentage of positive reactions to the histoplasmin skin test in white male military recruits between the ages of 17 and 21 years who had been lifetime residents of the counties represented (Reproduced with permission from Edwards LB et al: Am Rev Respir Dis 99(Part 2):1, 1969.)

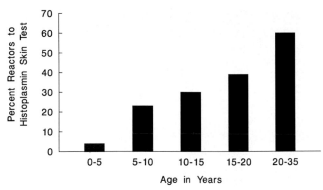

Figure 50–3. Percentage of positive reactors to the histoplasmin skin test by age in an endemic area (Louisville, Kentucky). The study included 1068 individuals.

PATHOGENESIS

Spores (conidia) from the mold (mycelial) phase of *H. capsulatum* reach the mucous membranes and lower airways of the respiratory tract by the air-borne route, and the primary infection is in the pulmonary parenchyma. In rare instances, the portal of entry may be the skin or intestinal mucosa. In the lower respiratory tract, the spores transform to the yeast phase of the fungus, which is susceptible to phagocytosis by macrophages. The yeast forms can persist in the macrophages of the nonimmune host as an infiltrate develops. Also, yeast-laden macrophages may be transported via lymphatics to peribronchial and mediastinal lymph nodes and other sites, where new foci of infection develop. It is likely that hematogenous dissemination occurs with the primary pulmonary infection, but extrapulmonary infection is rare in an immunocompetent host. If the host has impaired immune responses, especially infants and patients with impaired cell-mediated immunity (e.g., AIDS), the yeast seeds to extrapulmonary sites and disseminated disease becomes established. Competent hosts contain the infection in the primary pulmonary complex. These sites normally heal by calcification. The usual lesion of histoplasmosis is a tubercle-like granuloma.

The immune response to *H. capsulatum* infection depends on cellular immune mechanisms. The interval between the primary inoculation of the organism and skin test response to histoplasmin is about 6 weeks.

CLINICAL MANIFESTATIONS

Infection with *H. capsulatum* may invoke a wide spectrum of clinical features, extending from a totally asymptomatic infection, to a mild influenza-like illness, to an acute localized pneumonia, to extensive bilateral pulmonary infection progressing to extrapulmonary infection, which may affect one or more deep organs. The major determinants of clinical expression of disease are the size of *H. capsulatum*

inoculum and the immunocompetence of the host. Basically, histoplasmosis can be categorized as either pulmonary or extrapulmonary.

PULMONARY HISTOPLASMOSIS

The pulmonary infection may be of limited extent, insufficient to be recognized by radiograph and with no discernible signs or symptoms. This is referred to as *asymptomatic* infection. A residual pulmonary calcification may eventually be found at the site of the infection.

Acute pulmonary histoplasmosis may resemble an influenza-like illness with fever, cough, malaise, chest pain, sore throat, and headache. Pulmonary infiltrates and enlargement of hilar lymph nodes may be seen by radiographs (Fig. 50–4). The lesions may be localized infiltrates, lobar involvement, or bilateral diffuse lung infiltrates. Rales may or may not be heard, and the respiratory rate may be increased with severe involvement. Some patients may have erythema nodosum or erythema multiforme, possibly representing hypersensitivity to the infection.

Chronic pulmonary histoplasmosis is uncommon in infants and children. It resembles chronic tuberculosis with cavitation.

EXTRAPULMONARY HISTOPLASMOSIS

The most severe form of extrapulmonary histoplasmosis is one in which the organism is disseminated hematogenously to several deep organs, especially the reticuloendothelial system. *Acute disseminated histoplasmosis* is limited almost exclusively to infants and children younger than 2 years of age, adults older than 50 years of age, and patients who are immunocompromised as a result of cancer, immunosuppressive drugs, AIDS, or other compromising entities. The clinical features in the disseminated disease are usually fever, weight loss, hepatomegaly, splenomegaly, cough, diarrhea, mucosal ulcer, or skin lesions. Anemia, leukopenia, and thrombocytopenia may also occur, especially in infants (Leggiadro et al, 1988; Hughes, 1984; Johnson et al, 1988).

A *chronic* form of *disseminated histoplasmosis* is rarely encountered with ulcerative lesions of the oral mucosa or infections of the larynx, lungs, liver, spleen, heart, lymph nodes, adrenal glands, and other organs. In contrast to the acute disseminated form, the lesions of the chronic disease develop more slowly and persist for weeks or months without treatment.

Some unusual forms of histoplasmosis are meningitis, pericarditis, chorioretinitis, and pleural effusion. Pericardial and pleural effusion may occur without active fungal invasion of these sites and may be related to small adjacent lesions. The pathogenesis of chorioretinitis has not been well defined but may

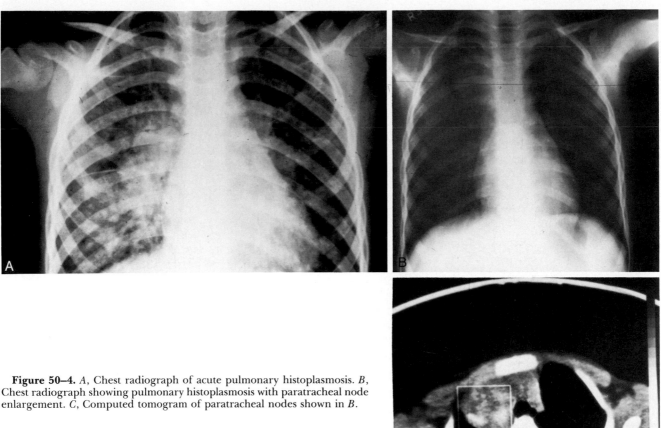

Figure 50–4. *A*, Chest radiograph of acute pulmonary histoplasmosis. *B*, Chest radiograph showing pulmonary histoplasmosis with paratracheal node enlargement. *C*, Computed tomogram of paratracheal nodes shown in *B*.

be due to a hypersensitivity reaction, with the retina as a target organ.

The AIDS epidemic has added a new dimension to histoplasmosis. The severe defect in cell-mediated immunity caused by the human immunodeficiency virus (HIV) renders the host highly susceptible to severe disseminated infection from *H. capsulatum*, even outside endemic areas. The clinical features are similar to those described above for the *acute disseminated histoplasmosis;* fever, weight loss, and splenomegaly are the most frequent manifestations (Johnson et al, 1988).

DIAGNOSIS

H. capsulatum is not a component of the usual microbial flora of humans, so its presence in a lesion of the mucous membranes, skin, deep organs, or in body fluids signifies cause and effect. Thus, the isolation of the organism in culture is the most precise method for diagnosis. Although the organism can be cultured on standard mycologic media, such as brain-heart infusion agar and broth, incubation for 2 to 6

weeks is usually required before *H. capsulatum* can be identified. Specimens for culture depend on the infected site. Blood and bone marrow should be cultured with the disseminated types, sputum for pulmonary disease, and biopsy material from localized lesions. Failure to isolate the organism in culture does not rule out the diagnosis of histoplasmosis, because in some infected specimens the organism fails to grow in vitro.

Histologic examination of tissues provides a useful diagnostic aid. The bone marrow and biopsy specimens of tissue give the highest yield of positive results. Only the yeast form is found in tissues and body fluids. This form of the organism is about 3.0 μm in diameter, oval, and budding. It is found in the cytoplasm of histiocytes stained with polychrome stains such as Giemsa (see Fig. 50–1*B*). The cytoplasm retracts away from the yeast during the staining process, giving the false appearance of a capsule. Some of the yeast cells have a single polar bud with a chromatic mass located in the periphery. The Grocott-Gomori methenamine-silver nitrate stain is useful in locating these yeast forms.

The histoplasmin skin test becomes reactive 2 to 4 weeks after infection. About 90 per cent of normal immunocompetent individuals infected with *H. capsulatum* will develop reactions to skin tests. However, with the acute disseminated type only about 50 per cent will develop positive reactions, because this form usually occurs in immunocompromised patients. The main disadvantage of the histoplasmin skin test as a diagnostic aid is that the majority of young adults and older residents in endemic areas are positive reactors.

Serologic tests may be of some help, but no single method for antibody determination has been established as a national standard. Reagents for such tests have not been subjected to quality control and standardization. The complement-fixation tests usually detect antibody after 2 to 4 weeks of infection. Histoplasmin and yeast phase antigens are used. A titer of 1:8 or greater is suggestive of infection, but a fourfold increase is strong evidence of acute histoplasmosis. Antibodies to the yeast phase antigen correlate more closely with active infection than do antibodies to the histoplasmin (mycelial) antigen. Other methods such as radioimmunoassay, immunoprecipitation, and enzyme-linked immunoassay offer promise, but none has been adequately tested and standardized for general use. Recent studies show that the detection of *H. capsulatum* antigen by radioimmunoassay may be useful as a diagnostic test (Wheat et al, 1986), but here again confirmatory studies and standardization of reagents and methods are needed.

TREATMENT

The acute primary pulmonary form of histoplasmosis in a normal host rarely requires treatment because complete recovery occurs in the vast majority of cases. The clinical illness, if it occurs, is self-limited and resolves in 10 to 14 days. However, roentgenographic signs of pulmonary infiltrates may persist for longer periods of time, and hilar lymphadenopathy due to *H. capsulatum* infection may remain detectable for several months. Acute pulmonary histoplasmosis in a severely immunocompromised host (e.g., with AIDS), certain organ transplant recipients, cancer patients receiving chemotherapy, and patients with congenital immunodeficiency disorders require treatment with either amphotericin B or ketoconazole. Chronic pulmonary histoplasmosis with or without cavitation rarely occurs in children, but when it does, some of these patients require specific treatment. Lymphadenitis of the hilar, paratracheal, and mediastinal nodes requires treatment only if there is encroachment on a major vital structure. Pericarditis may occur, often without actual invasion of the pericardium or the heart with fungus. This noninvasive inflammatory response with sterile pericardial effusion does not require antifungal drugs. In the rare case with fungal invasion of the pericardium, antifungal drugs should be used.

The disseminated systemic form of histoplasmosis requires specific treatment whether in an immunocompetent or immunocompromised infant, child, or adult. Untreated, the prognosis is poor and the fatality rate is about 85 per cent, but with early treatment, 75 to 100 per cent will recover (Furcolow, 1963; Leggiadro et al, 1988).

Two drugs are currently used for the treatment of histoplasmosis. These are amphotericin B administered intravenously and ketoconazole given orally. Amphotericin B has been studied most thoroughly, and evidence to date indicates it is more effective than ketoconazole. However, amphotericin B is more toxic than ketoconazole. All cases of disseminated histoplasmosis of life-threatening intensity must be treated with intravenous amphotericin B, at least initially. Ketoconazole should be considered for use in patients who require treatment but who do not have life-threatening histoplasmosis. Ketoconazole may also be used as "maintenance" antifungal therapy following an initial course of amphotericin B. The simultaneous administration of ketoconazole has not been studied for histoplasmosis. Because such a combination is not likely to have therapeutic advantages, its use is not advised.

AMPHOTERICIN B

Amphotericin B is a polyene that binds to sterols in the cell membrane of *H. capsulatum*, thereby bringing about an increase in the permeability of the membrane and the leakage of cellular electrolytes and other constituents, resulting in death or inhibition of replication of the organism.

After some 30 years of use in medical practice, it is remarkable that so little is known about the optimal dosages and schedules for administration and duration of therapy with amphotericin B. Certain dogma has been accepted and to a great extent dictates guides to therapy. For example, unlike any other antimicrobial drug, the total amount of amphotericin B given over the course of therapy is used as a single figure to judge likelihood of toxicity. It has been suggested that a total dose of 25 to 35 mg/kg of body weight of amphotericin B should be administered for a course of treatment. Although adverse effects are very frequent in pediatric patients, with proper monitoring and some wisdom in the day-to-day administration, full courses of amphotericin B can be given and life-threatening adverse effects are rare.

Amphotericin B is prepared in a solution of 5 per cent dextrose in water, providing 0.1 mg/ml of solution. The drug should be administered within 24 hours after it is prepared. It can be delivered as an infusion through a needle in a peripheral vein or through a central venous access device. The time required to infuse the single daily dose can be titrated to the patient's tolerance, but it is advised to start with the first infusion over a period of 4 to 6 hours, because infusion reactions occur very frequently during the first several days of therapy and tend to diminish after 10 to 14 days of treatment. An amphotericin B infusion usually is never given more rapidly than over a 2-hour period. A few patients tolerate a 1-hour infusion well, but no one should have the drug given more rapidly than in 1 hour. How these infusion rates affect peak serum levels is not known, but it is reasonable to expect a higher peak level with the more rapid infusion.

Amphotericin B therapy is started with a very low initial dose. This serves to test for the immediate adverse effects that will likely occur. Usually 0.25 mg/kg is given over 4 to 6 hours without any premedication to mask fever and chills or other effects. This dose will provide no effective therapeutic level. If a patient's infection is very serious, one may move to a second dose within 6 to 8 hours after the initial infusion if it is well tolerated. Henceforth, one dose is given no more often than once a day. The dose is escalated in increments of 0.25 mg/kg/day until a dose of 0.5 to 1.0 mg/kg/day is achieved. With mild disease in a competent host, the 0.5 mg/kg dose may be adequate for the entire course. If the disease is extensive, especially in sites poorly penetrated by amphotericin B (e.g., cavities, spinal fluid) the dose of 1.0 mg/kg/day should be used until the infection is under control. After the disease is under control, the 1.0 mg/kg dose can be given every other day. At least 4 to 6 weeks of amphotericin B therapy is required for most patients with disseminated histoplasmosis. Patients with AIDS are the exception. In these patients, slow responses and frequent relapses are common. Furthermore, the immune defect is not reversible at this time. A reasonable approach at present is to achieve recovery from the infection with about 4 weeks of amphotericin B and then to place the patient on ketoconazole for an indefinite period (Johnson et al, 1988). Some experimental drugs that show promise for disseminated histoplasmosis are itraconazole and fluconazole (Graybill, 1988). However, further studies are needed to know the relative efficiencies and toxicities of these drugs in infants and children when compared with amphotericin B and ketoconazole.

The adverse effects of amphotericin B are frequent, and probably no patient receives a course of treatment without experiencing one or more side effects or toxicity. The frequent abnormalities associated with the infusion are fever, chills, headache, and phlebitis. Less frequent but important to recognize are hypotensive episodes. Other adverse effects are electrolyte imbalance, especially hypokalemia; renal toxicity; thrombocytopenia; anemia; hepatotoxicity; rashes; cardiac arrhythmias; hypocalcemia; vertigo; abdominal pain; and convulsions.

Patients must be monitored carefully. Laboratory tests recommended include hemoglobin, blood urea nitrogen, creatinine, potassium, calcium, transaminases, phosphorus, and platelet count at least every 3 days. If the creatinine exceeds 2.0 mg/dL, the dosage of amphotericin B should be reduced. This can usually be best accomplished by omitting one or more daily doses until the creatinine is at or near normal levels. When treatment with amphotericin B is essential for patients in renal failure, the dosage does not need to be changed from the standpoint of therapeutic serum levels of the drug because elimination is not altered with impaired renal function. In patients who have fever and chills associated with amphotericin B administration, these reactions can often be prevented or minimized with premedication. Studies have suggested that amphotericin B is a potent inducer of prostaglandin E_2 synthesis and that the administration of the inhibitor ibuprofen (10 mg/kg) orally 30 min before starting the infusion will reduce fever and chilling (Gigliotti et al, 1987). With severe reactions not controllable by ibuprofen, hydrocortisone, 0.5 mg/kg intravenously immediately before the infusion is started, may be necessary.

KETOCONAZOLE

Ketoconazole is an imidazole absorbed after oral administration to produce peak serum levels of about 3.5 μg/ml 1 to 2 hours after the usual dosage. The half-life is about 6 hours, and excretion is primarily through the biliary system. Absorption is reduced in patients with achlorhydria, so the use of antacids, H_2-blocking agents, and so on should be avoided with ketoconazole therapy.

Ketoconazole is administered in the dosage of 6 to 8 mg/kg once daily. The total daily dose should not exceed 400 mg. The efficacy and safety of ketoconazole have not been established for infants less than 2 years of age. The course of therapy for disseminated histoplasmosis has not been determined. In patients who have AIDS and histoplasmosis, ketoconazole should be continued indefinitely. In patients who do not have AIDS, a minimal course is probably 3 to 6 months.

Hepatotoxicity of the hepatocellular type has been associated with ketoconazole use. The liver damage is usually reversible if the drug administration is discontinued. This drug in high dosage may reduce the production of adrenal corticosteroids and gonadal steroids.

REFERENCES

Christie A and Peterson JC: Pulmonary calcification in negative reactors to tuberculin. Am J Public Health 35:1131, 1945.

Christie A and Peterson JC: Histoplasmin sensitivity. J Pediatr 29:417, 1946.

Darling ST: A protozoan general infection producing pseudo tubercles in the lungs and focal necrosis in the liver, spleen and lymph nodes. JAMA 46:1283, 1906.

De Monbreun WA: The cultivation and cultured characteristics of Darling's H. capsulatum. Am J Trop Med 14:93, 1934.

Dodd K and Tompkins EH: A case of histoplasmosis of Darling in an infant. Am J Trop Med 14:127, 1934.

Edwards LB, Acquaviva FA, and Livesay VT: An atlas of sensitivity to tuberculin, PPD-B and histoplasmin in the United States. Am Rev Respir Dis 99(Pt. 2):1, 1969.

Furcolow ML: Comparison of treated and untreated severe histoplasmosis. JAMA 183:813, 1963.

Gigliotti F, Shenep JL, Lott L, and Thornton D: Induction of prostaglandin synthesis as the mechanism responsible for the chills and fever produced by infusing amphotericin B. J Infect Dis 156:784, 1987.

Graybill JR: Histoplasmosis in AIDS. J Infect Dis 158:623, 1988.

Hughes WT: Hematogenous histoplasmosis in the immunocompromised child. J Pediatr 105:569, 1984.

Leggiadro RJ, Barrett FF, and Hughes WT: Disseminated histoplasmosis of infancy. J Pediatr Infect Dis 7:799, 1988.

Johnson PC, Khardori N, Najjar AF et al: Progressive disseminated histoplasmosis in patients with acquired immunodeficiency syndrome. Am J Med 85:152, 1988.

Wheat LJ, Kohler RB, and Tewari RP: Diagnosis of disseminated histoplasmosis by detection of *Histoplasma capsulatum* antigen in serum and urine specimens. N Engl J Med 314:83, 1986.

51

RICHARD F. JACOBS, M.D., and
ROBERT W. BRADSHER, M.D.

THE MYCOSES OTHER THAN HISTOPLASMOSIS

The majority of recognized pulmonary infections in children are due to viral and bacterial pathogens. However, with the continued epidemiologic risk of exposure to pathogenic dimorphic fungi, as well as aggressive treatment regimens for cancer and other diseases leading to subsequent host immunosuppression, the diagnosis and treatment of pulmonary mycoses in children have taken on an increasingly important place in modern medicine. Many clinicians would correctly suspect mycotic infection with a subacute or chronic pneumonia unresponsive to antibiotic therapy when common bacterial, mycobacterial, or viral causes have not been identified. Fungal infections are also becoming an increasingly important part of the differential diagnosis of opportunistic pulmonary infections in immunocompromised hosts.

The incidence of mycotic pulmonary infections has been increasing. This increase is only partly due to recognition secondary to improved diagnostic techniques. It has partly resulted from increasing urbanization with crowding in the inner-city areas and resultant exposure of a nonimmune population to pathogenic fungal organisms. The opportunistic invasion of fungal organisms in the lungs has been brought about by several potential factors: (1) selection of fungal organisms as flora by the widespread use of broad-spectrum antibiotics; (2) the induction of leukopenia by cytotoxic agents; (3) humoral and cell-mediated immunosuppression by cytotoxic and immunosuppressive therapy; (4) the widespread use of immunosuppressive drugs in patients with collagen-vascular diseases and in transplant recipients; (5) the increasing recognition that certain patients with intrinsic or acquired cell-mediated immune defects (acquired immune deficiency syndrome, or AIDS) are susceptible to fungi; and (6) enhancement of portals of entry for fungi into the body through direct mucosal toxicity (gastrointestinal) and surgical procedures performed on hospitalized children.

Mycotic infections cause significant morbidity and mortality in immunocompromised hosts. As current aggressive therapeutic modalities have lengthened the survival of patients with malignancies, organ transplantation, and inflammatory diseases, the incidence of mycotic infections has increased. In this select group of patients, the diagnosis and management of mycotic infections are often difficult, especially if the infection involves the lungs. The diagnosis of a pulmonary mycotic infection is made more difficult by the varied and often nonspecific clinical presentations. The confirmation of fungal pneumonia is often hindered by a lack of microbiologic data, which may require invasive procedures to establish histologic and culture-proven diagnoses. In certain of these patients, the morbidity and mortality from these invasive procedures are enhanced by the severity of the underlying disease, the potential for bleeding complications, and the current lack of expertise by pediatric subspecialists to perform these procedures in small children.

In general, the majority of pulmonary mycotic infections occur in two microbiologic and clinical groups (Table 51–1). As a general rule, different patient groups are at risk for infection due to opportunistic or dirmorphic pulmonary fungi. Primary pulmonary mycotic infections generally afflict otherwise healthy children who are exposed to the

The authors would like to thank Dr. Joanna Seibert for providing the radiographs displayed in this chapter.

Table 51–1. PULMONARY MYCOSES

Opportunistic	Primary Dimorphic Fungi
Aspergillosis	Histoplasmosis
Cryptococcosis	Blastomycosis
Candidiasis	Cryptococcosis
Mucormycosis	Coccidioidomycosis
Sporotrichosis	Paracoccidioidomycosis
Other rare fungi	Penicilliosis
Pseudoallescheria boydii	
Penicillium	
Fusarium	
Trichosporin	

pathogens in a particular endemic geographic or environmental setting and include blastomycosis, coccidioidomycosis, paracoccidioidomycosis, and histoplasmosis. The potential for these pathogenic pulmonary fungi to occur in immunocompromised patients with acquired immune deficiency syndrome (AIDS) and human immunodeficiency virus infection has been recognized. The opportunistic mycotic infections, such as aspergillosis, candidiasis, and cryptococcosis, are discussed in detail in the following sections. Other fungi may rarely infect the lungs, including the organisms causing zygomycosis, sporotrichosis, and phaeohyphomycosis, which are briefly discussed.

OPPORTUNISTIC PULMONARY MYCOSES

PULMONARY ASPERGILLOSIS

Allergic bronchopulmonary aspergillosis and aspergillomas are not aggressive infections and are not discussed. Invasive pulmonary aspergillosis occurs almost exclusively in immunocompromised patients, although there are sporadic case reports of systemic aspergillosis in normal hosts. The diagnosis of this disease may be difficult, because clinical manifestations of invasive disease are often subtle and culture confirmation may be inapparent or confused by the presence of other pathogens. Infection can assume many forms, including disseminated disease. Invasive pulmonary aspergillosis is often fatal despite treatment, unless the patient's immune function improves. The classic example is a febrile patient with neutropenic cancer with prolonged neutropenia. For a successful outcome, pulmonary infection with *Aspergillus* must be diagnosed and treated with amphotericin B without delay (Davies and Sarosi, 1985).

Cases of invasive aspergillosis in immunocompromised hosts are sporadic and usually hospital acquired. Small clusters of cases have occurred in hospitals, especially those undergoing renovation or new construction. In these environments, exposure to a large number of *Aspergillus* spores through environmental contamination due to ground breaking of sites significantly increases the risk of infection (Sarubbi et al, 1982).

Epidemiologically, two groups of patients are especially susceptible to invasive aspergillosis, those with hematologic malignancies and organ transplantation. Patients with acute myelogenous and acute lymphocytic leukemia are at particular risk for this infection. This is believed to be because of the malignant transformation of effective immune cells, as well as the cyclical neutropenia secondary to repeated doses of cytotoxic chemotherapy (Fisher et al, 1981). Although their risk is lower than that of leukemic patients, children with lymphoma or Hodgkin's disease are also susceptible to invasive aspergillosis. Among organ transplantation patients, those receiving cardiac and bone marrow transplants have a particularly high risk for *Aspergillus* infection, with reports ranging from 10 to 30 per cent (Sidransky and Pearl, 1961). Although they have a lower reported incidence of approximately 2.5 per cent, renal transplant recipients still have a predisposition to infection with *Aspergillus* (Masur et al, 1982).

Immunologically, neutropenia is an important risk factor for invasive aspergillosis. Both the absolute neutrophil count and the duration of neutropenia are significant risk factors for the incidence of infection (Gerson et al, 1984). In some studies, steroid therapy has been demonstrated to predispose patients to invasive pulmonary aspergillosis. In organ transplant recipients, intermittent high-dose courses of corticosteroids have been found to be a particularly important risk factor for invasive aspergillosis (Gustafson et al, 1983). Also emphasizing the importance of neutropenia in invasive aspergillosis is the observation that broad-spectrum antibiotic therapy alone or hypogammaglobulinemia is not considered a major risk factor for invasive aspergillosis (Gerson et al, 1984; Meyer et al, 1973).

The clinical signs of invasive pulmonary aspergillosis are nonspecific. The usual presentation includes fever and pulmonary infiltrates that do not respond to antibacterial therapy (Meyer et al, 1973). If symptoms are present, they are usually either subacute or chronic. Patients frequently exhibit dyspnea and a nonproductive cough. Although chest pain is a helpful symptom often indicating hemorrhagic pulmonary infarction that follows invasion of the fungus into vessels, these symptoms are usually difficult to elucidate in small children. Hemoptysis is rare, and physical findings are usually minimal. Pulmonary auscultatory changes are occasionally found, but only with far advanced disease in which diffuse pulmonary infiltrates are present (Williams et al, 1976). Adding to the difficulty in diagnosis is the fact that the signs and symptoms of invasive aspergillosis are often attributed to infection with other pathogens. Simultaneous bacterial or other fungal infections are associated with *Aspergillus* pneumonia in more than 50 per cent of the cases. The most common associated pathogens include *Candida* species, Enterobacteriaceae, and *Pseudomonas* species (Meyer et al, 1973). In one study in adults, more than 50 per cent of patients with aspergillosis had concomitant bacterial pneumonia caused by gram-negative bacilli (Orr et al, 1978). In immunocompromised patients, the combination of nonspecific symptoms and frequent isolation of other potentially pathogenic organisms makes the diagnosis of invasive pulmonary aspergillosis even more difficult. Because *Aspergillus* hyphae may invade blood vessels in the lungs, hematogenous dissemination should be expected. This complication almost always originates from a primary pulmonary focus, with some series describing as many as 24 per cent of patients with invasive pulmonary aspergillosis progressing to dissemination (Meyer et al, 1973).

No radiographic abnormality is specific for pulmonary aspergillosis. Chest radiographs are frequently described as having patchy infiltrates, necrotizing pneumonitis, miliary nodules, or frank lung abscesses (Fig. 51–1). A common early finding in *Aspergillus* pneumonia is a round, patchy infiltrate, which may be present in any lobe of the lungs. As the pulmonary process progresses, the pneumonia may enlarge or spread to other areas, eventually producing the wedge-shaped densities characteristic of pulmonary infarctions with the diagnostic crescent sign. Although not specific for invasive aspergillosis, this radiographic presentation suggests the diagnosis when it occurs in an appropriate clinical setting (Orr et al, 1978). With resolution of neutropenia, the area may cavitate and leave the appearance of a fungus ball (Przyjemski and Mattii, 1980). An occasional patient with proven pulmonary aspergillosis may have a normal chest radiograph as a result of an inadequate inflammatory response secondary to immunosuppression.

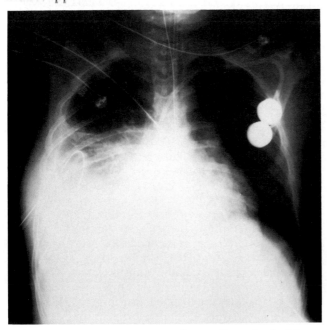

Figure 51–1. A posteroanterior chest radiograph of a 12-year-old girl with acute myelogenous leukemia and invasive aspergillosis. The radiographic description was a consolidated right lower lobe infiltrate with a parapneumonic effusion. A computed tomographic visualization of the chest revealed changes consistent with a right lower lobe intraparenchymal abscess. The abscess developed over time in conjunction with normalization of the patient's white blood cell count.

The definitive diagnosis of invasive pulmonary aspergillosis may require histopathologic identification of the fungus in tissue specimens. Sputum cultures in adults have been found to be notoriously insensitive as a test for aspergillosis. The fungus has been isolated from sputum in only 8 to 34 per cent of immunocompromised patients with proven pulmonary disease (Nalesnik et al, 1980). Because *Aspergillus flavus* has been isolated from as many as 16 per cent of immunologically normal individuals, positive sputum cultures do not prove the presence of invasive disease even in compromised hosts (Comstock et al, 1974). The presence of organisms in sputum is also not a specific indicator of invasive pulmonary disease. In one study of patients with leukemia and lymphoma, *Aspergillus* was isolated from the respiratory tract of 17 patients, but only 6, or 35 per cent, were later shown to have invasive pulmonary aspergillosis by pathologic examination (Fisher et al, 1981).

In an attempt to improve the sensitivity and specificity of cultures for *Aspergillus*, nasal swabs were used in a study of leukemic patients infected with *A. flavus*. Nasal cultures were only moderately sensitive (56 per cent) but very specific (99 per cent) as a test for invasive pulmonary aspergillosis (Aisner et al, 1979). In immunocompromised patients, any isolation of *Aspergillus* should be taken seriously, and multiple positive cultures should be considered as strong evidence of fungal infection (Davies and Sarosi, 1985). Attempts at serologic diagnosis of *Aspergillus* infection have demonstrated an unacceptable rate of false-negative results. Compounding the difficulty in obtaining positive antibody assays for this organism is the fact that an immunocompromised patient population may lack a normal antibody response (Fisher et al, 1981). Some investigators have attempted to identify fungal antigens in the serum of infected patients, and although a radioimmunoassay has shown moderate sensitivity and high specificity for this organism, further evaluation is currently needed before this, or any other, antigen assay can play a definitive role in the diagnosis of invasive pulmonary aspergillosis (Weiner et al, 1983). Flexible bronchoscopy with bronchial washings or bronchoalveolar lavage currently represents the initial diagnostic test of choice in these patients (Albelda et al, 1984). If this procedure is nondiagnostic, an open-lung biopsy may be required.

The optimal treatment for pulmonary aspergillosis requires early institution of antifungal therapy and correction of the underlying immunologic defects, especially neutropenia (Herbert and Bayer, 1981). Patients with invasive pulmonary aspergillosis should receive amphotericin B (Tables 51–2 and 51–3). Although no antifungal combination therapy has been proved superior to amphotericin B alone, the combinations of amphotericin B and 5-flucytosine or amphotericin B and rifampin have been suggested for potential synergistic activity. Although surgical resection of isolated pulmonary *Aspergillus* infections is not indicated in the treatment of critically ill

Table 51–2. ANTIFUNGAL THERAPY

Drug	Route	Dose (Per Day)
Amphotericin B (Fungizone)	IV	Schedule* (over 4–6 hours) test dose: 0.1 mg/kg (1 mg) 0.25 mg/kg 0.5 mg/kg 1.0 mg/kg
Flucytosine (Ancobon)	PO	100–150 mg/kg divided every 6 hours
Ketoconazole (Nizoral)	PO	3.3–6.6 mg/kg, single dose† Adult: 200–800 mg daily
Miconazole (Monistat)	IV	20–40 mg/kg divided every 8 hours (infuse over 30–60 minutes)
Investigational agents (itraconazole, fluconazole, SCH39304)	PO	To be determined. Greater absorption, potential central nervous system penetration.

*Single daily dose; 0.25 mg/kg given on the same day as the test dose. Following dose increments made on a daily basis dependent on severity of disease and tolerance of medication.

†Children 2 years old and younger—daily dose not established.

patients with uncontrolled disease, it may be considered for a few patients who have residual foci of infection after partial response to initial antifungal therapy. Patients with recalcitrant or relapsing aspergillosis in a well-defined lung segment or an aspergilloma causing massive hemoptysis may benefit from surgical resection of these lesions (Herbert and Bayer, 1981).

Untreated, invasive pulmonary aspergillosis is usually fatal in immunocompromised patients. Mortality rates in most series have been shown to be greater than 80 per cent (Rinaldi, 1983). This dismal figure has improved with early recognition, diagnosis, and intervention with antifungal chemotherapy. In a study of patients with leukemia and invasive pulmonary aspergillosis, when treatment was instituted within 4 days of initial detection of pulmonary infiltrates, a 50 per cent survival was obtained (Aisner et al, 1977). To treat invasive pulmonary aspergillosis effectively, a physician must maintain a high degree of suspicion for this organism in high-risk patients to allow the early, aggressive institution of diagnostic and therapeutic measures.

PULMONARY CRYPTOCOCCOSIS

Cryptococcus neoformans is a ubiquitous, saprophytic yeast found in soil contaminated by the feces of birds,

Table 51–3. ANTIFUNGAL TOXICITIES

Drug	Toxicities
Amphotericin B	Fever, chills, nephrotoxicity, anemia, hypokalemia, thrombophlebitis
Flucytosine	Netropenia with elevated serum levels. (If levels are not available, this agent should not be used.)
Ketoconazole	Nausea, vomiting, rare hepatotoxicity, testosterone synthesis blockade
Miconazole	Cardiac arrhythmias, cardiovascular collapse with rapid infusion
Itraconazole, fluconazole	Nausea, vomiting, dizziness

specifically pigeons. Organisms from the environment enter the host by inhalation of air-borne particles with deposition in the lungs. Although meningitis is the most serious form of this infection, most cryptococcosis in humans is localized in the lungs and may be subclinical. Dissemination occurs in a minority of patients, with most of these patients manifesting cryptococcal pneumonia at the time of presentation. Although various abnormalities of cell-mediated immunity render the host susceptible to cryptococcal infection, this fungal pneumonia is a cause of infection in normal hosts. Several reports have described pulmonary cryptococcosis in otherwise normal individuals or in individuals with chronic respiratory disease in the absence of immunosuppression (Lewis and Rabinovich, 1972). In contrast, an association between pulmonary cryptococcosis and Hodgkin's disease is well established (Littman and Walter, 1986). Patients being treated with corticosteroids are also known to have an increased risk of serious infection. *C. neoformans* has a predilection for patients with reticuloendothelial malignancies, as well as for transplant recipients on immunosuppressive drugs (Kaplan et al, 1977). This organism has become an important pathogen in patients with AIDS (Masur et al, 1985). In contrast to patients with invasive aspergillosis, patients with neutropenia or those receiving broad-spectrum antibiotic therapy are not at greater risk of pulmonary cryptococcosis (Goldstein and Rambo, 1962).

The most common presenting symptoms in children with pulmonary cryptococcosis are fever, malaise, pleuritic or nonpleuritic chest pain, weight loss, dyspnea, and night sweats. Cough has been found to be an uncommon symptom in some series, and hemoptysis remains an unusual finding (Kerkering et al, 1981). Cryptococcal involvement in the lungs may present in a totally asymptomatic patient who comes to a physician's attention because of an abnormal chest radiograph. If infection spreads to the central nervous system, headache is the main symptom.

Confusing to many physicians is the fact that *C. neoformans* may colonize the respiratory tract in normal hosts or those with chronic respiratory disease.

However, colonization is not usually appreciated in immunocompromised hosts because these patients develop clinical disease (Kaplan et al, 1977). Unlike infections in normal hosts, cryptococcal pneumonia in immunocompromised hosts may also involve multiple organs and can occur simultaneously with other respiratory pathogens such as *Escherichia coli*, *Klebsiella*, and other gram-negative organisms (Kaplan et al, 1977).

The radiologic presentation of patients with pulmonary cryptococcal disease includes various different abnormalities (Fig. 51–2*A* and *B*). The most common lesions seen are nodules or mass lesions with alveolar interstitial infiltrates. On occasion, a combination of rounded opacities and inflammatory infiltrates is seen. In a series by Kerkering, most of the immunocompromised patients with pulmonary cryptococcosis presented with nodular patterns, mass lesions, abscesses, or cavitary disease. Also seen were solitary coin lesions, multiple small, round opacities, and occasionally an alveolar or interstitial infiltrate (Kerkering et al, 1981). In children, cryptococcal disease has no focal predilection, with all lobes being equally involved. Although pulmonary fibrosis and cavitary lesions are uncommon, the presence of hilar lymph node enlargement, which can be seen in cryptococcal pulmonary disease, may make the distinction from tuberculosis difficult in children. As seen in immunocompromised patients with invasive pulmonary aspergillosis, pulmonary cryptococcosis can present with a normal chest radiograph.

The diagnosis of pulmonary cryptococcosis can be difficult. Identification of high-risk groups, including patients who have AIDS, organ transplantation with immunosuppressive therapy, cancer, and chronic pulmonary disease should be considered with a high index of suspicion for cryptococcal involvement. Sputum should be cultured if available, and the isolation of *C. neoformans* should lead to tests for disseminated disease. Although colonization of the tracheobronchial tree may occur in normal and immunocompromised patients (Tynes et al, 1968), isolation of *C. neoformans* with pulmonary involvement should be presumed to indicate infection. Early studies of normal hosts demonstrated a moderate rate of 19 to 23 per cent for cryptococcal isolation from sputum in adults (Lewis and Rabinovich, 1972). Later series of immunocompromised hosts have shown higher rates of *C. neoformans* recovery (Kerkering et al, 1981). Isolation of organisms may take several days, although the organism may grow on common bacteriologic media. In patients with pronounced pulmonary involvement, bronchoscopy with bronchial washings or bronchoalveolar lavage can provide valuable material for direct wet-preparation evaluation, cytocentrifugation preparations, fungal stains, and culture. Although open-lung biopsy with histopathologic examination of tissue may prove to be necessary, surveys have demonstrated that bronchoalveolar lavage can have a comparable yield. Tests for cryptococcal antigen in serum have been less successful for the diagnosis of pulmonary cryptococcosis. Conflicting reports have demonstrated moderate to low yields of serum cryptococcal antigen in pulmonary disease (Prevost and Newell, 1978), compared with approximately 95 per cent positivity when cerebrospinal

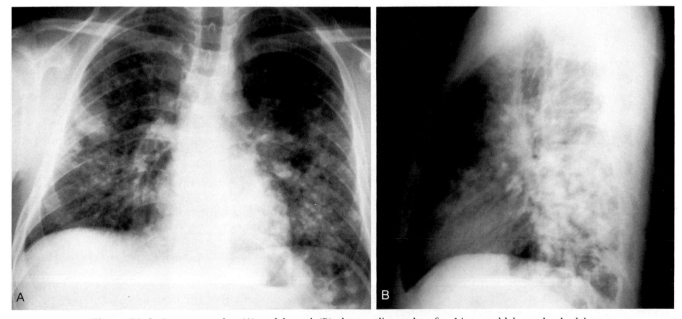

Figure 51–2. Posteroanterior *(A)* and lateral *(B)* chest radiographs of a 14-year-old boy who had been exposed to bird droppings in a barn and presented with sudden onset of fever, chills, and cough. He was diagnosed with cryptococcal pneumonia on the basis of a direct smear and culture following a flexible bronchoscopy and bronchoalveolar lavage. The radiographic description is a diffuse, patchy, parenchymal infiltrate in all lobes of the lung with maximal involvement in the lower lobes bilaterally.

fluid is analyzed in cryptococcal meningitis. Therefore, detection of cryptococcal antigen in serum is helpful when positive in immunocompromised patients, but a negative serologic test does not rule out the possibility of pulmonary cryptococcal disease. If pulmonary cryptococcosis is diagnosed in an immunocompromised patient, an evaluation for disseminated disease with cultures of urine, blood, cerebrospinal fluid, bone marrow, or biopsy material is indicated. Because of the increased risk of dissemination in immunocompromised patients, pulmonary disease due to *C. neoformans* should always be treated with antifungal drugs with a suspicion of dissemination (Kerkering et al, 1981).

Although prospective studies to determine the optimal combination of drugs, dosages, or length of therapy have been performed, amphotericin B and 5-flucytosine have been proved to be effective in cryptococcal meningitis (Bennett et al, 1979). The use of amphotericin B alone in cryptococcal pneumonia has been considered the mainstay of therapy. The use of oral imidiazole drugs such as ketoconazole have been successful in anecdotal reports of normal children with isolated pulmonary involvement (see Table 51–2). As with other pulmonary mycoses in immunocompromised patients, the prognosis for this infection depends on the presence or absence of dissemination. Early diagnosis and rapid initiation of therapy in patients with isolated pulmonary cryptococcosis contribute to an excellent prognosis. However, disseminated cryptococcal disease in immunocompromised patients may have a mortality as high as 50 per cent (Kerkering et al, 1981).

PULMONARY CANDIDIASIS

Of all the pulmonary mycoses in immunocompromised patients, candidal pneumonia can be the most difficult to diagnose and treat effectively because the organism routinely colonizes the upper respiratory tract, leading to positive cultures even without disease. Signs and symptoms of infection are nonspecific, and infected patients frequently have simultaneous infections with other pulmonary pathogens (Masur et al, 1977). Candidal pneumonia may manifest as a focal process in the lungs and may be easily missed by bronchoalveolar lavage or biopsy.

Candidal pneumonia usually occurs in immunocompromised patients but is also a frequent infection in neonates or patients on prolonged courses of broad-spectrum antibiotics. Children with leukemia and associated neutropenia are at high risk for candidal pneumonia or disseminated disease. Patients with increased susceptibility include those with reticuloendothelial malignancies, on steroid therapy, with depressed cell-mediated immunity including AIDS, and organ transplant recipients on immunosuppressive therapy (Masur et al, 1977).

The majority of children with candidal pneumonia are febrile and appear septic. The pulmonary findings may be due to any one of various pathologic processes. However, patients may be entirely asymptomatic or may have various degrees of dyspnea up to and including respiratory failure. Crackles on lung auscultation are a variable finding and are not specific for candidal pneumonia, especially considering the possibility of secondary infection with other organisms.

The radiographic findings of candidal pneumonia are nonspecific. Early in the course of infection, approximately half of patients have a normal chest radiograph. Various radiographic abnormalities appear as the disease progresses, but few of these lesions are attributable to candidal infection alone (Buff et al, 1982). Therefore, the chest radiographs in patients with disseminated candidal infection may reflect multiple pulmonary processes. In a study of 20 immunocompromised patients with isolated *Candida albicans* pneumonia, all patients had alveolar disease on radiography, with 11 of 20 demonstrating evidence of interstitial abnormalities and 16 of 20 with bilateral disease. Eight of 20 patients had patchy, poorly defined parenchymal infiltrates, and 8 others had strictly lobar disease. The remaining four patients in this series had unilateral lobar or segmental abnormalities (Buff et al, 1982). In this study, 5 of 20 patients had pleural effusions. The diagnosis of candidal pneumonia may be extremely difficult. Although isolation of *Aspergillus* species or *C. neoformans* from the sputum of immunocompromised hosts may have some diagnostic significance, the isolation of *Candida* species may simply reflect colonization secondary to an immunocompromised state or broad-spectrum antibiotic therapy. Isolation of *Candida* species from blood or urine cultures in patients who appear critically ill is indicative of sepsis. This type of overwhelming infection with a concomitant pulmonary infiltrate is very suspicious of candidal pneumonia.

Serologic tests are presently of no clinical value in the diagnosis of candidal pneumonia because assays for *Candida* antibodies are insensitive and unable to distinguish between deep infection and superficial colonization. Antigen assays have yielded better results in clinical trials, but these tests are time consuming and not widely available. Methods of detection of D-arabinitol by gas liquid chromatography and yeast mannan by radioimmunoassay both are promising but have not yet been confirmed in extensive clinical trials (de Repentigny and Reiss, 1984). Proof of candidal pneumonia requires tissue examination or evaluation of bronchoalveolar lavage or protected brush samples from bronchoscopy as direct evidence of tissue invasion. As with the other opportunistic fungal pneumonias, the best treatment for candidal infection is control of the patient's underlying disease state with alleviation of immunosuppression and concomitant administration of amphotericin B. Although an in vitro synergistic effect for amphotericin B plus 5-flucytosine has been demonstrated for most *Candida* species (Montgomerie et al, 1975), the possible benefit of combined therapy in pulmonary infections remains unproven. The prognosis of candidal pneumonia is uncertain, because too few patients have been diagnosed ante mortem to allow assessment of outcome for treated and untreated patients. However, it is well known that the overall morbidity and mortality of disseminated candidal infection is similar to that of gram-negative enteric bacterial infections, especially in patients with underlying immunosuppression.

DIMORPHIC FUNGI

Certain fungal infections are known as endemic mycoses because of particular geographic distribution patterns, including those due to *H. capsulatum, Blastomyces dermatitidis, Coccidioides immitis, Paracoccidioides brasiliensis,* and *Penicillium marneffei.* The latter two dimorphic fungi are primarily found in South and Central America (Restrepo et al, 1976) and in China and Southeast Asia (Deng et al, 1988), respectively, and do not cause infection in the United States. Histoplasmosis is common and is discussed in detail in Chapter 50. All of these organisms have some characteristics that will be outlined briefly.

The terminology of dimorphism indicates that the fungus exists in nature in a mycelial phase that converts to a ycast phase at body temperature. Unlike other fungi *(Candida, Aspergillus),* these organisms are not associated with colonization or contamination. Therefore, visualization of the yeast in or from tissue specimens or culture of organisms usually accomplished in the mycelial phase from clinical specimens gives a secure and reliable diagnosis (Davies and Sarosi, 1987). Other diagnostic studies of serology or skin tests range from being useless in a clinical setting for blastomycosis (Sarosi and Davies, 1979) to a helpful aid for diagnosis and for following effectiveness of therapy in coccidioidomycosis (Drutz and Catanzaro, 1978). Cross-reactivity between fungal antigens remains a difficult limiting factor for these studies.

These dimorphic fungi cause infection following inhalation of conidia into the pulmonary system (Drutz and Frey, 1985). As the host begins to mount its defenses, particularly with cellular immunity, transition to the yeast phase occurs with growth in the lung and at foci in various organs after hematogenous or lymphatic dissemination. After the development of immunity, which is noted in the majority of patients, inflammatory responses characterized by both granuloma formation and by suppuration with polymorphonuclear infiltration halt the growth at the initial and distant sites of infection. Endogenous reactivation may occur at either pulmonary or extrapulmonary sites (Goodwin and DesPrez, 1978; Laskey and Sarosi, 1978). Progressive primary infection in the absence of host defenses (infant, immunocompromised) may lead to miliary dissemination and death if untreated.

Cellular immunity is considered to be the primary host defense for these deep mycoses (Bradsher, 1984). Evidence includes lethal infections in experimental animal models with intact humoral immunity but deficient T lymphocyte activity. Conversely, patients with agammaglobulinemia do not have progressive infection with these mycoses. Lymphocyte reactivity to portions of the fungus has provided an in vitro marker of immunity in coccidioidomycosis (Cox et al, 1976; Barbee and Hicks, 1988), paracoccidioidomycosis (Musati et al, 1976), histoplasmosis (Alford and Cartwright, 1981), and blastomycosis (Bradsher et al, 1987) correlating with cure of the infection. Delayed hypersensitivity skin test reactions with fungal antigens are not helpful diagnostically in the endemic areas but have been useful in defining the epidemiology of these mycoses.

The treatment of these fungal infections is also similar. Many cases of histoplasmosis (Goodwin and DesPrez, 1978), coccidioidomycosis (Drutz and Catanzaro, 1978), and probably blastomycosis (Sarosi and Davies, 1979) are subclinical and require no antifungal therapy. Those patients with severe, life-threatening infections should receive amphotericin B therapy. The oral imidazole and triazole antifungal drugs are used for patients with illnesses in between those ends of the spectrum. Specific regimens for blastomycosis and coccidioidomycosis will be presented in the discussion of the causative organisms.

COCCIDIOIDOMYCOSIS

Primarily occurring in the southwestern United States, coccidioidomycosis is a relatively common infection whose incidence reportedly approaches that of varicella in the highest endemic areas. The lower Sonoran life zone including parts of California, Arizona, Texas, Nevada, New Mexico, and Mexico apparently supports growth from the mycelia and represent the infectious stage of the fungus. These arthrospores resist drying, which likely is the explanation for illness in microbiology laboratory workers or in persons outside the endemic area exposed to dust from endemic locations (Gehlbach et al, 1973). In humans, the fungus becomes a spherule containing ultimately large numbers of endospores. Budding does not occur with this fungus.

Susceptibility to primary infection is uniform, but certain groups have a greater risk of dissemination. Race is a factor, and Asians (particularly Filipino) are at highest risk for progressive disease, followed by blacks and Native Americans (Drutz and Catanzaro, 1978). Mexicans are reported to be only slightly more susceptible than whites to disseminated disease. The frequency of progressive disease is also higher in children 5 years or younger and adults 50 years or older. Pregnancy greatly increases the risk of fatal dissemination of primary infection (Vanbergen et al, 1976), and the later coccidioidomycosis is contracted in the gestation period, the greater the risk of dissemination. Although the fact is not surprising, immunosuppressive therapy or diseases such as HIV infection greatly increase the chance of disseminated disease.

The characteristic clinical picture of coccidioidomycosis is a flu-like illness with fever, cough, and chest pain, and transient rash is reported to be common in children. This may either be a maculopapular eruption or the classic lesions of erythema nodosum, which when associated with arthralgias is called *valley fever* (Smith, 1940).

Radiographic abnormalities are common but not diagnostic and range from patchy infiltrates to hilar adenopathy to pleural disease. Extrapulmonary disease means dissemination, and osseous, cutaneous, and articular sites are the most common. Meningitis may occur with or without other sites of dissemination and may be more common in young children to adolescents than other manifestations.

Diagnostic studies include skin tests with coccidioidin or spherulin, with the latter being a better antigenic stimulus. In the endemic area, positive skin tests are not diagnostic of acute infection (Drutz and Catanzaro, 1978). Antibody detection by complement fixation or precipitin is a useful measure of severity of disease and a guide to effectiveness of therapy.

Amphotericin B is given as a total dose of 15 to 40 mg/kg for serious coccidioidal infections and requires 6 to 8 weeks (Drutz and Catanzaro, 1978). Because of the nephrotoxicity, systemic symptoms, hypokalemia, and anemia associated with amphotericin B, many clinicians favor nontreatment when faced with a patient with only mild pulmonary illness. If the infection causes prolonged fever, mediastinal adenopathy, or disseminated lesions, therapy is considered. Ketoconazole, an orally absorbed imidazole antifungal agent, has been useful in skeletal, cutaneous, and other localized infection but not for meningitis with the commonly used lower doses (Brass et al, 1980). Other agents such as itraconazole and fluconazole are currently under clinical investigation. Meningitis due to *C. immitis* is the most difficult manifestation to treat. Intraventricular or intralumbar intrathecal therapy with amphotericin B is used in conjunction with systemic therapy.

BLASTOMYCOSIS

B. dermatitidis, like histoplasmosis and coccidioidomycosis, is associated with either epidemics of infection or endemic cases of infection (Sarosi and Davies, 1979). The majority of endemic cases occur in young adult to middle-aged persons, particularly men with significant occupational or recreational exposure to outdoor areas. Cases are most likely located in states surrounding the Mississippi and Ohio rivers, with the greatest numbers from Arkansas, Kentucky, Mississippi, North Carolina, Tennessee, Louisiana, and Wisconsin (Bradsher, 1987). Blastomycosis has been reported from other continents, so the *North American*

blastomycosis has been abandoned. Likewise, infection with *P. brasiliensis* should be known as *paracoccidioidomycosis* and not *South American blastomycosis*. The male-to-female ratio in large series has ranged from 4:1 to 15:1 for blastomycosis. Fewer than 80 endemic cases have been reported in children, with an estimate of fewer than 2 per cent of blastomycosis occurring during childhood (Steele and Abernathy, 1983).

In contrast to the endemic infections, epidemics of infection may involve children with a more equal distribution between boys and girls. A total of nine well-documented epidemics have been reported from North Carolina, Minnesota, Illinois, Wisconsin, and Virginia (Klein et al, 1987). Klein and co-workers reported infection in 47 of 89 children visiting an environmental camp and documented, for the first time, the point source for an epidemic of blastomycosis by isolating the organism from the soil (Klein et al, 1986). Another epidemic in children investigated by the same workers confirmed the isolation techniques with a second isolation from soil (Klein et al, 1987). Both instances of cultural confirmation used moist soil with high organic content associated with bodies of water. This association with lakes and rivers may simply be the greater potential for exposure because of increased recreational activities (Bradsher, 1987).

The organism is a thick-walled, budding yeast that may be microscopically found in sputum or in exudates of skin or other lesions after potassium hydroxide digestion of host cells. Cultures are uniformly positive if organisms are seen in specimens. Cytology examination of sputum may also allow the diagnosis of blastomycosis. The relative ease of diagnosis by smears or cultures is fortunate because other diagnostic studies are not helpful (Davies and Sarosi, 1987). Antibody studies by complement fixation or immunodiffusion precipitin bonds or with delayed hypersensitivity skin tests with blastomycin are not helpful. Patients with blastomycosis are just as likely to have antibodies to histoplasmin as they are to blastomycin (Sarosi and Davies, 1979). Newer techniques using enzyme immunoassay or immunodiffusion with yeast phase antigens are more promising but not clinically available.

Acute pneumonia may be confused with bacterial disease, whereas the more common picture of chronic pneumonia resembles tuberculosis (Fig. 51–3). Extrapulmonary infections are most likely to be in the skin and subcutaneous tissues, although bone, genitourinary, meningeal, or virtually all tissues may be sites of blastomycosis. Although immunosuppressed patients may be infected with this fungus, other fungal infections such as disseminated histoplasmosis or cryptococcal meningitis are much more likely to be opportunistic than blastomycosis.

Treatment of blastomycosis follows the same pattern as in coccidioidomycosis. When the choice was between amphotericin B and simple observation for spontaneous resolution of pneumonia, the toxicity of the antifungal agent made nontreatment an attractive

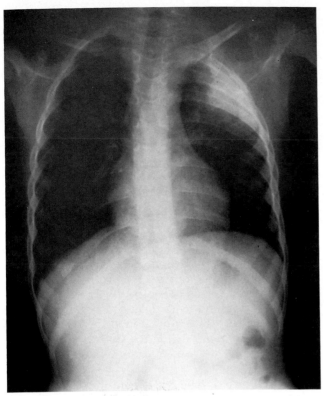

Figure 51–3. A posteroanterior chest radiograph of a 7-year-old boy from southern Arkansas who presented with fever, night sweats, mild lethargy, and a 5- to 10-pound weight loss over a period of 3 months. *Blastomyces dermatitidis* was isolated from bronchoalveolar lavage fluid. The radiographic description reveals an abnormal density in the left upper lobe consistent with localized, consolidated pneumonia.

option. With progressive infection or with extrapulmonary manifestation, therapy is indicated. Amphotericin B is effective at a total dose of 15 to 40 mg/kg over a 6- to 8-week regimen. Several studies have reported success rates of 80 per cent or higher with ketoconazole (Bradsher et al, 1985; National Institutes of Allergy and Infectious Diseases, 1985). Although endocrine effects of depressed testosterone levels may be noted with ketoconazole, the oral agent has been successfully used in children with blastomycosis. Itraconazole, an experimental triazole agent, is another oral antifungal with efficacy in this infection, including patients who have failed to respond or have suffered relapse after ketoconazole. As with the other systemic fungi, in very ill patients, amphotericin B remains the drug of choice, but switching to an oral imidazole after improvement may be appropriate. One difficulty with oral therapy is noncompliance. Some patients reported to have poor results with ketoconazole were those who did not take the drug as instructed. In patients with less than life-threatening infection with blastomycosis, ketoconazole taken for 6 months can be considered to be the drug of choice.

OTHER PULMONARY DIMORPHIC FUNGI

P. brasiliensis is distinguished from other dimorphic fungi by the geographic distribution in Latin America from Argentina to Mexico and by the multiple buds that may be seen from the yeast cells on direct smears of exudate (Restrepo et al, 1976). The infection follows the same pathophysiology as for blastomycosis. It is rarely found in persons younger than 30 years and manifests as pneumonia or focal lesions in the skin or mucous membranes. This fungus may be the most susceptible to ketoconazole, itraconazole, or other imidazole agents (Negroni et al, 1987; Restrepo et al, 1987).

Penicilliosis due to *P. marneffei* has been reported to follow a pattern very similar to histoplasmosis in that it is a dimorphic fungus that produces suppurative and granulomatous tissue reactions in normal persons but necrotic areas in anergic patients (Deng et al, 1988). It may present with either focal or disseminated disease but usually begins by a pulmonary portal of entry. The organism proliferates inside macrophages as does *H. capsulatum* and has a specific ecologic niche that is restricted to the Far East. Of the 22 reports in the literature, six were in children less than 20 years of age (Deng et al, 1988).

OTHER UNCOMMON PULMONARY MYCOSES

PULMONARY MUCORMYCOSES

Fungi of the order Mucorales can cause devastating pulmonary infection in immunocompromised hosts. *Rhizopus*, *Mucor*, and *Absidia* are most common, although in recent years *Fusarium*, *Cunninghamolla*, and *Saksenaea* have been reported as opportunistic infections in immunocompromised hosts. The clinical picture for these pulmonary mycoses closely resembles infection due to *Aspergillus*, with the same difficulty of diagnosis requiring histopathologic examination or examination by bronchoalveolar lavage (Kolbeck et al, 1985).

Epidemiologically, the same high-risk factors of organ transplantation, immunosuppressive therapy, chemotherapeutic regimens in oncology patients, and long-term administration of corticosteroids predispose to infection with these fungal elements. Specifically for mucormycosis, patients with ketoacidosis due to diabetes mellitus and those with insufficient peripheral vascular disease are at high risk for infection (Pennington, 1983). The clinical presentation of pulmonary mucormycoses is very similar to that of aspergillosis. The radiologic presentations most commonly seen with this group include parenchymal consolidation without a predilection for any particular lobe (Greene, 1980). A normal chest radiograph does not rule out mucormycosis in immunocompromised patients; upper respiratory tract involvement with sinusitis represents the most common manifestation of mucormycosis in this group.

Definitive diagnosis requires histologic demonstration of the fungus within lung parenchyma or on bronchoalveolar lavage. The organisms can be isolated from these cultures but may take 2 to 6 weeks for final identification. Stains of histopathologic sections or cytocentrifugation preparations on bronchoalveolar lavage fluid may prove to be important in differentiating the characteristic morphology of *Mucor* from that of other fungi (Williams et al, 1976). Phaeohyphomycosis due to organisms known as *Helminthosporium*, *Curvularia*, *Drechslera*, and *Bipolaris* may cause similar infections, but in normal persons. These organisms do not typically lead to the devastating effects noted with mucormycosis (Jay et al, 1988; Adam et al, 1986).

Control of the patient's underlying disease is the mainstay of therapy for disease due to mucormycosis. Amphotericin B is the drug of choice, but it has been difficult to show prolongation of life if the underlying disease persists (Lehrer, 1980). Amphotericin B is less effective against the Mucorales and select other fungal species because of variable in vitro sensitivities, which means that very high intravenous doses must be used. Surgical resection can be considered for patients with localized parenchymal disease in the lung, but its value is unproven. Pulmonary mucormycosis carries a dismal prognosis; only a few patients with early intervention, diagnosis, and treatment have survived.

SPOROTHRIX SCHENCKII

Pulmonary sporotrichosis is rare, even in immunocompromised patients (Wilson et al, 1967). *Sporothrix schenckii* is dimorphic but is the exception to the typical pattern described earlier for *Blastomyces* and others. The vast majority of cases of sporotrichosis are secondary to cutaneous inoculation rather than respiratory inhalation. Pulmonary infection may rarely occur as an isolated event or as a manifestation of dissemination from lymphocutaneous sites. Pulmonary involvement with this fungus is rare in children, and most case reports in adults are associated with alcoholism, sarcoidosis, and the use of corticosteroids.

Human pulmonary infections usually begin as a mild bronchitis with subsequent fever and cough (Beland et al, 1968). Chest radiographs of normal hosts usually show cavitary disease, but in immunocompromised patients linear or nodular patterns predominate. The diagnosis of pulmonary sporotrichosis relies on culture and histologic demonstration of the organism. Isolation from sputum is highly suggestive of infection but is not diagnostic because of its occasional role as a saprophyte (Lowenstein et al, 1978). On histologic examination, the small yeasts may be difficult to see on routine smears but if present may be diagnosed by direct fluorescent antibody staining of pathology specimens. Serologic tests are helpful in documenting pulmonary sporotrichosis of normal hosts, but their role in immunocompromised patients is undefined. Skin testing for delayed hypersensitivity is of doubtful value.

Treatment of pulmonary sporotrichosis can be difficult even in normal hosts, but amphotericin B remains the drug of choice (Parker et al, 1970). Ketoconazole is not effective, but newer imidazoles such as itraconazole may have promise in the therapy of sporotrichosis. For cavitary disease, a combination of amphotericin B and surgical resection may offer the best chance for cure. Even with this modality, the prognosis is uncertain because so few cases have been described even in adults.

OTHER FUNGAL PATHOGENS

A number of other saprophytic fungi have been shown to cause pulmonary infection in immunocompromised hosts. *Pseudoallescheria boydii* has been recovered from the lungs of patients who had leukemia and who presented with persistent fever, pleuritic chest pain, and hemoptysis (Winston et al, 1977). This pathogen has also been found in bone marrow transplant recipients with bilateral pneumonia and refractory fever. This infection differs from other fungal infections in its relative clinical resistance to amphotericin B, and miconazole or one of the imidazoles is the drug of choice (Gumbart, 1983).

Trichosporon has been isolated from autopsy material of transplant recipients and from patients with hematologic malignancies (Saul et al, 1981). A *Penicillium* species other than *P. marneffei* causing hemorrhagic pulmonary infarctions has been described in a rare patient with acute leukemia (Huang and Harris, 1963). *Fusarium*, another opportunist, has been encountered histologically in the lungs of a patient with non-Hodgkin's lymphoma (Young et al, 1978). All three of these fungi share the angioinvasive propensities of *Aspergillus*, and histologic and cultural distinction are necessary for diagnosis.

REFERENCES

Adam RD, Paquin ML, Petersen EA et al: Phaeohyphomycosis caused by the fungal genera *Bipolaris* and *Exserohilum*. A report of 9 cases and review of the literature. Medicine 65:203, 1986.

Aisner J, Murillo J, Schimpff SC et al: Invasive aspergillosis in acute leukemia: correlation with nose cultures and antibiotic use. Ann Intern Med 90:4, 1979.

Aisner J, Schimpff SC, and Wiernik PH: Treatment of invasive aspergillosis: relation of early diagnosis and treatment to response. Ann Intern Med 86:539–543, 1977.

Albelda SM, Talbot GH, Gerson SL et al: Role of fiberoptic bronchoscopy in the diagnosis of invasive pulmonary aspergillosis in patients with acute leukemia. Am J Med 76:1027, 1984.

Alford RH and Cartwright BB: Human lymphocyte blastogenesis induced by living and dead *Histoplasma capsulatum* yeasts and soluble yeast autolysate. Sabouraudia 19:85, 1981.

Barbee RA and Hicks MJ: Clinical usefulness of lymphocyte transformation in coccidioidomycosis. Chest 93:1003, 1988.

Beland JE, Mankiewicz E, and MacIntosh DJ: Primary pulmonary sporotrichosis. Can Med Assoc J 99:813, 1968.

Bennett JE, Dismukes WE, Duma RJ et al: A comparison of amphotericin B alone and combined with flucytosine in the treatment of cryptococcal meningitis. N Engl J Med 301:126, 1979.

Bradsher RW: Development of specific immunity in patients with pulmonary or extrapulmonary blastomycosis. Am Rev Respir Dis 129:930, 1984.

Bradsher RW: Water and blastomycosis: don't blame beaver. Am Rev Respir Dis 136:1324, 1987.

Bradsher RW, Balk RA, and Jacobs RF: Growth inhibition of *Blastomyces dermatitidis* in alveolar and peripheral macrophages from patients with blastomycosis. Am Rev Respir Dis 135:412, 1987.

Bradsher RW, Rice DC, and Abernathy RS: Ketoconazole therapy for endemic blastomycosis. Ann Intern Med 103:872, 1985.

Brass C, Galgiani JN, Campbell SC et al: Therapy of disseminated or pulmonary coccidioidomycosis with ketoconazole. Rev Infect Dis 2:656, 1980.

Buff SJ, McLelland R, Gallis HA et al: *Candida albicans* pneumonia: radiographic appearance. AJR 138:645, 1982.

Comstock GW, Palmer CE, Stone RW et al: Fungi in the sputum of normal men. Mycopathologia 54:55, 1974.

Cox RA, Vivas JR, Gross A et al: In vivo and in vitro cell-mediated immune responses in coccidioidomycosis. Am Rev Respir Dis 114:937, 1976.

Davies SF, Sarosi GA: Aspergillosis in the immunosuppressed patient. In Al-doory Y and Wagner GE (eds): Aspergillosis. Charles C Thomas, Springfield, Ill, 1985.

Davies SF and Sarosi GA: Serodiagnosis of histoplasmosis and blastomycosis. Am Rev Respir Dis 136:254, 1987.

Deng Z, Ribas JL, Gibson DW, and Connor DH: Infections caused by *Penicillium marneffei* in China and Southeast Asia: review of eighteen published cases and report of four more Chinese cases. Rev Infect Dis 10:640, 1988.

de Repentigny L and Reiss E: Current trends in immunodiagnosis of candidiasis and aspergillosis. Rev Infect Dis 6:301, 1984.

Drutz DJ and Catanzaro A: Coccidioidomycosis. State of the art. I. Am Rev Respir Dis 117:559, 1978.

Drutz DJ and Frey CL: Intracellular and extracellular defenses of human phagocytes against *Blastomyces dermatitidis*, candida and yeasts. J Lab Clin Med 105:737, 1985.

Fisher BD, Armstrong D, Yu B et al: Invasive aspergillosis: progress in early diagnosis and treatment. Am J Med 71:571, 1981.

Gehlbach SH, Hamilton JD, and Conant NF: Coccidioidomycosis. An occupational disease in cotton mill workers. Arch Intern Med 131:254, 1973.

Gerson SL, Talbot GH, Hurwitz S et al: Prolonged granulocytopenia: the major risk factor for invasive pulmonary aspergillosis in patients with leukemia. Ann Intern Med 100:345, 1984.

Goldstein E and Rambo ON: Cryptococcal infection following steroid therapy. Ann Intern Med 56:114, 1962.

Goodwin RA and DesPrez RM: Histoplasmosis. State of the art. Am Rev Respir Dis 117:929, 1978.

Greene R: Opportunistic pneumonias. Semin Roentgenol 15:50, 1980.

Gumbart CH: *Pseudallescheria boydii* infection after bone marrow transplantation. Ann Intern Med 99:193, 1983.

Gustafson TL, Schaffner W, Lavely GB et al: Invasive aspergillosis in renal transplant recipients: correlation with corticosteroid therapy. J Infect Dis 148:230, 1983.

Herbert PA and Bayer AS: Fungal pneumonia: invasive pulmonary aspergillosis. Chest 80:220, 1981.

Huang S and Harris LS: Acute disseminated penicilliosis. Am J Clin Pathol 39:167, 1963.

Jay WM, Bradsher RW, LeMay B et al: Ocular involvement in mycotic sinusitis caused by Bipolarina. Am J Ophthalmol 105:366, 1988.

Kaplan MH, Rosen PP, and Armstrong D: Cryptococcosis in a cancer hospital. Cancer 39:2265, 1977.

Kerkering TM, Duma RJ, and Shadomy S: The evolution of pulmonary cryptococcosis. Ann Intern Med 94:611, 1981.

Klein BS, Vergeront JM, DiSalvo AF et al: Two outbreaks of blastomycosis along rivers in Wisconsin. Am Rev Respir Dis 136:1333, 1987.

Klein BS, Vergeront JM, Weeks RJ et al: Isolation of *Bidermatitidis* in soil associated with a large outbreak of blastomycosis in Wisconsin. N Engl J Med 314:529, 1986.

Kolbeck PC, Makhoul RG, Bollinger RR et al: Widely disseminated *Cunninghamella* mucormycosis in an adult renal transplant pa-

tient: case report and review of the literature. Am J Clin Pathol 83:747, 1985.

Laskey WL and Sarosi GA: Endogenous reactivation in blastomycosis. Ann Intern Med 88:50, 1978.

Lehrer RI: Mucormycosis. Ann Intern Med 93:93, 1980.

Lewis JL and Rabinovich S: The wide spectrum of cryptococcal infections. Am J Med 53:315, 1972.

Littman ML and Walter JE: Cryptococcosis: current status. Am J Med 45:922, 1986.

Lowenstein M, Markowitz SM, Nottebart HC et al: Existence of *Sporothrix schenckii* as a pulmonary saprophyte. Chest 73:419, 1978.

Maddy KT: Observations on *Coccidioides immitis* found naturally growing in soil. Ariz Med 22:281, 1965.

Masur H, Cheigh JS, and Stubenbord WT: Infection following renal transplantation: a changing pattern. Rev Infect Dis 4:1208, 1982.

Masur H, Rosen PP, and Armstrong D: Pulmonary disease caused by *Candida* species. Am J Med 63:914, 1977.

Masur H, Shelhamer J, and Parrillo JE: The management of pneumonias in immunocompromised patients. JAMA 253:1769, 1985.

Meyer RD, Young LS, Armstrong D et al: Aspergillosis complicating neoplastic disease. Am J Med 54:6, 1973.

Montgomerie JZ, Edwards JE, and Guze LB: Synergism of amphotericin B and 5-fluorocytosine for *Candida* species. J Infect Dis 132:82, 1975.

Musati CC, Rezkallah MT, Mendes E et al: In vivo and in vitro evaluation of cell-mediated immunity in patients with paracoccidioidomycosis. Cell Immunol 24:365, 1976.

Nalesnik MA, Myerowitz RL, Jenkins R et al: Significance of *Aspergillus* species isolated from respiratory secretions in the diagnosis of invasive pulmonary aspergillosis. J Clin Microbiol 11:370, 1980.

National Institutes for Allergy and Infectious Diseases. Mycosis Study Group: Treatment of blastomycosis and histoplasmosis with ketoconazole: results of a prospective randomized clinical trial. Ann Intern Med 103:861, 1985.

Negroni R, Palmieri O, Korenk M et al: Oral treatment of paracoccidioidomycosis and histoplasmosis with itraconazole in humans. Rev Infect Dis 9:547, 1987.

Orr OD, Myerowitz RL, and Dubois PJ: Patho-radiologic correlation of invasive pulmonary aspergillosis in the compromised host. Cancer 41:2028, 1978.

Parker JD, Sarosi GA, and Tosh FE: Treatment of extracutaneous sporotrichosis. Arch Intern Med 125:858, 1970.

Pennington JE: Opportunistic fungal pneumonias: *Aspergillus, Mucor, Candida, Torulopsis*. In Pennington JE, (ed): *Diagnosis and Management*. New York, Raven Press, 1983.

Prevost E and Newell R: Commercial cryptococcal latex kit: clinical evaluation in a medical center hospital. J Clin Microbiol 8:529, 1978.

Przjemski C and Mattii R: The formation of pulmonary mycetomata. Cancer 46:1701, 1980.

Restrepo A, Gomez I, Robledo J et al: Itraconazole in the treatment of paracoccidioidomycosis: a preliminary report. Rev Infect Dis 9:551, 1987.

Restrepo A, Robledo M, Giraldo R et al: The gamut of paracoccidioidomycosis. Am J Med 61:33, 1976.

Rinaldi MG: Invasive aspergillosis. Rev Infect Dis 5:1061, 1983.

Sarosi GA and Davies SF: Blastomycosis. State of the art. Am Rev Respir Dis 120:911, 1979.

Sarubbi FA, Kopf HB, Wilson MB et al: Increased recovery of *Aspergillus flavus* from respiratory specimens during hospital construction. Am Rev Respir Dis 125:33, 1982.

Saul SH, Khachatoorian T, Poorsattar A et al: Opportunistic *Trichosporon* pneumonia. Arch Pathol Lab Med 105:456, 1981.

Sidransky H and Pearl MA: Pulmonary fungus infections associated with steroid and antibiotic therapy. Dis Chest 39:630, 1961.

Smith CE: Epidemiology of acute coccidioidomycosis with erythema nodosum ("valley fever"). Am J Public Health 30:600, 1940.

Steele RW and Abernathy RS: Systemic blastomycosis in children. Pediatr Infect Dis 2:304, 1983.

Tynes B, Mason KN, Jenning AE et al: Variant forms of pulmonary cryptococcosis. Ann Intern Med 69:1117, 1968.

Vanbergen WS, Fleury FJ, and Cheatle EL: Fatal maternal disseminated coccidioidomycosis in a nonendemic area. Am J Obstet Gynecol 124:661, 1976.

Weiner MH, Talbot GH, Gerson SL et al: Antigen detection in the diagnosis of invasive aspergillosis. Ann Intern Med 99:777, 1983.

Williams DM, Krick JA, Remington JS et al: Pulmonary infection in the compromised host. Am Rev Respir Dis 114:131, 1976.

Wilson DE, Mann JJ, Bennett JE et al: Clinical features of extracutaneous sporotrichosis. Medicine 46:265, 1967.

Winston DJ, Jordan MC, and Rhodes J: *Allescheria boydii* infections in the immunosuppressed host. Am J Med 63:830, 1977.

Young NA, Kwon-Chung KJ, Kubota TT et al: Disseminated infection by *Fusarium moniliforme* during treatment for malignant lymphoma. J Clin Microbiol 7:589, 1978.

52

ROBERT F. PASS, M.D.

CYTOMEGALOVIRUS

Cytomegalovirus (CMV), a member of the herpesvirus group, is of medical significance principally because it is the leading cause of congenital viral infection in the United States, and it can produce severe and even fatal disseminated infections in immunocompromised patients. Lower respiratory disease due to CMV has been encountered almost exclusively in hosts with impaired cell-mediated immunity and is characterized by diffuse pneumonitis, a prolonged course, and frequent co-infection by other opportunistic pathogens.

THE VIRUS

In electron micrographs, CMV cannot be distinguished from other herpesviruses. It is a relatively large particle approximately 200 nm in diameter (Wright et al, 1964; Sarov and Abody, 1975). An electron-dense core of approximately 64 nm is surrounded by a capsid of 162 capsomeres with icosahedral symmetry. The capsid is contained within the tegument or matrix, which is surrounded by a lipid envelope. The nucleocapsid contains double-stranded DNA of approximately 150×10^6 daltons or 240 kilobases (DeMarchi et al, 1978; Gelen et al, 1978). At the molecular level, CMV replication has been characterized by sequential transcription of mRNA encoding immediate early, early, and late proteins (DeMarchi et al, 1980; Wather and Stinski, 1982), similar to that described for herpes simplex virus (Honess and Roizman, 1974). The immediate early proteins appear to be necessary for further transcription of the viral DNA; early proteins include viral DNA polymerase, as well as other enzymes and regulatory proteins (Landini and Michelson, 1988). Late proteins include structural proteins required for assembly of intact virions (Landini and Michelson,

1988). Replication of CMV takes place relatively slowly, with an eclipse phase of 72 to 96 hours.

In vitro replication of CMV is restricted to human fibroblasts. Viral replication takes place in the nucleus, with the envelope acquired by budding through the nuclear membrane. Enveloped virus particles accumulate within the cytoplasm. In fibroblast monolayers, CMV produces a focal cytopathic effect characterized by cell rounding, eosinophilic perinuclear inclusions, and basophilic nuclear inclusions; multinucleate giant cells are sometimes seen (Smith and deHarven, 1974). The time course of development of cytopathic effect is variable, depending on the size of the inoculum and the viral strain. Changes in cell architecture are usually detectable by conventional light microscope within 1 to 10 days after inoculation.

EPIDEMIOLOGY

Seroepidemiologic studies of many culturally and geographically diverse groups have found CMV infection in every human population that has been studied (Krech et al, 1971; Pass, 1985). The prevalence of antibody to CMV increases with age, although the rate of seropositivity at any given age may vary widely according to race, socioeconomic status, and geographic area. In developing countries CMV is acquired earlier in life; studies in Africa and the South Pacific have reported seropositivity rates of almost 100 per cent among prepubertal children (Schopfer et al, 1978; Lang, 1975). In Western Europe and the United States, higher CMV prevalence earlier in life has been associated with lower socioeconomic status (Krech et al, 1971; Pass, 1985). No perennial or seasonal patterns in incidence of CMV infection have been observed. Humans are the only known reservoir of human CMV infection.

Initial acquisition of CMV is clinically silent in more than 95 per cent of cases (Griffiths and Baboonian, 1984; Stagno et al, 1982). After primary infection, normal adults and children excrete virus from multiple sites (saliva, urine, tears, cervix, semen) for months to years (Pass, 1985). By means of latency and reactivation or low-level persistent infection, excretion of CMV can occur many years after primary infection. Thus acquisition of CMV in the community likely occurs through contact with someone who is silently infected. Through large-scale longitudinal studies and analysis of DNA from CMV strains, situations associated with horizontal transmission of CMV have been identified. All these situations present daily opportunities for repeated close contact with secretions or body fluids that could contain virus. Toddlers in day nurseries often transmit CMV to each other and to their adult caretakers, including parents and day-care workers (Pass et al, 1984; Adler, 1985; Murph et al, 1986; Pass et al, 1986; Adler, 1988). Among adults with multiple sex partners, CMV infection is highly prevalent (Drew et al, 1981; Chandler et al, 1985), and restriction enzyme analysis of DNA from CMV isolates from sex partners has revealed similar restriction fragment profiles, evidence for transmission (Handsfield et al, 1985). Respiratory droplets or aerosols are not thought to be important means of spread of CMV.

Perinatal transmission of CMV from mother to baby occurs mainly through three routes and is important because it maintains a reservoir of infection within a population and because it has associated morbidity. Transplacental transmission of CMV results in congenital infection in around 1 per cent of live-born infants in the United States (Alford et al, 1980). Although most infected infants escape damage, 10 to 20 per cent develop central nervous system sequelae (Pass, 1987; Stagno et al, 1982). CMV is present in the cervix or vaginal secretions of up to 28 per cent of women late in pregnancy and can be transmitted to newborns during birth (Pass, 1987). Around 50 per cent of babies born to mothers excreting virus in the genital tract will acquire virus natally; these infants usually begin to excrete CMV between 3 weeks and 3 months of age.

In addition, CMV is shed in human milk and can be transmitted to breast-fed infants (Hayes et al, 1972; Stagno et al, 1980). In populations in which most mothers are seropositive and nurse their babies, infection rates of more than 50 per cent have been noted during the first year of life (Stagno et al, 1980). Children who acquire CMV perinatally or during the first year of life are likely to excrete virus in saliva or urine for years and can serve as a source of infection in the community.

Nosocomial transmission of CMV occurs through blood products and transplanted tissue (Pass and Stagno, 1988). Transfusion-acquired CMV in immunologically normal adults and children is usually asymptomatic but has been associated with a heterophil-negative mononucleosis or "postperfusion syndrome." In immunocompromised hosts, including small premature neonates, hospital-acquired CMV infection is a significant problem. A case report found evidence of cross-infection among newborns in a hospital nursery (Spector, 1983), but a prospective study in a newborn nursery could not document spread of CMV strains among patients or to personnel (Adler et al, 1986). Other studies of nurses, including those working with neonates and transplant recipients, have found no evidence of increased risk of CMV infection (Dworsky, et al, 1983; Balfour and Balfour, 1986), although one report suggested increased risk for nurses on intensive care units and teams handling intravenous blood (Friedman et al, 1984). In spite of the fact that CMV can remain infectious for hours on plastic surfaces (Faix, 1985) and that hospitalized children frequently shed virus, nonparenteral transmission in the hospital seems to be rare.

CLINICAL MANIFESTATIONS

Acquired CMV infection in normal hosts is usually asymptomatic. Less than 5 per cent of adults with primary CMV infection have heterophile antibody-negative mononucleosis syndrome. Cytomegalovirus mononucleosis was initially characterized by fever, hepatomegaly, adenopathy, and lymphocytosis with atypical lymphocytes (Klemola et al, 1969). In a study of 44 patients with heterophil antibody-negative mononucleosis, none of the 19 in whom CMV was the cause was less than 15 years of age (Klemola et al, 1970). As with Epstein-Barr virus, primary CMV infection in children is less likely to be symptomatic than in adults. A comparison of clinical features of CMV mononucleosis (diagnosed by IgM antibody) in adults and children reported that children were less likely than adults to have fever (43 versus 94 per cent) but were more likely to have cervical adenopathy, hepatomegaly, and lymphocytosis (Pannuti et al, 1985). The prominent features of CMV mononucleosis in 14 Brazilian children are shown in Table 52–1. Lower respiratory disease does not appear to be a feature of CMV mononucleosis in otherwise healthy

Table 52–1. FEATURES OF CMV MONONUCLEOSIS IN 14 PREVIOUSLY HEALTHY CHILDREN

Feature	No.	(%) Positive
Hepatomegaly	14	(100)
Lymphocytosis > 5000/mm³	13	(93)
Atypical lymphocytes > 1000/mm³	13	(93)
Cervical adenopathy	12	(86)
Splenomegaly	12	(86)
Elevated transaminase	11/13	(85)
Fever > 10 days	6	(43)
Exudative tonsillitis	3	(21)

Mean age 5.1 years. Diagnosis of acute CMW infection was made by detection of IgM antibody.

(From Pannuti CS, Vilas Boas LS, Angelo MJO et al: Cytomegalovirus mononucleosis in children and adults: differences in clinical presentation. Scand J Infect Dis 17:153, 1985.)

adults or children. In a review of 82 cases of CMV mononucleosis, pneumonitis was not described (Horwitz et al, 1986). A literature review found eight cases reported, but the diagnoses were made mostly by serology (Cohen and Corey, 1985). The occurrence of lower respiratory disease in nonimmunocompromised, nontransfused patients with CMV mononucleosis is so unusual that CMV should not be assumed to be the cause when these two problems coincide.

Recognition of pulmonary disease due to CMV requires knowledge of the clinical situations in which it is likely to occur and a critical approach to diagnosis. In most cases, lower respiratory disease due to CMV presents as tachypnea, a nonproductive cough, and bilateral diffuse interstitial pneumonitis. There is great variability in rapidity of onset, severity, duration of respiratory illness, and presence of associated signs of disseminated CMV infection such as fever, leukopenia, and hepatitis.

CONGENITAL INFECTION

Clinical manifestations of congenital CMV infection have been reviewed elsewhere (Hanshaw, 1983; Pass, 1987). More than 90 per cent of congenital CMV infections are clinically silent; among those patients who are symptomatic in the newborn period, the most common clinical and laboratory abnormalities are hepatosplenomegaly, petechiae, jaundice, small size for gestational age, inguinal hernias, microcephaly, direct hyperbilirubinemia, thrombocytopenia, and elevated transaminases. Pneumonitis appears to be a distinctly unusual manifestation of congenital CMV infection. However, inclusion-bearing cells are frequently found in the lungs at autopsy, even in the absence of clinical or histologic evidence of pneumonitis (Becroft, 1981). Because pneumonitis is infrequently observed in congenital CMV infection, other causes should be sought in any suspected case.

INFANTS

Cytomegalovirus pneumonitis has been encountered in small premature neonates who acquired the virus through blood transfusion (Table 52–2). Newborns who are born to seronegative mothers and receive blood from seropositive donors are at risk.

Yeager and colleagues (1981) found that 13.5 per cent of these newborns acquired CMV as compared with no infections when red blood cells from seronegative donors were used. Volume of blood transfused and number of donors seemed to be important risk factors. Nine of Yeager's 10 premature neonates with transfusion-acquired CMV had received blood from five or more donors, and CMV infection was not observed in seronegative infants who received less than 50 ml. Symptomatic infection was noted in newborns who weighed less than 1200 g at birth in Yeager's study and in a similar prospective study (Adler et al, 1983). Abnormalities associated with onset of CMV excretion in these patients have included findings much like those observed in neonates with congenital CMV infection—hepatosplenomegaly, elevated transaminases, petechiae, thrombocytopenia, and lymphocytosis. Lung involvement was indicated by appearance of new infiltrates on chest radiograph or deterioration in preexisting lung disease with increasing oxygen requirement. Yeager described four cases of pneumonia; three of the infants died. Adler described respiratory disease in two of three small premature neonates who died after transfusion-acquired CMV infection. In another study, the incidence of respiratory disease among preterm infants (< 2000 g) who acquired CMV postnatally was compared with controls matched for birth weight, gestational age, and date of birth (Sawyer et al, 1987). There was radiographic evidence of bronchopulmonary dysplasia in 75 per cent of infected infants as compared with 33 per cent of controls (p = 0.005). Infants with CMV required oxygen longer, were intubated longer, and were hospitalized longer. CMV must be considered an important cause of respiratory morbidity among premature newborns who are seronegative and acquire virus through transfusion.

The role of CMV as a pathogen in lower respiratory disease in term infants who acquire virus from a maternal source is more controversial. A report of two cases in 1976 suggested that CMV acquired during birth could cause pneumonia in young infants (Whitley et al, 1976). Two infants each had diffuse pneumonitis beginning at 1 month of age, and respiratory and radiologic abnormalities persisted for weeks. Cytomegalovirus was isolated from the cervix of each mother, and CMV was recovered from the upper respiratory tract of each infant. Although

Table 52–2. FREQUENCY OF CMV INFECTION AND PNEUMONIA IN INFANTS

Report	Patients	CMV Infected	Pneumonitis	Comment
Yeager et al, 1981	CMV seronegative infants given blood from seropositive donor(s)	10/74 (13.5%)	4/10 (40%)	3 fatalities
Adler et al, 1983	Neonatal intensive care unit	8/178 (4.5%)	3/8 (37.5%)	All 8 had birth weights <1100 g
Stagno et al, 1981	Infants <3 months of age with pneumonitis	21/104 (20.2%)	21/21 (100%*)	8/21 had other respiratory pathogens
Kumar et al, 1984	Infants born to CMV-excreting mothers	21/81 (25.9%)	3/21 (14.3%)	Respiratory symptoms resolved in 10–14 days

*Enrollment required radiographic evidence of diffuse, bilateral lower respiratory disease.

CMV appeared to be at least a contributing factor if not the principal cause of lower respiratory tract disease in these infants, by today's standards they were not adequately assessed for other common causes of diffuse lower respiratory disease such as *Chlamydia* or respiratory viruses. Stagno and colleagues (1981) reported results of a prospective study of 104 infants who were between 1 and 3 months of age and were hospitalized with pneumonitis; 21 were excreting CMV as compared with 3 of 97 (3 per cent) control infants (hospitalized for reasons other than pneumonia). A total of 44 infants in this study had evidence of infection by other respiratory pathogens including *Pneumocystis carinii* (by countercurrent immunoelectrophoresis), *Chlamydia trachomatis, Ureaplasma urealyticum,* enteroviruses, and various respiratory viruses; 8 of the CMV-infected infants were also infected with other agents. Further evidence associating CMV infection with lower respiratory disease in infants was reported by Kumar and associates (1984). They followed 81 neonates who were not CMV infected at birth and found that 21 acquired CMV during their first year of life; 16 of this group began to excrete CMV before 14 weeks of age. Seven infected infants had symptoms with onset of CMV excretion, including three with pneumonitis. It is likely that most of these infants acquired CMV from the maternal genital tract as they were born to mothers known to be infected with CMV. The infants were not viruric at birth; only one was breast-fed, and most began to excrete CMV 2 to 3 months after birth. Unfortunately, other respiratory pathogens were not rigorously sought, and therefore the etiologic role of CMV in the three cases of pneumonitis is unclear. Another report summarized results of follow-up of 60 infants who acquired CMV perinatally from the maternal genital tract at delivery or from mother's milk (Dworsky and Stagno, 1982). Four developed protracted pneumonitis temporally related to onset of CMV excretion; however, three of these had *C. trachomatis* infection as well. Although the temporal association between onset of CMV excretion and respiratory disease in infants exposed to virus natally suggests a causal role for CMV in some infants, there is no evidence that CMV acquired through mother's milk can result in lower respiratory tract disease in healthy term infants.

The most consistent pulmonary abnormality among CMV-infected infants with lower respiratory disease has been radiographic evidence of diffuse, bilateral, interstitial pneumonitis. Air trapping, diffuse atelectasis, and bronchial wall thickening have also been observed. Clinical findings are nonspecific and likely to be insidious. Most patients have tachypnea, nonproductive cough, and no fever. Diffuse rales are likely to be present with auscultation; expiratory wheeze has not been associated with CMV alone (Whitley et al, 1976; Stagno et al, 1981; Kumar et al, 1984; Dworsky and Stagno, 1982). The only clinical finding significantly associated with CMV as compared with other etiologies in Stagno's study was paroxysmal cough (Stagno, et al, 1981). Neither clinical nor radiographic findings allow one to distinguish pneumonitis due to CMV from that caused by other agents.

IMMUNOCOMPROMISED HOSTS

Frequently CMV is implicated as a cause of pneumonitis in immunocompromised patients, particularly transplant recipients (Table 52–3). Transplantation often combines use of immunosuppressive agents that significantly impair cell-mediated immunity with procedures that result in transmission of CMV. Both epidemiologic evidence from studies of risk factors for primary CMV infection and molecular studies of CMV strains recovered from donors and recipients indicate that CMV can be carried with renal, liver, and marrow grafts, resulting in primary infection during a time when the recipient is immunocompromised (Betts et al, 1975; Meyers et al, 1986; Rand et al, 1976; Chou, 1986; Singh et al, 1988). Among the various types of transplant recipients, CMV infection is most severe among those who have the greatest impairment of cellular immunity. Therefore, renal transplant recipients who receive well-matched kidneys (and thus minimal immunosuppression) usually handle CMV infections well, but among bone marrow recipients CMV remains a major cause of pulmonary disease including fatal pneumonia.

Although serologic or virologic evidence of CMV infection is commonly identified in transplant recipients, the occurrence of associated clinical manifestations is quite variable. Primary CMV infection in renal, cardiac, and liver transplant recipients, when symptomatic, has been heralded by fever, malaise, arthalgias, neutropenia, abnormal liver function test results, macular rash, and occasionally pneumonia (Meyers et al, 1986; Rand et al, 1976; Singh et al, 1988; Betts et al, 1977). The majority of primary infections in these patients have followed transplantation of an organ from a seropositive donor into a seronegative recipient; blood products have also been a source of primary CMV infection. Seroconversion, virus excretion, viremia, and symptoms usually occur between 4 and 8 weeks after transplantation. Similar symptoms associated with onset of CMV excretion have been encountered with reactivation of infection, though less frequently. The type and amount of immunosuppression used appear to influence both frequency and severity of CMV disease in recipients of renal, cardiac, and liver grafts. Use of antithymocyte globulin or OKT3 antibody have been associated with more severe CMV disease in renal (Pass et al, 1980) and liver graft recipients, respectively (Singh et al, 1988). In cardiac transplant recipients, both steroid dosage and antithymocyte globulin have been associated with greater risk of CMV infection and disease (Gorensek et al, 1988). Because centers vary in the proportion of patients who are seropositive before transplant, in screening for CMV infection in

Table 52–3. FREQUENCY OF CMV PNEUMONITIS IN IMMUNOCOMPROMISED PATIENTS, SELECTED REPORTS

Report	Patient Group	CMV Pneumonia	Comment
Betts et al, 1977	Renal transplant (RT) recipients with primary CMV infection	5/16 (31.3%)	Pneumonia temporally associated with onset of CMV excretion; infiltrates resolved in all 5.
Chatterjee et al, 1979	RT recipients	0/40 (0%)	3 had primary CMV infection.
Pass et al, 1980	RT recipients, seropositive pretransplant	5/67 (7.5%)	Only recipients of antithymocyte globulin had pneumonitis; 3 of 5 had other pulmonary pathogens.
Stover et al, 1985	Adults with AIDS	21/130 (16.2%)	86% mortality; 13 had *P. carinii* also.
Myers et al, 1986	Bone marrow transplant recipients	91/545 (16.7%)	85% mortality
Gorensek et al, 1988	Cardiac transplant recipients	5/34 (14.7%)	9 of 23 patients with posttransplant CMV infection were symptomatic; 5 had pneumonia.

organ and blood donors for seronegative recipients and in immunosuppressive regimens, there has been great center-to-center variability in the incidence of symptomatic CMV infection with associated pulmonary disease (see Table 52–3). There is evidence that transplant recipients with active CMV infection are at greater risk for infection by other opportunistic agents (Chatterjee et al, 1978), and apparent CMV pneumonia often includes co-infection with other pulmonary pathogens. Most renal, cardiac, and liver transplant recipients recover from CMV pneumonia, although fatalities have occurred.

Among bone marrow transplant recipients, CMV is the leading cause of lower respiratory tract disease and a major cause of morbidity and mortality (Meyers et al, 1986). Donor marrow and granulocyte transfusions are the major sources of virus for seronegative recipients. Acute graft-versus-host disease is an important risk factor for CMV infection and pneumonia. Patients undergoing bone marrow transplant for leukemias or other malignancies in which total-body irradiation is used have a greater risk of CMV pneumonia than patients who have aplastic anemia but are not irradiated (Meyers et al, 1986). Degree of donor/recipient histocompatibility is also a risk factor; CMV pneumonia is rare after transplantation of syngeneic marrow. Approximately 15 per cent of patients receiving allogeneic marrow for hematologic malignancy develop CMV pneumonia, with a case fatality rate of around 85 per cent (Meyers et al, 1986).

Among patients with the acquired immunodeficiency syndrome (AIDS), CMV has also proved to be a major cause of pulmonary disease. Three of the four homosexual men with AIDS initially described by Gottlieb had bronchial specimens positive for CMV (Gottlieb et al, 1981), as did three of Masur's 11 patients with community-acquired *P. carinii* pneumonia (Masur et al, 1981). An autopsy study of 54 patients who died with AIDS found lung to be the most common site of CMV infection as indicated by inclusion-bearing cells (Wallace and Hannah, 1987). Respiratory failure was thought to be a major cause of death in 31 of these patients; however, in only 2

was CMV the only identifiable pulmonary pathogen. A longitudinal study of 130 patients with AIDS found CMV pneumonia in 34, 13 of whom did not have evidence of coexisting *P. carinii* pneumonitis (Stover et al, 1985). Mortality in this study was similar to that observed in allogeneic marrow transplant, 75 per cent for CMV pneumonia and 92 per cent for CMV with *P. carinii*. In patients with AIDS, CMV also causes disseminated infection with severe retinitis and enteritis. In infants and children with AIDS, persistent interstitial pneumonitis has been a major clinical problem (Rogers et al, 1987). Not surprisingly, however, CMV infection is much less common than in adults with AIDS. More than 90 per cent of adults with AIDS have previously experienced CMV infection and are thus subject to reactivation of endogenous virus as the immune system fails. Although the prevalence of antibody to CMV among a cohort of pediatric AIDS patients has not been reported, we would expect only around 10 to 20 per cent to have acquired CMV during the first year of life. Although CMV does not seem to be the cause of the lymphoid interstitial pneumonitis reported in about 50 per cent of pediatric AIDS cases, a review of complications in 307 pediatric cases reported disseminated CMV infection in 19 per cent (Rogers et al, 1987).

Cytomegalovirus does not appear to cause pneumonia or disseminated infection among other immunocompromised patients with the frequency or severity noted in transplant recipients and patients with AIDS. A study of children with leukemia found viremia in 11 of 36 (30.5 per cent) known to have CMV infection, but only two had lower respiratory disease (Cox and Hughes, 1975).

PATHOLOGY AND PATHOGENESIS

Histologic examination of lung tissue from patients with CMV pneumonitis typically reveals interstitial edema and mononuclear cell infiltration with obliteration of alveolar spaces (Craighead, 1971). Pathologic changes are often focal but scattered through both lungs. Inclusion-bearing cells are rounded and enlarged, with large nuclear inclusions separated from the nuclear membrane, giving an owl's eye appearance (Fig. 52–1). Cytoplasmic inclusions are periodic acid-Schiff positive and located near the nucleus. Inclusions can be found in pneumocytes lining alveoli as well as in macrophages. The number of inclusion-bearing cells does not correlate with the degree of focal pathologic change. In patients with AIDS and CMV pneumonia, two distinct patterns of pulmonary pathology have been described (Wallace and Hannah, 1987). A pattern of diffuse alveolar damage was characterized by both exudative changes with interstitial edema and hyaline membrane and a proliferative phase with regenerating alveolar epithelium, interstitial inflammation, and fibrosis. Other patients had focal interstitial pneumonitis with focal mononuclear cell inflammation with or without fibrosis (Wallace and Hannah, 1987).

The precise mechanisms by which CMV causes pulmonary disease are not known. Autopsy pathology, experimental animal studies, and observations in humans suggest that both the virus's ability to infect and damage cells in the pulmonary parenchyma and its effect on host immune responses are important. As noted earlier, histologic evidence of CMV infection can be found in both alveolar pneumocytes and macrophages; in situ DNA hybridization and fluorescein-labeled monoclonal antibodies to CMV often reveal virus in many cells without overt cytopathology. Lytic infection of cells and the resulting inflammatory response likely result in diffuse alveolar damage and impaired gas exchange. Although it is tempting to speculate a role for immune-mediated damage, this does not seem consonant with observations that the most severe cases of CMV pneumonitis are observed in the most profoundly immunocompromised patients.

In addition to directly damaging pulmonary parenchymal cells, CMV appears to be able to impair

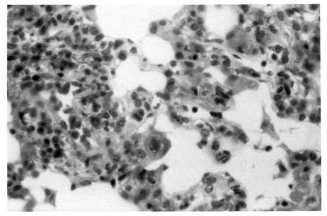

Figure 52–1. An open-lung biopsy specimen from an immunocompromised patient with cytomegalovirus (CMV) pneumonitis. A single enlarged cell, probably a pneumocyte, with a large intranuclear inclusion with a surrounding halo is readily apparent. There is abundant lymphoid interstitial infiltrate. Cytomegalovirus was isolated from the lung; there was no histologic or culture evidence of *Pneumocystis carinii*, fungi, bacteria, or other viral pathogens.

host immune responses to other pathogens. Combined infection of the lungs with other agents, particularly *P. carinii*, is often observed (Stagno et al, 1981; Meyers et al, 1986; Stover et al, 1985). In renal transplant patients, opportunistic fungal infections have been found to occur more often in patients with primary CMV infection (Chatterjee et al, 1978). In vitro studies indicate that CMV can infect both lymphocytes and monocytes and can interfere with their functions in blastogenesis and cytotoxicity (Rice et al, 1984; Schrier and Oldstone, 1986). Animal studies have shown increased susceptibility to bacterial and fungal pathogens after murine CMV infection and impaired function of both lymphocytes and phagocytic cells (Brody and Craighead, 1974; Shanley and Pesanti, 1980).

DIAGNOSIS

In approaching diagnosis of CMV pneumonitis, there are three questions that must be dealt with: (1) Does the patient have CMV infection? (2) Does the patient have pulmonary CMV infection? (3) Is CMV the cause of the current pulmonary disease? The first question is easily answered by the virology laboratory. The second can usually be addressed successfully with appropriate specimens. The third cannot always be answered clearly even with biopsy or autopsy material because other pathogens are often involved.

Cytomegalovirus should be considered as a possible cause of lower respiratory disease in any patient in one of the groups discussed in "Clinical Manifestations" who has clinical evidence of lower respiratory disease. Specimens of urine and blood should be submitted for virus culture, and serum should be tested for antibody. Although negative CMV cultures from urine and blood do not rule out pulmonary infection, they make it unlikely; patients with CMV pneumonitis are almost always viruric, and most will be viremic. Antibody results must be interpreted with caution. Infants may still have passively acquired maternal IgG antibody. Patients with primary infection can become symptomatic before seroconversion. Immunocompromised patients may have impaired antibody response in the presence of overwhelming CMV infection, or they could be agammaglobulinemic as in the case of some pediatric patients with AIDS and congenital immunodeficiencies. Testing for IgM antibody carries similar potential problems. Reliable assays for IgM antibody are not widely available. In immunocompromised patients, IgM antibody to CMV is not specific for primary infection; it has been detected in both cardiac and renal transplant recipients with reactivation infection. It obviously is important to know the patient's history regarding recent transfusions, as well as CMV antibody status of organ donors or blood donors.

Determining whether CMV is present in the lungs requires collection of material by bronchoalveolar lavage (BAL), bronchial washing, transbronchial biopsy, or open-lung biopsy. Experience in adults indicates that BAL and open-lung biopsy provide the best specimens of various pathogens (Springmeyer et al, 1986; Cordonnier et al, 1985); BAL appears to be equal in sensitivity to open-lung biopsy for diagnosis of *P. carinii* (McKenna et al, 1986). Unfortunately, data evaluating either technique in CMV infection in children are sparse. Expectorated sputum as well as specimens collected from the upper respiratory tract or from an endotracheal tube are not acceptable as indicators of lower respiratory tract CMV infection because the virus is so commonly found in the mouth and upper respiratory tract of patients with CMV infection. If BAL fluid and cells or lung biopsy is negative for CMV by staining with monoclonal antibody and virus culture, then CMV is unlikely to be the problem. However, even a positive result is not straightforward proof of causation. Craighead (1971) isolated CMV from lung tissue obtained at autopsy from 2 of 31 patients who died from cardiovascular causes and 2 of 13 who died from miscellaneous causes. If CMV can be isolated from lungs without pathologic evidence of pneumonitis, then how does one conclude that CMV is the cause of lower respiratory disease in a patient? In reaching a conclusion, the presence of risk factors (transfusion, seropositive organ donor/negative recipient), allogeneic marrow versus syngeneic, graft-versus-host disease, type of immunosuppression (antithymocyte globulin), and underlying disease (AIDS) must be considered along with virologic data. If a patient belongs to a group known to be commonly afflicted with CMV pneumonitis, is currently infected (viruric or viremic), and has a positive BAL or biopsy results and no other cause is found, then CMV should be considered the cause. In patients who have compromised cellular immunity and viremia or virus in the lower respiratory tract, CMV should be considered a contributing cause even if other etiologies are found. Because other pathogens frequently accompany CMV or produce similar patterns of disease, it is important that they be carefully sought. In fact, the decision to perform BAL or open-lung biopsy is usually prompted by the desire to identify other causes such as *P. carinii*, fungus, or mycobacteria.

A review of techniques used to detect CMV or measure antibody is beyond the scope of this discussion. In patients suspected of having CMV pneumonitis, any lung tissue available should be cultured for virus and histologically examined with antibody to CMV. In addition to the traditional detection of viral cytopathology in tissue culture, which may take weeks to complete, a newer rapid culture method that uses monoclonal antibody to CMV immediate early antigen should be used (Gleaves et al, 1984). This method appears to be sensitive and specific, and infected cells are easily identified in tissue in 24 to 48 hours (Fig. 52–2). Cells from BAL or biopsy specimens should also be examined with fluorescent antibody to CMV, which can provide same-day results

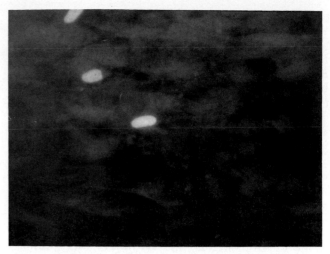

Figure 52–2. Cytomegalovirus-infected fibroblasts identified in tissue culture 24 hours after inoculation. Cells were stained with a fluorescein-labeled murine monoclonal antibody to CMV immediate early antigen.

(Hackman et al, 1985; Emanuel et al, 1986). Because procedures for collecting and testing specimens vary among virology laboratories, it is wise to discuss diagnostic problems with the laboratory before submitting specimens.

PREVENTION AND TREATMENT

Prevention of CMV infection in small, premature neonates and immunocompromised hosts is advantageous because of the frequency and severity of disease in these patients. The blood from donors and from recipients in these high-risk groups can be screened to prevent administration of blood products from a seropositive donor to a seronegative recipient, with its attendant risk of symptomatic infection (Yeager, 1981; Bowden, 1986). Use of frozen deglycerolized red blood cells also prevents transmission of CMV (Brady et al, 1984; Taylor et al, 1986). Both screening of blood for CMV and use of frozen deglycerolized red blood cells increase the cost of transfusions. Because of regional variability in the prevalence of antibody to CMV among donors and recipients, as well as variability in occurrence of disease with transfusion-acquired CMV infection, there is not yet a consensus among hospitals regarding prevention of transfusion-acquired CMV infection.

Screening of organ donors is even more problematic because of the scarcity of donors. Other approaches have been used to prevent CMV disease in transplant recipients, including active and passive immunization and prophylactic treatment with antiviral agents. Vaccination of renal transplant patients with a live, laboratory-adapted virus (Towne strain) decreased morbidity due to primary CMV infection but did not prevent infection (Plotkin et al, 1984). No CMV vaccines are currently available outside of very limited research protocols. Passive immunization with a CMV immune globulin preparation decreased the severity of primary CMV infection in renal transplant recipients (Snydman et al, 1987). In bone marrow transplant recipients there is also evidence for efficacy of prophylactic CMV immune globulin or immune plasma (Winston et al, 1987). Others have concluded that there is insufficient evidence, however, and further study is needed before prophylactic CMV immune globulin can be recommended for routine use (Bowden et al, 1986).

Chemoprophylaxis with acyclovir in seropositive bone marrow recipients has been associated with reduced risk of CMV reactivation, delayed onset of virus excretion, reduction in incidence of CMV pneumonitis, and decreased mortality (Meyers et al, 1988). Although acyclovir is effective in treatment of herpes simplex virus infections in normal and compromised hosts and for varicella-zoster virus infections in compromised hosts, it is much less active in vitro against CMV and has not been effective in treating CMV infections. At this time, limited experience precludes any broad recommendations for use of acyclovir to prevent reactivation of CMV in transplant recipients; however, the results presented by Meyers and colleagues suggest that chemoprophylaxis holds promise.

At this writing, no antiviral agents are licensed for use in CMV infections in normal or compromised hosts. A number of compounds have been used without notable success (Alford and Britt, 1985). A promising compound, 9-(1,3-dihydroxy-2-propoxymethyl) guanine (DHPG), has been shown to stop viremia and viruria in bone marrow transplant recipients and patients with AIDS (Shepp et al, 1985; Collaborative DHPG Treatment Study Group, 1986). These two studies also reported clinical improvement with treatment in CMV retinitis and gastroenteritis; unfortunately, patients with pneumonia did not respond as well. More encouraging results have been obtained in renal, hepatic, and cardiac transplant recipients, as well as in patients with solid tumors (Paya et al, 1988; Harbison et al, 1988; Watson et al, 1988). In these patients, immunosuppression is less severe or of shorter duration than in marrow transplant recipients and patients with AIDS, and treatment of CMV pneumonia was accomplished (Watson et al, 1988). DHPG has significant toxicity, including inhibition of spermatogenesis, gastrointestinal mucosal ulceration, and bone marrow depression, and has been studied almost exclusively in life-threatening infections. The ultimate clinical role of DHPG will be defined by further study.

REFERENCES

Adler SP: The molecular epidemiology of cytomegalovirus transmission among children attending a day care center. J Infect Dis 152:760, 1985.

Adler SP: Molecular epidemiology of cytomegalovirus: viral transmission among children attending a day care center, their parents, and caretakers. J Pediatr 112:366, 1988.

Adler SP, Baggett J, Wilson M et al: Molecular epidemiology of cytomegalovirus in a nursery: lack of evidence for nosocomial transmission. J Pediatr 108:117, 1986.

Adler SP, Chandrika T, Lawrence L, and Baggett J: Cytomegalovirus infection in neonates acquired by blood transfusions. Pediatr Infect Dis 2:114, 1983.

Alford CA and Britt WJ: Cytomegalovirus. In Fields BN, Knipe DM, Chanock RM, et al (eds): Virology. New York, Raven Press, 1985.

Alford CA, Stagno S, and Pass RF: Natural history of perinatal cytomegaloviral infection. Ciba Found Symp 30:477, 1980.

Balfour CL and Balfour HH: Cytomegalovirus is not an occupational risk for nurses in renal transplant and neonatal units. JAMA 256:1909, 1986.

Becroft DMO: Prenatal cytomegalovirus infection: epidemiology, pathology and pathogenesis. Perspect Pediatr Pathol 6:203, 1981.

Betts RF, Freeman RB, Douglas G, and Talley TE: Clinical manifestations of renal allograft derived primary cytomegalovirus infection. Am J Dis Child 131:759, 1977.

Betts RF, Freeman RB, Douglas RG et al: Transmission of cytomegalovirus infection with renal allograft. Kidney Int 8:387, 1975.

Bowden RA, Sayers M, Flournoy N et al: Cytomegalovirus immune globulin and seronegative blood products to prevent primary cytomegalovirus infection after marrow transplantation. N Engl J Med 314:1006, 1986.

Brady MT, Milam JD, Anderson DC et al: Use of deglycerolized red blood cells to prevent posttransfusion infection with cytomegalovirus in neonates. J Infect Dis 150:334, 1984.

Brody AR and Craighead JE: Pathogenesis of pulmonary cytomegalovirus infection in immunosuppressed mice. J Infect Dis 129:677, 1974.

Chandler SH, Holmes KK, Wentworth BB et al: The epidemiology of cytomegaloviral infection in women attending a sexually transmitted disease clinic. J Infect Dis 152:597, 1985.

Chatterjee SN, Fiala M, Weiner J et al: Primary cytomegalovirus and opportunistic infections. JAMA 240:2446, 1978.

Chou S: Acquisition of donor strains of cytomegalovirus by renal-transplant recipients. N Engl J Med 314:1418, 1986.

Cohen JI and Corey GR: Cytomegalovirus infection in the normal host. Medicine 64:100, 1985.

Collaborative DHPG Treatment Study Group: Treatment of serious cytomegalovirus infections with 9-(1,3-dihydroxy-2-propoxymethyl) guanine in patients with AIDS and other immunodeficiencies. N Engl J Med 314:801, 1986.

Cordonnier C, Bernaudin JF, Fleury J et al: Diagnostic yield of bronchoalveolar lavage in pneumonitis occurring after allogeneic bone marrow transplantation. Am Rev Respir Dis 132:1118, 1985.

Cox F and Hughes WT: Cytomegaloviremia in children with acute lymphocytic leukemia. J Pediatr 87:190, 1975.

Craighead JE: Pulmonary cytomegalovirus infection in the adult. Am J Pathol 63:487, 1971.

DeMarchi JM, Blankenship ML, Brown GD, and Kaplan AS: Size and complexity of human cytomegalovirus DNA. Virology 39:643, 1978.

DeMarchi JM, Schmidt CA, and Kaplan AS: Patterns of transcription of human cytomegalovirus in permissively infected cells. J Virol 35:277, 1980.

Drew WL, Mintz L, Miner RC et al: Prevalence of cytomegalovirus infection in homosexual men. J Infect Dis 143:188, 1981.

Dworsky ME and Stagno S: Newer agents causing pneumonitis in early infancy. Pediatr Infect Dis 1:188, 1982.

Dworsky ME, Welch K, Cassady G, and Stagno S: Occupational risk for primary cytomegalovirus infection among pediatric health-care workers. N Engl J Med 309:950, 1983.

Emanuel D, Peppard J, Stover D et al: Rapid immunodiagnosis of cytomegalovirus pneumonia by bronchoalveolar lavage using human and murine monoclonal antibodies. Ann Intern Med 104:476, 1986.

Faix RG: Survival of cytomegalovirus on environmental surfaces. J Pediatr 106:649, 1985.

Friedman HM, Lewis MR, Nemerofsky DM, and Plotkin SA: Acquisition of cytomegalovirus infection among female employees at a pediatric hospital. Pediatr Infect Dis 3:233, 1984.

Gelen JLMC, Walig C, Wertheim P, and Varder NJ: Human cytomegalovirus DNA. I. Molecular weight and infectivity. J Virol 26:813, 1978.

Gleaves CA, Smith TF, Shuster EA, and Pearson GR: Rapid detection of cytomegalovirus in MRC-5 cells inoculated with urine specimens by using low-speed centrifugation and monoclonal antibody to an early antigen. J Clin Microbiol 19:917, 1984.

Gorensek MJ, Stewart RW, Keys TF et al: A multivariate analysis of the risk of cytomegalovirus infection in heart transplant recipients. J Infect Dis 157:515, 1988.

Gottlieb MS, Schroff R, Schanker HM et al: *Pneumocystis carinii* pneumonia and mucosal candidiasis in previously healthy homosexual men. N Engl J Med 305:1425, 1981.

Griffiths PD and Baboonian C: A prospective study of primary cytomegalovirus infection during pregnancy: final report. Br J Obstet Gynecol 91:307, 1984.

Hackman RC, Myerson D, Meyers JD et al: Rapid diagnosis of cytomegaloviral pneumonia by tissue immunofluorescence with a murine monoclonal antibody. J Infect Dis 141:325, 1985.

Handsfield HH, Chandler SH, Caine VA et al: Cytomegalovirus infection in sex partners: evidence for sexual transmission. J Infect Dis 151:344, 1985.

Hanshaw JB: Cytomegalovirus. In Remington JS and Klein JO (eds): Infectious Diseases of the Fetus and Newborn Infant. Philadelphia, WB Saunders Co, 1983.

Harbison MA, De Girolami PC, Jenkins RL, and Hammer SM: Ganciclovir therapy of severe cytomegalovirus infections in solid-organ transplant recipients. Transplantation 46:82, 1988.

Hayes K, Danks DM, Gibas H, and Jack I: Cytomegalovirus in human milk. N Engl J Med 287:177, 1972.

Honess RW and Roizman B: Regulation of herpesvirus macromolecular synthesis. I. Cascade regulation of synthesis of three groups of viral proteins. J Virol 14:8, 1974.

Horwitz CA, Henle W, Henle G et al: Clinical and laboratory evaluation of cytomegalovirus-induced mononucleosis in previously healthy individuals. Report of 82 cases. Medicine 65:124, 1986.

Klemola E, von Essen R, Henle G, and Henle W: Infectious mononucleosis-like disease with negative heterophile agglutination test. Clinical features in relation to Epstein-Barr virus and cytomegalovirus antibodies. J Infect Dis 121:608, 1970.

Klemola E, von Essen R, Wager O et al: Cytomegalovirus mononucleosis in previously healthy individuals. Ann Intern Med 71:11, 1969.

Krech U, Jung M, and Jung F: Epidemiology. Cytomegalovirus Infections of Man. Basel, S Karger AG, 1971.

Kumar ML, Nankervis GA, Cooper AR, and Gold E: Postnatally acquired cytomegalovirus infections in infants of CMV-excreting mothers. J Pediatr 104:669, 1984.

Landini MP and Michelson S: Human cytomegalovirus proteins. In Melnick JL (ed): Progress in Medical Virology. Basel, S Karger AG, 35:152, 1988.

Lang DJ: The epidemiology of cytomegalovirus infections: interpretation of recent observations. In Krugman S and Gershon AA (eds): Infections of the Fetus and Newborn Infant. New York, Alan R Liss, Inc., 1975.

McKenna RJ, Campbell A, McMurtrey MJ, and Mountain CF: Diagnosis for interstitial lung disease in patients with acquired immunodeficiency syndrome (AIDS): a prospective comparison of bronchial washing, alveolar lavage, transbronchial lung biopsy, and open-lung biopsy. Ann Thorac Surg 41:318, 1986.

Masur H, Michelis MA, Greene JB et al: An outbreak of community-acquired *Pneumocystis carinii* pneumonia: initial manifestation of cellular immune dysfunction. N Engl J Med 305:1431, 1981.

Meyers JD, Flournoy N, and Thomas ED: Risk factors for cytomegalovirus infection after human marrow transplantation. J Infect Dis 153:478, 1986.

Meyers JD, Reed EC, Sheep DH et al: Acyclovir for prevention of cytomegalovirus infection and disease after allogeneic marrow transplantation. N Engl J Med 318:70, 1988.

Murph JR, Bale JF, Murray JC et al: Cytomegalovirus transmission in a Midwest day care center: possible relationship to child care practices. J Pediatr 109:35, 1986.

Pannuti CS, Vilas Boas LS, Angelo MJO et al: Cytomegalovirus mononucleosis in children and adults: differences in clinical presentation. Scand J Infect Dis 17:153, 1985.

Pass RF: Epidemiology and transmission of cytomegalovirus. J Infect Dis 152:243, 1985.

Pass RF: Congenital and perinatal infections due to viruses and toxoplasma. In Kretchmer N, Quilligan EJ, and Johnson JD (eds): Prenatal and Perinatal Biology and Medicine. Vol. 2. Disorders, Diagnosis and Therapy. New York, Harwood Academic Publishers, 1987.

Pass RF, Hutto C, Reynolds DW, and Polhill RB: Increased frequency of cytomegalovirus in children in group day care. Pediatrics 74:121, 1984.

Pass RF, Hutto C, Ricks R, and Gloud GA: Increased rate of cytomegalovirus infection among parents of children attending day-care centers. N Engl J Med 314:1414, 1986.

Pass RF and Stagno S: Cytomegalovirus. In Donowitz LG (ed): Hospital Acquired Infection in the Pediatric Patient. Baltimore, Williams & Wilkins Co, 1988.

Pass RF, Whitley RJ, Diethelm AG et al: Cytomegalovirus infection in patients with renal transplants: potentiation by antithymocyte globulin and an incompatible graft. J Infect Dis 142:9, 1980.

Paya CV, Hermans PE, Smith TF et al: Efficacy of ganciclovir in liver and kidney transplant recipients with severe cytomegalovirus infection. Transplantation 46:229, 1988.

Plotkin SA, Friedman HM, Fleisher GR et al: Towne vaccine-induced prevention of cytomegalovirus disease after renal transplants. Lancet 1:528, 1984.

Rand KH, Rasmussen LE, Pollard RB et al: Cellular immunity and herpesvirus infections in cardiac-transplant patients. N Engl J Med 296:1372, 1976.

Rice GPA, Schrier RD, and Oldstone MBA: Cytomegalovirus infects human lymphocytes and monocytes: virus expression is restricted to immediate-early gene products. Proc Natl Acad Sci USA 81:6134, 1984.

Rogers MF, Thomas PA, Starcher ET et al: Acquired immunodeficiency syndrome in children: report of the centers for disease control national surveillance, 1982 to 1985. Pediatrics 79:1008, 1987.

Sarov I and Abody I: The morphogenesis of human cytomegalovirus. Isolation and peptide characterization of cytomegalovirus and dense bodies. Virology 66:464, 1975.

Sawyer MH, Edwards DK, and Spector SA: Cytomegalovirus infection and bronchopulmonary dysplasia in premature infants. Am J Dis Child 141:303, 1987.

Schopfer K, Lauber E, and Krech U: Congenital cytomegalovirus infection in newborn infants of mothers infected before pregnancy. Arch Dis Child 53:536, 1978.

Schrier RD and Oldstone MBA: Recent clinical isolates of cytomegalovirus suppress human cytomegalovirus-specific human leukocyte antigen-restricted cytotoxic T-lymphocyte activity. J Virol 59:127, 1986.

Shanley JD and Pesanti EL: Replication of murine cytomegalovirus in lung macrophages: effect on phagocytosis of bacteria. Infect Immun 29:1152, 1980.

Shepp DH, Dandliker PS, de Miranda P et al: Activity of 9-[2-hydroxy-1-(hydroxymethyl)ethoxymethyl]guanine in the treatment of cytomegalovirus pneumonia. Ann Intern Med 103:368, 1985.

Singh N, Dummer JS, Kusne S et al: Infections with cytomegalovirus and other herpesviruses in 121 liver transplant recipients: Transmission by donated organ and the effect of OKT3 antibodies. J Infect Dis 158:124, 1988.

Smith JD and deHarven E: Herpes simplex virus and human cytomegalovirus replication in WI-38 cells. II. An ultrastructural study of viral penetration. J Virol 14:945, 1974.

Snydman DR, Werner BG, Heinze-Lacey B et al: Use of cytomegalovirus immune globulin to prevent cytomegalovirus disease in renal transplant recipients. N Engl J Med 317:1049, 1987.

Spector SA: Transmission of cytomegalovirus among infants in hospital documented by restriction-endonuclease-digestion analyses. Lancet 1:378, 1983.

Springmeyer SC, Hackman RC, Holle R et al: Use of bronchoalveolar lavage to diagnose acute diffuse pneumonia in the immunocompromised host. Infect Dis 154:604, 1986.

Stagno S, Brasfield DM, Brown MB et al: Infant pneumonitis associated with cytomegalovirus, chlamydia, pneumocystis, and ureaplasma: a prospective study. Pediatrics 68:322, 1981.

Stagno S, Pass RF, Dworsky ME et al: Congenital cytomegalovirus infection: the relative importance of primary and recurrent maternal infection. N Engl J Med 306:945, 1982.

Stagno S, Reynolds DW, Pass RF, and Alford CA: Breast milk and the risk of cytomegalovirus infection. N Engl J Med 302:1073, 1980.

Stover DE, White DA, Romano PA et al: Spectrum of pulmonary diseases associated with the acquired immune deficiency syndrome. Am J Med 78:429, 1985.

Taylor BJ, Jacobs RF, Baker RL et al: Frozen deglycerolized blood prevents transfusion-acquired cytomegalovirus infections in neonates. Pediatr Infect Dis 5:188, 1986.

Wallace JM and Hannah J: Cytomegalovirus pneumonitis in patients with AIDS. Findings in an autopsy series. Chest 92:198, 1987.

Wather MW and Stinski MF: Temporal patterns of human cytomegalovirus transcription: mapping of the viral RNA's synthe-sized at immediate early, early and late times after infection. J Virol 41:462, 1982.

Watson FS, O'Connell JB, Amber IJ et al: Treatment of cytomegalovirus pneumonia in heart transplant recipients with 9(1,3-dihydroxy-2-proproxymethyl)-guanine (DHPG). J Heart Transplant 7:102, 1988.

Whitley RJ, Brasfield D, Reynolds DW et al: Protracted pneumonitis in young infants associated with perinatally acquired cytomegaloviral infection. J Pediatr 89:16, 1976.

Winston DJ, Ho WG, Lin CH et al: Intravenous immune globulin for prevention of cytomegalovirus infection and interstitial pneumonia after bone marrow transplantation. Ann Intern Med 106:12, 1987.

Wright HT Jr, Goodheart CR, and Lielausis AL: Human cytomegalovirus. Morphology by negative staining. Virology 23:419, 1964.

Yeager AS, Grumet FC, Hafleigh EB et al: Prevention of transfusion acquired cytomegalovirus infections in newborn infants. J Pediatr 98:281, 1981.

53

MARC O. BEEM, M.D., EVELYN M. SAXON, B.S., and MARGARET A. TIPPLE, M.D.

CHLAMYDIAL INFECTIONS OF INFANTS

Chlamydiae are gram-negative bacteria that by virtue of certain metabolic deficiencies are obligately parasitic within eukaryotic cells. Two species are presently recognized within the genus, *Chlamydia psittaci* and *Chlamydia trachomatis*. A third group of chlamydial organisms that appears to be significantly different from these species is called the *TWAR group* organisms. *C. psittaci* strains, although widely distributed among lower animals, are only occasional, accidental causes of human illness and will not be discussed here. In contrast, *C. trachomatis* and TWAR, as presently known, are largely indigenous to humans, and their roles in human respiratory disease will be discussed.

CHLAMYDIA TRACHOMATIS

In industrialized countries, *C. trachomatis* exists mainly in a genital reservoir, spreading among adults through sexual contact and from infected mothers to their infants through birth contact. About 50 per cent of infants born vaginally to infected mothers acquire infection. Either the conjunctiva or the respiratory tract or both may serve as a portal of entry. However, it is from the respiratory tract that *C. trachomatis* can most consistently be recovered from natally infected infants, because positive nasopharyngeal cultures are the rule in infants with chlamydial conjunctivitis and are found in the absence of conjunctivitis as well. The chief illnesses related to *C. trachomatis* infections in infancy are conjunctivitis and pneumonia. About 60 per cent of infected infants develop conjunctivitis, 10 to 20 per cent develop pneumonia, and 10 to 15 per cent develop neither and so are judged to be asymptomatically infected.

CONJUNCTIVAL DISEASE

Inclusion conjunctivitis of neonates is a well-described entity. It usually becomes evident between 3 days and 3 weeks of age. When present, it provides the earliest clinical evidence of natally acquired infection, and it requires a full course of systemic treatment.

RESPIRATORY TRACT DISEASE

A spectrum of clinical entities may be related to chlamydial respiratory tract infection. The two well-established points on this spectrum, asymptomatic infection and a syndrome of afebrile pneumonia, lie

Table 53–1. CLINICAL CHARACTERISTICS OF CHLAMYDIAL PNEUMONIA OF INFANCY

Age of patient	2–12 weeks*
Onset	Gradual
Systemic manifestations	No fever*
	Minimal malaise
	Sometimes poor weight gain
Eye findings	Inclusion conjunctivitis (chronic phase)
Ear findings	Secretory otitis media
Respiratory findings	Tachypnea
	Cough (sometimes in staccato paroxysms)
	At auscultation: good breath sounds, inspiratory crepitant rales, absent or minimal expiratory wheezing
	On x-ray: hyperexpansion, diffuse and symmetrical interstitial-type infiltrates, scattered patches of airless lung, narrow upper mediastinal silhouette*

*Attributes considered essential to the diagnosis.

at the clinical extremes. Intermediate points, which may be aspects of evolving infection or entities unto themselves, include nasopharyngitis, secretory otitis media, bronchitis, and synergistic or additive interactions with other respiratory pathogens. Asymptomatic infection requires no elaboration except to note the long persistence of *Chlamydia* shedding by these infants and the resulting possibility that *C. trachomatis* may be coincidentally identified in the respiratory secretions of infants experiencing illness due to other causes. The salient features of chlamydial pneumonia of infants, summarized in Tables 53–1 and 53–2, are described in the paragraphs that follow.

Age at Onset

Chlamydial pneumonia is an illness of the first 3 months of life. Patients typically present at 3 weeks to 3 months of age but are sometimes younger. Indeed, there are reports of infants who have experienced ante-partum ascending infection and presented in the immediate neonatal period with evidence of both this infection and respiratory distress. However, in the single such case in the authors' experience as well as those reported by others, the infants have been prematurely born, and it is uncer-

Table 53–2. LABORATORY CHARACTERISTICS OF CHLAMYDIAL PNEUMONIA OF INFANCY

General	
Blood gas values	Pa$_{O_2}$ low, Pa$_{CO_2}$ normal
Blood eosinophil count	≥300 cells/mm³
Serum immunoglobulin levels	IgM always, IgG usually, and IgA sometimes elevated for age*
***Chlamydia*-specific**	
Culture	*C. trachomatis* in nasopharyngeal secretions*
Serologic	Sustained high or rising serum chlamydia antibody titer*†
	Chlamydia-specific IgA or IgM antibody*

*Attributes considered essential to diagnosis.
†By indirect microimmunofluorescence or similarly sensitive method.

tain whether their respiratory problems are attributable to prematurity, chlamydial infection, or both.

Mode of Onset

Patients with chlamydial pneumonia typically have a history of gradually evolving and worsening respiratory illness. Usually but not invariably there are upper respiratory tract signs, including nasal obstruction with or without discharge, sometimes beginning within a few days of birth. Gradually worsening cough and tachypnea follow, but days or even weeks may elapse before the diagnosis of pneumonia is considered.

Systemic Effects

A paucity of systemic effects is characteristic of chlamydial infections of infancy and contributes to the sometimes late recognition of chlamydial pneumonia. *C. trachomatis* respiratory tract infections are always afebrile, even in infants with extensive pneumonia. Indeed, the presence of fever in a patient in whom a diagnosis of chlamydial pneumonia is being considered should suggest either secondary infection (rare in our experience) or other cause of illness. Malaise is also minimal and, like the poor weight gain sometimes noted in infected infants, is seldom more than could be expected from the respiratory difficulties.

Eye and Ear Findings

About 50 per cent of infants with chlamydial pneumonia have either active inclusion conjunctivitis or a history of the disease. When present, conjunctivitis is usually in the chronic phase, with thickened, somewhat pale conjunctival epithelium and only modest conjunctival discharge. Some infants also have secretory otitis media.

Respiratory Tract Findings

Tachypnea with respiratory rates ranging from 40 to 80 breaths/min is common. Cough is also the rule; it sometimes occurs as staccato paroxysms that may be followed by vomiting or periods of apnea. On auscultation, breath sounds are well heard throughout the chest, inspiratory crackles are present and irregularly distributed, and expiratory wheezing is either absent or less than one would expect from the relatively good air exchange and the hyperexpansion evident on chest radiographs. In addition to symmetrical hyperexpansion, chest x-ray films show diffuse, symmetrically distributed, interstitial-type infiltrates; scattered patches of airless lung; and a narrowed upper mediastinal silhouette (Fig. 53–1). Additionally, a small amount of pleural reaction is sometimes seen.

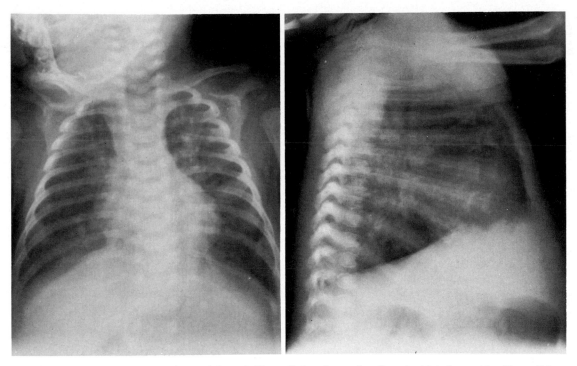

Figure 53–1. Anteroposterior and lateral films of the chest of a 6-week-old infant with chlamydial pneumonia. The lungs are hyperexpanded. Interstitial infiltrates and patches of airless lung are most dense toward the hilum but are present in all lung fields. The upper mediastinal silhouette is narrowed.

Laboratory Findings

General. An absolute blood eosinophilia is often but not invariably found. In one reported series of 41 infants, 71 per cent had peripheral blood eosinophil counts equal to or greater than 300 cells/mm³; in another series of 16 infants, 75 per cent had eosinophil counts equal to or greater than 400 cells/mm³. In spite of these findings and the probable identity of chlamydial pneumonia with a disease described by Botsztejn (1941) as "pertussoid eosinophilic pneumonia," it should be noted that normal eosinophil values are found in some patients. Serum immunoglobulin abnormalities are the rule. IgM levels are always elevated for age; IgG levels are high in most cases; IgA values are less consistently elevated; and IgE values are normal. Arterial blood gas analyses often show Pa_{O_2} values in the range of 50 to 60 mm Hg but Pa_{CO_2} values within normal limits.

Chlamydia-Specific. *C. trachomatis* can always be isolated from the nasopharyngeal secretions of untreated patients and may also but less consistently be recovered from conjunctival and rectal swabs. Serum antibodies to the organism are present at sustained high or rising titers when measured by a suitably sensitive test, such as the indirect microimmunofluorescent method. As a rule, chlamydia-specific IgM antibody when measured by the same method is also present, but this finding is not invariable. In addition, chlamydia-specific IgM antibody may sometimes be found in *C. trachomatis*–infected infants who do not have clinically evident respiratory tract involvement.

Clinical Course

Eleven patients whom we followed with expectant management provide some sense of the natural history of chlamydial pneumonia; they averaged 43 days of unimproved or worsening illness before recovery began (spontaneously in three patients and after the start of *Chlamydia*-specific antimicrobial treatment in eight). Once under way, recovery progresses to complete resolution of the immediate clinical and radiographic abnormalities. However, in follow-up studies of children 7 to 8 years after hospitalization and treatment for chlamydial pneumonia, an excess of mild, long-term pulmonary changes was observed. These consisted of limitations of expiratory airflow variables in pulmonary function tests and, by pulmonary histories, an excess of airway symptoms, including physician-diagnosed asthma in a third of the patients.

Diagnosis

The diagnosis of chlamydial pneumonia requires evidence that (1) the infant is infected with *C. trachomatis* and (2) the infection is etiologically rather than coincidentally related to the illness. Culture offers the most sensitive and specific method for identification of infection, except in patients who recently were or currently are being treated with antimicrobials that inhibit *C. trachomatis*. Chlamydiae should always be present in nasopharyngeal secretions. However, the demonstration of the organism at another body site (e.g., conjunctiva, rectum) gives indirect evidence of respiratory tract infection, because virtually all natally infected infants have chlamydiae in the respiratory tract. Direct immunofluorescence provides a practical alternative to culture for the detection of *C. trachomatis* in the nasopharyngeal and conjunctival secretions of infants. Serologic confirmation of *C. trachomatis* infection must be sought by a sensitive method such as indirect microimmunofluorescence or enzyme-linked immunosorbent assay and requires demonstration of a significant rise in *C. trachomatis* antibody titer or the demonstration of *C. trachomatis*-specific IgA or IgM antibody. The method used for the latter should rule out the possibility of false-positive reaction due to rheumatoid factor.

Because *C. trachomatis* may be found in the respiratory tract of infants who are asymptomatic or convalescing from prior chlamydial illness, a distinction must be made between chlamydial infections that are only coincidentally related to respiratory illness due to another cause and those that are responsible for the respiratory illness. Serum IgM values may be helpful when attempting to make this distinction in the individual case. Elevated IgM values, both total and *Chlamydia* specific, have been found to be significantly related to *C. trachomatis* infection and pneumonia. This relationship has been observed in a comparison between *Chlamydia*-positive and *Chlamydia*-negative infants with pneumonia and a comparison of infants who have *C. trachomatis* infection and pneumonia with infants who have *C. trachomatis* infection and conjunctivitis only or who are asymptomatically infected.

From a diagnostic viewpoint, the diagnosis of chlamydial pneumonia is most confidently given to infant illness with the attributes indicated by asterisks (*) in Tables 53–1 and 53–2. Complicating factors or alternative causes should be considered when these criteria are not fulfilled. However, from a therapeutic viewpoint, antichlamydial treatment should be included in the management of any infant who is of the appropriate age and is found to be infected with *C. trachomatis*, because incipient or future respiratory illness related to this infection cannot be ruled out.

Treatment

The central element of treatment is the systemic administration of a suitable antichlamydial drug. We have used erythromycin or sulfisoxazole in standard doses for body weight for a period of 14 days. Clinical improvement commonly begins between the third and fifth days of treatment, and infants are completely asymptomatic and normal on physical examination by the 14th day. Chest radiographs taken 1 month after completion of treatment usually appear normal. *C. trachomatis* can seldom be recovered from any body site after 2 days of treatment with erythromycin or 5 days of treatment with sulfisoxazole. However, after treatment, cultures of the nasopharyngeal aspirates of occasional patients again yield chlamydiae that, when tested, remain sensitive to the antimicrobial used. The factors accounting for such microbiologic relapses (e.g., poor compliance with treatment, inadequate duration of treatment, reinfection) are not known. Because these relapses are typically asymptomatic and eventually terminate spontaneously or coincidentally with treatment of another illness with a *Chlamydia*-effective antimicrobial, we do not monitor for them.

Hospitalization for initial stabilization and treatment is indicated for infants with respiratory distress or coughing paroxysms that significantly interfere with eating or sleeping. Hospitalization is particularly important for infants with periods of posttussive apnea. Chest physical therapy and suctioning decrease the frequency and duration of coughing episodes, and apneic spells seldom continue after this treatment is started. Other supportive measures include supplemental oxygen and parenteral fluids. On rare occasions, ventilatory assistance may be necessary.

C. trachomatis *and Other Respiratory Illnesses*

The relation of *C. trachomatis* to other respiratory diseases of infants and children is problematic. Efforts to isolate the organism from older infants and children with secretory otitis media or lower respiratory tract illnesses have either been entirely negative or have yielded a small number of positive results that could well represent coincidental sampling of a child who is a chronic carrier. *C. trachomatis* also appears to play a minor role in lower respiratory tract disease in immunocompromised patients. It is infrequently isolated from respiratory specimens of such patients, perhaps in part because of the antichlamydial activity of antibiotics often given to such patients for other reasons (e.g., trimethoprim-sulfamethoxazole). Additionally, chlamydial infections that have been identified by culture or serology in such patients have often been accompanied by other potential respiratory pathogens.

TWAR ORGANISMS

A group of *Chlamydia* described by Grayston and associates has been called *TWAR organisms*, after the specimen designations of the first isolates made in their laboratories. Serologic studies provide evidence that the organism is indigenous to humans, is global in distribution, and infects the majority of the population one or more times. The relation of serologically evident TWAR infection to age resembles that of *Mycoplasma pneumoniae*. TWAR antibody prevalence is low during the preschool years and then increases to levels of 40 to 60 per cent by the fourth decade of life.

RESPIRATORY DISEASE

In retrospective studies, TWAR organisms have been linked by serology to localized epidemics of mild pneumonia in teen-aged and young adult civilians as well as military trainees in Finland and Denmark. Futhermore, these organisms, rather than *C. psittaci*, are now considered to be the cause of pneumonia outbreaks noted in Scandinavian countries from 1981 to 1983. These cases were associated with complement-fixing antibody to *Chlamydia* and lacked epidemiologic evidence of an avian source of infection. In prospective studies of 386 university students with acute respiratory infections, serologic evidence of TWAR infection was found in 13 patients, and the organism was isolated from 8 of them. Of the 13 seropositive patients, 9 constituted 12 per cent of 76 students with pneumonia, 3 represented 5 per cent of 63 with bronchitis, and the other TWAR antibody-positive patient was 1 of 151 with a diagnosis of pharyngitis. The observed clinical illnesses have typically been mild, with fever, cough, localized inspiratory crackles on auscultation, focal areas of infiltrate on x-ray study of the chest, elevation of the sedimentation rate, and unremarkable white blood cell count. Pharyngitis sometimes preceded or accompanied the lower respiratory illness, and both biphasic (pharyngitis-pneumonia) and relapsing illnesses have been noted. Severe illnesses have occasionally been described, with pneumonia involving all areas of the lung and necessitating ventilatory support.

Diagnosis

Isolation and propagation of TWAR organisms requires skills and specific reagents that are not generally available. However, complement-fixing antibody with the *Chlamydia* group antigen at titer of $\geq$ 1:64 or that shows a fourfold rise in titer between paired specimens can be considered presumptive evidence of recent TWAR infection.

Treatment

The treatment of TWAR infection has not been specifically studied. However, based on experience with other chlamydial infections, tetracycline would be the preferred drug for children 9 years of age and older; for those less than 9 years of age, erythromycin is now considered the drug of choice.

REFERENCES

Chlamydia trachomatis

Arth C, Von Schmidt B, Grossman M, and Schachter J: Chlamydial pneumonitis. J Pediatr 93:447, 1978.

Attenburrow AA and Barker CM: Chlamydial pneumonia in the low birthweight neonate. Arch Dis Child 60:1169, 1985.

Beem M and Saxon E: *Chlamydia trachomatis* infections of infants. In Mardh P-A, Holmes KK, Oriel JD et al (eds): Chlamydial Infections. Amsterdam, Elsevier Biomedical Press, 1982.

Beem M, Saxon E, and Tipple M: Treatment of chlamydial pneumonia of infancy. Pediatrics 63:198, 1979.

Botsztejn VA: Die pertussoide, eosinophile pneumonie des sauglings. Ann Pediatr (Basel) 157:28, 1941.

Hammerschlag M, Chandler J, Alexander E et al: Erythromycin ointment for ocular prophylaxis of neonatal chlamydial infection. JAMA 244:2291, 1980.

Harrison R, Phil D, English M et al: *Chlamydia trachomatis* infant pneumonitis. Comparison with matched controls and other infant pneumonitis. N Engl J Med 298:702, 1978.

Ito JI, Comess KA, Alexander ER et al: Pneumonia due to *Chlamydia trachomatis* in an immunocompromised adult. N Engl J Med 307:95, 1982.

Mardh P-A, Johansson PJH, and Svenningsen N: Intrauterine lung infection with *Chlamydia trachomatis* in a premature infant. Acta Paediatr Scand 73:569, 1984.

Moncada JV, Schachter J, and Wofsy C: Prevalence of *Chlamydia trachomatis* lung infection in patients with acquired immune deficiency syndrome. J Clin Microbiol 23:986, 1986.

Paisley JW, Lauer BA, Melinkovich P et al: Rapid diagnosis of *Chlamydia trachomatis* pneumonia in infants by direct immunofluorescence microscopy of nasopharyngeal secretions. J Pediatr 109:653, 1986.

Radkowski MA, Kranzler JK, Beem MO et al: *Chlamydia* pneumonia in infants: radiography in 125 cases. AJR 137:703, 1981.

Schachter J: Chlamydiae. In Lennette EH (ed): Manual of Clinical Microbiology. 3rd ed. Washington, DC, American Society of Microbiology, 1980.

Schachter J, Grossman M, and Azimi PH: Serology of *Chlamydia trachomatis* in infants. J Infect Dis 146:530, 1982.

Schachter J, Holt J, Goodner E et al: Prospective study of chlamydial infection in neonates. Lancet 2:377, 1979.

Tipple M, Beem M, and Saxon E: Clinical characteristics of the afebrile pneumonia associated with *Chlamydia trachomatis* infection in infants less than 6 months of age. Pediatrics 63:192, 1979.

Weiss SG, Newcomb RW, and Beem MO: Pulmonary assessment of children after chlamydial pneumonia of infancy. J Pediatr 108:659, 1986.

TWAR Organisms

Campbell LA, Kuo C-C, and Grayston JT: Characterization of the new *Chlamydia* agent, TWAR, as a unique organism by restriction endonuclease analysis and DNA-DNA hybridization. J Clin Microbiol 25:1911, 1987.

Forsey T, Darougar S, and Treharne JD: Prevalence in human beings of antibodies to chlamydia IOL-207, an atypical strain of chlamydia. J Infect 12:145, 1986.

Grayston JT, Juo C-C, Wang S-P et al: A new *Chlamydia psittaci* strain, TWAR, isolated in acute respiratory tract infections. N Engl J Med 315:161, 1986.

Kleemola M, Saikku P, Visakorpi R et al: Epidemics of pneumonia caused by TWAR, a new *Chlamydia* organism, in military trainees in Finland. J Infect Dis 157:230, 1988.

Kuo C-C, Chen H-H, Wang S-P et al: Identification of a new group of *Chlamydia psittaci* strains called TWAR. J Clin Microbiol 24:1034, 1986.

Marrie TJ, Grayston JT, Wang S-P et al: Pneumonia associated with the TWAR strain of *Chlamydia*. Ann Intern Med 106:507, 1987.

Mordhorst CH, Wang S-P, and Grayston JT: Epidemic "ornithosis" and TWAR infection, Denmark 1976–85. In Oriel JD, Ridgway G, Schachter J et al (eds): Chlamydial Infections. Cambridge, England, Cambridge University Press, 1986.

Wang S-P and Grayston JT: Microimmunofluorescence serological studies with the TWAR organism. In Oriel JD, Ridgway G, Schachter J et al (eds): Chlamydial Infections. Cambridge, England, Cambridge University Press, 1986.

A. AVITAL, M.D., and
V. CHERNICK, M.D.

54

PSITTACOSIS (ORNITHOSIS)

One of the first accurate descriptions of psittacosis was made by Ritter (1880), who described an unusual and severe mini-epidemic of pneumonia that developed in his brother's house in Uster, Switzerland, after contact with tropical birds. He named the disease *pneumotyphus* and elegantly described the clinical presentation, epidemiology, pathologic findings, and natural history of the infection, which was later attributed to *Chlamydia psittaci*. At first only psittacine birds (parrots, parakeets, cockatiels, and others of the order of Psittaciformis) were thought to be the source of the human infection. However, the organism was shown to infect both wild and domesticated birds, such as pigeons, turkeys, chickens, ducks, canaries, and sea gulls, and therefore the more inclusive term *ornithosis* was suggested. Because the causative agent is *C. psittaci*, the generic name *psittacosis* is retained for the disease that affects humans.

ETIOLOGY

Chlamydiae were first considered to be large viruses because of their size and their obligatory intracellular parasitism. However, like other bacteria, they have a cell envelope structurally and chemically analogous to those of gram-negative bacteria. They contain both DNA and RNA, divide by binary fission, have ribosomes similar in size to those of bacteria (synthesize their own proteins, nucleic acids, and lipids), and are susceptible to a wide range of antibiotics. Two distinct species of *Chlamydia* are recognized:

1. *Chlamydia trachomatis*, which affects primarily the eyes and genital tract in humans, is inhibited by sulfonamides and produces iodine-staining cytoplasmic inclusions. Further differentiation of *C. trachomatis* includes three biotypes (mouse, lymphogranuloma venereum, trachoma) and 15 immunotypes. Diseases caused by this organism are discussed in Chapter 53.

2. *Chlamydia psittaci*, which affects mainly the lungs in humans, is not inhibited by sulfonamides and does not produce iodine-staining inclusions. There may be different serotypes of *C. psittaci*, because multiple infections in individual patients have been documented.

Grayston and associates (1986) reported the isolation of a new strain of *C. psittaci* called TWAR, after the laboratory designation of the first two isolates *TW*-183 and *AR*-39, which reflected the history of the first cases: *TaiWan* and *Acute Respiratory* disease. This strain appears to be more common in young adults; causes pneumonia, bronchitis, and pharyngitis; is apparently transmitted from human to human without any avian or mammalian host; and represents a new distinct strain of chlamydiae (Campbell, Kuo, and Grayston, 1987). The strain has been named *Chlamydia pneumoniae* and is probably the most common chlamydial infection in humans.

There are two morphologic forms of *Chlamydia*: the elementary body (EB) and reticulate body (RB) (Fig. 54–1). The EB is the infectious form; it is smaller, spherical, 0.2–0.4 μm in diameter, and it has a rigid wall that permits extracellular survival. It attaches to the target host and infects it. The RB is a larger (0.6–1.0 μm diameter) intracellular form that synthesizes its own DNA, RNA, and proteins but still needs high-energy phosphate bonds from the host cells. It divides by binary fission and produces many progeny, which mature into infectious elementary bodies that are released from the host cells.

PATHOGENESIS

C. psittaci can be detected in blood, tissues, secretions from the eyes and nostrils, feathers, and feces of infected birds. Affected birds demonstrate nonspecific signs of disease. They may have a subclinical infection or suffer from apathy, shivering, weakness, eye discharges, and diarrhea. The death rate in affected flocks may reach 30 per cent. The agent can be shed for prolonged periods by asymptomatic birds or birds that have recovered from the infection. It remains viable in dried feces, bird feathers, and dust from the surroundings. Birds may show a latent stage of infection with relapse when environmental conditions are adverse, especially when the birds are crowded, wet, chilly, and malnourished. Intercurrent infections often spread during shipment, explaining the outbursts of epidemics after importations of pet birds from remote countries (South America, Australia, and the Far East).

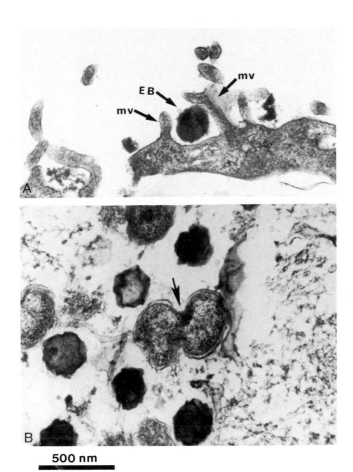

Figure 54–1. *A,* An elementary body *(EB)* being engulfed by microvilli (× 50,000). *B,* A reticulate body *(arrow)* dividing by binary fission within the cell (× 50,000). (Courtesy of Rossanna Peeling, Ph.D., and Dr. Robert Brunham.)

C. psittaci gains access to the human body through the respiratory tract, rapidly enters the blood, and is transported to the reticuloendothelial cells of the liver and the spleen where it replicates. It then invades the lung and other organs by the hematogenous route. Rarely, the organism is transmitted by handling infected plumage, bird bite, or person to person.

INCIDENCE

Psittacosis occurs as outbreaks when flocks are infected or as isolated cases from infected pet birds. It is an uncommon infection in children but should be suspected in any child with respiratory illness who has a history of contact with birds.

CLINICAL MANIFESTATIONS

The signs and symptoms of psittacosis in humans vary greatly from an asymptomatic infection to severe and fatal pneumonia. The incubation period ranges from 1 to 3 weeks, after which the disease begins abruptly or insidiously, with sore throat, anorexia, weakness, malaise, myalgia, and headache. Chills and a nonproductive cough are common. Epistaxis, hemoptysis, or chest pain due to pleuritic or pericardial inflammation may occur. Confusion and disorientation are common. A diffuse headache (sometimes more frontal) may dominate the picture, and when it is associated with fever and even minimal pulmonary signs and symptoms should raise the suspicion of psittacosis (Braude, Davis, and Fierer, 1986). Fever is generally high, with temperatures reaching 39° to 40°C, and is sometimes accompanied by a relative bradycardia. A faint, macular, rose-colored eruption (Horder's spots) may be present. Physical findings over the chest may be surprisingly few, with only fine crackles, whereas the chest radiograph may show significant changes (Davis, Dulbecco, Eisen et al, 1973). Signs of meningeal irritation are extremely rare, but coma, encephalitis, convulsions, and death may occur, with typical inclusions in the meninges (Walton, 1954). Inflammatory heart disease, with myocarditis, pericarditis, subacute endocarditis, and congestive heart failure have been reported. Hepatitis and icterus, with or without formation of hepatic granulomas, erythema nodosum, or erythema multiforme may occur (Joklik, Willett, Amos et al, 1988). Disseminated intravascular coagulopathy, acute renal failure, and shock may develop (Byron, Walls, and Mair, 1979; Van Berkel, Dik, Van Der Meer et al, 1985). Acute placentitis and spontaneous abortion in wives of sheep farmers have been attributed to *C. psittaci* of sheep origin (Wong, Gray, Buxton et al, 1985). Reactive arthritis (Cooper and Ferriss, 1986), Stevens-Johnson syndrome (South, Wreghitt, and Caul, 1985), thrombophlebitis of the lower extremities, and pulmonary infarction have also been reported.

The differential diagnosis includes bacterial pneumonia, mycoplasma pneumonia, legionnaires' disease, influenza, encephalitis, typhoid fever, Q fever, primary coccidioidomycosis, and tuberculosis.

PATHOLOGY

The initial inflammatory reaction in the human lung is an intra-alveolar polymorphonuclear exudate resembling a bacterial infection. Later it becomes lymphocytic and mononuclear in the alveoli and interstitium. Edema, necrosis, and hemorrhage may occur. Pulmonary macrophages containing basophilic cytoplasmatic inclusion bodies are pathognomonic and are called LCL bodies after their discoverers (Levinthal, Coles, and Lillie). The tracheobronchial epithelium is generally spared. The liver may show intralobular focal necrosis with elementary bodies in Kupffer cells. Basophilic inclusion bodies may be seen in the cytoplasm of all the tissues involved.

DIAGNOSIS

A careful epidemiologic history must be taken, even though some patients appear to have had no contact with birds. Leukopenia may be present early in the disease (25 per cent of patients), and leukocytosis may appear during convalescence. Mild proteinuria may occur. The sedimentation rate is usually normal, and cold agglutinins are absent. The cerebrospinal fluid (CSF) is generally normal. Chest radiographs vary, commonly showing patchy infiltrates in the lower lobes or interstitial pneumonitis without any distinctive pattern (Macfarlane, Miller, Smith et al, 1984). Pleural effusions are uncommon, even though pathologically there is pleural involvement.

In the first stages, *C. psittaci* can be recovered from blood, throat swabs, and sputum, where it persists until convalescence. The chlamydiae can be inoculated intraperitoneally into mice, the yolk sac of embryonated hen eggs, or cell tissue cultures (HeLa 229 cells or McCoy cells irradiated or treated with 5-iododeoxyuridine [IUDR] or cycloheximide). Cultivation of the organism may pose a threat to laboratory personnel and should be performed only in specialized facilities. The organism can be seen as large intracytoplasmic inclusions within the infected cells and can be stained with Giemsa stain.

Serologic tests are widely used for the diagnosis of psittacosis, especially the complement fixation (CF) test that uses a heat-stable chlamydial antigen prepared from infected chick embryos. A fourfold rise in CF titers can be shown between acute and convalescent serum samples. Maximum titers range from 1:32 to 1:256 during the third to fifth week of the illness and then diminish slowly. The rise in titer may be delayed by therapy. A single titer of 1:16 or greater can be considered as presumptive evidence of the disease in a patient with a compatible clinical picture. The antigen used for the CF test measures antibody responses to all chlamydiae and therefore is not specific for psittacosis. There may be also a cross-reaction with *Coxiella burnetii* or *Brucella*. Other tests include a radioisotope precipitation technique, an immunofluorescent test, and an enzyme-linked immunosorbent assay (ELISA) method. Antibodies to TWAR strain can be tested by microimmunofluorescence.

TREATMENT AND PROPHYLAXIS

Recommended therapy includes tetracycline (2 to 3 g/day for patients older than 8 years) or erythromycin ethylsuccinate (30 mg/kg/day for patients younger than 8 years). The treatment is usually continued for 3 weeks to prevent relapse. Generally there is a clinical improvement within 1 to 3 days of treatment. The patients should be observed carefully for extrapulmonary complications, such as myocarditis, endocarditis, and liver dysfunction. Experience with erythromycin, chloramphenicol, and rifampin is limited. Without treatment, the mortality rate may reach 20 per cent. After the introduction of tetracycline, the mortality rate fell to less than 1 per cent. Respiratory isolation is required during the acute phase of the disease, especially for patients with severe coughing. Patients may shed the organism in sputum for years. Bed linens and clothes should be disinfected, and the suspected pet should be sacrificed.

The use of tetracycline in the food of domestic animals and turkeys is effective both prophylactically and therapeutically. Vaccines against ornithosis have so far proved to be of little use. Pregnant women who live or work on sheep farms should avoid contact with lambing ewes and newborn lambs, even if the animals seem healthy, because of the increased risk of placentitis and abortion (Johnson, Matheson, Williams et al, 1985; Wong, Gray, Buxton et al, 1985).

REFERENCES

Braude AI, Davis CE, and Fierer J: Infectious diseases and medical microbiology. 2nd ed. Philadelphia, WB Saunders Co, 1986.

Byron NP, Walls J, and Mair HJ: Fulminant psittacosis. Lancet 1:353, 1979.

Campbell LA, Kuo CC, and Grayston JT: Characterization of the new *Chlamydia* agent, TWAR, as a unique organism by restriction endonuclease analysis and DNA-DNA hybridization. J Clin Microbiol 25(10):1911, 1987.

Cooper SM and Ferriss JA: Reactive arthritis and psittacosis. Am J Med 81:555, 1986.

Davis BD, Dulbecco R, Eisen HN et al: Microbiology. 2nd ed. New York, Harper & Row, 1973.

Grayston JT, Kuo CC, Wang SP et al: A new *Chlamydia psittaci* strain, TWAR, isolated in acute respiratory infections. N Engl J Med 315:161, 1986.

Johnson FWA, Matheson BA, Williams H et al: Abortion due to infection with *Chlamydia psittaci* in a sheep farmer's wife. Br Med J 290:592, 1985.

Joklik WK, Willett HP, Amos DB et al: Zinsser microbiology. 19th ed. East Norwalk, Conn, Appleton & Lange, 1988.

Macfarlane JT, Miller AC, Smith RWH et al: Comparative radiographic feature of community acquired legionnaires' disease, pneumococcal pneumonia, mycoplasma pneumonia, and psittacosis. Thorax 39:28, 1984.

Ritter J: Beitrag zur Frage des Pneumotyphus (Eine Hausepidemie in Uster [Schweiz] betreffend.) Deutsches Archiv für Klinische Medizin (Munich) 25:53, 1880.

South M, Wreghitt TG, and Caul EO: Stevens-Johnson syndrome associated with psittacosis. J Infect 11:173, 1985.

Van Berkel M, Dik H, Van Der Meer JWM et al: Acute respiratory insufficiency from psittacosis. Br Med J 290:1503, 1985.

Walton KW: The pathology of a fatal case of psittacosis showing intracytoplasmic inclusion in the meninges. J Path & Bact 68:565, 1954.

Wong SY, Gray ES, Buxton D et al: Acute placentitis and spontaneous abortion caused by *Chlamydia psittaci* of sheep origin: a histological and ultrastructural study. J Clin Pathol 38:707, 1985.

55

Q FEVER

Q (for query) fever was first reported as a distinct febrile illness by Derrick in Australia in 1937 after an outbreak in slaughterhouse workers. The causative organism, *Coxiella burnetii*, was subsequently isolated from a specimen obtained from Derrick by Burnet and Freeman (1937) in Australia and independently from a tick by Davis and Cox (1938) in the United States.

EPIDEMIOLOGY

Q fever, which occurs as a geographically widespread zoonosis, is associated with both sporadic and epidemic disease (Marmion and Stoker, 1958; Hart, 1973; D'Angelo et al, 1979; Sawyer et al, 1987). *C. burnetii* is maintained in nature in two infectious cycles involving domestic animals and wildlife (Fig. 55–1). Although not well described, the cycle in widely disseminated feral animals appears to involve numerous species of arthropod vectors, particularly ticks, which have been shown to transmit the organism transovarially as well as to other animals. No clear association has been shown, however, between this wildlife cycle and the domestic cycle, although the wildlife cycle may serve as a reservoir in nonendemic areas (Marmion and Stoker, 1958; Hart, 1973).

The domestic cycle is far more important as a source of human infection. Q fever antibodies have been found in cattle or sheep in all endemic areas (McKiel, 1964; Wisniewski and Krumbiegel, 1970; Ferris et al, 1973). Infected animals show no evidence of infection, but organisms are excreted in large quantities in their milk and feces, and their placenta is heavily infected. *C. burnetii*, unlike other rickettsiae, is highly resistant to desiccation, and transmission by aerosol inhalation is likely with an infectious dose as low as a single organism. Transmission by arthropod vectors in the domestic cycle may be less significant.

Inhalation appears to be a much more important route of infection for humans than ingestion of milk, and unlike in other human rickettsial diseases tick-borne transmission appears to be unimportant in Q fever (Marmion and Stoker, 1958; Krumbiegel and Wisniewski, 1970). This association of Q fever with domestic animals almost certainly accounts for the higher reported incidence in men whose occupation involves the handling of domestic animals, particularly at parturition. Recent serosurveys in Canada show dairy herd reactor rates of greater than 80 per cent (Lang, 1988). Most epidemic disease can be accounted for by exposure to infected domestic animals, in persons handling cattle or sheep such as farmers or dairyworkers, in persons handling animal products such as slaughterhouse and tannery person-

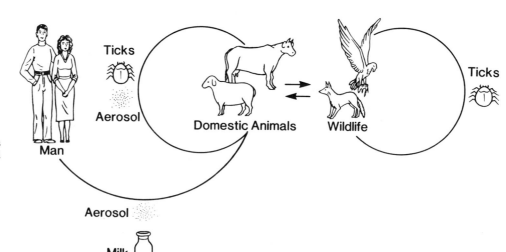

Figure 55–1. Infectious cycles of *Coxiella burnetii* in nature and their relationship to humans.

nel, and in medical research personnel involved in studies with pregnant sheep (McLean et al, 1960; Wisniewski and Krumbiegel, 1970; Schachter et al, 1971; Curet and Paust, 1972; Gross et al, 1972; Ferris et al, 1973; Meiklejohn et al, 1981). Disease in laboratory workers handling infected material has been reported as well (Johnson and Kadull, 1966). The epidemiology of sporadic endemic disease, however, is less clear (Clark et al, 1951). Residential and travel exposures have been implicated, and the ability of the organism to be transmitted over long distances from infective sources makes source tracing difficult (Lumio et al, 1981). Nevertheless, a large number of cases remain unexplained, and other vehicles such as human milk should be considered potential sources of Q fever in certain populations (Herbert et al, 1965; Krumbiegel and Wisniewski, 1970).

Marrie and colleagues (1988) showed a strong association with rural residence and exposure to parturient cats, especially stillborn kittens, with the acquisition of Q fever in Maritime Canada suggesting that small mammals and domestic pets may play a large role in sporadic cases and small epidemics. Such findings have been supported by observations on the epidemiology of Q fever in Europe (Aitken et al, 1987).

THE ORGANISM

C. burnetii, a member of the family Rickettsiaceae, is a small pleomorphic intracellular organism sharing properties with the gram-negative bacteria. It differs from other *Rickettsia* in resistance to physical and chemical agents, DNA base composition, unique phase variation, and possibly differentiation of endospores (McCaul and Williams, 1981). Intrastrain variation in phase I lipopolysaccharide structure appears to be responsible for the observed phase variation analogous to the smooth-rough transition of gram-negative bacteria (Stoker and Fiset, 1956). Recent isolates are in phase I, and high antibody titers to phase I organisms have been associated with chronic infection in humans (Fiset and Ormsbee, 1968). Interstrain variation in phase I lipopolysaccharide structure has been demonstrated, and subtypes appear to be associated with chronic infection (Hackstadt, 1986). Differences in restriction endonuclease digestion patterns of the plasmid DNA found in isolates from acute and chronic infection appear to be correlated with the interstrain variation in phase I lipopolysaccharide (Samuel et al, 1985). Other biologic differences exist, but their clinical relevance is unclear.

CLINICAL DISEASE

Although asymptomatic infection may be common, the usual presentation in adults is as an acute febrile systemic illness following an incubation period of 1 to 4 weeks (Eschar et al, 1966; Brown, 1973). Although the infection is frequently said to be "flu-like," with abrupt onset of fever, chills, headache, and myalgia with or without a nonproductive cough or other respiratory symptoms, Meiklejohn and associates (1981) have noted several features that are atypical for influenza and other viral respiratory disease, particularly an excessively high fever and rigors in the absence of significant respiratory symptoms. Nevertheless, pneumonitis is a major component of the clinical presentation, and abnormal radiologic findings were present on admission in 87 per cent of one series of hospitalized patients (Millar, 1978). Also, Q fever accounted for nearly 10 per cent of one series of patients with atypical pneumonia (Marrie et al, 1982). The most common radiologic findings in such cases are multiple round segmental consolidations and linear atelectasis. Rash, adenopathy, and arthritis in Q fever, again unlike in other rickettsial infections, are characteristically absent. Hepatitis with elevation of the serum glutamic-oxaloacetic transaminase is common, but clinical jaundice is rare (Dupont et al, 1971). Headache is a prominent feature of the acute illness. Although the cerebrospinal fluid is virtually always normal, there have been occasional case reports of meningitis/encephalitis with Q fever (Brooks et al, 1986). Thus, the major differential diagnostic considerations in the adult are influenza, brucellosis, tularemia, *Mycoplasma* or viral respiratory infection, and psittacosis. Although other clinical syndromes such as gastroenteritis have been reported, they are rare (Eschar et al, 1966; Marrie et al, 1982).

The acute clinical syndrome in infants and children has not been well described. In one series, however, the second largest group of patients included children between the ages of 5 months and 5 years (Wisniewski and Krumbiegel, 1970). Richardus and colleagues (1985) reported a series of 18 cases of Q fever in children younger than 3 years of age in the Netherlands. Clinical manifestations of pneumonia were present in only four at the time of hospital admission, and the radiologic findings that are typical in adults were largely absent. Nonspecific findings of fever, malaise, and anorexia were more common. Several cases of Q fever in children have been associated with rash, which may be more common in childhood (Herbert et al, 1965). Serologic evidence of congenital *C. burnetii* infection has been reported, although clinical infection was inapparent at birth, and late effects were unknown (Giroud et al, 1968; Fiset et al, 1975).

Chronic Q fever usually manifests as culture-negative subacute endocarditis (Turck et al, 1976), and there is usually evidence of prior valvular damage or a prosthetic valve. Rash and other manifestations of immune complex disease may also be present (Kimbrough et al, 1979). Infection can persist at other sites, and several cases of subclinical chronic Q fever have been reported (Fergusson et al, 1985). Although primarily a disease of adults, Q fever endocarditis has been reported in a 6-year-old child (Jones and Pitcher, 1980).

DIAGNOSIS

The diagnosis of Q fever may be made by inoculation of animals or embryonated eggs with infected tissue or by examination of post-mortem or biopsy material, but the usual method of diagnosis is serologic (Urso, 1974; Peirce et al, 1979). Complement fixation (CF) and agglutination are the usual serologic tests, although indirect fluorescent-antibody tests and enzyme-linked immunosorbent assay of comparable sensitivity and specificity have been reported (Peter et al, 1987). Specific IgM antibody and a serologic rise in phase II antigens in the CF test usually indicate acute infection (Fiset and Ormsbee, 1968; Murphy and Magro, 1980; Dupuis et al, 1985). High titers of phase I antibody have been associated with chronic infection, endocarditis, and granulomatous hepatitis (Turck et al, 1976). Result of the Weil-Felix agglutination of *Proteus* antigens is negative in Q fever, unlike in other rickettsial diseases.

Q fever should be considered in the differential diagnosis of all granulomatous diseases. Characteristic fibrin-ring "doughnut" granulomas, consisting of a central clear lipid area surrounded by leukocytes and rimmed by eosinophilic fibrinoid material, are highly suggestive of Q fever. The presence of undiagnosed granulomatous disease or the characteristic granulomas should prompt a serologic investigation for Q fever (Travis et al, 1986; Srigley et al, 1985).

TREATMENT

Tetracycline is probably the antimicrobial of choice, although chloramphenicol would be appropriate for children less than 8 years of age. Erythromycin, trimethoprim-sulfamethoxazole, and combination therapy using lincomycin or doxycycline have also been used (Turck et al, 1976; Kimbrough et al, 1979). Comparative efficacy trials, however, are not available. Combination therapy with rifampin may be useful, and in vitro studies suggest that the quinolones may be useful as well (Yeaman et al, 1987). Early treatment diminishes the serologic response, and successful treatment of chronic Q fever should be associated with a decline in phase I antibodies (Murphy and Field, 1970). Nevertheless, antimicrobial treatment appears to be less satisfactory for Q fever than for other rickettsial diseases.

PREVENTION

Avoidance of contact with infected cattle and sheep or ingestion of raw milk appears to be the only practical means of prevention. Other domestic animals, especially parturient cats, may also pose an increased risk. Exposure to infected wild animals is less likely to be preventable. Although human and animal vaccines have been developed, their role in prevention is at present unclear (Kishimoto et al, 1979). Research groups, particularly hospital-based groups using pregnant ewes, should exercise extreme care in the transportation and maintenance of animals in order to limit transmission of *C. burnetii* infection to humans.

REFERENCES

Aitken ID et al: Q fever in Europe: current aspects of aetiology, epidemiology, human infection, diagnosis and therapy. Infection 15:323, 1987.

Brooks RG et al: Encephalitis caused by *Coxiella burnetii*. Ann Neurol 20:91, 1986.

Brown GL: Clinical aspects of 'Q' fever. Postgrad Med J, 49:539, 1973.

Burnet FM and Freeman M: Experimental studies on the virus of "Q" fever. Med J Aust 2:299, 1937.

Clark WH et al: Q fever in California. Am J Hyg 54:319, 1951.

Curet LB and Paust JC: Transmission of Q fever from experimental sheep to laboratory personnel. Am J Obstet Gynecol 114:566, 1972.

Davis GE and Cox HR: A filter-passing infectious agent isolated from ticks. 1: Isolation from *Dermacentor andersoni*, reactions in animals, and filtration experiments. Public Health Rep 53:2259, 1938.

D'Angelo LG et al: Q fever in the United States, 1948–1977. J Infect Dis 139:613, 1979.

Derrick EH: "Q" fever, a new entity: clinical features, diagnosis and laboratory investigation. Med J Aust 2:281, 1937.

Dupont HL et al: Q fever hepatitis. Ann Intern Med 74:198, 1971.

Dupuis G et al: Immunoglobulin responses in acute Q fever. J Clin Microbiol 22:484, 1985.

Eschar J et al: Syndromes of Q fever. JAMA 195:146, 1966.

Fergusson RJ et al: Subclinical chronic Q fever. Q J Med 57:669, 1985.

Ferris DH et al: Epidemiologic investigations of Q fever in a major milkshed region of the United States of America. J Hyg Epidemiol Microbiol Immunol 17:375, 1973.

Fiset P and Ormsbee RA: The antibody response to antigens of *Coxiella burnetii*. Zentralbl Bakteriol Parasitenk Infektionskr Hyg Abt I Orig 206:211, 1968.

Fiset P et al: Immunologic evidence of human fetal infection with *Coxiella burneti*. Am J Epidemiol 101:65, 1975.

Giroud A et al: Inapparent maternal infection by *Coxiella burnetii* and fetal repercussions. Teratology 1:257, 1968.

Gross PA et al: Epidemiology of a Q fever outbreak in Los Angeles County, 1966. HSMHA Health Rep 87:71, 1972.

Hackstadt T: Antigenic variation in the phase I liposaccharide of *Coxiella burnetii* isolates. Infect Immun 52:337, 1986.

Hart RJC: The epidemiology of Q fever. Postgrad Med J 49:535, 1973.

Herbert FA et al: Q fever in Alberta—infection in humans and animals. Can Med Assoc J 93:1207, 1965.

Johnson JE III and Kadull PJ: Laboratory-acquired Q fever—a report of fifty cases. Am J Med 41:391, 1966.

Jones RWA and Pitcher DW: Q fever endocarditis in a 6-year-old child. Arch Dis Child 55:312, 1980.

Kimbrough RC III et al: Q fever endocarditis in the United States. Ann Intern Med 91:400, 1979.

Kishimoto RA et al: Q fever: diagnosis, therapy, and immunoprophylaxis. Milit Med 144:183, 1979.

Krumbiegel ER and Wisniewski HG: II. Consumption of infected raw milk by human volunteers. Arch Environ Health 21:63, 1970.

Kumar A et al: Human milk as a source of Q-fever infection in breast-fed babies. Indian J Med Res 73:510, 1981.

Lang GH: Serosurvey on the occurence of *Coxiella burnetii* in Ontario cattle. Can J Public Health 79:56, 1988.

Lumio J et al: Q fever in Finland: clinical, immunological and epidemiological findings. Scand J Infect Dis 13:17, 1981.

Marmion BP and Stoker MGP: The epidemiology of Q fever in Great Britain. Br Med J 2:809, 1958.

Marrie TJ et al: Exposure to parturient cats: a risk factor for acquisition of Q fever in Maritime Canada. J Infect Dis 158:101, 1988.

Marrie TJ et al: Q fever in Maritime Canada. Can Med Assoc J 126:1295, 1982.

McCaul TF and Williams JC: Developmental cycle of *Coxiella burnetii*: structure and morphogenesis of vegatative and sporogenic differentiations. J Bacteriol 147:1063, 1981.

McKiel JA: Q fever in Canada. Can Med Assoc J 91:573, 1964.

McLean DM et al: Q fever infections in an Ontario family. Can Med Assoc J 83:1110, 1960.

Meiklejohn G et al: Cryptic epidemic of Q fever in a medical school. J Infect Dis 144:107, 1981.

Millar JK: The chest film findings in 'Q' fever—a series of 35 cases. Clin Radiol 29:371, 1978.

Murphy AM and Field PR: The persistence of complement-fixing antibodies to Q-fever (*Coxiella burnetii*) after infection. Med J Aust 1:1148, 1970.

Murphy AM and Magro L: IgM globulin response in Q fever (*Coxiella burnetii*) infections. Pathology 12:391, 1980.

Peirce TH et al: Q fever pneumonitis. West J Med 130:453, 1979.

Peter O et al: Comparison of enzyme-linked immunosorbent assay and complement fixation and indirect fluorescent-antibody tests for detection of *Coxiella burnetii* antibody. J Clin Microbiol 25:1063, 1987.

Richardus JH et al: Q fever in infancy: a review of 18 cases. Pediatr Infect Dis 4:369, 1985.

Samuel JE et al: Correlation of plasmid type and disease caused by *Coxiella burnetii*. Infect Immun 49:775, 1985.

Sawyer LA et al: Q fever: current concepts. Rev Infect Dis 9:935, 1987.

Schachter J et al: Potential danger of Q fever in a university hospital environment. J Infect Dis 123:301, 1971.

Srigley JR et al: Q fever: the liver and bone marrow pathology. Am J Surg Pathol 9:752, 1985.

Stoker MGP and Fiset P: Phase variation of the Nine Mile and other strains of *Rickettsia burnetii*. Can J Microbiol 2:310, 1956.

Travis LB et al: Q fever: a clinicopathologic study of five cases. Arch Pathol Lab Med 110:1017, 1986.

Turck WPG et al: Chronic Q fever. Q J Med 45:193, 1976.

Urso RP: The pathologic findings in rickettsial pneumonia. Am J Clin Pathol 64:335, 1974.

Wisniewski HG and Krumbiegel ER: I. Q fever in the Milwaukee area cattle. Arch Environ Health 21:58, 1970.

Wisniewski HG and Krumbiegel ER: III. Epidemiological studies of Q fever in humans. Arch Environ Health 21:66, 1970.

Yeaman MR et al: In vitro susceptibility of *Coxiella burnetii* to antibiotics, including several quinolones. Antimicrob Agents Chemother 31:1079, 1987.

56

WILLIAM A. HOWARD, M.D.

TULAREMIA

Tularemia is primarily a septicemic disease of rodents; it may be transmitted to humans by the handling of infected material or by the bite of certain insect vectors. The disease is generally considered to be fatal to the animal hosts, but of 39 rabbits trapped during the study of one epidemic, 15 were found to possess agglutinating antibodies to the causative organism. Tularemia was first described in ground squirrels in Tulare County, California, in 1912 by McCoy of the United States Public Health Service, and the first human case was described by Wherry in 1914.

INCIDENCE

Tularemia probably has worldwide distribution and is found in all those parts of the United States and Canada where rodents and small game abound. The disease is also reported regularly in Europe and the USSR and is endemic in northern Sweden. Sporadic cases are the rule, although the disease may appear occasionally in epidemic form, as in the outbreak in Vermont in 1968, when 72 cases were identified, and in the group of 38 cases that occurred in Utah in 1971. From 1960 through 1968, a total of 2594 cases were reported in the United States, with 23 deaths, a marked drop from the peak incidence of 2291 cases reported in 1939. Most recent figures show a median of 271 cases yearly from 1982 to 1986, with a decline to 168 cases in 1986 and 188 cases in 1987. In the first 42 weeks of 1989, there were 129 cases reported, compared with 157 cases for a similar period in 1988. The majority of cases are now reported from the central states, both northern and southern, with relatively few from the Mountain and Pacific states, representing a major shift in geographic distribution from the western to the central and eastern parts of the country. Missouri, Arkansas, and Oklahoma have accounted for almost three quarters of the cases reported in the past 2 years. A special susceptibility to tularemia is noted among laboratory workers handling the infecting agent.

ETIOLOGY

The disease is caused by *Francisella tularensis (Pasteurella tularensis)*, a nonmotile, gram-negative, coccoid bacillus, 0.3 to 0.7 μ in length. The organism is readily destroyed by heating at 56°C for 10 minutes and by most disinfectants, including chlorine at one part per million in drinking water. This fragility probably accounts for the rarity of the gastrointestinal, oropharyngeal, and glandular varieties of the disease in the United States, where potentially infected foods are nearly always cooked before being eaten and chlorination of water is the rule.

PATHOGENESIS

Although *F. tularensis* is usually found in rodents, including rabbits and hares, the organism may infect deer, foxes, coyotes, woodchucks, sheep, skunks, squirrels, opossums, water rats, cats, dogs, and many other animals. Birds and quail may also harbor *F. tularensis*. The disease is transmitted from animal to animal by several species of ticks of the family Ixodidae, including the rabbit tick *(Haemaphysalis leporispalustris)*, the brown dog tick *(Rhipicephalus sanguineus)*, as well as species of the genera *Ixodes* and *Amblyomma*. *Ixodes dammini*, the tick responsible for the transmission of the infective agent of Lyme disease, has been implicated as a possible vector in tularemia.

Transmission from animals to humans may also be mediated by members of the family Ixodidae, most commonly the American dog tick *(Dermacentor variabilis)*, the Rocky Mountain wood tick *(D. andersoni)*, the Pacific coast tick *(D. occidentalis)*, and the southern lone star tick *(Amblyomma americanum)*. In the tick, the infection is perpetuated by transmission through the egg, and the organism is present in both the gut and hemocele. The deer fly *(Chrysops discalis)* transmits tularemia in the northwestern United States, and other tabanid flies probably are responsible for the spread of the disease in the USSR. In Russia, the common mosquitoes *Aedes aegypti* and *Culex apicalis* have been implicated as vectors. To date, mosquito transmission has not been reported in this country, but with the recognized mosquito population of the United States, it remains a distinct possibility. *F. tularensis* has survived for 50 days in *Anopheles maculipennis*. Squirrel and rabbit fleas may also be vectors in occasional instances. In the Utah epidemic, there was some evidence that biting gnats of the genus *Culicoides* were implicated in the rodent-to-human transmission.

Naturally acquired infection is almost always obtained by handling infected small game, primarily rabbits. Rarely, it may be caused by the bite of an infected tick or by crushing a tick on the skin. The organism seems able to penetrate the unbroken skin, and a remarkably small number of bacteria (10 to 50) are regularly capable of causing the infection in experimental subjects. Person-to-person transmission has not been recorded, but laboratory infections are common.

F. tularensis is an intracellular parasite, and recent evidence indicates that host resistance to tularemia, like host resistance to various other intracellular bacteria, may be dependent primarily on a cellular immune response, humoral factors (circulating antibody) appearing to be of secondary importance. Recovery usually results in lifelong immunity.

CLINICAL MANIFESTATIONS

Tularemia has been more prevalent during the fall and winter months, coincident with the hunting season. However, with the increase in the number of cases apparently transmitted by arthropods, an increasing incidence is being observed during the summer months, when these vectors are most prevalent. The incubation period of the disease is nearly always less than 2 weeks and usually less than 1 week.

Depending on the portal of entry and the mode of infection, six clinical types are described: (1) ulceroglandular (most common), (2) oculoglandular, (3) oropharyngeal, (4) pulmonic, (5) glandular, and (6) intestinal (typhoidal). There obviously may be some overlapping, and some reports indicate that a high percentage of patients, regardless of the type of clinical appearance, have roentgenographic evidence of lung involvement.

In naturally occurring infections, mostly from handling infected animals, approximately 90 per cent are of the ulceroglandular type, whereas laboratory infections are almost always of the pneumonic variety. In natural infections, the onset is abrupt, with chills, temperature as high as 105 or 106°F, (40.6 or 41.1°C), headache, and vomiting. Evidence of the portal of entry may not be present for the first 24 hours, although there may be regional lymphadenopathy. The initiating lesion begins as a localized inflammatory area 2 to 3 cm in diameter with a central papule. The lesion progresses to central necrosis, with abscess formation and ulceration. The regional lymph nodes become enlarged, firm, reddened, and tender and may undergo abscess formation, requiring surgical drainage. Other systemic symptoms include generalized muscle aches and pains, prostration, sweating, and somnolence. Skin rashes, varying from macules and papules to petechiae, may be present. Hepatosplenomegaly may be noted. Variations occur, depending on the portal of entry, and ulcers may be found on the tonsils, pharynx, or conjunctiva. Corneal ulcers have also been reported.

Many patients have both clinical and roentgenographic evidence of pulmonary involvement, often with an associated hilar adenopathy (Fig. 56–1). In diagnosing obscure pulmonary lesions, one should consider tularemia, because the portal of entry may not be obvious and primary lesions may not be found.

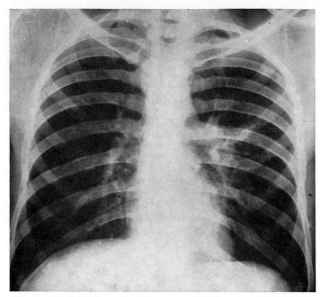

Figure 56–1. Tularemia. (Courtesy of Walter T Hughes, M.D.)

Infection acquired by laboratory workers is nearly always of the pulmonic variety. Respiratory symptoms include dry cough, sore throat, substernal discomfort, and pleuritic pain. Physical signs may include those of bronchopneumonia. Roentgenographic findings may be indicative of patchy bronchopneumonia, pleural effusion, peribronchial thickening, and nodular infiltration. Residual changes include fibrosis and an apparent increase in calcification.

The oropharyngeal type usually results from the ingestion of contaminated food or water and may involve more than one member of the family because there is a common source of infection. This form produces the characteristic ulcerations in the mouth, throat, or tonsils, with cervical adenitis and occasionally exudate or pseudomembrane on the tonsils.

Eye involvement causes lacrimation, photophobia, itching and swelling of the eyelids, and enlargement of the preauricular lymph nodes. Rarely, corneal ulcers may cause permanent impairment of vision.

DIAGNOSIS

The presence of tularemia usually may be suspected when the patient gives a history of contact with some sort of small wild animal, usually a rabbit, especially with the classic appearance of the ulceroglandular form of the disease. The leukocyte count may be as high as 14,000 to 16,000 cells/mm³ at onset, and the erythrocyte sedimentation rate and C-reactive protein level are usually slightly elevated. Laboratory confirmation may be obtained by the isolation of the causative agent from material from ulcers or buboes cultured on glucose-cystine blood agar. Animal inoculation is also an effective way of establishing the diagnosis. Unfortunately, both methods carry a high degree of risk to laboratory personnel and are

not normally recommended. Blood drawn early in the disease and 3 to 4 weeks after onset may be used for comparative complement fixation, fluorescent antibody studies, hemagglutination inhibition, and antibody-neutralizing studies. Enzyme-linked immunosorbent assay (ELISA) has been recommended most recently as a definitive diagnostic procedure. An elevated titer can be significant in the first week of the disease, and increases in consecutive serum samples further substantiate the diagnosis of tularemia. Initially, IgG and IgM antibodies are present in approximately equal amounts, but later, IgG antibodies increase in proportion, so that after 2 to 3 years IgG values are more than twice those of IgM. This finding may be of help in deciding whether the titer of a single serum sample is of recent or long-standing duration.

The intradermal skin test for tularemia is a valuable diagnostic tool, because the result will be positive in the first 7 to 14 days of the disease and is often positive on the first day the patient presents to the physician. The test is evidence of the development of delayed hypersensitivity, suggesting that cell-mediated immunity plays a prominent part in development of host resistance. The reaction may be read in 48 to 72 hours; induration measuring greater than 5 mm indicates a positive response. Such a test rarely causes a rise in the agglutination titer, and the skin reaction may continue to be positive for many years.

The ulceroglandular form of the disease must be differentiated from lymphadenitis due to pyogenic organisms, from infectious mononucleosis, and from other infections that produce an initial skin lesion followed by regional lymph node involvement, such as sporotrichosis, plague, and anthrax. The rarer oropharyngeal form must be distinguished from herpes simplex mucous membrane involvement, herpangina, and the oral manifestations of blood dyscrasias. Pneumonic involvement resembling tularemia may occur in *Mycoplasma* infections, tuberculosis, brucellosis, sepsis, rat-bite fever, Q fever, psittacosis, relapsing fever, histoplasmosis, and *Salmonella* infections.

PATHOLOGY

In addition to the local lesion, pathologic findings include enlarged regional lymph nodes that contain focal lesions with central suppurative necrosis, characteristically bordered by a granulomatous infiltrate consisting of epitheloid cells and multinucleated giant cells of the foreign body type. In addition, there are focal necrotic lesions in various organs throughout the body, especially the liver, spleen, kidneys, lungs, and bone marrow. Polymorphonuclear leukocytes are plentiful in the center of these lesions, whereas in older lesions evidence of fibrosis is usually present.

COMPLICATIONS

Involvement of the respiratory tract occurs most commonly and includes bronchopneumonia, chronic bronchitis, and pleural effusion. Encephalitis and meningitis have been reported, and painful arthritis may occur. Other rare complications include thrombophlebitis, osteomyelitis, peritonitis, and pericarditis.

PREVENTION

Tularemia is most effectively prevented by the avoidance of contact with infected wild game and with various insect vectors. One should reject for use and destroy by burying or burning any game with evidence of liver involvement, such as abscesses or spots. Vaccine prophylaxis has been used in laboratory workers but is rarely indicated for children. The killed vaccine does not appear to prevent local infection, but it may prevent the resulting systemic infection or may modify the severity of the disease. The viable attenuated vaccine seems to offer protection against respiratory challenge in experimental subjects and appears to be the material of choice. The causative agent is not destroyed by digestive processes in the stomach, and successful trials or an oral attenuated vaccine in both monkeys and humans suggest that this might eventually become the vaccine of choice for individuals at high risk of infection. In spite of the routine use of vaccines in laboratory workers, there are now more than 200 cases of tularemia recorded in this group.

TREATMENT

Streptomycin is the most effective drug in the treatment of tularemia. It is bactericidal at concentrations of 1.9 μg/ml; if the strain is resistant to the drug, it will remain resistant regardless of concentration. Dosage in children should be 20 to 40 mg/kg/day in divided doses, the total dose not to exceed 1 to 2 g daily. Treatment is continued for 7 to 10 days. Relapses have not been observed with this plan of therapy. The later in the course of the disease that streptomycin is started, the slower will be the response. Signs of ototoxicity and nephrotoxicity should be monitored.

The tetracyclines are also effective drugs in the treatment. Because tetracyclines are bacteriostatic, relapses are common if they are begun too early in the course of the disease, before host immune response has been initiated. Relapses respond promptly, however, to a second course of the drug. Tetracyclines are used in a dosage of 20 to 40 mg/kg/day in divided doses orally, or 12 to 20 mg/kg/day intramuscularly or intravenously, for at least 10 days. Gentamicin has also been found to be effective in dosages of 4 to 6 mg/kg/day. This drug is bactericidal against *F. tularensis* and is effective against a spectrum of pulmonary pathogens that do not respond to antibiotic therapy; it may be useful in unresponsive pneumonias in areas where tularemia

is endemic. Chloramphenicol, in dosages of 50 mg/kg/day orally or intramuscularly, may be used when the other drugs are for any reason contraindicated. A brief increase to 100 mg/kg/day may be required for severe infections.

For the individual case, general supportive measures are used for fever and pain, including administration of acetaminophen or acetylsalicylic acid, analgesics, and sedatives. Local treatment is largely symptomatic, with emphasis on the maintenance of cleanliness. Surgical intervention, with the drainage of suppurative processes, may be necessary but may be accompanied by systemic reactions. Isolation is generally not considered necessary, although exudates and dressings should be handled with rubber gloves. Ocular lesions may be treated with saline soaks, and topical atropine may be used for corneal ulcers.

Untreated, the majority of patients recover in 6 to 8 weeks but experience a rather protracted convalescence. Suitable antibiotic therapy greatly shortens both the duration and severity of the infectious process.

REFERENCES

Anderson RA: Oculoglandular tularemia. J Iowa Med Soc 60:21, 1970.
Archer VW, Blackford SD, and Wissler JE: Pulmonary manifestations in human tularemia. JAMA 104:895, 1935.
Brooks GP and Buchanan TM: Tularemia in the United States. J Infect Dis 121:359, 1970.
Buchanan TM, Brooks GF, and Brachman PS: The tularemia skin test. Ann Intern Med 74:336, 1971.
Burroughs AL, Holdenried R, Longanecker DB, and Meyer KF: A field study of latent tularemia in rodents with a list of all known naturally infected vertebrates. J Infect Dis 76:115, 1945.
Carlsson HE, Lindberg AA, Lindberg G et al: Enzyme-linked immunosorbent assay for immunological diagnosis of human tularemia. J Clin Microbiol 10:615, 1979.
Faust EC and Russell PF: Tularemia. In Faust EC and Russell PF (eds): Clinical Parasitology. 7th ed. Philadelphia, Lea & Febiger, 1964.
Gould SE, Hinerman DL, Batsakis JG, and Beamer PR: Diagnostic patterns in diseases of the reticulo-endothelial system: tularemia. Am J Clin Pathol 41:419, 1964.
Hughes WT: Tularemia in children. J Pediatr 62:495, 1963.
Klock LE, Olsen PF, and Fukushima T: Tularemia epidemic associated with the deer fly. JAMA 226:149, 1973.
Ljung O: Intradermal and agglutination tests in tularemia. Acta Med Scand 160:149, 1958.
Ljung O: The intradermal test in tularemia. Acta Med Scand 160:135, 1958.
Mason WL, Eigelsbach HT, Little SF, and Bates JH: Treatment of tularemia, including pulmonary tularemia, with gentamycin. Am Rev Respir Dis 121:39, 1980.
Miller RP, and Bates JH: Pleuropulmonary tularemia—a review of 29 cases. Am Rev Respir Dis 99:31, 1969.
Morbidity and Mortality Weekly Reports: 25:209, 1976; 36:840, 1988; 37:344, 1988.
Overholt EL, Tigertt WD, Kadall PJ, and Ward MK: An analysis of forty-two cases of laboratory acquired tularemia. Am J Med 30:785, 1961.
Pankey GA: Tularemia. In Gellis SS and Kagan BM (eds): Current Pediatric Therapy 7. Philadelphia, WB Saunders Co, 1976.
Parker RT, Lister LM, Bauer RE et al: Use of chloramphenicol in experimental and human tularemia. JAMA 143:7, 1950.
Saslaw S, Eigelsbach HT, Wilson HE et al: Tularemia vaccine study. I. Intracutaneous challenge. Arch Intern Med 107:689, 1961.

57

WILLIAM L. ALBRITTON, M.D., Ph.D.

VARICELLA PNEUMONIA

Varicella-zoster virus (VZV) is one of five herpesviruses causing disease in humans and is the causative agent of chickenpox (varicella) and shingles (zoster). The virus measures 180 to 200 nm, is enveloped, contains double-stranded DNA, and is indistinguishable morphologically from the other human herpesviruses: herpes simplex virus (HSV), cytomegalovirus (CMV), Epstein-Barr virus (EBV), and human herpesvirus-6. Like other herpesviruses, VZV has a tendency to infect tissue of neuroectodermal origin and remains latent after primary infection. Infection with VZV resembles HSV infections in that there is a clearly recognizable primary infection syndrome (chickenpox) and a reactivation infection syndrome (zoster). Although VZV appears to be a single virus, recent studies at the molecular level reveal small variations in DNA (Oakes et al, 1977; Richards et al, 1979; Straus et al, 1983). The significance of these variations, however, is unknown, and our present understanding of the epidemiology and clinical manifestations of pulmonary disease associated with VZV infections require consideration of only a single virus. Several excellent reviews of VZV infections are available (Weller, 1983; Straus et al, 1988; Preblud et al, 1984).

EPIDEMIOLOGY

Primary infection with VZV results in a clinically recognizable generalized disease—chickenpox—in nearly 90 per cent of susceptible patients, unlike primary HSV infections, which are largely subclinical (Gordon, 1962). Chickenpox in temperate climates is a disease of childhood, with 80 per cent of cases occurring in the first decade of life and only 1.8 per cent in patients more than 20 years of age (Preblud and D'Angelo, 1979). In tropical climates, however, chickenpox occurs less commonly in childhood, resulting in a larger susceptible adult population (Maretic and Cooray, 1963).

Pneumonia as a complication was reported in 0.8 per cent of one series, making it less common as a complication of varicella than of other childhood diseases such as scarlet fever, pertussis, measles, and diphtheria (Bullowa and Wishik, 1935). The majority of the pneumonias and other reported complications in this series, however, were pyogenic and represented secondary infections. The incidence of primary varicella pneumonia since the introduction of antibiotics and routine immunization for common childhood infections is not known. Although only 1.8 per cent of cases of chickenpox occurred in patients more than 20 years of age, 25 per cent of the deaths occurred in this population (Preblud and D'Angelo, 1979; Preblud, 1981). One study on deaths due to chickenpox in infants reported a four times higher death/case ratio for children less than 1 year of age compared with children 1 to 14 years old, with the most common complication listed on death certificates as pneumonia (Preblud et al, 1985). Primary varicella pneumonia appears to occur with increased frequency and severity in adults (Fitz and Meiklejohn, 1956; Weinstein and Meade, 1956; Krugman et al, 1957; Mermelstein and Freireich, 1961; Gordon, 1962; Triebwasser et al, 1967), pregnant women (Harris and Rhoades, 1965; Geeves et al, 1971; Duong and Munns, 1979), neonates (Meyers, 1974), and immunocompromised patients (Feldman et al, 1975; Dolin et al, 1978; Atkinson et al, 1980).

Reactivation disease due to VZV also results in a clinically recognizable localized zoster, shingles. Progression of shingles to a generalized disease that may be indistinguishable from primary varicella is a serious complication in immunocompromised patients (Feldman et al, 1973; Dolin et al, 1978). Although clusters of zoster cases have been reported, all studies to date can be explained by our current concept that zoster occurs after reactivation of a latent infection following primary chickenpox (Hope-Simpson, 1965). Restriction endonuclease analysis of viral DNA from patients with varicella and zoster supports this hypothesis (Straus et al, 1983, 1984). Reactivation is more common with increasing age and with immunosuppression. The period of latency appears to be shortened with early primary infections, especially when primary infection occurs in utero (Baba et al, 1986; Guess et al, 1985).

CLINICAL FEATURES

PRIMARY VARICELLA PNEUMONIA

Primary varicella pneumonia appears to be a manifestation of a progressive varicella syndrome. It occurs in the absence of underlying disease and more commonly in adults than children with chickenpox. The onset of pneumonitis is usually 2 to 5 days after the appearance of the rash but may occur before the rash. As would be expected, evidence of involvement of other viscera, such as hepatitis, arthritis, myocarditis, and encephalitis, may be found (Ey et al, 1981). The spectrum of pneumonia varies widely from asymptomatic radiologic findings to a rapidly fatal disease. Cough, dyspnea, cyanosis, and tachypnea are common clinical findings in most series. In the absence of secondary bacterial infection, the radiologic picture is that of a diffuse nodular pulmonary infiltrate (Conte et al, 1970). In nonfatal cases, resolution of the pneumonia coincides with resolution of the skin lesions. The primary pathologic respiratory condition appears to be an abnormal ventilation-perfusion relationship due to unstable alveoli and reduced surfactant (Finucane et al, 1970). Pulmonary embolism has been described in the acute disease (Glick et al, 1972), and multiple pulmonary calcifications may be found as a late complication following varicella pneumonia (Raider, 1971). The spectrum of visceral involvement other than pneumonia also appears to vary considerably in primary VZV infections, leading to some confusion in the differentiation of mild Reye syndrome from varicella hepatitis.

Although primary varicella pneumonia probably occurs no more commonly in pregnant women than in the nonpregnant adult population, it appears to be associated with increased maternal morbidity and mortality and an adverse outcome for the fetus. Harris and Rhoades (1965) reported maternal mortality at 41 per cent and fetal mortality at 48 per cent. The largest number of cases was reported in the third trimester, and therefore the overall maternal mortality was highest in this group. A later prospective study of 43 pregnancies complicated by varicella demonstrated a 20 per cent morbidity, with four of nine women having pneumonia (Paryani and Arvin, 1986). There was only one death, and 1 of 11 infants born to mothers with first-trimester varicella showed evidence of the congenital varicella syndrome. There are no clear explanations for the increased severity of chickenpox in pregnancy. Reports of zoster in pregnancy do not show increased severity or evidence of dissemination (Brazin et al, 1979; Paryani and Arvin, 1986). Although varicella in pregnancy is relatively uncommon, as many as 5 to 16 per cent of adult women of childbearing age in the United States were shown in one seroepidemiologic study to be susceptible to chickenpox (Gershon et al, 1976). The higher susceptibility occurred in immigrant populations from tropical countries.

Primary varicella pneumonia may also occur as part of a fatal progressive varicella syndrome in infants born to mothers who have onset of chickenpox rash within 4 days before delivery (Meyers, 1974; Brunell, 1983). The onset of disease in neonates typically occurs 5 to 10 days post partum, suggesting that transmission to the fetus has occurred just before onset of clinical disease in the mother rather than at the time of maternal exposure. The severity of disease in the newborn would appear to be due to the viremic spread to the fetus and subsequent delivery before the appearance of protective or modifying maternal antibodies (Gershon, 1975; Enders, 1984). Pathologic findings are similar to those of progressive varicella in an older child or adult. Maternal varicella in the first trimester may be associated with congenital anomalies, but pulmonary disease is uncommon (McKendry and Bailey, 1973; Srabstein et al, 1974; Frey et al, 1977).

Finally, primary varicella pneumonia occurs in immunocompromised patients. In a group of 77 children who had cancer and who developed varicella, 32 per cent of those receiving chemotherapy had visceral dissemination and 7 per cent died (Feldman et al, 1975). All fatalities were associated with primary varicella pneumonia. No fatalities or disseminated infections occurred in patients who were in remission and not undergoing chemotherapy. Status and type of malignancy were not correlated with dissemination in this study, although lymphopenia (<500 cells/mm^3) appeared to be associated with dissemination. In a smaller study, 15 of 31 immunocompromised children who developed varicella showed evidence of dissemination (Morgan and Smalley, 1983). Two clinical patterns of dissemination were noted: (1) severe multisystem involvement, characterized by a predictable clinical sequence of fever, rash, and severe abdominal or back pain followed by elevation of serum transaminase levels and subsequent multisystem involvement, including pneumonitis, encephalitis, and hepatitis and (2) a mild clinical syndrome with elevated transaminase and mild interstitial pneumonitis but without abdominal or back pain. Immunosuppressed patients who have had chickenpox do not appear to be at increased risk on reexposure, with the possible exception of recipients of bone marrow transplants. Severe varicella has been reported in children with renal transplants, but varicella pneumonia has not been a complication (Feldhoff et al, 1981). Viremia and delayed development of interferon in vesicular fluid have been associated with progressive varicella in high-risk patients (Myers, 1979).

DISSEMINATED ZOSTER

In addition to the increased risk of progressive disease and primary varicella pneumonia in patients with malignant disease and varicella, patients undergoing treatment for malignant disease are at high risk of developing zoster. In one study, the incidence of zoster in children with acute lymphocytic leukemia was 122 times the incidence in children without an underlying malignancy (Guess et al, 1985). Patients with Hodgkin's disease or bone marrow transplants are at exceptionally high risk, with over 50 per cent of cases occurring within a year after diagnosis or transplant (Feldman et al, 1973; Atkinson et al, 1980). Unlike the reported increase in incidence of zoster with advancing age in the normal population, zoster appears to be as prevalent in children with malignant disease as in adults; the overall incidence of zoster in children with cancer is about 9 per cent. Of the high-risk patients such as those with Hodgkin's disease, 30 to 50 per cent show evidence of generalized cutaneous dissemination, and 10 per cent of these show significant visceral involvement, including pneumonitis. The mortality rate for disseminated zoster in immunosuppressed patients is 3 to 5 per cent, with virtually all reported cases showing pulmonary involvement. Unlike varicella, zoster occurred much more frequently in patients with lymphoreticular malignancies. In more than 75 per cent of such patients, zoster occurred during remission of the underlying disease.

Although it would appear from the foregoing discussion that varicella and zoster in cancer patients account for most varicella fatalities, only 16 per cent of varicella deaths reported in one series were associated with an underlying malignant disease (Preblud, 1981).

DIAGNOSIS

A diagnosis of varicella or varicella pneumonia is usually made on the basis of clinical examination and chest radiographs (Fig. 57–1). Laboratory confirmation of VZV infection occasionally is important, however, in clinical situations in which the presentation is atypical. Severe atypical vesicular disease in a hospitalized patient and exposure of a susceptible child with malignant disease to a patient with an atypical vesicular rash are examples of situations in which laboratory diagnosis may be helpful in management. Similarly, the decision to use antiviral chemotherapy may depend on laboratory diagnosis. In such situations, viral isolation, detection of viral particles or antigen in vesicular fluid, and serologic procedures have been useful. Before the global eradication of smallpox, examination of vesicular fluid by electron microscopy could differentiate severe varicella from smallpox by the presence of herpes-like virus particles (Fig. 57–2). The inability to distinguish the various herpesviruses on morphologic grounds makes this method of less value, because disseminated HSV infections may resemble varicella or disseminated zoster. Nevertheless, electron microscopy is useful in distinguishing herpes (including varicella) from other vesicular rashes such as those produced by enteroviruses, *Mycoplasma*, and other agents. Counterimmunoelectrophoresis has been useful in the rapid detection of VZV antigen in vesicular fluid (Frey et al, 1981), but specific antiserum is not yet commercially available. Although viral isolation or immunofluorescent detection of early virus antigen is definitive, the virus is labile and the time necessary

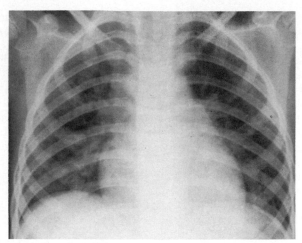

Figure 57–1. Typical varicella pneumonia. The patient is a 6-year-old female admitted in relapse 4 months after an initial diagnosis of acute lymphocytic leukemia with lymphomatous syndrome. She underwent intensive chemotherapy, and just before discharge, while she was still in profound marrow suppression, she was inadvertently exposed to a child with chickenpox. Zoster immune globulin (ZIG) was not available, and despite receiving plasma from an adult convalescent from zoster, she developed varicella 19 days after exposure. Progressive varicella was noted 4 days after the onset of a rash, and she was admitted to the hospital, where chest radiographs showed multiple bilateral nodular densities with diffuse streaking compatible with varicella pneumonia. Vesicular fluid from the skin showed numerous herpes-like virus particles. Resolution occurred with the rash, and she was discharged 8 days after admission. (Courtesy of Dr. Martin Reed.)

for detection of a cytopathic effect is relatively long, making viral isolation difficult and of little value in the diagnosis of acute infections.

A large number of serologic tests have been developed for the diagnosis of VZV infections as a result of the lack of sensitivity of the common serologic tests such as complement fixation (CF) for this purpose. The CF test is of little value in determining the immune status to varicella, because CF antibody declines to undetectable levels within several years of primary infection in most normal individuals and may fail to rise sufficiently for detection of seroconversion in immunosuppressed patients. Determination of immune status is occasionally important for both (1) assessing the risk of developing progressive disease on exposure in a patient with malignant disease who is undergoing therapy and (2) managing hospital staff who are exposed to patients with varicella or zoster.

Fluorescent antibody to membrane antigen (FAMA) (Brunell et al, 1969), indirect immunoperoxidase antibody technique (Gerna et al, 1979), and radioimmunoassay (Arvin and Koropchak, 1980) all have been used with excellent results in experimental laboratories but have not yet been used widely in general clinical virology laboratories. A skin test has been proposed to monitor susceptibility in hospital personnel when sensitive serologic testing is not available, but commercial antigen is not available (Steele et al, 1982).

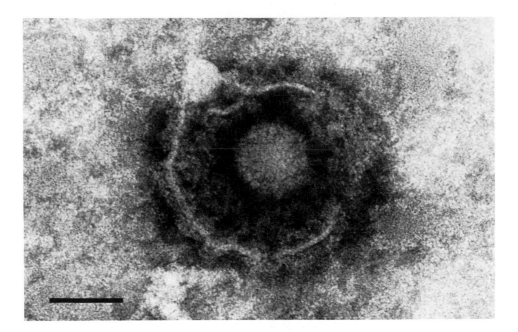

Figure 57–2. Typical herpeslike virus particle seen in vesicular fluid from a patient with varicella. This is an enveloped full particle, showing a full nucleocapsid surrounded by a lipid envelope. Such particles are approximately 180 nm in diameter, and the nucleocapsid contains doublestranded DNA (× 280,000; bar = 100 nm). (Courtesy of Paul Hazelton.)

TREATMENT

Nonspecific supportive measures are important in the treatment of primary varicella pneumonia and disseminated zoster with pulmonary involvement. When indicated, oxygen and ventilation should be used early, and considering the presence of unstable alveoli, the early use of positive end-expiratory pressure may be indicated.

Specific antiviral therapy has not been adequately evaluated in pneumonia due to VZV. In one randomized, double-blind, placebo-controlled trial of human leukocyte interferon in the treatment of varicella in children with cancer, progression of infection and complications were significantly less in patients receiving interferon (Arvin et al, 1978). Parenteral antiviral chemotherapy with newer agents such as adenine arabinoside and acyclovir appears promising in trials including largely immunosuppressed patients with cutaneous disseminated zoster or generalized HSV infection (Whitley et al, 1976; Prober et al, 1982; Balfour, 1984). Acyclovir appeared better than vidarabine in one study of the treatment of VZV infections in immunocompromised patients (Shepp et al, 1986). Other agents in similar trials have not been promising (Schimff et al, 1974). Such studies have not specifically addressed the question of efficacy in children with primary varicella pneumonia or the pulmonary disease of disseminated zoster. Future controlled trials will be necessary to answer this important question, particularly as it applies to nonimmunosuppressed patients.

PREVENTION

Several studies have shown that convalescent zoster immune globulin (ZIG)* or plasma (ZIP) is effective

*ZIG is currently available for distribution in North America through the Red Cross.

in preventing or modifying varicella if given soon after exposure (Brunell et al, 1969; Brunell et al, 1972; Gershon et al, 1974; Judelsohn et al, 1974; Balfour and Groth, 1979; Orenstein et al, 1981). High-risk susceptible patients, such as immunosuppressed patients with malignancy, newborns of mothers with onset of varicella within 5 days of delivery, premature infants, and pregnant women near term, should receive passive protection. The value of ZIG or ZIP in adults or in early pregnancy has not been established; the use of immune serum globulin (ISG), which has been shown to modify varicella in family contacts (Ross, 1962), may be more appropriate in such patients. Intravenous gamma globulin has been shown to provide serum levels of antibody comparable to ZIG (Paryani et al, 1984). ZIG, ZIP, and ISG are of no value in treating established varicella or zoster.

Active immunization of high-risk patients with a live attenuated varicella-zoster vaccine has been reported. Its use at present in North America is limited to high-risk patients with malignant disease, and many questions are yet unanswered regarding its potential usefulness in other high-risk patients and in the population at large. A supplement to the October 1986 issue of Pediatrics is devoted entirely to the current status of varicella vaccine, with an accompanying editorial by Plotkin (1986). Although a mild varicella-like illness has been reported in immunosuppressed vaccine recipients (Brunell et al, 1987), the long-term protective immunity in vaccine recipients (Asano et al, 1985) and the potential for combination vaccines (Brunell et al, 1988) appear promising. The risk of zoster in children with leukemia who received vaccine appears to be less than the risk in similar children who acquired natural varicella infections (Brunell et al, 1986).

Hospitalization of children with varicella pneumonia requires exceptional precautions. Nosocomial varicella can be easily demonstrated, and we see several patients every year who acquire varicella in the hospital, despite isolation precautions, from patients admitted with chickenpox or zoster. Hospital transmission can be a major problem on oncology wards, and admission of patients with varicella or zoster should be avoided if at all possible. In most hospitals, the usual respiratory precautions and infection control procedures will at best only limit and will not prevent transmission. A rational approach to hospital infection control of VZV infections has been presented by Myers and colleagues (1982).

REFERENCES

Arvin AM and Koropchak CM: Immunoglobulins M and G to varicella-zoster virus measured by solid-phase radioimmunoassay: antibody responses to varicella and herpes zoster infections. J Clin Microbiol 12:367, 1980.

Arvin AM et al: Human leukocyte interferon in the treatment of varicella in children with cancer: a preliminary controlled trial. Antimicrob Agents Chemother 13:605, 1978.

Asano Y et al: Long-term protective immunity of recipients of the OKA strain of live varicella vaccine. Pediatrics 75:667, 1985.

Atkinson K et al: Varicella-zoster virus infection after marrow transplantation for aplastic anemia or leukemia. Transplantation 29:47, 1980.

Baba K et al: Increased incidence of herpes zoster in normal children infected with varicella-zoster virus during infancy: community-based follow-up study. J Pediatr 108:372, 1986.

Balfour HH: Intravenous acyclovir therapy for varicella in immunocompromised children. J Pediatr 104:134, 1984.

Balfour HH and Groth KE: Zoster immune plasma prophylaxis of varicella: a follow-up report. J Pediatr 94:743, 1979.

Brazin SA et al: Herpes zoster during pregnancy. Obstet Gynecol 53:175, 1979.

Brunell PA: Fetal and neonatal varicella-zoster infections. Semin Perinatol 7:47, 1983.

Brunell PA: Prevention of varicella by zoster immune globulin. N Engl J Med 280:1191, 1969.

Brunell PA et al: Prevention of varicella in high risk children: a collaborative study. Pediatrics 50:718, 1972.

Brunell PA et al: Varicella-zoster immunoglobulins during varicella, latency and zoster. J Infect Dis 132:49, 1975.

Brunell PA et al: Risk of herpes zoster in children with leukemia: varicella vaccine compared with history of chickenpox. Pediatrics 77:53, 1986.

Brunell PA et al: Varicella-like illness caused by live varicella vaccine in children with acute lymphocytic leukemia. Pediatrics 79:922, 1987.

Brunell PA et al: Combined vaccine against measles, mumps, rubella, and varicella. Pediatrics 81:779, 1988.

Bullowa JGM and Wishik SM: Complications of varicella: their occurrence among 2,534 patients. Am J Dis Child 49:927, 1935.

Conte P et al: Viral pneumonia. Roentgen pathological correlations. Radiology 95:267, 1970.

Dolin R et al: Herpes zoster-varicella infections in immunosuppressed patients. Ann Intern Med 89:375, 1978.

Duong CM and Munns RE: Varicella pneumonia during pregnancy. J Fam Pract 8:277, 1979.

Enders G: Varicella-zoster virus infection in pregnancy. Prog Med Virol 29:166, 1984.

Ey JL et al: Varicella hepatitis without neurologic symptoms or findings. Pediatrics 67:285, 1981.

Feldhoff CM et al: Varicella in children with renal transplants. J Pediatr 98:25, 1981.

Feldman S et al: Herpes zoster in children with cancer. Am J Dis Child 126:167, 1973.

Feldman S et al: Varicella in children with cancer: seventy-seven cases. Pediatrics 56:388, 1975.

Finucane KE et al: The mechanism of respiratory failure in a patient with viral (varicella) pneumonia. Am Rev Respir Dis 101:949, 1970.

Fitz RH and Meiklejohn G: Varicella pneumonia in adults. Am J Med Sci 232:489, 1956.

Frey HM et al: Congenital varicella: case report of a serologically proved long-term survivor. Pediatrics 59:110, 1977.

Frey HM et al: Rapid diagnosis of varicella-zoster virus infections by countercurrent immunoelectrophresis. J Infect Dis 143:274, 1981.

Geeves RB et al: Varicella pneumonia in pregnancy with varicella neonatorum: report of a case followed by severe digital clubbing. Aust NZ J Med 1:63, 1971.

Gerna G et al: Antibody to early antigens of varicella-zoster virus during varicella and zoster. J Infect Dis 140:33, 1979.

Gershon AA: Infections of the Fetus and the Newborn Infant. New York, Alan R Liss, Inc, 1975.

Gershon AA et al: Zoster immune globulin: a further assessment. N Engl J Med 290:243, 1974.

Gershon AA et al: Antibody to varicella-zoster virus in parturient women and their offspring during the first year of life. Pediatrics 53:692, 1976.

Glick N et al: Recurrent pulmonary infarction in adult chickenpox pneumonia. JAMA 222:173, 1972.

Gordon JE: Chickenpox, an epidemiologic review. Am J Med Sci 224:362, 1962.

Guess HA et al: Epidemiology of herpes zoster in children and adolescents: a population-based study. Pediatrics 76:512, 1985.

Harris RE and Rhoades ER: Varicella pneumonia complicating pregnancy. Obstet Gynecol 25:734, 1965.

Hope-Simpson RE: The nature of herpes-zoster: a long-term study and a new hypothesis. Proc R Soc Med 58:9, 1965.

Judelsohn RG et al: Efficacy of zoster immune globulin. Pediatrics 53:476, 1974.

Krugman S et al: Primary varicella pneumonia. N Engl J Med 257:843, 1957.

McKendry JBJ and Bailey JD: Congential varicella associated with multiple defects. Can Med Assoc J 108:66, 1973.

Maretic Z and Cooray MPM: Comparisons between chickenpox in a tropical and a European country. J Trop Med Hyg 66:311, 1963.

Mermelstein RH and Freireich AW: Varicella pneumonia. Ann Intern Med 55:456, 1961.

Meyers JD: Congenital varicella in term infants: risk reconsidered. J Infect Dis 129:215, 1974.

Morgan ER and Smalley LA: Varicella in immunocompromised children. Am J Dis Child 137:883, 1983.

Myers MG: Viremia caused by varicella-zoster virus: association with malignant progressive varicella. J Infect Dis 140:229, 1979.

Myers MG et al: Hospital infection control for varicella zoster virus infection. Pediatrics 70:199, 1982.

Oakes JE et al: Analysis by restriction enzyme cleavage of human varicella-zoster virus DNAs. Virology 82:353, 1977.

Orenstein WA et al: Prophylaxis of varicella in high-risk children: dose-response effect of zoster immune globulin. J Pediatr 98:368, 1981.

Paryani SG and Arvin AM: Intrauterine infection with varicella-zoster virus after maternal varicella. N Engl J Med 314:1542, 1986.

Paryani SG et al: Varicella-zoster antibody titers after the administration of intravenous immune serum globulin or varicella zoster immune globlin. Am J Med 76:124, 1984.

Plotkin SA: Varicella vaccine: a point of decision. Pediatrics 78:705, 1986.

Preblud SR: Age-specific risks of varicella complications. Pediatrics 68:14, 1981.

Preblud SR and D'Angelo LJ: Chickenpox in the United States, 1972–1977. J Infect Dis 140:257, 1979.

Preblud SR et al: Deaths from varicella in infants. Pediatr Infect Dis 4:503, 1985.

Preblud SR et al: Varicella: clinical manifestations, epidemiology and health impact in children. Pediatr Infect Dis 3:505, 1984.

Prober CG et al: Acyclovir therapy of chickenpox in immunosuppressed children—a collaborative study. J Pediatr 101:622, 1982.

Raider L: Calcification in chickenpox pneumonia. Chest 60:504, 1971.

Richards JC et al: Analysis of the DNAs from seven varicella-zoster virus isolates. J Virol 32:812, 1979.

Ross AH: Modification of chickenpox in family contacts by administration of gamma globulin. N Engl J Med 267:369, 1962.

Schimff SC et al: Cytosine arabinoside for localized herpes zoster in patients with cancer: failure in a controlled trial. J Infect Dis 130:673, 1974.

Shepp DH et al: Treatment of varicella-zoster virus infection in severely immunocompromised patients. N Engl J Med 314:208, 1986.

Srabstein JC et al: Is there a congential varicella syndrome? J Pediatr 84:239, 1974.

Steele RW et al: Varicella zoster in hospital personnel: skin test reactivity to monitor susceptibility. Pediatrics 70:604, 1982.

Straus SE (moderator): Varicella-zoster virus infections: biology, natural history, treatment, and prevention. Ann Intern Med 108:221, 1988.

Straus SE et al: Genome differences among varicella-zoster virus isolates. J Gen Virol 64:1031, 1983.

Straus SE et al: Endonuclease analysis of viral DNA from varicella and subsequent zoster infections in the same patient. N Engl J Med 311:1362, 1984.

Triebwasser JH et al: Varicella pneumonia in adults. Medicine 46:409, 1967.

Weinstein L and Meade RH: Respiratory manifestations of chickenpox. Arch Intern Med 98:91, 1956.

Weller TH: Varicella and herpes zoster. N Engl J Med 309:1362, 1983.

Whitley RJ et al: Adenine arabinoside therapy of herpes zoster in the immunosuppressed. N Engl J Med 294:1193, 1976.

58

ROSA LEE NEMIR, M.D., and
VICTOR CHERNICK, M.D.

MEASLES AND GIANT CELL PNEUMONIA

Measles is the most common contagious exanthematous disease of childhood. It has been known since ancient times and continues to cause serious problems in many parts of the world. With the use of measles vaccine, a dramatic decline in both morbidity and mortality has been achieved in countries such as the United States and Great Britain. However, there has been a recent increase in the number of measles cases in the United States, particularly in children older than 10 years of age (Markowitz et al, 1989).

Measles pneumonia, caused by the measles virus alone, may occur early in the disease. More commonly, pneumonia may occur later, after the rash fades, in association with secondary viral or bacterial invaders. Bronchitis, laryngotracheitis, and even bronchiolitis may be manifestations of a severe attack of measles. The acute inflammatory process throughout the bronchial tree may produce special symptoms of laryngeal obstruction, resulting in the clinical and alarming picture of croup. Tracheolaryngitis is a part of the measles infection; therefore, accurately speaking, clinical "croup" in measles represents tracheolaryngitis of increased severity. The ensuing discussion includes measles pneumonia, the leading cause of death from measles, and a related entity, giant cell pneumonia.

MEASLES PNEUMONIA

PATHOLOGY

All epithelial cells of the respiratory tract from the nasal mucosa to the bronchioles are inflamed (Fig. 58–1). Hyperplasia of the lymphoid tissue is seen. There is an interstitial pneumonia with peribronchial infiltration by mononuclear cells (Fig. 58–2). Two types of giant cells are found: large multinucleated syncytial cells containing inclusion bodies and Warthin-Finkeldey cells, found in the lymph nodes and the reticuloendothelial system, probably formed by the clumping and fusion of lymphoid cells, and rarely showing inclusion bodies. Epithelial multinucleated cells are seen in "giant cell" pneumonia; Warthin-Finkeldey cells are pathognomonic for measles. Warthin-Finkeldey cells were first described in the tonsils and appendix; they have subsequently been found in lymph nodes throughout the respiratory and gastrointestinal tracts and in the spleen, thymus, and bone marrow.

The alveoli may become filled with the syncytial giant cells, and these, together with desquamated, degenerative cells, may line the alveolar wall like a hyaline membrane (Fig. 58–3). In some instances, obstructions to bronchioles may occur, resulting in hyperaeration and bullae.

PATHOGENESIS

Measles is a respiratory disease, beginning with infection in the upper respiratory tract and the conjunctivae. The infectious droplets from the nasopharyngeal secretions of a patient with an acute infection lodge on the respiratory epithelium of the new host. The virus invades the blood stream, pro-

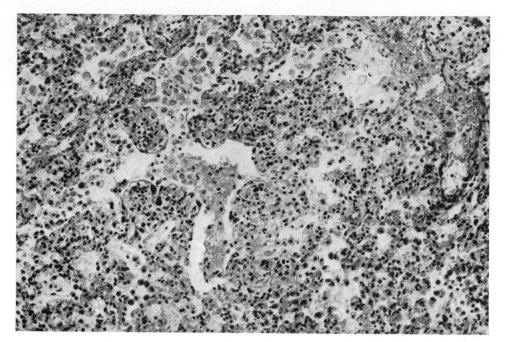

Figure 58–1. Measles pneumonia. Section of a lung showing extensive interstitial inflammation. Desquamated bronchial epithelium, giant cells, and mononuclear cells are present in the alveoli and ducts (hematoxylin and eosin, × 150). (Courtesy of Dr. Renata Dische.)

ducing a viremia. As the virus progresses to the reticuloendothelial system, generalized lymphadenopathy develops. This first viremia was demonstrated by Enders, Katz, and Medearis (1959), who inoculated monkeys with measles virus from tissue culture. They recovered the virus from the blood within 5 to 7 days after inoculation. Using blood from patients with measles to inoculate monkeys, Sergiev and associates (1960) recovered the virus as early as the third day. There is a short period of decrease in virus titer in the blood after inoculation, followed by a demonstrable viremia (the second viremia) starting 6 to 11 days before the appearance of the rash and persisting for a day or two after the appearance of the rash. The prodromal signs of measles—fever, coryza, and conjunctivitis—usually

occur 10 to 12 days after the initial infection and during this second viremia.

Measles virus may be cultured from the respiratory tract during the early prodromal period of respiratory infection. Tracheobronchitis is usually found at this time, and pneumonia occasionally occurs. Roentgenograms taken during the first days of the rash show increased hilar markings that correlate with the peribronchial infiltration present in the first few days of the posteruptive stage of measles.

During the eruptive stage of measles, the inflamed epithelial lining of the respiratory tract with its disturbed physiology is ripe for secondary bacterial infection and the consequent development of bacterial complications. Accumulated bronchial secretions, desquamated giant cells, and epithelial cells often fill

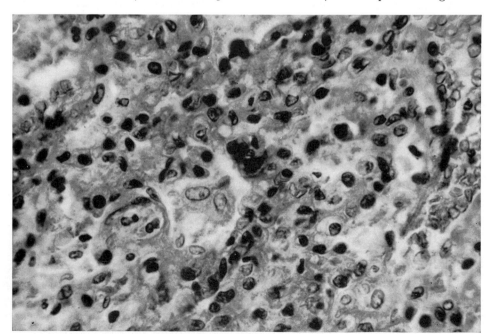

Figure 58–2. Measles pneumonia. Alveolar septa infiltrated by mononuclear cells (hematoxylin and eosin, × 500). (Courtesy of Dr. Renata Dische.)

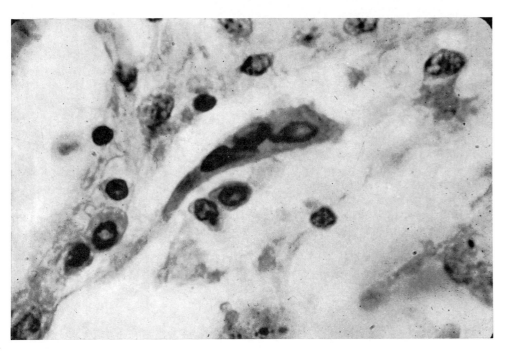

Figure 58–3. Measles pneumonia. Giant cell lining alveolus (hematoxylin and eosin, × 1500). (Courtesy of Dr. Renata Dische.)

the lumina of the bronchi and produce obstruction of the bronchial tree, thus promoting areas of atelectasis, areas of hyperaeration, and the growth of bacterial pathogens in pulmonary tissues, resulting in superimposed bacterial pneumonia.

INCIDENCE

The frequency of *pulmonary complications* varies from epidemic to epidemic and from country to country and currently is heavily influenced by the extensive use of measles virus vaccine, which was licensed for use in 1963.

The dramatic decline in measles in the United States from 400,000 cases in 1963 to about 3000 cases in 1981 is a testimonial to the efficacy of the measles virus vaccine and its implementation. Many other countries have been equally successful. In 1969, 85 to 95 per cent protection was achieved in two epidemics in Great Britain, and in Poland in 1968, the lowest mortality rate from measles in the past 20 years (0.3:100,000) was reported and attributed to the widespread use of measles vaccination.

Epidemics in developed countries are still occurring despite the availability of measles vaccine for immunization. In Canada, such an epidemic in Winnipeg in 1973 affected 688 children, 73 of whom had previously been immunized, some before 1 year of age. In the United States, several reports may be cited. One epidemic reported in Aberdeen, South Dakota, between October of 1970 and mid-January of 1971 resulted in 292 cases (patients 1 to 14 years of age). From one group in this area, pneumonia was diagnosed in more than a third of the patients, three of whom died. Another epidemic, reported from the Naval Hospital in Great Lakes, Illinois, in the winter of 1974, listed 32 naval recruits 17 to 27 years of

age, admitted for acute measles; 50 per cent had measles pneumonia. The third epidemic occurred in St. Louis during the winter and spring of 1970–1971; of the estimated 10,000 cases, 44 per cent were vaccine failures. A fourth measles outbreak in the winter of 1980 was of unusual interest because the source cases resulted from "importation" into the United States (Westchester County, New York) by persons arriving from Portugal and Venezuela. There were 116 reported patients, mostly 10 years of age and over, one half of whom had previously received measles vaccine. Only one person, an adult, developed pneumonia. By contrast, a fifth epidemic in southern Texas in 1981 largely affected infants under 15 months of age (42 of the 94 cases). Pneumonia was a frequent complication, occurring in 16 per cent, all of whom were less than 2 years of age. One patient with pneumonia died (Morbidity, 1981).

Recent outbreaks of measles in the United States (>6000 cases in 1986 and a major outbreak in 1989) have prompted a reevaluation of current immunization policy (Morbidity, 1989). The majority of cases occurred in children older than 10 years of age and in college students (Markowitz et al, 1989).

In many underdeveloped countries, measles is still a common and serious disease. Morley (1962) reported on a large group of Nigerian children ill with measles (1283 over a 3-year period) in which approximately half had bronchopneumonia, 28 per cent of whom died; Morley attributed the high fatality rate in part to the severe malnutrition in these children. Many observers in Africa have called attention to the frequency with which measles precipitates kwashiorkor. Bwibo (1970), during a 5-year period (1963–1968) in Uganda, also related the high mortality rate from measles (8.6 to 13.5 per cent) to severe malnutrition. Half of the 83 deaths in this series were complicated by bronchopneumonia. The severity of measles with high incidence of pneumonia among the Canadian North American Indian children has led to intensified efforts at immunization with measles vaccine (Houston et al, 1979).

Similarly, the epidemiologic change in the United States, with more frequent infections of high school and college youths, will redirect public health efforts toward eradication. In 1989, the American Academy of Pediatrics revised its measles immunization policy to recommend two doses of vaccine, the first at 15 months of age and the second on entrance to middle or junior high school (Committee on Infectious Diseases Report, 1989). It remains to be seen whether this policy will be effective in reducing the number of outbreaks seen recently in the United States.

FACTORS AFFECTING SUSCEPTIBILITY AND SEVERITY

A study of the effect of malnutrition on the antibody response to live attenuated measles vaccine was made in 20 malnourished children and 20 matched healthy controls (Chandra, 1975). Serum and IgA antibody levels were studied. In the malnourished group, the time of first appearance of secretory IgA antibody was delayed and the maximum level reached was lower. These findings suggest that impaired antibody response may contribute to the severity and fatality of measles infection. Further studies by Whittle and colleagues (1977) in South African children showed depression of cell-mediated immunity during measles; these researchers emphasize the special relevance of this observation in malnourished children. The adverse effect of dehydration and malnutrition on patients with measles has frequently been emphasized by reports of the disease in the tropics and often described in patients who died of measles.

Previously unexposed and isolated populations are highly susceptible to measles infection. Such infection is frequently severe, with an associated high mortality rate, chiefly due to pulmonary complications.

Christensen and associates (1952–1953), reporting on the measles epidemic in southern Greenland in 1951, noted that half of the pulmonary complications developed early in the course of disease, in direct connection with the rash, and during the prodromal period; the other half developed late in the disease. Fatalities from measles pneumonia largely occur late in the course of the disease and are due to secondary bacterial infection. Antibiotic therapy is effective against these complications. The decline in mortality rate before measles immunization resulted, in large measure, from control of these late bacterial infections. There were only 20 deaths from measles (all causes) in the United States in 1974, compared with 552 in 1959.

Patients with immunologic deficits, whether genetic or related to disease, may have severe and often fatal measles. One illustration of severe measles is a report of a boy with dysgammaglobulinemia who developed disseminated measles following attenuated measles vaccine and died of giant cell pneumonia 7 weeks later (Mawhinney et al, 1971). Patients with leukemia and lymphoma have increased susceptibility to infection by the measles virus because of lowered resistance, which is a function of their disease and of their therapy, whether they are receiving antimetabolites, chemotherapy, or irradiation. Many deaths from measles pneumonia in leukemic patients have been reported (Gray et al, 1987; Kernahan et al, 1987). In addition, measles pneumonia is now looming as an important and severe complication in children with human immunodeficiency virus (HIV) infection (Lauzon et al, 1985) (see also Chapter 74).

RESPIRATORY SYMPTOMS AND SIGNS

Inflammation of the conjunctivae and mucous membranes of the nasopharynx may occur even at the time of the initial invasion by the virus, with mild transient respiratory symptoms and the horizontal red lines in the conjunctivae described by Papp (1956). In general, however, the first signs of measles infection occur later, during the prodromal period, after an average incubation period of 10 to 12 days. These signs include profuse mucoserous nasal discharge, sneezing, excessive tearing and photophobia, a mild irritating cough, Koplik spots, and some fever. As the rash develops, the fever mounts and the inflammation in the tracheobronchial tree progresses. Cough increases and often develops a "barking" quality. Transient crackles and rhonchi may be heard in the lungs.

Most patients recover within a few days, although a mild cough may linger for a while. In some patients, a recrudescence of the disease or an increasing severity of the initial symptoms is noted, with increase in the fever. These patients must be carefully examined for evidence of complications, such as encephalitis, otitis media, lymphadenitis, sinusitis, and pulmonary disease—either bronchitis, tracheobronchitis, bronchiolitis, or pneumonia. Excessive mucoid and mucopurulent secretions may be found in the posterior pharyngeal spaces. A hoarse voice or barking cough may call attention to increased infection in the larynx. Physical findings suggesting obstruction of bronchi, either partial or complete, may be obtained. Hyperresonance and decreased breath sounds suggest areas of hyperaeration and large bullae. These areas may clear quickly if they are due to endobronchial obstruction by mucoid secretions and desquamated epithelial material, but they remain longer if they are also associated with bronchopneumonia and peribronchial inflammation. Similarly, complete obstruction with segmental collapse may clear readily or remain longer, depending on the underlying disease.

Bacterial pneumonia during the course of measles may be detected not only by means of laboratory aids but also by clinical observations of the patients. An increase in respiratory distress and areas of consolidation, for example, found on examination of the lungs, suggest the presence of bacterial pneumonia in measles.

DIAGNOSIS

When pneumonia occurs during the typical clinical picture of measles, there is usually no difficulty in making the diagnosis. In most instances, when the diagnosis of measles is not clear, laboratory and immunologic aids, including tests for immunodeficiency, may be helpful.

Measles

Antibody formation in measles can be measured by the hemagglutination inhibition test, by measurement of complement-fixing antibodies, which appear within 2 to 3 days, and by measurement of neutralizing antibodies, which appear as the rash begins to subside, often as early as the fourth day after the rash has appeared.

The measles epidemic in Greenland in 1951, a virgin area for measles infection, furnished a unique opportunity for the study of antibody titers. Bech (1962) showed that one third of 71 patients had complement-fixing antibodies on the first day after the onset of exanthem. Within a short time, the titers reached high levels; on the second day after the rash appeared, the majority had titers of 1:32 to 1:512.

The usual antibody response, however, may be suppressed in patients who are debilitated or have long-standing disease, notably leukemia. Determination of antibody titer may differentiate immune persons from nonimmune. Bech found a more rapid rise in antibody level in immune persons after exposure to measles. A neonate receives transplacental antibodies from an immune mother; these antibodies usually persist for the first 5 months of life (Krugman et al, 1965).

Fluorescent antibody technique may enable us to make an early presumptive diagnosis. It may be helpful when the disease is atypical, in experimental work, when a retrospective or necropsy diagnosis of the origin is to be made, or in the clarification of the agent of giant cell pneumonia.

In the prodromal period of measles, typical multinucleated giant cells, sometimes containing inclusion bodies, may be demonstrated in smears from nasal secretions and from nasal, conjunctival, and buccal tissue, including areas over Koplik spots (Tompkins and Macaulay, 1955). The appearance of these giant epithelial cells before the exanthem may be of diagnostic assistance. They rapidly decrease, disappearing on the fifth to seventh day, although they may be found in the urine some days later. The specificity of these cells in nasal secretions has been established for humans (Mottet and Szanton, 1961);

similar cells have been found in dogs with distemper. The practicality and usefulness of this test were demonstrated in Africa, where the dark-pigmented skin of patients made recognition of exanthem and diagnosis more difficult and where early diagnosis to prevent spread of infection was also important (Lightwood and Nolan, 1970).

Measles Pneumonia

Measles pneumonia of viral origin alone occurs early in the course of the disease. Later, bacterial infection may produce symptoms of pulmonary disease. Certain tests are diagnostically helpful, such as white blood cell counts, bacterial cultures, erythrocyte sedimentation test, and roentgenograms. For example, the white blood cell count shifts from the usual leukopenia with slight lymphocytosis to a leukocytosis with an increase in polymorphonuclear cells as secondary bacterial infections occur. The most common bacterial invaders of the respiratory tract are staphylococci, hemolytic streptococci, pneumococci, and Hemophilus influenzae. These were reported as etiologic agents by Weinstein and Franklin (1949) in their study of 163 children with measles, 25 per cent of whom had pneumonia. Recent reports include respiratory viruses, especially the adenovirus and herpesvirus (Kaschula et al, 1983).

A roentgenogram of the chest is essential in the diagnosis of pulmonary complications in measles (Fig. 58–4). Because the tracheobronchial tree (Figs. 58–5 and 58–6) and bronchopulmonary lymph nodes are always infected in measles, it is logical to assume that the chest roentgenogram will show some evidence of this involvement.

Our experience on the Pediatric Service at Bellevue Hospital is that the majority of chest roentgenograms show a picture commonly seen in viral pneumonia (Fig. 58–7). There are increased bronchovascular markings radiating out from the hilar areas, especially into the lower lobes, and enlargement of the bronchopulmonary nodes in the hilar areas. These radiographic findings may persist several weeks after the patient has recovered clinically from measles. Rarely, pronounced enlargement in the superior mediastinum, similar to that in childhood tuberculosis, is seen.

When bronchopneumonia becomes established, the areas of increased density may coalesce. Patchy areas of unequal aerations with blebs and atelectasis may appear and disappear; emphysematous blebs may also be a complication. These findings, which are not specific for measles, are also found in other viral bronchopneumonias. Segmental collapse occasionally occurs, but it usually clears as the infection subsides.

The radiologic lung changes of 897 patients from Manchester, England, seen from January of 1948 to June of 1955 were categorized by Fawcitt and Parry (1957). In addition to the aforementioned findings,

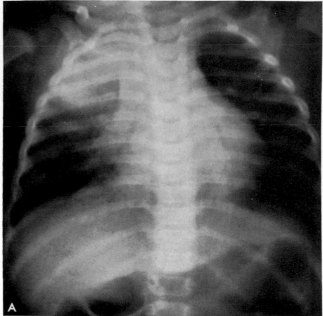
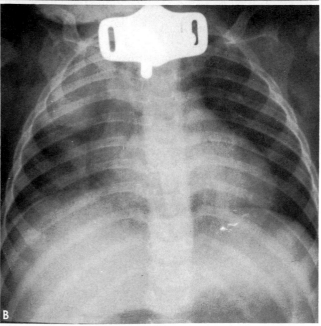

Figure 58–4. *A,* A chest radiograph taken on admission 3 days after an onset of measles rash, showing homogeneous density in the right upper lobe and some prominence of the right root. *B,* A chest radiograph taken 3 days after admission and 2 days after tracheostomy. Respiratory distress was relieved, although the right upper lobe pulmonary shadow remains.

they reported hilar gland enlargement in 63 per cent.

At present, with antibiotics readily available, the majority of pulmonary lesions are due to measles virus alone. Roentgenographic evidence of superimposed bacterial pulmonary infection will vary, depending on the type of invading organism.

A persisting pulmonary shadow in the roentgenogram that does not coincide with the criteria for a bacterial pneumonia (negative bacterial cultures and so on) may be due to a collapsed segment or lobe of

the lung, secondary either to the measles infection or to tuberculous bronchopulmonary nodes; or it may represent a tuberculous pulmonary infiltrate. Tuberculosis cannot be ruled out on the basis of a negative tuberculin skin reaction alone. The skin reaction to tuberculin is greatly decreased during the period of active measles infection; therefore, a tuberculin test should be repeated 3 to 6 weeks later.

GIANT CELL PNEUMONIA

Giant cell interstitial pneumonia was first described by Hecht, who in 1910 reported autopsy findings in 27 children. In 19 of these cases there was a history of measles. Clinically, the disease cannot be distinguished from other pneumonias. The diagnosis depends solely on the histologic examination of lung tissue.

The nature of the etiologic agent has remained obscure until recently. In many cases, the patient has had measles immediately preceding the pneumonia. In the absence of clinical evidence of measles, the disease has been referred to as Hecht's pneumonia.

The most valuable contribution in elucidating the cause of this disease was made by McCarthy and associates (McCarthy et al, 1958; Mitus et al, 1962). A virus indistinguishable from the measles virus was isolated at autopsy from each of three cases of giant cell pneumonia. There had been no clinical manifestations of measles in these patients. All had other serious illnesses, such as cystic fibrosis, leukemia, and Letterer-Siwe disease. This report suggests that in cases of giant cell pneumonia occurring in the course of other serious disease, but with no clinical measles, the host response to the measles infection is altered. The reason for this atypical host response is not clear, although it has been reported in patients already affected with chronic debilitating disease and with impaired immune response.

Laboratory diagnostic methods now available for the detection of measles virus may permit the clinical recognition of giant cell pneumonia. It is especially important to make this diagnosis in order to choose therapy and prevent measles in contacts, because the virus may persist and be a source of contagion for considerable periods after the initial infection. The survival of two patients who received large doses of gamma globulin at the time of exposure suggests that this material may be of value in the modification of subsequent measles pneumonitis. Furthermore, it is possible that large quantities of antibody administered intravenously in the form of measles-convalescent plasma may mitigate this condition. In children with acute leukemia, measles infection may present as a mild disease with a typical course or as a fatal giant cell pneumonia; therefore, it is important to offer these children protection. Administration of attenuated live measles vaccine of Enders to children with acute leukemia is contraindicated. The use of large doses of gamma globulin for passive immuni-

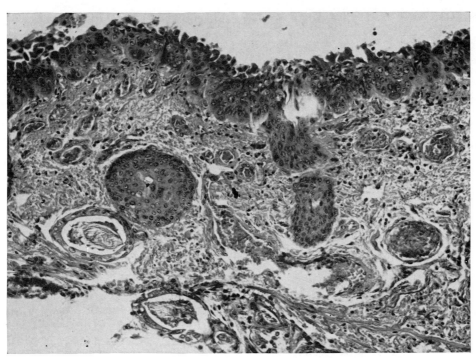

Figure 58–5. Measles tracheitis (× 150).

zation is preferable. Patients with leukemia in remission for at least 3 months can be given live virus vaccine (Morbidity, 1989).

Giant cell pneumonia is now known to affect children with underlying disease of the reticuloendothelial or hematopoietic system, children treated with antimetabolites, those with altered immune states, and children with acquired immune deficiency syndrome (AIDS) or AIDS-related complex (Clinicopathologic Exercises, 1988).

Giant cell pneumonia has been reported to be associated with paramyxovirus infections. Respiratory syncytial virus, influenza type 3 virus, and others have been found in immunocompromised children dying of giant cell pneumonia.

COMPLICATIONS

Obstructive lesions in the diseased lower respiratory tract may lead to *mediastinal emphysema*, although this is not a common complication. Three of the 897

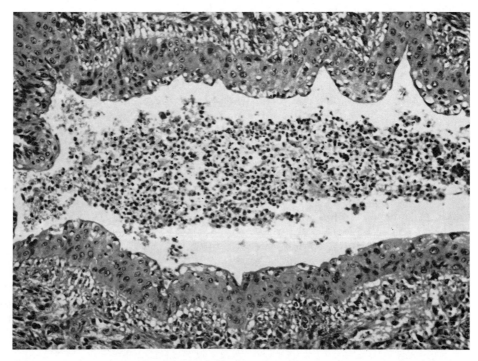

Figure 58–6. Extensive bronchitis and squamous cell metaplasia seen in autopsy material of a patient who died of measles pneumonia (× 150).

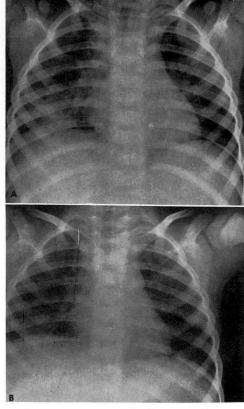

Figure 58–7. *A,* Four days after admission, pulmonary infiltration is seen in the right base above the diaphragm. There are also mottled soft lesions of irregular size in the right lung near the hilus and in the left upper lobe. *B,* There is complete clearing of the lungs 6 days later.

patients studied by Fawcitt and Parry (1957) had emphysema, and other references are occasionally found in the literature.

The mechanism for the development of mediastinal emphysema has been described by Macklin and Macklin (1944). Rupture of diseased alveoli with blebs and the coalescence of adjacent blebs into large bullae form the framework for pulmonary interstitial emphysema. The trapped air follows the path of least resistance and proceeds along the sheaths of blood vessels and adjacent bronchi, either toward the mediastinum and along the structures upward to the mediastinum and around the heart, the usual route, or peripherally to the pleura, producing a pneumothorax.

Atelectasis in single or multiple lobes of the lungs occurs in patients of all ages with measles, although less frequently than in patients with pertussis. Fawcitt and Parry (1957) obtained roentgenographic evidence of atelectasis in 28.4 per cent of the patients in their series, practically all of whom were more than 1 year of age. If atelectasis persists for a time and secondary bacterial infection occurs, bronchiectasis may be the ultimate outcome (see Chapter 25). A patient with long-standing atelectasis should be considered a potential candidate for bronchiectasis. If clinical signs and impairment of health corroborate

the suspicion of lung damage, bronchograms should be obtained.

With the possible exception of staphylococcal infections, *empyema* is a rare complication now that broad-spectrum antibiotic therapy is available. In contrast, in the 1937 pathologic study by Degen of 100 cases of measles, empyema was described in 13 per cent and pleurisy in 27 per cent. In this same study, four patients were described as having exudative pericarditis.

The deleterious effect of measles on active tuberculosis has been common knowledge. On the Children's Tuberculosis Ward at Bellevue Hospital before 1960, there were many instances of tuberculous meningitis, bronchogenic spread of tuberculosis, and miliary tuberculosis following measles. The importance of isoniazid (INH) therapy to "cover" this period of greater susceptibility needs to be emphasized. It is suggested that INH be given to children who have measles and are known to be positive tuberculin reactors and are not receiving therapy (see Chapter 48). At present, however, the spread of tuberculous disease associated with measles that was seen two or more decades ago, before the widespread use of INH, is very rare.

A second effect of measles and the administration of measles vaccine on tuberculosis is the suppression of tuberculin sensitivity as measured by the tuberculin reaction (Helms and Helms, 1958; Starr and Berkovich, 1964; Brody et al, 1964). Clinically, we are quite familiar with this phenomenon. Considerable variation in time occurs in the return of tuberculin sensitivity, ranging from 10 days to 5 weeks, with an average of 18 days after the onset of the rash.

TREATMENT

Symptomatic care of patients with measles should be carefully supervised; whenever complications arise, close observation and appropriate specific therapy must be provided. Bendz and Engström (1953), for example, reported the risk of asphyxiation in measles encephalitis. Cough may require medication, but we are cautious in the use of codeine mixtures. Humidified atmosphere is helpful for tracheitis. Patients with signs of obstructive laryngotracheitis should be observed closely, preferably in a hospital, where tracheostomy may be done if the symptoms of increased respiratory distress and restlessness suggest impending serious obstruction.

There is no specific treatment for measles interstitial pneumonia. Humidity and oxygen therapy are used as indicated for anoxia. Routine antibiotic therapy as a preventive measure is not desirable; in fact, its use may result in possible harm from superimposed infection. Bacterial cultures in severely ill patients should be taken early in the course of disease so that the results may be used as a guide to therapy in the event of complications.

The treatment of bacterial pneumonia is described in Chapter 19. Careful and repeated cultures of the nasopharynx and blood help to determine the choice of therapeutic agents.

PREVENTION

Nonimmune persons known to have been exposed within a period of 4 days should be protected with gamma globulin.

Extensive use of measles virus vaccine in a worldwide program has shown that measles immunization is safe, effective, and long lasting. Krugman (1977), in a 10-year follow-up of children immunized with live measles vaccine, observed clinical protection against measles and a rise in protective antibody titer when these children were exposed in epidemics even 8½ years later. Many studies in this country and elsewhere have reflected the high level of immunity (95 to 98 per cent) obtained from live measles vaccination. It is hoped that a concerted, well-designed worldwide immunization program will continue to be attempted in an effort to eradicate this disease. It is now clear that a single-dose immunization for measles will not eradicate the disease. In recent measles outbreaks in the United States, two thirds of patients had been previously immunized. It remains to be seen how effective a two-dose vaccination program will be in eradicating this disease. Moreover, it is likely that certain susceptible populations will have to receive the vaccine earlier than 15 months of age and then be revaccinated if we are to totally eliminate measles in infants.

ATYPICAL MEASLES PNEUMONIA (IN CHILDREN PREVIOUSLY IMMUNIZED WITH KILLED MEASLES VIRUS VACCINE)

The dramatic results achieved in the control of measles can be attributed to the use of measles vaccine. Two vaccines were licensed for use in the United States in 1963: live attenuated measles virus vaccine (Edmonston B type) and formalin-inactivated alum-precipitated vaccine, which is now no longer used. This latter killed measles vaccine (KMV) originally was given to patients in whom live virus was postulated to have a possible harmful effect, e.g., children receiving immunodepressant drugs, such as corticosteroids or antimetabolites, and children who were acutely ill or infected with disease that would be affected adversely by live measles virus, such as tuberculosis.

Withdrawal of KMV followed a report by Rauh and Schmidt in 1965. They described the findings in 125 children immunized 2½ years previously with KMV when they were intimately exposed in an epidemic of clinical measles. Fifty-four of these children developed some form of measles, predominantly a modified form. Most surprising was the *atypical measles* seen in eight (6.4 per cent) of those infected. The atypical features were an unusual (in appearance, location, and progression) rash, severe pneumonia, and the absence of catarrhal symptoms and conjunctivitis that are commonly noted in patients with measles. The rash progressed from the extremities toward the body (caudocephalad) rather than following the usual sequence of face to body and extremities (cephalocaudad). Such a rash may be confused with that of Rocky Mountain spotted fever (Nieburg et al, 1980).

Similar reports of small numbers of these atypical measles cases continued to appear in the United States, Canada, and Sweden. In the cases reported from the three countries, more than half the patients had pneumonia, a much higher incidence than in natural measles infection. Three patients who failed to develop a rash had atypical measles pneumonia as confirmed by increase in antibody titer to measles.

These atypical reactions to measles infection have been attributed to delayed hypersensitivity and to Arthus reaction. Administration of KMV results in delayed hypersensitivity to measles virus antigen and to specific serum antibodies. With the passage of time, vaccinated persons may lose more of their protective antibody than of their virus hypersensitivity. When they are subsequently exposed to wild measles virus, an exaggerated Arthus type reaction occurs in the pulmonary mucous membranes; this explains the severe and frequent atypical pneumonia. Bellanti and colleagues (1969), in a comparative study of children receiving attenuated and inactivated measles vaccines, reported a difference in antibody responses. Recipients of inactivated measles virus showed a reduced amount of nasal secretory gamma A antibody but adequate production of serum antibodies. The differences in the antibody response of the respiratory tract may account for the altered or atypical response of a child receiving inactivated vaccine to measles virus infection. An Arthus-like phenomenon is observed locally in skin reactions of persons vaccinated with KMV upon retesting with live measles virus.

A histopathologic and serologic study of 17 adolescents with atypical measles syndrome (and pneumonia) 14 years after vaccination with KMV indicated an inadequate production of antibody to hemolysin (protein F) (Annunziato et al, 1982). This antibody acts to prevent cell-to-cell spread of paramyxovirus. Absence of antibody to protein F resulted because killed measles vaccine lacked the protein F antigen (Norrby et al, 1975). This phenomenon is probably the major reason that recipients of KMV may develop atypical measles.

CLINICAL FEATURES

The onset is abrupt after exposure to measles virus, usually during epidemics. High fever, cough, headache, myalgia, and abdominal pain usually precede the rash by 2 or 3 days. Unlike in typical measles, the rash appears first on the palms and soles and in the creases of the body and spreads to the trunk, often sparing the face. As mentioned, the progression of the rash is caudocephalad instead of cephalocaudad. The exanthem is maculopapular with petechial and purpuric lesions, sometimes also vesicular without progression to crusting; it is occasionally urticarial. Edema of the extremities is often observed. Pulmonary symptoms and signs soon develop and suggest pneumonia, which can be confirmed by roentgenographic findings. Although the pneumonia is usually severe, all patients recover, and the pleural effusion that may occur clears within a short time. The acute illness usually subsides within 4 to 7 days.

LABORATORY FINDINGS

White blood cell counts are low, ranging from 2700 to 10,000 cells/mm³. The differential count varies, sometimes showing a mild eosinophilia of 4 to 13 per cent and returning to normal in 4 to 6 days. The platelet count is normal, but occasional elevation of the erythrocyte sedimentation rate is found. The nasopharyngeal cultures show normal flora. Pleural fluid from one patient (Young et al, 1970) was straw colored and sterile and contained some eosinophils.

ROENTGENOGRAPHIC FINDINGS

Evidence of pneumonia is chiefly that of a lobular infiltration, but more diffuse and segmental lesions are occasionally seen. Hilar adenopathy is a common finding, as is pleural effusion (Fulginiti et al, 1967; Young et al, 1970; Annunziato et al, 1982). In general, these pulmonary lesions clear completely, but Young and associates (1970) found that some of their patients had residual nodular lesions measuring 1.5 to 4 cm that remained for many months—one for 30 months. A number of subsequent reports have described residual pulmonary nodules lasting for many months following atypical measles illness, one for 14 months (Laptook et al, 1978; Margolin and Gandy, 1979; Sherkow, 1980). These nodular radiologic sequelae gradually disappear. The finding of calcification in one of three such patients, described by Mitnick and colleagues (1980), posed a critical diagnostic problem, that of ruling out the possibility of tuberculosis.

TREATMENT

No specific treatment is required once the diagnosis is clarified. Antibiotics and antipyretics given early in the disease do not alter its course.

PREVENTION

Because KMV is no longer available, this type of atypical measles pneumonia should gradually disappear.

It is important, however, to appreciate that atypical measles syndrome may occur many years after vaccination. Recurrence 14 years later in 17 adolescents was reported by Annunziato and co-workers (1982). Thus, Fulginiti and colleagues (1980), who reported two adolescents with atypical measles syndrome 16 years after vaccination with KMV, suggest counseling such vaccinees on their potential susceptibility.

REFERENCES

Adams JM and Imagawa DT: The relationship of canine distemper to human respiratory disease. Pediatr Clin North Am 4:193, 1957.

Akhtar M and Young I: Measles giant cell pneumonia in an adult following long-term chemotherapy. Arch Pathol 96:145, 1973.

Annunziato D, Kaplan MH, Hall WW et al: Atypical measles syndrome: pathologic and serologic findings. Pediatrics 70:203, 1982.

Archibold WR, Weller RO, and Meadow SR: Measles pneumonia and the nature of the inclusion-bearing giant cells: a light and electron microscope study. J Pathol 103:27, 1971.

Baratta RO, Ginter MC, Price MA et al: Measles (rubeola) in previously immunized children. Pediatrics 46:397, 1970.

Barkin RM: Measles mortality; analysis of the primary cause of death. Am J Dis Child 129:307, 1975.

Barsky P: Measles: Winnipeg, 1973. Can Med Assoc J 110:931, 1974.

Beale AJ: A rapid cytological method for the diagnosis of measles. J Clin Pathol 12:335, 1959.

Bech V: Studies on the development of complement fixing antibodies in measles patients. J Immunol 83:267, 1959.

Bech V: Measles epidemics in Greenland. Am J Dis Child 103:252, 1962.

Bellanti JA, Sanga RL, Kluntinis B et al: Antibody responses in serum and nasal secretions of children immunized with inactivated and attenuated measles-virus vaccines. N Engl J Med 280:628, 1969.

Bendz P and Engström CG: Risk of death from asphyxiation in measles encephalitis. Am J Dis Child 86:772, 1953.

Black FL, Woodall J, and Pinheiro De P: Measles vaccine reactions in a virgin population. Am J Epidemiol 89:168, 1969.

Blake FG and Trask JD Jr: Studies on measles. II. Symptomatology and pathology in monkeys experimentally infected. J Exp Med 33:413, 1921.

Bolande RP: Inclusion-bearing cells in the urine in certain viral infections. Pediatrics 24:7, 1959.

Breitfeld V, Hashida Y, Sherman FE et al: Fatal measles infection in children with leukemia. Lab Invest 28:279, 1973.

Brodsky AL: Atypical measles. Severe illness in recipients of killed measles virus vaccine upon exposure to natural infection. JAMA 222:1415, 1972.

Brody JA and McAlister R: Depression of tuberculin sensitivity following measles vaccination. Am Rev Respir Dis 90:607, 1964.

Brody JA, Overfield T, and Hammes LM: Depression of the tuberculin reaction by viral vaccines. N Engl J Med 271:1294, 1964.

Buser F: Side reaction to measles vaccination suggesting the Arthus phenomenon. N Engl J Med 277:250, 1967.

Bwibo NO: Measles in Uganda. An analysis of children with measles admitted to Mulago Hospital. Trop Geogr Med 22:167, 1970.

Carlstrom G: Neutralization of canine distemper virus by serum of patients convalescent from measles. Lancet 273:344, 1957.

Chandra RK: Reduced secretory antibody response to live attenuated measles and poliovirus vaccines in malnourished children. Br Med J 2:583, 1975.

Christensen PE et al: An epidemic of measles in Southern Greenland, 1951. Acta Med Scand 144:430, 1952–1953.

Clinicopathologic Exercises, Case 34–1988. N Engl J Med 319:495, 1988.

Committee on Infectious Diseases Report: Measles: reassessment of the current immunization policy. Am Acad Pediatr News, July, 1989.

Cooch JW: Measles in U.S. Army recruits. Am J Dis Child 103:264, 1962.

Coovadia HM, Wesley A, Brian P et al: Immunoparesis and outcome on measles. Lancet 1:619, 1977.

Corkett EU: The visceral lesions in measles. Am J Pathol 21:905, 1945.

Crawford K, Joseph JM, Mellin H et al: From the National Communicable Disease Center. Current status of measles in the United States. J Infect Dis 121:234, 1970.

DeBuse PJ, Lewis MG, and Mugerwa JW: Pulmonary complications of measles in Uganda. J Trop Pediatr 16:197, 1970.

DeCarlo J Jr and Startzman HH Jr: The roentgen study of the chest in measles. Radiology 63:849, 1954.

Degen JA: Visceral pathology in measles: a clinicopathologic study of 100 fatal cases. Am J Med Sci 194:104, 1937.

Dover AS, Escobar JA, Dueñas AL, and Leal EC: Pneumonia associated with measles. JAMA 234:612, 1975.

Dudgeon JA: Measles vaccines. Br Med Bull 25:153, 1969.

Enders JF: Development of attenuated measles-virus vaccines. Am J Dis Child 103:335, 1962.

Enders JF, Katz SL, and Medearis DN: Recent advances in knowledge of the measles virus. In Perspective in Virology. Vol I. New York, John Wiley & Sons, Inc, 1959.

Enders JF, McCarthy K, Mitus A, and Cheatham WJ: Isolation of measles virus at autopsy in cases of giant-cell pneumonia without rash. N Engl J Med 261:875, 1959.

Escobar JA, Dover AS, Dueñas A et al: Etiology of respiratory tract infections in children in Cali, Colombia. Pediatrics 57:123, 1976.

Fawcitt J and Parry HE: Lung changes in pertussis and measles in childhood. A review of 1894 cases with a follow-up study of the pulmonary complications. Br J Radiol 30:76, 1957.

Finkeldey W: Über Riesenzellbefunde in den Gaumenmandeln, zugleich ein Beitrag zur Histopathologie der Mandelveranderungen im Maserninkubationsstadium. Virchows Arch [A] 281:323, 1931.

Fulginiti VA and Arthur JH: Altered reactivity to measles virus: skin test reactivity and antibody response to measles virus antigens in recipients of killed measles virus vaccine. J Pediatr 75:609, 1969.

Fulginiti VA and Helfer RE: Atypical measles in adolescent siblings 16 years after killed measles virus vaccine. JAMA 244:804, 1980.

Fulginiti VA, Eller JJ, Downie AW, and Kempe CH: Altered reactivity to measles virus. Atypical measles in children previously immunized with inactivated measles virus vaccines. JAMA 202:1075, 1967.

Garcia AGP: Fetal infection in chickenpox and alastrium with histopathological study of the placenta. Pediatrics 32:895, 1963.

Gordon JE, Jansen AAJ, and Ascoli W: Measles in rural Guatemala. J Pediatr 66:779, 1965.

Gray MM, Glass S, Eden OB et al: Mortality and morbidity caused by measles in children with malignant disease attending four major treatment centres: a retrospective review. Br Med J 295:19, 1987.

Hecht V: Die Riesenzellenpneumonia im Kindesalter, eine historische-experimentelle Studie. Beitr Pathol Anat Allg Pathol 48:263, 1910.

Helms S and Helms P: Tuberculin sensitivity during measles. Acta Tuberc Scand 35:166, 1958.

Hers JF: Fluorescent antibody techniques in respiratory viral diseases. Am Rev Respir Dis 88:316, 1963.

Hong Kong Measles Vaccine Committee: Two-year follow-up study of measles vaccine antibodies. Med J Aust 1:532, 1970.

Houston CS, Weiler RL, and Habbick BF: Severity of lung disease in Indian Children. Can Med Assoc J 120:116, 1979.

Houston CS, Weiler RL, and MacKay RW: Native children's lung. J Can Assoc Radiol 30:218, 1979.

Janigan DT: Giant cell pneumonia and measles: an analytical review. Can Med Assoc J 85:741, 1961.

Jones OR: Measles: a case of emphysema correspondence. Am Rev Respir Dis 87:597, 1963.

Josan R, Suciu O, Iepureau A, and Marina M: On the gravity of the complications of measles after the epidemic that occurred in the winter of 1968–1969 in patients hospitalized in the infectious disease clinic of Cluj. Pediatria (Bucur) 19:41, 1970.

Karelitz S, Berliner UC, Orange M et al: Inactivated measles virus vaccine. Subsequent challenge with attenuated live virus vaccine. JAMA 184:684, 1963.

Karzon DT, Rush D, and Winkelstein W Jr: Immunization with inactivated measles virus vaccine: effect of booster dose and response to natural challenge. Pediatrics 36:40, 1965.

Kaschula RO, Druker J, and Kipps A: Late morphologic consequences of measles: a lethal and debilitating lung disease among the poor. Rev Infect Dis 5:395, 1983.

Kemahan J, McQuillin J, and Craft AW: Measles in children who have malignant disease. Br Med J 295:15, 1987.

Koffler D: Giant cell pneumonia. Arch Pathol 78:267, 1964.

Kohn JL and Koiransky H: Roentgenographic reexamination of the chests of children from six to ten months after measles. Am J Dis Child 41:500, 1931.

Kohn JL and Koiransky H: Relation of measles and tuberculosis in young children. A clinical and roentgenographic study. Am J Dis Child 44:1187, 1932.

Krugman S: Present status of measles and rubella immunization in the United States: a medical progress report. J Pediatr 90:1, 1977.

Krugman S, Giles JP, Friedman H, and Stone S: Studies on immunity to measles. J Pediatr 66:471, 1965.

Laptook AWE, Nussbaum M, and Shenker IR: Pulmonary lesions in atypical measles. Pediatrics 62:42, 1978.

Lauzon D, Delage G, Brochu P et al: Pathogens in children with severe combined immunodeficiency disease or AIDS. Can Med Assoc J 135:33, 1985.

Lennon RG, Isacson P, and Rosales T: Skin tests with measles and poliomyelitis vaccines in recipients of inactivated measles virus vaccine. Delayed dermal hypersensitivity. JAMA 200:275, 1967.

Levine AS, Graw RG Jr, and Young RC: Management of infections in patients with leukemia and lymphoma: current concepts and experimental approaches. Semin Hematol 9:141, 1972.

Levitt LP, Case GE, Neill JS et al: Determination of measles immunity after a mass immunization campaign. Public Health Rep 85:261, 1970.

Lightwood R and Nolan R: Epithelial giant cells in measles as an aid in diagnosis. J Pediatr 77:59, 1970.

McCarthy K: Measles. Br Med Bull 15:201, 1959.

McCarthy K, Mitus A, Cheatham W, and Peebles TC: Isolation of virus of measles from three fatal cases of giant cell pneumonia. Am J Dis Child 96:500, 1958.

McConnell EM: Giant-cell pneumonia in an adult. Br Med J 2:289, 1961.

McCormick JB, Halsey N, and Rosenberg R: Measles vaccine efficacy determined from secondary attack rates during a severe epidemic. J Pediatr 90:13, 1977.

Macklin MT and Macklin CC: Malignant interstitial emphysema of the lungs and mediastinum as an important occult complication in many respiratory diseases and other conditions: an interpretation of the clinical literature in the light of laboratory experience. Medicine 23:281, 1944.

McLean DM, Best JM, Smith PA et al: Viral infections of Toronto children during 1965. II. Measles encephalitis and other complications. Can Med Assoc J 94:905, 1966.

McLean DM, Kettyls GDM, Kingston J et al: Atypical measles following immunization with killed measles vaccine. Can Med Assoc J 103:743, 1970.

Margolin F and Gandy TK: Pneumonia of atypical measles. Pediatr Radiol 131:653, 1979.

Markowitz LE, Preblud SR, Orenstein WA et al: Patterns of transmission in measles outbreaks in the United States 1986–1987. N Engl J Med 320:75, 1989.

Mawhinney H, Allen IV, Beare JM et al: Dysgammaglobulinemia complicated by disseminated measles. Br Med J 2:380, 1971.

Meadow SR, Weller RO, and Archibald RWR: Fatal systemic

measles in a child receiving cyclophosphamide for nephrotic syndrome. Lancet 2:876, 1969.

Miller DL: Frequency of complications of measles, 1963. Br Med J 2:75, 1964.

Mitnick J, Becker MH, Rothberg M, and Genieser NB: Nodular residua of atypical measles pneumonia. Am J Roentgenol 134:257, 1980.

Mitus A, Enders JF, Craig JM, and Holloway A: Persistence of measles virus and depression of antibody formation in patients with giant-cell pneumonia after measles. N Engl J Med 261:882, 1959.

Mitus A, Holloway A, Evans AE, and Enders JF: Attenuated measles vaccine in children with acute leukemia. Am J Dis Child 103:413, 1962.

Morbidity and Mortality Weekly Reports: 24:2, 1976; 30:18, 1981; 30:288, 1981; 38:205, 1989; and 38:456, 1989.

Morley DC: Measles in Nigeria. Am J Dis Child 103:230, 1962.

Morley DC: Severe measles in tropics I. Br Med J 1:297, 1969.

Mottet NK and Szanton V: Exfoliated measles giant cells in nasal secretions. Arch Pathol 72:434, 1961.

Nader PR, Horwitz MS, and Rousseau J: Atypical exanthem following exposure to natural measles. Eleven cases in children previously inoculated with killed vaccine. J Pediatr 72:22, 1968.

Naruszewicz-Lesiuk D: Measles in Poland in the years 1962–1968 as viewed against the background of the epidemiologic situation throughout the world. Przegl Epidemiol 24:1, 1970. (Pol.)

Neel JV, Centerwall WR, Chagnon NA, and Casey HL: Notes on the effect of measles and measles vaccine in a virgin-soil population of South American Indians. Am J Epidemiol 91:418, 1970.

Nieburg PI, D'Angelo LJ, and Herrmann KL: Measles in patients suspected of having Rocky Mountain spotted fever. JAMA 244:808, 1980.

Norrby E: Hemagglutination by measles virus: a simple procedure for production of high potency antigen for hemagglutination-inhibition (HI) tests. Proc Soc Exp Biol Med 111:814, 1962.

Norrby E, Enders-Ruckle G, and ter Meulen V: Difference in the appearance of antibodies to structural components of measles virus after immunization with inactivated and live virus. J Infect Dis 132:262, 1975.

Norrby E, Lagercrantz R, and Gard S: Measles vaccination. IV. Responses to two different types of preparations given as a fourth dose of vaccine. Br Med J 1:813, 1965.

Norrby E, Lagercrantz R, and Gard S: Measles vaccination. V. The booster effect of purified hemagglutinin in children previously immunized with this product of formalin-killed vaccine. Acta Paediatr Scand 55:73, 1966.

Norrby E, Lagercrantz R, and Gard S: Measles vaccination. VI. Serological and clinical follow-up analysis 18 months after a booster injection. Acta Paediatr Scand 55:457, 1966.

Olson RW and Hodges GR: Measles pneumonia. Bacterial suprainfection as a complicating factor. JAMA 232:363, 1975.

Panum PL: Observations during the epidemic of measles on the Faroe Islands in the year 1846. (Translated by Mrs. AS Hatcher, United States Public Health Service.) Medical Classics 3:829, 1939.

Papp K: Expériences prouvant que la voie d'infection de la rougeole est la contamination de la muqueuse conjonctivale. Rev Immunol 20:27, 1956.

Pinkerton H, Smiley WL, and Anderson WAD: Giant-cell pneumonia with inclusions. Pediatrics 10:681, 1952.

Pneumonia in atypical measles (editorial). Br Med J 2:235, 1971.

Rauh LW and Schmidt R: Measles immunization with killed virus vaccine. Am J Dis Child 109:232, 1965.

Ristori C, Boccardo H, Borgono JM, and Armijo R: Medical importance of measles in Chile. Am J Dis Child 103:236, 1962.

Rossipal E, Falk W, and Zanger J: Atypical measles with giant cell pneumonia under treatment with chlorambucil (author's translation). Verh Dtsch Ges Pathol 56:388, 1972.

Schaffner W, Schluederberg AES, and Byrne EB: Clinical epidemiology of sporadic measles in a highly immunized population. N Engl J Med 279:783, 1968.

Scott FFMcN and Bononno DE: Reactions to live-measles-virus vaccine in children previously inoculated with killed-virus vaccine. N Engl J Med 227:248, 1967.

Sergiev PG, Ryazantseva NE, and Shroit IG: The dynamics of pathological processes in experimental measles in monkeys. Acta Virol 4:265, 1960.

Shah KJ, Lewis MJ, Cameron AH et al: Giant cell pneumonia complicating acute lymphocytic leukemia in remission. Ann Radiol 20:79, 1977.

Sherkow L: Pulmonary residuum 14 months after skin rash and pneumonia. JAMA 243:65, 1980.

Sherman FE and Ruckle G: In vivo and in vitro cellular changes specific for measles. Arch Pathol 65:587, 1959.

Siegel MM, Walter TC, and Ablin AR: Measles pneumonia in childhood leukemia. Pediatrics 60:38, 1977.

Siegal M, Fuerst HT, and Peress NS: Comparative fetal mortality in maternal virus diseases: a prospective study in rubella, measles, mumps, chickenpox and hepatitis. N Engl J Med 274:768, 1966.

Starr S and Berkovich S: Effects of measles, gamma-globulin-modified measles, and vaccine measles on tuberculin test. N Engl J Med 270:386, 1964.

Steele BT: Measles in Auckland, 1971–72. NZ J Med 77:293, 1973.

Stokes J Jr, Maris EP, and Gellis SS: Chemical, clinical, and immunological studies in the products of human plasma fractionation. XI. The use of concentrated normal human serum gamma globulin (human immune serum globulin) in the prophylaxis and treatment of measles. J Clin Invest 23:531, 1944.

Tompkins V and Macaulay JC: A characteristic cell in nasal secretions during prodromal measles. JAMA 157:711, 1955.

Warthin AS: Occurrence of numerous large giant cells in the tonsils and pharyngeal mucosa in the prodromal stage of measles. Report of four cases. Arch Pathol 11:864, 1931.

Weinstein L: Failure of chemotherapy to prevent the bacterial complications of measles. N Engl J Med 253:679, 1955.

Weinstein L and Franklin W: The pneumonia of measles. Am J Med Sci 217:314, 1949.

Weintraub PS, Sullender WM, Lombard C et al: Giant cell pneumonia caused by parainfluenza type 3 in a patient with acute myelomonocytic leukemia. Arch Pathol Lab Med 111:569, 1987.

Whittle HC, Dossetor A, Oduloju A et al: Cell-mediated immunity during natural measles infection. J Clin Invest 62:678, 1977.

Young LW and Ross DW: Radiological case of the month. Giant cell pneumonia. Am J Dis Child 134:511, 1980.

Young LW, Smith DI, and Glasgow LA: Pneumonia of atypical measles. Residual nodular lesions. Am J Roentgenol 110:439, 1970.

Zweiman B, Pappagianis D, Maibach H, and Hildreth EA: Effect of measles immunization on tuberculin hypersensitivity and in vitro lymphocyte reactivity. Int Arch Allergy 40:834, 1971.

59

BARBARA J. LAW, M.D.

PERTUSSIS

Pertussis in English means "violent cough." The Chinese word for pertussis or whooping cough translated into English means "100-day cough." Both translations provide a terse yet accurate description of the nature of the illness caused by *Bordetella pertussis*, which is a uniquely adapted respiratory pathogen.

EPIDEMIOLOGY

The change in incidence of pertussis over the last 5 decades bears witness to the critical role of immunization in the control of this troublesome disease (Cherry et al, 1988; Cherry, 1984; Geller, 1984). Before the vaccine was introduced, the reported annual incidence of pertussis in England and Wales was 230 per 100,000 population. By the 1970s, this rate had decreased to 0.5 to 20 per 100,000 per year, with the variation reflecting cyclic epidemic activity. During the same decade, however, growing public concern over the safety and effectiveness of pertussis vaccine led to a reduction in the proportion of infants immunized before the age of 2 years from 77 to 30 per cent. Subsequently, two major and long-lasting epidemics of pertussis occurred between 1977 and 1979 and 1982 and 1983, during which the annual attack rate exceeded 100 per 100,000 population. A similar pattern of increased incidence following discontinuation of pertussis immunization programs has been documented in both Japan and Sweden (Romanus et al, 1987). In the United States, 1500 to 5000 cases are reported yearly for an annual incidence of 0.5 to 1.5 per 100,000 population (CDC, 1987). In reviewing incidence data for pertussis, it must be remembered that reported cases account for only 18 to 20 per cent of the actual incidence (Cherry, 1984).

Pertussis is primarily a disease of young infants and children. More than 50 per cent of reported cases in the United States occur in children younger than 1 year of age and 80 per cent in children younger than 5 years of age. In England and Wales, the peak incidence occurs in children between the ages of 2 and 4 years.

Pertussis is unique among respiratory infections in that the attack rate is higher in females than in males, with reported male to female ratios of 0.9:1. The excess of females relative to males increases with age. Racial origin is not a factor in the incidence of pertussis. The disease occurs throughout the world and is a major cause of morbidity and mortality in developing countries, where annual rates as high as 200 to 500 per 100,000 population have been reported (WHO, 1979). There is no evidence for seasonality in the occurrence of pertussis.

The pattern of occurrence of pertussis is one of endemic activity, with cyclic periodic epidemics occurring on average every 3.3 years and lasting 12 to 18 months. Before the widespread use of vaccine, pertussis-related deaths in infants exceeded those from measles, scarlet fever, polio, diphtheria, and meningitis combined. The decline in deaths due to pertussis has been dramatic, and the decline actually preceded the decrease in attack rate. The overall case fatality rate is 0.5 per cent, but 70 to 90 per cent of deaths occur in infants aged 1 year or less.

Pertussis is one of the most highly communicable diseases, with attack rates up to 90 per cent among exposed individuals who are susceptible. The infectivity period extends from 7 days after exposure until 3 weeks following the onset of paroxysms. Following close contact with an infected individual, the organism enters through the respiratory tract. The incubation period is usually 7 days but may range between 5 and 21 days. *B. pertussis* affects only humans. Because prolonged asymptomatic carriage (carrier state) does not occur, the disease is perpetuated within the community by person-to-person contact. Naturally occurring disease produces a lifelong immunity, but vaccine-induced protection against infection is of limited duration. Among adults exposed to pertussis more than 12 years after their last dose of vaccine, the attack rate is more than 50 per cent. The disease in older children and adults is often mild and may go unrecognized as pertussis, as will be discussed later. These groups serve as important ongoing reservoirs for *B. pertussis* in the community (Biellik et al, 1988; Thomas and Lambert, 1987; Mertsola et al, 1983; Bass and Stephenson, 1987).

PATHOLOGY

In pertussis, the entire mucosal lining of the respiratory tract is congested, edematous, and infiltrated by cells. Characteristic lesions consist of necrosis of basilar midzonal portions of bronchial epithelium with clumps of organisms in the cilia of the bronchial and tracheal epithelium (Mallory and Horner, 1912). The presence of pneumonia is indicated both by the polymorphonuclear leukocytic infiltration of the bronchial walls and by the peribronchial collar of mononuclear cells (Fig. 59–1). The alveolar walls are thickened and are also infiltrated by mononuclear cells. Viscous mucus, so characteristic of pertussis, may fill the bronchi or bronchioles. Atelectasis is common, and distention of alveoli with bleb formation occurs often. Early in the disease, edema and hemorrhage may be found in the parenchyma. Terminal pneumonia may be produced by *B. pertussis* alone or in combination with secondary bacterial invaders, the last accounting for pus, cellular debris, and mucus within the alveolus. The interstitial pneumonia of pertussis is similar to that of influenza and other viral infections. The enlargement of tracheal and bronchial lymph nodes, if present, is not impressive clinically or roentgenographically and does not approach that seen in primary tuberculosis.

PATHOGENESIS

To understand the pathogenesis of pertussis, it is important to distinguish between infection and disease. The former refers to the attachment and multiplication of the organism within the host, whereas the latter refers to the damage to the host. Although pertussis as a syndrome may be caused by *B. parapertussis* and *B. bronchiseptica*, the overwhelming majority of cases are caused by *B. pertussis*. Thus subsequent discussion pertains only to *B. pertussis*.

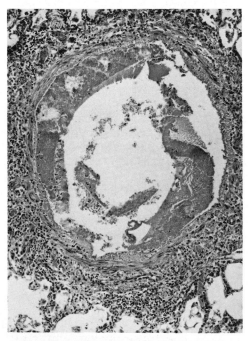

Figure 59–1. Necrotizing bronchitis (× 100).

B. pertussis is a highly selective pathogen in that it attaches only to ciliated cells of the respiratory tract. Attachment is thought to be mediated by the cell surface filamentous hemagglutinin antigen (FHA), although pertussis toxin (PT) may also play a role (Tuomanen and Weiss, 1985). Once attached, the organisms multiply and spread over the epithelial cell surface. The process is a noninvasive one, and bacteremia does not accompany pertussis. During growth of pertussis organisms, toxins are produced that result in the disease commonly known as whooping cough (Pittman, 1979, 1984). In the past, a variety of toxins had been characterized, and it was uncertain which were most important in disease production. It is now apparent that PT mediates most of the effects associated with the disease. The toxin has two subunits, A and B. The latter binds specifically to targets in receptor cells, presenting the active A subunit to the site of enzyme action within the cell membrane. The toxin mediates adenosine diphosphate (ADP)-ribosylation of a regulatory protein in the cytoplasmic membrane. This activity results in an alteration of the physiologic function of the target cells, which include lymphocytes, leukocytes, myocardial cells, and pancreatic islet cells. Measurable physiologic outcomes include lymphocytosis, an increase in host susceptibility to histamine and serotonin, a beta-adrenergic blockade-like effect, and an increase in insulin activity with a drop in serum glucose concentration. Within the respiratory tract, the result of toxin activity is manifest both by a mild inflammatory response with peribronchial lymphoid hyperplasia and by an increase in the amount of mucus covering the ciliary surfaces. The latter may result from both an increase in mucus production as well as a decrease in clearance due to altered ciliary function. Ultimately, the bronchioles may become plugged by the thick, tenacious mucus, resulting in areas of obstruction and collapse. Subsequently, bronchopneumonia may develop owing either to primary *B. pertussis* infection or to a secondary bacterial invader, most frequently *Streptococcus pneumoniae*, *Haemophilus influenzae*, *Staphylococcus aureus* or *Streptococcus pyogenes*. Hypoxemia accompanied by cyanosis probably occurs by more than one mechanism, including ventilation-perfusion mismatch and apnea (Southall et al, 1988). It is still not clear whether the central nervous system damage that occurs is directly toxin mediated or is secondary to anoxia. It is likely that the paroxysms of coughing are also mediated by toxin, although there is no direct evidence for this. Of note, the changes in cellular function are irreversible, and thus recovery is seen only when the epithelial cells regenerate, which explains, at least in part, the lack of effect of antibiotics on the natural course of the disease process.

CLINICAL FEATURES

The natural history of pertussis encompasses three distinct clinical stages. During the initial catarrhal stage, which lasts for 1 to 2 weeks, the symptoms are similar to those of the common cold and include coryza, sneezing, lacrimation, conjunctival injection, malaise, slight cough, and occasionally a low-grade fever. The paroxysmal stage, which lasts 2 to 4 weeks, is marked by an increase in both the frequency and severity of cough. Various stimuli, including eating and drinking, crying, talking, and sudden loud noises, may induce paroxysms of coughing. These consist of multiple, forceable hacking coughs over a 15- to 20-sec period during which there are no or few inspirations. The characteristic whoop at the end of a paroxysm is caused by the sudden inrush of inspired air through a narrowed glottis. During the paroxysm, there may be cyanosis, neck-vein distention, bulging eyes, lacrimation, tongue protrusion, and salivation. Vomiting may follow. Fever is usually minimal or absent. Aside from the paroxysms, there are few characteristic physical findings during this phase unless a complication occurs. The appearance of fever along with a deterioration in respiratory status usually indicates the occurrence of a secondary bacterial pneumonia. During the convalescent stage, which lasts up to several weeks, there is a gradual improvement that is marked primarily by a decrease in the frequency of paroxysms. The cough may persist for several months with intermittent exacerbations of severity often associated with intercurrent respiratory tract infections.

Variations from this clinical picture are more often the rule than the exception for infants (Sotomayor et al, 1985), especially those younger than 6 months of age, adolescents, and adults. In infants, the characteristic whoop is often absent; they may present with apnea, choking spells, or feeding difficulty. Among both adolescents and adults, the disease may occur as a nonspecific upper respiratory tract infection associated with a more severe and prolonged cough than usual.

COMPLICATIONS

The severity of pertussis and its complications vary inversely with age. Younger children, especially those less than 6 months of age, are more likely to be hospitalized and develop complications, especially pneumonia (Robinson et al, 1981). The frequency of hospitalization for pertussis varies depending on how case finding is performed. In a large study of 94 British health authorities from whom 70 per cent of pertussis cases were reported, the hospitalization rate was 9.6 per cent overall but 60 per cent for infants less than 6 months old and 28 per cent for infants 6 to 11 months old (Miller and Fletcher, 1976). Among all cases reported to the Centers for Disease Control in Atlanta during 1982 and 1983, 49 per cent of patients were hospitalized (1984). This higher incidence may reflect a bias toward reporting more severe cases. In this group, 77 per cent of infants younger than 6 months old were hospitalized, as opposed to 59 per cent of 6 to 11 month olds and 28 per cent of 1 to 4 year olds.

The most frequent and troublesome complication of pertussis is the development of bronchopneumonia. Bronchopneumonia occurs in 0.8 to 2 per cent of all cases and 16 to 20 per cent of all hospitalized patients. The pneumonia may be primary due to *B. pertussis* or secondary due to another respiratory tract pathogen. The prognosis for survival is significantly lower in the presence of pneumonia. Of the seven deaths reported in the United States between 1979 and 1981, all occurred in infants younger than 1 year of age who were hospitalized and had pneumonia. From 1976 to 1983, there were 62 pertussis-related deaths in the United Kingdom and Wales. Fifty-nine per cent were associated with pneumonia, with the remainder distributed between central nervous system complications and cardiovascular problems. Other respiratory complications include otitis media, bronchitis, laryngitis, hilar adenitis, and atelectasis. Activation of latent tuberculosis has been associated with pertussis (Feigin and Cherry, 1987).

Nonrespiratory complications may occur secondary to the pressure effects of severe repeated cough, including subconjunctival hemorrhage, herniation, rectal prolapse, subdural hematoma, subcutaneous emphysema, and rarely mediastinal emphysema. Traumatic ulceration of the frenulum of the tongue may also take place during violent coughing. Central nervous system complications include seizures, encephalitis, squint, and deafness. The anoxia associated with the paroxysmal phase may also cause central nervous system damage, including paralysis, deafness, blindness, and mental retardation. In addition, protracted illness may result in weight loss and other nutritional disturbances.

Long-term follow-up studies of patients who have had whooping cough suggest that there is neither long-term impairment in pulmonary function nor increased bronchial reactivity (Johnston et al, 1983, 1986; Britten and Wadsworth, 1986). The frequency of acute respiratory infections does appear to increase in children who have had whooping cough. Whether this increase is due to a predetermined increased susceptibility to respiratory infections or a direct effect of past whooping cough is unknown. Other researchers have found a slight compromise in pulmonary function among children who have had pertussis infection, but this disadvantage disappeared after the age of 7 years (Swansea Research Unit, 1985).

The occurrence of bronchiectasis as a late complication of pertussis pneumonia was seen in the past and was most likely related to an associated chronic pulmonary collapse. This complication is seen rarely in modern times (Cherry, 1984; Biering, 1956).

DIAGNOSIS

A high index of clinical suspicion is imperative in the diagnosis of pertussis, especially for infants and adults in whom the characteristic features of the illness may be lacking. A history of exposure to pertussis lends support to the same diagnosis as a cause of an obvious pulmonary disease. This suspicion may be heightened by a history of inadequate pertussis immunization before the onset of illness. It must be remembered, however, that illness may also occur in individuals who have completed the primary series of immunizations and have received one or more boosters. Of note, in immunized individuals, the illness is usually much less severe. A peripheral lymphocytosis, with values up to 100,000/mm³, often accompanies pertussis and is a nonspecific clue to diagnosis. The lymphocytes are normal in appearance.

Cultural isolation of B. pertussis from respiratory secretions is the only way to make a diagnosis of pertussis with absolute certainty. Unfortunately, the sensitivity of culture is low for many reasons. Culture positivity is highest early in the illness, which is when clinical suspicion is low. During the catarrhal phase, 95 to 100 per cent of cultures will be positive if taken. During the paroxysmal phase, there is a rapid decline in culture positivity from 94 per cent in the third week of illness to 44 per cent in the fourth week and less than 20 per cent thereafter. Even when present in respiratory secretions, the organism may not be recovered because of its susceptibility to environmental conditions, especially drying. It is essential that specimens be obtained from the proper site using the correct swabs, transported in appropriate media as quickly as possible, and cultured on appropriate selective media.

The nasopharynx is the optimal site for specimen collection (Marcon et al, 1987). Cotton swabs should be avoided because they lead to a loss of organisms (Ross and Cumming, 1981). Dacron swabs are preferable, but calcium alginate swabs are also acceptable. When swabs are used, they should be either plated at the bedside onto appropriate media or placed immediately in transport media and sent as quickly as possible to the microbiology laboratory. Alternatively, a nasopharyngeal aspirate can be obtained by suction, using an appropriate sized feeding catheter. The entire feeding catheter can then be packaged to avoid leakage and sent to the laboratory intact. The small bore of the tubing helps to prevent the specimen from drying between the bedside and the laboratory (Wort, 1983). Selective media for culture of B. pertussis include either Bordet-Gengou (potato-glycerol-blood) or Regan-Lowe media (oxoid charcoal agar, horseblood, cephalexin). Bordet-Gengou medium must be made fresh at the time of sample collection; in contrast, Regan-Lowe medium has a shelf life of 8 weeks. In one comparative study, Regan-Lowe was more sensitive for recovery of B. pertussis than Bordet-Gengou (Regan and Lowe, 1977). A nonblood-containing medium with a long shelf life has been described by Japanese workers but has not yet been tested in North America (Aoyama et al, 1986).

Given the problems of culturing B. pertussis, various nonculture-dependent, rapid diagnostic methods have been developed. The one used most extensively employs a direct fluorescent antibody (DFA) method to detect the presence of B. pertussis organisms, whether viable or not, in respiratory secretions. The test has been found to be more sensitive than culture by some investigators (Onorato and Wassilak, 1987; Hakansson et al, 1984) and less sensitive by others (Gilligan and Fisher, 1984; Steketee et al, 1988). Sensitivity varies depending on the stage of illness and at best is 60 to 70 per cent (Marcon et al, 1987; Gilligan and Fisher, 1984). The specificity of DFA is generally good (86 to 95 per cent). An enzyme-linked immunosorbent assay (ELISA) method has been used to examine nasopharyngeal secretions from patients with respiratory tract infections for IgA antibodies to FHA and PT (Granstrom, Askelof, and Granstrom, 1988). Of 100 patients with respiratory tract infections, 54 were confirmed to have pertussis by a combination of culture and serologic response. The sensitivity of culture alone was 54 per cent, whereas that for nasal IgA directed against FHA was 70 per cent, and against PT was 52 per cent. IgA antibodies against one or both antigens were detected in 81 per cent of infected patients. Specificity of the test was 100 per cent. These results are promising, but the test is not yet available on a widespread basis.

The demonstration of an increase in antibodies between the acute and the convalescent stages either to the whole pertussis organism (agglutinins) or to specific antibodies to pertussis antigens (including FHA and PT) has also been used to establish a diagnosis of pertussis. In one investigation, an ELISA method for detecting a rise in IgA and IgG antibodies to FHA, PT, or both between the acute and the convalescent periods had a sensitivity of 88 per cent, as opposed to 45 per cent for a rise in neutralizing antibodies to PT among 90 patients with culture-confirmed pertussis (Granstrom, Wretlind, Salenstedt, and Granstrom, 1988). IgM antibodies were found in only one third of the patients. Unfortunately, the need to obtain specimens during the convalescent period 4 to 6 weeks after the initial presentation has limited the practical clinical utility of serologic diagnosis. Lawrence and Paton (1987), however, established a diagnosis of pertussis in 67 per cent of 1240 patients using an ELISA method to detect antibody to whole B. pertussis cells in a single serum sample obtained during acute illness. Thus with more sensitive techniques, serodiagnosis may prove more useful.

In conclusion, to establish a diagnosis of pertussis, it is essential to have a high clinical suspicion, to obtain nasopharyngeal secretions as early as possible in the disease for culture as well as for DFA and, if available, for IgA antibody to FHA and PT antigens. A serum sample taken during acute illness should also be obtained when it is essential that the diagnosis be made. Subsequent collection of a specimen during convalescence 4 to 6 weeks later with testing preferably by ELISA for IgG or IgA antibody to PT and FHA should further increase the diagnostic yield.

ROENTGENOGRAPHIC DIAGNOSIS

There are no characteristic roentgenographic features of pertussis infection. The most frequent abnormalities are consolidation, collapse, and hilar lymphadenopathy. Bellamy and colleagues (1987) reviewed the radiographs of 238 patients admitted to hospital with pertussis. Abnormalities were found in 63 (26 per cent) and included consolidation in 79 per cent, lymphadenopathy in 35 per cent, and collapse in 14 per cent. Among those with consolidation, 72 per cent had peribronchial infiltrates, 32 per cent had lobar and sublobar patterns, and 12 per cent had bronchopneumonia. The right lung was involved three times as often as the left, with the right lower lobe and middle lobe being the most frequently involved. Of 22 patients with lymphadenopathy, the unilateral tracheobronchial gland was involved in 16 (72 per cent). Repeat radiographs in 34 of the 175 patients whose chest radiograph was initially normal showed abnormalities developing in 18 per cent, including four with evidence of consolidation and two with collapse. Of 63 patients with initially abnormal films, 32 (52 per cent) had follow-up radiographs. When present, collapse never persisted longer than 1 month. Consolidation had resolved in 22 out of 26 patients by 1 month after the illness. In one patient, a repeat radiograph was not done until 12 weeks after presentation, by which time consolidation had resolved. In three patients, minor residual changes were still present 5 to 34 days after the initial admitting radiograph, but improvement was noted in all three.

These results suggest a lower frequency of roentgenographic abnormalities associated with pertussis than did earlier reports (Nicholson, 1949; Fawcitt and Parry, 1957), in which abnormalities were described in 43 to 89 per cent of the cases. In the older studies, radiographs were obtained more frequently, and lateral as well as lordotic views were included for many of the cases, which may have accounted for an increased number of abnormalities being detected. Conversely, it is also possible that, in modern times, radiologic abnormalities are less frequent either because of milder clinical disease, which in turn may be related to more extensive immunization coverage, or because of earlier introduction of antibiotics, which could affect the incidence of secondary pneumonia. At least two other reports confirm a lower incidence (18 to 23 per cent) of radiographic abnormalities (Bennett, 1973; Robinson et al, 1981). Despite the differences in the prevalence of abnormalities, published studies agree that the clinical features of illness do not correlate with the likelihood of abnormalities being present on chest radiographs. Thus it could be concluded that for patients admitted to hospital, radiographs should be obtained in the majority of cases to rule out minor degrees of consolidation or collapse.

DIFFERENTIAL DIAGNOSIS

During the catarrhal phase of pertussis, the differential diagnosis is large and includes all viruses that infect the respiratory tract (influenza, parainfluenza, respiratory syncytial virus, adenovirus, rhinovirus, coronavirus) as well as bacterial bronchitis.

Pertussis in its typical paroxysmal form is easily identified. Difficulty may arise when the disease is modified by the partial protection of past immunization. In very young infants, the whoop is usually absent; paroxysmal cough in such patients should arouse suspicion. The pattern of cough may help to distinguish pertussis from infantile pneumonitis caused by Chlamydia trachomatis. In chlamydia, there is a repetitive, staccato cough, but usually there are inspirations between coughs. In pertussis, however, there are few or no inspirations between coughs during a paroxysm. Some patients with extensive bronchopneumonia and interstitial pneumonia unassociated with B. pertussis may also have paroxysmal spasmodic cough without whoop or vomiting. These patients usually have extensive physical findings in the lungs, consisting of many scattered crackles, and suffer from much respiratory difficulty. They continue to be quite ill between the bouts of coughing, with rapid and often shallow respirations.

Occasionally, a patient with enlarged tuberculous bronchopulmonary glands has a paroxysmal spasmodic cough similar to that noted in pertussis; there may also be an associated collapse of a segment of the lung. The presence of a whoop in pertussis and a barking, metallic cough in tuberculosis may aid in diagnosis. Cyanosis, rather than suffusion of the face, is more commonly associated with the paroxysmal coughing of the tuberculous child, and vomiting is rare. In addition to a diagnostic test for B. pertussis, tuberculin tests and a chest roentgenogram are valuable aids in the differential diagnosis of these two conditions. A clinical history of exposure to either pertussis or tuberculosis should also be sought.

Noninfectious conditions that may be confused with the paroxysmal stage of pertussis include aspirated foreign body, severe asthma, and cystic fibrosis (Sant'Agnese, 1955).

It was thought that adenovirus could cause a "pertussis syndrome." Although adenovirus has been isolated from autopsy specimens (Collier et al, 1966) as well as from nasopharyngeal secretions of some patients with a pertussis-like illness, the association is not a proven one. Adenovirus can also be isolated from up to 5 per cent of asymptomatic children and may reflect prolonged excretion from previous illness or asymptomatic carriage. However, adenoviruses may be associated with severe respiratory infections, especially in native North American Indian children. A fourfold or greater rise in antibodies to adenovirus in paired serum specimens from the acute and the convalescent stages would help to establish the diagnosis.

TREATMENT

Erythromycin remains the treatment of choice for pertussis. As noted previously, antimicrobial therapy does not affect the natural history of infection but does diminish infectivity. Given in doses of 50 mg/kg/day, erythromycin leads to eradication of the organism in 3 to 4 days. The recommended duration of therapy is 14 days (Bass, 1986).

When intercurrent bacterial infections are suspected, an antibiotic selected in accordance with the clinician's best judgment may be used until bacterial cultures, viral studies, and other aids to diagnosis clarify the etiologic pathogen. Empiric antibiotics for secondary bacterial pneumonia should be active against pneumococcus, *S. aureus*, and both ampicillin-resistant and ampicillin-sensitive *H. influenzae*.

In the past, hyperimmune pertussis gamma globulin has been given to seriously ill patients, but controlled studies failed to establish the efficacy of this therapy (Balagtas et al, 1971).

General supportive medical care is extremely important for infants hospitalized with pertussis. The demonstration that hypoxemia can occur in such infants in the absence of a paroxysm or apnea indicates that vital signs and possibly oxygen saturation should be monitored closely. Efforts should be made to avoid stimuli that trigger paroxysms. Careful attention should be paid to providing adequate fluids and maintaining nutrition, especially in infants with a prolonged course.

Adjuncts to antibiotics that have been studied include corticosteroids and beta-adrenergic agents, such as salbutamol. Evidence suggests that both may lead to a reduction in the frequency and severity of paroxysms, but further clinical evaluation is required (Bass, 1985).

Hospitalized patients in whom pertussis is suspected or documented should be nursed with respiratory isolation precautions until 7 days of erythromycin therapy have been received or until the diagnosis of pertussis has been ruled out. If antibiotics are contraindicated, precautions should be continued until 3 weeks after the start of paroxysms.

PREVENTION

Antibacterial prophylaxis with erythromycin, in the same dosage and duration as for treatment of established infection, is recommended for close contacts of patients with pertussis who are younger than 1 year of age as well as for unimmunized close contacts younger than 7 years of age.

A thorough discussion of the issues involving the use of the current whole-cell pertussis vaccine as well as the investigational acellular pertussis vaccines is beyond the scope of this chapter. Interested readers are referred to the report of the task force on pertussis and pertussis immunization by Cherry and colleagues (1988). The best available way of preventing pertussis is still with a primary series and two booster doses of the whole-cell pertussis vaccine. Most reported estimates of current vaccine effectiveness vary from 80 to 95 per cent (Fine and Clarkson, 1987). Unlike natural disease, which provides lifelong protection against both pertussis infection and disease, the vaccine-induced protection is limited and does not prevent infection. Nevertheless, the vaccine is very effective in decreasing the severity of the disease. In a cost-benefit analysis, it was shown that for every dollar spent on vaccine, $11.10 were saved in terms of the cost associated with pertussis disease and complications including hospitalization. A subsequent reanalysis to incorporate increases in vaccine costs still showed a saving of $3.10 for every dollar spent (Hinman and Koplan, 1984). Although there is a lower rate of transient local and systemic reactions, such as fever, associated with the acellular vaccine, it is not known whether the frequency of severe neurologic reactions will be lower relative to the whole-cell vaccine. Furthermore, it is not yet known whether the new acellular pertussis vaccine will be as effective or more effective than the whole-cell vaccine.

REFERENCES

Aoyama T, Murase Y, Iwata T et al: Comparison of blood-free medium (cyclodextrin solid medium) with Bordet-Gengou medium for clinical isolation of *Bordetella pertussis*. J Clin Microbiol 23:1046, 1986.

Balagtas RC, Nelson KE, Levin S et al: Treatment of pertussis with pertussis immune globulin. J Pediatr 79:203, 1971.

Bass JW: Pertussis. Current status and prevention. Pediatr Infect Dis J 4:624, 1985.

Bass JW: Erythromycin for treatment and prevention of pertussis. Pediatr Infect Dis J 5:154, 1986.

Bass JW and Stephenson SR: The return of pertussis. Pediatr Infect Dis J 6:141, 1987.

Bellamy EA, Johnston IDA, and Wilson AG: The chest radiograph in whooping cough. Clin Radiol 38:39, 1987.

Bennett NM: Whooping cough in Melbourne. Med J Aust 2:481, 1973.

Biellik RJ, Patriarca PA, Mullen JR et al: Risk factors for community- and household-acquired pertussis during a large-scale outbreak in Central Wisconsin. J Infect Dis 157:1134, 1988.

Biering A: Childhood pneumonia, including pertussis pneumonia and bronchiectasis. A follow-up study of 151 patients. Acta Pediatr 45:348, 1956.

Britten N and Wadsworth J: Long term respiratory sequelae of whooping cough in a nationally representative sample. Br Med J 292:442, 1986.

Centers for Disease Control: Pertussis. Morbid Mortal Wkly Rpt 36:168, 1987.

Cherry JD: The epidemiology of pertussis and pertussis immunization in the United Kingdom and the United States: a comparative study. In Lockhart JD (ed): Current Problems in Pediatrics. Chicago, Year Book Medical Publishers, Inc, 1984.

Cherry JD, Brunell PA, Golden GS, and Karzon DT: Report of the task force on pertussis and pertussis immunization—1988. Pediatr 81(Suppl):939, 1988.

Collier AM, Conner JD, and Irving WR: Generalized type 5 adenovirus infection associated with the pertussis syndrome. J Pediatr 69:1073, 1966.

Fawcitt J and Parry HE: Lung changes in pertussis and measles in childhood. A review of 1894 cases with a follow-up study of the pulmonary complications. Br J Radiol 39:76, 1957.

Feigin RD and Cherry JD: Pertussis. In Feigin RD and Cherry JD (eds): Textbook of Pediatric Infectious Diseases. Philadelphia, WB Saunders Co, 1987.

Fine PEM and Clarkson JA: Reflections on the efficacy of pertussis vaccines. Rev Infect Dis 9:866, 1987.

Geller RJ: The pertussis syndrome: a persistent problem. Pediatr Infect Dis J 3:182, 1984.

Gilligan PH and Fisher MC: Importance of culture in laboratory diagnosis of Bordetella pertussis infections. J Clin Microbiol 20:891, 1984.

Granstrom G, Askelof P, and Granstrom M: Specific immunoglobulin A to Bordetella pertussis antigens in mucosal secretion for rapid diagnosis of whooping cough. J Clin Microbiol 26:869, 1988.

Granstrom G, Wretlind B, Salenstedt C-R, and Granstrom M: Evaluation of serologic assays for diagnosis of whooping cough. J Clin Microbiol 26:1818, 1988.

Hakansson S, Sundin CG, Granstrom M, and Gastrin B: Diagnosis of whooping cough—a comparison of culture, immunofluorescence and serology with ELISA. Scand J Infect Dis 16:281, 1984.

Hinman AR and Koplan JP: Pertussis and pertussis vaccine: reanalysis of benefits, risks and costs. JAMA 251:3109, 1984.

Johnston IDA, Bland JM, Ingram D et al: Effect of whooping cough in infancy on subsequent lung function and bronchial reactivity. Am Rev Respir Dis 134:270, 1986.

Johnston IDA, Lambert HP, Anderson HR, and Patel S: Respiratory morbidity and lung function after whooping cough. Lancet 2:1104, 1983.

Lawrence AJ and Paton JC: Efficacy of enzyme-linked immunosorbent assay for rapid diagnosis of Bordetella pertussis infection. J Clin Microbiol 25:2102, 1987.

Mallory FB and Horner AA: The histological lesion in the respiratory tract. J Med Res 27:115, 1912.

Marcon MJ, Hamoudi AC, Cannon HJ, and Hribar MM: Comparison of throat and nasopharyngeal swab specimens for culture diagnosis of Bordetella pertussis infection. J Clin Microbiol 25:1109, 1987.

Mertsola J, Ruuskanen O, Eerola E, and Viljanen MK: Intrafamilial spread of pertussis. J Pediatr 103:359, 1983.

Miller CL and Fletcher WB: Severity of notified whooping cough. Br Med J 1:117, 1976.

Mortimer Jr EA: Pertussis. In Evans AS and Feldman HA (eds): Bacterial Infections of Humans. Epidemiology and Control. New York, Plenum Medical Book Co, 1982.

Nicholson DP: Pulmonary collapse in pertussis. Arch Dis Child 24:29, 1949.

Onorato IM and Wassilak SGF: Laboratory diagnosis of pertussis: the state of the art. Pediatr Infect Dis J 6:145, 1987.

Pertussis—United States, 1982 and 1983: Morbid Mortal Wkly Rpt 33:573, 1984.

Pittman M: Pertussis toxin: the cause of the harmful effects and prolonged immunity of whooping cough. A hypothesis. Rev Infect Dis 1:401, 1979.

Pittman M: The concept of pertussis as a toxin-mediated disease. Pediatr Infect Dis J 3:467, 1984.

Regan J and Lowe F: Enrichment medium for the isolation of Bordetella. J Clin Microbiol 6:303, 1977.

Robinson DA, Mandal BK, Ironside AG, and Dunbar EM: Whooping cough—a study of severity in hospital cases. Arch Dis Child 56:687, 1981.

Romanus V, Jonsell R, and Bergquist S-O: Pertussis in Sweden after the cessation of general immunization in 1979. Pediatr Infect Dis J 6:364, 1987.

Ross PW and Cumming CG: Isolation of Bordetella pertussis from swabs. Br Med J 283:403, 1981.

Sant'Agnese PA di: The pulmonary manifestations of fibrocystic disease of the pancreas. Dis Chest 27:654, 1955.

Sotomayor J, Weiner LB, and McMillan JA: Inaccurate diagnosis in infants with pertussis. An eight-year experience. Am J Dis Child 139:724, 1985.

Southall DP, Thomas MG, and Lambert HP: Severe hypoxaemia in pertussis. Arch Dis Child 63:598, 1988.

Steketee RW, Burstyn DG, Wassilak SGF et al: A comparison of laboratory and clinical methods for diagnosing pertussis in an outbreak in a facility for the developmentally disabled. J Infect Dis 157:441, 1988.

Swansea Research Unit of the Royal College of General Practitioners: Respiratory sequelae of whooping cough. Br Med J 290:1937, 1985.

Thomas MG and Lambert HP: From whom do children catch pertussis? Br Med J 295:751, 1987.

Tuomanen E and Weiss A: Characterization of two adhesions of Bordetella pertussis for human ciliated respiratory-epithelial cells. J Infect Dis 152:118, 1985.

World Health Organization Statistical Record: Infectious diseases: cases. Geneva, WHO, 1979.

Wort AJ: Bacteriologic diagnosis of pertussis. Lancet 1:766, 1983.

60

STUART P. ADLER, M.D., and
GILBERTO E. RODRIGUEZ, M.D.

SALMONELLA PNEUMONIA

Salmonella are gram-negative bacterial rods belonging to the family Enterobacteriaceae. There are three species: Salmonella typhi (one serotype), Salmonella choleraesuis (one serotype), and Salmonella enteritidis (more than 2200 known serotypes). Previous convention referred to each serotype of S. enteritidis as if it were a species, i.e., Salmonella typhimurium, although the correct nomenclature is S. enteritidis serotype typhimurium. Identification of the salmonella within the family Enterobacteriaceae is based on a series of biochemical properties, including the ability to ferment specific sugars, such as glucose and manose but not lactose or sucrose (Buchanan and Gibbons, 1974). Subclassification of the salmonella within species and serotypes is based on a detailed analysis of two major antigens, the somatic (O) antigens, which are lipopolysaccharide components of the cell wall, and the flagellar (H) antigens, which are proteins. Each of the three species of salmonella produces distinctly different clinical illnesses and associated characteristic pulmonary manifestations. We therefore discuss individually the clinical illness and pulmonary complications caused by each of the three salmonella species.

EPIDEMIOLOGY

S. enteritidis and *S. choleraesuis* are pathogens of animals. These organisms have been recovered from almost all animal species, and although human-to-human transmission frequently occurs, most outbreaks of infections are associated with contaminated food products, especially beef, pork, and dairy products. *S. typhi*, however, infects only humans naturally; hence acquisition of this infection takes place either by direct contact with a chronic carrier or by ingestion of food or liquids contaminated with human feces.

Although the incidence of typhoid fever due to *S. typhi* has decreased steadily over the last 4 decades to less than 400 cases per year in North America, the incidence of nontyphoidal salmonella infections has increased by 28 per cent over the last 10 years (Summary, 1986).

Between 500 and 1000 salmonella isolates are reported each week to state and local health departments, but it is estimated that less than 1 per cent of all infections are reported. Nontyphoidal salmonella infections occur most frequently during the warmweather months, with the peak incidence in the United States being in late August. The age distribution for all isolates (excluding *S. typhi* and *S. choleraesuis*) is always highest for infants approximately 2 months of age. There is a rapid decrease in the incidence of salmonella infection through early childhood, but this lower level remains fairly constant from age 6 years through adulthood. In spite of the fact that there are more than 2200 known serotypes of *S. enteritidis*, only nine strains of *S. enteritidis* as well as *S. typhi* account for more than 70 per cent of the isolates. *S. typhi* accounted for only 2.0 per cent of isolates in 1980 (Human, 1981).

Tragically, typhoid fever continues to pose serious public health problems in Third World countries, where there is little chance of implementing the public health measures necessary for containment. With the emergence of *S. typhi* strains that are resistant to antibiotics, prevention by vaccination is the most promising method for the control of the disease.

PATHOGENESIS OF NONPULMONARY SALMONELLA INFECTION

A large number of organisms (10^6 to 10^9) must be ingested for any salmonella species, including *S. typhi*, to produce clinical disease, but asymptomatic infections can occur with ten to 100 times fewer organisms. In patients with reduced host defenses, symptomatic infections may occur with the ingestion of only a few organisms. For example, one third of a group of children with cystic fibrosis became ill after ingesting porcine pancreatin containing less than two organisms per 100-g tablet (Lipson and Meikle, 1977). Most ingested salmonella are rapidly killed by stomach acids (pH 2.0). Viable organisms that pass into the small intestine replicate, resulting in either asymptomatic infection with transient excretion of organisms in the stool or symptomatic infection, such as acute gastroenteritis, typhoidal fever, or bacteremia. The frequency of bacteremia is variable, depends on the causative organism, and may lead to localized infection at any body site, including the lung. Localized infection is characterized by an inflammatory response of predominantly polymorphonuclear cells. The pathogenesis of gastroenteritis is thought to result from a direct invasion of the mucosal surface by the bacteria plus an enterotoxin-like effect upon the intestinal transport mechanisms.

Certain groups of patients with underlying systemic disease appear to have reduced defenses against salmonella infection, especially the suppurative complications of bacteremia. These include patients who have malnutrition or malignancies; those receiving immunosuppressive therapy, such as corticosteroids; and those with sickle hemoglobinopathies or malaria. Patients with sickle cell anemia have a defect in the alternate complement pathway that may account for their increased susceptibility to salmonella bacteremia (Hand and King, 1978).

S. typhi penetrates the intestinal mucosa and replicates in the intestinal lymph follicles (Hook, 1961; Hornick et al, 1970). The lymph follicle becomes hyperplastic, and a mononuclear cell infiltrate develops. Bacteria eventually reach the mesenteric lymph nodes, with subsequent migration into the thoracic duct and blood stream. Organisms are cleared by the reticuloendothelial system in the bone marrow, liver, and spleen. Circulating endotoxins—lipopolysaccharides of the bacterial cell wall—probably contribute to fever and the characteristic systemic symptoms of typhoid fever, although the exact mechanism is unknown.

Whereas salmonella bacteremia occurs less frequently than the recovery of organisms from stool, *S. typhi*, *S. choleraesuis*, and two serotypes of *S. enteritidis*—dublin and paratyphoid A—are isolated much more commonly from blood than from fecal cultures. The frequency of blood isolates for these organisms is ten to 60 times higher than for other serotypes (Blaser and Feldman, 1981). *S. choleraesuis*, for example, is seldom found in the stool and rarely causes gastroenteritis, but bacteremia, suppurative focal infection, and pneumonia are common with this organism. *S. enteritidis* bacteremia occurs most frequently in infants less than 2 months of age and in the elderly (older than 60 years). The organisms most frequently associated with bacteremia are also most likely to be associated with pulmonary disease.

IMMUNITY

The morbidity and mortality of salmonella infections depend not only on the dose, route of inoculation, and virulence of the salmonella serotype but also on the host's genotype and ability to mount an immune response.

Salmonella species are included in the category of facultative intracellular organisms because they can survive within the cells of the reticuloendothelial system. Cell-mediated immunity is important in controlling infection by other intracellular organisms, such as *Listeria monocytogenes* and *Mycobacteria tuberculosis*, and appears also to be important in controlling infections caused by *S. typhi*.

Enteric fever in animal models suggests that the early phase of the immune response consists primarily of phagocytosis by resting macrophages. These macrophages are then activated by lymphokines produced by T lymphocytes. The response of T lymphocytes and macrophages to salmonella in humans has not been studied.

In addition to cell-mediated immunity, antibody, polymorphonuclear leukocytes, and complement are undoubtedly also important. Numerous reports demonstrate the high degree of protection conferred by specific antibody against specific salmonella serotypes (Rowley et al, 1964; Hochadel and Keller, 1977; O'Brien et al, 1979; Akeda et al, 1981).

Present whole-cells typhoid vaccines are 70 per cent effective in preventing typhoid fever. However, they contain lipopolysaccharide (LPS) that elicits local or systemic reactions, or both, in most recipients. The immunity they provide does not persist for more than 3 to 5 years (Hornick et al, 1970; Cvjetanovic, 1973).

More promising is work being done with the Vi Antigen (Vi for virulence), the capsular polysaccharide of *S. typhi*. Antibodies to the Vi surface antigen are more effective than those against O or H antigens in confirming protection against lethal infection with Vi-positive strains in mammals (Robbins et al, 1984). Several *Salmonella* vaccines are now under trial (Forrest, 1988; Clements, 1987; Dougan et al, 1987). Both live attenuated organisms and specific bacterial antigen (Vi) vaccines are protective (Mohandas et al, 1989; Tacket et al, 1988; Acharya et al, 1987). Studies have shown that in humans the antibody response is not critical. Protection associates best with cell-mediated immunity to specific *Salmonella* antigens (Murphy et al, 1989; Tackett et al; Levine et al, 1987).

PULMONARY DISEASE IN SALMONELLA INFECTIONS

Lower respiratory tract complications of salmonella infections are often secondary to bacteremia following colonization of the intestinal tract. However, there is some evidence suggesting that salmonella may sometimes be transmitted to humans by airborne particles. Netter (1950), Varela and Ochoa (1953), and Datta and Pridie (1960) cultured salmonella from the nose, pharynx, and sputum of humans. Salmonella organisms have also been isolated from tonsils of asymptomatic children (Hormaeche et al, 1940; Varela and Olarte, 1942). These observations suggest that the portal of entry is the respiratory tract. Further evidence is provided by Darlow and Bale (1959), who showed that flushing of a lavatory pan could produce aerosolized particles sufficiently small to be inhaled into the pulmonary alveoli. Bate and James (1958) reported a dust-borne salmonella epidemic. In this outbreak, dust-borne organisms kept alive an epidemic of *S. enteritidis*, serotype *typhimurium*, that required a children's hospital ward to close for fumigation eight different times in 11 months. The source of salmonella was eventually determined to be heavily infected dust in the bag of a vacuum floor polisher.

Experimental pneumonia has been produced in animal models after inhalation of aerosolized salmonella (Trillat and Kaneko, 1921; Darlow et al, 1961). Abscess formation has been common. One hundred times fewer bacteria are required to initiate infection by the respiratory route than by the percutaneous, conjunctival, or oral route.

A third mechanism involved in salmonella-induced pneumonia is aspiration of infected vomitus or meconium, which may cause focal inflammation and lung abscess. We treated a full-term newborn infant for salmonella pneumonia. The infant was born by vaginal delivery to a febrile mother in whom salmonella amnionitis was demonstrated. *S. enteritidis* serotype *kentucky* was isolated from blood, stool, and amniotic fluid cultures. The infant became febrile and on the second day of life developed pneumonia grequiring ventilatory assistance. Blood, stool, and multiple endotracheal cultures grew the same salmonella serotype found in his mother. The infant was successfully treated with ampicillin. Because salmonella pneumonia is an uncommon complication of salmonellosis, even in neonates, we suspect that this infant's pulmonary disease was acquired from aspirated amniotic fluid.

Salmonella typhi

Typhoid fever is a preventable disease that does not exist except in areas of poor sanitation. It is typically a disease of childhood and early adult life, occurring most commonly between the ages of 15 and 30 years. It is rare in infants, in whom the mortality rate is high. The clinical course in children over the age of 2 years is similar *but usually less severe* than in adults.

The respiratory tract is usually involved in typhoid fever. However, it is mild and frequently confined to coryza, pharyngitis, and manifestations of bronchitis.

Bronchitis is reported to occur during the first week of illness in more than 80 per cent of children with the disease. It is most commonly manifested by cough alone. More severe manifestations include gross rales, transmitted rhonchi, and chest pain aggravated by coughing. Nose bleed (epistaxis), at times severe, was present at some stage of the disease, usually early, in 21 per cent of 360 patients (one third were children) reported from Louisiana (Stuart and Pullen, 1946).

In rare cases, bronchopneumonia appears during the second week, manifested by fine rales, altered breath sounds, and purulent, sometimes blood-tinged sputum. It is usually associated with septicemia. Chest pain and cyanosis may become prominent. Neither the physical nor the radiographic findings differentiate salmonella pneumonia from other pulmonary infections. *S. typhi* infection of the lung and pleura may occur without septicemia or gastrointestinal manifestations (Olutola and Familusi, 1985). Not uncommonly, typhoid pneumonia is hemorrhagic. *S. typhi* causes vascular endothelial damage in many sites, so pulmonary arteritis, pulmonary embolism, and pulmonary infarction often occur. Lung abscess and pleural effusion are other pulmonary complications of typhoid fever that are rare in children.

Before the antibiotic era, the typhoid bacillus was often isolated in pure form at autopsy of patients with lobar pneumonia and typhoid fever. However, *Streptococcus pneumoniae* may occur as a secondary invader responsible for the lobar consolidation.

Typhoid pneumonia and typhoid lung abscess may also occur several decades after the initial infection (De Matteis and Armani, 1967). Whether such late infections represent a reactivation of a dormant typhoid lesion, as suggested by Saphra and Winter (1957), is uncertain. There is one report of *S. typhi* causing an abscess in a tuberculous pulmonary cavity (Hahne, 1964).

S. enteritidis

S. enteritidis is responsible for the majority of cases of salmonellosis in the United States but is rarely responsible for significant pulmonary disease. In a review of 7779 cases of salmonellosis (Saphra and Winters, 1957), lobar pneumonia or bronchopneumonia occurred in only 85. Most of the patients were elderly or immunocompromised. Of the 85 cases of pulmonary disease, 41 were caused by either *S. choleraesuis* or *S. enteritidis* serotype *paratyphi C*. Serotypes *paratyphi A* and *B* also cause a clinical syndrome whose course resembles that of a mild, atypical typhoid fever with malaise, bradycardia, leukopenia, and fever, although splenomegaly and rose spots are often absent. The fever may be continuous or spiking with a duration of 1 to 3 weeks. As in typhoid fever, coryza, pharyngitis, and bronchitis are commonly seen. Salmonella pneumonia occurs most frequently in adults with malignancy, especially lymphoma, Hodgkin's disease, leukemia, or lung cancer (Berke-ley and Mangels, 1985; Olutola and Familusi, 1985; Canney et al, 1985).

Acute salmonella pleural effusion, as the presenting manifestation, has been ascribed to *S. enteritidis* serotypes *paratyphi B* (Annamalai et al, 1969) and *typhimurium* (Burney et al, 1977). *S. enteritidis*, serotype *oranienburg*, has been reported to cause chronic empyema after a penetrating gunshot wound (Bokra, 1958).

Epidemics of paratyphoid and typhoid fever may coexist, and the infections may even occur simultaneously in the same patient.

S. choleraesuis

S. choleraesuis is more invasive than *S. enteritidis* and is responsible for more cases of localized infection (Saphra and Wasserman, 1954; Saphra and Winter, 1957). Bullowa (1928) first reported lobar pneumonia due to *S. choleraesuis* (then called *S. suispestifer*) in which the bacterium was isolated in cultures of blood and sputum and at post mortem by lung puncture. Harvey (1937) reviewed and described 71 cases, in approximately one third of which there was pleuropulmonary disease, mainly bronchopneumonia, pleural effusion, empyema, and, rarely, lobar pneumonia. The average age of the 24 patients with bronchopneumonia was 19 years, and ten of them died. Goulder and co-workers (1942) reported six cases of sporadic *S. choleraesuis* infection in children ages 2 to 9 years, two of whom developed pneumonia. Saphra and Wasserman (1954) reviewed 329 cases of *S. choleraesuis* infections. In 32 (10 per cent), pneumonia, empyema, or both occurred, with positive cultures from blood, sputum, or pleural fluid.

DIAGNOSIS

The diagnosis of pulmonary disease due to any of the salmonellas requires isolation of the organism from pleura, pleural fluid, or pulmonary tissue as well as radiographic or clinical evidence of a pneumonic process. Recovery of the organism from the stool, the blood, or a site of focal lesions does not establish that the pulmonary disease is caused by salmonella. This finding is especially true for children, in whom 75 per cent of lower respiratory tract disease is probably due to respiratory viruses. Given the very low incidence in children of pulmonary complications with *S. enteritidis*, the simultaneous occurrence of viral pneumonia and salmonella gastroenteritis would be more likely than pneumonia caused by salmonella. In one study, five of six 2-month-old infants with bacteremia (one with salmonella) and lower respiratory tract disease had a concomitant respiratory viral infection (Zullar et al, 1973). Recovery of salmonella from tracheal aspirates is seldom attempted in children, although the presence of polymorphonuclear cells, abundance of gram-negative organisms on smear, and the growth of salmonella from a tracheal aspirate with concomitant pulmonary disease would be adequate to establish the diagnosis of salmonella pneumonia. A presumptive diagnosis of salmonella pneumonia should be made in the febrile child with clinical or radiographic evidence, or both, of pneumonia if either *S. typhi* or *S. choleraesuis* is recovered from the stool or blood. Because these two organisms usually produce bacteremia, a positive stool culture in a symptomatic child should be considered presumptive evidence of systemic or pulmonary infection, or both. Antibiotic therapy is necessary in these situations.

Serologic studies are not reliable for the diagnosis of salmonella infection, particularly with pulmonary complications. Only 50 per cent of untreated patients demonstrate a fourfold rise in specific agglutinins against salmonella H and O antigens. Antibiotic therapy decreases antibody responses in infected patients (Hoffman et al, 1975).

Typhoid fever pneumonia has recently been described in adult acquired immune deficiency syndrome (AIDS) patients. As this disease continues to become more common in children, it is expected that typhoid pneumonia will be seen more frequently in the pediatric AIDS population. Accurate diagnosis of this pneumonia will become more critical. Antibodies to the Vi antigen are more sensitive and more specific for *S. typhi* infection and should be of great help in the diagnosis. However, their measurement is not widely available.

TREATMENT

Antibiotic therapy reduces the likelihood of recovery of salmonella from blood, urine, sputum, and, in the case of *S. typhi*, stool. Hence all appropriate cultures should be obtained before the institution of antibiotic therapy. Any salmonella pleural effusion must be surgically drained. If empyema is present, it should be continuously drained with a large chest tube until cultures are sterile and the drainage of pleural fluid has ceased.

Because salmonella rapidly becomes resistant to many antibiotics and because antibiotic therapy does not shorten the carrier state, antibiotics should be used only if *S. enteritidis* has been recovered from blood, urine, or sputum or if *S. typhi* or *S. choleraesuis* has been isolated from any body site. Ampicillin, 200 to 400 mg/kg/day IV q 6 hr, is the preferred antibiotic unless the organism is resistant to that drug. At the Medical College of Virginia, 10 per cent of all salmonella isolates are resistant to ampicillin. All of these isolates (with one exception) have been sensitive to chloramphenicol and trimethoprim-sulfamethoxazole. There is adequate clinical experience to justify the use of these drugs in the treatment of salmonella infections other than gastroenteritis. Chloramphenicol is given at a dosage of 100 mg/kg/day intravenously every 6 hours. Trimethoprim-sulfamethoxazole should be administered orally every 6 hours in dosages of 10 to 20 mg/kg/day of trimethoprim and 50 to 100 mg/kg/day of sulfamethoxazole. Antibiotic therapy is continued for at least 14 days, depending on the rate of resolution of pulmonary symptoms. Organisms from areas outside the United States may be resistant to these drugs. We have recently encountered a 24-day-old Laotian infant with salmonella bacteremia caused by a salmonella species that was resistant to ampicillin, chloramphenicol, and trimethoprim-sulfamethoxazole. In such a situation, one of the cephalosporins may be used, provided that the organism is sensitive to that drug. Even though all salmonella species are sensitive in vitro to the aminoglycosides (gentamicin, tobramycin, and amikacin), these drugs are not efficacious when used alone. For *S. enteritidis*, stool cultures will remain positive in spite of systemic antibiotic therapy. Thus stool culture cannot be used as a guide to duration or efficacy of antibiotic therapy.

REFERENCES

Acharya IL, Lowe CU, Thapa R et al: Prevention of typhoid fever in Nepal with the Vi capsular polysaccharide of *Salmonella typhi*. A preliminary report. N Engl J Med 317:1101, 1987.
Akeda H, Mitsuyama M, Tatsukawa K et al: The synergistic contribution of macrophages and antibody to protection against *Salmonella typhimurium* during early phase infection. J Microbiol 123:209, 1981.
Annamalai A, Shreekumar S, and Muthukumaran R: Empyema in enteric fever due to *Salmonella paratyphi B*. Dis Chest 55:72, 1969.
Bate JG and James U: *Salmonella typhimurium* infection dustborne in a children's ward. Lancet 2.713, 1958.
Berkeley D and Mangels J: Salmonella pneumonia in a patient with carcinoma of the lung. Am J Clin Pathol 74:476, 1980.
Blaser MJ and Feldman RA: From the Centers for Disease Control. Salmonella bacteremia: reports to the Centers for Disease Control, 1968–1979. J Infect Dis 143:743, 1981.
Bokra ST: Chronic empyema due to *Salmonella oranienburg*; complication of old chest wound. Can Med Assoc J 78:599, 1958.
Buchanan RE and Gibbons NE (eds): Bergey's Manual of Determinative Bacteriology. 8th ed. Baltimore, Williams & Wilkins Co, 1974.
Bullowa JGM: Bacillus suispestifer (hog cholera) infection of the lung. Med Clin North Am 12:691, 1928.
Burney DP, Fisher RD, and Schaffner W: *Salmonella* empyema: a review. Southern Med J 70:375, 1977.
Canney PA, Larson SN, Hay JH, and Yussuf MA: Case report: salmonella pneumonia associated with chemotherapy for non-Hodgkin's lymphoma. Clin Radiol 36:459, 1985.
Clements JD: Use of attenuated mutants of *Salmonella* as carriers for delivery of heterologous antigens in the secretory immune system. Lancet 2:1165, 1987.
Cvjetanovic B: Typhoid fever and its prevention. Public Health Rev 2:229, 1973.
Darlow HM and Bale WR: Infective hazards of water closets. Lancet 1:1196, 1959.
Darlow HM, Bale WR, and Carter GB: Infection of mice by the respiratory route with *Salmonella typhimurium*. J Hyg (Camb) 59:303, 1961.
Datta N and Pridie RB: An outbreak of infection with *Salmonella typhimurium* in a general hospital. J Hyg (Camb) 58:229, 1960.
DeMatteis A and Armani G: *Salmonella typhi* pneumonia without intestinal lesions. J Pathol Bacteriol 94:464, 1967.
Dougan G, Hormaeche CE, and Maskell DJ: Live oral *Salmonella* vaccines: potential use of attenuated strains as carriers of heterologous antigens to the immune system. Parasite Immunol 9:151, 1987.

Forrest BD: The development of bivalent vaccine against diarrhea disease. Southeast Asian Journal of Tropical Medicine & Public Health 19:449, 1988.

Goulder NE, Kingsland MF, and Janeway CA: Salmonella suispestifer infection in Boston. N Engl J Med 226:127, 1942.

Hahne OH: Lung abscess due to *Salmonella typhi*. Am Rev Respir Dis 89:566, 1964.

Hand WL and King NL: Serum opsonization of salmonella in sickle cell anemia. Am J Med 64:388, 1978.

Harvey AM: *Salmonella suispestifer* infection in human beings. Arch Intern Med 59:118, 1937.

Hochadel JF and Keller KF: Protective effects of passively transferred immune T- or B-lymphocytes in mice infected with *Salmonella typhimurium*. J Infect Dis 135:813, 1977.

Hoffman TA, Ruiz CJ, Counts GW et al: Waterborne typhoid fever in Dade County, Florida: clinical and therapeutic evaluations of 105 bacteremic patients. Am J Med 59:481, 1975.

Hook EW: Salmonellosis: certain factors influencing the interaction of salmonella and the human host. Bull NY Acad Med 37:499, 1961.

Hormaeche E, Peluffo CA, and Aleppo PL: Las salmonelas en patologia infantil. Arch Paediat Uruguay 11:8, 1940.

Hornick RB, Greisman SE, Woodward TE et al: Typhoid fever: pathogenesis and immunologic control. N Engl J Med 283:686, 1970.

Human salmonella isolates—U.S., 1980, 1981. Morbid Mortal Wkly Rep 30:377, 1981.

Le Chevalier B, Jehan A, Brun J, and Vergnaud M: Pleuropulmonary localizations of non-typhoid salmonella. Rev Pneumo Clin 41:320, 1985.

Levine MM, Herrington D, Murphy JR et al: Safety, infectivity, immunogenicity, and in vivo stability of two attenuated auxotrohic mutant strains of *Salmonella typhi*, 541. J Clin Invest 79:888, 1987.

Lipson A and Meikle H: Porcine pancreatin as a source of salmonella infection in children with cystic fibrosis. Arch Dis Child 52:562, 1977.

Mohandas V, Cherian T, Sridharan G et al: Immune response of infants and preschool children to typhoid vaccine given intradermally or subcutaneously. Br Med J 298:162, 1989.

Murphy JR, Wasserman SS, Bagar S et al: Immunity to *Salmonella typhi*: considerations relevant to measurement of cellular immunity in typhoid-endemic regions. Clin Exp Immunol 75:228, 1989.

Netter E: Observations on the transmission of salmonellosis in man. Am J Public Health 40:929, 1950.

O'Brien AD, Scher J, Campbell GH et al: Susceptibility of CBA/N mice to infection with *Salmonella typhimurium*: influence of the x-linked gene controlling B-lymphocyte function. J Immunol 123:720, 1979.

Olutola PS and Familusi JB: *Salmonella typhi* pneumonia without gastrointestinal manifestations. Diagn Imaging Clin Med 54:263, 1985.

Robbins JD and Robbins JB: Reexamination of the protective role of the capsular polysaccharide (Vi antigen) of salmonella typhi. J Infect Dis 150:436, 1984.

Rowley D, Turner KJ, and Jenkin CR: The basis for immunity to mouse typhoid III, cell-bound antibody. Aust J Exp Biol Med Sci 42:237, 1964.

Saphra I and Wasserman M: *Salmonella choleraesuis*: clinical and epidemiological evaluation of 329 infections identified between 1940 and 1954 in New York Salmonella Center. Am J Med Sci 228:525, 1954.

Saphra I and Winter JW: Clinical manifestations of salmonellosis in man. An evaluation of 7779 human new infections identified at the New York Salmonella Center. N Engl J Med 256:1128, 1957.

Stuart BM and Pullen RL: Typhoid: clinical analysis of three hundred and sixty cases. Arch Intern Med 78:629, 1946.

Summary of notifiable diseases United States, 1986: U.S., 1986, 1987. Morbid Mortal Wkly Rep 35:3, 1987.

Tacket CO, Ferreccio C, Robbins JB et al: Safety and immunogenicity of two *Salmonella typhi* Vi capsular polysaccharide vaccines. J Infect Dis 154:392, 1986.

Tacket CO, Levine MM, and Robbins JB: Persistence of antibody titres three years after vaccination with Vi polysaccharide vaccine against typhoid fever. Vaccine 4:307, 1988.

Trillat A and Kaneko R: Activité de l'infection par voie aesienne. CR Acad Sci (Paris) 173:109, 1921.

Varela G and Ochoa AA: *Salmonella panama y Escherichia coli* 055 en la garganta de nenes lactantes. Rev Inst Salub Enferm Trop Mex 13:331, 1953.

Varela G and Olarte G: Investigation de salmonellas en las amigdales. Rev Inst Salub Enferm Trop Mex 3:289, 1942.

Zullar LM, Krause HE, and Mufson MA: Microbiologic studies on young infants with lower respiratory tract disease. Am J Dis Child 126:56, 1973.

61

MORTON N. SWARTZ, M.D., and
MARK S. PASTERNACK, M.D.

LEGIONNAIRES' DISEASE AND OTHER RELATED PNEUMONIAS

During the 1970s, a group of sporadic and outbreak-associated pneumonias previously undefined as to etiology were found to be due to infection with several "new" species of bacteria. The first and most important of these species to be identified was *Legionella pneumophila*, the causative agent of legionnaires' disease. Other genetically or phenotypically related organisms subsequently characterized have also been designated as *Legionella* species, and the clinical syndromes (usually pneumonia) they produce have been loosely termed *legionellosis*.

The clinical importance of legionnaires' disease stems from its frequency of occurrence, the difficulty in establishing a diagnosis by conventional bacteriologic techniques (Gram stain and culture of sputum), the specific antimicrobial therapy required (erythromycin), and high mortality if untreated (about 15 per cent). Of the approximately 2.5 million cases of pneumonia occurring annually in the United States, about two thirds can be defined by routine microbiologic techniques and represent the common bacterial pneumonias (Sullivan et al, 1972; Fraser, 1980). The other one third comprises the group of "atypical pneumonias," which usually go undiagnosed as to etiology. The best available estimates indicate that from 2 to 4 per cent (roughly 25,000 cases) of such undiagnosed pneumonias in the United States are cases of legionnaires' disease, representing an approximate incidence of 12 cases per 100,000 population per year (Foy et al, 1979; Helms et al, 1981a).

In the 14 years since its initial recognition in 1976, legionnaires' disease has been described predominantly in middle-aged adults and only rarely in infants and children.

INFECTIONS DUE TO *Legionella pneumophila*

EPIDEMIOLOGY

Legionnaires' disease was brought to the attention of the medical profession and the public dramatically by the outbreak that occurred among persons attending the American Legion Convention in Philadelphia in July 1976. In that outbreak, there were 221 cases: 182 of the victims had attended the convention or had spent some time in the lobby of the headquarters hotel, and the other 39 (cases of "Broad Street pneumonia") had walked on Broad Street, which abuts the main entrance to the hotel (Fraser et al, 1977). Epidemiologic analysis, emphasizing particularly the exposure of individuals in the hotel lobby and on the street adjacent to the lobby, suggested airborne spread of the etiologic agent. A previously undescribed gram-negative bacillus, *L. pneumophila*, was isolated by guinea pig inoculation of lung tissue from several patients with fatal pneumonia (McDade et al, 1977). Although *L. pneumophila* was not isolated from environmental samples, circumstantial evidence suggested that spread of the agent had occurred through the air-circulating system. Once the etiologic agent had been isolated and laboratory cultivation had been achieved, it was possible to develop an indirect fluorescent antibody (IFA) test. Use of this serologic test then provided proof that the microorganism isolated from the inoculated guinea pigs had been responsible for the illness now known as legionnaires disease. Animal (and/or egg) inoculation and fluorescent antibody tests have since proved helpful in the isolation and identification of additional *Legionella* species responsible for still other newer types of pneumonia.

With the use of principally serodiagnostic methods, two rather different types of disease due to *L. pneu-mophila* have been identified: legionnaires' disease, which is an acute pneumonia, and "Pontiac fever," which is a nonpneumonic, self-limited, febrile illness (Glick et al, 1978).

Legionnaires' Disease

The occurrence of legionnaires' disease may take two forms: *common source outbreaks* and *sporadic cases*. Between 1965, when the first known outbreak of legionnaires' disease occurred (Thacker et al, 1978)—diagnosed only retrospectively by serologic means following the epidemic at the American Legion convention—and late 1980, there were 20 identified outbreaks of legionellosis, 18 of legionnaires' disease, and two of Pontiac fever, involving approximately 1100 individuals (Blackmon et al, 1981). Most outbreaks of legionellosis have occurred in the summer months. An outbreak may occur as a sharply circumscribed explosive epidemic, as in Philadelphia in 1976; an ongoing epidemic with a persisting point source, as at the Wadsworth Veterans Administration Medical Center in Los Angeles, where 218 cases were identified between 1977 and 1981 (Meyer, 1983); or a seasonal upswing of cases in a hyperendemic area. Outbreaks have centered in hotels, at conventions, and among travelers; nosocomial outbreaks have been particularly prominent (Blackmon et al, 1981) (Table 61–1). Sites of soil excavation (Thacker et al, 1978) and air-conditioning systems (Dondero et al, 1980), either cooling towers or evaporative condensers (Cordes et al, 1980), have been clearly implicated as the sources of the airborne transmission of the infecting agent in several well-studied outbreaks. *L. pneumophila* has been found in various aqueous environments, such as streams, ponds, and lakes in the United States (Fliermans, 1981), and in water collected from faucets, shower heads, and air-conditioning systems. Although as yet no procedures have proved consistently effective in preventing the spread of *L. pneumophila* from its sources in nature or in preventing legionellosis, outbreaks have been interrupted by shutting down implicated water cooling towers and evaporative condensers (Glick et al, 1978; Dondero et al, 1980), hyperchlorinating potable water and changing shower heads (Tobin et al, 1980; Shands et al, 1981; Fisher-Hoch et al, 1981; Helms et al, 1988), and heating warm tap water to a higher temperature (Fisher-Hoch et al, 1981). Routine decontamination of potential sources of dissemination of *L. pneumophila*, such as cooling towers and evaporative condensers, is an important preventive measure. Water disinfectants, such as a quaternary ammonium compound (didecyldimethyl ammonium chloride) and calcium hypochlorite, are effective in vitro against *L. pneumophila*. Thermally altered lakes appear to provide particularly favorable habitats for the organism during the summer months. There, *L. pneumophila* proliferate intracellularly in protozoa, such as blue-green algae, *Acanthamoeba*, and *Tetrahymena* (Fields et al, 1984).

Table 61-1. SELECTED OUTBREAKS OF LEGIONELLOSIS

Location	Year	Month(s)	Number of Cases	Attack Rate (%)	Site	Source
			Legionnaires' Disease			
Washington, D.C.	1965	July–Aug	81	1.4	Hospital	Excavation
Philadelphia, PA	1974	Sept	11	2.9	Hotel	NE*
Philadelphia, PA	1976	July–Aug	221	4.0	Hotel	NE
Burlington, VT	1977	May–Dec	69†	NE	Community; hospital	NE
Los Angeles, CA	1977–81	Jan–Dec	218	0.5	Hospital	Potable water
Bloomington, IN	1978	Jan–Dec	39	0.1	Hotel–student union	NE
Atlanta, GA	1978	July	8	1.5	Country club	Evaporative condenser
New York, NY	1978	Aug–Sept	38	NE	City garment district	NE
Dallas, TX	1978	Aug–Sept	19	0.5	Convention	NE
Memphis, TN	1978	Aug–Sept	39	0.02–0.34	Hospital	Cooling tower
Jamestown, NY	1979	July	7	0.7	Factory	NE
Eau Claire, WI	1979	June–July	13	0.2	Hotel	Cooling tower
Iowa City, IA	1981	March–Dec	16	3.5	Hospital	Potable water
			"Pontiac Fever"			
Pontiac, MI	1968	July–Aug	144	95	Health department	Evaporative condenser
James River, VA	1973	July–Aug	10	100	Steam turbine	James River

*Not established.
†130 cases by late 1980.

By October 1979, 1005 cases of sporadic legionellosis due to *L. pneumophila* had been reported in the United States (England et al, 1981). Legionnaires' disease pneumonia occurred in 98 per cent of these. Most cases developed in the summer and fall months, but cases did appear all year round. Legionellosis has occurred in practically every state and in many countries around the world. The vast majority of sporadic cases appear to have been community acquired. Outbreak-associated and sporadic cases have features in common: increasing incidence with advancing age, greater risk among males than females, higher incidence in smokers than nonsmokers, prior travel, and exposure to construction and excavation as predisposing circumstances. Similarly, both forms are particularly associated with certain underlying conditions such as chronic bronchitis, cancer, treatment with immunosuppressive drugs, and chronic renal disease.

"Pontiac Fever"

Several outbreaks of this nonpneumonic, "flu-like" illness, characterized by chills, fever, myalgias, headache, cough, and sore throat, have occurred (see Table 61-1): the first among 144 employees and visitors in a health department facility in Pontiac, Michigan (Glick et al, 1978); another among ten workers who had cleaned a steam turbine condenser that was cooled by water circulated through it from the James River in Virginia (Fraser et al, 1979). In both outbreaks, there was an incubation period of about 36 hours (shorter than that in outbreaks of legionnaires' disease), a self-limited course with defervescence in 2 to 5 days, a lack of secondary cases, a lack of mortality, and an extremely high attack rate (95 to 100 per cent) among those exposed. These outbreaks, which occurred before the first identification of legionnaires' disease in 1976, were diagnosed retrospectively by serologic means on stored sera from the afflicted persons. Epidemiologic evidence implicated a faulty air-conditioning system in the Pontiac cases. *L. pneumophila* was subsequently isolated (after its identification in the outbreak at the American Legion convention in 1976) from the frozen, stored lung tissue of sentinel guinea pigs that had been exposed to the Pontiac facility and to aerosols generated from water in its evaporative condenser. Unexplained features of these outbreaks are the very short incubation period (usually associated with an inoculum that is large or has enhanced virulence) and the mild clinical manifestations. Pontiac fever was the clinical picture in 0.14 to 2.0 per cent of the 1005 cases of sporadic legionellosis in the United States (England et al, 1981). However, it is likely that most cases of Pontiac fever are not studied serologically and are ascribed to a viral etiology.

Evidence in the Population of Prior Exposure to *L. pneumophila*

In a control population of 1143 persons older than 45 years of age who lived in various areas of the United States (Atlanta, Washington, D.C., Houston, Rochester, N.Y.) and who were not acutely ill at the time, the overall prevalence of IFA (reciprocal titer of ≥64) was 1.7 per cent (Storch et al, 1979). Titers of ≥128 have been observed in 4 per cent of 116 employees of the Veterans Administration in an office building near Wadsworth Medical Center, in 5.7 per cent of 122 control subjects in a town close to Kingsport, Tennessee, that was the site of an outbreak of legionnaires' disease, and in 15 per cent of 110 volunteer subjects from an industry in Burlington, Vermont, where an outbreak had occurred among hospital patients (Storch et al, 1979). These findings may have reflected antibody prevalence in hyperendemic areas. Analogous seroepidemiologic surveys of unselected pediatric populations have not been reported.

BACTERIOLOGY

L. pneumophila was first isolated by guinea pig inoculation of material from the lungs of four persons who died of legionnaires' disease in the Philadelphia outbreak of 1976. The organism, a slow-growing, gram-negative, non–acid-fast bacillus, did not grow on blood agar plates or other routine bacteriologic media but did grow in the yolk sacs of embryonated eggs; it subsequently was found to grow on Mueller-Hinton agar supplemented with cysteine and hemoglobin (or ferric pyrophosphate) at 35°C (92°F). Buffered charcoal yeast extract (BCYE) agar has proved more helpful in primary isolation of the organism and in its laboratory cultivation (Blackmon et al, 1981). Special media (e.g., CYE–diphasic medium) are useful for isolation of *L. pneumophila* from blood. Isolation from blood can also be accomplished by plating centrifuged, lysed blood on CYE agar. Isolation from sputum and tracheal aspirates, in which normal flora constituents readily overgrow the more slowly growing *L. pneumophila,* is difficult. A selective medium consisting of CYE agar containing the antibiotics vancomycin, anisomycin, and polymyxin B has been developed for primary isolation of the organism from respiratory tract secretions (Edelstein and Finegold, 1979).

L. pneumophila shows little biochemical reactivity and is an obligate aerobe. It has a distinctive pattern of branched-chain fatty acids for a gram-negative bacillus.

There are 25 species in the genus *Legionella.* Fourteen species have been documented by culture to cause human disease (Thacker et al, 1988). The species *L. pneumophila* is comprised of 12 antigenically distinct serogroups; other species consist of one or two serogroups, totalling 41. In the aggregate, all the *L. pneumophila* serogroups account for about 80 per cent of *Legionella* infections (Reingold et al, 1984). *L. pneumophila* serogroup 1 is responsible for 50 per cent of cases of legionnaires' disease. *L. micdadei* (Pittsburgh pneumonia agent) has been implicated in 5 to 10 per cent of cases, and other species *(L. bozemanii, L. dumoffii, L. longbeachae)* (Table 61–2) each account for 2 or 3 per cent of cases.

Although the first isolation of *L. pneumophila* from legionnaires' disease was made in 1976, an atypical agent, initially thought to be a *Rickettsia* (designated OLDA), was isolated in 1947 by guinea pig inoculation from the blood of a laboratory worker with a febrile respiratory illness and has since been shown to belong to the same species (McDade et al, 1979). It seems quite clear that *L. pneumophila* and legionellosis have been around for a long time, antedating the introduction of modern air-conditioning technology.

PATHOGENESIS

The strong association of epidemic legionnaires' disease with environmental foci, such as air-conditioning systems, cooling towers, and soil excavation, has implicated inhalation of aerosolized bacteria as the primary route of infection. This hypothesis has been corroborated experimentally, because inhalation of aerosols containing *L. pneumophila* produced pneumonitis in guinea pigs and monkeys (Baskerville et al, 1981).

L. pneumophila is a facultative intracellular parasite. In tissue culture, the organism replicates exclusively within monocytes (Horwitz and Silverstein, 1980) but multiplies on cell-free complex media as well. The host defense mechanisms so important in other pyogenic infections—opsonization by antibody and complement, phagocytosis by granulocytes and macrophages, and lysis by oxygen-dependent lysosomal process—are ineffective against *L. pneumophila.* The bacilli are not lysed directly in the presence of specific antibody and complement. When opsonized in this fashion, they do adhere to and are phagocytosed by granulocytes and macrophages, yet they are not efficiently killed (Horwitz and Silverstein, 1981a, 1981b).

In the absence of specific antibody, the usual circumstance at initiation of clinical infection, phagocytosis of *L. pneumophila* is mediated by complement receptors on macrophages and monocytes (Payne and Horwitz, 1987). Phagocytosis of *L. pneumophila* by human monocytes, alveolar macrophages, and neutrophils occurs by a novel form of engulfment in which a pseudopod coils around the bacterium ("coiling phagocytosis") (Horwitz, 1984). Whether induction of this coiling phenomenon is a consequence of initial adherence of the organisms to complement receptors is unclear.

Various extracellular products, such as proteases and other hydrolytic enzymes, have been identified in *L. pneumophila* cultures (Meyer, 1983), but their role in the pathogenesis of infection is undefined. A peptide cytolytic toxin of approximately 1300 daltons has been isolated (Friedman et al, 1980). At concentrations that are nontoxic to granulocyte viability or phagocytosis, the cytotoxin interferes with the respiratory burst that normally accompanies phagocytosis (Friedman et al, 1982). Thus oxygen consumption, hexose monophosphate shunt activity, bacterial iodination, and killing of *Escherichia coli* are all inhibited. This effect on the hexose monophosphate shunt is highly selective, because soluble stimulators of this pathway are not inhibited by the cytotoxin (Lochner et al, 1985). This toxin may be important in the striking resistance of *L. pneumophila* to intracellular killing.

The interaction between *L. pneumophila* and macrophages shares key features with other intracellular pathogens, such as *Mycobacterium tuberculosis.* First, phagosomes containing the ingested *L. pneumophila* do not fuse with lysosomes (Horwitz et al, 1983) and

Table 61–2. CLASSIFICATION AND PROPERTIES OF LEGIONELLACEAE

	L. pneumophila	*L. micdadei*	*L. bozemanii*	*L. dumoffi*	*L. gormanii*	*L. longbeachae*
Properties						
Gram stain	−*	−	−	−	−	−
Ziehl-Neelsen stain	−†	−	−	−	−	−
Growth on blood agar	NG‡	NG	NG	NG	NG	NG
Growth on CYE agar§	+	+	+	+	+	+
Fluorescence‖	yellow-green	yellow-green	blue-white	blue-white	blue-white	yellow-green
Oxidase	+	±	−	−	−	weakly +
Catalase	+	+	+	+	+	+
Gelatinase	+	−	+	+	+	+
β-lactamase	+	−	+	+	+	+

*Faintly gram-negative from CYE agar.
†Not acid-fast by routine Ziehl-Neelsen stain from CYE agar.
‡No growth.
§Primary isolation on charcoal yeast extract agar.
‖CYE agar plates examined in the dark with long-wave ultraviolet light (366 nm).

so remain inaccessible to the myeloperoxidase-hydrogen peroxide-halide bactericidal system. Although the organisms are catalase positive, they are not intrinsically resistant to the oxygen-dependent microbicidal system (Locksley et al, 1982). Second, the growth of *L. pneumophila* is inhibited by *activated* macrophages (Horwitz and Silverstein, 1981c) but not by resting macrophages, indicating the importance of T cell-mediated immunity in the control of legionellosis. A possible explanation for this inhibition lies in the observation that interferon gamma-activated monocytes downregulate transferrin receptors and limit the availability of intracellular iron (Byrd and Horwitz, 1989). *L. pneumophila* has a distinct metabolic requirement for iron for extracellular (unable to grow on agar medium without iron supplementation) and, presumably, intracellular growth.

PATHOLOGY

Acute Pulmonary Changes

The gross appearance of the lungs in legionnaires' disease is that of a nodular bronchopneumonia that tends to become confluent (Carrington, 1979; Winn et al, 1979; Blackmon et al, 1981; Winn and Myerowitz, 1981). *Legionella* can also cause lobar pneumonia. The histopathologic findings in legionnaires' disease and in pneumonias due to other *Legionella* species are those of an acute fibrinopurulent pneumonia involving primarily the alveoli and terminal bronchioles. Whereas the alveolar inflammatory response consists of approximately equal numbers of neutrophils and macrophages, sometimes macrophages predominate in the periphery of an area of inflammation. Leukocytoclasis is a distinctive feature. In the majority of rapidly fatal cases, the alveolar and bronchiolar walls have remained intact. In a minority of cases, particularly later in the course of illness, necrosis of alveolar walls and microscopic abscesses occur (Winn and Myerowitz, 1981). Macroscopic abscesses have occasionally developed in fatal cases with extensive pneumonia. In some cases, the abscesses are undoubtedly due to superinfection with common pyogenic bacteria, but in other instances *L. pneumophila* has been demonstrated in the abscess by direct immunofluorescence and has been the only organism isolated on culture from the lesion (Lewin et al, 1979; Venkatachalam et al, 1979). The overall pathologic picture is similar to that of many of the pyogenic pneumonias; it differs considerably from that of pneumonia caused by influenza virus and *Mycoplasma pneumoniae*.

The microscopic pulmonary findings in legionnaires' disease differ from those in the common bacterial pneumonias in the frequent failure to demonstrate the etiologic agent in fixed sections with the usual tissue Gram stains. However, the organism has been demonstrated at times using the Gram stain on touch preparations of lung tissue (Winn and Myerowitz, 1981). The Dieterle stain, a silver impregnation method, has proved the most satisfactory for defining the organism in histologic sections (Chandler et al, 1977); but it is nonspecific, staining many types of bacteria and spirochetes as well. However, the finding of organisms in lung tissue sections that stain with Dieterle stain but fail to stain with tissue Gram stain strongly suggests the presence of a *Legionella* species. Confirmation would be provided by direct fluorescent antibody (DFA) staining of tissue sections.

On Dieterle stain, the organisms are concentrated in the alveoli, particularly within macrophages. Organisms are also found in the interstitial tissue in many patients, particularly those who have been immunosuppressed.

Pathologic Pulmonary Sequelae

Surgical and autopsy specimens from a group of well-documented cases of legionnaires' disease examined more than 2 weeks after the onset of the illness have shown intra-alveolar and interstitial fibrosis, changes seen in organizing pneumonias due to various etiologies (Blackmon et al, 1979; Winn and Myerowitz, 1981).

Pathologic Evidence of Extrapulmonary Involvement

Contiguous spread of *L. pneumophila* within the thorax to the pleural and pericardial spaces has been documented by DFA and direct isolation of the organism (Mayock et al, 1983; Kugler et al, 1983). Dissemination of *L. pneumophila* from the lung in at least a few cases has been indicated by the occurrence of bacteremia (Edelstein et al, 1979) and the demonstration of scattered organisms by DFA in lymph nodes, liver (Watts et al, 1980), kidney (Dorman et al, 1980), bone marrow (Weisenburger et al, 1980), spleen, heart (White et al, 1980), and brain (Cutz et al, 1982). In the liver and spleen, the bacilli were associated with cells of the reticuloendothelial system (Evans and Winn, 1981). In most instances, inflammatory reactions were absent in organs in which organisms were found.

CLINICAL FEATURES OF LEGIONNAIRES' DISEASE

Clinical Setting

Various factors appear to predispose an individual to the development of legionnaires' disease. These have been defined from studies of the Philadelphia and other outbreaks (Fraser et al, 1977; Blackmon et al, 1981), from review of the first 1000 sporadic cases of legionnaires' disease in the United States (England et al, 1981), and from evaluation of nosocomial (both epidemic and sporadic) legionellosis (England and Fraser, 1981). Risk factors in adults include smoking, alcohol consumption, chronic bronchitis or emphysema, renal failure and renal transplantation, cancer, and treatment with immunosuppressive drugs. Also males are more likely than females to contract legionnaires' disease.

Legionnaires' disease has been implicated by seroconversion to be responsible for only a small fraction of sporadic cases of pneumonia in otherwise normal infants and children, generally 0 to 1 per cent (Anderson et al, 1981; Muldoon et al, 1981; Orenstein et al, 1981), but a rate of 7 per cent was reported in a single small series (Fumarola et al, 1983). However, it has also been reported in association with trisomy 21 (Sturm et al, 1981), severe combined immunodeficiency (Cutz et al, 1982), chronic granulomatous disease (Peerless et al, 1985), steroid therapy (Cohen et al, 1979; Joly et al, 1986), acute lymphocytic leukemia (during induction chemotherapy [Gutzeit et al, 1986], relapse [Kovatch et al, 1984], remission [Ryan et al, 1979], as well as following bone marrow transplantation [Kugler et al, 1983]). In addition, children with chronic pulmonary disease such as cystic fibrosis (Katz and Holsclaw, 1982) and bronchial asthma (Beer et al, 1985) have had an increased prevalence of seropositivity to *Legionella* species by IFA compared to age-matched controls. Some controversy exists, however, as to whether such results reflect bona fide exposure to legionnella, or artifactual serologic cross-reactivity (Wang et al, 1987).

Age of Patients

Legionnaires' disease has occurred in individuals from 4.5 months of age (Fuchs et al, 1986) to the ninth decade of life. Increasing age is associated with a higher risk, and the highest risk is among persons 50 years of age and older (England et al, 1981). Only a small number of cases of legionnaires' disease have been reported in children. In the 1976 outbreak at the American Legion convention, one of the patients was a 3-year old child (Fraser et al, 1977). According to the summary of the first 1005 cases of sporadic legionellosis reported to the Centers for Disease Control (CDC), a total of ten cases occurred in persons 16 years old or younger (England et al, 1981). In a serologic survey (employing acute-phase and convalescent-phase serums) of 170 Iowa children and adolescents (0 to 19 years of age) with clinical diagnoses of pneumonia, four (2.4 per cent) had legionnaires' disease as judged by a fourfold or greater rise in IFA titer to 1:128 or higher (Renner et al, 1979). The youngest patient in this series was 5 years of age. In a study of pneumonia occurring in patients in a prepaid medical group practice in Seattle, no cases of legionnaires' disease were identified by a fourfold or higher titer rise among 167 patients (0 to 19 years of age) with pneumonia (Foy et al, 1979).

Serologic surveys of children with acute respiratory disease in other locations have had similar results. In Chicago, one of 23 pneumonia patients with paired serums available for analysis demonstrated an eightfold IFA titer rise to 1:2048, and in addition, an 11-month-old infant with bronchiolitis had an eightfold IFA titer rise to 1:128 (Muldoon et al, 1981). In Denver, no diagnostic seroconversions were observed among 52 children younger than 4 years of age with acute lower respiratory tract disease (Anderson et al, 1981). Among 110 children hospitalized with pneumonia (with paired serums available) in Los Angeles, only one diagnostic seroconversion occurred (Orenstein et al, 1981). A second child was reported as a possible case, with an acute IFA titer of 1:512 and a repeat titer of 1:128 drawn 8 months later.

The analysis of acute-phase serums in the incidence studies reported previously provide information regarding the prevalence of prior legionellosis. In a prospective evaluation of the incidence of legionnaires' disease among 191 children (age 6 days to 17 years) hospitalized in Los Angeles in 1979, 11 (5.7 per cent) had evidence of legionellosis (at some time) as judged by at least one reciprocal serum titer (IFA) of ≥ 128 (Orenstein et al, 1981). Despite the absence of documented acute *Legionella* pneumonia, annual follow-up testing of the Denver cohort revealed that 27 (52 per cent) of the 52 children had fourfold or greater rises of reciprocal IFA titers to ≥ 128.

On the basis of available clinical and epidemiologic

information, it appears that legionnaires' disease is not a common cause of pneumonia in children, at least not in Denver (Anderson et al, 1981), Chicago (Muldoon et al, 1981), Seattle (Foy et al, 1979), and Los Angeles (Orenstein et al, 1981). The high percentage of children in these three investigations with reciprocal IFA titers ≥ 128 (52, 30, 17, and 5.7 per cent, respectively) suggests that although legionnaires' disease is uncommon at this age, exposure to *L. pneumophila* with ensuing subclinical infection (or Pontiac fever) is not at all unusual. At present, one is unable to exclude the possibility that some of these serologic findings in population studies represent cross-reacting antibodies to other infectious agents.

Incubation Period

The incubation period of legionellosis is definable only on the basis of observations of outbreaks. The incubation period for legionnaires' disease ranges from 2 to 10 days, whereas that for Pontiac fever is about 36 hours (Glick et al, 1978; Fraser et al, 1979).

Prodrome

A nonspecific premonitory 24-hour "flu-like" illness consisting of fever (38–39°C [100.5–102.2° F]), malaise, anorexia, myalgias, and headache (with or without a dry cough) occurred commonly in the outbreak at the American Legion convention (Fraser et al, 1977; Tsai et al, 1979) and has often been observed in the group of patients described from the Wadsworth V.A. Hospital in Los Angeles (Kirby et al, 1978; Helms et al, 1984). In many other patients, the onset is more abrupt and without a distinct prodrome; in some nosocomial infections, the manifestations of the underlying illness may obscure the early nonspecific features of superimposed legionnaires' disease. Sore throat and coryza are rare.

Symptoms

The clinical features of the sporadic and epidemic forms of legionnaires' disease are very similar. Within 1 or 2 days of onset the patient is acutely ill, with high fever, usually over 39.4°C (103°F), repeated chills, nausea, vomiting, and nonproductive or minimally productive cough. Watery diarrhea without mucus, blood, or abdominal pain occurs in 40 to 55 per cent of patients, usually within the first 3 or 4 days of illness (Kirby et al, 1978, Tsai et al, 1979; Keys, 1980). Lethargy, unsteadiness, slurring of speech, confusion, and delirium (manifestations of toxic encephalopathy) are present in some patients and may initially suggest primary involvement of the nervous system. These changes are out of proportion to the extent of any hypoxia or metabolic derangements. Pleuritic chest pain develops in 15 to 40 per cent of patients (Kirby et al, 1978; Tsai et al, 1979; Keys, 1980). As the disease progresses, rigors continue, and pulmonary manifestations, such as dys-

pnea (50 per cent) and sputum production (50 per cent), become evident. The sputum produced is usually scanty and nonpurulent but sometimes is purulent (20 to 40 per cent) or bloody (37 per cent) (Kirby et al, 1978; Tsai et al, 1979). Extrapulmonic symptoms, especially those involving the gastrointestinal tract (particularly diarrhea) and central nervous system, are often prominent (Lees and Tyrell, 1978; Shetty et al, 1980; Brenner et al, 1981; Helms et al, 1984) and are more frequent among patients with legionnaires' disease than among patients with other pneumonias (Sharrar et al, 1979; Tsai et al, 1979; Kirby et al, 1980).

Signs

Patients commonly appear acutely ill. In many, fever reaches 40.5°C (105°F) or higher at the peak of illness. Kirby and associates (1978) observed relative bradycardia in the majority of patients in their series. Tachypnea and dyspnea vary with the extent of pulmonary consolidation and the height of fever. The major findings are in the lungs. Localized or diffuse medium inspiratory rales and rhonchi are noted on the second or third day of illness. In some patients, lobar consolidation can subsequently be detected.

Unusual Signs. Pretibial rash, in the form of tender macular erythema, is a very rare finding in legionnaires' disease (Helms et al, 1981b). In the original outbreak of Pontiac fever, 6 per cent of patients reported a rash, but its nature was not described (Glick et al, 1978). The occurrence of rash is of some interest because a related *Legionella* species (*L. micdadei*) has been implicated retrospectively in an epidemic of so-called pretibial fever, a febrile illness with an erythema nodosum-like rash (Hebert et al, 1980).

Obtundation, headache, and confusion are common features suggesting neurologic involvement in legionnaires' disease. Occasional instances of cerebellar involvement (ataxia, dysarthria, dysmetria), focal deficits, and seizures have occurred (Shetty et al, 1980; Johnson et al, 1984).

Laboratory Findings

A leukocytosis of 14,000 to 24,000 cells/mm³ with a shift to the left is present in most patients. Gram-stained smears of sputum are not remarkable, and smears of transtracheal aspirates show few neutrophils or bacteria. Hyponatremia has been noted in the majority of patients in one series (Kirby et al, 1978) but has not been observed as frequently in others. Mild abnormalities of liver function (elevated levels of glutamic-oxalacetic transaminase, lactic dehydrogenase, alkaline phosphatase, and serum bilirubin) are noted in about 40 per cent of patients. Urinary abnormalities (marked albuminuria, microscopic hematuria, pyuria) have been observed in some patients. Renal insufficiency or frank renal failure was observed in about 15 per cent of patients in the 1976 Philadelphia outbreak (Tsai et al, 1979). In some patients, renal failure was a consequence of shock, and in others it was observed before the development of shock and in the absence of therapy with nephrotoxic antibiotics (Tsai et al, 1979; Williams et al, 1980). Renal failure has also been observed in association with elevation of serum creatinine phosphokinase level, acute rhabdomyolysis, and myoglobinuria (Friedman, 1978; Posner et al, 1980).

When levels of serum and urine electrolytes and osmolalities were measured in several patients, they were found to be consistent with inappropriate secretion of antidiuretic hormone. This occurs in other types of pneumonia as well. Hypophosphatemia (≤ 2.5 mg/dl) was observed in the majority of patients at one institution (Kirby et al, 1978) but has not been a general finding. The explanation for this observation is unclear, but several suggestions have been offered: (1) hypophosphatemia is associated with bacteremia due to gram-negative bacilli, and bacteremia has been demonstrated to occur in legionnaires' disease; (2) hypophosphatemia occurs with respiratory alkalosis; and (3) hypophosphatemia occurs in chronic alcoholism.

The cerebrospinal fluid has been abnormal in some of the patients with legionnaires' disease who have had lumbar punctures. In about 20 per cent, a pleocytosis was observed, neutrophilic in about one third and mononuclear (or mixed) in the remainder (Johnson et al, 1984). The pleocytosis has been of a minor degree but in one instance reached 874 neutrophils/mm³.

Summary of Evidence for Extrapulmonary Involvement

The prominent clinical findings relating to the central nervous system and gastrointestinal tract, the occasional early development of acute rhabdomyolysis, and the laboratory abnormalities suggesting mild hepatic damage and varying degrees of renal damage are indicative of extrapulmonary involvement. A putative toxin produced by *L. pneumophila* has been invoked to account for such disparate effects. However, the occurrence of *L. pneumophila* bacteremia (documented in at least six patients) in the course of legionnaires' disease, along with the demonstration by DFA of the organism in liver, kidney, spleen, and myocardium in fatal cases, provides another possible explanation for some of the systemic findings (Meyer et al, 1980; Blackmon et al, 1981).

Clinically significant extrapulmonary focal infection occasionally complicates *Legionella* pneumonitis. In addition to the development of pleural space infection, *L. pneumophila* pericarditis with tamponade has been observed in a patient with legionnaires' disease (Mayock et al, 1983). Extrathoracic infections reported in conjunction with legionnaires' disease have included pyelonephritis (Dorman et al, 1980), defined at autopsy with cortical abscesses and acute tubulointerstitial nephritis; hemodialysis fistula infections with local inflammation and purulent collections (Kalweit et al, 1982); cutaneous abscess due to *L. micdadei* (Ampel et al, 1985); and perirectal abscess containing mixed flora including *L. pneumophila* serogroup 3 (Arnow et al, 1983).

Legionella has also been implicated in focal infections developing in the absence of pulmonary disease. Prosthetic valve endocarditis due to *L. pneumophila* and *L. dumoffii* has been reported in seven patients (Tompkins et al, 1988). These patients presented with a chronic illness 3 to 19 months after valve replacement, which included fever, night sweats, malaise, weight loss, mild congestive heart failure, and anemia without emboli or immune complex disease. *Legionella* infection was confirmed by valve, wound, or blood culture, as well as by high antibody titers to *L. pneumophila*. A case of *L. pneumophila* pericarditis (in the absence of pneumonia) was diagnosed serologically (Nelson et al, 1985). *L. pneumophila* has also been recovered from a wound, together with *Pseudomonas aeruginosa*, in a patient undergoing physical therapy in a Hubbard tank (Brabender et al, 1983).

RADIOLOGIC FEATURES

The principal radiologic changes in *L. pneumophila* pneumonia consist of patchy bronchopneumonic infiltrates, poorly marginated rounded opacities located either centrally or adjacent to pleural surfaces, lobar consolidation, or perihilar densities (Dietrich et al, 1978) (Fig. 61–1). The process commonly begins as patchy alveolar infiltrates involving one lobe, more

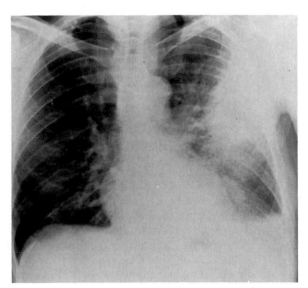

Figure 61–1. A chest roentgenogram of a 50-year-old man with fatal legionnaires' disease complicating aplastic anemia. There are a dense pleural-based consolidation in the left upper lobe and an ovoid area of consolidation in the left lower lobe adjacent to the cardiac apex. A left pleural effusion is present. The pneumonia rapidly progressed to involve most of the left lung and the right upper lobe. The indirect fluorescent antibody (IFA) titer for *Legionella pneumophila* rose from 1:64 to $\geq$ 1:1024. (Courtesy of Dr. P Stark.)

commonly a lower lobe, and then progresses, if untreated, to lobar or multilobar consolidation. At the peak of illness, when the radiologic changes are most marked, bilateral involvement and lobar consolidation are the most common findings. Pleural effusions occur in association with pulmonary infiltrates in up to one third of patients, but they are not usually extensive or prominent features. Rarely, a small pleural effusion is the first change noted on chest radiographs. Radiologic evidence of hilar adenopathy has been observed occasionally in association with pulmonary lesions. Progression of consolidation to cavitation, evident on radiologic or biopsy findings, has been observed in a small number of patients (Gump et al, 1979; Saravolatz, 1979; Keys, 1980; Edelstein et al, 1981). This progression has been the result either of a simultaneous infection (or superinfection) with a pyogenic organism or of tissue necrosis due to *L. pneumophila* itself. In the latter category, 27 cases of *L. pneumophila* lung abscess have been reported (Senécal et al, 1987). In most instances, this complication has occurred in nosocomial legionnaires' disease, predominantly in transplant recipients and in patients with systemic lupus erythematosus receiving corticosteroids, sometimes in combination with cytotoxic drugs.

DIAGNOSIS

Laboratory Methods

Differentiation on clinical grounds of sporadic cases of *L. pneumophila* pneumonia from other types of community-acquired and nosocomial pneumonias is difficult at best. Proper management requires the skilled use of appropriate serologic, staining (DFA), and culture techniques.

Culture of *L. pneumophila* from Clinical Specimens. The most sensitive and specific method for diagnosis of *Legionella* pneumonia is isolation of *L. pneumophila* from tracheal aspirates, sputum, pleural fluid, or lung biopsy specimens on BCYE agar. Isolation of *L. pneumophila* was possible within 3 to 7 days in 13 of 21 patients with legionnaires' disease (Edelstein et al, 1980). Isolation of *L. pneumophila* from blood cultures requires special media (Edelstein et al, 1979; Blackmon et al, 1981) or the use of lysis-centrifugation techniques. Properties of isolates (see Table 61–2) provide a provisional identification of *L. pneumophila*. For more definitive identification of an isolate, DFA staining or slide agglutination (by group-specific antibody) may be employed. Identification of an isolate as *Legionella* can be accomplished by using a commercially available DNA gene probe (containing ^{125}I-labeled complementary DNA, cDNA, to *Legionella* ribosomal RNA). As yet, the sensitivity of this DNA probe is not sufficient for reliable, direct diagnosis on specimens such as tracheal aspirates.

Direct Immunofluorescent Examination of Respiratory Secretions. Sputum or transtracheal aspirate specimens from patients with legionnaires' disease are usually thin and mucoid; as many as 25 per cent may be bloody. Gram-stained smears usually show only a few polymorphonuclear leukocytes, and *L. pneumophila* cannot be identified.

Direct immunofluorescent staining (Fig. 61–2) of clinical specimens can be performed rapidly and with high specificity (99 per cent), but sensitivity is low (25 to 80 per cent) compared with culture. The CDC no longer makes polyvalent antiserums available. Commercial products (polyclonal pooled conjugates) for *L. pneumophila* serogroups 1 through 6 and *L. micdadei* are available. Monoclonal antibodies with serogroup specificities have been produced. A species-specific monoclonal antibody recognizing an outer membrane protein of *L. pneumophila* serogroups 1 through 10 but not reacting with other *Legionella* species has been developed (Gosting et al, 1984).

With direct immunofluorescent staining of appropriate clinical specimens, cross-reactions are rarely noted, usually with *Pseudomonas* species, *Bacteroides fragilis*, and *E. coli*.

Serodiagnosis. The usual means to establish a diagnosis of legionnaires' disease has been the IFA test. A fourfold or greater reciprocal serum titer rise to ≥128 in patients with an appropriate illness is acceptable evidence of legionellosis. Three to 4 weeks

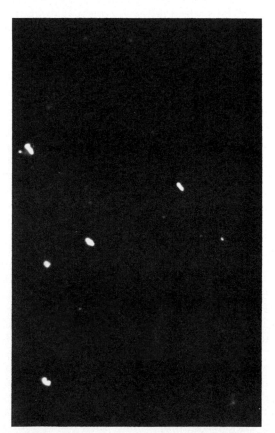

Figure 61–2. A lung biopsy specimen from a patient with legionnaires' disease stained using the direct fluorescent antibody technique. The bacilli are stained with fluorescent antibody to *Legionella pneumophila* and appear white. (Courtesy of the Bacteriology Laboratory of Massachusetts General Hospital.)

(sometimes as long as 6 weeks) are needed from the onset of illness until maximum antibody levels are achieved. Thus this method provides a diagnosis in retrospect rather than at the time of clinical presentation, when therapeutic decisions must be made. Furthermore, only 50 to 75 per cent of patients with epidemiologically or culturally confirmed legionnaires' disease have shown seroconversion. (McDade et al, 1977; Edelstein et al, 1980). A single reciprocal titer of ≥256 in the course of a compatible illness has been used as evidence for a presumptive diagnosis of legionnaires' disease. However, in hyperendemic areas for legionellosis such titers may reflect prior exposure to the microorganism rather than a current episode of legionnaires' disease. Twelve serogroups of *L. pneumophila* have been identified thus far, and they possess serogroup-specific as well as common antigens. Testing against all serogroups is necessary to identify all seroconverters, but this testing is not done currently even in large reference laboratories. Other serologic tests have been developed, such as enzyme-linked immunosorbent assay (ELISA) and microagglutination.

Cross-reactive antigens with other respiratory pathogens are rare. Occasional titer rises against *M. pneumoniae* have been observed in serums of patients with epidemic or sporadic legionnaires' disease and might represent simultaneous or secondary infections with these microorganisms (Blackmon et al, 1981). Rarely, unidirectional cross-reacting antibody developing during the course of legionnaires' disease has suggested a diagnosis of psittacosis until the IFA titer rise to *L. pneumophila* was observed to be substantially higher.

Antigen Detection. Antigenuria can be detected in patients with legionnaires' disease by ELISA or by solid-phase radioimmunoassay (Kohler et al, 1984). Specific serogroup 1 *L. pneumophila* antigen was detected in the urine of 14 of 16 patients (88 per cent) with legionnaires' disease during the first 3 days of symptomatic illness, and antigenuria persisted for at least 42 days. A radioimmunoassay and a newer latex particle agglutination test are commercially available.

Differential Diagnosis

The diagnosis should be strongly suspected in a patient who has high fever, recurring chills, a nonproductive cough, and a patchy bronchopneumonic infiltrate that has advanced to lobar consolidation, and whose sputum or transtracheal aspirate shows few, if any, neutrophils and no bacteria on Gram-stained smear. The diagnosis is even more likely in an individual who is immunosuppressed or smokes, or when the illness occurs during an outbreak of pneumonia (particularly in hospitals or among patients on hemodialysis) during the summer months. Extrapulmonary manifestations, in particular toxic encephalopathy, early unexplained renal failure, and diarrhea, may provide clues as to diagnosis, as may failure to respond to treatment with potent beta-lactam and aminoglycoside antibiotics. Recurring chills over several days in a patient who has lobar consolidation and whose respiratory secretions fail to indicate a bacterial pathogen is suggestive of legionnaires' disease. Although rigors are a feature of pneumococcal lobar pneumonia, they usually occur early in the disease; recurrent chills are uncommon in pneumococcal pneumonia unless a complication such as consolidation of another lobe, empyema, or endocarditis rapidly ensues.

Legionnaires' disease, especially in its early stages when there is little if any sputum production, closely resembles other types of "atypical" pneumonia. These include *M. pneumoniae* pneumonia particularly, psittacosis, tularemia, Q fever, and viral (influenza, parainfluenza, respiratory syncytial viruses, and adenovirus) pneumonias. Exposure to birds, to cattle or sheep, and to rabbits provides clues as to the diagnosis of psittacosis, Q fever, and tularemia, respectively. Antecedent upper respiratory symptoms would suggest viral or *mycoplasma* pneumonia rather than legionnaires' disease. Although the picture of toxic encephalopathy is sometimes prominent with legionellosis, it should be emphasized that confusion, delirium, and obtundation may be observed with influenza and *M. pneumoniae* infections and may be a consequence of hypoxia secondary to various pulmonary processes. The radiologic appearance of legionnaires' disease is not sufficiently distinctive to provide an etiologic diagnosis.

Difficult diagnostic problems may be presented by occasional patients with dual pulmonary infections, either mixed or sequential, involving *L. pneumophila* and other bacterial pathogens. In mixed infections with *Streptococcus pneumoniae* or *Klebsiella pneumoniae*, the more common microorganism has usually been identified first on Gram-stained smears or culture and has been the target for antimicrobial therapy (Kirby et al, 1980; Meyer et al, 1980). After initial improvement, clinical and radiologic worsening has led to reevaluation and demonstration of concurrent *L. pneumophila* infection. Superinfection with gram-negative bacilli has also occasionally complicated the course of legionnaires' disease.

TREATMENT

Recommendations for antimicrobial therapy of *L. pneumophila* pneumonia are derived from results of treatment of patients who became ill in the 1976 Philadelphia outbreak, from laboratory susceptibility test results, and from later clinical experience in the treatment of legionnaires' disease with erythromycin. Data from controlled comparative clinical trials involving different antibiotics are not available. Retrospective study of the outcome of cases occurring during the 1976 outbreak indicated that a lower mortality rate occurred among those patients treated with erythromycin or tetracycline than among those receiving cephalothin, aminoglycosides, penicillins, or chloramphenicol (Fraser et al, 1977). Subsequent clinical experience indicates that erythromycin is the drug of choice and is preferable to tetracycline, but a direct comparison of these two agents has not been made (Keys, 1980; Kirby et al, 1980).

Susceptibility testing of *L. pneumophila* has been determined in vitro (Table 61–3) and in protection tests of embryonated eggs and guinea pigs experimentally infected with the microorganism. On in vitro testing, erythromycin and rifampin are the most active agents. Although *L. pneumophila* is susceptible to gentamicin in vitro, *L. pneumophila* pneumonia does not respond to this antibiotic, perhaps because of the intracellular location of the bacteria and the failure of the aminoglycoside to penetrate tissue cells. *L. pneumophila* produces a beta-lactamase and is resistant to penicillin and ampicillin but shows susceptibility in vitro to low concentrations of cefoxitin. Tetracycline and its congeners appear to be inactivated by CYE agar and cannot be tested satisfactorily under these conditions. Testing of this drug's effects by Thornsberry and co-workers (1978) using supplemented Mueller-Hinton agar indicated that the minimal inhibitory concentration (MIC) for *L. pneumophila* of tetracycline was 5.2 μg/ml, whereas the MICs of erythromycin and rifampin were 0.18 and .01 μg/ml, respectively. When tested for effectiveness in preventing death of embryonated eggs inoculated with *L. pneumophila*, rifampin and erythromycin were much better than ampicillin, cephalothin, and oxytetracycline (Lewis et al, 1978). In a guinea pig model of legionnaires' disease produced by intratracheal inoculation of *L. pneumophila*, erythromycin, rifampin, doxycycline, and trimethoprim-sulfamethoxazole significantly reduced fatality rates (Edelstein et al, 1984). With rifampin, a distinctly higher rate of bacterial killing was observed. The quinolones ofloxacin and ciprofloxacin have been found to be active against *L. pneumophila*. In vitro and in the guinea pig model of *L. pneumophila* pneumonia, the activity of these quinolones appeared to be between that of rifampin and of erythromycin (Saito et al, 1986).

Erythromycin has been widely used in, and is the drug of choice for, the treatment of legionnaires' disease. The usual dose of erythromycin is 0.5 g either orally or intravenously every 6 hours for adults; the intravenous route is preferable for sicker patients or when adequate absorption via the oral route is uncertain. Erythromycin should be given at higher doses, 1.0 g intravenously every 6 hours, in adults who are more seriously ill or who fail to respond to the lower dose. Erythromycin, 50 mg/kg/day orally in four divided doses, has been successful in treatment of a 3-year-old child with *L. pneumophila* pneumonia (Sturm et al, 1981). Most patients respond with defervescence and general improvement within a few days (sometimes within 24 to 48 hours) of starting erythromycin therapy. Despite a prompt clinical response, relapse may occur if treatment is discontinued after 4 or 5 days without fever. Treatment should be continued for a minimum of 2 weeks, preferably for 3 weeks.

Rifampin, 600 mg/day orally in adults, has generally been used in combination with erythromycin in treatment of more severe cases of legionnaires' disease, particularly in immunologically compromised adults, or in patients in whom the response to initial therapy with erythromycin has been unsatisfactory. Rifampin is not used alone in the treatment of *L. pneumophila* pneumonia because of the rapid emergence of resistance of many bacterial species to this antimicrobial agent. Experience with quinolones has been limited to a few patients in whom its use has been in combination with erythromycin or rifampin. Thus its clinical efficacy cannot yet be evaluated.

COURSE AND PROGNOSIS

Infection with *L. pneumophila* may produce (1) asymptomatic seroconversion, (2) a benign self-limited illness without pneumonia, or (3) a moderately severe, even life-threatening pneumonia. The former two processes have not been associated with mortality, whereas the latter (legionnaires' disease) has had a significant case-fatality rate, particularly if untreated or inappropriately treated. In the 1976 outbreak in Philadelphia, the case-fatality rate was 15 per cent (Fraser et al, 1977). Nineteen per cent of the first 1005 reported cases of sporadic legionellosis were fatal (England et al, 1981). The case-fatality rate differs depending on the antibiotic treatment employed. In the 1976 Philadelphia outbreak, the rate was highest in those patients receiving cephalothin (48 per cent), intermediate in those receiving aminoglycosides (36 per cent) and ampicillin (24 per cent), and lowest in those receiving erythromycin (11 per cent). The overall case-fatality rate in the 65 nosocomially acquired cases reported from the Wadsworth V.A. Hospital in Los Angeles was 25 per cent (Kirby et al, 1980). In the Wadsworth V.A. Hospital

Table 61–3. IN VITRO ANTIBIOTIC SUSCEPTIBILITY OF *Legionella pneumophila*

Antimicrobial Agent	Minimum Inhibitory Concentration (MIC)* (μg/ml)
Penicillin	12.5
Ampicillin	3.5
Cephalothin	32.0
Cefazolin	73.5
Cefamandole	27.9
Cefoxitin	2.0
Gentamicin	0.3
Amikacin	0.5
Chloramphenicol	0.5
Trimethoprim	3.5
Erythromycin	0.1
Rifampin	0.1

*Geometric mean MIC of five clinical isolates on CYE agar after 72-hour incubation.

(Modified from Edelstein PH and Meyer RD: Susceptibility of *Legionella pneumophila* to twenty antimicrobial agents. Antimicrob Agents Chemother 18:403, 1980.)

group, both treatment with erythromycin and the use of immunosuppressive therapy (corticosteroids, cytotoxic drugs) influenced mortality rates. Among patients receiving erythromycin, the mortality rate was 13 per cent, in contrast to 55 per cent in those who had not received the antibiotic. Furthermore, among those patients who both were immunosuppressed and did not receive erythromycin, the mortality rate was 80 per cent. Among 87 cases of *L. pneumophila* pneumonia in Iowa between 1970 and 1980, the mortality rate was much higher among nosocomial infections (70 per cent) than in community-acquired infections (22 per cent) (Helms et al, 1984). Similarly, the mortality rate of patients treated with erythromycin (6 per cent) was much lower than the mortality rate of those who received penicillin (36 per cent) or a cephalosporin (32 per cent).

Although clinical improvement is usually evident within 2 to 3 days of initiation of erythromycin therapy, radiologic progression often continues for up to 5 days after starting treatment. Definite improvement in radiographic findings occurs within 2 weeks, and complete resolution occurs in 6 weeks to several months.

In addition to the severe forms of legionnaires' disease with high attendant mortality, milder forms exist. In the 1976 Philadelphia outbreak, 20 per cent of the patients were ambulatory (Sharrar et al, 1979). The clinical picture in such patients resembled that of *M. pneumoniae* pneumonia. In most patients with legionnaires' disease in that outbreak, the illness progressed over 2 or 3 days. In those who survived, the fever became remittent and subsided by lysis. Defervescence occurred about 4 days after instituting therapy with antibiotics that are now known to be ineffective, suggesting that the "untreated" course of mild illness may have a duration of about 8 days. However, the course of untreated legionnaires' disease in previously healthy individuals may sometimes be protracted.

INFECTIONS DUE TO OTHER *LEGIONELLA* SPECIES

Pittsburgh Pneumonia (Pneumonia Due to L. micdadei)

Clinical Features. Pittsburgh pneumonia, a pulmonary infection due to *L. micdadei*, was first identified in 1979 (Myerowitz et al, 1979; Rogers et al, 1979; Aronson et al, 1981; Winn and Myerowitz, 1981). It accounts for about 6 per cent of *Legionella* infections in the United States (Reingold et al, 1984). Patients who develop this form of pneumonia are almost always hospitalized patients, usually immunosuppressed or chronically ill, and frequently renal transplant recipients (Muder et al, 1983a). The clinical presentation is very similar to that of legionnaires' disease in the nosocomial setting. Patients with Pittsburgh pneumonia tend to be more compromised

than patients with legionnaires' disease: more immunosuppression, more surgery, and longer hospitalization before the onset of pneumonia. Dual infection with both *L. micdadei* and *L. pneumophila* have occurred in seven patients at one hospital (Muder et al, 1983b).

The radiologic findings are either patchy bronchopneumonic infiltrates in the middle or lower lung fields, circumscribed gross nodular infiltrates, or unilateral perihilar edema. Pulmonary cavitation has occurred in up to 20 per cent of cases.

The clinical course of surviving patients has been that of slow defervescence and even slower clearing of the radiologic abnormalities. In fatal cases, complications have included acute renal failure, disseminated intravascular coagulation, adult respiratory distress syndrome, and superinfection with pyogenic gram-negative bacilli. The case-fatality rate has been 12 to 40 per cent.

Erythromycin, rifampin, doxycycline, and trimethoprim-sulfamethoxazole are effective in reducing mortality in a guinea pig model of *L. micdadei* pneumonia (Pasculle et al, 1985). Erythromycin is effective therapy for *L. micdadei* pneumonia in humans (Muder et al, 1983b). A combination of trimethoprim-sulfamethoxazole and rifampin has been successful in two patients with *L. micdadei* pneumonia who failed to respond to erythromycin plus rifampin therapy (Rudin and Wing, 1984). Recovery is usually slow, with radiologic resolution taking at least several weeks. Recovery may be associated with organizing pneumonitis.

Pathology. The gross features are those of a patchy, hemorrhagic, lobular pneumonia, commonly involving peripheral areas of the lung (Winn and Myerowitz, 1981). Extension to a lobar distribution occasionally occurs. Necrosis of the center of consolidated areas is common. The acute intra-alveolar infiltrate predominantly consists of polymorphonuclear leukocytes with a variable admixture of alveolar macrophages. Numerous bacilli (demonstrated by Dieterle silver stain) are present, particularly within both polymorphonuclear leukocytes and macrophages.

Epidemiology. *L. micdadei* appears to share a common environmental niche with *L. pneumophila*. It has been detected in the water distribution system of a hospital with an endemic problem of *L. pneumophila* and *L. micdadei* infections (Muder et al, 1983a). It has been isolated from reservoirs of ultrasonic nebulizers used in hospitals and from shower heads.

Bacteriology. The microbiologic properties of *L. micdadei* are summarized in Table 61–2. Although phenotypically related and producing similar pneumonias, *L. micdadei* and *L. pneumophila* are genetically unrelated, as shown by DNA hybridization studies (Hebert et al, 1980).

Diagnosis. *L. micdadei*, unlike other *Legionella* species, sometimes stain with modified acid-fast stains applied to lung imprints and as faintly gram-negative bacilli on Gram stain. In the sputum of one patient with *L. micdadei* pneumonia, Kinyoun carbolfuchsin stain showed many acid-fast bacilli that reacted specifically with fluorescent antibody to *L. micdadei* (Hilton et al, 1986). In tissue sections, the organisms stain well with Dieterle silver stain and frequently stain with modified tissue acid-fast stains.

L. micdadei can be isolated from sputum on buffered CYE agar containing antibiotics (vancomycin, anisomycin, polymyxin) that inhibit contaminating flora. When nosocomial outbreaks involving both *L. pneumophila* and *L. micdadei* have occurred, dyes (bromthymol blue and bromcresol purple) have been added to selective media to provide presumptive visual identification of the two species in clinical and environmental specimens (Muder et al, 1983a).

Direct fluorescent antibody staining with specific antibody is useful for identification of *L. micdadei* in smears and tissue. Serologic evidence of infection can be provided by demonstration of seroconversion or a fourfold or greater rise in titer of specific antibody to *L. micdadei* on enzyme-linked immunosorbent or microagglutination assay.

Pneumonia Due to Legionella *Species other than* L. pneumophila *and* L. micdadei

Over the past decade, a dozen *Legionella* species in addition to *L. pneumophila* and *L. micdadei* have been found rarely to cause human disease. Among these are *L. bozemanii*, responsible for 20 sporadic cases of community-acquired pneumonia and an outbreak of five nosocomial pneumonias in immunocompromised patients (Parry et al, 1985); *L. longbeachae*, responsible for occasional cases of community-acquired pneumonia (McKinney et al, 1981); *L. dumoffii* (Lewallen et al, 1979); *L. wadsworthii* (Edelstein et al, 1982); *L. hackeliae* (Wilkinson et al, 1985a); *L. cincinnatiensis* (Thacker et al, 1988); and *L. maceachernii* (Wilkinson et al, 1985b), all isolated from patients (often immunocompromised) with pneumonia. Data on clinical efficacy of antimicrobial therapy are very limited, but erythromycin and rifampin appear to be the drugs of choice until more data are available.

L. feeleii has been implicated in an outbreak of Pontiac fever involving several hundred industrial workers in a plant in which a water coolant system for lubricating and cleaning grinding machines was the source of infection (Herwaldt et al, 1984).

REFERENCES

Ampel NM et al: Cutaneous abscess caused by *Legionella micdadei* in an immunosuppressed patient. Ann Intern Med 102:630, 1985.

Anderson RD et al: Infections with *Legionella pneumophila* in children. J Infect Dis 143:386, 1981.

Arnow PM et al: Perirectal abscess caused by *Legionella pneumophila* and mixed anaerobic bacteria. Ann Intern Med 98:184, 1983.

Aronson MD et al: *Legionella micdadei* (Pittsburgh pneumonia agent) infection in nonimmunosuppressed patients with pneumonia. Ann Intern Med 94:485, 1981.

Baskerville A et al: Experimental transmission of legionnaires' disease by exposure to aerosols of *Legionella pneumophila*. Lancet 2:1389, 1981.

Beer S et al: Serum antibodies to *Legionella* agents in bronchial asthma. Arch Dis Child 60:225, 1985.

Blackmon JA et al: Pulmonary sequelae of acute legionnaires' disease pneumonia. Ann Intern Med 90:552, 1979.

Blackmon JA et al: Legionellosis. Am J Pathol 103:429, 1981.

Brabender W et al: *Legionella pneumophila* wound infection. JAMA 250:3091, 1983.

Brenner DE et al: Early diagnosis of legionnaires' disease: distinctive neurological findings. Lancet 1:940, 1981.

Byrd TF and Horwitz MA: Interferon gamma-activated human monocytes downregulate transferrin receptors and inhibit the intracellular multiplication of *Legionella pneumophila* by limiting the availability of iron. J Clin Invest 83:1457, 1989.

Carrington CB: Pathology of legionnaires' disease. Ann Intern Med 90:496, 1979.

Chandler FW et al: Demonstration of the agent of legionnaires' disease in tissue. N Engl J Med 297:1218, 1977.

Cohen ML et al: Fatal nosocomial legionnaires' disease: clinical and epidemiologic characteristics. Ann Int Med 90:611, 1979.

Cordes LG et al: Legionnaires' disease outbreak at an Atlanta, Georgia, country club: evidence for spread from an evaporative condenser. Am J Epidemiol 111:425, 1980.

Cutz E et al: Disseminated *Legionella pneumophila* infection in an infant with severe combined immunodeficiency. J Pediatr 100:760, 1982.

Dietrich PA et al: The chest radiograph in legionnaires' disease. Radiology 127:577, 1978.

Dondero TT Jr et al: An outbreak of legionnaires' disease associated with a contaminated air-conditioning cooling tower. N Engl J Med 302:365, 1980.

Dorman SA et al: Pyelonephritis associated with *Legionella pneumophila*, serogroup 4. Ann Intern Med 93:835, 1980.

Edelstein PH and Finegold ST: Use of a semiselective medium to culture *Legionella pneumophila* from contaminated lung specimens. J Clin Microbiol 10:141, 1979.

Edelstein PH and Meyer RD: Susceptibility of *Legionella pneumophila* to twenty antimicrobial agents. Antimicrob Agents Chemother 18:403, 1980.

Edelstein PH et al: Isolation of *Legionella pneumophila* from blood. Lancet 1:750, 1979.

Edelstein PH et al: Laboratory diagnosis of legionnaires' disease. Am Rev Respir Dis 121:317, 1980.

Edelstein PH et al: Long term follow-up of two patients with pulmonary cavitation caused by *Legionella pneumophila*. Am Rev Respir Dis 124:90, 1981.

Edelstein PH et al: *Legionella wadsworthii* species nova: a cause of human pneumonia. Ann Intern Med 97:809, 1982.

Edelstein PH et al: Antimicrobial therapy of experimentally induced legionnaires' disease in guinea pigs. Am Rev Respir Dis 130:849, 1984.

England AC III and Fraser DW: Sporadic and epidemic nosocomial legionellosis in the United States: epidemiologic features. Am J Med 70:707, 1981.

England AC III et al: Sporadic legionellosis in the United States: the first thousand cases. Ann Intern Med 94:164, 1981.

Evans CP and Winn WC Jr: Extrathoracic localization of *Legionella pneumophila* in legionnaires' pneumonia. Am J Clin Pathol 76:813, 1981.

Fields BS et al: Proliferation of *Legionella pneumophila* as an intracellular parasite in the ciliated protozoan *Tetrahymena pyriformis*. Appl Environ Microbiol 47:467, 1984.

Fisher-Hoch SP et al: Investigation and control of an outbreak of legionnaires' disease in a district general Hospital. Lancet 1:932, 1981.

Fliermans CB: Ecological distribution of *Legionella pneumophila*. Appl Environ Microbiol 41:9, 1981.

Foy HM et al: Legionnaires' disease in a prepaid medical care group in Seattle, 1963–1975. Lancet 1:767, 1979.

Fraser DW: Legionnaires' disease: four summers' harvest. Am J Med 68:1, 1980.

Fraser DW et al: Legionnaires' disease: description of an epidemic of pneumonia. N Engl J Med 297:1189, 1977.

Fraser DW et al: Nonpneumonic, short-incubation-period legionellosis (Pontiac fever) in men who cleaned a steam turbine condenser. Science 205:690, 1979.

Friedman HM: Legionnaires' disease in non-legionnaires: a report of five cases. Ann Intern Med 88:294, 1978.

Friedman RL et al: Identification of a cytotoxin produced by *Legionella pneumophila*. Infect Immun 29:271, 1980.

Friedman RL et al: The effects of *Legionella pneumophila* toxin on oxidative processes and bacterial killing of human polymorphonuclear leukocytes. J Infect Dis 146:328, 1982.

Fuchs GJ et al: Fatal legionnaires' disease in an infant. Pediatr Infect Dis J 5:377, 1986.

Fumarola D et al: Letter to the editor. Lancet 1:361, 1983.

Glick TH et al: An epidemic of unknown etiology in a health department. I. Clinical and epidemiologic aspects. Am J Epidemiol 107:149, 1978.

Gosting LH et al: Identification of a species-specific antigen in *Legionella pneumophila* by a monoclonal antibody. J Clin Microbiol 20:1031, 1984.

Gump DW et al: Legionnaires' disease in patients with associated serious disease. Ann Intern Med 90:538, 1979.

Gutzeit MF et al: Fatal *Legionella* pneumonitis in a neutropenic leukemic child. Pediatr Infect Dis J 6:68, 1986.

Hebert GA et al: The rickettsia-like organisms TATLOCK (1943) and HEBA (1959): bacteria phenotypically similar to but genetically distinct from *Legionella pneumophila* and the WIGA bacterium. Ann Intern Med 92:45, 1980.

Helms CM et al: Legionnaires' disease among pneumonias in Iowa (FY1972–1978). J Iowa Med Soc 71:335, 1981a.

Helms CM et al: Pretibial rash in *Legionella pneumophila* pneumonia. JAMA 245:1758, 1981b.

Helms CM et al: Sporadic legionnaires' disease: clinical observations on 87 nosocomial and community-acquired cases. Am J Med Sci 288:2, 1984.

Helms CM et al: Legionnaires' disease associated with a hospital water system: a five-year progress report on continuous hyperchlorination. JAMA 259:2423, 1988.

Herwaldt LA et al: A new *Legionella* species, *Legionella feeleii* species nova, causes Pontiac fever in an automobile plant. Ann Intern Med 100:333, 1984.

Hilton E et al: Acid-fast bacilli in sputum: a case of *Legionella micdadei* pneumonia. J Clin Microbiol 24:1102, 1986.

Horwitz MA: Phagocytosis of the legionnaires' disease bacterium (*Legionella pneumophila*) occurs by a novel mechanism: engulfment within a pseudopod coil. Cell 36:27, 1984.

Horwitz MA and Silverstein SC: Legionnaires' disease bacterium (*Legionella pneumophila*) multiples intracellularly in human monocytes. J Clin Invest 66:441, 1980.

Horwitz MA and Silverstein SC: Interaction of the legionnaires' disease bacterium (*Legionella pneumophila*) with human phagocytes. I. *L. pneumophila* resists killing by polymorphonuclear leukocytes, antibody, and complement. J Exp Med 153:386, 1981a.

Horwitz MA and Silverstein SC: Interaction of the legionnaires' disease bacterium (*Legionella pneumophila*) with human phagocytes. II. Antibody promotes binding of *L. pneumophila* to monocytes but does not inhibit intracellular multiplication. J Exp Med 153:398, 1981b.

Horwitz MA and Silverstein SC: Activated human monocytes inhibit the intracellular multiplication of legionnaires' disease bacteria. J Exp Med 154:1618, 1981c.

Horwitz MA et al: The legionnaires' disease bacterium (*Legionella pneumophila* inhibits phagosome-lysosome fusion in human monocytes. J Exp Med 158:2108, 1983.

Johnson JD et al: Neurologic manifestations of legionnaires' disease. Medicine 63:303, 1984.

Joly JR et al: Legionnaires' disease caused by *Legionella dumoffii* in distilled water. Can Med Assoc J 135:1274, 1986.

Kalweit WH et al: Hemodialysis fistula infections caused by *Legionella pneumophila*. Ann Intern Med 96:173, 1982.

Katz SM and Holsclaw DS Jr: Serum antibodies to *Legionella pneumophila* in patients with cystic fibrosis. JAMA 248:2284, 1982.

Keys TF: Legionnaires' disease. A review of the epidemiology and clinical manifestations of a newly recognized infection. Mayo Clinic Proc 55:129, 1980.

Kirby BD et al: Legionnaires' disease: clinical features of 24 cases. Ann Intern Med 89:297, 1978.

Kirby BD et al: Legionnaires' disease: report of sixty-five nosocomially acquired cases and review of the literature. Medicine 59:188, 1980.

Kohler RB et al: Onset and duration of urinary antigen excretion in legionnaires' disease. J Clin Microbiol 20:605, 1984.

Kovatch AL et al: Legionellosis in children with leukemia in relapse. Pediatrics 73:811, 1984.

Kugler JW et al: Nosocomial legionnaires' disease: occurrence in recipients of bone marrow transplants. Am J Med 74:281, 1983.

Lees AW and Tyrrell WF: Severe cerebral disturbances in legionnaires' disease. Lancet 2:1336, 1978.

Lewallen KR et al: A newly identified bacterium phenotypically resembling, but genetically distinct from *Legionella pneumophila*: an isolate in a case of pneumonia. Ann Intern Med 91:831, 1979.

Lewin S et al: Legionnaires' disease—a cause of severe abscess-forming pneumonia. Am J Med 67:339, 1979.

Lewis VJ et al: In vivo susceptibility of the Legionnaires' disease bacterium to ten antimicrobial agents. Antimicrob Agents Chemother 13:419, 1978.

Lochner JE et al: Defective triggering of polymorphonuclear leukocyte oxidative metabolism by *Legionella pneumophila* toxin. J Infect Dis 151:42, 1985.

Locksley RM et al: Susceptibility of *Legionella pneumophila* to oxygen-dependent microbicidal systems. J Immunol 129:2192, 1982.

McDade JE et al: Legionnaires' disease: isolation of a bacterium and demonstration of its role in other respiratory disease. N Engl J Med 297:1197, 1977.

McDade JE et al: Legionnaires' disease bacterium isolated in 1947. Ann Intern Med 90:659, 1979.

McKinney RM et al: *Legionella longbeachae* species nova, another etiologic agent of human pneumonia. Ann Intern Med 94:739, 1981.

Mayock R et al: *Legionella pneumophila* pericarditis proved by culture of pericardial fluid. Am J Med 75:534, 1983.

Meyer RD et al: Legionnaires' disease: unusual clinical and laboratory features. Ann Intern Med 93:240, 1980.

Meyer RD: *Legionella* infections: a review of five years of research. Rev Infect Dis 5:258, 1983.

Muder RR et al: Pneumonia due to the Pittsburgh pneumonia agent: new clinical perspective with a review of the literature. Medicine 62:120, 1983a.

Muder RR et al: Simultaneous infection with *Legionella pneumophila* and Pittsburgh pneumonia agent. Clinical features and epidemiologic implications. Am J Med 74:609, 1983b.

Muldoon RL et al: Legionnaires' disease in children. Pediatrics 67:329, 1981.

Myerowitz RL et al: Opportunistic lung infection due to "Pittsburgh pneumonia agent." N Engl J Med 301:953, 1979.

Nelson DP et al: *Legionella pneumophila* pericarditis without pneumonia. Arch Intern Med 145:926, 1985.

Orenstein WA et al: The frequency of *Legionella* infection prospectively determined in children hospitalized with pneumonia. J Pediatr 99:403, 1981.

Parry MF et al: Waterborne *Legionella bozemanii* and nosocomial pneumonia in immunosuppressed patients. Ann Intern Med 103:205, 1985.

Pasculle AW et al: Antimicrobial therapy of experimental *Legionella micdadei* pneumonia in guinea pigs. Antimicrob Agents Chemother 28:730, 1985.

Payne NR and Horwitz MA: Phagocytosis of *Legionella pneumophila* is mediated by human monocyte complement receptors. J Exper Med 166:1377, 1987.

Peerless AG et al: *Legionella* pneumonia in chronic granulomatous disease. J Pediatr 106:783, 1985.

Posner MR et al: Legionnaires' disease associated with rhabdomyolysis and myoglobinuria. Arch Intern Med 140:848, 1980.

Reingold AL et al: *Legionella* pneumonia in the United States: the distribution of serogroups and species causing human infection. J Infect Dis 149:819, 1984.

Renner ED et al: Legionnaires' disease in pneumonia patients in Iowa. A retrospective seroepidemiologic study. 1972–1977. Ann Intern Med 90:603, 1979.

Rogers BH et al: Opportunistic pneumonia—a clinicopathological study of five cases caused by an unidentified acid-fast bacterium. N Engl J Med 301:959, 1979.

Rudin JE and Wing EJ: A comparative study of *Legionella micdadei* and other nosocomial acquired pneumonia. Chest 86:675, 1984.

Ryan ME et al: Legionnaires' disease in a child with cancer. Pediatrics 64:951, 1979.

Saito A et al: The antimicrobial activity of ciprofloxacin against *Legionella* species and the treatment of experimental *Legionella* pneumonia in guinea pigs. J Antimicrob Chemother 18:251, 1986.

Saravolatz LD et al: The compromised host and legionnaires' disease. Ann Intern Med 90:533, 1979.

Senécal J-L et al: Case report: *Legionella pneumophila* lung abscess in a patient with systemic lupus erythematosus. Am J Med Sci 30:309, 1987.

Shands KN et al: Potable water as a source of legionnaires' disease. Clin Res 29:260A, 1981.

Sharrar RG et al: Summertime pneumonias in Philadelphia in 1976: an epidemiologic study. Ann Intern Med 90:577, 1979.

Shetty KR et al: Legionnaires' disease with profound cerebellar involvement. Arch Neurol 37:379, 1980.

Storch G et al: Prevalence of antibody to *Legionella pneumophila* in middle-aged and elderly Americans. J Infect Dis 140:784, 1979.

Sturm R et al: Pediatric legionnaires' disease: diagnosis by direct immunofluorescent staining of sputum. Pediatrics 68:539, 1981.

Sullivan RJ et al: Adult pneumonia in a general hospital. Arch Intern Med 129:935, 1972.

Thacker SB et al: An outbreak in 1965 of severe respiratory illness caused by the legionnaires' disease bacterium. J Infect Dis 138:512, 1978.

Thacker WL et al: *Legionella cincinnatiensis* sp. nov. isolated from a patient with pneumonia. J Clin Microbiol 36:418, 1988.

Thornsberry C et al: In vitro activity of antimicrobial agents on legionnaires' disease bacterium. Antimicrob Agents Chemother 13:78, 1978.

Tobin J O'H et al: Legionnaires' disease in a transplant unit: isolation of the causative agent from shower baths. Lancet 2:118, 1980.

Tompkins LS et al: *Legionella* prosthetic-valve endocarditis. N Engl J Med 318:530, 1988.

Tsai TF et al: Legionnaires' disease: clinical features of the epidemic in Philadelphia. Ann Intern Med 90:509, 1979.

Venkatachalam KK et al: Legionnaires' disease—a cause of lung abscess. JAMA 241:597, 1979.

Wang EEL et al: False positivity of *Legionella* serology in patients with cystic fibrosis. Pediatr Infect Dis J 6:256, 1987.

Watts JC et al: Fatal pneumonia caused by *Legionella pneumophila* serogroup 3: demonstration of the bacilli in extrathoracic organs. Ann Intern Med 92:186, 1980.

Weisenburger DD et al: Legionnaires' disease. Am J Med 69:476, 1980.

White HJ et al: Extrapulmonary histopathologic manifestations of legionnaires' disease. Arch Pathol Lab Med 104:287, 1980.

Wilkinson HW et al: Second serogroup of *Legionella hackeliae* isolated from a patient with pneumonia. J Clin Microbiol 22:488, 1985a.

Wilkinson HW et al: Fatal *Legionella maceachernii* pneumonia. J Clin Microbiol 22:1055, 1985b.

Williams ME et al: Case report. Legionnaires' disease with acute renal failure. Am J Med Sci 279:177, 1980.

Winn WC Jr and Myerowitz RL: The pathology of the *Legionella* pneumonias: a review of 74 cases and the literature. Hum Pathol 12:401, 1981.

Winn WC Jr et al: Macroscopic pathology of the lungs in legionnaires' disease. Ann Intern Med 90:548, 1979.

62

WILLIAM A. HOWARD, M.D.

VISCERAL LARVA MIGRANS

Visceral larva migrans is the term applied to a clinical syndrome consisting of eosinophilia, hepatomegaly, and pneumonitis that results from the invasion of and prolonged migration through human viscera by nematode larvae that are normally parasitic to lower animals. Although aberrant human ascarid and hookworm larvae may occasionally produce the disease, the most common cause appears to be the dog ascarid, *Toxocara canis,* and possibly the cat ascarid, *T. cati.* The disease is widespread and apparently may occur anywhere that infected dogs are present, cases being reported from North and South America, England, and Europe. One Canadian report indicates that 43 per cent of stools of stray dogs tested were found to contain ova of *T. canis.*

ETIOLOGY

The etiologic agent, *T. canis* (and possibly *T. cati*), is a common parasite of dogs but is only accidentally infective to humans, who are unnatural hosts. *T. canis* in dogs produces lesions and symptoms similar to those of *Ascaris lumbricoides* infection in humans, to which it is related (both are members of the superfamily Ascaridoidea). The adult male Toxocara is approximately 4 to 6 cm long, but the female may be 10 cm or more in length. The ova of this parasite measure 75 by 85 μ and are passed unembryonated onto the soil in the feces of the infected animal. Although the dog and the cat are the most likely sources of human infection, it is possible that the fox is a natural host. True intestinal infection with adult worms in humans has not been substantiated.

PATHOGENESIS

The unembryonated ova of *T. canis* are passed onto the soil and under suitable conditions of temperature and humidity become embryonated and infective for the accidental intermediate human host, usually a small child with pica who is a dirt eater. The ingested, embryonated eggs pass through the stomach, and their larvae hatch in the upper levels of the small intestine. The freed larvae penetrate the intestinal wall and migrate through blood and lymph channels to the liver, lungs, brain, and other organs. In these areas, the larvae are attacked by a host-cell reaction of granulomatous nature, which effectively blocks their further migration. The larvae do not grow or molt but become encapsulated and remain alive and infective for indefinite periods. The term *paratenic* has been suggested to describe the intermediate host role of humans and also the many small mammals that serve as reservoirs of infection for the natural host. The larvae cannot complete their migration through the lungs to the tracheobronchial tree, so there is no opportunity for *T. canis* to mature in the human intestine. The liver-lung-trachea migration of Ascaris and Necator in humans should not be included in the term *visceral larva migrans*.

The immune response to such helminthic infections is caused primarily by, and operates against, larval migration stages in tissues. Lesions produced by various nematode larvae in tissues of immunologically responsive hosts are strikingly similar in different hosts and in different tissues, all resembling the eosinophilic granuloma. The tissue reaction, including the peripheral eosinophilia, is proportional in both intensity and promptness to the immune state and the degree of foreignness of the host. It has been suggested that the encapsulating granulomas may not be a host reaction but instead are under the control of the parasites and are induced by them to provide for their biologic needs during the long periods of survival (paratenesis).

CLINICAL MANIFESTATIONS

Clinical symptoms are derived primarily from the number and location of the granulomatous lesions and from the allergic response of the human host to the presence of the nematode larvae. Visceral larva migrans occurs primarily in the child younger than 4 or 5 years who has a history of pica and dirt eating and has ample opportunity for contact with dogs. The usual early signs and symptoms include mild anorexia, failure to gain weight, low-grade fever, anemia, eosinophilia, and hepatomegaly of varying degree. There may be evidence of bronchitis, pneumonitis, or asthma. More severe involvement may produce gross liver enlargement, abdominal pain, pains in muscles and joints, weight loss, high intermittent fever, severe pulmonary involvement, and various neurologic disturbances. The eye may be involved, with iritis, choroiditis, and ocular hemorrhage.

Relative eosinophilia is usually pronounced, ranging from 50 to 90 per cent, but unless it is more than 30 per cent, the diagnosis may be questionable. Leukocytosis is common and may be extreme, greater than 100,000 cells/mm.[3]

Hepatomegaly is an almost constant finding, because the liver is the first organ invaded and is usually most heavily involved; this finding is absent in only the mildest infections. Fever, regardless of degree, may be associated with profuse sweating.

Pulmonic involvement is manifested clinically as bronchitis, pneumonitis, or asthma in approximately 20 per cent of cases, but pulmonary infiltrates are found in as many as 50 per cent of those patients who have chest roentgenograms. These lesions may represent actual migration of larvae, because studies in fatal cases have shown larval granulomatoses in the lungs as well as in other tissues. An occasional patient may show severe pulmonary involvement with widespread pneumonia, high fever, and roentgenographic findings similar to those seen in miliary tuberculosis.

Neurologic disturbances are reported in severe cases. The author has observed a young black boy with epilepsy in whom a presumptive diagnosis of visceral larva migrans was made on the basis of a history of pica and dirt eating, close association with dogs, and a 56 per cent blood eosinophilia. Encephalitis has also been reported as occurring in *T. canis* infection.

Other laboratory findings in visceral larva migrans include hypergammaglobulinemia, which may involve any or all of the IgG, IgA, and IgM classes. Serum IgE levels above 900 IU/mm have been found in 60 per cent of the few patients tested. Anti-A and anti-B isohemagglutinins are usually elevated, sometimes to a striking degree. Levels of serum albumin are normal, but the sedimentation rate is elevated and albuminuria is common. Most liver function tests have been reported as normal or equivocal, with the exception of the cephalin flocculation test, which may be elevated. Transaminase levels may be elevated. The bone marrow shows a pronounced eosinophilia.

COMPLICATIONS

Eye involvement, occurring without the usual findings of eosinophilia and hepatomegaly, may prove serious. There may be iritis, choroiditis, retinal detachment, fibrous tumors, and keratitis. In some instances, the appearance of the eye may prompt suspicion of retinoblastoma, and occasionally diagnosis can be made only after removal of the eye.

Pica is associated not only with visceral larva migrans but also with lead poisoning, and the finding of refractory anemia, eosinophilia and abdominal pain may be part of either picture. Cases are reported in which both conditions have existed simultaneously, with disastrous results.

COURSE AND PROGNOSIS

The clinical course of visceral larva migrans may be divided into three stages. During stage I, usually lasting several weeks, increasing eosinophilia, low-grade fever, and episodes of bronchitis, pneumonia, and asthma occur. Stage II, lasting approximately 1 month, encompasses the cardinal signs of eosinophilia, hepatomegaly, pulmonary involvement, hypergammaglobulinemia, and intermittent high fever. This is followed by stage III, the period of recovery, which may last as long as 1 to 2 years, although eventual return to normal may be expected. A few patients die, either because of a massive involvement or because of a severe hypersensitivity reaction to the parasite.

DIAGNOSIS

The diagnosis of visceral larva migrans is based on the clinical history of pica, dirt eating, and adequate exposure to dogs plus the clinical findings of chronic sustained eosinophilia, hepatomegaly, and hypergammaglobulinemia. Additional findings may be referable to other organs involved, including the brain, eye, and lung. Accurate diagnosis is still most readily made by biopsy of a lesion, usually of the liver, and the finding of the typical nematode larva in an eosinophilic granuloma. Stool examination for ova and parasites is not helpful because the larvae rarely become mature in humans. Until recently, most serodiagnostic tests have lacked sufficient accuracy to be definitive in diagnosis, because the antigens used were prepared from adult worms and often gave false-positive reactions with *Ascaris* and other helminths.

The major antigen present in *T. canis* is contained in the embryonated egg and hatched larva and not in adult worms or unembryonated eggs. This antigen has proved useful in diagnosis when employed in the enzyme-linked immunosorbent assay (ELISA). It is specific for *Toxocara* and appears in high titer in almost all patients with visceral larva migrans. Occasional positive results have been noted in adults with no previous history of the disease. If cross reactivity to *Ascaris* appears to be a problem, it may be eliminated by adsorption with *Ascaris* antigen. The ELISA test is specially useful in ocular toxocariasis, in which results of other serologic tests may be negative.

Differential diagnosis should include the visceral lesions that may be produced by a number of other nematode worms, including *Ascaris lumbricoides, Ancylostoma braziliense, Ancylostoma caninum, Strongyloides stercoralis,* as well as immature stages of certain spiroid nematodes and filarial worms. Invasion of the liver by *Fasciola hepatica,* a nematode worm, or *Capillaria hepatica,* a trematode, might also be included. It is apparent that *T. canis* may be one cause of the picture of Löffler's syndrome, of transient pulmonary infiltrations and eosinophilia, but other diseases may also mimic such a picture. Also to be considered in the diagnosis are trichinosis, hepatitis, leukemia, familial eosinophilia, tropical eosinophilia, tuberculosis, asthma, lead poisoning, and the leukemoid reaction occurring in certain severe bacterial pneumonias.

TREATMENT

No satisfactory treatment for visceral larva migrans is recognized at present. Diethylcarbamazine (Hetrazan) in doses of 10 to 30 mg/kg/day for 14 days has been suggested but has proved disappointing and is no longer commercially available. Thiabendazole, successfully used in cutaneous larva migrans (creeping eruption) in a dosage of 25 to 100 mg/kg/day, has been used for the visceral form in a few cases with good results and apparent absence of any evidence of toxic effects. The usual dosage is 25 to 50 mg/kg/day in two to three divided doses for 7 to 10 days, with the course of treatment being repeated in 4 weeks. I have treated one patient in this manner, with rapid disappearance of symptoms and subsidence of the eosinophilia after 4 months. Adrenocorticosteroids in adequate dosage may be life saving for patients who are highly sensitive to the larval nematode, especially those with severe pneumonitis. Otherwise, treatment is primarily symptomatic and supportive, with stress on the correction of the anemia.

PREVENTION

Because pica is a very important risk factor, children with this problem should not be exposed to environments potentially contaminated with *T. canis* eggs, whether in homes or in outdoor areas. Appropriate anthelmintics should be administered to nursing bitches and puppies approximately 2 weeks post partum and then repeated weekly for 3 weeks. Thereafter, twice-yearly stool exminations of dogs are recommended, with treatment as indicated. Because such treatment does not destroy larval forms in somatic tissues, elimination of the worms from the intestinal tract does not prevent transmission of larvae to subsequent litters. The potential for transmission of *T. canis* or *T. cati* is another subject for parent education by appropriate persons, including the pediatrician.

REFERENCES

Aur RJA, Pratt CB, and Johnson WW: Thiabendazole in visceral larva migrans. Am J Dis Child 121:226, 1971.
Beaver PC: The nature of visceral larva migrans. J Parasitol 55:3, 1969.
Beaver, PC, Snyder CH, Carrera GM et al: Chronic eosinophilia due to visceral larva migrans. Pediatrics 9:7, 1952.
Brain L and Allen B: Encephalitis due to infection with *Toxocara canis*. Reports of a suspected case. Lancet 1:1355, 1964.
Chandra RK: Visceral larva migrans. Indian J Pediatr 30:388, 1963.
Cypress RH, Karol MH, Zidian JL et al: Larva-specific antibodies

in patients with visceral larva migrans. J Infect Dis 135:633, 1977.

Dafalla AA: The serodiagnosis of human toxocariasis by the capillary-tube precipitin test. Trans R Soc Trop Med Hyg 69:146, 1975.

de Savigny DH: In vitro maintenance of *Toxocara canis* larvae and a simple method for the production of Toxocara ES antigen for use in serodiagnostic tests for visceral larva migrans. J Parasitol 61:781, 1975.

Faust EC and Russell PF: Clinical Parasitology. Philadelphia, Lea & Febiger, 1964.

Friedman S and Hervade AR: Severe myocarditis with recovery in a child with visceral larva migrans. J Pediatr 56:91, 1960.

Galvin TJ: Experimental *Toxocara canis* infections in chickens and pigeons. J Parasitol 50:124, 1964.

Jacklin HN and Holt LB: Ocular localization in larva migrans. NC Med J 31:55, 1970.

Karpinski FE Jr, Everts-Saurez EZ, and Sawitz WG: Larval granulomatosis (visceral larva migrans). Am J Dis Child 92:34, 1956.

Patterson R, Huntley CC, Roberts M and Irons JS: Visceral larva migrans: immunoglobulins, precipitating antibodies and detection of IgG and IgM antibodies against *Ascaris* antigen. Am J Trop Med Hyg 24:465, 1975.

Schantz PM and Glickman LT: Toxocaral visceral larva migrans. N Engl J Med 298:436, 1978.

Seah SKK, Hucal G, and Law C: Dogs and intestinal parasites: a public health problem. Can Med Assoc J 112:1191, 1975.

Smith MHD and Beaver PC: Persistence and distribution of Toxocara larvae in the tissues of children and mice. Pediatrics 12:491, 1953.

Snyder CH: Visceral larva migrans. Pediatrics 28:85, 1961.

Vinke B: Application of haemagglutination test for visceral larva migrans in adult. Trop Geogr Med 16:43, 1964.

Woodruff AW and Thacher CKM: Infections with animal helminths. Br Med J 1:1001, 1964.

63

ALEXANDER O. TUAZON, M.D., and
HANS PASTERKAMP, M.D., F.R.C.P.(C)

HYDATID DISEASE OF THE LUNG (PULMONARY HYDATIDOSIS)

The lung is involved in two forms of human hydatidosis caused by the cystic larval stage of the tapeworm *Echinococcus*: cystic hydatid disease, caused by *Echinococcus granulosus*, which is worldwide in distribution, and alveolar hydatid disease, associated with *Echinococcus multilocularis*, which is commonly seen in the Northern Hemisphere.

The life cycles of these two species are similar. The first developmental stage is the tapeworm, which reaches sexual maturity only in the intestinal tract of its definitive mammalian host, usually a carnivore. Infective ova are released during defecation, contaminating fields, irrigated lands, and wells. *Echinococcus* eggs are extremely resistant to climatic conditions, and in northern regions will survive for at least 2 years. When eggs are swallowed by intermediate mammalian hosts, including humans, the outer shell is digested and the hexacanth embryos—the second developmental stage—are liberated. The embryos penetrate the intestinal wall with their hooklets and are distributed through the blood vessels to various parts of the body, mostly to the liver and lung, where they form the third developmental stage, the cystic larval stage or hydatid. Under ideal conditions, tapeworm heads, or protoscoleces, develop within the cyst. The cycle is completed when carnivores ingest viscera infected with fertile cysts, those containing protoscoleces.

CYSTIC HYDATID DISEASE

A pastoral and a sylvatic cycle are seen with *E. granulosus*. In the pastoral cycle, the definitive host is the dog, and the intermediate hosts are sheep, cattle, hogs, goats, horses, and camels. A sylvatic form of *E. granulosus* is found with the large deer-wolf cycle in Alaska and Canada, the wallaby-dingo cycle in Australia, and the sheep-jackal cycle in the Middle East. The sylvatic Alaskan-Canadian cycle forms a distinct clinical variety and will be discussed separately.

Classic, or pastoral, cystic hydatidosis is most commonly seen in the sheep- and cattle-raising areas of the Mediterranean, Middle East, South America, Russia, eastern Europe, India, Australia, and Africa. In North America, it is seen among the California Basque sheepherders, and in Utah, New Mexico, and Arizona, particularly among the native American populations.

Humans become infected from contaminated water and food or through close contact with infected dogs. Lung cysts develop when embryos pass through the liver, through lymphatic ducts bypassing the liver, by contiguous extension from the liver, or through the bronchi.

The hydatid slowly enlarges, and its rate of growth is dependent on the distensibility of the tissue and the age of the host. Pulmonary cysts grow fast, and they grow faster in children. At a size of 1 cm, three layers can be identified within the cyst: (1) an inner layer of germinal epithelium or endocyst that is responsible for formation of daughter cysts by endogenous vesiculation; (2) a middle noncellular, laminated layer or ectocyst; and (3) an adventitia or pericyst, an outer capsule of fibrous tissue, vasculature, giant cells, and eosinophils resulting from a weak host reaction. With time, brood capsules and daughter cysts may develop and disintegrate, liberating free scoleces or "hydatid sand."

E. granulosus is known to affect all age groups and any body cavity, organ, or site. Infection occurs mostly during childhood, though years may elapse before manifestations are seen. Neither sex is favored, and the slight differences in sex incidence are probably due to activity or occupation. Asymptomatic hydatidosis in family members is seen in 5 to 18 per cent of cases.

In cystic hydatid disease, 17 to 75 per cent of cases occur in children. It does not tend to occur in the very young but has been reported in a 2-year-old child. After the age of 4 years, there is even distribution throughout childhood. In Tunis, of 643 children with pulmonary hydatid cysts, the mean age was 5 years (2 to 15 years) (Chaouachi et al, 1988).

The liver and the lungs are most frequently affected, with the lung being more commonly affected in children (McIntyre, 1971; Chaouachi et al, 1988). Other tissues that may be affected are the brain, eye, heart, mediastinum, blood vessels, pleura, diaphragm, pancreas, spleen, endocrine glands, bone, and genitourinary tract. The central nervous system is affected more often in children than in adults.

CLINICAL FEATURES

Clinical manifestations are determined by cyst size, location, and the potential for impairment of vital structures. The slowly enlarging hydatid cyst is usually well tolerated. An awareness of symptoms is due to pressure from the enlarging cyst, secondary infection, and cyst rupture. The intact cyst is most commonly asymptomatic and may account for a third of all cases. In a study of South Australian children with pulmonary hydatidosis, McIntyre (1971) found 19 per cent to be asymptomatic.

The more common manifestations of pulmonary cysts are cough, chest pain, hemoptysis, fever, and malaise. Retarded growth patterns have been observed in a significant number of children. Other manifestations are sputum production, chest discomfort, loss of appetite, dyspnea, vomiting of cyst elements, dysphagia, and hepatic pain. Bronchospasm has been reported with relief of bronchial asthma after removal of the cyst (Bakir, 1967).

Little (1976) in Australia found that 13 per cent of the patients at one medical center presented as emergency cases because of complications of the disease. Complications may be mechanical, with hydatid growth affecting the bronchial tree or pleura; they may also occur as a result of hematogenous spread, infection, or allergic reaction. Cyst rupture, pneumothorax, atelectasis, bronchopleural fistula, empyema, residual cavity, bronchiectasis, secondary cysts, and superimposed infection have been reported. A rare complication is rupture into the cardiovascular system with dissemination or sudden death.

Up to 30 per cent of lung cysts may be complicated by rupture into the pleural space or bronchus that has been precipitated by coughing, sneezing, trauma, or increased abdominal pressure. Rupture is indicated by chills, fever, increased cough, mild hemoptysis, and change in appearance on radiographs. Coughing up of hydatid cyst elements, described as "coughing up grape skins," is diagnostic. Secondary hydatidosis in the pleura, acute asphyxia by bronchial obstruction, and allergic reactions, including anaphylaxis, may follow cyst rupture and leakage.

Bronchobiliary fistula occurs in 2 per cent of cases and is commonly, but not always, preceded by suppuration. The right side and posterior basal segment are most frequently affected. Pyrexia and weight loss may mimic malignancy, but bile expectoration is pathognomonic.

Rarer complications caused by the cysts' unusual location have been reported: arterial emboli, portal hypertension, systemic venous obstruction, paraplegia, pleural effusion, phrenic nerve paralysis, transitory paralysis of cervical sympathetic chain, lower extremity thrombophlebitis, and stress ulcer (Ayuso et al, 1981; Ozdemir and Kalaycioglu, 1983).

DIAGNOSIS

Awareness of the disease is most important. Lung involvement is very likely if there is a cyst present elsewhere in the body. Cystic hydatid disease is suspected on the basis of a history of current or previous residence in an endemic area, clinical observations, and radiographic evidence. In 10 per cent a diagnosis is suspected on routine radiographic study alone. A history of contact with possibly infected dogs may be obtained in only 29 to 48 per cent of cases.

Physical examination is rarely definitive. On rare occasions, a hydatid thrill (fluid wave) can be heard on auscultation while percussing a large cyst. Demonstration of scoleces and hooklets of the parasite in vomitus, stool, urine, or sputum is pathognomonic but is rarely observed and may be seen only during surgery. Needle aspiration is particularly dangerous, as leakage may induce anaphylactic shock.

Hepatic function may be abnormal in one half of patients with liver cysts. An increased specific serum IgE may be observed, but eosinophilia is more often absent than present and is completely unreliable in areas endemic for other parasites.

The basis for serologic tests is the formation of antibodies to the parasite that develop in the host tissue. False negative results may be found in 10 to

30 per cent of tests and are more common in children and with pulmonary cysts.

The Casoni skin test involves injection of hydatid fluid in the dermis, which produces an erythematous papule in 50 to 80 per cent of patients in less than 60 min. A Casoni test can be very helpful if strongly positive, but its positivity in known cases varies considerably from 38 to 81 per cent. False negative results, sometimes due to infected cysts, and false positive results occur in 30 per cent of those tested. The Casoni test remains positive for life. Serum antibody testing by complement-fixation is positive in 52 to 60 per cent, reverts to negative within 1 to 2 years after successful removal of the cyst, and will also presumably revert to negative sometime after death of a cyst. Thus when only live cysts are taken into account, the test is positive in 72 per cent. If both the Casoni skin test and complement-fixing antibodies are positive, 84 per cent of cases are detected. However, because of the low sensitivity and low specificity of the Casoni skin test and complement-fixation titers, most centers have discontinued using these tests.

Other diagnostic serologic tests, such as indirect hemagglutination, immunofluorescent antibody, and enzyme-linked immunosorbent assay (ELISA), have a sensitivity of 85 per cent for liver cysts and 50 per cent for lung cysts. Test findings such as fluorescent antibody, indirect hemagglutination, and latex agglutination may remain positive for about 10 years, but titers fall after successful removal of the cyst. Persistent titers, however, do not necessarily indicate a recurrence. Laboratory tests may be more sensitive in complicated cysts, but at present, no single test is infallible, and there is still no serologic test that can effectively rule out the disease. Thus disease awareness is most important.

The main diagnostic tool is the radiographic study, which is 98 to 100 per cent accurate. However, with miniature screening x-ray studies, only 40 per cent of cases are diagnosed. On occasion, inflammatory reactions and secondary infections may mask both closed and ruptured cysts, and the cysts are discovered after inflammation subsides.

On radiography, lung cysts are readily detected, and the possibility of hydatid cyst in an endemic area should always be considered. An unruptured cyst is seen as a round or oval homogenous lesion with a sharply defined smooth border surrounded by normal lung or a zone of atelectasis (Fig. 63–1). It may be located in the periphery, center, or hilum; may be single or multiple, unilateral or bilateral; and may be of various size. The final form depends on the location and neighboring structures. With an increase in size, bronchial dislocation occurs but no obstruction, as has been demonstrated by tomography or bronchography. On fluoroscopy, good elasticity of the cyst wall is demonstrable, and there is no interference with movement of the diaphragm.

As the cyst grows, air passages and surrounding vessels are eroded, producing bronchial air leaks into the cyst adventitia. The bronchial air leak is actually nonfunctional before rupture because of pressure of the endocyst against bronchial passages and may be demonstrated only during surgery. With varying stages of air dissection into the cyst, different classic radiologic signs may be seen. A pericystic emphysema is seen in preruptured cysts. A "meniscus sign" or "crescent sign" is a crescentic radiolucency above the homogenous cyst shadow on deep inspiration that is seen when air penetrates between adventitia and ectocyst. As air dissection continues, the parasite's membrane is torn, and some hydatid fluid flows out. An air-fluid level is seen within the cyst lumen as well as an air cup between ectocyst and adventitia, known as "double air-layer appearance" or Cumbo sign. With free connection to a bronchus, the cyst wall is detached from adventitia, crumbles, collapses, and floats on remaining cyst fluid. This result is seen on the radiograph as air between the collapsed floating cyst wall and the adventitia, known as "water lily sign" or Camellote sign. The adventitial wall does not collapse at once, so the obliteration of the cyst cavity is not an immediate outcome.

Cystic hydatidosis of the lung occurs most often in the form of a single unilocular cyst. Only about 7 to 38 per cent occur as multiple unilocular cysts. The inferior lobes are most commonly affected. In children, the ratio of unruptured to ruptured cysts is 3:1, which is the inverse of that in adults. Unlike in liver and spleen hydatid cysts, calcification of lung cysts is rare. A high right hemidiaphragm and right basal bronchiectasis are suggestive of bronchobiliary fistula. A tract on sinugram or bronchogram is diagnostic.

Computed tomography (CT) may aid in the diagnosis by determining the location, extent of involvement, and demonstration of the internal anatomy of the cyst. Simple hydatid cysts cannot be differentiated from water-density lung cysts of other etiology on CT, and complicated lesions may be confusing. The ability of CT, however, to demonstrate characteristic hydatid anatomy, such as detached or collapsed membrane and daughter cysts, allows specific diagnosis to be made (Saksouk et al, 1986).

Ultrasonography helps distinguish cystic lesions from solid tumors. Pathognomonic signs on ultrasonography are multiple daughter cysts within a cyst, separation of the laminated membrane from the wall of the cyst, and sonographically collapsed cysts (Pant and Gupta, 1987). A simple cyst with a thick wall in patients from an endemic area is suggestive. Abdominal ultrasonography is also recommended for liver cyst detection. Angiography can sometimes demonstrate a characteristic halo effect around the cyst and may help determine the number and location of cysts.

Differential diagnoses include abscess, hamartoma, pulmonary arteriovenous fistula, benign granuloma, malignant tumor, metastasis, and cysts of different origin. The presence of Cumbo sign is confirmatory.

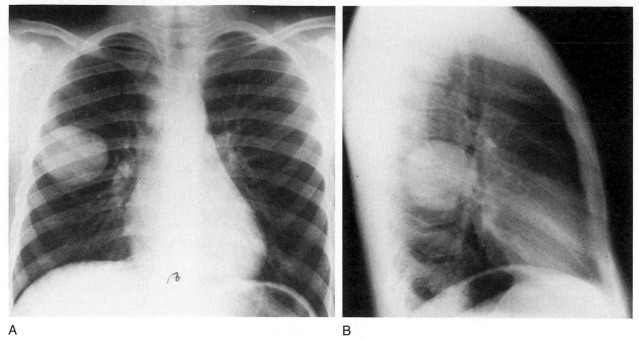

A   B

Figure 63–1. The posteroanterior *(A)* and lateral *(B)* chest radiographs from a 7.5-year-old girl with a cough of several months' duration show clearly a sharply circumscribed homogenous density in the superior segment of the right lower lobe at the periphery of the lung. The lesion was surgically excised and proved to be a hydatid cyst.

HISTOPATHOLOGY

Histopathology depends on the size of cyst, the time after rupture, and the allergic reactivity of the host. In unruptured hydatid cysts, minimal atelectasis and compression are seen. A strong allergic eosinophilic reaction in surrounding lung tissue can be found with a recently ruptured cyst. Cysts ruptured less than 10 days show reversible inflammatory infiltrates of lymphocytes or giant cell granulomata around parasite components. When the rupture is older than 10 days, severe fibrosis starts to develop, leading to dense scarring with subsequent tendency to bronchiectasis and superinfection.

TREATMENT

Spontaneous cure is possible after coughing out the cyst and its contents, but more commonly infection and toxemia from the residual cyst may follow. Up to two thirds of symptomatic patients may die without intervention. When possible, surgery is the recommended treatment for all cases, even when asymptomatic. The success of surgery is dependent on the size and location of the cyst and on the skill of the surgeon. It is important to perform surgery immediately after diagnosis because the weak adventitial reaction and occurring bronchial communications may lead to rupture with intrapulmonary dissemination. Only in the benign Alaskan-Canadian variant is conservative treatment recommended.

The aims of surgery are total eradication of the parasite with evacuation of the cyst and removal of

the endocyst, prevention of cyst rupture and consequent dissemination during the operation, and extirpation of the residual cavity. The lung parenchyma should be preserved and resection should be avoided in children if possible because the damaged lung parenchyma has great capacity for recovery. Lung resection may be done in cases with bronchiectasis, severe inflammation, and large or multiple cysts that have destroyed lung parenchyma.

The posterolateral approach is favored. Surgical techniques to eradicate the parasite may include puncture and aspiration of cyst in situ, excision of the entire cyst by enucleation, wedge resection, segmentectomy, lobectomy, or pneumonectomy.

Such surgical procedures as enucleation with or without obliteration of the residual cavity by sutures (capitonnage) and cystectomy are mainly used for uncomplicated cysts. Lobectomy or segmental resection is reserved for lung destroyed by large cysts or bronchobiliary and biliary-pleural fistulas. One favored procedure is subtotal cystopericystectomy with total extirpation of the parasite or its rests in ruptured cysts, followed by closure of bronchial leaks and washing with a scolicidal solution. Subtotal extirpation of the pericyst or adventitia is then performed, leaving the hilar portion in place, because total resection of the adventitia in its hilar pole carries with it some considerable risk. In many cases of cystic hydatid disease of the lung, Keystone (1988) has found it possible to eliminate the intact cyst by the use of positive pressure ventilation to force the cyst from the surgical opening in the lung.

Rupture and spillage may occur and may lead to dissemination and anaphylaxis, which may be fatal.

This complication, though uncommon even with spillage during surgery, is greatly feared. The differences in surgical techniques therefore reflect the desire to prevent spillage of viable cyst contents. Commonly, the operative field is protected with saline moistened gauzes, and the cysts are gently manipulated.

After extirpation of the parasite, bronchial fistulas are closed. To prevent recurrence, the residual cavity is injected with scolicidal agents, such as formalin, hypertonic saline, or absolute alcohol; silver nitrate has been used to freeze the cyst wall. Because of extremely grave complications with the use of formalin and hypertonic solutions, others have used hydrogen peroxide with good results. The residual cavity is then either obliterated by sutures or left open to communicate with the pleural space. Alternatively, the pericystic membrane is resected with repair of bronchial leakage. With a bronchobiliary fistula, the usually accompanying biliary hypertension is corrected, and the hepatic cavity is obliterated or drained. In cases with bronchobiliary fistula, the operative mortality is between 5 and 50 per cent.

The more common surgical complications in children include atelectasis, hydropneumothorax, wound infection, pleural reaction, and hemothorax. Other reported complications from surgery are chest infection, abscess, empyema, septic shock, bronchial rupture, pneumothorax, bronchobiliary fistula, biliary-pleural fistula, hemorrhage, massive aspiration, prolonged drainage, bronchiectasis, and allergic reactions, including anaphylactic shock and death with rupture. The perioperative morbidity rate is 3 to 10 per cent, and the mortality rate is 0 to 5 per cent. The recurrence rate is 0 to 5 per cent.

When surgery is impractical or impossible, mebendazole at a dose of 30 to 50 mg/kg/day for 1 to 6 months is recommended. Mebendazole interferes with uptake of glycogen by cestodes but is poorly absorbed and produces low blood concentrations of the drug. Alternatively, 50 to 100 mg/kg/day for 3 months may be used to achieve the necessary blood concentration. A peak therapeutic blood level of 80 ng/ml, measured by high-pressure liquid chromatography or radioimmunoassay, is recommended. Absorption is enhanced with meals, and mebendazole should therefore be taken with meals in three divided doses. Repeated courses may be necessary. Subjective improvement has been shown in 75 per cent of the cases studied, but no controlled studies have been done, and objective improvement and cure have been seen in only a few cases.

Adverse reactions to mebendazole may occur within the first month. Febrile and allergic reactions, alopecia, glomerulonephritis, and reversible leukopenia have been reported. With hepatobiliary disease, increased blood levels and toxicity have been observed. Monitoring of clinical status, liver function, renal function, and complete blood count should be done weekly for the first month and biweekly thereafter.

Preliminary studies with albendazole, a new benzimidazole derivative, have shown it to be more effective than mebendazole. Furthermore, high blood and tissue levels of the drug can be achieved. For those who are 10 years of age and older, 28-day courses separated by 14-day drug-free periods have been recommended.

PREVENTION AND FOLLOW-UP

Hydatid lung disease is preventable. Preventive measures include the use of veterinary taeniacides for dogs; the proper disposal of carcasses and entrails of animals to prevent dogs from gaining access to them; and proper hand, food, and drink care to prevent contamination from dog excrement.

Follow-up abdominal ultrasound should be done annually for 5 years or more. Chest radiographs and CT scans should be repeated after 2 or 3 years and at 5 years. A cyst cavity may remain, and serologic findings may be positive for several years.

SYLVATIC ALASKAN-CANADIAN VARIANT

Among the sylvatic cycles, the Alaskan-Canadian variety is clinically and morphologically distinct and has been named *E. granulosus var. canadensis*. It is seen in the tundra and northern coniferous forests of North America to the Great Lakes, mainly among the native population, including the Eskimo, Aleut, and other native American Indians, 75 per cent of whom live in areas where *E. granulosus* occurs. The wolf is the definitive host, and sometimes the dog, which ingests the tapeworm by eating the viscera of infected deer. Intermediate hosts are large deer, elk, reindeer, moose, and caribou. Pig, sheep, and cattle have been shown in experiments to resist the infection. Humans are not very suitable hosts.

The Alaskan-Canadian sylvatic infection is more benign; the cysts are smaller, more delicate, do not grow as rapidly, and produce fewer symptoms than the classic or pastoral *E. granulosus*. The risk of anaphylaxis with rupture is less, and the prospect for spontaneous cure without significant complications seems excellent.

Most commonly affected organs are the liver and the lung, with lung involvement in 61 per cent of the cases. Most cysts are simple, intact, and uninfected. The mean age for pulmonary cysts is younger than that for liver cysts. For pulmonary cysts, the mean age is 22 years (5 to 77 years), and for liver cysts, it is 65.3 years (24 to 96 years). In patients with lung cyst, 71 per cent are below the age of 20 years.

Only 6 to 8 per cent of cases are symptomatic, mostly because of cyst rupture, which may occur in some 26 per cent of patients. Cough, purulent expectoration, and hemoptysis are usual complaints. Serious complications are rare, and no cases of anaphylaxis or seeding have been seen in the Alaskan experience (Wilson et al, 1968; Pinch and Wilson, 1973).

Diagnosis is based on a history of residence in an endemic area, association with dogs, and routine radiographic study. Typically, a round or oval homogenous water-like density with clear-cut borders and no surrounding reaction is seen. Such classic signs as water lily and crescent sign are rare. Laboratory tests are of little value. Eosinophilia is positive in only 29 per cent of cases, hemagglutination in 10 per cent, and the Casoni test in 56 per cent. With cyst leak or rupture, test results are usually but not always positive.

The surgical risk is minimal. Extrusion of the intact vesicle is not appropriate, and an open wedge resection of adventitia with intact cyst is favored. Gentleness is very important. The bronchial stump should be closed, and the defect in the lung is obliterated. Alternatively, cystectomy may be performed.

Quite commonly, the cyst evacuates into the bronchi, and the symptoms disappear. Thus surgery is not recommended for the asymptomatic, and the patient is managed by observation. No serious morbidity and mortality have been reported with this approach.

ALVEOLAR HYDATID DISEASE

E. multilocularis is a cestode that differs morphologically and biologically in its larval and adult stages from *E. granulosus*. The usual definitive host is the fox, with dogs and cats acting as sources of human infection in endemic areas. Intermediate hosts are rodents and humans. The larval stage develops normally in rodents, but humans are unusual and poor intermediate hosts. The disease is usually found across much of the Soviet Union, central Europe, northern Japan, Alaska, and northern Canada. Human disease is rare in the Western Hemisphere, but the cestode is endemic in the north central United States and Canada.

The infection usually occurs during childhood. A case-control study has identified the following risk factors: having a lifetime pattern of dog ownership, tethering dogs near the house, and living in a house built directly on the tundra rather than on gravel or permanent foundations, thus allowing contact with contaminated dog feces (Stehr-Green et al, 1988). Other implicated factors are the drinking of unboiled melted snow and the skinning of foxes. The disease becomes manifest usually between the ages of 19 and 40 years but has been seen in those as young as 5 years. The mean age at diagnosis in Alaska is 53 years. The disease favors neither sex.

The larval cestode persists in its proliferative phase because of the inability of humans to provide the conditions necessary for normal development. Instead of developing a thick, laminated layer and growing into large, single cysts, the parasite has a thin, deficient ectocyst that grows and infiltrates into the surrounding tissues. The growing cyst may have several small, fluid-filled pockets containing protoscoleces. Because of its type of construction, this larval form is called an alveolar or multilocular hydatid. It provokes a severe host reaction and becomes surrounded by an inflammatory or granulomatous reaction, instead of the fibrous host response seen with *E. granulosus*. A central area of necrosis is always seen.

The cyst is slow growing, behaves like a malignancy, and has been mistaken for carcinoma, which it can mimic clinically and microscopically. The primary site of infection is the liver, where a dense honeycomb of small, multilocular cysts is formed. The cyst appears as a solid cancer-like growth that may cavitate and attain massive size. Through the inferior vena cava it may metastasize to distant organs. Alveolar hydatid disease of the lung is invariably a metastatic focus.

Diagnosis is based on history of exposure, elevated serologic titers, and characteristic changes on radiographic studies. Physical signs are confusing, and subjective symptoms may be mild, vague, and ill defined. Patients present usually with asymptomatic hepatomegaly. When symptoms are present, they are commonly related to the abdomen: mild epigastric and right upper-quadrant abdominal pain or distress, intermittent fever, and jaundice.

On radiologic examination, hepatomegaly and hepatic calcification are the most common findings. Typically, the diagnosis is made with abdominal radiographs that show scattered radiolucent areas surrounded with calcification, sometimes referred to as the "swiss-cheese" liver calcification pattern. This finding is pathognomonic, but at least 5 years of illness must elapse before calcification can be demonstrated. Without the characteristic radiographic study, the diagnosis is rarely made preoperatively.

Computed tomography and ultrasound will demonstrate an indistinct mass with a necrotic center. Serologic tests used are the same as that for *E. granulosus* but tend to produce more positive findings with high titers. Indirect hemagglutination titers decline markedly during the first year after radical surgical resection but not after chemotherapy. The EM2 ELISA test, using a semipurified homologous antigen fraction, is more sensitive and specific than tests using heterologous *E. granulosus* antigen fractions (Lanier et al, 1987). Results may still be positive, however, even when the parasite is no longer viable (Rausch et al, 1987). Needle biopsy confirms the diagnosis. There is no risk of anaphylaxis or spillage of protoscoleces because the tumor is essentially solid.

Treatment is by surgery. Early diagnosis is of fundamental importance to permit resection before infiltration becomes too extensive. However, many cases are undiagnosed until they are well advanced and the hepatic lesions are unresectable.

At surgery, liver invasion is often more extensive than suggested by the degree of calcification on the radiograph. Complete excision is the only hope. Cure is possible when partial hepatectomy or hepatic lobectomy can remove all multilocular cysts and still preserve enough organ function. Still, radical hepatic resection is curative in only 20 per cent of cases. Palliative measures are designed to ensure adequate bile drainage.

If surgery is unsuccessful or impractical, mebendazole is recommended at 40 mg/kg/day in divided doses for life, which may prevent progression of the primary lesion and metastasis and prolong life. Mebendazole's lethal effect on the larval cestode, however, has not been demonstrated conclusively. Albendazole has been shown to be effective in killing the larval cestode. Hepatic toxicity with the use of this drug can develop without warning, however, and does not seem to be dose related or likely due to hypersensitivity. Hepatic function should then be monitored the entire time the drug is administered. Monitoring should be done weekly during the first month and monthly thereafter.

Though not fulminating, the disease is ultimately fatal unless early surgical interference can remove the parasite cyst. Patients have survived at least 16 years after diagnosis. Death is due to liver failure, invasion of contiguous areas, and metastases to the lung, brain, and distant organs. The best means of preventing alveolar hydatid disease remains the control of the cestode in domestic animals, the primary source of human infection.

REFERENCES

Cystic Hydatid Disease

Aletras HA: Hydatid cyst of the lung. Scand J Thorac Cardiovasc Surg 2(3):218, 1968.

Ayuso LA, de Peralta GT, Lazaro RB et al: Surgical treatment of pulmonary hydatidosis. J Thorac Cardiovasc Surg 82(4):569, 1981.

Bakir F: Serious complications of hydatid cyst of the lung. Am Rev Respir Dis 96(3):483, 1967.

Borrie J and Shaw JHF: Hepatobronchial fistula caused by hydatid disease. The Dunedin experience 1952–79. Thorax 36(1):25, 1981.

Bouzid A, Nekmouche L, and Benallegue S: Les kystes hydatiques multifocaux de l'enfant. Chir Pediatr 27(1):33, 1986.

Chaouachi B, Nouri A, Ben Salah S et al: Les kystes hydatiques du poumon chez l'enfant. A propos de 643 cas. Pediatrie 43(9):769, 1988.

Dogan R, Yuksel M, Cetin G et al: Surgical treatment of hydatid cysts of the lung: report on 1055 patients. Thorax 44(3):192, 1989.

Door J, Houel J, Dor V et al: Le k, .e hydatique du poumon considerations anatomo-chirurgicales. A propos d'une observation recente chez un enfant et d'une statistique de plus de 500 cas operes. Ann Chir Thorac Cardiovasc 6(2):369, 1967.

Grunebaum M: Radiological manifestations of lung echinococcus in children. Pediatr Radiol 3(2):65, 1975.

Katz R, Murphy S, and Kosloske A: Pulmonary echinococcosis: a pediatric disease of the southwestern United States. Pediatrics 65(5):1003, 1980.

Keystone JS: Larval Tapeworm Infections: Nelson JD (ed): Current Therapy in Pediatric Infectious Disease. 2nd ed. Toronto, BC Decker, 1988.

Little JM: Hydatid disease at Royal Prince Alfred Hospital, 1964 to 1974. Med J Aust 1(24):903, 1976.

McIntyre A: Hydatid disease in children in South Australia. Med J Aust 1:1064, 1971.

Monies-Chass I, Wajsbort E, and Zveibil FR: Massive aspiration during surgery for a hydatid cyst of the lung. Anaesthetist 24(4):177, 1975.

Mottaghian H, Mahmoudi S, and Vaez-Zadeh K: A ten-year survey of hydatid disease (Echinococcus granulosus) in children. Prog Pediatr Surg 15:113, 1982.

Novick RJ, Tchervenkov CI, Wilson JA et al: Surgery for thoracic hydatid disease: a North American experience. Ann Thorac Surg 43(6):681, 1987.

Ozdemir A and Kalaycioglu E: Surgical treatment and complications of thoracic hydatid disease. Report of 61 cases. Eur J Respir Dis 64(3):217, 1983.

Ozer Z, Cetin M, and Kahraman C: Pleural involvement by hydatid cysts of the lung. Thorac Cardiovasc Surg 33(2):103, 1985.

Pant CS and Gupta RK: Diagnostic value of ultrasonography in hydatid disease in abdomen and chest. Acta Radiol 28(6):743, 1987.

Pinch LW and Wilson JF: Non-surgical management of cystic hydatid disease in Alaska. A review of 30 cases of Echinococcus granulosus infection treated without operation. Ann Surg 178(1):45, 1973.

Sadrieh M, Dutz W, and Navabpoor S: Review of 150 cases of hydatid cyst of the lung. Dis Chest 52(5):662, 1967.

Saksouk FA, Fahl MH, and Rizk GK: Computed tomography of pulmonary hydatid disease. J Comput Assist Tomogr 10(2):226, 1986.

Toumbouras M, Panagopoulos F, Spanos P, and Lazarides DP: Zur Chirurgie des Echinococcus Cysticus der Lunge im Kindesalter. Z Kinderchir 36(3):88, 1982.

Tuncel E: Pulmonary air meniscus sign. Respiration 46(1):139, 1984.

Webster GA and Cameron TWM: Epidemiology and diagnosis of echinococcosis in Canada. Can Med Assoc J 96:600, 1967.

Sylvatic Alaskan-Canadian Variant

Pinch LW and Wilson JF: Non-surgical management of cystic hydatid disease in Alaska. A review of 30 cases of Echinococcus granulosus infection treated without operation. Ann Surg 178(1):45, 1973.

Webster GA and Cameron TWM: Epidemiology and diagnosis of echinococcosis in Canada. Can Med Assoc J 96:600, 1967.

Wilson JF, Diddams AC, and Rausch RL: Cystic hydatid disease in Alaska. A review of 101 autochthonous cases of Echinococcus granulosus infection. Am Rev Respir Dis 98(1):1, 1968.

Alveolar Hydatid Disease

Lanier AP, Trujillo DE, Schantz PM et al: Comparison of serologic tests for the diagnosis and follow-up of alveolar hydatid disease. Am J Trop Med Hyg 37(3):609, 1987.

Rausch RL, Wilson JF, McMahon BJ, and O'Gorman MA: Consequences of continuous mebendazole therapy in alveolar hydatid disease—with a summary of a ten-year clinical trial. Ann Trop Med Parasitol 80(4):403, 1986.

Rausch RL, Wilson JF, Schantz PM, and McMahon BJ: Spontaneous death of Echinococcus multilocularis. Cases diagnosed serologically (by EM2 ELISA) and clinical significance. Am J Trop Med Hyg 36(3):576, 1987.

Schantz PM, Wilson JF, Wahlquist SP et al: Serologic tests for diagnosis and post-treatment evaluation of patients with alveolar hydatid disease (Echinococcus multilocularis). Am J Trop Med Hyg 32(6):1381, 1983.

Stehr-Green JK, Stehr-Green PA, Schantz PM et al: Risk factors for infection with Echinococcus multilocularis in Alaska. Am J Trop Med Hyg 38(2):380, 1988.

Thompson WM, Chisholm DP, and Tank R: Plain film roentgenographic findings in alveolar hydatid disease—Echinococcus multilocularis. Am J Roentgenol Radium Ther Nucl Med 116(2):345, 1972.

Webster GA and Cameron TWM: Epidemiology and diagnosis of echinococcosis in Canada. Can Med Assoc J 96:600, 1967.

Wilson JF, Davidson M, and Rausch RL: A clinical trial of mebendazole in the treatment of alveolar hydatid disease. Am Rev Respir Dis 118:747, 1978.

Wilson JF and Rausch RL: Alveolar hydatid disease. A review of clinical features of 33 indigenous cases of Echinococcus multilocularis infection in Alaskan Eskimos. Am J Trop Med Hyg 29(6):1340, 1980.

Wilson JF, Rausch RL, McMahon BJ et al: Albendazole therapy in alveolar hydatid disease. A report of favorable results in two patients after short-term therapy. Am J Trop Med Hyg 37(1):162, 1987.

64

WILLIAM A. HOWARD, M.D.

PULMONARY INFILTRATES WITH EOSINOPHILIA (LÖFFLER SYNDROME)

In 1932, Löffler described a group of patients with shadows of variable structures and fleeting density on chest roentgenograms, accompanied by a moderate eosinophilia (10 to 20 per cent) and mild systemic symptoms. This combination of symptoms was generally called Löffler syndrome and was presumed to be benign and of short duration, usually a matter of a few weeks. Although no etiologic agent was established, infection with *Ascaris lumbricoides* was known to be present in some of Löffler's cases. A year later, Weingarten reported the same pulmonary and blood findings in cases of tropical eosinophilia from India. Since that time, a number of other similar clinical pictures have been described, and the many variants are now often grouped together under the terms *eosinophilic pneumonopathy* or *pulmonary infiltrates with eosinophilia*, the PIE syndrome. The term *hypereosinophilic syndrome* has been proposed for the broad spectrum of disease states varying from Löffler's original syndrome to disseminated eosinophilic collagen disease and eosinophilic leukemia. Although Löffler syndrome remains as a diagnostic entity, it seems more appropriate to use the term *pulmonary infiltrates with eosinophilia* (PIE syndrome) as more indicative of current knowledge.

CLASSIFICATION

Crofton and associates (1952) proposed the following classification of this heterogeneous group, though it obviously goes far beyond Löffler's original concept.

Group I: Simple pulmonary involvement with eosinophilia, or Löffler's syndrome. This group is limited to those cases in which pulmonary infiltration persists for no more than 1 month, with mild or absent systemic symptoms.

Group II: Prolonged pulmonary eosinophilia. Here the duration is 2 to 6 months with definite symptoms and occasional recurrences but ultimate recovery. This type is not common in children.

Group III: Tropical eosinophilia (eosinophilic lung, Weingarten syndrome). This term is now reserved for those cases of eosinophilic pneumonia due to the presence of degenerating microfilariae found in eosinophilic granulomas in the lung in the absence of circulating adult filarial worms. The designation *occult filariasis* has been used for this form of the syndrome. Pulmonary symptoms may be mild, moderate, or severe, there is a characteristic marked eosinophilia, and without treatment, the course is prolonged.

Group IV: Pulmonary eosinophilia with asthma. Originally, this classification was made so that asthma with shifting pulmonary infiltrates could be included as an eosinophilic pneumopathy. It is now recognized that most such clinical pictures represent fungal infections with accompanying or superimposed allergic reactions to the causative fungus. The majority of these cases probably represent allergic bronchopulmonary aspergillosis.

Group V: Polyarteritis nodosa. This entity was recognized originally as being sometimes associated with eosinophilic lung disease with peripheral eosinophilia. This concept must now be enlarged to include the collagen vascular diseases as a group: systemic lupus erythematosus, eosinophilic granuloma, and other diseases associated with a disseminated vasculitis.

Taking into account new knowledge of the hypereosinophilic syndromes and more information concerning the role of the eosinophil in the inflammatory response, Neva and Ottesen (1978) have proposed a new classification based on etiology that would be applicable, in their opinion, to those conditions in which the eosinophil count exceeds 3000 cells/mm.[3] They suggest that hypereosinophilia be designated as parasitic, fungal, drug induced, vasculitic, or idiopathic, thus allowing for the variable manifestations of the syndrome due to the same etiologic agent, an eminently practical suggestion.

ETIOLOGY AND PATHOLOGY

In many instances of pulmonary infiltrates with eosinophilia, no specific etiologic agent can be determined. However, with a careful history and appropriate laboratory studies, it is possible to establish the correct diagnosis in the majority of patients.

Classic Löffler syndrome tends to occur in individuals with a personal or family history of allergy. Roentgenographic densities may be unilateral or bilateral, are usually located in the periphery of the lung, and are produced by infiltration of alveolar septa and alveolar spaces by eosinophils and histiocytes, without basement membrane damage. These shadows migrate and resolve spontaneously. Duration is 1 to 4 weeks, and the condition appears to be self-limited. This transient type appears to be due either to the migratory phase of parasitic nematodes, such as *Ascaris*, *Ancylostoma*, *Toxocara*, and *Trichuris*, or to drugs, including aspirin, penicillin, sulfonamides, imipramine, methyl phenidate, chlorpromazine, and nitrofurantoin (the list continues to grow).

The entity designated as prolonged pulmonary eosinophilia is distinguished from typical Löffler syndrome largely on the basis of duration. Peripheral eosinophilia and transient radiographic abnormalities may be present for as long as 6 months. The etiology appears to be the same, but symptoms are more severe and more prolonged, even though resolution or response to treatment may be similar.

Tropical eosinophilia (eosinophilic lung, Weingarten syndrome) is a specific hypereosinophilic syndrome occurring as a reaction to filarial infection. Evidence was largely circumstantial until microfilariae were identified in pulmonary nodules and lymph nodes, surrounded by necrotic tissue and eosinophilic leukocytes. These granulomatous lesions appear well within the lung parenchyma, and filariae cannot always be demonstrated. The larval forms of *Wuchereria bancrofti* and *Brugia malayi* have been identified as the causative agents when identification was possible. There is little or no filaremia, and the human host is able to sequester and contain the larval forms in the pulmonary parenchyma, much as happens in *Toxocara canis* infections. In each instance, the defense mechanism subjects the host to considerable tissue damage, with resulting development of the clinical picture of disease.

Asthma has been noted to be a part of many of the conditions associated with pulmonary eosinophilia, and in light of present knowledge it is difficult to find a reason to separate as a clinical entity those cases that manifest wheezing at some point in their course. However, asthma may assume a more prominent role in some situations, as in bronchopulmonary aspergillosis. Manifestations of this disease stem from noninvasive colonization of segments of the bronchi and bronchioles with *Aspergillus*, and perhaps other fungi such as *Candida*. Bronchi become dilated but are filled with inspissated mucus and exudate, which may lead to mucoid impaction and bronchiolitis obliterans. Parenchymal granulomas are seen occasionally, and bronchiectasis may be an end result without appropriate management. The growing fungi give rise to antigens that produce both reaginic (IgE) and IgG antibodies. The IgE level may be as high as several thousand IU per milliliter.

Pulmonary eosinophilia occurring with polyarteritis nodosa and other collagen vascular diseases is only one of the many manifestations of these systemic ailments, in which problems extend far beyond lung tissue abnormalities. Autoimmune phenomena, abnormalities of T and B cell function, and organ involvement, which characterize this large group of diseases, make it impractical to do more than mention them here as one other possible cause of pulmonary infiltrates with eosinophilia.

CLINICAL MANIFESTATIONS

In Löffler syndrome and the more prolonged forms of pulmonary infiltrates with eosinophilia, initial symptoms may be mild or absent. In the simplest forms, an occasional cough or wheeze may occur, and scattered moist rales and rhonchi may be heard. Pulmonary lesions appear as migratory infiltrates, which may give the appearance of pneumonia or atelectasis (Figs. 64–1, 64–2, and 64–3). The disappearing lesions leave no residua. When the disease is more prolonged, cough and dyspnea may appear and may be accompanied by mucoid sputum, malaise, fever, and even hemoptysis, suggesting tuberculosis. Asthma, if present, is related to the degree of lung involvement and only rarely to IgE-mediated atopic allergic responses, such as are seen in bronchopulmonary aspergillosis. Spontaneous exacerbations and remissions of both symptoms and signs may occur. Pulmonary function tests are more apt to show a restrictive pattern of lung disease with decreased vital capacity, and hypoxemia may occur during active phases of the disease. First-second vital capacity may be reduced when wheezing is a part of the picture.

In tropical eosinophilia, there is generally an insidious onset in an individual who gives a history of residence in an area endemic for human filariasis. There may be cough, wheeze, dyspnea, bronchitis, chest pain, fever, weight loss, and fatigue. The duration may be weeks or months, and remissions and recrudescences are common. Initial pulmonary function studies suggest an obstructive pattern, but a restrictive pattern develops in most individuals, along with evidence of impairment of diffusion. Affected patients may be quite ill and, if untreated, may develop chronic lung disease.

As indicated previously, when asthma is a major feature of pulmonary infiltrates with eosinophilia, one suspects fungal involvement of the lung, usually by some species of *Aspergillus*. Affected patients have elevated temperature, episodic wheezing, and chronic cough with expectoration of brown mucus plugs. Anorexia, malaise, and fatigue are present, as well as weight loss and night sweats. There are signs of chronic asthma with hyperinflation, and in advanced cases there may be clubbing of the fingers. A more detailed discussion of this entity and related fungal diseases is found elsewhere in this volume (Chapters 42 and 51).

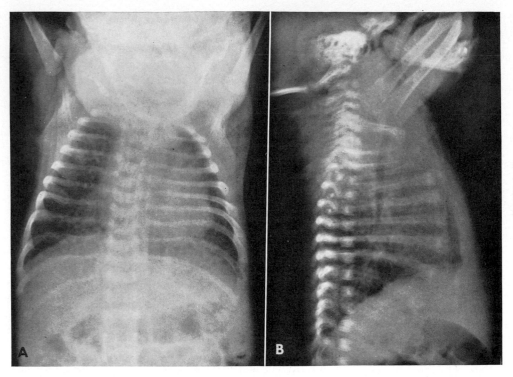

Figure 64–1. Radiograph, on admission of a child with Löffler syndrome. There is increased density at the base of the right lung. (Courtesy of John Kirkpatrick, M.D.)

DIAGNOSIS

Diagnosis depends on roentgenographic evidence of transient and migratory pulmonary infiltrations with eosinophilia and only mild systemic manifestations. A consideration of possible etiologic agents should include a careful history of recent drug ingestion and a careful search for parasites. Among those responsible besides *Ascaris* and *Toxocara* are the hookworms, *Strongyloides* infection, and other nematodes. If intestinal parasites are suspected, the diagnosis may not be definitive until positive identification of the offending agent can be made. The pulmonary phase of nematode infections may appear days or weeks before ova from adult worms can be detected in the stools. It is appropriate to examine stools for ova and parasites both at the time of the initial evaluation and at intervals of 2 to 4 weeks if necessary. Differentiation of Löffler syndrome from prolonged pulmonary eosinophilia is based primarily on observing the duration and severity of the disease, because the basic problem remains the same.

Eosinophil counts are usually quite high, up to 50 per cent in peripheral blood smears, and absolute eosinophil counts should exceed 3000 cells/mm^3 to sustain a diagnosis of pulmonary infiltrates with eo-

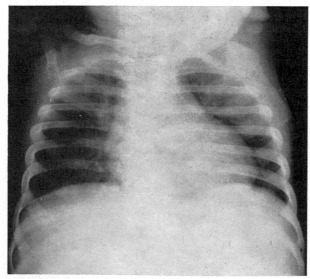

Figure 64–2. Radiograph taken 2 weeks after the radiograph shown in Figure 64–1. (Courtesy of John Kirkpatrick, M.D.)

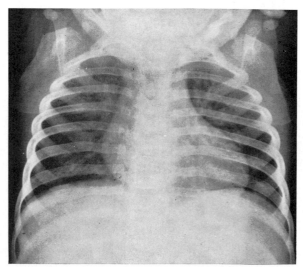

Figure 64–3. Radiograph taken 1 month after the one shown in Figure 64–2. There is an area of infiltration at the base of the right lung. (Courtesy of John Kirkpatrick, M.D.)

sinophilia. Immunoglobulin E levels are quite high, perhaps exceeding 10,000 IU/ml. If *Toxocara* is suspected and ova are not present in the stool, the enzyme-linked immunosorbent assay (ELISA) will show the presence of toxocaral antibodies and is sufficiently sensitive to differentiate *Toxocara* from *Ascaris*.

Tropical eosinophilia is suspected in those individuals who have resided in an area endemic for human filariasis and who have symptoms suggesting prolonged pulmonary eosinophilia but usually more severe and of longer duration. Diagnosis is made difficult because microfilariae cannot be found in the blood during either the day or the night. However, high titers of antifilarial antibodies can be detected in the patient's serum by complement-fixation, hemagglutination, and the more sensitive ELISA tests. Immunoglobulin E levels are generally in the range of 1000 to 5000 IU/ml but not as high as those seen in prolonged pulmonary eosinophilia. Peripheral eosinophilia is pronounced. Lung or lymph node biopsy may give a definitive diagnosis, but the yield is low, and the procedure seems unnecessary with the available laboratory aids. Diagnosis can also be confirmed by favorable response to treatment.

Ottesen and co-workers (1981) noted that patients with filarial infections develop specific IgE antibody, but when subsequently exposed to filarial antigen in vivo, they rarely manifest allergic reactions. Using the technique of histamine release from basophils, they were able to show that autologous serum blocked the release of histamine. Development of an IgG blocking antibody was shown to be a regular component of the immunologic response to chronic filarial infections. Subsequently, the same group (1985) demonstrated in patients with either microfilaremia or tropical pulmonary eosinophilia that up to 95 per cent of the blocking antibody activity was in the IgG4 fraction. Hussain, Grogyl, and Ottesen (1987) further showed that filarial antibody in patients with elephantiasis was largely of the IgG1 and IgG3 classes. Lal and Ottesen (1988) were able to show an enhanced diagnostic specificity by assessment of filaria-specific IgG4 antibody.

If bronchopulmonary aspergillosis is suspected and asthma is a regular part of the clinical picture, diagnosis can be made by identification of hyphae in the brown mucus plugs that are expectorated, and *Aspergillus* can be recovered on culture. Positive immediate skin-test reactions to *Aspergillus* are present, as well as Arthus-type reactions due to the presence of IgG precipitating antibodies. Roentgenographic findings may vary tremendously, from patchy areas of consolidations to proximal saccular bronchiectasis. Lung damage is enhanced by delayed recognition and treatment. Again, immunoglobulin E levels are high, and blood eosinophilia is pronounced.

TREATMENT

Typically, Löffler syndrome is self-limited, and treatment may not be necessary because it will have little or no effect on the pulmonary phase of the disease. Treatment of an identifiable underlying nematode infection is desirable, especially in those individuals with prolonged pulmonary eosinophilia, in which duration of symptoms is longer, remissions are common, systemic symptoms more severe, and there exists the possibility of some lung damage. *Toxocara* infections should be treated with thiabendazole, 25 to 50 mg/kg/day in divided doses for 7 to 10 days, with a repeat course in 4 weeks. Corticosteroid therapy may be indicated when symptoms are severe.

The response of microfilarial infections to diethylcarbamazine (Hetrazan) is both diagnostic and therapeutic. The large majority of patients show marked improvement or disappearance of symptoms after 7 to 10 days of treatment with 5 mg/kg/day in divided doses. Relapses may occur and may be retreated. The longer the duration of illness and the more severe the symptoms, the less likely there is to be a favorable response. Diethylcarbamazine, while effective, may require daily administration for as long as 2 to 3 weeks to achieve the maximum therapeutic effect. It often produces severe reactions, especially in individuals with heavier microfilarial loads, and compliance is often poor. This drug is not currently available. Kumaraswami and coworkers (1988) tried ivermectin, a semisynthetic macrolide antibiotic with a wide helminthicidal spectrum for parasites of animals that was shown to be effective in human onchocerciasis (Greene et al, 1985; Awadzi et al, 1986). It was found that a single dose of ivermectin in the range of 25 to 200 mg compared favorably with diethylcarbamazine with respect to parasite killing and side effects, with the obvious benefit of requiring only a single dose. They suggest that further investigation will be needed to determine the smallest effective dose and whether additional doses might enhance killing of adult worms. Corticosteroids will prove useful in controlling symptoms and are most useful in the more severely ill patients.

Bronchopulmonary aspergillosis is also best treated with corticosteroids, if long-term lung damage is to be avoided. Bronchodilators and physical therapy will also be useful in helping the patient clear the thick secretions from the chest. Anti-fungal agents are not usually very effective because of the difficulty of reaching the organisms in the viscid mucus in the respiratory tract.

REFERENCES

Awadzi K, Dadzie KY, and Schulz-Key H: The chemotherapy of onchocerciasis: XI. A double blind comparative study of ivermectin, diethylcarbamazine and placebo in human onchocerciasis in Northern Ghana. Ann Trop Med Parasitol 80:927, 1986.

Bell RJM: Pulmonary infiltrations with eosinophilia caused by chlorpropamide. Lancet 1:1249, 1964.

Crofton JW, Livingston JL, Oswald NC, and Roberts ATM: Pulmonary eosinophilia. Thorax 7:1, 1952.

Danaraj TJ, Pacheco G, Shanmugaratnam K, and Beaver PC: The etiology and pathology of eosinophilic lung (tropical eosinophilia). Am J Trop Med Hyg 15:183, 1966.

Greene BM et al: Efficacy of ivermectin and diethylcarbamazine in the treatment of onchocerciasis. N Engl J Med 313:133, 1985.

Hussain R, Grogyl M, and Ottesen EA: IgG antibody subclasses in human filariasis. J Immunol 139:2794, 1987.

Incaprera FP: Pulmonary eosinophila. Am Rev Respir Dis 84:730, 1961.

Kumaraswami V et al: Ivermectin for the treatment of Wuchereria bancrofti filariasis. JAMA 259:3150, 1988.

Lal RB and Ottesen EA: Enhanced diagnostic specificity in human filariasis by IgG$_4$ antibody assessment. J Infect Dis 158:1034, 1988.

Loeffler W: Zur Differential-Diagnose der Lungeninfiltrierungen. II. Ueber fluchtige Succedan-Infiltrate (mit Eosinophilie). Beitr Klin Tuberk 79:368, 1932.

Mark L: Loeffler's syndrome. Dis Chest 25:128, 1954.

Neva FA, Kaplan AP, Pacheco G et al: Tropical eosinophilia. J Allergy Clin Immunol 55:422, 1976.

Neva FA, and Ottesen EA: Tropical (filarial) eosinophila. N Engl J Med 298:1129, 1978.

Ottesen EA et al: Naturally occurring blocking antibodies modulate immediate hypersensitivity responses in human filariasis. J Immunol 127:2014, 1981.

Ottesen EA et al: Prominence of IgG4 in the IgG antibody response to human filariasis. J Immunol 134:2707, 1985.

Pepys J: Basic mechanisms in acute and chronic allergic lung disease. Immunol Allergy Pract 3:115, 1981.

Poh SC: The course of lung function in treated tropical pulmonary eosinophilia. Thorax 29:710, 1974.

Quinlan CD and Mitchell DM: The hypereosinophilic syndrome. J Ir Med Assoc 63:186, 1970.

Rutenberg AM, Rosales CL, and Bennett JM: An improved histochemical method for the demonstration of leukocyte alkaline phosphatase. Clinical application. J Lab Clin Med 65:698, 1965.

Scheer EH: Loeffler's syndrome. Arch Pediatr 68:407, 1951.

Weingarten RJ: Tropical eosinophilia. Lancet 1:103, 1933.

Wilson IC, Gambill JM, and Sandifer MG: Loeffler's syndrome occurring during imipramine therapy. Am J Psychiatry 119:892, 1963.

65

NATHAN L. KOBRINSKY, M.D., BSc. (Med), HILDA L. GRITTER, M.D., F.R.C.P.(C), and BRUCE SHUCKETT, M.D., F.R.C.P.(C)

LANGERHANS CELL HISTIOCYTOSIS

Langerhans cell histiocytosis (LCH), previously known as histiocytosis X, encompasses three rare conditions (eosinophilic granuloma of bone, Hand-Schüller-Christian disease, and Letterer-Siwe disease) that have in common an infiltration of tissues by histiocytes (Lichtenstein, 1953). The change in nomenclature reflects the central role played by the Langerhans cell (similar or identical to the Langerhans cell normally resident in skin) in these disorders (Chu et al, 1987).

Any of the tissues in which cells of the mononuclear phagocytic system (MPS) normally reside can be involved in LCH, including the skin (Langerhans cell), bone (osteoclast), liver (Kupffer cell), brain (microglial cell), blood (monocyte), spleen, thymus, lymph nodes, soft tissues, bone marrow (tissue macrophage), and lung (alveolar macrophage) (Basset et al, 1983). The following discussion focuses primarily on lung involvement in LCH. Readers interested in a more comprehensive discussion of the topic are referred to a review by Osband and Pochedly (1987).

Supported by the Children's Hospital of Winnipeg Research Foundation, Inc.

THE ROLE OF IMMUNE DYSFUNCTION IN THE GENESIS OF LANGERHANS CELL HISTIOCYTOSIS

For a long time, LCH was thought of as a neoplastic disorder. Superficially, this classification seems entirely reasonable: LCH may disseminate widely; produce destructive lesions in bone and other tissues; and run a rapidly progressive, lethal course. Furthermore, standard treatment strategies have evolved to include radiation therapy and chemotherapy—modalities used primarily in the treatment of cancer.

Despite these similarities, LCH demonstrates none of the histopathologic features of a malignant neoplasm: the histiocytic infiltration of tissues in LCH appears to be reactive rather than primary. There is compelling evidence that this process is immune mediated and that LCH results from an abnormality in immune regulation (Osband, 1987). The cells found in the lesions of LCH, including the Langerhans cell, monocytes, eosinophils, and lymphocytes, are all immunoreactive. Also LCH bears clinical and histopathologic similarities to various other immune-mediated disorders, including severe combined immune deficiency and graft-verses-host disease following bone marrow transplantation (Cedarbaum et al, 1972; Cedarbaum et al, 1974; Scott et al, 1975).

Evidence of immune dysfunction in LCH is considerable. Thymic dysplasia has been reported in 23 out of 28 patients (82 per cent) with LCH but in 0 out of 4 cases of malignant histiocytosis (Hamoudi et al, 1982). This study suggests that an abnormality in the T cell arm of the immune system may exist. In several studies of peripheral blood lymphocyte function performed at diagnosis or during remission, abnormal proliferative responses to mitogens were found in only 9 out of 63 cases (14 per cent) (Leikin et al, 1973; Nesbit et al, 1981; Thommesen et al, 1978; McLelland et al, 1987). Studies of lymphocyte subsets have, however, defined a seemingly consistent defect in the suppressor (T8) subset of peripheral blood T cells (Osband et al, 1981; Broadbent et al, 1984; Davies et al, 1983; Shannon et al, 1986). Whether this defect is primary or is secondary to damaged thymic epithelium is unknown. Abnormalities of immunoglobulins have also been reported in LCH (Leikin et al, 1973; Lahey et al, 1985). These abnormalities are not consistent and appear to be secondary rather than primary abnormalities.

PATHOLOGY

Pulmonary LCH is characterized pathologically by nodular or diffuse infiltrates, or both, consisting of histiocytes and variable numbers of eosinophils, plasma cells, and lymphocytes (Figs. 65–1 and 65–2). The infiltrate typically occurs in the interstices but may extend into the alveolae, particularly early in the course of the disease. The lesions occur near vessels, bronchioles, and pleurae. Cystic changes are often prominent, and the interstitium may show varying degrees of fibrosis and xanthomatous

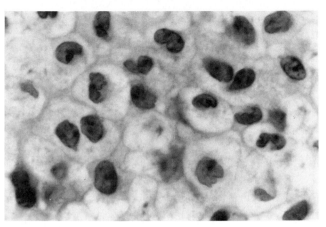

Figure 65–2. This higher power magnification emphasizes the irregular nuclei of the Langerhans cells, with prominent nucleoli and clefting (hematoxylin and eosin, original magnification × 100).

changes in the Langerhans cells, particularly if the process has been long-standing (Figs. 65–3, 65–4, 65–5, and 65–6). Arteritis or obliteration of small blood vessels, or both, may be evident (Kawanami et al, 1981). In a study of 51 cases of LCH, specific pathologic features, including cellular atypia and mitotic activity, were not found to correlate with disease outcome (Risdall et al, 1983).

Electron microscopy is essential in establishing the diagnosis of LCH by identifying the characteristic Langerhans cells. These cells are histiocytes that normally reside in the epidermis and dermis and are thought to play a central role in the pathogenesis of the disease. They are identified by characteristic intracytoplasmic rod-shaped structures called X bodies (or Birbeck granules) (Basset et al, 1978) (Fig. 65–7). Langerhans cells have been shown to react with OKT6 (Ortho Diagnostics)—an antibody that reacts with normal human thymocytes. Langerhans cells have also been shown to react with antibodies to S-100 protein and with a peanut lectin (Fig. 65–8). These techniques have been useful in establishing

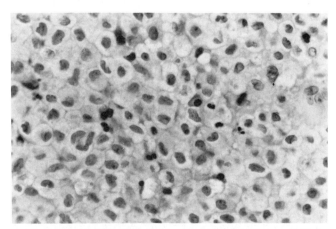

Figure 65–1. This classic infiltration of Langerhans cell histiocytosis demonstrates cells with abundant cytoplasm and large, irregular nuclei with prominent clefting and lobation. Several plasma cells are also noted (hematoxylin and eosin, original magnification × 40).

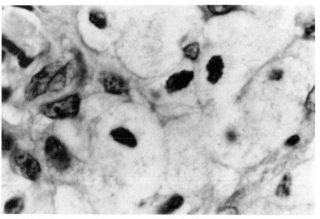

Figure 65–3. As the lesions of Langerhans cell histiocytosis age, the cells may undergo xanthomatous change, and the nuclear morphology becomes less striking. Large, bizarre Langerhans cells are noted adjacent to cells with more pyknotic nuclei and abundant cytoplasm (hematoxylin and eosin, original magnification × 100).

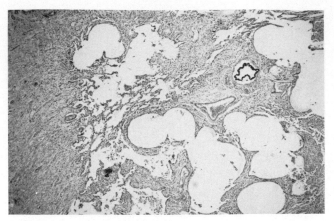

Figure 65–4. Lung involvement with Langerhans cell histiocytosis demonstrates irregular, cystic air spaces with an increase in the intervening interstitial tissue. The pleura shows marked thickening (hematoxylin and eosin, original magnification × 25).

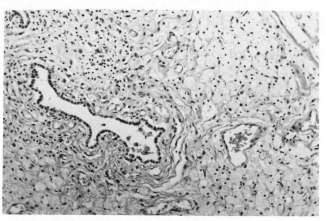

Figure 65–6. The pleura shows infiltration by large, xanthomatous cells. An air space lined by type II alveolar cells is noted in the center of the field (hematoxylin and eosin, original magnification × 100).

the diagnosis of LCH by immunochemical staining of fixed tissue and by the staining of cells obtained by bronchoalveolar lavage (Ree and Kadin, 1986; Soler et al, 1985; Chollet et al, 1984; Flint et al, 1986; Verea-Hernando et al, 1982).

In patients with known multifocal LCH, the appearance of an interstitial infiltrate on chest radiographs may be presumptive evidence of pulmonary involvement; however, the possibility of a superimposed opportunistic pneumonia cannot be excluded without a tissue diagnosis. Similarly, bronchoscopy with bronchoalveolar lavage may be adequate in establishing the diagnosis using immunohistochemical techniques; however, this approach may be suboptimal if infection is a major concern.

multifocal (Hand-Schüller-Christian) disease. Isolated or "primary" pulmonary involvement is distinctly unusual in children but common in young and middle-aged adults. In the discussion that follows, isolated eosinophilic granuloma of bone and congenital cutaneous LCH (a self-limited disorder confined to skin) are not considered (Marsh et al, 1983). Disseminated LCH with pulmonary involvent and primary pulmonary LCH are discussed separately.

DISSEMINATED LANGERHANS CELL HISTIOCYTOSIS

NATURAL HISTORY

In infants, LCH commonly involves the lung with widespread rapidly progressive (Letterer-Siwe) disease; in children, it involves the lung with chronic

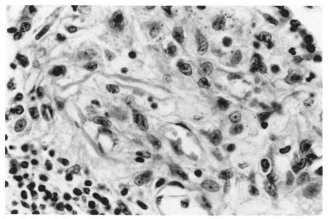

Figure 65–5. The interstitium contains inflammatory cells, mainly lymphocytes, and a population of cells with large, irregular nuclei and a variable amount of xanthomatous cytoplasm, which can be seen at the higher power magnification (hematoxylin and eosin, original magnification × 400).

Letterer-Siwe Disease

Children with LCH younger than 6 months of age typically present with widespread rapidly progressive (Letterer-Siwe) disease with involvement of skin, liver, spleen, lymph nodes, bone marrow, and lung (Berry and Becton, 1987). Lytic lesions of bone and diabetes insipidus, features of chronic multifocal (Hand-Schüller-Christian) disease, are rarely present. Clinical features may include fever, generalized seborrheic or hemorrhagic rash or both, pallor, icterus, hepatosplenomegaly, and lymphadenopathy.

Pulmonary involvement is usually evident on chest radiographs but rarely produces symptoms and may regress with time (Carlson et al, 1976). Some infants, however, develop a dry, nonproductive cough, cyanosis, and tachypnea. These symptoms may be due to histiocytic infiltration of the lung or, alternatively, to the development of an opportunistic interstitial or alveolar pneumonia, e.g., *Pneumocystis carinii*, histoplasmosis, atypical mycobacteria, *Aspergillus* or *Pseudomonas* secondary to underlying immune dysfunction (Komp et al, 1980; Komp, 1981). Over time, symptomatic lung involvement by LCH may lead to

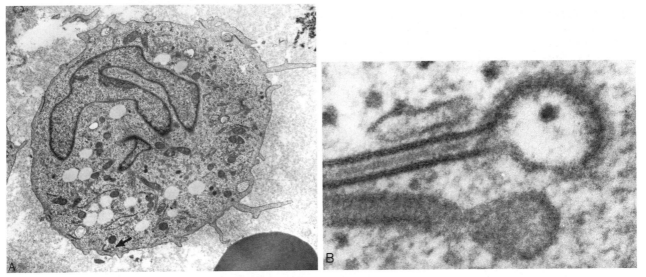

Figure 65–7. *A,* Electron microscopy shows the Langerhans cell to resemble a histiocyte with irregular plasma membranes; a lack of cell junctions; a large, irregular nucleus; and abundant cytoplasm. Birbeck granules can be identified at low power. *B,* The Birbeck granules (enlarged) demonstrate a cylindric structure with two membranes and a central zipper-like structure with a terminal swelling that forms a characteristic racquet shape. (Transmission electron micrograph, original magnification in *A* × 16,790; original magnification in *B* × 276,750).

failure to thrive from the increased work of breathing (Nondahl et al, 1986).

Hand-Schüller-Christian Disease

Children with LCH older than 6 months of age typically present with an isolated lesion of bone (eosinophilic granuloma) or multiple lesions of bone or other tissues or both (Hand-Schüller-Christian disease) (Berry and Becton, 1987). Bony lesions are often located in sites of active hematopoiesis, including the skull, axial skeleton, and proximal long bones. Clinical manifestations may include a localized or generalized seborrheic rash, bone pain, "floating" teeth (due to erosion of alveolar bone in the jaw), otitis media refractory to standard therapy, exophthalmos (from soft tissue infiltration), diabetes insip-

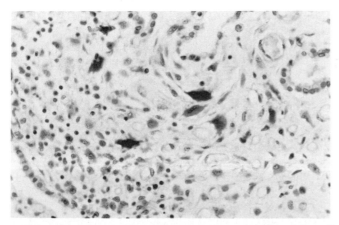

Figure 65–8. Langerhans cells demonstrate variable staining of S-100 protein. The cells with smaller nuclei and more abundant cytoplasm stain less well (S-100 immunoperoxidase, original magnification × 250).

idus (from infiltration of the hypothalamus), hepatosplenomegaly, lymphadenopathy, icterus, anemia, and thrombocytopenia.

Pulmonary involvement is common in children with multifocal LCH. In a review of 350 cases, pulmonary involvement was evident in 111 (32 per cent) (Lahey, 1983). Further, pathologic study confirms the presence of lung involvement in the majority of cases in which autopsies are performed (Komp et al, 1980; Komp, 1981). Signs and symptoms of pulmonary involvement may include fever, fatigue, weight loss, cough, tachypnea, cyanosis, clubbing, and hemoptysis. Recurrent spontaneous pneumothoraces are common in adults with LCH but are also recognized in children and adolescents (Gelfand and Sheiner, 1974). Pulmonary involvement may be clinically silent, regress with time, or slowly progress over years. Patients in the last category may eventually develop cor pulmonale and lung failure, or they may succumb to an overwhelming opportunistic pneumonia. Pulmonary involvement is the most common cause of death in long-term survivors (Komp et al, 1980; Komp, 1981).

Prognosis

For all children with multifocal LCH (Letterer-Siwe or Hand-Schüller-Christian variants), the clinical course may be exceedingly variable with periods of disease activity followed by prolonged or indefinite periods of quiescence. In a study of 92 patients by the Pediatric Oncology Group, the onset of last disease activity was 24 months or less for 55 per cent of cases (Berry et al, 1986). In this series, 25 (27 per cent) developed no disease progression after initial presentation; 53 (58 per cent) developed disease progression (primarily skin, bone, soft tissue, or diabetes insipidus) without organ dysfunction; and 14 (15 per cent) developed disease progression with organ dysfunction (hematopoietic in five, liver in seven, and lung in five). All patients with disease progression and organ dysfunction died (15 per cent). All other patients survived with varying degrees of morbidity during the study period (1974 to 1982). In another study of 70 patients, hematopoietic, liver, and lung dysfunction were also found to predict a poor outcome. Conversely, a patient with bone involvement with an absence of skin involvement was found to have a particularly good prognosis (Broadbent, 1986).

Late Effects

The long-term complications of the disease and its treatment are frequent (affecting more than 50 per cent of survivors) and severe. For example, in the Pediatric Oncology Group study, 27 (29 per cent) developed diabetes insipidus. Other reported late effects include deafness, mental retardation, short stature (from chronic disease, erosion of the axial skeleton, and growth hormone deficiency), hypogonadism, panhypopituitarism, scoliosis and paraplegia (from vertebral erosion and collapse), osteoarthritis, cirrhosis of the liver, gastrointestinal hemorrhage, liver failure, and the long-term pulmonary complications previously discussed (Komp et al, 1980; Komp, 1981; Braunstein and Kolher, 1981). At least 12 malignant neoplasms have been reported in long-term survivors of LCH—undoubtedly due to the effects of radiation therapy, chemotherapy, and perhaps the disease process itself. These include thyroid cancer (3), brain tumors (3), leukemia (2), lymphoma (1), hepatocellular carcinoma (2), and osteogenic sarcoma (1) (Matus-Ridley et al, 1983; Berry et al, 1986).

To summarize, the prognosis for LCH is poor if organ dysfunction (not just organ involvement) is present, namely, anemia, thrombocytopenia, jaundice, or clinically significant lung disease (Lahey, 1975; Lahey, 1983; Matus-Ridley et al, 1983). The prognosis is also poor if disease activity is unremitting despite optimal medical therapy (Berry et al, 1986). Late effects of the disease and its treatment are a major concern.

"PRIMARY" PULMONARY LANGERHANS CELL HISTIOCYTOSIS

Children

Although pulmonary involvement is present in approximately 32 per cent of cases of disseminated LCH in childhood, "primary" pulmonary LCH (or eosinophilic granuloma of the lung) is distinctly rare in patients under 15 years of age (Aftimos et al, 1974; Carlson et al, 1976; Hambleton et al, 1976; Berlow et al, 1982; Nondahl et al, 1986). In the 12 cases reported, the clinical features and the radiologic and pathologic findings are identical to those found in disseminated LCH except that extrapulmonary involvement is minimal or absent. Also the development of spontaneous pneumothoraces is uncommon. As with disseminated LCH, the clinical course is unpredictable: the disease may rapidly progress, spontaneously remit, or smolder for years with exacerbations and remissions, leading eventually to pulmonary fibrosis and a respiratory death.

Adults

In adults, primary pulmonary LCH is an uncommon but well-recognized entity. Since its first description by Farinacci in 1951, hundreds of cases have been reported (Farinacci et al, 1951; Smith et al, 1986; Basset et al, 1978; Prophet, 1982; Colby and Lombard, 1983; Marcy and Reynolds, 1985). In one series, LCH was found to be the cause of 17 out of 502 cases (3.4 per cent) of diffuse interstitial lung disease (Gaensler and Carrington, 1980).

Primary pulmonary LCH is a disease of young and middle-aged adults (20 to 40 years; mean of 32 years in one large series), although cases in the elderly have been reported (Colby and Lombard, 1983). Caucasians are primarily affected; blacks are rarely stricken, and Asians are virtually never affected (Prophet, 1982). This pattern is the opposite to that found in sarcoidosis, another granulomatous lung disease. Smoking is a strong risk factor for the development of pulmonary LCH (Friedman et al, 1981; Colby and Lombard, 1983). In one series of 320 patients, 80 per cent were smokers at the time of diagnosis, and 97 per cent were past or present smokers. This factor may explain the shift from a strong male predominance in earlier series to an almost equal sex distribution in later series because of the increased prevalance of smoking among women. Of interest in this regard, smoking has been shown to increase the number of alveolar macrophages obtained by bronchoalveolar lavage in control subjects and in patients with pulmonary LCH. Conversely, smoking has been shown to decrease the number of alveolar macrophages in patients with sarcoidosis, a disease in which smoking appears to be protective (Hance et al, 1986).

There are several distinctive features of primary pulmonary LCH in adults that are rare or undescribed in children. Adult patients develop recurrent, spontaneous pneumothoraces in approximately 20 to 25 per cent of cases (Lewis, 1964; Roland et al, 1964). Recurrent pleural effusions are also described (Winkler and Yam, 1980; Tittel and Winkler, 1981). Diabetes insipidus is present in approximately 7 to 10 per cent and bony lesions in 5 to 13 per cent of cases (Lewis, 1964; Friedman et al, 1981). Involvement of these extrapulmonary sites emphasizes the multisystem nature of the disease and the shortcomings of the designations *primary* and *multifocal*. The clinical features of adult pulmonary LCH are summarized in Table 65–1.

The outcome for adults with primary pulmonary LCH is variable and is largely unpredictable for the individual patient. Based on data obtained from an evaluation of 294 patients culled from two large series, 65 per cent stabilized or improved, 17 per cent deteriorated, and 18 per cent died of pulmonary disease (Basset et al, 1978; Colby and Lombard, 1983). Two cases of Hodgkin's disease of the lung and four cases of bronchogenic carcinoma have been reported in patients with previously diagnosed pulmonary LCH (Sajiad and Luna, 1982; Lombard et al, 1987). The significance of these associations is unknown but, at least for the cases of bronchogenic carcinoma, may reflect the commonality of smoking as a risk factor for the development of both diseases.

RADIOLOGIC FEATURES

At the time of initial presentation, extensive lung involvement may be evident from chest radiograph despite a lack of clinical symptoms. If LCH is suspected, a chest radiograph is therefore a mandatory part of the investigation.

Early in the course of the disease, a diffuse bilaterally symmetric linear and nodular interstitial pattern is evident. This pattern reflects the interstitial cellular infiltrate seen pathologically. The upper and midlung zones are most severely affected, and the costophrenic angles spared. This feature distinguishes LCH from other diffuse diseases of the lungs (Fraser and Paré, 1979). One study, limited to the pediatric age group, found no predilection of interstitial lung changes for any portion of the lung (Carlson et al, 1976) (Fig. 65–9). Differences in the chest radiographic findings of patients with primary or generalized pulmonary LCH were also not identified.

Cases have been described with perihilar alveolar density in a "butterfly" pattern suggestive of pulmonary edema (Fig. 65–10). This has been considered to be the first phase of lung involvement, representing alveolar infiltration by histiocytes and eosinophils before interstitial involvement (Weber et al, 1969).

Table 65–1. CLINICAL FEATURES OF PULMONARY LANGERHANS CELL HISTIOCYTOSIS IN ADULTS

Features	Per Cent (%)
Asymptomatic	14
Cough	58
Dyspnea	38
Chest pain	21
Fever	15
Weight loss	20
Fatigue	33
Hemoptysis	7
Pneumothorax	14
Diabetes insipidus	7
Bone lesions	8

(Adapted from Marcy T and Reynolds H: Lung 163:129, 1985.)

Others have not found such an alveolar pattern (Carlson et al, 1976).

As the disease progresses, increasing numbers of cysts develop, leading to a state known as honeycomb lung. Classically, honeycombing refers to multiple radiolucencies, each of which is less than 10 mm in diameter and can be traced through 360 degrees (Felson, 1966). Histologically, this process corresponds to an interstitial infiltrate of LCH in the walls of the primary pulmonary lobule. Honeycombing is considered characteristic of LCH particularly when seen in the upper lobes (Fraser and Pare, 1979) (Fig. 65–11).

With further progression, diffuse fibrosis occurs, usually in association with primary pulmonary LCH (Carlson et al, 1976). Larger cysts and bullae may be seen in the upper lobes along with linear densities representing fibrosis. Lung volumes are typically maintained in LCH, further differentiating it from other fibrotic lung diseases, such as fibrosing alveolitis (Fraser and Pare, 1979).

Pneumothorax is a feature associated with LCH and has been reported in up to 20 per cent of cases (Aftimos et al, 1974). Pneumothoraces may occur before interstitial changes are evident on chest radiographs (Carlson et al, 1976).

Hilar and mediastinal adenopathy, although rare in adults, have been described in children, and in one report, they preceded other manifestations of disease (Weber et al, 1969; Nakata et al, 1982) (Fig. 65–12). Cavitation of anterior mediastinal masses in LCH has also been reported (Abramson et al, 1987). Pleural effusion associated with LCH is considered rare but has been described in children (Matlin et al, 1972).

The clinical course of pulmonary LCH is extremely variable. Exacerbations and remissions are commonly reported and are certainly features of the disease in extrapulmonary sites. Nevertheless, in view of the known propensity of patients with LCH to develop opportunistic alveolar and interstitial pneumonias, clinical or radiologic deterioration, or both, may be due to infection rather than to disease activity. For this reason, a tissue diagnosis should be considered strongly if uncertainty exists. Further, in evaluating any new therapy, investigators must consider the possibility that clearing of an interstitial process on chest radiographs may in fact be due to the resolution of an infection rather than a response to therapy.

Concomitant involvement of lung and bone is not uncommon. The chest radiograph should therefore be assessed for lesions of the bony thorax and a complete skeletal survey performed routinely. Destructive punched out areas with well-defined borders and usually without marginal reactive sclerosis may be seen in membranous or long bones (Fig. 65–13). Vertebra plana is a characteristic feature of LCH, with flattening throughout of the vertebral centrum without anterior or posterior wedging (Edeiken, 1981) (Fig. 65–14). A [99m]technetium bone scan (sensitivity 67 per cent compared with standard radiog-

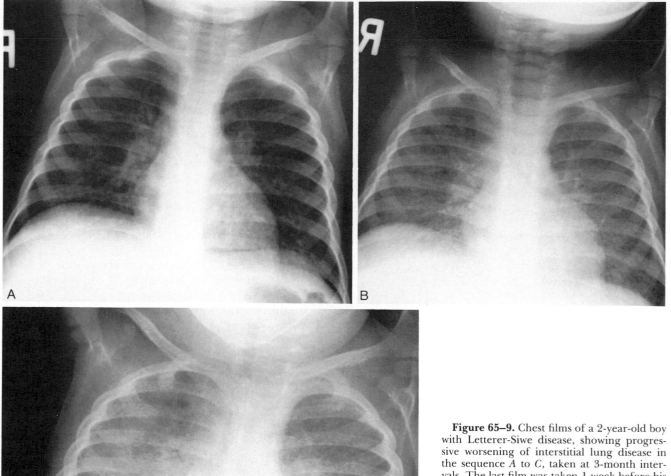

Figure 65–9. Chest films of a 2-year-old boy with Letterer-Siwe disease, showing progressive worsening of interstitial lung disease in the sequence *A* to *C*, taken at 3-month intervals. The last film was taken 1 week before his death. An autopsy demonstrated diffuse lung involvement by Langerhans cell histiocytosis and no evidence of superimposed infection.

raphy) may miss LCH lesions noted on the skeletal survey (Schaub et al, 1987).

The radiologic findings in 50 cases of adult pulmonary LCH are summarized in Table 65–2. In this series, sparing of the costophrenic angles was the only predictor of outcome and was associated with a good prognosis. Five patients died—two from pulmonary fibrosis and one from emphysema.

Differential Diagnosis

The differential diagnosis of a chronic diffuse interstitial process noted on chest radiographs would include infection (as discussed previously), sarcoidosis, allergic alveolitis, idiopathic pulmonary fibrosis, and lymphangiomyomatosis. Mediastinal and hilar adenopathy are uncommon features of LCH. If present, sarcoidosis should be considered. These entities may otherwise be difficult to distinguish on the basis of the chest radiograph appearance alone. The presence of extrapulmonary lytic lesions of bone with little or no sclerotic reaction noted on the skeletal survey strongly support the diagnosis of LCH.

EFFECTS ON PULMONARY FUNCTION

A mixed obstructive and restrictive pattern of functional impairment is noted in LCH (Colby and Lombard, 1983; Marcy and Reynolds, 1985). Early in the course of the disease, interstitial and alveolar

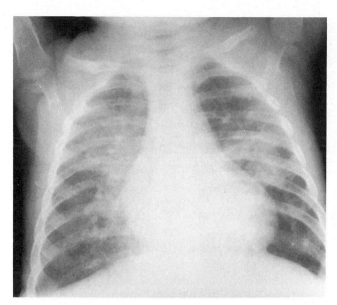

Figure 65–10. An 8-month-old native North American Indian boy with dermatitis, pyrexia, dyspnea, cyanosis, hepatosplenomegaly, diffuse lymphadenopathy, and failure to thrive. A skin biopsy confirmed the diagnosis of Langerhans cell histiocytosis, clinically the Letterer-Siwe variant. The chest radiograph shows perihilar densities with a "butterfly" pattern of alveolar infiltration. A fine nodular pattern is also seen diffusely throughout the lungs. These changes cleared with time.

aces. Pulmonary function tests reveal a decrease in vital capacity (VC) and an increase in residual volume (RV). Regional differences in compliance resulting from cyst formation may have variable effects on overall lung compliance (because of decreased recoil in the cyst wall). In general, however the FEV_1 is decreased. As the disease progresses further, fibrosis develops, which leads to a further decrease in lung compliance, an increase in dead-space ventilation, and a relative increase in the perfusion of poorly ventilated fibrotic tissues. The resultant ventilation-perfusion ($\dot{V}A/\dot{Q}$) mismatch may produce significant hypoxemia at rest. Stasis of secretions resulting from disruption of the mucociliary network leads to a further decrease in alveolar ventilation and predisposes to infection.

THERAPEUTIC STRATEGIES

Treatment of LCH remains unsatisfactory. Despite improvements in supportive care, morbidity and mortality figures remain unacceptably high, largely because of the lack of a consistently effective therapy. Furthermore, potentially new therapies are difficult to evaluate in a low-incidence disease with an extremely variable and a largely unpredictable clinical course (Lavin and Osband, 1987).

SUPPORTIVE CARE

Smoking

Smoking is a known risk factor for the development of pulmonary LCH in adults. Avoidance of

infiltration leads to impaired gas exchange (noted by a decreased DL_{CO}) and decreased lung compliance. These changes may be evident despite a normal chest radiographic appearance. As cyst formation develops and normal pulmonary architecture is disrupted, airway obstruction and increased dead-space ventilation (namely, preferential ventilation of cystic areas) become evident. These changes may lead to the formation of bullae and spontaneous pneumothor-

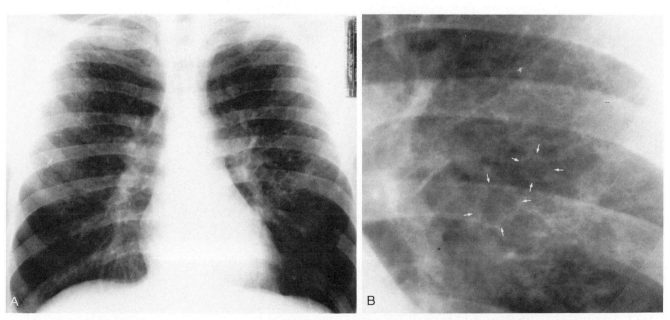

Figure 65–11. A 20-year-old male presenting with a 3-month history of exertional dyspnea and left-sided chest pain. *A*, Note the interstitial pattern in the mid and upper lung zones. *B*, A honeycomb pattern is demonstrated on the magnified view *(arrows)*. Langerhans cell histiocytosis was confirmed by lung biopsy. (Courtesy of Dr. Mark Rigby.)

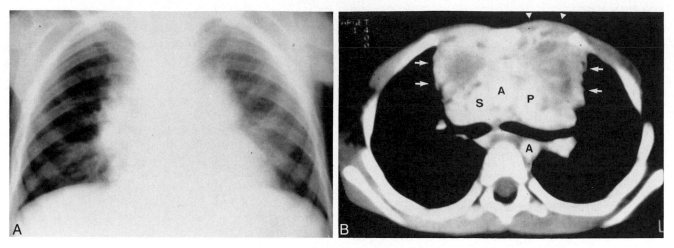

Figure 65–12. A 3-year-old boy with a 6-month history of pyrexia and wheezing. Lymphadenopathy of the neck and groin and diabetes insipidus were present. The chest radiograph shows hilar prominence and widening of the mediastinum *(A)*. A computed tomographic scan taken at a level just caudad to the carina *(B)* shows a large anterior mediastinal mass *(arrows)* with evidence of chest wall extension *(arrowheads)*. The superior vena cava *(S)*, ascending and descending thoracic aorta *(A)*, and pulmonary artery *(P)* are labeled. A biopsy specimen of the anterior mediastinal mass showed changes typical of Langerhans cell histiocytosis, clinically, the Hand-Schüller-Christian variant. (Courtesy of Dr. Alan Daneman.)

both active and passive smoking is therefore recommended.

Infection

Because of the known propensity for patients with LCH with pulmonary involvement to develop opportunistic alveolar and interstitial pneumonias, prophylactic treatment with trimethoprim-sulfamethoxazole (5 mg/kg/day trimethoprim and 25 mg/kg/day sulfamethoxazole or on three consecutive days weekly, taken orally) is recommended (Hughes et al, 1987;

Tubergen et al, 1986). This therapy will decrease the risk of *Pneumocystis carinii* pneumonia but will have no effect on the development of pneumonia due to viral or fungal organisms. Patients who demonstrate apparent disease progression clinically or radiologi-

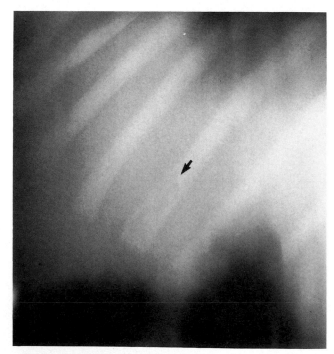

Figure 65–13. Tomogram of a lytic lesion *(arrow)*, involving the ninth rib in a 5-year-old boy with Langerhans cell histiocytosis.

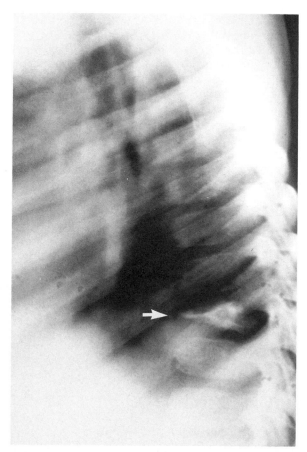

Figure 65–14. Vertebra plana of T9 *(arrow)* in a 5-year-old boy with Langerhans cell histiocytosis.

Table 65–2. RADIOLOGIC FINDINGS IN 50 CASES OF ADULT PULMONARY LANGERHANS CELL HISTIOCYTOSIS

Findings	Per Cent (%)
Reticulation	94
Micronodules (<2 mm)	92
Micronodules (2–5 mm)	40
Micronodules (5–10 mm)	12
Macronodules (>10 mm)	8
Cysts (<10 mm)	50
Cysts (>10 mm)	16
Bullae	4
Pneumothorax	14

(From Laronique J et al: Thorax 37:104, 1982.)

cally should be considered for fiberoptic bronchoscopy with bronchoalveolar lavage and transbronchial biopsy or an open-lung biopsy.

Pneumothorax

Patients who develop recurrent pneumothoraces may benefit from pleurodesis to eliminate the risk of recurrence.

Pulmonary Fibrosis

Fibrosis is often a feature of advanced pulmonary LCH. In an attempt to decrease the progression of pulmonary fibrosis, penicillamine was administered to five adult patients with advanced pulmonary LCH refractory to treatment with steroids, antimetabolites, and Vinca alkaloids. The dose of penicillamine used was 750 to 1000 mg/day, taken orally. All five patients improved symptomatically and demonstrated improvements in pulmonary function. Their chest radiographs, however, remained unchanged (Petheram et al, 1981). Penicillamine has been shown to inhibit the cross-linkage of polypeptides during collagen formation and to inhibit lysosomal enzyme activity (Friedman, 1977).

Colchicine (1.0 mg/day, taken orally, in adults) has been shown to decrease cirrhosis of the liver (Kershenobich et al, 1988). The mechanisms of action are not completely understood, although the drug is known to block mitosis and various functions of neutrophils, to decrease collagen formation, and to stimulate collagenase activity. Whether colchicine will also be effective in decreasing pulmonary fibrosis in LCH is unknown. Of interest in this regard, colchicine has been shown to decrease the raised levels of interleukin-1 in the peripheral blood mononuclear cells of patients with primary biliary cirrhosis (Kershenobich et al, 1984). Interleukin-1 is known to be produced by Langerhans cells (Saunder et al, 1984).

For patients with end-stage lung disease, heart-lung transplantation may be a possibility. Heart-lung transplantation has been performed successfully in children with cystic fibrosis and end-stage lung disease (Scott, 1988). Furthermore, there is a precedent for organ transplantation in LCH. Liver transplantation has been performed successfully in at least three children with LCH and end-stage liver disease (Esquivel, 1988). Two of the patients continue to do well postoperatively. The third patient has rejected two organ grafts because of noncompliance with the use of cyclosporin (used to prevent graft rejection). The use of cyclosporin has not been associated with disease exacerbation. For theoretic reasons (see subsequent discussion), cyclosporin may in fact prevent both graft rejection and disease recurrence.

"SPECIFIC" THERAPY

Corticosteroids

Steroids are effective in the treatment of LCH with bone, soft tissue, and skin involvement. They have also been shown to be effective in the treatment of lung involvement in both children and adults (Nondahl et al, 1986). A course of prednisone (2 mg/kg/day, taken orally) for 4 weeks with a subsequent taper over 8 weeks (with or without coincident treatment with a Vinca alkaloid) is recommended as initial therapy for patients with symptomatic pulmonary involvement.

Vinca Alkaloids

Vincristine (1.5 mg/m²; maximum 2.0 mg) or vinblastine (6.5 mg/m²) administered every 1 to 2 weeks intravenously is effective in the treatment of LCH with bone, soft tissue, and skin involvement. Efficacy in the treatment of liver and lung disease is unclear. Etoposide (VP-16-213) has been found to be effective, even in patients resistant to other therapies. The drug has not, however, been evaluated in a controlled trial. VP-16-213 is administered at a dosage of 100 to 150 mg/m² intravenously or 200 to 300 mg/m² taken orally for 3 days every 3 to 4 weeks (depending on peripheral blood count recovery) for a total of two to six courses (Starling, 1987; McLelland et al, 1987).

Antimetabolites

Methotrexate (20 to 25 mg/m²/week, taken orally) and 6-mercaptopurine (50 mg/m²/day, taken orally) have been shown to be effective in the treatment of LCH. Liver and pulmonary toxicities have, however, been described with these agents, and they are now considered second-line therapies (Starling, 1987).

Alkylating Agents

Chlorambucil (5 to 6 mg/m²/day, taken orally) and cyclophosphamide (90 to 150 mg/m²/day, taken orally) are generally less effective agents than the Vinca alkaloids in the treatment of LCH; furthermore, they carry the risk of second malignant neoplasms. For these reasons they are rarely used (Starling, 1987).

Radiation Therapy

Radiation therapy is often effective in controlling pulmonary LCH. The dose required is generally less than 1500 cGy, given in seven or eight fractions. This dose is below the limit of lung tolerance. Despite the feasibility of this approach, radiation therapy is usually restricted to the treatment of bone disease and only rarely employed for patients with visceral involvement. The long-term sequelae of pulmonary irradiation may include short stature, pulmonary fibrosis, osteogenic sarcoma, and nonlymphocytic leukemia (Cassady, 1987).

Thymic Extract (Suppressin)

Based on the finding of a suppressor cell defect in LCH, Osband and coinvestigators treated 17 patients with daily injections of a crude calf-thymic extract (suppressin) (Osband et al, 1981). In vitro correction of the immune defect was demonstrated in 12 patients (71 per cent). Since that time, 20 additional patients have been studied. The overall clinical response of 19 out of 37 (51 per cent) is comparable to that observed with conventional chemotherapy. A prospective randomized placebo-controlled trial is ongoing (Osband, 1987). Other clinical trials using thymic extracts have been less effective (Davies et al, 1983; Eckstein et al, 1984). The use of thymic extracts and synthetic thymic hormones for LCH remains controversial (McLelland et al, 1987).

FUTURE CONSIDERATIONS

Bone Marrow Transplantation

Bone marrow transplantation theoretically should be an extremely effective treatment for LCH. This approach should ablate all sites of active disease and correct the underlying immune defect. Generally, bone marrow transplantation would be available only for patients with an HLA-matched donor. Patients with extensive liver or lung involvement, or both, would not be good candidates. For patients without significant organ dysfunction, this approach would seem somewhat excessive (Komp, 1987). At least one child, an 11-year-old boy with chemotherapy-resistant progressive disease involving multiple bones, nodes, liver, and lungs, has successfully undergone bone marrow transplantation (Ringder et al, 1987).

Cyclosporin A

Cyclosporin is a potent immunosuppressive agent used primarily to treat aplastic anemia and other autoimmune disorders and to prevent graft rejection following kidney and liver transplantation. Cyclosporin acts mainly on cellular immunity and favors the expansion of antigen-specific, suppressor T cells (Kupiec-Weglinski et al, 1984). In view of the previously discussed suppressor cell deficiency in LCH,

there is theoretical justification for the use of this agent (McLelland et al, 1987). As previously discussed, at least three patients with LCH have undergone liver transplantation and have received cyclosporin in the posttransplant period to prevent graft rejection. Disease recurrence has not been observed while receiving the drug (Esquivel, 1988).

Alpha-interferon

Alpha-interferon has been used to treat two children (siblings) with advanced LCH with visceral involvement refractory to prednisone, vinblastine, 6-mercaptopurine, methotrexate, and doxorubicin (Jakobson et al, 1987). The drug was used as an immunomodulatory agent in view of the previously reported response to calf-thymic extract (Osband et al, 1981). The dose used was 1.3 million units intramuscularly daily (estimated 5×10^4 units/kg). After 10 weeks the interferon regimen was decreased to three times per week and was continued for 9+ and 21+ months. The therapy was well tolerated. Both children achieved complete and sustained remissions. This report is very exciting and will lead, it is hoped, to a prospective clinical trial in the near future.

REFERENCES

Abramson S et al: Cavitation of anterior mediastinal masses in children with histiocytosis X. Report of four cases with radiographic, pathologic findings and clinical follow-up. Pediatr Radiol 17:10, 1987.

Aftimos S et al: Primary pulmonary histiocytosis in an infant. Am J Dis Child 128:851, 1974.

Basset F and Ferrans V: The histiocytoses. Pathol Annu 2:27, 1983.

Basset F et al: Pulmonary histiocytosis X. Am Rev Respir Dis 118:811, 1978.

Basset F et al: The histiocytoses. Pathol Annu 2:27, 1983.

Berlow M et al: Diffuse pulmonary disease in a 2 1/2 year-old child. JAMA 248:875, 1982.

Berry D and Becton D: Natural history of histiocytosis X. Hematol Oncol Clin North Am 1:23, 1987.

Berry D et al: Natural history of histiocytosis X: a pediatric oncology group study. Med Pediatr Oncol 14:1, 1986.

Braunstein G and Kolher P: Endocrine manifestations of histiocytosis. Am J Pediatr Hematol Oncol 3:67, 1981.

Broadbent V: Favourable prognostic features in histiocytosis X: bone involvement and absence of skin disease. Arch Dis Child 61:1219, 1986.

Broadbent V et al: Spontaneous remission of multi-system histiocytosis-X. Lancet 1:253, 1984.

Carlson R et al: Pulmonary involvement by histiocytosis X in the pediatric age group. Mayo Clin Proc 51:542, 1976.

Cassady R: Radiation therapy in the management of histiocytosis-X. Hematol Oncol Clin North Am 1:123, 1987.

Cedarbaum S et al: Combined immunodeficiency manifested by Letterer-Siwe syndrome. Lancet 1:958, 1972.

Cedarbaum S et al: Combined immunodeficienct presenting as the Letterer-Siwe syndrome. J Pediatr 85:466, 1974.

Chollet S et al: Diagnosis of pulmonary histiocytosis X by immunodetection of Langerhans cells in bronchoalveolar lavage fluids. Am J Pathol 115:225, 1984.

Chu T et al: Histiocytosis syndromes in children. Lancet 1:208, 1987.

Colby T and Lombard C: Histiocytosis X in the lung. Hum Pathol 14:847, 1983.

Davies E et al: Thymic hormone therapy for histiocytosis-X. N Engl J Med 309:493, 1983.

Eckstein R et al: Influence on immune function parameters in histiocytosis-X of thymostimulin. Arzneimittleforsch 125:2611, 1984.

Edeiken J: Roentgen Diagnosis of Diseases of Bone. Vol 2, 3rd ed. Baltimore, Williams & Wilkins Co, 1981.

Esquivel C: Personal communication. Pacific Presbyterian Medical Center, 1988.

Farinacci C et al: Eosinophilic granuloma of the lung: report of two cases. US Armed Forces Med J 2:1085, 1951.

Felson B: Disseminated interstitial diseases of the lung. Ann Radiol (Paris) 9:325, 1966.

Flint A et al: Pulmonary histiocytosis X: immunoperoxidase staining for HLA-DR antigen and S-100 protein. Arch Pathol Lab Med 110:930, 1986.

Fraser R and Paré J: In Diagnosis of Diseases of the Chest. Vol 3, 2nd ed. Philadelphia, WB Saunders Co, 1979.

Friedman M: Chemical basis for pharmacological and therapeutic action of penicillamine. Ad Exp Med Biol 86B:649, 1977.

Friedman P et al: Eosinophilic granuloma of lung. Medicine 60:385, 1981.

Gaensler E and Carrington C: Open biopsy for chronic diffuse infiltrative lung disease: clinical, roentgenographic, and physiologic correlations in 502 patients. Ann Thorac Surg 30:411, 1980.

Gelfand E and Sheiner N: Pneumothorax in pulmonary eosinophilic granuloma. Can Med Assoc J 110:937, 1974.

Hambleton G et al: Pulmonary eosinophilic granuloma in a child. Arch Dis Child 51:805, 1976.

Hamoudi A et al: Thymic changes in histiocytosis. Am J Clin Pathol 77:169, 1982.

Hance A et al: Smoking and interstitial lung disease: the effect of cigarette smoking on the incidence of pulmonary histiocytosis X and sarcoidosis. Ann NY Acad Sci 465:643, 1986.

Hughes W et al: Successful intermittent chemoprophylaxis for *Pneumocystis carinii* pneumonitis. N Engl J Med 316:1627, 1987.

Jakobson A et al: Treatment of Langerhans cell histiocytosis with alpha-interferon. Lancet 2:1520, 1987.

Kawanami O et al: Pulmonary Langerhans' cells in patients with fibrotic lung disorders. Lab Invest 44:227, 1981.

Kershenobich D et al: Effect of colchicine on immunoregulatory T-lymphocytes and monocytes in patients with primary biliary cirrhosis (abstract). Clin Res 32:496, 1984.

Kershenobich D et al: Colchicine in the treatment of cirrhosis of the liver. N Engl J Med 318:1709, 1988.

Komp D: Long-term sequelae of histiocytosis-X. Am J Pediatr Hematol Oncol 3:165, 1981.

Komp D: Langerhans cell histiocytosis. N Engl J Med 316:747, 1987.

Komp D et al: Quality of survival in histiocytosis-X: a Southwest Oncology Group study. Med Pediatr Oncol 8:35, 1980.

Kupiec-Weglinski J et al: Sparing of suppressor cells: a critical action of cyclosporin. Transplantation 38:97, 1984.

Lahey M: Histiocytosis X—an analysis of prognostic factors. J Pediatr 87:184, 1975.

Lahey M: Prognostic factors in histiocytosis X. Am J Pediatr Hematol Oncol 3:57, 1981.

Lahey M: Histiocytosis X. In Kendig E and Chernick V (eds): Disorders of the Respiratory Tract in Children. 4th ed. Philadelphia, WB Saunders Co, 1983.

Lahey M et al: Hypergammaglobulinemia in histiocytosis-X. J Pediatr 107:572, 1985.

Laronique J et al: Chest radiological features of pulmonary histiocytosis X: a report based on 50 adult cases. Thorax 37:104, 1982.

Lavin P and Osband M: Evaluating the role of therapy in histiocytosis X: clinical studies, staging and scoring. Hematol Oncol Clin North Am 1:35, 1987.

Leikin S et al: Immunologic parameters in histiocytosis-X. Cancer 32:796, 1973.

Lewis J: Eosinophilic granuloma and its variants with special reference to lung involvement. Q J Med 33:337, 1964.

Lichtenstein L: Histiocytosis X-integration of eosinophilic granuloma of bone, "Letterer-Siwe Disease," and "Schuller-Christian Disease" as related manifestations of a single nosologic entity. Arch Pathol 56:84, 1953.

Lombard C et al: Pulmonary histiocytosis and carcinoma. Arch Pathol Lab Med 111:339, 1987.

McLelland J et al: Current controversies. Hematol Oncol Clin North Am 1:147, 1987.

Marcy T and Reynolds H: Pulmonary histiocytosis X. Lung 163:129, 1985.

Marsh W et al: Congenital self-healing histiocytosis-X. Am J Pediatr Hematol Oncol 5:227, 1983.

Matlin A et al: Pleural effusion in two children with histiocytosis X. Chest 61:33, 1972.

Matus-Ridley M et al: Histiocytosis X in children: patterns of disease and results of treatment. Med Pediatr Oncol 11:99, 1983.

Nakata H et al: Histiocytosis X with anterior mediastinal mass as its initial manifestation. Pediatr Radiol 197:280, 1982.

Nesbit M et al: The immune system and the histiocytosis syndromes. Am J Pediatr Hematol Oncol 3:141, 1981.

Nondahl S et al: A case report and literature review of "primary" pulmonary histiocytosis X of childhood. Med Ped Oncol 14:57, 1986.

Osband M: Immunotherapy of histiocytosis X. Hematol Oncol Clin North Am 1:131, 1987.

Osband M and Pochedly C (eds): Histiocytosis-X. (Hematol Oncol Clin North Am). Philadelphia, WB Saunders Co, 1987.

Osband M et al: Histiocytosis X: demonstration of abnormal immunity, T cell histamine receptor deficiency, and successful treatment with thymic extract. N Engl J Med 304:146, 1981.

Petheram I et al: Penicillamine in eosinophilic granuloma. Br J Dis Chest 75:410, 1981.

Prophet D: Primary pulmonary histiocytosis X. Clin Chest Med 3:643, 1982.

Ree H and Kadin M: Peanut agglutinin: a useful marker for histiocytosis X and interdigitating reticulum cells. Cancer 57:282, 1986.

Ringder O et al: Allogeneic bone marrow transplantation in a patient with chemotherapy-resistant progressive histiocytosis X. N Engl J Med 316:733, 1987.

Risdall R et al: Histiocytosis X (Langerhans cell histiocytosis): prognostic role of histopathology. Arch Pathol Lab Med 107:59, 1983.

Roland A et al: Recurrent spontaneous pneumothorax—a clue to the diagnosis of histiocytosis X. N Engl J Med 270:73, 1964.

Sajiad S and Luna M: Primary pulmonary histiocytosis X in two patients with Hodgkin's disease. Thorax 37:110, 1982.

Saunder D et al: Langerhans cell production of interleukin-I. J Invest Dermatol 82:605, 1984.

Schaub T et al: Radionuclide imaging in histiocytosis X. Pediatr Radiol 17:397, 1987.

Scott H et al: Familial opsonization defect associated with fatal infantile dermatitis, infections and hisiocytosis. Arch Dis Child 50:311, 1975.

Scott J: Preliminary report: heart-lung transplantation for cystic fibrosis. Lancet 2:192, 1988.

Shannon B et al: Lack of suppressor cell activity in children with active histiocytosis-X. Med Pediatr Oncol 14:111, 1986.

Smith M et al: "Primary" pulmonary histiocytosis X. Chest 65:176, 1986.

Soler P et al: Immunochemical characterization of pulmonary histiocytosis X cells in lung biopsies. Am J Pathol 118:439, 1985.

Starling K: Chemotherapy of histiocytosis-X. Hematol Oncol Clin North Am 1:119, 1987.

Thommesen P et al: Immunologic response assessed by lymphocyte transformation tests. Acta Radiol Oncol 17:524, 1978.

Tittel P and Winkler C: Chronic recurrent pleural effusion in adult histiocytosis-X. Br J. Radiol 54:68, 1981.

Tubergen D et al: Trimethoprim sulfa (TMZ) reduces infections during intensive chemotherapy of acute lymphoblastic leukemia (ALL) in children (abstract). Proc Am Soc Clin Oncol 5:157, 1986.

Verea-Hernando H et al: Langerhans cells in bronchoalveolar lavage in the late stages of pulmonary histiocytosis X. Chest 81:130, 1982.

Weber W et al: Pulmonary histiocytosis X. A review of 18 patients with reports of 6 cases. Am J Roentgenol 197:280, 1969.

Winkler C and Yam L: Pleural effusion in histiocytosis X. Arch Int Med 140:988, 1980.

66

BERNHARD H. SINGSEN, M.D., and
ARNOLD C. G. PLATZKER, M.D.

PULMONARY INVOLVEMENT IN THE RHEUMATIC DISORDERS OF CHILDHOOD

Until the etiology and pathogenesis of the so-called collagen diseases become known, any classification of this group of syndromes will be no more than descriptive. A number of terms have been employed, including *collagen (vascular) diseases, connective tissue diseases,* and *rheumatic diseases,* but none of these is totally adequate. However, it is increasingly evident that most rheumatic diseases are not primarily diseases of collagen or connective tissues.

The rheumatic diseases may be characterized as chronic or chronic-recurrent disorders of tissue inflammation with unknown pathogenesis. With rare exception, meticulous investigation has not revealed an infectious cause for the rheumatic disorders. Whipple's disease, some cases of Reiter syndrome and other "reactive arthropathies," and specific arthritis-associated viral diseases, such as hepatitis, rubella, and mononucleosis, have an infectious cause but are mediated through immunologic mechanisms. Many lines of evidence favor the chronic or recurrent presence of one or many antigens to stimulate the immune-mediated inflammation common to the rheumatic diseases. Favorite candidates for these unknown antigens are infectious agents, particularly undetected viral genomes, and long-departed viruses that have contributed genetic material to alter the host immunologic response.

A simplified schematic may help to explain the chronicity of inflammation characteristic of the rheumatic diseases. Figure 66–1 shows three major but normal activities: the fundamental reparative process from injury to healing, the phagocytosis by neutrophils of various foreign materials, and the stimulation of the immune system by antigens. Central to an understanding of chronic or recurrent rheumatic inflammation is the potential within the normal inflammatory system for amplification and reamplification. It is widely presumed that the persistence of

unrecognized antigens leads to the chronic inflammation that characterizes most of the rheumatic diseases. One can see from the schematic that this persistence leads to continuous Ag-Ab-C' formation, stimulates continuous phagocytosis and cellular toxicity, and thus constantly reamplifies the processes causing injury.

Most rheumatic diseases in children and adults exhibit serologic abnormalities, which result from antigenic stimulation of the humoral immune system (displayed on the right side of Fig. 66–1). These serologic changes suggest that the patients have an altered immunologic status, but it is important to stress that the observed abnormalities need not have either specific diagnostic or etiologic significance. As an example, much of the nephritis of systemic lupus erythematosus (SLE) is due to the deposition of soluble DNA–anti-DNA antibody–complement complexes in the kidney. However, it is not clear what causes the presence of soluble DNA or why it persists in the circulation. The injection of soluble DNA into normal experimental animals does not lead to the development of antinuclear antibodies (including anti-DNA antibodies) and does not cause nephritis. Further, although the presence of high titers of antinuclear antibodies (ANA) may be highly suggestive of SLE, their presence is by no means diagnostic of, or restricted to, this condition.

Table 66–1 shows the relative prevalence of ANA and rheumatoid factor (RF) in a survey of children with rheumatic disease. Evidence of altered immunologic status is present in all of the diseases tested, and the results highlight the lack of diagnostic specificity of RF or ANA.

The clinical features of the various rheumatic diseases are in many respects similar and often are described as "overlapping," much in the fashion that serologic features appear to overlap. It is true that many of the rheumatic diseases share gross, common denominators, but it is equally true that careful study, particularly of the clinical characteristics, allows delineation of the differences. As an example, the majority of rheumatic diseases exhibit arthritis at some time during the disease course. But careful

Deep appreciation is expressed to those who contributed to the preparation of materials for this manuscript: Fred Lee (radiology), Benjamin Landing (pathology), Virgil Hanson, Helen Kornreich, Bram Bernstein, and Karen Koster King (rheumatology), and Stuart Foster and Daisy Bautista (pulmonary physiology).

TISSUE INJURY, INFLAMMATION, AND IMMUNE MECHANISMS

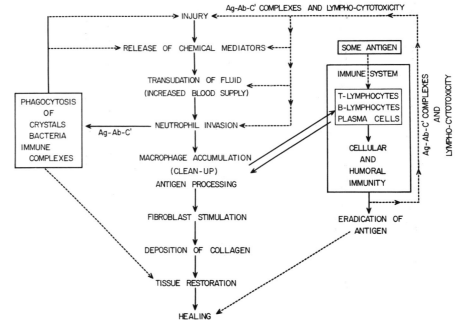

Figure 66–1. A simplified schematic showing three simultaneously occurring aspects of inflammation and healing, including the roles of cellular and humoral immunity, the process of phagocytosis, and the direct sequence of tissue healing. A major consequence of this system is the capability for chronic inflammation if antigens, immune complexes, or crystals are persistently or intermittently present. (Schematic designed by Virgil Hanson, M.D.)

examination and follow-up reveal marked differences—e.g., the chronic, slowly progressive, erosive changes of juvenile rheumatoid arthritis (JRA), contrasted with the nondestructive, recurrent synovitis of SLE, versus the early synovitis of childhood scleroderma and dermatomyositis. Similarly, investigation of JRA with HLA typing has further defined the pauciarticular subtypes of childhood arthritis (Schaller et al, 1976; Miller, 1979). As another example, mixed connective tissue disease (MCTD) is a distinct entity with typical but slowly evolving characteristics (Singsen et al, 1977). But here again, anti-ribonucleoprotein antibodies are not exclusive to MCTD (Notman et al, 1975), and further investigation may define subclasses of MCTD or additional "overlap" syndromes with special, but not exclusive, serologic characteristics.

More than 100 distinct syndromes are known to be associated with arthritis in childhood, including metabolic disorders and numerous miscellaneous conditions; some of these are listed in Table 66–2. The reader who desires an understanding of the pediatric rheumatic diseases beyond the scope of this chapter is referred to several excellent compendia of

the rheumatic disorders of childhood (Ansell, 1980; Kelly, 1980; Jacobs, 1982; Cassidy, 1982; Miller, 1986).

It is important to distinguish between the pediatric and adult forms of the rheumatic diseases. In some disorders, such as ankylosing spondylitis, the disease appears to be a continuum from child to adult, with earlier detection increasingly extending the diagnosis to younger age groups. But the pediatric rheumatic diseases are not just "little people's" versions of the adult form; examples of differences between children and adults are: the prevalence of linear and focal forms of scleroderma to the relative exclusion of the

Table 66–2. THE RHEUMATIC DISEASES OF CHILDHOOD

Systemic lupus erythematosus (SLE)
Scleroderma
Lyme disease
Dermatomyositis
Juvenile rheumatoid arthritis (JRA)
Mixed connective tissue disease (MCTD)
Wegener granulomatosis
Periarteritis nodosa
Systemic vasculitis
Postinfectious reactive arthritis
Henoch-Schönlein purpura
Stevens-Johnson syndrome
Kawasaki syndrome
Ulcerative colitis
Regional enteritis
Ankylosing spondylitis
Reiter syndrome
Psoriatic arthritis
Behçet syndrome
Sjögren syndrome
Familial Mediterranean fever (FMF)
Acute rheumatic fever
Sarcoidosis (see Chapter 49)

Table 66–1. RHEUMATOID FACTOR (RF) AND ANTINUCLEAR ANTIBODIES (ANA) IN CHILDHOOD

Diagnosis	Number of Patients	% Positive RF	% Positive ANA
Systemic lupus erythematosus	108	5	95
Juvenile rheumatoid arthritis	110	25	28
Dermatomyositis	20	0	55
Scleroderma	19	25	47
Ulcerative colitis	34	11	23
Mixed connective tissue disease	14	64	100
Controls	49	0	6

systemic form in childhood, the greater morbidity and mortality of childhood SLE, the prominence of pauciarticular JRA (often with iridocyclitis), and the unique histologic characteristics of vasculitis in childhood dermatomyositis. Therefore, it is not unreasonable to speculate that the type and severity of pulmonary involvement in the pediatric rheumatic diseases may differ also.

Investigations of pathologic pulmonary processes in the rheumatic diseases of childhood are few in number. There are no extensive studies of the pulmonary histopathology, nor, perhaps more important, are there published serial studies of pulmonary function over the course of most of the pediatric rheumatic diseases. It is hoped that this chapter will be a small step toward further knowledge in this area.

The mechanisms by which lung injuries occur in the rheumatic disorders are largely unknown, but some patterns are similar to the immune complex (IC) deposition associated with experimental glomerulonephritis. Brentjens and co-workers (1974) have found that daily injection of antigen in rabbits, to maintain maximal levels of antibody and IC, is associated with development of proliferative and membranous pneumonitis and pulmonary deposition of IgG, complement, fibrinogen, and antigen. Thus it appears likely that patterns of rheumatic lung injury will be understood to be related to type, amount, and duration of pulmonary antigen exposure (Gregory and Rich, 1946), type and amount of antibody response, and the physical characteristics of the immune complexes deposited in the lung (Hunninghake and Fauci, 1979). How immune complexes cause pulmonary damage is not clear. Immune complexes may activate complement, lead to the release of vasoactive amines, promote the generation of chemotactic factors, and interact with various lung macrophages and lymphoid tissues (Cochrane and Dixon, 1976; Hunninghake et al, 1978). Excellent reviews of pulmonary involvement in the rheumatic diseases of adults with particular detail regarding the systemic vasculitides are available (Hunninghake and Fauci, 1979; Mohsenifar et al, 1981).

Because the lung is highly vascular, and blood vessels are often immunologic targets, the lung may be quite vulnerable in the rheumatic disorders. The incidence of lung involvement varies according to whether one or more clinical, radiologic, physiologic, or histologic criteria are used for documentation. In the following sections, the diseases are presented roughly in the order of the likelihood and the severity of pulmonary involvement by the primary disease process. After the initial nine diseases, which are dealt with in detail, is a larger group of pediatric rheumatic diseases. We have not recognized pulmonary involvement, nor is it described in the pediatric literature, in diseases such as Henoch-Schönlein purpura, Kawasaki syndrome, and allergic (systemic) vasculitis. Yet, the nature of the pathologic processes of these entities suggests that pulmonary involvement might occur. When appropriate, pulmonary involvement in the adult presentation of a disease is described.

SYSTEMIC LUPUS ERYTHEMATOSUS

Systemic lupus erythematosus in children and adults demonstrates highly variable clinical and serologic manifestations. It is a diffuse and chronic inflammatory process of unknown etiology, characterized by the occurrence of multiple autoantibodies that participate in immunologically mediated tissue damage and that may affect any organ system. Establishing a diagnosis of SLE may be aided by the criteria for the classification of SLE of the American College of Rheumatology (Tau et al, 1982). Childhood SLE has been the subject of many excellent reports; those of Fish and colleagues (1977) and Emery (1986) are suggested for further review.

Awareness of pleuropulmonary involvement in SLE has existed since the nineteenth century, but little attention was paid to specific pulmonary manifestations until 1952 (Bagenstoss, 1952; Purnell et al, 1955). Since that time, investigation has expanded rapidly in three directions: pulmonary function studies, histopathology, and chest roentgenography. Segal and co-workers have published an excellent review of pulmonary involvement in SLE (1985). They propose a classification of disease-related manifestations that includes (1) pleurisy with and without effusion, (2) acute lupus pneumonitis, (3) diffuse interstitial disease, (4) pulmonary hypertension, (5) diaphragmatic dysfunction, (6) atelectasis, and (7) pulmonary hemorrhage.

In 1965, Huang and co-workers studied pulmonary function in 28 adults with SLE. Four groups were identified, including eight patients with past or present evidence of pleural involvement; nine with parenchymal disease; three patients with both pleural and parenchymal involvement; and eight with no past or present pulmonary disease. The high incidence of abnormal lung function was unexpected and included abnormal diffusing capacity for carbon monoxide (DL_{CO}) in 89 per cent of the patients tested. Forced vital capacity was abnormal in 79 per cent, inspiratory capacity was decreased in 87 per cent, and total lung capacity was decreased in 61 per cent. Most significantly, pulmonary function abnormalities were present in almost two thirds of the patients without current clinical or roentgenographic evidence of pulmonary disease.

Similar findings were reported by Gold and Jennings (1966), who suggested that the single-breath carbon monoxide determination (DL_{CO}) was the most sensitive indicator of pulmonary dysfunction in SLE. Grennan and co-workers (1978) observed a restrictive ventilatory defect in 41 per cent of 22 adults with SLE. Both this study and another by Gibson and co-workers (1977) confirmed the high frequency of clinically silent abnormalities of gas diffusion in SLE. Researchers have also debated, with inconclusive results, the contribution of cigarette smoking to observed dysfunction (Hunt et al, 1975; Chick et al, 1976). Unfortunately, serial studies of pulmonary function in SLE, from disease onset and over extended periods, have not been performed.

Gibson and co-workers (1977) have addressed the issue of "shrinking lungs" found in some patients with SLE. Seven of 30 patients, not selected for pulmonary involvement, had abnormally elevated diaphragms. Diaphragm function was assessed in five of these patients and was grossly abnormal in four. Thus diaphragm weakness, or immobility following extensive pleural adhesions, may be a cause of SLE-associated "shrinking lungs."

We have performed pulmonary function studies in 20 children with SLE (mean age at testing: 15.5 years). All patients with clinical or roentgenographic evidence of pulmonary disease at the time of study were excluded. The findings included abnormal Dl_{CO} in 25 per cent, pulmonary restrictive defects in 35 per cent, abnormal P_{O2} in 10 per cent, and an obstructive defect in 5 per cent. These results suggest that pulmonary abnormalities are less common in children with SLE or may merely reflect a shorter disease duration and less exposure to environmental hazards. Miller and associates (1988) have done pulmonary function tests in nine children with SLE and have shown that two thirds had abnormal forced vital capacities. Although eight children had no respiratory symptoms and seven had a normal pulmonary examination, chest radiographs were abnormal in five.

Numerous histopathologic descriptions of SLE with associated pulmonary disease are available, but the described changes lack specificity (Haupt et al, 1981). According to Purnell and associates (1955), interstitial pneumonitis, pleuritis with effusions, and atelectasis are the most common pathologic changes. Gross and co-workers (1971) observed bronchopneumonia, interstitial pneumonia, alveolar hemorrhage, and chronic pleural thickening in more than 50 per cent of cases in an autopsy series. Another major finding included the lack of significant interstitial fibrosis, despite the almost constant presence of interstitial thickening and inflammatory infiltrates. However, 100 per cent of their 44 patients had evidence of distal airway alterations, including bronchiolar dilation, alveolar simplification, and focal panacinar emphysema. It was speculated that these changes contribute to decreased diffusing capacity and to ventilation-perfusion inequalities. Only 19 per cent of the patients had pulmonary vascular lesions, in comparison with 40 per cent in another report by Fayemi (1975). Fayemi stressed that the correlation between clinical and pathologic findings is poor because primary histologic changes are commonly obscured by congestive heart failure, infection, and uremia.

Between 1961 and 1976, there were 21 deaths due to SLE in a clinic population of 130 lupus patients followed at the Children's Hospital of Los Angeles. Review of the pulmonary histopathology (in association with Benjamin Landing, M.D.) revealed many of the changes to be similar to those described in adults. It was striking that between 1971 and 1976, eight of ten SLE deaths occurred as a direct result of pulmonary compromise. Among the 21 children, pulmonary vascular lesions were uncommon, but unexpected hemosiderosis and alveolitis obliterans (mucoid or hyaline-like round collections within the alveolus) each occurred in one third of the cases. Acute bronchopneumonia was present in 57 per cent of the lungs reviewed.

Cultures were taken from the lungs at post-mortem examination in 15 cases, and all 21 were reviewed histologically for pathogens. The results, shown in Table 66–3, indicate that infection is a common denominator in childhood SLE pulmonary involvement and confirm the findings of several adult series. Staples and co-workers (1974) showed that infection rate and the number of disseminated infections increase in lupus patients with increasing steroid doses and with decreasing renal function. However, those patients with normal renal function who are receiving no or small dose steroid therapy also had a significantly higher infection rate than controls did. The authors suggested that a defect in neutrophil function was at least partially responsible. Other reports have described deep fungal infections (Sieving et al, 1975) and have related such occurrences to immunosuppressive therapy or SLE-related deficits in cell-mediated immunity (Paty et al, 1975).

The patterns encountered on chest roentgenograms of patients with SLE are widely varied, and their proper evaluation presents a formidable challenge to the radiologist and clinician. The implication of early roentgenographic studies was that patients with SLE commonly develop a primary lung disease, which may be called "lupus pneumonitis." Conversely, Dubois and Tuffanelli (1964) noted only a 0.9 per cent incidence of pulmonary involvement due to SLE, but 31 per cent of their patients had bacterial pneumonias as a secondary complication.

Table 66–3. PATHOGENS IN THE LUNGS OF 21 CHILDREN DYING FROM SLE

Pathogen	No. Children
Klebsiella aerobacter	5
Escherichia coli	4
alpha-hemolytic streptococcus	3
Candida albicans	3
Aspergillus species	3
cytomegalic inclusion virus	3
Pneumocystis carinii	3
alpha-hemolytic enterococcus	2
Staphylococcus epidermidis	2
Pseudomonas aeruginosa	1
Proteus mirabilis	1
Staphylococcus aureus	1
Cryptococcus neoformans	1
Allescheria boydii	1

Levin (1971) attempted to resolve this conflict with an evaluation of the clinical histories and chest roentgenograms of 111 patients with SLE. He noted that 38 patients had pleural involvement, and many of these had patchy atelectasis on the involved side. Superimposed pulmonary infection developed in 16 patients, and uremic pulmonary edema in four. True "lupus pneumonitis," as determined using roentgenographic criteria, developed in only three individuals (2.7 per cent); these patients were symptomatic, with dyspnea, cough, or chest pain, and showed patchy infiltration of small nodules (without evidence of congestive heart failure or pleuritis) on chest roentgenograms.

Drug-induced SLE should be mentioned briefly. In adults, there is a high frequency of pleuropulmonary disease in the hydralazine and procainamide-induced lupus syndromes, but pleuropulmonary involvement is not striking in most children with SLE induced by medications (chiefly anticonvulsants) (Singsen, Fishman, and Hanson, 1976). A lupus-like syndrome with associated pulmonary reaction following administration of nitrofurantoin (Selroos and Edgren, 1975) and the in vivo fixation of ANA to the pleura in procainamide-induced SLE (Chandrasekhar et al, 1978) have been described.

Holgate and co-workers (1976) observed four types of pleuropulmonary involvement in SLE, based on combined clinical and roentgenographic features: (1) episodic pleurisy with effusions but normal parenchyma; (2) pleuropericarditis with moderate cough or dyspnea and elevated or thickened hemidiaphragm; (3) frequent attacks of either episodic pleurisy or pleuropericarditis, but with persistent or progressive dyspnea; (4) progressive dyspnea with roentgenographic evidence of fibrosing alveolitis. Holgate and co-workers (1976), Grennan and colleagues (1978), and Gibson and associates (1977) were unable to correlate the type or degree of immunologic abnormalities, in a combined total of 82 SLE patients, with pulmonary abnormalities. Nonetheless, the participation of immune complex deposition in the pathogenesis of lupus lung is an attractive concept (Inoue et al, 1979).

The following case reports illustrate three types and degrees of SLE pulmonary involvement in children. An approach to diagnosis and therapy, which can, with some modification, be extended to pulmonary involvement in each of the childhood rheumatic diseases is then presented.

Case 1. A 4-year-old girl was first hospitalized with a 3-month history of progressive malaise, fever, arthralgias, and rash over the trunk and extremities. Examination revealed an anxious, febrile girl with an erythematous maculopapular eruption over the trunk and thighs. Moderate lymphadenopathy and hepatosplenomegaly were present. The lungs were clear, but tachypnea was present. The heart showed cardiomegaly and a grade II/VI systolic ejection murmur. Arthritis of the elbows, wrists, and knees was present.

Laboratory findings included a white blood cell count (WBC) of 11,800 cells/mm³, hemoglobin (Hgb) 8.8 g/100 ml, erythrocyte sedimentation rate (ESR) of 130 mm/hr, positive direct and indirect Coombs tests results, serum albumin level 2.9 g/100 ml, and serum globulin level 5.2 g/100 ml; serum (ANA) was 1:2560, and rheumatoid factor was 1:160. Serum IgG was 3525 mg/100 ml (normal: 550–1100 mg/100 ml), and the serum C3 was less than 10 mg/100 ml (normal: 60–140 mg/100 ml). Creatinine clearance was 47 ml/min/1.73 m². A urinalysis revealed 2+ proteinuria, 25 to 30 WBC/hpf, 75 to 100 red blood cell count (RBC)/hpf, and granular and hyaline casts. A chest roentgenogram showed moderate cardiomegaly with slightly increased pulmonary vascularity. An electrocardiogram and echocardiogram were both normal.

A diagnosis of SLE with renal disease and mild myocarditis was made, and prednisolone, 35 mg/day, and hydroxychloroquine, 100 mg/day, were started. A renal biopsy revealed histologic evidence of severe proliferative glomerulonephritis with diffuse, chronic interstitial nephritis. Diuretics were begun because of progressive edema and hypertension.

Three months later, the patient's serum C3 had returned to 133 mg/100 ml. The ANA was only 1:160. One episode of mild pneumonitis resolved following treatment with oral ampicillin. The next 18 months were marked by active nephritis and varying degrees of rash and arthritis. Despite continuous prednisolone therapy (15 to 40 mg every other day), serum C3 progressively fell to 30 mg/100 ml.

When she was 6.5 years old, the patient was readmitted with fever and headaches. The cerebrospinal fluid protein level was 30 mg/100 ml, but an electroencephalogram revealed mild, diffuse dysfunction. A second renal biopsy showed diffuse, proliferative lupus nephritis with positive immunofluorescence for IgG, M, A, E, C3, and fibrin. A urine protein determination was 4.1 gr/24 hr. Cyclophosphamide, 50 mg/day, was begun, and the prednisolone was increased to 30 mg/day; serum C3 and ANA levels slowly reverted to normal.

Four months and again 6 months after the second hospitalization, the patient was admitted because of fever and pneumonia. Cyclophosphamide was discontinued. Clinical and roentgenographic resolution of both episodes followed administration of intravenous cephalothin. Serum C3 and C4 levels were normal during both episodes, and the ANA test was negative. The ANA again became positive 4 months later and remained so for the rest of her illness. Active renal disease continued, with fluctuating serum C3 and C4 levels, proteinuria, and an active urine sediment.

At the age of 8, the patient developed fever and a left lower lobe pneumonia, which responded to intravenous cephalothin. Three months later, she developed *Haemophilus influenzae* cellulitis of the left arm, pericarditis, and central nervous system involvement with chorea. Intravenous ampicillin and dexamethasone, 1.5 mg every 6 hours, were successfully employed. A chest roentgenogram showed clear lung fields. Hypertension was present; serum blood urea nitrogen (BUN) level rose to 66 mg/100 ml and creatinine level to 1.5 mg/100 ml.

Several weeks later, the patient developed fever, cough, and chest pain. Mild cardiomegaly was present on chest roentgenogram. Myocarditis was detected 3 days later, and she received diuretics and antibiotics; dexamethasone was increased to 2.0 mg every 6 hours. On the following day, tachypnea, nasal flaring, grunting respirations, and bilateral rales were present. A chest roentgenogram revealed bilateral infiltrates suggestive of congestive heart failure (CHF), pneumonia, or pulmonary hemorrhage (Fig. 66–2). Arterial blood gas (ABG) determinations included pH

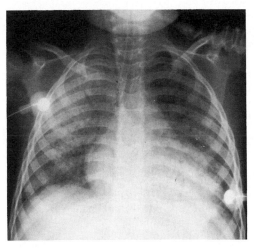

Figure 66–2. *Case 1.* A portable anteroposterior chest roentgenogram showing bilateral parenchymal infiltrates consistent with diffuse, intra-alveolar hemorrhage or edema. The heart is large in its transverse diameter. The small pneumomediastinum and interstitial emphysema in the neck present in the original film are not well reproduced.

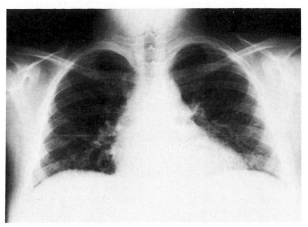

Figure 66–3. *Case 2.* A chest roentgenogram showing a poor inspiratory effort with resultant prominent cardiac silhouette. The lungs show diffuse reticular changes suggestive of chronic pulmonary fibrosis. There are no pleural effusions or acute infiltrates.

7.40, P_{O_2} 56, P_{CO_2} 30, and base excess −6. Increasing amounts of blood-tinged sputum were produced. Therapy for CHF was begun, and methylprednisolone, 500 mg, was given. Progressive respiratory distress occurred, and the patient was put on a respirator with FI_{O_2} 85 per cent, rate 20, positive end-expiratory pressure (PEEP) 4; ABG readings were pH 7.45, P_{O_2} 57, P_{CO_2} 37, base excess +2. Three days after detection of the myocarditis, rapid clinical deterioration occurred, and the patient expired following a cardiac arrest.

Post-mortem examination of the heart showed histologic changes caused by hypertension, focal vasculitis of the right side of the heart, mild epicarditis, and myocardial edema. In the lungs, there was massive alveolar hemorrhage with few residual aerated sacs. Focal necrotizing pneumonitis and increased interstitial inflammatory cell infiltrates were present. Panacinar edema, alveolar septal decrease, and fibrinoid swelling of arteriolar walls were all occasionally observed.

This case represents the apparent rapid onset of primary lupus pneumonitis leading to diffuse alveolar hemorrhage and death. Congestive heart failure and superimposed pulmonary infection were major diagnostic and therapeutic complications.

Case 2. A 9-year-old girl developed SLE manifested by skin rash, nephritis, and myocarditis with congestive heart failure that necessitated digitalis and diuretic therapy. Shortly thereafter, she was hospitalized with spiking fever, characteristic malar rash of SLE, malaise, and arthralgias. Laboratory findings included profuse proteinuria and an active urine sediment. The ANA was positive, and anti-DNA antibodies were present; serum C3 was below normal. There was no clinical or roentgenographic evidence of pulmonary disease.

Her course was marked by persistent hypocomplementemia (C3 and C4) and long periods of very active skin rash. Nephritis remitted 5 months after she was first seen and never recurred. Since the onset of SLE, this patient was troubled by relapsing but slowly progressive neurologic manifestations, including peripheral neuritis, mood swings, deterioration of fine motor coordination, episodes of psy-

chosis, and persistent headaches. One cerebrospinal fluid protein level was 76 mg/100 ml (normal: ≤ 45 mg/100 ml).

The neurologic manifestations and episodes of severe oropharyngeal rash necessitated the intermittent use of cyclophosphamide and continuous prednisolone in doses ranging from 7.5 to 90 mg/day. The patient is moderately cushingoid and has marked striae. Hypertension has not been a management problem, perhaps because of the absence of clinically evident renal disease.

Numerous chest roentgenograms have been obtained throughout the course of the disease. Slight thickening and prominence of lung markings were first observed a year after the hospitalization and have not subsequently changed (Fig. 66–3).

Pulmonary function studies were performed 5 years after the prominent lung markings first appeared; the results were as follows: vital capacity (VC) and its subdivisions are mildly to moderately reduced (Table 66–4). The functional residual capacity (FRC), residual volume (RV), and total lung capacity (TLC) show similar reductions in volume. The 1-sec forced vital capacity (FEV_1), although reduced, reflects the reduction in VC. Thus the 1-sec forced expiratory volume expressed as a percentage of the forced vital capacity (FEV_1/FVC) is normal. The maximal midexpiratory flow–volume curve (MMEF) has a normal configuration, with normal expired flow rates at all lung volumes. The closing volume (CV) and closing capacity are

Table 66–4. *CASE 2:* PULMONARY VALUES

	Normal Range	Predicted Mean	Measured (% pred.)
VC (L)	1.9–3.3	2.6	1.6 (64)
FRC (L)	1.0–2.1	1.5	0.9 (58)
RV (L)	0.4–1.1	0.7	0.5 (69)
TLC (L)	2.5–4.1	3.3	2.2 (65)
FEV₁ (L)	2.0–2.9	2.5	1.5 (61)
FEV₁/FVC (%)	72–100	86.0	87.0
MMEF (L/min)	122–258	190.0	109.0 (57)
CV (L)		0.2	0.3
CV/VC (%)		7.0	19.0
N₂ (40) (%)		1.5	0.5
DL_CO (ml/min/mm Hg)	12.1–25.3	18.7	12.0
P_O₂ (mm Hg)		97.0	82.0
P_CO₂ (mm Hg)	37–43		30.0
pH	7.37–7.43		7.40

increased. The distribution of ventilation as measured by the single-breath oxygen and the 40-breath nitrogen washout curve ($N_2(40)$) fall well within the normal limits. The single-breath diffusion capacity for carbon monoxide (DL_{CO}) is reduced from the predicted mean but is within one standard deviation. The P_{O_2} is within the normal range, and the P_{CO_2} and pH reflect a compensated respiratory alkalosis.

Pulmonary function testing during exercise revealed that oxygen consumption at rest is normal (Table 66–5); however, the CO_2 production expressed as a fraction of the oxygen consumption is elevated. Minute respiratory volume is increased as a function of respiratory rate. Wasted ventilation and the wasted ventilation–tidal volume ratio are within the normal range. After 6 min of exercise at 150 kg-m/min, there is moderate hypoxia and a threefold increase in the oxygen consumption. The respiratory quotient falls. Minute respiratory volume increases approximately threefold, and the respiratory rate doubles. Wasted ventilation increases, but the wasted ventilation–tidal volume ratio remains unchanged. Twelve min after the beginning of exercise and 6 min after the rate is increased to 250 kg-m/min, the patient experiences complete exhaustion. The arterial P_{O_2} has fallen further. The oxygen consumption has increased to four-and-one-half times above the baseline level, and there is balance of carbon dioxide production and oxygen consumption. Minute respiratory volume is now four times baseline levels. The respiratory rate is increased by 20 per cent from the first exercise load, and the heart rate is 178 beats/min. Wasted ventilation remains relatively unchanged, and the wasted ventilation–tidal volume ratio is also unchanged. Four minutes after cessation of exercise, the P_{O_2} has risen to the normal range, whereas the carbon dioxide tension remains markedly depressed.

This patient has moderately severe restrictive lung disease with intact airway function. The elevated closing volume and closing capacity may reflect basilar vascular congestion that is causing expiratory closure of the airway at relatively large lung volumes. The diffusing capacity is decreased, reflecting some reduction in the pulmonary capillary blood volume consistent with either moderate restrictive lung disease or complicating pulmonary vascular or interstitial lung disease. The magnitude of the patient's lung disorder is clarified by relatively low loads of exercise. At this point, she cannot reduce wasted ventilation by recruitment of further pulmonary vascular bed for gas exchange. This supports the speculation of pulmonary vascular or interstitial lung disease or abnormal matching of pulmonary ventilation and perfusion, or both.

This patient has slowly progressive chronic respiratory insufficiency with parenchymal fibrosis due to SLE, without known antecedent pulmonary infection or episodes of primary lupus pneumonitis.

Case 3. This 15-year-old girl developed SLE manifested by progressive weight loss, anorexia, fatigue, anemia, frequent epistaxis, and urinary frequency during 1 month. Physical examination revealed a thin female with arthritis but no rash; the lungs were clear. The blood pressure was 100/70. Laboratory data included Hgb 8.1 gm/100 ml, WBC 7200 cells/mm³, ESR 152 mm/hr. ANA level was 4+, including anti-DNA antibodies. Serum C3 level was less than 10 mg/100 ml, BUN level 67 mg/100 ml, and creatinine level 1.9 mg/100 ml; urinalysis showed 1 to 3 WBC/hpf and 15 to 20 RBC/hpf. A 24-hour urine determination for protein clearance contained 2.5 gr of protein.

On the day following hospitalization, pericarditis with tachycardia and fever were detected, and prednisolone, 15 mg every 6 hours, was begun. A chest roentgenogram revealed slight cardiomegaly but clear lung fields. Following several transfusions of packed red blood cells for severe anemia, a renal biopsy was performed and revealed diffuse lupus glomerulonephritis. Prednisolone was increased to 25 mg every 6 hours.

Seventeen days later, the patient developed severe chest pain, dyspnea, and orthopnea; there was no fever. Examination showed a heart rate of 160 beats/min, and respiratory rate was 60 breaths/min; breath sounds were diminished on the right, and bilateral crackles were present. The cardiac examination was normal, but the liver was descended 5 cm. A chest roentgenogram demonstrated cardiomegaly and a diffuse alveolar process with prominence on the right and posteriorly (Fig. 66–4A). Blood and sputum cultures were obtained. Intravenous antibiotics and hydrocortisone, 100 mg every 6 hours, were begun. Digitalis and diuretics were added because of apparent right-sided heart failure secondary to severe pneumonitis. Hydrocortisone was increased to 150 mg every 6 hours. Oxygen by mask was delivered at 10 L/min.

By the third day, the cardiac and respiratory rates were decreased, and dyspnea was less pronounced. A sputum smear for *Pneumocystis carinii* was negative. The next 4 days revealed further improvement in respiratory status, although roentgenographic evidence of clearing of infiltrates was delayed (Fig. 66–4B). Prednisolone was substituted at 25 mg every 6 hours, and oxygen was discontinued. All cultures were negative, and the intravenous antibiotics were stopped. The impression was that the patient had experienced severe, primary lupus pneumonitis with rapid improvement in response to large doses of corticosteroid.

Table 66–5. *CASE 2:* EXERCISE TEST RESULTS

		Exercise Load: 150 kg-m/min	Exercise Load: 250 kg-m/min	Recovery
Arterial blood	rest	6 min	6 min	4 min
O₂ tension (mm Hg)	86	72	64	88
CO₂ tension (mm Hg)	32	29		29
pH	7.43	7.42	7.41	7.41
O₂ consumption (L/min)	0.129	0.415	0.550	
R (CO₂/O₂)	1.03	0.87	0.98	
Minute vol. resp. (L/min)	11.9	32.9	45.3	
Resp. rate (breaths/min)	28.3	48.0	58.0	
Heart rate (beats/min)	100.0	148.0	178.0	
Wasted vent. (L)	0.17	0.28	0.29	
VD/VT	0.41	0.41	0.38	

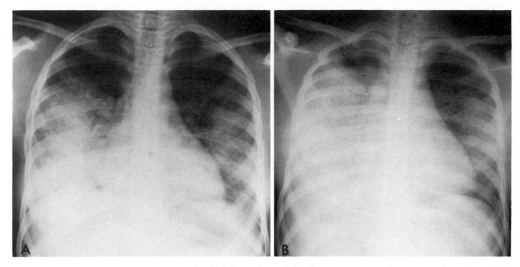

Figure 66–4. *Case 3. A,* The heart is slightly enlarged in the transverse diameter. There is a diffuse, bilateral alveolar process, which is more pronounced on the right. This pattern is not etiologically specific and may reflect hemorrhage, edema, or infection. *B,* There is no appreciable change in heart size. The bilateral alveolar infiltrates have progressed and the right diaphragm is obscured, despite the clinical evidence of improvement.

Shortly after this episode, cyclophosphamide was begun because of a severe peripheral neuropathy and active, diffuse lupus nephritis. The subsequent course included arthralgias, mild intermittent rash, and moderate fatigue, but was marked by a complete remission of active renal disease. The patient subsequently developed severe, recurrent hemorrhagic cystitis believed to be due to cyclophosphamide therapy. She continued to have a positive ANA, anti-DNA antibodies, and hypocomplementemia, despite the absence of clinically significant disease. No further episodes of pulmonary involvement occurred.

Pulmonary function studies were performed 5 years later to assess whether significant functional sequelae existed (Table 66–6). The patient had smoked two to three cigarettes per day for 4 years and seven per day during the previous year. The VC and its subdivisions fall within the normal range, as do the FRC, RV, and TLC. The FEV_1/FVC and the maximal expiratory flow, measured at all lung volumes, are normal. The CV and closing capacity fall within the predicted range, and the indices of uniformity of alveolar ventilation—the single-breath oxygen test and the 40-breath nitrogen washout test—suggest a normal distribution of ventilation. The DL_{CO}, measured by the single-breath method is reduced but falls just within one standard deviation below the predicted mean. Exercise stress testing, in this patient and in others with SLE, is usually the most sensitive index of impaired ventilation and gas exchange. Thus exercise testing should be utilized to monitor the progress of lung disease and the response to therapy. Arterial blood has normal oxygen tension, a mild uncompensated metabolic acidosis, and an acute respiratory alkalosis.

Although the lung volumes, mechanics of ventilation, and distribution of ventilation are within the normal range predicted for the patient, she does have a reduced diffusing capacity, even when normalized to alveolar volume, and a mildly reduced Pa_{O_2}. She has a 4-year history of smoking but no evidence of small airways disease, although the contour of the MMEF suggests reduction in expired flow at low lung volumes. The arterial blood gas, although reflecting marked hyperventilation, has an acceptable oxygen tension and a normal alveolar-arterial oxygen difference. Arterial blood gases and wasted ventilation both at rest and during graded exercise should be measured to determine whether there is evidence of underlying interstitial disease.

DIAGNOSTIC AND THERAPEUTIC CONSIDERATIONS

Three broad classifications of SLE pulmonary disease in childhood can be delineated: (1) mild to moderate progressive impairment in pulmonary function without clinical symptoms or significant roentgenographic findings (Case 2); (2) slow progression of pulmonary symptoms with roentgenographic findings; and (3) rapid onset of severe pulmonary distress. The first type should be watched closely, with an awareness that worsening function may predispose to later infection. The latter two types will be treated as different in degree only. It has been reported that pulmonary function abnor-

Table 66–6. *CASE 3:* PULMONARY VALUES

	Normal Range	Predicted Mean	Measured (% pred.)
VC (L)	1.9–3.3	2.6	2.2 (84)
FRC (L)	1.0–2.1	1.5	1.3 (83)
RV (L)	0.4–1.1	0.7	0.7 (90)
TLC (L)	2.5–4.1	3.3	2.8 (86)
FEV_1 (L)	2.0–2.9	2.5	1.9 (77)
FEV_1/FVC (%)	72–100	86.0	91.0
MMEF (L/min)	122–258	190.0	155.0 (82)
CV (L)		0.2	0.2
CV/VC (%)		7.0	10.0
N_2 (40) (%)		1.5	1.0
DL_{CO} (ml/min/mm Hg)	12.1–25.3	18.7	12.7 (68)
P_{O_2} (mm Hg)		95.0	114.0
P_{CO_2} (mm Hg)		37–43	28.0
pH		7.37–7.43	7.42

malities in SLE are responsive to corticosteroids (Venizelos and Al-Bazzaz, 1981). However, because many pulmonary function test changes in SLE do not appear to progress to clinically significant abnormalities, one should be cautious in treating isolated laboratory changes. In view of the autopsy findings in childhood SLE that reveal a high incidence of lung infection, infection must be ruled out before corticosteroids are prescribed for the pediatric patient with SLE.

Pulmonary disease management should always start with a comprehensive assessment of general SLE disease activity. Falling serum complement levels and increasing titers of ANA or anti-DNA antibody suggest increased disease activity, as do increased rash, arthralgia, myalgia, and evidence of internal organ derangement. In this setting, persistent low-grade fever, or spiking fever, is common. However, fever may be absent if the patient is receiving moderate to large doses of corticosteroids.

The rapid onset of fever, cough, and tachypnea is almost invariably due to infection, and following appropriate bacterial, fungal, and viral cultures, broad-spectrum antibiotics should be started. Three rapidly occurring exceptions to this rule should be noted. Spontaneous hemothorax is a rare complication of primary SLE pulmonary involvement (Mulkey and Hudson, 1974). The presence of frothy, blood-tinged sputum usually suggests alveolar hemorrhage due to SLE (Case 1) (Gould and Soriano, 1975) and may respond to intravenous methylprednisolone pulse therapy, 30 mg/kg/day up to a maximum of 1.0 gm/day, for up to 3 days, or to immunosuppressive drugs. If dyspnea and chest pain are prominent findings, primary SLE pneumonitis (Case 3) should be considered. In this rare situation, a combination of antibiotics and increased doses of corticosteroids are appropriate. In these latter circumstances, the potential for secondary infection is great, and the patient should be watched carefully. Only rarely is plasma pheresis indicated for treatment of nonresponsive, severe SLE pulmonary disease.

Exceptional diagnostic difficulty may be encountered in those children with a rapid onset of symptoms who do not respond to antibiotics within 72 hours and in those who have the slow progression (days to weeks) of pulmonary symptoms and roentgenographic findings. In our experience, results of cultures from these patients are commonly negative or contradictory, and accurate interpretation of chest roentgenograms is extremely difficult. Frequently, when a child becomes rapidly ill with major pulmonary manifestations, the concomitants of pneumonia, uremia, cardiomegaly due to myocarditis, pericarditis, or fluid retention, pulmonary edema, and mild to moderate pleuritis may combine to make roentgenographic distinctions difficult. At this point, a multidisciplinary team approach, including specialists in cardiology, radiology, nephrology, infectious diseases, pulmonary diseases, and rheumatology, should be mandatory.

The temptation to change or continue antibiotics, to markedly increase corticosteroid doses, or to add immunosuppressive agents should be tempered by the knowledge that any course may lead to pulmonary or systemic superinfection. Use of flexible fiberoptic bronchoscopy for bronchoalveolar lavage has been of value in the diagnosis of pulmonary infection, especially opportunistic infection, such as *Candida* and *P. carinii* in the immunocompromised patient. This procedure has the advantage that it can be performed without the use of general anesthesia. When this less-invasive procedure is not informative, then lung biopsy may be strongly considered. Percutaneous or open lung biopsy (Bandt et al, 1972; Gaensler et al, 1964), endobronchial brush biopsy (Fry and Manalo-Estrella, 1970), and transbronchoscopic lung biopsy (Anderson et al, 1970) all have their proponents, but none of these procedures is without significant risk.

It is critically important to recognize the several possible causes of prolonged bleeding in SLE. Abnormalities of prothrombin time or partial thromboplastin time and thrombocytopenia are common. In addition, abnormal template bleeding times are common, even when coagulation parameters are normal. All four tests should be performed before biopsy.

SCLERODERMA

Scleroderma (systemic sclerosis) is the rheumatic disease most frequently associated with severe pulmonary involvement. However, the prevalence of pulmonary disease in children may be lower than that in adults because a different spectrum of scleroderma is encountered. Scleroderma is usually divided into two major categories, progressive systemic sclerosis (PSS) and "localized" scleroderma. Morphea and linear scleroderma are the major subdivisions of "localized" scleroderma. Discussions of scleroderma in adults suggest that PSS is more prevalent than localized forms (Tuffanelli and Winkelmann, 1961; Medsger, 1989); the opposite appears true in children (Dabich et al, 1974; Singsen, 1986). One large 15-year experience includes 48 children with scleroderma. Thirteen (27 per cent) had PSS, 19 had predominantly linear scleroderma (40 per cent), and 16 (33 per cent) developed morphea (Kornreich et al, 1977). The clinical course of PSS in children is similar to that in adults and includes the slow but relentless progression of major internal organ involvement, most predominantly in the heart, intestines, kidneys, and lungs. Raynaud phenomenon, severe skin changes, and articular disability also occur but are not life threatening (D'Angelo et al, 1969).

The typical histologic finding in childhood scleroderma is extensive fibrosis with hyperplasia of connective tissue, perhaps resulting from overproduction of collagen; impressive vascular and inflammatory lesions may be also evident (Hanson, 1985).

Alveolitis, producing large numbers of lymphocytes and macrophages and increased percentages of neutrophils and eosinophils, can be documented by bronchoalveolar lavage, particularly early in the disease course (Owens et al, 1986). Microvascular damage, perhaps related to endothelial cell abnormalities, now appears central to the pathogenesis of scleroderma (Le Roy, 1985). Serologic abnormalities, including the presence of rheumatoid factor, ANA, and antibodies to DNA and elevated immunoglobulin levels, occur in between one quarter and one half of adults and children with scleroderma (Kornreich et al, 1977); these findings may also relate to the pathogenesis of the disease.

Pulmonary involvement in childhood PSS has received little attention because the findings are generally considered identical with those found in adults. In autopsy series, the lungs are affected in almost 90 per cent of adults with PSS (D'Angelo et al, 1969); the predominant histologic changes consist of interstitial and peribronchial fibrosis, subpleural cystic changes, and pleural thickening (Weaver, Divirtie, and Titus, 1968; D'Angelo et al, 1969).

Pulmonary involvement is fourth in frequency in scleroderma, behind skin, peripheral vascular, and esophageal disease, and lung disease is emerging as a leading cause of death, because the renal prognosis has improved because of early and aggressive antihypertensive therapy. However, lung involvement in scleroderma is remarkable because of the common dissociation of clinical, radiologic, functional, and histologic findings. Pulmonary disease, confirmed by biopsy findings, is well known to antedate the skin findings on which a diagnosis of scleroderma is often based (McCarthy et al, 1988).

Vascular lesions may be prominent and may include intimal proliferation and medial hypertrophy of small pulmonary arteries and arterioles. In early lesions, material rich in acid mucopolysaccharides is increased in the intima of small muscular arteries. Small-vessel change appears to be an early component of PSS but later may be difficult to distinguish from the chronic effects of pulmonary or systemic hypertension. Young and Mark (1978), in an autopsy series of 30 patients, noted that pulmonary fibrosis and pulmonary arterial disease could not be correlated, and that fibrosis was not a constant finding. Arterial involvement correlated better with severe right ventricular hypertrophy than with fibrosis. They described three patients whose marked vascular disease led to rapidly progressive respiratory failure. Extensive vascular sclerosis may be a late finding in PSS, particularly in association with pulmonary hypertension and cor pulmonale (Trell and Lindstrom, 1971).

The vascular changes of PSS have been postulated to be pathogenetically related to Raynaud phenomenon, because vascular change in renal vessels has been detected in response to peripheral cold challange (Guttadauria et al, 1979). Furst and co-workers (1981) demonstrated decreases in pulmonary perfusion, measured by [81]M-krypton scan, following cold challenge to the hands. They also showed increased pulmonary uptake of gallium-67, suggestive of inflammatory cells in the lungs, in six of nine patients with early PSS. All patients demonstrated abnormal levels of circulating immune complexes by Raji cell, polyethylene glycol assays, or both, but results of neither assay correlated with changes seen on lung scan. Conversely, however, Shuck and co-workers (1985) were not able to confirm the occurrence of either pulmonary vasospasm or transient pulmonary hypertension during episodes of Raynaud phenomenon in PSS. Both severe Raynaud phenomenon and smoking increase susceptibility to rapid deterioration in lung function in scleroderma (Peters-Golden et al, 1984).

Impairment of carbon monoxide diffusing capacity is usually the earliest physiologic abnormality and frequently can be found before clinical or roentgenographic evidence of pulmonary disease (Greenwald et al, 1987). In many cases, decreased lung compliance and reduced vital capacity develops as the scleroderma progresses, and these restrictive changes may be related to interstitial and peribronchial fibrosis. Guttadauria and co-workers (1979) classified 44 PSS patients by type of pulmonary function abnormality and found 29 per cent with restrictive disease, 27 per cent with obstructive disease, and 42 per cent with small airways disease. One patient (2 per cent) had an abnormality of DL_{CO} only. These investigators suggest, in contrast to others, that small airways disease often precedes gas diffusion abnormalities in PSS. Other investigators report difficulty, even with sensitive exercise studies, in detecting gas exchange abnormalities in PSS patients who have known pulmonary vasculitis (Mohsenifar et al, 1981).

Obstructive lung disease, including reduced maximal breathing capacity and increased residual volume, may become prominent late in the disease course. Exertional dyspnea is the most common symptom of PSS lung involvement (47 to 80 per cent of patients) but is rarely the presenting complaint. Dyspnea may remain stable, may progress slowly with increased exercise intolerance, or may be associated with a rapidly fatal course. Tightness of the skin of the chest is not a cause of dyspnea, but pulmonary fibrosis commonly causes decreased lung compliance and increased work of breathing. Cough is not common unless PSS is associated with a respiratory tract infection, and chest pain due to PSS lung disease is very rare. Fine, bibasilar inspiratory crackles are the most frequent auscultatory finding; clubbing is less frequently seen than with other causes of interstitial fibrosis. These changes rarely appear to be the dominant cause of death unless pulmonary hypertension leads to cor pulmonale and cardiac failure. Another late complication of chronic interstitial inflammation and fibrosis of the lung is terminal bronchiolar carcinoma. The underlying inflammation and fibrosis may be associated with PSS or may be idiopathic (Spain, 1957).

It may be convenient to discern three types of pulmonary involvement in PSS: (1) predominant lung fibrosis with a slow obliteration of the vascular bed and slowly progressive cor pulmonale, (2) combined pulmonary parenchymal and vascular lesions, and (3) predominant pulmonary vascular involvement associated with rapidly lethal right ventricular failure (Trell and Lindstrom, 1971).

Chest roentgenograms may reveal linear or nodular densities with accentuation in the lower lung fields (Weaver, Divirtie, and Titus, 1968) or, in approximately one fourth of patients with PSS, may exhibit a more diffuse pattern of fibrosis. Cardiomegaly, vascular congestion, and pleural thickening are also frequently observed abnormalities. Spontaneous pneumothorax, occasionally seen, is presumed due to intrapleural rupture of a cyst. Roentgenographic signs of pulmonary fibrosis are not, according to Guttadauria and co-workers (1979), well correlated with respiratory symptoms, skin changes, or involvement of other organ systems. The following is an illustrative case.

Case 4. This 18-year-old girl first developed "arthritis" at 4 years of age and had the onset of progressive systemic sclerosis at 6 years. The initial skin involvement, Raynaud phenomenon, and dysphagia were treated with prednisone, 2.5 mg three times per day for 2 months, without improvement. Growth failure was noted before steroid therapy and persisted after steroids were discontinued. At age 10 years she underwent a skin biopsy that revealed increased fibrosis with reduced cellularity of the dermis; atrophic sweat glands surrounded by "constricting" collagen fibers were present. A chest roentgenogram demonstrated very little subcutaneous tissue, marked emphysema, and severe interstitial fibrosis. Cysts were present in both lower lung fields.

By age 18, the patient was suffering from shortness of breath, dyspnea on exertion, alternating constipation and diarrhea, and severe Raynaud phenomenon. Examination revealed generalized atrophic skin with variable hypopigmentation and hyperpigmentation. She had poor chest expansion, intercostal and supracostal retractions, mild nasal flaring, and fine crackles at both bases. The cardiac and abdominal findings were not remarkable. Generalized muscle wasting and numerous severe flection contractures were evident.

Laboratory results included negative ANA and RF, normal CBC, BUN, and creatinine, and severely abnormal barium enema findings; the chest roentgenogram revealed advanced parenchymal fibrosis. Serial pulmonary function studies were performed during the final 2 years of her disease course.

Various therapies, including D-penicillamine and corticosteroids, were employed without success. Her course was marked by progressive cough, shortness of breath, and dyspnea on exertion, and the continuous administration of oxygen was required by her twentieth year. Because of long-standing hypercapnia, oxygen was maintained at only 30 per cent to prevent loss of O_2 drive to ventilation; arterial blood gases at this time included: pH 7.37, P_{CO_2} 55, P_{O_2} 75, base excess −9. The patient developed pneumonia, cor pulmonale, and congestive heart failure, which responded well to intravenous gentamicin and methicillin, diuretics, and oral Lanoxin. The chest roentgenogram

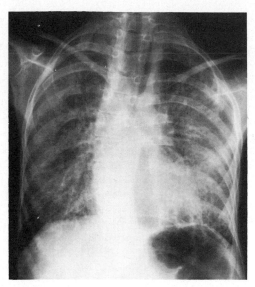

Figure 66–5. *Case 4.* An advanced case of scleroderma lung with chronic pulmonary fibrosis in a reticulated honeycomb pattern more prominent in the lower lobes. The heart is minimally enlarged, gaseous distention of the proximal and distal thirds of the esophagus is present, and there is a moderate right convex scoliosis.

revealed progressive fibrosis (Fig. 66–5); severe hypoxia and hypercapnia were also present.

She was rehospitalized after a spontaneous right pneumothorax. Thoracotomy and insertion of a chest tube were performed. Partial lung expansion occurred, but during the next 2 months, all attempts to remove the chest tube were followed by reaccumulations of air in the right thorax. A right-sided empyema developed, in addition to progressive weakness and severe decubitus ulcers due to immobility. She exhibited advancing psychiatric disability with disassociation from events around her. Strength, endurance, and respiratory status continued to deteriorate, but a chest roentgenogram showed no cardiomegaly and only a 10 per cent right pneumothorax. The patient experienced a sudden cardiorespiratory arrest and died at the age of 20.

Results of one series of pulmonary function tests are listed in Table 66–7. The VC and its subdivisions are severely attenuated. The RV, FRC, and TLC are markedly reduced as a reflection of the reduction in VC. The FEC_1 is moderately reduced, but it falls well within the normal range when expressed as a percentage of the FVC. Maximal

Table 66–7. *CASE 4:* PULMONARY VALUES

	Normal Range	Predicted Mean	Measured (% pred.)
VC (L)	2.6–4.2	2.6	0.6 (21)
FRC (L)	1.2–2.7	1.6	0.7 (46)
RV (L)	0.5–1.3	0.7	0.5 (64)
TLC (L)	3.3–5.2	3.4	1.0 (30)
FEV_1 (L)	2.5–3.8	2.4	1.5 (20)
FEV_1/FVC (%)	72–100	89.0	91.0
MMEF (L/min)	166–302	177.0	63.0 (35)
CV (L)			
CV/VC (%)			
N_2 (40) (%)			
DL_{CO} (ml/min/mm Hg)	15.0–31.3	14.7	2.2
P_{O_2} (mm Hg)		93.0	57.9
P_{CO_2} (mm Hg)		37–43	30.5
pH		7.37–7.43	7.39

expiratory flow, measured at all lung volumes, falls within the normal range when corrected for the reduction in vital capacity. The carbon monoxide diffusing capacity reveals a major reduction in transport of carbon monoxide into the pulmonary capillary blood.

This patient has such marked restrictions of the lung volume and pulmonary capillary blood volume that her ability to diffuse carbon monoxide into the alveolar capillary blood is drastically reduced.

There is no well-accepted treatment for PSS or for its pulmonary component, although numerous agents have been tried, including corticosteroids, immunosuppressive drugs, para-aminobenzoic acid, chelating agents, calcium channel blockers, and vasodilating agents. Steen and colleagues (1985) have shown that D-penicillamine treatment is associated with significant improvement in the DL_{CO}, absence of progression of dyspnea or parenchymal fibrosis, and reduction of skin thickening in scleroderma. The results are preliminary but occasion cautious optimism.

CREST SYNDROME

The CREST syndrome variant of scleroderma consists of calcinosis, Raynaud phenomenon, esophageal dysfunction, sclerodactyly, and telangiectasias (Medsger, 1989). Initial reports of the CREST syndrome stressed its benign prognosis in comparison with progressive systemic sclerosis, but prolonged evaluation reveals slowly developing gastrointestinal involvement, pulmonary hypertension, Sjögren syndrome, and biliary cirrhosis. Thus its distinguishing features are onset with Raynaud phenomenon, extensive calcinosis, and profuse telangiectasia. CREST syndrome has not been specifically reported in children, but its features are similar to "acrosclerosis" and to some forms of focal scleroderma of childhood (Hanson, 1985; Singsen, 1986).

Pulmonary involvement in the CREST syndrome was described by Salerni and co-workers (1977). They found ten of 120 patients to have pulmonary hypertension; exertional dyspnea occurred in all ten. These patients commonly exhibited tricuspid regurgitation, enlarged pulmonary arteries, and congestive heart failure; six of the ten died of pulmonary hypertension. Chest roentgenograms and post-mortem studies did not reveal interstitial pulmonary fibrosis, but the DL_{CO} was diminished in five of ten patients tested. Steen and colleagues (1985) performed pulmonary function tests in 88 adults with the CREST syndrome and found that only 25 (28 per cent) had no abnormalities. Pulmonary fibrosis was found on chest roentgenogram in 37 per cent of patients, and calcific pulmonary granulomata were detected in 67 per cent.

DERMATOMYOSITIS

Childhood dermatomyositis is a chronic inflammatory disease primarily of skin and muscle, but it also may have significant internal organ involvement. Dermatomyositis in childhood, a syndrome distinct from the adult form of the disease, is a systemic angiopathy (Banker and Victor, 1966). Proximal muscle weakness and a characteristic erythematous or violaceous rash around the eyes and over the malar eminences, the extensor surfaces of the elbows and knees, and the metacarpophalangeal and proximal interphalangeal joints are the most common presenting features. Laboratory findings include elevated serum muscle enzymes and characteristic electromyographic changes. Histologic changes on muscle biopsy may include muscle fiber degeneration, sarcolemmal nuclear proliferation, mononuclear cell infiltrates around muscle fibers, and vascular changes including prominent perivascular infiltrates and the occlusion of small vessels by intimal proliferation and fibrin thrombi.

Several large series of childhood dermatomyositis suggest that prognosis has significantly improved in the past 20 years (Sullivan et al, 1972; Hanson, 1976). In all probability, this is due to the sustained use of corticosteroids for as long as clinical or serologic evidence of muscle disease persists and to an increased awareness of the potential for life-threatening internal organ involvement, particularly in the gastrointestinal tract (Banker and Victor, 1966) and heart and lungs (Singsen, Goldreyer, Stanton, and Hanson, 1976; Singsen et al, 1978). Childhood dermatomyositis is a diffuse or systemic vasculopathy, and thus inflammatory vascular changes may be found in many major organs at some time during the disease course.

Diffuse interstitial pulmonary fibrosis is a well-documented complication of adult polymyositis and dermatomyositis. The incidence of histologically confirmed pulmonary fibrosis (fibrosing alveolitis) is estimated to vary from 5 to 10 per cent (Frazier and Miller, 1974; Salmeron et al, 1981; Schwartz et al, 1976). However, Songcharoen and co-workers (1980) found seven of 15 patients to have pulmonary fibrosis, their patients were abnormal by clinical criteria (six of seven), chest radiographs (six of seven), or pulmonary function tests (five of five).

The clinical presentation may be one of acute onset of fever, dyspnea, and cough or may be insidious with only mild, slowly progressive symptoms, such as nonproductive cough and dyspnea on exertion. Bibasilar crackles are the most common physical finding; clubbing is not usually seen. Roentgenograms usually reveal slowly developing diffuse interstitial fibrosis. This pattern is occasionally noted by accident in an adult with dermatomyositis and no pulmonary symptoms. Other infrequent radiographic findings include patchy alveolar infiltrates, spontaneous pneumothorax or pneumomediastinum, and decreased lung volumes. One retrospective analysis of 105 adults with polymyositis showed 10 per cent (ten patients) to have radiographic evidence of interstitial pulmonary disease. Eight of these ten had pulmonary function testing, and all eight were abnormal with a mean total lung capacity of 67 per cent and a mean vital capacity of 60 per cent (Salmeron et al, 1981).

Restrictive defects and diminished DL_{CO} are typical pulmonary function abnormalities in most patients tested, but these frequently do not progress. Histologic examination of involved lungs may reveal alveolar septal thickening and fibrosis, with the infiltration of chronic inflammatory cells. Vasculitis is usually not a feature, but cyst formation, perhaps due to dissolution of alveolar septal walls, has been observed (Hyun and co-workers, 1962). In patients whose pulmonary disease responds to corticosteroids, the histologic features include interstitial round cell infiltrates, alveolar epithelial hyperplasia, desquamation, and fibrosis. Patients with unresponsive disease have demonstrated predominantly fibrosis (Schwartz et al, 1976; Salmeron et al, 1981). Various investigators differ as to the efficacy of corticosteroid therapy (Camp et al, 1972; Frazier and Miller, 1974), but particularly in the patient with an acute onset or early chronic fibrosis, a trial of corticosteroids appears warranted (Weaver, Brundage, Nelson, and Bischoff, 1968).

In childhood dermatomyositis, roentgenographic evidence of pulmonary fibrosis has been reported in four children (Dubowitz and Dubowitz, 1964; Gwinn and Lee, 1975; Singsen et al, 1977), with histologic confirmation in two. Spontaneous pneumothorax has occurred in three cases, including one as a terminal event (Park and Nyhan, 1975; Singsen et al, 1977). It has been suggested that pneumothorax may be a complication of the basic angiopathic and inflammatory disease process.

The most common types of pulmonary involvement are thoracic muscle weakness, impaired swallowing, and poor airway toilet in children with active early dermatomyositis, or rarely in those with end-stage disease. In both situations, aspiration pneumonia and hypoventilation with secondary hypostatic pneumonia can occur (Bitnum et al, 1964). In patients with acute-onset dermatomyositis and active muscle disease, vigorous therapy with corticosteroids should be pursued to improve strength. Methotrexate is an effective treatment for steroid-resistant dermatomyositis but may be associated with opportunistic infections or, rarely, drug-induced pneumonia (Batist and Andrews, 1981).

Case 5. This 21-year-old woman was well until age 12 years, when she developed rash, anorexia, and weight loss. The rash was red and scaly over the metacarpophalangeal and proximal interphalangeal joints; a violaceous discoloration of the upper eyelids was also present. The following 6 months were marked by progressive proximal weakness of the quadriceps, neck, and abdominal flexors. A muscle biopsy revealed fiber degeneration, sarcolemmal nuclear proliferation, and vascular intimal thickening with perivascular infiltration of chronic inflammatory cells. Serum muscle enzyme levels were elevated.

The institution of prednisolone therapy led to almost complete resolution of the rash and muscle weakness over 4 months. Prednisolone doses, varying from 5 to 15 mg/day, were required during the next 4 years to maintain control of the dermatomyositis. Numerous complications occurred during the course of the disease, including vasculitis of the fingertips and progressive Raynaud phenomenon, which began when she was 14 and resulted in the autoamputation of several fingertips. Progressive generalized calcinosis was first detected at age 15. At age 18, perforation of the nasal septum occurred; a biopsy of the adjacent mucosa revealed vasculitis, fibrosis, and chronic inflammatory infiltrates.

At age 18, she developed a nonproductive cough, and chest examination revealed fine, bibasilar crackles. Serial chest roentgenograms from 14 to 18 years were reviewed and showed "progressive interstitial markings" suggestive of slowly increasing pulmonary fibrosis.

A spontaneous left pneumothorax occurred when she was 19 in association with an exacerbation of the Raynaud phenomenon and worsening vasculitis of several fingertips. The patient was not receiving corticosteroids at this time. Thoracotomy, for chest tube placement and open-lung biopsy, was performed. The lung revealed histologic evidence of pleural and interstitial fibrosis with focal, subpleural chronic pneumonitis. Irregular patterns of aeration, centrilobular emphysema, and perivascular fibrosis were present, but no obliterative vascular lesions were observed. Prednisolone, 5 mg four times per day, was begun, and over the next 6 weeks resolution of the pneumothorax and decrease in the vasculitis of the fingertips were observed.

The subsequent 2 years of her disease course included numerous complications, including severe muscle atrophy and flection contractures, limited exercise tolerance, recurrent pneumonia and pneumothoraces, and an unexplained episode of abdominal pain without evidence of gastrointestinal involvement. Depression and withdrawal from reality occurred, and several episodes of psychosis responded poorly to medication and psychotherapy. An elevated cerebrospinal fluid protein level and an electroencephalogram showing diffuse slowing were suggestive of cerebral dysfunction, perhaps due to dermatomyositis. However, the patient resisted further hospitalization or corticosteroid therapy. The pulmonary fibrosis slowly advanced, as could be seen on a chest roentgenogram taken when she was 21 (Fig. 66–6). The following month, the patient died at home from cardiorespiratory failure. No post-mortem examination was performed.

The data from serial pulmonary function studies are

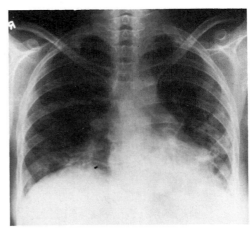

Figure 66–6. *Case 5.* Dermatomyositis with chronic pulmonary fibrosis of 2 years' duration. The heart is normal in size, and soft tissue calcifications are present in both axillae. Interstitial thickening and cystic changes are bilateral and most pronounced at the bases.

shown in Table 66–8. The VC and its subdivisions are severely reduced. FRC, RV, and TLC are within one standard deviation of the mean, with the RV equal to the mean predicted value. The FEV₁, expressed as a percentage of the FVC, is normal, as is the maximal expiratory flow measured at all lung volumes. Distribution of ventilation falls within the normal range. The DL_{CO}, measured by the steady state method, is less than 50 per cent of predicted, even when corrected for alveolar volume. There is moderate arterial hypoxia, an enlarged alveolar-arterial oxygen difference, and a marked acute and chronic alveolar hyperventilation in the face of a mild metabolic acidosis.

This patient had a very severe, restrictive lung disorder, compromised alveolar volume and alveolar surface area, and reduced alveolar capillary blood volume resulting in hypoxia.

JUVENILE RHEUMATOID ARTHRITIS

There are more than 100 medical conditions known to be associated with arthritis in children. Among these, juvenile rheumatoid arthritis (JRA) is the most well known, afflicting perhaps 175,000 children in the United States alone. The terms *JRA, juvenile arthritis,* and *Still disease* are frequently used interchangeably by physicians, but *Still disease* should be reserved for the acute systemic onset–type associated with spiking fever, typical rash, and various organ derangements. The remaining two groups within the classification of JRA are polyarticular and pauciarticular disease, both defined after a minimum 3-month observation period. Until causes and subtle differential diagnostic points are better understood, some children with arthritis associated with inflammatory bowel disease, ankylosing spondylitis, psoriatic arthritis, Reiter syndrome, and various postinfectious reactive arthropathies will undoubtedly continue to be included in surveys of children with JRA (Brewer, 1986). The interested reader is referred to several excellent monographs in this fascinating field (Ansell, 1980; Schaller and Hanson, 1977; Miller, 1979; Cassidy, 1985; Jacobs, 1982).

Lung involvement in children with JRA is exceptionally rare and is largely limited to those with a

systemic onset (Jacobs, 1982). Pneumonitis and pleuritis may accompany early systemic manifestations and are most frequently associated with myocarditis or pericarditis. Occasionally, asymptomatic pleural involvement will be an incidental finding on chest roentgenogram (Jayson, 1976); one child with symptomatic pleural effusions that improved following thoracentesis has been reported (Gewanter and Baum, 1981). Athreya and co-workers (1980) reported eight of 191 children with JRA to have pleuropulmonary manifestations; six of these eight had systemic onset. Five presented with cough, four with chest pain, and seven with dyspnea, tachypnea, or both. All had both pericardial and pleural effusions. Five patients had evidence of interstitial pulmonary disease; the four of these who were tested had decreases in VC. Other researchers have reported single cases of JRA with associated pulmonary arteritis and cor pulmonale (Jordan and Synder, 1964), fatal pulmonary amyloidosis (Romicka and Maldyk, 1975), JRA with recurrent pneumonitis (Yousefzadeh and Fishman, 1979), lymphoid interstitial pneumonia (Lovell et al, 1984), and JRA that developed following long-standing idiopathic pulmonary hemosiderosis (Smith, 1966).

Pulmonary function in JRA has been the subject of a preliminary study by Wagener and colleagues (1981). Ten of 16 children younger than 18 years of age had abnormal pulmonary function values. Five had abnormal forced expiratory flow (FEF)₇₅%. This study did not include longitudinal design or assess responses to therapy.

Lung involvement in adults with rheumatoid arthritis (RA) is relatively common. The five major types recognized include pleural effusions, pleural and pulmonary rheumatoid nodules, perhaps with high titers of rheumatoid factor, obstructive bronchiolitis (Collins et al, 1976), Caplan syndrome (Turner-Warwick and Evans, 1977), and diffuse interstitial pneumonitis with fibrosis (Martel et al, 1968; Steinberg, 1975). Hakela (1988) has reviewed 57 patients with rheumatoid arthritis who were hospitalized for diffuse interstitial lung fibrosis. Eight had largely reversible disease related to gold or penicillamine treatment, but the remaining 49 patients showed a poor prognosis, with a median survival of 3.5 years and a 5-year survival rate of 39 per cent.

Pleural effusions may be transient and asymptomatic or can be associated with pleural granulomas (Martel et al, 1968). Other complications of RA, as noted by MacFarlane and co-workers (1978), include a higher frequency of bronchitis and bronchiectasis at autopsy than in matched controls. In their discussions of adult RA, these authors also stressed the possible occurrence of acute bronchiolitis, the increased frequency of acute empyema, and the presence of solitary cavitary pulmonary rheumatoid nodules that may cause hemoptysis or simulate malignancy. Patients with RA and "shrinking lung" and one patient with upper lobe fibrosis have also been described.

Table 66–8. *CASE 5:* PULMONARY VALUES

	Normal Range	Predicted Mean	Measured (% pred.)
VC (L)	2.6–4.2	3.3	1.3 (38)
FRC (L)	1.2–2.7	2.0	1.4 (71)
RV (L)	0.5–1.3	0.9	1.1 (116)
TLC (L)	3.3–5.2	4.2	2.3 (55)
FEV₁ (L)	2.5–3.8	3.1	1.2 (38)
FEV₁/FVC (%)	72–100	86.0	87.0
MMEF (L/min)	166–302	234.0	78.0 (33)
CV (L)		0.3	
CV/VC (%)		8.0	
N₂ (40) (%)		1.5	1.3
DL_{CO} (ml/min/mm Hg)	15.0–31.3	23.1	8.1
P_{O_2} (mm Hg)		93.0	62.0
P_{CO_2} (mm Hg)		37–43	25.0
pH		7.37–7.43	7.45

Rheumatoid interstitial lung disease appears to closely resemble idiopathic pulmonary fibrosis, with parallels including the overproduction of local immunoglobulin, immune complex deposition, and neutrophil-mediated oxidant injury. Additionally, synovitis may be related to the disruption of articular collagen fibers via specific proteolytic attack by an active collagenase. Weiland and co-workers (1987) have performed pulmonary lavage of rheumatoid arthritis patients and have isolated an active neutrophil collagenase that could contribute to their developing interstitial lung disease.

Historical and clinical findings are frequently of little value in diagnosing rheumatoid interstitial lung disease, but in one study a combination of chest roentgenogram and DL_{CO} testing found one third of 30 adults to be abnormal (Popper et al, 1972). Subsequently, Frank and co-workers (1973) demonstrated abnormalities of diffusion in 41 per cent of 41 consecutive adult RA patients. All eight patients who were biopsied had interstitial fibrosis, even the several who were asymptomatic and had normal chest roentgenograms. Thus patients appeared to have clinically mild disease and to progress slowly. These findings suggest that lung disease in JRA might also have its origins early in the course of the disorder. Laitinen and co-workers (1975) evaluated pulmonary function in 129 RA patients and suggested that restrictive changes develop early in the disease, whereas decreased diffusing capacity is associated with more advanced "rheumatoid lung." Oxholm and colleagues (1982) studied 144 adult RA patients and found DL_{CO} to be reduced below the predicted mean in all cases; they suggested inflammatory vascular changes in the lung as a cause, even when other extra-articular manifestations could not be seen. Geddes and associates (1979) carried out an excellent study of 100 patients, with controls matched for age, sex, and smoking habits, which suggests that airway disease may be the most common form of lung involvement in RA. Scott and co-workers (1987) have suggested an association between the B cell alloantigen HLA-DR-4 and significant reductions in FEV_1/FVC in patients with rheumatoid arthritis. These changes appeared to develop irrespective of smoking status.

An increasing number of medications in common use for RA can also produce pulmonary complications: diffuse interstitial lung disease sometimes occurs with use of gold (Scott et al, 1981). Gold therapy-induced pneumonitis in RA was studied in 17 patients by Partanen and co-workers (1987), and they found a striking homogeneity of major histocompatability markers (HLA-A3, B-35, and B-40 alleles), suggesting that those at risk of pulmonary complications of gold therapy could be identified. Acute obliterative bronchiolitis and bronchitis have been associated with penicillamine (Epler et al, 1979; Penny et al, 1982), and there have been various pleural and parenchymal reactions to several chemotherapeutic agents that may be employed for RA and other rheumatic disorders (Green, 1977). Pulmonary infiltrates, presumably due to a hypersensitivity reaction, have also been reported in association with treatment with several nonsteroidal anti-inflammatory drugs (Buscaglia et al, 1984).

One additional form of progressive, severe pulmonary impairment should also be recognized. In both adults and children, marked thoracolumbar spine and sternoclavicular joint disease may lead to severe thoracic cage deformities and restrictive pulmonary defects.

Case 6. This 6-year-old girl had a 3-year history of polyarticular JRA following a systemic onset. Despite previous therapy with aspirin, gold, and corticosteroids, she had become nonambulatory owing to severe lower extremity joint disease. Poor weight gain was observed, and cricoarytenoid joint involvement was associated with partial vocal cord paralysis. Moderate scoliosis (convex to the right), dorsal kyphosis, and a bell-shaped rib cage were seen (Fig. 66–7).

Because of active synovial inflammation, marked muscle wasting, severe flection contractures, and respiratory insufficiency, this child received intensive in-patient rehabilitation for 8 months. Indomethacin and ibuprofen were added to her therapeutic regimen. Efforts to achieve ambulation were successful, but progressive weight bearing was associated with rapid advancement of the scoliosis from 10 degrees to 85 degrees and marked decrease in respiratory reserve. Placement of a Harrington rod was considered, but the patient was judged an unacceptable operative risk; in addition, the osteoporotic spine appeared too frail to retain the rod.

D-Penicillamine was substituted for weekly intramuscular gold therapy, without success. However, a Milwaukee brace arrested the progression of the kyphoscoliosis. The addition of oral chlorambucil led to a marked reduction in joint disease activity, increased exercise tolerance, and improved pulmonary function.

Results of pulmonary function studies are listed in Table 66–9. The VC and its subdivisions are greater than two standard deviations below the predicted mean. The FEV_1/FVC is normal, as is the maximal expiratory flow

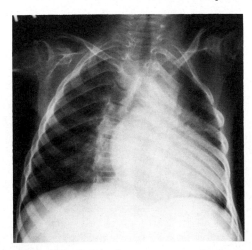

Figure 66–7. *Case 6.* The bones are severely demineralized. Right convex scoliosis is present, and the heart is moderately enlarged and projected to the left. The rib cage is noticeably bell shaped. A severe pectus carinatum cannot be appreciated in this view. The lung fields are clear.

Table 66–9. *CASE 6:* PULMONARY VALUES

	Normal Range	Predicted Mean	Measured (% pred.)
VC (L)	0.7–1.1	0.9	0.35 (38)
FRC (L)	0.3–0.7	0.5	
RV (L)	0.2–0.4	0.3	
TLC (L)	0.9–1.4	1.2	
FEV$_1$ (L)	0.7–1.0	0.8	0.3 (42)
FEV$_1$/FVC (%)	72–100	86.0	100.0
MMEF (L/min)	22–114	46.0	47.0 (104)
CV (L)			
CV/VC (%)			
N$_2$ (40) (%)			
DL$_{CO}$ (ml/min/mm Hg)			
P$_{O_2}$ (mm Hg)		100.0	69.0
P$_{CO_2}$ (mm Hg)		37–43	34.0
pH		7.37–7.43	7.39

volume curve, after correction for the reduction in VC. A resting arterial blood sample reveals mild reduction in the P$_{O_2}$, increased alveolar-arterial oxygen difference, and a compensated alveolar hyperventilation.

This patient has severe restrictive lung disease but normal airway function. Her maximal expiratory flow rates at all lung volumes are reduced, but they are normal when corrected for the degree of lung restriction. The restrictive lung disease is so severe that alveolar volume and probably pulmonary perfusion have been compromised. Thus the patient has mild hypoxia despite sustained alveolar hyperventilation. These findings are all attributed to the severe chest wall deformity and scoliosis resulting from the arthritis.

ANKYLOSING SPONDYLITIS

Ankylosing spondylitis (AS) in children is being recognized with increasing frequency. AS is characterized by the predominance of large joint and lower extremity involvement, prevalence in boys, and presence of HLA-B27 in up to 80 per cent of cases. The diagnostic criteria for adult AS do not apply to children because young patients have (1) late or asymptomatic development of sacroiliac joint disease by either clinical or radiographic evaluation; (2) infrequency of limited chest expansion; and (3) a relative rarity, even with long follow-up, of obvious spinal involvement (Bernstein et al, 1979).

Pulmonary disease in children with AS has not been documented, but lung involvement in adults with ankylosing spondylitis is well known. The reported incidence is between zero and 30 per cent. Most frequently the disease is detected as upper lobe fibrosis (Appelrouth and Gottlieb, 1975). Lung disease in AS may progress from spotty linear apical shadows to nodules that coalesce or cavitate (nontuberculous fibrocavitary disease).

Rosenow and colleagues (1977) found that 28 of 2080 adults with AS (1.3 per cent) had pleuropulmonary manifestations, including five who developed pulmonary aspergillomas. Thickening of the apical and nonapical pleura and, rarely, calcification were observed, but pleural effusion was rare. In none of these cases did pulmonary disease precede arthritis.

Apical fibrobullous disease usually began unilaterally but eventually was bilateral and without predilection for one lung or the other. The lung disease is usually without cough, pain, dyspnea, or hemoptysis and is rarely associated with clubbing. Pneumothorax is also rare, as is bronchopleural fistula following thoracotomy. The most consistent pulmonary function test changes in adult AS have been decreased VC and TLC and increased RV. These may be due to decreased thoracic wall compliance. Serial and therapeutic response studies are not available.

MIXED CONNECTIVE TISSUE DISEASE

Rheumatologists have long recognized unusual overlap syndromes characterized by features of several rheumatic diseases. In 1972, however, Sharp and co-workers first described mixed connective tissue disease (MCTD) as a unique entity that exhibited overlapping clinical features of SLE, dermatomyositis, and scleroderma and distinctive serologic findings, including high titers of speckled ANA and antibody against a ribonucleoprotein antigen (RNP). The clinical features of MCTD include a high frequency of Raynaud phenomenon, arthritis, sausage-shaped fingers, and rashes suggestive of SLE, dermatomyositis, and scleroderma (Sharp and Singsen, 1989).

It is now recognized that rheumatoid arthritis, renal disease in 15 to 40 per cent of patients, and thyroiditis may also occur in MCTD. Treatment includes nonsteroidal anti-inflammatory or remittive agents for arthritis. In addition, MCTD is not as steroid sensitive as originally thought, may require immunosuppressives, and frequently evolves to include many scleroderma-like features.

In 1973, a brief report described an 11-year-old girl with MCTD (Sanders et al, 1973). Fourteen children with MCTD were subsequently investigated and their serologic findings compared with those from 127 children with other rheumatic diseases (Singsen et al, 1977). The children with MCTD (median age, 10.5 years) are similar to their adult counterparts, but exhibit more frequent arthritis, significant cardiac (64 per cent) and renal (43 per cent) involvement, and severe thrombocytopenia (43 per cent). The larger and more prolonged doses of corticosteroids required in these children and the death of four from hemorrhage or septicemia may suggest a more severe prognosis in childhood MCTD.

Approximately 62 children with MCTD have now been reported. We are aware of its association with Sjögren syndrome (Fraga et al, 1978) and pulmonary hypertension (Rosenberg et al, 1979), and detailed histologic descriptions are available (Singsen et al, 1980). Widespread proliferative vascular disease is the hallmark of MCTD; silent involvement of most organs is probable; and pulmonary disease may be one of the worst, and most common, late complications of MCTD.

Harmon and associates (1976) evaluated 24 adult patients with MCTD through histories of unexplained dyspnea, physicial examination, chest roentgenograms, and pulmonary function tests. Thirteen of the 24 patients had no symptoms, but only four were negative for all parameters. Five of the 13 had abnormal pulmonary function test values, one had only an abnormal chest roentgenogram, and three had abnormal pulmonary function test values and chest roentgenograms. Thus nine of 13 asymptomatic patients (69 per cent) had pulmonary disease. The remaining 11 symptomatic patients all had abnormal pulmonary function test values and chest roentgenograms. The abnormal pulmonary function tests always included decreased DL_{CO} and, frequently, reduced lung volumes. The chest roentgenograms revealed diffuse infiltrates and occasional volume loss or pleural disease; these findings were similar to the roentgenographic findings of Silver and co-workers (1976). Of the 24 fully evaluated patients, 20 (84 per cent) had pulmonary disease.

In an extension of Harmon's early studies, Sullivan and co-investigators (1984) have now prospectively evaluated pulmonary involvement in 34 patients with MCTD. Only 33 per cent were asymptomatic, whereas 58 per cent developed dyspnea, 42 per cent had evidence of pleural disease, and 24 per cent had cough. Of 11 patients with negative findings from their medical histories and physical examinations, 8 (73 per cent) had abnormal pulmonary function tests, chest radiographs, or both. Overall, 29 out of 34 (85 per cent) had pulmonary involvement. Right-heart catheterization showed pulmonary hypertension in 11 of 15 (73 per cent), and its presence could not be predicted by pulmonary function tests, gallium scanning, or exercise testing. At least one abnormality was found at pulmonary function testing in 85 per cent of the cases. Many patients appeared to show significant improvement with corticosteroid or cyclophosphamide treatment, or both. In addition to reductions in DL_{CO}, MCTD patients may also demonstrate decreased lung volumes and abnormal frequency dependence of compliance in the presence of normal total airways resistance, suggesting the presence of small airways disease (Derderian et al, 1985).

Pulmonary hypertension in MCTD is now described in children (Jones et al, 1978; Rosenberg et al, 1979); it may be related to proliferative vascular changes, thrombus formation, or both, and may respond to steroids or immunosuppressives (Wiener-Kronish et al, 1981).

Case 7. This 15-year-old girl had a 7-month history of arthralgias and swelling of the hands, substernal chest pain, shortness of breath, malar rash, malaise, and a 20-pound weight loss. She was first thought to have SLE, and prednisolone was prescribed, 5 mg three times per day.

Further history revealed Raynaud phenomenon, chronic constipation, and dysphagia. Physical examination showed the skin to be clear; arthritis was present at the wrists, knees, and ankles, as were "sausage fingers" and mild digital vasospasm. The lungs were clear, and the cardiac findings were normal.

Laboratory data included a white blood cell count of 4200/mm³. Creatinine phosphokinase was 464 IU (normal: 0–100); a speckled ANA, titer 1:256, was detected. Antibody against ribonucleoprotein was present in a titer of $1:2.0 \times 10^7$. A barium esophagogram showed diminished peristalsis and dilation of the distal third, and a barium enema revealed pseudodiverticula at the hepatic and splenic flexures. A chest roentgenogram and ventilation-perfusion lung scan were both interpreted as normal. A diagnosis of MCTD was considered confirmed because of overlapping clinical and laboratory features of SLE, dermatomyositis, and scleroderma.

Hydroxychloroquine, 400 mg/day, and prednisone, 40 mg/day, were effective in controlling the disease activity. Seven months later the patient was receiving prednisone, 15 mg/day, and had no respiratory or articular complaints. She continued to have Raynaud phenomenon, intermittent myalgias, and dysphagia.

Results of pulmonary function studies are listed in Table 66–10. The VC and its subdivisions, although reduced from predicted values, fall within one standard deviation of the mean. The FRC and RV approximate the mean predicted value; the TLC is reduced but is within one standard deviation of the mean. The FEV_1/FVC is normal, as is the maximal expiratory flow rate when measured at all lung volumes. The distribution of ventilation, measured by the single-breath oxygen test, and 40-sec nitrogen washout test result are normal. The CV also falls within the normal range. The DL_{CO} is reduced. A resting arterial blood sample has normal oxygen tension and alveolar-arterial oxygen difference and reveals a partially compensated alveolar hyperventilation.

This patient has mild restrictive lung disease and evidence of interstitial disease. The shortness of breath experienced might be due in greater part to the interstitial rather than the restrictive component. Thus measurement of ventilation and blood gases during exercise should be valuable for assessment of the pulmonary response to therapy.

SJÖGREN SYNDROME

Sjögren syndrome (SS) primarily affects adult women, is the second most common autoimmune

Table 66–10. *CASE 7:* PULMONARY VALUES

	Normal Range	Predicted Mean	Measured (% pred.)
VC (L)	2.4–4.1	3.3	2.5 (78)
FRC (L)	1.2–2.7	1.9	1.6 (81)
RV (L)	0.5–1.3	0.9	0.6 (70)
TLC (L)	3.2–5.1	4.2	3.2 (76)
FEV₁ (L)	2.5–3.7	3.1	2.2 (72)
FEV₁/FVC (%)	72–100	86.0	93.0
MMEF (L/min)	163–299	231.0	226.0 (98)
CV (L)		0.2	0.2
CV/VC (%)		7.9	7.0
N₂ (40) (%)		1.5	0.5
DL_{CO} (ml/min/mm Hg)	14.8–30.8	22.8	14.3
P$_{O_2}$ (mm Hg)		97.0	106.0
P$_{CO_2}$ (mm Hg)	37–43		32.0
pH		7.36–7.43	7.45

syndrome after rheumatoid arthritis, and is probably the result of lymphocyte-mediated destruction of exocrine glands (Moutsopoulos et al, 1980). Sjögren (sicca) syndrome may occur alone (primary) or in combination with almost any other rheumatic disorder (secondary). Both the primary and the secondary forms are extremely immunoreactive. Common manifestations include dry eyes, dry mouth with oral ulcerations and dental caries, salivary gland swelling, difficulty swallowing, vulvovaginitis, and gastrointestinal abnormalities. The Schirmer test for tear production and the lip biopsy for accessory salivary glands are both diagnostically helpful. In 25 per cent of adults the lymphoproliferative process involves extraglandular sites, such as muscles, kidneys, lungs, and nervous system. Lymphoma and pseudolymphomatous transformation are both increased in Sjögren syndrome.

Athreya and associates (1977) reported two children with Sjögren syndrome and reviewed three other case reports. None of these patients was uniquely different from adults with SS. One should consider that "recurrent mumps" in children and recurrent benign parotitis of adolescence may actually be early manifestations of sicca syndrome.

Cough, dyspnea, recurrent pneumonitis, and pleural effusion have been the most common pulmonic features of Sjögren syndrome in adults, according to Strimlan and co-workers (1976). They reviewed 343 patients and found pulmonary involvement in 31 (9 per cent). Diffuse infiltrations were the most common roentgenographic pattern, followed by pleural effusions. As previously noted by Karlish (1969), 18 patients who underwent pulmonary function testing demonstrated restrictive ventilatory patterns or a low carbon monoxide diffusing capacity, or both. Diffuse interstitial fibrosis is a common late finding. Papathanasiou and co-workers (1986) have demonstrated, by pulmonary function testing, that diffuse interstitial lung disease develops in 38 per cent of primary SS patients and in 12 per cent of secondary SS patients. However, the clinical impact was minimal, most often seen as dry cough or mild dyspnea, and was negligibly different from that found in control subjects.

BEHÇET DISEASE

Behçet disease (syndrome) is a clinical triad of relapsing iritis, ulcers of the mouth, and genital ulcers, which may be associated with systemic manifestations, such as arthritis, thrombophlebitis migrans, erythema nodosum, meningoencephalitis, and arterial aneurysms (O'Duffy, 1981). It has few serologic markers, and responses to all forms of treatment have been inconsistent and temporary. Behçet disease is rare in children, with a peak of onset in the third decade, but 15 per cent of reported patients have some evidence of disease before 18 years of age (Chajek and Fainara, 1975).

Cadman and co-investigators (1976) reported one case of pulmonary involvement and reviewed 12 others. They found that pulmonary abnormalities were not isolated but rather accompanied disease exacerbations elsewhere. Massive hemoptysis and pulmonary hemorrhage were the most common findings (10 of 13) and caused death in four patients. These manifestations appear to be causally related to peripheral thrombophlebitis, widespread vasculitis, superior vena cava thrombosis, and pulmonary emboli. Histologic evidence of pulmonary vasculitis has also been observed. The most common chest roentgenographic finding is diffuse infiltration. We are not aware that pulmonary function studies in Behçet disease have been performed. Treatment of these rare pulmonary complications has usually not been successful.

WEGENER GRANULOMATOSIS

Wegener granulomatosis (WG) is a necrotizing, granulomatous vasculitis that occurs in a localized form that involves the upper and lower respiratory tract or in a more common form that includes renal involvement (Wolff et al, 1974). Controversy exists as to whether midline granuloma, limited WG, and generalized WG are separate clinicopathologic entities or represent an interrelated disease spectrum. The former view is supported by the apparently differing responses to therapy (Schechter et al, 1976). However, the similarity of many clinical and histologic features of WG to other vasculitic, granulomatous, or infectious disorders may cause diagnostic difficulty (Fauci and Wolff, 1973). Isreal and co-workers (1977) further suggest that "benign lymphocytic angiitis and granulomatosis of lung" and "lymphomatoid granulomatosis" can both be distinguished from Wegener granulomatosis via clinical and immunologic assessment. The first-named disease is quite corticosteroid sensitive, and the second is usually rapidly fatal in spite of any form of treatment.

Rhinorrhea, sinus pain, fever, arthralgias or arthritis, cough, hemoptysis, and skin rashes or ulcerations are the most commonly occurring signs and symptoms of WG. Renal involvement usually occurs late in the disease course rather than as an initial finding, but once begun it may progress rapidly to death. The histologic findings are widely varied but characteristically include necrotizing granulomas with or without vasculitis. Almost all organ systems can be involved, although the nasopharynx, sinuses, kidneys, skin, joints, and lungs predominate (Wolff et al, 1974).

Wegener granulomatosis is rare in children. Several dozen patients under the age of 16 years have been described (Roback et al, 1969; Moorthy et al, 1977; Baliga et al, 1978); however, knowledge of WG is now widespread, and thus many isolated cases may remain unreported.

Pulmonary involvement in WG may begin with fever, persistent cough, chest pain, or hemoptysis or may first be detected on observation of infiltrates on the chest roentgenogram of the asymptomatic patient. The roentgenographic pattern has no characteristic localization of lesions and may reveal multiple or solitary nodular densities or infiltrates. Lesions may vary in size from less than 1 to more than 10 cm and may have vague or sharply demarcated borders. The lesions may be unilateral or bilateral, may cavitate, and frequently are transient and fleeting. However, associated atelectasis, pleural effusions, mediastinal lymph node enlargement, and calcification of lesions are rare (Landman and Burgener, 1974).

The prognosis for Wegener granulomatosis has dramatically improved in the past decade, although renal failure remains a possible cause of death. Previously, corticosteroids were the primary form of therapy but appeared responsible only for doubling the mean duration of survival to 12 months. Numerous investigators have described the advantages of cytotoxic therapy for WG (Isreal and Patchefsky, 1975; Reza et al, 1975; Cupps and Fauci, 1981; Jacobs, 1982). Cyclophosphamide, the most impressive agent used so far, induced remission in all ten patients from one study (Reza et al, 1975). The mean duration of remission was 38 months; two patients were disease free for 7 years, and the one case that relapsed responded to a second course of therapy. However, cyclophosphamide is very toxic and should be used only by those experienced in its administration (Cupps and Fauci, 1981; Batist and Andrews, 1981). Chlorambucil has also been used with success and may be indicated as a first cytotoxic drug because of its fewer side effects (Isreal and Patchefsky, 1975). The following case illustrates the protean nature of WG, an excellent response to cyclophosphamide, and late findings of pulmonary function studies.

Case 8. This 12-year-old female had a 5-month history of fatigue, weight loss, progressive cough, gingival inflammation, and a slowly enlarging submandibular mass. There was no dyspnea or hemoptysis. Physical examination revealed generalized granulomatous inflammation of the mouth, obstruction of the left nose with a mass, and a 7 by 7 cm mass in the right submandibular area. The skin showed occasional small nodules on the legs; the lungs were clear to percussion and auscultation.

Results of laboratory determinations included a normal chest roentgenogram, absence of serum ANA and RF, normal serum creatinine, BUN and quantitative immunoglobulin levels, and a normal 24-hour urine determination for protein and creatinine clearance.

A skin biopsy from the left leg demonstrated a necrotizing dermal granuloma consistent with Wegener granulomatosis; there was no evidence of vasculitis. One month later the onset of hematuria and diminished creatinine clearance prompted a percutaneous renal biopsy, which revealed extracapillary proliferative and necrotizing glomerulonephritis without evidence of granulomas or vasculitis. Cultures of all biopsy specimens were negative for tuberculosis and other pathogens.

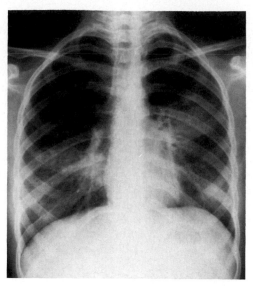

Figure 66–8. *Case 8.* The heart is small, and the left border is obscured by a lingular, segmental infiltrate. Patchy infiltrates are also present in the left upper and right middle lung zones, where cystic pneumatoceles or cavities are seen.

Prednisolone and cyclophosphamide were started when progressive respiratory distress occurred owing to upper airway insufficiency. Serial chest roentgenograms revealed progressive hilar prominences, perihilar infiltrates, and diffuse, enlarging nodules. Several weeks later pneumonia developed, antibiotics were begun, and cyclophosphamide and prednisolone were discontinued. Following resolution of the pneumonia, cyclophosphamide was restarted and given without further complications. One year later, the patient was in total remission except for residual bronchial stenosis, which required repeated dilations.

After the patient had been free of disease and receiving no medications for 2 years, a chest roentgenogram demonstrated multiple cavitations with accompanying infiltrates of the left perihilar and midlung regions; lingular and right middle lobe infiltrates were also present (Fig. 66–8).

Pulmonary function studies were performed at this time; the results are listed in Table 66–11. The VC and its subdivisions are moderately reduced, as are the FRC, RV, and TLC. However, the helium gas dilution method utilized to measure these parameters may significantly underestimate the size of these compartments in patients with obstructive airways disease. The FEV_1 is reduced to a larger

Table 66–11. *CASE 8:* PULMONARY VALUES

	Normal Range	Predicted Mean	Measured (% pred.)
VC (L)	2.6–4.4	3.5	2.3 (66)
FRC (L)	1.3–2.9	2.1	1.4 (69)
RV (L)	0.5–1.4	1.0	0.8 (83)
TLC (L)	3.4–5.5	4.6	3.1 (69)
FEV_1 (L)	2.7–4.0	3.3	1.7 (51)
FEV_1/FVC (%)	72–100	86.0	68.0
MMEF (L/min)	75–311	243.0	92.0 (38)
CV (L)		0.2	
CV/VC (%)		7.0	
N_2 (40) (%)		1.5	4.0
DL_{CO} (ml/min/mm Hg)	15.7–32.7	24.2	190.0 (78)
P_{O_2} (mm Hg)		97.0	97.0
P_{CO_2} (mm Hg)	37–43		30.0
pH	7.37–7.43		7.43

degree than the VC. Thus the FEV_1 expressed as a percentage of the forced vital capacity is reduced. There is a marked reduction in the MMEF rate and the expiratory flow rate measured at all lung volumes. The peak inspiratory flow rate is also reduced. The phase IV closing volume measurement is indeterminate owing to a marked slope in the phase III component and absence of an alveolar plateau.

Uniformity of ventilation (single-breath oxygen test) and the N_2 washout (40) are abnormal. The single-breath DL_{CO} falls within the normal range when corrected for the reduction in alveolar volume. Arterial blood reveals moderate hyperventilation and a normal arterial oxygen tension. The alveolar-arterial oxygen difference is within the normal range. After bronchodilator inhalation, there is moderate improvement in the VC and the FEV_1/FVC. Midmaximal end-expiratory flow rates and the maximal expiratory flow rates measured at all lung volumes also improve. There was no evidence at pulmonary function testing of interstitial lung disease; however, exercise testing was not performed.

This girl has mild to moderate restrictive lung disease and reversible obstructive airways disease. Although the restrictive component is consistent with Wegener granulomatosis, the reversible airway obstructive disease is atypical and might not be related to this disorder.

There is no evidence from this study of pulmonary vasculitis, which might be demonstrable only with measurement of ventilation, ventilatory dead space, and arterial blood gases during exercise.

VASCULITIS SYNDROMES

Numerous classifications of the vasculitides have been described. The disease patterns most probably represent a continuum of pathologic changes ranging from necrosis and granuloma formation to various forms of angiitis, with the clinical presentation relating to the size and location of affected vessels. Table 66–12 is an extensive but by no means inclusive list of the vasculitides (with references), several of which are described elsewhere in this test. Cupps and Fauci (1981) have published an excellent monograph describing the vasculitis syndromes in detail.

PERIARTERITIS NODOSA

Periarteritis nodosa (PAN) is a disease of inflammation and necrosis of medium and small muscular arteries, which may also be known as polyarteritis because of the relative rarity of nodular lesions. Almost any organ in the body can be affected, but the kidneys, heart, and lungs are most frequent, with liver, spleen, gastrointestinal tract, adrenals, testes, brain, and peripheral nerves somewhat less commonly involved. The cause is not known, but PAN has been reported following drug exposure and is believed to have a hypersensitivity etiology. Clinical manifestations are varied but may include fever, weight loss, arthritis, abdominal pain, renal disease, and hypertension. Cutaneous disease is also common (Cupps and Fauci, 1981).

Table 66–12. THE MAJOR VASCULITIDES, WITH REFERENCES

Vasculitis	Reference(s)
Periarteritis nodosa	Alarcon-Segovia and Brown, 1964; Winkelmann and Ditto, 1964; Frohnert and Sheps, 1967; Levin, 1970; Melam and Patterson, 1971; Arms et al, 1972; Reimold et al, 1976; Magilavy et al, 1977; Cupps and Fauci, 1981.
Henoch-Schönlein purpura	Hanson, 1985; Emery, 1988.
Wegener granulomatosis*	Roback et al, 1969; Fauci and Wolff, 1973; Wolff et al, 1974; Isreal and Patchefsky, 1975; Reza et al, 1975; Schechter et al, 1976; Landman and Burgener, 1974; Fauci et al, 1983; Jacobs, 1982.
Stevens-Johnson syndrome	Rallison et al, 1961.
Erythema nodosum	Gorin, 1988.
Takayasu arteritis	Warshaw and Spach, 1965; Bonventre, 1974.
Churg-Strauss vasculitis	Lanham et al, 1984; Wishnick et al, 1982.
Goodpasture syndrome	See Chapter 36.
Idiopathic pulmonary hemosiderosis	See Chapter 36.
Temporal arteritis (giant cell arteritis)	Healy, 1989.
Serum sickness	Cupps and Fauci, 1981.
Hypersensitivity angiitis, "systemic vasculitis"	Cupps and Fauci, 1981.
Kawasaki syndrome	Hicks and Melish, 1986.

*See discussion of this disease earlier in this chapter.

In childhood, PAN is rare but well described, occurring as a form resembling the adult disease course and as infantile polyarteritis (Dabich et al, 1974; Reimold et al, 1976; Magilavy et al, 1977). In older children, differentiation from other rheumatic disorders may be difficult, and if muscle or testicular biopsies are not helpful, the diagnosis is occasionally not made until autopsy. The prognosis is guarded, death being commonly associated with heart or renal failure or marked central nervous system or gastrointestinal disease. Reimold and associates (1976) suggest that a combination of corticosteroids and immunosuppressives may improve prognosis but stress that the rarity of childhood PAN makes any treatment regimen difficult to evaluate.

Polyarteritis in infants is an uncommon illness that usually manifests with signs suggestive of a viral illness. However, the disease persists, and cardiac involvement then predominates; pericarditis, aneurysms, coronary thromboses, and myocardial infarcts are commonly found. Pulmonary disease is rare in infantile polyarteritis. Several studies suggest that the histopathology of infantile PAN and Kawasaki syndrome are very similar and that the two illnesses are closely linked (Landing and Larson, 1977; Hicks and Melish, 1986).

Pulmonary involvement in the vasculitides, particularly in PAN, has been classified histopathologically (Alarcon-Segovia and Brown, 1964) and clinically

(Arms et al, 1972) and has been discussed in terms of therapeutic response (Levin, 1970). In adult PAN, respiratory disease was noted in 24 per cent of patients in one series (Winkelmann and Ditto, 1964) and in 38 per cent in another (Frohnert and Sheps, 1967). In both reports, chest roentgenogram findings were not consistent or diagnostic, in contrast to the report of Levin (1970), and neither group of investigators could clearly link prognosis to the presence or absence of pulmonary involvement. Few studies of pulmonary function in the vasculitides are available. Many investigators concur that the incidence of secondary pulmonary infection is low in affected patients, except in the terminal stages of illness, but superimposed pulmonary edema of cardiac or renal origin appears frequently.

Pulmonary involvement in children with PAN has been documented in isolated case reports but is probably quite rare (Levin, 1970; Melam and Patterson, 1971; Reimold et al, 1976). Use of both prednisone and azathioprine has been reported to lead to improvement of respiratory symptoms in some cases.

Investigators concur that immune-complex or cell-mediated hypersensitivity to usually unrecognized antigens plays a dominant role in the vasculitides. Animal models to study hypersensitivity pneumonitis are being developed and so far suggest abnormalities in cellular immunoregulatory mechanisms (Schuyler et al, 1987). Only rarely, such as in serum sickness and Stevens-Johnson syndrome, can a specific etiologic agent be identified. However, a number of postinfectious "reactive arthropathies" have been associated with vasculitic manifestations. They follow anicteric hepatitis and *Mycoplasma*, *Streptococcus*, *Shigella*, *Salmonella*, meningococcal, and *Yersinia* infections, among others. In our experience, affected patients can be quite ill but usually recover rapidly (perhaps requiring steroids) without sequelae. We have studied lung function in several children with Stevens-Johnson syndrome and detected severe impairment of gas exchange during the acute phase of illness, with the subsequent development of pulmonary interstitial fibrosis and chronic obstructive lung disease.

Other than polyarteritis, Wegener granulomatosis, Löffler and Goodpasture syndromes, and idiopathic pulmonary hemosiderosis, the primary vasculitides are only rarely associated with pulmonary disease. The character of the histopathologic changes in the primary vasculitides suggests that pulmonary disease might occur, but in our clinical experience with children, it has been rare.

SUMMARY

A majority of the rheumatic diseases can and do involve the pulmonary system at some time during their course. The most common initial events appear to be pleural inflammation, vasculitis, or granulomatous parenchymal involvement, frequently resulting in slowly progressive interstitial fibrosis. However, pulmonary function studies in adults with various rheumatic diseases frequently suggest that initial pulmonary impairment may occur silently, without obvious antecedent respiratory tract events. The same is probably true for the childhood rheumatic diseases.

Most childhood rheumatic diseases are associated with, or are suspected to cause, defects in humoral or cell-mediated immunity, or both. In addition, many children with rheumatic diseases are receiving corticosteroids or immunosuppressive agents. For these reasons, it is imperative that infection be the first consideration when any sudden change in respiratory status occurs. Complete cultures should always be taken and appropriate antimicrobial therapy should be begun, unless exceptionally clear-cut evidence points to a noninfectious cause. The addition of, or change in the doses of, corticosteroids or immunosuppressives usually should occur only after appropriate culture findings are known to be negative.

It is not clear what role chronic pulmonary impairment plays in the apparently increased incidence of lung infections in the childhood rheumatic diseases. Detailed serial pulmonary function studies and correlation with immune and pulmonary infectious status, and medications in use in the childhood rheumatic diseases are important areas for further study.

RHEUMATIC PNEUMONIA

Acute rheumatic fever (ARF) in children, the center of much attention and study some decades ago, has been steadily declining in frequency (Taranta, 1989). However, it has not been entirely conquered. Several new outbreaks of ARF in the United States have been observed, perhaps related to changes in streptococcal serotype.

Unfortunately, there is no pathognomonic sign or test for rheumatic pneumonia, and thus its diagnosis and treatment are subjects of controversy. According to Scott and co-workers (1959), the lung is involved to varying degrees in ARF. Reporting on 87 children who died between 1919 and 1954 during an active attack of ARF, these investigators found 54 cases of rheumatic pneumonia, an overall incidence of 62 per cent. More than one third of these (39 per cent) had only slight pulmonary involvement; half (54 per cent) showed moderate pulmonary disease. However, Griffith and co-workers in 1946 noted an 11.3 per cent incidence of rheumatic pneumonia based on an autopsy analysis of 119 fatal cases of ARF from 1046 patients at the U.S. Naval Hospital. The experience of Neuberger and colleagues (1944) with post-mortem material was similar; they found an incidence of 12.7 per cent among 63 patients, some with quiescent and others with active rheumatic fever.

Rheumatic pneumonia is rare today. Yet in July 1981, a 13-year-old girl was admitted to Bellevue Hospital in New York City with acute carditis, hep-

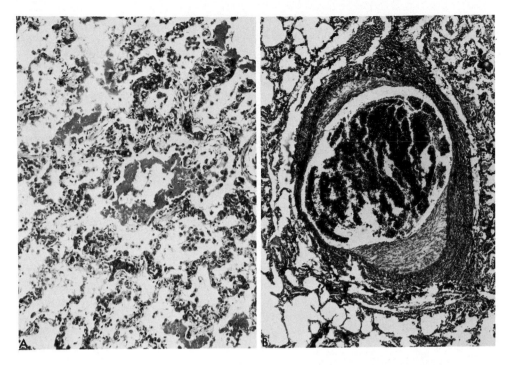

Figure 66–9. A 4-year-old girl was admitted to the hospital with acute arthritis and active carditis. She was treated with digitalis and salicylates and improved. Three months later, fever, substernal pain, and pericarditis developed. Crackles were also heard in the chest. She was in acute respiratory distress and died 4 months after admission. The lungs showed some pathologic features described in rheumatic pneumonia. *A*, Hyaline membranes and congestion (× 150). *B*, Arterial thrombus, organized (× 30).

atomegaly without edema, left-ankle swelling, and rheumatic pneumonia. She recovered within 10 days from this, her second attack of ARF. The first attack, 4 years previously, was appropriately treated by prophylactic penicillin.

It is difficult to differentiate rheumatic pneumonia from congestive heart failure; it is often impossible without pathologic evidence. Indeed, pulmonary edema and rheumatic pneumonia may coexist, as has been described by Mahajan and colleagues (1973) in an Indian patient with "uncommon manifestations of rheumatic fever." The autopsy report of this child demonstrated rheumatic pneumonia, with associated bilateral pulmonary edema.

PATHOLOGY

The first histologic description of rheumatic pneumonia was made by Naish in 1928. Grossly, the lungs are larger than normal, with dark red areas due to unilateral or bilateral scattered hemorrhages; are elastic and resilient on palpation; and have a consistency comparable to India rubber (Hadfield, 1938). On microscopic examination, the following are found: hemorrhage, necrosis of alveolar walls, arteriolitis and vasculitis with occasional thrombosis, hyaline membrane lining of alveoli and alveolar ducts, and alveolar proliferation of mononuclear fibroblast cells. The pleura may show a fibrinous exudate, usually without effusion. Unfortunately, none of these lesions is pathognomonic.

Many pathologists have attempted to describe rheumatic pneumonitis. Scott and co-workers (1959) thought that the most satisfactory criterion for diagnosis was a focal mononuclear, fibrinous, intra-alveolar or intraductal exudate containing protein-rich fluid. Lustock and Kuzma (1956) observed unusual bronchiolar changes, in which the epithelial cells were desquamated and often stripped completely from the bronchi, and eosinophilic granular necrosis of the lamina.

One explanation for the lung changes in ARF was advanced by Rich and Gregory (1943), who attributed them to a hypersensitivity phenomenon leading to arteriolar damage. They were able to reproduce pathologic lesions of the heart in animals identical with those seen in the lungs of patients with rheumatic pneumonitis. Van Wijk (1984) and Jensen (1946) suggested that the pneumonia seen in ARF has an allergic basis, wherein there is capillary endothelial injury, and a hyaline membrane then develops following capillary injury, with the seepage of fibrinogen into the alveoli, where it is converted to fibrin (Fig. 66–9).

In 1972, Grunow and Esterly described the pathology in 24 patients dying of acute rheumatic fever between 1949 and 1970. Pulmonary arteriolitis, seen in four cases, was complicated in three of these by acute pneumonia. One third of the 24 patients, 3 to 25 years of age, showed thromboemboli in arteries and arterioles. In only two was there evidence of nonrheumatic lung disease. Influenza virus was cultured from one, and another specimen suggested possible cytomegalic inclusion disease.

CLINICAL FEATURES

The predominant pulmonary symptoms in ARF are dyspnea, tachypnea, tachycardia (usually out of proportion to fever and the general appearance of illness), persistent cough, and blood-streaked sputum. Pleuritic chest pain, restlessness, and cyanosis

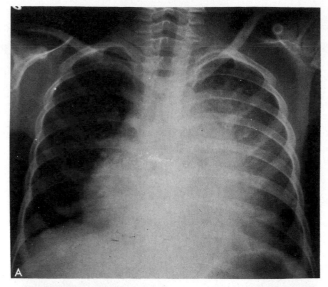

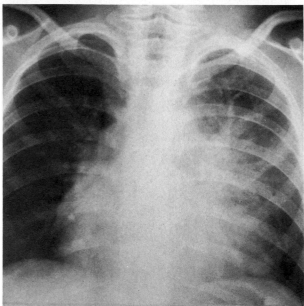

Figure 66–10. *A,* A chest roentgenogram, taken 24 hours after the onset of symptoms, shows a fuzzy-edged, homogeneous, nonsegmental infiltrate in the middle third of the lung. The cardiac silhouette is enlarged. *B,* The right diaphragm and costophrenic angle are clear 20 days later. The infiltrate in the left midlung shows some clearing at the periphery. The cardiac silhouette is smaller, but the left border remains obscured by a mottled infiltrate with increased bronchovascular markings.

may develop. The presence, degree, and duration of fever are variable. The onset of pneumonia may be insidious, simulating an upper respiratory tract infection, or may occur as an acute attack of dyspnea. Rheumatic pneumonia may rarely precede other signs of rheumatic infection, as suggested by Rubin and Rubin (1961).

Seldin and colleagues (1947) found that pneumonia may occur at any time from 4 days to 12 months after the onset of ARF. Griffith and co-workers suggest the following classification: (1) primary acute pneumonitis, as a initial manifestation of rheumatic

fever; (2) secondary acute pneumonitis, occurring during the polycyclic course of rheumatic fever; and (3) subclinical pneumonitis, in which the pulmonary involvement may be overlooked entirely. There are few symptoms or signs. Thus, for example, a history of pneumonia of unknown etiology was significantly more common in 279 Denver schoolchildren who had had rheumatic fever than in 556 control subjects who did not (Wedum, 1981).

Roentgenograms of the chest in rheumatic fever may show the rapid appearance and disappearance of hazy-edged densities, which may be peripheral, central, in the left midlung, the right upper lobe, or they may be bilateral. Pleurisy is commonly transitory. Radiographs may reveal increased bronchovascular markings, homogenous segmental densities, or even small, soft, mottled infiltrates. Lobar involvement is rare and usually transitory. The lung apices and bases are usually clear.

The list of diseases simulating rheumatic pneumonitis is long; among them are viral illnesses, congestive heart failure, bacterial pneumonia, and Löffler pneumonia (reacting to antigens other than *Streptococcus*). The greatest difficulty in diagnosis lies in distinguishing between viral pneumonitis and pulmonary edema, especially with associated carditis. Figure 66–10 is an example of rheumatic pneumonitis as the initial manifestation of ARF.

Rheumatic pneumonitis may have a guarded prognosis, particularly if it presents as widespread pulmonary disease during the initial attack. Chronic interstitial fibrosis may develop late in the course of rheumatic fever.

REFERENCES

Rheumatic Diseases

Alarcon-Segovia D and Brown AL: Classification and etiologic aspects of necrotizing angiitides: an analytic approach to a confused subject with a critical review of the evidence for hypersensitivity in polyarteritis nodosa. Mayo Clin Proc 39:205, 1964.

Anderson HA, Fontana RS, Sanderson DR, and Harrison EG: Transbronchoscopic lung biopsy in diffuse pulmonary disease: results in 300 cases. Med Clin North Am 54:951, 1970.

Ansell BM: Rheumatic disorders in childhood. In Clinics in Rheumatic Diseases. Philadelphia, WB Saunders Co, 1976.

Ansell BM: Rheumatic Diseases in Childhood. Boston, Butterworth's, 1980.

Appelrouth D and Gottlieb NL: Pulmonary manifestations of ankylosing spondylitis. J Rheumatol 2:446, 1975.

Arms RA, Dines DE, and DeRemee RA: Pulmonary vasculitides: importance of the clinical and pathologic differentiation. Minn Med 55:871, 1972.

Athreya BH, Doughty RA, Bookspan M et al: Pulmonary manifestations of juvenile rheumatoid arthritis: a report of eight cases and review. Clin Chest Med 1:361, 1980.

Athreya BH, Norman ME, Myers AR, and South MA: Sjögren's syndrome in children. Pediatrics 59:931, 1977.

Bagenstoss AH: Visceral lesions in disseminated lupus erythematosus. Proc Mayo Clin 27:412, 1952.

Baliga R, Chang C, Bidani AK et al: A case of generalized Wegener's granulomatosis in childhood: successful therapy with cyclophosphamide. Pediatrics 61:286, 1978.

Bandt PD, Blank N, and Castellino RA: Needle diagnosis of pneumonitis. JAMA 220:1578, 1972.

er BO and Victor M: Dermatomyositis (systemic angiopathy) of childhood. Medicine 45:261, 1966.

ST IN THE RHEUMATIC DISORDERS OF CHILDHOOD 913

Banker BO and Victor M: Dermatomyositis (systemic angiopathy) of childhood. Medicine 45:261, 1966.

Batist G and Andrews JL: Pulmonary toxicity of antineoplastic drugs. JAMA 246:1449, 1981.

Bernstein BH, Singsen BH, Lorber A et al: Juvenile ankylosing spondylitis: are adult criteria appropriate? Arthritis Rheum 22:593, 1979.

Bitnum S, Daeschner EW, Travis LB et al: Dermatomyositis. J Pediatr 64:101, 1964.

Bonventre MV: Takayasu's disease, revisited. NY State J Med 74:1960, 1974.

Brentjens JR, O'Connell DW, Pawlowski IB et al: Experimental immune complex disease of the lung: the pathogenesis of a laboratory model resembling certain human interstitial lung diseases. J Exp Med 140:105, 1974.

Brewer EJ: Pitfalls in the diagnosis of juvenile rheumatoid arthritis. Pediatr Clin North Am 33:1015, 1986.

Buscaglia AJ, Cowden FE, and Brill H: Pulmonary infiltrates associated with naproxen. JAMA 251:65, 1984.

Cadman EC, Lundberg WB, and Mitchell MS: Pulmonary manifestations in Behçet's syndrome. Arch Intern Med 136:934, 1976.

Camp AV, Lane DJ, and Mowat AG: Dermatomyositis with parenchymal lung involvement. Br Med J 1:155, 1972.

Cassidy JT: Juvenile rheumatoid arthritis. In Kelley WN, Harris ED, Ruddy S, and Sledge CB (eds): Textbook of Rheumatology. 2nd ed. Philadelphia, WB Saunders Co, 1985.

Cassidy JT (ed): Textbook of Pediatric Rheumatology. New York, John Wiley & Sons, Inc, 1982.

Chajek T and Fainara M: Behçet's disease. Report of 41 cases and review of the literature. Medicine 54:179, 1975.

Chandrasekhar AJ, Robinson J, and Barr L: Antibody deposition in the pleura: a finding in drug-induced lupus. J Allergy Clin Immunol 61:399, 1978.

Chick TW, DeHoratins RJ, Skipper BE, and Messner RP: Pulmonary dysfunction in systemic lupus erythematosus without pulmonary symptoms. J Rheumatol 3:262, 1976.

Clausen KP and Bronstein H: Granulomatous pulmonary arteritis: a hypereosinophilic syndrome. Am J Clin Pathol 62:82, 1974.

Cochrane CG and Dixon FJ: Antigen-antibody complex induced disease. In Miescher PA and Muller-Eberhard HJ (eds): Textbook of Immunopathology. 2nd ed, vol 1. New York, Grune & Stratton, Inc, 1976.

Collins RL, Turner RA, Johnson AM et al: Obstructive pulmonary disease in rheumatoid arthritis. Arthritis Rheum 19:623, 1976.

Cupps TR and Fauci AS: The Vasculitides. Philadelphia, WB Saunders Co, 1981.

Dabich L, Sullivan DB, and Cassidy JT: Scleroderma in the child. J Pediatr 85:770, 1974.

D'Angelo WA, Fries JF, Masi AT, and Shulman LE: Pathologic observations in systemic sclerosis (scleroderma): a study of fifty-eight autopsy cases and fifty-eight matched controls. Am J Med 46:428, 1969.

Derderian SS, Tellis CJ, Abbrecht PH et al: Pulmonary involvement in mixed connective tissue disease. Chest 88:45, 1985.

Dubois EL and Tuffanelli DL: Clinical manifestations of systemic lupus erythematosus. JAMA 190:104, 1964.

Dubowitz LM and Dubowitz V: Acute dermatomyositis presenting with pulmonary manifestations. Arch Dis Child 39:293, 1964.

Emery H: Clinical aspects of systemic lupus erythematosus in childhood. Pediatr Clin North Am 33:1177, 1986.

Emery H: Henoch-Schönlein purpura. In Hicks RV (ed): Vasculopathies of childhood. Littleton, Mass, PSG Publishing Co, Inc, 1988.

Epler GR, Snider GL, Gaensler EA et al: Bronchiolitis and bronchitis in connective tissue disease. JAMA 242:528, 1979.

Fauci AS, and Wolff SM: Wegener's granulomatosis: studies in eighteen patients and a review of the literature. Medicine 52:535, 1973.

Fauci AS, Haynes BF, Katz P, and Wolff SM: Wegener's granulomatosis: prospective clinical and therapeutic experience with 85 patients for 21 years. Ann Intern Med 98:76, 1983.

Fayemi AO: The lung in systemic lupus erythematosus: a clinicopathologic study of 20 cases. Mt Sinai J Med 42:110, 1975.

Fish AJ, Blau EB, Westberg NG et al: Systemic lupus erythematosus within the first two decades of life. Am J Med 62:99, 1977.

Forrester RM, Lees VT, and Watson GH: Idiopathic pulmonary haemosiderosis and rheumatoid arthritis. Br Med J 1:1403, 1966.

Fraga A, Gudino J, Ramos-Niembro F, and Alarcon-Segovia D: Mixed connective tissue disease in childhood: relationship with Sjögren's syndrome. Am J Dis Child 132:263, 1978.

Frank ST, Weg JG, Harkleroad DE, and Firch RF: Pulmonary dysfunction in rheumatoid disease. Chest 63:27, 1973.

Frazier AR and Miller RD: Interstitial pneumonitis in association with polymyositis and dermatomyositis. Chest 65:403, 1974.

Frohnert PP and Sheps SG: Long-term follow-up study of periarteritis nodosa. Am J Med 43:8, 1967.

Fry WA and Manalo-Estrella P: Bronchial brushing. Surg Gynecol Obstet 130:67, 1970.

Furst DE, David JA, Clements PJ et al: Abnormalities of pulmonary vascular dynamics and inflammation in early progressive systemic sclerosis. Arthritis Rheum 24:1403, 1981.

Gaensler EA, Moister VB, and Hamm J: Open lung biopsy in diffuse pulmonary disease. N Engl J Med 270:1319, 1964.

Geddes DM, Webley M, and Emerson PA: Airways obstruction in rheumatoid arthritis. Ann Rheum Dis 38:222, 1979.

Gewanter HL and Baum J: The use of tolmetin sodium in systemic onset juvenile rheumatoid arthritis. Arthritis Rheum 24:1316, 1981.

Gibson GJ, Edmonds JP, and Hughes GRV: Diaphragm function and lung involvement in systemic lupus erythematosus. Am J Med 63:926, 1977.

Gold WM and Jennings DB: Pulmonary function in patients with systemic lupus erythematosus. Am Rev Respir Dis 93:556, 1966.

Gorin L: Erythema nodosum. In Hicks RV (ed): Vasculopathies of Childhood. Littleton, Mass, PSG Publishing Co, Inc, 1988.

Gould DB and Soriano RZ: Acute alveolar hemorrhage in lupus erythematosus. Ann Intern Med 83:836, 1975.

Green MR: Pulmonary toxicity of antineoplastic agents. West J Med 127:292, 1977.

Greenwald GI, Tashkin DP, Gong H et al: Longitudinal changes in lung function and respiratory symptoms in progressive systemic sclerosis. Am J Med 83:83, 1987.

Gregory JE and Rich AR: The experimental production of anaphylactic pulmonary lesions with the basic characteristics of rheumatic pneumonitis. Bull Johns Hopkins Hosp 78:1, 1946.

Grennan DM, Howie AD, Moran F, and Buchanan WW: Pulmonary involvement in systemic lupus erythematosus. Ann Rheum Dis 37:536, 1978.

Gross M, Esterly JR, and Earle RH: Pulmonary alterations in systemic lupus erythematosus. Am Rev Respir Dis 105:572, 1971.

Guttadauria M, Ellman H, and Kaplan D: Progressive systemic sclerosis: pulmonary involvement. Clin Rheum Dis 5:151, 1979.

Gwinn JL and Lee FA: Radiological case of the month: dermatomyositis with interstitial lung disease and soft tissue calcification. Am J Dis Child 129:703, 1975.

Hakala M: Poor prognosis in patients with rheumatoid arthritis hospitalized for interstitial lung fibrosis. Chest 93:115, 1988.

Hanson V: Dermatomyositis, scleroderma and polyarteritis nodosa. In Ansell BM (ed): Clinics in Rheumatic Disease. Philadelphia, WB Saunders Co, 1976.

Hanson V: Systemic lupus erythematosus, dermatomyositis, scleroderma and vasculitides in childhood. In Kelley WN, Harris ED, Ruddy S, and Sledge CB (eds): Textbook of Rheumatology. 2nd ed. Philadelphia, WB Saunders Co, 1985.

Harmon C, Wolfe F, Lillard S et al: Pulmonary involvement in mixed connective tissue disease (MCTD). Arthritis Rheum 19:801, 1976.

Haupt HM, Moore GW, and Hutchins GM: The lung in systemic lupus erythematosus. Analysis of the pathologic changes in 120 patients. Am J Med 71:791, 1981.

Healy LA: Polymyalgia rheumatica and giant cell arteritis. In McCarty DJ (ed): Arthritis and Allied Conditions. 11th ed. Philadelphia, Lea & Febiger, 1989.

Hicks RV and Melish ME: Kawasaki syndrome. Pediatr Clin North Am 33:1151, 1986.

Holgate ST, Glass DN, Haslam P et al: Respiratory involvement in systemic lupus erythematosus: a clinical and immunological study. Clin Exp Immunol 24:385, 1976.

Huang CT, Hennigar GR, and Lyons HA: Pulmonary dysfunction in systemic lupus erythematosus. N Engl J Med 272:288, 1965.

Hunninghake GW and Fauci AS: Pulmonary involvement in the collagen vascular diseases. Am Rev Respir Dis 119:471, 1979.

Hunninghake GW, Gallin JI, and Fauci AS: Immunologic reactivity of the lung: the in vivo and in vitro generation of a neutrophil chemotactic factor by alveolar macrophages. Am Rev Respir Dis 117:15, 1978.

Hunt R, Turner R, Collins R, and McLean R: Cardiopulmonary manifestations of systemic lupus erythematosus. Arthritis Rheum 18:524, 1975.

Hyun BH, Diggs CL, and Toone EC: Dermatomyositis with cystic fibrosis (honeycombing) of the lung. Dis Chest 42:451, 1962.

Inoue T, Kanayama Y, Ohe A et al: Immunopathologic studies of pneumonitis in systemic lupus erythematosus. Ann Intern Med 91:30, 1979.

Isreal HL and Patchefsky AS: Treatment of Wegener's granulomatosis of lung. Am J Med 58:671, 1975.

Isreal HL, Patchefsky AS, and Saldana MJ: Wegener's granulomatosis, lymphomatoid granulomatosis, and benign lymphocytic angiitis and granulomatosis of lung. Ann Intern Med 87:691, 1977.

Jacobs JC: Pediatric Rheumatology for the Practitioner. New York, Springer-Verlag, 1982.

Jayson M IV (ed): Still's Disease: Juvenile Chronic Polyarthritis. New York, Academic Press, 1976.

Jones MB, Osterholm RK, Wilson RB et al: Fatal pulmonary hypertension and resolving immune-complex glomerulonephritis in mixed connective tissue disease. Am J Med 65:855, 1978.

Jordan JD and Snyder CH: Rheumatoid disease of the lung and cor pulmonale. Am J Dis Child 108:174, 1964.

Karlish AJ: Lung changes in Sjögren's syndrome. Proc Roy Soc Med 62:1042, 1969.

Kelly V (ed): Brennemann's Practice of Pediatrics. Vol III. New York, Harper & Row Publishers, Inc, 1980.

Kornreich HK, King KK, Bernstein BH et al: Scleroderma in childhood. Arthritis Rheum 20:343, 1977.

Laitinen O, Nissila M, Salorrine Y, and Aalto P: Pulmonary involvement in patients with rheumatoid arthritis. Scand J Respir Dis 56:297, 1975.

Landing BH and Larson EJ: Are infantile periarteritis nodosa with coronary artery involvement and fatal mucocutaneous lymph node syndrome the same? Comparison of 20 patients from North America with patients from Hawaii and Japan. Pediatrics 59:651, 1977.

Landman S and Burgener F: Pulmonary manifestations in Wegener's granulomatosis. Am J Roentgenol 122:750, 1974.

Lanham JG, Elkon KB, Pusey CD, and Hughes GR: Systemic vasculitis with asthma and eosinophilia: a clinical approach to the Churg-Strauss syndrome. Medicine 63:65, 1984.

Le Roy EC: Scleroderma (systemic sclerosis). In Kelley WN, Harris ED, Ruddy S, and Sledge CB (eds): Textbook of Rheumatology. 2nd ed. Philadelphia, WB Saunders Co, 1985.

Levin DC: Pulmonary abnormalities in the necrotizing vasculitides and their rapid response to steroids. Radiology 97:521, 1970.

Levin DC: Proper interpretation of pulmonary roentgen changes in systemic lupus erythematosus. Am J Roentgenol 111:510, 1971.

Lovell D, Lindsley C, and Langston C: Lymphoid interstitial pneumonia in juvenile rheumatoid arthritis. J Pediatr 105:947, 1984.

McCarthy DS, Baragar FD, Dingra S et al: The lungs in systemic sclerosis (scleroderma): a review and new information. Sem Arthritis Rheum 17:276, 1988.

McCombs RP: Systemic "allergic" vasculitis: clinical and pathological relationships. JAMA 194:1059, 1965.

MacFarlane JD, Dieppe PA, Rigden BG, and Clark TJH: Pulmonary and pleural lesions in rheumatoid disease. Br J Dis Chest 72:288, 1978.

Magilavy DB, Petty RE, Cassidy JT, and Sullivan DB: A syndrome of childhood polyarteritis. J Pediatr 91:25, 1977.

Martel W, Abell MR, Mikkelson WM, and Whitehouse WM: Pulmonary and pleural lesions in rheumatoid disease. Radiology 90:641, 1968.

Medsger TA: Systemic sclerosis (scleroderma), localized scleroderma, eosinophilic fasciitis, and calcinosis. In McCarty DJ (ed): Arthritis and Allied Conditions. 11th ed. Philadelphia, Lea & Febiger, 1989.

Meislin AG and Rothfield NF: Systemic lupus erythematosus in childhood. Pediatrics 42:37, 1968.

Melam H and Patterson R: Periarteritis nodosa: a remission achieved with combined prednisone and azathioprine therapy. Am J Dis Child 121:424, 1971.

Miller JJ III (ed): Juvenile Rheumatoid Arthritis. Littleton, Mass, PSG Publishing Co, Inc, 1979.

Miller ML (ed): Pediatric rheumatology. Pediatr Clin North Am 33(5), 1986.

Miller RW, Magilavy DB, Bock GH et al: Pulmonary function abnormalities in pediatric patients with systemic lupus erythematosus. Immunol and Allergy Prac 10:143, 1988.

Mohsenifar Z, Tashkin DP, Levy SE et al: Lack of sensitivity of measurements on V_D/V_T at rest and during exercise in detection of hemodynamically significant pulmonary vascular abnormalities in collagen vascular disease. Am Rev Respir Dis 123:508, 1981.

Moorthy AV, Chesney RW, Segar WE, and Groshong T: Wegener granulomatosis in childhood: prolonged survival following cytotoxic therapy. J Pediatr 91:616, 1977.

Moutsopoulos HM, Chused TM, Mann DL, et al: Sjögren's syndrome (sicca syndrome): Current issues. Ann Intern Med 92:212, 1980.

Mulkey D and Hudson L: Massive spontaneous unilateral hemothorax in systemic lupus erythematosus. Am J Med 56:570, 1974.

Notman DD, Kurata N, and Tan EM: Profiles of antinuclear antibodies in systemic rheumatic diseases. Ann Intern Med 83:464, 1975.

O'Duffy D: Behçet's disease. In Kelley WN, Harris ED, Ruddy S, and Sledge CB (eds): Textbook of Rheumatology. 2nd ed. Philadelphia, WB Saunders Co, 1985.

Owens GR, Paradis IL, Gryzan S et al: Role of inflammation in the lung of systemic sclerosis: comparison with idiopathic pulmonary fibrosis. J Lab Clin Med 107:253, 1986.

Oxholm P, Madsen EB, Manthorpe R, and Rasmussen FV: Pulmonary function in patients with rheumatoid arthritis. Scand J Rheumatol 11:109, 1982.

Papathanasiou MP, Constantopoulos SH, Tsampoulas et al: Reappraisal of respiratory abnormalities in primary and secondary Sjögren's syndrome: a controlled study. Chest 90:371, 1986.

Park S and Nyhan WL: Fatal pulmonary involvement in dermatomyositis. Am J Dis Child 129:723, 1975.

Partanen J, van Assendelft AHW, Koskimies S et al: Patients with rheumatoid arthritis and gold-induced pneumonitis express two high-risk major histocompatibility complex patterns. Chest 92:277, 1987.

Paty JG, Sienknecht CW, Townes AS et al: Impaired cell-mediated immunity in systemic lupus erythematosus (SLE): a controlled study of 23 untreated patients. Am J Med 59:769, 1975.

Penny WJ, Knight RK, Rees AM et al: Obliterative bronchiolitis in rheumatoid arthritis. Ann Rheum Dis 41:469, 1982.

Peters-Golden M, Wise RA, Schneider P et al: Clinical and demographic predictors of loss of pulmonary function in systemic sclerosis. Medicine 63:221, 1984.

Popper MS, Bogdonoff ML, and Hughes RL: Interstitial rheumatoid lung disease: a reassessment and review of the literature. Chest 62:243, 1972.

Purnell DC, Bagenstoss AH, and Olsen AM: Pulmonary lesions in disseminated lupus erythematosus. Ann Intern Med 42:619, 1955.

Rallison ML, Carlisle RE, Lee RE et al: Lupus erythematosus and Stevens-Johnson syndrome. Am J Dis Child 101:725, 1961.

Reimold EW, Weinberg AG, Fink CW, and Battles ND: Polyarteritis in children. Am J Dis Child 130:534, 1976.

Reza MJ, Dornfeld L, Goldberg LS et al: Wegener's granulomatosis: long-term follow-up of patients treated with cyclophosphamide. Arthritis Rheum 18:501, 1975.

Roback SA, Herdman RC, Hoyer J, and Good RA: Wegener's granulomatosis in a child: observations on pathogenesis and treatment. Am J Dis Child 118:608, 1969.

Romicka A and Maldyk E: Pulmonary lesions in the course of

rheumatoid arthritis in children. Bull Polish Med Sci XV/III:263, 1975.

Rosenberg AM, Petty RE, Cumming GR, and Koehler BE: Pulmonary hypertension in a child with mixed connective tissue disease. J Rheumatol 6:700, 1979.

Rosenow EC, Strimlan CV, Muhm JR, and Ferguson RH: Pleuropulmonary manifestations of ankylosing spondylitis. Mayo Clin Proc 52:641, 1977.

Salerni R, Rodnan GP, Leon DF, and Shaver JA: Pulmonary hypertension in the CREST syndrome variant of progressive systemic sclerosis (scleroderma). Ann Intern Med 86:394, 1977.

Salmeron G, Greenberg SD, and Lidsky MD: Polymyositis and diffuse interstitial lung disease: a review of the pulmonary histopathologic findings. Arch Intern Med 141:1005, 1981.

Sanders DY, Huntley CC, and Sharp GC: Mixed connective tissue disease in a child. J Pediatr 83:642, 1973.

Schaller JG: Ankylosing spondylitis of childhood onset. Arthritis Rheum 20:398, 1977.

Schaller JG and Hanson V (eds): Proceedings of the first ARA conference on the rheumatic diseases of childhood. Arthritis Rheum 20:145, 1977.

Schaller JG, Ochs HD, Thomas ED et al: Histocompatibility antigens in childhood-onset arthritis. J Pediatr 88:929, 1976.

Schechter SI, Bole GG, and Walker SE: Midline granuloma and Wegener's granulomatosis: clinical and therapeutic considerations. J Rheumatol 3:241, 1976.

Schuyler M, Subramanyan S, and Hassan MO: Experimental hypersensitivity pneumonitis: transfer with cultured cells. J Lab Clin Med 109:623, 1987.

Schwartz MI, Matthay RA, Sahn SA et al: Interstitial lung disease in polymyositis and dermatomyositis: analysis of six cases and review of the literature. Medicine 55:89, 1976.

Scott DL, Bradby GVH, Aitman TJ et al: Relationship of gold and penicillamine therapy to diffuse interstitial lung disease. Ann Rheum Dis 40:136, 1981.

Scott TE, Wise RA, Hochberg MA, and Wigley FM: HLA-DR-4 and pulmonary dysfunction in rheumatoid arthritis. Am J Med 82:765, 1987.

Segal AM, Calabrese LH, Ahmad M et al: The pulmonary manifestations of systemic lupus erythematosus. Semin Arthritis Rheum 14:202, 1985.

Selroos O and Edgren J: Lupus-like syndrome associated with pulmonary reaction to nitrofurantion. Acta Med Scand 197:125, 1975.

Sharp GC and Singsen BH: Mixed connective tissue disease. In McCarty DJ (ed): Arthritis and Allied Conditions. 11th ed. Philadelphia, Lea & Febiger, 1989.

Sharp GC, Irvin WS, Tan EM et al: Mixed connective tissue disease—an apparently distinct rheumatic disease syndrome associated with a specific antibody to an extractable nuclear antigen (ENA). Am J Med 52:148, 1972.

Shuck JW, Oetgen WJ, and Tesar JT: Pulmonary vascular response during Raynaud's phenomenon in progressive systemic sclerosis. Am J Med 78:221, 1985.

Sieving RR, Kaufman CA, and Watanakunakorn C: Deep fungal infection in systemic lupus erythematosus—three cases reported, literature reviewed. J Rheumatol 2:61, 1975.

Silver TM, Farber SJ, Bole GG, and Martel W: Radiological features of mixed connective tissue disease and scleroderma–systemic lupus erythematosus overlap. Radiology 120:269, 1976.

Singsen BH: Scleroderma in childhood. Pediatr Clin North Am 33:1119, 1986.

Singsen BH, Bernstein BH, Kornreich HK et al: Mixed connective tissue disease (MCTD) in childhood: a clinical and serological survey. J Pediatr 90:893, 1977.

Singsen BH, Fishman L, and Hanson V: Antinuclear antibodies and lupus-like syndromes in children receiving anticonvulsants. Pediatrics 57:529, 1976a.

Singsen BH, Goldreyer B, Stanton R, and Hanson V: Childhood polymyositis with cardiac conduction defects. Am J Dis Child 130:72, 1976b.

Singsen BH, Swanson VL, Bernstein BH et al: A histological evaluation of mixed connective tissue disease in childhood. Am J Med 68:710, 1980.

Singsen BH, Tedford JS, Platzker ACG, and Hanson V: Sponta-

neous pneumothorax: a complication of juvenile dermatomyositis. J Pediatr 92:771, 1978.

Smith BS: Idiopathic pulmonary haemosiderosis and rheumatoid arthritis. Brit Med J 1:1403, 1966.

Songcharoen S, Raju SF, and Pennebaker JB: Interstitial lung disease in polymyositis and dermatomyositis. J Rheumatol 7:353, 1980.

Spain DM: The association of terminal bronchiolar carcinoma with chronic interstitial inflammation and fibrosis of the lungs. Am Rev Tuberc 76:59, 1957.

Staples PJ, Gerding DN, Decker JO, and Gordon RS: Incidence of infection in systemic lupus erythematosus. Arthritis Rheum 17:1, 1974.

Steen VD, Owens GR, Fino GJ et al: Pulmonary involvement in systemic sclerosis (scleroderma). Arthritis Rheum 28:759, 1985.

Steen VD, Owens GR, Redmond C et al: The effect of D-penicillamine on pulmonary findings in systemic sclerosis. Arthritis Rheum 28:882, 1985.

Steinberg CL: Rheumatoid lung disease: granulomas, fibrosis, pulmonary effusion. NY State J Med 75:854, 1975.

Strimlan CV, Rosenow EC, Divertie MB, and Harrison EG: Pulmonary manifestations of Sjögren's syndrome. Chest 70:354, 1976.

Sullivan DB, Cassidy JT, Petty RE, and Burt A: Prognosis in childhood dermatomyositis. J Pediatr 80:555, 1972.

Sullivan WD, Hurst DJ, Harmon CE et al: A prospective evaluation emphasizing pulmonary involvement in patients with mixed connective tissue disease. Medicine 63:92, 1984.

Tan EM, Cohen AS, Fries JM et al: The 1982 revised criteria for the classification of systemic lupus erythematosus. Arthritis Rheum 25:1271, 1982.

Trell E and Lindstrom C: Pulmonary hypertension in systemic sclerosis. Ann Rheum Dis 30:390, 1971.

Tuffanelli DL and Winkelmann RK: Systemic scleroderma: a clinical study of 727 cases. Arch Dermatol 84:359, 1961.

Turner-Warwick M and Evans RC: Pulmonary manifestations of rheumatoid disease. Clin Rheum Dis 3:549, 1977.

Venizelos PC and Al-Bazzaz F: Pulmonary function abnormalities in systemic lupus erythematosus responsive to glucocorticoid therapy. Chest 79:702, 1981.

Wagener JS, Taussig LM, DeBenedetti C et al: Pulmonary function in juvenile rheumatoid arthritis. J Pediatr 99:108, 1981.

Warshaw JB and Spach MS: Takayasu's disease (primary aortitis) in childhood: case report with review of literature. Pediatrics 35:620, 1965.

Weaver AL, Brundage BH, Nelson RA, and Bischoff MB: Pulmonary involvement in polymyositis: report of a case with response to corticosteroid therapy. Arthritis Rheum 11:765, 1968b.

Weaver AL, Divertie MB, and Titus JI: Pulmonary scleroderma. Dis Chest 54:490, 1968a.

Wedgwood RJ, and Schaller J: Diseases of connective tissue. In Nelson WE, Vaughan VC, and McKay RJ (eds): Textbook of Pediatrics. Philadelphia, WB Saunders Co, 1969.

Weiland JE, Garcia JGN, Davis WB, and Gadek JE: Neutrophil collagenase in rheumatoid interstitial lung disease. J Appl Physiol 62:628, 1987.

Wiener-Kronish JP, Solinger AM, Warnock ML et al: Severe pulmonary involvement in mixed connective tissue disease. Am Rev Respir Dis 124:499, 1981.

Winkelmann RK and Ditto WB: Cutaneous and visceral syndromes of necrotizing or "allergic angiitis": a study of 38 cases. Medicine 43:59, 1964.

Wishnick MM, Valensi Q, Doyle EF et al: Churg-Strauss syndrome: development of cardiomyopathy during corticosteroid treatment. Am J Dis Child 136:339, 1982.

Wolff SM, Fauci AS, Horn RG, and Dale DC: Wegener's granulomatosis. Ann Intern Med 81:513, 1974.

Young RH and Mark GJ: Pulmonary vascular changes in scleroderma. Am J Med, 64:998, 1978.

Yousefzadea DK and Fishman PA: The triad of pneumonitis, pleuritis, and pericarditis in juvenile rheumatoid arthritis. Pediatr Radiol 8:147, 1979.

Rheumatic Pneumonia

Griffith GC, Phillips AW, and Asher C: Pneumonitis occurring in rheumatic fever. Am J Med Sci 212:22, 1946.

Grunow WA and Esterly JR: Rheumatic pneumonitis. Chest 61:298, 1972.

Hadfield G: The rheumatic lung. Lancet 2:710, 1938.

Jensen CR: Non-suppurative post-streptoccal (rheumatic) pneumonia. Arch Intern Med 77:237, 1946.

Lustock MJ and Kuzma JF: Rheumatic fever pneumonitis: a clinical and pathological study of 35 cases. Ann Intern Med 44:337, 1956.

Mahajan CM, Bidwai PS, Walia BNS, and Berry JN: Some uncommon manifestations of rheumatic fever. Indian J Pediatr 40:102, 1973.

Naish AE: The rheumatic lung. Lancet 2:10, 1928.

Neubuerger KT, Geever EF, and Rutledge EK: Rheumatic pneumonia. Arch Pathol 37:1, 1944.

Rich AR and Gregory JE: Experimental evidence that lesions with the basic characteristics of rheumatic carditis can result from anaphylactic hypersensitivity. Bull Johns Hopkins Hosp 73:239, 1943.

Rubin EH and Rubin M: Rheumatic fever pneumonia. In Thoracic Diseases. Philadelphia, WB Saunders Co, 1961.

Scott RF, Thomas WA, and Kissane JM: Rheumatic pneumonitis: pathologic features. J Pediatr 54:60, 1959.

Seldin DW, Kaplan HS, and Bunting H: Rheumatic pneumonia. Ann Intern Med 26:496, 1947.

Taranta A: Rheumatic fever. In McCarty DJ (ed): Arthritis and Allied Conditions. 11th ed. Philadelphia, Lea & Febiger, 1989.

Van Wijk E: Rheumatic pneumonia. Acta Paediatr 35:108, 1948.

Wedum BG: Rheumatic fever in school children of Denver, Colorado. Public Health Rep 96:157, 1981.

67

FELICIA B. AXELROD, M.D.

FAMILIAL DYSAUTONOMIA

In 1949, five children were reported with "central autonomic dysfunction with defective lacrimation." Since then, more than 500 patients with familial dysautonomia, or Riley-Day syndrome, have been diagnosed. In order to provide a background for discussion of the pulmonary manifestations, a brief general description of the disease is first presented.

GENETICS

Familial dysautonomia is an inherited disorder resulting from the expression of an autosomal recessive gene. In studies of the inheritance pattern of patients in America and in Israel, it was found that the disease occurred predominantly in Jews of Ashkenazi origin. This suggests that the mutation took place after the migration of the Jews from Spain to central and eastern Europe at the end of the fifteenth century. In this population, the disease incidence is approximately 1:3600, indicating a carrier rate of 1:30 Ashkenazi Jews.

PATHOLOGY

The primary pathologic defect is neurologic. The sympathetic and sensory ganglia are small, with a diminished number of neurons. Degenerative changes are not prominent in sensory spinal ganglia, but there tend to be fewer neurons in older patients. Surviving sympathetic neurons have a higher than normal content of immunoreactive tyrosine hydroxylase. The submucosal neurons and axons in the tongue are poorly organized and reduced in number, and the fungiform and circumvallate papillae, in which the taste buds are normally found, are rudimentary. Sural nerve biopsies have revealed a thin nerve with very few nonmyelinated fibers and a considerable reduction in small-diameter myelinated fibers. These fibers subserve pain detection. Within the kidneys, glomerulosclerosis worsens with age and vascular autonomic terminals cannot be demonstrated.

Familial dysautonomia is believed to represent a developmental arrest of unmyelinated and small-diameter myelinated neuronal populations. Slow, progressive degeneration may also be occurring. The role of nerve growth factor is under investigation.

CLINICAL MANIFESTATIONS

The symptoms of familial dysautonomia are protean, and there is considerable variation among individuals. A relatively typical history is that of an infant who shortly after birth is recognized to have problems with sucking or swallowing. Other presenting symptoms may be frequent unexplained fevers and slow motor and physical development. Respiratory infections are common. Feeding problems usually become less frequent by 1 to 2 years of age and are replaced in prominence by the "dysautonomic crisis": attacks of vomiting, fever, hypertension, excessive sweating, and a blotchy erythema that lasts hours or days. A relative insensitivity to pain predisposes to burns, fractures, corneal abrasions, and other types of trauma. An older dysautonomic indi-

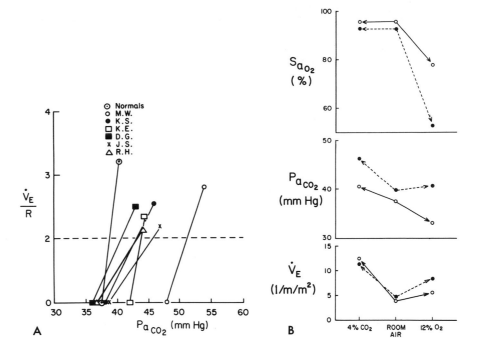

Figure 67–1. *A,* The relation between partial pressure of arterial CO_2 (Pa_{CO_2}) and the increase in minute ventilation. The average of the results in five control subjects is presented as one line; the dysautonomic responses are presented individually. The smaller slope in dysautonomia indicates that a greater change in Pa_{CO_2} is necessary to produce a corresponding increase in minute ventilation. *B,* Average values for arterial oxygen saturation (Sa_{O_2}), Pa_{CO_2}, and minute ventilation ($\dot{V}E$) in five control subjects *(solid line)* and in six dysautonomic patients *(broken line)* while breathing, respectively, room air, 4 per cent CO_2 in air, and 12 per cent O_2. (Reproduced with permission from Filler J et al: Respiratory control in familial dysautonomia. J Pediatr 66:509, 1965.)

vidual may often be recognized by a peculiar pinched face with a transverse mouth, an awkward gait, short stature, nasal speech, and exotropia. Kyphoscoliosis occurs in the majority of patients.

DIAGNOSIS

The most distinctive clinical sign is the *absence or marked diminution of overflow tearing.* When this is supported by other evidence of autonomic and sensory disturbance, such as postural hypotension, absence of patellar jerks, decreased pain sensation, history of feeding difficulties, and poor taste discrimination, the diagnosis is virtually assured. There are, in addition, three simple objective signs that aid in confirming the diagnosis.

Histamine Test. In a normal child, intradermal injection of histamine, 1:1000 (1:10,000 may be more distinctive in infants), produces intense pain and erythema followed within minutes by the development of a central wheal surrounded by the axon flare, a zone of erythema 2 to 6 cm in diameter, which is maintained for more than 10 minutes. In a dysautonomic individual, the pain is greatly reduced and there is no axon flare. No false-negative responses have been observed in patients older than 3 months (dysautonomics with a normal flare), and the only false-positive reactions requiring serious consideration occur in other peripheral congenital sensory neuropathies.

Methacholine (Mecholyl) Test. The instillation of methacholine, 2.5 per cent, or pilocarpine, 0.0625 per cent, into the conjunctival sac produces miosis in almost all cases of familial dysautonomia and has no observable effect on the normal pupil. This reaction is a sign of parasympathetic denervation and will be produced in any condition with such denervation.

Absence of Fungiform Papillae on the Tongue. This unusual sign is associated with markedly impaired taste discrimination. To date, there have been only three reported cases of familial dysautonomia in which fungiform papillae have been clinically visible.

RESPIRATORY PROBLEMS

FUNCTIONAL DEFECTS

Patients have a decreased sensitivity to breathing increased concentrations of carbon dioxide in the air (4 per cent CO_2). With hypercapnia, the minute ventilation does not increase as much as in a normal child, and respiratory acidosis results. When exposed to moderate hypoxia (12 per cent oxygen inhalations), normal persons respond with a slight increase in minute ventilation and only a moderate fall in oxygen saturation, without visible disturbance to the subject. In dysautonomic individuals, the oxygen saturation rapidly falls to a very low level, despite an appropriate increase in minute ventilation. Cyanosis results, as well as syncope and convulsions in some instances (Fig. 67–1). The systemic hypotension that complicates hypoxia in dysautonomic individuals probably contributes to the dramatic symptoms.

The abnormal response to hypoxia and the insensitivity to hypercapnia may help explain the following alarming clinical situations. During a flight on a commercial airplane with a pressurized cabin, a 12-year-old dysautonomic boy became comatose and convulsive. At a later date, this same boy was admitted to the hospital, comatose, with pneumonia; his Pa_{CO_2}

was 75 mm Hg and his Pa_{O_2} was 48 mm Hg. Several dysautonomic youngsters have drowned during underwater swimming. In one such instance, the child was demonstrating his breath-holding ability!

Abnormal breathing patterns become evident during sleep. The occasional deep respirations noted in normal individuals are infrequent, and periods of apnea of 15 seconds and longer have been noted.

PULMONARY DISEASE

Recurrent pneumonias are frequent. Repeated aspiration is probably the major factor in producing pulmonary disease. The disturbance in swallowing has been clearly demonstrated by cineesophagrams. Dysautonomic children have difficulty in forming a bolus of food and then in directing the food properly. It can be misdirected into the trachea, eustachian tubes, or nasopharynx (Fig. 67–2).

Dysfunction is also present at the cardiac-esophageal junction. Gastroesophageal reflux can be overt or subtle. The entire clinical spectrum has been seen, from regurgitation with obvious aspiration to noctur-

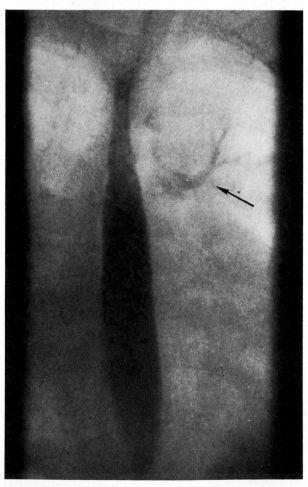

Figure 67–2. A posteroanterior view of a barium swallow in a dysautonomic patient. Note the barium that has been aspirated into the upper (left) stem bronchus *(arrow)*. (Courtesy of Dr. Melvin Becker.)

nal episodes of wheezing, apnea, or iron deficiency anemia secondary to chronic esophagitis.

Repeated pulmonary aspiration, secondary to either misdirection during eating or gastroesophageal reflux, results in chronic pulmonary disease (i.e., atelectasis and bronchiectasis). Diffuse fibrosis may occur in the absence of a history of recurrent pneumonia. Vital capacity is reduced, perhaps as a result of general muscle weakness, poorly coordinated breathing, or scoliosis.

Culture results may be confusing because the offending organisms may not be the usual pathogens. Gastrointestinal flora such as *Escherichia coli* are common etiologic agents. In severely ill children, blood gases must be monitored to detect CO_2 accumulation, which may require assisted ventilation. Suctioning may help children who accumulate a lot of secretions in the nasopharynx and have difficulty in expectorating.

For a child who aspirated frequently in infancy and becomes congested after eating or drinking milk products, dietary elimination of milk is suggested. However, supplemental calcium and vitamin D should be provided. When aspiration regularly accompanies feeding, a feeding gastrostomy may be necessary if thickening of feedings is not sufficient to prevent aspiration.

Feeding therapy is an important adjunct to helping a child abandon primitive feeding patterns such as the tongue thrust. It also helps in developing better oral coordination, normal chewing, and improved jaw control. Such therapy allows some children eventually to be weaned from gastrostomy tubes and to eat more normally without risk of aspiration. Fundoplication is indicated for patients with gastroesophageal reflux.

Bronchiectasis is generally treated with vigorous chest physiotherapy, and postural drainage is emphasized. For patients who cannot expectorate or seem to be reaspirating their own bronchial secretions, suctioning is used. When a child is old enough to cooperate, efforts should be made to improve coordination of breathing. Incentive spirometers or positive-pressure respirators are prescribed.

Four patients who suffer from frequent apneic episodes have had tracheostomy to permit mechanical ventilation during sleep.

The pulmonary pathologic condition is generally diffuse, and lobectomy is rarely indicated.

Scoliosis of variable degree occurs in 95 per cent of dysautonomic individuals over the age of 10 years. On occasion, it is so severe as to further limit an already compromised pulmonary function (Fig. 67–3). Cor pulmonale may complicate the final stages of decompensation.

PROGNOSIS

Increasing numbers of patients with familial dysautonomia are reaching adulthood. Three women with dysautonomia have given birth to normal in-

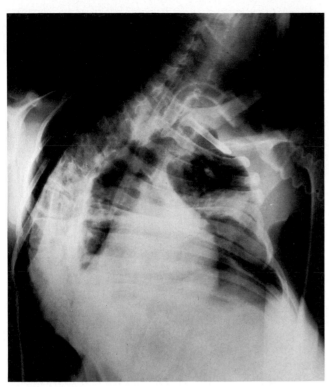

Figure 67–3. A posteroanterior view of severe scoliosis in a 21-year-old male with dysautonomia. Chronic atelectasis and fibrosis are apparent in the left lung. A tracheostomy was required for adequate ventilation.

fants. Pulmonary disease continues to be the most common cause of death, with aspiration pneumonias the prominent cause in young children and sepsis secondary to bronchiectatic disease in adolescents. Death due to renal failure is becoming more common as the number of adult patients increases.

TREATMENT

Treatment of familial dysautonomia with pulmonary complications is generally the same as for any disorder complicated by acute and chronic pulmonary disease. Such treatment is adequately described elsewhere in this book. There are a few distinctive features, however, that deserve emphasis. The frequency of subtle clinical signs warrants a high index of suspicion for atelectasis and pneumonia. Fever, shaking chills, loss of appetite, fainting spells, or listlessness may be the only warning signs. Tachypnea and auscultatory abnormalities may not be present because of poor chest excursion. Cyanosis is a late sign and portends a poor prognosis. Radiographic examination should be performed if pneumonia is suspected, and antibiotics should be given until results of cultures are known.

During general anesthesia, careful attention must be given to avoid hypoxia and hypercapnia. The serious complication of hypotension, followed by cardiac arrest, may be prevented by adequate hydra-

tion before surgery and monitoring of arterial blood pressure. Gas anesthetics are preferred because they can be rapidly titrated as dictated by blood pressure readings. Volume expanders and vasopressors such as neostigmine may be necessary.

Activity at high altitudes and underwater swimming should be prohibited. During flying, precautions should be taken to have oxygen available. It may be advisable to instruct parents in mouth-to-mouth resuscitation, a simple way to assist ventilation mechanically.

REFERENCES

Axelrod FB and Abularrage JJ: Familial dysautonomia. Prospective study of survival. J Pediatr 101:234, 1982.

Axelrod FB and Pearson J: Sensory and autonomic disorders. In Rimoin D and Emery A (eds): Principles and Practices of Medical Genetics. Edinburgh, Churchill Livingstone, 1981.

Axelrod FB, Donnenfeld RF, Danziger F, and Turndorf HT: Anesthesia in familial dysautonomia. Anesthesiology 68:153, 1988.

Axelrod FB, Iyer K, Fish I, et al: Progressive sensory loss in familial dysautonomia. Pediatrics 67:517, 1981.

Axelrod FB, Nachtigal R, and Dancis J: Familial dysautonomia: diagnosis, pathogenesis and management. Adv Pediatr 21:75, 1974.

Axelrod FB, Porges RF, and Sein ME: Neonatal recognition of familial dysautonomia. J Pediatr 110:946, 1987.

Axelrod FB, Schneider KM, Ament ME et al: Gastroesophageal fundoplication and gastrostomy in familial dysautonomia. Ann Surg 195:253, 1982.

Breakefield X and Schwartz J: Altered nerve growth factor in fibroblasts from patients with familial dysautonomia. Proc Natl Acad Sci USA 77:1154, 1980.

Brunt PW and McKusick VA: Familial dysautonomia—a report of genetic and clinical studies, with a review of the literature. Medicine 49:343, 1970.

Dancis J and Smith AA: Current concepts: familial dysautonomia. N Engl J Med 274:207, 1966.

Edelman NH, Cherniack NS, Lahini S et al: Effects of abnormal sympathetic nervous function upon the ventilatory response to hypoxia. J Clin Invest 49:1153, 1970.

Filler J, Smith AA, Stone S, and Dancis J: Respiratory control in familial dysautonomia. J Pediatr 66:509, 1965.

Gyepes MT and Linde LM: Familial dysautonomia: the mechanism of aspiration. Radiology 91:471, 1968.

Maayan CH, Kaplan E, Shachar SH et al: Incidence of familial dysautonomia in Israel 1977–1981. Clin Genet 32:106, 1987.

Moses SW, Rotem Y, Jagoda N et al: A clinical, genetic and biochemical study of familial dysautonomia in Israel. Isr J Med Sci 3:358, 1967.

Pearson J and Pytel B: Quantitative studies of sympathetic ganglia and spinal cord intermediolateral gray columns in familial dysautonomia. J Neurol Sci 39:47, 1978.

Pearson J, Axelrod F, and Dancis J: Current concepts of dysautonomia: neuropathological defects. Ann NY Acad Sci 228:288, 1974.

Pearson J, Brandeis L, and Goldstein M: Tyrosine hydroxylase immunoreactivity. Science 206:71, 1979.

Pearson J, Gallo G, Gluck M, and Axelrod F: Renal disease in familial dysautonomia. Kidney Int 17:102, 1980.

Riley CM, Day RL, Greely D McL, and Langford WS: Central autonomic dysfunction with defective lacrimation. Pediatrics 3:468, 1949.

Smith AA and Dancis J: Response to intradermal histamine in familial dysautonomia—a diagnostic test. J Pediatr 63:889, 1963.

Smith AA, Dancis J, and Breinin G: Ocular responses to autonomic drugs in familial dysautonomia. Invest Ophthalmol 4:358, 1965.

68

BYUNG HAK PARK, M.D.

CHRONIC GRANULOMATOUS DISEASE OF CHILDHOOD

Fatal (chronic) granulomatous disease of childhood (Good et al, 1968) was first described by Berendes and colleagues (1957) and Bridges and co-workers (1959) as a distinct clinical entity of unknown cause. This disease is characterized by recurrent infections with low-grade pathogens, formation of suppurative granulomas, and normal humoral and cellular immunity. The usual onset of symptoms is early in life (one patient died at 6 days of age), the disease is generally chronic (the oldest patient we know is 33 years old), and the outcome was previously thought to be fatal—the result of overwhelming infection.

Since the original report, similar cases have been described using various names: progressive septic granulomatous disease (Carson et al, 1965), chronic granulomatous disease (Baehner and Nathan, 1967), and congenital dysphagocytosis (Macfarlane et al, 1968). We use *chronic granulomatous disease* (CGD) clinically for purposes of relieving parental apprehension.

Eighty-three years after Mechnikoff's theory of phagocytosis (1883), Holmes, Quie, Windhorst, and Good (1966) clearly demonstrated in patients with CGD that a defect in phagocytic function is a major cause of the inadequacy in host defense against invading organisms. Thus, major advances in the original theory of phagocytosis as well as in the understanding of the pathogenesis of CGD were made, and this disease became a unique "experiment of Nature" for the study of phagocytosis.

The respiratory tract is almost always involved in CGD, presenting complex clinical manifestations.

CLINICAL FEATURES

The hallmark of this disease is the occurrence, in the same lesions, of septic purulent inflammation due to catalase-positive, low-grade pyogenic bacteria (Table 68–1) and the formation of granulomas.

The clinical problems seen early in life in CGD include infection of the skin, persistent purulent rhinitis, and lymphadenopathy in a well-nourished infant of otherwise normal appearance (Table 68–2).

Johnston and Baehner (1971) reviewed data on 92 patients with CGD, including four new ones. Marked lymphadenopathy was noted in 87 patients, and in 79 of these the lymph nodes suppurated and drained pus. Pneumonitis or pneumonia occurred in 80 patients. Hepatomegaly was found in 77 patients, and splenomegaly in 68; these findings were noted in all but three patients who reached the age of 6 years. Of the 85 patients whose age at onset of disease was known, 84 had their first symptoms by age 2 years. There were 45 reported deaths, 34 before the age of 7 years. Overwhelming pulmonary disease was the primary cause of death in 21 of 38 patients in whom the cause of death was stated. Septicemia led to death in 11 patients.

The skin lesion is characterized by granulomatous eruption surrounding impetigo; it progresses slowly to suppuration. The healing process is also extremely slow, resulting in granulomatous nodules that may persist for months. These lesions may be found in any part of the body, the face and neck being the more frequent sites.

Purulent rhinitis and otitis are characteristic clinical features of this disease. They occur very frequently and represent recurrent clinical problems. With adequate local and systemic antibiotic therapy, the lesion of the external nostrils clears up slowly, only to recur within a few days after the treatment is discontinued.

Lymphadenitis, another common clinical feature,

Table 68–1. A CLASSIFICATION OF BACTERIA ACCORDING TO THE BACTERICIDAL CAPACITY OF LEUKOCYTES FROM PATIENTS WITH FATAL GRANULOMATOUS DISEASE

Bacteria that are not killed (catalase-positive)
Coagulase-positive staphylococci
Escherichia coli
Aerobacter aerogenes
Paracolon hafnia (Klebsiella)
Serratia marcescens

Bacteria that are killed (catalase-negative)
Lactobacillus acidophilus
Streptococcus viridans
Diplococcus pneumoniae
Streptococcus faecalis

Table 68–2. CLINICAL FEATURES OF FATAL GRANULOMATOUS DISEASE

Recurrent infections with low-grade pathogens starting early in life.
Chronic suppurative granulomatous lesions of the skin and lymph nodes.
Hepatosplenomegaly—parenchymatous granuloma and liver abscess.
Progressive pulmonary disease—granulomatous infiltration, abscess, empyema.
Granulomatous septic osteomyelitis.
Pericarditis.
Normal cellular and humoral immune response.
Familial occurrence.

occurs in the majority of patients during the course of the disease. It is characteristically chronic, suppurative, and granulomatous and very often requires surgical drainage. Swelling and induration of cervical, axillary, and inguinal lymph nodes are most frequently seen, but involvement of hilar and mesenteric lymph nodes also occurs with great frequency.

In the common form of this disease, the family history usually reveals strong evidence of X-linked recessive inheritance (Bridges et al, 1959; Carson et al, 1965; Windhorst et al, 1967, 1968; Baehner and Nathan, 1968).

On physical examination, hepatosplenomegaly is observed in the majority of patients. An increase in the anteroposterior diameter of the chest can be found in patients with chronic fibrotic lungs.

The most prominent pulmonary lesions include an extensive infiltration of the lung parenchyma and prominent hilar adenopathy demonstrable on roentgenogram (Fig. 68–1). In addition, bronchopneumonia, often combined with lobar pneumonia, pleural effusion, pleural thickening, pulmonary abscess, and atelectasis of the right middle lobe, may

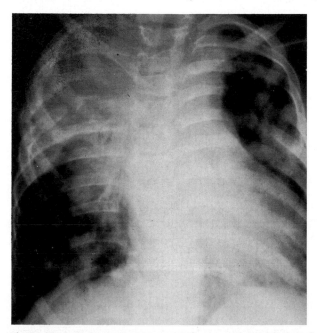

Figure 68–1. A chest roentgenogram from a patient with chronic granulomatous disease, showing extensive involvement of the right lung. This patient died of the overwhelming infection.

be present. An extensive reticulonodular infiltration often leads to pulmonary insufficiency and death.

The pneumonia characteristically begins as a hilar infiltration; it is bronchial, either unilateral or bilateral, or is basilar. In spite of extensive antibiotic treatment, these lesions regress very slowly over a period of weeks to months or frequently progress to involve an entire lobe (Figs. 68–2 and 68–3). An unusual manifestation of pulmonary involvement frequently observed in these patients is so-called encapsulated pneumonia (Wolfson et al, 1968). This pneumonia is characteristically seen on roentgenogram as a homogenous, discrete, relatively round lesion; it may occur singly or in groups of two to three infiltrates (see Fig. 68–2A). The size and contour of the lesions may change within a few days or remain unchanged for weeks or months. Discoid atelectasis, thickening of the bronchi, air bronchogram, "honeycombing," and loss of lobar volume are occasionally observed. When underlying reticulation of the lungs persists, the pulmonary function may be correspondingly impaired.

Hepatic abscess, mesenteric lymphadenitis, osteomyelitis, and oophoritis are also frequent manifestations. Anemia is often present and may be an early sign of parenchymal infection.

LABORATORY FINDINGS

Early attempts to identify the common organisms associated with parenchymal granulomatous infiltration (mycobacteria, fungi, and others) failed to produce conclusive results. Although organisms usually considered to be true high-grade bacterial, viral, or fungal pathogens rarely cause the lesions, the organisms frequently associated with the lesions are generally low-grade pyogenic pathogens (see Table 68–1). It is striking that those organisms infecting the patients and causing clinical illness can be grouped together as catalase-producing organisms.

Immunologic study has revealed normal or slightly elevated circulating immunoglobulins, vigorous antibody responses to active immunization, and normal cellular immunity.

This paradoxical situation, i.e., the apparent deficiency of host defense against infection despite normal immunity, has provoked an extensive search for the mechanism underlying deficiency of bodily defense. The first major breakthrough in this clinical dilemma was made by Holmes, Quie, Windhorst, and Good (1966), who reported that the leukocytes of patients with CGD failed to kill ingested bacteria (Fig. 68–4). In the course of their studies, these investigators showed that bacteria ingested by the phagocytic cells of these patients are actually protected from antibiotics present in high concentrations outside phagocytes (Holmes, Quie, Windhorst et al, 1966). The exhaustive studies by Quie and associates (1967) and Kaplan and colleagues (1968) established that CGD leukocytes were unable to kill a number of

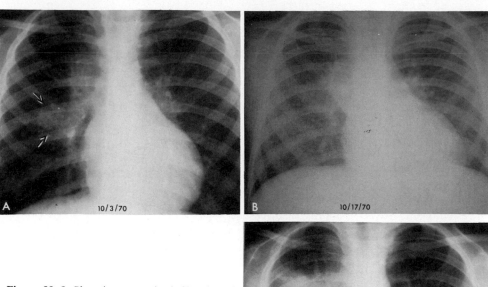

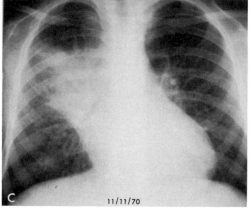

Figure 68–2. Chronic progressive infiltration of the right lung despite intensive antibiotic therapy. The right upper lobe was resected to control the infection. *A,* An early stage of infiltration with typical "encapsulated pneumonia" *(arrows). B* and *C,* Progression of the lesion.

organisms that are usually associated with the lesions but that catalase-negative organisms, which cause little clinical difficulty in these patients, are killed in a normal manner by their leukocytes (see Table 68–1).

The demonstration of the bactericidal defect in the leukocytes of patients with CGD led Holmes and co-workers (1967) to study the metabolic response of leukocytes during phagocytosis. It was clearly shown that the leukocytes of patients with CGD have deficiencies of the metabolic stimulation associated with phagocytosis. Associated with the diminished bactericidal capacity is a decrease in iodide binding of

organisms ingested by CGD leukocytes (Klebanoff and White, 1969; Pincus and Klebanoff, 1971). Iodination of bacteria appears to require the myeloperoxidase present in lysosomal granules plus hydrogen peroxide, and this combination is bactericidal in a cell-free system. A defect in superoxide dismutase activity has been reported in the leukocytes of patients with CGD (Curnutte et al, 1975).

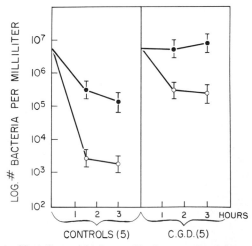

Figure 68–4. Bactericidal test of leukocytes. *Staphylococcus aureus* 502A was incubated with leukocytes, and the number of surviving bacteria was determined by a colony count at intervals. *Closed circles,* no antibiotics were added; *open circles,* penicillin and streptomycin were added at 5 min of incubation; *CGD,* chronic granulomatous disease. The number of patients or controls is shown in parentheses.

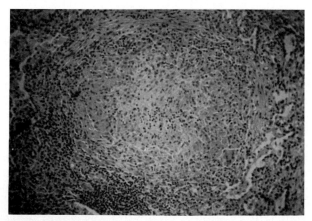

Figure 68–3. A typical granuloma of lung tissue removed from the patient shown in Figure 68–2 (magnification approximately × 400).

Baehner and Nathan (1967, 1968) and Baehner and Karnovsky (1969) reported that the leukocytes of patients with CGD have a deficiency of nicotinamide-adenine dinucleotide (NADH) oxidase and fail to reduce nitroblue tetrazolium (NBT) dye during phagocytosis. Holmes and co-workers (1970), however, did not find the NADH oxidase deficiency. Hohn and Lehrer (1975) described a defect of nicotinamide-adenine dinucleotide phosphate (NADPH) oxidase deficiency, which in my view also may be secondary to the abnormality of the metabolic changes produced by a more fundamental abnormality.

Cytochrome b is located predominantly within the plasma membrane, rapidly incorporated into phagocytic vacuoles during phagocytosis, and thus plays a pivotal role in the respiratory burst leading to bactericidal function. Segal and Jones (1980) reported that cytochrome b was absent in neutrophils of the X-linked form of CGD. In contrast, cytochrome b was present in neutrophils of CGD with the autosomal form of inheritance but was unable to be reduced on stimulation. Weening and colleagues (1985) reported a family with autosomal form of CGD in which cytochrome b was less than 4 per cent of normal. Somatic cell hybridization was performed between monocytes from the affected boy in this family with monocytes from either a cytochrome b negative male patient with X-linked CGD or a cytochrome b positive male patient with the autosomal form of CGD. In both combinations, the monocyte hybrids showed NBT reduction activity. This observation suggests that the defect in this latter family is genetically distinct from those in the other two forms of CGD.

Glutathione peroxidase of the leukocytes was, however, found to be deficient in female patients (Holmes et al, 1970). The glucose-6-phosphate dehydrogenase (G6PD) of leukocytes from male patients has been reported to be less stable at 4 and 38°C than the G6PD of normal leukocytes (Bellanti et al, 1970), but this abnormality is probably secondary rather than primary.

Some patients with CGD may have red cells with a very rare Kell system phenotype (Giblett et al, 1971). Transfusion of such patients may stimulate the formation of antibodies against all of the common antigens of the Kell system, making it extremely difficult to find a subsequent blood donor. The majority of patients with CGD, however, do not have red cells with this peculiar Kell phenotype. The patient originally described as having this rare blood type (McLeod Kell phenotypes) did not have manifestations of CGD (Allen et al, 1961).

Two studies by Marsh and colleagues (1975) reported that neutrophils from male patients with CGD lacked what they called Kx antigen. This Kx antigen was also absent in the red cells of McLeod Kell phenotype. They postulated that this lack of Kx antigenic molecule in the membrane might be linked to the metabolic abnormality of CGD neutrophils.

However, a report by Branch and colleagues (1986) casts some doubt about this contention. These researchers found that the Kx antigen was also absent in normal neutrophils as well.

Quie and co-workers (1967) presented electron microscopic evidence that phagocytosis of bacteria by CGD leukocytes was not accompanied by the vigorous degranulation that occurs in normal leukocytes. However, evidence that granule lysis is normal in the patients' leukocytes has been presented by others (Kauder et al, 1968; Baehner and Karnovsky, 1969; Elsbach et al, 1969; Ulevitch and co-workers, 1974). Some reports indicate that the kinetics of degranulation may be abnormal (Gold et al, 1974).

Even though no satisfactory explanation, at the enzymatic level, for the metabolic abnormalities observed in CGD has been forthcoming, diminished hydrogen peroxide production by CGD cells appears to be of major importance in the bactericidal defect. The enzyme responsible for the transfer of ions from reduced pyridine nucleotide to NBT dye seems to be localized in the granules of the cytoplasm (Park, 1971). This enzyme is present and normal in the granules of the leukocytes from patients with CGD. The failure of NBT dye reduction by the leukocytes of these patients may, in fact, be due to an anomaly in the rupture of the particular granule containing this enzyme. Delayed granule rupture and release of myeloperoxidase may also be a crucial factor in the bactericidal defect. A strikingly reduced activity of an enzyme in the plasma membrane of the neutrophils has been described in male patients with CGD by Segal and Peters (1976). This enzyme, located in the plasma membrane of normal neutrophils, reduces NBT dye when NADH is present at lower, more physiologic levels than are customarily used for the NADH-dependent oxidase assay. The study of the relation of this enzyme and its activation to the Kx antigen would be of great interest.

INHERITANCE

At present, at least four separate groups of patients with the leukocyte bactericidal defect have been identified. The first is the group described by Berendes and colleagues (1957) and subsequently by others; this group represents the classic form of this disease. Males are selectively involved, and the mothers as well as approximately half the sisters and all the maternal grandmothers of affected patients are detectable as carriers. In both the bactericidal tests and the NBT test, the leukocytes of carriers (of the defect) were shown to fall between the leukocytes of patients with CGD and normal controls (Windhorst et al, 1967, 1968). However, other reports indicate that the carriers may have various degrees of abnormality ranging from near normal to the level of CGD (Biggar et al, 1976). This is what would be predicted if random inactivation of one or the other X chromosome of somatic cells (Lyon's hypothesis) occurs in the neutrophils of patients with CGD.

In the second group, the defect appears to be inherited as an autosomal recessive trait, and both male and female patients with this defect have now been defined (Azimi et al, 1968; Baehner and Nathan, 1968; Quie et al, 1968; Chandra et al, 1969; Malawista and Gifford, 1975). These patients present a clinical picture similar to that of the first group but often somewhat less severe. Holmes and colleagues (1970) reported that leukocyte glutathione peroxidase was deficient in two such patients, whereas the parents of one of these families had glutathione peroxidase values approximately half that of normal. Matsuda and co-workers (1976) reported glutathione peroxidase deficiency in a male patient with chronic granulomatous disease. Cytochrome b studies mentioned earlier indicate three genetically distinct groups: (1) X linked, cytochrome b negative; (2) autosomal, cytochrome b positive; and (3) autosomal, cytochrome b negative. Roger-Pokara and colleagues (1986) reported successful cloning of a gene for CGD. Thus, the molecular basis for inheritance of CGD may soon be elucidated.

The third group is represented by the cases originally described by Ford and colleagues (1962) and studied by Rodey and associates (1970). The latter group reported that a bactericidal activity of leukocytes was defective in females with lipochrome histiocytosis. Levels of glutathione peroxidase in the leukocytes of these patients were normal (Holmes, unpublished data). The finding that the patients were female and that the mother did not show leukocyte functional deficiencies established that this disease is not of X-linked inheritance. Although these findings are compatible with an autosomal recessive inheritance, they did not establish a mendelian nature for this cellular defect.

The fourth form is represented by the patients reported by Cooper and co-workers (1970) and by Gray and associates (1973); in these patients, a complete absence of G6PD was associated with defective bactericidal activity of the leukocytes. The mode of inheritance of this defect is not clear, but it probably represents an inborn error transmitted as an autosomal recessive trait.

DIAGNOSIS

History and physical examination reveal the characteristic clinical features of chronic granulomatous disease. By the use of a simple screening test (Park and Good, 1970), it is now possible to make a prompt presumptive diagnosis. In this test, the total absence of reduced NBT dye in the leukocytes is observed in each of the four groups of patients thus far defined. This initial screening test should be followed by a more elaborate functional and metabolic study of the leukocytes. The demonstration of a defect in bactericidal function of leukocytes establishes the diagnosis

(Windhorst et al, 1968). Nakamura and colleagues (1987) obtained a monoclonal antibody to cytochrome b of human neutrophils. Immunocytochemical studies showed total absence of cytochrome b in CGD neutrophils. This method may be a useful addition to our diagnostic armamentarium.

TREATMENT

The new knowledge of granulomatous disease is useful in making the diagnosis at an early stage of the disease. Recognition of the bacteria in the lesions as potential pathogens permits an appreciation of the significance of low-grade pyogenic pathogens in each infection. This knowledge of the potential causative organisms facilitates the prompt use of appropriate antibiotics and chemotherapy at an earlier time than was previously possible. Because of this progress in diagnosis and treatment, the disease is much better managed and not nearly as lethal as it once was. Nonetheless, chronic granulomatous disease continues to have a high mortality owing to occurrence of overwhelming infection.

Treatment with gamma globulin, leukocyte transfusion, vitamin A to facilitate degranulation, and methylene blue to initiate pentose pathway activity in leukocytes has been tried without clinical benefit. Continuous administration of nafcillin has been advocated, and some clinical benefit has been ascribed to this prophylactic antibiotic regimen (Philippart et al, 1972). However, we have chosen not to give continuous antibiotic therapy to our patients with CGD, primarily because gram-negative bacteria and fungi have usually been responsible for infections leading to hospitalization and requiring specific antibiotic therapy or surgical excision, or both. Two of the three deaths in CGD patients that I know of since 1966 were due to pulmonary infections with *Aspergillus*, and the third was due to disseminated *Pseudomonas* infection. Early surgical drainage, excision of extending lesions, and at times even radical surgery can be helpful and may be necessary for clinical management of the infections. Close supervision of patients, early recognition of the characteristic symptoms and signs of each infection, and prompt initiation of specific antibiotic therapy constitute the most effective present-day treatment of this group of diseases. It was reported that sulfisoxazole could partially correct the functional abnormality of the leukocytes of patients with CGD (Johnston et al, 1975). Prolonged treatment using trimethoprim-sulfamethoxazole, although it does not correct the cellular defect as was originally thought, has been clinically useful (Pyesmany and Cameron, 1975). Quie and Belani (1987) suggested that judicial use of corticosteroids may be of value in treating progressive restrictive pulmonary disease associated with fungal infection in patients with CGD.

Ideally, correction of the inborn error of metabolism by cellular engineering, for example by using bone marrow transplantation, should cure this disease. Although not clearly documented, this approach has been claimed by Hobbs (unpublished data) to work and, with perfection of bone marrow transplantation, could become the treatment of choice. At present, however, the risks of marrow transplantation seem too great for treatment of this disease, which is usually well managed these days if the responsible physician understands the disease and the organisms likely to cause trouble and is available to provide vigorous antibiotic therapy or chemotherapy when needed.

REFERENCES

Allen FHJ, Krabbe SMR, and Corcoran PA: A new phenotype (McLeod) in the Kell blood group system. Vox Sang 6:555, 1961.

Azimi PH, Bodenbender JG, Hintz RL, and Kontras SB: Chronic granulomatous disease in three female siblings. JAMA 206:2865, 1968.

Baehner RL, and Karnovsky ML: Deficiency of reduced nicotinamide-adenine dinucleotide oxidase in chronic granulomatous disease of childhood. Science 162:1277, 1968.

Baehner RL, and Karnovsky ML: Degranulation of leukocytes in chronic granulomatous disease. J Clin Invest 48:187, 1969.

Baehner RL, and Nathan DG: Leukocyte oxidase. Science 155:835, 1967.

Baehner RL, and Nathan DG: Quantitative nitroblue tetrazolium test in chronic granulomatous disease. N Engl J Med 278:971, 1968.

Bellanti JA, Cantz BE, and Schlegel RJ: Accelerated decay of glucose-6-phosphate dehydrogenase activity in chronic granulomatous disease. Pediatr Res 4:405, 1970.

Berendes H, Bridges RA, and Good RA: A fatal granulomatosis of childhood. Minn Med 40:309, 1957.

Biggar WD, Buron S, and Holmes B: Chronic granulomatous disease in an adult male: a proposed X-linked defect. J Pediatr 88:63, 1976.

Branch DR, Gaidulis L, and Lazar GS: Human granulocytes lack red cell Kx antigen. Br J Haematol 62:747, 1986.

Bridges RA, Berendes H, and Good RA: A fatal granulomatosis disease of childhood. Am J Dis Child 97:387, 1959.

Carson JM, Chadwick DL, Brubacker CA et al: Thirteen boys with progressive septic granulomatosis. Pediatrics 35:405, 1965.

Chandra RK, Cope WA, and Soothill JR: Chronic granulomatous disease. Lancet 2:71, 1969.

Cooper MR, DeChatelet LR, McCall CE et al: Leucocyte G-6-PD deficiency. Lancet 2:110, 1970.

Curnutte JH, Kipnes RS, and Babior BM: Defect in pyridine nucleotide dependent superoxide production by a particulate fraction from the granulocytes of patients with chronic granulomatous disease. N Engl J Med 293:628, 1975.

Elsbach P, Zucker-Franklin D, and Sansaricq C: Increased lecithin synthesis during phagocytosis by normal leukocytes and by leukocytes of a patient with chronic granulomatous disease. N Engl J Med 280:1319, 1969.

Ford DK, Price GE, Charles FAC, and Vassar PS: Familial lipochrome pigmentation of histiocytes with hyperglobulinemia, pulmonary infiltration, splenomegaly, arthritis and susceptibility to infection. Am J Med 33:478, 1962.

Giblett ER, Klebanoff SJ, Pincus SH et al: Kell phenotypes in chronic granulomatous disease: a potential transfusion hazard. Lancet 1:1235, 1971.

Gold SB, Hanes DM, Stites DP, and Fudenberg HH: Abnormal kinetics of degranulation in chronic granulomatous disease. N Engl J Med 291:332, 1974.

Good, RA: Progress toward a cellular engineering. JAMA 214:1289, 1970.

Good RA, Quie PG, Windhorst DB et al: Fatal (chronic) granulomatous disease of childhood. Semin Hematol 5:215, 1968.

Gray GR, Stamatoyannopoulos G, Naiman SC et al: Neutrophil dysfunction, chronic granulomatous disease and nonspherocytic haemolytic anemia caused by complete deficiency of glucose-6-phosphate dehydrogenase. Lancet 2:530, 1973.

Hohn DC and Lehrer RI: NADPH oxidase deficiency in X-linked chronic granulomatous disease. J Clin Invest 55:707, 1975.

Holmes B, Page AR, and Good RA: Studies of the metabolic activity of leukocytes from patients with a genetic abnormality of phagocytic function. J Clin Invest 46:1422, 1967.

Holmes B, Park BH, Malawista SE et al: Chronic granulomatosis disease in females. N Engl J Med 283:217, 1970.

Holmes B, Quie PG, Windhorst DB, and Good RA: Fatal granulomatous disease of childhood. Lancet 1:1225, 1966.

Holmes B, Quie PG, Windhorst DB et al: Protection of phagocytized bacteria from the killing action of antibiotics. Nature (London) 210:1131, 1966.

Johnston RB and Baehner RL: Chronic granulomatous disease: correlation between pathogenesis and clinical findings. Pediatrics 48:730, 1971.

Johnston RB and McMurray JS: Chronic familial granulomatosis. Am J Dis Child 114:370, 1970.

Johnston RB, Wilfert CM, Buckley RH et al: Enhanced bactericidal activity of phagocytes from patients with chronic granulomatous disease in the presence of sulphisoxazole. Lancet 1:824, 1975.

Kaplan EL, Laxdal T, and Quie PG: Studies of polymorphonuclear leukocytes from patients with chronic granulomatous disease of childhood. Pediatrics 41:591, 1968.

Karnovsky ML: The metabolism of leukocytes. Semin Hematol 5:156, 1968.

Kauder E, Kahle LL, Moreno H, and Parten JC: Leukocyte degranulation and vacuole formation in patients with chronic granulomatous disease of childhood. J Clin Invest 47:1753, 1968.

Klebanoff SJ and White LR: Iodination defect in the leukocytes of a patient with chronic granulomatous disease of childhood. N Engl J Med 280:460, 1969.

Macfarlane PS, Speirs AL, and Sommerville RG: Fatal granulomatous disease of childhood and benign lymphocytic infiltration of the skin (congenital dysphagocytosis). Lancet 1:844, 1968.

Malawista SE and Gifford RH: Chronic granulomatous disease of childhood (CGD) with leukocyte glutathione peroxidase (LGP) deficiency in a brother and sister: a likely autosomal recessive inheritance. Clin Res 23:416a, 1975.

Marsh WL, Oyen R, Nichols ME, and Allen FH Jr: Chronic granulomatous disease and the Kell blood groups. Br J Haematol 29:247, 1975.

Marsh WL, Uretsky C, and Douglas SD: Antigens of the Kell blood group system on neutrophils and monocytes: their relation to chronic granulomatous disease (CGD). J Pediatr 87:1117, 1975.

Matsuda I, Oka Y, Taniguchi N et al: Leukocyte glutathione peroxidase deficiency in a male patient with chronic granulomatous disease. J Pediatr 88:581, 1976.

Mechnikoff E: Untersuchungen uber die mesodermalen Phagocyten einiger Wirbeltiere. Biol Central Bl 3:560, 1883.

Nakamura M, Murakami M, Koga T et al: Monoclonal antibody 7D5 raised to cytochrome 558 b of human neutrophils: immunocytochemical detection of the antigen in peripheral phagocytes of normal subjects, patients with chronic granulomatous disease, and their carrier mother. Blood 69:1404, 1987.

Park BH: The use and limitation of NBT reduction test as a diagnostic aid. J Pediatr 78:376, 1971.

Park BH and Good RA: NBT test stimulated. Lancet 2:616, 1970.

Philippart AI, Colodny AH, and Baehner RL: Continuous antibiotic therapy in chronic granulomatous disease: preliminary communications. Pediatrics 50:923, 1972.

Pincus SH and Klebanoff SJ: Quantitative leukocyte iodination. N Engl J Med 284:744, 1971.

Pyesmany AF and Cameron DL: Septrin-induced stimulation of granulocyte metabolism in chronic granulomatous disease (CGD) (abstract). Pediatr Res 7:143, 1975.

Quie PG and Belani KK: Corticosteroids for chronic granulomatous disease. J Pediatr 111:393, 1987.

Quie PG, Kaplan EL, Page AR et al: Defective polymorphonuclear leukocyte function and chronic granulomatous disease in two female children. N Engl J Med 279:967, 1968.

Quie PG, White JG, Holmes B, and Good RA: In vitro bactericidal capacity of human polymorphonuclear leukocytes. J Clin Invest 46:668, 1967.

Rodey GE, Holmes B, Park BH et al: Leukocyte function in lipochrome histiocytosis. Am J Med 49:322, 1970.

Roger-Pokora B, Kunkel LM, Monaco AP et al: Cloning the gene for an inherited human disorder—chronic granulomatous disease—on the basis of its chromosomal location. Nature 322:32, 1986.

Segal AW and Jones OTG: Absence of cytochrome b reduction in stimulated neutrophils from both female and male patients with chronic granulomatous disease. FEBS Lett 110:111, 1980.

Segal AW and Peters TJ: Characterization of the enzyme defect in chronic granulomatous disease. Lancet 1:1363, 1976.

Ulevitch RJ, Henson P, Holmes B, and Good RA: An in vitro study of exocytosis of neutrophil granule enzymes in chronic granulomatous disease neutrophils. J Immunol 112:1383, 1974.

Weening RS, Corbeel L, deBoer M et al: Cytochrome b in an autosomal form of chronic granulomatous disease. J Clin Invest 75:915, 1985.

Windhorst DB, Holmes B, and Good RA: A newly defined X-linked trait in man with demonstration of the Lyon effect in carrier females. Lancet 1:737, 1967.

Windhorst DB, Page AR, Holmes B et al: The pattern of genetic transmission of the leukocyte defect in fatal granulomatous disease of childhood. J Clin Invest 47:1026, 1968.

Wolfson J, Quie PG, Laxdal SD, and Good RA: Roentgenologic manifestations in children with a genetic defect of polymorphonuclear leukocyte function. Radiology 91:37, 1968.

69

CARL ALEXANDER-REINDORF, M.D., MELVIN E. JENKINS, M.D., and ADEKUNLE D. ADEKILE, M.B., B.S.

THE LUNGS IN SICKLE CELL DISEASE

Sickle cell disease is relatively new to the western world, having been first clinically described in the early part of the twentieth century (Herrick, 1910). The past three decades have witnessed a remarkable accumulation of knowledge and understanding of the biochemical basis and clinical picture of this protean illness.

The exact origin of the sickle cell gene is still unknown. Haplotype analyses in various sickle cell populations have indicated that there are four independent origins of the sickle cell mutations: two in West Africa (Benin and Senegal), one in Central Africa (Bantu), and the fourth in Saudi Arabia and some East Indian populations (Saudi) (Serjeant, 1989). Sickle cell disease conforms to an autosomal recessive mode of inheritance, with sickle cell trait representing the heterozygous condition. Each child of two parents with the trait will therefore have a 25 per cent probability of inheriting the homozygous state (SS), or sickle cell anemia. Approximately 50 per cent demonstrate the trait (AS), and another 25 per cent possess entirely normal hemoglobin (AA). Restriction enzyme analysis of DNA from fetal blood samples, amniotic fluid, or chorionic villi has made prenatal diagnosis of sickle cell anemia at 12 to 16 weeks of gestation fairly routine (Bank, 1985).

One of the restriction enzymes used for this analysis is Mst-II. When the sickle gene is present, the mutation at the sixth codon of the beta gene (B6), consisting of a single nucleotide change (GAG to GGG), abolishes one Mst-II site on the beta-globulin chain. Thus, a single 1.35-kb fragment of DNA is obtained instead of the 1.15 and the 0.20-kb fragments of normal hemoglobin A gene. This is transcribed biochemically into the substitution of valine for glutamic acid. Because of the great variability in the manifestations of the disease, even prenatal diagnosis of sickle cell anemia cannot predict who will suffer from the associated pulmonary complications.

Other abnormal hemoglobins, such as hemoglobin C and that in thalassemia, are also transmitted as autosomal recessives. These genes in heterozygous alleles can combine with the sickle cell gene to produce variant forms of sickle cell disease. In general, the variant forms are associated with less severe anemia. However, sickle cell–hemoglobin C disease (SC) is beset by many complications, such as retinopathy and pregnancy-related problems, which are more frequent than in homozygous sickle cell anemia.

There currently are approximately 1.8 million black Americans with clinically detectable AS hemoglobin, an incidence of between 6 and 12 per cent (Scott-Emaukpor, 1976). On the basis of reports of AS frequencies, homozygous sickle cell disease (SS) should afflict 1 in 144 to 1 in 600 blacks in the United States. Sickle cell hemoglobin predominates in each red cell in the homozygous state. The qualitative aberration of SS hemoglobin determines its effects on body structure and tissues. The pathogenesis of sickle cell disease results from deoxygenation-dependent polymerization of hemoglobin S with the formation of spindle-shaped liquid crystalline bodies called tactoids. The final product is a viscous gel that deforms the red blood cell and makes it rigid. Gelation is being intensively studied because it is undoubtedly the basis of sickling of erythrocytes, which leads to increased viscosity of the blood and impairs circulation to vital tissues (Dean and Schechter, 1978).

From a clinical point of view, sickle cell disease is characterized by recurrent "crises," which in children are often precipitated by infections, especially those involving the respiratory, urinary, and gastrointestinal systems. These crises may be classified as follows:

1. Vaso-occlusive or painful crisis, which results from vascular stasis.

2. Hemolytic crisis, which occurs when red cells break down at a more rapid rate than the steady-state hemolysis of SS disease.

3. Aplastic crisis, in which bone marrow suppression occurs, usually secondary to a viral infection, thus compromising the hyperactive marrow needed to partially compensate for chronic hemolysis in SS disease.

4. Sequestration crisis, which results from massive erythrostasis of visceral organs and leads to shock and death if not treated promptly.

The lungs, as the obligatory organs of oxygen (O_2) entry and carbon dioxide (CO_2) exit, bear the huge burden of helping to compensate for the chronic tendency toward tissue hypoxia in sickle cell anemia. At the same time, like other organs, the lungs are vulnerable to vaso-occlusive phenomena brought on by the sickling process itself. In this connection, it must be emphasized that the homozygous sickle cell condition (SS) and some of its allelic variants frequently produce disease. The heterozygous state (AS) is benign under almost all circumstances.

In this chapter, the adverse effects of homozygous sickle cell disease on the lungs are presented in the context of biochemical, pathophysiologic, and clinical derangements.

DERANGEMENTS OF PULMONARY FUNCTION

Hypoxemia, which is unrelated to the hemoglobin level, is the hallmark of the pulmonary function abnormality in sickle cell patients of all age groups. This observation was first documented by Klinefelter in 1942 and has since been confirmed by other investigators (Sproule et al, 1958; Young et al, 1981). Numerous attempts have been made to elucidate the pathophysiologic basis of this phenomenon. Fowler and associates (1957) studied normal subjects, patients with sickle cell anemia, and patients with other types of anemia. All SS patients had reduced arterial oxygen saturation and showed an increased alveolar-arterial (A-a) O_2 tension gradient. The A-a gradient fell toward normal when the the patients breathed mixtures with low concentrations of O_2 (15.6 per cent), suggesting that increased admixture of unsaturated blood may be responsible for the hypoxemia. These investigators also found that sickle hemoglobin consistently showed a slower uptake of O_2 than nor-

mal hemoglobin under the same experimental conditions, with a resultant displacement of the dissociation curve of oxyhemoglobin to the right of normal.

Sproule and colleagues (1958) attempted to clarify the cause of the increased A-a O_2 tension gradient in sickle cell patients by determining alveolar and arterial O_2 tensions at three levels of oxygenation, i.e., with the patient breathing low O_2 concentrations, room air, and 100 per cent O_2. The premise was that if desaturation was due to hypoventilation, no appreciable increase in the gradient would exist at any level of oxygenation, and any observed increase in the gradient would therefore be due to either a diffusion defect or venoarterial admixture. Diffusion defect and venoarterial admixture can be differentiated by measuring the effective A-a gradient at a minimum of two levels of oxygenation. Low levels of inspired O_2 exaggerate the effects of impaired diffusion and minimize the effects of ventilation-perfusion mismatching. If ventilation-perfusion mismatching is the problem, its effects would be eliminated by the administration of 100 per cent O_2. However, 100 per cent O_2 would not eliminate hypoxemia due to the right-to-left shunt. These investigators confirmed the presence of hypoxemia in the majority of patients but determined that diffusion defects were not the major factors in desaturation. Although it was evident that a minor loss of diffusing capacity had occurred in most sickle cell patients, the most important mechanism producing desaturation was right-to-left shunt within the pulmonary parenchyma, probably resulting from episodes of pneumonia and/or thromboembolic phenomena.

Using more sophisticated methods, Femi-Pearse and co-workers (1970) performed pulmonary function studies, including the measurement of single-breath diffusing capacity for carbon monoxide (DL_{CO}), membrane diffusing capacity (DM), and pulmonary capillary volume (V_c) in normal subjects and patients with sickle cell disease. In the sickle cell–hemoglobin S (SS-Hb) patients, the mean values for vital capacity (VC) and total lung capacity (TLC) were 80 and 83 per cent of predicted normal values, respectively. In the sickle cell–hemoglobin C (SC-Hb) patients, the mean VC was 88 per cent of normal and the average TLC was 94 per cent. No evidence of airway obstruction or abnormality in the distribution of inspired gas was detectable in these patients. Compared with normal subjects, the mean DL_{CO} in both SS-Hb and SC-Hb patients was significantly decreased. When correction was made for hemoglobin levels, the values of DL_{CO} were within the normal range in the SC-Hb group but disproportionately high in the SS-Hb group. The mean values for DM in both groups were significantly decreased. There was a significant increase in V_c in the SS-Hb patients but not in the SC-Hb patients (Table 69–1). It was postulated that in some SS-Hb patients, despite low hemoglobin levels, a chronically expanded pulmonary capillary bed may serve a compensatory role to maintain an appropriate level of DL_{CO}. The cause of

Table 69–1. PULMONARY DIFFUSING CAPACITY AND ITS SUBDIVISION IN NORMAL SUBJECTS AND IN TEN PATIENTS WITH SICKLE CELL DISEASE

Subjects	Hb (g/100 ml)	$D_{L_{CO}}$* (ml/min/mm Hg)	D_M (ml/min/mm Hg)	V_c (ml)
Normal subjects†	13.9 ± 0.14	29 ± 0.75	65 ± 1.6	67 ± 2.1
SS-Hb disease				
WT	7.1	23	47	70
KR	7.8	20	39	89
JW	8.8	22	48	69
HW	7.2	32	66	92
SM	6.5	20	41	77
HD	7.8	27	45	95
Mean ± SE	7.5 ± 0.32	24 ± 1.9	48 ± 3.9	82 ± 4.7
SC-Hb disease				
JJ	12.5	22	40	
AC	13.2	21	39	65
ER	12.5	21	50	48
MH	12.9	23	49	57
Mean ± SE	12.8 ± 0.17	22 ± 0.48	45 ± 2.9	52 ± 3.5

*Measured at alveolar P_{O_2} of 120 mm Hg.
†30 normal subjects studied, with means ± SE.
(Reproduced with permission from Femi-Pearse D, Gazioglu KM, and Yu PN: Pulmonary function studies in sickle cell disease. J Appl Physiol 28:574, 1970.)

the reductions in VC and TLC in these patients cannot be satisfactorily explained, but previous episodes of pulmonary embolization may have led to the development of restrictive impairment of respiratory function. In a similar study by Young and co-workers (1976), most subjects exhibited restrictive lung disease, with low TLC and VC, and D_M was decreased in 67 per cent of SS-Hb patients; these investigators postulated that part of the decrease in pulmonary function is related to the anemia of SS disease.

In addition to measuring lung volumes, carbon monoxide transfer factor or diffusing capacity, D_M, and V_c, Miller and Serjeant (1971) recorded anthropometric data (stature, sitting height, and chest diameters) in patients with SS. Not only was the thorax short relative to body stature, but the lateral chest diameter was narrower than expected in healthy subjects of the same ethnic origin (Table 69–2). Thus, there appears to be a reduction in the volume of the thorax and lungs relative to body size, causing a corresponding reduction in TLC/VC. Transfer factor was also significantly reduced in both sexes, probably as a consequence of anemia, small lungs, and low D_M.

Most studies have assessed mainly adult sickle cell patients. However, Wall and co-workers (1979) investigated pulmonary function in children age 7 to 13 1/2 years (Table 69–3). They found lung volumes and expiratory flow to be comparable with those of an appropriate normal (AA) control group. However, the abnormal $D_{L_{CO}}$ and mild hypoxemia described in adults with sickle cells were also documented in children by these researchers. They reported that the restrictive defect of lung function noted in older patients appears to follow recurrent pulmonary thromboembolism and pneumonias and progressively develops with age. Indeed, the one child in their sample whose lung volume was slightly decreased had had three documented bouts of pneumonia.

The role of the cardiovascular status in SS patients with documented hypoxemia is not clear. Cor pulmonale is occasionally found in SS patients. Oppenheimer and Esterly (1971) described post-mortem evidence of pulmonary hypertension in one SS patient. Although cardiomegaly is detected radiologically in most SS patients, cardiac catheterization values are essentially normal (Sproule et al, 1958). This observation, therefore, does not support the possi-

Table 69–2. AGE, ANTHROPOMETRY, AND HEMOGLOBIN CONCENTRATION IN SICKLE CELL ANEMIA

	Males (16)		Females (9)	
	Mean	*SD*	*Mean*	*SD*
Age (years)	28.2	8.7	27.8	10.9
Hemoglobin (g/100 ml)	7.7	1.6	7.7	1.1
Weight (kg)	57.0	7.0	55.4	8.3
Stature (m)	1.747	0.054	1.644	0.077
Sitting height (m)	0.841	0.031	0.806	0.035
Sitting height/stature	0.48	0.02	0.49	0.02
Lateral chest diameter (cm)	24.1	1.7	23.0	1.1
Anteroposterior chest diameter (cm)	17.6	1.4	16.5	1.8

(Reproduced with permission from Miller GJ and Serjeant GR: An assessment of lung volume and gas transfer in sickle cell anemia. Thorax 26:309, 1971.)

Table 69–3. LUNG VOLUMES AND EXPIRATORY FLOWS IN CHILDREN WITH SICKLE CELL ANEMIA (SS-Hb), NORMAL BLACK CONTROL CHILDREN AND NORMAL WHITE CHILDREN

	SS-Hb					Control Children			
	Actual Values		% of Values in Control Children	% of Values in White Children		Actual Values		% of Values in White Children	
	Mean	SD		Mean	SD	Mean	SD	Mean	SD
TLC	2.61	0.71	98	78	9	2.66	0.59	80	9
VC	2.00	0.54	93	79	9	2.15	0.47	85	9
RV	0.61	0.24	120	76	25	0.51	0.22	63	18
RV/TLC (%)	23	7	121	—	—	19	3	—	—
FRC	1.38	0.49	110	81	17	1.26	0.28	76	9
PEF (min)	297	73	91	92	10	327	68	100	11
FEV$_1$	1.68	0.42	90	78	9	1.86	0.42	85	8
FEV$_1$/VC (%)	84	5	98	—	—	87	5	—	—
FEF$_{25-50\%}$, 2 (min)	122	41	85	80	20	144	37	95	21
V$_{max50}$, 2 (sec)	2.60	0.98	98	83	21	2.73	0.57	86	10
V$_{max50}$, TLC/sec	1.03	0.36	98	107	38	1.05	0.21	108	22

(Reproduced with permission from Wall MA, Platt OS, and Strieder DJ: Lung function in children with sickle cell anemia. Am Rev Respir Dis 120:211, 1979.)

bility that cardiac enlargement in SS patients is often due to cor pulmonale. The abnormal cardiac findings in SS disease are probably secondary to the high cardiac output, which has been estimated to increase to 50 to 150 per cent above normal.

In studies involving 66 sickle cell disease patients at rest and during treadmill walking, Young and colleagues (1988) found that the patients had restrictive ventilatory defects, decreased lung compliance, and uneven ventilation-perfusion ratios. These abnormalities created an increased A-a O$_2$ tension difference that caused hypoxemia. They found that during treadmill walking the patients showed decreased work tolerance caused by impaired O$_2$ delivery. Furthermore, the anaerobic threshold that was reached earlier by patients with the sickle cell disease, when compared with healthy subjects, might account for the limitations in the patients' work capacity. They concluded that because O$_2$ transport in these patients is inadequate to support even moderate work, care must be taken to prevent patients with sickle cell anemia from performing heavy workloads for fear of inducing vaso-occlusive (painful) crises.

PULMONARY INFARCTION

Wollestein and Kreidel (1928) described an autopsy finding in a 4-year-old patient with sickle cell disease as "a wedge-shaped area of organized pneumonia," perhaps the first description of pulmonary infarction in sickle cell disease. However, the first report of the presence of thromboemboli in the pulmonary vessels of patients with sickle cell anemia was made by Steinberg (1930), who noted marked congestion of capillaries and larger vessels and the presence of serum in some alveoli. Today, pulmonary infarction is accepted as the primary component of a substantial portion of the cases of acute and chronic lung disease in patients with sickle cell anemia.

INCIDENCE

It has been postulated that the majority of acute pulmonary episodes simulating pneumonia in sickle cell disease are, in reality, infarcts (Margolies, 1951). In one study, 28 per cent of SS patients over the age of 2 years had microscopic organized pulmonary thromboemboli (Margolies, 1951). In another study, however, pulmonary infarction was documented by angiography or lung scan in only 1 of 69 subjects (Reynolds, 1965); 40 per cent of the patients in this study had radiographically demonstrable pulmonary infiltrates. Likewise, only 3 of 166 SS patients in another study had infarcts, although 45 per cent had acute pulmonary infiltrates (Barrett-Connor, 1971a). Pulmonary infarction is, however, a common complication of the last trimester of pregnancy in sickle cell–HbC patients (Edington, 1957; Karayalcin et al, 1972). The precise frequency of pulmonary infarction in SS disease has not been determined, but pulmonary infarcts are life threatening and must be detected and treated early.

CLINICAL FEATURES

The classic clinical features of pulmonary infarction are chest pain, dry cough, dyspnea, generalized weakness, and palpitation. Less often, hemoptysis with rusty sputum is encountered. Dullness to percussion and crepitant rales may be elicited. There occasionally is tenderness over the involved region of the chest wall (Karayalcin et al, 1972). The frequency of painful vaso-occlusive crises involving the thorax and the increased susceptibility of SS patients to pulmonary infection make the diagnosis of pulmonary thromboembolism difficult. Also, angiography, which is sometimes used for the diagnosis of pulmonary infarction, is hazardous in sickle cell disease because hypertonic dyes in themselves can induce sickling.

PATHOLOGY

Although Wollestein and Kreidel (1928) and Steinberg (1930) earlier reported wedge-shaped areas representing infarcts of the lungs, it was the detailed autopsy findings of Diggs and Barreras (1967) that systematically documented the pathologic features of pulmonary infarction in sickle cell disease. These researchers studied 62 patients with sickle cell anemia and 10 subjects with variant forms of sickle cell disease, e.g., SC and sickle cell–thalassemia (S-thal). There were multiple pulmonary lesions, but emboli and infarcts were observed in only 1 of the 32 children who had sickle cell anemia who were less than 10 years of age. Fresh and organized pulmonary emboli were demonstrated in 60 per cent of older patients, with gross infarcts in 40 per cent.

Oppenheimer and Esterly (1971) found autopsy evidence of thromboemboli in nearly 66 per cent of SS patients. The degree of organization and the frequency of thromboemboli increased with age. Proliferation of the arterial intima was noted in the pulmonary vessels, but associated morphologic evidence of pulmonary hypertension was observed only once. Pulmonary infarcts were encountered in one infant, three children, and four adults, all of whom had thromboemboli. In all but the two youngest infants, peribronchial lymph nodes displayed follicular differentiation. Shelley and Curtis (1958) reported eight additional instances of pulmonary vascular occlusion in patients with SS disease, in whom emboli of cellular marrow elements were the basis of the lesions in most individuals.

PATHOGENESIS

It has been proposed that intravascular sickling leads to increased blood viscosity and local stasis, with resultant ischemia and infarction producing in situ thrombosis (Moser and Shea, 1957). Circumstances that favor increased sickling in the pulmonary vascular system include low venous P_{O_2} and a high extraction of O_2 from the blood in this condition (Walker et al, 1979). Young and colleagues (1981) also suggested that in situ thrombosis from distorted red cells in hypoxemic pulmonary arteries and capillaries was the basis of infarction. For reasons that are unclear, pulmonary embolism rarely follows thrombophlebitis in sickle cell disease (Barrett-Connor, 1973; Heller et al, 1979).

COMPLICATIONS AND PROGNOSIS

Pulmonary infection is often superimposed on pulmonary infarction in SS disease. Infection may lead to hilar adenopathy, which may on rare occasion result in bronchial obstruction from direct compression. The infarction itself may initiate serosanguineous pleural effusion or may progress to hemorrhage in the affected segment. Acute pulmonary infarction is fatal in 10 to 12 per cent of patients with sickle cell anemia. In the others, it resolves spontaneously within about 2 weeks (Reynolds, 1965; Barrett-Connor, 1971a). The prognosis ultimately depends on the extent of the infarction. When severe, impairment of O_2 supply usually damages adjacent areas, further extending infarction, tissue necrosis, and life-threatening hypoxemia.

TREATMENT

The treatment of pulmonary infarction in sickle cell anemia must be individualized and is primarily supportive. Use of anticoagulants such as heparin and low-molecular-weight dextran has been recommended in the absence of specific contraindications (Barrett-Connor, 1973). However, there are no firm data to show that anticoagulants are of therapeutic benefit in pulmonary infarction. In adults at Howard University Hospital in Washington, D.C., partial exchange transfusions have been useful (Castro, 1981). In children, packed red cell transfusions are indicated for severe anemia and extensive or protracted acute pulmonary disease associated with significant pulmonary insufficiency (Pearson and Diamond, 1971).

Associated infection must be vigorously treated. The choice of antibiotics is based on assessment of the clinical presentation and identification of causative organisms. When associated in situ thrombosis follows pneumonia with consequent anoxia, fever, and prolongation of the course of the infection, anticoagulant therapy together with antibiotic therapy may hasten resolution of the pneumonia.

Supportive treatment consists of analgesics, hydration, and O_2. It is important to avoid the use of narcotic analgesics, which inhibit the respiratory center. Steroid therapy may aggravate the predilection for thrombosis in SS disease and must therefore be used with caution when indicated.

PREVENTION

Because pulmonary infarction is the result of in situ aggregation of sickled erythrocytes in hypoxemic pulmonary arterioles, it is reasonable to assume that prevention of sickling can prevent pulmonary infarction. It has been demonstrated, for example, that erythrostasis can be prevented in pregnant patients with sickle cell disease by monthly blood transfusions during the third trimester (Castro, 1981).

A large number of chemical agents that reduce gelation of deoxygenated sickle hemoglobin are being assessed for therapeutic effects. They can be categorized into three main groups: (1) those that inhibit polymerization of sickle hemoglobin by disrupting intermolecular bonding; (2) those that inhibit polymerization by decreasing the concentration of deoxygenated hemoglobin S; and (3) those that interact with erythrocyte membranes.

Regardless of the availability of these newer antisickling agents, the appropriate agent or combination of drugs that will prevent infarcts has not yet been clinically studied sufficiently to predict effectiveness. In the mean time, physicians who treat children must become familiar with newer agents and should select a drug that seems to fit the individual need of the patient. In time, a more satisfactory preventive regimen may emerge.

PNEUMONIAS

Bacterial infection, not crisis, is the leading cause of morbidity and mortality in children with sickle cell anemia (Porter and Thurman, 1963; Charache and Richardson, 1964; Barrett-Connor, 1971b). Patients with other variants of sickle cell disease, especially sickle cell–hemoglobin C disease, are also at an increased risk for infection, although the risk is not as pronounced as in the homozygous condition (Barrett-Connor, 1971b; Young et al, 1981). The greatest hazard of life-threatening infection is in patients less than 4 years of age, and pneumonia is the most common infection (Scott and Ferguson, 1966; Barrett-Connor, 1971b, 1973; Bromberg, 1974; Tsou and Katz, 1977; Young et al, 1981). It has been estimated that pneumonia is 100 to 300 times more common in patients with sickle cell anemia than in the general population (Barrett-Connor, 1971b). Reindorf and colleagues (1989), who studied the records of children with sickle cell anemia, found that those children with gallstones had more than the expected morbidity owing to repeated respiratory tract infection including pneumonia.

MECHANISM OF INFECTION

Pyogenic organisms (e.g., pneumococci, beta-hemolytic streptococci, *Hemophilus influenzae*) can gain access to the body through the respiratory tract. After the organisms cross the normal integument, the initial defense is provided by surface phagocytes, which in the lungs are the alveolar macrophages (Gee and Smith, 1981).

Once in the blood stream, the bacteria are taken up mainly by the reticuloendothelial (lymphoid-macrophage) system, primarily in the liver and spleen, and by phagocytes in the capillaries of organs, especially the lungs. Once the phagocytic cells have ingested the bacteria, antigens are passed along to the lymphoid cells, which recognize them as foreign and initiate the production of specific antibody. The bactericidal activity of the serum against gram-negative bacteria is dependent primarily on antibody, complement, and lysozymes. Although there are also bactericidal factors against gram-positive organisms, the major killing effect is attributed to leukocyte phago-

cytosis in the presence of opsonins (specific antibody, complement, and other heat-labile factors).

ABNORMALITIES OF THE IMMUNE SYSTEM IN SICKLE CELL DISEASE

Integument and Phagocytosis

Evidence that a defective integument contributes to infection in sickle cell disease is lacking. It has been proposed, however, that the increased susceptibility of sickle cell patients to *Salmonella* bacteremia results from a pathologic condition secondary to sickling in the gastrointestinal tract (Roberts and Hilburg, 1965). In the lungs, subclinical thrombi, fluid-filled alveoli, and congestion also afford supportive media for bacterial multiplication and, at the same time, impair surface phagocytosis. Moreover, phagocytosis is impaired at reduced P_{O_2} (Green, 1968), which also occurs in sickle cell disease.

Metabolic abnormalities have also been described in the polymorphonuclear leukocytes of sickle cell patients who have repeated infections. These abnormalities include a failure to demonstrate three processes: stimulation of respiratory CO_2, consumption of O_2, and oxidation of formate during phagocytosis. These findings, which signify impairment of degranulation and intracellular killing of bacteria, were absent in polymorphonuclear leukocytes from patients with sickle cell trait, splenectomized patients, and normal individuals (Dimitrov et al, 1972).

The bactericidal process in neutrophils and monocytes depends on the generation of hydrogen peroxide, which in turn is dependent on the ready availability of O_2 in the presence of either NADH or NADPH oxidases. Therefore, bactericidal action of these cells is reduced under relatively anaerobic conditions. Patients with SS disease develop the sickling phenomenon when the blood P_{O_2} falls to between 35 and 45 mm Hg, causing focal areas of hypoxia in the lungs that impair the bactericidal capacity of leukocytes. Pneumococci, salmonellae, and shigellae all grow under anaerobic conditions; thus, sickle cell patients are particularly susceptible to infection with these organisms (Craddock, 1973).

Complement System

Winkelstein and Drachman (1968) studied the serum opsonizing activity for pneumococci with a phagocytic test using normal peripheral leukocytes incubated in serum from patients with sickle cell anemia and in normal serum. Heat-labile serum opsonizing activity for pneumococci was found to be markedly deficient in serum from SS patients, in whom the mean phagocytosis was 6.5 per cent, compared with a mean value of 35.1 per cent in normal control children under the same conditions. Serum opsonizing activity for salmonellae was similar in both groups.

Johnston and associates (1973) found that sera from sickle cell patients promoted normal phagocytosis of pneumococci if the bacteria had previously been sensitized with an excess of antibody but that a deficiency emerged when the amount of antibody added to the experimental system was decreased. The abnormality could not be attributed to a deficiency of antibody or complement components. However, under conditions that prevented activation of C1 and the classic complement sequence, the sera did not fully activate to fix the essential opsonin C3 to the microorganism by the alternate pathway. When specific pneumococcal antibody is deficient, SS patients may be unable to phagocytize the organisms normally on first encounter. The basic cause of this deficiency in sickle cell disease is unknown.

The Spleen and Immunoglobulins

The spleen plays a critically important role in host defense against many infections in childhood. Its lymphoid tissue produces opsonizing antibody (Ellis and Smith, 1966) as well as other immunoglobulins, especially in response to small doses of intravenously administered particulate antigens (Rowley, 1950a, b). The spleen's reticuloendothelial system is responsible for clearing particulate foreign material including bacteria from the blood of nonimmune individuals (Schulkind et al, 1967).

The majority of children with hemoglobin SS develop clinical enlargement of the spleen by the time they are 3 years of age. However, in late childhood (6 to 8 years), the size of the spleen regresses as a result of recurrent infarction and fibrosis. Pearson and co-workers (1969) showed that even though clinically enlarged, the spleen in a young SS child is functionally inactive. This state is usually reversible by transfusions of normal red cells (Pearson et al, 1970). The condition should be suspected if a peripheral blood smear shows the presence of red cells with whole nuclei, with nuclear fragments (Howell-Jolly bodies), with precipitated masses (Heinz bodies), and with pitted and distorted membranes (Crosby, 1959). Deficient splenic function greatly increases the risk of repeated infections, especially pneumonias.

Low immunoglobulin M (IgM) levels have been described following splenectomy in children (Schumacher, 1970; Wasi et al, 1977). Evans and Reindorf (1968) found no decrease in the mean serum immunoglobulin concentrations in children with SS disease. However, the range of serum IgM concentrations was low in some adult patients. Gavrilis and associates (1974) measured serum immunoglobulin concentrations in patients with sickle cell disease syndromes (SS, SC, S-Thal) and correlated the levels with splenic size as determined by ^{99m}technetium sulfur colloid scanning. These observations support the theory of a relationship between immunoglobulin deficiency, pulmonary infections in sickle cell disease, and spleen size. From a functional point of view, therefore, most children with SS disease behave like

splenectomized children and exhibit the same susceptibility to severe bacterial infections, especially pneumococcal. On the other hand, splenic function is relatively normal in sickle cell trait, hemoglobin S–thalassemia, and hereditary persistence of fetal hemoglobin. Splenic function is poor in SC disease, but not to the same degree as in SS disease (Pearson et al, 1969).

Humoral and Cellular Immune Defect

Lack of splenic function per se does not completely explain the increased susceptibility to infections in children with sickle cell anemia. For example, fulminant bacterial infections are not common in adults with sickle cell anemia, even though most of these adult patients develop autosplenectomy as a result of multiple previous spleen infarctions.

Reindorf and colleagues, in collaborative studies in Washington, D.C., and in Los Angeles, found that in patients with sickle cell anemia thymosin alpha-1 (TA-1) was elevated: 1050 to 1362 pg/ml in SS patients, but 563 to 614 pg/ml in AA volunteers. The thymosins are a family of hormone-like peptides originally isolated from the epithelial framework of the thymus gland. The first thymosin to be isolated, sequenced, and synthetized is TA-1. It is generally depressed in primary immune deficiency diseases. However, elevated levels of TA-1 are found in the presence of immunodeficiencies associated with acquired immune deficiency syndrome (AIDS) and also in patients with multiple sclerosis, T-cell leukemias, and Brazilian pemphigus foliaceus. Furthermore, they found in the same group of patients that the cytotoxic/suppressor cells (OKT8) were increased disproportionately to the helper/inducer cells (OKT4) such that the helper/suppressor ratio was reversed.

ROLE OF IRON AND OTHER RED CELL BREAKDOWN PRODUCTS

Various factors predispose SS patients to the accumulation of iron and other products of red cell breakdown. These include chronic hemolysis, frequent blood transfusions, and increased intestinal absorption of iron (Erlandson et al, 1962). Iron compounds have been shown to promote growth, multiplication, and virulence of several bacterial organisms both in vivo and in vitro (Weinberg, 1966). Iron overload also inhibits the killing and digestion of phagocytized bacteria (Gladstone and Walton, 1971) and blocks the reticuloendothelial system (Gabrielli and Holmgren, 1967; Caroline, Rosner, and Kozinn, 1969; Caroline, Kozinn, Feldman et al, 1969).

Masawe and Nsanzumuhire (1973) examined blood from patients with sickle cell anemia, those with severe iron deficiency anemia, and normal controls for the capacity to support bacterial growth. The specimens from patients with sickle cell anemia yielded more colonies than specimens from controls. These investigators used whole blood samples and discounted the role of other components in the serum that might support bacterial growth. They concluded, however, that increased iron levels in SS patients contribute significantly to the susceptibility of SS patients to bacterial infections.

ETIOLOGIC ORGANISMS

The fact that SS patients are unusually susceptible to more than one type of bacteria was first demonstrated by Eeckels and colleagues (1967). These investigators examined the distribution of hemoglobin genotypes in a group of black children with acute generalized bacterial infections including pneumonia. After ruling out salmonellae, the major causative organisms were pneumococci, coliforms, staphylococci, and *H. influenzae.* The pneumococcal group was of highest prevalence in SS patients. Several reports attest to a high frequency of fulminating pneumococcemia in sickle cell disease (Fernbach and Burdine, 1970; Kabins and Lerner, 1970; Dymet and Donowho, 1971; Seeler et al, 1972; Overturf et al, 1979).

Barrett-Connor (1971b) reported the largest and most sharply defined series of patients with sickle cell disease complicated by pneumonia. In about half of patients, cultures were negative. In the remaining half, *Streptococcus pneumoniae* accounted for almost 60 per cent of bacteremias. If positive blood cultures are considered along with positive sputum and nasopharyngeal cultures, *S. pneumoniae* is responsible for more than 80 per cent of pneumonia in SS disease. *H. influenzae* and other gram-negative organisms account for most of the remaining infectious agents. It is not known whether there is a higher risk of mycoplasmal pneumonia in sickle cell anemia, but when it occurs, this type of pneumonia tends to be unusually severe (Shulman et al, 1972).

Earlier reports suggested increased morbidity and mortality from tuberculosis in sickle cell disease (Diggs and Ching, 1934; Carroll and Evans, 1949), but in a review of 250 infections in 166 sickle cell patients, Barrett-Connor (1971b) did not find active tuberculosis to be more common or more severe than in patients without hemoglobinopathy. There is also no evidence that sickle cell patients are more prone to viral pneumonia than the general population. Young and co-workers (1981) have demonstrated an increased frequency of sarcoidoisis in patients with hemoglobinopathies.

CLINICAL PRESENTATION OF PNEUMONIA IN SICKLE CELL DISEASE

As previously pointed out, pneumonia in sickle cell disease at any age is usually caused by pneumococci.

The basis for this profound susceptibility to pneumococcal infections has been discussed. The disease is much more severe and resolution is slow, the average duration of fever being 10 to 12 days despite appropriate antibiotic treatment. There are at least two explanations for the slow response of SS patients to therapy. First, the regional hypoxia in inflamed and consolidated lungs probably promotes local sickling and vaso-occlusion, thus delaying resolution of the inflammation (Bromberg, 1974). Second, access of antibiotics to the areas of inflammation might be compromised by the presence of subclinical pulmonary thrombi and infarcts. Pneumococcemia in sickle cell disease is not infrequently associated with a Shwartzman-like reaction resulting in disseminated intravascular coagulation. The process is often very fulminant and may be rapidly fatal (Kabins and Lerner, 1970; Seeler et al, 1972).

Adolescents and adults with sickle cell disease are very frequently hospitalized for what has been described as "acute chest syndrome," the components of which are fever, chest pain, cough, and pulmonary infiltrates. The pulmonary problem can be confused with a severe bacterial pneumonia, pulmonary infarction, or both (Barrett-Connor, 1973; Bromberg, 1974; Charache et al, 1979; Young et al, 1981). In small children, infarction of the ribs can be confused with acute chest syndrome. However, lung scan or flow studies using ^{99m}technetium can define the infarcted rib cage.

DIFFERENTIATION OF PNEUMONIA FROM PULMONARY INFARCTION

Thromboembolic phenomena with or without infarction are rare in children (Barrett-Connor, 1971a, 1973; Young et al, 1981). Ninety per cent of bacteremic pneumonia occurs in children 3 years of age or younger. Pulmonary infarction, however, has not been documented in any patient younger than 12 years (Barrett-Connor, 1973), probably because the pulmonary changes that predispose sickle cell patients to infarction, such as recurrent pneumonia, subclinical thrombi, and pulmonary vessel narrowing from intimal proliferation, take years to develop. Pregnancy significantly accentuates the risk of infarction (Reynolds, 1965), which is a serious complication of the latter stages of gestation in SC patients (Edington, 1957).

Blood cultures are positive in less than 10 per cent of cases of lobar pneumonia with or without hemoglobinopathy (Barrett-Connor, 1973), but when positive the culture is of diagnostic importance. Culture of a pathogen from sputum or the nasopharynx is helpful, but unless the sputum is purulent or the growth is very heavy, the pathogen cannot necessarily be implicated as the cause of pneumonia (Barrett-Connor, 1973; Tsou and Katz, 1977).

Chest roentgenograms are sometimes helpful. Infarction is usually confined to the lower lobes, whereas lobar pneumonia occurs with the greatest frequency in the middle and upper lobes (Figs. 69–1 and 69–2); Reynolds, 1965; Diggs and Barreras, 1967; Tsou and Katz, 1977).

The ventilation-perfusion scan has been used in the differentiation of pulmonary infection from infarction. However, when there is a corresponding shadow on chest x-ray film or an abnormality on the xenon ventilation scan, the ventilation-perfusion scan, even if positive, is not reliable in the diagnosis of vascular occlusion (Fig. 69–3). The gallium scan, which may be positive in untreated pneumonia and sarcoidosis and negative in infarction, may be a more helpful differential diagnostic tool (Young et al, 1981).

Although leukocytosis with a shift to the left may suggest pneumonia in a patient without hemoglobin-opathy, it does not help differentiate infection from infarction in sickle cell disease. White cell counts of 20,000 to 50,000 cells/mm^3 are common in sickle cell crisis without detectable evidence of infection. Jaundice may complicate lobar pneumonia or pulmonary infarction in persons without hemoglobinopathy. However, in sickle cell anemia, jaundice significantly greater than the usual low-grade icterus strongly suggests pulmonary infarction. Barrett-Connor (1973) observed a total serum bilirubin level greater than 5 mg/100 ml in four of five patients with bacterial pneumonia. This increase may result from the microangiopathic hemolytic anemia that complicates pulmonary infarction. Other signs of microan-

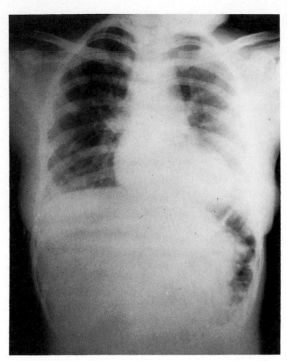

Figure 69–2. Pulmonary infarction. A chest radiograph of an 18-year-old female with leg pains and abdominal pain who developed severe dyspnea and chest pain 4 days after the initiation of antibiotic therapy. Differentiation of the left lung infiltrate from the pneumonia is not possible.

giopathy are seen in the peripheral blood smear in pulmonary infarction, including marked poikilocytosis, blister cells, helmet cells, and fragmented and/or triangular cells (Barreras et al, 1968; Karayalcin et al, 1972).

Result of the nitroblue tetrazolium (NBT) test, which is based on the reduction of NBT to formazan by normal polymorphonuclear leukocytes, is said to be positive in infection and negative in infarction (Walters and Reddy, 1974). A high leukocyte alkaline phosphatase value may suggest pneumonia, although this value can also increase in vascular occlusion (Young et al, 1981). Fibrinogen levels are markedly elevated in patients with sickle cell anemia and infection but are normal in asymptomatic patients and in patients with painful crisis only (Green et al, 1968).

TREATMENT OF PNEUMONIA IN SICKLE CELL DISEASE

Antibiotics

Pneumonia is best treated with antibiotics and/or antimicrobials as indicated by results of stained smears of bronchoalveolar secretions and blood cultures. Because most pneumonias complicating sickle cell disease are pneumococcal, however, it is advisable to institute prompt antibiotic therapy with intravenous penicillin G, 250,000 units/kg/day IV every 6 hours, after obtaining the appropriate cultures. Ampicillin, 200 mg/kg/day IV every 6 hours, can also be

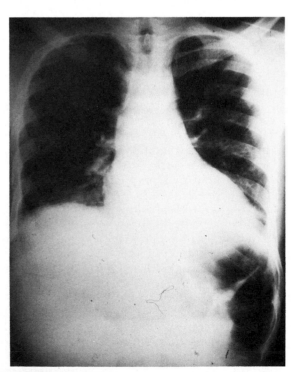

Figure 69–1. Left lower lobe pneumonia. A chest radiograph of a 19-year-old patient with chest pain, dyspnea, jaundice, and fever. Note the left lower lobe infiltrate and the obliteration of the costophrenic angle.

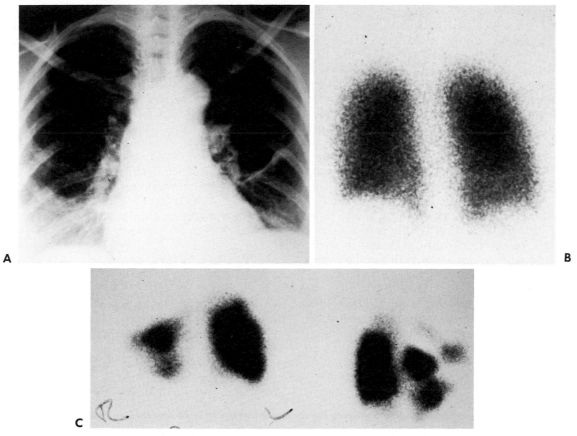

Figure 69–3. Lung scan in the diagnosis of early pulmonary infarct in sickle cell disease. *A*, A chest radiograph of a dyspneic patient with sickle cell disease. *B*, The ventilation-diffusion study is normal (anterior view). *C*, The perfusion study, however, reveals irregular uptake in the right lung (anterior view—*left*; right posterior oblique view—*right*). The normal ventilation-diffusion study together with abnormal perfusion uptake indicates infarction but is not diagnostic.

used as the initial therapy, especially because it is also effective against most strains of *H. influenzae* and salmonellae. A high titer of cold hemagglutinins would suggest mycoplasmal infection, for which erythromycin is the drug of choice.

Supportive Treatment

Analgesics should be administered for pleuritic pain and/or the pain of concurrent vaso-occlusive crisis. O_2 is indicated if the patient is markedly dyspneic. Charache and associates (1979) advocate that Pa_{O_2} be monitored in all sickle cell patients with pulmonary infiltrates. If the Pa_{O_2} is less than 70 mm Hg, O_2 should be given and the measurement should be repeated. Persistent hypoxemia despite O_2 administration should lead to a consideration of immediate partial exchange transfusion.

Packed red cell transfusion is recommended for severe anemia or a protracted course of infection. In Howard University Hospital, repeated packed red cell transfusions, at a rate of 10 ml/kg, are administered until the hemoglobin level reaches 11 to 12 g/dL (Uy and Scott, 1978).

The demonstrated reversal of functional asplenia by blood transfusion in SS children with splenomeg-

aly suggests an acceptable rationale for using transfusion in such children with pneumococcal bacteremia. However, Pearson and co-workers (1970) point out that because of the fulminant nature of pneumococcal sepsis, it is unlikely that transfusion can act quickly enough to be of clinical benefit.

Optimal hydration must be assured. Parenteral hydration is usually mandatory. Because of the increased risk of congestive heart failure in severe anemia, care must be taken not to produce fluid overload.

Patients with pneumococcal bacteremia must be monitored very closely. A decrease in platelet count, low fibrinogen level, and a prolonged activated partial thromboplastin time indicate disseminated intravascular coagulation and the possible need for heparin therapy. A significant decrease in serum pH necessitates rapid correction of metabolic acidosis with sodium bicarbonate or another clinically useful buffer.

PROPHYLAXIS

Surveillance studies have established that 14 of the more than 80 types of pneumococci are responsible for 75 per cent of pneumococcal disease. A polyvalent vaccine has been developed against these 14 types, and pneumococcus immunization has undergone clinical trials over the past few years in several centers. Amman and colleagues (1977) showed that sickle cell patients respond to immunization with the pneumococcal polysaccharide much like healthy control subjects. However, several children have contracted pneumococcal sepsis or meningitis after vaccination (Ahonkhai et al, 1979; Giebink et al, 1979; Minor et al, 1979; Overturf et al, 1979). We have also encountered three failures (two from type 23 and one from type 6A pneumococcus) in Howard University Hospital. Boyer and associates (1981) found an increase in IgG isohemagglutinins against A and B red blood cells in adults immunized with the pneumococcal vaccine. These researchers caution against its use in women of child-bearing age because of the theoretical danger of ABO incompatibility in neonates.

Penicillin prophylaxis has been advocated for young children with sickle cell disease; however, it has not been convincingly satisfactory (Barrett-Connor, 1973). There is also the possibility that resistant pneumococcal strains may emerge with the prolonged use of penicillin prophylaxis (Finland, 1971).

FAT EMBOLISM

Fat embolization of the lungs is being recognized with increasing frequency in sickle cell disease. Shelley and Curtis (1958) were the first to document fat embolism in children with SS disease. Lehmann and McNathin (1928) found various degrees of fat embolism at autopsy in the lungs of 37 of 50 adults with SS disease. Vance (1931), on the other hand, could find minimal fat embolism in only 7 of 82 normal patients. In normal individuals, fat embolism usually occurs in association with fractures of long bones. In sickle cell disease, fat embolization seems to arise from medullary centers of the bone after necrosis of the fatty marrow. The necrotic marrow then becomes embolized via the medullary veins.

SIGNS AND SYMPTOMS

The signs and symptoms of fat embolization include a triad of pyrexia, neurologic disorders, and respiratory abnormalities. Excruciating pain is the most common symptom. It is often localized, usually to the back or legs, interfering with walking. The pain can be so severe that the patient may scream uncontrollably, groan, or lash about. When the pain causes nausea and vomiting as well as profuse sweating, fat embolism may simulate a myocardial infarction. Neurologic findings are common and include (1) inability to verbalize in response to questions, (2) stupor, semicoma, or disorientation, and (3) global aphasia or hemiparesis with urinary incontinence.

Respiratory symptoms such as shortness of breath, wheezing, and tachypnea are prominent. Respirations may occasionally become shallow or stertorous. Rhonchi are common. Other general features such as pyrexia and petechiae of the conjunctivae and skin can mimic a disseminated infection. Fundoscopy reveals refractile bodies (i.e., fat emboli). Fat droplets may also be demonstrated in the sputum and urine.

Because of the protean manifestations of multiple fat emboli, a wide range of diagnoses must be considered, such as conversion hysteria, cerebral thrombosis, subacute bacterial endocarditis, septic shock, cortical vein thrombosis, cerebral edema, and overwhelming pneumonia. The possibility of fat emboli must be kept in mind in patients with sickle cell disease who suffer sudden severe back pain, tachycardia, respiratory distress, or loss of consciousness.

PATHOLOGY

In fat embolization, a liquid oil enters the circulating blood and is transported in globules large enough to obstruct the lumens of blood vessels in different parts of the body (Vance, 1931). In fat embolism occurring in sickle cell disease, necrotic bone marrow, including several bony spicules in many of the large, medium, and small pulmonary arteries, can be detected. Sections of vertebra, rib, and sternum show hyperplasia and numerous foci of fresh necrosis. Microscopic examination of the lungs shows numerous small fragments of both necrotic and well-preserved bone marrow in the small pulmonary arteries. There is also widespread fat embolization of the capillaries. The visceral pleurae are covered with numerous petechial hemorrhages (Ober, 1959). Hemorrhagic infarcts may also occur.

According to Diggs (1965), fat emboli are more common in patients with SC disease than in those with SS anemia. Wade and Stevenson (1941) described necrotic bone marrow in tissues during crisis. Although bone marrow necrosis is probably common, the condition is underdiagnosed because painful bones are seldom aspirated. It is reasonable to assume, however, that necrotic bone marrow can result from the infarction of vaso-occlusive crisis and may be dislodged and enter the venous circulation, with devastating systemic consequences.

MANAGEMENT

At present, treatment of fat embolism is basically preventive. It consists of avoiding chilling, dehydration, or infections that can precipitate vaso-occlusive crisis. Alcohol, heparin, clofibrate, emulsifying agents, and steroids all have been tried. In fat embolism, petechiae are manifestations of thrombopenia, and platelet counts therefore, must be monitored during any vaso-occlusive crisis. Exchange blood transfusions have also been advocated for the management of fat embolism in sickle cell patients

(Castro, 1981). A truly effective treatment regimen has not yet been developed, however.

SUMMARY

The lungs are frequently targets of pathologic insults in homozygous sickle cell disease and some of its variants. Impairment in pulmonary function in SS children has been detailed in this chapter. Vaso-occlusive phenomena brought on by intravascular sickling may lead to symptomatic pulmonary crises, single or multiple pulmonary infarcts, and, very rarely, pulmonary fat emboli. Pulmonary infarcts are uncommon in young children with sickle cell disease. Actually, the pneumonias constitute the bulk of acute and recurrent lung disease in SS children. Pneumococcal organisms predominate, but others such as *H. influenzae* are also encountered more often than in normal children. Mycoplasmal pneumonia, when contracted by SS children, runs a more prolonged course. A number of immune incompetencies in children with SS disease make early, vigorous treatment of acute pulmonary infections mandatory and also make some forms of prophylaxis more rational. The pneumococcal vaccine, for example, despite its limitations, is recommended for SS children older than 2 years. In the future, more research and clinical study must be directed toward the lungs as important target organs for the pathogenic consequences of sickle cell disease in children.

REFERENCES

Ahonkhai VI, Landesman SH, Fikrig SM et al: Failure of pneumococcal vaccine in children with sickle cell disease. N Engl J Med 301:26, 1979.

Amman AJ, Addiego J, Wara DW et al: Polyvalent pneumococcal polysaccharide immunization of patients with sickle cell anemia and patients with splenectomy. N Engl J Med 297:897, 1977.

Bank A: Genetic disorders of hemoglobin synthesis. Hosp Pract 20:109, 1985.

Barreras L, Diggs LW, and Bell A: Erythrocyte morphology in patients with sickle cell anemia and pulmonary emboli. JAMA 203:569, 1968.

Barrett-Connor E: Acute pulmonary disease and sickle cell anemia. Am Rev Respir Dis 104:159, 1971a.

Barrett-Connor E: Bacterial infection and sickle cell anemia. Medicine 50:96, 1971b.

Barrett-Connor E: Pneumonia and pulmonary infarction in sickle cell anemia. JAMA 224:997, 1973.

Boyer KM, Theeraunthichai J, Vogel LC et al: Antibody response to group B streptococcus type III and AB blood group antigens induced by pneumococcal vaccine. J Pediatr 98:374, 1981.

Bromberg PA: Pulmonary aspects of sickle cell anemia. Arch Intern Med 133:652, 1974.

Caroline L, Kozinn PJ, Feldman E et al: Infection and iron overload in Thalassemia. Ann NY Acad Sci 165:148, 1969.

Caroline L, Rosner R, and Kozinn PS: Elevated serum iron, low unbound transferrin and candidiasis in acute leukaemia. Blood 34:441, 1969.

Carroll DS and Evans JW: Roentgen findings in sickle cell anemia. Radiology 53:834, 1949.

Castro O: Personal communication, Washington DC, 1981.

Charache S: Management of sickle cell disease in pregnant patients. Obstet Gynecol 55:407, 1980.

Charache S and Richardson SN: Prolonged survival of a patient with sickle cell anemia. Arch Intern Med 133:844, 1964.

Charache S, Scott JC, and Charache P: Acute chest syndrome in adults with sickle cell anemia. Arch Intern Med 139:67, 1979.

Chmel H and Bertles JF: Hemoglobin S-C disease in a pregnant woman with crisis and fat embolism syndrome. Am J Med 58:563, 1975.

Craddock PR: Bacterial infection in sickle cell disease. N Engl J Med 288:1301, 1973.

Crosby WH: Normal functions of the spleen relative to red blood cells: a review. Blood 14:399, 1959.

Dean J and Schechter AN: Sickle cell anemia: molecular and cellular basis of therapeutic approaches. N Engl J Med 299:752, 1978.

Diggs LW: Sickle cell crisis. Am J Clin Pathol 44:1, 1965.

Diggs LW: Pulmonary lesions in sickle cell anemia. Blood 34:734, 1969.

Diggs LW and Barreras L: Pulmonary emboli vs. pneumonia in patients with sickle cell anemia. Memphis Med J 42:375, 1967.

Diggs LW and Ching RE: Pathology of sickle cell anemia. South Med J 27:839, 1934.

Dimitrov NW, Douwes FR, Bartolotta B et al: Metabolic activity of polymorphonuclear leukocytes in sickle cell disease. Acta Haematol 47:283, 1972.

Dymet PG and Donowho EM: Fatal pneumococcemia and sickle cell anemia. South Med J 64:758, 1971.

Edington GM: The pathology of sickle cell haemoglobin-C. disease and sickle cell anemia. J Clin Pathol 10:182, 1957.

Eeckels R, Gatti F, and Renoirte AM: Abnormal distribution of hemoglobin genotypes in Negro children with severe bacterial infections. Nature 216:382, 1967.

Ellis EF and Smith RT: The role of the spleen in immunity: with special reference to the post-splenectomy problem in infants. Pediatrics 37:111, 1966.

Erlandson ME, Walsen B, Stern G et al: Studies on congenital hemolytic syndromes. IV. Gastrointestinal absorption of iron. Blood 19:359, 1962.

Evans HE and Reindorf C: Serum immunoglobulin levels in sickle cell disease and thalassemia major. Am J Dis Child 116:586, 1968.

Femi-Pearse D, Gazioglu KM, and Yu PN: Pulmonary function studies in sickle cell disease. J Appl Physiol 28:574, 1970.

Fernbach DJ and Burdine JA: Sepsis and functional asplenia. N Engl J Med 288:691, 1970.

Finland M: Increased resistance in the pneumococcus. N Engl J Med 284:212, 1971.

Fowler NO, Smith O, and Greenfield JC: Arterial blood oxygen in sickle cell anemia. Am J Med Sci 234:449, 1957.

Gabrielli E and Holmgren H: Studies on the blockage of the reticulo-endothelial system. Acta Pathol Microbiol Scand 31:205, 1967.

Gavrilis P, Rothenberg SP, and Guy R: Correlation of low serum IgM levels with absence of functional splenic tissue in sickle cell disease syndromes. Am J Med 57:542, 1974.

Gee BJ and Smith GJW: Lung cells and disease. Basics Respir Dis 9:1, 1981.

Giebink GS, Schiffman G, Petty K, and Quie PG: Vaccine type pneumococcal pneumonia: occurrence after vaccination in an asplenic patient. JAMA 241:2736, 1979.

Gladstone GP and Walton E: The effect of iron and haematin on the killing of staphylococci by rabbit polymorphs. Br J Exp Pathol 52:452, 1971.

Green GM: Pulmonary clearing of infectious agents. Ann Rev Med 19:315, 1968.

Heller P, Best WR, Nelson RB, and Becktel J: Clinical implications of sickle cell trait and glucose 6-phosphate dehydrogenase deficiency in hospitalized black male patients. N Engl J Med 300:1001, 1979.

Herrick JB: Peculiar elongated and sickle-shaped red blood corpuscles in a case of severe anemia. Arch Intern Med 6:517, 1910.

Hutchinson RM: Fat embolism in sickle cell disease. J Clin Pathol 26:620, 1973.

Johnston RB, Newman SL, and Struth AG: An abnormality of the alternate pathway of complement activation in sickle cell disease. N Engl J Med 288:803, 1973.

Kabins SA and Lerner C: Fulminant pneumococcemia and sickle cell anemia. JAMA 211:467, 1970.

Karayalcin G, Imram M, and Rosner F: "Blister cells": association with pregnancy, sickle cell disease and pulmonary infarction. JAMA 219:1727, 1972.

Klinefelter HP: The heart in sickle cell anemia. Am J Med Sci 203:34, 1942.

Lehmann EP and McNathin RF: Fat embolism, incidence at postmortem. Arch Surg 17:79, 1928.

Margolies MP: Sickle cell anemia: a composite study and survey. Medicine 30:357, 1951.

Masawe AE and Nsanzumuhire H: Growth of bacteria in vitro in blood from patients with severe iron deficiency anemia and from patients with sickle cell anemia. Am J Clin Pathol 59:706, 1973.

Miller GJ and Serjeant GR: An assessment of lung volume and gas transfer in sickle cell anemia. Thorax 26:309, 1971.

Minor D, Schiffman G, and McIntosh LS: Response of patients with hodgkin's disease to pneumococcal vaccine. Ann Intern Med 90:887, 1979.

Morrison JC and Wiser WL: The use of prophylactic partial exchange transfusion in pregnancies associated with sickle cell hemoglobinopathies. Obstet Gynecol 48:516, 1976.

Moser KM and Shea JG: The relationship between pulmonary infarction, cor pulmonale, and the sickle cell states. Am J Med 27:561, 1957.

Ober WB, Bruno MS, Simon RM, and Weiner L: Hemoglobin S-C disease with fat embolism: report of a patient dying in crisis: autopsy findings. Am J Med 27:647, 1959.

Oppenheimer EH and Esterly JR: Pulmonary changes in sickle cell disease. Am Rev Respir Dis 103:858, 1971.

Overturf GD, Field R, and Edmonds R: Death from type 6 pneumococcal septicemia in a vaccinated child with sickle cell disease. N Engl J Med 300:143, 1979.

Pearson HA and Diamond LK: The critically ill child: sickle cell disease crises and their management. Pediatrics 48:629, 1971.

Pearson HA, Cornelius EA, Schwartz AD et al: Transfusion-reversible functional asplenia in young children with sickle cell anemia. N Engl J Med 283:334, 1970.

Pearson HA, Spencer RP, and Cornelius EA: Functional asplenia in sickle cell anemia. N Engl J Med 281:923, 1969.

Porter FS and Thurman WG: Studies of sickle cell disease, diagnosis in infancy. Am J Dis Child 106:35, 1963.

Reindorf CA, Nwaneri RU, Worrel RG et al: The significance of gallstones in children with sickle cell anemia. J Natl Med Assoc, 1990, in press.

Reindorf CA, Shacks S, Naylor P et al: Unpublished data, Washington DC and Los Angeles, 1987.

Reynolds J: The Roentgenological Features of Sickle Cell Disease and Related Hemoglobinopathies. Springfield, Ill, Charles C Thomas, 1965.

Roberts AR and Hilburg LE: Sickle cell disease with salmonella osteomyelitis. J Pediatr 66:877, 1965.

Rowley DA: The effect of splenectomy on the formation of circulating antibody in the adult male albino rat. J Immunol 64:289, 1950a.

Rowley DA: The formation of circulating antibody in the splenectomized human being following intravenous injection of heterologous erythrocytes. J Immunol 65:515, 1950b.

Schulkind ML, Ellis EF, and Smith RT: Effect of antibody upon clearance of I^{125} labelled pneumococci by the spleen and liver. Pediatr Res 1:178, 1967.

Schumacher MJ: Serum immunoglobulin and transferrin levels after childhood splenectomy. Arch Dis Child 45:114, 1970.

Scott RB and Ferguson AD: Studies in sickle cell anemia. XXVII: Complications in infants and children in the United States. Clin Pediatr 5:403, 1966.

Scott-Emuakpor AB: Genetic aspects of sickle cell disease. In Scott RB (ed): International Aspects of Sickle Cell Disease. Washington, DC, Howard University Center for Sickle Cell Disease, 1979.

Seeler P, Metzger W, and Mufson M: *Diplococcus pneumoniae* infections in children with sickle cell disease. Am J Dis Child 123:8, 1972.

Serjeant GR: Geography and the clinical picture of sickle cell disease. In Whitten CF and Bertles JF (eds): Ann NY Acad Sci 565:109, 1989.

Shelley WM and Curtis EM: Bone marrow and fat embolism in sickle cell anemia and sickle cell hemoglobin C disease. Bull Johns Hopkins Hosp 103:8, 1958.

Shulman ST, Bartlett J, Clyde WA, and Ayoub EM: The unusual severity of mycoplasmal pneumonia in children with sickle cell disease. N Engl J Med 287:164, 1972.

Sproule BJ, Halden ER, and Miller WF: A study of cardiopulmonary alterations in patients with sickle cell disease and its variants. J Clin Invest 37:486, 1958.

Steinberg B: Sickle cell anemia. Arch Pathol 9:876, 1930.

Tsou E and Katz S: Sickle cell lung disease. Am Fam Physician 16:128, 1977.

Uy C and Scott RB: Guidelines for Care of Patients with Sickle Cell Disease. Washington DC, Howard University Publication, 1978.

Vance BM: The significance of fat embolism. Arch Surg 23:426, 1931.

Wade LJ and Stevenson LD: Necrosis of the bone marrow with fat embolism in sickle cell anemia. Am J Pathol 17:47, 1941.

Walker BK, Ballas SK, and Burka ER: The diagnosis of pulmonary thromboembolism in sickle cell disease. Am J Hematol 7:219, 1979.

Wall MA, Platt OS, and Strieder DJ: Lung function in children with sickle cell anemia. Am Rev Respir Dis 120:210, 1979.

Walters TR and Reddy BN: Sickle cell anemia and the NBT test. J Clin Pathol 27:783, 1974.

Wasi C, Wasi P, and Thongcharoen P: Serum immunoglobulin levels in thalassemia and the effects of splenectomy. Lancet 2:237, 1971.

Weinberg ED: Metallic ions in host-parasite interactions. Bacteriol Rev 30:136, 1966.

Winkelstein JA and Drachman RH: Deficiency of pneumococcal serum opsonizing activity in sickle cell disease. N Engl J Med 279:459, 1968.

Wollestein M and Kreidel KV: Sickle cell anemia. Am J Dis Child 36:998, 1928.

Young RC, Wright P III, and Banks DD: Lung function abnormalities occurring in sickle cell hemoglobinopathies: a preliminary report. J Natl Med Assoc 68:201, 1976.

Young RC, Castro O, Baxter RP et al: The lung in sickle cell disease: a clinical overview of common vascular infections and other problems. J Natl Med Assoc 73:19, 1981.

Young RC, Rachal RE, Reindorf CA et al: Lung function in sickle cell hemoglobinopathy patients compared with healthy subjects. J Natl Med Assoc 80:509, 1988.

70

DANIEL C. SHANNON, M.D., and
DOROTHY H. KELLY, M.D.

SIDS AND APNEA OF INFANCY

Sudden death occurs at all ages. In adults it is frequently the result of cardiac arrhythmia, especially ventricular fibrillation; in adolescents it is often accidental; and in infants, although it can follow arrhythmia or accident, it is generally unexplained and is called *sudden infant death syndrome* (SIDS). There may be pathologic effects in various organs, such as inflammation of the respiratory tract, but the degree is insufficient to explain death. In the past, sudden infant death was attributed to suffocation from thymic enlargement (Lee, 1842) or anaphylaxis due to milk protein (Parish et al, 1960; Peterson and Good, 1963), associations that were later proved false. We have now entered a period of careful quantitative chemical and morphometric analyses of various tissues in order to test hypotheses.

Abnormal cardiac conduction and abnormal regulation of breathing aggravated by infection have been proposed as likely causes of SIDS. In general, the hypothesis is that infants who die suddenly, unexpectedly, and without a sufficient cause being found at post-mortem examination share an abnormality in the autonomic regulation of cardiovascular and/or respiratory activity that can be triggered or exaggerated by a stimulus such as inflammation of the respiratory tract; this is generally called the *apnea hypothesis*.

This chapter discusses the contributions that epidemiologists and pathologists have made to our understanding of SIDS and presents the observations that sleep and cardiorespiratory physiologists have made about a high-risk state called *apnea of infancy* (AoI), which is generally heralded by sudden onset of apnea with cyanosis or pallor prompting resuscitative efforts by parents or caretakers.

PATHOLOGY

Following the suggestion that histologic abnormalities of the His bundle might predispose to lethal conduction disturbances (James, 1968), several investigators have now shown that the structure of the conduction system from the sinoatrial node through the His bundle does not deviate in unexpected death

from that seen after expected death in infancy (Valdes-Dapena et al, 1973; Lie et al, 1976). Structures of other components of the cardiovascular control system, e.g., carotid and aortic baroreceptors, stellate ganglia, and central vagal nuclei, have not been systematically examined. Some evidence suggests that the central vagal nuclei might be affected (Takashima, Armstrong, Becker, and Bryan, 1978). Although there is no histologic evidence that suggests death due to a rhythm disturbance in most infants, there are isolated reports of death due to QT syndrome (Maron et al, 1976; Smith et al, 1979; Southall et al, 1979) and to Wolff-Parkinson-White syndrome (Keeton et al, 1977; Southall et al, 1979). One unconfirmed report calls attention to the possibility that beat-to-beat regulation of cardiac repolarization (QT versus RR interval) may be defective in some SIDS victims (Sadeh et al, 1987).

Most recent efforts have focused on searching for evidence of the anatomic expression of the apnea hypothesis, either by examining the carotid body and brain stem, the structures responsible for regulation of normoxia and normocarbia, or by searching for indirect evidence of hypoxia in the brain, blood vessels, heart, liver, adrenal glands, and brown fat. Acute hypoxia affects primarily the organs with the greatest energy requirements, the heart and brain. This may explain the observation of focal coronary artery and myocardial necrosis in the hearts of infants who are stillborn or who die shortly after birth or are victims of SIDS (DeSa, 1979) and of brainstem gliosis in SIDS (Naeye, 1976; Takashima, Armstrong, Becker, and Bryan, 1978). At first it seems surprising that gliosis from hypoxia might affect the brainstem and not the cerebral cortex. Myers (1973) has shown in primates, however, that asphyxia first alters histologic features of the watershed zones, particularly in the brainstem in the region of nuclei that regulate autonomic function. Astroglial proliferation in the brainstem (Naeye, 1976; Kinney et al, 1983) around the nucleus of the solitary tract, dorsal motor nucleus of the vagus, and nucleus ambiguus (Takashima, Armstrong, Becker, and Bryan, 1978; Takashima, Armstrong, Becker, and Huber, 1978) may represent the basis for abnormal breathing activity or may follow hypoxia. Such a pathologic feature is evident not only in SIDS victims who manifest other signs of hypoxia but also in preterm infants who experience

Supported by USPH Grant #RO1 HD11965.

Table 70–1. PERCENTAGE OF SMALL (<2 μm) MYELINATED VAGAL FIBERS (MVF) IN SIDS VICTIMS

	No. Subjects	Average No. MVF	Average % MVF < 2 μm
SIDS infants	22	24,003	7.24
Controls	14	30,062	18.7

(Data from Sachis PN, Armstrong DL, Becker LE, and Bryan AC: The vagus nerve and sudden infant death syndrome: a morphometric study. J Pediatr 98:278, 1981.)

prolonged apnea spells and in infants who die of cyanotic heart disease (Takashima, Armstrong, Becker, and Bryan, 1978; Takashima, Armstrong, Becker, and Huber, 1978). Whether these findings represent cause or effect, they have focused attention on defective autonomic regulation of respiration and/or cardiac output as a critical factor in explaining SIDS.

If apnea is the consequence of defective control of breathing, structural alterations might be anticipated in the neuromuscular components of the control system. Only the brainstem and carotid bodies have been examined by two or more groups of investigators, and the vagus nerve by one. As previously noted, brainstem astrogliosis has been confirmed. There is less agreement that the carotid body is histologically abnormal. Cole and associates (1979) have reported glomus cells to be smaller and chemoreceptor granules fewer in six SIDS victims; their control population, however, was inadequate to draw firm conclusions. Naeye, Fisher, Ryser, and Whalen (1976) found increased glomus volume in 23 per cent of SIDS victims whose pulmonary arteries were excessively muscular. This finding is consistent with evidence for increased volume of chemoreceptor cells in humans (Saldana et al, 1973) and various animals (Edwards et al, 1971) who have resided at high altitude and have therefore experienced chronic hypoxia. However, Naeye, Fisher, Ryser, and Whalen (1976) also found that glomus volume was significantly reduced in another 63 per cent of SIDS victims who had less consistent evidence of chronic hypoxia. The actual glomus volumes in these subjects were comparable to volumes in those dying from other causes examined by Dinsdale and colleagues (1977). Therefore, the histologic and histochemical features of the carotid body must be extensively studied before these preliminary findings can be accepted. An exciting but unconfirmed observation is a paucity of small myelinated nerve fibers in the cervical vagus (Sachis et al, 1981) (Table 70–1).

Smooth muscle in small pulmonary arteries but not in renal arteries is thicker (Naeye, Whalen, Ryser, and Fisher, 1976) and extends farther into the periphery of the lung (Williams et al, 1979) in SIDS victims than in infants who die of accidents. Although thickening can occur with hypoxia and increased pulmonary artery pressure or flow (Levin et al, 1978), extension appears to be more specific for chronic or repeated alveolar hypoxia. One study was unable to

confirm the presence of thicker pulmonary arteries (Kendeel and Ferris, 1977), but observer bias or the wide variance inherent in the point-count method may have affected the results. The degree of muscle hyperplasia appears to correlate with the extent of astrogliosis in the brainstem (Fig. 70–1). As impedance to flow of blood through the pulmonary circulation increases, thickening of right ventricular muscle would be expected, but evidence for this alteration in SIDS is divergent (Guntheroth, 1973; Naeye, Whalan, Ryser, and Fisher, 1976). The right ventricular weights in hearts of SIDS victims were similar to those of controls in two separate blinded studies, but Naeye, Whalan, Ryser, and Fisher (1976) found the weights in controls to be significantly less, which may explain why they concluded that the right ventricle in SIDS victims was hypertrophied.

Intrathoracic petechiae, originally considered evidence for airway obstruction (Beckwith, 1970), probably indicate sustained perimortal hypoxia (Guntheroth, 1973).

Other changes that might reflect recurrent or chronic hypoxia, such as increased periadrenal brown fat, hepatic erythropoiesis, adrenal medullary depletion, increased fat-laden cells in the cerebrospinal fluid, fatty metamorphosis around the tapetum, and failure of regression of reticulodendritic spines in the reticular formation, are controversial or unconfirmed (Naeye, 1974; Gadsdon and Emery, 1976; Naeye, 1976; Valdes-Dapena et al, 1976; Emery and Dinsdale, 1978; Quattrochi et al, 1980). For example, Valdes-Dapena and associates (1976) found an increased percentage of multilobular fat cells (brown fat) in the perirenal pannus, but only in those infants who died at 5.1 months or older, an age by which most SIDS deaths have already occurred.

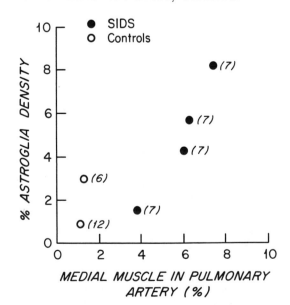

Figure 70–1. The percentage of area in brainstem sections occupied by astroglia compared with the percentage of area in pulmonary arteries occupied by smooth muscle in victims of sudden infant death syndrome (SIDS) (28) and controls (18). (Data from Naeye RL: Brain-stem and adrenal abnormalities in the sudden infant death syndrome. Am J Clin Pathol 66:526, 1976.)

Recognizing that apnea could follow acute dynamic airway obstruction, Pinkham and Beckwith (1970) examined the larynx, identified local necrosis of the vocal cords, and suggested that such a finding might support the hypothesis that airway obstruction was a factor. However, a more careful extensive study by Cullity and Emery (1975) found equal incidences of ulceration or necrosis in victims of SIDS and sudden deaths of recognized cause. Another unconfirmed study suggests that mucous glands occupy a higher than expected percentage of the vestibular folds in SIDS victims (Fink and Beckwith, 1980); however, two of ten controls had cystic fibrosis, which affects mucous gland structure and may have biased the results, although the bias might be expected to obscure differences because of increased mucous glands in these subjects.

The potential role played by apparently minor infections is discussed in the sections entitled "Pathology" and "Infection and Immunity."

There are, then, subtle changes in several organs, particularly the brain and lungs in about two thirds of cases of SIDS. These changes antedate death by at least several weeks and can be interpreted as evidence of hypoxia-ischemia that occurred without symptoms in most infants. The relative contributions of ventilatory and circulatory failure to these changes have not been resolved. Likewise, the primary or secondary role of gliosis around brainstem nuclei that regulate ventilation and circulation in such failure must be elucidated. The lack of these changes in a third of cases suggests that SIDS has several causes.

INFECTION AND IMMUNITY

Between 40 and 75 per cent of SIDS victims have evidence of mild respiratory tract infections (Beckwith, 1970). The seasonality of deaths due to SIDS may be linked to the increased likelihood of infection and parallels that of deaths due to recognized causes (Kraus and Borhani, 1972). Thus, winter with its attendant increase in respiratory infections is associated with an increased risk of infant deaths, both sudden and expected. Collectively, various studies have reported an association of SIDS with the full range of respiratory viruses isolated from secretions (Gold et al, 1961; Nelson et al, 1975; Ogra et al, 1975; Roberts, 1975; Tapp et al, 1975; Bonser et al, 1978; Scott et al, 1978). However, neither viremia nor increased interferon level has been identified (Seto and Carver, 1978). Only respiratory syncytial virus has been associated with episodic apnea (Bruhn et al, 1977). If this association is related to hypoxemia during the infection, it may be significant that this study was performed in Denver, Colorado, where normal Pa_{O_2} is 75 mm Hg; on the other hand, apnea might also represent an abnormal response to nasal obstruction or to airway irritation.

Arnon and colleagues (1978) found *Clostridium botulinum* organisms and/or toxin in 4.3 per cent of SIDS victims in 1977 in Los Angeles and concluded that *C. botulinum* accounted for these deaths. However, most infants with botulism present with constipation, weakness, and cranial nerve deficits and would not be considered SIDS victims if they died of ventilatory failure (Arnon et al, 1977). The origin of the organisms and toxin is unknown (Arnon et al, 1979), but one report calls attention to the presence of *C. botulinum* organisms in the stools of asymptomatic infants and those with other clinical syndromes (Thompson et al, 1980).

Amnionitis in preterm births is associated with SIDS (Naeye, 1977), and the risk of death due to SIDS in preterm infants is increased severalfold. If the association with infected decidua is confirmed, it would suggest that intrauterine septicemia, a recognized cause of hypoxia-ischemia, might be responsible for altered brainstem structure and function.

Few studies have reported systematic examination of immunologically active tissues. There is a suggestion that splenic germinal centers are increased and that the thymus is depleted in those who die with infection (Sinclair-Smith et al, 1976; Borzanji and Emery, 1977), but not in those who do not. Levels of immunoglobulins G, A, M, and E in serum and immunofluorescence to these major immunoglobulin classes in lung tissue are comparable in SIDS victims and controls (Ogra et al, 1975; Turner et al, 1975); however, six of the eight SIDS victims in one study had no evidence of secretory component in bronchial tissue, whereas all eight controls had this component (Ogra et al, 1975). This observation must be pursued, because it suggests a mechanism for systemic penetration of potent antigens that might trigger anaphylaxis.

Summary. Mild infection contributes to infant deaths of known cause as well as those due to SIDS; in both groups, infection is associated with a male preponderance. The mechanism by which mild infection triggers acute ventilatory or circulatory failure is unknown. Two possibilities are suggested by published data. Depletion of vagal innervation may predispose to an altered response to irritation similar to that in preterm infants (Fleming et al, 1978), or a defect in production or degradation of the secretory component of IgA may predispose to anaphylaxis.

CHEMISTRY AND TOXICOLOGY

Alterations in chemistry have not explained SIDS. Electrolyte composition and levels of creatinine, urea nitrogen, and protein in vitreous humor (Hillman et al, 1980) and concentrations of divalent cations of calcium, magnesium, copper, zinc, and selenium in plasma (Blumenfeld et al, 1979; Hillman et al, 1980) and liver (Lapin et al, 1976) in SIDS victims are similar to those in infants who die of known cause. Magnesium deficiency causes death in weanling rats (Caddell, 1978) but apparently is not responsible for SIDS (Blumenfeld et al, 1979; Hillman et al, 1980).

Exploring the hypothesis that abnormal regulation of blood glucose might promote hypoglycemia as infants extend nocturnal sleeping, Naeye and colleagues (1980) found in 26 SIDS victims that neither plasma cortisol nor growth hormone level was reduced and that in those SIDS victims with nonlethal infection, plasma insulin concentration was reduced. Hypoglycemia is therefore not a likely cause of SIDS. Nevertheless, individual case reports attest to sudden death with a metabolic basis. One such infant apparently died of Addison's disease at 9 months of age (Russell et al, 1977); in another, fatal apnea occurred during a bicarbonate infusion (Buchanan et al, 1978). Post-mortem artifact probably explains elevation of 25-hydroxyvitamin D (Hillman et al, 1980), further refuting the hypothesis that hypocalcemic tetany is a cause of SIDS.

Although serum analysis of 130 cases of SIDS failed to identify toxic levels of ethanol, barbiturate, salicylate, organic bases, or opiates (Smialek and Monforte, 1977), several reports have now confirmed an association between narcotic addiction in mothers, particularly to methadone and cocaine, and sudden death in their infants (Rajegowda et al, 1978; Chavez et al, 1979; Finnegan, 1979; Chasnoff et al, 1985). Even when socioeconomic factors are controlled, the risk is increased 4.8-fold, to 24.7:1000 live births (Chavez et al, 1979). These infants are primarily boys, are full term but small for gestational age, and die without detectable amounts of drugs in body fluids (Rajegowda et al, 1978). These data suggest that methadone may produce its effect even after clearance from the circulation, that methadone bound in brain may be important, or that maternal addiction is associated with another unmeasured risk factor. Olsen and Lees (1980) have shown that brainstem regulation of breathing is depressed in babies with measurable quantities of methadone in plasma and that this depression, although improved, continues after the drug has been cleared from plasma at several weeks of age.

On the basis of observations by McCandless and Hodgkin (1977) that altered breathing control in Leigh's subacute necrotizing encephalopathy might be due to defects in thiamine-dependent pathways of energy production in the brainstem, altered thiamine metabolism has been proposed as a cause of SIDS (Read, 1978). Davis and colleagues (1980) found elevated thiamine and folate levels in plasma but no pyridoxal or vitamin B_{12} in 121 SIDS victims compared with 26 controls. On the other hand, Peterson and associates (1981), comparing post-mortem levels of erythrocyte transketolase in 20 SIDS victims and 17 infants dying of other causes with levels measured in 22 live controls, found no significant differences.

An unconfirmed study has reported elevated fetal hemoglobin levels in SIDS victims (Giulian et al, 1987) after 5 weeks of age. Other studies (Roe et al, 1986; Duran et al, 1986; Harpey et al, 1987) have reported sudden deaths secondary to medium-chain acyl coenzyme A dehydrogenase deficiency. However, these are most frequent after 6 months of age, a time at which 95 per cent of all SIDS cases have already occurred.

Finally, many studies have now associated prenatal smoking in mothers with SIDS in their infants (Steele and Langworth, 1966; Bergman and Wiesnes, 1976; Naeye, Ladis, and Drage, 1976). The risk of SIDS is highest in black mothers who smoke. Smoking, in turn, has been associated with placenta previa, abruption, preterm births, and inadequate weight for gestational age (Comstock et al, 1971; Butler et al, 1972; Oakley et al, 1978). In addition, carboxyhemoglobin level in infants is 80 per cent higher than in their smoking mothers and is associated with structural alteration in placental and umbilical arteries (Comstock et al, 1971).

Summary. There is confirmation that methadone and cocaine addiction as well as cigarette smoking is associated with increased risk of SIDS, but none of these factors has been proved causal. Methadone may be related through its effects on brainstem regulation of breathing. Smoking and maternal cocaine use are associated with SIDS, but the physiologic effects of various components of cigarette smoke and metabolic products of cocaine on the fetus and infant are largely unknown.

EPIDEMIOLOGY

The promise of an epidemiologic investigation of SIDS is that it will define one or more characteristics that might uniquely describe infants at risk, suggest causality, and permit prospective identification. Achievement has fallen short of that hope, in part because of inadequate study design and in part because of limitations inherent in the methods. In an ideal study design, subjects and controls are alike in all but the characteristic to be compared; lacking that ideal, they should be matched in order to increase the power of observed differences, i.e., the likelihood that observed differences are both statistically significant and clinically meaningful. Given comparable subjects and controls, data must be collected prospectively. Retrospective comparison increases the risks of subjective bias and incomplete ascertainment. Multivariate analysis should be applied in order to ferret out discriminant variables; cluster analysis should be employed to better visualize the relationship of one variable to another. Finally, results should be supported by independent assessment of comparable groups, preferably in separate geographic areas.

Several limitations of epidemiologic investigations of SIDS must be understood before one examines published data. First, by chance alone, 1 in 20 variables compared will be significantly different at the 5 per cent level, yielding false clues. Second, one assumes that among the variables compared are those that will best discriminate at-risk and control infants, but the key variables may not have been analyzed or were not available. Third, if SIDS is due to more than one cause, the variables found to distinguish at-risk infants will be a collage of characteristics of the several underlying diseases, each with different sex ratios, age distributions, or seasonal variations. Finally, for each distinguishing variable there may be a converse interpretation; for instance, an unequal sex ratio may mean a higher risk for one or increased protection for the other or both.

We will discuss those variables that have been reported according to whether they existed during pregnancy, during labor and delivery, in the neonatal period, or at the time of death. We will judge as *confirmed* those characteristics identified in two or more independent, controlled studies in which ascertainment of that characteristic was 90 per cent or greater, and as *suggestive* those findings identified in one such study in which ascertainment was less than 90 per cent. In only two epidemiologic studies of SIDS were data collected prospectively for the purpose of discovering variables associated with SIDS (Naeye, Ladis, and Drage, 1976; Biering-Sorensen et al, 1978, 1979). In the majority of study reports there was no clear statement that retrospective examination of records or interview of parents was performed without the interviewer's knowledge of their group designation; in only two studies were the data collected without this bias (Naeye, Ladis, and Drage, 1976; Arsenault, 1980).

Various characteristics confirmed as significantly different during pregnancy, labor, and delivery and in the home environment both before and after birth all support the conclusion that an at-risk state of altered physiology is seriously affected by the psychosocial milieu. As we will see, there are also subtle structural expressions of these alterations. The risk of SIDS is increased if the mother is younger than 20 years of age (Steele and Langworth, 1966; Froggatt et al, 1971; Kraus and Borhani, 1972; Biering-Sorensen et al, 1978, 1979; Peterson et al, 1979; Arsenault, 1980), unmarried (Kraus and Borhani, 1972; Spiers and Wang, 1976; Biering-Sorenson et al, 1979; Peterson et al, 1979), or poor (Protestos et al, 1973; Spiers and Wang, 1976; Biering-Sorenson et al, 1979); delayed or even failed to seek prenatal care (Kraus and Borhani, 1972; Naeye, Ladis, and Drage, 1976; Peterson et al, 1979); had a short interpregnancy interval (Spiers and Wang, 1976; Carpenter et al, 1977); was ill during the pregnancy (Froggatt et al, 1968; Naeye, Ladis, and Drage, 1976); had experienced previous fetal loss (Protestos et al, 1973; Naeye, Ladis, and Drage, 1976; Arsenault, 1980); smoked cigarettes (Steele and Langworth, 1966; Bergman and Wiesnes, 1976; Naeye, Ladis, and Drage, 1976; Oakley et al, 1978); or abused narcotics (Rajegowda et al, 1978; Chasnoff et al, 1985). The risk is also increased if the father is younger than 20 years old (Froggatt et al, 1971; Biering-Sorensen et al, 1979) or of low social or economic level (Cooke and Welch, 1964; Froggatt et

al, 1971; Kraus and Borhani, 1972). Independent of economics, ethnicity is important. In the United States, where the overall risk is about 2.0:1000 births (Peterson, 1966; Kraus and Borhani, 1972; Peterson, 1972; Standfast et al, 1979), Orientals experience the lowest risk (0.51:1000), and American Indians (5.93) (Kraus and Borhani, 1972), Alaskan natives (4.5) (Fleshman and Peterson, 1977), and poor blacks (5.04) (Valdes-Dapena et al, 1968) the highest. Similar variation is observed in comparing other countries; the rate in Denmark is 0.92 (Biering-Sorenson et al, 1979), in Ireland 2.8 (Froggatt et al, 1971), and in Tasmania, where the rate among Maori is nearly twice that of infants of European stock, 2.98 (Grice and McGlashan, 1978). Interpretation of the meaning of these observations and of their interrelationships is complicated by the fact that discriminant or cluster analyses are incomplete or not available. Furthermore, controls have generally been chosen for their health. One study of deaths among infants discharged from a newborn intensive care unit suggests that low socioeconomic level, youth, lack of marriage, and being nonwhite are maternal factors that also increase the risk of death due to known causes such as congenital defects (Kulkarni et al, 1978). Two other studies found that there were no differences in social and economic factors between SIDS victims and infants who died of recognized causes (Cameron and Watson, 1975; McWeeny and Emery, 1975). Thus, many of the previously listed associations appear to lack specificity. Social and economic instability in parents seems to increase the likelihood of infant death, whether due to SIDS or not. Perhaps these factors reflect inadequate intellectual and economic resources that lead to delayed recognition of illness. Alternatively, some infants whose deaths are explained at autopsy may share the pathophysiology that characterizes SIDS.

Three studies showed differences in maternal blood groups; however, there is disagreement over what is different, an increase in type O (Arsenault, 1980) or an increase in type B (Steele and Langworth, 1966; Naeye, Ladis, and Drage, 1976). Ascertainment was less than 50 per cent in each of the studies citing type B increase. Furthermore, interethnic A and B gene frequencies are so different that these results are not interpretable without controlling for ethnic origin. Even among Eskimo of various origins the frequency of the B gene is highly variable, being 18 per cent in Point Barrow and 0 in Thule (Mourant et al, 1976). It might be especially significant that blacks have a higher frequency of B gene and lower frequency of A gene than whites of Northern European origin. Perhaps Froggatt and associates (1968) failed to find a difference in blood groups in Northern Ireland because the population there is ethnically homogeneous and nonblack.

Although there is only a suggestion that third-trimester bleeding and maternal sedation or anesthesia play a role (Protestos et al, 1973), there is agreement that a number of abnormal characteristics of birth and delivery predicate increased risk. Preterm birth (Peterson, 1966; Richards and McIntosh, 1972; Protestos et al, 1973; Naeye, Ladis, and Drage, 1976; Naeye, Messmer, Spech, and Merritt, 1976; Spiers, 1976) and low birth weight for gestational age (Kraus and Borhani, 1972; Arsenault, 1980) both increase risk. Apgar scores tend to be lower (Naeye, Ladis, and Drage, 1976; Carpenter et al, 1977), and resuscitative efforts with oxygen and ventilatory support are more frequently required (Protestos et al, 1973; Naeye, Ladis, and Drage, 1976). Being second or third in birth order carries a higher risk than being first. Infants who are products of multiple-birth pregnancies carry special risks (Froggatt et al, 1971; Protestos et al, 1973; Carpenter et al, 1977; Arsenault, 1980), but Cooke and Welch (1964) also observed more twins than expected among those with known causes of death. Being the lighter-weight twin carries no increased risk of SIDS (Froggatt et al, 1971), but being the second twin born does (Standfast et al, 1980). Triplets are at even greater risk (8.3:1000). Several twin pairs, both dizygous and monozygous, have died on the same day (Cooke and Welch, 1964; Froggatt et al, 1971; Arsenault, 1980). Among 32 twin pairs recorded (Cooke and Welch, 1964; Strimer et al, 1969; Froggatt et al, 1971; Richards and McIntosh, 1972; Peterson et al, 1980), three pairs were found dead together. Even though the denominator is certainly an underestimate, this observation is striking and indicates the probability of a strong environmental influence acting against an abnormal physiologic background in these infants. Taken together with epidemiologic and pathologic observations, these data suggest that perinatal hypoxia either results from an underlying autonomic defect or causes the physiologic instability that predisposes to SIDS.

Few neonatal problems that are common to SIDS infants have surfaced in various studies, but there does appear to be an increased incidence of feeding difficulties (Naeye, Ladis, and Drage, 1976; Carpenter et al, 1977). Unconfirmed observations show head molding, hypotonicity, and jitteriness to be less common than expected.

Most investigators have focused on events surrounding the time of death and in the preceding weeks. Infants tend to die asleep, at night, in any position (Froggatt et al, 1971; Biering-Sorenson et al, 1979), between 1 and 4 months of age, and during winter months (Peterson, 1966; Steele and Langworth, 1966; Froggatt et al, 1971; Peterson, 1972; Peterson et al, 1980). Likewise, summer months, the awake state, and age over 6 months appear to be protective. No study has compared the proportion who die during sleep with the amount of time that an infant sleeps at various ages. In comparing age at death to cause of death (SIDS versus recognized cause), Kraus and Borhani (1972) noted that the peak age of death due to either SIDS or other causes was 1 to 3 months of age for all infants born during 2-month periods, with two exceptions; for those born in May and June, there was no peak month of death, and for those born in July and August, age at death peaked at 4 to 5 months, overlapping the deaths of infants born during September and October. Thus, summer and fall are sparing, and winter's risks increase the chances of death during the early months of life from SIDS as well as recognized causes.

There is general agreement that SIDS victims tend to have mild respiratory or gastrointestinal symptoms in the preceding week (Froggatt et al, 1971; Richardson and McIntosh, 1972; Biering-Sorensen et al, 1979) and that some require admission to hospital in the interval from birth to death (Froggatt et al, 1968, 1971; Biering-Sorensen et al, 1979). In various studies, however, 25 to 75 per cent were free of such symptoms or history at the time of death. Poor weight gain after birth was found in one study (Naeye, Ladis, and Drage, 1976) but was not significant in another (Froggatt et al, 1971). In comparison with siblings, afflicted infants have been described by their parents as less active, less responsive, and having an unusual cry (Stark and Nathanson, 1975; Naeye, Ladis, and Drage, 1976; Golub and Corwin, 1982). These recollections could be affected by fading and sad memories of the dead or by positive reinforcement of the living. It is tempting to relate an abnormal cry to altered brainstem function, especially because there are no adequate explanations of laryngeal abnormalities.

Nearly all investigators (eight of those reviewed here) agree that maleness is a risk. Kraus and Borhani (1972) and McWeeny and Emery (1975) have observed similar male-to-female ratios among infants who died of known causes. This correlation, then, may reflect a natural protection of females from adversity and may have no special relevance to SIDS. As previously stated, when SIDS victims are stratified for presence or absence of infection, the increased proportion of boys is found only in the group manifesting infection.

Prompted by a theory that anaphylaxis to milk protein might be causative, several investigators have explored the possibility that breast milk might be protective. Two investigations have failed to find a difference in death rate between breast-fed infants and bottle-fed infants (Steele and Langworth, 1966; Froggatt et al, 1971). Similarly, Biering-Sorensen and colleagues (1978) found no difference in the age at death between Danish bottle-fed and breast-fed babies and no change in death rate between 1956 and 1971, when feeding infants on breast milk alone declined from 52 to 25 per cent.

Summary. Epidemiologic studies have confirmed or suggested various associations between SIDS and events that occur during gestation, labor, delivery, and the neonatal and immediate premortal periods. Definitive discriminative and cluster analyses have not been reported. When the most discriminative variables were evaluated prospectively in two studies, SIDS was found to have occurred in only 1 per cent of those at highest risk (Naeye, Ladis, and Drage,

1976; Carpenter et al, 1977). Furthermore, many of the associations that have been described are true for both SIDS and deaths due to recognized causes. Thus, infants who die of recognized causes share certain pathobiologic and psychosocial features with those who die of SIDS. Furthermore, because SIDS is probably one outcome of several diseases, one cannot be certain how various epidemiologic features should be attributed. Evidence suggests that the preponderance of afflicted boys is related to infection. The striking risk among infants born to methadone-addicted mothers suggests a mechanism of death based on the effects of narcotics on brainstem regulation of breathing. Observed ethnic differences need to be discriminated from attendant social factors in order to better define the nature of the increased risk in blacks and American Indians and the very low risk in Japanese and Danes.

GENETICS

As previously mentioned, the risk of SIDS is increased in twins, especially the second born (Standfast et al, 1980), but is independent of zygosity (Speer, 1973). In some families there is aggregation of SIDS, with risks of 2.1 per cent in subsequent siblings of SIDS infants who were singleton births and 4.2 per cent in survivors of twins (Cooke and Welch, 1964). Although this pattern does not follow mendelian inheritance, it suggests either nonmendelian factors or the presence of a strong environmental influence during gestation or postnatal life. A number of twin pairs, both monozygous and dizygous, have died or have experienced AoI within hours of each other (Cooke and Welch, 1964; Speer, 1973; Peterson et al, 1980), strengthening the argument for potent environmental factors. The rate of SIDS in infants whose families have had two or more previous SIDS is approximately 19 per cent (Oren et al, 1987). We have seen six families who experienced three or more SIDS deaths, suggesting a genetic or repeated environmental influence in some families.

Several studies have now focused on the possibility of abnormalities in respiratory pattern and control that might be shared by parents or siblings of the lost infant. At this time, their conclusions appear to be divergent. Kelly and associates (1980) found that siblings have more periodic breathing when they sleep, but Hoppenbrouwers and colleagues (1980) found siblings to have less short apnea at various ages during the first 6 months of life. Although the second group of investigators did not analyze their data for periodic breathing, the associated apnea should have been registered by computer analysis. Perhaps the difference is that the first group carried out their investigation in the subjects' homes and the second in a hospital laboratory, where sleep might have been disturbed. In one family in which the father and three of five adult sons manifested obstructive sleep apnea, one of the 14 grandchildren

died of SIDS (Strohl et al, 1978). There is no way to test the statistical significance of this association.

Explorations of chemoreceptor control in parents of SIDS victims have yielded mixed results. Zwillich and associates (1980), comparing parents of one SIDS victim or even parents of one SIDS and one AoI victim to controls, found no difference in ventilatory response during carbon dioxide rebreathing, but Schiffman and colleagues (1980) have observed diminished responses in parents of SIDS victims, especially when inhaling against added inspiratory resistance. Normalizing these data for body surface area to permit intergroup comparison shows that controls in the Schiffman study exhibited a more brisk response than controls in the Zwillich study, whereas the parents of SIDS victims had similar responses. This difference, however, would not account for the second observation, that the ventilatory response to carbon dioxide during inspiratory loading increased in controls and decreased in parents of SIDS victims. Finally, Zwillich and associates (1980) found no alteration in hypoxic ventilatory chemosensitivity. In an attempt to answer this question more critically, we selected for subjects parents whose infants had documented blunting of the ventilatory response to carbon dioxide (Shannon et al, 1977), four of whom had died and had been diagnosed as SIDS victims at post-mortem examination (Shannon and Kelly, 1977). For controls, we selected twice as many adults of similar age who had no history of apnea or SIDS in their families (Kanarek et al, 1981). The ventilatory responses to carbon dioxide rebreathing and to progressive hypoxia were similar in subjects and controls collectively and when segregated by sex.

Summary. No data support a genetic influence in general in SIDS. Although SIDS occurs repeatedly in some families, even in association with abnormal breathing control in the infants, there is no confirmed evidence that this defect is transmitted genetically. Because SIDS probably encompasses many disease states, future investigations should focus on parents of infants whose physiologic defect is known.

CARDIOVASCULAR ABNORMALITIES

The chief hypotheses propose that cardiovascular failure results either from exaggeration of a normal reflex response, such as the diving reflex (Angell-James and Daley, 1972) or the laryngeal chemoreflex (Downing and Lee, 1975; Harding et al, 1975), or from qualitative defects in cardiovascular control (Ferrer and Jesse, 1977; Keeton et al, 1977; Takashima, Armstrong, Becker, and Bryan, 1978). The former possibility is discussed in "Apnea and Respiratory Control."

Although previous reports suggested a defective His bundle (Ferrer and Jesse, 1977; Valdes-Dapena et al, 1980), the heart muscle and the conduction system from the sinoatrial node through the His bundle are generally normal when tissues are compared with those obtained from age-matched controls (Valdes-Dapena et al, 1973, 1980).

Arrhythmias rank high as a cause of sudden death in adults (Liberthson et al, 1974), but they appear to account for only a small fraction of SIDS cases. Prolongation of the QT interval has indeed been identified before death or resuscitation, but in only four cases (Maron et al, 1976; Smith et al, 1979). An optimistic report that suggested a familial defect in 14 per cent of parents of SIDS victims (Maron et al, 1976) has been followed by several better-controlled studies that found no such association (Kukolich et al, 1977; Steinschneider, 1978). In adults, prolongation beyond 0.5 sec has been associated with a tendency to fatal ventricular arrhythmia (Liberthson et al, 1974), perhaps owing to reentry of a depolarizing current during this vulnerable period. The mechanism may be an imbalance of control between the right and left stellate ganglia (Schwartz et al, 1975). The QT interval in one series of 21 AoI cases and three infants who later died of SIDS was not prolonged (Kelly et al, 1977). Nor is this electrical interval prolonged in siblings of SIDS victims (Williams et al, 1979). In fact, the corrected QT interval may be shorter in the AoI cases, particularly during active sleep, in which the average interval is 0.416 sec, compared with 0.435 sec in normal infants, suggesting an increase in catecholamine activity (Haddad, Epstein, Epstein et al, 1979). The dynamic relationship of changes in the RR interval to the QT interval has been evaluated by computer from 5000 consecutive heartbeats in 10 SIDS victims and 29 matched controls. In 5 of 10 SIDS victims there was minimal change in QT, with RR intervals increasing the likelihood of blocked conduction or a reentrant rhythm (Sadeh et al, 1987). Likewise, Wolff-Parkinson-White syndrome has also been identified in SIDS and AoI by the finding of aberrant conduction bundle or electrocardiographic (ECG) characteristics (Keeton et al, 1977; Lipsitt et al, 1979; Southall et al, 1979). Several other infants have presented with sudden collapse and with ECG evidence of sinoatrial node block and junctional escape patterns (Maron et al, 1976; Keeton et al, 1977).

If defective autonomic cardiovascular control predisposes to SIDS, abnormalities in cardiac rate or variability would be expected.

Descriptions of heart rate and, more importantly, of heart rate variability in normal infants as a function of age and environment (hospital or home) are just becoming available (Katona and Egbert, 1978; Haddad et al, 1980; Leistner et al, 1980; Southall et al, 1980). Average heart rate at any postnatal age varies with gestational age at birth (Katona and Egbert, 1978); a 12-week-old preterm infant at home has a mean rate of 141 beats/min compared with 123 beats/min for a 12-week-old full-term baby. The latter value is comparable to 125 beats/min for 12-week-old full-term infants studied in the laboratory. Thus, although gestational age at birth and postnatal age

influence heart rate, the laboratory environment does not appear to alter average heart rate in normal full-term babies. Heart rate variability in a full-term infant exceeds that in a preterm infant, according to Southall and colleagues (1980) who studied heart rates in the first weeks of life using a 24-hour in-hospital recording; neonatal heart rate is slightly higher and the range is greater in active sleep than in quiet sleep. These observations may be related to increased catecholamine levels in active sleep (Haddad, Epstein, Epstein et al, 1979).

Do values in SIDS or AoI victims differ from these norms? Increase in heart rate during sleep has been identified in the first 6 months of life in both AoI victims (Leistner et al, 1980) (Fig. 70–2) and in siblings of SIDS victims (Harper et al, 1978) compared with normal babies, but the increases were generally only a few beats per minute. These small differences would not explain increased vulnerability to death but do point to altered autonomic function. Leistner and co-workers (1980) found heart rate variability as well as beat-to-beat variability in rate to be less in AoI victims than in normal infants during both active and quiet sleep at various ages up to 4 months. On the other hand, the range of heart rate variability following controlled exposure to white noise was greater in one infant who later died of SIDS than in 24 control infants who survived infancy (Salk et al, 1974). These findings suggest an altered state of cardiovascular control. In an attempt to identify an abnormality in heart rate regulation in utero, Hoppenbrouwers and colleagues (1979) analyzed fetal heart rate recordings from 20 infants who subsequently died of SIDS but found no differences in rate or pattern compared with those in 20 infants matched for date of birth, gestational age, and weight. These observations suggest that infants with AoI represent a subset of SIDS victims, i.e., that in the majority of infants who later die of SIDS, heart rate patterns in utero are normal. However, lack of abnormal patterns on fetal monitoring does not rule out their development after birth. Alternatively, the methods used by Hopperbrouwers and colleagues may not have been sufficiently sensitive, and computer analysis of fetal heart rate data similar to that used by Leistner and associates (1980) on such data from infants might uncover differences in beat-to-beat variability.

Summary. A few infants with SIDS and AoI have well-defined defects in cardiac electrophysiology. In others, recent data suggest that autonomic cardiac repolarization is altered. Further research is needed to determine whether this difference represents an altered level of activity in a normal autonomic system, perhaps in response to hypoxia, or whether a branch of the autonomic system itself is defective.

APNEA AND RESPIRATORY CONTROL

Because sudden death without obvious cause implies cessation of autonomic regulation of cardiovas-

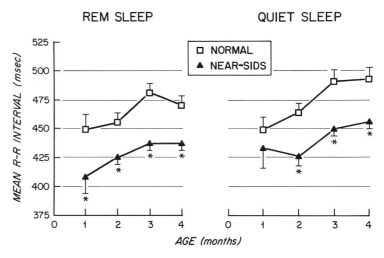

Figure 70–2. The average R–R interval from > 5000 consecutive beats in 12 apnea of infancy (AoI) patients compared with 12 age- and sex-matched normal controls during rapid eye movement (REM) sleep and quiet sleep at monthly intervals. Vertical bars are ± the standard error of the mean. The * represents significance at p < 0.05. (Data from Leistner HL et al: Heart rate and heart rate variability during sleep in aborted sudden infant death syndrome. J Pediatr 97:51–55, 1980.)

cular or respiratory activity or both, it is important to understand how normal control mechanisms maintain ventilation and prevent or terminate apnea. It is even more pertinent because several investigators have identified abnormal breathing patterns or control mechanisms in infants who later died of SIDS.

REGULATION OF SKELETAL MUSCLES OF RESPIRATION

This is a rapidly evolving area of research. Here we review only those features that are cited as important to understanding episodic apnea or hypoventilation. The respiratory control system guards against hypoxemia and hypercapnia, changing frequency and tidal volume by varying the timing of inspiratory or expiratory flow in response to metabolic demands or variations in impedance to airflow. Successful regulation involves the cooperation of innervated skeletal muscles in the upper airway and thorax acting on the passive elements in the lung so that air moves in and out of alveoli, supplying oxygen and removing carbon dioxide in proportion to needs. These muscles act under the influence of the peripheral (carotid body) and central medullary chemoreceptors in concert with vagally mediated volume feedback against the background of activity arising from the pontomedullary pacemakers (Wang and Ngai, 1964; Wyman, 1977). Lack of carotid body influence is associated primarily with modest alveolar hypoventilation, lack of increased ventilation during hypoxia (Purves, 1966; Lugliani et al, 1971), and prolonged voluntary breath-holding (Davidson et al, 1974). Lack of medullary chemoreception is accompanied by life-threatening hypoventilation during sleep. In humans, lack of vagal afferent activity would be expected to abolish the Hering-Breuer inflation reflex, cough reflex, and laryngeal chemoreflex, as well as other important autonomic reflexes. However, a clinical syndrome with these features has not been described.

Both upper airway and chest wall muscles increase

inspiratory activity in response to hypercapnia and mild hypoxia (Onal et al, 1981; Patrick et al, 1981). Studies by Megirian and associates (1980) in awake rats highlight the importance of selective entrainment of airway muscles by hypoxia and hypercapnia. The studies by Orem and co-workers (1977) of cats define the accompanying changes in airway resistance, which declines a fraction of a second before inspiration and becomes maximal at end-expiration. During expiration, activation of the cricothyroid, thyroarytenoid, and lateral cricoarytenoids narrows the glottic opening. Thus, the upper airway muscles prepare for inspired airflow just before the diaphragm and intercostals are activated and stabilize lung volume by narrowing the airway at end-expiration. The latter would be a particularly useful mechanism in a young infant with a relatively compliant chest wall. During air breathing, activation of the posterior cricoarytenoid muscles spreads the cords, and during hypoxia, laryngeal constrictor muscles dominate, particularly during expiration, thus increasing expiratory flow resistance. During hypercapnia, the muscles that open the larynx are activated during both inspiration and expiration so that both inspiratory and expiratory flow resistance are minimized (Megirian et al, 1980).

Phillipson (1978) has cited a number of changes associated with normal sleep that increase the likelihood of apnea, hypoventilation, and hypoxia. Inhibition of skeletal muscle tone and of the gamma motoneuron system during active sleep (Henderson-Smart and Read, 1978) can promote recession of the tongue and pharyngeal constrictors, resulting in a tendency to obstruction and reliance on the diaphragm alone to generate airflow. Nevertheless, obstructive sleep apnea in adults occurs primarily in stage 1 and stage 2 sleep; in fact, such adults seldom enter stage 3 or 4 or rapid eye movement (REM) sleep (Weitzman et al, 1980). Chemical regulation of breathing in dogs is less effective during active sleep (Phillipson et al, 1976), and upper airway resistance increases owing to change in tone of both skeletal and smooth muscles (Sullivan et al, 1979). Similarly, the ventilatory response to carbon dioxide in infants is reduced during active sleep, but the difference is not statistically significant (Fagenholz et al, 1976). In infants, such changes would increase vulnerability to inadequate ventilation because (1) the hypopharynx is shallow, (2) the tongue and epiglottis are more cephalad, (3) the mandible is more mobile (Tonkin, 1975), and (4) the rib cage is relatively more compliant than in a child; this latter effect may account for the decline in functional residual capacity (FRC) and P_{O_2} associated with active sleep in newborns (Martin et al, 1979). FRC, which provides a reservoir of oxygen, is low in infants compared with children or adults and decreases rapidly during apnea (Henderson-Smart and Read, 1978). This may be the result of the very compliant chest wall, of a time dependence of small-airway resistance, or of failure of glottic closure during expiration (Orem et al, 1977). Thus, there are several physiologic alterations and sites of anatomic vulnerability that appear during sleep even in a normal infant, any of which could predispose to inadequate maintenance of pulmonary gas exchange. Upper airway muscles lose tone and can narrow the nasopharynx, hypopharynx, or larynx, increasing resistance to airflow. Loss of tone in intercostal muscles, along with the reduction in tone of upper airway muscles, can result in reduction of FRC, paradoxical chest movements, a lower reservoir of oxygen in alveoli, hypoxemia, and vulnerability to rapid decline in P_{O_2} during apnea.

APNEA AND SIDS

In most deaths, apnea represents the last in a series of exhausting events. The apparent lack of such preceding events in SIDS suggests that apnea may be related primarily to defective control rather than to muscle fatigue. Prolonged apnea, defined here as lack of breathing long enough to be associated with pallor or cyanosis or with duration of 15 sec or longer, occurs more frequently than normal in AoI cases (Thoman et al, 1978; Stein et al, 1979; Southall et al, 1980), some of whom died days to months later of SIDS (Steven, 1965; Steinschneider, 1972; Guilleminault et al, 1975; McNamara, 1976; Steinschneider and Rabuzzi, 1976; Cornwell et al, 1978; Southall et al, 1980; Oren et al, 1987). Similarly excessive short apnea of 3 to 5 sec (Monod et al, 1976; Guilleminault, Ariagno, Korobkin et al, 1979) and periodic apnea (Steinschneider and Rabuzzi, 1976; Guilleminault, Ariagno, Forno et al, 1979; Kelly and Shannon, 1979) (Fig. 70–3) (Table 70–2) as well as mixed apnea (Guilleminault, Ariagno, Korobkin et al, 1979) have been observed in these infants. Mixed apnea is really central apnea with a few obstructed breaths when ventilation resumes.

One can conclude that these abnormal breathing patterns are associated with an increased risk of SIDS in some infants. The patterns can be interpreted to mean either that one or more components of the ventilatory control system are abnormal, that the system is normal but is responding excessively, or that the system has failed because of an altered chemical environment or exaggeration of airway obstruction during sleep.

Abnormal Regulatory System

Chemical Abnormalities. If the regulatory system itself is abnormal, apnea could represent failure at any level, from phasic output from respiratory centers for activation of various upper airway or chest wall muscles to the feedback of chemical or mechanical signals. In some patients there is evidence of a defect in one or more of these control components, manifested by hypoventilation and insufficient increase in ventilation during exposure to hypercapnic (Shannon and Kelly, 1977; Shannon et al, 1977) (Fig. 70–4) or hypoxic (Brady et al, 1978; Hunt et al, 1981) gas mixtures. Observations in other patients indicate that a defect in control of upper airway skeletal muscle results in partial airway obstruction (Steinschneider and Rabuzzi, 1976; Guilleminault, Ariagno, Forno et al, 1979; Guilleminault, Ariagno, Korobkin et al, 1979). The latter observation may explain the abnormal crying that has been described in SIDS victims when they have been sleeping. Arousal, which relies in part on reflex responses to rising P_{CO_2} or falling P_{O_2}, may be defective in infants with AoI (Hunt, 1981).

Mechanical Abnormalities. Other evidence suggests that the response to airway obstruction rather than its occurrence might characterize some infants at risk. Perhaps the most commonly occurring airway obstruction in normal infants accompanies nasopharyngitis. Infants with AoI have prolonged apnea more frequently during nasopharyngitis than when they are healthy (Steinschneider, 1975). On the other hand, normal infants who have nasopharyngitis at 1 to 3 months of age have short apnea (less than 10 sec) less frequently in active sleep but more frequently in quiet sleep than those who are healthy (Gould et al, 1980). Normal infants also have difficulty responding to nasal occlusion; in one study, 44 per cent of 6-week-old infants struggled but failed to establish an oral airway when the nostrils were pinched for 25 sec; this was especially evident during active sleep (Swift and Emery, 1973). The physiologic basis for the failure to maintain adequate oral ventilation during occlusion in both normal and at-risk infants is unknown. This mechanism was first suggested as a cause of SIDS by Anderson and Rosenblith (1971). Because of the observation that death with infection is linked to maleness, it is important to determine whether there are sex differences in the response to nasal obstruction.

Although there is no published evidence associating these abnormalities in the same infants with AoI, there are data from other diseases that suggest this possibility. Adults and children (Glenn et al, 1980) and some infants with central hypoventilation syn-

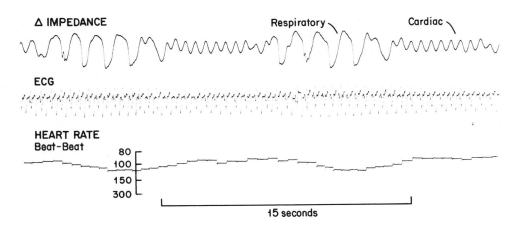

Figure 70–3. Periodic pattern of apnea seen in home recordings of an apnea of infancy (AoI) baby. The upper trace is transthoracic impedance; note the impedance change from cardiovascular activity during apnea. The middle trace is the electrocardiogram *(ECG)*. The lower trace is the instantaneous heart rate. Note changes in the heart rate that coincide with apnea occurring for a period of 15 sec.

drome (Shannon, 1980) manifest quiet-sleep hypoventilation, markedly reduced or absent chemical regulation of breathing, and obstructive sleep apnea. A similar or less severe defect could explain the observations in some infants with AoI (Shannon and Kelly, 1977; Shannon et al, 1977). We have also observed unexplained intermittent stridor and obstruction during sleep in one of our original patients who had hypoventilation and who died (Shannon and Kelly, 1977) and in several similar but unreported patients who have survived. The possible explanations for this association of findings are several. A defect in the brainstem respiratory center that coordinates innervation of upper airway and chest wall muscles (Onal et al, 1981; Patrick et al, 1981) and their responses to chemical stimulation might be at fault. As noted previously, histologic features of the brainstem are altered in SIDS and there are suggestions of structural abnormalities in carotid bodies and vagus nerves. Alternatively, the alteration in tone of one or more airway skeletal muscles that occurs during sleep could increase airflow resistance and promote hypoventilation in normal infants or cause markedly increased resistance and obstructive apnea in infants born with marginal chemoreceptor control. A similar mechanism has been thought to explain hypoventilation in patients who have adenoid hypertrophy and in whom the degree of obstruction alone was insufficient to provoke ventilatory failure (Ingram and Bishop, 1970). Finally, it should be noted that intermittent stridor may be due to laryngospasm from seizure (Nelson and Ray, 1968) or to gastroesophageal reflux (Herbst

et al, 1978; Carson et al, 1980; Leape and Ramenofsky, 1980).

No published data have so far explained how defects in chemoreceptor regulation of breathing or faulty activation of upper airway muscles in a sleeping infant might cause lethal apnea. Either would cause hypoxemia, which if severe enough should promote gasping and arousal to a state in which breathing would improve and hypoxemia would be relieved. Lack of such a response suggests that progressive hypoxia promotes a positive rather than a negative feedback effect. Positive feedback, manifested by ventilatory depression, has been described in sleeping preterm infants (Rigatto et al, 1975), in newborn lambs with carotid body denervation (Shannon, 1980), and in children with congenital central hypo-

Table 70–2. PERCENTAGE OF SLEEP TIME DURING WHICH PERIODIC APNEA OCCURS IN INFANTS WITH AoI

		Periodic Apnea (%)		
	No.	Mean	Median	No. with > 2% Periodic Apnea
AoI infants	32	4.9	1.8	15*
Controls	32	0.5	0.4	0

*Note that about one half of the SIDS subjects cannot be distinguished from controls using this criterion.

(Data from Kelly and Shannon, 1979.)

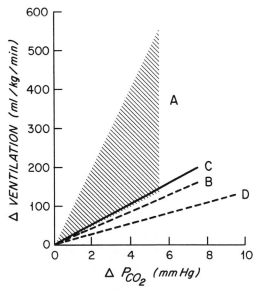

Figure 70–4. The change in ventilation plotted against the change in alveolar P_{CO_2} during quiet sleep while breathing 4 per cent CO_2. *A* and *B* represent results from Shannon and associates (1977), *C* and *D* from Olsen and Lees (1980). *A* indicates the range of values obtained from normal infants aged 1 to 8 months; *B* is the mean value for 30 apnea of infancy (AoI) infants; *C* is the mean for 4 normal controls (birth to 6 weeks); and *D* is the mean for 9 infants (birth to 6 weeks) born to methadone-addicted mothers. Note that the wide range of normality limits the usefulness of this test in discriminating illness from normality.

ventilation (CCHS) (Shannon, 1980). In each instance, progressive hypoxia induced by breathing a gas mixture at FI_{O_2} 0.15 caused a progressive fall in P_{O_2}. In one patient with CCHS, breathing 15 per cent oxygen caused acute cor pulmonale and a precipitous decline in cardiac output. Baker and McGinty (1977) observed bradycardia and hypoventilation in quiet sleep and sudden death in 10-day-old kittens raised in a 10 per cent oxygen environment.

Normal Regulatory System

Reflex Apnea. Reflex apnea is one component of the response to several common stimuli, such as water in or around the nose or larynx. An exuberant response to each has been cited as a possible cause of SIDS (Wolf, 1966; Downing and Lee, 1975; Johnson et al, 1975; Harding et al, 1975). Interest in the laryngeal chemoreceptors stems from the observation that lethal apnea can result from application of nonphysiologic fluids even though the airway is open and from the suggestion that reflux of gastric contents can cause apnea as well as aspiration pneumonia (Herbst et al, 1978; Carson et al, 1980; Leape and Ramenofsky, 1980). However, there are no published data that describe a similar fatal laryngeal reflex in human infants, nor is there proof of an association with gastroesophageal reflux or even agreement on the definition of abnormal gastroesophageal reflux. Apnea is also a component of the aortic baroreceptor reflex (Talman et al, 1980) and the Bezold-Jarisch reflex (right atrial stretching) (Dawes and Comroe, 1954).

Abnormal Chemical Environment. Hypoventilation and apnea can occur with a normal regulatory system when the chemical environment is altered. The best-documented examples are of ventilatory failure due to opiates. As described previously, infants of methadone-addicted mothers continue to hypoventilate and fail to increase ventilation appropriately with hypercapnia even after they have cleared methadone from plasma, and the incidence of SIDS in infants of methadone-addicted mothers is increased tenfold. Central hypoventilation has also been described in a number of infants with Hirschsprung disease and/or ganglioneuroblastoma. These infants are also at risk of sudden death (Haddad et al, 1978; Hunt et al, 1978; Bower and Adkins, 1980). This latter observation suggests, as observed by Haddad and associates (1980), that altered serotonin production might be a factor and that serotonin is normally involved as a neurotransmitter in the regulation of breathing, especially during quiet sleep.

Abnormal Airway Structure. Sleep-related changes in airway muscle tone might explain sleep-related obstructive apnea, which occurs in various clinical conditions. In infants with adenoid hypertrophy, obstruction occurs when the soft palate and tongue relax and appose, especially during sleep; in those with myelomeningocele, obstruction can result from sleep-related paralysis of vocal cord abduction

(Holinger et al, 1978); in Down syndrome, it may be related to midfacial hypoplasia (Loughlin et al, 1980). In adults, obstructive apnea may follow relaxation of the genioglossus (Remmers et al, 1978; Strohl et al, 1978) or change in configuration of the pharyngeal constrictors (Weitzman et al, 1978). Life-threatening apnea durig sleep has also been described in association with partial airway obstruction, as encountered with an aberrant innominate artery (Berdon et al, 1969; Mustard et al, 1969; Koivikko et al, 1976) or adenoid hypertrophy (Guilleminault et al, 1976). Investigations of breathing control in these patients have rarely been performed, but in the few reported patients with adenoid hypertrophy, chemoreceptor regulation was defective months to years after relief of obstruction (Ingram and Bishop, 1970).

Structure-Function Relationships

In five infants who had AoI and who later died of SIDS, we have found that pulmonary vascular smooth muscle extended abnormally into vessels accompanying alveoli (Williams et al, 1980) (Fig. 70–5). We have recently found the same changes in two others. Thus, all seven infants who were recognized as having AoI and who later died of SIDS manifest this marker of repeated alveolar hypoxia, which was seen in two thirds of SIDS victims examined by Naeye, Whalen, Ryser, and Fisher (1976) and by Williams and colleagues (1979).

The evidence from pathologic examination and physiologic investigation of infants with AoI, some of whom died of SIDS, suggests the following hypothesis: Some infants, born with the inability to vary the tonic and phasic activity of upper airway and

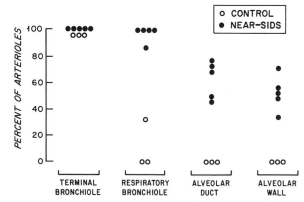

PERCENT OF VESSELS FULLY MUSCULARIZED AT SUCCESSIVE LEVELS OF THE AIRWAYS

Figure 70–5. The percentage of small pulmonary arteries (< 200 μm diameter) that contain a circumferential layer of smooth muscle in five victims of SIDS who were first identified as apnea of infancy (AoI) babies, compared with the percentage in three controls who died owing to congenital defects not associated with chronic hypoxia. Vessels were landmarked by their proximity to identifiable airways. At least 15 vessels were examined at each site by the method of Williams and associates (1979). As noted in their original study, no controls had pulmonary artery smooth muscle beyond the level of the respiratory bronchiole.

thoracic respiratory muscles in response to mechanical and chemical stimuli, are prone to abnormal ventilatory patterns that promote repeated alveolar hypoxia and consequent arterial hypoxemia. These patterns are exaggerated because of either partial obstruction of the upper airway or inadequacy of the ventilatory pump, either of which can occur during sleep even in normal infants. Alveolar hypoxia stimulates pulmonary vasoconstriction and, after repeated episodes, pulmonary vascular smooth muscle hyperplasia. Arterial hypoxemia-ischemia leads to other changes, perhaps including astrogliosis of the brainstem, a site that is particularly vulnerable in neonatal primates (Myers, 1973). This brainstem abnormality promotes hypoventilation and hypoxemia, which in turn cause further brainstem injury, constituting a life-threatening positive feedback loop. As pulmonary vascular muscularity increases, pulmonary vasoconstriction becomes more intense and right ventricular afterload becomes sufficient to promote cardiac failure and even more severe tissue hypoxia. This second positive feedback loop, acting in concert with the first, may be responsible for death. This sequence of events would explain the striking increase in death rate among infants of methadone-addicted mothers. Alternatively, excess responsiveness of the pulmonary circulation to only modest reductions in alveolar P_{O_2} would initiate a similar series of events. These proposed mechanisms would explain death only in those SIDS victims who have pathologic evidence of repeated or chronic hypoxia.

FAMILY COUNSELING

After the sudden death of an infant, medical personnel from clerks to physicians must be aware that parents need calm support and a diagnosis as soon as it is made at post-mortem examination, preferably within 24 hours. Most questions about the infant's history, especially about the hours preceding death, are not pertinent before a diagnosis is available. These will only cultivate the parents' guilt and promote unhealthy anxiety. It is true that a small percentage of such deaths are due to accident (Beckwith, 1970; Kraus and Borhani, 1972; Peterson et al, 1979) or even to child abuse (Berger, 1979), but even these events are best discussed with the parents after their acute grief reaction has subsided.

Parents generally respond with disbelief, denial, hostility or anger, self-reproach, and guilt and often comment that the infant's death has confirmed previous fears (Smialek, 1978). Fathers respond more frequently with denial, intellectualization, and involvement in activities outside the home (Mandell et al, 1980). Although fathers feel an urgency to have another child, mothers fear it, perhaps explaining their subsequent difficulty in conceiving (Mandell and Wolfe, 1975) and the high miscarriage rate in the first year following the death of their babies. These are all part of the usual grief response. If the sudden death of an infant occurs in the hospital, medical personnel will express similar notions and concerns (Friedman et al, 1979) and, like bereaved parents and children, need emotional support. A caring person who is comfortable in that supportive role, particularly a physician, can best guide family or hospital staff through the grieving process (Merritt et al, 1975). In addition to the physician, parent groups, usually sponsored by the National Foundation for Sudden Infant Death or the Guild for Infant Survival, provide support to many families.

EVALUATION AND CARE OF PATIENTS WITH APNEA OF INFANCY

The term *apnea of infancy* best describes our current state of ignorance while calling physicians' attention to the high-risk status of some infants. An infant who experiences a spell of apnea sufficiently frightening to prompt resuscitative efforts by parents or caretakers deserves a diagnostic evaluation so that rational therapy and an accurate prognosis can be given. It is beyond the scope of this review to specify the many conditions of primarily respiratory, cardiac, and neurologic origin that first manifest as apnea and cyanosis or pallor, but once these conditions are eliminated from consideration, a number of infants are still likely to have the more subtle conditions described in the preceding discussions of cardiovascular and respiratory dysfunctions. In about a third, we find no abnormalities; in two thirds, treatment of apnea must be supportive rather than curative.

For those with a pathologic cause of partial airway obstruction that worsens during sleep, such as adenoid hypertrophy or anomalous innominate artery, surgical correction may be sufficient but may not be curative. An underlying defect in breathing regulation may persist (Ingram and Bishop, 1970). For those few with congenital central hypoventilation, mechanical ventilatory support during sleep is necessary (Shannon et al, 1976). There are no data to indicate the outcome for a population of untreated infants who manifest apnea beyond the immediate newborn period. However, in full-term infants who manifested apnea in the newborn period during a 10-year collaborative study ending in 1966, 5 per cent of those who had only one spell and 44 per cent of those who had more than one died (Naeye, 1979). Infection doubled these risks. We believe that these data warrant vigorous treatment of idiopathic apnea. We have found that in full-term neonates with AoI, theophylline at serum concentrations averaging 11 µg/ml eliminates both the observed spells and the laboratory abnormalities of prolonged apnea and periodic breathing (Kelly and Shannon, 1981). This is similar to our previous observation in preterm infants (Shannon et al, 1975) and has been supported by others (Uauy et al, 1975; Davi et al, 1978; Demarquez et al, 1978; Dietrich et al, 1978). For all other infants, we recommend electronic monitoring until the clinical problem resolves (Kelly et al, 1978). In our home monitoring program, parents learn to perform cardiopulmonary resuscitation and to use the electronic monitor that detects heart rate and respiratory movements by impedance change. In the first weeks at home after a patient's discharge, parents benefit from daily psychosocial as well as medical support from trained personnel. After that crucial period, these supports can be tailored to the needs of individual families. In our experience and that of others, about two thirds of infants with either idiopathic sleep apnea or unexplained AoI experience at least one more spell of apnea of 20 sec or longer with cyanosis or pallor (Berdon et al, 1969; Guilleminault, Ariagno, Korobkin et al, 1979). Although we do not yet have objective proof that the assessment of these events by individual parents is accurate, we are certain that in this group of infants, particularly those with repeat spells, there are infants at high risk for SIDS (Shannon and Kelly, 1977).

Use of such monitoring devices in the home as a means of alerting parents to events that might lead to hypoxia or even death (prolonged apnea or bradycardia) has been advocated by some (Steinschneider, 1976; Kelly et al, 1978; American Academy, 1978; United States DHHS, 1987) and adversely criticized by others (Lucey, 1978; Nelson, 1978). Critics are concerned about excessive use, cost, psychosocial trauma, and the accuracy and reliability of available devices. Impedance monitoring, which is the most tested and the most appropriate of available methods for home use, suffers from the potential for two false-negative indications. First, if the threshold of impedance sensitivity is below the impedance change that accompanies each heartbeat and the alarm is set on a 20-sec delay, an alarm will not signal apnea until impedance change due to circulatory pulsations falls below threshold or heartbeats cease for 20 sec. In order to avoid this, most manufacturers have set the impedance threshold at 0.2 ohm, so that breaths that are accompanied by an impedance change of 0.2 to 5.0 ohms can be distinguished from heartbeats that produce a change of 0.03 to 0.1 ohm. However, the impedance change that would be expected to accompany increased stroke volume during bradycardia is unknown. This is important because such a change might exceed 0.2 ohm and so might be falsely registered as a breath. Newer monitors have been programmed to exclude cardiogenic artifact. Second, if obstructive apnea is accompanied by continued respiratory efforts, the apnea alarm might be delayed even until all breathing movements have ceased for 20 sec. Under these conditions, heart rate tends to decrease more quickly than during central apnea. A heart rate monitor would alert the caretaker to the infant's distress. Until a better method is available, we continue to use and to recommend a combined cardiorespiratory monitor.

Parents agree with critics that using these devices on their infants at home is stressful, but they consider the available alternatives to be less acceptable (Cain et al, 1980). Most have judged that the stress is related to their infant's medical condition rather than to the devices and report that their anxiety markedly diminishes by the end of the first month of monitoring if an appropriate support system is available.

If use of these devices is controlled and recommended by trained medical personnel who offer a 24-hour-a-day support program, parents sustain tolerable stress, the outcome is usually excellent, and the costs are acceptable.

CONCLUSIONS

Most deaths in the first year of life after the neonatal period occur suddenly and unexpectedly. A disproportionate number of deaths occur in infants raised in poor socioeconomic conditions; this is true of both those who exhibit a post-mortem cause and those who do not (SIDS). In both groups, mild infection appears to trigger death, an occurrence that especially characterizes sudden death in infant boys. The most striking increase in risk occurs in babies born to methadone-addicted mothers.

Subtle alterations in several organs, particularly smooth muscle hyperplasia of the pulmonary circulation and astrogliosis of the brainstem, have been identified in two thirds of unexplained deaths, findings that suggest repeated hypoxia. We do not understand how these findings are related or whether they represent cause or effect.

Studies of pathophysiology have been limited to AoI and siblings of SIDS victims, a few of whom have later died. These infants manifest abnormal breathing patterns, excess periodic apnea, short apnea, and prolonged apnea, which is best identified during sleep and indicates both central neurogenic as well as obstructive causes. Other infants hypoventilate and have blunted ventilatory responses to carbon dioxide breathing and to low oxygen breathing. A recent report indicates that hypercapnic and hypoxic arousal may be defective. Still other infants have been identified as having heart rate and ECG alterations that indicate increased sympathetic activity. At this time, there are no data to indicate how or whether these pathophysiologic mechanisms are related in the same infant.

It should be noted that a small percentage of apnea episodes can be explained by identifiable alterations in cardiovascular rhythm or by a seizure disorder.

After death, psychosocial support of parents, children, and medical personnel is paramount. Similarly, while an infant with AoI requires monitoring, support of the parents is crucial.

REFERENCES

American Academy of Pediatrics, Task Force on Prolonged Apnea: Prolonged apnea. Pediatrics 61:651, 1978.

Anderson RB and Rosenblith JF: Sudden unexpected death syndrome. Biol Neonate 18:395, 1971.

Angell-James JE and Daley M deB: Reflex respiratory and cardiovascular effects of stimulation of receptors in the nose of the dog. J Physiol 220:673, 1972.

Arnon SS, Midura TF, Clay SA et al: Infant botulism: epidemiological, clinical and laboratory aspects. JAMA 237:1946, 1977.

Arnon SS, Midura TF, and Damus K: Intestinal infection and toxin production by *Clostridium botulinum* as one cause of sudden infant death syndrome. Lancet 1:1273, 1978.

Arnon SS, Midura TF, Damus K et al: Honey and other environmental risk factors for infant botulism. J Pediatr 94:331, 1979.

Arsenault PS: Maternal and antenatal factors in the risk of sudden infant death syndrome. Am J Epidemiol 111:278, 1980.

Baker TL and McGinty DJ: Cardiopulmonary failure during active sleep in kittens: implications for sudden infant death. Science 198:419, 1977.

Beckwith JB: Observations of the pathological anatomy of the sudden infant death syndrome. In Bergman AB, Beckwith JB, and Ray CG (eds): Proceedings of the Second International Conference on Causes of Sudden Death in Infants. Seattle, University of Washington Press, 1970.

Berdon WE, Baker DH, Bordink J, and Mellins R: Innominate artery compression of the trachea in infants with stridor and apnea. Radiology 92:272, 1969.

Berger D: Child abuse simulating "near-miss" sudden infant death syndrome. J Pediatr 95:554, 1979.

Bergman AB and Wiesnes LA: Relationship of passive cigarette-smoking to sudden infant death syndrome. Pediatrics 58:665, 1976.

Biering-Sorensen F, Jorgensen T, and Hilden J: Sudden infant death in Copenhagen 1956–1971. I. Infant feeding. Acta Paediatr Scand 67:129, 1978.

Biering-Sorensen F, Jorgensen T, and Hilden J: Sudden infant death in Copenhagen 1956–1971. II. Social factors and morbidity. Acta Paediatr Scand 68:1, 1979.

Blumenfeld TA, Mantell CH, Catherman RL, and Blanc WA: Postmortem vitreous humor chemistry in sudden infant death syndrome and in other causes of death in childhood. Am J Clin Pathol 71:219, 1979.

Bonser RSA, Knight BH, and West RR: Sudden infant death syndrome in Cardiff. Association with epidemic influenza and with temperature 1955–1974. Int J Epidemiol 7:335, 1978.

Borzanji AA and Emery JL: Quantitative study of the lymphatic tissue and germinal centers in the spleen in infants dying from unexpected causes (cot deaths). Histopathology 1:445, 1977.

Bower RJ and Adkins JC: Ondine's curse and neurocristopathy. Clin Pediatr 19:665, 1980.

Brady JP, Ariagno RL, Watts JL et al: Apnea hypoxemia and aborted sudden infant death syndrome. Pediatrics 62:686, 1978.

Bruhn FW, Mokrohisky ST, and McKintosh K: Apnea associated with respiratory syncytial virus infection in young infants. J Pediatr 90:382, 1977.

Buchanan N, Pettifor JM, Cane RD, and Bill PLA: Infantile apnoea due to profound hypocalcemia associated with Vitamin D deficiency. S Afr Med J 53:766, 1978.

Butler NR, Goldstein H, and Ross EM: Cigarette smoking in pregnancy. Its influence on birth weight and maternal mortality. Br Med J 2:127, 1972.

Caddell JL: Exploring the magnesium deficient weanling rat as an animal model for the sudden infant death syndrome: physical, biochemical, electrocardiographic and gross pathologic changes. Pediatr Res 12:1157, 1978.

Cain LP, Kelly DH, and Shannon DC: Parent's perceptions of the psychological and social impact of home monitoring. Pediatrics 66:37, 1980.

Cameron JM and Watson E: Sudden death in infancy in inner North London. J Pathol 117:55, 1975.

Carpenter RG, Gardner A, McWeeny PM, and Emery JL: Multistage scoring system for identifying infants at risk of unexpected death. Arch Dis Child 52:606, 1977.

Carson JA, Tunell WP, and Smith EI: Pediatric gastroesophageal reflux: age-specific indications for operation. Am J Surg 140:768, 1980.

Chasnoff IJ, Burns WJ, Schnoll SH, and Burns KA: Cocaine use in pregnancy. N Engl J Med 313:666, 1985.

Chavez CJ, Ostrea EM, Stryker JC, and Smialek Z: Sudden infant death syndrome among infants of drug-dependent mothers. J Pediatr 95:407, 1979.

Cole S, Lindenberg LB, Galioto FM et al: Ultrastructural abnormalities of the carotid body in sudden infant death syndrome. Pediatrics 63:13, 1979.

Comstock GW, Shah FE, Meyer MB, and Abbey H: Low birth weight and neonatal mortality rate related to maternal smoking and socioeconomic status. Am J Obstet Gynecol 11:53, 1971.

Cooke RT and Welch RG: A study in cot death. Br Med J 2:1549, 1964.

Cornwell AC, Weitzman ED, and Marmarou A: Ambulatory and in-hospital continuous recording of sleep state and cardiorespiratory parameters in near-miss for the sudden infant death syndrome and control infants. Biotelemetry 5:113, 1978.

Cullity GJ and Emery JL: Ulceration and necrosis of vocal cords in hospital and unexpected child deaths. J Pathol 115:27, 1975.

Davi MJ, Sankaran K, Simons KJ et al: Physiologic changes induced by theophylline in the treatment of apnea in preterm infants. J Pediatr 92:91, 1978.

Davidson JT, Whipp BJ, Wasserman K et al: Role of the carotid bodies in breathholding. N Engl J Med 290:819, 1974.

Davis RE, Icke GH, and Hilton JMN: High thiamine levels in sudden infant death syndrome. N Engl J Med 303:462, 1980.

Dawes GS and Comroe JH: Chemoreflexes from the heart and lungs. Physiol Rev 34:167, 1954.

Demarquez JL, Brachet-Lierman A, Paty J et al: Traitment preventif des apnees du premature par la theophylline. Arch Fr Pediat 35:783, 1978.

DeSa DJ: Coronary arterial lesions and myocardial necrosis in stillbirths and infants. Arch Dis Child 54:918, 1979.

Dietrich J, Krauss AN, Reidenberg M et al: Alterations in state in apneic preterm infants receiving theophylline. Clin Pharm Ther 24:474, 1978.

Dinsdale F, Emery JL, and Gadsdon DR: The carotid body—a quantitative assessment in children. Histopathology 1:179, 1977.

Downing SE and Lee JC: Laryngeal chemosensitivity; a possible mechanism for sudden infant death. Pediatrics 55:640, 1975.

Duran M, Hofkamp M, Rhead WJ et al: Sudden child death and healthy affected family members with medium-chain acyl-coenzyme A dehydrogenase deficiency. Pediatrics 78:1052, 1986.

Edwards C, Heath D, Harris P et al: The carotid body in animals at high altitude. J Pathol 101:231, 1971.

Emery JL and Dinsdale F: Structure of periadrenal brown fat in childhood in both expected and cot deaths. Arch Dis Child 53:154, 1978.

Fagenholz SA, O'Connell K, and Shannon DC: Chemoreceptor function and sleep state in apnea. Pediatrics 58:31, 1976.

Ferrer PL and Jesse ML: Prolonged QT index in "near-miss" sudden death in infancy. Clin Res 25:64A, 1977.

Fink BR and Beckwith JB: Laryngeal mucous gland excess in victims of sudden infant death. Am J Dis Child 134:144, 1980.

Finnegan LP: In utero opiate dependence and sudden infant death syndrome. Clin Perinatol 6:163, 1979.

Fleming PJ, Bryan AC, and Bryan MH: Functional immaturity of pulmonary irritant receptors and apnea in newborn preterm infants. Pediatrics 61:515, 1978.

Fleshman JK and Peterson DR: The sudden infant death syndrome among Alaskan natives. Am J Epidemiol 105:555, 1977.

Friedman GR, Granciosi RA, and Drake RM: The effects of observed sudden infant death syndrome (SIDS) on hospital staff. Pediatrics 64:538, 1979.

Froggatt P, Lynas MA, and Marshall TK: Sudden death in babies: epidemiology. Am J Cardiol 22:457, 1968.

Froggatt P, Lynas MA, and Marshall TK: Epidemiology of sudden unexpected death in infants (cot death). Report of a collaborative study in Northern Ireland. Ulster Med J 40:116, 1971.

Gadsdon DR and Emery JL: Fatty change in the brain in perinatal and unexpected death. Arch Dis Child 51:42, 1976.

Giulian GG, Gilbert ES, and Moss RL: Elevated fetal hemoglobin levels in sudden infant death syndrome. N Engl J Med 316:1122, 1987.

Glenn WW, Haak B, Saski C, and Kirchner J: Characteristics and surgical management of respiratory complications accompanying pathologic lesions of the brain stem. Ann Surg 191:655, 1980.

Gold E, Carver DH, Heineberg H et al: Viral infection. A possible cause of sudden unexplained death in infants. N Engl J Med 264:53, 1961.

Golub H and Corwin M: Infant cry: a clue to diagnosis. Pediatrics 69:197, 1982.

Gould JB, Lee AFS, Cook P, and Morelock S: Apnea and sleep state in infants with nasopharyngitis. Pediatrics 65:713, 1980.

Grice AC and McGlashan ND: Sudden death in infancy in Tasmania (1970–1976). Med J Aust 2:177, 1978.

Guilleminault C, Ariagno RL, Forno LS et al: Obstructive sleep apnea and near-miss for SIDS. I. Report of an infant with sudden death. Pediatrics 63:837, 1979.

Guilleminault C, Ariagno R, Korobkin R et al: Mixed and obstructive sleep apnea and near-miss for sudden infant death syndrome. II. Comparison of near-miss and normal control infants by age. Pediatrics 64:882, 1979.

Guilleminault C, Eldridge FL, Simmons FB, and Dement WC: Sleep apnea in eight children. Pediatrics 58:23, 1976.

Guilleminault C, Perarta R, and Souquet M: Apneas during sleep in infants: possible relationship with sudden infant death syndrome. Science 190:677, 1975.

Guntheroth WG: The significance of pulmonary petechiae in crib death. Pediatrics 52:601, 1973.

Haddad GG, Epstein MAF, Epstein RA et al: The QT interval in aborted sudden infant death syndrome infants. Pediatr Res 13:136, 1979.

Haddad GG, Epstein RA, Epstein MAF et al: The R-R interval and RR variability in normal infants during sleep. Pediatr Res 14:809, 1980.

Haddad GG, Kronrad E, Epstein RA et al: Effect of sleep state on the QT interval in normal infants. Pediatr Res 13:139, 1979.

Haddad GG, Mazza NM, Defendini R et al: Congenital failure of automatic control of ventilation, gastrointestinal motility and heart rate. Medicine 57:517, 1978.

Harding R, Johnson P, Johnston BE et al: Cardiovascular changes in newborn lambs during apnea induced by stimulation of laryngeal receptors with water. J Physiol 256:35, 1975.

Harding R, Johnson P, Johnston BE et al: Cardiovascular changes in new-born lambs during apnea induced by stimulation of laryngeal receptors with water. J Physiol (London) 256:35P, 1976.

Harper RM, Leake B, Hoppenbrouwers T et al: Polygraphic studies of normal infants and infants at risk for the sudden infant death syndrome: heart rate and variability as a function of state. Pediatr Res 12:778, 1978.

Harpey JP, Charpentier C, Coude M et al: Sudden infant death syndrome and multiple acyl-coenzyme A dehydrogenase deficiency, ethylmalonic-adipic aciduria, or systemic carnitine deficiency. J Pediatr 111:881, 1987.

Henderson-Smart DJ and Read DJ: Depression of intercostal and abdominal muscle activity and vulnerability to asphyxia during active sleep in the newborn. In Guilleminault C and Dement W (eds): Sleep Apnea Syndromes. New York, Alan R Liss, Inc, 1978.

Herbst JJ, Book LS, and Bray PF: Gastroesophageal reflux in the "near-miss" sudden infant death syndrome. J Pediatr 92:73, 1978.

Hillman LS, Erickson M, and Haddad JG: Serum 25-hydroxyvitamin D concentrations in sudden death syndrome. Pediatrics 65:1137, 1980.

Holinger PC, Holinger LD, Reichert TJ, and Holinger PH: Respiratory obstruction and apnea in infants with bilateral abductor vocal cord and paralysis meningomyelocoele, hydrocephalus and Arnold-Chiari malformation. J Pediatr 92:368, 1978.

Hoppenbrouwers T, Hodgman JE, McGinty D et al: Sudden infant death syndrome: sleep apnea and respiration in subsequent siblings. Pediatrics 66:205, 1980.

Hoppenbrouwers T, Zanini B, and Hodgman JE: Intrapartum fetal heart rate and sudden infant death syndrome. Am J Obstet Gynecol 133:217, 1979.

Hunt CE: Abnormal hypercarbic and hypoxic sleep arousal responses in near-miss SIDS. Pediatr Res 15:462, 1981.

Hunt CE, McCulloch K, and Brouillette RI: Diminished hypoxic ventilatory responses in near-miss SIDS. J Appl Physiol 50:1313, 1981.

Hunt CE, Matalon SV, Thompson TR et al: Central hypoventilation syndrome. Am Rev Respir Dis 118:23, 1978.

Ingram RH and Bishop JB: Ventilatory response to carbon dioxide after removal of chronic upper airway obstruction. Am Rev Respir Dis 102:645, 1970.

James TN: Sudden death in babies: new observations in the heart. Am J Cardiol 22:479, 1968.

Johnson P, Salisburg DM, and Storey AT: Apnoea induced by stimulation of sensory receptors in the larynx. In Bosma JF and Showacre J (eds): Development of Upper Respiratory Anatomy and Function. Washington, DC, U.S. Government Printing Office, 1975.

Kanarek DJ, Kelly DH, and Shannon DC: Ventilatory chemoreceptor response in parents of children at risk for sudden infant death syndrome. Pediatr Res 15:1402, 1981.

Katona PG and Egbert JR: Heart rate and respiratory rate differences between pre-term and full-term infants during quiet sleep; possible implications for sudden infant death syndrome. Pediatrics 62:91, 1978.

Keeton BR, Southall E, Rutter N et al: Cardiac conduction disorders in six infants with "near-miss" sudden infant deaths. Br Med J 2:600, 1977.

Kelly DH and Shannon DC: Periodic breathing in infants with near-miss sudden infant death syndrome. Pediatrics 63:355, 1979.

Kelly DH and Shannon DC: Treatment of apnea and excessive periodic breathing in the full term infant. Pediatrics 68:183, 1981.

Kelly DH, Shannon DC, and Liberthson RR: The role of QT interval in the sudden infant death syndrome. Circulation 55:633, 1977.

Kelly DH, Shannon DC, and O'Connell K: Care of infants with near-miss sudden infant death syndrome. Pediatrics 61:511, 1978.

Kelly DH, Walker AM, Cahen L, and Shannon DC: Periodic breathing in siblings of sudden infant death syndrome victims. Pediatrics 66:515, 1980.

Kendeel SR and Ferris JAJ: Apparent hypoxic change in pulmonary arterioles and small arteries in infancy. J Clin Pathol 30:481, 1977.

Kinney HC, Burger PC, Harrell FE, and Hudson RP: "Reactive gliosis" in the sudden infant death syndrome. Pediatrics 72:181, 1983.

Koivikko A, Puhakka HJ, and Vilkki P: Innominate artery compression syndrome. Otorhinolaryngology 38:187, 1976.

Kraus JF and Borhani NO: Post-neonatal sudden unexplained death in California—a cohort study. Am J Hyg 95:497, 1972.

Kukolich M, Telsey A, Ott J, and Mitulsky AG: Sudden infant death syndrome; normal QT interval on ECGs of relatives. Pediatrics 60:51, 1977.

Kulkarni P, Hall RT, Rhodes PG, and Sheehan MB: Postneonatal infant mortality in infants admitted to a neonatal intensive care unit. Pediatrics 62:178, 1978.

Lapin CA, Morrow G, Chuapil M et al: Hepatic trace elements in sudden infant death syndrome. J Pediatr 89:607, 1976.

Leape LL and Ramenofsky ML: Surgical treatment of gastroesophageal reflux in children. Am J Dis Child 134:935, 1980.

Lee CA: On the thymus gland, its morbid affections, and the diseases that arise from its abnormal enlargement. Am J Med Sci 3:135, 1842.

Leistner HL, Haddad GG, Epstein RA et al: Heart rate and heart rate variability during sleep in aborted sudden infant death syndrome. J Pediatr 97:51, 1980.

Levin DL, Hyman AI, Heymann MA, and Rudolph AM: Fetal hypertension and the development of increased pulmonary vascular smooth muscle: a possible mechanism for persistent pulmonary hypertension of the newborn infant. J Pediatr 92:265, 1978.

Liberthson RR, Nagel EL, Hirschman JC et al: Pathophysiologic observations in prehospital ventricular fibrillation and sudden cardiac death. Circulation 49:790, 1974.

Lie JT, Rosenberg HS, and Erickson EE: Histopathology of the conduction system in the sudden infant death syndrome. Circulation 53:3, 1976.

Lipsitt LP, Sturner WO, Oh W et al: Wolff-Parkinson-White and sudden infant death syndromes (letter). N Engl J Med 300:1111, 1979.

Loughlin G, Wynne J, Victoria B et al: Intermittent upper airway obstruction during sleep causing accelerated pulmonary hypertension in Down's syndrome (abstract). Chest 78:529, 1980.

Lucey JF: False alarms in the nursery. Pediatrics 61:665, 1978.

Lugliani R, Whipp BJ, Seard C et al: Effect of bilateral carotid body resection on ventilatory control at rest and during exercise in man. N Engl J Med 285:1105, 1971.

McCandless DW and Hodgkin WE: Subacute necrotizing encephalomyelopathy (Leigh's disease) (editorial). Pediatrics 60:635, 1977.

McNamara J: Abnormal polygraphic findings in near-miss sudden infant death. Lancet 2:689, 1976.

McWeeny PM and Emery JL: Unexpected postneonatal deaths (cot deaths) due to recognizable disease. Arch Dis Child 80:191, 1975.

Mandell F and Wolfe LC: Sudden infant death syndrome and subsequent pregnancy. Pediatrics 56:774, 1975.

Mandell F, McAnulty E, and Reece RM: Observations of paternal response to sudden unanticipated infant death. Pediatrics 65:221, 1980.

Maron BJ, Clark CE, Goldstein RE, and Epstein SE: Potential role of QT interval prolongation in sudden infant death syndrome. Circulation 54:423, 1976.

Martin RJ, Okken A, and Rubin D: Arterial oxygen tension during active and quiet sleep in the normal neonate. J Pediatr 94:271, 1979.

Megirian D and Sherrey J: Respiratory functions of the laryngeal muscles during sleep. Sleep 3:289, 1980.

Megirian D, Ryan AT, and Sherrey JH: An electrophysiological analysis of sleep and respiration of rats breathing different gas mixtures: diaphragmatic muscle function. Electroencephalogr Clin Neurophysiol 50:303, 1980.

Merritt TA, Bauer WI, and Hasselmeyer EG: Sudden infant death syndrome: the role of the emergency room physician. Clin Pediatr 14:1095, 1975.

Monod N, Curzi-Dascalova L, Guidasci S, and Valenzuela S: Pauses respiratoires et sommeil chez le nouveau-né et le nourrisson. Rev Encephalogr Neurophysiol Clin 6:105, 1976.

Mourant AE, Kopec AC, and Domaniewska-Sobczak K: The Distribution of the Human Blood Groups and Other Polymorphisms. 2nd ed. London, Oxford University Press, 1976.

Mustard WT, Bayliss CE, Fearon B et al: Tracheal compression by the innominate artery in children. Ann Thorac Surg 8:312, 1969.

Myers RE: Threshold values of oxygen deficiency leading to cardiovascular and brain pathological changes in term monkey fetuses. In Bruley DF and Bicher HI (eds): Oxygen Transport to Tissue. New York, Plenum, 1973.

Naeye RL: Hypoxemia and the sudden infant death syndrome. Science 136:837, 1974.

Naeye RL: Brain-stem and adrenal abnormalities in the sudden infant death syndrome. Am J Clin Pathol 66:526, 1976.

Naeye RL: Placental abnormalities in victims of the sudden infant death syndrome. Biol Neonate 32:189, 1977.

Naeye RL: Neonatal apnea: underlying disorders. Pediatrics 63:515, 1979.

Naeye RL, Fisher R, Rubin R, and Demers IM: Selected hormone levels in victims of the sudden infant death syndrome. Pediatrics 65:1134, 1980.

Naeye RL, Fisher R, Ryser M, and Whalen P: Carotid body in sudden infant death syndrome. Science 91:567, 1976.

Naeye RL, Ladis B, and Drage JS: Sudden infant death syndrome. Am J Dis Child 130:1207, 1976.

Naeye RL, Messmer J, Spech TT, and Merritt TA: Sudden infant death syndrome: temperament before death. J Pediatr 88:511, 1976.

Naeye RL, Whalen P, Ryser M, and Fisher R: Cardiac and other abnormalities in the sudden infant death syndrome. Am J Pathol 82:1, 1976.

Nelson DA and Ray CD: Respiratory arrests from seizure disorders in the limbic system. Arch Neurol 19:198, 1968.

Nelson KE, Greenberg MA, Mufson AM, and Moses VK: The sudden infant death syndrome and epidemic viral disease. Am J Epidemiol 101:423, 1975.

Nelson NM: Who will monitor the monitor (editorial)? Pediatrics 61:663, 1978.

Oakley JR, Tavare CJ, and Stanton AN: Evaluation of the Sheffield system for identifying children at risk from unexpected death in infancy. Arch Dis Child 53:649, 1978.

Ogra PL, Ogra SS, and Coppola PR: Secretory component and sudden infant death syndrome. Lancet 2:387, 1975.

Olsen GD and Lees MH: Ventilatory response to carbon dioxide of infants following chorionic prenatal methadone exposure. J Pediatr 96:983, 1980.

Onal E, Lopata M, and O'Connor TD: Diaphragmatic and genioglossal electromyographic responses to CO_2 rebreathing in humans. J Appl Physiol 50:1052, 1981.

Orem J, Netick A, and Dement WC: Increased upper airway resistance to breathing during sleep in the cat. Electroencephalogr Clin Neurophysiol 43:14, 1977.

Oren J, Kelly D, and Shannon DC: Identification of a high risk group for SIDS among infants who were resuscitated for sleep apnea. Pediatrics 77:495, 1986.

Oren J, Kelly DH, and Shannon DC: Familial occurrence of sudden infant death and apnea of infancy. Pediatrics 80:355, 1987.

Parish WE, Barrett AM, Coombs RRA et al: Hypersensitivity to milk and sudden death in infancy. Lancet 2:1106, 1960.

Patrick GB, Rubin SB, Strohl KP, and Altose MD: Comparison of alae nasi and diaphragmatic activity during hypoxia, hypercapnia and resistive loading in normal subject (abstract). Am Rev Respir Dis 123:187, 1981.

Peterson DR: Sudden unexpected death in infants; an epidemiologic study. Am J Epidemiol 81:478, 1966.

Peterson DR: Sudden unexpected deaths in infants. Incidence in two climatically dissimilar metropolitan communities. Am J Epidemiol 95:95, 1972.

Peterson DR, Chinn NM, and Fisher LD: The sudden infant death syndrome: repetitions in families. J Pediatr 97:265, 1980.

Peterson DR, Labbe RF, vanBelle G, and Chinn NM: Erythrocyte transketolase activity and sudden infant death. Am J Clin Nutr 34:65, 1981.

Peterson DR, vanBelle G, and Chinn NM: Epidemiologic comparisons of the sudden infant death syndrome with other major components of infant mortality. Am J Epidemiol 110:699, 1979.

Peterson RDA and Good RA: Antibodies to cow's milk proteins—their presence and significance. Pediatrics 31:209, 1963.

Phillipson EA: Control of breathing during sleep. Am Rev Respir Dis 118:909, 1978.

Phillipson EA, Murphy E, and Kozar LF: Regulation of respiration in sleeping dogs. J Appl Physiol 40:688, 1976.

Pinkham JR and Beckwith JB: Vocal cord lesions in sudden infant death syndrome. In Bergman AB, Beckwith JB, and Ray CG (eds): Proceedings of the Second International Conference on Causes of Sudden Death in Infants. Seattle, University of Washington Press, 1970.

Protestos CD, Carpenter RD, McWeeny PM, and Emery JL: Obstetric and perinatal histories of children who died unexpectedly (cot death). Arch Dis Child 48:835, 1973.

Purcell M: Response in the newborn to raised upper airway resistance. Arch Dis Child 51:602, 1976.

Purves MJ: The effects of hypoxia in the newborn lamb before and after denervation of the carotid chemoreceptors. J Physiol 185:60, 1966.

Quattrochi JJ, Baba N, Liss L, and Adrion W: Sudden infant death syndrome (SIDS): a preliminary study of reticular dendritic spines in infants with SIDS. Brain Res 181:245, 1980.

Rajegowda BK, Kandall SR, and Falciglio H: Sudden unexpected death in infants of narcotic-dependent mothers. Early Hum Devel 2:219, 1978.

Read DJC: The etiology of the sudden infant death syndrome: current ideas on breathing and sleep and possible links to deranged thiamine neurochemistry. Aust NZ J Med 8:322, 1978.

Remmers JE, deGroot WJ, and Sauerland EK: Pathogenesis of upper airway occlusion during sleep. J Appl Physiol 44:931, 1978.

Richards IDG and McIntosh HT: Confidential inquiry into 226 consecutive infant deaths. Arch Dis Child 47:697, 1972.

Rigatto H, Brady JP, and de la Toree Verduzco R: Chemoreceptor reflexes on preterm infants. I. The effect of gestational and postnatal age on the ventilatory response to inhalation of 100% and 15% oxygen. Pediatrics 55:604, 1975.

Roberts PF: Thymic dysplasia, persistence of measles virus and unexpected infant death. Arch Dis Child 50:401, 1975.

Roe CR, Millington DS, Maltby DA, and Kinnebrew P: Recognition of medium-chain acyl-CoA dehydrogenase deficiency in asymptomatic siblings of children dying of sudden infant death or Reye-like syndromes. J Pediatr 108:13, 1986.

Russell MA, Opitz JM, Viseskul C et al: Sudden infant death due to congenital adrenal hypoplasia. Arch Pathol Lab Med 101:168, 1977.

Sachis PN, Armstrong DL, Becker LE, and Bryan AC: The vagus nerve and sudden infant death syndrome: a morphometric study. J Pediatr 98:278, 1981.

Sadeh D, Shannon DC, Abboud S et al: Altered cardiac repolarization in some victims of sudden infant death syndrome. N Engl J Med 317:1501, 1987.

Saldana MJ, Salem LE, and Travezan R: High altitude hypoxia and chemodectomas. Hum Pathol 4:251, 1973.

Salk L, Grellong BA, and Dietrich J: Sudden infant death. Normal cardiac habituation and poor autonomic control. N Engl J Med 291:219, 1974.

Schiffman PL, Westlake RE, Santiago TV, and Edelman NH: Ventilatory control in parents of victims of sudden infant death syndrome. N Engl J Med 302:486, 1980.

Schwartz PJ, Periti M, and Malliani A: The long QT syndrome. Am Heart J 89:378, 1975.

Scott DJ, Gardner PS, McQuillin J et al: Respiratory viruses and cot death. Br Med J 2:12, 1978.

Seto DSY and Carver DH: Circulating interferon in sudden infant death syndrome. Proc Soc Exp Biol Med 157:378, 1978.

Shannon DC: Pathophysiologic mechanisms causing sleep apnea and hypoventilation in infants. Sleep 3:343, 1980.

Shannon DC and Kelly D: Impaired regulation of alveolar ventilation and the sudden infant death syndrome. Science 197:367, 1977.

Shannon DC, Gotay F, Stein IM et al: Prevention of apnea and bradycardia in low birth weight infants. Pediatrics 55:589, 1975.

Shannon DC, Kelly DH, and O'Connell K: Abnormal regulation of ventilation in infants at risk for sudden infant death syndrome. N Engl J Med 297:747, 1977.

Shannon DC, Marsland DW, Gould JB et al: Central hypoventilation during quiet sleep in two infants. Pediatrics 57:343, 1976.

Sinclair-Smith C, Dinsdale F, and Emery J: Evidence of duration and type of illness in children found unexpectedly dead. Arch Dis Child 51:424, 1976.

Smialek JE and Monforte JR: Toxicology and sudden infant death. J Forensic Sci 22:757, 1977.

Smialek Z: Observations on immediate reactions of families to sudden infant death. Pediatrics 63:160, 1978.

Smith TA, Mason JM, Bell JS, and Francisco JT: Prolongation of the Q-T interval in a victim of sudden infant death syndrome: cause or effect? South Med J 72:522, 1979.

Southall DP, Arrowsmith WA, Oakley JR et al: Prolonged QT interval and cardiac arrhythmias in two neonates: sudden infant death syndrome in one case. Arch Dis Child 54:776, 1979.

Southall DP, Richards J, Brown DJ et al: 24-hour tape recordings of ECG and respiration in the newborn infant with findings related to sudden death and unexplained brain damage in infancy. Arch Dis Child 55:7, 1980.

Speer L: Aborted crib death? JAMA 223:1512, 1973.

Spiers PS: Previous fetal loss and risk of sudden infant death syndrome in subsequent offspring. Am J Epidemiol 103:355, 1976.

Spiers PS and Wang L: Short pregnancy interval, low birth weight and the sudden infant death syndrome. Am J Epidemiol 104:15, 1976.

Standfast S, Jereb S, and Janerich DT: The epidemiology of sudden infant death in upstate New York. JAMA 241:1121, 1979.

Standfast SJ, Jereb S, and Janerich DT: The epidemiology of sudden infant death in upstate New York. II. Birth characteristics. Am J Public Health 70:1061, 1980.

Stark RE and Nathanson SN: Unusual features of cry in infant dying suddenly and unexpectedly. In Bosma JF and Showacre J (eds): Development of Upper Respiratory Anatomy and Function. Bethesda, National Institutes of Health, 1975.

Steele R and Langworth JT: The relationship of antenatal and postnatal factors to sudden unexpected death in infancy. Can Med Assoc J 94:1165, 1966.

Stein IM, White A, Kennedy JL Jr et al: Apnea recordings of healthy infants at 40, 44, 52 weeks post conception. Pediatrics 63:724, 1979.

Steinschneider A: Prolonged apnea and the sudden infant death syndrome: clinical and laboratory observations. Pediatrics 50:646, 1972.

Steinschneider A: Nasopharyngitis and prolonged sleep apnea. Pediatrics 56:967, 1975.

Steinschneider A: A re-examination of the apnea monitoring business. Pediatrics 58:1, 1976.

Steinschneider A: Sudden infant death syndrome and prolongation of the QT interval. Am J Dis Child 132:688, 1978.

Steinschneider A and Rabuzzi DD: Apnea and airway obstruction during feeding and sleep. Laryngoscope 86:1359, 1976.

Steven LH: Sudden unexplained death in infancy. Am J Dis Child 110:243, 1965.

Strimer R, Adelson L, and Oseasohn R: Epidemiologic features of 1,134 sudden unexpected infant deaths. JAMA 209:1493, 1969.

Strohl KP, Saunders NA, Feldman NT, and Hallett M: Obstructive sleep apnea in family members. N Engl J Med 299:969, 1978.

Sullivan CE, Zamel N, Kozar LF et al: Regulation of airway smooth muscle tone in sleeping dogs. Am Rev Respir Dis 119:87, 1979.

Swift PGF and Emery JL: Clinical observations on response to nasal occlusion in infancy. Arch Dis Child 48:947, 1973.

Takashima S, Armstrong D, Becker L, and Bryan AC: Cerebral hypoperfusion in the sudden infant death syndrome? Brainstem gliosis and vasculature. Ann Neurol 4:257, 1978.

Takashima S, Armstrong D, Becker LE, and Huber J: Cerebral white matter lesions in sudden infant death syndrome. Pediatrics 62:155, 1978.

Talman WT, Perrone MH, and Reis DJ: Evidences for L-glutamate as the neurotransmitter of baroreceptor afferent nerve fibers. Science 209:813, 1980.

Tapp E, Jones DM, and Tobin JOH: Interpretation of respiratory tract histology in cot deaths. J Clin Pathol 28:899, 1975.

Thoman EB, Freese MP, Becker PT et al: Sex differences in the autogeny of sleep apnea during the first year of life. Physiol Behav 20:699, 1978.

Thompson JA, Glasgow LA, Warpinski JR, and Olson C: Infant botulism: clinical spectrum and epidemiology. Pediatrics 66:936, 1980.

Tonkin S: Sudden infant death syndrome; hypothesis of causation. Pediatrics 55:650, 1975.

Turner JK, Baldo BA, Carter RF, and Kerr HR: Sudden infant death syndrome in South Australia: measurement of serum IgE antibodies to three common allergens. Med J Aust 2:855, 1975.

Uauy R, Shapiro DL, Smith B, and Warshaw JB: Treatment of severe apnea in prematures with orally administered theophylline. Pediatrics 55:595, 1975.

United States Department of Health and Human Services: Infantile Apnea and Home Monitoring. Report of a Consensus Development Conference sponsored by the National Institutes of Health. NIH Publication No. 87-2905, 1987.

Valdes-Dapena M, Amazon K, Gillane MM et al: The question of right ventricular hypertrophy in sudden infant death syndrome. Arch Pathol Lab Med 104:184, 1980.

Valdes-Dapena M, Birle LJ, McGovern JA et al: Sudden unexpected death in infancy: a statistical analysis of certain socioeconomic factors. J Pediatr 73:387, 1968.

Valdes-Dapena MA, Gillane MM, and Catherman R: Brown fat retention in sudden infant death syndrome. Arch Pathol Lab Med 100:547, 1976.

Valdes-Dapena MA, Greene M, Basavanard N et al: The myocardial conduction system in sudden death in infancy. N Engl J Med 289:1179, 1973.

Wang SC and Ngai SH: General organization of central respiratory mechanisms. In Fenn WO and Rahn H (eds): Handbook of Physiology. Section 3: Respiration. Vol 1. Washington, DC, American Physiological Society, 1964.

Weitzman ED, Kahn E, and Pollack CP: Quantitative analysis of sleep and sleep apnea before and after tracheostomy in patients with the hypersomnia–sleep apnea syndrome. Sleep 3:407, 1980.

Weitzman ED, Pollack CP, and Borowiccki B: The hypersomnia–sleep apnea syndrome: site and mechanism of upper airway obstruction. In Guilleminault C and Dement WC (eds): Sleep Apnea Syndromes. New York, Alan R Liss, Inc, 1978.

Williams A, Vawter G, and Reid L: Increased muscularity of the pulmonary circulation in victims of sudden infant death syndrome. Pediatrics 63:18, 1979.

Williams AJ, Shannon DC, Rabinovitch M et al: Pulmonary vascular muscle hyperplasia associated with impaired ventilatory control in sudden infant death syndrome (SIDS). Am Rev Respir Dis 121:419, 1980.

Wolf S: Sudden death and the oxygen conserving reflex. Am Heart J 71:840, 1966.

Wyman RJ: Neural generation of the breathing rhythm. Am Rev Physiol 39:417, 1977.

Zwillich C, McCullough R, Guilleminault C et al: Respiratory control in the parents of sudden infant death syndrome victims. Ventilatory control in SIDS parents. Pediatr Res 14:762, 1980.

71

MARIANNA M. HENRY, M.D., and
THOMAS F. BOAT, M.D.

LUNG INJURY CAUSED BY PHARMACOLOGIC AGENTS

Numerous drugs can cause pulmonary or pleural reactions, or both, in children. The most frequent offenders are certain chemotherapeutic agents used in the treatment of childhood neoplasms (Table 71–1), although the toxic effects of other agents are increasingly recognized (Table 71–2). Diffuse interstitial pneumonitis and fibrosis constitutes the most frequent clinical syndrome. Hypersensitivity lung disease, noncardiogenic pulmonary edema, pleural effusion, bronchiolitis obliterans, and alveolar hemorrhage are also encountered.

Table 71–1. CYTOTOXIC DRUGS

	Incidence (%)	Mortality	Clinical Syndromes
Antibiotics			
Bleomycin	2–40	10% (> 550 mg)	IP/PF, H, P Eff
Mitomycin	3–12	50%	IP/PF, PE, P Eff
Alkylating agents			
Cyclophosphamide	1	40%	IP/PF, PE, B
Chlorambucil	*	—	IP/PF
Busulfan	4	—	IP/PF, P Eff
Melphalan	*	—	IP/PF
Nitrosureas			
Carmustine	20–30	—	PF
Antimetabolites			
Methotrexate	8	1%	IP/PF, H, PE, P Eff
Azathioprine	*	—	IP/PF
6-Mercaptopurine	*	—	IP/PF
Cytosine arabinoside	*	—	IP/PF, PE

*Infrequent case reports.
IP/PF, interstitial pneumonitis/pulmonary fibrosis; H, hypersensitivity lung reaction; P Eff, pleural effusion; PE, pulmonary edema (noncardiogenic); B, bronchospasm; PF, pulmonary fibrosis.

Although some drug-induced pulmonary damage is reversible, persistent and even fatal dysfunction may occur. Lung reactions occasionally are temporally remote from exposure to chemotherapeutic agents. Depending on the agent involved, the reaction may or may not be dose related. The mechanism of toxicity is thought to be direct injury to lung cells in most cases, but immunologic and central nervous system–mediated mechanisms seem to play a role in the toxicity of certain agents. Identified risk factors associated with cytotoxic drug therapy vary, but in general include cumulative dose, age of the patient, prior or concurrent radiation, oxygen therapy, and use of other toxic drugs. Most reactions to noncytotoxic drugs appear to develop idiosyncratically. When patients are treated with several potentially toxic drugs or with a toxic drug plus irradiation to the chest or high concentrations of oxygen, the specific offenders often cannot be identified. There is little if any evidence that children are more susceptible to drug-related pulmonary injury, and in fact they may be less susceptible to some agents such as bleomycin.

The clinical presentation of drug-induced lung disease often includes fever, malaise, dyspnea, and a nonproductive cough. Radiologic studies almost always demonstrate diffuse alveolar and/or interstitial involvement. Segmental or lobar disease, particularly if unilateral, should suggest another diagnosis. Abnormal pulmonary function values, either obstructive or restrictive, may be found before appearance of roentgenographic lesions. Hypoxemia is an early and clinically important functional consequence. Pathologic features do not distinguish among most drugs and most often consist of interstitial thickening with chronic inflammatory cell infiltrate in the interstitial

Table 71–2. NONCYTOTOXIC DRUGS

	Recorded Cases or Incidence	Mortality	Clinical Syndromes
Nitrofurantoin	> 500 adult 8 pediatric	8%	H, IP/PF, B, AH, P Eff
Sulfasalazine	17 adult	1 case	H, BO, FA, B
Diphenylhydantoin	6 adult 3 pediatric	0	H
Carbamazepine	2 adult 4 pediatric	0	H, B
Penicillamine	24 adult 1 pediatric	50% (AH, BO)	H, DA, BO, AH
Gold	> 60 adult 1 pediatric	2 cases	H, IP/PF
Amiodarone	5%	5–10%	IP/PF

H, hypersensitivity lung reaction; IP/PF, interstitial pneumonitis/pulmonary fibrosis; B, bronchospasm; AH, alveolar hemorrhage; P Eff, pleural effusion; BO, bronchiolitis obliterans; FA, fibrosing alveolitis; DA, diffuse alveolitis.

or alveolar compartment, fibroblast proliferation, fibrosis, and hyperplasia of type II pneumocytes, which contain enlarged hyperchromatic nuclei. With hypersensitivity reactions, the interstitial infiltrate includes substantial numbers of eosinophils. Other diagnoses, such as infection, pulmonary hemorrhage, lung disease related to an underlying disorder, and radiation damage must be considered in patients with suspected drug-induced lung injury.

CYTOTOXIC DRUGS

ANTIBIOTICS

Bleomycin

Bleomycin is a mixture of peptide antibiotics obtained from *Streptomyces verticillus*. Although the drug is active against squamous cell carcinoma and testicular tumors, its major use in children is to treat Hodgkin's disease and other lymphomas. Because of the high frequency of pulmonary reactions and the utility of bleomycin for generating animal models of lung fibrosis, this agent has been studied more thoroughly than others. Pulmonary damage develops in two distinct patterns, most commonly progressive fibrosis and uncommonly an acute hypersensitivity reaction.

Pulmonary disease secondary to bleomycin occurs in approximately 4 per cent of all patients receiving the drug, although the reported incidence is as great as 40 per cent. The frequency of reactions in children is not well documented because relatively few children receive this agent. Risk of lung disease depends largely on the cumulative dose. Significant lung damage rarely occurs in adults at cumulative doses less than 150 mg. When more than 283 mg/m² is administered, 50 per cent of adult patients develop severe pneumonitis. Pulmonary damage is more severe in elderly than in young patients, but gender does not appear to influence toxicity. Slow intravenous administration results in less lung disease than intramuscular injection or an intravenous bolus. The combination of radiotherapy or high inspired oxygen concentrations and bleomycin produces more lung injury than either alone. Pulmonary toxicity to relatively small quantities of bleomycin has been reported during combination drug therapy.

Pulmonary injury due to bleomycin occurs by direct injury to cells as well as by secondary immunologic reactions. Direct toxicity may be mediated by oxidant injury, either through the production of reactive oxygen metabolites or through inactivation of antioxidants. Bleomycin also generates factors, possibly leukotriene B$_4$, which are chemotactic for polymorphonuclear leukocytes. These inflammatory cells may participate in oxidant and perhaps proteolytic injury to lung cells. Bleomycin promptly increases collagen synthesis by fibroblasts. Collagen synthesis declines 1 to 2 weeks after exposure, perhaps as a result of release of a suppressive factor by alveolar macrophages.

Bleomycin-induced lung disease can begin insidiously. Asymptomatic patients may have decreases in arterial oxygen saturation and carbon monoxide diffusing capacity (DL$_{CO}$). As the illness progresses, there is a decline in vital capacity and total lung capacity, characteristic of restrictive lung disease. In both interstitial pneumonitis and hypersensivity lung reactions, patients typically present with a dry hacking cough and dyspnea; these signs occur only on exertion in mild cases, but profound respiratory distress accompanies advanced illness. Fever suggests a hypersensitivity reaction. Physical examination reveals tachypnea and fine crackles. Chest roentgenograms in symptomatic patients most commonly demonstrate diffuse linear densities. A widespread reticulonodular or alveolar pattern may also be seen. Biopsy specimens usually reveal interstitial pneumonitis and fibrosis and extensive alveolar damage. There is a decrease in type I pneumocytes and a subsequent hyperplasia of type II cells. In contrast to lesions caused by alkylating agents, this lesion is most prominent in subpleural and basilar regions.

Patients receiving bleomycin should be monitored by serial determinations of DL$_{CO}$. Therapy of bleomycin-induced pneumonitis consists largely of supportive measures. Withdrawal of the drug at the onset of toxicity must be considered. Careful monitoring of oxygen therapy to avoid excessive exposure is imperative. Although a portion of the cellular inflammatory element resolves with cessation of therapy, much of the fibrotic damage is irreversible. The use of steroids is controversial; when administered early in the course of disease, they may be beneficial. In the few patients exhibiting hypersensitivity reactions, corticosteroids have a definite role.

Mitomycin

Mitomycin is an antibiotic that is metabolized to an alkylating agent. Its major uses are in treatment of carcinomas of the cervix, colon, rectum, pancreas, and bladder. Although it is useful in treating some lymphomas and leukemias, mitomycin is rarely used in pediatrics.

Three to 12 per cent of patients receiving mitomycin develop lung disease. However, many of the affected patients have also received other drugs known to cause pulmonary symptoms. Most cases develop within 6 months of institution of therapy; there is no obvious relationship to dose.

Patients with mitomycin pulmonary toxicity typically present with dyspnea and nonproductive cough. Fever is uncommon. Pulmonary decompensation may be acute, but symptoms usually appear gradually. A restrictive ventilatory defect with fibrosis is most common, but noncardiogenic pulmonary edema may occur. Chest roentgenograms are normal or demonstrate a fine reticulonodular pattern. Pleural effusion occurs infrequently. The pathologic picture is identical to that of pulmonary damage from other alkylating agents. The mortality with mitomycin-associated lung damage approaches 50 per cent. Several patients have improved after withdrawal of the drug, and dramatic improvement has been reported after introduction of corticosteroids.

ALKYLATING AGENTS

Cyclophosphamide

Cyclophosphamide is widely used in the treatment of leukemias, lymphomas, and nonmalignant illnesses. It frequently produces severe alopecia and hemorrhagic cystitis. Although pulmonary toxicity is uncommon, it does produce severe and even fatal lung damage. Mechanisms of pulmonary injury include oxidative processes as well as activation and recruitment of immunocompetent cells with presumed immunotoxicity. Acute IgE-mediated systemic reactions have been reported, including angioedema and bronchospasm.

Little is known about the relationship of dose, duration, and frequency of administration to the appearance of parenchymal disease. Pulmonary reactions have occurred following total doses between 0.15 and 50 g. Pulmonary disease may begin during, shortly after (weeks), or long after (years) cyclophosphamide therapy. Remote interstitial pneumonitis

and fibrosis have been observed in two adolescents who were treated with the drug in early childhood. The most striking feature in these cases was chest wall deformity secondary to failure of lung growth during the adolescent growth spurt (Fig. 71–1).

The onset of pulmonary toxicity is usually subacute rather than insidious as with other alkylating agents. Dry cough and dyspnea herald the onset; malaise, anorexia, and weight loss follow. Physical examination reveals tachypnea and diffusely diminished breath sounds. Adventitious breath sounds are uncommon. Chest roentgenograms may show diffuse bilateral infiltrates, sometimes with pleural thickening. Pulmonary function testing reveals hypoxemia and restrictive lung disease. Biopsy and port-mortem specimens show interstitial fibrosis, alveolar exudates, and atypical alveolar epithelial cells. Withdrawal of the drug, supportive therapy, and corticosteroids are recommended treatment. The disease may be progressive and even fatal despite therapeutic intervention.

Cyclophosphamide also may predispose to toxicity when medications such as bleomycin, azathioprine, and carmustine are used subsequently.

Chlorambucil

Chlorambucil is used in the treatment of leukemias, some lymphomas, and nephrosis. Several well-documented reports indicate that the drug produces pulmonary toxicity, albeit rarely. Little is known concerning the dose or duration of therapy necessary to produce lung damage. Patients developing lung disease have received the drug both intermittently and continuously. Duration of therapy before onset of disease ranges from months to several years.

Patients develop cough, dyspnea, fatigue, and weight loss that appears 6 months to 3 years after initiation of therapy and progressively worsens. Physical examination reveals tachypnea and fine bibasilar crackles. Chest roentgenograms demonstrate a diffuse interstitial infiltrate. Pulmonary function tests indicate restrictive lung disease accompanied by a defect in DL_{CO}. At the cellular level, the lesion is characterized by alveolar epithelial cell dysplasia, interstitial mononuclear cell infiltrates, and fibrosis. As with other drug-induced toxicities, a number of atypical type II pneumocytes are also seen. In one case, partial recovery of lung function followed prednisone therapy.

Other Alkylating Agents

Busulfan (Myleran) is used to treat chronic myelogenous leukemia, which occurs occasionally in childhood. Four per cent of adult patients undergoing long-term treatment with this drug develop interstitial pneumonitis and fibrosis. Subclinical pulmonary changes are noted at autopsy in up to one half. One child died secondary to pulmonary toxicity. As with chlorambucil, pulmonary injury is usually not evident

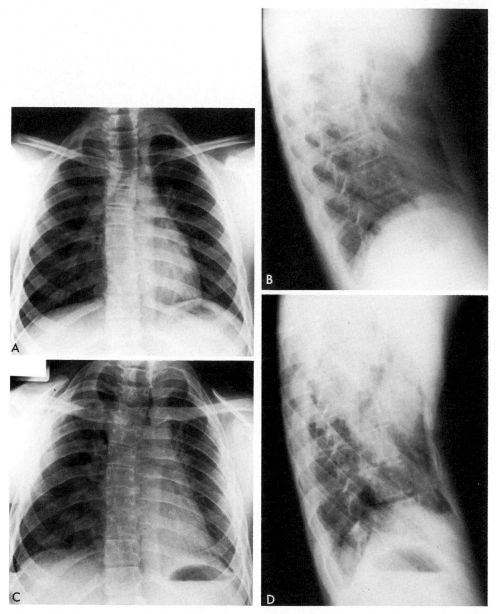

Figure 71–1. Posteroanterior and lateral chest roentgenograms, taken at ages 15 years and 19 years, of a patient successfully treated with cyclophosphamide, 25 to 50 mg daily for 4 years, between the ages of 4 and 8 years (total dose 42 g). Radiation therapy was applied to the cervical and upper mantle regions, excluding the lung fields. Pulmonary symptoms, including cough, tachypnea, and reduced exercise tolerance, were noted at 14 years of age. Lung biopsy specimen of the right lower lobe at age 15 showed interstitial inflammation and fibrosis. A and B, Chest roentgenograms taken at age 15 showed linear interstitial markings and reduced lung volume, as demonstrated by a marked narrowing of the anteroposterior diameter. Vital capacity was 35 per cent, and total lung capacity was 48 per cent of predicted. C and D, At 19 years, interstitial markings were more prominent, and lung volumes had diminished further. The anteroposterior diameter had narrowed markedly, and pleural thickening, fluid, or both were prominent at both lung apices. A small spontaneous pneumothorax was present in the right lower thorax. Vital capacity was 14 per cent and total lung capacity was 27 per cent of predicted.

for many months after initiation of treatment. Radiation and previous cytotoxic therapy are risk factors. The clinical syndrome is similar to that produced by the other alkylating agents. Treatment consists of discontinuation of busulfan and a carefully monitored course of corticosteroids. Efficacy of corticosteroids is unproven, but a trial is indicated because of the poor prognosis.

Melphalan is used primarily in the treatment of multiple myelomas and hence is employed infrequently in pediatrics. Although overt toxicity is unusual, the frequency of epithelial changes and fibrosis at autopsy may be as high as 50 per cent. Bronchial epithelial cell proliferation has been an unusual finding. Otherwise, the pathologic changes are typical for alkylating agents and may be reversible with discontinuation of the drug. One variation in presentation is the occurrence of a productive rather than a dry cough.

NITROSUREAS

Carmustine

Carmustine, also called BCNU, is a synthetic antineoplastic compound. Its major use is in the therapy of lymphomas and gliomas.

The incidence of BCNU pulmonary toxicity is quite variable; 20 to 30 per cent of treated patients develop some lung disease. The total dose administered, duration of therapy, and preexistence of lung disease are the most accurate predictors of pulmonary toxicity. Most patients with symptomatic respiratory disease have received large cumulative doses (greater than 777 mg/m^2). When the cumulative dose exceeds 1500 mg/m^2, there is a 50 per cent probability of lung disease. Patients with toxicity also appear to have received the drug over a shorter period, irrespective of the total dose given. The onset of pulmonary symptoms has been noted between 30 and 371 days after institution of therapy, sometimes after BCNU has been discontinued. Young patients reportedly are at greater risk, but this may be the result of relatively higher doses and increased numbers of therapy cycles because of greater general tolerance. Gender, race, and tumor type have no obvious predisposing effect. Radiation therapy may be synergistic.

Patients with BCNU pulmonary toxicity exhibit much the same clinical picture as that described for bleomycin. Histologic findings are also similar, with alveolar exudates, dysplasia of alveolar epithelium, interstitial fibrosis, and pleural thickening. The disease is fatal in approximately 15 per cent of those affected.

Therapy is essentially supportive. When steroids are administered concomitantly with BCNU, no protection from subsequent pulmonary toxicity occurs. However, corticosteroids may offer some benefit in the treatment of early stages of acute disease.

ANTIMETABOLITES

Methotrexate

Methotrexate (4-aminopteroylglutamic acid) is an antimetabolite used in the treatment of several childhood malignancies, notably leukemias and osteogenic sarcoma as well as nonmalignant conditions. Unlike most other chemotherapeutic agents, methotrexate causes mild and most often reversible lung disease.

As many as 10 per cent of patients treated with methotrexate develop some degree of pulmonary toxicity, but ascertainment of its effects is complicated by the frequent use of combination therapy. In some series, however, no patient treated with high doses of methotrexate demonstrated signs of lung disease clinically, radiographically, or by pulmonary function testing. Total dose and route of administration do not relate to the development of pulmonary toxicity. Daily rather than intermittent methotrexate administration may increase the incidence of lung disease. Leucovorin rescue does not protect. Methotrexate toxicity has been reported to occur days to years after administration. Gender and age do not affect predisposition. The major mechanism of toxicity is a hypersensitivity reaction, although typical cytotoxic reactions occur. Pulmonary injury is unusual in several respects: (1) Recovery may occur in the presence of continued therapy, (2) reinstitution of the drug may not result in recurrent symptoms, (3) fatal noncardiogenic pulmonary edema has occurred after intrathecal administration, and (4) acute pleuritic symptoms have been reported.

Disease usually begins slowly with a prodrome of headache and malaise, followed by dyspnea and dry cough. Physical examination reveals tachypnea, diffuse crackles, cyanosis, and occasionally skin eruptions. Laboratory studies may show a mild peripheral eosinophilia. Hypoxemia and a decreased DL_{CO} occur in most patients. Chest roentgenograms may be normal or may demonstrate diffuse alveolar filling and reticulonodular or linear interstitial densities (Fig. 71–2). There appears to be a predilection for the midlung zones as well as the bases. Pleural effusion and hilar adenopathy are rare findings. Histopathologic findings are remarkable for a prominent mononuclear interstitial infiltrate and often an accompanying tissue eosinophilia.

Therapy consists of withdrawal of methotrexate and administration of steroids. Many patients exhibit transient illness and recover completely without having to stop methotrexate therapy. Radiologic abnormalities usually resolve completely with time. Although patients eventually become asymptomatic, abnormalities of pulmonary function may persist for many months. Mortality is low, approximately 1 per cent.

Azathioprine

Azathioprine is an immunosuppressive agent that is used for various clinical situations including renal

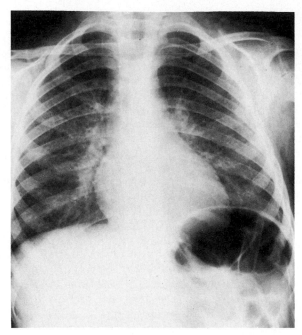

Figure 71–2. A posteroanterior chest roentgenogram of a 5.5-year-old child with acute lymphocytic leukemia, taken 3 months after treatment with methotrexate was initiated. This film was obtained soon after the appearance of cough and dyspnea. It shows both linear interstitial densities and an alveolar infiltrative pattern, most prominent in the middle and lower lung zones. A lung biopsy specimen showed typical interstitial and alveolar pneumonitis. No evidence was found for an infectious cause or for leukemic infiltration.

transplantation, inflammatory bowel disease, and autoimmune disorders. A small number of cases of dose-related toxicity have been reported in adults, largely after renal transplantation. Fever and hypoxemia are major presenting manifestations. Lung biopsy specimens reveal diffuse alveolar damage including hyaline membranes and interstitial pneumonitis with fibrosis. Eosinophilia and immune deposits have not been found. Improvement following withdrawal of the drug or treatment with corticosteroids or Cytoxan has been reported. Progressive deterioration and death have occurred in about one half of patients.

6-Mercaptopurine and Cytosine Arabinoside

Scattered case reports have linked pulmonary dysfunction to 6-mercaptopurine and cytosine arabinoside. In addition, an autopsy study of patients who had leukemia and who received cytosine arabinoside within 30 days of death demonstrated significant pulmonary edema for which there was no obvious other explanation in most instances.

Other Cytotoxic Agents

Procarbazine, VM-26, and vinca alkaloids (vinblastine and vindesine) have been associated with pulmonary injury, but in all cases other agents may have contributed. Reactions to procarbazine have been of the hypersensitivity type.

NONCYTOTOXIC DRUGS

Nitrofurantoin

Nitrofurantoin is an antimicrobial agent used widely in the prophylaxis of urinary tract infections. Significant pulmonary reactions are relatively common; more than 500 cases have been reported.

Pulmonary reactions occur in two distinct clinical patterns. In the more common acute presentation, patients report the abrupt onset of fever, cough, and dyspnea usually within hours to 2 weeks after initiation of therapy. Rash and flu-like symptoms may occur. Diffuse fine crackles and, rarely, wheezes are noted on chest examination. Bilateral interstitial or alveolar infiltrates with or without pleural effusion are characteristically present on chest x-ray; however, chest radiographs may be normal. Physiologic abnormalities include hypoxemia, evidence of a restrictive ventilatory defect, and a reduced DL_{CO}. Eosinophilia, leukocytosis, and an elevated sedimentation rate may accompany the reaction. Symptoms and chest radiographic abnormalities usually resolve within several days after withdrawal of the drug. Pulmonary histopathology associated with the acute syndrome has not been well defined, as patients improve rapidly after withdrawal of nitrofurantoin, making biopsy unnecessary.

In the less common chronic presentation, patients develop the insidious onset of cough, dypsnea, and fatigue after months to years of nitrofurantoin therapy. A lupus-like syndrome has also been reported. Crackles are heard, and diffuse, usually interstitial infiltrate is present on chest radiographs. Pleural effusion is less common than in the acute reaction. Physiologic abnormalities are similar to those found in the acute reaction but are often more severe. Eosinophilia, elevated gamma globulin and hepatic enzymes, and positive reactions for antinuclear antibodies are often found. Pulmonary histopathology typically reveals an interstitial pneumonitis with a variable amount of fibrosis. Desquamative interstitial pneumonia has also been reported in two adults on long-term nitrofurantoin therapy. Treatment includes permanent withdrawal of the drug and supportive measures. Corticosteroids have been used with apparent benefit in some patients; however, controlled studies to evaluate efficacy are not available. Resolution of symptoms, physiologic dysfunction, and radiographic abnormalities requires weeks to months and may be incomplete. Approximately 8 per cent of adult cases with the chronic syndrome are fatal.

Nitrofurantoin may injure the lungs by several mechanisms. The findings of eosinophilia, an elevated sedimentation rate, positive antinuclear antibodies, and an enhanced blastogenic response of lymphocytes from some patients in the presence of nitrofurantoin support a role for a hypersensitivity reaction. The drug may also damage the lungs by promoting the production of toxic oxygen species. Nitrofurantoin induces the production of superoxide and hydrogen peroxide in aerobic cultures of rat lung microsomes and is cytotoxic to rat lung parenchymal cells. Parenchymal cell injury is reduced by antioxidants and accelerated by hyperoxia, supporting a role for oxidant mechanisms. Modulation of lung injury by antioxidants has also been found in an in vivo rat model.

Sulfasalazine

Sulfasalazine, a combination of sulfapyridine and 5-aminosalicylic acid, is used primarily in the treatment of ulcerative colitis. Adverse reactions occur in approximately 20 per cent of recipients and include fever, nausea, vomiting, rash, and blood dyscrasias. Pulmonary reactions are uncommon. Diagnosis of drug-related lung disease may be particularly troublesome, as ulcerative colitis can be associated with various lung disorders including bronchitis, interstitial pneumonitis, alveolitis, and pulmonary vasculitis. Patients experiencing drug-related illness report the acute onset of fever, cough, dyspnea, and chest pain 1 to 6 months into therapy. Fine crackles are usually present. Chest radiographs reveal bilateral alveolar densities. Eosinophilia is often present. Pulmonary function tests reveal hypoxemia and evidence of obstructive and occasionally restrictive lung disease. Histopathologic lesions include interstitial pneumonitis with fibrosis, fibrosing alveolitis, and bronchiolitis obliterans. Discontinuation of the drug usually results in resolution of symptoms and radiographic abnormalities in several weeks to months. Corticosteroids may accelerate improvement, although their effectiveness is not well established. One fatality has been reported.

Diphenylhydantoin and Carbamazepine

The anticonvulsant agents diphenylhydantoin and carbamazepine have been associated rarely with acute pulmonary disease as part of a generalized hypersensitivity reaction. Clinical manifestations consistently include fever, cough, dyspnea, and rash occurring 3 to 6 weeks (14 months in one patient) after initiation of therapy. Crackles are heard, and bilateral interstitial or alveolar infiltrate with hilar adenopathy is seen in some instances on chest radiographs. Associated findings include eosinophilia, elevated liver enzymes, hypoxemia with a restrictive pattern of lung function, and reduced DL_{CO}. Cell counts from bronchoalveolar lavage reveal a lymphocyte predominance, and lung biopsy shows an interstitial pneumonitis possibly with mild fibrosis. Rapid improvement over days to weeks follows discontinuation of the drug. Resolution may be hastened by corticosteroid administration.

Penicillamine

Penicillamine, a chelating agent, is commonly used to treat Wilson disease, cystinuria, and lead poisoning and, occasionally, in the management of rheumatoid arthritis and primary biliary cirrhosis. Nonpulmonary toxic reactions are sufficiently severe in 25 per cent of patients to require discontinuation of therapy. A conclusive association between this agent and lung disease is problematic because of the occurrence of similar lung disorders in the underlying diseases. Twenty-five cases of well-documented penicillamine-associated lung disease are reported. Several patterns have been described: diffuse alveolitis (3 cases), hypersensitivity lung disease (3 cases), alveolar hemorrhage with or without associated acute glomerulonephritis, similar to Goodpasture syndrome (7 cases), and obstructive airway disease characterized pathologically as bronchitis, bronchiolitis, and bronchiolitis obliterans (12 cases). Cough and dyspnea develop progressively over several weeks but may begin abruptly in hypersensitivity reactions and in association with hemoptysis. Duration of therapy before the onset of symptoms tends to be short in patients with hypersensitivity reactions (< 2 months), intermediate in those with diffuse alveolitis and bronchiolitis obliterans (3 to 19 months), and prolonged in patients with alveolar hemorrhage (2 to 7 years). Elevation of the sedimentation rate, increased serum IgE, and eosinophilia may be present. Chest x-ray films show diffuse alveolar or interstitial infiltrate, hyperinflation alone, or no changes. Hypoxemia and severe obstructive lung disease with or without a component of restriction are usually identified. Discontinuation of the drug and corticosteroid therapy are warranted in most cases. Diffuse alveolitis and hypersensitivity lung disease generally improve using this approach, although some patients have residual lung disease. Response to corticosteroids has been disappointing in most cases of bronchiolitis obliterans and alveolar hemorrhage. Plasmapheresis and immunosuppressive agents have been used with apparent success in two patients with Goodpasture-like syndrome.

Gold

Gold compounds are used chiefly in the therapy of rheumatoid arthritis. Pulmonary reactions are uncommon, and diagnosis is difficult because of the occurrence of lung disease in rheumatoid arthritis. Pulmonary reactions to gold do occur in patients treated for other disorders not associated with lung disease such as other arthritides and pemphigus foliaceus. Cough and progressive shortness of breath develop over days to weeks. Symptoms begin after 1 to 4 months of therapy. Crackles are present, and chest radiographs show diffuse alveolar and/or interstitial infiltrates. Eosinophilia is found in approximately 40 per cent of patients, and the sedimentation rate is usually elevated. Lung function tests reveal hypoxemia, a reduced DL_{CO}, and restrictive lung disease. Lung histopathology reveals widened alveo-

Table 71–3. ADDITIONAL DRUGS ASSOCIATED WITH HYPERSENSITIVITY LUNG DISEASE

Sulfadimethoxine	Methylphenidate
Penicillin	Imipramine
Isoniazid	Dantrolene
Para-aminosalicylic acid	Hydralazine
Cromolyn sodium	Mecamylamine
Nonsteroidal anti-inflammatory agents*	Chlorpropamide

*Includes fenoprofen, naproxen, sulindac.

lar septa, interstitial infiltrate with lymphocytes and plasma cells, and a variable amount of fibrosis. Proliferation of type II pneumocytes may be a prominent feature. A lymphocyte predominance in bronchoalveolar lavage fluid has been found in several patients. Withdrawal of gold therapy is associated with improvement or resolution of lung disease over weeks to months. Improvement appears to be hastened by the addition of corticosteroid therapy and may be dramatic early in the course of illness. The prognosis for survival is good; however, a substantial number of patients have residual restrictive lung disease.

The mechanism of gold-induced lung injury is unknown. Cell-mediated hypersensitivity is supported by the finding of gold-induced blastogenesis of lymphocytes from blood and bronchoalveolar lavage fluid. Peripheral lymphocytes from two patients with gold-associated lung disease also elaborated lymphokines after in vitro exposure to gold. These factors were not released by lymphocytes from patients who had rheumatoid arthritis and no lung disease and who were treated with gold.

Amiodarone

Amiodarone is used in the treatment of serious cardiac rhythm disturbances. Pulmonary toxicity is the most serious complication of therapy. Approximately 5 per cent of patients develop drug-related lung disease. Risk factors for the development of lung disease are not well defined but may include total daily dose, as most adult patients who develop lung disease are maintained on more than 400 mg daily. The majority of patients insidiously develop cough, dyspnea, weight loss, weakness, and, in some instances, pleuritic chest pain and fever during the first year of therapy. Approximately one third of patients may have a more acute onset of these symptoms. Chest examination reveals crackles and, occasionally, a pleural friction rub. Diffuse interstitial or alveolar infiltrate is typically present on chest x-ray films. Pleural effusion is uncommon. Laboratory findings include leukocytosis, elevated hepatic enzymes, and a high sedimentation rate. Physiologic abnormalities include hypoxemia, restrictive lung disease, and impairment of diffusion. Lung biopsy reveals infiltration of alveolar septa with lymphocytes, plasma cells and histiocytes, patchy fibrosis, hyperplasia of type II pneumocytes, and intra-alveolar foamy macrophages representing lysosomal accumulation of phospholipids. Foamy macrophages also

can be recovered in bronchoalveolar lavage fluid. Although their presence is not pathognomonic of drug-induced injury, it has been suggested that their absence makes the diagnosis unlikely. Discontinuation of the drug results in immediate symptomatic improvement in most patients and in resolution of physiologic and radiographic abnormalities over several months. The role of corticosteroid therapy is not defined. Recurrence of symptoms has been observed in some patients as steroid doses are tapered. Alternative approaches for patients who must remain on amiodarone because of life-threatening refractory dysrhythmias are limited. Reinstitution of amiodarone therapy at lower doses after resolution of pulmonary disease alone or in combination with low-dose corticosteroid therapy has been successful in a few patients.

The mechanism by which amiodarone causes lung injury is unknown. Direct toxicity is supported by the finding that amiodarone injures cultured pulmonary endothelial cells at concentrations equivalent to those reported in lung tissues of toxic patients. It has been suggested that cellular accumulation of phospholipid may also directly injure lung cells. Disordered immune mechanisms are suggested by a marked reduction in the normal ratio of helper to suppressor T lymphocytes derived from bronchoalveolar lavage.

OTHER AGENTS

Acute respiratory deterioration has been observed when the antifungal agent *amphotericin B* is administered to potentially septic, neutropenic patients being given leukocyte transfusions. Patients develop the acute onset of hemoptysis, dyspnea, and hypoxemia in association with the appearance of new infiltrates on chest radiographs. Alveolar hemorrhage is seen in lung biopsy specimens. In one study, this syndrome occurred in approximately 60 per cent of courses of combined therapy as compared with 6 per cent of similar patients treated with leukocyte transfusions alone. A second, retrospective study has not confirmed the increased risk of respiratory deterioration; however, differences in patient population and study design may account for this discrepancy.

The parenteral administration of *fat emulsions* (e.g., Intralipid) to infants has been associated with lipid accumulation in pulmonary capillaries and small muscular arteries. Physiologic alterations in human and animal studies include transient hypoxemia, decreased diffusing capacity, and pulmonary hypertension. Potential mechanisms include alterations in pulmonary blood flow or production of vasoactive

Table 71–4. NONCYTOTOXIC DRUGS ASSOCIATED WITH NONCARDIOGENIC PULMONARY EDEMA

Aspirin*	Heroin*	Lidocaine
Propoxyphene*	Methadone*	Haloperidol
Hydrochlorothiazide	Naloxone	Ethchlorvynol*

*Pulmonary edema associated with overdose.

Table 71–5. DRUGS ASSOCIATED WITH IMPAIRMENT OF MUCOCILIARY CLEARANCE

Aspirin	General anesthetics
Opiates	N-acetylcysteine
Ethanol	Anticholinergic agents

prostaglandins. Adverse cardiopulmonary responses to lipid administration are not recognized frequently in clinical practice.

Several other drugs have been implicated sporadically in the development of hypersensitivity lung disease (Table 71–3).

Drugs producing a clinical syndrome consistent with noncardiogenic pulmonary edema are listed in Table 71–4. Some are associated with this clinical syndrome only after an overdose.

A number of drugs impair airway mucociliary clearance (Table 71–5). One of these agents, N-acetylcysteine, is used as an aerosolized mucolytic agent in the treatment of cystic fibrosis and in the bronchoscopic lavage of tenacious mucus plugs. Although its effects on mucociliary clearance after acute administration appear to be transient, repeated use of this agent is potentially deleterious. Contrary to the effects of other anticholinergic agents, the atropine analogue ipratropium has not been found to impair mucociliary clearance.

CONCLUSION

Lung injury caused by pharmacologic agents is recognized increasingly as a significant clinical problem. Lung disease caused by cytotoxic agents is particularly troublesome in that chronicity is the rule and death is a frequent outcome. Precise information about risk factors is required to bolster predictive capabilities for patients using these drugs. Additional information is needed about mechanisms of injury in order to develop more specific interventions. Finally, more sensitive and widely available diagnostic approaches and monitoring schemata are important if early intervention is to be of value.

REFERENCES

General Reviews

Bedrossian CWM: Pathology of drug-induced lung diseases. Semin Respir Med 4:98, 1982.

Cooper JAD Jr, White DA, and Matthay RA: Drug induced pulmonary disease I. Cytotoxic drugs. II. Noncytotoxic drugs. Am Rev Respir Dis 133:321, 1986; 133:488, 1986.

Wanner A: Clinical aspects of mucociliary transport. Am Rev Respir Dis 116:73, 1977.

Specific Cytotoxic Drugs

Alvarado CS, Boat TF, and Newman AJ: Late-onset pulmonary fibrosis and chest deformity in two children treated with cyclophosphamide. J Pediatr 92:443, 1978.

Bedrossian CWM, Sussman J, Cronklin RH, and Kahan B: Azathioprine-associated interstitial pneumonitis. Am J Clin Pathol 82:148, 1984.

Case records of the Massachusetts General Hospital: Case 41-1980. N Engl J Med 303:927, 1980.

Clark JG, Kostal KM, and Marino BA: Bleomycin-induced pulmonary fibrosis in hamsters. J Clin Invest 72:2081, 1983.

Clark JG, Overton JE, Marino BA et al: Collagen biosynthesis in bleomycin-induced pulmonary fibrosis in hamsters. J Clin Med 96:943, 1980.

Cooper JAD, Merril WW, and Reynolds HY: Cyclophosphamide modulation of bronchoalveolar cellular populations and macrophage oxidative function. Am Rev Respir Dis 134:108, 1986.

Jones AW: Bleomycin lung damage: the pathology and nature of the lesion. Br J Dis Chest 72:321, 1978.

Moseley PL, Shasby DM, Brady M, and Hunninghake GW: Lung parenchymal injury induced by bleomycin. Am Rev Respir Dis 130:1082, 1984.

St Clair EW, Rice JR, and Snyderman R: Pneumonitis complicating low-dose methotrexate therapy in rheumatoid arthritis. Arch Intern Med 145:2035, 1985.

Samuels ML, Johnson DE, Holoye PY et al: Large-dose bleomycin therapy and pulmonary toxicity. A possible role of prior radiotherapy. JAMA 235:1117, 1976.

Shen AS, Haslett C, Feldstein DC et al: The intensity of chronic inflammation and fibrosis after bleomycin is directly related to the severity of acute injury. Am Rev Respir Dis 137:564, 1988.

Wall MA, Wohl ME, Jaffe N, and Strieder DJ: Lung function in adolescents receiving high-dose methotrexate. Pediatrics 63:741, 1979.

Specific Noncytotoxic Drugs

Broughton RA and Wilson HD: Nitrofurantoin pulmonary toxicity in a child. Pediatr Infect Dis 5:466, 1986.

Chamberlain DW, Hyland RH, and Ross DJ: Diphenylhydantoin-induced lymphocytic interstitial pneumonia. Chest 90:458, 1986.

De Swert LF, Ceuppens JL, Teuwen D et al: Acute interstitial pneumonitis and carbamazepine therapy. Acta Paediatr Scand 73:285, 1984.

Evans RB, Ettensohn DB, Fawaz-Estrup F et al: Gold lung: recent developments in pathogenesis, diagnosis, and therapy. Semin Arthritis Rheum 16:196, 1987.

Holmberg L and Boman G: Pulmonary reactions to nitrofurantoin—447 cases reported to the Swedish Adverse Drug Reaction Committee 1966–1976. Eur J Respir Dis 62:180, 1981.

Kumar A, Bhat A, Gupta DK et al: D-penicillamine-induced acute hypersensitivity pneumonitis and cholestatic hepatitis in a patient with rheumatoid arthritis. Clin Exp Rheumatol 3:337, 1985.

Louie S, Gamble CN, and Cross CE: Penicillamine associated pulmonary hemorrhage. J Rheumatol 13:963, 1986.

Martin WJ and Rosenow EC: Amiodarone pulmonary toxicity—recognition and pathogenesis (parts 1 and 2). Chest 93:1067, 1988; 93:1242, 1988.

Matloff DS and Kaplan MM: D-penicillamine-induced Goodpasture's-like syndrome in primary biliary cirrhosis—successful treatment with plasmapheresis and immunosuppressives. Gastroenterology 78:1046, 1980.

Teague WG, Sutphen JL, and Fechner RE: Desquamative interstitial pneumonitis complicating inflammatory bowel disease of childhood. J Pediatr Gastroenterol Nutr 4:663, 1985.

Wang KK, Bowyer BA, Fleming CR, and Schroeder KW: Pulmonary infiltrates and eosinophilia associated with sulfasalazine. Mayo Clin Proc 59:343, 1984.

Yousem SA, Colby TV, and Carrington CB: Lung biopsy in rheumatoid arthritis. Am Rev Respir Dis 131:770, 1985.

JOANNA R. FIRTH, M.D., STEPHEN J. McGEADY, M.D.,
and DAVID S. SMITH, M.D.

72

PULMONARY HEMORRHAGE AND MASSIVE HEMOPTYSIS

Life-threatening intrapulmonary hemorrhage occurs in pediatric patients with or without massive hemoptysis. Whether or not hemoptysis is present depends on the age of the patient (e.g., hemoptysis is not encountered in neonates) and the location and extent of the bleeding. Unfortunately, most of the general literature on severe intrapulmonary hemorrhage concerns experiences in adults. The pediatric literature on this topic consists of isolated case reports of uncommon entities and discussions of hemorrhage in a particular age group, such as neonates, or as a complication of a disease entity, such as cystic fibrosis (CF). In addition to the paucity of comprehensive pediatric reviews, the subject is made more difficult by modification during the years of the relative frequency of the causes of massive intrapulmonary hemorrhage. The advent of antibiotics and the relative availability of health care in developed countries have nearly eliminated pulmonary abscess and chronic bronchitis with bronchiectasis as causes of massive pulmonary bleeding, but CF has emerged simultaneously as an important cause because more children with CF now survive longer. Among third-world populations, however, inflammatory lung disease remains prevalent and is a major cause of serious hemoptysis (Conlan et al, 1983).

The underlying causes of massive intrapulmonary hemorrhage may be classified as (1) congenital or acquired abnormalities of the cardiovascular and pulmonary systems, (2) infectious conditions and their complications, (3) immunologically mediated diseases, (4) neoplasms, and (5) miscellaneous causes (Table 72–1). The relative frequency of each cause varies with the age group. Consideration here is limited to hemorrhage originating in the lungs and airways and excludes bleeding secondary to upper airway lesions and hematemesis that may be mistaken for hemoptysis. Also excluded are diffuse coagulation disorders (e.g., disseminated intravascular coagulopathy, or DIC), which may affect the lung.

CAUSES OF HEMORRHAGE

NEONATAL PERIOD

Pulmonary hemorrhage in neonates has been reported to occur in 0.7 to 3.8 per 1000 live births (Yeung, 1976) and to be present in 6 to 10 per cent of neonates at post-mortem examination (Keenan and Altshuler, 1975). This frequently fatal complication is seen in infants of all sizes, although premature infants are affected most often. Onset of bleeding from the lungs may occur almost immediately after delivery or as late as 14 days of age (Esterly and Oppenheimer, 1966).

The principal causes of this entity in neonates are judged to be *abnormalities of the cardiovascular system*, on the basis of studies by Cole and co-workers (1973). In evaluating 12 neonates with pulmonary "hemorrhage," these authors established that the intrapulmonary blood actually represents pulmonary edema fluid with hematocrit level and protein content considerably different from those of the infant's blood. The common predisposing factor in their 12 infants was left ventricular failure. These investigators emphasized that diverse underlying pulmonary disorders, including hyaline membrane disease, oxygen toxicity, bacterial pneumonia, and sequelae of mechanical ventilation or aspiration, may precipitate left ventricular failure by rendering the infant asphyxic and leaving the lung more prone to bleeding as a result of direct tissue injury. Nonpulmonary disorders associated with neonatal intrapulmonary bleeding include kernicterus, intracranial hemorrhage, and hypothermia. The association of central nervous system (CNS) insults with the development of pulmonary edema has been suggested to reflect a common effect of hypoxia on the two systems (Keenan and Altshuler, 1975). It has been shown experimentally, however, that severe CNS injury may directly affect cardiac function, causing increased left ventricular end-diastolic pressure. Coagulation defects are found in some infants with extensive intrapulmonary bleeding but are believed by most investigators to be secondary to the hemorrhage rather than causative (Cole et al, 1973; Trompeter et al, 1975).

The significance of *infectious conditions* and their complications as causes of intrapulmonary hemorrhage in neonates is believed by most researchers to lie in their precipitation of left heart failure or infliction of pulmonary tissue injury. Yeung (1976), however, has described massive intrapulmonary

Table 72–1. CAUSES OF PULMONARY HEMORRHAGE AND MASSIVE HEMOPTYSIS IN PEDIATRIC PATIENTS

Category	Neonatal Period	Infancy	Childhood	Adolescence
Congenital or acquired cardiopulmonary abnormalities	Left ventricular failure with: Hyaline membrane disease, Oxygen toxicity, Bacterial pneumonia, Aspiration, Kernicterus, Intracranial hemorrhage, Prematurity, Other problems, e.g., congenital cardiac lesions	Bronchogenic cysts, Gastroenteric cysts	Pulmonary sequestration, Bronchogenic cysts, Congenital arteriovenous fistula (may be part of Osler-Weber-Rendu syndrome)	Congenital cardiac lesions: Tetralogy of Fallot, Eisenmenger complex, Pulmonic valve stenosis, Mitral valve stenosis, Various shunting procedures for pulmonic stenosis, Congenital pulmonary vein stenosis, Pulmonary arterial stenosis, Pulmonary embolism, Pulmonary sequestration
Infections and their complications	Bacterial pneumonia, Sepsis (?disseminated intravascular coagulation)	Pulmonary abscess (uncommon)	Pulmonary abscess—bacterial, Mycoses: Mucormycosis—opportunistic organism, Intracavitary aspergillosis (fungus ball) associated with preexisting pulmonary disease, e.g., cystic fibrosis, Allergic bronchopulmonary aspergillosis (occasionally seen in asthmatics), Parasitic diseases, e.g., paragonimiasis	Cystic fibrosis, Bronchiectasis
Immunologically mediated diseases	Not reported	Uncommon	Goodpasture syndrome, Immune complex-mediated glomerulonephritis, Allergic bronchopulmonary aspergillosis, Henoch-Schönlein purpura	Goodpasture syndrome, Systemic lupus erythematosus, Periarteritis nodosa, Wegener's granulomatosis, Henoch-Schönlein purpura
Neoplasms Malignant	Not reported	(Uncommon) Primary, Metastatic: Sarcoma, Wilms tumor, Osteogenic sarcoma	Bronchial adenoma—carcinoid, cylindroma, mucoepidermoid	Bronchial adenoma, Sarcoma
Benign	Not reported	Angiomas	Hemangioma	Hemangioma
Miscellaneous causes	Congenital hyperammonemia	Heiner syndrome, Pulmonary compression injury	Idiopathic pulmonary hemosiderosis, Heiner syndrome, Retained foreign body, Pulmonary compression injury	Pulmonary compression injury, Pulmonary alveolar proteinosis, Retained foreign body

hemorrhage with sepsis and has proposed a primary role for DIC in precipitating these hemorrhages.

Immunologically mediated disorders and *neoplastic lesions* are not reported to cause intrapulmonary hemorrhage in neonates.

As for *miscellaneous* causes, some neonates with congenital hyperammonemia have presented with intrapulmonary bleeding. The reason for this association is unclear but may involve ammonia toxicity of the vascular endothelium (Sheffeld et al, 1976).

INFANCY

Congenital *cardiopulmonary anomalies* occasionally cause pulmonary hemorrhage in infancy. Both bronchogenic and gastroenteric cysts have been reported to cause massive hemoptysis during this period (MacPherson et al, 1973; Chong et al, 1976; McCracken, 1979). Initial symptoms of these malformations are usually those of compression or infection, but the early signs may be overlooked. Bronchogenic cysts are prone to become infected and bleed when vessel walls are eroded. Gastroenteric cysts, which are actually enteric duplication cysts occurring within the thorax, are lined by gastric mucosa, the acid peptic secretions of which may erode the cyst wall and adjacent structures, including bronchial walls and blood vessels. Systemic–pulmonary arterial fistulas may form and rupture into an airway with resultant massive bleeding (MacPherson et al, 1973).

Infectious processes are not a common cause of hemoptysis in infancy. A lung abscess may erode large vessels with resultant massive bleeding at any age, but abscesses are uncommon today (McCracken, 1979). Fungal and parasitic infections likewise are uncommon causes of intrapulmonary hemorrhage in infancy.

Since its initial description in 1981, acquired immune deficiency syndrome (AIDS) has reached epidemic proportions in the United States and is expected to continue its course. More than 75 per cent of the pediatric AIDS cases in the United States have occurred in children infected by perinatal transmission of the human immunodeficiency virus, and most of these children become symptomatic within the first 2 years of life (Barbour, 1987). Because AIDS destroys the immune system, children are prone to become infected by various opportunistic organisms, some of which produce pulmonary infections. To date, the most common pathogen producing pneumonia in AIDS patients has been *Pneumocystis carinii*. Although this organism is not associated with pulmonary hemorrhage, the AIDS epidemic is just beginning, and other pathogens that do produce this complication may yet emerge.

Immunologically mediated diseases are uncommon in infants and have only rarely been reported to cause pulmonary hemorrhages in this age group.

Congenital angiomas are benign *neoplasms* that often manifest in infancy. Within the airway, these vascular malformations are most commonly located in the subglottic area but may also be found in the lungs. Angiomas are symptomatic by the age of 6 months in almost 90 per cent of cases. These lesions manifest most often with symptoms of obstruction, although they have been reported to produce massive intrapulmonary bleeding (Gilbert et al, 1953). Primary pulmonary malignancies, almost exclusively sarcomas, are quite rare in infancy (Glenn et al, 1975); however, metastases to the lung from extrapulmonary tumors occur, principally from Wilms tumor and osteogenic sarcoma (Glenn et al, 1975). Rarely, primary or metastatic tumors produce massive intrapulmonary bleeding in infants (Kay and Reed, 1953).

Among the *miscellaneous causes* of pulmonary hemorrhage is Heiner syndrome, which occurs most often in infancy. Characterized by recurrent pulmonary infiltrations, iron deficiency anemia, and the presence of precipitating antibodies to milk proteins, this entity is considered by some to be related to idiopathic pulmonary hemosiderosis (IPH). Hemosiderin-laden macrophages in the bronchial washings attest to the intrapulmonary bleeding, and massive hemorrhage may occur. The finding of precipitating antibodies to cow's milk proteins in the blood of patients has suggested an immunologic mechanism for Heiner syndrome, but this theory remains unproven (Boat et al, 1975). Affected patients usually improve and have fewer pulmonary hemorrhages when milk and milk products are eliminated from their diets. IPH occurs during infancy but is encountered more commonly in young children (Matsaniotis et al, 1968). Despite their propensity to produce bleeding, congenital clotting factor deficiencies alone do not cause intrapulmonary bleeding (Donaldson and Kisker, 1974).

CHILDHOOD

The congenital *cardiopulmonary malformations* associated with intrapulmonary hemorrhage during childhood include pulmonary sequestration. This anomaly consists of a segment of embryonic cystic pulmonary tissue, usually seen as a triangular density on chest roentgenogram, located in the lower lobes and nourished by a systemic arterial blood supply. Intralobar and extralobar variations in the pleural covering of the abnormal tissue have been described. The extralobar type of sequestration, located outside the visceral pleura, is more likely to manifest during childhood. The sequestration is not functional and is prone to infection. Hemorrhage may ensue as the infectious process erodes blood vessels. Bronchogenic cysts, discussed previously, may go undiagnosed until early or middle childhood; however, the complications of these cysts are similar regardless of age. Congenital arteriovenous fistula may produce massive intrapulmonary bleeding during childhood. Only 20 cases of this anomaly have been reported in children, however, indicating that the onset of symptoms is usually delayed until adult life (Bosher et al, 1963). Some patients with pulmonary arteriovenous fistulas have familial hemorrhagic telangiectasia (Osler-Weber-Rendu disease), and telangiectases of the skin should be sought in a child with unexplained intrapulmonary bleeding (Hodgson and Kaye, 1963). Bleeding occurs when these malformations break down (Masson et al, 1974). The clinical features of pulmonary arteriovenous malformations have been reviewed in depth (Burke et al, 1986). Congenital and acquired cardiac or pulmonary vascular lesions are uncommon causes of massive pulmonary bleeding during childhood but become more important during adolescence (Haroutuman and Neill, 1972). One report, however, describes hemoptysis in a 3-

year-old having congenital unilateral absence of the pulmonary artery, indicating that this complication may occur (Taguchi et al, 1987).

Infections of several types are associated with severe intrapulmonary hemorrhage during childhood. Pulmonary abscess can be associated with profuse bleeding, usually with massive hemoptysis, but as noted, these lesions are not common today in developed nations. Such abscesses may develop as sequelae to sepsis, pneumonia, or CF or as complications of foreign body aspiration. *Staphylococcus aureus* and other aerobic organisms are usually responsible for abscess formation, although some reports have implicated anaerobic organisms (McCracken, 1979). Symptoms of fever, toxicity, and pyoptysis usually antedate the intrapulmonary bleeding and hemoptysis associated with these lesions. Mycotic infections are rare causes of pulmonary hemorrhage. Implicated mycoses include the invasive forms of aspergillosis and phycomycosis. These represent opportunistic infections and generally occur only in children who are severely debilitated, immunodeficient, or immunosuppressed. The principal clinical manifestation of intracavitary aspergillosis (fungus ball) may be hemoptysis, usually of small amount. Occasionally, however, erosion of major vessels with massive bleeding occurs. Fungus ball occurs almost exclusively as a complication of existing pulmonary disease, such as CF (Mearns et al, 1967; Berger et al, 1972; Wood et al, 1976). Allergic bronchopulmonary aspergillosis (ABPA) is another manifestation of *Aspergillus* infection associated with intrapulmonary bleeding, although usually of small amount. Patients with this syndrome have asthma and present with recurrent pulmonary infiltrations and eosinophilia; thus they may also have symptoms of pneumonia or hemoptysis. Although ABPA is usually considered a complication of asthma in adults two of three patients in one report were less than 10 years of age at onset of symptoms (Imbeau et al, 1977, 1978). Other infectious conditions producing massive hemoptysis in adults include tuberculosis and bronchiectasis; in children, however, they are very seldom responsible for intrapulmonary hemorrhage (Lincoln and Sewell, 1963). Paragonimiasis is a parasitic lung-fluke disease contracted by eating infected crustacea. Found widely in Asia and Africa, this parasite often infects children and adolescents. The major manifestation is cough with blood-stained sputum, which may be intermittent or persistent. In some instances, massive hemoptysis occurs (Nwokolo, 1972). In areas where *Echinococcus granulosus* is endemic, hydatid cysts formed by this organism in the lungs may erode bronchi and produce hemoptysis (Kalani et al, 1986); similarly, amebic liver abscesses produced by *Entamoeba histolytica* may erode into the lungs and cause hemoptysis. Large-scale shifts of populations due to political upheaval in endemic areas may eventuate in the spread of these parasitic infections to parts of the world where they are not normally found (Fischer et al, 1980).

Immunologically mediated diseases are not common causes of intrapulmonary hemorrhage in children. Although Goodpasture syndrome, with massive hemoptysis, has been reported during childhood (O'Connell et al, 1964), this disorder is more common in adolescents and is discussed more fully later in the chapter. An entity with the appearance of Goodpasture syndrome has been reported in two children; it has been called *immune complex-mediated glomerulonephritis with pulmonary hemorrhage* and is differentiated from Goodpasture syndrome by the presence of circulating immune complexes rather than antibasement membrane antibodies (Loughlin et al, 1978). Asthma, considered an immunologically mediated disease, is mentioned here mainly to emphasize that uncomplicated asthma is *not* associated with pulmonary hemorrhage. Wheezing associated with severe pulmonary hemorrhage and/or hemoptysis must be regarded as indicative of another entity, such as a retained foreign body, or as a complication of asthma (e.g., allergic bronchopulmonary aspergillosis) (Marks, 1971; Imbeau et al, 1978). Henoch-Schönlein purpura is a diffuse vasculitis believed to be immunologically precipitated. It manifests most often in childhood with the triad of purpura, arthritis, and abdominal pain (Weiss and Naidu, 1979). There are two case reports of fatal pulmonary hemorrhage in patients with this purpura (Jacome, 1967; Weiss and Naidu, 1979), and one of a 10-year-old successfully treated with prednisone. Wegener granulomatosis is not common in young people, but at least 17 cases in persons younger than 16 years have been described (Roback et al, 1969; Leatherman et al, 1982).

Pulmonary hemosiderosis with hemoptysis associated with cow's milk sensitivity is noted in childhood (Levy et al, 1985).

Primary bronchial and pulmonary *neoplasms* occur infrequently during childhood. Bronchial adenomas are the most common, but fewer than 25 cases are reported. Despite the designation as adenomas, these are malignant neoplasms of three histologic types: carcinoid, cylindroma, and mucoepidermoid adenoma. The carcinoid type constitutes the majority of bronchial adenomas but does not produce the carcinoid syndrome of flushing and hyperperistalsis in children. Bronchial adenoma is a highly vascular lesion, and hemoptysis, which may be alarming in amount, occurs in 50 per cent of cases (Verska and Conolly, 1968). Other types of primary malignant bronchopulmonary tumors are quite uncommon during childhood, although both carcinoma and sarcoma are reported (Nitu et al, 1974). Benign neoplasms, including papillomas, fibromas, and angiomas, occur during childhood but are more likely to cause obstructive symptoms than bleeding (Gilbert et al, 1953; Dehner, 1975).

Three *miscellaneous causes* of severe intrapulmonary bleeding rank among the most important etiologies during childhood. The first is primary idiopathic pulmonary hemosiderosis (IPH), which manifests most often during childhood (Soergel, 1962; Levy et al, 1978). In IPH there is pulmonary hemorrhage, which may be massive, together with pulmonary infiltrations and iron deficiency anemia. The cause of IPH, as the name suggests, is unknown. Death from exsanguinating hemorrhage or respiratory failure is common in this disease (Thaell et al, 1978; Sprince and Mark, 1979). The diagnosis of primary pulmonary hemosiderosis necessitates the demonstration of hemosiderin-laden macrophages in bronchial or gastric aspirates and the ruling out of other causes of intrapulmonary hemorrhage. Among the conditions to be excluded are pulmonary hemosiderosis with precipitating antibodies to milk (Heiner syndrome), which is more common in infancy, and Goodpasture syndrome, in which antibasement membrane antibody is found (Thomas and Irwin, 1975). Some authorities believe that a lung biopsy is necessary for the diagnosis of IPH, whereas others maintain that demonstration of hemosiderin-laden macrophages and rigorous exclusion of other causes are sufficient to establish the diagnosis (Soergel, 1962).

The second miscellaneous cause of pulmonary hemorrhage in childhood is a retained intrabronchial foreign body, particularly part of a plant. In our experience this is an often overlooked cause of unexplained severe intrapulmonary hemorrhage and hemoptysis in a child. Because considerable time can elapse between the aspiration of the foreign body and the onset of hemoptysis, the history may not be helpful (Williams and Phelan, 1969; Marks, 1971). The anatomic lesion in hemoptysis secondary to foreign body retention involves hyperplasia of the bronchial vessels with development of tortuosity and varicosities. Bronchiectasis may also develop. These vessels are prone to rupture and bleed massively (Moore, 1951). Wheezing after foreign body aspiration may lead to the mistaken diagnosis of asthma, so we reemphasize here that uncomplicated asthma is *not* associated with intrapulmonary hemorrhage or significant hemoptysis. Awareness of the ability of a retained foreign body to produce wheezing, intrapulmonary hemorrhage, and even massive hemoptysis is critical, both because the bleeding is potentially lethal and because surgical resection of the involved bronchopulmonary segment is curative (Marks, 1971).

The third miscellaneous cause of pulmonary hemorrhage in children, regardless of age, is pulmonary compression injury. This may occur from exposure to a blast (acceleration), from a fall, or from an automobile crash (deceleration). The rib cage of the child, being quite flexible, need not sustain fractures in order for pulmonary compression to occur. When compression does occur, if the glottis is closed, there is a sudden violent increase in intra-alveolar pressure, resulting in severe tissue disruption. Extensive hemorrhage into the lung may occur. The pulmonary tissue changes include edema, hemorrhage, and atelectasis, a combination often referred to as "wet lung" (Moghissi, 1971).

ADOLESCENCE

Congenital or acquired *cardiovascular and pulmonary abnormalities* are an important cause of intrapulmonary bleeding during adolescence. Hemorrhages are prone to develop with anomalies producing pulmonary arterial obstruction, lesions leading to increased bronchial circulation, or conditions associated with pulmonary venous congestion. Although present from birth, these lesions characteristically produce pulmonary hemorrhage only in the second decade of life. The specific lesions most often associated with intrapulmonary bleeding are as follows: Eisenmenger complex; conditions in which pulmonic stenosis is corrected by a shunting procedure, such as tetralogy of Fallot and pulmonic stenosis; pulmonary arterial or venous obstruction; and mitral valve stenosis (Haroutuman and Neill, 1972). Pulmonary embolism, although uncommon in younger children, is encountered during adolescence and may cause intrapulmonary hemorrhage. Pregnancy and use of oral contraceptives are known to predispose adolescent girls to pulmonary emboli as they do adult women. Among malformations of the lungs, pulmonary sequestration complicated by intrapulmonary hemorrhage (described under "Childhood") may manifest during adolescence (Symbas et al, 1969). Intrapulmonary arteriovenous malformations, as noted, are most commonly discovered in adults. They are reported during adolescence, however, and may produce intrapulmonary hemorrhage (Bosher et al, 1963).

Intrapulmonary bleeding in chronic *infection* is a complication whose frequency is related to the duration of the infection; thus, it becomes more common with advancing age. During adolescence, massive hemoptysis may appear in patients with chronic bronchitis, bronchiectasis, and particularly CF. The basic lesion in hemorrhage associated with chronic infection occurs because the blood vessels of involved bronchopulmonary segments become enlarged and tortuous and supporting connective tissue is lost. Intravascular pressure may simultaneously be increased. The infectious process may erode the vessel walls, producing acute bleeding or leading to fragile systemic-pulmonary arterial fistulas (Liebow et al, 1979). Massive hemorrhage secondary to chronic infection is generally recurrent. Severe bleeding in patients with CF or bronchiectasis has been said to indicate a grave prognosis (Holsclaw et al, 1970), although a recent report disputes this traditional concept (Stern et al, 1978). As noted earlier, longer survival has led to the emergence of those with CF as a group of patients who are quite prone to severe intrapulmonary bleeding (Case Records of Massachusetts General Hospital: Case 6, 1984). A literature review of this complication of CF notes that a mortality of up to 11 per cent can accompany major pulmonary bleeding (Porter et al, 1983). Pulmonary abscess has the same risks and etiologies during adolescence as at other ages. The fungal and parasitic infections cited as causes of hemorrhage in children may likewise produce intrapulmonary hemorrhage during adolescence.

Immunologically mediated diseases, including Goodpasture syndrome, systemic lupus erythematosus (SLE), polyarteritis nodosa (PAN), Wegener granulomatosis, and Behçet disease, may cause intrapulmonary hemorrhage during adolescence. Goodpasture syndrome predominantly afflicts young males. The pathologic features consist of intrapulmonary hemorrhage and a proliferative glomerulonephritis. Massive hemoptysis often occurs, and fully half of patients with Goodpasture syndrome succumb to asphyxia during pulmonary hemorrhages (Fishman, 1976). Circulating antibasement membrane antibody can be demonstrated in the serum of 90 per cent of patients with this syndrome, and the remainder have antibody at the site of the lesion (Thomas and Richard, 1975). Immunofluorescent staining of a lung or kidney biopsy specimen from the patient or of monkey kidney overlaid with the patient's serum demonstrates a characteristic linear pattern of immunoglobulin and complement deposition along the alveolar or glomerular basement membrane; the definitive diagnosis depends on this demonstration. Goodpasture syndrome represents a cytotoxic or Gell and Coombs type II immunopathologic reaction (Coombs and Gell, 1975).

Pulmonary hemorrhage in SLE and PAN is described in individual case reports (Kuhn, 1972; Gould and Soriano, 1975; Eagen et al, 1978) and in small series (Abud-Mendoza et al, 1985) but seems to be uncommon. Both of these conditions are thought to be caused by deposition of circulating immune complexes in blood vessel walls with subsequent complement fixation and inflammatory cell infiltration; ensuing vascular wall damage is believed to lead to pulmonary hemorrhage. Immunofluorescent studies of the involved tissue in immune complex diseases demonstrate a granular or "lumpy-bumpy" pattern of deposition of immunoglobulin and complement. SLE, PAN, and the entity of immune complex-mediated glomerulonephritis and pulmonary hemorrhage, described previously, are examples of immune complex-mediated or Gell and Coombs type III immunopathologic reactions (Coombs and Gell, 1975). It has been found that inflammation of the pulmonary vessels, particularly the capillaries, may coincide with, follow, or precede evidence of vasculitis in other organs. In addition, pulmonary capillaritis may be difficult to diagnose because the unique structure of the lung allows inflammatory cells, extravasated blood, and debris to diffuse away from an injured vessel into the air spaces (Mark and Ramirez, 1985). Thus, some cases of unexplained hemoptysis may actually be undiagnosed pulmonary capillaritis as a prodrome of one of the vasculitic diseases described earlier.

Wegener granulomatosis is a severe granulomatous vasculitis involving the upper and lower respiratory tract and the kidneys; it is thought to be immunolog-ically caused. Damage to vascular walls from the granulomatous lesions may lead to intrapulmonary hemorrhage. It has been proposed that the conditions causing alveolar hemorrhage known or suspected to be on an immune basis be considered as a group (Leatherman, 1987). This group would include (1) antibasement membrane disease, (2) vasculitides, (3) idiopathic rapidly progressive glomerulonephritis, (4) chemical or drug-related conditions, and (5) idiopathic pulmonary hemosiderosis. Although instructive, this grouping does not lessen the diagnostic or therapeutic challenge for the clinician.

Neoplasms are also uncommon during adolescence, bronchial adenomas being the type likely to cause intrapulmonary hemorrhage. Thymoma has been reported in late teen years, with erosion of blood vessels by the tumor or by the radiation therapy for tumor regression, causing hemoptysis (Ludmerer and Kissane, 1982).

Miscellaneous causes of pulmonary hemorrhage during adolescence include traumatic pulmonary compression and idiopathic pulmonary hemosiderosis, described previously, and a condition only rarely reported to cause intrapulmonary hemorrhage, pulmonary alveolar proteinosis (Bhagwat et al, 1970). In patients with Ehlers-Danlos syndrome, hemoptysis is observed rarely. The mechanism in these patients is not known (Ayres et al, 1981).

In occasional cases of massive pulmonary hemorrhage, a specific precipitating cause of the bleeding is not identified despite considerable search by the physician. This disorder has been called "essential hemoptysis" if blood is coughed up (Selecky, 1978).

EVALUATION OF PULMONARY HEMORRHAGE

Evaluation of massive pulmonary hemorrhage depends on the age of the child and is influenced by the physician's knowledge of the underlying cause of bleeding. If the basic cause is unknown, the physician must determine it in order to formulate therapy. If the underlying cause is known (e.g., CF), a more limited evaluation in an attempt to localize the bleeding site may be adequate. Patients with intrapulmonary bleeding are critically ill; attention must be given to airway patency and vital signs, and unnecessary manipulation must be avoided throughout the evaluation (American Thoracic Society, 1966).

Evaluation in neonates is directed at determination of the basic problem. As indicated previously, causes of neonatal pulmonary hemorrhage are almost invariably conditions that produce hypoxia and left ventricular failure. Evaluation for these conditions is discussed at length in neonatology texts. In an infant, child, or adolescent, the history, with emphasis on the type and duration of symptoms and approximate volume of blood lost through hemoptysis, helps to define the severity of the current situation. History may also reveal the presence and type of coexisting systemic disease. The physical examination provides information on the current respiratory and circulatory status of the patient and may help to uncover the underlying disease process that produced the intrapulmonary bleeding.

Of laboratory studies and other procedures, only the blood count and posteroanterior and lateral chest roentgenograms should be routine in assessment of these patients. The causes of intrapulmonary bleeding are so diverse that a physician's knowledge of the underlying disease process, the results of these basic studies, and a patient's clinical status will dictate what further studies and procedures are indicated.

Despite this need for individualization, it is helpful to consider the assets and limitations of the techniques available for assessment. *Direct laryngoscopy and bronchoscopy* may be used to differentiate upper from lower respiratory tract bleeding. Bronchoscopy, particularly if performed while the patient is actively bleeding, can often determine whether the intrapulmonary hemorrhage is focal or diffuse and may localize the bleeding to a particular bronchopulmonary segment (Jokinen et al, 1977; Bredin et al, 1978; Selecky, 1978). *Angiograms* outlining the bronchial and/or pulmonary vessels can be most helpful in localizing pulmonary bleeding. These studies may define the underlying cause of the bleeding by showing dilated tortuous bronchial vessels, increased numbers of vessels, and bronchopulmonary anastomoses; the procedure sometimes demonstrates the bleeding site itself (Bredin et al, 1978). Angiograms may be considered for any patient in whom bronchoscopy demonstrates focal or even unilateral intrapulmonary hemorrhage. These studies are particularly important if surgical resection of the bleeding focus is anticipated, as they may localize the diseased pulmonary segment(s) and prevent needless removal of healthy tissue. *Bronchography* has a limited application in evaluation of this type of pulmonary problem; it is primarily helpful in the diagnosis of bronchiectasis (Pursel and Lindskog, 1961; Forrest et al, 1976). Except in adolescents with CF and in patients with retained foreign bodies, bronchiectasis seldom causes pulmonary hemorrhage in the pediatric age group (Holsclaw et al, 1970). During periods of active bleeding there may be dilution and washing out of the contrast material, limiting the usefulness of bronchography. In the past decade, the technologic advances in diagnostic imaging have been impressive. Computed tomography (CT), magnetic resonance imaging (MRI), and improved ultrasonography all have contributed to greatly improved diagnosis. The application of these imaging techniques to the diagnosis of the cause of intrathoracic bleeding, however, remains to be fully demonstrated. One survey in adults with hemoptysis of multiple causes compared CT studies with standard chest roentgenograms. It concluded that although the CT often provided additional information, there was seldom any impact on the clinical management of the patient (Haponik et al, 1987). In situations such as a suspected intra-bronchial radiolucent foreign body or a neoplastic lesion, CT is able to demonstrate the defect in the airway. Because MRI provides soft tissue contrast that is superior to CT, this imaging technique should be even more helpful in similar situations. Case reports of high-quality CT providing significant information in the diagnosis of bronchopulmonary sequestrations (Chan et al, 1988) or demonstrating an anomalous location of these lesions or of the blood supply (Baker et al, 1982) suggest that the potential of these modalities is great. The use of the imaging technique must be individualized to the suspected problem.

Radionuclide scans are particularly useful in detecting perfusion defects associated with pulmonary emboli. The use of scanning to determine the site of bleeding has recently been extended to infusion of ^{99m}technetium-labeled sulfur colloid, with the scan demonstrating the site of extravasation. This is a rapid and noninvasive method (Winzelberg et al, 1982).

Bronchoscopy remains an essential part of evaluation in massive hemoptysis, because a single site of bleeding is often responsible and can be identified by bronchoscope. Debate continues over whether rigid bronchoscopy or the flexible fiberoptic bronchoscope is preferable. The use of the larger rigid bronchoscope in a patient with severe bleeding has been recommended because of its greater size and ability to permit suctioning of blood (Noseworthy and Anderson, 1986). Some reports, however, have recommended use of the flexible fiberoptic bronchoscope, noting that it is able to evaluate the airway farther out than the rigid scope (Saw et al, 1976). Some authors have even recommended the use of the rigid scope initially, followed by the flexible instrument if the bleeding source remains undiagnosed. Most authorities agree that bronchoscopy should be carried out initially in massive bleeding, followed by arteriography if bronchoscopy fails to demonstrate the site of the lesion and/or to delineate the blood supply (Muthuswamy et al, 1987; Noseworthy and Anderson, 1986) and possibly as part of definitive treatment.

MANAGEMENT

The greater likelihood that patients with massive intrapulmonary bleeding will succumb as a result of asphyxiation rather than exsanguination emphasizes the need for continued close attention to airway maintenance (American Thoracic Society, 1966). Equipment for emergency intubation, large catheters with a reliable source of suction, supplemental oxygen, and the means for ventilatory assistance may be needed in management of these patients. Massive intrapulmonary bleeding may also result in hypovolemia; thus, a secure intravenous line that is large enough to permit administration of whole blood should be in place.

The management of intrapulmonary hemorrhage depends on its cause. Patients with diffuse alveolar bleeding associated with systemic illness are managed expectantly while the underlying disease is treated. Because alveolar bleeding does not easily gain access to the central airways, these patients do not usually have massive hemoptysis (Leatherman, 1987). Patients with massive hemoptysis are most likely to have a single focus of bleeding, necessitating a much more aggressive approach. All significant intrapulmonary bleeding is potentially fatal and should be managed in an intensive care unit.

NEONATES

Management of pulmonary "hemorrhage" in neonates takes into account that the origin of this blood is most often pulmonary edema fluid. Some authors recommend comparison of hematocrit measurements in the bloody fluid within the airway and the peripheral blood to demonstrate that the fluid is indeed edema rather than hemorrhage (Trompeter et al, 1975). An infant may be in severe distress when the frothy blood is first noted in the nose or mouth or may progress to respiratory failure. Assisted ventilation is usually needed, and the survival of several infants with intrapulmonary bleeding after treatment with intermittent positive-pressure ventilation (IPPV) and later continuous positive airway pressure (CPAP) has been reported (Cole and Entress, 1974; Trompeter et al, 1975). Blood loss may be significant, so careful replacement with packed red blood cells is sometimes needed. The left heart failure and whatever conditions may have precipitated the failure (e.g., hypoxia, acidosis, sepsis, intracranial hemorrhage) are treated, when possible, by means of standard therapy. The prognosis for neonates with intrapulmonary bleeding has not been good, although more recent researchers employing IPPV in treatment have reported improved survival (Trompeter et al, 1975).

OLDER INFANTS, CHILDREN, AND ADOLESCENTS

If the cause or location of the intrapulmonary bleeding is not known, the evaluation should proceed without hesitation, because exacerbations of bleeding are unpredictable and may lead to fulminant deterioration of a patient's condition. The greatest hazard of hemoptysis is based on the risk of aspiration and asphyxia. Although most reports on massive hemoptysis have emphasized the need for surgical resection of the bleeding focus (Noseworthy and Anderson, 1986; Garzon et al, 1982; Conlan et al, 1983), the effectiveness of more conservative therapy is well established in those who cannot tolerate surgery (Bobrowitz et al, 1983). General measures that have been recommended include periodically positioning the patient so that clots may be coughed up and lowering the head of the bed to facilitate tracheobronchial clearance of blood. Lowering of the head may not be tolerated by all patients, however, because some are dyspneic and feel comfortable only with their head elevated 30 to 40 degrees. The benefits of head lowering are probably not worth the anxiety it provokes in these patients. Dyspnea may be alleviated somewhat by administration of oxygen. Children or adolescents with intrapulmonary hemorrhage may become agitated, and the question of sedation invariably arises. Sedatives should be avoided or used sparingly for two reasons: (1) They may suppress the cough reflex, which is protective in that it helps clear blood from the airways, and (2) the agitation may signal hypoxia and as such is an important clinical sign, warning a physician of the urgent need for intervention.

Several traditional remedies for massive pulmonary bleeding are mentioned because they seem to confer no benefit in treating intrapulmonary bleeding. These include the application of ice bags to the chest wall over the area of suspected bleeding and various pulmonary collapse-inducing procedures. The induction of pulmonary collapse, in particular, is contraindicated because it further reduces the already compromised number of functioning pulmonary units.

A number of treatments recommended for massive hemoptysis appear to be helpful in at least temporarily controlling the bleeding. When a bleeding site has been localized to a bronchopulmonary segment by bronchoscopy, lavage of that segment with iced saline via the bronchoscope may bring about cessation of the bleeding. Iced saline lavage was reported to produce hemostasis in 23 patients with massive hemoptysis (Conlan et al, 1983). This therapy is thought to be effective by causing vasoconstriction of the bronchial vessels that are usually the source of severe bleeding. The use of intravenous vasopressin (Pitressin) has been recommended in treating massive hemoptysis. Although this treatment was formerly believed to be ineffective, two reports have recommended that administering 0.2 units/min (total dose 10 units) of vasopressin intravenously is helpful in controlling massive hemoptysis (Magee and Williams, 1982; Noseworthy and Anderson, 1986). This treatment causes vasoconstriction of the systemic circulation and is thought to be effective primarily as a temporizing or stabilizing maneuver until more definitive therapy can be provided.

Two procedures have proved helpful in managing selected patients with intrapulmonary hemorrhage. In unilateral bleeding, the insertion of a balloon-tipped (Fogarty) catheter into the affected bronchus during bronchoscopy has been reported (Gottlieb and Hillberg, 1975; Gourin and Garzon, 1975; Saw et al, 1976). The balloon is inflated, and the catheter is left in place. Adequate respiration is maintained in the opposite lung, and tamponade is provided at the bleeding site as the blockaded bronchus fills with blood. The catheter is left inflated in place for 24 hours, after which the balloon is deflated and the catheter is left for several hours longer. If bleeding does not recur, the catheter is removed; if there is further bleeding, the balloon is reinflated (Saw et al, 1976). This technique provides short-term control of bleeding and might be used in patients who could not tolerate immediate surgery or in whom surgery is not possible at all. Fogarty catheter insertion can be carried out in conjunction with diagnostic bronchoscopy if there is concern about the patient's stability and, thus, need entail no additional manipulation. It has been noted that placement of the Fogarty catheter in the right main stem bronchus for right upper lobe bleeding may result in the balloon being displaced upward into the trachea, where it precludes air exchange, or downward into the right lower lobe, where it is ineffective (Garzon et al, 1982). Right upper lobe bleeding is best managed by intubating the left main stem bronchus with a cuffed tube and inflating the cuff of the tube. This isolates the left lung and permits respiration to occur.

The second technique suggested for management of intrapulmonary hemorrhage is selective embolic occlusion of the bronchial or pulmonary vessels, leading to a focal hemorrhage, with glass microspheres (Boushy et al, 1971), small pledgets of absorbable gelatin sponge (Shuster and Fellows, 1977), or polyvinyl alcohol sponge (Fellows et al, 1979). Detachable latex balloons filled with silicone polymer have also been used to occlude vessels (Tress et al, 1983). The procedure necessitates identification of the vessel responsible for the hemorrhage by selective bronchial or pulmonary arteriography. When identification is certain, the embolizing material is selectively injected into the vessel through the catheter. This procedure is not without risk. If the arteries to the spinal cord arise anomalously from the bronchial vessels, embolization could produce a transverse myelitis with resulting paraplegia. Alternatively, dislodging the catheter from the bronchial vessel during injection of the embolizing material could lead to systemic embolization, resulting in CNS or coronary arterial occlusion. Despite these potential hazards, the procedure has been reported to be effective in treatment of patients with massive hemoptysis. This technique seems particularly suited to patients with advanced pulmonary disease such as CF or a noncorrectable cardiac or vascular anomaly, in whom surgery for the intrapulmonary hemorrhage is impractical. Some authors state that occlusion by embolization is temporary and that vessels so occluded recanalize. This seems particularly likely to happen when gelatin sponge is used as the embolizing substance (Magilligan et al, 1981). Despite this risk of delayed recurrence, the embolization is a worthwhile temporizing procedure in unstable patients or poor surgical candidates. Another technique is electrocoagulation with alternating current and a bipolar electrode. It appears to be a reliable and safe technique to gain localized obliteration and yet maintain the distal flow (Brunelle et al, 1985).

Despite the development of these new techniques for management of intrapulmonary hemorrhage, surgical resection of a bleeding focus remains the procedure of choice when feasible (Magilligan et al, 1981). In our experience, the majority of previously healthy children and adolescents who present with unexplained intrapulmonary hemorrhage are found to have a long-overlooked foreign body. It is often of plant origin and was aspirated when the child fell into grass or shrubbery while playing years before. In such patients, attempts are made to establish a diagnosis without delay and then embark on either surgical resection of the bronchopulmonary segment or transbronchial removal of the foreign body. If transbronchial removal is attempted, it must be recognized that massive bleeding may ensue. Provision for that eventuality must be made (Rees, 1985).

REFERENCES

Abud-Mendoza C, Diaz-Jonanen E, and Alac'on-Segovia D: Fatal pulmonary hemorrhage in systemic lupus erythematosus. Occurrence without hemoptysis. J Rheumatol 12:558, 1985.

American Thoracic Society, Committee on Therapy: The management of hemoptysis. Am Rev Respir Dis 93:471, 1966.

Ayres J et al: Hemoptysis and nonorganic upper airways obstruction in a patient with previously undiagnosed Ehlers-Danlos syndrome. Br J Dis Chest 75:309, 1981.

Baker EL, Gore RM, and Moss AA: Retroperitoneal pulmonary sequestration: computed tomography findings. AJR 138:956, 1982.

Ballard RA, Vinocur B, Reynolds JW et al: Transient hyperammonemia of the preterm infant. N Engl J Med 299:920, 1978.

Barbour SD: Acquired immunodeficiency syndrome of childhood. Pediatr Clin North Am 34:247, 1987.

Berger I, Phillips WL, Shenker IR et al: Pulmonary aspergillosis in childhood. Clin Pediatr 11:78, 1972.

Bhagwat AG, Wentworth P, and Cohen PC: Observations in the relationship of desquamative interstitial pneumonia and pulmonary alveolar proteinosis in childhood. Chest 58:326, 1970.

Boat TF, Polmar SH, Whitman V et al: Hyperreactivity to cow milk in young children with pulmonary hemosiderosis and cor pulmonale secondary to nasopharyngeal obstruction. J Pediatr 82:23, 1975.

Bobrowitz ID, Ramakrishna S, Shim YS et al: Comparison of medical vs. surgical treatment of major hemoptysis. Arch Intern Med 143:1343, 1983.

Bosher LH, Blake DA, and Byrd BR: An analysis of the pathologic anatomy of pulmonary A-V aneurysms with particular reference to the applicability of local excision. Surgery 45:449, 1963.

Boushy SF, Helgason AH, and North LB: Occlusion of the bronchial arteries by glass microspheres. Am Rev Respir Dis 103:249, 1971.

Bredin CP, Richardson PR, King T et al: Treatment of massive hemoptysis by combined occlusion of pulmonary and bronchial arteries. Am Rev Respir Dis 117:969, 1978.

Brunelle F et al: Successful electrocoagulation of an internal mammary artery in a child. Pediatr Radiol 15:251, 1985.

Burke CM et al: Pulmonary arteriovenous malformation: A critical update. Am Rev Respir Dis 134:334, 1986.

Case records of The Massachusetts General Hospital. New Engl J Med 310:375, 1984.

Chan CK, Hyland RH, Gray RR et al: Diagnostic imaging of intralobar bronchopulmonary sequestration. Chest 93:189, 1988.

Chong SH, Morrison L, Shaffney L, and Crowe JE: Intrathoracic gastrogenic cysts and hemoptysis. J Pediatr 88:554, 1976.

Cole VA and Entress A: Continuous positive airway pressure in infants. Lancet 1:505, 1974.

Cole VA, Normand A, Reynolds E et al: Pathogenesis of hemorrhagic pulmonary edema and massive pulmonary hemorrhage in the newborn. Pediatrics 51:175, 1973.

Conlan AA, Hurwitz SS, Krige L et al: Massive hemoptysis. J Thorac Cardiovasc Surg 85:120, 1983.

Coombs RRA and Gell PGH: Classification of allergic reactions responsible for clinical hypersensitivity and disease. In Gell PGH, Coombs RRA, and Lachmann PJ (eds): Clinical Aspects of Immunology. London, Blackwell Scientific Publications, 1975.

Dehner LP: Mediastinum, lungs, and cardiovascular system. In Dehner LP (ed): Pediatric Surgical Pathology. St. Louis, CV Mosby Co, 1975.

Donaldson VH and Kisker CT: Blood coagulation in hemostasis. In Nathan DG and Oski FA (eds): Hematology of Infancy and Childhood. Philadelphia, WB Saunders Co, 1974.

Eagen JW, Memoli VA, Roberts JL et al: Pulmonary hemorrhage in SLE. Medicine 57:545, 1978.

Esterly JR and Oppenheimer EH: Massive pulmonary hemorrhage in the newborn. J Pediatr 69:3, 1966.

Fellows K, Khaw K, Schuster S et al: Bronchial artery embolization in cystic fibrosis. J Pediatr 95:959, 1979.

Fischer GW, McGrew GL, and Bass JW: Pulmonary paragonimiasis in childhood. JAMA 243:1360, 1980.

Fishman AP: Pulmonary hemorrhage in Goodpasture's syndrome. N Engl J Med 295:1430, 1976.

Forrest J, Sagel S, and Omell G: Bronchography in patients with hemoptysis. Am J Roentgenol 126:597, 1976.

Garzon AA, Cerruti MM, Golding ME et al: Exsanguinating hemoptysis. J Thorac Cardiovasc Surg 84:829, 1982.

Gilbert JG, Mazzarella LA, and Feit LJ: Primary tracheal tumors in the infant and adult. Am Arch Otolaryngol 58:1, 1953.

Glenn W, Liebow P, and Lindskog G: Mediastinum tumors. In Glenn WW, Liebow A, and Lindskog G (eds): Thoracic and Cardiovascular Surgery with Related Pathology. New York, Appleton-Century-Crofts, Inc, 1975.

Godman G and Chung J: Wegener's granulomatosis: pathology and review of the literature. Arch Pathol 58:533, 1954.

Gottlieb LS and Hillberg R: Endobronchial tamponade therapy for intractable hemoptysis. Chest 67:482, 1975.

Gould DB and Soriano RZ: Acute alveolar hemorrhage in lupus erythematosus (letter). Ann Intern Med 83:836, 1975.

Gourin A and Garzon AA: Control of hemorrhage in emergency pulmonary resection for massive hemoptysis. Chest 68:120, 1975.

Haponik EF, Britt EJ, Smith PL et al: Computed chest tomography in the evaluation of hemoptysis. Impaction diagnosis and treatment. Chest 91:80, 1987.

Haroutuman LV and Neill CA: Pulmonary complications of congenital heart disease: hemoptysis. Am Heart J 84:540, 1972.

Heiner DC, Sears JW, and Kniker WFS: Multiple precipitins to cows' milk in chronic respiratory disease. Am J Dis Child 103:634, 1962.

Hodgson CH and Kaye RL: Pulmonary arteriovenous fistula and hereditary hemorrhagic telangiectasia. Dis Chest 43:449, 1963.

Holsclaw DS, Grand RJ, and Shwachman H: Massive hemoptysis in cystic fibrosis. J Pediatr 76:829, 1970.

Hooper P et al: Pseudohemoptysis from isoetharine. N Engl J Med 308:1602, 1983.

Imbeau S, Cohen M, and Reed CE: Allergic bronchopulmonary aspergillosis in infants. Am J Dis Child 131:1127, 1977.

Imbeau SA, Nichols D, Flaherty D et al: Allergic bronchopulmonary aspergillosis. J Allergy Clin Immunol 62:243, 1978.

Jacome AF: Pulmonary hemorrhage and death complicating anaphylactoid purpura. South Med J 60:1003, 1967.

Jokinen K, Palva F, and Nuutinen J: Hemoptysis. A bronchological evaluation. Ann Clin Res 9:8, 1977.

Kalani BP et al: Hydatid disease presenting with hemoptysis and multiple cysts in lungs, liver and spleen. Ann Trop Paediatr 1:61, 1986.

Kay S and Reed WG: Chorioepithelioma of the lung in a female infant seven months old. Am J Pathol 29:555, 1953.

Keenan WJ and Altshuler WB: Massive pulmonary hemorrhage in a neonate. J Pediatr 86:466, 1975.

Kuhn C: Systemic lupus erythematosus in a patient with ultrastructural lesions of the pulmonary capillaries previously reported in the review as due to IPH. Am Rev Respir Dis 106:931, 1972.

Leatherman JL et al: Pulmonary hemorrhage and glomerulonephritis. Am J Med 72:401, 1982.

Leatherman JW: Immune alveolar hemorrhage. Chest 91:891, 1987.

Levy J et al: Hemoptysis and anemia in a three year old boy. Ann Allergy 55:439, 1985.

Levy M, Cayroche P, Chang AWC et al: L'hemosiderose pulmonaire chez l'enfant. Arch Fr Pediatr 35:382, 1978.

Liebow A, Hales MR, and Lindskog G: Enlargement of the bronchial arteries and their anastomoses with the pulmonary arteries in bronchiectasis. Am J Pathol 25:211, 1979.

Lincoln EM and Sewell EM: Tuberculosis in Children. New York, McGraw-Hill Book Co, Inc, 1963.

Loughlin G, Taussig LM, Murphy SA et al: Immune complex-mediated glomerulonephritis and pulmonary hemorrhage simulating Goodpasture's syndrome. J Pediatr 93:181, 1978.

Ludmerer KM and Kissane JM: Massive hemoptysis in a young man with myasthenia gravis and thymoma. Am J Med 73:914, 1982.

McCracken GH: Lung abscess in childhood. Hosp Pract 13:35, 1979.

MacPherson RJ, Reed MH, and Ferguson CC: Intrathoracic gastrogenic cysts: a cause of lethal pulmonary hemorrhage in infants. J Can Assoc Radiol 24:362, 1973.

Magee G and Williams MH: Treatment of massive hemoptysis with intravenous pitressin. Lung 160:165, 1982.

Magilligan DJ, Ravipati S, Zayat P et al: Massive hemoptysis: control by transcatheter bronchial artery embolization. Ann Thorac Surg 32:392, 1981.

Mark EJ and Ramirez JF: Pulmonary capillaritis and hemorrhage in patients with systemic vasculitis. Arch Pathol Lab Med 5:413, 1985.

Marks MB: Significance of recurrent hemoptysis in allergic asthma. Clin Pediatr 10:479, 1971.

Masson RG, Altose MD, and Mazack RL: Isolated bronchial telangiectasia. Chest 65:450, 1974.

Matsaniotis N, Karpouzas J, Apostolopoulou E et al: Idiopathic pulmonary haemosiderosis in children. Arch Dis Child 43:307, 1968.

Mearns M, Longbottom J, and Batlen J: Precipitating antibodies to Aspergillus fumigatus in cystic fibrosis. Lancet 1:538, 1967.

Moghissi K: Laceration of the lung following blunt trauma. Thorax 26:223, 1971.

Moore BP: Bronchiectasis with unsuspected foreign body. Br Med J 2:1259, 1951.

Muthuswamy PP, Akbik F, Franklin C et al: Management of major or massive hemoptysis in active pulmonary tuberculosis by bronchial arterial embolization. Chest 92:77, 1987.

Nitu Y, Kubota H, Hasegawa S et al: Lung cancer (squamous cell carcinoma) in adolescence. Am J Dis Child 127:128, 1974.

Noseworthy TW and Anderson BJ: Massive hemoptysis. Can Med Assoc J 135:1097, 1986.

Nwokolo C: Outbreak of paragonimiasis in Eastern Nigeria. Lancet 1:32, 1972.

O'Connell EJ, Dower JC, Burke EC et al: Pulmonary hemorrhagic-glomerulonephritis syndrome. Am J Dis Child 108:302, 1964.

Porter PK et al: Massive hemoptysis in cystic fibrosis. Arch Intern Med 143:387, 1983.

Pursel SE and Lindskog GE: Hemoptysis: a clinical evaluation of 105 patients examined consecutively on a thoracic surgical service. Am Rev Respir Dis 84:329, 1961.

Rees JR: Massive hemoptysis associated with foreign body removal. Chest 8:475, 1985.

Roback SA, Herdman RC, Hoyer J, and Good RA: Wegener's granulomatosis in a child. Am J Dis Child 118:608, 1969.

Sarnoff SJ and Berglund E: Neurodynamics of pulmonary edema. Am J Physiol 170:588, 1952.

Saw EC, Gottlieb LS, Yokozama T et al: Flexible fiberoptic bronchoscopy and endobronchial tamponade in the management of massive hemoptysis. Chest 70:589, 1976.

Selecky PA: Evaluation of hemoptysis through the bronchoscope. Chest 73(suppl):741, 1978.

Sheffeld LJ, Danks DM, Hammond JW et al: Massive pulmonary hemorrhage as a presenting feature in congenital hyperammonemia. J Pediatr 88:450, 1976.

Shuster S and Fellows K: Management of major hemoptysis in patients with cystic fibrosis. J Pediatr Surg 12:889, 1977.

Soergel K: Idiopathic pulmonary hemosiderosis and related syndromes. Am J Med 32:499, 1962.

Sprince NL and Mark EJ: Idiopathic pulmonary hemosiderosis in case records of Massachusetts General Hospital. N Engl J Med 301:201, 1979.

Stankiewicz JA et al: Embolization and treatment of massive hemoptysis in patients with cystic fibrosis. Ear Nose Throat J 64:180, 1985.

Stern RC, Wood RE, Boat TF et al: Treatment and prognosis of massive hemoptysis in cystic fibrosis. Am Rev Respir Dis 117:825, 1978.

Symbas PN, Hatcher ER, Abbott OA et al: An appraisal of pulmonary sequestration: special emphasis on unusual manifestations. Am Rev Respir Dis 99:406, 1969.

Taguchi T et al: Isolated unilateral absence of left pulmonary artery with peribronchial arteriovenous malformations showing recurrent hemoptysis. Pediatr Radiol 17:316, 1987.

Thaell JF, Griepp PR, Stubbs SE et al: Idiopathic pulmonary hemosiderosis: two cases in a family. Mayo Clin Proc 53:113, 1978.

Thomas HM and Irwin RS: Classification of diffuse intrapulmonary hemorrhage. Chest 68:483, 1975.

Thomas HM and Richard RS: Classification of diffuse intrapulmonary hemorrhage. Chest 68:484, 1975.

Trento A, Estner S, Griffith B et al: Massive hemoptysis in patients with cystic fibrosis: three case reports and a protocol for clinical management. Ann Thorac Surg 39:254, 1985.

Tress BM, Thomson KR, ApSimon HT et al: Treatment of caroticocavernous fistulae with detachable balloons introduced by percutaneous catheterization. Med J Austral 1:373, 1983.

Trompeter R, Yu V, Aynsley-Green A et al: Massive pulmonary hemorrhage in the newborn infant. Arch Dis Child 50:128, 1975.

Ullah MI: Potential hazard of nebulised salbutamol in patients with haemoptysis. Br Med J 286:844, 1983.

Verska JJ and Conolly JE: Bronchial adenomas in children. J Thorac Cardiovasc Surg 55:411, 1968.

Wakefield SJ et al: Abnormal cilia in Polynesians with bronchiectasis. Am Rev Respir Dis 121:1003, 1980.

Weiss VF and Naidu M: Fatal pulmonary hemorrhage in Henoch-Schönlein purpura. Cutis 23:687, 1979.

Williams HE and Phelan PD: The "missed" inhaled foreign body in children. Med J Aust 1:625, 1969.

Winter JH: Haemoptysis and aspirin ingestion. Lancet 1(8339):1441, 1983.

Winzelberg G, Wholey MH, and Sachs M: Scintigraphic localization of pulmonary bleeding using technetium Tc 99m sulfur colloid: a preliminary report. Radiology 143:757, 1982.

Wood RE, Boat TF, and Doershuk CF: Cystic fibrosis. Am Rev Respir Dis 113:833, 1976.

Yeung CY: Massive pulmonary hemorrhage in neonatal infection. Can Med Assoc J 114:135, 1976.

73

ARNOLD M. SALZBERG, M.D., JAMES W. BROOKS, M.D., and THOMAS M. KRUMMEL, M.D.

DISORDERS OF THE RESPIRATORY TRACT DUE TO TRAUMA

The occurrence of thoracic trauma in infants and children is exceedingly rare and is usually confined to automobile accidents, the battered child syndrome, and falls from a considerable height. Stab and bullet wounds are rare. Nevertheless, the complete spectrum of chest trauma has been recorded, including pneumothorax, hemothorax, destruction of the integrity of the chest wall and diaphragm, thoracic visceral damage, and combined thoracoabdominal injuries (Fig. 73–1).

As in adults, the significance of thoracic trauma parallels the pulmonary, cardiac, and systemic dysfunction that follows, and in the pediatric age group, because of chest wall resiliency, physiologic aberrations can occur with trauma that does not fracture or penetrate. The interruption of satisfactory respiration and circulation secondary to chest injury is frequently complicated by blood loss and hypotension, and all three factors must be quickly reversed for survival. Shock from hemorrhage can usually be managed through intelligent, arithmetic specific re-placement, which is monitored by serial determinations of blood pressures, hematocrit, central venous pressure, blood gases, and, if necessary, blood volume, and by pulmonary artery catheterization with a Swan-Ganz catheter for more precise information relating to pulmonary capillary wedge pressures and cardiac output. Restoration of the normal cardiopulmonary function fundamentally depends on a clear airway, intact chest and diaphragm, and unrestricted heart-lung dynamics. This condition can in most instances be accomplished by maneuvers other than thoracotomy.

STERNAL FRACTURES

Fractures of the sternum in infancy and childhood follow high-compression crush injuries and are usually associated with other thoracic and orthopedic problems elsewhere.

On physical examination there is local tenderness,

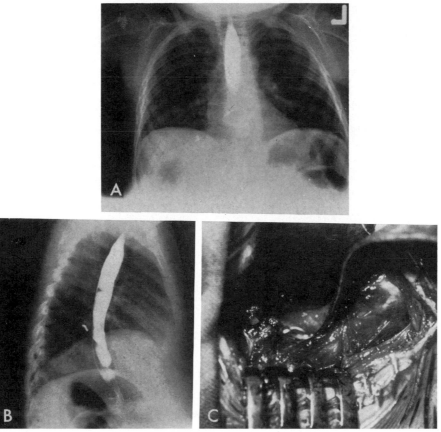

Figure 73–1. The posterior chest wall of this 8-year-old boy was penetrated by an object that was apparently accelerated by a power mower operating 8 feet away. *A* and *B*, Posteroanterior and lateral chest films with barium in the esophagus demonstrate an opaque foreign body in the posterior mediastinum. *C*, Through an extrapleural approach a curved nail, seen just below the stump of the resected rib and lying on the aorta, was removed from the posterior mediastinum.

ecchymosis, and sometimes a peculiar concavity or paradoxical respiratory movement, but the sternal segments usually are well aligned, without much displacement. Dyspnea, cyanosis, tachycardia (or arrhythmia), and hypotension may be evidence of an underlying contusion of the heart.

Cardiac tamponade and acute traumatic myocardial damage must be ruled out by various studies, including serial electrocardiograms, echocardiograms, sonography, and careful monitoring of venous blood pressure. If the bony deformity is minimal, appropriate posture will suffice. Markedly displaced fragments are reduced under general anesthesia by the closed or open technique in order to prevent a traumatic pectus excavatum. Violent paradoxical respirations can be controlled by operative fixation or, preferably, by assisted mechanical respiration through an artificial airway.

RIB FRACTURES

Rib fractures are unusual in children because of the extreme flexibility of the osseous and cartilaginous framework of the thorax. Crush and direct blow injuries are the usual etiologic factors. In addition, manual compression of the lateral chest wall, rickets, tumors, and osteogenesis imperfecta have been incriminated. Multiple fractures of the middle ribs can be seen in the battered child syndrome (Fig. 73–2). The upper ribs are protected by the scapula and related muscles, and the lower ones are quite resilient.

Violence to the chest wall may produce pulmonary and cardiac lacerations and contusions, various pneumothoraces, and hemothorax. Critical respiratory distress may also follow multiple anterior rib fractures, in which the integrity of the thoracic cage is destroyed and the involved chest becomes flail (Fig. 73–3). The unsupported area of the chest wall moves inward with inspiration and outward with expiration, and these paradoxical respiratory excursions inexorably lead to dyspnea (Fig. 73–4). The explosive expiration of coughing is dissipated and made ineffectual by the paradoxical movement and intercostal pain. In effect, the ideal preparation for the respiratory distress syndrome—airway obstruction, atelectasis, and pneumonia—has been established.

The clinical picture includes local pain that is aggravated by motion. Tenderness is elicited by pressure applied directly over the fracture or elsewhere on the same rib. The fracture site may be edematous

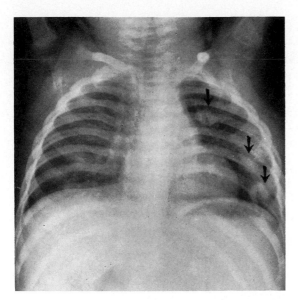

Figure 73–2. Multiple fractures of the left fourth and fifth ribs and fracture of the left clavicle in a battered child.

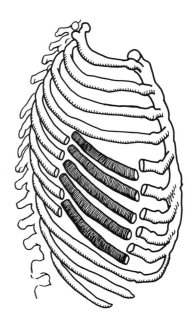

FRACTURED RIBS

Figure 73–3. An illustration of five ribs broken in two places, with loss of chest wall stability and resultant paradoxical or "flail chest" wall.

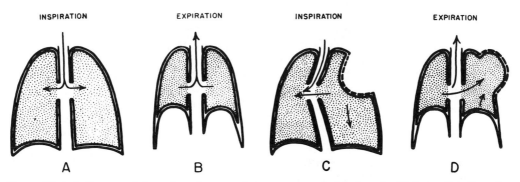

NORMAL RESPIRATION   PARADOXICAL MOTION

INSPIRATION   EXPIRATION   INSPIRATION   EXPIRATION

A   B   C   D

Figure 73–4. A diagram of the action of a normal chest compared with that of a "flail chest" during phases of the respiratory cycle.

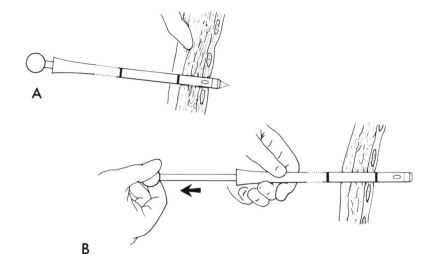

Figure 73–5. The trocar technique of chest tube insertion.

and ecchymotic. The clinical manifestations may range from these minimal findings with simple, restricted fractures to the severest form of ventilatory distress with a flail chest and lung injury.

Chest roentgenograms demonstrate the extent and displacement of the fractures and underlying visceral damage.

Treatment of the uncomplicated fracture involves control of pain in order to permit unrestricted respiration. Displacement requires no therapy. With severe fractures, alleviation of pain and restoration of cough are important and can be provided by analgesics, physiotherapy, and intermittent positive-pressure breathing mechanisms. Thoracentesis and insertion of intercostal tubes should be done promptly for pneumothorax and hemothorax, and shock should be managed by appropriate replacement therapy and oxygen (Figs. 73–5 and 73–6).

Paradoxical respiratory excursions with flail chest must be promptly brought under control to help prevent the respiratory distress syndrome, which may be the morbid pulmonary complication (Fig. 73–7).

TRACHEOSTOMY IN CHEST WALL INJURY

Controlled mechanical respiration through an endotracheal tube has been used for paradox and respiratory insufficiency. In spite of vigorous ther-

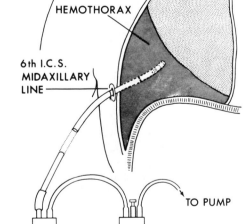

Figure 73–6. The classic setup for closed drainage of pleural space.

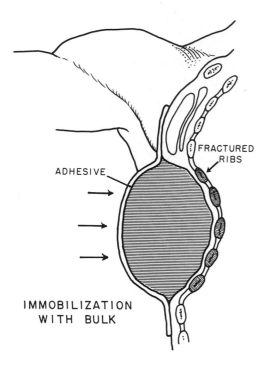

Figure 73–7. Bulky dressings applied as temporary stabilization for "flail chest" wall.

apy, secretions cannot be avoided; they are treated using tracheal catheterization and bronchoscopy. Tracheostomy, then, becomes useful in providing an avenue for the control of profuse secretions, diminishing the dead space, and bypassing an obstructed airway (Fig. 73–8). Mechanical respiration can be applied and maintained through the tracheostomy for several weeks.

During the first year of life, however, tracheostomy is a morbid operation and should be avoided if possible. Secretions may be difficult to aspirate, and the small tracheostomy tube easily becomes plugged; distal infection, often with staphylococci, is poorly handled by such young patients, and withdrawal of the tracheostomy tube at times is a precarious and unpredictable adventure. Nevertheless, even in this age group, and certainly later, tracheostomy can be mandatory and life saving in specific instances of chest trauma.

The decision for tracheostomy in cases of chest

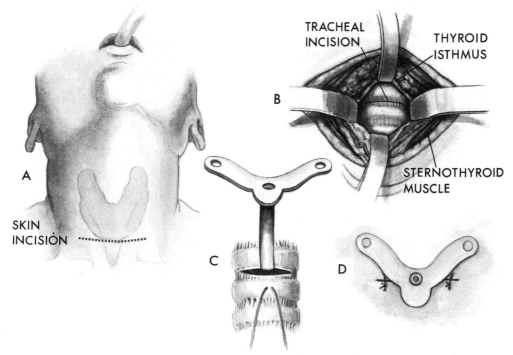

Figure 73–8. Techniques of tracheostomy performed over an oral endotracheal tube. Note the transverse skin incision in *A* and the suture on the lower tracheal flaps to facilitate subsequent tube changes *(C)*.

injury can often be made if there is (1) a mechanically obstructed airway that cannot be managed more conservatively and (2) flail chest. The unstable, paradoxical chest wall movement can be controlled for long periods by assisted positive-pressure respirations through a short, uncuffed Silastic tracheostomy tube.

Often, however, the decision for tracheostomy is first considered in the presence of minimal dyspnea. In this situation, use of blood gas studies can augment the clinical impression and intercept clinical respiratory failure. Serial measurements of pH and arterial carbon dioxide tension are a satisfactory chemical guide to imminent ventilatory distress and the need for and efficiency of assisted or controlled mechanical respiration, because the finding of normal values rules out the presence of anoxia.

TRAUMATIC PNEUMOTHORAX

Traumatic tension and open pneumothorax are rare in infants and children, in whom a very mobile mediastinum would compound the cardiorespiratory distress usually encountered in such injuries. Both types of injuries are formidable and require specific maneuvers to reverse a malignant chain of events.

The creation of a tension pneumothorax in which intrapleural pressures approach or exceed atmospheric pressures requires a valvular mechanism through which the amount of air entering the pleural space exceeds the amount escaping it. The positive intrapleural pressure is dissipated by a mediastinal shift, which compresses the opposite lung in the presence of ipsilateral pulmonary collapse and angulates the great vessels entering and leaving the heart. Intrapleural tension can be increased by traumatic hemothorax, and respiratory exchange and cardiac output are critically diminished by this form of mediastinal tamponade.

The etiologic possibilities, in addition to chest wall and lung trauma, include rupture of the esophagus, pulmonary cyst, emphysematous lobe, and postoperative bronchial fistula. These latter sources of tension pneumothorax almost always require thoracotomy for control.

The clinical findings may include external evidence of a wound, tachypnea, dyspnea, cyanosis with hyperresonance, absence or transmission of breath sounds, and dislocation of the trachea and apical cardiac impulse. The hemithoraces may be asymmetric, the involved side being the larger.

A confirmatory radiograph is comforting but often cannot be afforded in this thoracic emergency. Fiberoptic transillumination may be helpful. Plastic needle aspiration or chest tube insertion is indicated for a tension pneumothorax or a pneumothorax exceeding 25 per cent. Prompt relief and pulmonary expansion can be anticipated if the source of the intrapleural air has been controlled. Obviously, a traumatic valvular defect in the chest wall can be occluded. If the pulmonary air leak persists or recurs, the possibility of further tension pneumothorax is circumvented by the insertion of one or more intercostal tubes connected to water-seal drainage with mild suction. Most instances of traumatic tension pneumothorax require tube drainage for permanent decompression, although the needle is indispensable for emergency management. Stubborn bronchopleural fistulas that continue to remain widely patent despite adequate intercostal tube deflation may close after a therapeutic pneumoperitoneum. If this fails, thoracotomy may be required.

An open, sucking pneumothorax in which atmospheric air has direct, unimpeded entrance into and exit from a relatively free pleural space is a second, equally urgent thoracic emergency (Fig. 73–9). This access is almost invariably accomplished through a large traumatic hole in the chest wall. Ingress of air during inspiration and egress during expiration produce an extreme degree of paradoxical respiration and mediastinal flutter, which is partially regulated by the size of the chest wall defect in comparison with the circumference of the trachea. If a considerable segment of chest wall is absent, more air is exchanged at this site than through the trachea, because the pressures are similar. Inspiration collapses the ipsilateral lung and drives its alveolar air into the opposite side. During expiration, the air returns across the carina. In addition, the mediastinum becomes a widely swinging pendulum compressing the uninjured lung on inspiration and the lung on the injured side during expiration (Fig. 73–10). Obviously, under these circumstances, little effective ventilation is taking place because of the tremendous increase in the pulmonary dead space and the decrease in tidal exchange. A totally ineffective cough completes the clinical picture.

The diagnosis is readily made by inspection of the thoracic wound and the peculiar sound of air going into and coming out of the chest.

The emergency management of this critical situation is prompt occlusion of the chest wall defect by bulky sterile dressings (Fig. 73–11) and measures to prevent conversion of this open pneumothorax into an equally aggravating tension pneumothorax, which can occur if the underlying lung has been traumatized. In this regard, Haynes (1952) has emphasized the importance of simultaneous pleural decompression by closed intercostal tube drainage. After systemic stabilization, more formal surgical débridement, reconstruction, and closure can be done in the operating room.

Subcutaneous emphysema usually results from injury to the pulmonary ventilatory system (Fig. 73–12). The possibility of gastrointestinal tract injury or gas-forming bacilli must not be overlooked.

HEMOTHORAX

Blood in the pleural cavity is perhaps the most common sequela of thoracic trauma, regardless of type. The source of the bleeding is either systemic (high pressure) from the chest wall or pulmonary (low pressure). Hemorrhage from pulmonary vessels

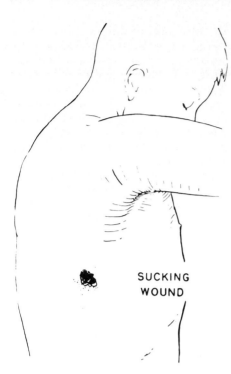

Figure 73–9. An open pneumothorax due to a traumatic chest wall defect allowing ingress and egress of air into and from the pleural cavity.

SUCKING
WOUND

NORMAL RESPIRATION   OPEN PNEUMOTHORAX

INSPIRATION   EXPIRATION   INSPIRATION   EXPIRATION

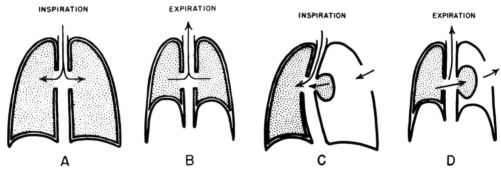

A   B   C   D

Figure 73–10. Changes in the normal respiratory pattern brought about by an open, sucking thoracic wall injury.

Figure 73–11. A temporary occlusive chest wall dressing applied to a sucking wound with underwater intercostal chest tube drainage. Once the period of emergency is over, operative débridement and closure of the chest wound is necessary.

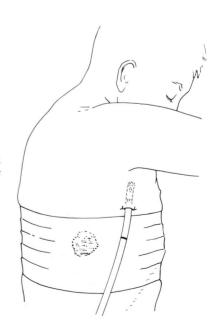

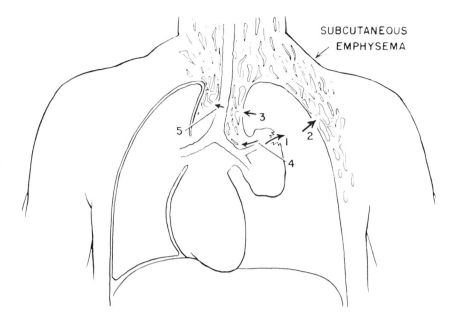

Figure 73–12. Subcutaneous emphysema resulting from an injury to the pulmonary system.

is usually self-limiting unless major tributaries have been transected.

Intrapleural blood eventually clots and becomes organized fibrous tissue (fibrothorax) (Fig. 73–13). Before this development, pulmonary compression and mediastinal displacement with reduced vital capacity and atrial filling can occur. With the development of a fibrothorax, the changes in cardiorespiratory dynamics become chronic as the lung becomes incarcerated and the chest wall is immobilized. Finally, empyema from secondary contamination is always a threat when the pleural space is filled with blood.

The immediate findings are those of blood loss compounded by respiratory distress and perhaps hemoptysis. The trachea and apical impulse are dis-

located, the percussion note is flat, and the breath sounds are indistinct. The actual diagnosis is confirmed by thoracentesis after adequate radiographic studies, if time allows.

It has been established that aspiration of a hemothorax and expansion of the underlying lung do not instigate additional bleeding. Accordingly, the local management of hemothorax is prompt, continuous, and total evacuation without air replacement. The dead space is abolished, and without it empyema cannot occur. Such evacuation is best accomplished by insertion of a chest tube (see Fig. 73–6). Clotting is circumvented, and pulmonary function is restored by pulmonary expansion. Further extensive bleeding must be controlled by operation. Obviously, systemic resuscitation has not been overlooked.

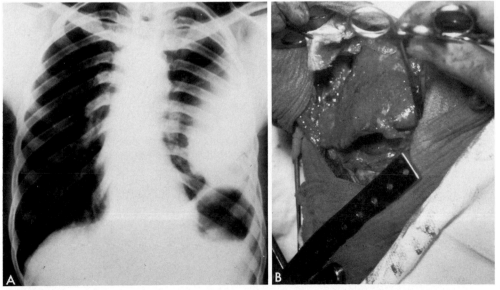

Figure 73–13. *A,* A clotted hemothorax. *B,* Operative decortication of the pleural peel of an improperly treated hemothorax.

Clotting, loculation, and infection may supervene despite vigorous initial therapy. A rare patient eventually requires decortication.

TRACHEOBRONCHIAL TRAUMA

Rupture of the trachea or bronchus in infants and children is usually preceded by a severe compression injury of the chest or a sharp blow to the anterior part of the neck. This discontinuity of a major airway is characterized by intrathoracic tension phenomena; later, stricture at the site of rupture leads to loss of lung function by sepsis and atelectasis.

Rapidly progressive interstitial emphysema, pneumomediastinum, tension pneumothorax, and hemoptysis are fairly specific. Upper rib fractures usually occur on the involved side but certainly are not constant in children with partial tracheal or bronchial transection.

Conventional chest roentgenograms and the air tracheobronchogram can suggest the diagnosis in the presence of a compatible clinical picture, but bronchoscopic demonstration of the rupture is always necessary. The diagnosis may not be suspected during the acute phase of smaller transections of major or minor bronchi but becomes obvious when late stricture with distal atelectasis and chronic pneumonitis is related retrospectively to a history of fairly severe chest trauma.

The initial management of bronchial rupture is concerned with the maintenance of a patent airway and decompression of the pleura and mediastinum by one or more intercostal tubes connected to closed drainage. Confirmatory endoscopy and elective bronchoplasty within several months are followed by little or no loss of pulmonary function distal to the narrowed segment (Weisel and Jake, 1953; Mahaffey et al, 1956). Emergency bronchoscopy and immediate repair of the defect are preferred to a course of delayed recognition and repair, because morbidity can thus be circumvented.

Severe lacerations of the trachea can be immeasurably helped by bypassing the glottis with an artificial airway during the acute phase while preparing the patient for emergency tracheal repair. Smaller tears may heal spontaneously with tracheostomy alone; others result in stricture and require later tracheorrhaphy.

PULMONARY COMPRESSION INJURY (TRAUMATIC ASPHYXIA)

Explosive blasts compress a child's flexible ribs, sternum, and cartilages against the lungs with a sudden, violent increase in intra-alveolar pressure. Alveolar disruption, interstitial emphysema, and pneumothorax may follow if the glottis is closed when the compression occurs. Distribution of this force to the great, valveless veins of the mediastinum and jugular system leads to venous distention, extravasation of blood, purplish edema of the head, neck, and upper extremities, and possible central nervous system changes due to intracerebral edema and petechial hemorrhages ("traumatic asphyxia"). The pulmonary contusion is represented pathologically by edema, hemorrhage, and atelectasis.

Clinically, there may be dyspnea, cough, chest pain, hemoptysis, hypoxia, hypercarbia, and mental confusion. The face and the neck can be grotesquely swollen, with crepitus and submucous and subconjunctival hemorrhage (Fig. 73–14). There need not be evidence of external trauma or fractured ribs in

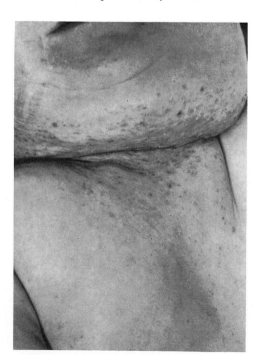

Figure 73–14. Subcutaneous hemorrhage and emphysema of the face and chest in an infant involved in an automobile accident. There were bilateral pulmonary contusions but no fractured ribs.

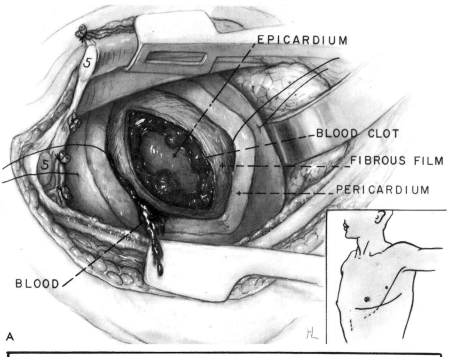

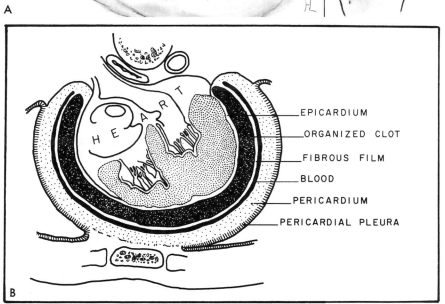

Figure 73–15. A traumatic cardiac tamponade relieved by an open thoracotomy 5 days following trauma and after two partially relieving pericardioocenteses.

a child, and accordingly, the indication for chest roentgenogram is merely the possible history of a blast, acceleration (fall), or deceleration (automobile) injury. Unilateral or bilateral pulmonary hematoma, hemothorax, pneumothorax, and pneumomediastinum can be encountered.

With mild injuries, the subcutaneous emphysema and purplish hue gradually and spontaneously disappear over several days. Patients with more serious blast injuries are treated initially for anoxia and hypotension, and attention is then directed to the wet lung, atelectasis, and pleural complications. Rapid progression of the mediastinal and subcutaneous emphysema indicates a serious disruption of the trachea, bronchi, or lungs and may require intercostal tube drainage or even thoracotomy.

POSTTRAUMATIC ATELECTASIS (WET LUNG)

With pulmonary contusion from any source, production of tracheobronchial secretions is stimulated, but elimination is impeded by airway obstruction, pain, and depression of cough. The addition of hemorrhage to these accumulated secretions produces atelectasis in the damaged lung and inevitable infection—a syndrome aptly called wet lung.

The clinical findings are dyspnea and cyanosis, an incessant, unproductive cough with wheezing and audible rattling, and gross rhonchi and rales. Chest roentgenograms show varying degrees of unilateral and bilateral atelectasis.

The syndrome demands vigorous treatment to

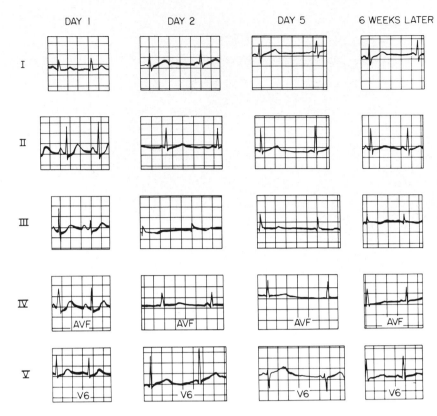

Figure 73–16. An electrocardiogram of a 15-year-old male admitted for blunt chest wall trauma after an automobile accident. Note the progressive ST and T changes with marked depression immediately after the accident. There was an improvement in the ST segment and a flattening of the T waves on day 2 and a reversal to normal in later tracings. (Courtesy of Dr. C McCue.)

avoid morbidity and mortality. Such preventive treatment should be started, in all instances of chest trauma, by frequent changes of position, insistence on coughing, small amounts of depressant drugs, oxygen, humidification, antibiotics, mechanical ventilation, diuretics, intravenous colloid, and minimal hydration. If a child with chest trauma will not cough, tracheal catheterization, popularized by Haight (1938), should be instituted before the appearance of early signs of the wet lung syndrome. Failure of this step should be followed in quick succession by bronchoscopy and an endotracheal tube insertion or tracheostomy if endoscopic aspiration is required too frequently. Spencer (1964) has emphasized the advantages of endoscopy through the tracheal stoma.

The adult respiratory distress syndrome that occurs after critical illness, surgery, or trauma with congestion, edema, hemorrhage, pneumonia, and pulmonary fibrosis is rarely, if ever, encountered in pediatric practice.

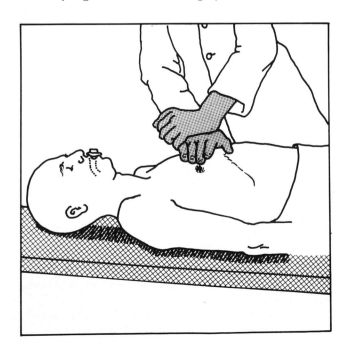

Figure 73–17. External cardiac massage.

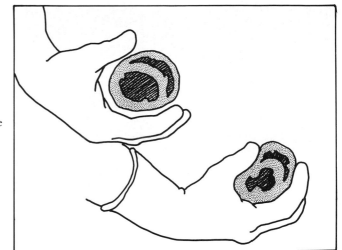

Figure 73–18. Internal cardiac massage: one handed technique for neonates and infants.

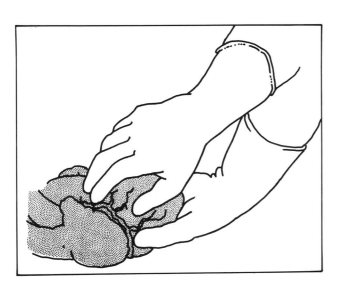

Figure 73–19. Internal cardiac massage: bimanual technique for older children and adults.

Figure 73–20. Electrode application for external cardiac defibrillation.

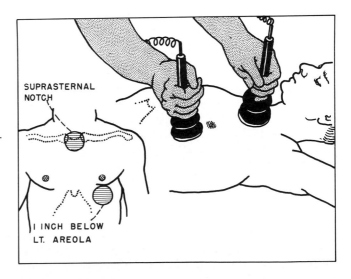

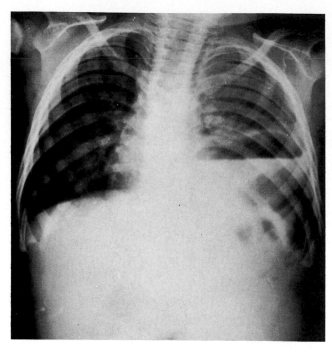

Figure 73-21. A blunt traumatic rupture of the left hemidiaphragm that went unrecognized. Death occurred 1 hour later from acute gastric dilation of the intrathoracic stomach (same physiologic effects as tension pneumothorax).

CARDIAC TRAUMA

Cardiac wounds should be suspected after penetration of any part of the chest, lower part of the neck, or upper part of the abdomen. The possibility of heart injury also exists in the presence of blunt trauma to the anterior or left hemithorax with laceration by fractured sternum or ribs or severe compression between the sternum and the vertebral column. Blood loss with perforation varies between exsanguination, either internal or external, and minimal bleeding with or without acute cardiac tamponade. Tamponade usually follows trauma to the myocardium with both pleura intact. The hemopericardium cannot decompress into the pleura or externally, because the pericardial wound is dislocated from the soft tissue wound of entrance by the pericardial blood. The resulting increase in intrapericardial pressure constricts the heart and great veins, and the venous return and cardiac output are critically impaired.

The physical findings with acute tamponade are often classic. The veins of the neck and upper extremity may be distended. The heart sounds are distant and perhaps inaudible. The systolic pressure is depressed, the pulse pressure is narrow, and the pulse rate is relatively slow in spite of the lowered blood pressure.

The elevation of venous pressure is a valuable laboratory finding. Fluoroscopy demonstrates an inactive cardiac silhouette whose margins may not be widened. Sonography may be helpful.

With this clinical picture, emergency needle aspiration of the pericardial sac through a subxiphoid approach should be performed in addition to systemic resuscitation while the operating suite is being prepared. Aspiration of small amounts of blood can restore cardiopulmonary dynamics (Fig. 73-15).

Nonpenetrating trauma can produce various degrees of myocardial contusions ranging from a small area of edema to a ruptured chamber. The chest pain and tachycardia may be difficult to evaluate without evidence of cardiac failure. Serial electrocardiograms and cardiac enzyme determinations are essential for the diagnosis of myocardial damage secondary to trauma (Fig. 73-16).

Penetrating trauma may injure myocardial chambers or coronary arteries and may require closure of the myocardial chambers or even coronary bypass surgery in pediatric patients.

The treatment can follow the standard regimen for coronary occlusion, with the exclusion of anticoagulants, and complete rehabilitation can be anticipated. Late complications include chronic constrictive pericarditis, congestive heart failure, and ventricular aneurysm.

In this regard, physicians attending an acutely injured child in the emergency ward must be prepared to institute prompt external cardiac massage (Fig. 73-17), internal cardiac massage (Figs. 73-18 and 73-19), or cardiac defibrillation (Fig. 73-20).

INJURIES TO THE ESOPHAGUS

Perforation of the esophagus in the pediatric age group can occur in the delivery room from extreme positive-pressure resuscitation or aspiration with a stiff catheter. In later infancy and childhood, rupture can follow ingestion of lye or a solid foreign body, esophagoscopy, or dilatation. Spontaneous rupture proximal to an esophageal web has been described. As in adults, stab and gunshot wounds can perforate the esophagus.

Clinically, hyperthermia, hypotension, and chest and neck pain mirror the mediastinitis. Pneumome-

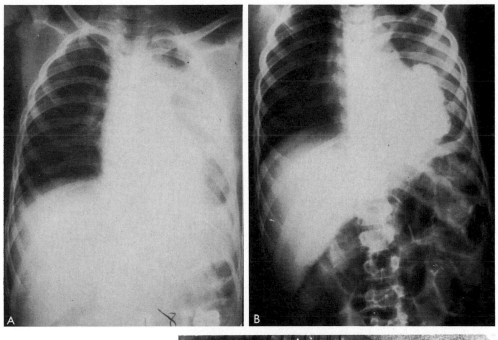

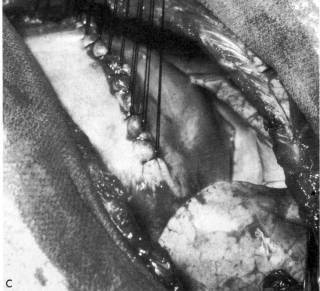

Figure 73–22. A blunt traumatic rupture of the left hemidiaphragm (A), with barium swallow confirmation (B) and final closure at operation (C).

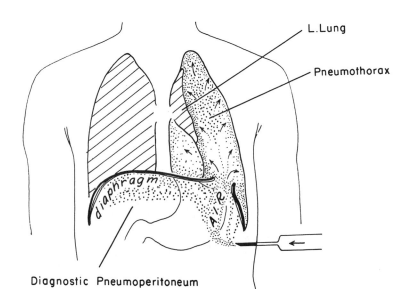

Figure 73–23. Diagnostic pneumoperitoneum in a suspected rupture of the diaphragm.

diastinum, tension pneumothorax, subcutaneous emphysema, and hematemesis may be encountered.

Plain chest roentgenograms followed by a contrast esophagram and thoracentesis may demonstrate the tension sequelae, esophageal defect, and perhaps high-acid fluid.

The tension pneumothorax must quickly undergo decompression followed promptly by closure of the esophageal defect, mediastinal drainage, and massive doses of antibiotics.

THORACOABDOMINAL INJURIES

In infants and children, combined injury to the thorax and abdomen, including diaphragm rupture, is usually preceded by a violent traffic accident or other form of sudden, jolting impact. Splenic and hepatic lacerations commonly occur with minimal external evidence of injury and need not be associated with fractured ribs or soft tissue mutilation.

The clinical signs of upper abdominal tenderness, rigidity, and rebound tenderness almost uniformly accompany lower chest trauma and are explained by the abdominal distribution of the intercostal nerves. Therefore, peritoneal irritation, of itself, is not conclusive evidence of a combined or abdominal injury. Careful repeated examinations correlated with laboratory data are necessary for the diagnosis of intra-abdominal perforation or hemorrhage in the presence of chest trauma. Aspiration of the peritoneum may have a place and perhaps should be used more often.

Diaphragm rupture can occur with minimal soft tissue injury, and there may be chest pain, dyspnea, and hypotension. On inspection, the involved chest wall lags during inspiration, and percussion can be dull or hyperresonant (Fig. 73–21). Chest roentgenograms may not show fractured ribs but almost invariably demonstrate abnormality or absence of the diaphragmatic shadow on the affected side. There is usually mediastinal shift to the right, because in 90 per cent of cases the posterolateral left leaf of the diaphragm is torn in a radial manner (Fig. 73–22). At times, a spontaneous pneumoperitoneum is seen. Diagnostic pneumoperitoneum may improve the radiologic diagnoses of rupture of the diaphragm (Fig. 73–23).

The preliminary management of combined thoracoabdominal injuries must provide an adequate airway and circulation, gastric decompression, and evaluation and control of other injuries. Intra-abdominal hemorrhage and perforation with thoracic and abdominal soiling is an obvious indication for immediate exploration. Ideally, a ruptured diaphragm should be repaired as soon as systemic stabilization has been achieved.

REFERENCES

Avery EE, Morch ET, and Benson DW: Critically crushed chests. J Thorac Surg 32:291, 1956.

Berry FB: Chest injuries. Surg Gynecol Obstet 70:413, 1940.
Besson A and Saegesser F: Color Atlas of Chest Trauma and Associated Injuries, Vol 1 and 2. Oradell, NJ, Medical Economics Co., 1983.
Betts RH: Thoraco-abdominal injuries: report of twenty-nine operated cases. Ann Surg 122:793, 1945.
Bickford BJ: Chest injuries in childhood and adolescence. Thorax 17:240, 1962.
Blades B and Salzberg AM: The importance of tracheostomy in acute ventilatory distress. Milit Surg 114:184, 1954.
Blane CE, White SJ, Wesley JR, and Coran AE: Immediate traumatic pulmonary pseudocyst formation in children. Surgery 90:872, 1981.
Burke J and Jacobs TT: Penetrating wounds of the chest. Ann Surg 123:363, 1916.
Burke JF: Early diagnosis of traumatic rupture of bronchus. JAMA 181:682, 1962.
Carter BN and Guiseffi J: Tracheostomy—a useful procedure in thoracic surgery, with particular reference to its employment in crushing injuries of the thorax. J Thorac Surg 21:495, 1951.
Carter R, Wareham EE, and Brewer LA III: Rupture of the bronchus following closed chest trauma. Am J Surg 104:177, 1962.
Childress ME and Grimes OF: Immediate and remote sequelae in traumatic diaphragmatic hernia. Surg Gynecol Obstet 113:573, 1961.
Daughtry DC: Thoracic Trauma. Boston, Little, Brown & Co, 1980.
DeBakey ME (ed): The Year Book of General Surgery (1963–1964 Year Book Series). Chicago, Year Book Medical Publishers, Inc, 1964.
Edwards HC: Surgical Emergencies in Children. Baltimore, William Wood and Co, 1963.
Ellerton DG, McGough EC, Rasmussen B et al: Pulmonary artery monitoring in critically ill surgical patients. Am J Surg 128:791, 1974.
Fagan CJ and Swischuk LE: Traumatic lung and paramediastinal pneumatoceles. Radiology 120:11, 1976.
Flavell G: An Introduction to Chest Surgery. London, Oxford University Press, 1957.
Fraser J: Surgery of Childhood. Vol II. New York, William Wood and Co, 1926.
Fryfogle JD: Discussion of paper by R. L. Anderson: rupture of the esophagus. J Thorac Surg 24:369, 1952.
Graivier L and Freeark RJ: Traumatic diaphragmatic hernia. Arch Surg 86:33, 1963.
Greening R, Kynett A, and Hodes PJ: Unusual pulmonary changes secondary to chest trauma. Am J Roentgenol 77:1059, 1957.
Haight C: Intratracheal suction in the management of postoperative pulmonary complications. Ann Surg 107:218, 1938.
Haynes BW Jr: Dangers of emergency occlusive dressing in sucking wounds of the chest. JAMA 150:1404, 1952.
Howell JF, Crawford ES, and Jordan GL: Flail chest: analysis of 100 patients. Am J Surg 106:628, 1963.
Johnson J: Battle wounds of the thoracic cavity. Ann Surg 123:321, 1946.
Keshishian JM and Cox PA: Diagnosis and management of strangulated diaphragmatic hernias. Surg Gynecol Obstet 115:626, 1962.
Kilman JW and Charnock E: Thoracic trauma in infancy and childhood. J Trauma 9:863, 1969.
Levy JL Jr: Management of crushing chest injuries in children. South Med J 65:1040, 1972.
Lindskog GE: Some historical aspects of thoracic trauma. J Thorac Cardiovasc Surg 42:1, 1961.
Lucido JL and Wall CA: Rupture of diaphragm due to blunt trauma. Arch Surg 86:989, 1963.
Mahaffey DE, Creech O Jr, Boren HG, and DeBakey ME: Traumatic rupture of the left main bronchus successfully repaired eleven years after injury. J Thorac Surg 32:312, 1956.
Mahour GH, Lynn HB, and Sanderson D: Rupture of the bronchus. J Pediatr Surg 2:263, 1967.
Maloney JV Jr and McDonald L: Treatment of trauma to thorax. Am J Surg 105:484, 1963.
Melzig EP, Swank M, and Salzberg AM: Acute blunt traumatic

rupture of the diaphragm in children. Arch Surg 111:1009, 1976.

Nealon TF and Ching NPH: Trauma to the chest. In Sabiston DC and Spencer FC (eds): Gibbon's Surgery of the Chest. 3rd ed. Philadelphia, WB Saunders Co, 1976.

Paulson DL: Traumatic bronchial rupture with plastic repair. J Thorac Surg 22:636, 1951.

Pearl M, Milstein M, and Rook GD: Pseudocyst of the lung due to traumatic nonpenetrating lung injury. J Pediatr Surg 8:967, 1973.

Perry JF and Galway CF: Chest injury due to blunt trauma. J Thorac Cardiovasc Surg 49:684, 1965.

Pilcher RS: Trachea, bronchi, lungs and pleura. In Brown JJM (ed): Surgery of Childhood, Baltimore, Williams & Wilkins Co, 1963.

Ransdell HT Jr, McPherson RC, Haller JA Jr et al: Treatment of flail chest injuries with a piston respirator. Am J Surg 104:22, 1962.

Richardson WR: Thoracic emergencies in the newborn infant. Am J Surg 105:524, 1963.

Santos GH and Mahendra T: Traumatic pulmonary pseudocysts. Ann Thorac Surg 27:359, 1979.

Schwartz A and Borman JB: Contusion of the lung in childhood. Arch Dis Child 36:557, 1961.

Segal S: Endobronchial pressure as an aid to tracheobronchial aspiration. Pediatrics 35:305, 1965.

Shaw J: Pulmonary contusion in children due to rubber bullet injuries. Br Med J 4:764, 1972.

Shaw RR, Paulson DL, and Kee JL Jr: Traumatic tracheal rupture. J Thorac Cardiovasc Surg 42:281, 1961.

Smyth BT: Chest trauma in children. J Pediatr Surg 14:41, 1979.

Sorsdahl OA and Powell JW: Cavitary pulmonary lesions following nonpenetrating chest trauma in children. Am J Roentgenol 95:118, 1965.

Spencer FC: Treatment of chest injuries. Curr Probl Surg January 1964.

Stevens E and Templeton AW: Traumatic nonpenetrating lung contusion. Radiology 85:247, 1965.

Strug LH, Glass B, Leon W et al: Severe crushing injuries of the chest. A simple method of stabilization. J Thorac Cardiovasc Surg 39:166, 1960.

Swenson O: Pediatric Surgery. 2nd ed. New York, Appleton-Century-Crofts, Inc, 1962.

Taylor SF: Recent Advances in Surgery. Boston, Little, Brown & Co, 1946.

Thomas PS: Rib fractures in infancy. Ann Radiol (Paris) 20:115, 1977.

Warden JD and Mucha SJ: Esophageal perforation due to trauma in the newborn. Arch Surg 83:813, 1961.

Webb WR: Chest injuries. J La State Med Soc 116:1, 1964.

Weisel W and Jake RJL: Anastomosis of right bronchus to trachea 46 days following complete bronchial rupture from external injury. Ann Surg 137:220, 1953.

White M and Dennison WM: Surgery in Infancy and Childhood, A Handbook for Medical Students and General Practitioners. Edinburgh, E & S Livingstone, Ltd, 1958.

White PD and Glenby BS: In Brahdy L and Kahn S (eds): Trauma and Disease. Philadelphia, Lea & Febiger, 1937.

Williams JR and Stembridge VA: Pulmonary contusion secondary to nonpenetrating chest trauma. Am J Roentgenol 91:284, 1964.

Zollinger RW, Creedon PJ, and Sanguily J: Trauma in children in a general hospital. Am J Surg 104:855, 1962.

74

LAURA S. INSELMAN, M.D.

PULMONARY DISORDERS IN PEDIATRIC ACQUIRED IMMUNE DEFICIENCY SYNDROME

ETIOLOGY

The acquired immune deficiency syndrome (AIDS) is caused by the human immunodeficiency virus, HIV-1, which was previously known as human T cell lymphotropic virus/lymphadenopathy-associated virus (HTLV-III/LAV-1). The HIV-1 is a lymphotropic retrovirus, which, through the actions of its enzyme, reverse transcriptase, enables DNA to be synthesized from RNA. Other lymphotropic retroviruses include HTLV-I, HTLV-II, and HTLV-V, which cause leukemia and lymphoma in humans; HTLV-IV and HIV-2, which cause a less severe AIDS-like syndrome in humans; and the simian viruses, STLV-I, which causes lymphoma, and STLV-III, which causes AIDS in primates. Infection with several human retroviruses can occur simultaneously, and infection with a retrovirus is lifelong.

Retroviruses contain several genes that are responsible for replication and serologic differentiation. These genes include "env" (envelope), which produces envelope proteins; "gag" (group associated), which synthesizes core antigens; "pol" (polymerase), which codes for reverse transcriptase production; "LTR" (long terminal repeat sequence), which is responsible for transcription and regulation of the viral genes; and one viral replicating regulator, "tat" (transactivation of transcription). HIV-1 has four additional genes that control viral synthesis and infectivity: "nef" (negative factor), "vif" (virion infectivity factor), "rev" (regulator of expression of virion proteins), and "vpu" (viral protein U). The human retroviruses differ in their env, gag, LTR, and tat proteins, although all have a p24 gag protein. Serologically, HIV-1 is identified by the p24 gag, gp41 env, and gp160/120 env proteins. The envelope proteins of HIV-1 and HIV-2 differ, which helps to distinguish the two viruses.

Cells infected with a retrovirus become multinucleated, or syncytial, and incorporate contiguous noninfected cells into the syncytium. Cellular death occurs with infection with HIV-1 and HIV-2, whereas the other four human lymphotropic viruses transform and immortalize infected cells to reproduce indefinitely.

EPIDEMIOLOGY

In humans, AIDS is transmitted by exposure to virus-containing body fluids through sexual contact, contaminated needles, and blood and blood products and by transplacental infection to the fetus from an infected mother. Approximately 75 per cent of pediatric AIDS cases are acquired perinatally, and an additional 20 per cent of childhood infections result from transfusions by blood and blood products (Curran et al, 1988). The remaining 5 per cent have unidentifiable risk factors at present.

DEFINITION

A spectrum of seroconversion, laboratory data abnormalities, persistent generalized lymphadenopathy, and AIDS itself characterizes HIV infection. The presence of AIDS depends on the status of laboratory documentation of HIV infection and the occurrence of a specific indicator disease, as defined by the Centers for Disease Control (1987a, 1987c). Unique features of AIDS in children under the age of 13 years include the presence of lymphocytic interstitial pneumonitis, pulmonary lymphoid hyperplasia, unexplained recurrent pyogenic bacterial infections, failure to thrive, parotid gland enlargement, encephalopathy with microcephaly and loss of developmental milestones, and a possible fetal AIDS syndrome characterized by growth failure and craniofacial anomalies. Pediatric HIV infection, as defined by the Centers for Disease Control, excludes the adolescent age group.

PULMONARY DISORDERS

Pulmonary disorders in pediatric AIDS include the "noninfectious" interstitial pneumonitides, particularly lymphocytic interstitial pneumonitis, and infection with opportunistic organisms, most frequently *Pneumocystis carinii* and cytomegalovirus (Table 74–1). In contrast, opportunistic infections and Kaposi's sarcoma cause the majority of pulmonary disease in adult AIDS patients. In addition, pyogenic bacterial

Table 74–1. PULMONARY DISORDERS IN PEDIATRIC HIV INFECTION

Interstitial Pneumonitis ("noninfectious")
  Lymphocytic interstitial pneumonitis
  Desquamative interstitial pneumonitis
  Chronic interstitial pneumonitis

Opportunistic Pneumonia* ("infectious")
  BACTERIA
    Branhamella catarrhalis
    Enterobacter aerogenes
    Escherichia coli
    Haemophilus influenzae type b
    Klebsiella sp
    Legionella pneumophila
    Mycobacterium avium-intracellulare
    Mycobacterium tuberculosis, Mycobacterium bovis
    Mycoplasma pneumoniae
    Proteus mirabilis
    Pseudomonas aeruginosa
    Salmonella typhimurium
    Staphylococcus aureus
    Staphylococcus epidermidis
    Streptococcus pneumoniae
    Streptococcus viridans

  VIRUSES
    Adenovirus
    Cytomegalovirus
    Epstein-Barr virus
    Herpes simplex virus
    Influenza viruses
    Measles virus
    Respiratory syncytial virus
    Varicella-zoster virus

  FUNGI
    Aspergillus niger
    Candida albicans
    Candida (Torulopsis) glabrata

  PROTOZOA
    Pneumocystis carinii
    Toxoplasma gondii

Diffuse Alveolar Damage
Immunoblastic Sarcoma

*Only those opportunistic organisms recorded in the literature on pediatric AIDS are listed.

pneumonia is more likely to occur in children, whereas mycobacterial disease appears to be more frequent in adults. These apparent differences in AIDS in children and adults are not readily explained but may be a result of differences in the technique of obtaining culture material from each age group and in defining and reporting the diseases. In addition, immunodeficient children may be unable to respond adequately to pyogenic bacteria on initial exposure, whereas antibodies to these organisms are often present in adults before the onset of the immunodeficiency and allow a sufficient immunologic anamnestic response on later reexposure.

INTERSTITIAL PNEUMONITIDES

Lymphocytic Interstitial Pneumonitis

Lymphocytic interstitial pneumonitis (LIP) causes approximately half of the reported pulmonary disease in children with AIDS (Rogers et al, 1987), is an indicator disease for the diagnosis of pediatric AIDS, and is observed only occasionally in adults with the syndrome. It is part of a spectrum of lymphoid lesions that cause pulmonary proliferation of lymphocytes and are also characteristic of pediatric AIDS. These lesions most likely represent variable responses of the lung to an injury, which could be HIV in whole or in part or another as yet unidentified agent. Included in this group of lesions are pulmonary lymphoid hyperplasia (PLH), which is associated with nodules of lymphocytes and plasma cells around bronchioles and in alveolar septa; hyperplasia of bronchus-associated lymphoid tissue (BALT); and a systemic polymorphic polyclonal B cell lymphoproliferative disorder (PBLD), which is characterized by nodules of immature and mature lymphocytes and plasma cells in the lungs and other organs.

The most frequently occurring lesion in this spectrum is LIP, which is distinguished by lymphoid nodules, giant cells, and a uniform dense infiltration of alveolar septa with lymphocytes, plasma cells, histiocytes, and immunoblasts, resulting in marked distortion of normal pulmonary structure. The lymphocytes in this infiltrate are both B and T cells, with the T8 subset predominating. Although an infectious organism has not been established in its etiology, genetic components of HIV-1 and Epstein-Barr virus have been identified in LIP in pediatric AIDS.

The clinical course of LIP is characteristically insidious, with an initial mild cough and dyspnea. Adventitious breath sounds, chest retractions, tachypnea, and fever are present but with less frequency than in pulmonary opportunistic infections. In addition, mild hypoxemia, clubbing, generalized lymphadenopathy, and parotitis are more likely to occur in LIP and PLH than in infections with opportunistic organisms. Interstitial fibrosis, honeycomb lung, and respiratory failure can ensue. A diffuse reticulonodular interstitial pattern, which is bilateral and more dense in the lower lung fields, is seen on radiographs in LIP (Figs. 74–1 and 74–2), whereas chest radiographs in PLH have progressively enlarging diffuse nodules and hilar and mediastinal adenopathy. Restrictive lung disease, impaired diffusion, and arterial hypoxemia, particularly with exercise, are present with pulmonary function testing.

Definitive diagnosis is made by histologic examination of lung tissue obtained by open-lung biopsy. In addition, the magnitude of the increase in serum IgG levels, which characterizes HIV infection, can help identify LIP. IgG levels in the 3000 to 5000 mg per cent range are likely to be associated with LIP, whereas lower values are more characteristic of other pulmonary disorders (Rubinstein et al, 1986).

The course of the disease waxes and wanes, but temporary clinical, laboratory, and radiographic improvement can occur with corticosteroid therapy (prednisone 2 mg/kg/day orally in one to two divided doses; hydrocortisone 10 mg/kg/day or methylprednisolone 2 mg/kg/day intravenously or intramuscu-

larly in four divided doses) (Table 74–2). Rubinstein and colleagues (1988) have utilized a 2- to 4-week course of daily corticosteroids when arterial oxygen tensions are ≤60 mm Hg. Following a 20-mm Hg increase in arterial oxygen tension, the steroid dose is tapered and changed to an alternate-day regimen, with subsequent maintenance of oxygenation, radiographic improvement, and no apparent adverse effects.

Desquamative Interstitial Pneumonitis

Desquamative interstitial pneumonitis (DIP) is characteristic of pediatric AIDS and is usually associated with either LIP or a pulmonary opportunistic infection. It is a response to lung injury and can proceed to interstitial fibrosis, honeycomb lung, and respiratory failure, features that are similar to those of LIP. However, normal pulmonary morphology is preserved. A sparse interstitial infiltration of lymphocytes and plasma cells occurs, with intra-alveolar proliferation of macrophages and monocytes, cuboidal metaplasia of alveolar epithelial type II cells, and absence of viral inclusions and lymphoid nodules. The macrophages may have iron-containing inclusions, although these round or oval bodies are not pathognomonic of DIP.

The onset and course of DIP are insidious, with dyspnea, tachypnea, nonproductive cough, bilateral basilar rales, cyanosis, and clubbing. Triangular areas of ground-glass haziness spreading from the hila to the lung bases are present on radiographs, although 10 per cent of patients have normal chest radiographs. Restrictive lung disease, diminished diffusing capacity, and arterial hypoxemia at rest and with exercise are observed with pulmonary function testing and can occur even if clinical manifestations of DIP are absent.

Histologic examination of lung tissue obtained by open-lung biopsy is necessary for a definitive diagnosis. The presence of the iron-containing inclusions, which stain blue-gray with hematoxylin and eosin and are periodic acid–Schiff stain positive, helps in the diagnosis. Corticosteroid therapy is more likely to ameliorate the clinical, radiographic, and histologic manifestations of DIP than of LIP, at least in non-AIDS individuals. However, because DIP occurs less frequently in pediatric AIDS than does LIP and is often present with LIP, the natural course of DIP and the effect of corticosteroids are not known at present. Dosages and treatment schedule with corticosteroids are the same as those for LIP. The few children with AIDS diagnosed with DIP have died (Joshi and Oleske, 1986).

Chronic Interstitial Pneumonitis

A chronic interstitial pneumonitis has been described in several children with HIV infection. Its characteristics include intra-alveolar proliferation of macrophages and interstitial fibrosis, features similar

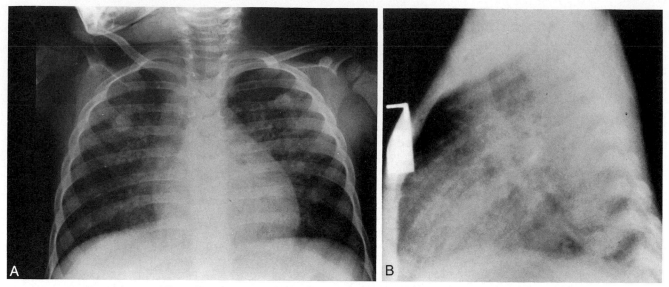

Figure 74–1. Diffuse bilateral interstitial infiltrates on posteroanterior *(A)* and lateral *(B)* views of biopsy-proven lymphocytic interstitial pneumonitis in a 2.5-year-old girl with acquired immune deficiency syndrome (AIDS).

to those of DIP and LIP. Bronchiolar destruction with peribronchiolar interstitial infiltration of lymphocytes, plasma cells, and macrophages also occurs. The pneumonitis is not associated with opportunistic or viral infections, and its clinical course and radiographic changes are similar to those observed with LIP. T8 and T11 lymphocytes predominate in the infiltrate, although T4 and B lymphocytes also occur. Treatment consists of corticosteroids, with clinical, radiographic, and immunologic improvement at least 2 to 3.5 years later in the two children described (Kornstein et al, 1986). Dosages and treatment regimen with corticosteroids are the same as those for LIP.

OPPORTUNISTIC INFECTIONS

Pneumocystis carinii Pneumonia

Pneumonia caused by *Pneumocystis carinii* is the most frequently occurring pulmonary infection in pediatric AIDS, with an incidence approaching 55 per cent (Rogers et al, 1987). *P. carinii* is a protozoan parasite that, although typically localized to the lungs in non-AIDS infection, can cause extrapulmonary disease in AIDS. In immunocompetent children, a latent infection with *P. carinii* can result in low levels of antibody to the parasite, with subsequent development of clinical disease when associated with stress

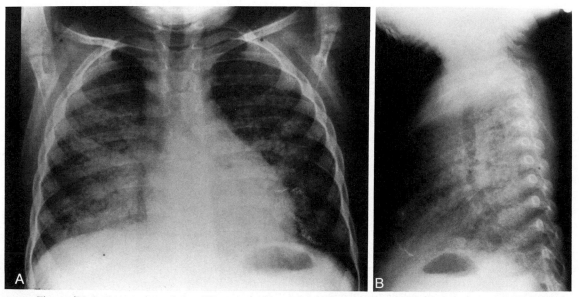

Figure 74–2. Progression of the diffuse reticulonodular infiltrates on posteroanterior *(A)* and lateral *(B)* views 7 months later in the child in Figure 74–1.

Table 74–2. DRUG TREATMENT OF LUNG DISEASE IN PEDIATRIC HIV INFECTION

Drug	Lung Disease	Possible Adverse Effects	Drug Interactions
Corticosteroids	Lymphocytic, desquamative, and chronic interstitial pneumonitides; diffuse alveolar damage	Pituitary-adrenal suppression, myopathy, hypokalemic alkalosis, edema, osteoporosis, growth inhibition, cataracts, peptic ulcer, behavioral disturbances	Enhances action of neuromuscular blocking agents; decreased action with phenytoin, barbiturates, rifampin
Pentamidine isethionate (Pentam 300)	*Pneumocystis carinii* pneumonia	Hypo- or hyperglycemia, gastrointestinal disturbances, transient hypotension, tachycardia, hepatotoxicity, reversible nephrotoxicity, pancreatitis, diabetes mellitus, granulocytopenia, megaloblastic anemia, hypocalcemia; intravenous administration increases incidence of adverse effects	None known
Trimethoprim-sulfamethoxazole (Septra, Bactrim, TMP-SMX)	*Pneumocystis carinii* pneumonia	Gastrointestinal disturbances, stomatitis, dermatitis, fever, hepatotoxicity, irreversible nephrotoxicity, neurotoxicity, pancytopenia; HIV increases incidence of fever, malaise, dermatitis, and pancytopenia; decrease dose in G6PD deficiency or liver or renal disease; contraindicated under the age of 2 months	Enhances action of phenytoin, oral anticoagulants, diuretics, methotrexate; bone marrow suppression prevented by leucovorin
9-(1,3-dihydroxy-2-propoxymethyl) guanine (DHPG, ganciclovir, cytovene)	Cytomegalovirus pneumonia, infection with herpes simplex and varicella-zoster viruses	Dermatitis, reversible leukopenia, eosinophilia, thrombocytopenia, gastrointestinal disturbances, nephrotoxicity, psychosis, disorientation, hepatitis, phlebitis at infusion site	Increased adverse effects with zidovudine
Clofazimine (Lamprene)	Nontuberculous mycobacterial infection	Gastrointestinal disturbances; anticholinergic effect; ichthyosis; red-brown color of skin, cornea, tears, retina, urine	None known
Ansamycin (Rifabutin)	Nontuberculous mycobacterial infection	Hepatotoxicity, red-orange color of secretions, bone marrow suppression	Possibly similar to rifampin
Ribavirin (Virazole)	Respiratory syncytial virus infection	Bronchospasm, dermatitis, conjunctivitis	Decreased action with zidovudine
Vidarabine (Vira-A)	Infection with herpes simplex and varicella-zoster viruses	Gastrointestinal disturbances, neurotoxicity, bone marrow suppression, thrombophlebitis	Increased adverse effects with allopurinol, increases serum theophylline levels
Amphotericin B (Fungizone)	Fungal infections	Gastrointestinal disturbances, anaphylaxis, nephrotoxicity, seizures, hypokalemia, hypomagnesemia, thrombophlebitis at infusion site; reversible anemia, chills, fever, and vomiting during infusions	Decreased action with miconazole; increased adverse effects with corticosteroids, flucytosine; increased nephrotoxicity with aminoglycosides, curariform drugs, cyclosporine
Flucytosine (Ancobon)	Fungal infections	Gastrointestinal disturbances, hepatotoxicity, pancytopenia, dermatitis	Increased adverse effects with amphotericin B
Amantadine hydrochloride (Symmetrel)	Influenza A virus infection	Gastrointestinal disturbances, orthostatic hypotension, congestive heart failure, dermatitis, lethargy, insomnia, dizziness, psychosis, urinary retention; decrease dose in renal disease	Increased adverse effects with hydrochlorothiazide-triamterene, anticholinergic agents, glycopyrrolate, ipratropium

Table continued on following page

Table 74–2. DRUG TREATMENT OF LUNG DISEASE IN PEDIATRIC HIV INFECTION *Continued*

Drug	Lung Disease	Possible Adverse Effects	Drug Interactions
Acyclovir sodium (Zovirax)	Infection with herpes simplex and varicella-zoster viruses	Nephrotoxicity, hepatotoxicity, neurotoxicity, pancytopenia, thrombophlebitis, metabolic encephalopathy, headache, vertigo, nausea, dermatitis, irritation at infusion site, crosses placenta	Increased adverse effects with probenecid, interferon, zidovudine
Pyrimethamine (Daraprim)	*Toxoplasma gondii* infection	Folic acid antagonist with bone marrow suppression, teratogenic in animals	Bone marrow suppression prevented by leucovorin
Sulfadiazine, trisulfapyrimidine	*Toxoplasma gondii* infection	Nephrotoxicity, acute hemolytic anemia, pancytopenia, hepatotoxicity, dermatitis, serum sickness	Potentiates action of oral anticoagulants, oral hypoglycemic agents, phenytoin
Zidovudine (Retrovir, AZT)	Human immunodeficiency virus infection	Macrocytic anemia, neutropenia, myalgia, skeletal muscle atrophy, nausea, headache, insomnia, gastrointestinal disturbances, hepatotoxicity, fever, seizures, dermatitis, nail pigmentation	Decreased action with ribavirin; increased action with probenecid, acyclovir, acetaminophen, nonsteroidal anti-inflammatory agents, narcotics

or acquired immunodeficiency. Airborne spread of the organism can also occur.

The onset of *P. carinii* pneumonia in pediatric AIDS is acute, and respiratory failure can rapidly ensue. High fever, tachypnea, a nonproductive cough, rales, flaring of nasal alae, cyanosis, and hypoxemia are usually present. Bilateral diffuse alveolar and interstitial infiltrates, which spread peripherally from the perihilar and lower lung fields, are seen radiographically (Fig. 74–3). Hilar adenopathy, hyperexpansion, unilateral infiltrates, lobar infiltrates, air bronchograms, a honeycomb pattern, pneumothoraces, and endobronchial lesions may also be present. The chest radiograph can appear normal

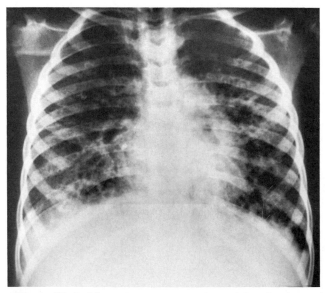

Figure 74–3. Bilateral perihilar and lower lobe alveolar and interstitial infiltrates of *Pneumocystis carinii* identified in bronchoalveolar lavage fluid in a 4.5-year-old girl with acquired immune deficiency syndrome (AIDS). Hyperexpansion of the lungs is also present.

even with severe respiratory distress or with abnormal gallium lung scan findings. Restrictive lung disease, decreased diffusing capacity, and arterial hypoxemia at rest and with exercise characterize the results of pulmonary function testing.

P. carinii causes an intra-alveolar inflammation. Initially, isolated cystic forms of the organism occur in alveolar septa without the appearance of clinical disease. The cysts subsequently proliferate within intra-alveolar macrophages, and alveolar epithelial type II cells desquamate. Clinical disease may now be present. A diffuse desquamative alveolitis then occurs, with a pathognomonic intra-alveolar foamy eosinophilic exudate composed of macrophages, cysts, and sporozoites. Trophozoites attach to alveolar epithelial cells, causing alveolar capillary membrane thickening, and interstitial inflammation and fibrosis, hyaline membranes, and focal alveolar hemorrhage also occur. At this stage, clinical and radiographic evidence of disease is present.

P. carinii is recognized histologically as thick-walled cysts composed of one to eight oval bodies called sporozoites and as thin-walled extracysts called trophozoites. Wright, Giemsa, and polychrome methylene blue stains identify sporozoites and trophozoites. The thick cyst walls also stain purple-violet with toluidine blue O and brown-black with Gomori methenamine silver stains. Although histologic examination of lung tissue obtained by open-lung biopsy provides a definitive diagnosis, stains of bronchoalveolar lavage fluid can identify the organism in approximately 80 per cent of patients (Stover et al, 1984). In addition, stains of respiratory secretions and sputum, indirect immunofluorescence of sputum using monoclonal antibodies, and DNA hybridization can be utilized for diagnosis.

Additional diagnostic studies include measurements of a *P. carinii* antigen, determined by latex particle agglutination; *P. carinii* IgG antibody, determined by enzyme-linked immunosorbent assay (ELISA); and serum lactate dehydrogenase (LDH) levels. Although LDH is increased in both *P. carinii* pneumonia and LIP, with values of 600 to 920 and 340 to 465 units/L, respectively, in children (Silverman and Rubinstein, 1985), the levels are highest during active *P. carinii* infection, decrease with apparent improvement, and increase again with subsequent relapse. A persistently elevated level of LDH indicates a poor prognosis. *P. carinii* pneumonia is also associated with increased LDH levels in bronchoalveolar lavage fluid.

Treatment includes pentamidine isethionate (4 mg/kg/dose, maximum 56 mg/kg total dose, intravenously or intramuscularly once daily) or trimethoprim-sulfamethoxazole (TMP-SMX) (20 mg TMP/kg/day, maximum 320 mg/day, and 100 mg SMX/kg/day, maximum 1600 mg/day, orally or intravenously in four divided doses) (see Table 74–2). The drugs are prescribed for at least 14 days and often longer because of frequent recurrence of disease. TMP-SMX (5 mg TMP/kg/day and 25 mg SMX/kg/day orally in two divided doses) or aerosolized pentamidine can also be administered prophylactically. The frequent occurrence of skin rashes, pancytopenia, and fever with use of TMP-SMX in HIV infection often necessitates discontinuation of the drug. The bone marrow suppression of TMP-SMX caused by antifolate activity of these two drugs may be circumvented by the addition to the regimen of leucovorin, a folate compound that is not affected by the actions of TMP-SMX (Fischl et al, 1988). Corticosteroids, eflornithine, and combined therapy of trimetrexate and leucovorin and of trimethoprim and dapsone are investigational drugs that may prove effective in the treatment of *P. carinii* pneumonia.

Cytomegalovirus Pneumonia

Cytomegalovirus (CMV) pneumonia is the second most frequently occurring pulmonary infection in pediatric AIDS. Acquired, rather than congenital, CMV infection must be present in pediatric AIDS for CMV to be considered an opportunistic organism. Acquired CMV infection, which must begin after age 1 month, occurs by exposure to virus-containing body fluids, including urine, stool, breast milk, saliva, cervical secretions, semen, blood leukocytes, and transplanted organs or tissues. The CMV infection is rarely transmitted by the airborne route. A latent infection and secretion of the virus can occur, and CMV can be present without clinical manifestations or pathologic alterations. Subsequent immunodeficiency or stress can eventually result in clinical disease.

The onset of CMV pneumonia is insidious and is characterized by fever, tachypnea, dyspnea, a nonproductive cough, rales, and hypoxemia. Diffuse interstitial and occasionally lobar infiltrates are evident on radiographs (Fig. 74–4). Cytomegalovirus causes primarily a diffuse or focal interstitial pneu-

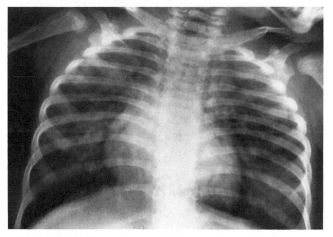

Figure 74–4. Bilateral interstitial markings in a 14-month-old boy with disseminated cytomegalovirus infection and growth of human immunodeficiency virus (HIV) in the blood.

monia with little intra-alveolar consolidation. Cytomegaly with both intranuclear viral and cytoplasmic mucopolysaccharide inclusions is characteristic of this DNA herpesvirus and occurs in interstitial and endothelial cells, desquamated alveolar epithelial cells, and alveolar macrophages. Focal alveolar hemorrhage and proteinaceous exudates may be present, but necrosis is unusual.

Stains and cultures of respiratory secretions, bronchoalveolar lavage fluid, or lung tissue obtained by open-lung biopsy is utilized in the diagnosis of CMV pneumonia. The coarse, basophilic cytoplasmic inclusions are identified with Gomori methenamine silver, hematoxylin and eosin, and periodic acid-Schiff stains, whereas the purple-staining intranuclear inclusions encircled by a halo are recognized with hematoxylin and eosin stain. Examination of lavage fluid identifies CMV in approximately 80 per cent of patients (Stover et al, 1984). In addition, DNA-hybridization and monoclonal antibody studies of lung tissue may help in the diagnosis. Complement fixation, ELISA, indirect fluorescence, and anticomplement and macroglobulin immunofluorescence are serologic antibody tests that are also utilized.

Cytomegalovirus pneumonia waxes and wanes in its course, is difficult to treat, and can be fatal. The drug, ganciclovir or DHPG, causes transient improvement of CMV pneumonia. Its dose is 6.0 to 7.5 mg/kg/day intravenously in two to three divided doses for 10 to 21 days (see Table 74–2). Multiple doses of CMV immune globulin prevent the onset of clinical CMV infection in non-AIDS individuals and may also prove effective in HIV infection.

Mycobacterial Lung Infections

Both tuberculous and nontuberculous mycobacteria cause pulmonary disease in HIV infection, although their clinical, radiographic, and histologic features differ from those occurring in non-HIV infection. The most frequently identified mycobacteria are *Mycobacterium avium-intracellulare*, particularly strains 4, 6 and 8, and *Mycobacterium tuberculosis*.

Nontuberculous Mycobacteria. *M. avium-intracellulare* is a ubiquitous organism that can cause cervical lymphadenitis in otherwise healthy children. Its usual portal of entry is the gastrointestinal tract. However, airborne spread can also occur but has not been a documented means of transmission in humans.

Disseminated disease resulting from *M. avium-intracellulare* occurs in children with HIV. Although *M. avium-intracellulare* has been identified in lungs in pediatric HIV infection, it is frequently accompanied by another opportunistic organism. Initially, anorexia, weight loss, fever, abdominal pain, and malabsorption occur with *M. avium-intracellulare* infection, and these nonspecific systemic manifestations may be incorrectly attributed to HIV. Progressive dyspnea, a productive or nonproductive cough, fevers, and night sweats subsequently occur, but severe respiratory distress and adventitious lung sounds are infrequent. Pulmonary symptoms may be mild, and isolation of *M. avium-intracellulare* from respiratory secretions may be the only indication of infection in the lung. Chest radiograph findings are usually normal (Fig. 74–5) or may reveal another simultaneous infection. Histologic changes can be minimal or, more likely, associated with atypical granulomas composed of macrophages laden with acid-fast bacilli but without giant cells, epithelioid cells, or caseation necrosis.

Definitive diagnosis depends on growth of the organism in culture from respiratory secretions, sputum, gastric washings, bronchoalveolar lavage and pleural fluids, and lung tissue. Gastric washings can have falsely positive stains in certain areas of the United States as a result of the occurrence of nontuberculous mycobacteria in drinking water. The presence of atypical granulomas on histologic examination of lung tissue helps to confirm the diagnosis.

Disease resulting from *M. avium-intracellulare* is frequently diagnosed only in a post-mortem examination, which likely reflects its insidious course, initial confusion with HIV itself, and frequent association with other fatal illnesses. Except for *M. kansasii*, nontuberculous mycobacteria are difficult to treat and eradicate with chemotherapy. Therapy for *M. avium-intracellulare* includes a 6- to 24-month course of isoniazid (10 to 15 mg/kg/day, maximum 300 mg/day, orally or intramuscularly once daily); ethambutol (15 to 25 mg/kg/day, maximum 1.5 g/day, orally once daily); and two drugs that are under investigation, clofazimine (2 to 5 mg/kg/day, maximum 300 mg/day, orally in one to three divided doses) and Ansamycin (5 mg/kg/day, maximum 300 mg/day, orally in one to two divided doses) (see Table 74–2). *M. kansasii* can be treated with a 15-month course of isoniazid and ethambutol (same doses as for *M. avium-intracellulare*) and rifampin (10 to 20 mg/kg/day, maximum 600 mg/day, orally once daily), with the optional addition of streptomycin (20 to 40 mg/kg/day, maximum 1 g/day, intramuscularly twice weekly) for the first 3 months.

Tuberculous Mycobacteria. Although the onset of tuberculosis can occur following the diagnosis of AIDS, it frequently predates AIDS by years and can be an indication of HIV infection in an individual who is at increased risk for acquiring AIDS. Both pulmonary and extrapulmonary tuberculosis appear with increased frequency in HIV infection.

The majority of reported cases of tuberculosis with HIV infection have been in adults. However, as the number of cases of pediatric AIDS continues to rise, particularly in those who are at increased risk for acquisition of *M. tuberculosis*, it is likely that tuberculosis will be diagnosed more frequently in pediatric HIV infection.

Adults with HIV and tuberculosis frequently have hilar or mediastinal adenopathy; middle or lower lobe infiltrates; and a fourfold increase in the incidence of extrapulmonary disease, particularly lymphatic and miliary tuberculosis. These features contrast with those of tuberculosis in non–HIV-infected individuals, which are usually associated with apical, cavitary lesions in the lungs. These characteristics of tuberculosis in HIV infection are similar to those of tuberculosis in the immunocompetent child, thus reflecting the relative inability of both the immunocompetent young child and the HIV-infected individual to prevent the development of systemic tuberculosis.

Pulmonary tuberculosis in AIDS may be misdiagnosed as *P. carinii* pneumonitis because of the atypical radiographic changes present with *M. tuberculosis* and the occurrence of tuberculin skin test anergy. However, the hilar and mediastinal adenopathies associated with pulmonary tuberculosis are characteristic of neither *P. carinii* pneumonitis nor HIV itself.

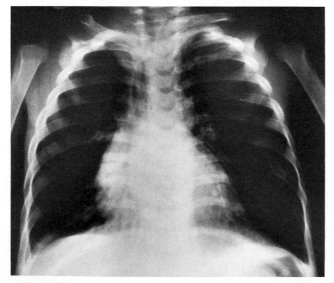

Figure 74–5. Normal chest radiograph of a 2-year-old girl with acquired immune deficiency syndrome (AIDS) and growth of *Mycobacterium avium-intracellulare* in the lungs at autopsy. Previously, *Pneumocystis carinii* was identified on a lung biopsy specimen, and *Torulopsis glabrata* grew in a tracheal aspirate. (Courtesy of Dr. Haesoon Lee.)

Definitive diagnosis of *M. tuberculosis* depends on identification of the organism. Histologically, granulomas can be well formed or atypical without giant cells, epithelioid cells, or caseation necrosis. However, in contrast to non-HIV infection, tuberculosis can still be present with HIV if granulomas and acid-fast bacilli are absent.

In addition, nucleic acid hybridization with DNA probes is a rapid screening test that can be utilized to identify the presence of tuberculous as well as nontuberculous mycobacteria in sputum in untreated individuals within 3 to 4 hours of obtaining the specimen. Subsequent confirmatory cultures are necessary for isolation of the organism and drug susceptibility testing. Additional diagnostic studies, particularly if culture results are negative, can include ELISA testing for antibody to antigen 5 of *M. tuberculosis* and a radioactive-labeled gallium lung scan.

To identify exposure to or disease with *M. tuberculosis* in HIV infection, Mantoux tuberculin skin testing with 5 tuberculin units (TU) of purified protein derivative (PPD) is recommended. Although HIV-induced anergy can cause a negative or doubtful tuberculin skin test reaction, 40 per cent of patients with both *M. tuberculosis* and HIV have positive reactions (Chaisson et al, 1987). A Mantoux tuberculin skin test reaction with an induration of 5 mm or more in an HIV-infected individual is considered indicative of the occurrence of tuberculous infection or disease (Centers for Disease Control, 1989b). Regardless of the result of the Mantoux skin test, if clinical HIV infection occurs, a chest radiograph and evaluation for extrapulmonary tuberculosis should be performed (Snider et al, 1987; Centers for Disease Control, 1987b, 1989b). If radiographic evidence of tuberculosis is present or the Mantoux skin test is positive, or both, further diagnostic studies are indicated to evaluate the occurrence of tuberculous infection or disease. In addition, individuals presenting with tuberculous infection or disease should be evaluated for HIV risk factors, and, if these are present, HIV testing should be considered. HIV testing should also be considered for individuals with severe or unusual manifestations of tuberculosis.

Chemotherapy for *M. tuberculosis* with HIV infection is the same as for non-HIV infection. The drugs should be prescribed when acid-fast bacilli are present in an individual with or at increased risk for HIV infection (Centers for Disease Control, 1989b). However, the duration of drug therapy for treatment of tuberculosis in HIV infection is not standardized at present. Antituberculous drugs are prescribed for at least 9 months, including a minimum of 6 months following culture conversion, as documented by three cultures with negative findings (Snider et al, 1987; Centers for Disease Control, 1987b, 1989b). Longer regimens may be necessary, including the use of isoniazid indefinitely. If isoniazid or rifampin cannot be utilized because of drug toxicity or resistance, therapy is frequently extended to at least 18 months, with a minimum of 12 months after *M. tuberculosis*

no longer grows in culture. In general, patients with *M. tuberculosis* and HIV respond well to antituberculous chemotherapy.

Regardless of age, individuals with HIV and tuberculin skin test conversions without evidence of tuberculous disease have an increased risk for developing tuberculosis and should receive a minimum 1-year course of prophylactic isoniazid (Snider et al, 1987; Centers for Disease Control, 1987b, 1989b). This prophylactic regimen is particularly important in children because a positive tuberculin skin test reaction in the pediatric age group indicates recent exposure to *M. tuberculosis* and increased risk of developing disease.

Asymptomatic children with HIV who have negative tuberculin skin test reactions and no evidence of clinical or radiographic tuberculous disease but are at increased risk for developing tuberculosis should receive the Calmette-Guérin bacillus (BCG) vaccine. Because the vaccine utilizes a live attenuated bacillus and can cause BCG sepsis in immunodeficient individuals, administration of the vaccine is not recommended for HIV-infected children who are symptomatic from HIV or at low risk for developing tuberculosis (Centers for Disease Control, 1988).

LUNG DISEASE WITH OTHER OPPORTUNISTIC ORGANISMS

An increased incidence of severe life-threatening pulmonary infections occurs in pediatric AIDS with organisms not usually considered opportunistic in immunocompetent individuals (see Table 74–1). The presence of disease with certain viruses, bacteria, and fungi provides criteria for the diagnosis of pediatric HIV infection, particularly pyogenic bacterial infections resulting from *Streptococcus pneumoniae* or *Haemophilus influenzae* (Centers for Disease Control, 1987a, 1987c). Several of these pulmonary infections can occur simultaneously. In addition to disease of other organs, such as gastroenteritis, dermatitis, meningoencephalitis, and bone and joint disease, which may be associated with a particular organism, nonspecific signs and symptoms of respiratory distress appear and include fever, dyspnea, adventitious lung sounds, hypoxemia, and cough. The cough may be productive of sputum in certain infections after the age of 6 years. Characteristic radiographic changes occur with some of these organisms (Fig. 74–6), and these lung infections can be fatal despite antimicrobial therapy.

For details of specific techniques for the diagnosis of these organisms, the reader is referred to the chapters describing these infectious agents. Special techniques, such as DNA-hybridization studies of lung tissue for Epstein-Barr virus and varicella-zoster virus, are now available. Cultures of respiratory secretions may grow viruses in only 60 per cent of respiratory infections proved viral by other methods (Kauffman, 1989). Therefore, lung disease due to

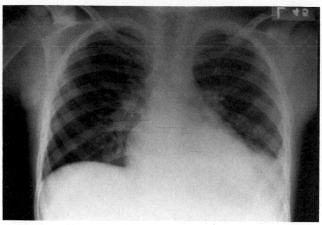

Figure 74–6. Left lower lobe infiltrate and pleural effusion in a 6-year-old girl with acquired immune deficiency syndrome (AIDS). Radiograph and respiratory symptoms cleared with antibiotic therapy, suggesting the presence of a bacterial pneumonia.

certain viruses may still occur despite negative culture findings. In addition, Epstein-Barr virus, CMV, herpes simplex virus, and adenovirus can be present in the respiratory tract without causing clinical or laboratory evidence of lung disease. Culture of bronchoalveolar lavage fluid can identify fungi in 80 per cent of patients with AIDS (Stover et al, 1984). Smears of lung tissue will help in identification of protozoan infections. However, protozoa cannot be cultured in vitro.

Ribavirin (6 g diluted with 180 ml water and aersolized with a SPAG-2 generator for 12 to 20 hours/day for 3 to 7 days) can be utilized to treat infections with respiratory syncytial virus (see Table 74–2). Amantadine hydrochloride (5 to 8 mg/kg/day, maximum 200 mg/day, orally in two divided doses) provides therapy for influenza A virus (see Table 74–2). Infections with herpes simplex and varicella-zoster viruses can be treated with acyclovir sodium (45 mg/kg/day as a 2-hour infusion intravenously or orally in three divided doses for 5 to 7 days), vidarabine (10 mg/kg/day as a 6-hour infusion intravenously for 5 days), or ganciclovir (see "Cytomegalovirus Pneumonia" for doses) (see Table 74–2).

Fungal pneumonias are treated with a 6-week course of amphotericin B (0.25 mg/kg/day as a 6-hour infusion intravenously, increasing the dose by 0.25 mg/kg/day every 2 to 3 days, maximum 1 mg/kg/day or 30 to 35 mg/kg total dose) (see Table 74–2). Amphotericin B can also be combined with flucytosine (150 mg/kg/day orally in four divided doses) for treatment of a lung infection resulting from *Candida* (see Table 74–2).

Pulmonary toxoplasmosis is treated with pyrimethamine (2 mg/kg/day for 3 days, then 1 mg/kg/day, maximum 25 mg/day, orally in two divided doses) and either sulfadiazine or trisulfapyrimidine (120 to 150 mg/kg/day, maximum 4 g/day, orally in four divided doses) (see Table 74–2). Folinic acid, or leucovorin (1 mg/kg/day, maximum 10 mg/day, orally or parenterally in one dose), is added to prevent pyrimethamine-induced hematologic toxicity. The drugs are prescribed for at least 3 to 4 weeks but may be continued indefinitely with HIV infection.

DIFFUSE ALVEOLAR DAMAGE

Diffuse alveolar damage (DAD) occurs as a result of injury to the lung, which, in AIDS, is likely to be a combination of opportunistic infection, increased ambient oxygen, and mechanical ventilation. It causes an interstitial pneumonitis with damage to both alveolar epithelial and capillary endothelial cells. It has an acute onset and course, usually results in respiratory failure, and, although its mortality rate is 50 to 90 per cent depending on its etiology, it is 100 per cent fatal in the few children reported with DAD and HIV (Joshi et al, 1985). It can appear on radiographs as pulmonary edema, segmental atelectasis, interstitial infiltrates, and honeycomb lung pattern.

During the first 7 days after the lung injury, an exudative phase occurs, with interstitial and intraalveolar edema; proliferation of lymphocytes, plasma cells, and histiocytes in alveolar septa; sloughing of alveolar epithelial cells; and destruction of the alveolar capillary membrane. Hemorrhage and atelectasis also occur, and hyaline membranes containing protein, fibrin, and necrotic epithelial cells form within the acini. Toward the end of this phase, alveolar epithelial type II cells multiply in a reparative response.

An organizing, or proliferative, phase occurs during the next 7 days, with occlusion of the acinus by proliferating fibroblasts within the hyaline membranes and organization of fibrous tissue. If death does not occur, gradations of destruction and remodeling of alveoli ensue, with fibrosis and honeycomb lung pattern. The exudative and organizing phases may overlap, and recovery or death can occur at either phase.

A diagnosis of DAD is made by histologic examination of lung tissue obtained by open-lung biopsy. Drug therapy includes corticosteroids (see "Lymphocytic Interstitial Pneumonitis" for doses).

IMMUNOBLASTIC SARCOMA, KAPOSI'S SARCOMA

Immunoblastic sarcoma of the lung has been reported in one child with AIDS and was characterized by multiple tumor nodules with penetration into bronchial walls and surrounding pleura (Zimmerman et al, 1987). Tumor nodules were also present in the spleen, liver, kidney, and adrenal glands.

Kaposi's sarcoma occurs in approximately 4 per cent of patients with pediatric HIV infection as a disseminated malignancy of the lymph nodes, thymus, and spleen (Rogers et al, 1987; Buck et al, 1983). However, it has not been reported in the lungs of children with HIV infection.

LABORATORY EVALUATION

Immunologic

Alterations in cell-mediated immunity, immuno-globulin formation and function, and phagocytosis can be caused by HIV (Table 74–3). These alterations predispose the patient to infection with opportunistic organisms and the development of malignancies. For example, *P. carinii*, *Toxoplasma gondii*, mycobacteria, Cryptococcus neoformans, and CMV cause disease in the presence of dysfunctional monocytes.

Although polyclonal hypergammaglobulinemia is characteristic of HIV infection, hypogammaglobulin-emia can also occur in children. Lymphopenia is not present as frequently in children as it is in adults with HIV. A reversed helper-to-suppressor T lymphocyte ratio can also occur with tuberculosis and acute infections with other viruses. However, unlike HIV, the number of T4 cells is normal, and the number of T8 cells is increased with *M. tuberculosis* and other viruses. After several months of antituber-culous chemotherapy or during convalescence from the viral infection, the ratio returns to normal.

The diagnosis of AIDS is only made definitively by the growth of or histologic evidence of HIV-1 in tissue (Figs. 74–4 and 74–7). The occurrence of HIV should be evaluated in the presence of an unex-

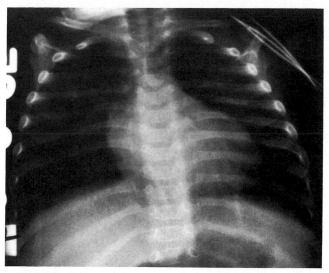

Figure 74–7. Normal lung parenchyma with hyperexpansion in a 7-month-old boy with clinical and immunologic evidence of human immunodeficiency virus (HIV) infection and growth of HIV in the lungs at autopsy.

plained interstitial pneumonitis, a pulmonary oppor-tunistic infection, or other findings suggestive of HIV infection, such as failure to thrive; unintentional weight loss; generalized lymphadenopathy; parotid gland enlargement; recurrent fever, infection, or diarrhea; clubbing; thrombocytopenia; hepatosple-nomegaly; generalized dermatitis; and encephalopa-thy with dementia and loss of developmental mile-stones.

Table 74–3. IMMUNOLOGIC ABNORMALITIES IN PEDIATRIC HIV INFECTION

Blood
T lymphocyte
  Decreased number of helper (CD4) T lymphocytes*
  Reversed helper (CD4)/suppressor (CD8) T lymphocyte ratio†
  Absolute lymphopenia‡
  Impaired cytotoxicity
  Presence of cutaneous anergy
B lymphocyte
  Polyclonal hyper-§ or hypogammaglobulinemia‖
  Loss of function in vitro
  Decreased lymphoproliferative responses to mitogens
  Decreased antibody response to immunization
  Presence of serum antibody to HIV-1, cytomegalovirus,
    hepatitis B virus, herpes simplex virus, varicella-zoster
    virus, Epstein-Barr virus, toxoplasma
Monocyte
  Impaired chemotaxis
  Impaired cytotoxicity
  Decreased serum interleukin-1 and interleukin-2 levels
Miscellaneous
  Presence of serum antigen and antibody to HIV-1
  Presence of HIV-1 cellular DNA
  Decreased plasma thymulin level
  Impaired activity of natural killer null lymphocytes
  Presence of circulating immune complexes

Bronchoalveolar Lavage Fluid
  Increased number of total and suppressor (CD8) T lymphocytes
  Decreased number of helper (CD4) T lymphocytes
  Reversed helper (CD4)/suppressor (CD8) T lymphocyte ratio†
  Increased IgG and IgA levels
  Decreased number of macrophages

*<400/mm³
†<1.0
‡<1500/mm³
§>2 SD for age
‖<2 SD for age

Pulmonary

The presence, type, and severity of pulmonary disease in pediatric AIDS can be evaluated as outlined in Figure 74–8. A localized infiltrate on a chest radiograph usually indicates a bacterial or viral in-fection, whereas a diffuse interstitial pattern is more likely to occur with nonbacterial infections, such as *P. carinii*; CMV and other viruses; or with LIP and DIP.

With the possible exception of tuberculosis, the pulmonary disorders in pediatric AIDS may not be readily distinguished both clinically and radiograph-ically from one another and from other lung infec-tions. In general, the opportunistic pneumonias have a more acute onset and a more rapid course than do the interstitial pneumonitides. However, they are differentiated definitively only by histologic or micro-biologic studies, or both.

PROGNOSIS

The two most frequently identified pulmonary disorders in pediatric AIDS are LIP and *P. carinii* pneumonia. Although a relatively more favorable short-term prognosis exists for LIP, both diseases are receiving new therapeutic approaches. However, the

CLINICAL MANIFESTATIONS OF LUNG DISEASE

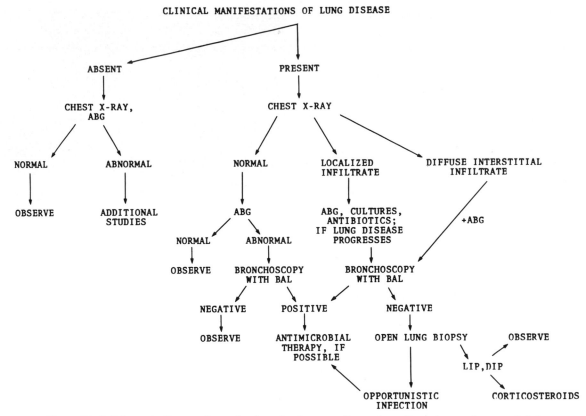

Figure 74–8. Schematic diagram for evaluation of pulmonary disease in pediatric human immunodeficiency virus (HIV) infection. *ABG,* arterial blood gas studies; *BAL,* bronchoalveolar lavage; *LIP,* lymphocytic interstitial pneumonitis; *DIP,* desquamative interstitial pneumonitis.

immunodeficiency of AIDS is, at present, progressive and fatal, and pulmonary disease remains the most frequent cause of death.

Although zidovudine is available for treatment of selected individuals with AIDS, other drugs are still under investigation and have not been released for widespread use in children.* Therapy in children includes sequential intravenous infusions of gammaglobulin in an attempt to provide more optimal humoral immunity on exposure to new antigens, and, if respiratory failure occurs, assisted ventilation, positive end-expiratory pressure, supplemental oxygen, and other supportive measures, as indicated. It is hoped that more effective treatment and prevention of transmission will halt the progress of death from this syndrome.

REFERENCES

Barnes DW and Whitley RJ: Antiviral therapy and pulmonary disease. Chest 91:246, 1987.
Buck BE, Scott GB, Valdes-Dapena M, and Parks WP: Kaposi sarcoma in two infants with acquired immune deficiency syndrome. J Pediatr 103:911, 1983.

---

*The types of drugs and doses mentioned in this chapter are current as of November 1989. Because these drugs and doses change rapidly, the reader is advised to verify the therapy current for the particular disease.

Calvelli TA and Rubinstein A: Intravenous gamma-globulin in infant acquired immunodeficiency syndrome. Pediatr Infect Dis J 5:S207, 1986.
Centers for Disease Control: Classification system for human immunodeficiency virus (HIV) infection in children under 13 years of age. Morbidity and Mortality Weekly Report 36:225, 1987a.
Centers for Disease Control: Diagnosis and management of mycobacterial infection and disease in persons with human immunodeficiency virus infection. Ann Intern Med 106:254, 1987b.
Centers for Disease Control: Revision of the CDC surveillance case definition for acquired immunodeficiency syndrome. Morbidity and Mortality Weekly Report 36:3S, 1987c.
Centers for Disease Control: Use of BCG vaccines in the control of tuberculosis: a joint statement by the ACIP and the Advisory Committee for Elimination of Tuberculosis. Morbidity and Mortality Weekly Report 37:663, 1988.
Centers for Disease Control: Guidelines for prophylaxis against *Pneumocystis carinii* pneumonia for persons infected with human immunodeficiency virus. Morbidity and Mortality Weekly Report 38:1, 1989a.
Centers for Disease Control: Tuberculosis and human immunodeficiency virus infection: recommendations of the Advisory Committee for the Elimination of Tuberculosis (ACET). Morbidity and Mortality Weekly Report 38:236, 1989b.
Chaisson RE, Schecter GF, Theuer CP et al: Tuberculosis in patients with the acquired immunodeficiency syndrome. Clinical features, response to therapy, and survival. Am Rev Respir Dis 136:570, 1987.
Chayt KJ, Harper ME, Marselle LM et al: Detection of HTLV-III RNA in lungs of patients with AIDS and pulmonary involvement. JAMA 256:2356, 1986.
Collaborative DHPG Treatment Study Group: Treatment of serious cytomegalovirus infections with 9-(1,3-dihydroxy-2-propoxymethyl) guanine in patients with AIDS and other immunodeficiencies. N Engl J Med 314:801, 1986.

Curran JW, Jaffe HW, Hardy AM et al: Epidemiology of HIV infection and AIDS in the United States. Science 239:610, 1988.

DeLorenzo LJ, Huang CT, Maguire GP, and Stone DJ: Roentgenographic patterns of *Pneumocystis carinii* pneumonia in 104 patients with AIDS. Chest 91:323, 1987.

Dorsky DI and Crumpacker CS: Drugs five years later: acyclovir. Ann Intern Med 107:859, 1987.

Fauci AS: The human immunodeficiency virus: infectivity and mechanisms of pathogenesis. Science 239:617, 1988.

Fischl MA, Dickinson GM, and La Voie L: Safety and efficacy of sulfamethoxazole and trimethoprim chemoprophylaxis for *Pneumocystis carinii* pneumonia in AIDS. JAMA 259:1185, 1988.

Gallo RC and Wong-Staal F: A human T-lymphotropic retrovirus (HTLV-III) as the cause of the acquired immunodeficiency syndrome. Ann Intern Med 103:679, 1985.

Gorelkin L, Chandler FW, and Ewing EP Jr: Staining qualities of cytomegalovirus inclusions in the lungs of patients with the acquired immunodeficiency syndrome: a potential source of diagnostic misinterpretation. Hum Pathol 17:926, 1986.

Hanshaw JB: Cytomegalovirus infections. In Feigin RD and Cherry JD (eds): Textbook of Pediatric Infectious Diseases. 2nd ed. Philadelphia, WB Saunders Co, 1987.

Hirsch MS: Azidothymidine. J Infect Dis 157:427, 1988.

Ho DD, Pomerantz RJ, and Kaplan JC: Pathogenesis of infection with human immunodeficiency virus. N Engl J Med 317:278, 1987.

Ho M: Cytomegalovirus. In Mandell GL, Douglas RG Jr, and Bennett JE (eds): Principles and Practice of Infectious Diseases, 3rd ed. New York, Churchill Livingstone, Inc, 1990.

Joshi VV and Oleske JM: Pulmonary lesions in children with the acquired immunodeficiency syndrome: a reappraisal based on data in additional cases and follow-up study of previously reported cases. Hum Pathol 17:641, 1986.

Joshi VV, Kauffman S, Oleske JM et al: Polyclonal polymorphic B-cell lymphoproliferative disorder with prominent pulmonary involvement in children with acquired immune deficiency syndrome. Cancer 59:1455, 1987.

Joshi VV, Oleske JM, Minnefor AB et al: Pathologic pulmonary findings in children with the acquired immunodeficiency syndrome: a study of ten cases. Hum Pathol 16:241, 1985.

Katzenstein A-LA and Askin FB: Chronic interstitial pneumonia, interstitial fibrosis, and honeycomb lung. In Bennington JL (ed): Surgical Pathology of Non-Neoplastic Lung Disease. Philadelphia, WB Saunders Co, 1982a.

Katzenstein A-LA and Askin FB: Diffuse alveolar damage. In Bennington JL (ed): Surgical Pathology of Non-Neoplastic Lung Disease. Philadelphia, WB Saunders Co, 1982b.

Kauffman RS: Viral pneumonia. In Pennington JE (ed): Respiratory Infections: Diagnosis and Management. 2nd ed. New York, Raven Press, 1989.

Kornstein MJ, Pietra GG, Hoxie JA, and Conley ME: The pathology and treatment of interstitial pneumonitis in two infants with AIDS. Am Rev Respir Dis 133:1196, 1986.

Kovacs JA, Ng VL, Masur H et al: Diagnosis of *Pneumocystis carinii* pneumonia: improved detection in sputum with use of monoclonal antibodies. N Engl J Med 318:589, 1988.

Pifer LLW, Woods DR, Edwards CC et al: *Pneumocystis carinii* serologic study in pediatric acquired immunodeficiency syndrome. Am J Dis Child 142:36, 1988.

Piot P, Plummer FA, Mhalu FS et al: AIDS: an international perspective. Science 239:573, 1988.

Pitchenik AE and Rubinson HA: The radiographic appearance of tuberculosis in patients with the acquired immune deficiency syndrome (AIDS) and pre-AIDS. Am Rev Respir Dis 131:393, 1985.

Rankin JA, Collman R, and Daniele RP: Acquired immune deficiency syndrome and the lung. Chest 94:155, 1988.

Rogers MF, Ou C-Y, Rayfield M et al: Use of the polymerase chain reaction for early detection of the proviral sequences of human immunodeficiency virus in infants born to seropositive mothers. N Engl J Med 320:1649, 1989.

Rogers MF, Thomas PA, Starcher ET et al: Acquired immunodeficiency syndrome in children: report of the Centers for Disease Control national surveillance, 1982 to 1985. Pediatrics 79:1008, 1987.

Rubinstein A, Bernstein LJ, Charytan M et al: Corticosteroid treatment for pulmonary lymphoid hyperplasia in children with the acquired immune deficiency syndrome. Pediatr Pulmonol 4:13, 1988.

Rubinstein A, Morecki R, Silverman B et al: Pulmonary disease in children with acquired immune deficiency syndrome and AIDS-related complex. J Pediatr 108:498, 1986.

Sankary RM, Turner J, Lipavsky A et al: Alveolar-capillary block in patients with AIDS and *Pneumocystis carinii* pneumonia. Am Rev Respir Dis 137:443, 1988.

Sanyal SK, Mariencheck WC, Hughes WT et al: Course of pulmonary dysfunction in children surviving *Pneumocystis carinii* pneumonitis. A prospective study. Am Rev Respir Dis 124:161, 1981.

Seligmann M, Pinching AJ, Rosen FS et al: Immunology of human immunodeficiency virus infection and the acquired immunodeficiency syndrome. An update. Ann Intern Med 107:234, 1987.

Shannon KM and Ammann AJ: Acquired immune deficiency syndrome in childhood. J Pediatr 106:332, 1985.

Silverman BA and Rubinstein A: Serum lactate dehydrogenase levels in adults and children with acquired immune deficiency syndrome (AIDS) and AIDS-related complex: possible indicator of B cell lymphoproliferation and disease activity. Effect of intravenous gammaglobulin on enzyme levels. Am J Med 78:728, 1985.

Snider DE Jr, Hopewell PC, Mills J, and Reichman LB: Mycobacterioses and the acquired immunodeficiency syndrome. Am Rev Respir Dis 136:492, 1987.

Snydman DR, Werner BG, Heinze-Lacey B et al: Use of cytomegalovirus immune globulin to prevent cytomegalovirus disease in renal-transplant recipients. N Engl J Med 317:1049, 1987.

Stover DE, Zaman MB, Hajdu SI et al: Bronchoalveolar lavage in the diagnosis of diffuse pulmonary infiltrates in the immunosuppressed host. Ann Intern Med 101:1, 1984.

Walzer PD: *Pneumocystis carinii*. In Mandell GL, Douglas RG Jr, and Bennett JE (eds): Principles and Practice of Infectious Diseases, 3rd ed. New York, Churchill Livingstone, Inc, 1990.

Wong-Staal F and Gallo RC: Human T-lymphotropic retroviruses. Nature 317:395, 1985.

Young KR Jr, Rankin JA, Naegel GP et al: Bronchoalveolar lavage cells and proteins in patients with the acquired immunodeficiency syndrome. An immunologic analysis. Ann Intern Med 103:522, 1985.

Zimmerman BL, Haller JO, Price AP et al: Children with AIDS—is pathologic diagnosis possible based on chest radiographs? Pediatr Radiol 17:303, 1987.

75

CARL E. HUNT, M.D., and
ROBERT T. BROUILLETTE, M.D.

DISORDERS OF BREATHING DURING SLEEP

Respiratory disorders during sleep, in the absence of any primary lung dysfunction, are related to abnormalities or deficiencies in the control of breathing. Although a contributing abnormality in peripheral chemoreceptors may be present in some instances, in general these respiratory control deficits originate within the central nervous system. The respiratory control centers are located in the brainstem, but specific morphologic abnormalities have not been identified and correlated with any of the primary (congenital) respiratory control disorders known to occur in children, except in part as related to Arnold-Chiari malformation.

Respiratory control disorders are state dependent and typically cause significant clinical symptoms only during sleep. Whereas obstructive sleep apnea may occur or even be predominant in rapid eye movement (REM) sleep, alveolar hypoventilation is characteristically no worse in REM sleep than in periods of awakeness and is associated with significant hypoventilation only in quiet sleep.

Apnea of prematurity, apnea of infancy, and sudden infant death syndrome all have known or hypothesized abnormalities that affect the control of breathing, but these important entities are discussed in other chapters. In this chapter, we discuss those respiratory control disorders that are not simply related to delays in maturation (albeit potentially life-threatening delays) but rather are related to congenital or acquired abnormalities that will result in substantial morbidity and mortality if not diagnosed and treated in a timely and appropriate manner. These disorders include abnormalities in neuromuscular control of upper airway patency and abnormalities in chemical drive that result in alveolar hypoventilation.

OBSTRUCTIVE SLEEP APNEA

Pharyngeal airway obstruction during sleep occurs in infants and children as well as in adults. When frequent and severe obstruction is present, such obstructive sleep apnea (OSA) may cause sleep disturbance, behavioral abnormalities, growth failure,

and cor pulmonale. Most commonly, OSA in children is due to hypertrophy of the tonsils, adenoids, or both and can be cured by surgical removal of the obstructing tissue.

Tonsillectomy and adenoidectomy have been surgical procedures for more than 2000 and 120 years, respectively (Paradise, 1983). Two developments in the 1960s have influenced current clinical practice toward relieving or bypassing sleep-related airway obstruction. The first was the recognition that enlarged tonsils and adenoids could cause hypoventilation and cor pulmonale (Menashe et al, 1965; Noonan, 1965). The second was Gastaut's report the following year on OSA in adults (Gastaut et al, 1966).

PATHOGENESIS

Obstructive sleep apnea occurs when the upper airway collapses during inspiration. The pharyngeal airway, unlike the nasal, tracheal, and laryngeal airways, is not well supported by a bony or cartilaginous skeleton. When subjected to negative pressure during inspiration, the pharynx tends to collapse. Normally, the brainstem areas that control breathing activate both the inspiratory pressure-generating muscles, such as the diaphragm, and the upper airway dilating muscles, such as the genioglossus. The coordinated contraction of these two muscle groups allows the unimpeded flow of air into the lungs. When resistance to inspiratory airflow increases or when activation of pharyngeal dilator muscles decreases, negative inspiratory pressure may collapse the airway (Remmers et al, 1978; Brouillette and Thach, 1979). Both functional and anatomic factors may tilt the balance toward airway collapse (Bradley and Phillipson, 1985).

Sleep is the most obvious functional factor that predisposes to OSA. The mechanism is thought to be a reduction of airway-maintaining muscular activity in sleep compared with wakefulness, particularly during REM sleep. Other factors that may depress airway-maintaining activity include narcotics, sedatives, alcohol, and some brainstem lesions, particularly those associated with perinatal asphyxia or Arnold-Chiari malformation.

1004

Anatomic factors predispose to OSA by increasing inspiratory resistance, thereby lowering the negative pressure within the upper airway. In adults with OSA, pharyngeal narrowing has not been as obvious and has generally required computed tomography (CT) scanning or other specialized techniques for its demonstration. In most children, however, an anatomic lesion that narrows the upper airway and increases airway resistance can be identified (Table 75–1). Premature infants often have obstructive components to their apneas (Roberts et al, 1982). It is not known whether this obstruction is due to the immaturity of the central nervous system control of airway patency, to the narrow upper airway, or to both.

CLINICAL FEATURES AND DEFINITION

The triad of loud snoring, difficulty breathing during sleep, and sleep-related breathing pauses as reported by the parents characterizes most children with clinically significant OSA (Brouillette et al, 1984). Although some snoring may be present in 9 to 27 per cent of normal children (Brouillette et al, 1984), loud snoring, difficulty breathing, and obstructive apneas are much more unusual. Other findings and sequelae in pediatric OSA are listed in Table 75–2 (Brouillette et al, 1982; Frank et al, 1983; Guilleminault et al, 1981).

Most children with OSA are initially seen by physicians during wakefulness. These patients may look quite normal while awake yet have severe problems breathing while asleep. It is thus essential that the physician ask the parents about sleep-related complaints and examine the child during sleep.

Definition. There are no universally accepted, minimum diagnostic criteria for OSA in children concerning frequency and duration of obstructive apnea. Rather, OSA is best regarded as the extreme manifestation of a spectrum of sleep-related pharyngeal airway obstructive problems. Between children with perfectly normal breathing and those with severe, prolonged, and frequent obstructive apneas are many who snore as a manifestation of a partial obstruction

Table 75–1. ANATOMIC FACTORS PREDISPOSING TO OBSTRUCTIVE SLEEP APNEA

Adenotonsillar hypertrophy
Micrognathia
Down syndrome
Craniofacial abnormalities
Allergic rhinitis
Upper respiratory infection
Choanal atresia or stenosis
Nasal foreign body
Deviated nasal septum
Chronic use of nasal decongestants
Velopharyngeal flap
Cleft palate repair
Macroglossia
Obesity

Table 75–2. CLINICAL FINDINGS IN PEDIATRIC OBSTRUCTIVE SLEEP APNEA

Sleep-related
Loud snoring
Difficulty breathing during sleep
Breathing pauses reported by parents
Sweating during sleep
Enuresis
During Wakefulness
Mouth breathing
"Adenoid facies"
Chronic rhinorrhea
Difficulty swallowing
Pectus excavatum
Sequelae
Cor pulmonale
Failure to thrive and poor appetite
Systemic hypertension
Frequent respiratory infections
Polycythemia
Hypersomnolence
Hyperactivity
Pathologic shyness and social withdrawal
Delayed development and learning problems

of the airway. Furthermore, some children have constant, severe partial airway obstruction during sleep with few or no complete obstructions. Thus we diagnose OSA (1) when episodes of partial or complete airway obstruction during sleep result in hypoxemia ($Sa_{O_2} < 90$ per cent) and hypercarbia ($Pa_{CO_2} > 45$ mm Hg); and (2) when sleep-related asphyxia and sleep deprivation result in clinically significant effects, such as failure to thrive, cor pulmonale, or neurobehavioral disturbance.

DIAGNOSIS

The evaluation of a child with possible obstructive sleep apnea should be directed at answering three questions. Does the child have a clinically significant sleep-related breathing problem? Is this problem due to upper airway obstruction? What is the site and mechanism of obstruction?

The history and physical examination are most helpful in determining the clinical significance of the problem and in putting all other tests in perspective. A standardized history for sleep-related breathing can be helpful (Brouillette et al, 1984). The presence and extent of failure to thrive need to be ascertained. In many children, no further testing will be necessary. It is reasonable to proceed to tonsillectomy, adenoidectomy, or both if a child has loud snoring; difficulty breathing during sleep; repetitive obstructive apneas; large tonsils or adenoids; and no other neuromuscular, craniofacial, or cardiopulmonary disorders.

Polygraphic monitoring during natural sleep allows quantitation of the number and duration of obstructive apneas, the severity of partial airway obstruction, and the degree of hypercarbia and hypoxemia (Figs. 75–1 and 75–2). Sedatives should not be used as they predispose the patient to upper airway collapse, thus invalidating the study and placing the patient at risk

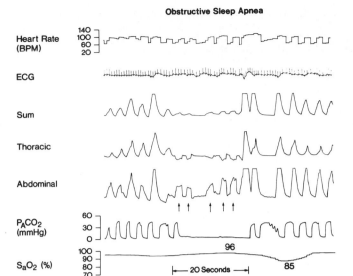

Figure 75–1. This polygraphic tracing shows an 18-sec obstructive apnea in a 5-year-old girl with large tonsils and adenoids and a past history of subglottic stenosis. Five obstructed inspirations are indicated by upward arrows. Note the inward thoracic and outward abdominal movements, by respiratory inductive plethysmography. Sa_{O_2} begins to decrease about 15 sec after the onset of the apnea. The marked sinus arrhythmia is characteristic of obstructive sleep apnea. Fluoroscopy showed intermittent complete obstruction at the tonsillar level.

(Hershenson et al, 1984). Adequate information can usually be obtained without esophageal pressure monitoring.

Fluoroscopy can be of value. The site and mechanism of obstruction can be identified radiographically. A standard lateral neck radiograph during wakefulness will show enlarged tonsils, adenoids, or both and rule

Sleep-Related Partial Airway Obstruction

Figure 75–2. This polygraphic tracing, from the same patient shown in Figure 75–1, demonstrates the noninvasive diagnosis of sleep-related partial upper airway obstruction. Hypercarbia (PA_{CO_2} = 51 mm Hg) indicates alveolar hypoventilation. Paradoxical movement of the chest and abdomen during inspiration (*I*) accompanied by loud snoring indicates pharyngeal partial airway obstruction as the cause of hypoventilation.

out other lesions. In difficult or complex cases, upper airway fluoroscopy during natural sleep has been exceptionally helpful in identifying the site of obstruction (Felman et al, 1979; Fernbach et al, 1983). If fluoroscopy is not available, lateral neck radiographs of the sleeping child during inspiration and expiration may be adequate (Fig. 75–3). These images provide the surgeon with information on how best to treat the obstruction. During normal sleep, the walls of the pharyngeal airway move very little with inspiration and expiration. However, when the airway is obstructed, the normal balance between negative inspiratory pressure and pharyngeal dilator muscles is lost. The pharynx below an obstructing lesion (for instance, the adenoids) collapses on inspiration because of excessive negative pressure. Conversely, the pharynx above an obstructing lesion (subglottic stenosis, for example) widens because inspiratory activation of pharyngeal dilators is not opposed by negative inspiratory pressure. The specific fluoroscopic findings, however, are highly variable from patient to patient.

TREATMENT

As adenotonsillar hypertrophy is the predominant anatomic cause of OSA in childhood, tonsillectomy and adenoidectomy are the mainstays of treatment (Brouillette et al, 1982; Frank et al, 1983; Guilleminault et al, 1981). Nasal continuous positive airway pressure (CPAP) may effectively relieve OSA in premature neonates (Miller et al, 1985) and is now a recommended treatment for adult OSA (Sullivan et al, 1981). Only a few pediatric cases have been treated with nasal CPAP (Guilleminault, 1987; Schmidt-Nowara, 1984). Nasopharyngeal intubation has been recommended as a diagnostic technique, as a preoperative stabilizing procedure, and as a long-term treatment. One study indicates good results treating pediatric OSA by continuously insufflating air into the nasopharynx (Klein and Reynolds, 1986). Various craniofacial operations are available for specific conditions, but careful postoperative monitoring is needed to be certain that the airway obstruction is truly resolved (Guilleminault et al, 1981). Weight loss may be of significant benefit in children who are obese. Tracheostomy remains an effective therapy but will seldom be necessary because most upper airway obstructive problems in children can be corrected surgically.

ALVEOLAR HYPOVENTILATION

In addition to the abnormalities in neuromuscular control of upper airway patency already discussed, other conditions occur in children in which there is no upper airway obstruction but in which central inspiratory drive (chemical drive) is insufficient, thus resulting in hypoventilation. Although the terminol-

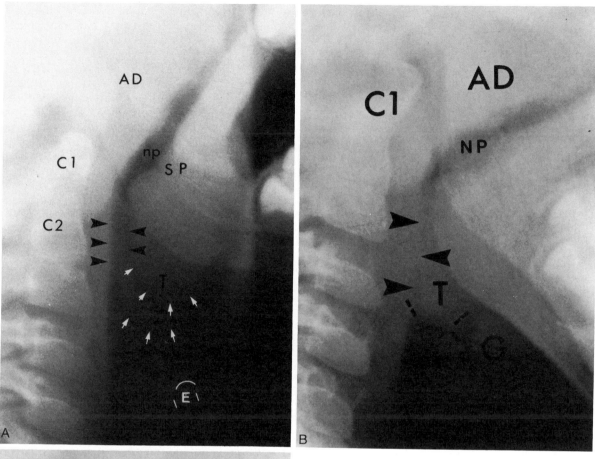

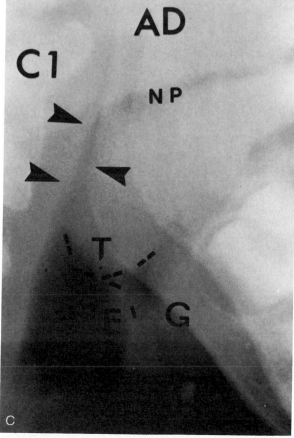

Figure 75–3. Lateral airway radiographs of a 3-year-old girl with obstructive sleep apnea. *A*, A standard lateral airway radiograph, obtained with the patient upright and awake, shows the entire upper airway to be patent. Moderately enlarged tonsils *(T) (white arrows)* are surrounded by air. The airway posterior to the tonsils is patent *(black arrowheads)*. *B*, A radiograph obtained during an inspiratory effort with the patient asleep and supine shows obstruction of the pharyngeal airway at the tonsillar level. The black arrowheads show the tonsillar to posterior pharyngeal apposition. Lack of an air-tissue interface suggests complete obstruction. Note the widening of the retropharyngeal soft tissues below the tonsils. *C*, During expiration with the patient asleep and supine, the airway *(black arrowheads)* appears patent behind the tonsils. *AD*, adenoids; *C1* and *C2*, cervical vertebrae; *NP*, nasopharynx; *SP*, soft palate; *E*, epiglottis; *T*, tonsil; *G*, tongue; *H*, hyoid.

ogy that has evolved is somewhat misleading, these deficits in chemical drive are collectively referred to as *alveolar hypoventilation*, with the term *central hypoventilation syndrome* (CHS) reserved for the most severe form. These alveolar hypoventilation conditions (Table 75–3) may be congenital or acquired, with considerable interpatient variation in severity.

Alveolar hypoventilation should be suspected clinically whenever there is a history of sleep-related cyanosis or hypoventilation without snoring or of unexplained cor pulmonale. Although primary lung disease can generally be excluded by the medical history and the confirmation of normal awake ventilation, this exclusion may be difficult if the alveolar hypoventilation has already resulted in significant cor pulmonale. If cor pulmonale is present, primary lung or other primary neuromuscular abnormalities can be excluded only by demonstrating that respiratory center output is deficient or that voluntary respiratory control can achieve spontaneous tidal breaths that are of a sufficient volume and frequency to result in acceptable levels of P_{O_2} and P_{CO_2}. The deficit in respiratory control does not affect the voluntary control of breathing but rather the automatic control of breathing that is regulated in the brainstem. This brainstem deficiency in automatic control results in deficient or absent ventilatory and arousal responsiveness to hypercarbia and hypoxia.

The rate and depth of breathing are normally controlled automatically to maintain appropriate CO_2 and O_2 levels. Alveolar hypoventilation occurs when the output from the brainstem centers is deficient. Children with alveolar hypoventilation typically have normal respiratory rates associated with shallow breathing (hypopnea); these rates tend to be relatively invariable during sleep and are not responsive to the progressive asphyxia that occurs consequent to the hypopnea (Fig. 75–4). In contrast, however, some children with brainstem structural lesions may hypoventilate because of low respiratory rate rather than tidal volume. In selected children with Arnold-Chiari malformation or acquired CHS secondary to a brain tumor, for example (Fig. 75–5), we have observed significant alveolar hypoventilation that is caused by very low respiratory frequency (bradypnea) in the presence of normal or even increased tidal volumes.

The chemoreceptor deficits evident during sleep are also present while awake. It is only during quiet sleep, however, that one is totally dependent on these automatic respiratory control systems and thus only during quiet sleep that most such deficits become clinically significant. The only exception to the sleep dependency of hypoventilation in CHS is the most severely affected CHS patient who also has a deficient ventilatory drive while awake and during REM sleep, albeit always with intact voluntary or conscious control of breathing.

TRANSIENT

The significant sleep-related asphyxia occurring with severe OSA can result in blunting of hypercarbic and hypoxic ventilatory responses that persists temporarily after treatment of the OSA. Now that OSA is a recognized problem in children, it is unusual for long-standing, severe, sleep-related asphyxia to occur, and transient alveolar hypoventilation should thus be uncommon in the future. Nonetheless, we have previously observed alveolar hypoventilation following complete resolution of the obstruction. We assumed initially that these children had a central respiratory control deficit associated both with impaired neuromuscular airway patency and decreased chemical drive; subsequently, however, the residual alveolar hypoventilation has resolved in virtually all instances and can thus be explained by temporary blunting of hypercarbic-hypoxic ventilatory drive rather than by a congenital respiratory center deficit.

CONGENITAL

In the most severely affected infants, congenital deficits may be evident in the first hours of life, even

Table 75–3. CAUSES OF ALVEOLAR HYPOVENTILATION IN CHILDREN

Transient	Generally associated with severe obstructive sleep apnea; progressively resolves once the obstruction has been eliminated.
Congenital	
A. Alveolar hypoventilation	Mild-moderate in severity. Responds to treatment with respiratory stimulants. Age at diagnosis variable.
B. Central hypoventilation syndrome (CHS)	Severe hypoventilation, with onset of symptoms typically in neonatal period or early infancy.
C. Arnold-Chiari malformation	Associated with multiple other brainstem abnormalities.
Late-onset CHS	Underlying abnormality likely congenital in origin, but symptoms not manifest until later childhood.
Acquired	Related to a structural lesion in brainstem: Trauma Infection Tumor Infarct Asphyxia

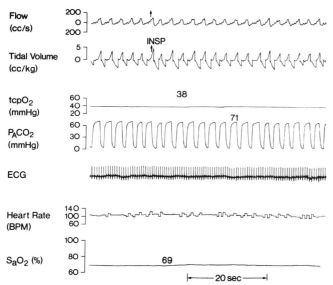

Figure 75–4. This tracing from a 2.5-year-old girl shows the typical breathing pattern during quiet sleep in idiopathic congenital central hypoventilation syndrome. Note the regular shallow breathing (hypopnea). Tidal volume averaged only 2.9 cc/kg, and respiratory rate was stable at 22 breaths per min, resulting in a $\dot{V}_I$ of only 64 cc/kg/min. As final proof of the central respiratory control deficit, the progressive hypercarbia and hypoxemia failed to stimulate ventilation or arousal.

in the delivery room. Congenital deficits may be of familial origin (Fuchs and Kummer, 1980; Moore et al, 1976). In adults (Block, 1980), alveolar hypoventilation may be associated with obesity, upper airway obstruction, or both and may be responsive to respiratory stimulants. Similarly, we have observed some children with normal awake ventilation and sleep-

Central Hypoventilation: Bradypnea

A.

B.

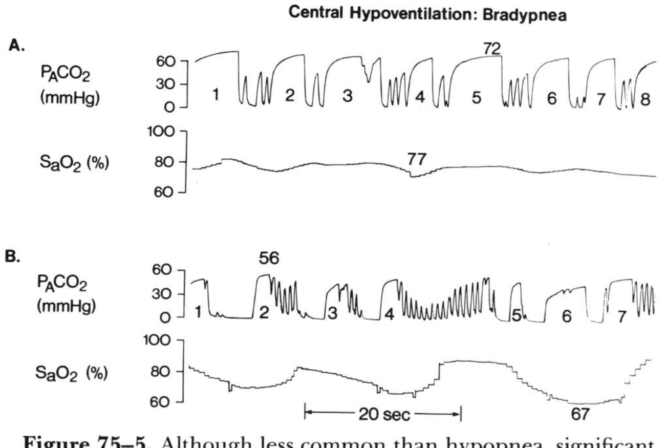

Figure 75–5. Although less common than hypopnea, significant hypoventilation and hypoxemia due to low respiratory rate (bradypnea) can also occur despite normal to increased tidal volumes. Expirations are numbered on the Pa_{CO_2} channel. *A*, A 14-month-old child with Chiari II malformation, myelomeningocele, and brainstem dysfunction. During sleep, tidal volume averaged 12 cc/kg, but the respiratory rate was only 5 to 10 breaths per min and was unresponsive to progressive hypercarbia and hypoxemia. *B*, A 12-year-old boy with medullary astrocytoma, which also caused severe alveolar hypoventilation due to bradypnea without hypopnea.

related hypopnea associated with decreased hypercarbic-hypoxic ventilatory sensitivity who have responded to treatment with theophylline or other respiratory stimulants. Although the two classic literary references for respiratory control disorders in adults, Ondine's curse and pickwickian syndrome (Block, 1980; Comroe, 1975), are also appropriate for certain children, we do not encourage the use of these terms because they are not correct literary references, are physiologically imprecise, and may have negative connotations for parents.

The severe form of alveolar hypoventilation, CHS, is not cured by respiratory stimulants and requires mechanical ventilatory support (Table 75–4). Following the initial report of a well-studied adult with CHS (Ratto et al, 1955), the occurrence of CHS in children was recognized, and the first detailed example of congenital CHS with symptoms since birth was reported in 1970 (Mellins et al, 1970). Although a precise estimate of the frequency of congenital CHS is still not possible, it is certainly not a rare diagnosis in the modern neonatal intensive care unit environment and with the sophisticated technologies available in pediatric sleep laboratories. Based on personal communications and individual case reports, a very rough estimate of at least 50 new cases of congenital CHS in infants annually in the United States appears reasonable. Reports of collective and individual experience with CHS in children, especially congenital CHS, have now substantially increased the number of reported cases (Guilleminault et al, 1982; Brouillette et al, 1988).

Apnea is actually quite uncommon in congenital CHS, but the extent of hypopnea can be very substantial. In infants, we have observed tidal volumes that measure even less than anatomic dead space (approximately 2 ml/kg). Basal respiratory rates tend to be normal but are unresponsive to the progressive sleep asphyxia. The extent of hypopnea is state dependent (Fleming et al, 1980). Depending on the severity of the deficit in metabolic control of breathing, hypopnea may be evident only during stages 3 and 4 of quiet sleep; hypopnea may also occur during REM sleep in more severely affected patients but generally to a lesser extent than in quiet sleep. In the most severely affected patients, typically with

Table 75–4. PRIMARY CHARACTERISTICS OF CONGENITAL CENTRAL HYPOVENTILATION SYNDROME (CHS)

Absent or negligible ventilatory and arousal sensitivity to hypercarbia.

Variable deficiency in hypoxic ventilatory responsiveness, with absent or negligible hypoxic arousal responsiveness.

Ventilation normal during wakefulness and rapid eye movement (REM) sleep except in severely affected patients, but hypopnea during quiet sleep leads to progressive hypercarbia and hypoxia.

Hypoventilation during wakefulness generally associated with absent or negligible ventilatory sensitivity to hypoxia.

Generally unresponsive to respiratory stimulants.

symptoms first evident in the delivery room or new-born nursery, variable degrees of hypopnea also occur during wakefulness. Even in the most severely affected congenital CHS patients, however, normal alveolar ventilation can be achieved by voluntary or conscious control of breathing. A unique characteristic of CHS, which likely differentiates between the milder forms of alveolar hypoventilation responsive to respiratory stimulants and the more severe forms, is the associated deficiency in arousal responsiveness. In most patients, there is no arousal response from sleep regardless of the extent of hypopnea-induced asphyxia, and during wakefulness there is no perception of asphyxia. Thus dyspnea does not appear to be an achievable experience in CHS patients. In addition to the pathophysiologic significance of this arousal deficit, there is also an important clinical correlate. In CHS patients, the absence of tachypnea or respiratory distress does not preclude the presence of severe respiratory acidosis or hypoxia.

Congenital CHS is of unknown etiology. The fundamental abnormality most likely resides in the brainstem respiratory control centers, which would explain the constellation of ventilatory and arousal deficits that occur. Whether the basic abnormality is morphologic or related to a neurotransmitter remains to be determined. Magnetic resonance imaging has been unhelpful thus far in identifying a morphologic correlate of the functional deficits associated with congenital CHS (Weese-Mayer et al, 1988). Neuropathologic studies of CHS patients have thus far not revealed a morphologic abnormality except in two infants, one with a generalized loss of medullary neurons in the region of the brainstem respiratory control centers (Liu et al, 1978) and a second with absence of the external arcuate nucleus (Folgering et al, 1979). Except for one report of a possible link between central nervous system dopamine activity and CHS (Hedner et al, 1987), there is no direct evidence to date that CHS is a neurotransmitter abnormality.

Congenital CHS may occur as a more generalized neurologic abnormality than suggested by just the brainstem respiratory control abnormality. Seizure disorders are relatively common, and developmental delay and mild cerebral atrophy have been observed (Weese-Mayer et al, 1988); although these associations have been assumed to be secondary to prior hypoxic-ischemic events, not all such patients have had major identifiable asphyxic crises.

Central hypoventilation syndrome can occur with generalized neurologic dysfunction, such as in pyruvate dehydrogenase deficiency (Johnston et al, 1984) and Leigh disease (Dooling and Richardson, 1977). In addition, CHS may be associated with hypothalamic dysfunction syndrome (duRivage et al, 1985). Abnormalities in cranial nerve nuclei may also be associated, and we have evaluated one patient who also had Möbius syndrome. Brainstem auditory responses may be abnormal (Beckerman et al, 1986). Some patients have had varying degrees of generalized autonomic nervous system dysfunction (Haddad et al, 1978) or dysautonomia (Frank et al, 1981). A number of patients have had an associated neurocristopathy, a term describing lesions resulting from maldevelopment of neural crest tissue (Bolande, 1974). Several patients, for example, have had ganglioneuromas (Frank et al, 1981; Hunt et al, 1978), and some patients have had a neuroblastoma (Bower and Adkins, 1980). As the most common neurocristopathy, Hirschsprung's disease has occurred in a number of CHS patients (Haddad et al, 1978; O'Dell et al, 1987; Poceta et al, 1987; Stern et al, 1981). Although it is not currently possible to accurately calculate the actual incidence of Hirschsprung's disease in congenital CHS, our experience to date suggests that 10 to 15 per cent may be a reasonable estimate.

Congenital alveolar hypoventilation may also occur in Arnold-Chiari malformation (see Table 75–3). Although the brainstem deficiency in the control of breathing may be manifest only as a deficiency in the respiratory pattern (Ward et al, 1986), approximately 13 per cent of children with Arnold-Chiari malformation (McClone et al, 1985) have severe hindbrain dysfunction associated with variable degrees of alveolar hypoventilation (Bokinsky et al, 1973; Oren, Kelly, Todres, and Shannon, 1986; Papasozomenos and Roessman, 1981; Weese-Mayer et al, 1988). In such patients, other brainstem abnormalities are characteristically present, including but not restricted to deficient sucking and swallowing reflexes and vocal cord paralysis. As already mentioned, the anatomic lesions in such children may result in hypoventilation secondary to severe bradypnea without hypopnea (see Fig. 75–5) rather than to the hypopnea without bradypnea (see Fig. 75–4) that characteristically occurs in CHS.

LATE-ONSET CENTRAL HYPOVENTILATION SYNDROME

Late-onset CHS has also been observed in some children (see Table 75–3). Although an underlying congenital brainstem abnormality is likely present in most if not all instances, significant hypoventilation becomes evident only as a consequence of an intercurrent illness, such as pneumonia, or as associated with cor pulmonale. We have also observed late-onset CHS associated with idiopathic hypothalamic dysfunction (duRivage et al, 1985; Moss et al, 1986).

ACQUIRED

Alveolar hypoventilation can also be acquired in an individual with previously normal control of breathing following an event resulting in brainstem injury (see Table 75–3). Although not specifically reported in children, an infarct can result in alveolar hypoventilation. Severe asphyxia can result in CHS

(Brazy et al, 1987; Leech and Alford, 1977; Volpe, 1987). Encephalitis (Brouillette et al, 1986; Jensen et al, 1988; Mellins et al, 1970) and other infectious encephalopathies (Liebhaber et al, 1977) can also result in CHS. Brainstem tumors are another cause of CHS in children (see Fig. 75–5). Posttraumatic CHS has also been reported (Quera-Salva and Guilleminault, 1987). Trauma to the upper cervical cord resulting in quadriplegia and respiratory paralysis, however, is not included as an acquired cause of CHS because brainstem respiratory control centers are normal; only the connection between these centers and the muscles of respiration is deficient.

DIAGNOSIS

The diagnosis of alveolar hypoventilation is suggested by the medical history and by the examination of the patient during sleep. All other disorders that could explain hypoventilation should be excluded, such as primary lung problems, airway obstruction, phrenic nerve paralysis, diaphragmatic abnormalities, neuropathy, and myopathy. To confirm the diagnosis and to assess its severity, a sleep laboratory evaluation is necessary. Wakefulness, REM sleep, and quiet sleep all need to be assessed during the polysomnogram. Invasive blood gas determinations are generally unnecessary in the assessment of alveolar hypoventilation; even sampling from an indwelling arterial line may potentially alter the patient's state. Fortunately, the extensive development of noninvasive blood gas technologies has virtually eliminated the need for invasive sampling. We rely primarily on end-tidal P_{CO_2} and pulse oximeter measurements of O_2 saturation for noninvasive blood gas assessments.

The polysomnogram also should include measurements of tidal volume. The documentation of spontaneous resting tidal volumes and noninvasive blood gas values across all states is sufficient to establish the presence and severity of alveolar hypoventilation. The most important objective observation in CHS is the inability to increase respiratory frequency, tidal volume, or both regardless of the severity of the progressive hypercarbia and hypoxia that occur. Further, it is characteristic for CHS patients to fail to arouse from sleep regardless of the magnitude of the hypercarbic or hypoxic stimulus. Challenges with hypercarbic and hypoxic gas mixtures, however, are unnecessary because the ventilatory and arousal responses to hypercarbia and hypoxia will already have been documented during the polysomnogram recordings of spontaneous ventilation.

TREATMENT

All known or suspected respiratory stimulants have been evaluated in children with alveolar hypoventilation. Theophylline is a central stimulant that may be very beneficial in the milder forms of alveolar hypoventilation (Hunt et al, 1983); only limited clinical experience with caffeine is available, but the respiratory stimulation is probably equivalent and the extent of the side effects less (Bairam et al, 1987). Progesterone has been very effective in some children with alveolar hypoventilation (Orenstein et al, 1977; Skatrud et al, 1980); its mechanism is unknown. Methylphenidate (Putnam et al, 1973) and pemoline have also been beneficial in a few selected children with alveolar hypoventilation, but they require precise titration to achieve the necessary respiratory stimulant effect without causing sleep deprivation. Naloxone has been utilized, based on the unproven hypothesis that endorphins might be associated with CHS, but except for possible help in one patient, it (Moss et al, 1986) has had no apparent clinical efficacy. Almitrine is a peripheral chemoreceptor stimulant that can significantly enhance hypoxic ventilatory drive, but trials in children with CHS have shown no apparent long-term efficacy (Oren, Newth, Hunt et al, 1986). Doxapram may normalize alveolar ventilation in some CHS children (Hunt et al, 1979), but no effective and practical enteral preparation is available in the United States, and the nonspecific adrenergic stimulation and resultant nonrespiratory stimulant effects may be incompatible with successful long-term use. Behavioral modification or training has been suggested as an effective treatment (Schlaefke and Burghardt, 1983) and is certainly an intriguing concept; to date, however, no effective and sustained benefits have been reported.

Oxygen alone may be an effective treatment in selected children with only mild or moderate alveolar hypoventilation; oxygen therapy has not been reported in children but has been effective in certain adults (McNicholas et al, 1982). In children with CHS who are unresponsive to supplemental O_2 or to any pharmacologic intervention, however, mechanical ventilatory support will be necessary, at least during sleep. Rocker beds have had some limited success in adults (Barlow et al, 1980) and may be worthy of evaluation in selected children; it is unlikely, however, that rocker beds will be practical for long-term use and unclear whether there are many patients whose defect is too severe to respond to medication yet not severe enough to require positive pressure ventilation or diaphragm pacing. Intermittent negative pressure, either by an iron lung or using a cuirass, has been very effective in some patients but is not suitable for younger children and is relatively cumbersome and impractical for long-term use. Nasal CPAP or nasal intermittent positive-pressure breathing (IPPB) (Ellis et al, 1987) has also been useful in individual children. None of these relatively noninvasive methods for mechanically enhancing or supporting ventilation during sleep will be practical or effective if awake ventilatory support is also necessary. If employed to improve ventilation during sleep, frequent surveillance is required to document appropriate noninvasive blood gas values and absence of cor pulmonale.

In the most severe forms of CHS, none of the aforementioned means of mechanical ventilatory support will be successful. In such children, the only remaining treatment options are positive-pressure home ventilators and diaphragm pacing. Home ventilators have been utilized very successfully in children with CHS (Oren et al, 1987). A tracheostomy is essential but may be plugged while the child is awake if continuous ventilatory support is not necessary. Although comprehensive and extensive home care programs are necessary, safe and effective long-term home ventilatory care with low morbidity and mortality can be achieved.

Since the initial report of diaphragm pacing in 1951, clinical experience with it in adults has been extensive (Glenn et al, 1988). During the past 20 years, there has been a gradually increasing amount of successful experience with diaphragm pacing in children (Brouillette et al, 1983; Ilbawi et al, 1985). We have now utilized diaphragm pacing in 26 children with CHS, with the oldest survivor now having been paced for more than 11 years (Hunt et al, 1988). Our current experience with diaphragm pacing, based on 96 patient-years, does document a need for periodic replacement of at least some of the implanted components, with the mean time to failure of any implanted component of 56 months (Weese-Mayer et al, 1989). However, there have been no problems with chronic nerve damage secondary to the electrical stimulation (Brouillette et al, 1988), and the overall quality of life achieved with pacing has been excellent. The advantages of diaphragm pacing are the most dramatic in children who require awake as well as sleeping ventilatory support; daytime pacing permits substantially greater mobility and, if supplemental O_2 is not necessary, allows participation in age-appropriate daytime activities, including regular school attendance. In adults, another advantage of pacing is the likelihood that the tracheostomy can be removed; in children, however, decannulation has generally not been feasible, at least before 5 to 6 years of age (Hunt et al, 1988).

FOLLOW-UP

The increasing awareness of CHS as a diagnostic consideration in children, the development of sophisticated sleep laboratory facilities, the ready availability of noninvasive blood gas monitoring, and the ability to implement comprehensive and effective home care programs have all contributed to substantially improved morbidity and mortality in CHS children. Timely diagnosis and establishment of a home care program should avoid the initial development of cor pulmonale, and effective long-term surveillance combining home-based noninvasive blood gas monitoring and periodic sleep laboratory evaluations should eliminate the risk for unfavorable hemodynamic trends. Except for congenital CHS patients with associated abnormalities, long-term morbidity appears to be primarily related to cor pulmonale.

There is no evidence to date that infants with congenital CHS will later outgrow the respiratory control deficiency. There is, however, a tendency for predictable changes to occur in the overall adequacy of automatic control of breathing. We have observed a number of congenital CHS infants with initially normal or at least adequate awake ventilation who gradually develop a need for continuous ventilatory support as infancy progresses, independent of the treatment provided. At approximately 2 years of age, however, there is a trend toward improvement in spontaneous ventilation; awake ventilation may normalize, and the sleep deficit may improve. The mechanism for this potential later stabilization is no better understood than is the etiology of CHS itself. Except for one child (Oren et al, 1987), however, no congenital CHS patient has been successfully weaned from ventilatory support on a long-term basis, and even this child has persistent moderate sleep-dependent hypoventilation. Thus although the later stabilization in automatic control of respiration that may occur is encouraging and the extent of ventilator or pacemaker support may decrease over time, congenital CHS patients do not appear to have the potential for full recovery of automatic ventilatory control. Nevertheless, with appropriate long-term surveillance and prevention of cor pulmonale, the long-term outlook can be very encouraging.

COR PULMONALE

The diagnosis and management of cor pulmonale in children are discussed in Chapters 38 and 46. The crucial point to emphasize is that a respiratory control disorder should be considered in any patient with unexplained cor pulmonale (Hunt and Brouillette, 1982; Noonan, 1965; Sofer et al, 1988). In children with CHS, the urgency for prompt diagnosis and the primary focus of subsequent treatment and long-term surveillance are all related to the prevention of cor pulmonale. In primary CHS without major associated abnormalities, the long-term mortality risk is directly correlated with the development of cor pulmonale.

We have no evidence to suggest that patients with respiratory control disorders have an increased susceptibility to cor pulmonale. We therefore assume that any unfavorable hemodynamic trend is proof of insufficient ventilation. The sleep laboratory evaluation should confirm this insufficiency and its resolution; prolonged evaluation is sometimes necessary to include the worst periods of hypoventilation, especially if they occur during wakefulness. The development of cor pulmonale or any unfavorable trend in this regard thus requires the introduction of more effective treatment of the chronic hypopnea or upper airway obstruction.

EFFECTS OF CHRONIC LUNG DISEASE

Disorders of breathing during sleep may also occur in children with chronic lung disease even though no underlying respiratory control abnormality is present. To understand these interrelationships among chronic lung disease, sleep, and respiratory control, it is first necessary to review the effects of sleep on ventilation and respiratory control in normal subjects.

In normal subjects, ventilation is less in quiet sleep than in wakefulness, CO_2 responsiveness is somewhat less, and minute volume is less at any given level of CO_2 (Gothe et al, 1981; Phillipson, 1978). Hypoxic responsiveness appears to be undiminished during sleep compared to wakefulness (Phillipson et al, 1978), but the absence of any sleep-related decrease is not as certain in young children as it is in adults. These differences, however, do not greatly affect overall patterns of breathing, ventilation, or oxygenation in normal subjects. In adults, for example, the normal sleep-related decrease in alveolar ventilation typically results in Pa_{CO_2} increases of 2 to 8 mm Hg, Pa_{O_2} decreases of 3 to 11 mm Hg, and Sa_{O_2} decreases of 2.0 per cent (Phillipson et al, 1977; Shepard, 1985). As measured in infants and adults, the respiratory pattern is known to be more periodic or irregular in sleep than in wakefulness, but the effect on Sa_{O_2} is negligible.

These clinically insignificant nocturnal decreases in ventilation and gas exchange that occur in normal children may be significantly exacerbated in the presence of chronic lung disease and may result in nocturnal desaturation. A number of factors are likely to be involved in the development of significant nocturnal desaturation. First, the shape of the oxyhemoglobin dissociation curve is an important consideration. Whereas baseline Pa_{O_2} is on the horizontal portion of the curve in normal subjects, it will be on the steep portion of the curve in the presence of significant chronic lung disease, thus resulting in larger Sa_{O_2} decreases than would be expected based on the absolute decrease in Pa_{O_2} occurring with tidal breathing or with the normal brief apneas or hypopneas present during sleep. Second, any reductions in thoracic gas volume or functional residual capacity associated with lung disease will result in larger Sa_{O_2} decrements consequent to respiratory pauses than would be the case in normal children. Third, the relative impairments in chest wall and airway mechanics normally occurring during REM sleep may aggravate the baseline abnormalities present during wakefulness. Fourth, if excessive secretions are part of the chronic lung disease, the generally modest decrease in mucociliary clearance during sleep may be of greater clinical significance. Finally, because the hypoxic ventilatory drive is intact, the hypoxia-induced increases in ventilatory drive may lead, at least in adults, to Cheynes-Stokes breathing with periods of apnea during non-REM sleep (Phillipson, 1978). Even though classic Cheynes-Stokes breathing is un-

usual in children, marked oscillations in the respiratory control system might well occur and result in marked periodic fluctuations in tidal volume and respiratory pattern.

The severe sleep-related asphyxia that can occur in CHS does not lead to sleep deprivation or any of its clinical consequences because impaired arousal is an integral component of the respiratory control deficit. In children with obstructive sleep apnea, however, many of the associated clinical symptoms are actually caused by the sleep deprivation occurring consequent to the presence of significant sleep-related asphyxia with intact sleep arousal responses. Similar clinical symptoms can appear in children with chronic lung disease for the same reasons: significant sleep-related asphyxia and an intact respiratory control system. In addition to the neurobehavioral consequences of sleep deprivation that will occur in both patient groups (see Table 75–2), the sleep deprivation will also lead to blunted hypercarbic and hypoxic ventilatory responsiveness (Bowes et al, 1980; Phillipson, 1978; White et al, 1983). Although secondary blunting of arousal responsiveness will lead to less sleep deprivation, this response is maladaptive because increased severity and duration of nocturnal desaturation will result.

Some clinical studies illustrate the nocturnal respiratory problems that can occur in patients with chronic lung disease. Adults with chronic obstructive lung disease have significant episodes of desaturation during sleep, and disordered breathing (apnea, hypopnea) is common (Wynne et al, 1979). In adults with chronic obstructive pulmonary disease, sleep (especially REM) resulted in significantly greater maximum Pa_{CO_2} increases and Pa_{O_2} decreases than in control subjects, and progressive nocturnal increases in pulmonary artery pressure occurred (Coccagna and Lugaresi, 1978). In children with moderate asthma, there was greater variability in Sa_{O_2} during sleep and a greater maximum decrease in Sa_{O_2} compared with normal children, despite theophylline treatment (Chipps et al, 1980). In a group of 16 children with chronic bronchial asthma, Sa_{O_2} decreases were greater and more frequent than in normal children, and nocturnal desaturation was worse when the asthma was unstable (Smith and Hudgei, 1980). In children and young adults with cystic fibrosis, sleep-related decreases in Sa_{O_2} (especially in non-REM sleep) were greater than in control subjects and contributed significantly to the development and progression of cor pulmonale (Francis et al, 1980).

In summary, the minimal decreases in ventilation, in ventilatory drive, and in Sa_{O_2} that can occur during sleep in normal subjects can be aggravated significantly by chronic lung disease. Whether related to mechanical changes or to exaggerated alterations in respiratory drive, the resultant nocturnal desaturation in the presence of intact sleep arousal mechanisms can result in marked sleep deprivation. The secondary blunting of arousal responsiveness that then occurs will minimize the neurobehavioral sequelae but will be the cause of progressive worsening of the nocturnal desaturation. Effective palliation in such children must be directed at documenting the full extent of nocturnal desaturation and assessing the potential benefits of nocturnal O_2 therapy or respiratory stimulants.

REFERENCES

Bairam A, Boutroy M, Badonnel Y, and Vert P: Theophylline versus caffeine: comparative effects in treatment of idiopathic apnea in the preterm infant. J Pediatr 110(4):636, 1987.

Barlow P, Bartlett D Jr, Hauri P et al: Idiopathic hypoventilation syndrome: importance of preventing nocturnal hypoxemia and hypercapnia. Am Rev Respir Dis 121:141, 1980.

Beckerman R, Meltzer J, Sola A et al: Brain-stem auditory response in Ondine's syndrome. Arch Neurol 43:698, 1986.

Block AJ: Respiratory disorders during sleep, Part I. Heart Lung 9(6):1011, 1980.

Bokinsky GE, Hudson LD, and Weil JV: Impaired peripheral chemosensitivity and acute respiratory failure in Arnold-Chiari malformation and syringomyelia. N Engl J Med 288:947, 1973.

Bolande RP: The neurocristopathies. Hum Pathol 5:409, 1974.

Bower R and Adkins J: Ondine's curse and neurocristopathy. Clin Pediatr 19:665, 1980.

Bowes G, Woolf GM, Sullivan CE, and Phillipson EA: Effect of sleep fragmentation on ventilatory and arousal responses of sleeping dogs to respiratory stimuli. Am Rev Respir Dis 122:899, 1980.

Bradley TD and Phillipson EA: Pathogenesis and pathophysiology of the obstructive sleep apnea syndrome. Med Clin North Am 69(6):1169, 1985.

Brazy JE, Kinney HC, and Oakes WJ: Central nervous system structural lesions causing apnea at birth. J Pediatr 111:163, 1987.

Brouillette RT and Thach BT: A neuromuscular mechanism maintaining extrathoracic airway patency. J Appl Physiol 46:772, 1979.

Brouillette RT, Fernback SK, and Hunt CE: Obstructive sleep apnea in infants and children. J Pediatr 100(1):31, 1982.

Brouillette RT, Hanson D, David R et al: A diagnostic approach to suspected obstructive sleep apnea in children. J Pediatr 105(1):10, 1984.

Brouillette RT, Hunt CE, and Gallemore GE: Respiratory dysrhythmia: a new cause of central alveolar hypoventilation. Am Rev Respir Dis 134:609, 1986.

Brouillette RT, Ilbawi MN, and Hunt CE: Phrenic nerve pacing in infants and children: a review of experience and report on the usefulness of phrenic nerve stimulation studies. J Pediatr 102(1):32, 1983.

Brouillette RT, Ilbawi MM, Kembka-Walden L, and Hunt CE: Stimulus parameters for phrenic nerve pacing in infants and children. Pediatr Pulmonol 4:33, 1988.

Chipps BE, Mak H, Schuberth KC et al: Nocturnal oxygen saturation in normal and asthmatic children. Pediatrics 65(6):1157, 1980.

Coccagna G and Lugaresi E: Arterial blood gases and pulmonary and systemic arterial pressure during sleep in chronic obstructive pulmonary disease. Sleep 1(2):117, 1978.

Comroe JH: Retrospectroscope—Frankenstein, Pickwick, and Ondine. Am Rev Respir Dis 111:689, 1975.

Dooling EC and Richardson EP: Ophthalmoplegia and Ondine's curse. Arch Ophthalmol 95:1790, 1977.

duRivage SK, Winter RJ, Brouillette RT et al: Idiopathic hypothalamic dysfunction and impaired control of breathing. Pediatrics 75(5):896, 1985.

Ellis ER, McCauley VB, Mellis C, and Sullivan CE: Treatment of alveolar hypoventilation in a six-year-old girl with intermittent positive pressure ventilation through a nose mask. Am Rev Respir Dis 136:188, 1987.

Felman AH, Loughlin GM, Leftridge CA et al: Upper airway obstruction during sleep in children. Am J Radiol 133:213, 1979.

Fernbach SK, Brouillette RT, Riggs TW, and Hunt CE: Radiologic evaluation of adenoids and tonsils in children with obstructive sleep apnea: plain films and fluoroscopy. Pediatr Radiol 13:258, 1983.

Fleming PJ, Cade D, Bryan MH, and Bryan AC: Congenital central hypoventilation and sleep state. Pediatr 66(3):425, 1980.

Folgering H, Kuyper F, and Kille JF: Primary alveolar hypoventilation (Ondine's curse syndrome) in an infant without external arcuate nucleus. Bull Eur Physiopathol Respir 15:659, 1979.

Francis PWJ, Muller NL, Gurwitz D et al: Hemoglobin desaturation. Am J Dis Child 134:734, 1980.

Frank Y, Kravath RE, Inoue K et al: Sleep apnea and hypoventilation syndrome associated with acquired nonprogressive dysautonomia: clinical and pathological studies in a child. Ann Neurol 10(1):18, 1981.

Frank Y, Kravath RE, Pollak CP, and Weitzman ED: Obstructive sleep apnea and its therapy: clinical and polysomnographic manifestations. Pediatrics 71:737, 1983.

Fuchs J and Kummer F: Familiare Storung der zentralen Atemregulation. Prax Pneumol 34:615, 1980.

Gastaut H, Tassinari CA, and Duron B: Polygraphic study of the episodic diurnal and nocturnal (hypnic and respiratory) manifestations of the Pickwick syndrome. Brain Res 1:167, 1966.

Glenn WWL, Brouillette RT, Fodstad DH et al: Fundamental considerations in pacing of the diaphragm for chronic ventilatory insufficiency. PACE 11:2121, 1988.

Gothe B, Altose MD, Goldman MD, and Cherniack NS: Effect of quiet sleep on resting and CO_2-stimulated breathing in humans. J Appl Physiol 50(4):724, 1981.

Guilleminault C: Obstructive sleep apnea syndrome and its treatment in children: areas of agreement and controversy. Pediatr Pulmonol 3:429, 1987.

Guilleminault C, Korobkin R, and Winkle R: A review of 50 children with obstructive sleep apnea syndrome. Lung 159:275, 1981.

Guilleminault C, McQuitty J, Ariagno RL et al: Congenital central hypoventilation syndrome in six infants. Pediatrics 70:684, 1982.

Haddad GG, Mazza NM, Defendini R et al: Congenital failure of automatic control of ventilation, gastrointestinal motility and heart rate. Medicine 57(6):517, 1978.

Hedner J, Hedner T, Breese GR et al: Changes in cerebrospinal fluid homovanillic acid in children with Ondine's curse. Pediatr Pulmonol 3:131, 1987.

Hershenson M, Brouillette RT, Olsen E, and Hunt CE: The effect of chloral hydrate on genioglossus and diaphragmatic activity. Pediatr Res 18(6):516, 1984.

Hunt CE and Brouillette RT: Abnormalities of breathing control and airway maintenance in infants and children as a cause of cor pulmonale. Pediatr Cardiol 3:249, 1982.

Hunt CE, Brouillette RT, and Hanson D: Theophylline improves pneumogram abnormalities in infants at risk for sudden infant death syndrome. J Pediatr 3(6):969, 1983.

Hunt CE, Brouillette RT, Weese-Mayer DE et al: Diaphragm pacing in infants and children. PACE 11:2135, 1988.

Hunt CE, Inwood RJ, and Shannon DC: Respiratory and nonrespiratory effects of doxapram in congenital central hypoventilation syndrome. Am Rev Respir Dis 119:263, 1979.

Hunt CE, Matalon SV, Thompson TR et al: Central hypoventilation syndrome. Am Rev Respir Dis 118:23, 1978.

Ilbawi MN, Idriss FS, Hunt CE et al: Diaphragmatic pacing in infants: techniques and results. Ann Thorac Surg 40(4):323, 1985.

Jensen TH, Hansen PB, and Brodersen P: Ondine's curse in Listeria monocytogenes brain stem encephalitis. Acta Neurol Scand 77:505, 1988.

Johnston K, Newth CJL, Sheu K-FR et al: Central hypoventilation syndrome in pyruvate dehydrogenase complex deficiency. Pediatrics 74(6):1034, 1984.

Klein M and Reynolds LG: Relief of sleep related oropharyngeal airway obstruction by continuous insufflation of the pharynx. Lancet 1:935, 1986.

Leech RW and Alvord EC: Anoxic-ischemic encephalopathy in the human neonatal period. Arch Neurol 34:109, 1977.

Liebhaber M, Robin ED, Lynne-Davies P et al: Reye's syndrome complicated by Ondine's curse. West J Med 126(2):110, 1977.

Liu M, Loew JM, and Hunt CE: Congenital central hypoventilation syndrome: a pathological study of the neuromuscular system. Neurology 28:1013, 1978.

McClone D, Dias L, Kaplan WE, and Sommers MW: Concepts in the management of spina bifida. Concepts Pediatr Neurosurg 5:97, 1985.

McNicholas WT, Carter JL, Rutherford R et al: Beneficial effect of oxygen in primary alveolar hypoventilation with central sleep apnea. Am Rev Respir Dis 125:773, 1982.

Mellins RB, Balfour HH, Turino GM, and Winters RW: Failure of automatic control of ventilation (Ondine's curse). Medicine 49(6):487, 1970.

Menashe VD, Farrehi C, and Miller M: Hypoventilation and cor pulmonale due to chronic upper airway obstruction. J Pediatr 67:198, 1965.

Miller MJ, Carlo WA, and Martin RJ: Continuous positive pressure selectively reduces obstructive apnea in preterm infants. J Pediatr 106:91, 1985.

Moore GC, Zwillich CW, Battaglia JD et al: Respiratory failure associated with familial depression of ventilatory response to hypoxia and hypercapnia. N Engl J Med 295(16):861, 1976.

Moss IR, Cataletto M, and Winnik GE: Primary central alveolar hypoventilation in a child: early diagnosis during acute illness; trials with respiratory stimuli; studies related to endorphins. Pediatr Pulmonol 2(2):114, 1986.

Noonan JA: Reversible cor pulmonale due to hypertrophied tonsils and adenoids: studies in two cases. Circulation 32 (Suppl II):II–164, 1965.

O'Dell K, Staren E, and Bassuk A: Total colonic aganglionosis (Zuelzer-Wilson syndrome) and congenital failure of automatic control of ventilation (Ondine's curse). J Pediatr Surg 22(11):1019, 1987.

Oren J, Kelly DH, and Shannon DC: Long-term follow-up of children with congenital central hypoventilation syndrome. Pediatrics 80(3):375, 1987.

Oren J, Kelly DH, Todres D, and Shannon DC: Respiratory complications in patients with myelodysplasia and Arnold-Chiari malformation. Am J Dis Child 140:221, 1986.

Oren J, Newth CJL, Hunt CE et al: Ventilatory effects of almitrine bismesylate in congenital central hypoventilation syndrome. Am Rev Respir Dis 134:917, 1986.

Orenstein DM, Boat TF, Stern RC et al: Progesterone treatment of the obesity hypoventilation syndrome in a child. J Pediatr 90(3):477, 1977.

Papasozomenos S and Roessman U: Respiratory distress and Arnold-Chiari malformation. Neurology 31:97, 1981.

Paradise JL: Tonsillectomy and adenoidectomy. In Bluestone CD and Stool SE (eds): Pediatric Otolaryngology. Philadelphia, WB Saunders Co, 1983.

Phillipson EA: Control of breathing during sleep. Am Rev Respir Dis 118:909, 1978.

Phillipson EA, Kozar LF, Rebuck AS, and Murphy E: Ventilatory and waking responses to CO₂ in sleeping dogs. Am Rev Respir Dis 115:251, 1977.

Phillipson EA, Sullivan CE, Read DJS et al: Ventilatory and waking responses to hypoxia in sleeping dogs. J Appl Physiol 44:512, 1978.

Poceta JS, Strandjord TP, Badura RJ, and Milstein JM: Ondine curse and neurocristopathy. Pediatr Neurol 3(6):370, 1987.

Potsic WP, Pasquariello PS, Baranak CC et al: Relief of upper airway obstruction by adenotonsillectomy. Otolaryngol Head Neck Surg 94:476, 1986.

Putnam JS, Kaufman LV, Michaels RM et al: Methylphenidate therapy in primary alveolar hypoventilation. Chest 64(1):137, 1973.

Quera-Salva MA and Guilleminault C: Post-traumatic central sleep apnea in a child. J Pediatr 110(6):906, 1987.

Ratto O, Biscoe WA, Morton JW, and Comroe JH Jr: Anoxemia secondary to polycythemia and polycythemia secondary to anoxemia. Am J Med 19:958, 1955.

Remmers JE, deGroot WJ, Sauerland EK, and Anch AM: Pathogenesis of upper airway occlusion during sleep. J Appl Physiol 44:931, 1978.

Roberts JL, Mathew OP, and Thach BT: The efficacy of theophylline in premature infants with mixed and obstructive apnea and apnea associated with pulmonary and neurologic disease. J Pediatr 100:968, 1982.

Schlaefke ME and Burghardt F: Training of central chemosensitivity in infants with sleep apnea. In Schlaefke ME, Koepchen HP, and See WR (eds): Central Neurone Environment. Berlin, Springer-Verlag, 1983.

Schmidt-Nowara WW: Continuous positive airway pressure for long term treatment of sleep apnea. Am J Dis Child 138:82, 1984.

Shepard JW: Gas exchange and hemodynamics during sleep. Med Clin North Am 69(6):1243, 1985.

Simmons FB and Hill MW: Hypersomnia caused by upper airway obstruction. Ann Otol 83:670, 1974.

Skatrud JB, Dempsey JA, Bhansali P, and Irvin C: Determinants of chronic carbon dioxide retention and its correction in humans. J Clin Invest 65:813, 1980.

Smith TF and Hudgei DW: Arterial oxygen desaturation during sleep in children with asthma and its relation to airway obstruction and ventilatory drive. Pediatrics 66(5):746, 1980.

Sofer S, Weinhouse E, Tal A et al: Cor pulmonale due to adenoidal or tonsillar hypertrophy or both in children: noninvasive diagnosis and follow-up. Chest 93:119, 1988.

Stern M, Hellwege HH, Gravinghoff L, and Lambrecht W: Total aganglionosis of the colon (Hirschsprung's disease) and congenital failure of automatic control of ventilation (Ondine's curse). Acta Paediatr Scand 70:121, 1981.

Sullivan CE, Issa FG, Berthon-Jones M et al: Reversal of obstructive sleep apnoea by continuous positive airway pressure applied through the nares. Lancet 1:862, 1981.

Volpe J: Hypoxic-ischemic encephalopathy: neuropathology and pathogenesis. In Volpe J: Neurology of the Newborn. 2nd ed. Philadelphia, WB Saunders Co, 1987.

Ward SL, Jacobs RA, Gaites EP et al: Abnormal ventilatory patterns during sleep in infants with myelomeningocele. J Pediatr 109:631, 1986.

Weese-Mayer DE, Brouillette RT, Naidich TP et al: Magnetic resonance imaging and computerized tomography in central hypoventilation. Am Rev Respir Dis 137:393, 1988.

Weese-Mayer DE, Morrow AS, Brouillette RT et al: Phrenic nerve pacing in infants and children: a life table analysis of implanted components. Am Rev Respir Dis 139:974, 1989.

White DP, Douglas NJ, Pickett CK et al: Sleep deprivation and the control of ventilation. Am Rev Respir Dis 128:984, 1983.

Wynne JW, Block AJ, Hemenway J et al: Disordered breathing and oxygen desaturation during sleep in patients with chronic obstructive lung disease (COLD). Am J Med 66:573, 1979.

INDEX

Note: Numbers in *italics* refer to illustrations; numbers followed by (t) indicate tables.